TEXTBOOK OF
ADULT EMERGENCY MEDICINE

SECOND EDITION

EDITED BY

Peter Cameron MB BS MD FACEM
Professor of Emergency Medicine, The Alfred Hospital, Prahran, and Monash University, Clayton, Victoria, Australia

George Jelinek MB BS MD DipDHM FACEM
Professor and Chairman, University of Western Australia; Department of Emergency Medicine, Sir Charles Gairdner Hospital, Nedlands, Western Australia, Australia

Anne-Maree Kelly MB BS MD MClinEd FACEM
Professor and Director of Emergency Medicine, Western Hospital, and Director of the Joseph Epstein Centre for Emergency Medicine Research, Footscray, Victoria, Australia

Lindsay Murray MB BS FACEM
Senior Lecturer in Emergency Medicine, University of Western Australia; Emergency Physician and Clinical Toxicologist, Sir Charles Gairdner Hospital, Nedlands, Western Australia; Medical Director, Western Australian Poisons Information Centre, Australia

Anthony F. T. Brown MB ChB FRCP FRCS (Ed) FACEM FFAEM
Associate Professor, Senior Staff Specialist, Department of Emergency Medicine, Royal Brisbane and Women's Hospital, Brisbane, Queensland, Australia

John Heyworth MB FRCS FFAEM
Consultant, Accident and Emergency Department, Southampton General Hospital, Southampton, UK

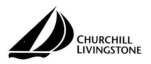

CHURCHILL LIVINGSTONE

EDINBURGH LONDON NEW YORK OXFORD PHILADELPHIA ST LOUIS SYDNEY TORONTO 2004

CHURCHILL LIVINGSTONE
An imprint of Elsevier Limited

First edition 2000
Second edition 2004
    Reprinted 2005

ISBN 0 443 07289 2

British Library Cataloguing in Publication Data
A catalogue record for this book is available from the British Library

Library of Congress Cataloguing in Publication Data
A catalogue record for this book is available from the Library of Congress

Note
Medical knowledge is constantly changing. Standard safety precautions must be followed, but as new research and clinical experience broaden our knowledge, changes in treatment and drug therapy may become necessary or appropriate. Readers are advised to check the most current product information provided by the manufacturer of each drug to be administered to verify there commended dose, the method and duration of administration, and contraindications. It is the responsibility of the practitioner, relying on experience and knowledge of the patient, to determine dosages and the best treatment for each individual patient. Neither the Publisher nor the authors assumes any liability for any injury and/or damage to persons or property arising from this publication.

The Publisher

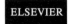
Printed in China

Preface to first edition

Emergency Medicine has developed into the most exciting area of medical practice. Apart from the immediacy and unpredictability of managing acutely ill patients, emergency practice allows the clinician to use a broad range of skills and work in a team environment.

New treatments for respiratory and cardiovascular disease, new systems of care for trauma and psychiatric disorders, necessitate higly sophisticated healthcare at the 'front door'. Attempts to restrain healthcare costs by better use of hospital beds also demand trained professionals to assess emergency patients on arrival. The community now expects immediate access to skilled personnel in emergencies. The recent emphasis on continuity of care for patients from community to hospital and back into the community underlines the importance of Emergency Medicine in new healthcare systems.

Emergency Medicine has grown from the Emergency Room to the Emergency Department. In Australasia, it is the fastest growing medical specialty with more than 800 trainees. The UK has seen a similar rapid expansion. In the United States it has the most popular residency training programmes. Doctors working in Emergency Medicine in Europe and Asia are finally achieving specialist status.

The genesis of this book was the need for a definitive textbook of adult emergency medicine, based on current practice in Australia, New Zealand and the United Kingdom. Many areas of Emergency Medicine are changing rapidly and it is likely that at the time of publication, practice will have developed further. Not all subjects are covered with equal emphasis. This is deliberate in that, for example, there are excellent texts on fracture management. In other areas such as trauma management, we have tried to give basic principles, together with references for further reading.

The layout of the sections has been carefully designed to make it easy to use, with essential information summarized in a clear and concise way. The inclusion of a section on controversies aims to highlight areas of varying practice, change or ongoing research.

The book is aimed principally to meet the needs of doctors in training in Emergency Medicine. In addition, it will be an important resource for general practitioners, specialist emergency and critical care nurses, residents and medical students rotating through an emergency term.

This text is a collaborative effort, involving 113 contributors from Australia, New Zealand, the United Kingdom and the United States of America. Individual contributions have been edited to conform with a consensus style and approach. Material within the text should therefore follow current management in the United Kingdom, New Zealand and Australia. It is anticipated that this book will help develop a common management approach to emergency patients and promote the specialty of Emergency Medicine.

Many people have been involved in the production of this work; the Editors are extremely grateful to them all. We would particularly like to thank our partners, children and friends who have endured the long months of the hard work involved in the development of this book. For their excellent secretarial assistance and manuscript preparation, we thank Mimi Morgan, Celina Everton, Lien Wright and Janet Carr. We are very grateful to the individual contributors for the enthusiasm with which they embraced the task and their generosity in giving their time. Finally, we would like to thank the production staff at Harcourt Brace, particularly Janice Urquhart.

P. C.   2000
G. J.
A-M. K.
L. M.
J. H.
A. B.

Preface to second edition

The specialty of emergency medicine continues to evolve and the spectrum of practice continues to expand. Training programs for emergency doctors and nurses are increasingly popular and new graduates are finding attractive job opportunities. Many countries around the world are now developing emergency medicine specialty training programs similar to those in the UK, Australasia and the USA. The improved training and consequent improvement in patient access to expert emergency care is having a profound effect on the delivery of care in these emergency medical systems.

The gradual shift away from hospital-based medicine towards team-based community care has led to an increasing role for the specialty of emergency medicine in delivering medical care. Hospital in the Home programs, short stay medicine and community care coordination are now seen as part of modern day emergency medicine. Diagnostic and social dilemmas are resolved in the emergency department rather than requiring use of a hospital bed. Several therapies previously requiring admission are now commenced in the emergency department and continued on an outpatient basis. The result is that emergency medicine incorporates a much larger component of what was traditionally seen as inpatient medicine. Resuscitation techniques and intensive monitoring are also most appropriately initiated in the emergency department to ensure optimal outcomes. Covering the whole of emergency medicine practice in a one volume text is not possible, so we have attempted to identify major components of the core body of specialist knowledge.

The first edition of the *Textbook of Adult Emergency Medicine* has proven to be a useful reference for doctors and nurses involved in the practice of emergency medicine. Readers told us that they have found the presentation easy to follow with a consistent approach to diagnosis and treatment of emergency presentations, so we have tried to maintain this approach. Since publication of the first edition, there have been continuing advances in the diagnostic and treatment regimens of many areas of emergency medicine. We have incorporated these advances into the second edition. We have also tried to fill some of the gaps in coverage from the first edition. As a result we have significantly expanded the toxicology section and introduced an orthopaedic section.

The second edition has been a major effort by the many contributors from Australasia, UK, USA, Hong Kong and beyond. Where possible, we actively sought practising clinicians with expert knowledge of a topic area, as we believe this strategy ensures relevance and practicality of information provided. We sincerely thank all of the authors for their efforts. The editors welcome feedback from readers to help ensure that the content remains accurate and relevant. We would like to thank readers for the valuable feedback on the first edition that has been used to shape the second edition.

Preparation of manuscripts requires a considerable team of people, we wish to thank Ms Lien Wright and Roz Jaworski. Special thanks should also go to Ms Mimi Morgan for coordinating the project along with the editorial team at Elsevier.

P. C.
G. J.
A-M. K.
L. M.
A. B.
J. H.

2004

Contributors

Jonathan Abrahams BSc MPH
Assistant Director Policy, Emergency
Management Australia, Dickson, ACT,
Australia

Nicholas Adams MB BS FACEM
Staff Specialist, Emergency Department,
The Alfred Hospital, Prahran, Victoria,
Australia

Peter Aitken MB BS FACEM
Staff Specialist, Emergency Medicine,
Townsville General Hospital,
Townsville, Queensland, Australia

Sylvia Andrew-Starkey MB BS
FACEM
Emergency Department, Caboolture
Hospital, Caboolture, Queensland,
Australia

Philip Aplin MB BS FACEM
Senior Staff Specialist, Emergency
Department, Flinders Medical Centre,
Bedford Park, South Australia

Michael Ardagh MB BS MD FACEM
Professor of Emergency Medicine,
Christchurch School of Medicine,
Christchurch, New Zealand

Richard Ashby MB BS BHA FRACGP
FRACMA FACEM FIFEM
Executive Director Medical Services,
Royal Brisbane & Women's Hospital,
Queensland, Australia

Neil Banham MB BS FACEM
Emergency Physician, Fremantle
Hospital, Fremantle; Director,
Emergency Department, Rockingham
Kwinana District Hospital,
Rockingham, Western Australia

Jack Bergman MBChB DipRACOG
FACEM MBA
Consultant; Health Risks, Victorian
Managed Insurance Authority and
Emergency Physician, Epworth Hospital
and St Vincent's Hospital, Melbourne,
Australia

Stephen Bernard MB BS FACEM
Deputy Director of Intensive Care,
Intensive Care Unit, Dandenong
Hospital, Victoria, Australia

David Bradt MD MPH FACEM
FAFPMH FAAEM
Staff Specialist, Royal Melbourne
Hospital, Parkville, Victoria, Australia

George Braitberg MB BS FACEM
FACMT
Departments of Medicine & Emergency
Medicine, University of Melbourne,
Austin & Repatriation Medical Centre,
Heidelberg, Victoria, Australia

Richard Brennan MB BS MPH
FACEM FIFEM
Health Director, International Rescue
Committee, New York, USA

Edward Brentnall MB BS Dip
Obstetrics(RCOG) FRACGP FACEM
Consultant Emeritus in Emergency
Medicine, Box Hill Hospital, Victoria,
Australia

Jennifer G. Brookes MB BS FACEM
Emergency Department, St Vincent's
Hospital, Fitzroy, Victoria, Australia

Anthony F. T. Brown MBChB FRCP
FRCS(Ed) FACEM FFAEM
Associate Professor, Senior Staff
Specialist, Department of Emergency
Medicine, Royal Brisbane Hospital,
Brisbane, Queensland, Australia

Sheila Bryan MB BS BSc (Hons)
FACEM MRACMA, Dip Venereology
Specialist, Royal Women's Hospital,
Carlton, Victoria, Australia

Michael Bryant MB BS MBus
MRACMA FACEM
Clinical Director, Department of
Emergency Medicine, Western Hospital,
Footscray, Victoria, Australia

Michael Cadogan BA MA MB ChB
Specialist Registrar, Department of
Emergency Medicine, Royal Brisbane
Hospital, Queensland, Australia

Peter Cameron MB BS MD FACEM
Professor, Emergency Medicine,
Monash University, The Alfred
Hospital, Prahran, Victoria, Australia

Tony Celenza MB BS MClinEd
FACEM FFAEM
Senior Lecturer in Emergency
Medicine, University of Western
Australia

Betty Chan MB BS FACEM PhD
Emergency Physician & Clinical
Toxicologist, Prince of Wales Hospital,
Randwick, New South Wales, Australia

Matthew Chu MB BS(Hons) FACEM
Director of Emergency Medicine,
Canterbury Hospital, Central Sydney
Area Health Service, Sydney, New
South Wales, Australia

Michael Coman MB BS FACEM
Staff Specialist, Sunshine Hospital, St
Albans, Victoria, Australia

Roslyn Crampton MB BS(Hons)
Staff Specialist in Emergency Medicine,
Director of Clinical Training, Westmead
Hospital, New South Wales, Australia

David Cruse MB BS FACEM
Emergency Physician, Joondalup Health
Campus, Joondalup; Clinical Senior
Lecturer, University of Western
Australia, Australia

Frank Daly MB BS FACEM
Emergency Physician & Clinical
Toxicologist, Royal Perth Hospital,
Perth; Clinical Senior Lecturer,
University of Western Australia

Andrew Dawson MB BS FRACP FRCP
Professor, Clinical Pharmacology,
University of Newcastle; Senior Staff
Specialist, Department of Clinical
Toxicology & Pharmacology, Hunter
Area Health, New South Wales,
Australia

Andrew Dent MB BS FACEM FRCS
Director, Emergency Department, St
Vincent's Hospital, Fitzroy, Victoria,
Australia

Stuart Dilley MB BS FACEM
Director, Emergency Department, The
Angliss Hospital, Upper Ferntree Gully,
Victoria, Australia

Jenny Dowd MD BS FRANZCOG
Specialist, Royal Women's Hospital,
Carlton, Victoria, Australia

Rob Dowsett MB BS FACEM
Director of Emergency Medicine &
Clinical Toxicologist, Westmead
Hospital, Wentworth, New South
Wales, Australia

Martin Duffy MB BS FACEM
Staff Specialist, Department of
Emergency Medicine, St Vincent's
Hospital, Sydney, New South Wales,
Australia

Robert Dunn MB BS FACEM
Associate Professor & Director of
Emergency Medicine, Royal Adelaide
Hospital, Adelaide, South Australia

Linas Dziukas MB BS MD FRACP
FACEM
Emergency Physician, The Alfred
Hospital, Prahran, Victoria, Australia

David Eddey MB BS DipRACOG
FACEM
Director of Emergency Medicine, The
Geelong Hospital, Geelong, Victoria,
Australia

Robert Edwards MB BS FACEM
Staff Specialist in Emergency Medicine,
Westmead Hospital, Wentworth, New
South Wales, Australia

Gregory Emerson MBChB DipObs
DipDHM FACEM
Staff Specialist, Department of
Emergency Medicine, Royal Brisbane
Hospital, Herston, Queensland; Visiting
Medical Officer, Wesley Centre for
Hyperbaric Medicine, Queensland,
Australia

Karen Falk MB BS(Hons) FRACR
Radiologist, Sydney X-Ray, Randwick
CT and MRI, Randwick, New South
Wales, Australia

Daniel Fatovich MB BS FACEM
Specialist in Emergency Medicine,
Royal Perth Hospital, Perth, Western
Australia; Clinical Associate Professor,
University of Western Australia

Mark Fitzgerald ASM MB BS FACEM
MRACMA
Director of Emergency Services, The
Alfred Hospital, Prahran, Victoria,
Australia

Peter Freeman MB BS FACEM
Director, Emergency Medicine,
Auckland City Hospital, Auckland, New
Zealand

James Galbraith MB BS FRACO
FRACS
Ophthalmology Department, Royal
Melbourne Hospital, Parkville, Victoria,
Australia

G Michael Galvin BSc MB BS
DTM&H FACEM
Emeritus Consultant in Emergency
Medicine, Fremantle Hospital,
Fremantle, Western Australia

Corinne Ginifer MB BS DipRACOG
DA(UK) FACEM
Staff Specialist, Emergency Medicine,
North West Regional Hospital, Burnie,
Tasmania, Australia

Robert Gocentas MB BS FACEM
The Emergency and Trauma Centre,
The Alfred Hospital, Prahran, Victoria,
Australia

Andis Graudins MB BS, PhD,
FACEM
Senior Lecturer, Department of
Medicine, University of New South
Wales;
Consultant Emergency Physician and
Clinical Toxicologist,
Prince of Wales Hospital, Randwick,
New South Wales, Australia

Tim Gray MB BS FACEM
Staff Specialist, Emergency Department,
The Royal Melbourne Hospital,
Parkville, Victoria, Australia

Dale Hanson BM BS DipRACOG
MRACMA FRACGP FACEM
Staff Specialist, Mackay Base Hospital,
Queensland, Australia

Roger Harris MB BS FACEM
Emergency Physician, Royal North
Shore Hospital, St Leonards, New
South Wales, Australia

Richard Harrod MB BS FACEM
Staff Specialist, Emergency Department,
The Royal Melbourne Hospital,
Parkville, Victoria, Australia

Taj Hassan MB BS MRCP DA FRCS
Consultant, Accident and Emergency
Medicine, Leeds General Infirmary,
Leeds, UK

James Hayes MB BS FACEM
Staff Specialist, The Northern Hospital,
Epping, Victoria, Australia

Mel Herbert FACEP
Associate Professor, Department of
Emergency Medicine, LAC & USC
Medical Center, California, USA

Ruth Hew MB BS FACEM
Staff Specialist, Department of
Emergency Medicine, Sunshine
Hospital, St Albans, Victoria, Australia

Sue Ieraci MB BS FACEM
Director of Emergency Medicine,
Liverpool Hospital, Liverpool, New
South Wales, Australia

Geoff Isbister BSc MB BS FACEM
Lecturer, Discipline of Clinical

Pharmacology, University of Newcastle, Newcastle; Clinical Toxicologist & Emergency Physician, Newcastle Mater Hospital, Newcastle, New South Wales, Australia

Trevor Jackson MB BS FACEM
Staff Specialist, Department of Emergency Medicine, Sir Charles Gairdner Hospital, Perth, Western Australia

George Jelinek MB BS MD DipDHM FACEM
Professor and Chairman of Emergency Medicine, University of Western Australia; Department of Emergency Medicine, Sir Charles Gairdner Hospital, Nedlands, Western Australia

Tony Joseph MB BS FACEM
Emergency Physician, Royal North Shore Hospital, University of Sydney, St Leonards, New South Wales, Australia

David Kaufman FRACS FRACO
Ophthalmology Department, Royal Melbourne Hospital, Parkville, Victoria, Australia

Anne-Maree Kelly MD MClinED FACEM
Professor/Director of Emergency Medicine, Western Hospital and Director of the Joseph Epstein Centre for Emergency Medicine Research, Footscray, Victoria, Australia

Marcus Kennedy MB BS FRACGP DA(UK) DipIMC(Ed) FACEM
Director, Emergency Medicine, Royal Melbourne Hospital, Victoria, Australia

Fergus Kerr MB BS FACEM MPH
Emergency Physician & Clinical Toxicologist, Emergency Department, Austin Hospital, Heidelberg, Victoria, Australia

Diane King MB BS FACEM
Emergency Department, Flinders Medical Centre, Bedford Park, South Australia

Jonathan Knott MB BS FACEM
Staff Specialist, Emergency Department, Royal Melbourne Hospital, Victoria, Parkville, Australia

Ian Knox MB BS FACEM
Specialist in Emergency Medicine, The

Wesley Hospital, Toowong, Queensland, Australia

Zeff Koutsogiannis MB BS FACEM
Staff Specialist, Department of Emergency Medicine, Western Hospital, Footscray, Victoria, Australia

Sashi Kumar MB BS DLO AMC FACEM
Senior Specialist, Deputy Director, Department of Emergency Medicine, Canberra Hospital, Canberra, ACT, Australia

Mary Lanctot RN MSNCEN FNP-C
Department of Emergency Medicine, LAC & USC Medical Center, California, USA

Deborah Leach MB BS FACEM
Emergency Department, Box Hill Hospital, Box Hill, Victoria, Australia

Marian Lee MB BS DCH FACEM
Staff Specialist, Emergency Department, Mount Druitt Hospital, New South Wales, Australia

David Lightfoot MB BS FACEM
Staff Specialist, Department of Emergency Medicine, Western Hospital, Footscray, Victoria, Australia

Mark Little MB BS FACEM MPH&TM DTM&H(Lon)
Emergency Physician & Clinical Toxicologist, Department of Emergency Medicine, Sir Charles Gairdner Hospital, Nedlands, Western Australia

Lewis Macken MB BS FACEM
Staff Specialist, Department of Emergency Medicine, Director of Emergency Medicine Training, Royal North Shore Hospital, New South Wales, Australia

Hamish Maclaren MA(Hons) BSc MB ChB MRCGP FACEM
Honorary Senior Lecturer in Emergency Medicine and Distance Learning, University of Auckland, New Zealand; Rural Practitioner, Aberfoyle Medical Centre, Aberfoyle, UK

Andrew Maclean MB BS FACEM
Director, Emergency Department, Box Hill Hospital, Box Hill, Victoria, Australia

John Maguire MB BS DipObs RACOG FACEM
Director, Division of Emergency Medicine, John Hunter Hospital, New South Wales, Australia

Paul Mark MB BS DipRACOG FACEM DipDHM MRACMA
Executive Director, Clinical Services, Fremantle Hospital & Health Service, Fremantle; Clinical Senior Lecturer, University of Western Australia

Suzanne Mason MB BS FRCS FFAEM MD
Senior Clinical Lecturer/Honorary Consultant, Medical Care Research Unit, University of Sheffield, UK

Alastair McGowan OBE FRCP FRCS FRCA FFAEM
Consultant in Emergency Medicine, St James's University Hospital, Leeds; President, Faculty of A&E Medicine, Leeds, UK

Alastair Meyer Bsc(Hons) BMedSci MB BS FACEM
Director, Department of Emergency Medicine, Royal Hobart Hospital, Hobart, Tasmania, Australia

Vanessa Morgan MB BS FRACP
Dermatology Department, Royal Melbourne Hospital, Parkville, Victoria, Australia

David Mountain MB BS FACEM
Emergency Physician, Department of Emergency Medicine, Sir Charles Gairdner Hospital, Nedlands; Clinical Senior Lecturer, University of Western Australia

Lindsay Murray MB BS FACEM
Senior Lecturer in Emergency Medicine, University of Western Australia; Emergency Physician and Clinical Toxicologist, Sir Charles Gairdner Hospital, Nedlands; Medical Director, Western Australian Poisons Information Centre, Australia

Sandra Neate MB BS DipRACOG DA FACEM
Staff Specialist, Emergency Department, St Vincent's Hospital, Fitzroy, Victoria, Australia

Fiona Nicholson MB BS FACEM
Staff Specialist, Emergency Department,
Royal Melbourne Hospital, Parkville,
Victoria, Australia

Debra O'Brien MB BS FACEM
Director, Emergency Medicine, Sir
Charles Gairdner Hospital, Nedlands:
Clinical Senior Lecturer, University of
Western Australia

Ken Ooi MB BS FACEM
Staff Specialist, Department of
Emergency Medicine, Western Hospital,
Melbourne, Victoria, Australia

Helen Parker MB BS FACEM
DMJ(Clin)
Staff Specialist, Department of
Emergency Medicine, Western Hospital,
Footscray, Victoria; Division of Clinical
Forensic Medicine, Victorian Institute
of Forensic Medicine, Southbank,
Victoria, Australia

John Pasco MB BS FACEM DA(UK)
Dip RACOG BSc(Hons) DipEd
Emergency Department, The Geelong
Hospital, Geelong, Victoria, Australia

Scott Pearson MB BS FACEM
Staff Specialist, Emergency Medicine,
Christchurch Hospital, Christchurch,
New Zealand

Stephen Priestley MB BS FACEM
Director, Department of Emergency
Medicine, Sunshine Hospital, St Albans,
Victoria, Australia

Michael Ragg MB BS FACEM
Staff Specialist, The Geelong Hospital,
Geelong, Victoria, Australia

Tim Rainer MD BSc MRCP
Trauma and Emergency Centre, Prince
of Wales Hospital, Shatin, Hong Kong

Drew Richardson MB BS(Hons)
FACEM
Emergency Department, The Canberra
Hospital, Garran, ACT; Associate
Professor of Road Trauma &
Emergency Medicine, The Canberra
Clinical School, University of Sydney,
New South Wales, Australia

Peter Ritchie MB BS DipEpitBiostats
FACEM
Staff Specialist, Emergency Department,

The Royal Melbourne Hospital,
Parkville, Victoria, Australia

Ian Rogers MB BS FACEM
Director, Post Graduate and Medical
Education and Coordinator of the
Centre for Medical Education and
Research, Sir Charles Gairdner Hospital;
Clinical Senior Lecturer, University of
Western Australia, Australia

Pamela Rosengarten MB BS FACEM
Director, Emergency Medicine, Monash
Medical Centre, Clayton, Victoria,
Australia

John Ryan FRCS Ed(A&E) FFAEM
DCH DipSportsMed
Consultant in Emergency Medicine, St
Vincent's University Hospital, Elm
Park, Dublin, Ireland

Sharmeen Safih MB BS FACEM
Staff Specialist, Department of
Emergency Medicine, Waikata Hospital,
Hamilton, New Zealand

Robert A Scott MBChB FRCP FACEM
Staff Specialist, Department of
Emergency Medicine, Royal Brisbane
Hospital, Queensland, Australia

Andrew Singer MB BS FACEM
Clinical Director of Emergency
Medicine, The Canberra Hospital,
Woden, ACT, Australia

David Smart BMedSci MB BS(Hons-1)
Dip DHM FACEM FACTM FAICD
Department of Diving and Hyperbaric
Medicine, Royal Hobart Hospital,
Hobart, Tasmania, Australia

David Spain MB BS FRACGP FACEM
Senior Staff Specialist, Emergency
Department, Gold Coast Hospital,
Southport, Queensland, Australia

Peter Sprivulis MB BS FACEM
Staff Specialist, Department of
Emergency Medicine, Fremantle
Hospital, Fremantle, Western Australia

Alan C Street MB BS FRACP
Deputy Directory, Victorian Infectious
Diseases Service, Royal Melbourne
Hospital, Parkville, Victoria, Australia

Roger Swift MB BS FACEM
Staff Specialist, Sir Charles Gairdner
Hospital, Nedlands, Western Australia

Janet Talbot-Stern BA MA MD
FACEM FACEP
Senior Staff Specialist, Royal Prince
Alfred Hospital, Sydney; Clinical Senior
Lecturer, Department of Surgery,
University of Sydney, New South Wales,
Australia

David Taylor MD MPH DRCOG
FACEM
Director of Emergency Medicine
Research, Department of Emergency
Medicine, Royal Melbourne Hospital,
Parkville, Victoria, Australia

James Taylor MB BS FACEM
Director, Department of Emergency
Medicine, Sandringham Hospital,
Sandringham, Victoria, Australia

Graeme Thomson MB BS FACEM
Department of Emergency Medicine,
Monash Medical Centre, Clayton,
Victoria, Australia

Gino Toncich MB BS(Hons) Dip
Anaes MBA FACEM
Staff Specialist, Emergency Department,
Royal Melbourne Hospital, Parkville,
New South Wales, Australia

Steven Troupakis MB BS DipRACOG
FACEM
Staff Specialist, Emergency Medicine,
Monash Medical Centre, Clayton,
Victoria, Australia

George Varigos MB BS FRACP
Dermatology Department, Royal
Melbourne Hospital, Parkville, Victoria,
Australia

John Vinen MB BS MHP FACEM
FIFEM
Director, Emergency Support Services,
Royal North Shore Hospital, St
Leonards, New South Wales,
Australia

Andrew Walby MB BS FACEM
Staff Specialist, Department of
Emergency Medicine, Western Hospital,
Footscray, Victoria, Australia

Mark Walland MB BS FRANZCO
FRACS
Ophthalmology Department, Royal
Melbourne Hospital, Parkville, Victoria,
Australia

Richard Waller MB BS BMedSci
FACEM
Staff Specialist, Emergency Department,
The Royal Melbourne Hospital,
Parkville, Victoria, Australia

Bryan Walpole MB BS FRCS FACEM
DTM&H
Medical Officer, Australian National
Antarctic Expedition, Macquarie Island,
Tasmania, Australia

Jeff Wassertheil OstJ MB BS FACEM
MRACMA
Director of Emergency Medicine,
Peninsula Health Care Network,
Victoria, Australia

Ian Whyte MB BS FRACP
FRCP(Edin)
Professor, Discipline of Clinical
Pharmacology, School of Population
Health Sciences, Faculty of Medicine
and Health Sciences, University of
Newcastle; Senior Staff Specialist &
Director, Department of Clinical
Toxicology and Pharmacology,
Newcastle Mater Misericordiae
Hospital, New South Wales, Australia

Garry Wilkes MB BS FACEM
Director, Emergency Medicine,
Bunbury Health Service, Western
Australia

Aled Williams MbChB MRCGP
FACEM MPH&TM
Staff Specialist, Department of
Emergency Medicine, Sir Charles
Gairdner Hospital, Nedlands, Western
Australia

Simon Wood MB BS DipPaed (NSW)
FACEM
Emergency Physician, Joondalup
Health Campus, Joondalup, Western
Australia

Peter Wright MB BS FACEM
Staff Specialist, Maroondah Hospital,
Victoria, Australia

Peter Wyllie MB BS FACEM
Staff Specialist, Emergency Medicine,
Liverpool Hospital, Liverpool, New
South Wales, Australia; Staff Specialist,
Emergency Medicine, Sutherland
Hospital, Caringbah, New South Wales,
Australia

Anusch Yazdani MB BS FRANZCOG
Staff Specialist Gynaecology, Mater
Hospitals Complex, South Brisbane,
Queensland, Australia

Kim Yates MBChB MMedSc FACEM
Emergency Medicine Specialist, North
Shore Hospital, Takapuna, Auckland,
New Zealand

Simon Young MB BS FACEM
Director, Emergency Department,
Royal Children's Hospital, Parkville,
Victoria, Australia

Allen Yuen MB BS(Hons) FRACGP
FACEM
Director of Emergency Medicine,
Epworth Hospital, Richmond, Victoria;
Senior Lecturer ACEM, Australia

Allen Yung MB BS OAM FRACP
Specialist in Infectious Diseases, Royal
Melbourne Hospital, Parkville, Victoria,
Australia

Salomon Zalstein MB BS BMedSci
FACEM
Staff Specialist, Royal Melbourne
Hospital, Parkville, Victoria, Australia

Contents

SECTION 1
Resuscitation 1
Editor: Anthony F.T. Brown

1.1 Basic life support 2
Stephen Bernard

1.2 Advanced life support 6
John E. Maquire

1.3 Advanced airway
management 15
Stephen Bernard

1.4 Cerebral resuscitation after
cardiac arrest 20
Stephen Bernard

1.5 Shock 23
Robert A. Scott

1.6 Ethics of resuscitation 33
Michael W. Ardagh

SECTION 2
Trauma 39
Editor: Peter Cameron

2.1 Trauma overview 40
Peter Cameron, David Yates

2.2 Neurotrauma 47
Marcus Kennedy, Angelo Annunziata

2.3 Spinal trauma 52
Jeff Wassertheil

2.4 Facial trauma 65
Lewis Macken, Ron Manning

2.5 Abdominal trauma 71
Garry J. Wilkes

2.6 Chest trauma 76
Markc Fitzgerald, Robert Gocentas

2.7 Limb trauma 80
Richard Harrod

2.8 Radiology in major trauma 86
Tony Joseph, Roger Harris, Karen Falk

2.9 Trauma in pregnancy 102
Steven Troupakis

2.10 Trauma in the elderly 105
Peter Ritchie

2.11 Wound care and repair 109
Richard Waller

2.12 Burns 123
Tim Gray

SECTION 3
**Orthopaedic
emergencies** 129
Editors: Anne-Maree Kelly,
Anthony F.T. Brown

3.1 Injuries of the shoulder 130
Anne-Maree Kelly

3.2 Fractures of the humerus 132
Timothy Hudson Rainer

3.3 Dislocations of the elbow 136
Timothy Hudson Rainer

3.4 Fractures of the forearm 138
Peter Wright

3.5 Hand injuries 142
Peter Freeman

3.6 Pelvic injuries 148
Michael Cadogan

3.7 Hip injuries 152
Michael Cadogan

3.8 Knee injuries 157
Michael Cadogan

3.9 Femur injuries 159
Michael Cadogan

3.10 Tibia and fibula injuries 165
Michael Cadogan

3.11 Ankle joint injuries 168
Michael Cadogan

3.12 Foot injuries 171
Michael Cadogan

SECTION 4
Cardiovascular 177
Editor: Anne-Maree Kelly

4.1 Chest pain 178
Michael Bryant

4.2 Ischaemic heart disease: acute
coronary syndromes 182
Corinne Ginifer

4.3 Assessment and management of
acute pulmonary oedema 193
David Lightfoot

4.4 Arrhythmias 197
Alastair D. McR. Meyer

4.5 Pulmonary embolism 210
Peter Cameron

4.6 Pericarditis, cardiac tamponade
and myocarditis 215
James Hayes

CONTENTS

4.7 Heart valve emergencies 223
Marian Lee

4.8 Peripheral vascular disease 231
Tajek B. Hassan, Jack Bergman

4.9 Hypertension 237
Marian Lee

4.10 Aortic dissection 242
Michael Coman, Dale Hanson

4.11 Aneurysms 248
Roger Swift

SECTION 5
Respiratory 253
Editor: Anthony F.T. Brown

5.1 Oxygen therapy 254
David R. Smart

5.2 Upper respiratory tract 265
Ken Ooi

5.3 Asthma 271
Anne-Maree Kelly

5.4 Community-acquired
pneumonia 275
Garry J. Wilkes

5.5 Chronic obstructive airways
disease 286
Martin Duffy

5.6 Pneumothorax 291
Janet Talbot-Stern

5.7 Pleural effusion 296
Suzanne Mason

5.8 Haemoptysis 300
Stuart Dilley

SECTION 6
Digestive 303
Editor: Anne-Maree Kelly

6.1 Dysphagia 304
Graeme Thomson

6.2 Bowel obstruction 306
Kim Yates

6.3 Hernia 309
Andrew Dent

6.4 Gastroenteritis 311
Corinne Ginifer, Simon Young

6.5 Haematemesis and
melaena 316
Peter Wyllie, Sue Ieraci

6.6 Peptic ulcer disease and
gastritis 322
Stuart Dilley

6.7 Biliary tract disease 326
Andrew Walby

6.8 Pancreatitis 329
Michael Bryant

6.9 Acute appendicitis 332
Andrew Dent

6.10 Inflammatory bowel
disease 335
Kim Yates

6.11 Acute liver failure 338
John M. Ryan

6.12 Rectal bleeding 341
Scott J. Pearson, Peter J. Aitken

6.13 Perianal conditions 344
Andrew Dent

SECTION 7
Neurology 347
Editor: Anne-Maree Kelly

7.1 Headache 348
Anne-Maree Kelly

7.2 Stroke and transient ischaemic
attacks 352
Phillip Aplin

7.3 Subarachnoid haemorrhage 361
Pamela Rosengarten

7.4 Altered conscious state 365
Ruth Hew

7.5 Seizures 371
Garry J. Wilkes

SECTION 8
Infectious diseases 379
Editor: Peter Cameron

8.1 Approach to undifferentiated fever
in adults 380
Allen Yung, Jonathan Knott

8.2 Meningitis 386
Andrew Singer

8.3 Septic arthritis 392
Trevor Jackson

8.4 Osteomyelitis 394
Trevor Jackson

8.5 Urinary-tract infection 396
Salomon Zalstein

8.6 Skin and soft-tissue
infections 403
John Vinen

8.7 Hepatitis 410
Deborah Leach

8.8 HIV/AIDS 417
Alan C. Street

8.9 Antibiotics in the ED 424
David McD. Taylor, John Vinen

8.10 Needlestick injuries 434
Fiona Nicholson, Alan C. Street

SECTION 9
Genitourinary 439
Editor: George Jelinek

9.1 Acute renal failure 440
Nicholas Adams, Linas Dziukas

9.2 The acute scrotum 453
Gino Toncich

9.3 Renal colic 457
Fiona Nicholson

SECTION 10
Endocrine 461
Editor: Anthony F.T. Brown

10.1 Diabetes mellitus 462
Michael Ragg

10.2 Thyroid and adrenal
emergencies 467
Andrew Maclean, Pamela Rosengarten

10.3 Alcoholic ketoacidosis 471
Michael Ragg

CONTENTS

SECTION 11
Metabolic 475
Editor: Lindsay Murray

11.1 Acid-base disorders 476
Robert Dunn

11.2 Electrolyte disturbances 481
John Pasco

SECTION 12
Haematology 493
Editor: Lindsay Murray

12.1 Blood transfusion 494
Hamish Maclaren

12.2 Neutropenia 499
Hamish Maclaren

12.3 Haemophilia 501
Hamish Maclaren

12.4 Anaemia 503
Hamish Maclaren

12.5 Thrombocytopenia 511
Simon Wood

SECTION 13
Rheumatology 515
Editor: Anthony F.T. Brown

13.1 Rheumatological
emergencies 516
Shameen Safih

SECTION 14
Dermatology 527
Editor: Anthony F.T. Brown

14.1 Emergency dermatology 528
George Varigos, Vanessa Morgan

SECTION 15
Eyes 535
Editor: Peter Cameron

15.1 Ocular emergencies 536
David V. Kaufman, James K. Galbraith,
Mark J. Walland

SECTION 16
Dental 545
Editor: Peter Cameron

16.1 Dental emergencies 546
Sashi Kumar

SECTION 17
ENT 549
Editor: Peter Cameron

17.1 Ears, nose and throat 550
Sashi Kumar

SECTION 18
**Obstetrics and
gynaecology** 555
Editor: Anthony F.T. Brown

18.1 Emergency delivery 556
Stephen Priestley

18.2 Ectopic pregnancy and bleeding
in early pregnancy 561
Sheila Bryan

18.3 Bleeding after the first trimester
of pregnancy 564
Jenny Dowd, Sheila Bryan

18.4 Abnormal vaginal bleeding in
the non-pregnant patient 567
Mel E. Herbet, Mary L. Lanctot

18.5 Pelvic inflammatory
disease 570
Sheila Bryan

18.6 Pelvic pain 572
Michael Cadogan, Anusch Yazdani,
James Taylor

SECTION 19
Psychiatric emergencies 579
Editor: George Jelinek

19.1 Mental state assessment 580
Sylvia Andrew-Starkey

19.2 Distinguishing medical from
psychiatric causes of mental
disorder presentations 584
David Spain

19.3 The violent patient 590
Jennifer G. Brookes

19.4 Deliberate self
harm/suicide 597
Antonio Celenza

SECTION 20
Crisis intervention 603
Editor: George Jelinek

20.1 Crisis intervention in the
emergency department 604
Jennifer G. Brookes, Deborah S. Leach

20.2 Death and dying 608
Bryan Walpole

20.3 Sexual assault 612
Ian Knox, Roslyn Crampton

20.4 Domestic violence 619
Sandra Neate

SECTION 21
Pain relief 625
Editor: Anthony F.T. Brown

21.1 Pain relief in emergency
medicine 626
Daniel M. Fatovich, Anthony F.T. Brown

SECTION 22
Ultrasound 635
Editor: George Jelinek

22.1 Emergency department
ultrasound 636
Tony Joseph

SECTION 23
Research methodology 647
Editor: George Jelinek

23.1 Research methodology 648
David McD. Taylor

CONTENTS

SECTION 24
Emergency medicine and the law 659
Editor: George Jelinek

24.1 Mental health and the law: the Australasian and UK perspectives 660
David Eddey, Suzanne Mason

24.2 The coroner: the Australasian and UK perspectives 667
Simon Young, Helen Parker

24.3 Consent and competence: the Australasian and UK perspectives 674
Edward Brentnall, G. Michael Galvin, Helen L. Parker

SECTION 25
Emergency medical systems 681
Editor: George Jelinek

25.1 Prehospital emergency medicine 682
Stephen Bernard

25.2 Retrieval 686
Salomon Zalstein

25.3 Medical issues in disasters 694
Richard J. Brennan, David A. Bradt, Jonathan Abrahams

25.4 Triage 702
Drew Richardson

25.5 Refugee health 706
Aled Williams, Mark Little

25.6 Emergency department observation wards 710
Aled Williams

SECTION 26
Administration 713
Editor: George Jelinek

26.1 Emergency department staffing 714
Sue Ieraci

26.2 Emergency department layout 716
Matthew W. G. Chu, Robert Dunn

26.3 Quality assurance/quality improvement 720
Diane King

26.4 Business planning 723
Richard H. Ashby

26.5 Accreditation, specialist training and recognition in Australasia 726
Allen Yuen, Andrew Singer

26.6 Specialist recognition and training in emergency medicine: the UK view 731
Alastair McGowan

26.7 Complaints 733
Allen Yuen

26.8 Clinical risk management in the emergency department 739
John Vinen

SECTION 27
Environmental 747
Editor: Lindsay Murray

27.1 Heat-related illness 748
Ian Rogers, Aled Williams

27.2 Hypothermia 752
Ian Rogers

27.3 Dysbarism 756
Gregory M. Emerson

27.4 Radiation accidents 763
Paul D. Mark

27.5 Near-drowning 769
David Mountain

27.6 Electric shock and lightning injury 774
Daniel M. Fatovich

27.7 Anaphylaxis 779
Anthony F.T. Brown

27.8 Altitude illness 784
Ian Rogers, Debra O'Brien

SECTION 28
Toxicology 789
Editor: Lindsay Murray

28.1 General principles in the management of drug overdose 790
Lindsay Murray

28.2 Antihistamine and anticholinergic poisoning 797
Andis Graudins

28.3 Cardiovascular drugs 800
Betty Chan, Lindsay Murray

28.4 Central nervous system drugs 806
George Braitberg, Fergus Kerr

28.5 Colchicine 820
Lindsay Murray, Roger Harris

28.6 Paracetamol 823
Andis Graudins

28.7 Salicylate 827
Andis Graudins

28.8 Theophylline 830
Lindsay Murray

28.9 Carbon monoxide 833
David C. Cruse

28.10 Cyanide 837
George Braitberg

28.11 Corrosive ingestion 840
Rob Dowsett

28.12 Drugs of abuse 844
Frank Daly

28.13 Methaemoglobinaemia 854
Robert Edwards

28.14 Pesticides 857
Ian Whyte, Andrew Dawson

28.15 Hydrofluoric acid 865
Andis Graudins

28.16 Iron 869
Zeff Koutsogiannis

28.17 Hypoglycaemic drugs 872
Lindsay Murray, Mark Little

28.18 Lithium 874
Lindsay Murray

28.19 Ethanol 877
Mark Little, Lindsay Murray

28.20 Snakebite 881
George Jelinek, Peter Sprivulis

28.21 Spider bite 885
George Jelinek, Geoff Isbister

28.22 Marine envenoming and poisoning 890
Neil Banham, Mark Little

Index 895

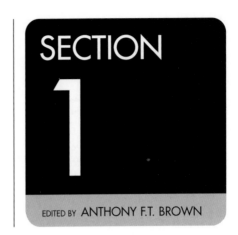

RESUSCITATION

1.1 Basic life support 2

1.2 Advanced life support 6

1.3 Advanced airway management 15

1.4 Cerebral resuscitation after cardiac arrest 20

1.5 Shock 23

1.6 Ethics of resuscitation 33

1.1 BASIC LIFE SUPPORT

STEPHEN BERNARD

ESSENTIALS

1 The patient with sudden cardiac arrest requires a bystander to institute the 'chain of survival', including immediate call to emergency medical services and the performance of bystander cardiopulmonary resuscitation.

2 Current survival rates for pre-hospital cardiac arrest are low, however, strategies for improvement are increasingly being implemented.

3 Early defibrillation is life-saving and is now regarded as a part of basic life support.

4 Co-responders with ambulance services, such as fire fighters, may provide early defibrillation.

5 Early defibrillation may be delivered by untrained bystanders or minimally trained security staff (public access defibrillation).

INTRODUCTION

The patient with sudden cardiac arrest requires a bystander to initiate a number of actions in rapid sequence for there to be any hope of successful resuscitation. These steps are known as the 'chain of survival'.[1] After the first step, a call to ambulance, the bystander needs to institute basic life support (BLS) whilst awaiting the arrival of the emergency medical services (EMS). The BLS procedures may be undertaken by personnel with little or no medical training and are applicable in the patient who has become unconscious as a result of airway obstruction, respiratory arrest or cardiac arrest. In general, BLS includes interventions that involve minimal training in the use of equipment, but also now include the

application of a semi-automatic external defibrillator (SAED), if one is available close to the site of the cardiac arrest.

DEVELOPMENT OF PROTOCOLS

It is important that the guidelines for BLS be nationally consistent. To achieve this, many countries have established national expert committees to advise the community, ambulance services and medical profession on BLS guidelines. Table 1.1.1 shows the national associations that make up the International Liaison Committee on Resuscitation (ILCOR). This group meets every 6 years to review the BLS guidelines and to consider changes to these guidelines. The most recent revision of BLS guidelines occurred in 2000.[2] Subsequently, each national committee may determine regional variations to these guidelines to take into account local practices.

One of the major considerations of changes to protocols for these committees is the feasibility of these protocols to be implemented by personnel with minimal training. The major handicap to consideration of the protocols is the relative paucity of good scientific evidence for the strategies that have been taught over many years.

Table 1.1.1
American Heart Association
Australian Resuscitation Council
European Resuscitation Council
Heart and Stroke Foundation of Canada
Inter-American Heart Foundation
New Zealand Resuscitation Council
Resuscitation Council of Southern Africa

INITIAL EVALUATION

A flow chart for the initial evaluation of the collapsed patient is shown in Figure 1.1.1. This flow chart commences with the recognition that a patient has collapsed. The initial steps are as follows:

Check for dangers

As the patient is approached, the bystander should immediately consider any dangers that may be associated with

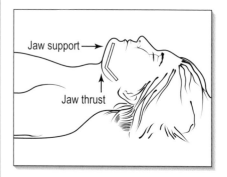

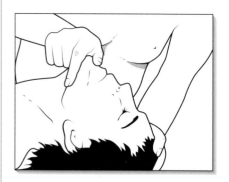

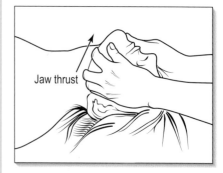

Fig. 1.1.1 Diagram of head tilt, jaw thrust (courtesy Australian Resuscitation Council).

2

the collapse of the patient. For example, the patient may have been electrocuted and there could be further casualties if the power source is not switched off prior to patient contact.

In the case of a motor-vehicle accident where a patient is unconscious, there is the risk of additional injury from further collisions involving passing vehicles and another bystander should be tasked to direct traffic at the scene. There may also be a risk of fire if fuel has leaked onto hot engine parts or there is an electrical fault. Therefore, the ignition should be switched off, and it is advised that unconscious patients should be immediately removed from vehicles prior to the arrival of emergency medical services, whilst taking care to minimize movement of the neck. It is considered that the risk of injury from a sudden fire or explosion exceeds that of moving an unconscious patient prior to immobilization of the cervical spine with a hard collar.

In the case of a patient who has collapsed in a confined space, the possibility of poisoning with carbon monoxide or a similar toxic gas should be considered, and the scene not entered until it can be made safe by emergency services.

Check for response

The patient who has collapsed must be quickly assessed to determine whether there is coma, indicating possible cardiac arrest or just a simple fall. This is assessed by a gentle 'shake and shout', followed by an examination of the motor and verbal response of the patient.

If the patient is unresponsive, cardiac arrest due to ventricular fibrillation should be suspected and emergency medical services telephoned immediately ('call first'). Alternatively, if the collapse is due to suspected airway obstruction (choking) or inadequate ventilations (drowning, hanging, etc.), then resuscitation should be commenced for approximately 1 minute prior to the calling of emergency medical services ('call fast').

Airway

If the unconscious patient has collapsed in a prone position, then he/she should be placed on his/her side in the coma

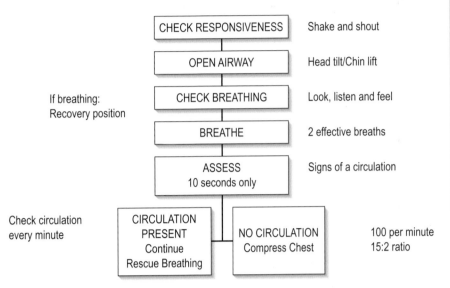

ADULT BASIC LIFE SUPPORT

CHECK RESPONSIVENESS — Shake and shout

OPEN AIRWAY — Head tilt/Chin lift

CHECK BREATHING — Look, listen and feel

If breathing: Recovery position

BREATHE — 2 effective breaths

ASSESS 10 seconds only — Signs of a circulation

Check circulation every minute

CIRCULATION PRESENT Continue Rescue Breathing

NO CIRCULATION Compress Chest — 100 per minute 15:2 ratio

Send or go for help as soon as possible according to guidelines

Fig. 1.1.2 BLS algorithm (courtesy of ILCOR).

position (see Fig. 1.1.2) and an assessment of the airway should be made. Alternatively, if the patient has collapsed and is supine, the airway may be checked in that position.

One exception to this initial step is if the unconscious patient has been retrieved from near drowning. In this setting, the initial step of rolling onto the side to allow assessment of airway and facilitate airway clearance has been practised by surf life-savers for many years and is still recommended by some authorities as the initial position for patient assessment.

The airway is checked with visual inspection, careful forward movement of the jaw ('jaw thrust') and sweeping out any foreign material or vomitus with a finger. In general, 'noisy breathing is obstructed breathing', although an exception to this rule might include the patient with severe asthma who has such a low tidal volume that there are no sounds from the upper airway.

If the airway is obstructed with a foreign body, there are a number of manoeuvres that have been described as helpful in this setting. In North America, the Heimlich manoeuvre is endorsed as the technique of choice. However, this technique is associated with some signi-

ficant complications, including intra-abdominal injuries. In Australia, the recommended technique for clearing an airway that is completely obstructed by a foreign body includes back blows and lateral chest thrusts.

In a study comparing standard chest compressions and Heimlich manoeuvre on cadavers with a simulated complete airway obstruction, the mean peak airway pressure was significantly lower with abdominal thrusts compared to chest compressions.[3] This study concluded that standard chest compressions have the potential of being more effective than the Heimlich manoeuvre for the management of complete airway obstruction by a foreign body in an unconscious patient.

Breathing

Adequate respirations are assessed by visually inspecting movement of the chest wall. In cases of cardiac arrest, infrequent, deep (agonal) respirations may continue for some minutes.

If the patient is found to have inadequate or absent breathing on initial assessment, then expired air resuscitation, mouth-to-mask or assisted ventilation with a bag/valve/mask will be required. On the other hand, if the initial assessment of the unconscious patient reveals adequate respirations, the victim should be turned and maintained in a recovery position.

Circulation

Previously, it was recommended that a bystander attempt to palpate a pulse in order to diagnose cardiac arrest and, if absent, commence external cardiac massage (ECM). However, it is now recognized that the pulse check is quite inaccurate in this setting.[4] Since cardiac arrest may be presumed if breathing is absent and is very unlikely if breathing is adequate, this step has now been deleted from BLS assessment.

CARDIOPULMONARY RESUSCITATION

If cardiac arrest is diagnosed, and the EMS has been summoned, the bystander should now commence CPR, using both expired air resuscitation (EAR) and ECM until a defibrillator arrives.

Expired air resuscitation

Since first described in 1958, EAR has become the standard in BLS for patients who have absent or inadequate respirations. However, there is often considerable reluctance for bystanders to perform EAR due to the perceived difficulty and contact with saliva resulting in the possibility of cross-infection.

It has been demonstrated in animal models that some ventilation occurs during chest compressions and it has been proposed that EAR may be withheld in patients who have cardiac arrest. In a study of 520 patients with pre-hospital cardiac arrest, bystanders were given instructions by ambulance dispatchers to perform EAR plus ECM or ECM alone.[5] There was a trend towards better survival to hospital discharge in the ECM only group compared with the EAR plus ECM (14.6% vs. 10.4%), however, this difference was not statistically significant (P=0.18). In this study, response times for EMS were very short (mean 5 minutes), consequently, the role of EAR in EMS areas where response times are longer remains uncertain.

There are a number of simple pieces of equipment that may be used as an alternative to EAR. These include mouth-to-mask and bag/valve/mask, with or without an oral-pharyngeal airway. This equipment has the advantage that there is no possible cross-infection risk, however, some training in the use of these devices is required. Within BLS, Guidelines 2000 recommends specific tidal volumes in bag/valve mask ventilation.[2] Whichever technique of assisted ventilation is used, adequate tidal volume is assessed by the rise of victim's chest, whether there is any distension of the stomach, and by listening and feeling for air being exhaled from the patient's mouth.

The use of supplemental oxygen has previously not been considered as part of BLS, however, some advisory committees within ILCOR are now incorporating oxygen use within BLS training. Although there are little data on the effect on outcome, it is intuitive that supplemental oxygen during CPR would increase the oxygen content of the blood and oxygen delivery to vital organs.

External cardiac compressions

External cardiac massage was first described in 1960. Subsequently, ECM has been adopted as the standard of care for patients with cardiac arrest. However, there is debate as to whether ECM generated blood flow via a 'cardiac pump' mechanism or a 'thoracic pump'. The thoracic pump theory had been supported by early transthoracic echocardiographic studies during CPR showing that the cardiac valves remained open during the relaxation phase of ECM. There had also been observations that 'cough CPR' resulted in some blood flow. It was presumed that the changes in intra-thoracic pressure led to forward blood flow and that valves in the venous system prevented back flow.

However, more recent studies of trans-oesophageal echocardiography during CPR in humans[6] has found that during the compression phase, the left ventricle is compressed; the mitral valve remains closed and the aortic valve opens only at the end of compression. During the relaxation phase, the mitral valve opens and the left ventricle is filled. These findings suggest that blood flow during ECM is a result of cardiac compression, at least early in the course of ECM.

Whatever the predominant mechanism of blood flow, ECM results in only 15%-20% of cardiac output in the adult, mainly owing to the relative rigidity of the chest wall. Consequently, there is progressive metabolic acidosis during CPR and very few adults survive when ECM has been given for more than 30 minutes.

The current recommended rate for ECM is 100 per minute, to ensure the delivery of a minimum of 60 compressions per minute. The sternum should be depressed at least 4 cm in the adult with compression being approximately 50% of the cycle. Pauses in chest compressions result in a prolonged decrease in mean arterial blood pressure, therefore, it is recommended that two breaths for every 15 compressions be delivered without a pause in chest compressions if there are two rescuers.

DEFIBRILLATION

Semi-automatic external defibrillation (SAED) is now considered part of BLS.[7] The SAED devices are extremely sensitive and specific for the correct diagnosis of ventricular fibrillation or ventricular tachycardia and are simple for bystanders to use with minimal training. Following the switching on of the device and the application of the pads, the SAED will request confirmation of coma and absent respirations, and advise the bystander to 'stand clear'. The bystander is then advised to press a button to deliver a shock.

There are four situations that have been proposed where non-medical personnel could use a SAED. First, the SAED may be used by first responders such as fire services who co-respond with ambulance services. For example, Ontario, Canada, has implemented an extensive programme to introduce rapid defibrillation across that state.[8] The use of fire department first responders resulted in 92.5% of cardiac arrest patients being defibrillated in under 8 minutes compared with 76.7% under the previous system (*P*<0.001). Survival to hospital discharge improved from 3.9% (183/4690 patients) to 5.2% (85/1614 patients) (*P*=0.03). This study demonstrated that an inexpensive, multifaceted system optimization approach to rapid defibrillation can lead to significant improvements in survival after cardiac arrest in a large system. In Melbourne, Australia, a study of a fireservice first responder programme found that the mean time to defibrillation was reduced from a mean of 7.1 minutes for ambulance services to 6.0 minutes for the combined approach.[9] However, this study did not have the power to assess the impact on patient outcomes.

Second, the SAED may be placed in a public area for use by designated personnel such as security staff who undergo a short training programme. In places such as casinos[10] and a large football stadium,[11] this approach has been shown to be effective.

Third, the SAED may be placed in a public area for use by personnel with no previous training at all in the use of an SAED. For example, at Chicago airport, there were defibrillators placed in strategic locations with signs advising of the correct use of the SAED.[12] Over a 2-year period, there were 21 patients with cardiac arrests, of whom 18 had an initial rhythm of ventricular fibrillation. A defibrillator was applied by a 'good Samaritan' bystander in 14/18 patients with ventricular fibrillation and 11 were successfully resuscitated, with 10 patients alive and well at 1 year.

However, most cardiac arrests occur in the home and it is estimated that the widespread implementation of this approach to all public areas would be very costly and result in relatively few lives saved.[13]

An SAED may be placed in the home of a patient who is at increased risk of sudden cardiac death for use by a partner or relative who (hopefully) would witness the cardiac arrest. Clinical trials are required to assess the cost-effectiveness of this approach prior to widespread implementation.

SUMMARY

Basic life support for the patient with sudden cardiac arrest has been described as a 'chain of survival' and includes recognition of cardiac arrest, a call to emergency medical services, the performance of EAR and ECM, and early defibrillation using a semi-automatic external defibrillator.

Current research explores the cost-effective means of delivering early defibrillation using public access defibrillation by personnel with no previous training, first responders with minimal training such as security personnel, co-responders

with ambulance services (such as fire fighters) or even defibrillators in the homes of high-risk patients.

CONTROVERSIES

❶ The cost-effectiveness of widespread training programmes to teach bystanders to perform cardiopulmonary resuscitation is uncertain.

❷ Expired air breathing may not be required early in cardiopulmonary resuscitation.

❸ The exact mechanism by which external chest compressions generate blood flow is uncertain. In any case, external chest compressions are minimally effective, and few patients survive prolonged chest compressions.

❹ Outcomes from public access defibrillation and first-responder programmes will need to demonstrate that these programmes are cost-effective.

REFERENCES

1. Cummins RO, Ornato JP, Thies WH, Pepe PE 1991 Improving survival from sudden cardiac arrest: The 'chain of survival' concept. A statement for health professionals from the advanced cardiac life-support subcommittee and the emergency cardiac care committee, American Heart Association. Circulation 83: 1832–47
2. American Heart Association in Collaboration with the International Liaison Committee on Resuscitation (ILCOR) 2000 Guidelines 2000 for cardiopulmonary resuscitation and emergency cardiovascular care. Resuscitation 46(1–3): 1–448
3. Langhelle A, Sunde K, Wik L, Steen PA 2001 Airway pressure with chest compressions versus Heimlich manoeuvre in recently dead adults with complete airway obstruction. Resuscitation 48: 185–7
4. Eberle B, Dick WF, Schneider T, Wisser G, Doetsch S, Tzanova I 1996 Checking the carotid pulse check: accuracy of first responders in patients with and without a pulse. Resuscitation 33: 107–16
5. Hallstrom A, Cobb L, Johnson E, Copass M 2000 Cardiopulmonary resuscitation by chest compression alone or with mouth to mouth ventilation. New England Journal of Medicine 342: 1546–53
6. Mair P, Furtwaengler W, Baubin M 1993 Aortic valve function during cardiopulmonary resuscitation. New England Journal of Medicine 329: 1965–6
7. Marenco JP, Wang PJ, Link MS, Homoud MK, Estes NA 2001 Improving survival from sudden cardiac arrest: the role of the automated external defibrillator. Journal of the American Medical Association 285: 1193–200
8. Stiell IG, Wells GA, Field BJ, et al 1999 Improved out-of-hospital cardiac arrest survival through the inexpensive optimization of an existing defibrillation program. Journal of the American Medical Association 281: 1175–81.
9. Smith KL, McNeill JJ, Emergency Medical Response Steering Committee 2002 Cardiac arrests treated by ambulance paramedics and fire fighters. Medical Journal of Australia 177: 305–9
10. Valenzuela T, Roe TJ, Nichol G, et al 2000 Outcomes of rapid defibrillation by security officers after cardiac arrests in casinos. New England Journal of Medicine 343: 1206–9
11. Wassertheil J, Keane G, Fisher N, Leditschenke JF 2000 Cardiac arrest at the Melbourne Cricket Ground and Shrine of Remembrance using a tiered response strategy – a forerunner to public access defibrillation. Resuscitation 44: 97–104
12. Caffrey SL, Willoughby PJ, Pepe PE, Becker LB 2002 Public use of automated external defibrillators. New England Journal of Medicine 347: 1242–7
13. Pell JP, Sirel JM, Marsden AK, Ford I, Walker NL, Cobbe SM 2002 Potential impact of public access defibrillators on survival after out of hospital cardiopulmonary arrest: retrospective cohort study. British Medical Journal 325: 515–20

1.2 ADVANCED LIFE SUPPORT

JOHN E. MAGUIRE

ESSENTIALS[1]

1 Follow international resuscitation guidelines.

2 Perform cardiopulmonary resuscitation (CPR) without interruption for pulseless patients (except when analyzing the rhythm or applying defibrillation shocks).

3 Defibrillate ventricular fibrillation (VF) and pulseless ventricular tachycardia (VT) until reverted to a stable, perfusing rhythm.

4 Obtain, maintain and protect an airway and provide adequate oxygenation and ventilation.

5 Give intravenous boluses of adrenaline (epinephrine).

6 Correct reversible causes of cardiac arrest.

INTRODUCTION

The patient in cardiac arrest is the most time-critical medical crisis an emergency physician is likely to manage. The interventions of basic life support (BLS) and advanced life support (ALS) have the greatest probability of success when applied immediately, but become less effective with the passing of time, and after only a short interval without treatment are ineffectual.

In 1993, Larsen et al[2] calculated the time intervals from collapse to the initiation of BLS, defibrillation and other ALS treatments, and analyzed their effects on survival from out-of-hospital cardiac arrest. When all three interventions were immediately available the survival was 67%, and this figure declined by 2.3% per minute of delay to BLS, a further 1.1% per minute to defibrillation and 2.1% per minute to other ALS interventions. Without treatment the decline in survival

rate was the sum of the three coefficients, or 5.5% per minute.

The importance of rapid treatment of cardiac arrest has led clinicians to develop a systems management approach, represented by the concept of the 'chain of survival', which has become a widely accepted model for the emergency medical services (EMS) systems.[3] The chain of survival idea maintains that more people survive sudden cardiac arrest when a sequence of events occurs as rapidly as possible. This sequence is:

- early access to the EMS system
- early BLS
- early defibrillation
- early advanced care.

A weakness in any link of the chain reduces the probability of patient survival, and all of the links must be connected. By convention, ALS involves continuation of BLS as appropriate, with the addition of defibrillation, invasive airway and vascular access techniques, and the administration of pharmacologic agents.

AETIOLOGY AND INCIDENCE OF CARDIAC ARREST

The commonest cause of adult sudden cardiac arrest is ischaemic heart disease.[4,5] Other causes of cardiac arrest include respiratory failure, drug overdose, metabolic derangements, trauma, hypothermia, immersion and hypovolaemia. While ALS guidelines are universally applicable, in these situations specific modifications may be appropriate.[4,5]

The incidence of sudden cardiac death (within 24 hours of the onset of symptoms) in the USA has been estimated as 1.24/1000/year.[6] In western metropolitan Melbourne, Australia, in 1995 the incidence of cardiac arrest notified to ambulance was approximately 0.72/1000/year.[7] In 20 communities from developed nations worldwide an average

of 0.62/1000/year received attempted resuscitation after out-of-hospital cardiac arrest.[6]

ADVANCED LIFE SUPPORT GUIDELINES AND ALGORITHMS

In 1997 the International Liaison Committee on Resuscitation (ILCOR), with delegates from Australia, Canada, Europe, South Africa and the USA published an advisory statement on ALS, *The Universal ALS Algorithm*,[1] based largely on the belief that valid scientific evidence supports only three interventions as unequivocally effective in adult cardiac resuscitation:

- basic CPR
- defibrillation if the dysrhythmia is VF or pulseless VT
- tracheal intubation.[1]

The algorithm (Fig. 1.2.1) recommends a specific sequence in which the above interventions should be performed, and prompts consideration of other therapies and potentially reversible causes of cardiac arrest. It is uncomplicated, concise, easy to memorize and adapt into poster format and is readily applied to the clinical situation. The guidelines and algorithm were ratified by the European Resuscitation Council (ERC) in Copenhagen, in June 1998 and published as *The 1998 European Resuscitation Council guidelines for adult advanced life support*.[8]

In 2000, the American Heart Association (AHA) convened the International Guidelines 2000 Conference on CPR and Emergency Cardiac Care (ECC). Following this conference, the *International Guidelines 2000 for CPR and ECC* were developed and published.[5] These guidelines represent a consensus of expert individuals and resuscitation councils and similar organizations from many countries,

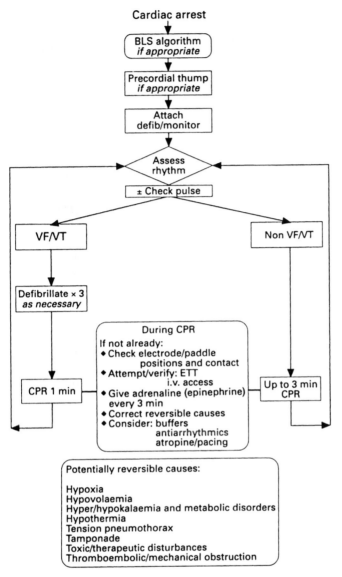

Fig. 1.2.1 Algorithm for advanced life support management. BLS - Basic life support. Reproduced with permission from *British Journal of Anaesthesia* 1997; 79:172–177.

RESUSCITATION

becoming universal in both inclusion of scientifically proven therapies and widespread acceptance, and have substantially simplified the management of cardiac arrest. Nevertheless, our resuscitation knowledge is still incomplete and many of the ALS techniques that we currently use are not supported by scientifically rigorous evidence.[10] Rigid adherence to guidelines is neither practical nor advisable and they should be interpreted with common sense. Individuals with specialist knowledge should take the opportunity to modify them according to the level of their expertise and the specific clinical situation or environment in which they practice.

CONFIRMATION OF CARDIAC ARREST RHYTHM AND INITIATION OF ALS

BLS is only a temporary and inefficient substitute for normal cardiorespiratory function. ALS is almost always necessary to produce return of spontaneous circulation (ROSC) after circulatory arrest. The purpose of BLS is to maintain the patient as effectively as possible until drugs and equipment, particularly a defibrillator, are available.[4, 5, 8]

The point of entry to the ALS algorithm is dependent upon the circumstances of the cardiac arrest. In many situations, such as out-of-hospital cardiac arrest, BLS will already have been initiated and should continue while the monitor/defibrillator is being prepared. When the patient is being monitored at the time of cardiac arrest, diagnosis should be swift and the defibrillator attached without delay.

For the rescuer with a manual defibrillator the critical decision is whether or not the rhythm present is VF/VT.[4] Nearly 70% of patients with an out-of-hospital cardiac arrest are in VF at the time of arrival of EMS personnel with a monitor/defibrillator.[11] Most eventual survivors come from this group.[3, 4]

VF is a pulseless, chaotic, disorganized dysrhythmia characterized by an undulating, irregular pattern that varies in

cultures and disciplines. The underlying principles that assisted decision-making when developing the guidelines were that additions to existing guidelines had to pass a rigorous evidence-based review, and revisions or deletions occurred because of:

- lack of evidence to confirm effectiveness
  and/or
- additional evidence to suggest harm or ineffectiveness
  and/or
- evidence that superior therapies had become available.

The guidelines include a version of the Universal ALS Algorithm and several other algorithms that expand on more specific areas of ALS assessment and management, and are a very valuable and clinically useful adjunct to the Universal ALS Algorithm.[5]

In 2002 the Australian Resuscitation Council published *Protocols for Adult Advanced Life Support*, which are succinct and include a slightly modified version of the Universal ALS Algorithm.[9]

The most exciting and clinically relevant advances in ALS over the last decade have been the development of guidelines and algorithms that are amplitude and morphology with a ventricular waveform of more than 150/minute.[1] Pulseless VT is characterized by broad, bizarrely shaped ventricular complexes associated with no detectable cardiac output. By definition the rate is greater than 100/minute and is usually well in excess of 150.

The absence of a detectable cardiac output in the presence of a coordinated electrical rhythm is called electro-mechanical dissociation (EMD) or pulseless electrical activity (PEA).[9]

Asystole is identified by the absence of any cardiac electrical activity. Occasionally asystole is incorrectly diagnosed because:

❶ **ECG leads may be broken or disconnected.** The presence of electrical artifact during external chest compression indicates that the leads are connected and probably intact.

❷ **Lead sensitivity may be inappropriate.** The sensitivity should be increased to maximum: an accompanying increase in the size of electrical artifact will confirm that the sensitivity selection is functioning.

❸ **On occasions VF has a predominant axis.** If this is at right angles to the selected monitor lead even coarse VF may cause minimal undulation in the baseline and resemble asystole. At least two leads should be selected in succession before asystole is diagnosed, preferably leads at right angles, such as II and aVL.

If there is any difficulty in diagnosing the rhythm in a patient with cardiac arrest the VF/VT protocol should be followed.[5,8]

DEFIBRILLATION

The only proven effective treatment for VF is electrical defibrillation.[1, 10, 12] When a defibrillator is available, it should be brought immediately to the side of the person in cardiac arrest and, if the dysrhythmia is VF/VT, defibrillation should be attempted without delay.

The chances of defibrillation restoring a sustained, perfusing rhythm, and also

of a long-term favourable outcome are optimal for as little as 90 seconds after cardiac arrest and decline rapidly there-after as myocardial high-energy phosphate stores are consumed.[4, 8, 9] BLS may be expected only to slow further myocardial deterioration, but is critical to the maintenance of cerebral circulation. Effective BLS will sustain the cerebral circulation at viable levels for 5–10 minutes or more. However, restoration of an effective spontaneous circulation provides the only means of completely reversing the effects of ischaemia and should be achieved as rapidly as possible.[8] Defibrillation should only ever be delayed by the commencement or continuation of BLS if this can be expected to improve the cellular biochemistry of the myocardium or if restoration of some cerebral circulation is essential.[1, 4, 8]

All of the resuscitation guidelines referred to previously stress the importance of minimum delay in the administration of defibrillating shocks.[1, 5, 8, 9] Furthermore, the ILCOR, ERC and ARC guidelines and algorithms qualify the commencement of BLS with the statement – 'if appropriate'.[1, 8, 9] This approach is justified because:

* the prospects of successful defibrillation decrease relatively rapidly over a few minutes after cardiac arrest
* BLS is unlikely to improve the odds of successful defibrillation
* modern defibrillators have very rapid charge times: three shocks of appropriate energy levels can be given within 30 seconds by a trained and well-equipped team.[1, 8]

Technique

For defibrillation to be successful, a critical myocardial mass must be depolarized synchronously to interrupt the fibrillation and allow recapture by a single pacemaker. The technique used must minimize transthoracic impedance in order to maximize the probability of success.[4, 11, 12, 13]

Reducing transthoracic impedance

Transthoracic impedance is reduced by:

* paddles of 10–13 cm in diameter for adults. Smaller paddles allow too concentrated a discharge of energy and may cause focal myocardial damage.[11, 12] Larger paddles may not be able to contact the chest over their entire area and/or may cause more current to be conducted through non-myocardial tissues.[11, 13]
* conductive electrode paste or pads reduce impedance by 30%.[11] Care should be taken to ensure that there is no contact between the paddles either directly or through electrode paste or defibrillation pads, as this will result in current arcing across the chest wall.[11–13]
* pressure of about 5 kg on each paddle.[11]
* defibrillation in expiration.[13]
* repeated countershocks with a short interval between.[11, 13]

Paddle placement

There are two widely accepted positions for the defibrillation paddles that optimize current delivery to the heart. The most convenient is the antero-apical position, where one paddle is placed to the right of the sternum just below the clavicle, and the other is centred lateral to the normal cardiac apex in the anterior or midaxillary line (V5-6 position). An alternative is the anteroposterior position with the anterior paddle placed over the precordium or apex and the posterior paddle on the back in the left or right infrascapular region. Paddles are often labelled sternum and apex, which is irrelevant for transthoracic defibrillation, but allows correct orientation of rhythms detected by the paddles for synchronized cardioversion.[4, 11, 12, 13]

Defibrillation should not be attempted over ECG electrodes or medicated patches, and placement of paddles over the breast tissue in female patients should be avoided.[4, 12] If the patient has an implanted pacemaker module or cardioverter defibrillator, the paddles should be placed at least 12–15 cm away from the module and pulse generator respectively. Pacemaker function should be checked as soon as practicable following successful defibrillation.[11, 12]

Technical problems

If attempted defibrillation is not accompanied by skeletal muscle contraction, care should be taken to ensure good contact and that the defibrillator is turned on, charged, develops sufficient power and is in asynchronous mode. The majority of defibrillator problems are due to operator errors or faulty care and maintenance.[12] The operational status of defibrillators should be checked regularly and a stand-by machine should be available when possible.

Timing and energy of shocks

When using a conventional defibrillator with a damped monophasic sinusoidal waveform (see below) the first shock is given with an energy level of 200 joules (J), which represents the best compromise between the probability of success and the risk of myocardial damage.[12] If the first attempt at defibrillation is unsuccessful, a shock of the same energy is repeated. If still unsuccessful a third shock is given, this time at 360 J.[4,5,9,11,12] The paddles need not be removed from the chest while being recharged and CPR need not be recommenced between these initial shocks, unless there is a delay exceeding 20 seconds in recharging the defibrillator.[9] With modern defibrillators it is possible to administer three shocks within 60 seconds.

The carotid pulse should be palpated if, after a defibrillating shock, an ECG rhythm compatible with cardiac output is obtained. However, if the monitor indicates persistent VF then additional shocks in the sequence of three can be administered without a further pulse check. After a defibrillating shock there is typically a delay of several seconds before an ECG trace of diagnostic quality is obtained. Additionally, even when defibrillation is successful, there is often a temporary impairment of cardiac function associated with a weak, or difficult to palpate, central pulse for seconds to minutes. It is important to recognize these phenomena and allow for them rather than hastily conclude that defibrillation has been unsuccessful or that EMD has developed.[4,12]

COMPLICATIONS OF DEFIBRILLATION

- Skin burns can occur; these are usually superficial.
- Skeletal muscle injury or thoracic vertebral fractures are possible, though are uncommon.
- Myocardial injury and post-defibrillation dysrhythmias can happen with cumulative high-energy shocks.[11,12]
- Health-care providers can receive electrical injuries due to electrical contact with the patient during defibrillation. These range from paraesthesiae to deep partial thickness burns. Cardiac arrest is a theoretical possibility. The operator should ensure that all rescue personnel are clear of the patient before delivering a defibrillation shock. A particular concern should be to ensure that the patient, rescuers and equipment are dry before defibrillation is attempted, especially outdoors or around a swimming pool area.[11,12]

DEVELOPMENTS IN DEFIBRILLATION

Automated external defibrillators

Automated external defibrillators (AEDs) were first introduced in 1979 and have become standard equipment in many EMS systems primarily for use outside of the hospital. The AED is attached by two connecting cables to adhesive pads that are placed on the patient's chest in the standard antero-apical positions for defibrillation. An internal microprocessor analyses the ECG signal and, if VF/VT are detected, causes the AED to display an alarm and either delivers a shock (automatic) or advises the operator to do so (semi-automatic).[11,12]

AEDs are highly accurate with some models demonstrating 100% specificity and 90–92% sensitivity for coarse VF.[12] Although their precision is less for fine VF and least for VT, their accuracy overall is comparable to that of experienced cardiologists.[11] Several EMS systems equipped with AEDs have shown that they can deliver the first shock up to 1 minute faster than when using conventional defibrillators and rates of survival to hospital discharge are equivalent to those achieved when first responders used manual defibrillators.[3]

The major advantage of AEDs over conventional defibrillators is their simplicity, which has markedly reduced the skill required to defibrillate a patient in cardiac arrest. This decreases the time and expense of initial training and continuing education, and increases the number of persons who can operate the device.[3,11,12] Members of the public have been trained to use AEDs in a variety of community settings and have demonstrated that they can retain skills for up to 1 year.[3] Encouraging results have been produced when AEDs have been placed with community responders, such as fire fighters, police officers, security guards at large public assemblies and public transportation vehicle crews.[3,11]

Current-based defibrillation

Conventional defibrillators are designed to deliver a specified number of joules (J). However, depolarization of myocardial tissue is accomplished by the passage of electrical current through the heart, and clinical studies have determined that the optimal current is 30–40 amperes (A).[11,13] At a fixed energy, the current delivered is inversely related to the transthoracic impedance and a standard energy dose of 200 J delivers about 30 A to a patient with average transthoracic impedance. In patients with greater than average impedance, the current generated may be inadequate, whereas a patient with smaller than average impedance may sustain myocardial damage from excessive current flow.[11,12,13]

Some newer defibrillators automatically measure transthoracic impedance and then predict and adjust the energy delivered to avoid inappropriately high or low transmyocardial currents. These devices have defibrillation success rates comparable to conventional defibrillators while cumulatively delivering less energy. The decreased energy should result in less myocardial damage and may reduce post-defibrillation complications.[4, 11, 12, 13]

New defibrillator waveforms

Most conventional defibrillators use a damped monophasic sinusoidal waveform, which is a single pulse lasting for 3–4 ms. Many studies over the last decade have shown that biphasic (bidirectional) truncated transthoracic shocks are as effective at lower energies as standard damped sine wave shocks and result in fewer post-defibrillation ECG abnormalities.[4,11,12,13] In a recent review, the reviewers concluded that lower-energy biphasic shocks, delivered without an increase in energy, achieved clinical outcomes equivalent to those of monophasic shocks with increasing energy levels, in out-of-hospital cardiac arrest.[14] Defibrillators using biphasic waveforms with impedance compensation are now available and will likely become the standard in the near future. Research is still needed to determine the optimal biphasic waveform and energy levels for first and subsequent shocks, but the potential advantages are equivalent or more effective external defibrillation with a reduction in myocardial injury produced by the defibrillatory shocks.[5]

FAILURE OF DEFIBRILLATION, EMD AND ASYSTOLE

Most patients who will survive cardiac arrest are successfully defibrillated by one of the first three shocks and even if this first sequence is unsuccessful, the best chance for restoring a perfusing rhythm is still defibrillation.[4] However, at this stage it is necessary to recommence BLS in an attempt to restore some myocardial and cerebral perfusion and maintain cellular viability. Additionally, efforts should be made to secure advanced airway management and ventilation, and to institute vascular access for administration of drugs.

Potentially reversible causes or aggravating factors of cardiac arrest (Fig. 1.2.1) should be considered and specific therapy commenced as indicated.

These interventions should occur during the 1 minute period of CPR, although it is unlikely that even a highly trained team will be able to complete all of these aspects of management within this interval. Further opportunities will occur with subsequent cycles.[4]

The ECG rhythm is then reassessed and if VF persists the next sequence of three defibrillating shocks is started without delay. These shocks are all at 360 J, or its equivalent if the defibrillator is current-based or uses a biphasic waveform.[4, 11, 12, 13]

If VF/VT is definitely excluded at the time of initial or later rhythm analysis, defibrillation is not appropriate and may be deleterious.[4, 11, 12] These patients will have EMD or asystole and the prognosis for these rhythms is much less favourable than for VF/VT. There are some situations where EMD or asystole may have been provoked by conditions that are treatable. The common causes are listed in Figure 1.2.1 and may be recalled under the headings of the four Hs and four Ts. Apart from treating potentially remediable conditions the management of EMD and asystole is largely the application of other ALS therapies and the continuation of BLS.[1, 4, 5, 8,]

OTHER ALS INTERVENTIONS

Except for defibrillation, no single ALS intervention has been scientifically proven to enhance patient outcome,[10, 15] although the ILCOR considers that there is valid scientific evidence to support tracheal intubation as unequivocally effective.[11] Many clinicians maintain that ALS has an incremental benefit compared with defibrillation alone.[3, 15, 16] While there are some data to support this contention, it remains impossible to prove.[10]

Advanced airway management

No randomized controlled studies exist that demonstrate the life-saving effect of endotracheal intubation compared to basic airway management.[15, 16] However, intuitively some benefit would be expected.

Direct expired air resuscitation and bag/valve-mask ventilation are less effective than ventilation via an endotracheal tube and provide no protection against aspiration, which is found in 28% of patients examined by the coroner after failed resuscitation from cardiac arrest.[16, 17 18] Also, EMS systems that use endotracheal intubation report higher survival rates than systems that do not.[15, 17]

Endotracheal intubation is the gold standard for advanced management of the airway during cardiac arrest. It provides a clear and secure airway, allowing ventilation, oxygenation, suction and administration of medications if indicated.[1,16,17,18] Attempts at intubation should not interrupt BLS for longer than 15–20 seconds. If intubation is not accomplished within that time, additional attempts should be delayed until the cycle of CPR following the next sequence of three defibrillation shocks, or with EMD and asystole until after a further 3 minutes of CPR.[4, 8, 9]

Ventilation and oxygenation

During cardiac arrest, carbon dioxide (CO_2) production and delivery to the pulmonary circulation is limited by the relatively low cardiac output achieved during CPR. As a consequence, relatively low minute volumes are sufficient to achieve adequate CO_2 excretion and prevent hypercapnia. This situation may be altered if CO_2-producing buffers such as sodium bicarbonate are administered, and relative increases in minute ventilation are required to prevent the development of respiratory acidosis.[4]

Several animal studies and evidence from humans in cardiac arrest indicate that, when the airway is patent, spontaneous gasping can provide sufficient ventilation during CPR to maintain normal arterial CO_2 levels. Similarly, chest compression alone provides some pulmonary ventilation and gas exchange, which can approach normal values with active compression–decompression CPR. Ventilation may actually be unnecessary during the first few minutes of CPR, although under conditions of prolonged cardiac arrest, it is essential for survival.[10, 19] In most cardiac arrest situations, a tidal volume of 400–500 mL (5–6 mL/ kg) is sufficient to clear CO_2 during CPR and will cause a visible rise and fall of the patient's chest.[18]

Cardiac arrest and CPR cause an increase in dead space and a reduction in lung compliance that may compromise gas exchange. As adequate oxygenation is of paramount importance in cardiac arrest, the aim should be to provide a fractional inspired oxygen concentration (FIO_2) of 1.0.[4, 18]

Tidal volumes of 400–500 mL and FIO_2 approaching 1.0 are attainable using self-inflating bag/valve/mask and intubation devices, which remain the mainstay of ventilation in ALS.[4, 8, 18]

Drug therapy

No drug used in resuscitation has been shown to improve long-term survival in humans after cardiac arrest.[10, 15, 20, 21] Despite this knowledge, a number of pharmacotherapeutic agents continue to be employed, largely for historical reasons based on theoretical, retrospective or anecdotal evidence of efficacy.[10, 20]

Adrenaline (epinephrine)

Actions The beneficial actions of adrenaline (epinephrine) in cardiac arrest are due to its α-adrenergic effects, whereas the β-adrenergic activity appears, at best, to be unimportant and may be detrimental. A series of experiments have demonstrated that adrenaline (epinephrine) maintains tone in intrathoracic arteries, preventing their collapse during external chest compression, and also increases resistance in non-cerebral and non-coronary arteries. These actions result in decreased blood flow to non-cerebral and non-coronary vessels, increased aortic blood pressure and increased perfusion of the cerebral and coronary vascular beds.[22]

Indications and dose Adrenaline (epinephrine) is recommended in VF/VT cardiac arrest if there is no ROSC after the first three attempts at defibrillation. It is recommended in EMD and asystole after commencement of CPR. The standard adult dose is 1 mg intravenously (IV) every 3 minutes.[1, 4, 5, 8, 20, 21]

For a number of years there has been considerable interest in high-dose adrenaline, usually defined as amounts in excess of 45 μg per kg every 5 minutes. However, no prospective randomized clinical trials in humans have demonstrated a significant improvement in survival to hospital discharge for adult patients treated with either standard-dose or high-dose adrenaline.[4, 10, 15, 16, 20]

Potential complications Particularly in higher doses adrenaline (epinephrine) may increase myocardial oxygen requirements, induce myocardial contraction band necrosis and predispose to tachy-dysrhythmias. After ROSC it can produce severe hypertension. Tissue necrosis occurs commonly after extravasation.[4, 18, 21, 22]

Vasopressin

Actions Vasopressin is an endogenous peptide hormone synthesized in the hypothalamus and secreted from the posterios pituitary in response to a variety of osmotic and non-osmotic stimuli. The principal physiologic effects of vasopressin are direct vasoconstriction of the systemic circulation, mediated by V_1 receptors on vascular smooth muscle and renal water retention, mediated by renal V_2 receptors. During the last decade research has indicated that vasopressin may be an important hormone during cardiac arrest and levels of vasopressin during CPR are significantly higher in eventual survivors than in those who do not survive. A possible advantage of vasopressin during cardiac arrest and CPR is that it produces vasoconstriction in non-vital tissues while preserving blood flow to the coronary and cerebral circulations.[23]

Indications and dose The AHA in the International Guidelines 2000 recommend that vasopressin is an effective vasopressor and can be used as an *alternative* to epinephrine for the treatment of adult shock-refractory VF.[5] The ERC and ARC do not include vasopressin in their recently published algorithms.[8, 21] Although there are still insufficient clinical data to support the

use of vasopressin as a first-line drug in the management of cardiac arrest, reports to date are promising and further research may well provide definitive information in the near future.[23] The dose currently recommended by the AHA is an i.v. bolus of 40 U administered once during an episode of cardiac arrest.[5]

Potential complications The beneficial effect of vasopressin on the cerebral circulation during CPR may increase the risk of cerebral oedema or haemorrhage after ROSC. Vasopressin has a relatively long half-life (10–20 minutes) and persistent vasoconstriction following ROSC may exacerbate myocardial ischaemia and interfere with left ventricular function. Vasopressin also exerts a procoagulant effect on platelets.[23]

Lidocaine

Actions Lidocaine is a Vaughan–Williams class IB agent that depresses myocardial excitability by blocking sodium channels without extending action potential duration. In animal models it also has an antifibrillatory action.

The role of lidocaine in assisting resuscitation from refractory VF is contentious. Several experimental studies in animals have shown that it increases the defibrillation threshold (the energy required for defibrillation).[12, 18] Other studies have shown no effect, or a decrease in the defibrillation threshold.[4, 24] A recently reported retrospective observational study of outcome from cardiac arrest with sustained VF, compared the survival of patients who received lidocaine with those who received no lidocaine. This study showed a significant increase in ROSC in the lidocaine group but there was no difference in the rate of hospital discharge between the two groups.[25] Controlled prospective trials of lidocaine and alternative antifibrillatory drugs are still needed.[4, 20]

Indications and dose Lidocaine cannot be recommended as first-line therapy in cardiac arrest, but may be considered if multiple DC shocks and adrenaline have failed to revert VF/VT.

It can also be used to help prevent reversion to VF/VT after successful defibrillation.[5, 12, 20, 21] The initial bolus dose is 1–1.5 mg/kg with an additional bolus of 0.5 mg/kg after 5–10 minutes if indicated.[4, 5, 21]

Potential complications Cardiovascular effects include hypotension, bradydysrhythmias and asystole. Neurological toxicity causes central nervous system (CNS) excitation with anxiety, tremor and convulsions followed by CNS depression.[4, 20, 21]

Amiodarone

Actions Amiodarone is a class III agent that has some class I activity and weak non-competitive β-blocking effects. Amiodarone lowers the defibrillation threshold and has a potent antifibrillatory effect. Its broad spectrum of antidysrhythmic activity and minimal adverse haemodynamic effects make it a potentially useful agent, but its value during cardiac arrest has not been extensively explored.[20, 24]

Indications and dose Amiodarone cannot be recommended as first-line therapy in cardiac arrest, but may be considered if multiple DC shocks and adrenaline have failed to revert VF/VT. The initial dose is 5 mg/kg given as a slow intravenous infusion over 5–15 minutes. This may be repeated if indicated.

Potential complications Cardiovascular effects include hypotension and bradycardia.[24]

Atropine

Actions Atropine antagonizes parasympathetic nervous effects on the heart by blocking cholinergic muscarinic receptors, leading to increased sinoatrial and atrioventricular automaticity and rate of conduction.[5, 20, 21] Atropine may be effective when increased vagal tone results in a haemodynamically significant bradyasystole but its effect on EMD or asystole caused by prolonged, widespread myocardial ischaemia is negligible.[24]

Indications and dose Atropine may be considered in bradyasystolic cardiac arrest that does not respond to initial CPR and adrenaline (epinephrine). The dose is 3 mg, which is considered to be the vagolytic dose.[4, 5, 8, 20]

Potential complications Adverse effects include tachycardia, CNS excitement and delirium, which are usually regarded as benign.[21, 24]

Magnesium

Actions Magnesium is an essential electrolyte that may be depleted by diuretics, severe diarrhoea and alcohol abuse. Hypomagnesaemia may cause cardiac dysrhythmias.[5, 21] Several case reports and trials have yielded contradictory results concerning the effect of magnesium in cardiac arrest, and there is little to support its routine use at present.[10, 20, 24]

Indications and dose Magnesium may be considered in refractory VF/VT, particularly if hypokalaemia is present, and is an agent of choice in torsades de pointes. The initial dose is 5 mmol (2.5 mL of 49.3% solution) given over 1 minute, which may be repeated if indicated and followed by an infusion of 20 mmol over 4 hours.[5, 20, 21]

Potential complications Adverse effects include hypotension and heart block. Muscle weakness and paralysis may occur if excessive quantities are administered.[5, 21]

Calcium

Actions Calcium is a divalent cation essential to neuromuscular function. Human studies have shown that its pharmacotherapeutic effects in cardiac arrest are negligible and may be adverse.[5, 20]

Indications and dose Calcium should not be administered unless there is evidence that cardiac arrest is caused or exacerbated by hyperkalaemia, hypocalcaemia or overdose of calcium-channel-blocking drugs.[4, 5, 21] The dose is 5–10 mL of 10% calcium chloride or three times that dose of 10% calcium gluconate.[5, 21]

Potential complications Calcium may increase the damage caused by profound ischaemia of myocardial and cerebral cells.[5, 20, 21] Extravasation causes tissue necrosis.[21]

Sodium bicarbonate

Actions Sodium bicarbonate ($NaHCO_3$) is an alkalinizing agent that, theoretically, reverses the metabolic acidosis associated with profound ischaemia. However, provided CPR is effective, acidosis does not develop rapidly or severely in otherwise healthy individuals during cardiac arrest.[4, 20, 21] There is no strong clinical evidence supporting the administration of alkalinizing agents in cardiac arrest.[4, 15, 20] Some benefits have been reported, particularly when the dose can be titrated to avoid alkalosis and with concurrent use of adrenaline (epinephrine).[16, 20] It is probably unwise to completely abandon $NaHCO_3$ therapy for all patients with cardiac arrest, and an objective reappraisal is needed to define its role.[10, 20]

Indications and dose Sodium bicarbonate is unnecessary in brief resuscitations when the patient has been previously well but can be considered if cardiac arrest exceeds 10–15 minutes duration.[20, 21] It should also be considered when cardiac arrest occurs in a patient with a preexisting profound acidosis or in special circumstances, such as tricyclic antidepressant overdose and hyperkalaemia.[5, 21]

Potential complications Adverse effects of $NaHCO_3$ include alkalosis, hyperosmolality and CO_2 production, causing paradoxical intracellular acidosis.[4, 5, 21]

VASCULAR ACCESS AND DRUG DELIVERY DURING CARDIAC ARREST

The ideal route of drug delivery combines rapid and easy vascular access with quick delivery to the central circulation. Central venous cannulae deliver drugs rapidly to the central circulation but require considerable technical proficiency to insert during CPR and some methods of insertion interfere with defibrillation and CPR, which is unacceptable.[4, 20] The most appropriate method of vascular access will usually be via a peripheral venous cannula. When drugs are administered by this route the extremity should be elevated and a 20 mL bolus of IV fluid should follow the agent to facilitate delivery to the central circulation.[4, 20]

Intratracheal deposition is an alternative route, and during cardiac arrest tracheal intubation often precedes venous access.[4, 20] If there is a delay in achieving vascular access most ALS drugs, including adrenaline (epinephrine), lidocaine and atropine, may be safely administered through the endotracheal tube.[5, 20] The ideal dose and dilution of drugs given by this route is uncertain but current recommendations are to use two to three times the standard IV dose diluted in 10 mL of normal saline. This solution should be delivered via a catheter placed beyond the tip of the endotracheal tube and followed by five ventilations to aid dispersion.[4, 20, 26]

Crystalloid solutions are preferred as the standard vehicle of drug delivery as administration of glucose-containing solutions during CPR may contribute to post-arrest hyperglycaemia, which is detrimental to cerebral recovery.[26]

HAEMODYNAMIC MONITORING DURING CPR

Researchers and clinicians have proposed and measured numerous physiological parameters as a means of monitoring the effectiveness of resuscitation during cardiac arrest. The techniques for measuring these parameters are usually invasive, technically difficult and time consuming to establish and maintain, thereby limiting their utility in sudden and unexpected cardiac arrest.[27]

Numerous animal and clinical experiments indicate that measurement of end-tidal CO_2 ($ETCO_2$) may be an effective and informative method of determining the progress of CPR.[10, 27] The normal $ETCO_2$ is 4–5% and typically falls to less than 1% at the onset of cardiac arrest. With effective CPR, the $ETCO_2$ rises to between one-quarter and one-third of normal and ROSC is associated with a rise to normal or supranormal levels over the next minute. These changes parallel proportionally similar alterations in cardiac output.[27]

An $ETCO_2$ of less than 1% during attempted resuscitation from cardiac arrest is an indication of ineffective CPR. This may be due to inadequate ventilation due to airway obstruction or oesophageal intubation, or due to the cardiac output being less than expected because of poor technique or causes such as hypovolaemia, pulmonary embolism or pericardial tamponade. A sharp rise in $ETCO_2$ may be the first indication of ROSC.[27]

End-tidal CO_2 measured immediately after commencement of CPR may also have a prognostic value in out-of-hospital cardiac arrests as it is higher in patients who have had a short interval of cardiac arrest, as compared with those who have had a longer period prior to the initiation of resuscitation. There is also evidence that patients who are eventually resuscitated have a higher $ETCO_2$ during CPR than those who will never have ROSC. Caution should be exercised in interpreting $ETCO_2$ following adrenaline (epinephrine), as this agent causes a decrease in $ETCO_2$, which is not necessarily a poor prognostic indicator.[27]

DISCONTINUING ALS

With the introduction of effective EMS systems, initiation of ALS for patients with out-of-hospital cardiac arrest moved from the institution into the community. Research indicates that the vast majority of patients who survive out-of-hospital cardiac arrest have ROSC before arrival at the emergency department (ED). In 18 papers published between 1981 and 1995, only 33 (0.6%) of 5444 patients who were transported to an ED still in cardiac arrest after unsuccessful pre-hospital resuscitation, survived to hospital discharge.[28] Twenty-four of the surviving patients arrived in the ED in VF and 11 of these patients had their initial arrest in the ambulance en route to the hospital or had temporary ROSC before arrival at the ED.

In 1993 a recommendation was made that after out-of-hospital cardiac arrest in the normothermic patient, resuscitation should cease if there is no ROSC after 25 minutes of ALS.[29] The two exceptions to this practice are if the cardiac arrest occurs in the presence of ambulance personnel, or the patient demonstrates persistent VF. These recommendations were applied and considered to be valid in a prospective study in the same year.[30]

Early in the resuscitation of patients with in-hospital cardiac arrest there are no absolute predictors of futility but some variables are associated with a greater or lesser chance of survival to discharge. Ventricular tachydysrhythmias, commencement of resuscitation within 5 minutes and ROSC within 15 minutes are all linked to better outcomes. Pre-existing conditions such as metastatic cancer, renal failure, sepsis, acute cerebrovascular accident and cardiogenic shock are all linked to poor outcome. Age is not an independent predictor of outcome and this has also been confirmed in out-of-hospital cardiac arrest.[31, 32] Resuscitation efforts lasting more than 30 minutes without ROSC appear to be so uniformly unsuccessful that they should be abandoned except in unusual circumstances.[10, 32]

PROGNOSIS AFTER CARDIAC ARREST

The prognosis for survival after an out-of-hospital cardiac arrest fluctuates from community to community. Some of the variation is due to differences in EMS systems but much is also due to diverse research methodology and data reporting. In King County, Washington, where a sophisticated EMS system has been in place for over two decades, survival to hospital discharge was between 15% and 20% from 1976 to 1987. These figures are in contrast to US national rates of survival, which were estimated to be from 1% to 3% in a 1991 report from the

AHA.[3] In 1987–88 in Perth, Australia survival was 22.7% of 231 cases of out-of-hospital cardiac arrest due to VF[33] and in western metropolitan Melbourne in 1995 the survival rate for all arrest dysrhythmias was 3%.[7] In a 1996 meta-analysis of 36 articles published between 1973 and 1992 describing 41 EMS systems in six countries, survival varied from 0% to 21% with an overall mean survival of 8%.[34]

Prognosis for survival from in-hospital cardiac arrest is only marginally better with survival to hospital discharge averaging 13.8% of 12961 patients described in reports published between 1961 and 1984.[31] In a further seven reports published between 1978 and 1989, 11% of 1804 patients survived to hospital discharge.[32]

UNIFORM REPORTING IN CARDIAC ARREST RESEARCH

Cardiac arrest research and the interpretation of available data has often been hampered by inconsistent methodology and reporting. An important initiative has been the recognition of the need for uniform, internationally recognized definitions and guidelines for reporting of cardiac arrest data. During the last few years a number of templates have been developed to include the most relevant variables for describing and comparing cardiac arrest research results. These are referred to as Utstein style guidelines or templates after Utstein Abbey, near Stavanger, Norway, where expert researchers and clinicians gathered in 1990.[35]

REFERENCES

1. Kloeck W, Cummins R, Chamberlain L 1997 The universal ALS algorithm. Resuscitation 34: 109–11

2. Larsen MP, Eisenberg MS, Cummins RO, Hallstrom AP 1993 Predicting survival from out-of-hospital cardiac arrest: a graphic model. Annals of Emergency Medicine 22: 1652–8
3. Cummins RO, Ornato JP, Thies WH, Pepe PE 1991 Improving survival from sudden cardiac arrest: the 'chain of survival' concept: a statement for health professionals from the Advanced Cardiac Life Support Subcommittee and the Emergency Cardiac Care Committee, American Heart Association. Circulation 83: 1832–47
4. Robertson CE 1997 Advanced life support guidelines. British Journal of Anaesthesia 79: 172–7
5. The American Heart Association in collaboration with the International Liaison Committee on Resuscitation 2000 Guidelines 2000 for cardiopulmonary resuscitation and emergency cardiovascular care: a consensus on science. Circulation 102(Suppl. 8): I1–I384
6. Becker LB, Smith DW, Rhodes KV 1993 Incidence of cardiac arrest: a neglected factor in evaluating survival rates. Annals of Emergency Medicine 22: 86–91
7. Bernard S 1998 Outcome from prehospital cardiac arrest in Melbourne Australia. Emergency Medicine 10: 25–29
8. Advanced Life Support Working Group of the European Resuscitation Council 1998 The 1998 European Resuscitation Council guidelines for adult advanced life support. Resuscitation 37: 81–90
9. Australian Resuscitation Council February 2002 Protocols for adult advanced life support. Revised Policy Statement P.S. 11.2.1
10. Maguire JE 1997 Advances in cardiac life support: sorting the science from the dogma. Emergency Medicine 9(Suppl 4): 1–21
11. Truong JH, Rosen P 1997 Current concepts in electrical defibrillation. Journal of Emergency Medicine 15: 331–8
12. Bossaert LL 1997 Fibrillation and defibrillation of the heart. British Journal of Anaesthesia 79: 172–7
13. Kerber RE 1993 Electrical treatment of cardiac arrhythmias: defibrillation and cardioversion. Annals of Emergency Medicine 22: 296–301
14. Cummins RO, Hazinski MF, Kerber RE, et al 1998 Low-energy biphasic waveform defibrillation: evidence-based review applied to emergency cardiovascular care guidelines: a statement for healthcare professionals from the American Heart Association Committee on Emergency Cardiovascular Care and the subcommittees on Basic Life Support, Advanced Cardiac Life Support, and Pediatric Resuscitation. Circulation 97: 1654–67
15. Pepe PE, Abramson NS, Brown CG 1994 ACLS-Does it really work? Annals of Emergency Medicine 23: 1037–41
16. Ornato JP, Paradis N, Bircher N, et al 1996 Future directions for resuscitation research. III. External cardiopulmonary resuscitation advanced life support. Resuscitation 32: 139–58
17. Pepe PE, Zachariah BS, Chandra NC 1993 Invasive airway techniques in resuscitation. Annals of Emergency Medicine 22: 393–403
18. Gabbott DA, Baskett PJF 1997 Management of the airway and ventilation during resuscitation. British Journal of Anaesthesia 79: 159–71
19. Idris AH 1996 Reassessing the need for ventilation during CPR. Annals of Emergency Medicine 27: 569–75
20. Vincent R 1997 Drugs in modern resuscitation. British Journal of Anaesthesia 79: 188–97
21. Australian Resuscitation Council February 2002 Medications in adult cardiac arrest. Revised Policy Statement P.S. 11.4
22. Paradis NA, Koscove EM 1990 Epinephrine in cardiac arrest: a critical review. Annals of Emergency Medicine 19: 1288–301
23. Barlow M 2002 Vasopressin. Emergency Medicine 14: 304–14
24. Jaffe AS 1993 The use of antiarrhythmics in advanced cardiac life support. Annals of Emergency Medicine 22 (pt 2): 307–16
25. Herlitz J, Ekstrom L, Wennerblom B, et al 1997 Lidocaine in out-of-hospital ventricular fibrillation. Does it improve outcome? Resuscitation 33: 199–205
26. Gonzalez ER 1993 Pharmacologic controversies in CPR. Annals of Emergency Medicine 22: 317–23
27. Ornato JP 1993 Hemodynamic monitoring during CPR. Annals of Emergency Medicine 22: 289–95
28. Brennan RJ, Luke C 1995 Failed prehospital resuscitation following out-of-hospital cardiac arrest: are further efforts in the emergency department warranted? Emergency Medicine 7: 131–8
29. Bonnin MJ, Pepe PE, Timball KT, et al 1993 Distinct criteria for termination of resuscitation in the out-of-hospital setting. Journal of the American Medical Association 269: 1457–62
30. Pepe PE, Brown CG, Bonnin MJ, et al 1993 Prospective validation of criteria for on-scene termination of resuscitation efforts after out-of-hospital cardiac arrest. Annals of Emergency Medicine 22: 884–5
31. McGrath RB 1987 In-house cardiopulmonary resuscitation after a quarter of a century. Annals of Emergency Medicine 16: 1365-8
32. Jastremski MS 1993. In-hospital cardiac arrest. Annals of Emergency Medicine 22: 113–7
33. Jacobs IG, Oxer HF 1990 A review of pre-hospital defibrillation by ambulance officers in Perth, Western Australia. Medical Journal of Australia 153: 662–4
34. Nichol G, Destsky AS, Stiell IG, et al 1995 Effectiveness of emergency medical services for victims of out-of-hospital cardiac arrest: a meta-analysis. Annals of Emergency Medicine 27: 700–10
35. Dick WF 1997 Uniform reporting in resuscitation. British Journal of Anaesthesia 79: 241–52

CONTROVERSIES

❶ Acceptance of universal guidelines and algorithms.

❷ The role of new technologies in defibrillation.

❸ The need for ventilation as initial therapy in cardiac arrest.

❹ The role of vasopressors in ALS.

❺ When is CPR futile?

1.3 ADVANCED AIRWAY MANAGEMENT

STEPHEN BERNARD

ESSENTIALS[1]

1 Intubation of the trachea in the emergency department usually requires the use of drugs for sedation and neuromuscular relaxation to facilitate placement of an endotracheal tube.

2 Clinical checks for tracheal placement may be inaccurate, and capnography or an air aspiration device should be used for confirmation.

3 If visualization of the vocal cords at laryngoscopy is difficult, a failed intubation drill should be followed to avoid patient hypoxaemia.

INTRODUCTION

Appropriate airway management is the initial step in the resuscitation of the patient with critical illness. Basic airway manoeuvres include jaw thrust, chin lift and finger sweeps to clear the airway, together with expired air or bag/valve/mask breathing for ventilation. Advanced airway management includes endotracheal intubation (ETI) to provide a secure airway and allow assisted ventilation. In many emergency departments, advanced airway management is undertaken by an appropriately trained emergency physician rather than an anaesthetist.[1] This chapter details the equipment, drugs and techniques that may be used in advanced airway management in the emergency department (ED).

Patients with respiratory arrest require immediate ETI and ventilation with oxygen. Although a trial of non-invasive ventilation may be used initially in conscious patients with severe hypoxaemia or hypercapnoea,[2] this may be unsuccessful and ETI will be required. Patients with a decreased conscious state

and/or depression of the cough reflex may require ETI for airway protection to minimize the risk of aspiration pneumonitis. In patients with severe head injury, ETI and controlled hyperventilation may be required for the short-term treatment of intracranial hypertension.[3] Finally, ETI may be indicated as part of general anaesthesia in combative patients who require investigations and/or procedures.

There are additional challenges to urgent intubation of the critically ill or injured patient in the ED compared with elective intubation in the operating room. Details of current medications, previous anaesthetics and allergies may not be available. There may be inadequate time for a complete clinical assessment of the upper airway or thorough consultation with the patient and/or family. In patients with coma following severe head injury, the status of the cervical spine will be uncertain even if initial imaging is normal.

RAPID SEQUENCE INTUBATION

Unless the patient is deeply comatose or in cardiac arrest, ETI will require the use of sedative and neuro-muscular blocking drugs to facilitate laryngoscopy and placement of the endotracheal tube. Rapid sequence intubation (RSI) is the technique of choice when definitive airway management is required in the ED, to minimize hypoxaemia or the risk of aspiration of vomitus.[4] Possible exceptions include patients with upper airway obstruction or severe facial trauma, where alternate initial techniques, such as awake intubation or awake tracheostomy, may be preferred (see later).

Careful preparation for RSI is required. If time and patient condition allow, a history should be sought of current medication, allergies and time of last meal. A careful examination of the upper airway is required, looking for

anatomical features that may predict difficult intubation.[5]

The conscious, cooperative patient should receive explanation and reassurance. Preoxygenation with 100% oxygen by mask is commenced using a non-rebreathing circuit. Optimal pre-oxygenation requires tidal volume breathing for 3–5 minutes using 10 litres/minute oxygen flow.[6] A pillow under the head is essential, unless the patient has suspected spinal column injury, in which case the neck must be immobilized in an anatomically neutral position.[7] Reliable intravenous access is required, as well as equipment for suctioning the airway.

Appropriate monitoring includes continuous ECG and pulse oximetry. The blood pressure should be measured, either invasively using an intra-arterial cannula or non-invasively using an automated blood-pressure monitoring device. Capnography must be prepared for end-tidal CO_2 ($ETCO_2$) measurement following intubation.

The required drugs should be chosen and will depend on operator preference and the clinical situation. In general, a narcotic and benzodiazepine are used in combination with a rapid-onset neuromuscular blocking drug.[8] Details of the indications, dosages and side effects of the commonly used drugs for rapid sequence intubation are shown in Table 1.3.1. These must be drawn up, checked and the syringes clearly labelled. A spare laryngoscope must be available, in case of failure of the first and the appropriate size ETT opened, lubricated and the cuff checked. Another ETT (one size smaller) should be immediately available. At least two assistants will be required, one to assist the operator with the drugs and equipment, and another to provide cricoid pressure following the induction of sedation and muscle relaxation. Further equipment in case of difficult intubation should be immediately available (see later).

When all preparations are complete,

Table 1.3.1 Drugs commonly used in RSI

Drug	Dose	Action	Onset (min)	Duration (min)
Premedication agents				
Atropine	0.02 mg/kg	Vagal blockade	1	30
Lidocaine	1.5 mg/kg	Decreases ICP	1	30
Fentanyl	1.5 µg/kg	Analgesic	2	30
Morphine	0.15 mg/kg	Analgesic	4	120
Midazolam	0.05 mg/kg	Anxiolytic	2	30
Vecuronium	0.01 mg/kg	Defasciculation	2	10
Induction agents				
Thiopental	1–5 mg/kg	Rapid-onset sedation Decreases ICP	0.5	10
Methohexital	1.0 mg/kg	Rapid-onset sedation	0.5	5
Midazolam	0.05–0.1 mg/kg	Rapid-onset sedation	2	10
Diazepam	0.1 mg/kg	Rapid-onset sedation	2	20
Ketamine	1 mg/kg	Dissociative state	2	20
Propofol	1–2 mg/kg	Sedation	1	10
Fentanyl	10–20 µg/kg	Sedation, analgesic	1	20
Muscle relaxants				
Suxamethonium	1.5 mg/kg	Depolarizing MR	0.5	5
Vecuronium	0.2 mg/kg	Non-depolarizing MR	2	40
Rocuronium	1.0 mg/kg	Non-depolarizing MR	1	30
Mivacurium	0.2 mg/kg	Non-depolarizing MR	0.5	20
Atracurium	0.5 mg/kg	Non-depolarizing MR	3	30
Pancuronium	0.1 mg/kg	Non-depolarizing MR	3	40

ICP, intracranial pressure
MR, muscle relaxant
RSI, rapid sequence intubation

premedication with adjunctive agents such as atropine, a benzodiazepine and/or a narcotic are administered as clinically indicated. The sedative drug is then given and, as consciousness is lost, the muscle relaxant (usually suxamethonium) is given with cricoid pressure applied. Following fasciculations and the loss of muscle tone, laryngoscopy is performed and the larynx sighted. The endotracheal tube is then placed through the vocal cords into the trachea, the cuff inflated and the ETT is secured with tapes. Cricoid pressure must be maintained until the ETT position is checked and secured.

Clinical methods of ensuring tracheal position include sighting the passage of the ETT through the vocal cords, misting of the ETT during exhalation, auscultation of breath sounds in the lung fields and palpation of the ETT cuff in the suprasternal notch by the squeeze test.[9] However, when visualization of the vocal cords has been difficult, these clinical tests may be misleading and confirmatory tests will be required. Although capnography is regarded as the gold standard for confirmation of tracheal placement, during cardiac arrest there may be inadequate delivery of carbon dioxide to the lungs and hence a false-negative reading. In this setting, the use of an oesophageal detector device (ODD) has been shown to be more accurate.[10]

After intubation, an orogastric or nasogastric tube should be inserted and chest X-ray taken to exclude right main bronchus intubation and confirm placement of the orogastric or nasogastric tube in the stomach. As the drugs used for sedation and muscle relaxation wear off, further drugs for the maintenance of sedation and paralysis will be required. Appropriate monitoring of vital signs, pulse oximetry and capnography with visual and audible alarms must be maintained at all times. Humidification of the inspired oxygen is desirable using a disposable filter. If the patient is placed on mechanical ventilation, the $PaCO_2$ should be checked to ensure adequate ventilation and to confirm correlation with $ETCO_2$. The unconscious patient requires eye care, pressure area care, temperature control and catheterization of the urinary bladder.

Hypotension following intubation must be treated promptly, especially in patients with neurological injury.[11] The causes include vasodilator and/or negative inotropic effects of the sedative drug(s) and/or positive pressure ventilation decreasing venous return and cardiac output. Treatment consists of a fluid challenge and/or inotrope administration, depending on the clinical setting. Rarely, hypotension may be due to tension pneumothorax occurring after the commencement of positive-pressure ventilation. Hypertension usually indicates inadequate sedation and should be treated with supplemental sedation.

In patients with severe head injury, the following additional measures need to be considered. As there is the possibility of cervical spine instability, an assistant must hold the head in the neutral position, which increases the difficulty in visualizing the larynx. Also, laryngoscopy may raise intracranial pressure, however, the benefit of lidocaine at 1.5 mg/kg as premedication is uncertain.[12] In hypotensive patients, thiopentone or propofol must be used cautiously in small doses, if at all.

The technique of RSI is not advised for patients with upper airway pathology and impending upper airway obstruction. Following the administration of a muscle relaxant, the larynx may not be visualized and ventilation of the apnoeic patient may be impossible, the 'can't intubate, can't ventilate' situation. In these patients, an initial awake technique may be performed instead. Alternatively, an inhalational anaesthetic agent or intravenous propofol is utilized, as their effects will rapidly be reversed and spontaneous respirations resume if intubation is impossible.

DIFFICULT INTUBATION

The intubation of the trachea under direct vision may be easy or difficult, depending on the view of the larynx during laryngoscopy. This has been classified into Grades 1-4 by Cormack and Lehane.[13] In Grade 1 laryngoscopy, there is a clear view of the entire laryngeal aperture. In Grade 2, only the posterior part of the larynx is visible. In Grade 3, only the epiglottis is able to be visualized and in Grade 4 only the soft palate is seen. A difficult intubation is defined as a Grade 3 or 4 view at laryngoscopy.

Difficult intubation may be anticipated in the presence of pathological disorders such as congenital facial and upper airway disorders, maxillofacial and airway trauma, airway tumours and abscesses, or cervical spine immobility. There may also be anatomical reasons for Grade 3-4 laryngoscopy and a range of clinical tests have been proposed that may predict difficulty in visualization of the larynx, including relative tongue/pharyngeal size, atlanto-occipital joint mobility and a thyromental distance < 6 cm. However, these are unlikely to be clinically useful in the emergency setting.[14]

When the larynx is not visualized, attempts at blind placement of the ETT into the trachea are unlikely to be successful and repeated attempts at intubation result in patient hypoxaemia. Failed intubation drills have been described for use in the operating theatre[15,16] and a failed intubation drill more suitable for use in the ED is shown in Figure 1.3.1.

Initial simple manoeuvres to visualize the larynx include the addition of pillows to further flex the neck (unless cervical spine injury is suspected), the use of a straight laryngoscope blade[17] and backward/upward/rightward external pressure (BURP) on the thyroid cartilage.[18] If the larynx is still unable to be visualized, blind placement of a gum elastic bougie and subsequent placement of the ETT by rail-roading the ETT over the bougie should be attempted as the initial manoeuvre.[19] If resistance to ETT passage at the larynx occurs, rotation of the ETT through 90° in an anti-clockwise direction may be helpful.[20]

If these initial steps are unsuccessful, oxygenation must be maintained using a bag/valve/mask with a Guedel's airway and alternative equipment suitable for use in the ED should be prepared for

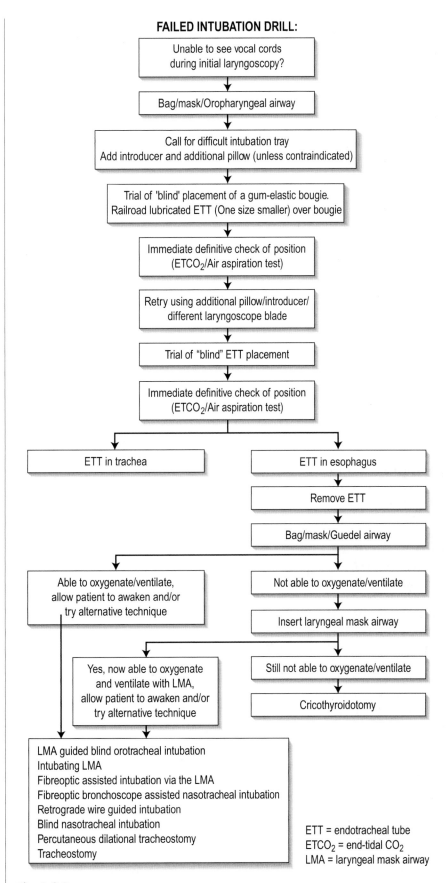

FAILED INTUBATION DRILL:

Unable to see vocal cords during initial laryngoscopy?

Bag/mask/Oropharyngeal airway

Call for difficult intubation tray
Add introducer and additional pillow (unless contraindicated)

Trial of 'blind' placement of a gum-elastic bougie.
Railroad lubricated ETT (One size smaller) over bougie

Immediate definitive check of position
(ETCO$_2$/Air aspiration test)

Retry using additional pillow/introducer/
different laryngoscope blade

Trial of "blind" ETT placement

Immediate definitive check of position
(ETCO$_2$/Air aspiration test)

ETT in trachea

ETT in esophagus

Remove ETT

Bag/mask/Guedel airway

Able to oxygenate/ventilate,
allow patient to awaken and/or
try alternative technique

Not able to oxygenate/ventilate

Insert laryngeal mask airway

Yes, now able to oxygenate
and ventilate with LMA,
allow patient to awaken and/or
try alternative technique

Still not able to oxygenate/ventilate

Cricothyroidotomy

LMA guided blind orotracheal intubation
Intubating LMA
Fibreoptic assisted intubation via the LMA
Fibreoptic bronchoscope assisted nasotracheal intubation
Retrograde wire guided intubation
Blind nasotracheal intubation
Percutaneous dilational tracheostomy
Tracheostomy

ETT = endotracheal tube
ETCO$_2$ = end-tidal CO$_2$
LMA = laryngeal mask airway

Fig. 1.3.1

use.[21,22] A summary of these devices is given below. However, if oxygenation and ventilation is considered unsatisfactory during the failed intubation drill, immediate cricothyroidotomy is indicated.

THE LARYNGEAL MASK AIRWAY

The laryngeal mask airway (LMA) is now used routinely for airway management during elective general anaesthesia. During a failed intubation drill, the LMA may be superior to bag/mask and oral airway for oxygenation and ventilation of the patient.[23] However, there has been a limited role for the LMA in the ED for two reasons. First, if pulmonary compliance is low or airway resistance is high, there will be a leak around the cuff of the LMA when peak inspiratory pressures exceed 20–30 mmHg. Second, there is a potential risk of aspiration pneumonitis, since the airway remains unprotected. To minimize the risk of aspiration pneumonitis, further developments of the LMA now include a modified cuff to improve the seal and a drainage tube to provide access to the gastrointestinal tract (the ProSeal ™).[24]

THE INTUBATING LARYNGEAL MASK AIRWAY

The LMA may be also used to assist in blind orotracheal intubation, either using a 6 mm ETT passed through the LMA, or an intubating LMA that has been developed for this purpose. Preliminary reports of the intubating LMA indicate a high success rate in the prehospital setting,[25] ED[26] and operating theatre.[27]

THE OESOPHAGEAL TRACHEAL COMBITUBE (COMBITUBE™)

The oesophageal tracheal combitube combines the functions of the oesophageal obturator airway and a conventional ETT and may be useful in the failed intubation algorithm. A 97% success rate for oxygenation and ventilation of patients undergoing elective anaesthesia[28] and a 91% success rate for successful insertion and ventilation by paramedics in cardiac arrest patients has been reported.[29] However there are little data on emergency department use of this device.

THE LARYNGEAL TUBE AIRWAY

The laryngeal tube airway (Airway Management Device ™) combines the functions of the LMA and an oesophageal obturator airway and consists of a tube placed in the oesophagus with a proximal cuff that inflates in the oropharynx to form a seal for ventilation and a distal cuff that inflates to seal the oesophagus and prevent aspiration of vomitus and/or insufflation of the stomach. Evaluation of the laryngeal tube airway in emergency medicine is limited to a manikin study, which found that adequate ventilation at the first insertion attempt was possible in 96%.[30]

BLIND NASOTRACHEAL INTUBATION

Blind nasotracheal intubation (BNTI) is a technique that is now rarely used in the operating theatre,[31] but may occasionally be useful in the ED, either as the initial technique of choice, or as part of a failed intubation drill. Requirements for successful BNTI include spontaneous respirations and depressed gag/cough reflexes. Contraindications include coagulopathy, fractured base of skull, maxillary fractures, upper airway obstruction or suspected laryngeal injury.

To perform BNTI, high-flow oxygen is administered by mask and the nares checked to assess size and patency. The nares are prepared with a pledget soaked in local anaesthetic and vasoconstrictor such as 5 ml of lidocaine 2% with adrenaline (epinephrine) 1:100 000. After several minutes, the pledget is removed and sterile lubricant applied. Local anaesthetic may also be applied by spray to the pharynx and larynx. If required and clinically appropriate, sedation using midazolam 1–2 mg may be administered. An ETT of one size less than the predicted oral size is passed via the nose to the pharynx and advanced slowly to the larynx, with the operator listening for breath sounds. To facilitate entry into the larynx, the head may need to be flexed, extended or rotated, the ETT rotated clockwise through 90°, and/or a suction catheter used to guide the ETT. When the ETT passes into the trachea, spontaneous respirations through the ETT confirm placement. However, complications of BNTI including epistaxis, injuries to the turbinates, perforation of the posterior pharynx, laryngospasm and injuries to the larynx currently limit enthusiasm for this technique.[32]

RETROGRADE INTUBATION

The technique of retrograde intubation may be useful in the ED when other techniques fail and time allows.[33] The cricothyroid membrane is punctured by a needle/cannula and a guide wire is passed through the cannula cephalad. This is brought out through the mouth using Magill's forceps. An ETT is placed over a special bougie that is passed over the guide wire through the larynx. Resistance will be felt when the ETT reaches the larynx. When the level of the cricothyroid is reached, the guide-wire is removed and the ETT passed further into the trachea.

FIBRE-OPTIC BRONCHOSCOPE ASSISTED INTUBATION

The fibre-optic bronchoscope may assist in the intubation of the patient where RSI fails or is contraindicated.[34] If the patient is awake, the nasal passage and upper airway should have topical anaesthetic applied as for BNTI. Initially, a well lubricated ETT is introduced nasally and passed to the posterior pharynx. The bronchoscope is then passed through the

ETT and the vocal cords visualized. The suction port may be used to clear any secretions. The bronchoscope is then advanced into the trachea and the ETT is railroaded over the bronchoscope. Following removal of the bronchoscope, the patient is ventilated with oxygen. If a LMA has been used during a failed intubation drill, this may be used to guide the bronchoscope with the ETT already placed over it.

The use of the fibre-optic bronchoscope in the ED is limited by several factors. The bronchoscope and light source must be immediately available for use during a failed intubation drill. The larynx may be difficult to visualize in the presence of blood, vomitus or secretions. Finally, the equipment is expensive to purchase and maintain.

CRICOTHYROIDOTOMY

Cricothyroidotomy is an essential skill for the emergency physician and must be considered immediately in cases of 'can't intubate-can't ventilate'.

To perform cricothyroidotomy, a small vertical incision is made over the cricothyroid membrane and artery forceps are used for blunt dissection to the cricothyroid membrane. The artery forceps are then passed into the trachea and the cricothyroid membrane opened horizontally. A size 6 mm ETT is passed through the opening into the trachea, the cuff is inflated and bag/valve ventilation commenced.

Alternatively, there are proprietary kits that allow a cricothyroidotomy tube to be passed over a guide-wire using the Seldinger technique. In this approach, the cricothyroid membrane is punctured with a needle/cannula mounted on a syringe and free aspiration of air confirms placement in the airway. The cannula is advanced as the needle is withdrawn and a guidewire is passed through the cannula down the trachea. The cannula is removed and a dilator passed along the guide-wire. Finally, a 4.5–6 mm cricothyroidotomy tube mounted on a dilator is passed along the guide-wire and placed in the trachea. The position of the crico-

thyoidotomy tube must be carefully checked, since misplacement in the mediastinum, anterior to the trachea is possible.

In children, puncture of the cricothyroid membrane with a 14 gauge needle/cannula and insufflation with oxygen is preferred, as injury to the tracheal mucosa at the level of the cricothyroid may lead to tracheal stenosis. In adults, placement of a too large tube (>6 mm) through the cricothyroid membrane is also considered unsatisfactory in the longer term because of possible stricture occurring at the level of the cricoid. Therefore, conversion of the cricothyroidotomy to a sub-cricoid tracheostomy is generally undertaken at the earliest time it is safe and convenient.

TRACHEOSTOMY

Compared with cricothyroidotomy, a surgical tracheostomy is more time-consuming and difficult to perform in the ED, although it is recommended in suspected direct laryngeal trauma when an emergency airway is needed. Pretracheal dissection requires adequate lighting, instruments and diathermy. Percutaneous dilatational tracheostomy may be performed without these requirements, however, there is little published experience with this technique in the ED.

REFERENCES

1. Nayyar P, Lisbon A 1997 Non-operating room emergency airway management and endotracheal practices: a survey of anaesthesiology program directors. Anesthesia and Analgesia 85: 62–8
2. Hillberg RE, Johnson DC 1997 Non-invasive ventilation. New England Journal of Medicine 337: 1746–52
3. Fessler RD, Diaz FG 1993 The management of cerebral perfusion pressure and intracranial pressure after severe head injury. Annals of Emergency Medicine 22: 998–1003
4. Sakles JC, Laurin EG, Rantapaa AA, Panacek EA 1998 Airway management in the emergency department: a one-year study of 610 tracheal intubations. Annals of Emergency Medicine 31: 325–32
5. Karkouti K, Rose DK, Ferris LE, et al 1996 Inter-observer reliability of ten tests used for predicting difficult intubation. Canadian Journal of Anaesthesia 43: 554–9
6. Nimmagadda U, Chiravuri SD, Salem R, Jospeh NJ, Wafai Y, Crystal GJ, El-Orbany MI 2001 Preoxygenation with tidal volume and deep breathing techniques: The impact of duration of

breathing and fresh gas flow. Anesthesia and Analgesia 92: 1337–41
7. Suderman VS, Crosby ET, Lui A 1991 Elective oral intubation in cervical spine-injured adults. Canadian Journal of Anaesthesia 38: 785–9
8. Morris J, Cook TM 2001 Rapid sequence induction: a national survey of practice. Anaesthesia 56: 1090–7
9. Pollard RJ, Lobato EB 1995 Endotracheal tube location verified reliably by cuff palpation. Anesthesia and Analgesia 81: 135–8
10. Bozeman WP, Hexter D, Liang HK, Kelen GD 1996 Esophageal detection device versus detection of end tidal carbon dioxide levels in emergency intubation. Annals of Emergency Medicine 27: 595–9
11. Chesnut RM 1997 Avoidance of hypotension: conditio sine qua non of successful severe head-injury management. Journal of Trauma 42: S4–S9
12. Robinson N, Clancy M 2001 In patients with head injury undergoing rapid sequence intubation, does pretreatment with intravenous lignocaine lead to an improved neurological outcome? A review of the literature. Emergency Medicine 18: 453–7
13. Cormack RS, Lehane J 1984 Difficult intubation in obstetrics. Anaesthesia 39: 1105–11
14. Yentis SM 2002 Predicting difficult intubation-worthwhile exercise or pointless ritual? Anaesthesia 57: 105–9
15. Practice Guidelines for the management of the difficult airway 1993 A report by the American Society of Anesthesiologists Task Force on Management of the Difficult Airway Anesthesiology 78: 597–602

16. Jansenns M, Harstein G 2001 Management of difficult intubation. European Journal of Anaesthesiology 18: 3–12
17. Henderson JJ 1997 The use of paraglossal straight blade laryngoscopy in difficult tracheal intubation. Anaesthesia 52: 552–60
18. Knopp RK 2002 External laryngeal manipulation: A simple intervention for difficult intubations. Annals of Emergency Medicine 40: 38–40
19. Moscati R, Jehle D, Christiansen G, D'Aprix T, Radford J, Connery C, Billittier A 2000 Endotracheal tube introducer for failed intubations: a variant of the gum elastic bougie. Annals of Emergency Medicine 36: 52–6
20. Dogra S, Falconer R, Latto IP 1990 Successful difficult intubation. Tracheal tube placement over a gum elastic bougie. Anaesthesia 45: 774–6
21. Levitan RM, Kush S, Hollander JE 1999 Devices for difficult airway management in academic emergency departments: Results of a national survey. Annals of Emergency Medicine 33: 694–8
22. Morton T, Brady S, Clancy M 2000 Difficult airway equipment in English emergency departments. Anaesthesia 55: 485–88
23. Tobias J 1996 The laryngeal mask airway: A review for the emergency physician. Pediatric Emergency Care 12: 370–3
24. Keller C, Brimacombe J, Kleinsasse A, Brimacombe L 2002 The laryngeal mask airway ProSeal™ as a tempory ventilatory device in grossly and morbidly obese patients before laryngoscope-guided tracheal intubation. Anesthesia and Analgesia 94: 737–40
25. Mason AM 2001 Use of the intubating laryngeal mask airway in pre-hospital care: a case report. Resuscitation 51: 91–95
26. Rosenblatt WH, Murphy M 1999 The intubating laryngeal mask: Use of a new ventilating-intubating device in the emergency department. Annals of Emergency Medicine 33: 234–8
27. Ferson DZ, Rosenblatt WH, Johansen MJ, et al 2001 Use of the intubating LMA-Fastrach in 254 patients with difficult to manage airways. Anaesthesiology 95: 1175–81
28. Gaitini LA, Vaida SJ, Mostafa S, et al 2001 The Combitube in elective surgery. Anaesthesiology 94: 79–82
29. Lefrancois DP, Dufour DG 2002 Use of the esophageal tracheal combitube by basic emergency medical technicians. Resuscitation 52: 77–83
30. Genzwuerler HV, Hilker E, Hohner E, Kuhnert-Frey B 2000 The laryngeal tube: a new adjunct for airway management. Prehospital Emergency Care 4: 168–72
31. Collins PD, Godkin RA 1992 Awake blind nasal intubation-A dying art. Anaesthesia and Intensive Care 20: 225–7
32. Tintinalli JE, Claffey J 1981 Complications of nasotracheal intubation. Annals of Emergency Medicine 10: 142–4
33. Dhara SS 1992 Retrograde intubation: A facilitated approach. British Journal of Anaesthesia 69: 631–3
34. Mlinek EJ, Clinton JE, Plummer D, et al 1990 Fibreoptic intubation in the emergency department. Annals Emergency Medicine 19: 359–62

1.4 CEREBRAL RESUSCITATION AFTER CARDIAC ARREST

STEPHEN BERNARD

ESSENTIALS[1]

1 Brain injury following global cerebral ischaemia is common following out-of-hospital cardiac arrest and is associated with high morbidity and mortality rates.

2 Reperfusion of the ischaemic brain results in glutamate-mediated calcium influx into cells, with biochemical cascades to cell death.

3 A number of pharmacological interventions have failed to improve neurological outcome in human randomized controlled trials.

4 Prospective, controlled trials indicate that induced hypothermia (33°C) for 12–24 hours after resuscitation from cardiac arrest is an effective treatment for anoxic neurological injury.

5 There is some evidence that hypotension and/or hyperglycaemia are deleterious to the injured brain and should be promptly treated.

INTRODUCTION

Prolonged cardiac arrest causing global cerebral ischaemia may lead to permanent neurological injury, despite effective cardiopulmonary resuscitation. Many patients who suffer out-of-hospital cardiac arrest remain comatose in the emergency department (ED) and the neurological injury accounts for much of the disability and death following hospital admission.[1, 2] This chapter details the pathophysiology of anoxic neurological injury and current cerebral resuscitation treatment strategies.

DEFINITION

Cerebral resuscitation involves the use of pharmacological or other strategies to minimize injury to the brain following a prolonged ischaemic insult.[3]

PATHOPHYSIOLOGY

The brain is highly dependant on an adequate supply of oxygen and glucose for aerobic metabolism. When cerebral oxygen delivery falls below 20 mL/100 g brain/minute, anaerobic glycolysis predominates with a marked decrease in the generation of adenosine triphosphate. After 3–6 minutes of complete cerebral ischaemia, the supply of adenosine triphosphate is exhausted and cellular metabolism ceases. The failure of the sodium/potassium transmembrane pump leads to persistant depolarization of the cell membrane and allows the equilibration of intracellular and extracellular ions, with the shift of sodium and water leading to cell swelling.[4] In addition, hydrogen ions with lactate ions are generated and the resulting intracellular metabolic acidosis is toxic to intracellular enzyme systems. The pH shift is partly dependant on the concentration of glucose, with hyperglycaemia leading to an intracellular acidosis.

THE REPERFUSION INJURY

Following reperfusion, additional injury occurs.[5] The intracellular levels of glutamate, an excitatory neurotransmitter released from presynaptic terminals, increase dramatically during reperfusion. The glutamate activates ion channel complexes including N-methyl-D-aspartate receptors and α-amino-3-hydroxy-5-methyl-4-isoxazole propionic acid receptors. When activated, these ion channels increase calcium conductance from the extracellular to intracellular fluid. In addition, glutamate activates G-protein associated metabotropic receptors, inducing changes in phospho-inositol metabolism resulting in the production of inositol triphosphate. This acts as a second messenger, which releases further calcium from stores within mitochondria and endoplasmic reticulum.

Multiple biochemical cascades are initiated by calcium influx into cells, leading to the production of oxygen free-radicals and the activation of degradative enzymes, including proteases, endonucleases, phospholipases and xanthine oxidase. Phospholipase activation results in lipid peroxidation, which causes cell membrane destruction and neuronal death. Activated phospholipase A_2 generates arachidonic acid, which mediates injury by several mechanisms, including the uncoupling of oxidative phosphorylation, inactivation of membrane Na/K-ATPase and increased release of glutamate. Activated proteases (calpains) degrade cytoskeletal and regulatory proteins.

Intracellular iron also plays an important role in free-radical production. Iron is usually maintained in a ferric state and is sequestered to intracellular proteins. During ischaemia, iron is reduced to the soluble ferrous form and reacts with peroxide, generating damaging hydroxyl free-radicals.

The generation of free-radicals activates an upregulation of adhesion molecules in the leucocytes, endothelium and platelets. These adhesion molecules mediate leucocyte adhesion and extravasation into brain parenchyma, with increased cerebral ischaemia by causing microvessel occlusion with leucocyte-platelet complexes. There is also experimental evidence of marked activation of blood coagulation without endogenous fibrinolysis and platelet activation during reper-

fusion after cardiac arrest.[6] In addition, vasoconstriction may occur secondary to the production of thromboxane A_2 and prostaglandin $F_{2\alpha}$ from arachidonic acid.

Ischaemia is also a stimulus for nitric oxide synthase activation. Nitric oxide synthase converts L-arginine to nitric oxide, a potent mediator of excitotoxic injury. The nitric oxide may combine with superoxide to form peroxynitrite radicals, which are potent activators of lipid peroxidation. Other proposed actions of nitric oxide include DNA damage, increased glutamate release and microvascular vasodilatation.

Finally, some neurones which survive the initial anoxic insult proceed to programmed cell death (apoptosis). After reperfusion, this delayed neuronal death may occur at different rates, varying from 6 hours for neurones in the striatum to 7 days for hippocampal CA1 neurones. Apoptosis is characterized by cellular and nuclear shrinkage, chromatin condensation and DNA fragmentation. The complex bichemical pathways for this phenomenon are currently under investigation.[7]

CEREBRAL HAEMODYNAMICS AFTER REPERFUSION

After restoration of a spontaneous circulation, cerebral haemodynamics may remain abnormal.[8] Following an initial hyperaemia, cerebral blood flow decreases, despite normal mean arterial blood pressure, whilst cerebral metabolic rate for oxygen increases. Thus, there may be continuing cerebral ischaemia for 12–24 hours following resuscitation from prolonged cardiac arrest. Cerebral oxygen supply/demand is also adversely affected by systemic hypoxaemia, raised intracranial pressure and/or seizure activity.

PHARMACOLOGICAL INTERVENTIONS

As much of the neurological injury seen following ischaemic injury occurs after reperfusion, there has been considerable

interest and research into pharmacological interventions that alter the above metabolic pathways and ameliorate the reperfusion injury.[3,9]

A number of drugs that have shown improved neurological outcome in animal models of global cerebral ischaemia have undergone large randomized controlled human trials, including thiopentone,[10] a corticosteroid[11] and the calcium antagonists, lidoflazine[12] and nimodipine.[13] However, none of these showed improved neurological or overall outcome. Magnesium has been shown to improve neurological outcome in patients resuscitated from in-hospital cardiac arrest;[14] however a study of patients with anoxic neurological injury after resuscitation from out-of-hospital cardiac arrest showed no benefit.[15]

Currently, there is some interest in the possible role of thrombolytic drugs during and after cardiac arrest with the goal of decreasing cerebral microcirculatory fibrin formation and improving cerebral blood flow.[6]

INDUCED HYPOTHERMIA

Induced hypothermia is theoretically beneficial after cardiac arrest and resuscitation. Hypothermia decreases cerebral oxygen demand without decreasing cerebral oxygen supply and potentially decreases the reperfusion injury by reducing the production of oxygen free-radicals after reperfusion.

Two prospective, controlled human studies have suggested improved outcome using moderate hypothermia in comatose survivors of prehospital cardiac arrest.[16,17] In one study, 43 patients were randomized to induced hypothermia (IH) at 33°C for 12 hours and 34 patients were maintained at normothermia.[16] Hypothermia was induced in the ED using ice-packs and neuromuscular blockade. At hospital discharge, 21/43 (49%) in the IH group had a good outcome compared with 9/34 (26%) in the control group (P=0.046). Following multivariate analysis for differences at baseline, the odds ratio for good outcome in the hypothermic group was 5.25 (95% confidence intervals 1.47 to 18.76: P=0.011). There were no apparent adverse effects of IH such as sepsis, lactic acidosis or coagulopathy.

A second clinical trial of induced hypothermia was conducted in Europe.[17] This study enrolled 273 comatose survivors of pre-hospital cardiac arrest, with 136 patients undergoing IH (33°C for 24 hours), and 137 patients maintained at normothermia. Hypothermia was induced in the ED using a refrigerated air mattress. At 6 months, 55% of the IH patients had good outcome, compared with 39% of normothermic controls (odds ratio 1.4, 95% confidence interval 1.08 to 1.81). The complication rate did not differ between the two groups.

However, these two studies also demonstrated that surface cooling had significant limitations. First, surface cooling is a slow method of decreasing core temperature, with 0.9°C/hour using ice packs[16] and 0.5°C/hour using forced cold air cooling.[17] Second, covering the patient with ice packs or cooling blankets during resuscitation is inconvenient and impractical for medical and nursing staff. Finally, the use of ice packs or refrigerated units (for forced air cooling) limit the use of these techniques to the hospital environment.

Since there is evidence from animal studies that outcome may be improved if cooling is initiated during or immediately after return of spontaneous circulation,[3] current research focuses on the development of techniques for the induction of hypothermia that may be feasible in the out-of-hospital setting.

One approach, which has been recently studied in 16 patients who were resuscitated from out-of-hospital cardiac arrest, is the use of a cooling helmet.[18] However, this technique is also a relatively slow, with the target core temperature of 34°C only reached after 180 minutes.

An alternative approach is the use of large volume, ice-cold (4°C) intravenous fluid.[19] In a recent study of 22 patients who had been resuscitated from out-of-hospital cardiac arrest, a rapid intravenous infusion of large-volume (30 mL/kg) lactated Ringers solution at 4°C was shown to be an effective and safe technique for the induction of mild hypothermia. This therapy decreased core temperature by 1.7°C over 25 minutes and there were improvements in mean arterial blood pressure, as well as acid-base and renal function. There were no apparent complications of this therapy such as pulmonary oedema. If subsequent studies confirm this finding, this approach may be applicable to the out-of-hospital environment.

OTHER INTERVENTIONS

Animal studies of anoxic brain injury have suggested that outcome may be improved if elevated blood pressure is maintained in the post-resuscitation period and it seems reasonable to provide elevated mean arterial blood pressure after cardiac arrest.[20] Hyperglycaemia is also associated with worse outcome following cerebral ischaemia and should also be corrected.[21]

CEREBRAL MONITORING

Recent developments in cerebral resuscitation include the use of invasive and non-invasive neurological monitoring to detect persistant cerebral ischaemia. Currently, monitoring for neurological deterioration after global or focal ischaemic injury is largely clinical, with observation of pupil reactivity, level of conscious state and the development or progression of focal neurologic signs. However, any change in clinical signs due to an increase in cerebral ischaemia may be delayed, with irreversible damage occuring before appropriate intervention. Thus, there is considerable interest in newer methods of non-clinical monitoring of the central nervous system.

The monitoring of cerebral perfusion pressure equating to the mean arterial blood pressure (MAP) minus the intracranial pressure (ICP) may give an estimation of cerebral oxygen delivery. Although increased ICP may occur after global ischaemia,[22] there are little data on ICP monitoring in adults following prolonged cardiac arrest.

Cerebral oxygen delivery may also be estimated by the continuous or intermittent measurement of jugular venous oxygen saturation. However, this technique does not appear to provide useful information that alters management.[23]

Other neurological monitoring techniques that are currently being evaluated include near infra-red spectroscopy, cerebral microdialysis and the direct continuous measurement of cerebral blood flow using jugular venous thermodilution.

SUMMARY

In patients with prolonged cardiac arrest and global cerebral ischaemia, neurological injury is mainly related to the time interval between cardiac arrest and the return of spontaneous circulation. Comatose patients should be intubated and have assisted ventilation with supplemental oxygen to protect the airway and assure adequate oxygenation and ventilation. Following the return of spontaneous circulation, a normal or elevated mean arterial blood pressure should be maintained using fluid and/or vasoactive drug therapy. In addition, hyperglycaemia should be promptly corrected with insulin therapy. Since adult out-of-hospital cardiac arrest often occurs in the setting of an ischaemic coronary syndrome, the usual cardiac care for this, such as the use of aspirin, heparin and thrombolysis, may be required.

There is now evidence that mild hypothermia for 12–24 hours following resuscitation is beneficial. The optimal technique for the induction of hypothermia is yet to be determined, however, preliminary evidence suggests that the rapid infusion of large-volume (30 mL/kg), ice-cold (4°C) intravenous fluid has advantages compared with surface cooling. Other pharmacologic and non-pharmacologic interventions are yet to be proven.

Admission to an intensive care unit will be required for most patients with anoxic brain injury following resuscitation for out-of-hospital cardiac arrest for further supportive care.

CONTROVERSIES

❶ The biochemical pathways of neuronal death following ischaemia and reperfusion are complex and require further study.

❷ Induced hypothermia is the only neuroprotective therapy that has shown benefit in clinical studies of global anoxic neurological injury.

❸ Future studies will focus on techniques for the rapid induction of hypothermia either in the ambulance or the emergency department.

REFERENCES

1. Bernard SA 1998 Outcome from prehospital cardiac arrest in Melbourne, Australia. Emergency Medicine 10: 25–9
2. Edgren E, Hedstrand U, Kelsey S, et al 1994 Assessment of neurological prognosis of comatose survivors of cardiac arrest. Lancet 343: 1055–9
3. Safar P, Behringer W, Bottinger BW, Stertz F 2002 Cerebral resuscitation potentials for cardiac arrest. Critical Care Medicine 30: S140–S144
4. Ebmeyer U, Katz LM 2001 Brain energetics after cardiopulmonary cerebral resuscitation. Current Opinion in Critical Care 7: 189–94
5. White BC, Grossman LI, ONeil BJ, et al 1996 Global brain ischemia and reperfusion. Annals of Emergency Medicine 27: 588–94
6. Bottinger BW, Martin E 2001 Thrombolytic therapy during cardiopulmonary resuscitation and the role of coagulation activation after cardiac arrest. Current Opinion in Critical Care 7: 176–83
7. Morita-Fujimura Y, Fujimura M, Yoshimoto T, Chan PH 2001 Superoxide during reperfusion contributes to caspase-8 expression and apoptosis after transient focal stroke. Stroke 32: 2356–61
8. Oku K, Kuboyama K, Safar P, et al 1994 Cerebral and systemic arteriovenous oxygen monitoring after cardiac arrest: Inadequate cerebral oxygen delivery. Resuscitation 27: 141–52
9. Gisvold SE, Stertz F, Abramson NS, et al. 1996 Cerebral resuscitation after cardiac arrest: Treatment potentials. Critical Care Medicine 24: S69–S80.
10. The Brain Resuscitation Clinical Trial Study Group 1986 Randomized clinical study of thiopentone loading in comatose survivors of cardiac arrest. New England Journal of Medicine 314: 397–410
11. The Brain Resuscitation Clinical Trial Study Group 1989 Glucocorticoid treatment does not improve neurologic recovery following cardiac arrest. Journal of the American Medical Association 262: 3427–30
12. Brain Resuscitation Clinical Trial II Study Group 1991 A randomized clinical study of a calcium-entry blocker (lidoflazine) in the treatment of comatose survivors of cardiac arrest. New England Journal of Medicine 324: 1225–31
13. Roine RO, Kaste M, Kinnamen A, et al 1990 Nimodipine after resuscitation from out-of-hospital ventricular fibrillation: A placebo-ciontrolled double-blind randomized trial. Journal of the American Medical Association 264: 3171–7
14. Thel MC, Armstrong AL, McNulty SE, et al 1997 Randomised trial of magnesium in in-hospital cardiac arrest. Lancet 350: 1272–6
15. Fatovich DM, Prentice DA, Dobb GJ 1997 Magnesium in cardiac arrest (the MAGIC trial). Resuscitation 35: 237–41
16. Bernard SA, Gray TW, Buist MD, Jones BM, Silvester W, Gutteridge GA, Smith K 2002 A randomised, controlled trial of induced hypothermia in comatose survivors of prehospital cardiac arrest. New England Journal of Medicine 346: 557–63
17. The Hypothermia after Cardiac Arrest Study Group 2002 Mild therapeutic hypothermia to improve the neurological outcome after cardiac arrest. New England Journal of Medicine 346: 549–56
18. Hachimi-Idrissi S, Corne L, Ebinger G, Michotte Y, Huyghens L 2001 Mild hypothermia induced by a helmet device: a clinical feasibility study. Resuscitation 51: 275–81
19. Bernard SA, Buist M, Monteiro O, Smith K 2003 Induced hypothermia using large volume, ice-cold intravenous fluid in comatose survivors of out-of-hospital cardiac arrest: A preliminary report. Resuscitation 56: 9–13
20. Safar P, Kochanek P 2000 Cerebral blood flow promotion after prolonged cardiac arrest. Critical Care Medicine 28: 3104–6
21. Longstreth WT, Inui TS 1984 High glucose levels on hospital admission and poor neurologic recovery after cardiac arrest. Annals of Neurology 15: 59–63
22. Morimoto Y, Kemmotsu O, Kitami K, Matsubara I, Tedo I 1993 Acute brain swelling after out-of-hospital cardiac arrest: Pathogenesis and outcome. Critical Care Medicine 21: 104–9
23. Van der Hoeven JG, DeKoning J, Compier EA, Meinders AE 1995 Early jugular bulb monitoring in comatose patients after an out-of-hospital cardiac arrest. Internal Care Medicine 21: 567–77

1.5 SHOCK

ROBERT A. SCOTT

ESSENTIALS

1 The three broad categories of shock include disorders of cardiac rate or rhythm; volume or vascular resistance problems; and myocardial pump dysfunction.

2 Hypotension, although characteristic of shock, should be considered a late finding.

3 Hypovolaemia, and hence volume resuscitation, should be carefully considered and excluded in every patient with undiagnosed shock.

4 The mortality following cardiogenic shock is improved by revascularization strategies, including angioplasty and coronary artery bypass grafting. Thrombolyis has no proven benefit but lysis may be supplemented with intra-aortic balloon counterpulsation where available.

5 Cyclo-oxygenase inhibitors, opioid antagonists and cytokine inhibitors confer little additional benefit in septic shock over fluid resuscitation, the use of inotropes and appropriate antibiotics or surgery. Activated protein C has been shown to improve mortality in severe sepsis and severe organ dysfunction.

DEFINITION

Shock is a clinical syndrome where tissue perfusion, and hence oxygenation, is inadequate to maintain normal metabolic function.[1] Insufficient ATP (adenosine triphosphate) is generated intracellularly to maintain the function and structural integrity of tissues. This causes a switch to anaerobic metabolism, resulting in an oxygen debt and tissue acidosis.[2]

The clinical recognition of shock may be difficult, particularly at the extremes of age. Pre-existing disease and the use of medications modify the compensatory mechanisms that protect vital organ perfusion. The emergency management of shock requires a high clinical suspicion and early, aggressive resuscitation.

23

SOURCES OF SHOCK

Shock is due to malfunction of the cardio-vascular system for which there may be more than one contributing mechanism. A simple classification recognizes three broad categories:

❶ Disorders of cardiac rate or rhythm
❷ Volume or vascular resistance problems
   a. volume loss - 'empty tank' (Table 1.5.1)
   b. altered vascular resistance - 'inappropriately sized tank' (Table 1.5.2)
❸ Myocardial pump dysfunction (Table 1.5.3).

This classification is not exhaustive and contributing causes may feature in more than one category.

Table 1.5.1. Examples of volume loss contributing to shock:

Blood loss (haemorrhagic shock)
External
– trauma
– gastrointestinal tract bleeding

Concealed
– haemothorax
– haemoperitoneum
– ruptured abdominal aortic aneurysm
– ruptured ectopic pregnancy

Loss of plasma
– Burns
– Exfoliative dermatitis

Loss of fluid and electrolytes
External
– vomiting
– diarrhoea
– excessive sweating
– urinary losses
– adrenal insufficiency (aldosterone deficiency)
– diabetes mellitus
– diabetes insipidus
– diuretics
– renal disease

Concealed
– pancreatitis
– ascites
– bowel obstruction
– peritonitis
– splanchnic ischaemia

Table 1.5.2. Examples of shock resulting from altered vascular resistance:

Septic shock

Anaphylactic shock

Spinal neurogenic shock

Vasodilator drugs or toxins

Adrenal insufficiency (cortisol deficiency)

Central nervous system injury

Prolonged shock from any cause

Table 1.5.3. Examples of myocardial dysfunction resulting in shock:

Primary cause of myocardial dysfunction (cardiogenic shock)
Acute myocardial infarction
Cardiac contusion
Cardiomyopathy
Congestive heart failure
Myocarditis
Ruptured ventricular septum or free wall
Acute valvular dysfunction
– aortic insufficiency
– chordae tendineae rupture
– papillary muscle dysfunction
– prosthetic valve thrombus/dysfunction
– severe aortic stenosis

Secondary causes of myocardial dysfunction
Obstructive causes
– tension pneumothorax
– pericardial disease (tamponade, constriction)
– pulmonary vascular disease (thromboembolism, pulmonary hypertension)
– atrial myxoma
– left atrial mural thrombus
– obstructive valvular disease (aortic, mitral)
Drugs
Systemic toxins or myocardial depressant factors

PATHOPHYSIOLOGY

The consequences of shock are cellular injury and death occurring by common mechanisms.[3] Shock and reperfusion cause intracellular calcium overload, producing ATP reduction, diastolic dysfunction and decreased contractile forces in excitable tissues. Calcium overload is also related to free-radical oxidative damage, degradation of cell ionic pumps, and the destruction of cytosol, nuclear and mitochondrial macromolecules.

The accumulation of hydrogen ions downregulates catecholamine receptors, resulting in a reduction in catecholamine effectiveness and a decrease in intracellular energy production. Shock also causes a catabolic state, with increased circulating catecholamines, angiotensins, glucagon and corticosteroids. Metabolism becomes glycolysis dependent, and circulating glucose, lactic acid, free fatty acids and triglycerides increase.

Oxygen consumption is defective in some tissues in shock. Many causes are responsible, including physical barriers to diffusion such as dysfunctional endothelium, and interstitial and intracellular oedema, as well as metabolic dysfunction. In humans, most shock states result in flow-dependent oxygen uptake. However, the role of supranormal oxygen delivery in therapy has yet to be resolved.

Prolonged shock results in myocardial dysfunction. An early compensatory increase in heart rate is common. Diastolic dysfunction has also been described where active ventricular relaxation is impaired through the disruption of ATP-dependent sarcoplasmic reticular calcium ion uptake. Circulating catecholamines are initially increased, but ultimately in decompensated shock the heart fails, owing partly to circulating myocardial depressant factors described in haemorrhagic and septic shock.

Organ blood flow changes are important in shock, as shock raises the threshold at which vital organ blood flow decreases. These and other specific pathophysiologic changes are discussed later.

DIAGNOSIS OF SHOCK

- Hypotension is a sentinel clinical sign, defined as a systolic blood pressure <90 mmHg or a reduction of >30 mmHg in a previously hypertensive patient. However, a low blood pressure should be considered a late finding. Aggressive management aims to prevent the development of hypotension.

- Tachycardia is usually present, but may be masked by drugs or advanced age. The trend with serial observation is more significant than absolute values. Bradycardia may occur, for instance, in catastrophic haemorrhage from a ruptured ectopic pregnancy, or following an inferior myocardial infarction (MI).
- An abnormal respiratory rate of <10 or >29 per minute depends on the cause, such as narcotic overdose or early septicaemia, but may also be part of the shock syndrome.
- Core temperature may be low, normal or elevated, and will be affected by age, environment, volume status, coexisting disease and drug therapy.
- SaO_2 should be measured to detect early hypoxaemia.
- The mental state reflects cerebral perfusion and may range from normal to confused or coma.
- The peripheral circulation usually reveals venoconstriction, decreased peripheral temperature, diaphoresis and pallor. Capillary return may be prolonged beyond 4 seconds. Peripheral or central cyanosis is a late sign. However, spinal neurogenic shock and sepsis may lead to warm, dry skin as a consequence of vasodilatation.
- Urine output is the most useful bedside monitor of the adequacy of end-organ perfusion. Levels below 0.5 mL/kg/h indicate underperfusion.

EMERGENCY DEPARTMENT MONITORING

The presence and progress of shock may be monitored in the emergency department (ED) by careful recording of repeated clinical assessment:

- vital signs, including temperature, pulse, respirations and blood pressure
- ECG
- pulse oximetry
- urine output.

Invasive monitoring in the ED may also include:

- intra-arterial blood pressure monitoring via the non-dominant radial artery
- central venous pressure (CVP) monitoring via the subclavian or internal jugular veins. Trends in CVP may be followed in response to volume loading, but should be interpreted in relation to the other observed parameters
- end-tidal CO_2 in ventilated patients.

Pulmonary artery catheterization, gastric tonometry, Doppler cardiac output studies and other more sophisticated investigations are best performed in an integrated intensive care environment.

Lactate measurements are an objective marker of the presence and severity of shock. Bedside lactate analysis is now available. Normal levels are <2 mmol/L, and levels of >4 mmol/L are associated with increased mortality. Similarly, base deficit (BD) is a useful indicator of hypoperfusion and may be used to assess the adequacy of resuscitation. BD levels reflect the volume of fluid required, the presence and severity of intra-abdominal haemorrhage and mortality. It may also be used to identify compensated shock and to predict transfusion requirements, the need for ICU and the length of stay. The incidence of adult respiratory distress syndrome (ARDS), multiple organ failure, renal failure and coagulopathy all increase with rising levels of BD.[4,5]

INITIAL EMERGENCY MANAGEMENT OF THE SHOCKED PATIENT

- The airway and ventilation are assessed and supported. Supplemental high-flow oxygen is given. Tracheal intubation should be considered for the standard indications of airway protection, airway maintenance, airway creation and the need for ventilatory support (see Chapter 1.3).
- External haemorrhage should be controlled with direct pressure while

intravenous access is obtained with large-bore peripheral cannulae. Cardiac rhythm and pulse oximetry (SaO_2) should be monitored. A fluid challenge may be given after drawing blood for investigations, including a bedside glucose level, and arterial blood gases are measured.
- Vital signs are recorded and any available history obtained, followed by a directed physical examination. Observations should be continued regularly.
- A chest X-ray, ECG and other emergency investigations are performed, e.g. bedside ultrasound to exclude pericardial tamponade, assess cardiac filling and ventricular function, or to seek intra-abdominal free fluid.

MANAGEMENT OF SPECIFIC SHOCK SYNDROMES

The following shock syndromes are discussed in detail.

- Hypovolaemic shock
- Cardiogenic shock
- Septic shock
- Neurogenic shock.

Hypovolaemic shock

Table 1.5.4 provides a guide to the pathophysiologic responses to acute haemorrhage. They relate to sympathetically mediated vasoconstriction and the release of endogenous catabolic hormones. Total peripheral resistance increases at the arteriolar level, venous capacitance increases, and blood flow to the brain and heart is maintained at the expense of renal, splanchnic, skin and muscle blood flow.[1] Cerebral vascular autoregulation maintains cerebral blood flow and oxygen transport down to a mean blood pressure of 50–60 mmHg, below which acidosis and brain ischaemia develop, followed by a progressive fall in cerebral perfusion pressure and coma. Lung parenchymal water increases with decreasing surfactant and alveolar collapse. Pulmonary dysfunction develops through

Table 1.5.4 Estimated volume losses in a 70 kg man at initial presentation

	Class I	Class II	Class III	Class IV
Blood loss (mL)	Up to 750	750–1500	1500–2000	>2000
Blood loss as a % of blood vol.	Up to 15	15–30	30–40	>40
Pulse rate per min	<100	>100	>120	>140
Blood pressure (mmHg)	Normal	Normal	Decreased	Decreased
Pulse pressure	Normal or increased	Decreased	Decreased	Decreased
Respiratory rate per min	14–20	20–30	30–40	>35
Urine output (mL/h)	>30	20–30	5–15	Negligible
Mental status	Minimal alteration	Mildly anxious	Anxious, confused	Confused, lethargic
Fluid replacement	Crystalloid	Crystalloid	Crystalloid and blood	Crystalloid and blood

multiple insults at the microvascular and cellular level.[4]

Renal perfusion is decreased and glomerular filtration rate falls with intra-renal shunting of blood flow. Pancreatic blood flow may decrease to as little as 15% of normal, which may persist post resuscitation.[1] A myocardial depressant factor has been isolated from the pancreas. Splanchnic blood flow is significantly reduced, with some preservation of mucosal circulation. Hypoperfusion may persist after the hypotension is corrected, which contributes to a failure of gut barrier function, leading to bacterial translocation and contributing to the development of multiple organ failure.[1,4]

Clinical presentation

Signs and symptoms: The pulse rate, blood pressure, pulse pressure, respiratory rate, urine output and mental status change are detailed in Table 1.5.4. Neck veins will be flat as a consequence of low central venous pressure, where cardiac function is normal. A specific cause for blood volume loss must be sought (see Table 1.5.1).

Investigations:
- Bedside glucose estimation, arterial blood gases and serum lactate
- Full blood examination, haematocrit, coagulation profile, blood group and cross-match
- Urea, creatinine, electrolytes and liver function tests
- β-HCG in females of childbearing age
- Chest X-ray and 12-lead electrocardiogram.

Additional studies will be indicated in specific situations, and all tests are repeated serially according to the clinical picture.

Diagnosis Hypovolaemia, and hence volume resuscitation, should be carefully considered in every patient presenting with undiagnosed shock.

Therapy

- General supportive care is provided as described previously, with supplemental oxygen, cervical spine immobilization in trauma, and early endotracheal intubation and mechanical ventilation for airway or respiratory failure or progressive shock.
- The Trendelenburg position provides no consistent effect on systemic vascular resistance or venous return. Passive leg raising is more effective in increasing left ventricular end-diastolic volume, stroke volume and cardiac output, but these effects are transient.[6]
- Application of the pneumatic antishock garment (PASG or MAST suit) results in a minimal autotransfusion effect. There is no evidence that it improves recovery in bleeding trauma patients and it has no place in the management of hypovolaemic shock.[7]
- External haemorrhage is controlled with firm direct pressure.
- Intravenous access is gained with two 14 g cannulae, and fluid warmers and infusers capable of rapid delivery are employed.
- O-negative or type-specific blood must be transfused as soon as possible in patients presenting with class III or IV haemorrhage. Surgical consultation is also urgently required.
- Efforts to return blood pressure to normal in bleeding trauma patients may be counter-productive and occasionally harmful. Contemporary resuscitation practice, in the absence of evidence for the effectiveness of currently recommended resuscitation protocols, might best be regarded as experimental.[7] Patients with class I or II haemorrhagic shock or non-haemorrhagic hypovolaemic shock should continue to receive warmed crystalloid. Timely restoration of perfusion and oxygen delivery should be the primary objective in bleeding patients presenting in rural and remote communities, in the elderly and in those with controlled haemorrhage. In those patients with uncontrolled haemorrhage following penetrating truncal trauma, in close proximity to facilities capable of definitive care, less aggressive fluid resuscitation, pending prompt surgical intervention, may be used.[8]
- There is little evidence supporting the continued use of colloids in the resuscitation of critically ill or injured patients.[8]
- A clinical role for hypertonic saline (HS) has yet to be defined as significant advantages of HS over standardized crystalloid solutions are unproven. HS may improve

outcomes in a subgroup of patients with shock and traumatic brain injury and has been recommended as the initial fluid of choice in haemorrhaging battlefield casualties.[8] There are no current definitive recommendations concerning the use of modified haemoglobin or perfluorocarbon blood substitutes.[8]

- Tension pneumothorax, cardiac tamponade and myocardial contusion should always be considered in the hypotensive trauma patient, although such patients should be assumed to be hypovolaemic until proven otherwise.
- Continuous monitoring and reassessment should take place in the ED pending definitive care and admission. Early ICU involvement should be considered.

Cardiogenic shock

Definition

Cardiogenic shock is the inability of the heart to deliver sufficient blood to the tissues to meet resting metabolic demands,[9] i.e. a systolic blood pressure of <90 mmHg or ≥30 mmHg below basal levels for at least 30 minutes; alternatively, a significant arteriovenous oxygen difference and a cardiac index of <2.2 L/min/m² where pulmonary capillary wedge pressure is >15 mmHg are seen. There is clinical evidence of poor tissue perfusion in the form of oliguria, cyanosis and altered mentation. Failure to respond to correction of hypoxaemia, hypovolaemia, arrhythmias and acidosis is a requirement for the diagnosis.[9]

Aetiology

The commonest cause of cardiogenic shock is MI or ischaemia, resulting in at least 40% dysfunctional myocardium (see Table 1.5.3).

Epidemiology

Cardiogenic shock complicates 6–20% of patients with acute myocardial infarction (AMI). The mortality rate exceeds 80%. It is the commonest cause of in-hospital post-infarct mortality, and there has been no change in its incidence or prognosis since the early 1970s.[9,10] Ten per cent of patients present already in established cardiogenic shock, while 90% develop it during admission.[11]

Older patients with anterior AMI, previous AMI, angina or congestive heart failure are at greater risk. One-quarter of patients will have reinfarcted. There is also a significant incidence of diabetes mellitus. There is a higher prevalence of patients with multivessel disease and persistent occlusion of the infarct-related artery. Patients with an occluded left anterior descending artery also have an increased incidence, termed the 'left main shock syndrome', with a mortality approaching 100%.[12] Only aggressive revascularization within 12 hours of symptom onset makes any difference to these patients.

In a series of 231 patients with cardiogenic shock, 214 presented with symptoms and/or signs of left ventricular failure: 42% received thrombolysis, 26% had percutaneous transcoronary angioplasty (PTCA), and 8% had emergency coronary artery bypass grafting (CABG). The overall mortality rate was 66%. Mortality in patients given intravenous thrombolytics was 61%, compared to 71% in those not receiving lysis. This was not statistically significant. Over 53% of patients with inferior AMI died, compared to 67% of those with anterior infarctions.[13]

Pathophysiology

The clinical consequences of pump dysfunction have been well described.[9,14] The activation of the sympathetic nervous and renin-angiotensin systems contributes to the failure to increase or a fall in myocardial oxygen demand, which contributes to infarct expansion, and further decreases in contractility, coronary perfusion pressure and oxygen extraction. Systolic dysfunction results in an increase in end-systolic volumes and falls in ejection fraction, stroke volume and cardiac output. Diastolic dysfunction is also well described. Systemic hypoperfusion and selective vascular redistribution lead to organ failure and metabolic acidosis.

Clinical presentation

Signs and symptoms These vary with the cause. Non-specific findings are similar to those described under hypovolaemic shock.

- Jugular venous pressure is frequently elevated, but is a non-specific finding as it is also seen in the following conditions:
  – pericardial tamponade
  – constrictive pericarditis
  – pulmonary hypertension
  – right ventricular infarction
  – superior vena caval obstruction
  – tension pneumothorax
  – tricuspid valve insufficiency or stenosis.
- Blood pressure may be within normal limits as a result of compensatory mechanisms, which also produce tachycardia and a narrowed pulse pressure.
- Signs of pulmonary venous congestion are common, but may be absent in pure right ventricular infarction.
- Precordial examination may demonstrate a dyskinetic apex beat or thrill. A fourth heart sound suggests decreased ventricular compliance, and third sound increased ventricular diastolic pressure. Murmurs common in systole may be due to mitral regurgitation or, rarely, rupture of the ventricular septum.

Investigations

- 12-lead ECG. Leads V4R and V7-9 are indicated in suspected right ventricular and posterior infarction, respectively
- Chest X-ray
- Full blood examination and film
- Bedside blood glucose, urea and creatinine, electrolytes, liver-function tests, calcium, magnesium and phosphorus levels
- Serial CK (creatine kinase), CKMB (creatine kinase, muscle-brain), myoglobin and troponin I or T levels, depending on local availability
- Blood-gas estimation, except in candidates for lysis or revascularization.

Bedside echocardiography should be available to all patients who present with undiagnosed shock, as an extension of the physical examination. Pericardial effusion or tamponade may be excluded and global systolic function or wall motion abnormalities confirmed. The presence of hypovolaemia with a hyperkinetic heart and small right-side chambers, or right ventricular dysfunction may also be ascertained.[15]

Diagnosis Cardiogenic shock must be considered in any patient presenting with a primary or secondary cause for cardiac dysfunction (see Table 1.5.3) in the presence of symptoms and signs of hypoperfusion despite optimizing circulating volume following a fluid challenge.

Therapy

- Initial care and monitoring should be provided, as described earlier.
- Tracheal intubation should be considered for airway stabilization and ventilatory support in the presence of worsening hypoxia.
- Tension pneumothorax should be excluded.
- Arrhythmias considered as contributory to the presence of cardiogenic shock should be treated according to ACLS principles.
- Hypovolaemia must be sought and corrected in all patients. A 250 mL aliquot of 0.9% saline should be given cautiously as a bolus and the response assessed. Further boluses may be indicated. Volume loading to maintain right atrial filling pressures is essential in inferior MI with right ventricular (RV) involvement. CVP monitoring may be indicated, although it is of limited value in the presence of pulmonary oedema.
- Persistence of the shock state following adequate fluid challenge in the presence of end-organ dysfunction is an indication for inotropic support.
- Dobutamine is a β_1-adrenergic agonist with some β_2 effects that, although weak, lead to increased contractility, cardiac output, stroke volume and heart rate (at the higher end of the dose range). Peripheral vasodilatation is also produced and coronary and collateral blood flow augmented.[9,16] Dobutamine is indicated at 2–20 µg/kg/min in patients with an SBP of 90–100 mmHg. It is the preferred inotrope in RV infarction and may be commenced by the peripheral route in the absence of central venous access. Tachycardia must be avoided, and obstructive cardiac lesions contraindicate its use.
- Dopamine is the endogenous precursor of noradrenaline, with dose-dependent effects[16] as listed below:
  - 1–2 µg/kg/min: Increases renal plasma flow, glomerular filtration rate (GFR) and sodium excretion via dopamine-1 and dopamine-2 receptors. This effect is no longer valid.
  - 2–10 µg/kg/min: Significant inotropic effects at the β-adrenoreceptor increase cardiac output.
  - >10 µg/kg/min: Increasing peripheral vasoconstriction through α-adrenergic stimulation.

Dopamine is useful as an inotropic agent when SBP is less than 90 mmHg in order to restore perfusion pressure to vital organs. It may increase the risk of arrhythmias and cause tissue necrosis following local extravasation. Its beneficial effects on renal blood flow in low dosage are debatable.

- Adrenaline (epinephrine) is a potent α and β_1 agonist and a moderate β_2 agonist: 0.04–0.1 µg/kg/min produces increased heart rate and contractility with unchanged or lowered peripheral vascular resistance. Higher doses produce α-receptor mediated vasoconstriction. Adrenaline (epinephrine) is indicated in profound hypotension accompanying cardiogenic shock, and in those unresponsive to dobutamine and dopamine.
- Noradrenaline (norepinephrine) is the main neurotransmitter at sympathetic postganglionic fibres, producing β_1- and potent α_1- and α_2-agonist effects. It is indicated in severe cardiogenic shock to increase perfusion pressure. Its peripheral vasoconstricting effects may be counterbalanced by a vasodilator. The early use of noradrenaline (norepinephrine) in profound undifferentiated shock helps restore vital organ perfusion while awaiting the effects of fluid loading, and allows the introduction of other inotropes or vasodilators. The starting dose is 0.5–10 µg/min. Myocardial oxygen consumption is increased, with the risks of myocardial ischaemia and compromised ventricular function.

- Systolic blood pressure should remain at least 100 mmHg. A minimum value of 60 mmHg is suggested for mean arterial pressure (MAP). The use of pressors in cardiogenic shock has not been shown to improve survival.[11]
- Vasodilators are indicated when peripheral and organ perfusion fails to respond to restoration of blood pressure alone. Glyceryl trinitrate is the vasodilator of choice in myocardial ischaemia, in a dose range of 10–200 µg/min. Sodium nitroprusside may be used when pulmonary oedema occurs in the absence of ischaemia. The dose range is 0.5–2.0 µg/kg/min, to a maximum of 10 µg/kg/min.
- MI must be sought and active management pursued dependent primarily on local facilities and expertise. Thrombolytic therapy in cardiogenic shock following AMI results in inadequate exposure of occlusive thrombus to the thrombolytic[17]. Intra-aortic balloon counterpulsation increases aortic diastolic pressure and cardiac output with no increase in oxygen demand and may be combined with thrombolytics, but when used alone confers no survival advantage unless revascularization is contemplated. Complications include leg ischaemia, dissection, thromboembolism and thrombocytopenia.[11]

Early transfer and revascularization confers a survival advantage in patients with MI and cardiogenic shock.[9,10,13,18]

Early revascularisation of the infarct-related artery by percutaneous trans-coronary angioplasty (PTCA) or coronary artery bypass grafting (CABG) is the only intervention that decreases mortality.[11] The greatest benefit is in those less than 75 years, with the optimal management of those over this age remaining unclear.[17] If catheterization facilities are unavailable, thrombolytics should be given to eligible patients while emergent transfer to an interventional facility is arranged.

Cardiac tamponade should be excluded by transthoracic echocardiography in the following patient groups:

- Blunt or penetrating cardiac trauma
- Pericarditis due to infection such as TB or viral, radiation, connective tissue disorders
- Uraemia
- Anticoagulant use
- Aortic dissection
- Iatrogenic, e.g. CVP insertion
- Pneumopericardium from barotrauma, gas-forming infection, Valsalva, PEEP, cocaine.

Coexistent hypovolaemia may mask the clinical signs of tamponade, such as a full JVP rising on inspiration (Kussmaul's sign). Volume loading is indicated with inotropic support until pericardiocentesis under echo-control or surgical pericardiotomy can be performed;

Aortic dissection should be considered in patients with risk factors, e.g. Marfan's syndrome, Ehlers-Danlos syndrome, bicuspid aortic valve, aortic coarctation, Ebstein's anomaly, hypertension in pregnancy and cocaine use.

Other causes of cardiogenic shock presenting to the emergency physician have been reviewed extensively.[14]

In summary, those patients with large infarctions and a resting tachycardia should be identified early and stabilized with inotropic and/or vasodilator agents when indicated. Intra-aortic balloon counterpulsation should be instituted urgently while emergent revascularization is contemplated. Patients managed outside centres with interventional capabilities should be considered for thrombolytics where eligible.[19]

Disposition

Patients presenting with cardiogenic shock require admission to CCU or ICU, depending on the requirement for ventilation, invasive monitoring or active management of myocardial ischaemia. Direct transfer from the ED to the catheter laboratory or operating theatre, or transfer to a tertiary centre, may be indicated.

Septic shock

Definitions

The following definitions were formulated at the consensus conference of the American College of Chest Physicians and Society of Critical Care Medicine (ACCP-SCCM) in 1992[20]:

- Bacteraemia: the presence of viable bacteria in the blood, usually confirmed by positive blood culture.
- Sepsis: clinical evidence of infection, accompanied by a systemic response, including two or more features from the following:
  - tachypnoea, RR >20/min or P_aCO_2 <32 mmHg (4.3 kPa)
  - where the patient is mechanically ventilated, minute ventilation >10 L/min
  - tachycardia >90 beats/min
  - hyper- or hypothermia, core or rectal temperature >38°C or <36°C and/or elevation or reduction in the leucocyte count >12000 cells/μL or <4000 cells/μL, or 10% or more bands.
- Systemic inflammatory response syndrome (SIRS): the presence of a severe clinical insult accompanied by two or more of the systemic responses outlined above.
- Severe sepsis: hypoperfusion (altered mentation, lactic acidosis and/or oliguria), hypotension or organ dysfunction associated with sepsis.
- Septic shock: sepsis accompanied by hypotension, systolic BP <90 mmHg or 40 mmHg or more below normal baseline and perfusion abnormalities despite adequate fluid resuscitation. Refractory septic shock is present when hypotension lasts >1 hour, despite adequate volume

replacement and high-dose vasopressor use.
- Multiple organ dysfunction syndrome (MODS): a syndrome of altered organ function in an acutely ill patient requiring intervention to maintain homoeostasis.

Debate surrounds these criteria, which, although still employed, should not form the sole basis for the clinical diagnosis of sepsis. Symptoms and signs that lead the clinician to suspect sepsis are as follows[21]:

Clinical signs:
- Fever/hypothermia
- Unexplained tachycardia
- Unexplained tachypnoea
- Signs of peripheral vasodilatation
- Unexplained shock
- Changes in mental state.

Laboratory parameters:
- Leucocytosis/neutropenia
- Unexplained lactic acidosis
- Unexplained alteration in renal or liver function tests
- Thrombocytopenia/disseminated intravascular coagulation
- Increased procalcitonin levels
- Increased cytokines, c-reactive protein levels.

Aetiology

Infection of bacterial, viral or fungal origin is the precursor of septic shock, which may complicate up to 50% of bacteraemic episodes.[22] Typically in Gram-negative sepsis, *Escherichia coli*, Klebsiella, *Pseudomonas aeruginosa*, Enterobacter, Acinetobacter, Proteus, Serratia, Aeromonas, Xanthomona, Citrobacter, Achronobacter, Salmonella or Shigella species are responsible.

The pathogenic mechanisms in septic shock have been well reviewed.[23,24] A nidus of infection is formed through multiplication of micro-organisms, which may invade the bloodstream or proliferate locally, releasing various mediators consisting of structural components and exotoxins into the circulation. Such mediators in turn stimulate plasma precursors or cells to release further endogenous mediators of sepsis. More than 100 mediators have been identified, including tumour necrosis factor-α (TNFα), interleukin-1 and interleukin-6, which are the most extensively studied. The effects of mediator release include direct organ injury, hepatic failure, disseminated intravascular coagulation (DIC), vasodilatation, altered capillary permeability, myocardial depression, endothelial cell dysfunction and leucocyte aggregation.

Circulatory changes

Nitric oxide overproduction in the peripheral vasculature causes the loss of vascular control seen in septic shock.[25] The vasodilatation and decreased systemic peripheral vascular resistance may be masked by hypovolaemia. Capillary blood flow is reduced, and decreased deformability of red and white blood cells underlies microvessel plugging, resulting in a potential trap for bacterial overgrowth in the microcirculation.[26]

Cardiac dysfunction

Ventricular dilatation with decreased ejection fraction is the commonest finding in septic shock, associated with a reduced stroke volume that is compensated for by an increase in heart rate to maintain or increase cardiac index.[27] This ventricular dilatation is necessary, and usually reverses in 7–10 days in patients who survive. Decreased right ventricular (RV) function and increased pulmonary artery pressure are associated with a poor outcome. As in decreased left ventricular function, circulating mediators have been implicated, as poor RV performance is not entirely explained by raised pulmonary vascular resistance.

Mortality

Reported mortality ranges from 20% to 80%. Patients admitted to the ICU with hypotension associated with sepsis have a mortality rate of over 50%.

High-risk groups

These include the young and the old, those with burns, alcohol dependence, chronic renal failure, diabetes mellitus, immunosuppression, chronic cardiorespiratory disease, infection, malnutrition and the multiply injured.

Clinical presentation

Signs and symptoms

- Early: tachypnoea, tachycardia, temperature instability, oliguria, altered mental state, peripheral vasodilatation;
- Late: reduced capillary refill, hypotension, further altered mental status and reduction in urine output, evidence of myocardial dysfunction, metabolic acidosis;
- Evidence of genitourinary, respiratory or gastrointestinal infection. Many other sites are possible, including iatrogenic sources such as CVP lines and indwelling catheters. A careful secondary survey following resuscitation is essential.

Investigations

- Full blood examination, urea, creatinine, electrolytes, bedside glucose, coagulation profile, and β-HCG in females of reproductive age.
- Arterial blood gases, arterial or venous lactate.
- Two sets of blood cultures, including a set through any indwelling cannulae or central venous lines. Consider arterial blood cultures in the immunosuppressed, e.g. intravenous drug users, and cultures through a pre-existing arterial line.
- Urinalysis, microscopy, Gram stain and culture.
- Chest X-ray and 12-lead electrocardiogram.
- Additional studies as indicated by the clinical situation, likely source of sepsis and search for possible foci of infection.

Diagnosis This is made utilizing ACCP-SCCM definitions. More than one cause for shock may exist in the same patient. Volume depletion must be treated with an appropriate fluid challenge.

Therapy

- Initial care is provided as outlined previously during the primary survey.

Early airway control with mechanical ventilation is necessary to optimize oxygenation and ventilation.

- Volume replacement should commence with 250 mL boluses of 0.9% saline titrated against observed parameters, and frequent clinical reassessment. CVP line insertion should be performed rapidly in the ED under strict asepsis if expertise is immediately available. Trends in CVP response to fluid infusion should be followed, rather than absolute values, in conjunction with other monitored parameters. CVP is of least value in the presence of myocardial dysfunction or elevated pulmonary artery pressures. An intra-arterial blood pressure monitoring line should be inserted in addition.
- Persistent hypotension and/or signs of organ hypoperfusion are indications for inotropic support. Dopamine is used commonly in higher doses, but is a weak vasoconstrictor in septic shock.[28] There is no role for low-dose dopamine in improving renal function. The early use of noradrenaline is recommended where hypotension is severe, SBP 70 mmHg or less, and the response to dopamine is suboptimal. Noradrenaline may preserve vital organ perfusion while volume is replaced and hypoxaemia corrected. It may effectively optimize renal blood flow and renal vascular resistance.[29]
- Oxygen consumption is maintained in haemorrhagic and cardiogenic shock by an ability to increase oxygen extraction where oxygen delivery is extremely low.[30] This ability is impaired in septic shock. Thus, oxygen delivery aims to reverse hyperlacticacidaemia to increase survival rates. The use of dobutamine is only advocated in patients with adequate central pressures, in order to increase cardiac index and hence oxygen delivery and consumption. However, routinely maintaining supranormal oxygen

delivery is no longer recommended.[28]

- The combination of noradrenaline and dobutamine appears to be more appropriate to the goals of septic shock therapy and effects on the splanchnic circulation.[29] The effects of vasopressin on the abnormal sympathetic function in sepsis is subject of further study.[28]
- The source of infection must be identified where possible, collections of pus drained and intravenous antibiotic therapy instituted as soon as practicable. This may have to precede complete specimen collection in life-threatening cases. A suggested regimen, which can be modified in the context of previous infections where microbiological information is available in the patient's chart, or according to local recommendations, may include[31]:

Immunocompetent adult:

Di(flu)cloxacillin 2 g IV 4–6 hourly PLUS gentamicin 4–6 mg/kg IV daily (tailor dose to age and renal function of patient).

If hypersensitive to penicillin: cephalothin 2 g IV 6 hourly or cephazolin 2 g IV 8 hourly.

Neutropenic patients:

$<0.5\times10^9/L$ or $<1\times10^9/L$ + predicted decline to $<0.5\times10^9/L$ + fever $> 38°C$. Empirical regimens should cover *Pseudomonas aeruginosa*.

Gentamicin 4–6 mg/kg daily PLUS either ceftazidime 1 g IV 8 hourly OR ticarcillin+clavulanate 3.1 g IV 6 hourly.

Cefpirome, cefepime or piperacillin + tazobactam may be substituted for ceftazidime or ticarcillin+clavulanate. Alternatively monotherapy with ceftazidime, cefpirome, cefepime, imipenem or meropenem in maximal dosage is equally effective.

Vancomycin should not be used in febrile neutropenics unless the patient is in shock, is known to be colonized with methicillin-resistant *Staphylococcus aureus* (MRSA) or has clinical evidence of a catheter infection from a unit with a high incidence of MRSA infection: vancomycin 1 g 12 hourly IV.

Appropriate antibiotic therapy confirmed by in-vitro testing reduces mortality by 50%, and should always be discussed with infectious disease specialists and microbiologists. Further advice on condition-specific antibiotic regimes is available elsewhere.[31]

- Sodium bicarbonate is not recommended for the treatment of lactic acidosis.[28]
- Corticosteroids should only be given for adrenal insuffciency, or if the patient is already receiving corticosteroids.[32] Corticosteroids in low dosage have also been found to be beneficial in a sub-set of patients with refractory septic shock.[28]
- Cyclo-oxygenase inhibitors such as ibuprofen have no significant effect on outcome.[29] Opioid antagonists in high dosage reverse low SBP and mean arterial pressure, but have no effect on survival.[32] The use of prostaglandins, pentoxifylline, N-acetylcysteine, selenium, anti-thrombin III, immunoglobulins, growth hormone and granulocyte colony stimulating factor in non-neutropenics is currently unsupported and is not recommended.[33]
- The use of cytokine inhibitors has not been associated with improvement in mortality rates in severe sepsis or septic shock. Inhibition of nitric oxide synthesis by methylene blue and the use of opioid antagonists are subject of further study.[28]
- The use of activated protein C has been associated with a relative reduction in the risk of death of 20%. Despite a significantly increased bleeding risk, this compound has been approved by the US FDA for use in those with severe sepsis at high risk of death, with an APACHE score of ≥25 or significant organ dysfunction, especially refractory dysfunction or multiorgan dysfunction.[28]

Disposition

Patients presenting to the ED with septic shock will require ICU admission for intensive therapy and monitoring. Clinical assessment, urine output and serial lactate levels are the best indicators of the effectiveness of therapy, which should see lactate levels decrease within 24 hours.[28]

Neurogenic shock

Definition

The term spinal neurogenic shock has been used to represent all phenomena surrounding physiologic or anatomic transection of the spinal cord that results in temporary loss or depression of all or most spinal reflex activity below the level of the lesion. Arterial hypotension may or may not be part of such phenomena.[34]

Pathophysiology

Low thoracic lesions result in loss of lower extremity sympathetic tone and subsequent venous pooling. Upper thoracic lesions result in venous pooling in the lower extremities and the abdominal viscera. Cervical lesions result in the absence of intrinsic cardiovascular sympathetic tone, with loss of thoraco-lumbar vascular tone.

One in three patients with a complete cervical-cord injury requires support for their hypotension. The presence of hypotension has no implications regarding the degree of completeness of cord injury or prognosis.

Clinical features

- This is a diagnosis of exclusion in the injured patient. Hypotension should be accompanied by flaccidity and areflexia distal to the suspected level of the lesion. There should be no compensatory tachycardia or peripheral pallor, sweating or vasoconstriction.
- Tension pneumothorax and cardiac tamponade must always be considered, and hypovolaemic shock, which may be masked and should be excluded by appropriate fluid challenge and investigations, such as abdominal ultrasound or CT

scanning for possible intra-abdominal or retroperitoneal blood loss.

Therapy

- Supportive therapy should be instituted to airway, ventilation and circulation, as indicated.
- Atropine 0.5–1 mg is given to counter unopposed parasympathetic vagal tone to a maximum dose of 3 mg, if bradycardia and symptomatic hypotension are present.
- Euvolaemia should be assessed with a fluid challenge: 250–1000 mL aliquots of 0.9% saline are given and the clinical response followed.
- If the above measures fail to return blood pressure and measurable signs of perfusion to normal, consider pharmacologic vasoconstriction. Ephedrine 5–10 mg IV, or phenylephrine 0.2–1 mg IV may be used. Noradrenaline (norepinephrine) at 2–5 μg/min titrated to response is used in refractory cases providing other causes of hypotension such as haemorrhage, tamponade, pneumothorax, etc., have been excluded.

Disposition

Patients should be cared for in an ICU or a dedicated spinal injury unit, depending on other injuries and local facilities.

CONCLUSION

The aetiology of shock in patients presenting to the emergency department is varied. Hypovolaemia should be sought in all cases, although specific management will depend on the underlying cause.

REFERENCES

1. Peitzman AB, Billiar TR, Harbrecht BG, Udekwu AO, Kelly E, Simmons RL 1995 Haemorrhagic shock. Current Problems in Surgery 32: 925–1012

CONTROVERSIES

❶ There is currently no evidence to support the use of colloids over crystalloids in shock management.

❷ The overall benefits of hypertonic fluids in shock are yet to be confirmed by prospective clinical studies.

❸ The use of fluid restriction until early surgery, although accepted in the management of penetrating truncal trauma, requires further evaluation in the blunt trauma patient.

❹ Corticosteroids have shown some benefit in certain subgroups of patients with severe sepsis and septic shock

❺ Only activated protein C can be currently recommended as adjunctive therapy in severe sepsis associated with organ failure

2. Fiddian-Green RG, Haglund U, Gutierrez G, Shoemaker WC 1993 Goals for the resuscitation of shock. Critical Care 21: S25–S31
3. Kline JA. Shock. In: Rosen P, Barkin R (eds) 1998 Emergency Medicine, Concepts and Clinical Practice. Mosby Year Book Inc., St. Louis, pp 86–106
4. Britt LD, Weireter LJ Jr, Riblet JL, Asensio JA, Maull K 1996 Priorities in the management of profound shock. Surgical Clinics of North America 76: 985–97
5. Davis JW, Parks JN, Kaups KL, Gladen HE, O'Donnell-Nicol S 1996 Admission base deficit predicts transfusion requirements and risk of complication. Journal of Trauma 41: 769–74
6. Terai C, Anada H, Matsushima S, Kawakami M, Okada Y 1996 Effects of Trendelenburg versus passive leg-raising autotransfusion in humans. Intensive Care Medicine 22: 613–4
7. Roberts IA, Evans P, Bunn F, Kwan I, Crowhurst E 2001 Is the normalisation of blood pressure in bleeding trauma patients harmful? Lancet 357: 385–7
8. Tremblay LN, Rizoli SB, Brennerman FD 2001 Advances in fluid resuscitation of hemorrhagic shock. Journal Canadien de Chirurgie 44: 172–9
9. Califf RM, Bengston JR 1994 Cardiogenic shock. Current concepts. New England Journal of Medicine 330: 1724–30
10. Domanski MJ, Topol EJ 1994 Cardiogenic shock: current understandings and future research directions. American Journal of Cardiology 74: 724–6
11. Prieto A, Eisenberg J, Thakar RK 2001 Non-arrhythmic complications of acute myocardial infarction. Emergency Medical Clinics of North America 19: 397–415
12. Quigley RL, Milano CA, Smith LR, White WD, Rankin JJ, Glover DD 1993 Prognosis and management of anterolateral myocardial infarction in patients with severe left main disease and shock: the left main shock syndrome. Circulation 88: 1165–70
13. Whitman JJ, Boland J, Sleeper LA, et al 1995 Current spectrum of cardiogenic shock and effect of early revascularisation on mortality. Circulation 91: 873–81
14. Rodgers KG 1995 Cardiovascular shock. Emergency Medical Clinics of North America 13: 793–810
15. Plummer D 1995 Other applications of ultrasound. In: Heller M, Jehle D (eds) Ultrasound in emergency medicine. WB Saunders, Philadelphia, pp 184–95
16. Barnard MJ, Linter SPK 1993 Acute circulatory support. British Medical Journal 307: 35–41
17. McPherson JA, Gibson RS 2001 Reperfusion therapy for myocardial infarction. Emergency Medical Clinics of North America 19: 433–49
18. Stomel RJ, Rasak M, Bates ER 1994 Treatment strategies for acute myocardial infarction complicated by cardiogenic shock in a community hospital. Chest 105: 997–1002
19. Brown M, D'Haem C, Berkompes D 1998 Emergency Medical Clinics of North America 16: 565–81
20. Bone RC, Balk RA, Cerra FB, et al 1992 Definitions for sepsis and organ failure and guidelines for the use of innovative therapies in sepsis. Chest 101: 1644–55
21. Matot I, Sprung CL 2001 Definition of sepsis in Guidelines for the Management of Severe Sepsis and Septic Shock. Intensive Care Medicine 27 Suppl 1: S3–S9.
22. Dunn DL 1994 Gram-negative sepsis and sepsis syndrome. Surgical Clinics of North America 74: 621–35
23. Baxter F 1997 Septic shock. Canadian Journal of Anaesthesia 44: 59–72
24. Parrillo JE 1993 Pathogenetic mechanisms of septic shock. New England Journal of Medicine 328: 1471–7
25. Brady AJB, Poole-Wilson PA 1993 Circulatory failure in septic shock. Nitric oxide: too much of a good thing? British Heart Journal 70: 103–10
26. Hinshaw LB 1996 Sepsis/septic shock: participation of the microcirculation: an abbreviated review. Critical Care Medicine 24: 1073–8
27. Bunnell E, Parrillo JE 1996 Cardiac function during septic shock. Clinics in Chest Medicine 17: 237–48
28. Fitch JJ Gossage JR 2002 Optimal management of septic shock. Postgraduate Medicine 111: 53–66.
29. Vincent JL 2001 Haemodynamic support in septic shock. Intensive Care Medicine 27 Suppl 1: S80–S92.
30. Edwards JD 1993 Management of septic shock. British Medical Journal 306: 1661–4
31. Severe sepsis 2000 Therapeutic Guidelines: Antibiotic Version 11. Therapeutic Guidelines Limited. State of Victoria: 159–68
32. Wessner WH, Casey LC, Zbilut JP 1995 Treatment of sepsis and septic shock: a review. Heart and Lung 24: 380–92
33. Carlet J 2001 Immunological therapy in sepsis. Intensive Care Medicine 27 Suppl 1: S93–S103.
34. Pate Atkinson P, Atkinson JLD 1996 Spinal shock. Mayo Clinic Proceedings 71: 384–9

1.6 ETHICS OF RESUSCITATION

MICHAEL W. ARDAGH

ESSENTIALS

1 Ethical deliberation may be aided by considering the four principles of: respect for patient autonomy; beneficence; non-maleficence and justice.

2 During deliberation, if the ethical principles seem to be competing the relative benefits and harms of the application of each should be considered.

3 During resuscitation, urgency and impaired patient competence conspire against adequate consideration of these principles, especially non-maleficence and respect for patient autonomy.

4 Resuscitation can be harmful in a number of ways. These should be considered when assessing the balance of benefit and harm of any resuscitation endeavour.

5 All medical interventions need some form of consent, including resuscitation, despite the urgency and the impaired patient competence. Of the consent options available, presumed consent is the one most commonly employed. Presumed consent using professional substituted judgement is a model that best respects patient autonomy.

6 The practice of resuscitation procedures, particularly endotracheal intubation, on the newly dead is common and valuable. Some form of consent is required for this to occur, but currently there is no suitable model. Presumed consent would be appropriate if the practice was explicit and if the public was well informed. In so doing those who would not consent are protected by the opportunity to decline. Until then, practising on the newly dead is ethically wrong.

INTRODUCTION

A working definition of ethics is the study of morality. It is reasonable to describe moral behaviour as that which is 'the right thing to do'. Thus, medical ethical deliberation is the process of determining what is the right thing to do when considering any of the dilemmas that arise in medical practice.

The approach to these dilemmas may vary according to the philosophical perspective adopted.[1] Although there are a variety of models describing moral decision making, only a pragmatic overview will be given here. In general terms one may adopt a utilitarian approach, which values the positive balance of good over bad brought about by any action, or a deontological approach, which values actions that adhere to overriding moral principles. However, moral philosophers have recognized that moral principles may compete against each other when specific actions are considered. Moral principles should be honoured, but when they are competing, in a given circumstance, we should then consider the relative balances of good and bad that ensue from the application of each principle. In other words, we have a composite philosophy wherein the principles and the consequences of their application could both be considered.

Beauchamp and Childress[2] have recently developed this further into a practical framework for medical ethical deliberation. They describe four principles that should be honoured in medical decision making. When these principles compete, the relative balance of good and bad should be considered. These principles are: respect for patient autonomy, beneficence, non-maleficence and justice.

RESPECT FOR PATIENT AUTONOMY

Autonomy is the patient's moral right to determine his or her own destiny. It is a principle that has grown in stature in recent years. The realization of the importance of informed consent is a consequence of this.

Although the principle of respect for patient autonomy remains sound, there are many occasions in resuscitation medicine where the patient's competence is impaired, as he or she is unable to receive information, undertake rational deliberation or express a decision free from coercion. Although we still endeavour to respect the patient's autonomy, we will struggle to define what the patient's autonomous wishes would be, if he or she was not impaired. This will be discussed further later in the chapter.

BENEFICENCE

Beneficence is the principle of acting in a way that benefits the patient. Historically, this and non-maleficence have been the overriding governing principles in medical practice. When these principles are enforced without due consideration of, or in contradiction to, the patient's perceived or expressed wishes, the action is termed paternalistic. When the principle of respect for patient autonomy is not honoured, the patient is deprived of a fundamental right and is treated as less worthy by being reduced to a position where he or she is considered incapable of self-governance. This harm to the patient needs to be considered when the relative benefits and harms of any action are considered.

NON-MALEFICENCE

Non-maleficence, or the principle of avoiding harm in therapeutic endeavours, is an established maxim attributed to Hippocrates. Although this is an obvious and common sense principle, we will commonly tolerate some harm, for example when delivering chemotherapy for cancer, or undertaking surgery that is known to have certain complications, because consideration of the other principles tells us our actions are right.

The principles of beneficence and non-maleficence risk being poorly considered because they 'go without saying'. However, we should be reasonably certain of the benefits and harms of our interventions before they may be considered right. For example, the performance of gastric lavage on a non-consenting patient after a trivial overdose several hours earlier is ethically unjustifiable as there is insufficient benefit to override our principles of respect for autonomy and non-maleficence. In order to consider the benefits and harms, information is required regarding the outcomes of our interventions, and to this end research becomes an ethical necessity to provide the evidence upon which to judge competing principles.

JUSTICE

The principle of justice is an essential balance to the first three principles, which apply primarily to the individual. Justice, or the concept of fairness, is best addressed by questioning whether there are others who might be adversely affected by a particular action. For example, in a mass casualty incident the performance of a hopeless resuscitation may be unjust (in addition to harming the patient) as it deprives another of resuscitation facilities.

APPLICATION OF THESE PRINCIPLES TO RESUSCITATION MEDICINE

There are two components of resuscitation medicine that conspire against adequate consideration of the principles outlined by Beauchamp and Childress. The first of these is urgency and the second is the impaired ability of the patient to make reasonable autonomous decisions.

Urgency may be a barrier to the application of these principles in any given case. It is often appropriate to perform resuscitation assuming these deliberations might occur more fully when time permits, rather than withhold resuscitation on the basis of limited deliberation.

The impaired competence of patients undergoing resuscitation complicates the principle of respect for autonomy, as the patient is commonly impaired in his or her ability to receive information, comprehend it, consider it in context and make a rational decision on the basis of this consideration. It is common practice not to seek or to ignore the wishes of the patient, and instead to presume that resuscitation is the right thing to do based on arguments of beneficence and non-maleficence.

Thus, it is generally perceived that consent is not required for resuscitation because resuscitation brings benefit and prevents harm, and because the patient is not in a position to give or withhold consent. Although this approach does not usually mean that bad things are done, from an ethical perspective it is fundamentally flawed. Resuscitation may be harmful in a number of ways and some form of consent must be obtained, just as for any other medical intervention.

THE HARMS OF RESUSCITATION[3]

The benefits of resuscitation include the avoidance of death and the restoration of good health. The harms of resuscitation, may be of the following five types:

❶ The first is if resuscitation is unnecessary because the patient's condition is insufficiently serious to justify it. As a consequence, the harm includes pain and other discomfort to the patient, iatrogenic illness and unnecessary use of limited resources, thereby depriving others in need of these resources. In resuscitation medicine the extent of overtreatment may be difficult to predict, as it is hard to know whether the patient would survive intact without the treatment. The most promising way of minimizing this harm is to have senior staff present during a resuscitation to draw upon their experience.

❷ The second harm of resuscitation is if it is unsuccessful because the patient's condition is too far advanced. When resuscitation will not produce the desired effects because the patient is too sick, there is the potential for a great number of harms. Harms to the patient include physical discomfort, loss of dignity, a prolonged death, and survival with an unacceptable quality of life. Harms to the family include the psychological discomfort of surrogate pain and loss of dignity, unfulfilled hope, loss of control of a loved one's destiny, the cost of lost earnings while at the bedside, and the cost of supporting a disabled survivor. The harms to the health workers include frustration and sadness at lack of success, guilt at inflicting harm, and the cost of being unable to treat others waiting for resources. The harms to the community include the loss of resources to treat others, the deception that resuscitation offered hope, and the worry that death must be preceded by a loss of dignity.

❸ The third harm of resuscitation is if it is unkind because it brings about an outcome with which the patient or their family is unhappy. Resuscitation may condemn the patient to a quality of life below that considered acceptable. This is potentially a tragic harm, with an ongoing burden from which the patient and their carers may have no means of escape.

❹ The fourth harm of resuscitation is if it is unwise because it diverts resources from alternative healthcare activities that would bring more benefit to other patients. Resuscitation is a significant user of resources: if it is futile and beneficial healthcare activities cannot proceed for lack of resources, then resuscitation is causing significant harm.

❺ Finally, resuscitation is harmful if it is against the patient's wishes. A preconceived 'do not resuscitate' order written by or negotiated with the patient, or consent declined by a competent patient, must be honoured, in keeping with the ethical principle of respect for autonomy. However, preconceived orders must be carefully considered as they relate to the situation in which the patient finds him or herself. For example, a written signed and witnessed statement (often called an advance directive, or living will) declining resuscitation from cardiac arrest means that the patient should not be resuscitated from cardiac arrest: it does not mean that the patient has declined resuscitation from haemorrhagic shock. Similarly, a 'no intensive care' directive does not mean the patient has declined aggressive treatment for pulmonary oedema with a nitrate infusion and continuous positive airway pressure ventilation. Although such directives may occasionally apply specifically to the patient's illness, on other occasions they may not. In the setting of some form of an advance directive, three questions should be considered: 1) Did the patient make this decision based on well informed deliberation? 2) Is the context they find themselves in now what they had in mind when they made the decision? If not, how closely does it relate to what they had in mind? 3) Since they made this decision, is there any indication they might have changed their mind? If the answers to these questions suggest some doubt as to how applicable the advance directive is to this resuscitation, at this time, then it should be considered an indication

of the patient's wishes, rather than morally binding.

These harms of resuscitation must be considered when weighing the relative merits of the principles of respect for patient autonomy, beneficence, non-maleficence and justice.

An ill-considered approach will lead to underrepresentation of patient autonomy in these deliberations, and an inadequate appreciation of the extent of the harm that may ensue from resuscitation efforts.

FUTILITY[4]

The concept of futility has been widely discussed in the medical literature, with particular emphasis on resuscitation medicine. Regrettably, discussions of the harms of resuscitation have become stalled by attempts to define futility. The word is derived from the Latin *futilis*, meaning 'that which easily pours or melts'. The current usage stems from the story in which the daughters of the King of Argos murdered their husbands and were then condemned to collect water for eternity in leaking buckets. To arrive at your destination with an empty bucket when the intention of the journey was to bring water is undoubtedly a futile endeavour. However, futility in medicine is much more difficult to define. Some emphasize physiological futility, meaning the inability to produce a physiological objective, for example if CPR produces no pulse, or transfusion produces no blood pressure. The proponents of this definition suggest that it has the least risk of unilaterally imposed physician value judgements. Others consider futility in terms of quantitative or qualitative measures. A quantitative estimate of futility is one in which an intervention is considered futile if it has failed in, for example the last 100 times attempted. The qualitative component describes futility if the patient's resultant quality of life falls below a threshold considered minimal by general professional judgement. It is unlikely that there will ever be agreement as to what physiological measure or quality of outcome measures are most appropriate, and what threshold

measure separates futility from benefit. Although these arguments are interesting, it is unfortunate that they have taken on more importance than they merit. Futility defines the absence of acceptable benefit for any given intervention, whereas reasonable ethical deliberation demands we consider the ratio of benefit and harm. If there is no benefit, any harm at all would make the benefit-harm ratio unfavourable. However, even if the endeavour is not futile and brings about measurable benefit, this does not necessarily mean that the endeavour is the right thing to do, as the amount of harm that ensues, as defined above, may outweigh any benefit. It is the benefit-harm balance, as assessed by considering the four ethical principles and the five types of harm described above, that has the most relevance in determining whether to start or stop resuscitation.

CONSENT, WITHHOLDING AND WITHDRAWING RESUSCITATION

Consent must be obtained for any medical intervention, including resuscitation. Informed consent, as is appropriate for elective surgery, may be inappropriate during resuscitation owing to the urgency of the treatment and impaired patient competence. However, if informed consent is not relevant, other forms of consent still are. The two most common forms of consent employed in resuscitation scenarios, where there is both urgency and impaired patient competence, are presumed consent and proxy consent. Presumed consent uses the concept that a reasonable patient under similar circumstances – or this patient if he or she were able to – would consent to the resuscitation endeavours proposed. This form of consent has merit and is commonly employed, but occasionally attracts criticism as being a form of medical paternalism, in that it may be perceived to be respecting the principle of beneficence, as the resuscitators perceive it, while ignoring respect for patient autonomy.

Proxy consent involves obtaining consent for resuscitation from a family member or other person who is perceived to be able to speak on behalf of the patient. Proxy consent avoids the criticism of medical paternalism as the decision is taken out of the physician's hands, but it suffers as a model as the decision maker may be unable to adequately receive information, understand it, and deliberate over it during a hurried and rapidly evolving resuscitation. In addition, the proxy may not reflect the views of the patient. There may be occasional circumstances where the proxy declines resuscitation because of some financial or other benefit that would accrue from the patient's death. More commonly, proxies have a tendency to demand more resuscitation than the patient would have wanted, for fear of becoming responsible for their death. When this form of consent is used there is greater scope for the harms of resuscitation. A modification of proxy consent that better addresses the issue of respect for patient autonomy is proxy consent with substituted judgement. This involves not asking what the proxy would want done for the patient, but instead what the proxy thinks the patient would want done. In other words, it attempts to see the resuscitation from the patient's perspective as viewed by the proxy.

A modification of presumed consent is presumed consent using professional substituted judgement.[5] This means the resuscitators gathering as much information about the patient as they possibly can to attempt to understand how the patient would view this decision. This usually involves speaking with the patient's loved ones. Then, with some knowledge of the likely outcome of the resuscitation proposed, based on previous experience and a knowledge of the medical literature, they can exercise their moral imagination by asking 'Would I want this treatment if I was this patient?' In this way the patient's autonomy is as best respected as it can be under difficult circumstances, by combining a knowledge of the harms and benefits of the resuscitation with an appreciation of this balance from the patient's perspective. If

presumed consent using professional substituted judgement is employed and the answer to the question is 'No', then the resuscitation cannot proceed. To resuscitate without regard for the patient's explicit or perceived wishes is a harmful disrespect for their autonomy. Often, and appropriately, a decision to proceed will be made on the basis of a perceived marginal benefit over harm. This balance is made more appealing by the alternative of certain death if resuscitation is not undertaken. However, the balance is dynamic, with a clearer view of the likely benefits and harms emerging as the patient responds to the resuscitation. If the treatment does not procure the hoped-for benefits, all concerned should be willing to minimize the ongoing harms of resuscitation by withdrawing treatment as the balance becomes more unfavourable.

The concept of withholding and withdrawing treatment is somewhat misdirected in that it implies a need for permission to stop the intervention, whereas the precedent in medicine is to obtain permission to proceed. It is wrong to withhold a resuscitation endeavour because of the concern that the life-saving treatment cannot be withdrawn at a later date if things are not going well. When resuscitation is withheld a small but significant number of patients may miss out on an opportunity for a good outcome had the resuscitation been offered to them. Similarly, it is wrong to be unable to withdraw treatment because of the ill-conceived concept that once resuscitation has begun it must continue.

By employing professional substituted judgement, the resuscitators should recognize when the balance of benefit and harm becomes unfavourable from the patient's perspective. At this point they have a moral obligation to withdraw resuscitation as they can no longer presume the patient's consent. By appreciating the benefits and harms of resuscitation, the use of professional substituted judgement to view these from the patient's perspective, and by a commitment to stop resuscitation when we cannot presume the patient's consent, we will minimize the harms of resuscitation medicine.

PRACTISING RESUSCITATION PROCEDURES ON THE NEWLY DEAD[6]

Practising resuscitation procedures – most commonly endotracheal intubation – on patients who have died after an unsuccessful resuscitation is a common practice in many parts of the world. However, some view this with a repugnance that can be rationally argued. Others would propose that the benefit of this practice to subsequent patients outweighs any repugnance felt by others who witness it, or any harm done to the recently deceased. However, like all other interventions in medicine, this procedure requires permission before it may proceed. Informed consent may be obtained from the terminally ill for permission to perform procedures after they die, but this has limited relevance to the practice as it occurs in many emergency departments. Implied consent argues that consent is implicit in the fact that the patient used the emergency services and, therefore, is agreeable to all that this entails, including being used for teaching. Implied consent criteria are commonly used for those who present of their own volition for non-invasive medical care. However, patients who die in the emergency department most often do not present of their own volition, but instead are brought in by others, usually ambulance staff, in a state of impaired competence. Furthermore, implied consent confers the right to administer treatment that the patient would reasonably expect at the time of presentation. Therefore, if a patient's attendance is non-voluntary with impaired competence or with ignorance of the procedure, he or she cannot imply consent and we cannot infer it.

Construed consent is a modification of implied consent, suggesting that if consent was obtained for a procedure it can be construed for a related procedure. If we concede that a form of consent (presumed consent, as suggested above) is obtained to intubate a patient during resuscitation, may we construe that consent also applies to intubation after death? There is a superficial logic to this, as to perform the same procedure on the same patient with the same equipment one minute before and one minute after death seems a continuum of the same therapeutic relationship. However, on close analysis there is a difference sufficiently significant to render previous consent null and void. The consent to resuscitate is based on a contract between medical staff and patient dedicated to helping the patient. When the objective is no longer to help the patient the previous contract is irrelevant and a new one must be entered. To proceed to intubate the deceased under the old contract is a violation of the trust inherent in the previously formed therapeutic relationship. An appreciation of this violation contributes to the repugnance of the procedure.

Presumed consent is appropriate when impaired competence renders the patient unable to give informed consent. Although it is likely that most would consent to postmortem procedures for the benefit of medical staff and subsequent patients, presumed consent does disadvantage the minority who would not. Formal application of a presumed consent rule for performing procedures on the recently dead mandates that the community should be well informed, so that individuals have the opportunity to explicitly decline consent if they so desire.

Proxy consent has also been argued in relation to this procedure. However, when proxy consent rules have been enforced the procedure tends not to occur, because staff are uncomfortable about obtaining consent in this way, or because relatives decline consent in an effort to protect their loved one from further harm.

The value of practising endotracheal intubation and other procedures on the newly dead is well argued and, therefore, there is a cost if it is disallowed. However, the current pervading policy of 'don't

ask, don't tell' is ethically unjustifiable. If we presume a patient's consent and do not ask, we are obliged to tell. The significant minority that would not consent are thereby protected by an opportunity to decline. Therefore, to proceed with presumed consent we must have a well informed public, and preferably a statute to formalize consent. An extrapolation of this, which is the most convincing solution, is called 'mandated choice', which proposes a process whereby, as a matter of public policy, individuals must choose on a variety of issues and these choices are recorded on, for example, their driving licence. This process informs and honours individual choice, gives the significant minority the opportunity to decline, and avoids deception. However, in the absence of a suitably informed public from whom we can presume consent, or a mandated choice, we do not have permission to proceed with postmortem resuscitation practice. Therefore, to do so is ethically wrong.

CONCLUSION

Emergency medicine abounds with clinical dilemmas requiring ethical deliberation. Such deliberation may be influenced by theories regarding the consequences of action, theories based on moral principles, or some combination of these two. Beauchamp and Childress[2] present a model for deliberation based on the principles of respect for autonomy, nonmaleficence, beneficence and justice. Although this model frequently will not provide an answer beyond dispute, it does allow a rational examination of the important issues so that our consequent actions will at least be better directed than they might otherwise have been.

Resuscitation medicine demands such deliberation despite the pressure of urgency and the common impairment of patient competence. Patient autonomy must be respected by employing a suitable consent process, such as the use

of presumed consent using professional substituted judgement. In this way we can attempt to honour the patient's autonomy by viewing the benefits and harms of resuscitation from their perspective. Often, particularly in the early stages of resuscitation, the relative benefits and harms may be difficult to establish and the patient's perspective may be difficult to formalize. It is appropriate to continue with resuscitation until these variables become more clear. However, as soon as there is a negative answer to the question 'Would I want this done if I was this patient, knowing what I know about the patient and knowing what I know about the likely outcome?', the resuscitators have a moral obligation to stop resuscitation.

CONTROVERSIES

❶ Performing resuscitation procedures where a poor outcome is expected or where there may be reasons to suspect that the patient may not wish to be resuscitated.

❷ Withholding resuscitation procedures on the basis of an argument of futility.

❸ Practising procedures on the newly dead.

REFERENCES

1. Beauchamp TL 1991 Philosophical Ethics. An Introduction to Moral Philosophy, 2nd edn. McGraw-Hill, New York
2. Beauchamp TL, Childress JF 1994 Principles of Biomedical Ethics, 4th edn. Oxford University Press, New York
3. Ardagh M 1997 Preventing harm in resuscitation medicine. New Zealand Medical Journal 110: 113–5
4. Ardagh MW 2000. Futility has no utility in resuscitation medicine. Journal of Medical Ethics 26: 393–6
5. Ardagh MW. 1999 Resurrecting autonomy during resuscitation - the concept of professional substituted judgement. Journal of Medical Ethics 25(5): 375–8
6. Ardagh M 1997 May we practise endotracheal intubation on the newly dead? Journal of Medical Ethics 23: 289–94

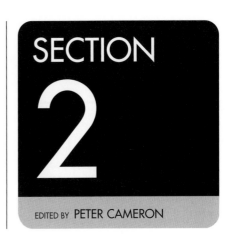

SECTION

2

EDITED BY PETER CAMERON

TRAUMA

2.1 Trauma overview 40

2.2 Neurotrauma 47

2.3 Spinal trauma 52

2.4 Facial trauma 65

2.5 Abdominal trauma 71

2.6 Chest trauma 76

2.7 Limb trauma 80

2.8 Radiology in major trauma 86

2.9 Trauma in pregnancy 102

2.10 Trauma in the elderly 105

2.11 Wound care and repair 109

2.12 Burns 123

2.1 TRAUMA OVERVIEW

PETER CAMERON • DAVID YATES

ESSENTIALS

1 Trauma remains the leading cause of death from 1 to 40 years of age in Australasia, UK, and the USA.

2 Improvements in trauma care systems have resulted in fewer patients dying from avoidable factors.

3 Initial management of trauma patients involves a team approach. A primary survey (ABCDE) is followed by a secondary survey involving head-to-toe examination.

4 Airway management requiring endotracheal intubation should be performed using a rapid sequence induction technique.

5 Classic concepts regarding clinical signs in traumatic shock may underestimate blood volume loss.

6 Sedation should not be used in agitated major trauma victims unless reversible causes for agitation have been excluded.

7 Audit of trauma systems is essential to improve outcomes.

INTRODUCTION

Trauma is the leading cause of death from 1 to 40 years of age in the USA, Australasia and UK. It is an even greater problem in developing countries where the majority of death and disability occurs.[1] Trauma deaths peak between the ages of 15 and 30, and therefore contribute significantly to the number of years of life lost in the population. In North America, more years of life are lost as a result of trauma (27.6%) than from cancer (16.7%) or heart disease (12.5%). Deaths from unintentional injury are much more common than suicide or homicide, even in the USA. However, in the USA, homicide causes more deaths than suicide in the <24 age group, this differs from other Western countries. Suicide now causes more deaths than MVAs in regions such as Australasia and Hong Kong.[2,3]

Injury morbidity affects a much larger group. For every death there are at least 10 serious non-fatal injuries, many causing long-term morbidity. The financial cost of this is enormous, and estimates range as high as $13.3 billion annually for Australia and $180 billion in the USA. The social cost is greater, as most victims are young and are major contributors to society through their work, family and organizational involvement.

There have been significant improvements in injury mortality and morbidity in most Western countries as a result of a systematic approach to trauma care. The majority of these have resulted from prevention strategies, including seatbelt legislation, drink-driving legislation, improved road engineering, motor cycle and cycle helmet use, and road safety and workplace injury awareness campaigns. The spectacular success of these interventions should be contrasted with the numerous reports over the last 20 years which have highlighted the ineffectiveness of medical care of trauma victims. However, changes both in system configuration and in individual patient management have brought about improvements in the survival rate of those who are seriously injured.

Civilian interest in injury morbidity and mortality was initially most evident in the USA because of the high incidence of urban violence and road trauma. Research into systems of trauma care began with epidemiological work by Trunkey and others[4] examining trauma deaths. The concept of a trimodal distribution of trauma deaths was developed. Trunkey proposed that about 50% of deaths occurred within the first hour as a result of major blood vessel disruption or massive CNS/spinal cord injury. This could only be improved by prevention strategies. A second more important group (from the therapy perspective) accounted for about 30% of the deaths and included patients with major truncal injury causing respiratory and circulatory compromise. The remaining 20% of patients were said to die much later from adult respiratory distress syndrome, multiple organ failure, sepsis and diffuse brain injury. Trunkey initially identified the second group as most likely to benefit from improvements in trauma system organization, and it is a tribute to the effectiveness of such schemes that the number of patients dying from avoidable factors within the first few hours of injury has generally declined. In some systems it is reported to be as low as 3%, but generally is probably nearer to 10–15%.[5,6]

Improvements in trauma system provision have resulted in a redistribution of the three groups proposed by Trunkey, and it is now generally accepted that far fewer than 30% are included in the second group.

Trauma care systems have been developed to ensure a multidisciplinary approach and a continuum of care, from the roadside, through hospital care to rehabilitation. Whereas initial work focused on the need for centres of expertise and trauma management, it is now accepted that the prehospital phase is of critical importance. Accurate triage of the patient to the closest most appropriate facility is essential. High-risk patients should be taken to a hospital capable of managing critically ill trauma patients.[7] Table 2.1.1 lists some predictors of life-threatening injury. Using these as a triage tool without modification will result in significant overtriage, that is, many more patients with non-threatening injuries will be triaged. Overtriage is minimized if abnormal vital signs and overt major injury are used as the triage criteria. Sensitivity is still greater than 85%. If mechanism is used as a triage tool

Table 2.1.1 Major trauma victims at high risk of life-threatening injury

Vital signs	Mechanism
Glasgow Coma Score ≤13 or Systolic blood pressure <90 or Respiratory rate <10 or >29 Trauma score <14	Evidence of high speed impact Falls 6 m or more Crash speed 60 kph or more 50 cm deformity of automobile Rearward displacement of front axle Passenger compartment intrusion 40 cm on patient side of car – 50 cm on opposite side of car Ejection of patient Rollover Death of same-car occupant Pedestrian hit at 30 kph or more
Injury Penetrating injury to chest, abdomen, head, neck and groin Some significant injury to two or more body areas. Severe injury to head/neck or trunk Two or more proximal long bone fractures Burns of >15% or face or airway	**Demographics** Age <5 or >55 Known cardiac or respiratory disease (lower the threshold of severity resulting in trauma centre care)

RESUSCITATION BAY FLOOR PLAN

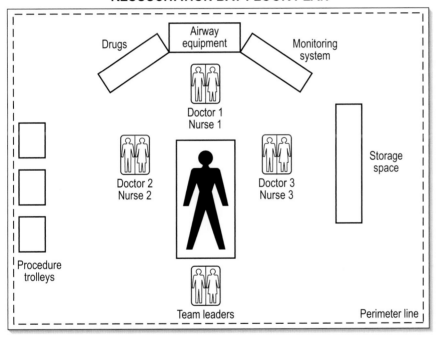

Fig. 2.1.1 The layout of a typical trauma resuscitation bay. Reproduced with permission Colin T Myers, et al 1993 Trauma teams: order from chaos. Emergency Medicine 5: 34.

then documented high speed and prolonged extrication time appear to be the most significant factors.[8]

Identifying weaknesses in such a system is always difficult because of the delay between cause and effect. Inappropriate management does not usually lead to immediate death: for example, a period of hypoxia may result in organ failure many hours later. Another difficulty is the relatively low incidence of death. Although this is of course to be welcomed, it does make statistical analysis more difficult when the 'adverse event' occurs uncommonly. Careful audit of the entire trauma process and accurate measurement of 'input' (i.e. injury severity) and 'output' (i.e. death or quality of survival) is essential if the process of trauma care is to be reviewed.

INITIAL MANAGEMENT

Seamless integration with the prehospital personnel should ensure that the hospital is 'on standby' to receive the major trauma victim. The trauma team should be in attendance in the resuscitation area and the patient brought directly to a prepared bay, the layout of which is illustrated in Figure 2.1.1. The general approach is to perform a primary survey to secure the airway/cervical spine, breathing and circulation. This is followed by a brief assessment of disability (neurological) and complete exposure of the patient. Life-threatening problems are thus identified and managed immediately. This is followed by a secondary survey involving a head-to-toe examination.

In most departments, parallel processing of the patient will occur simultaneously with management of ABCDE problems. The doctor and nurse team charged with protecting the airway immediately set about their task while the team leader obtains a brief history from the ambulance personnel and, if possible, the patient. The cervical spine is carefully controlled while the airway is being secured. The procedure doctor and the nurse team attend to i.v. access, blood tests, urinary catheter and other procedures. At this early stage of assessment and resuscitation the general philosophy should be to assume the worst and protect against all possible adverse events. Treatment is, therefore, designed to protect the patient against unforeseen consequences of the injury, rather than being focused on evident abnormalities. Although this approach can appear to be overly aggressive and unnecessary – and indeed in some circumstances can be rather frightening for the patient – careful reassurance from attending staff will usually gain approval and praise. It is, however, important that this 'better safe than sorry' approach is not taken to extremes. Senior staff must be able to assess risk and avoid a situation where inexperienced personnel keep uninjured patients aggressively splinted for hours on end, so that the treatment itself becomes a cause of further injury.

TRAUMA 2

The role of the various team members is shown in Table 2.1.2. In some facilities all these functions may have to be performed by one or two personnel, in which case a sequential rather than a parallel process will occur.

AIRWAY

It should be assumed that hypoxia is present in all patients who have sustained multiple injuries. Early expert airway intervention is essential. Every patient should receive initial supplemental oxygen via a well-fitting face mask. This includes those few patients who might later be found to have chronic obstructive airways disease. Concerns regarding pre-existing dependence on hypoxic drive can be addressed once the initial trauma resuscitation has been completed.

If the airway is clear and protected, the neck should be immobilized with a semirigid collar, tape and side support. If airway manoeuvres are necessary, it is often better to use manual inline immobilization without a collar, ensuring

Table 2.1.2 Team roles

Team leader	Overview Resuscitation Assessment Communication Ambulance Referrals Investigations Other team members Primary survey Secondary survey
Airway doctor	Control of airway Inline immobilization of cervical spine Ventilation Gastric tube
Procedure doctor	Intravenous access/bloods Intercostal catheter Urinary catheter ABG/Art line
Nurses	Airway nurse Procedure nurse Scout nurse Documentation/ coordinator Relatives
Radiographer	

minimal neck movement with constant vigilance. This is not the time for an inexperienced operator. Indeed, the entire management of an obstructed airway in a trauma patient should be undertaken by an experienced senior clinician with significant anaesthetic experience. The first priority is to clear the upper airway by direct visualization, suction, and removal of any foreign bodies. Insertion of an oropharyngeal or nasopharyngeal airway and the jaw thrust manoeuvre are usually successful in clearing an upper airway obstruction. Insertion of a nasopharyngeal airway can be hazardous in patients with a cribriform plate fracture. The direction of insertion (backwards not upwards) is important. Chin lift is not recommended because it may cause additional movement of the cervical spine.

Early endotracheal intubation should be undertaken if the patient is apnoeic, has an unrelieved upper airway obstruction, has persistent internal bleeding from facial injuries, has respiratory insufficiency due to chest or head injuries, or the potential for airway compromise (such as from facial burns or seizures). Intubation may also be necessary for procedures such as CT scan, or for the management of confused or disturbed patients.

The following course of action is recommended for the emergency intubation of the major trauma victim:

- Skilled personnel (anaesthetist or emergency physician with appropriate anaesthetic experience).
- Fully equipped resuscitation area (suction, oxygen, drugs, monitoring equipment).
- The following sequence is suggested:
  - Preoxygenate with bag/valve/ mask using 100% oxygen
  - Sedation (e.g. fentanyl/midazolam)
  - Manual immobilization (without cervical collar)
  - Cricoid pressure
  - Suxamethonium (1.5 mg/kg)
  - Visualize cords by direct laryngoscopy
  - Insert endotracheal tube (using introducer if necessary)
  - Monitor gas exchange using pulse oximeter and capnograph

  - Once endotracheal tube position is confirmed give non-depolarizing muscle relaxant (e.g. vecuronium) and sedation.

Any operator undertaking emergency intubation of major trauma victims (MTVs) should be prepared for a difficult intubation. When there is a high risk of difficult intubation and there is sufficient time, other techniques may be used, such as fibreoptic intubation. These are not appropriate as first-line emergency techniques. If the cords cannot be visualized and ETT inserted within 30 seconds (try holding *your* breath for 30 seconds), then bag/mask ventilation should be resumed. If ventilation is possible then there is no urgency; if ventilation is not possible a second attempt at ETT insertion should be made. If this is unsuccessful then a surgical airway using a cricothyroidotomy should be created. A laryngeal mask airway may also be useful as a temporary measure. More recently, the intubating laryngeal mask has proved useful. Gum elastic bougie and fibreoptic techniques may be helpful for difficult airways. (See Figure 1.3.1 Failed Intubation Drill.)

Cricothyroidotomy is the surgical airway of choice in an emergency because it is a relatively easy technique compared to tracheostomy, can be performed in a matter of seconds, has a low complication rate in adults, and requires only a scalpel, forceps and ETT. A cricothyroidotomy using a large-bore needle may be used as a temporary measure, especially in children, but will not allow adequate ventilation in adults, as it results in CO_2 accumulation. A number of proprietary kits are available. It must be emphasized that a needle cricothyroidotomy does not protect the airway from aspiration.

VENTILATION

Once the airway is secure the patient should be ventilated to maintain oxygenation and P_aCO_2 levels between 32 and 35 mmHg (4.3–4.7 kPa). There is evidence that severe hypocarbia (<32 mmHg) may be harmful to the cerebral circulation by causing cerebral vasoconstriction.[9,10] Conversely, hypercarbia will produce cerebral vasodilatation with a resultant increase in ICP. Although modest hypocarbia was advocated until relatively recently, it has been found that this does not confer any significant benefit. The objective should be to maintain normocarbia. Arterial blood gases should be monitored closely, but capnography should only be used as a guide as there are frequently gross discrepancies. Ventilatory rates should be approximately 10–14 breaths per minute, with a tidal volume of 10 mL/kg (lean mass). (See Chapter 2.2 Neurotrauma.)

PARALYSING AGENTS

Suxamethonium (1.5 mg/kg) is the drug of choice for intubation because of its fast onset, short duration and relative guarantee of complete relaxation. Because it is a depolarizing muscle relaxant it has the disadvantage of transiently increasing ICP and intraocular pressure. It will also cause release of potassium from damaged tissues (e.g. burns/crush injury), but this is not an issue in injuries in the first 24–48 hours. Experimentally it has been shown that the rise in ICP caused by suxamethonium is short-lived and not as significant as that caused by prolonged attempts at intubation and gagging. The rise in ICP can be lessened if adequate sedation (e.g. midazolam) is used. Some operators also premedicate with a non-depolarizing agent prior to the use of suxamethonium. The use of a non-depolarizing agent for intubation has never gained favour, mainly because of the slow onset. Newer agents such as rocuronium have a much faster onset (60 seconds), but are still not as good. For ongoing paralysis non-depolarizing agents such as vecuronium are favoured because of the low incidence of histamine release and other haemodynamic side effects.

SEDATION

Sedation may be necessary in the MTV for the following reasons:

- Preparation for endotracheal intubation
- In the agitated patient
- In association with analgesics for pain relief.

The major risk with these agents is that in patients with hypovolaemia the loss of sympathetic drive and relaxation of vascular smooth muscle may result in sudden hypotension. Of the commonly used sedative drugs, thiopentone is the most likely to cause hypotension; however, if titrated (50 mg aliquots) it may be used successfully. It is effective in reducing ICP rises associated with intubation, and has a very short duration of action. Midazolam is very likely to cause hypotension even with small doses (0.5 mg), but it is also useful in reducing ICP. Fentanyl is not as effective in sedating the patient and reducing ICP, but may be used in relatively high doses (100–500 μg) without causing hypotension. Etomidate (0.2–0.3 mg/kg) is increasingly used in the USA and Asian centres such as Hong Kong because of the rapid onset, short duration and minimal haemodynamic effects. Ketamine should not be used in the head-injured patient because of its potential to cause a rise in ICP. It is very effective in producing a dissociative state in patients without neurotrauma, which may allow fracture manipulation and other procedures. Enfluorane and halothane should also be avoided for this reason.

Pain or discomfort (such as a distended bladder) may be expressed as agitation in the obtunded patient, and giving sedatives alone will increase the problem. It is, therefore, important to assess the cause of agitation/anxiety before treatment is given.

CIRCULATION

Shock is a clinical syndrome in which the perfusion of vital organs is inadequate to maintain function. Blood loss is the major cause of shock in the MTV. Other uncommon causes of shock also need to be considered:

- **Cardiogenic shock.** This may be pre-existent (e.g. AMI causing accident, drugs causing reduced cardiac compensation and hypovolaemia) or secondary to injury, i.e. myocardial contusion, valvular/septal injury or pericardial tamponade.
- **Neurogenic shock.** This results from loss of sympathetic tone. It may be caused by central brain-stem injury and vasomotor instability, or spinal cord injury and interruption of descending sympathetic tracts. It is characterized by bradycardia, but this may also occur in profound hypovolaemic states (see below).
- **Anaphylactic shock** and **septic shock** may coexist with hypovolaemic shock.
- **Pulmonary embolus** and **tension pneumothorax** will cause sudden severe disruption to the circulation.

CLINICAL PRESENTATION

The initial stages of hypovolaemia are difficult to detect. Although four stages of blood loss have been described (see Table 1.5.4), the distinction made on blood pressure and pulse is usually not clear cut. The cardiovascular response to simple haemorrhage is modified by the presence of tissue injury. Although most major trauma victims have a combination of both, it should be appreciated that those who present with pure blood loss (for example after a stab wound) will often have maintained their blood pressure but may have a bradycardia despite blood loss due to a vagal response. Tissue injury will result in a tachycardia. Hence a normal blood pressure and pulse may be found in patients who have lost a significant amount of blood through a mixture of tissue injury and major blood vessel disruption. Of course, once a very large amount of blood has been lost (30–40% of blood volume), the blood pressure and pulse will become abnormal. An intravenous infusion of even a relatively small amount of fluid to such a patient may bring the recordings back to normal despite persisting hypovolaemia.

The picture is further complicated in older patients, and particularly in those who are receiving vasoactive drugs. The absolute values are less important than the trends.

MONITORING

All patients who have sustained injury that could be associated with significant blood loss (however remote the possibility) must be carefully monitored. In the initial phase, measurement of the parameters listed in Table 1.5.4 will give some information about vital organ perfusion. However, more invasive monitoring will be required if hypovolaemia is severe or sustained. Central venous pressure can be useful to detect changes in venous capacitance, and the response of the CVP to a fluid challenge is a useful test. Blood pressure is most accurately measured by an indwelling arterial catheter. The acid-base status should be checked frequently. Transoesophageal echo (TOE) or suprasternal ultrasound can be used to measure aortic blood flow velocity. The advantage of TOE is that causes of shock, such as myocardial/valvular dysfunction, pericardial effusion and aortic transection, can be identified.

MANAGEMENT

Venous access

It is essential to gain good venous access at the earliest phase in resuscitation. This is usually via two large-bore (>16g) peripheral cannulae. If there are no upper arm veins then the femoral vein is the next choice. Subclavian and internal jugular veins are hard to access during resuscitation. Cutdowns of the saphenous veins and cubital fossa may also be used. The intraosseous route is not useful in adults.

Fluids

Class I and II haemorrhage can usually be managed without blood transfusion, unless there is ongoing blood loss. Initial treatment is with crystalloid or colloid. There is no convincing evidence that one

is superior to the other, although for acute blood loss where rapid intravascular expansion is required, some would argue that it makes sense to use a fluid that stays in the intravascular space. In the UK and Australasia the ready availability of polygelatins led to increased usage compared to the USA, where crystalloids have been more commonly used. The Cochrane Collaboration has reviewed this topic and favours the use of crystalloids. If crystalloids are given then three times as much fluid will be required.[11] Given that there have been reported adverse events associated with colloid infusion, there is growing consensus that crystalloids should be the fluid of first choice. Hypertonic crystalloid has also been suggested, however available data are inconclusive and more research is required.

For class III and IV haemorrhage blood transfusion should commence immediately, initially using O-negative blood and changing to group-specific or cross-matched blood as it becomes available. There is no evidence that whole blood is superior to packed cells and replacement of clotting factors, unless the blood is fresh (less than 1–2 days). The availability of fresh blood is extremely limited.

Filters

Micropore blood filters slow the transfusion and do not appear to decrease complications from blood transfusion in the MTV.

Hypothermia

This is common in MTVs because of exposure and the use of cold intravenous fluids. Crystalloid/colloid infusions are usually at room temperature, although some centres prewarm fluids in blanket cupboards and microwave ovens. It is important to monitor this, as temperatures can fluctuate wildly. Blood is stored at 4°C and it is important to warm it; however, traditional blood warmers are cumbersome and slow to set up unless this can be done in anticipation. The use of the more expensive rapid infusion blood warmers is justified in trauma reception centres. There is growing consensus that a mild degree of hypothermia is

probably not harmful and may well be cerebroprotective. Rapid active rewarming may cause worse outcomes in the context of isolated severe head injury.[12] However, severe hypothermia less than 32°C will interfere with coagulation, decrease myocardial contractility and predispose to arrhythmias.

Coagulation factors

There is little evidence for the use of clotting factors if the total haemorrhagic loss is less than 5 litres. In the clinical situation, where there is evidence of ongoing blood loss after the replacement of five to six units, clotting factors should be replaced, as a blood loss of twice this volume would be anticipated. Coagulopathy is usually dilutional, but pre-existing problems such as liver disease and warfarinization should be looked for. Platelets should also be given if more than 10 units of blood are transfused. Although controversial, it is reasonable to give four units of fresh frozen or freeze-dried plasma for every six units of blood transfused. Haematologists have traditionally asked for evidence of coagulopathy before issuing clotting factors; however, in a rapidly deteriorating MTV requiring massive transfusion there is little logic in waiting for a coagulation result that reflects the situation 30–60 minutes previously.

MAST suit

Once popular, these devices are now very rarely used. A number of complications have been reported and, importantly, no therapeutic benefit has been demonstrated.[13] There may be some value in applying the MAST suit to patients who have an unstable pelvic fracture associated with massive internal bleeding, but the advent of external fixators that can be applied in the resuscitation area of the emergency department has largely removed this last indication.

HYPOTENSIVE RESUSCITATION

Recently increasing attention has been paid to the potential harm in overaggressive resuscitation of patients prior to definitive treatment of the cause of the bleeding. A number of studies have shown that in major trauma victims with penetrating injuries to the trunk, vigorous fluid resuscitation prior to operation actually results in worse outcomes.[14,15] This concurs with vascular surgical protocols, where it is acknowledged that outcomes are improved by limiting fluid resuscitation prior to the repair of leaking aneurysms. Logically, if the blood pressure is higher, more blood loss will occur. Therefore, more dilution of clotting factors, increased usage of blood products for replacement, hypothermia, coagulopathy, ARDS, sepsis, etc., will result. Conversely, if there is no perfusing pressure to vital organs then irreversible injury to those organs may occur.

The essential point in this debate is that the most important determinant of outcome in MTVs is the time to definitive surgery. There is certainly no point in delaying surgery 'to normalize the intravascular volume'. The relevance of penetrating injury studies to blunt trauma is unclear. However, where there is a cause of bleeding that can be ligated, this should be performed as soon as possible. This principle applies to bony injury (using fixation) as well as spleen, liver and other sources of bleeding. If there is no surgically remediable bleeding point, the physiological status should be returned to normal as soon as possible to prevent long-term complications from prolonged ischaemia to bowel and other organs.

NEXT STEPS

By this stage the trauma patient will have been received into a well organized resuscitation area and the first life-saving procedures will have been initiated by an integrated and skilled team of doctors and nurses. Any immediately life-threatening conditions can be expected to have been identified and dealt with. Constant vigilance and reassessment is essential. Other occult injuries may be present in those patients identified with serious injuries.

While the trauma team leader continues to review the situation in the light of a constantly changing clinical scenario, and hopefully the provision of more biomechanical data from the site of the incident, he or she should also be beginning to consider the next steps. The first of these is the calling in of other experts. Whereas it will have been clear that an airway doctor will be an essential part of the initial resuscitation team, it may be some minutes before it is known which other skills are required. Usually orthopaedic surgeons and neurosurgeons are near the top of the list. General surgery is not required as often as is commonly supposed,[16] although general surgeons are often useful in coordinating ongoing care. Whichever specialty is required, the patient's emergency problems demand experience, therefore, 'if in doubt, refer up'.

Radiographs are required at this stage. The initial films should be limited to those that will have a direct bearing on immediate management. These are:

- Cervical spine lateral view
- Chest AP view
- Pelvis AP view.

Ideally, the resuscitation room should have an integrated X-ray facility, but if this is not available portable films should be obtained. It is not appropriate to transfer a multiply injured unstable patient to a separate X-ray facility.

Subsequent chapters deal with individual trauma problems, but it is essential that throughout the patient's stay in hospital a single clinician has overriding responsibility for his or her care. In the resuscitation area this is the 'team leader', who may be from any discipline. Handover to the clinician responsible for ongoing care must be comprehensive, timed and well documented.

TRAUMA AUDIT

Trauma kills people in a variety of ways. Hence no one department in a hospital will see a large number of deaths. Many die before they reach hospital, some in the emergency department and others scattered through the inpatient specialties and in intensive care. Hence from any one clinician's perspective trauma is not an outstanding problem. However, when looked at from a public health perspective it is clearly a major issue, not least because some of the deaths are avoidable. Identifying these, and the much more difficult-to-define group of patients who survive but whose outcome is not as good as expected, is a major problem.

Just as cancers have been 'staged' in order to help to identify individual prognosis and aid collective review, so it is important to measure the severity of injury. Unfortunately, this is more complicated than in the cancer patient because of the multitude of injuries sustained by trauma victims.

The most important variables to measure are the extent of the anatomical injury, the degree of physiological derangement that results, age, and the previous well-being of the patient. All these have a direct effect on outcome and must, therefore, be measured before any comment can be made about the process of care. Outcome itself must also of course be measured. This is relatively easy in terms of mortality: the general accepted definition is death within 31 days of the incident. However, disability is a much more difficult issue, and currently there are no universally accepted measurement tools. The functional independence measure used in MTOS,[17] the Glasgow Outcome Scale,[18] GOSE[19] and the SF36[20] (Short Form - 36 Questions) are the best available tools.

Trauma audit was first formalized by Champion at the Washington Hospital Centre in the 1970s. The TRISS[21] system is now widely used, but there have been many proposals for its modification.

Most current trauma systems are now audited using some variation of the TRISS methodology. This combines measurement of anatomical injury using the Abbreviated Injury Scale and the Injury Severity Score, together with the Revised Trauma Score to measure physiological derangement. A probability of survival can be calculated by reference to large databanks with known outcomes which contain a range of these scores.

CONTROVERSIES

❶ The number of MTVs necessary for a hospital to maintain high quality trauma care.

❷ The degree to which potential MTVs should be overtriaged to ensure that patients with major trauma are received at major trauma centres. There may be a greater risk in bypassing hospitals to take patients to a trauma centre depending on distance and injury type. There is also the issue of deskilling of personnel from non-trauma centres and what effect this has on overall system outcomes.

❸ The degree to which MTVs should be managed by protocol versus clinical judgement. Increasingly clinicians are being asked to follow protocols in these critical situations. This prevents some adverse outcomes but may cause over-investigation and treatment.

❹ The role of hypotensive resuscitation in blunt trauma has not been defined. Where victims have prolonged delays to theatre or the bleeding is not surgically correctable, then hypotensive resuscitation may cause more complications.

❺ The role of controlled hypothermia in head injured patients.

Perhaps more importantly, the comparative performance of hospitals or the change in a single hospital's performance over time can be determined by bringing together the probability of survival of a number of patients and comparing them with the actual survival. Anonymous league tables can then be developed with the objective of identifying features of the best hospitals associated with high survival rates (and vice versa).

REFERENCES

1. Center for disease control, National Center for Injury Prevention and Control: WISQARS Atlanta, http://webapp.cdc.gov
2. Nantulya WM, Reich MR 2002 The neglected epidemic: road traffic injuries in developing countries. British Medical Journal 324: 1139–41
3. Australian Bureau of Statistics, http://www.abs.gov.au/austats
4. Trunkey DD 1983 Trauma. Scientific American 249(2): 28–35
5. Cales RH, Trunkey DD 1985 Preventable trauma deaths. A review of trauma care systems development. Journal of the American Medical Association 254: 1059–63
6. Roy PD 1987 The value of trauma centres: a methodologic review. Canadian Journal of Surgery 30: 17–22
7. Eastman AB, Lewis FR, Champion HR, Mattox KL 1987 Regional trauma system design: critical concepts. American Journal of Surgery 154: 79–87
8. Palanca S, Taylor D, Bailey M, Cameron PA 2002 Mechanisms of motor vehicle accidents that predict major injury. Journal of Emergency Medicine (in press)
9. Pickard JD, Czosnyka M 1993 Management of raised intracranial pressure. Journal of Neurology, Neurosurgery and Psychiatry 56: 845–58
10. Fortune JB, Feustel PJ, Graca L, Hasselbarth J, Kuehler DH 1995 Effect of hyperventilation, mannitol, and ventriculostomy drainage on cerebral blood flow after head injury. Journal of Trauma, Injury, Infection and Critical Care 39(6): 1091–9
11. Alderson P, Schierhout G, Roberts I, Bunn F Colloids versus crystalloids for fluid resuscitation in critically ill patients (Cochrane review). In: The Cochrane Library, Issue 3, 2002 Oxford: Update Software
12. Clifton GL, Miller ER, Sung RN, et al 2001 Lack of effect of induction of hypothermia after acute brain injury. New England Journal of Medicine 344: 556–63
13. Mattox KL, Bickell W, Pepe I, Burch J, Feliciano D 1989 Prospective MAST study in 911 patients. Journal of Trauma 29: 1102–12
14. Bickell WH, Wall MJ, Pepe PE, et al 1994 Immediate versus delayed fluid resuscitation for hypertensive patients with penetrating torso injuries. New England Journal of Medicine 331: 1105–9
15. Civil IDJ 1993 Resuscitation following injury: an end or a means? Australian and New Zealand Journal of Surgery 63: 921–6
16. Cameron PA, Dziukas L, Hadj A, Clark P, Hooper S 1995 Patterns of injury from major trauma in Victoria. Australian and New Zealand Journal of Surgery 65: 830–4
17. Champion HZ, Copes WS, Sacco WJ, et al 1990 The Major Trauma Outcome Study: establishing natural norms for trauma care. Journal of Trauma 30: 1356–65
18. Jennett B, Bond M 1975 Assessment of outcome after severe brain damage. Lancet 1: 480–4
19. Teasdale GM, Pettigrew LE, Wilson JT, Murray G, Jemett B 1998 Analysing outcome of severe head injury: a review and update on advancing the use of the Glasgow Outcome Scale. Journal of Neurotrauma 15: 587–97
20. Garratt AM, Ruta DA, Abdulher MI, Buckingham JK, Russell IT 1993 the SF36 Health Survey Questionnaire: an outcome measure suitable for routine use within the NHS? British Medical Journal 306: 1440–4
21. Boyd CR, Tolson MA, Copes WS 1987 Evaluating trauma care. The TRISS method. Journal of Trauma 27: 370–8

FURTHER READING

ATLS Manual, American College of Surgeons
Skinner D, Driscoll P 1999 ABC of Major Trauma, 3rd edn. BMJ Publishing, London

2.2 NEUROTRAUMA

MARCUS P KENNEDY • ANGELO ANNUNZIATA

ESSENTIALS

1 Neurotrauma is associated with the majority of trauma deaths.

2 A detailed history of the mechanics of the trauma experienced is invaluable.

3 Secondary brain injury is a major and potentially preventable cause of mortality and long-term morbidity.

4 Cerebral cellular dysfunction secondary to trauma is a result of both primary and secondary mechanisms and involves sodium, calcium and potassium shifts across the cell membrane, the development of oxygen free radicals, and lipid peroxidation.

5 There are two features of prime importance to resuscitation in patients suffering neurotrauma: maintenance of airway/ventilation, and maintenance of cerebral perfusion pressure.

6 Inline stabilization of the cervical spine during rapid sequence induction and orotracheal intubation is the preferred method for gaining definitive airway control in the head-injured patient.

7 Current emergency department and neurosurgical practice involves the use of CT scanning to investigate mild, moderate and severe head injury

INTRODUCTION

Neurotrauma is a common feature in the presentation of multisystem trauma, particularly that associated with motor vehicle accidents and falls. Over 50% of trauma deaths are associated with head injury. The implications for the health system are enormous, with an annual rate of hospital admission associated with head trauma exceeding 300 per 100 000 population. The long-term sequelae of moderate and severe neurotrauma are a major health resource drain, and the morbidities associated with mild brain injury are becoming clearer.

Advances in preventative strategies, trauma systems, resuscitative therapies and rehabilitation management have improved outcomes. However, neurotrauma remains a serious health issue, often affecting the productive youth of society.

DEFINITION

Neurotrauma may be classified according to severity as minimal, mild, or moderate or potentially severe (Table 2.2.1).[1] The usefulness of such classifications lies within the implied approaches to investigation and therapy, but there is clearly a continuum of injury within the spectrum of neurotrauma.

Table 2.2.1 Neurotrauma severity

Minimal
No loss of consciousness and
Glasgow Coma Score (GCS) 15, and
Normal alertness and memory, and
No neurological deficit, and
No palpable depressed fracture or other sign of skull fracture

Mild
Brief (<5 minutes) loss of consciousness, or
Amnesia for event, or
GCS 14, or
Impaired alertness or memory.
No palpable depressed fracture or other sign of skull fracture

Moderate or potentially severe
Prolonged (>5 minutes) loss of consciousness, or
Persistent GCS <14, or
Focal neurological deficit, or
Post-traumatic seizure, or
Intracranial lesion on CT scan, or
Palpable depressed skull fracture

CLASSIFICATION OF PRIMARY INJURY IN NEUROTRAUMA

- Skull fracture
- Concussion
- Contusion
- Intracranial haematoma
- Diffuse axonal injury
- Penetrating injury.

Skull fracture

The significance of skull fracture is generally not the specific bony injury but rather the associated neurotrauma. Fractures in the region of the middle meningeal artery in particular may be associated with acute extradural haemorrhage. Fractures involving the skull base and cribriform plate may be associated with CSF leak and the risk of secondary infection. Depressed skull fractures may compress underlying structures, cause secondary brain injury and require surgical elevation. Injury to underlying structures may result in secondary epilepsy.

Concussion

Concussion is a transient alteration in cerebral function, usually associated with loss of consciousness and often followed by rapid and complete recovery. The proposed mechanism is a disturbance in the function of the reticular activating system. Post-concussive syndromes, including headache and mild cognitive disturbance, are not uncommon.[2, 3] Symptoms, particularly headache, are usually short-lived but may persist. 'Second impact syndrome' describes a greater risk of significant reinjury following an initial injury causing a simple concussion. It is likely to be due to diffuse cerebral swelling.[4] In animal models concussion may be associated with modest short-term increases in intracranial pressure and disturbances in cerebral cellular functions.[5]

Contusion

Cerebral contusion is bruising of the brain substance associated with head trauma. The most common mechanism is blunt trauma. Forces involved are less than those required to cause major shearing injuries, and often occur in the absence of skull fracture. The associated morbidity is related to the size and site of contusion, and coexistent injury. Larger contusions may be associated with haematoma formation, secondary oedema or seizure activity. The most common sites for contusions are the frontal and temporal lobes.[6]

Intracranial haematoma

Extradural

Extradural haematoma (EDH) is uncommon but classically associated with fracture of the temporal bone and injury to the underlying middle meningeal artery. Haemorrhage subsequently occurs, stripping the dura from the skull, expanding to cause a rise in intracranial pressure and eventually uncal herniation and death. Haemorrhage may be from vessels other than the middle meningeal artery (e.g. brisk arteriolar or venous bleeding). Signs will depend on the site of the haematoma.

Subdural

Subdural haematomata (SDH) may have an acute, subacute or chronic course. It generally follows moderate head trauma with loss of consciousness. In the elderly SDH may be associated with trivial injury, and in children with shaking (abuse) injury. Haemorrhage occurs into the subdural space, slowly enlarging to cause a space-occupying collection whose functional implications will vary according to location. Acute subdural haemorrhage carries a high mortality risk (>50%),[7] similar to acute EDH. Subacute and chronic SDH is associated with a degree of cerebral dysfunction, headache or other symptomatology, and is associated with a significantly lower mortality (of the order of 20%).[7]

Intracerebral

As with cerebral contusion, the most common sites of intracerebral haemorrhage associated with trauma are the temporal and posterior frontal lobes. Functional expression is variable depending on site. Intracerebral haemorrhage may progress from an initial contusion or be secondary. Symptom development and complications may be delayed as the size of the haemorrhage increases over time.

Subarachnoid and intraventricular haemorrhage

Subarachnoid blood is relatively common after major head injury. Intraventricular haemorrhage may also be evident. As in non-traumatic settings, the presence of subarachnoid blood may lead to cerebral vasospasm and secondary ischaemic brain injury.

Diffuse axonal injury

Diffuse axonal injury (DAI) is the predominant mechanism of injury in neurotrauma, occurring in up to 50% of patients.[8]

Shearing and rotational forces on the axonal network may result in major structural and functional disturbance at a microscopic level. Disturbance to important communicative pathways sometimes results in significant long-term morbidity, despite non-specific or minimal changes on CT scanning. The exact pathogenesis of diffuse axonal injury is incompletely understood. Specific injury in the regions of the corpus callosum and midbrain has been proposed; however, DAI is believed to be the mechanism for persistent neurological deficits seen in head-traumatized individuals with normal CT scans.[9]

Penetrating injury

Penetrating neurotrauma is characterized by high levels of morbidity and mortality. This is true particularly of gunshot wounds and, to a lesser degree, of stab wounds. Exposure of cerebral tissue through large compound wounds, or through basilar skull structures, is associated with a dismal outlook. Penetrating injury in the periorbital and pernasal regions is associated with high risk of infection.

PATHOGENESIS

Primary brain injury occurs as a result of the forces and disruptive mechanics of the original incident. Secondary brain injury is due to a complex interaction of factors and typically occurs within 2–24 hours post injury.[10] A principal mechanism of secondary injury is cerebral hypoxia due to impaired oxygenation or impaired cerebral blood flow.

Cerebral blood flow is dependent on cerebral perfusion pressure, systemic blood pressure and intracranial pressure. Intracranial pressure may be raised as a result of the mass effect of the haemorrhage, or from generalized cerebral oedema.

Cerebral vasospasm further decreases cerebral blood flow in patients in whom significant subarachnoid haemorrhage has occurred.

Cellular dysfunction is a result of both primary and secondary mechanisms and involves sodium, calcium, magnesium and potassium shifts across the cell membrane, the development of oxygen free radicals, lipid peroxidation and glutamate hyperactivity. Excessive release of excitatory neurotransmitters and magnesium depletion also occur.[11]

PRESENTATION

History

A detailed history of the mechanics of the trauma is essential. This should be followed by consideration of time courses, prehospital care, presedative and prerelaxant neuromuscular function, and episodes and duration of hypotension or other decompensation. A history of previous health problems, allergies, medications and social setting is desirable.

Primary survey

As with all trauma patients the initial assessment and therapy must be directed at maintenance of airway, ventilation and circulatory adequacy. Early assessment of neurological disturbance is important (e.g. AVPU: alert, response to verbal stimuli, response to painful stimuli, or unresponsive). Simultaneous protection of the cervical spine by immobilization is fundamental. This management should commence in the prehospital setting and the level of care be maintained.

Inline stabilization of the cervical spine during rapid sequence induction and orotracheal intubation is the preferred method for gaining definitive airway control in the head-injured patient.

The greatest risk to the patient with a moderate-to-severe head injury is deficient cerebral perfusion due to systemic hypotension.

Secondary survey

A full secondary survey, including log-roll, should follow.

Specific examination

Clinical assessment of the neurological status of head-injured patients commences with formal documentation of the Glasgow Coma Score (GCS) (Table 2.2.2). The maximum score is 15 and the minimum 3. The GCS has been incorporated into other assessment scales in trauma (Trauma Score, Revised Trauma Score) and in TRISS estimation of probability of survival.

Coma may be defined in terms of the Glasgow Coma Scale, in which patients:

- Fail to show eye opening in response to pain
- Fail to obey commands

Table 2.2.2 Glasgow Coma Score

Best motor response

Obeys command	6
Localizes to pain	5
Withdraw to pain	4
Abnormal flexion to pain	3
Abnormal extension to pain	2
Nil	1

Best verbal response

Oriented	5
Confused	4
Uses inappropriate words	3
Makes incomprehensible sounds	2
Nil	1

Eye opening

Spontaneously	4
To verbal command	3
To pain	2
Nil	1

- Make at best only incomprehensible sounds.
  Eye-opening response = 1
  Best motor response = 5
  Best verbal response = 2.
  Total GCS = 8

Examination of pupillary responses, particularly in the unconscious patient, is important as an indicator of increasing intracranial pressure; a non-responsive dilated pupil indicating ipsilateral herniation. However, a more common cause of abnormal pupil reactions in head injury is the presence of direct ocular trauma.

A general neurological examination, including reflexes and fundoscopy, should be performed, the degree to which cooperation is possible and lateralization of signs being particularly important.

Consideration of the preinjury mental state is important, particularly where drug or alcohol intoxication is possible.

RESUSCITATION IN NEUROTRAUMA

There are two features of prime importance to resuscitation in patients suffering neurotrauma:

❶ Maintenance of airway and ventilation
❷ Maintenance of cerebral perfusion pressure.

With elevation of intracranial pressure and loss of autoregulation of cerebral circulation, relatively higher systemic blood pressures are required. The practice of minimal volume resuscitation has no place in the patient with serious neurotrauma. Standard approaches to the management of hypovolaemia in head-injured patients should be adopted. The use of hypertonic solutions in resuscitation (including hypertonic saline) has been adopted in some centres, with favourable outcomes for head injured patients.[12] More recent studies suggest no improvement in outcome.

Indications for intubation and ventilation of the neurotrauma patient are inadequate ventilation or gas exchange (hypercarbia, hypoxia, apnoea); inability

to maintain airway integrity (protective reflexes); a combative or agitated patient; and the need for transport where the status of the airway is potentially unstable (interhospital, to CT, to angiography, etc.).

MILD HEAD INJURY

Investigation

In head injury associated with loss of consciousness or amnesia and a GCS of 14–15, CT scanning will demonstrate a relevant positive scan (i.e. cerebral contusion, haematoma, oedema, pneumocephalus) in 7–12%, and a subsequent craniotomy rate of 1–3%.[13-16]

On the weight of research evidence current emergency department investigation of mild head injury should include CT scanning in all patients in this group.[1,17-20] Despite considerable research in this area, reliable risk stratification is difficult. Stratification of high-risk discriminators within the GCS 14–15 group has not been definitively achieved. Certain high-risk groups, such as the intoxicated, elderly (>65 years), anticoagulated or demented patients, warrant CT scanning after minor, presumed or possible head injury.

A prospective cohort study of 3121 patients has identified five high-risk criteria for neurosurgical intervention in patients with GCS 13–15 and mild head injury. They were failure to reach GCS 15 within 2 hours, suspected open skull fracture, any sign of basal skull fracture, vomiting (two or more episodes) or age greater than 65 years. The same study identified amnesia before impact and high-risk mechanism as predictors of clinically significant injury.[21] A recent study in the New England Journal of Medicine[22] showed that 6.3% of patients with one of the following findings had an abnormal CT scan: headache, vomiting, age >60 years, drug or alcohol intoxication, short term memory deficits, physical evidence of trauma above the clavicles, or seizure.

While coagulation disturbance was not included, it is advisable to have a reduced threshold for scanning those on aspirin, warfarin or with a coagulopathy (see also Chapter 2.8 Radiology in Major Trauma).

Recommendations in regard to a 'safe' period of observation, need for hospital admission or predictive value of injury mechanism are not consistent. Rural and isolated settings present logistic difficulties in the management of this group. Careful observation for a prolonged period is a reasonable alternative, and early neurosurgical consultation together with a low threshold to transfer to a neurosurgical centre is prudent.

Cervical spine X-ray is indicated if the patient has neck pain, neurological abnormality, altered conscious state, intoxication or significant distracting injury.

Management and disposition

All patients with mild head injury must be counselled appropriately and discharged with written advice in the care of a responsible adult. Specific advice must be provided regarding expected duration of symptoms, possible risks or delayed complications, and reasons for representation to the emergency department (Table 2.2.3). Information should also be given about the second impact syndrome and exclusions from sporting activity.

Follow-up by local medical officer should be arranged and neuropyscho-logical assessment may be warranted for high-risk groups. Patients should be cautioned about making major life, occupational and financial decisions until they are free of post-concussive symptoms.

In minimal and mild head injury a normal CT scan and the absence of neurological abnormality are reasonable criteria for patient discharge.[10] In the presence of these criteria the persistence of mild symptoms is common, e.g. mild headache, nausea, occasional vomiting.

In adults such symptoms may be treated with mild analgesics (paracetamol, aspirin) and antiemetics (metoclopramide, prochlorperazine) and the patient discharged when comfortable.

Currently there is no drug to treat the primary pathology in mild and minor head injury.[23]

MODERATE-TO-SEVERE HEAD INJURY

Investigation

Urgent CT scanning is the investigation of choice in moderate-to-severe neurotrauma; however, other investigation and therapy may take priority in the patient with multisystem trauma, particularly in the presence of unresponsive haemorrhagic shock.

In the absence of a CT scan a skull X-ray may provide some useful information (e.g. in the detection of radio-opaque foreign bodies), but should not delay consultation with a neurosurgeon or early transfer to an appropriate facility.

Cervical spine X-ray is indicated in all patients with moderate to severe neurotrauma. A significant proportion of patients with severe head injury will have cervical spine fractures.

Management

Priority in the management of moderate to severe neurotrauma is given to the maintenance of the airway and an adequate cerebral perfusion pressure (CPP). Hypotension (SBP<90) and hypoxia (Pa O2 < 60 [8kPa]) should be corrected immediately.[24] Control or modification of intracranial pressure (ICP) has a place in the emergency management of neurotrauma. Avoidance of secondary brain injury and associated cerebral swelling is the mainstay of such therapy, and the use of the head-up position, mannitol and hyperventilation is indicated in some situations.

Intracranial pressure monitoring is generally indicated in patients with severe head injury (GCS <8) who remain comatose. Institutional variability exists in methods for measurement, as do specific indications for monitoring.

Elevation of the head of the bed to 30° will decrease ICP modestly without altering CPP.

Mannitol (0.5–1.0 g/kg IV) and hyperventilation to induce hypocapnia (30–35 mmHg [4–4.7 kPa]) may both produce short-term reduction in ICP. Mannitol causes an osmotic dehydration, which is non-selective. Complications of mannitol therapy include fluid overload, hyperosmolality, hypovolaemia and rebound cerebral oedema. Contraindications to mannitol therapy include preexisting hypovolaemia, serum osmolarity >320 mmol/L and renal failure.

Hypocarbia decreases cerebral blood flow (and ICP) through vasoconstriction which, if extreme, may decrease CPP to the point of exacerbation of secondary brain injury.[25] Routine use of hyperventilation in head injury is contraindicated.

Table 2.2.3 Patient advice

General advice following head injury
The patient should read and understand these instructions.
1. Rest comfortably at home in the company of a responsible adult for the next 12–24 hours.
2. Resume normal activity after feeling recovered.
3. Drink clear fluids and consume a light diet only for the first 6–12 hours (a normal diet may be commenced as desired after that).
4. Mild pain killers (such as paracetamol) may be taken for headache as directed by the doctor.
5. Following head injury a small number of patients develop ongoing symptoms, such as recurrent mild headache, concentration difficulties, difficulty with complex tasks, mood disturbance, etc. If you notice such problems, consult your local doctor for appropriate referral.
6. Avoid exposure to activities that may create risk of further head injury within the next 2 weeks.
7. If you do not understand these instructions and advice, check with emergency department staff before your discharge or consult your local doctor.
8. If you require a certificate for work please make this clear to emergency department staff.

Report immediately the following problems:
1. Persistent vomiting (more than twice).
2. Persistent drowsiness – unable to be woken up completely.
3. Confusion or disorientation or slurred speech.
4. Increased headache (not relieved by standard doses of paracetamol).
5. Localized weakness or altered sensation or incoordination.
6. Blurred or double vision.
7. Seizures, fits or convulsions.
8. Neck stiffness.

Both osmotic diuresis and hyperventilation should be used with care, and preferably in consultation with neurosurgeons.

Anticonvulsant prophylaxis (phenytoin 15–18 mg/kg IV over 30–60 minutes) is indicated for the prevention of seizures within the first week after injury.[26] Seizures are managed acutely using standard therapies and guidelines (including benzodiazepines and phenytoin). The use of barbiturates, endotracheal intubation and mechanical ventilation may be indicated for status epilepticus or seizures that are refractory to therapy.

Antibiotic prophylaxis is indicated for compound fractures (flucloxacillin 1g 6 hourly IV, or cephalothin 1 g 6 hourly IV). Tetanus immunoprophylaxis is given as part of routine wound care.

Steroid therapy has had varied support and is not recommended as routine: there is little evidence to support it and the side effects may be significant.[27]

There has been considerable interest and experimental endeavour with regard to cerebral protection and salvage therapies. Examples include the use of adrenocorticotrophic hormone analogues, calcium antagonists superoxide dismutase, glutamate antagonists, free radical scavengers and ciclosporin A.[28] Definitive outcomes of trials are awaited. General supportive therapy, including maintenance of thermoregulation, hydration, pressure care and nutrition, must be addressed.

Disposition

Patients with moderate-to-severe neurotrauma require hospital admission, preferably under the care of a neurosurgeon in a specialized neurosurgical unit or ICU. Rehabilitation and social readjustment is a focus of therapy from early in the clinical course.

Interhospital transfer of patients with significant neurotrauma requires the attendance of skilled transfer staff and the maintenance of level of care during transfer. Airway management must anticipate the potential for the patient to deteriorate en route. The presence of pneumocephalus precludes unpressurized (high) altitude flight. The use of tele-radiology and neurosurgical consultation will be of value in the management of the remote head-injured patient.

Prognosis

The level of residual neurological impairment is a function of the severity of the degree of trauma and quality of care. Worse outcome is associated with prolonged pre-hospital time, delay of transfer to appropriate facility, admission to inappropriate facility and delay in definitive surgical treatment. [29]

Overall mortality in severe head injury is in the order of 35%. A lower GCS at presentation is associated with worse outcome. Approximately half the patients who remain comatose with GCS <9 for longer than 6 hours will die.[9] Acute subdural haematoma and diffuse axonal injury producing persistent coma are associated with the vast majority of neurotrauma deaths. Early neurologic abnormalities are, however, not reliable prognostic factors, and an initial period of maximally aggressive therapy is indicated in patients with closed neurotrauma.

CONTROVERSIES

❶ Intracranial pressure monitoring has not been shown to improve outcome from major head injury.

❷ The role of CT scanning in minor head injury has become more widespread. While it is increasingly accept that CT is indicated, the timing or urgency of the investigation is controversial. Further studies are required to define descriminators and high-risk markers as guides to the most rational application of this investigation.

❸ Consideration should be given to referral of all patients with minor or worse head injury for neuropyschological assessment on discharge in order to facilitate recovery and resumption of normal activities.

REFERENCES

1. Stein S, Ross S 1993 Minor head injury: a proposed strategy for emergency management. Editorial. Annals of Emergency Medicine 22(7): 1193–6
2. Lahaye PA, Gade GF, Becker DP 1991 Injury to the cranium. In: Moore EE, Mattox KL, Feliciano DV (eds) Trauma, 2nd edn. Emergency Department, Appleton & Lange, Norwalk, p. 247
3. Ponsford J, Willmott C, et al 2000 Factors influencing outcome following mild traumatic brain injury in adults, JINS 6: 568–79
4. McCory P 2001 Does second impact syndrome exist? Clinical Journal of Sport Medicine 11(3): 144–9
5. Goldman H, Hodgson V, Morehead M et al 1990 A rat model of closed head injury. Journal of Neurotrauma 8: 129
6. Javid M 1974 Head injuries. New England Journal of Medicine 291(17): 890
7. Povlishock JT 1993 Pathobiology of traumatically induced axonal injury in animals and man. Annals of Emergency Medicine 22: 980
8. Meythaler JM, Peduzzi JD, Eleftheriou E, et al 2001 Current concepts: Diffuse axonal injury - associated traumatic brain injury. Archives of Physical Medicine and Rehabilitation 82: 1461–71
9. Statham PF, Andrews PJ 1996 Central nervous system trauma. In: Baillière's Clinical Neurology 5(3): 501
10. Kay A, Teasdale MB 2001 Head injury in the United Kingdom. World Journal of Surgery 25(9): 1210–20
11. Morris JA, Limbird TJ, MacKenzie E 1991 Rehabilitation of the trauma patient. In: Moore EE, Mattox KL, Feliciano DV (eds) Trauma, 2nd edn. Emergency Department, Appleton & Lange, Norwalk, p. 247
12. Vassar MJ, Fischer RP, O'Brien PE, et al 1993 A multicenter trial for resuscitation of injured patients with 7.5% sodium chloride. The effect of added dextran 70. The Multicenter Group for the Study of Hypertonic Saline in Trauma Patients. Archives of Surgery 128: 1003–11
13. Shackford S, Waid S, et al 1992 The clinical utility of computed tomographic scanning and neurological examination in the management of patients with minor head injuries. Journal of Trauma 33(3): 385–94
14. Stein S, Ross SJ 1992 Mild head injury: a plea for routine early CT scanning. Trauma 33(1): 11–3
15. Richards KA, Lukin WG, Jones P 1997 Minor head injuries. (Royal Brisbane Hospital, personal communication. Unpublished data)
16. Lenninger BE, Kreutzer JS, Hill MR 1991 Comparison of minor and severe head injury emotional sequelae using the MMPI. Brain Injury 5(2): 199–205
17. The management of acute neurotrauma in rural and remote locations 1992 Neurosurgical Society of Australasia, The Royal Australasian College of Surgeons
18. Victorian Road Trauma Committee 1997 Report of the Consultative Committee on Road Traffic Fatalities. Victorian Institute of Forensic Pathology, Royal Australasian College of Surgeons
19. McAllister TW 1992 Neuropsychiatric sequelae of head injuries. Psychiatric Clinics of North America 15(2): S395–S413
20. Bullock R, Chesnut RM, et al 1996 Guidelines for the management of severe head injury. European Journal of Emergency Medicine 2: 109-127
21. Steil I, Wells G, et al 2001 The Canadian CT rule for patients with minor head injury. Lancet 357: 1391–6
22. Haydel MJ, Preston CA, Mills TJ, et al 2000 Indications for computed tomography in patients with minor head injury. New England Journal of Medicine 343: 100–5
23. McCrory P 2001 New treatments for concussion:

The next millenium beckons. Clinical Journal of Sport Medicine 11(3): 190–3
24. Chesnut RM, Marshall LF, Klauber MR, et al 1993 The role of secondary brain injury in determining outcome from severe head injury. Journal of Trauma 34: 216–22
25. Fortune JB, Fenstel PJ, Graca L, Husselbarth J, Kuehler DH 1995 Effect of hyperventilation,

Mannitol and ventriculostomy drainage on cerebral blood flow after head injury. Journal of Trauma, Injury, Infection and Critical Care 39(6): 1091–9
26. Temkin NR, Dikmen SS, Wilensky AJ, et al 1990 A randomised, double blind study of phenytoin for the prevention of post-traumatic seizures New England Journal of Medicine 323: 497–502

27. Pitts LH 1995 Neurotrauma and trauma systems. New Horizons 3: 546–8
28. Clausen T, Bullock R 2001 Medical treatment and neuroprotection in traumatic brain injury Current Parmaceutical Design 7: 1517–32
29. Atkinson L, Merry G 2001 Advances in neurotrauma in Australia 1970–2000. World Journal of Surgery 25: 1224–9

2.3 SPINAL TRAUMA

JEFF WASSERTHEIL

ESSENTIALS

1 Cervical spine injury can be confidently eliminated in conscious clear headed patients using clinical examination criteria alone.

2 Physical examination alone does not assist in the diagnosis of unstable vertebral injury unless deformity is gross.

3 A lack of neurological symptoms and signs does not eliminate spinal column injury or spinal cord at risk.

4 A patient can be ambulant and still have a major vertebral injury, even a potentially unstable one.

5 Spinal cord injury may not be associated with a vertebral injury as seen on plain X-ray. This situation is termed a SCIWORA (spinal cord injury without radiological abnormality) and is more common in children.

6 The natural history of spinal cord injury may lead to progressively increasing symptoms commencing some hours after the incident.

7 Magnetic resonance imaging is evolving as the imaging modality of choice in patients with neurological signs.

8 The likelihood of significant vertebral injury in unconscious trauma victims is 10%; 2% of all trauma victims with significant altered conscious state have a spinal cord injury.

INTRODUCTION

Spinal cord injury is one of the most disabling, causing major and irreversible physical and psychological disability to the patient and permanently affecting their lifestyle. The emotional, social and economic consequences affect the individual, family, friends and society in general.

Motor vehicle accidents, falls and sporting injuries – notably diving and water sports – are the major causes of acute spinal cord injury in Australia.[1-3] Road traffic accidents account for about half of all spinal injuries. Despite the work to minimize spinal injuries in contact sports such as rugby, serious spinal cord injuries still occur.[1,2] Spinal injuries occur mostly in young people. However, minor falls in the elderly or low impact injuries in people with pre-existing bony pathology can also cause spinal cord damage.[3] Spinal cord injury due to pathological vertebral fractures may be the first presentaion of malignancy.

Observations from two studies[4,5] suggest that possibly preventable neurological deterioration may be due to one or more of the following:

- The injury not being recognized initially, e.g. not being specifically examined for, occult and masked by other injuries
- The onset of the secondary effects of the spinal cord injury involving oedema and/or ischaemia
- Aggravation of the initial spinal cord lesion by inadequate oxygenation and/or hypotension
- Aggravation of the initial spinal cord lesion by inadequate vertebral immobilization.

PATHOPHYSIOLOGY

Level of vertebral injury

The level of neurologic injury in patients who sustain spinal injuries is variously reported. In studies from Victoria and New South Wales [5,6] distribution of the level of injuries was cervical 60%, thoracic 30%, lumbar 4% and sacral 2%.

Spinal cord injuries occur most commonly at the level of the 5th, 6th and 7th cervical vertebrae, largely because of the greater mobility of these regions. The C5-6 and C6-7 levels account for almost 50% of all subluxation injury patterns in blunt cervical spine trauma. [7]

Associated injuries

There are three noteworthy observations [4,6] from associated injuries in patients with spinal injury:

❶ Approximately 8–10% of patients with a vertebral fracture have a secondary fracture of another vertebra, often at a distant site. These secondary fractures are usually associated with the more violent mechanisms of injury, such as ejection or rollover. Secondary injuries are usually relatively minor and stable, e.g. fractures of the vertebral processes, but occasionally they may be major and may also be associated with neurological damage. Therefore, when 'thinking spine', it is important to 'think whole spine' and, in particular, to attempt to avoid rotation of the vertebral column.

❷ Owing to the mechanism of injury, many patients with spinal injuries often have other associated injuries, including head, intrathoracic or intra-abdominal injuries, which may modify priorities in management.[3,6]

❸ Patients may complain of pain from other injuries, and hence a back or neck injury may go unnoticed. Pain may often not be a significant feature despite severe vertebral column damage. Furthermore, spinal pain may take some time to become apparent because of other pathological processes modifying pain, such as swelling and inflammation.

NEUROLOGICAL INJURIES

Primary spinal cord damage
(Fig. 2.3.1)

Transverse spinal cord syndrome
The spinal cord is completely damaged transversely across one or more adjacent spinal segments. No motor or autonomic information can be transmitted below the damaged area, and ascending sensory stimuli from below the damaged spinal segments are blocked. The manifestations are: total flaccid paralysis, total anaesthesia, total analgesia, and usually areflexia below the injured segment.

The transverse cord syndrome can be incomplete, with partial paralysis, reduced sensation and pain sensibility below the injured part.

The term 'sacral sparing' implies that some sensibility with or without motor activity in the areas supplied by the sacral segments is preserved in an otherwise complete transverse cord syndrome. The presence of sacral sparing implies an incomplete injury, as some neurological transmission through the injured segments is preserved. It will be recalled that spinothalamic and corticospinal transmission to and from sacral segments are located

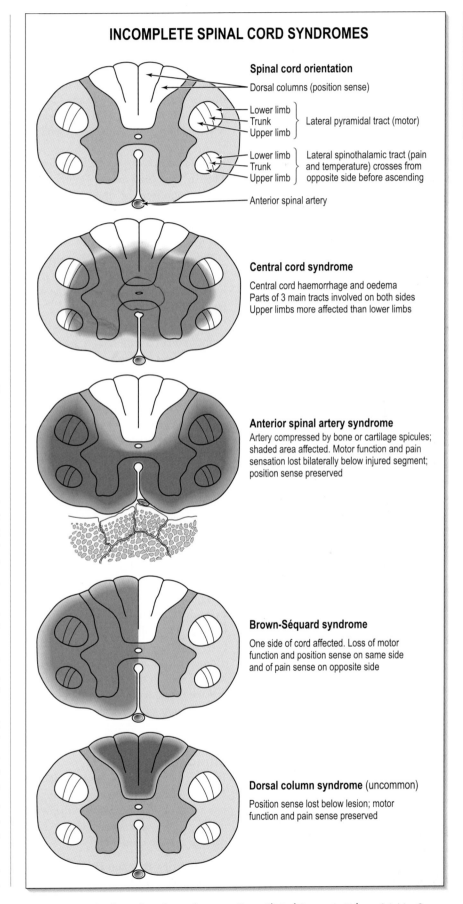

INCOMPLETE SPINAL CORD SYNDROMES

Spinal cord orientation
Dorsal columns (position sense)
Lower limb
Trunk — Lateral pyramidal tract (motor)
Upper limb
Lower limb
Trunk — Lateral spinothalamic tract (pain and temperature) crosses from opposite side before ascending
Upper limb
Anterior spinal artery

Central cord syndrome
Central cord haemorrhage and oedema
Parts of 3 main tracts involved on both sides
Upper limbs more affected than lower limbs

Anterior spinal artery syndrome
Artery compressed by bone or cartilage spicules; shaded area affected. Motor function and pain sensation lost bilaterally below injured segment; position sense preserved

Brown-Séquard syndrome
One side of cord affected. Loss of motor function and position sense on same side and of pain sense on opposite side

Dorsal column syndrome (uncommon)
Position sense lost below lesion; motor function and pain sense preserved

Fig. 2.3.1 Spinal cord and syndromes. (From Clinical Symposia Volume 34, No. 2, 1998. Comprehensive Management of Spinal Cord Injury, Plate 11 p.17. Redrawn with permission courtesy of Novartis Pty Ltd, Basel, Switzerland.)

in the outermost parts of the spinal cord, and are, therefore, immediately adjacent to the origin of the spinal cord's blood supply.

Acute central cervical cord syndrome

The central part or grey matter of the spinal cord is injured. Transmission in the outer rim of the spinal cord is essentially intact but impaired. The signs of this injury are:

- Motor function: there will be weakness in both upper and lower limbs, with weakness marked in the upper limbs.
- Sensation: there is sensory loss in both upper and lower limbs, which is more severe in the upper limbs.
- Reflexes are variable.

This is frequently caused by a hyperextension injury and is typically seen in older patients with cervical spondylosis. In this situation the cord is compressed between posterior osteophytes and the intervertebral disc in front and the ligamentum flavum behind.

Acute anterior cervical cord syndrome

The anterior half of the spinal cord, the region supplied by the anterior spinal artery, is damaged. There is motor loss or paralysis below the level of the injured segment(s). Spinothalamic transmission is impaired and thus there is analgesia with loss of temperature sensation and coarse touch. As the dorsal columns are relatively intact, there is some preservation of joint position, vibration sense and fine touch. In the context of an acute cord injury the patient may not interpret dorsal column preservation in terms of joint position sense or light touch. Dorsal column function may be manifested as preservation of vague and poorly localized sensation in the extremities.

These injuries are frequently the result of flexion-rotation or vertical compression injuries.

Brown-Séquard syndrome

This syndrome is a functional cord hemisection with dissociated sensory loss. One half of the cord is damaged. In a pure Brown-Séquard lesion ipsilateral motor function is impaired, as is light touch, joint position sense and vibration. Contralateral spinothalamic sensation – that is, pain and temperature – is impaired, whereas ipsilateral sensation is relatively preserved. Reflexes are variable.

Posterior cord syndrome

This is an uncommon injury that causes contusion or disruption to the dorsal columns. This leads to impaired or disrupted proprioception, vibration and fine touch sensation.

This syndrome is usually the result of penetrating trauma to the back or a hyperextension injury in association with fractures of the vertebral arch.

Spinal cord concussion

This diagnosis implies a temporary cessation of spinal cord neurological function. In this instance there is a near full recovery of cord function within 48 hours. The patient will be first assessed as suffering from either a complete or an incomplete spinal cord injury, and will then recover within the above time period. The patient has suffered an injury to the spinal cord that has been enough to temporarily cease electrical activity in the injured spinal segment, with no, or very little, mechanical or anatomical injury to the cord, such as haemorrhage or contusion. It is the pattern of recovery over a day or two that allows the diagnosis to be made. Unfortunately, this constitutes less than 1% of all spinal cord injuries.

In all the incomplete spinal cord syndromes, the location of cord pressure or damage vary in terms of incompleteness and segmental level(s) of cord injury, so will the range of symptoms and signs.

Secondary spinal cord damage

It is often believed that most spinal cord damage occurs at the time of injury, but it may occur subsequent to the initial injury.[9] This secondary spinal cord damage may be caused by:

- **Inappropriate manual handling.**[5,6] Subsequent mishandling causing

significant movement at the site of the primary vertebral injury, causing spinal cord damage. Exacerbation of injury leading to spinal cord damage can be prevented by careful handling of the patient. It is important to be aware of the possibility of a spinal cord injury and protect the spine until the diagnosis has been excluded. This involves standard cervical inline immobilization, whole-spine immobilization using a spine board, or Jordan frame and 'log roll' for moving the patient.

- **Hypoxia and hypotension.**[9,10] These aggravate the primary injury, causing progressive neurological deterioration by mechanisms similar to those that cause secondary brain damage in head injury.
- **Acute response to injury.**[9,10] Intrinsic metabolic changes in the previously undamaged spinal cord at the region of the initial vertebral injury may also cause secondary deterioration due to oedema, haemorrhage and the release of metabolically active substances from damaged neurons. The culmination of the pathophysiological processes leads to cord ischaemia and oedema, thereby promoting further neurological damage.

The oedema and haemorrhage tend to resolve in 10–14 days,[11-13] with some improvement in neurological function. Resolving oedema results in local segmental recovery. However, residual ischaemic change in secondarily affected spinal cord adjacent to the primarily injured segments does occur, producing permanent neurologic deficit.

AUTONOMIC NERVOUS SYSTEM EFFECTS OF SPINAL CORD DAMAGE

The whole of the sympathetic nervous system and the pelvic parasympathetic outflow is transmitted in the spinal cord. In an injury higher than the upper thoracic vertebrae there is significant impairment of total body sympathetic and pelvic parasympathetic functions. The extent and severity of autonomic dysfunction is dependent upon the segmental level(s) and extent or completeness of the neurological insult.

Direct effects

Direct effects include manifestations related to the cardiovascular, gastrointestinal, urogenital and thermoregulatory systems.

Cardiovascular effects

In complete quadriplegia sympathetic denervation causes relaxation of resting vasomotor tone, resulting in generalized systemic vasodilatation. It is recognized by dry extremities with variable warmth and colour during initial assessment. In males, penile engorgement or priapism may be present. Owing to the peripheral vasodilatation there is a drop in total peripheral resistance, with consequent hypotension (neurogenic shock). Under normal circumstances this would result in a baroreceptor response in order to achieve compensation. However, as the effector arm of the sympathetic nervous system is paralysed, the normal compensatory effects of tachycardia and vasoconstriction do not occur. The vagus nerve carrying parasympathetic supply to the heart is unopposed, with resultant bradycardia. The higher and more complete the spinal cord injury, the more extensive the autonomic dysfunction.

The usual symptoms and signs of the shock process in response to hypovolaemia cannot occur, as tachycardia and vasoconstriction are mediated by the sympathetic nervous system, which has been interrupted by the high spinal cord lesion.

Gastrointestinal

Following spinal cord injury a paralytic ileus develops. This is usually self-limiting and recovers over a 3–10-day period. Paralysis of sphincters occurs at the lower end of the oesophagus and at the pylorus; as a consequence, passive aspiration of the stomach content, especially of fluid, is a potential problem. Furthermore, owing to thoracic and abdominal wall muscle paralysis, the capacity to cough and hence clear the airway is diminished. In quadriplegia and high paraplegia, occult fluid aspiration due to passive regurgitation of retained gastric content may not be recognized. The airway, therefore, requires close observation and active protection. A nasogastric tube must be inserted and gastric contents drained.

Urinary

Urinary retention is partly the consequence of acute bladder denervation and, in the early post injury phase, due to spinal shock. Catheter insertion is required to prevent overdistension of the bladder in order to optimize bladder recovery. It also permits measurement of urinary output.

Thermoregulatory

Following cervical or upper thoracic spinal cord injury, the spinal patient effectively becomes poikilothermic. In a cold environment they are unable to vasoconstrict to conserve heat, or shiver to generate heat. The patient is already peripherally vasodilated, which promotes loss of heat and lowering of body temperature. In the warm environment, although the patient is already peripherally vasodilated, the capacity to sweat is sympathetically controlled and therefore lost.

SPINAL SHOCK[8,13–15]

Spinal shock is often confused with the neurogenic shock of sympathetic interruption. They are different entities. Complete separation of the spinal cord from the brain abolishes voluntary movement and sensory perception and causes changes in cord physiology and reflex activity. Acute cord confusion is a simple explanation of the resulting pathophysiology. Spinal shock is manifested by the transient cessation of cord activity in the normal cord below the injury. The cord distal to the injury is unable to function as one would expect from a newly created upper motor neurone lesion. Spinal shock may last for a few hours to several weeks, depending on the segmental level and extent of the cord injury. During this period both somatic and autonomic reflexes below the injured segments disappear. Spinal shock has been attributed to the sudden loss of descending facilitatory impulses from higher centres. Recovery from spinal shock is heralded by the return of the Babinski response, followed by the perineal reflexes. In quadriplegia and high paraplegia, as the cord recovers from spinal shock, either recovery of function (depending on the degree of injury resolution at the injury site) occurs or more commonly spasticity develops. If the cord injury is at the conus medullaris or the cauda equina, unless recovery occurs, a lower motor neuron pattern with areflexia remains.

VERTEBRAL INJURY[1,8,11–18]

Cervical spine fractures

Cervical spine injuries may result from one or combinations of the following mechanisms:

- Hyperflexion
- Hyperextension
- Flexion–rotation
- Vertebral compression
- Lateral flexion
- Vertebral compression
- Lateral flexion
- Distraction.

Hyperflexion

Hyperfelxion produces the following injuries:

- Simple stable wedge fracture
- A fracture with an anterior teardrop
- Bilateral anterior subluxation
- Clay shoveler's fracture
- Bilateral facet dislocation.

Radiographs may demonstrate an associated anterior disc space narrowing and a widened interspinous distance. Bilateral dislocations are evidenced by a displacement of greater than 50% of a vertebral body width of the vertebrae above over the vertebrae below. Oblique views of the cervical spine provide better visualization of the facet joints.

Flexion injuries can cause a vertebral body fracture with an antero-inferior extrusion tear drop fracture. This is often associated with retropulsion of a vertebral body fracture fragment or fragments into the spinal canal.

The clay shoveler's fracture is a particular spinous process fracture. It is produced by a sudden load on a flexed spine, with resulting avulsion of the C6, C7 or T1 spinous process.

Hyperextension

On X-ray, anterior widening of disc spaces, prevertebral swelling, avulsion of the anteroinferior corner of a vertebral body by the anterior longitudinal ligament, subluxation and crowding of the spinous processes are features of the hyperextension injury. Encroachment of the canal by an extruded disc or a posterior osteophyte may occur in patients with osteoarthritis of the cervical spine.

Flexion–rotation

This is responsible for unilateral facet dislocation or forward subluxation of the cervical spine. On lateral films this injury should be suspected when the vertebra above is displaced on the vertebra below by up to 25%. The injury is functionally stable by virtue of the locked facet and an intact contralateral facet joint. On the AP projection this injury is suggested by angulation of the spine at the level of injury of 11° or more, with the vertebrae above the injury angled towards the locked facet. This appears as a step in spinous process alignment.

Vertical compression

This is the mechanism responsible for burst fractures. The intervertebral disc is disrupted and driven into the vertebral body below. In addition, disc material may be extruded anteriorly into prevertebral tissues and posteriorly into the spinal canal. The vertebral body may be comminuted to varying degrees, with fragments being extruded anteriorly and posteriorly into the spinal canal.

Lateral flexion

This may produce uncinate fractures, isolated pillar fractures, transverse process injuries and lateral vertebral compression.

Distraction

These injuries may result in gross ligamentous and intervertebral disc disruption. The hangman's fracture may also occur by combined distraction and hyperextension mechanisms.

C1 - the atlas

Fractures of the atlas comprise 4% of cervical spine injuries. Mechanisms of injury generally involve hyperextension or compression. Around 15–20% of fractures may be associated with a C2 injury, and 25% may be associated with a lower cervical injury. The Jefferson fracture is a blowout fracture of the ring. Other fractures include isolated injuries of the posterior arch, the anterior arch, and the lateral mass.

C2 - the axis

Axis fractures comprise 6% of cervical spine injuries, with an association of concurrent C1 injury in 80% of cases.

X-rays are examined for odontoid subluxation. This diagnosis is suggested when the space between the anterior arch of the atlas and the odontoid is greater than 5 mm.

Three types of odontoid fracture are described:

- Type 1 is an avulsion of the odontoid tip. It is generally a stable injury and accounts for 5–8% of odontoid fractures.
- Type 2 injury is a fracture through the base of the dens and is generally unstable. It comprises 55–70% of odontoid injuries and is unstable. In younger children the epiphysis may be present and be confused with a type 2 fracture.
- Type 3 is a subdental fracture of the odontoid extending into the vertebral body. It comprises 30–35% of odontoid fractures.

Other fractures of the odontoid include avulsion fractures of the lower anterior margin of the body due to a hyperextension injury. A hangman's fracture is a bilateral neural arch fracture of C2. It is a hyperextension injury and is associated with prevertebral soft tissue swelling, anterior subluxation of C2 on C3, and avulsion of the anteroinferior corner of C2.

C3–C7

Examination of the lateral cervical spine film is as previously described. In particular, attention should be directed to the prevertebral soft tissue shadow, which should have a thickness less than 5 mm at C3 and less than one vertebral body width at C6. Children normally have a prevertebral space thickness two-thirds of the C2 body width. As this distance varies with ventilation, lateral cervical films should be performed in inspiration.

Fractures are defined as unstable when:

- The anterior and all of the posterior elements are disrupted.
- There is more than 3 mm overriding of the vertebral body above over the vertebral body below.
- The angle between two adjoining vertebrae is greater than 11°.
- The height of the anterior border of a vertebral body is less than two-thirds of the posterior border.

Fractures of thoracic spine

Hyperflexion is the principal mechanism of injury to the thoracic spine, with resultant wedging of vertebral bodies. Owing to the rigidity of the thoracic cage and the associated costovertebral articulations, most thoracic spine injuries are stable. However, internal stabilization may be necessary where kyphosis is pronounced.

Thoracolumbar spine

Fractures of the thoracolumbar spine comprise 40% of all vertebral fractures responsible for neurologic deficit. Most are flexion or hyperflexion-rotation injuries. Similar findings to those described in cervical spine injuries may be evident on X-ray. Plain films may demonstrate facet joint disruption, evidence of interspinal ligament disruption, posterior bony fragments protruding into the spinal canal, and burst fragments at the superior surface of the vertebral body. These fractures are generally unstable.

Lumbar spine

Injuries similar to those previously described do occur in the lumbar spine. Three specific injuries of the lumbar spine merit further discussion and are broadly considered posterior distraction injuries of the vertebral arch. They constitute a group known as seatbelt injuries, produced when a hyperflexion force is applied to a person wearing a lap-only type seatbelt.[17] In unrestrained persons a flexion injury generally flexes the spine around a point through the anterior spinal column, typically causing a wedge compression fracture of the body. In the restrained person the point of flexion is moved forward to the anterior abdominal wall. This change in momentum forces converts the hyperflexion mechanism to one of distraction. These injuries are caused by deceleration from high speed, as seen in head-on road traffic accidents or in aircraft crashes.

Plain film radiology remains the first-line imaging study. Suggestive findings include:

- A vacant or empty appearance of the vertebral body on the AP film
- Discontinuity in the cortex of the pedicles or spinous processes on the AP view
- Fracture, with or without dislocation in the lateral view, that may be subtle.

Computer tomography (CT) or magnetic resonance imaging (MRI) scanning is of value in further delineating architectural disruption. However, the exact nature of the fracture complex may be difficult to delineate on axial images, as the fractures are often orientated parallel to the scanning plane.

These injuries are often associated with concurrent intra-abdominal visceral injuries.

Chance fractures

These are characterized by an oblique or horizontal splitting of the spinous process and neural arch, and extending the superior posterior aspect of the vertebral body into and damaging the intervertebral disc.

Horizontal fissure fracture

This fracture is very similar to the chance fracture, with the exception of the fracture line, which extends horizontally through the vertebral body to its anterior aspect.

Smith fracture

This spares the posterior spinous process. The fracture line involves the superior articular processes, the arch and a small posterior fragment of the superior posterior aspect of the vertebral body. Although the spinous process is intact, the posterior ligaments are disrupted.

SPINAL CORD INJURY MANAGEMENT

Patients presenting with a potential spinal cord injury are managed in keeping with the approach for any major trauma patient. Therefore, a standard approach of primary survey,[20] resuscitation, secondary survey and definitive management is adopted.

Primary survey

Airway

Assessment of the airway is vital in the management of suspected spinal cord injury, especially when the cervical spine is involved. Passive regurgitation and aspiration of fluid stomach contents may occur as a result of blunting or absence of cough, gag and vomiting responses. This is especially so with higher cervical injuries. Therefore, the insertion of a nasogastric tube is of vital importance in minimizing the likelihood of aspiration. In quadriplegia and high paraplegia, unopposed vagal action owing to functional total or near-complete sympathectomy predisposes the patient to bradycardia on vagal stimulation of the pharynx. It is important that such patients have ECG monitoring and that atropine be immediately available to block these effects. Pretreatment with atropine prior to manipulation of the upper airway is a consideration.

Breathing

Ventilation may be affected by the level of cord injury, aspiration and primary lung injury. In the absence of major airway obstruction and flail chest the presence of paradoxical breathing is considered highly suggestive of cervical spine injury. Paradoxical breathing occurs because of loss of motor tone and paralysis of thoracic muscles innervated by thoracic spinal segments. Diaphragmatic action results in a negative intrapleural pressure. As a consequence of chest wall paralysis the tendency is for the soft tissues of the thorax to 'cave in', producing paradoxical chest wall movement. The diaphragm needs to undertake the full work of breathing, including overcoming added resistance to ventilation caused by paradoxical chest wall movement. In addition to standard respiratory status assessment, continuous pulse oximetry and assessment of vital capacity is necessary. Early intubation should be considered if vital capacity is inadequate or falling.

Ventilation may be reduced for several reasons:

- The diaphragm may simply fatigue and require assisted ventilation.
- A progressively ascending spinal cord injury owing to either further primary damage or secondary ascending spinal cord oedema may encroach upon the third to fifth cervical segments.
- The same segments may be involved with the initial injury, and thus the diaphragm may itself be partially paralysed.
- The consequences of coexisting chest trauma must also be taken into consideration, as respiration may be embarrassed by the natural progression of thoracic cage, pulmonary or intrapleural injuries.

Circulation

The impact of functional sympathectomy will depend upon the level and completeness of the neurological injury. Complete injuries above T1, and perhaps T4, can be expected to have clinically significant manifestations of neurogenic shock. The clinical signs are bradycardia due to unopposed vagal action, peripheral vasodilatation, and cessation of sweating. Peripheral vasodilatation is responsible for variable cutaneous manifestations. Initially, flushing can be expected; however, the skin may be pale or cyanosed, and its temperature elevated, reduced or within normal limits. The state of the above signs is dependent upon perfusion pressure, adequacy of oxygenation and the ambient temperature.

Priapism in a trauma patient is due to penile vasodilatation and is regarded as a highly suggestive sign of spinal cord injury.

Circulatory status is best assessed by conscious state, urine output and venous pressure monitoring. In the early phases of management, close urine output monitoring is of major importance. Early insertion of the urinary catheter allows measurement of urine output, may assist in identifying occult renal tract injury, and also prevents undesirable bladder overdistension.

Volume resuscitation in the resuscitative phase of the primary survey is undertaken in keeping with usual practices. With the exception of perhaps diving injuries, hypotensive trauma victims should be considered as intravascular volume depleted and bleeding until proven otherwise. Standard initial volumes of resuscitation fluid will not adversely affect the haemodynamic welfare. Owing to peripheral vasodilatation, these patients are relatively intravascular volume depleted and, therefore, volume preloading is appropriate. However, unnecessary volume overloading in an attempt to substantially raise systolic blood pressure will lead to acute pulmonary oedema.

Disability

Spinal cord injury has an association with significant head trauma.[25] In patients with altered conscious state due to head trauma, the early brief assessment of mental state and pupillary reflexes is important. All trauma victims with altered conscious state require spinal immobilization until spinal cord or unstable vertebral injury is excluded on physical examination and investigation.

In patients with injuries at or above T4 bilateral Horner's syndrome may be present, with relative pupillary constriction.

Exposure

As a spinal cord injury may be one of several injuries, the patient should be fully exposed in keeping with a routine approach to patients with multisystem trauma.

The secondary survey

The definitive diagnosis of a spinal cord injury is made from the findings on secondary survey. Two specific injury entities need to be considered, skeletal and neurological.

A head-to-toe clinical examination is conducted in keeping with the standard conventions used in examining any victim of major trauma. The following outlines the specific points of clinical examination pertinent to spinal injury.

Head and neck

An examination of the cervical spine is conducted while maintaining immobilization. Palpation of the spine posteriorly may demonstrate generalized tenderness owing to diffuse muscular spasm. However, the point of maximal tenderness should be determined. In hyperextension injuries the prevertebral and paravertebral muscles are often contused. This is a helpful sign when evaluating hyperextension-hyperflexion injuries in patients who were in stationary vehicles hit from behind. Longitudinal pressure to the head increases cervical pain. Such patients should be considered to have a higher likelihood of a significant vertebral injury.

The neck should be examined for swelling and bruising. Deformity will be noted if a dislocation with significant displacement is present. It should be remembered that significant bony and soft tissue injury frequently occurs without any major findings on external examination.

Prolonged immobilization of the cervical spine with rigid pre-hospital rescue collars and other rigid immobilization devices may unnnecessarily add to patient discomfort and the need for

ongoing spinal nursing. Reasons for this include times to definitive radiological assessment and awaiting for a window of opportunity to ensure vertebral stability. The cervical spine can be cleared of significant vertebral injury during the early phase of the clinical examinination using screening clinical examination criteria alone. The United States National Emergency X-Radiography Utilisation Study (NEXUS) identified a combination of clinical criteria that can be applied to identify a low-risk patient that can be managed without the need for cervical spine radiology[21] (Fig. 2.3.2).

An examination of the upper airway is required. A prevertebral haematoma can cause obstruction; the gag reflex may be blunted; airway protection may be embarrassed owing to paralysis of muscles below the neck, resulting in inefficient gag and cough. The patient will have gastric stasis and is at considerable risk of fluid aspiration.

The torso

The patient should either be lifted or rolled on to the side using a formal spinal-lifting technique, so that the back can be examined. The spine is examined for alignment, swelling, bruising and abrasion. Deformity is generally not a feature, except in the presence of major dislocation or disruption.

The rise and fall of the chest is noted. Paradoxical movement is a sign of thoracic cage muscular paralysis, and will be more pronounced the higher the segmental level of injury. Careful examination of the thorax, abdomen and pelvis is required. Owing to analgesia and anaesthesia, serious injury may be masked in both quadriplegia and high paraplegia. Significant vertebral injury to the thoracic and lumbar spines is associated with major injuries to the thoracic, abdominal and pelvic organs.

The abdomen is specifically assessed for an evolving paralytic ileus.

Neurological assessment

A thorough examination of the peripheral nervous system is required. It is strongly recommended that both motor and sensory examinations be undertaken in accordance with the following convention. Examine motor, sensory and reflexes components independently. Examination begins at the head, and then progresses across the shoulders. The upper limbs are then examined. The torso evaluation begins from just below the clavicles, extending inferiorly to the groins; each lower limb is then assessed. Finally, the saddle area and pelvic floor are assessed.

This approach reduces the likelihood of an incorrect diagnosis of paraplegia by finding a 'pseudo' neurological level of injury just below the clavicles when upper limbs have not been examined. It is, therefore, important that the upper limbs be assessed before examining the torso.

Motor function

Muscle power is assessed in terms of neurological segments and not muscle groups. Muscle power in each segment is graded from 0 to 5 in the following manner.

Power grade	Clinical finding
Grade 0/5	No movement
Grade 1/5	Flicker
Grade 2/5	Movement present, but not a full range against gravity
Grade 3/5	Full range of movement against gravity with no added resistance
Grade 4/5	Full range of movement against gravity with added resistance but with reduced power
Grade 5/5	Normal power

It is often impossible to assess power grades in certain segments owing to the patient's injuries. The upper limbs are the most easily examined. The strength of a cough provides some information as to the state of thoracic and abdominal musculature.

In the emergency setting the state of the pelvic muscles is determined through a rectal examination by assessing rectal tone and requesting the patient to tighten the sphincter on the examiner's gloved finger.

Sensory function

Dorsal column sensation is assessed using a piece of cotton wool and testing

According to the NEXUS Low-Risk Criteria, cervical spine radiography is indicated for trauma patients unless they exhibit ALL of the following criteria:

1. No posterior midline cervical spine tenderness
   and
2. No evidence of intoxication
   and
3. Normal level of alertness
   and
4. No focal neurological deficit
   and
5. No painful distracting injuries

Explanations:
  These are for purposes of clarity only. There are not precise definitions for the individual NEXUS Criteria, which are subject to interpretation by individual physicians.

1. Midline posterior bony cervical spine tenderness is present if the patient complains of pain on palpation of the posterior midline neck from the nuchal ridge to the prominence of the first thoracic vertebra, or if the patient evinces pain with direct palpation of any cervical spinous process.

2. Patients should be considered intoxicated if they have either of the following: a) a recent history by the patient or an observer of intoxication or intoxicating ingestion; or b) evidence of intoxication on physical examination such as odour of alcohol, slurred speech, ataxia, dysmetria or other cerebellar findings, or any behaviour consistent with intoxication. Patients may also be considered to be intoxicated if tests of bodily secretions are positive for drugs (including but not limited to alcohol) that affect level of alertness.

3. An altered level of alertness can include any of the following: a) Glasgow Coma Scale score of 14 or less; b) disorientation to person, place, time, or events; c) inability to remember 3 objects at 5 minutes; d) delayed or inappropriate response to external stimuli; or e) other.

4. Any focal neurologic complaint (by history) or finding (on motor or sensory examination).

5. No precise definition for distracting painful injury is possible. This includes any condition thought by the clinician to be producing pain sufficient to distract the patient from a second (neck) injury. Examples may include, but are not limited to: a) any long bone fractures; b) a visceral injury requiring surgical consultation; c) a large laceration, degloving injury, or crush injury; d) large burns: or e) any other injury producing acute functional impairment. Physicians may also classify any injury as distracting if it is thought to have the potential to impair the patient's ability to appreciate other injuries.

Fig. 2.3.2 NEXUS Low-Risk Criteria.

for light touch. Spinothalamic sensation is assessed using a pin or sharp object. Although proprioception, vibration and temperature can be assessed, these are not essential and adds little to the emergency examination. When testing with a sharp object a hypodermic injection needle or a trocar stylet must not be used: these are engineered to stab the skin as painlessly as possible, therefore, they cause trauma and are unreliable.

The general convention described below should be followed. Sensory examination begins on the face that, as it is supplied by the trigeminal nerve and bypasses the spinal cord, can act as a reference point. It is an important axiom based on anatomy, that 'in the absence of head injury or local facial injury, sensation to the face is always normal in pure spinal cord injury' (the trigeminal nerve comes from above the spinal cord). It is recommended that examination of the head, neck and upper torso is performed as follows. Start by examining the C2 dermatome laterally on the neck behind the mandible and beneath the ear. Extend examination on to the top of the shoulder, thus assessing the C3, C4 and C5 dermatomes. In the upper limbs examine the dermatomes in segmental order. This should include T2 on the upper medial aspect of the arm. Then carry on examining the torso in the midclavicular plane or at the outer border of the surface marking of the rectus sheath.

Reflexes

Reflexes are examined in keeping with usual examination practices. Superficial abdominal reflexes should be noted. The anal and bulbocavernosus reflexes are important in assessing sacral segments.

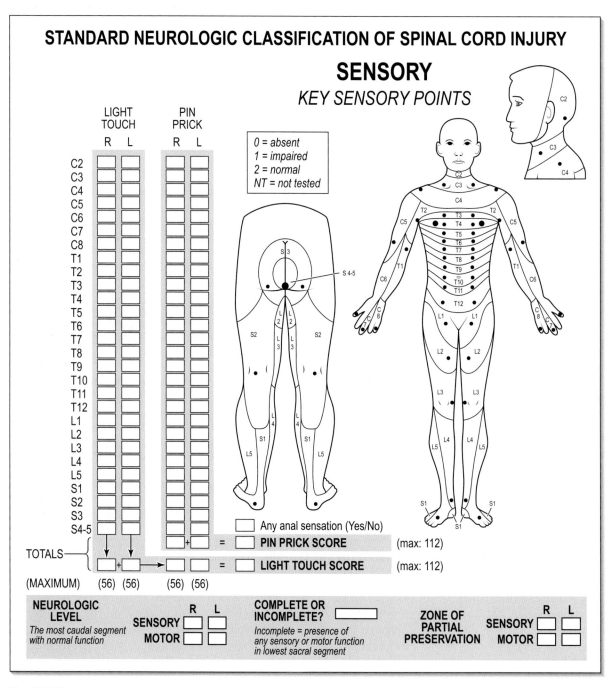

Fig. 2.3.3(a)

DOCUMENTATION CONVENTIONS

Two of the pitfalls in the management of any neurological injury are terminology and documentation. The following convention is recommended.

Motor function is recorded either using segmental terminology in written format, or on a muscle chart (Fig. 2.3.3).

It will be impossible to chart every segment accurately, but motor power in the upper and lower limbs should be able to be confidently recorded. Power should be graded using the 0–5/5 system.

Sensation is recorded more descriptively. Normaesthesia, hyperaesthesia, hypoaesthesia and anaesthesia are the descriptors for dorsal column function and testing for light touch. Normalgesia, hyperalgesia, hypoalgesia and analgesia are used in describing pain perception. These are recorded on sensory charts or described according to the following two examples.

In a patient with a transverse spinal cord syndrome, incomplete below C6 and complete below T1, the sensation is described as:

- Normaesthesia and normalgesia to C5
- Hypoalgesia and hypoaesthesia below C5
- Anaesthesia and analgesia below T1.

In a patient with an acute central cervical cord syndrome below C6, with total segmental paralysis in the C6-C8 segments and with some involvement of C5, the sensation might be described as:

- Normaesthesia and normalgesia to C4
- Hypoalgesia and hypoaesthesia below C4
- Anaesthesia and analgesia below C5
- Hypoalgesia and hypoaesthesia below T1.

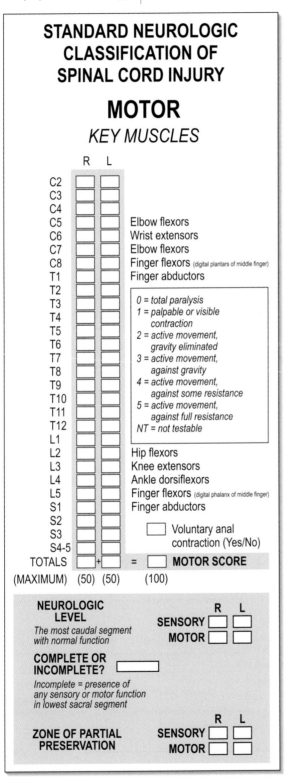

Fig. 2.3.3(b)

REFLEXES

	R	L	
C5-6			Biceps
C7-8			Triceps
L2-4			Knee jerk
S1			Ankle jerk
			Plantars ↑/↓

0	absent
+	reduced
++	normal
+++	increased
NT	not testable

Fig. 2.3.3(c)

UNCONSCIOUS PATIENTS

As previously mentioned, the definitive diagnosis of spinal cord injury is a secondary survey consideration and thus reasoned primarily from symptoms and physical findings. There is no pathognomonic sign of a spinal cord injury in an unconscious patient. The following should alert the examiner to the possibility of a coexisting spinal cord injury in an unconscious trauma victim:[8,13–15]

❶ Paradoxical breathing or chest wall movement (diaphragmatic breathing) in the absence of a major airway obstruction, stove-in or large flail chest suggests a cervical cord injury.

❷ Priapism in the unconscious trauma victim suggests quadriplegia or high to midthoracic paraplegia.

❸ Preserved facial grimace in the absence of a response to painful stimuli in the limbs.*

❹ Lower limb flaccidity in the presence of normal upper limb tone suggests paraplegia.*

❺ Observed upper limb movement in the absence of lower limb movement suggests paraplegia.*

❻ The combination of the persistent bradycardia and hypotension despite volume challenge.

*Where this is accompanied by a flaccid rectal sphincter there is an increased likelihood of spinal-cord injury.

Investigation

General investigations are those for multi-system trauma and are tailored to the patient's needs, as determined from primary and secondary surveys (see Chapter 2.8, Radiology in Trauma). The following summarizes key points in medical imaging of spinal trauma (Fig. 2.3.4):

• Initial evaluation must include a supine cross-table lateral film. The sensitivity of this film is reported as varying between 65% and 85%.

• In the early phase of management, the cervicothoracic junction must be displayed in at least one of a lateral, swimmers lateral or if necessary 30° oblique views.

• Bony definition is best demonstrated by CT. CT demonstrates detail of bony injury, extent of spinal canal embarrassment by displacement of fracture fragments, dislocated or subluxated vertebrae. CT is indicated in patients with abnormal or inadequate plain films requiring further evaluation or normal films but unexplained traumatic neck pain in circumstances when there is an increased risk for fracture or cord injury.[22,23]

• The role of MRI in spinal injury continues to evolve. It is recommended as the investigation of choice in the presence of neurological signs or if other imaging modalities are suggestive of significant subluxation due to ligamentous disruption without

Medical Imaging Considerations

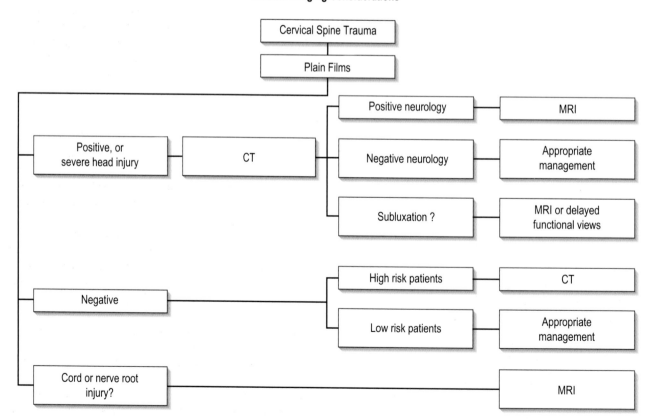

Fig. 2.3.4 Imaging Consideration Algorithm.

fracture. In addition to bony detail, MRI clearly demonstrates the cause of compression, the extent of cord injury and oedema. It may provide valuable information in the integrity of ligamentous and soft tissue structures, the state of intervertebral discs, integrity of vascular supply and the extent of extradural haematoma (Fig. 2.3.5). It is indicated as the investigation of choice in evaluating spinal cord injury without radiological abnormality (on plain X-ray) or SCIWORA. Although MRI is limited by its availability outside major trauma services, by the logistics of access and by resuscitation needs, it has allowed decisions to be made without the need for other invasive modalities.[23,24]

Management

General

The general management is in keeping with the approach to any victim of major trauma.

Analgesia and medications

Owing to the variable physiology of the peripheral circulation due to vascular tone denervation and sympathetic efferent interruption, the absorption of subcutaneous and intramuscular medications

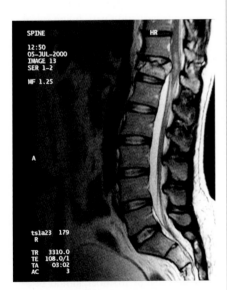

Fig. 2.3.5 MRI scan of acute central cord syndrome.

is unreliable. It is recommended that analgesia be provided by continuous intravenous infusion, with careful monitoring of vital signs. For similar reasons and where possible, all other medications are administered by the intravenous route.

Specific

Temperature In complete quadriplegia the patient has been rendered poikilothermic by the interruption of efferent sympathetic activity. Attention is directed to ensuring that the core temperature remains within the normal range. Such patients will demonstrate a core body temperature in keeping with changes in ambient temperature.

Immobilization Patients should remain in immobilization devices until spinal trauma has been excluded and splinting of specific injuries can be effected. However, they do not need to be left in the devices applied by prehospital care providers: these are structured to provide rigid immobilization for initial stabilization and transport. Nor should they be left tied to spine boards or wrapped in extrication devices, as these are uncomfortable and can cause unwanted cutaneous pressure injuries. Tight webbing and wraps can interfere with respiratory excursion. In general the prehospital devices are removed and replaced with more appropriate ones for the emergency department environment.

Corticosteroids – methylprednisolone Several centres prefer to use high-dose methylprednisolone [26,27] in the early management of patients with neurological injury. In Australia, spinal cord injury is not listed as an indication for high-dose methylprednisolone. Therefore, the decision to use high-dose corticosteroids should be made in conjunction with the specialist services, either the major trauma service or spinal injuries service that will be managing continuing care. If used, treatment must be commenced within 8 hours from the time of injury. The total treatment period should be for 24 hours if treatment is commenced

within 3 hours of injury and 48 hours if commenced between 3 and 8 hours.

The use of methylprednisolone is not without complication. It is contraindicated in patients with heavily contaminated open injuries, other heavily contaminated situations such as perforated bowel and established sepsis. It is relatively contraindicated in diabetes mellitus. Prophylactic measures such as for acute peptic ulceration and monitoring of blood glucose should be instituted.

A guideline for the use of methylprednisolone in acute spinal cord injury is presented in Figure 2.3.6.

Advanced airway management Early endotracheal intubation and assisted ventilation should be considered in patients with quadriplegia and high paraplegia. Regular assessment of respiratory status is undertaken and includes continuous pulse oximetry and frequent vital capacity measurement, in order to detect fatigue.

Blind nasal or endoscopic-assisted intubation under local anesthetic are the preferred modes of non-emergency intubation. The use of suxamethonium is acceptable for a rapid sequence intubation in the emergency setting. The hyperkalaemia associated with denervation is a concern in injuries more than 10–12 hours old (see Chapter 1.3, Advanced airway management).

Intravenous fluids After resuscitation fluids have been administered, haemorrhage controlled, ongoing losses replaced and fluid required for oedema responses to injury considered, routine maintenance fluids are all that is needed.

Paralysis of the sympathetic nervous system, and hence the compensatory mechanisms for intravascular volume depletion, necessitates a heightened suspicion of ongoing bleeding, the signs of which may be dramatic or subtle. Progressive hypotension is a key sign. Paradoxically, the heart rate may rise progressively from a bradycardia of 50–60 beats per minute to more normally acceptable rates. It is uncertain by which mechanism this pseudo or relative tachycardia of quadriplegia occurs.

Methylprednisolone for Acute Spinal Cord Injury

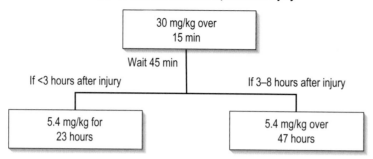

These doses may be approximated to the nearest 0.5 gram. For example, a 70 kg patient requiring 24 hours of treatment would need:

Calculation	Actual Dose
30 (mg/kg) x 70 (kg) = 2100mg followed by;	2g (1 x 2g or 2 x 1g or 4 x 500mg vials) followed by;
5.4 mg/kg/h x 70 (kg) = 8694mg	8.5g (4 x 2g + 1 x 500mg or 8.5 x 1g or 17 x 500mg vials) over 23 hours

Fig. 2.3.6

One thought is that with progressive hypotension and brain-stem hypoperfusion the vagal effects are switched off by the brain stem, thus allowing the heart rate to rise towards a more normal or denervated range. The skin may develop patchy or blotchy cyanosis. This is due to a sluggish peripheral circulation and thus locally elevated levels of deoxygenated or desaturated haemoglobin.

Inotropic support is often unnecessary.[11,6] However, satisfactory cerebral perfusion is essential. In the patient with a previously normal minimental state examination, deterioration may suggest intracranial hypoperfusion due to either intracranial trauma or the neurogenic shock process. Chronotropic and vasoconstrictor agents are occasionally required. These are more likely to be necessary in older patients, or those suffering from hypertension who are now relatively hypotensive despite volume loading. Chronotropic agents are occasionally required for patients prescribed β-blocker, peripheral and central vasodilator drugs. Likewise, patients with established cerebrovascular disease may require higher perfusion pressures than the resting pressure of the quadriplegic.

The degree of these physiological effects on the circulation will depend upon the site and completeness of the injury. Spinal-cord injury below the sympathetic outflow will have little effect on the circulation; complete spinal-cord injury above the thoracic outflow will produce a total body sympathectomy. A complete spinal-cord injury in the midthoracic segments should result in preserved vasomotor function in the head, neck and upper limbs. Cardiac reflexes should also be relatively well preserved. Vasomotor tone to the abdominal cavity, pelvis and lower limbs will be paralysed. Likewise, incomplete lesions will have a varying affect depending on the site and completeness of the injury. Careful establishment of the segmental level and degree of spinal cord injury on secondary survey will assist in anticipating the likely extent of autonomic dysfunction.

The denervated lung is intolerant of volume overloading. Therefore, careful monitoring of fluid balance, including urine output and, in circumstances of low urine flow, central venous pressure, is required.

Skin protection Pressure areas and decubitus ulceration are difficult problems to manage. Pressure relief and protection of bony prominences are important concerns from the outset. Hourly pressure lifts should be implemented as soon as practicable: patients should not remain on hard unpadded surfaces for longer than necessary.

REFERRAL-DISPOSITION

Patients with a spinal cord injury should be referred to a centre with facilities for optimal management as soon as practicable. Specific treatments such as immobilization, specific therapy and transport considerations should be discussed with the continuing care provider or spinal injuries unit prior to initiation of the transfer. If transport is delayed, it is appropriate that the spinal injuries unit be involved and contribute to the patient's initial management, especially in areas of specific management, as soon as possible, even if transfer is to be delayed by several days.

OTHER TREATMENTS

The use of hyperbaric oxygen and naloxone in minimizing spinal injury has

CONTROVERSIES

❶ The best intubation technique in critically ill trauma patients with probable cervical spine injury. Rapid sequence induction with inline spinal immobilization is preferred in this situation.

❷ The role of corticosteroids in preventing secondary injury from spinal cord trauma. There are varying protocols in different countries. Although used, spinal cord injury is not listed as an indication for steriod therapy in Australia. Because of this some centres recommend that patients be given the option and formally consent to receive high-dose methylprednisolone. In the case of a patient who is unable to make a decision, family member should be approached if practicable.

been considered in the acute management of spinal cord injuries. Naloxone appears to have little place in mangement.[26] The value of hyperbaric oxygen therapy is at present uncertain and logistically difficult.

The best outcomes in patients with a potential spinal cord injury are optimized by suspecting the injury in trauma victims and preventing secondary injury.

REFERENCES

1. Rotem TR, Lawson JS, Wilson FW, et al 1998 Severe spinal cord injuries related to rugby union and league football in New South Wales, 1984–1996. Medical Journal of Australia 168: 379–81
2. Yeo JD 1998 Rugby and spinal injury: what can be done? Medical Journal of Australia 168: 372–3
3. Lowery D, Marlena M, Browne B, Tigges S, et al 2001 Epidemiology of cervical spine injury victims. Annals of Emergency Medicine 38: 12–6
4. Seleki BR, et al 1986 Experience with spine injuries in NSW. Australian and New Zealand Journal of Surgery 56: 567–76
5. Toscano J 1988 Prevention of neurological deterioration before admission to a spinal cord injury unit. Paraplegia 26: 143–50
6. Superspeciality Service Subcommittee of the Australian Health Ministers Advisory Council. Guidelines for acute spinal cord injury services. Australian Institute of Health, A.G.P.S. 1990
7. Goldberg W, Mueller C, Panacek E, Tigges, et al 2001 Distribution and patterns of blunt cervical spine injury. Annals of Emergency Medicine 38: 12–16
8. Swain A, Dove J, Baker H 1991 Trauma of the spine and spinal cord. ABC of major trauma. BMJ Publishing, London, pp 38–44
9. Young W 1993 Secondary injury mechanisms in acute spinal cord injury. Journal of Emergency Medicine 11: 13–22
10. Anderson DK, Hall ED 1993 Pathophysiology of spinal cord trauma. Annals of Emergency Medicine 22: 987–92
11. Cloward RB 1980 Acute cervical spine injuries. CIBA Clinical Symposia 32(1)
12. Donovan WH, Bedbrook G 1982 Comprehensive management of spinal cord injury. CIBA Clinical Symposia 34(2)
13. Grundy D, Swain A 2001 ABC of Spinal Cord Injury, 4th edn. BMJ Publishing, London
14. American College of Surgeons 1997 Spine and spinal cord trauma. Advanced trauma life support student manual. American College of Surgeons, pp 215–30
15. Trauma Committee, Royal Australasian College of Surgeons 1992 Spine and spinal cord trauma. Early management of severe trauma course manual. Royal Australasian College of Surgeons, pp 157–68
16. Chandramohan K 1992 The emergency care of spinal trauma. Emergency Medicine 203–14
17. Domeier RM, Rawden WE, Evans MD, et al 1997 Prehospital clinical findings associated with spinal injury. Prehospital Emergency Care 1: 11–5
18. Schwartz GR, Wright SW, Fein JA, et al 1997 Paediatric cervical spine injury sustained in falls from low heights. Annals of Emergency Medicine 30(3): 249–52
19. Rogers LF 1971 The roentgenographic appearance of transverse or Chance fractures of the spine: the seat belt fracture. Australian Journal of Radiology 111: 844–8
20. Holley J, Jorden R, Jackson M 1989 Airway management in patients with unstable cervical spine fractures. Annals of Emergency Medicine 18: 1237–9
21. Hoffman JR, Mower W, Wolfson AB, et al 2000 Validitiy of a set of clinical criteria to rule out injury to the cervical spine in patients with blunt trauma. New England Journal of Medicine 343: 94–9
22. Blackmore CC, Emerson SS, Mann FA, Koepsell TD 1999 Cervical imaging in patients with trauma: determination of risk to optimise use. Radiology 211: 759–65
23. The Royal Australian and New Zealand College of Radiologists 2001 Imaging Guidelines 4th edn, RANZCR
24. Demiatridias D, Charakambides K, Chahwan S, et al 2000 Nonskeletal cervical spine injuries: epidemiology and diagnostic pitfalls. Journal of Trauma 48: 724–7
25. Neifeld GL, Keene JG, Hevesy G, et al 1988 Cervical injury in head trauma. Journal of Emergency Medicine 6: 203–7
26. Bracken MB, Shepard MJ, Collins WFJ, et al 1990 A randomised controlled trial of methylprednisolone or naloxone in the treatment of acute spinal cord injury. Results of the second National Acute Spinal Cord Injury Study. New England Journal of Medicine 322: 1405
27. Bracken MB, Collins WF, Freeman DF, et al 1984 Efficacy of methylprednisolone in acute spinal cord injury. Journal of the American Medical Association 251: 45–52
28. Brown D 2000 Guidelines for the use of methylprednisolne in acute spinal cord injury. Victorian Spinal Cord Service Austin & Repatriation Medical Centre, Melbourne

FURTHER READING

Burke DC, Burley HY, Ungar GH 1985 Data on spinal injuries Part 1. Collection and analysis of 325 consecutive cases. Australian and New Zealand Journal of Surgery 55: 3–12
Taskforce on Appropriateness Criteria for Imaging and Treatment Decisions 1995 Appropriateness criteria for imaging and treatment decisions. Musculoskeletal injury. Cervical spine trauma. American College of Radiology MS 2.1–2.9

2.4 FACIAL TRAUMA

LEWIS MACKEN • RON MANNING

ESSENTIALS

1 Facial trauma is a common problem in the emergency department, usually occurring as part of a multisystem injury.

2 Facial injuries that do not threaten the airway or risk life-threatening haemorrhage can usually be assessed and managed as part of the secondary survey.

3 Early diagnosis of facial injuries is vital, as late diagnosis may lead to compromised function and an unsatisfactory cosmetic outcome.

4 Plain radiography should be the initial radiological study; facial CT views assist with the precise delineation of facial fractures.

5 Penetrating trauma to the face is rarely fatal, but may result in significant morbidity. Attention to early airway intervention is vital after penetrating injuries, especially in patients with gunshot wounds to the face.

INTRODUCTION

Facial trauma is defined as injury to the facial soft tissues (including the ear) and bony skeleton. This covers a wide spectrum of injuries.[1] Patients with facial trauma are frequently seen in the emergency department as a result of motor vehicle accidents, interpersonal violence, contact sports, falls and animal bites. Facial injuries often occur as part of a multisystem injury: as many as 70% of motor vehicle accident victims have facial trauma as one component of their injuries,[2,3] and up to 60% of patients with facial trauma have associated injuries of other systems.[4,5]

Management of blunt and penetrating trauma to the face can be challenging. Facial trauma may result in airway compromise or life-threatening haemorrhage. At the same time, attention must be given to preserving long-term cosmesis and the normal functions of sight, speech and mastication.[6] After immediate resuscitation and stabilization, management of facial injuries requires a knowledge of clinical and radiographic anatomy, the injuries commonly associated with facial injury, and an awareness of treatment methods for the differing injuries to the face.[7,8] Consultation should be sought when the injury threatens the restoration of normal function or appearance.

HISTORY

The evaluation should commence with the history, with emphasis given to the mechanism of injury. This will help to suggest those injuries that are likely to be present. Respiratory and haemodynamic observations, and quantification of prehospital blood loss, are important components of the history.

EXAMINATION

The physical examination involves evaluation of all facial areas by inspection, palpation and assessment of function. Inspection of the face may reveal deformity, loss of normal symmetry, changes in contour, and localized areas of swelling. Skull-base fractures may be suggested by periorbital or postauricular bruising, and the ears must be inspected to exclude haemotympanum or CSF otorrhoea. Gentle systematic palpation of the facial skeleton should follow, assessing for tenderness, and feeling for asymmetry, bony margin irregularities, abnormal motion or crepitus. Specific attention should be given to the supraorbital and infraorbital margins, the zygomas, nasal bones, maxilla and mandible.[1] Mobility associated with midfacial maxillary fractures is assessed by grasping the anterior maxilla with the thumb and index finger of one hand, while stabilizing the forehead at the nasal bridge with the

other.[6] Ophthalmological evaluation includes inspection for enophthalmos or exophthalmos, and globe injury, and assessment of pupillary responses, visual acuity, visual fields, extraocular movements, and inquiry for diplopia. Although eye injury is an infrequent complication of blunt trauma, subjective impairment in visual acuity remains the most sensitive single predictor of eye injury,[9] and examination that reveals the presence of an afferent pupillary defect or a nonreactive pupil is the most important factor in predicting the severity of eye injury.[10] The nose should be inspected for the presence of any septal deviation, haematoma (more common in children) or CSF rhinorrhoea. Oral examination is necessary to look for loose, broken or missing teeth, malocclusion of dentition, soft tissue lacerations and contusions.[11] Examination of the mandible includes assessment of the temporomandibular joint in the open and closed positions.

Assessment of the function of facial structures is the final component of the examination of the face. Malocclusion, often identified by the presence of a new gap between the occlusal surfaces of the teeth when the patient closes the jaws, is a sensitive indicator of maxillary or mandibular fracture.[6,8] Similarly, pain on biting on a tongue depressor, loss of bite strength and limitation of jaw movement are strongly suggestive of a fracture; the patient should be asked if the bite has subjectively changed. Motor function of the facial nerve should be assessed, and all three branches of the trigeminal nerve should be evaluated. Commonly encountered symptoms and signs are hyperaesthesia or paraesthesia of the upper lip or upper alveolar margin, suggesting fracture of the maxilla causing injury to the alveolar branches of the infraorbital nerve. Sensory changes in the lower lip and lower alveolar margin suggest fracture through the mandibular canal, causing inferior alveolar nerve injury (a branch of the mandibular nerve).[8]

RADIOGRAPHIC EXAMINATION

When the patient's condition permits, plain radiography should be the initial

study performed. The most useful X-ray views for facial bones are Water's (occipitomental) view, which allows visualization of the maxilla, maxillary sinuses, inferior margins and floors of the orbits, and zygomatic bones;[1] posteroanterior (PA) view of the face and skull, which shows the outline of the mandible, but superimposition of the zygoma and mastoid processes obscures the heads of the mandibular condyles;[12] Towne's view (PA view of the mandible) shows the ascending rami and subcondylar regions;[6] submentovertex ('jug-handle') views demonstrate the zygomatic arches;[8] and true lateral views. The best X-ray for suspected fracture of the mandible is the OPG (orthopantomogram) view. Aspiration of teeth or fractured dental segments should be excluded by review of a chest X-ray. X-rays should also be considered to help determine the presence of retained radio-opaque foreign bodies within the wounds.

In interpreting facial X-rays the examiner should look for signs of loss of bony integrity, which, except for zygomatic arch fractures, will show as a disturbance of the continuity of the bony margins, rather than as a complete fracture line.[13] Also, indirect signs suggestive of anatomical disruption should be sought: opacity or air-fluid level within the sinuses, herniation of orbital soft tissue, and subcutaneous air.[1]

Facial CT views have been shown to assist in the precise delineation of facial fractures, especially of the upper and middle thirds of the face.[14,15] CT offers the advantages of clearly displaying soft tissues and showing their relation to the bony skeleton; allowing axial and coronal views and sagittal reconstruction; and clearly showing the degree of skeletal distortion, displacement and comminution.[12]

IMMEDIATE MANAGEMENT IN THE EMERGENCY DEPARTMENT

It is important to prioritize injuries in the management of the patient with facial trauma because facial injuries that do not threaten the airway or risk life-threatening haemorrhage can usually be assessed and managed as part of the secondary survey. Proper attention should be given to potentially more significant head, chest and abdominal injuries before a non-life-threatening facial injury is thoroughly evaluated, no matter how impressive and disfiguring the facial injury appears.[8] The association of facial injury with cervical spine or cord injury is questionable, especially if vehicular trauma was not the cause.[16] Patients with clinically significant head injuries (especially Glasgow Coma Score (GCS) of <9) are at greater risk of having cervical spine injuries than those with evidence of facial trauma;[17,18] intracranial injuries are more frequently associated with facial fractures than are cervical spine injuries.[19]

Airway management

Asphyxia due to upper airway obstruction is the major cause of death from facial trauma. The airway must be rapidly assessed, respiratory obstruction relieved and an adequate airway established.[6] Signs of partial airway obstruction include tachycardia, tachypnoea, restlessness, fighting to sit up, noisy respirations, stridor, and supraclavicular and intercostal retractions. This may lead to complete obstruction. An unobstructed airway in the presence of facial trauma should be closely monitored because increasing oedema and persistent bleeding may later compromise airway patency.[8,20]

Fractures of the mandible and maxilla with displacement posteriorly or inferiorly, together with displaced soft tissues, blood, secretions or other foreign material, may lead to airway embarrassment.[7,8,13] Simple airway measures such as chin lift and jaw thrust should be performed, and the mouth immediately examined. Any loose foreign material, such as food, broken dentures or teeth, or bone fragments, should be removed and blood clots suctioned.[7,8] If anterior traction on the fractured mandible or on the mobile segment of the maxilla (performed by inserting two fingers behind the soft palate and lifting the middle third of the face forwards and upwards)[13] fails to relieve posterior pharyngeal obstruction and does not establish unobstructed ventilation, a definitive airway must be placed. Rapid sequence orotracheal intubation can usually be performed. Awake fibreoptic intubation is an option, but the presence of persistent bleeding makes the procedure technically difficult. Standard drills for anticipated intubation difficulties should be at hand, and equipment for performing a cricothyroidotomy and transtracheal jet ventilation should be available. A surgical airway may be lifesaving when anatomical disruption makes intubation difficult.[20] A tracheostomy performed under local anaesthesia in the operating theatre is often the safest option in a stable patient with significant midfacial injuries in whom airway difficulties are expected.

Control of haemorrhage

Traumatic facial haemorrhage can be massive, difficult to manage, and potentially life-threatening in approximately 5% of patients with midfacial fractures.[21] Bleeding from midface trauma mainly originates from branches of the external carotid artery (with branches of the internal carotid artery also supplying the nose). Most haemorrhage can be controlled with direct pressure, anterior nasal packs, and Foley balloon catheters (12–14g Foley catheters with 10 mL balloons inflated and taped under tension to the side of the face) placed in the posterior nasopharynx.[8,22] Care must be taken with nasal instrumentation: the incidence of associated skull-base fractures is more common with orbital wall or rim fractures than with more inferiorly located facial fractures. Also, a skull-base fracture is more likely in the presence of multiple facial fractures (the presence of three or more facial fractures is associated with a skull-base fracture incidence of up to 33%).[23] Attempts to clamp bleeding vessels in the emergency department should be avoided because of the associated risks of damaging important structures, such as the facial nerve, parotid duct or lacrimal apparatus.[1] If simple measures fail to arrest the bleeding, operative reduction of the fractures, especially of the maxilla, and possible ligation of bleeding vessels should be undertaken, with angiography and selective embolization considered as a last resort if all other measures fail.

Disposition

After initial stabilization, immediate treatment of most facial injuries is mainly supportive. Most fractures requiring operative management are dealt with on a delayed basis, when soft tissue swelling is resolving. However, it is important that injuries be diagnosed, as undiscovered injuries may lead to compromised function.[1] Thorough documentation of injuries is important for medicolegal reasons, as well as for optimal patient care. Facial injuries are frequently due to personal assault, and so later litigation is often likely. Polaroid photographs stored in the patient's notes are ideal, and drawings of injuries and their dimensions should also be recorded.

SPECIFIC INJURIES

Soft tissue injuries

Soft tissue injuries include abrasions, contusions, lacerations, avulsion injuries and burns. The aim of treatment is to preserve appearance and function. The management of soft-tissue facial injuries involves consideration of how the wound should be repaired, and whether it should be repaired in the emergency department.[1] Possible reasons for delayed wound closure are more urgent coexisting injuries, severe crush injuries, the presence of a foreign body, severely contaminated wounds, and an underlying fracture. In these cases the wound should be irrigated, haemostasis achieved, and the wound covered with normal saline-soaked gauze.

Soft-tissue injuries that usually require repair in the operating theatre include ocular or significant eyelid injury; parotid gland or duct injury; facial nerve injury (injuries to the cheek between the tragus of the ear and a line drawn vertically through the pupil may be associated with damage to the facial nerve, parotid gland or duct);[1,5] nasolacrimal apparatus injury; alveolar process wounds and significant tooth injuries; lacerations with significant tissue loss or contamination or requiring exact anatomical closure; or where difficulties with patient cooperation are expected.[6] Careful consideration is required before areas of special concern are repaired in the emergency department, e.g. the lips and perioral area; tongue and oral cavity; nose; ears; periorbital structures; and eyebrows. If the wound is closed in the emergency department, careful attention must be given to thorough cleansing. This can be effectively achieved with pulsatile wound irrigation with normal saline, and abrasions containing dirt or other foreign bodies must be scrubbed to prevent traumatic tattooing of the dermis. If the wound is gaping, or if structures deeper than the skin and the subcutaneous layer are involved, then multiple-layer repair is usually advisable. This helps to prevent deep tissue space collections and produces a better cosmetic result, with less scar depression or widening.[11] Systemic antibiotics are not required for most facial wounds. However, antibiotics must be given for bites and grossly contaminated wounds, and should be considered for wounds that extend into the oral cavity, nose and paranasal sinuses; wounds with exposed nasal or ear cartilage; crush wounds and wounds with considerable oedema; and for immunologically compromised patients.[11] Tetanus immunity should be assessed. Paediatric wounds should be covered with a sterile nonadherent dressing, and large forehead lacerations may benefit from the application of a pressure dressing to minimize haematoma formation. Most facial wounds require only the application of a water-soluble ointment, which encourages re-epithelialization and limits crust formation;[24,25] most adult wounds can be left uncovered.

Facial fractures

Common facial fractures involve the nasal bones (45%), mandible (13%), zygoma (13%), orbital floor (3%), and maxilla (2%).[26] The facial skeleton is constructed to allow applied force to be dispersed via a series of small bone fractures, thus protecting the skull and intracranial contents.[6] The maxilla and mandible require three times the amount of applied force to cause a fracture than do the nasal bones.[1,27] Diagnosis of a facial fracture involves a combination of inspection, palpation and radiographic examination. Fractures other than nondisplaced fractures of the nose, zygomatic arch or maxilla will require acute maxillofacial surgical review. All fractures should be managed initially with elevation of the patient's head, if associated injuries allow this, and the application of ice.

Mandible

The horseshoe shape of the mandible disperses applied force, which leads to fractures occurring at vulnerable sites regardless of the point of impact, and a high incidence of multiple fractures. Common sites of fracture are the condylar neck and angle, and the body at the level of the first or second molar.[28,29] Fractures of the mandibular body are often compound and usually demonstrate point tenderness, malocclusion and abnormal range of motion, with interference with normal mastication. The integrity of the dental arch must be assessed.

Radiographic diagnosis is most easily made with a panoramic view; this demonstrates the condylar region more clearly than other facial views. Most fractures will require some form of immobilization. Complications of mandibular fractures include chin paraesthesia or hypoaesthesia, delayed union, non-union, infection and malocclusion.[30]

Zygomatic arch

Isolated fractures of the zygomatic arch are uncommon and are more commonly part of a more extensive zygomatic fracture. An isolated fracture may be evidenced by a depression over the arch initially, point tenderness, and limited or painful mouth opening owing to impingement on the coronoid process of the mandible by the fractured arch. The zygomatic arches are best seen by submentovertex X-ray views. Surgical reduction is required for cosmetic reasons, or to correct restricted mandibular range of motion.[12]

Zygomatic complex

Blunt trauma to the zygoma more commonly results in fractures at the articulations of the zygomatic bones with the frontal bone, maxilla and zygomatic process of the temporal bone. Separation at the zygomaticofrontal suture, the zygomaticotemporal suture, and at the zygomaticomaxillary suture or infraorbital rim produces the tripod or tripartite fracture. Frequently, the lateral wall of the maxillary sinus and the lateral and central portions of the orbital floor (not to be confused with the orbital blowout fracture) will also fracture as part of the zygomaticomaxillary complex fracture.

Clinical signs of a tripod fracture include flattening of the cheek initially (due to depression of the fracture segment); this is best seen by standing behind and above the patient, but it is soon replaced by significant swelling. Other signs are hypoaesthesia/hyperaesthesia or paraesthesia in the distribution of the infraorbital nerve; asymmetry of the ocular levels; palpable step defect of the inferior orbital margin; and circumorbital and subconjunctival ecchymoses.[1,5] Diplopia is often also present, and 10–20% of these fractures are accompanied by an ocular injury.[8] The Waters' (occipitomental) X-ray view will usually display zygoma complex fractures adequately. A maxillary antrum air-fluid level or evidence of herniation of the orbital contents is often present on X-ray. CT scan evaluation of these injuries is usually necessary and all patients will require referral.

Orbital floor fractures

Fracture of the orbital floor may occur as part of a zygomaticomaxillary fracture, or as an isolated injury – the less common orbital blowout fracture. This is a fracture of the orbital floor without fracture of the orbital margin. An increase in intraorbital pressure, as delivered by a fist or a small ball, is transmitted to within the orbit and the relatively weak orbital floor is disrupted, with possible herniation of the contents into the maxillary sinus.[1] Very rarely a supraorbital rim fracture may be part of a frontal sinus fracture, a lateral orbital wall fracture may be associated with a fracture of the zygoma, and a medial orbital wall fracture may occur with a nasoethmoidal fracture.[7] Clinical examination in cases of fracture of the orbital floor may reveal enophthalmos, a difference in pupillary levels, diplopia and impairment of upward gaze, and infraorbital hypoaesthesia/hyperaesthesia or paraesthesia.[5] An irregular edge to the orbital rim may be evident on palpation. The integrity and function of the eye must be documented to exclude associated injury. Radiographic examination may show emphysema of the orbit, displaced bony fragments in the maxillary sinus or the 'hanging drop' sign of herniated contents within the maxillary sinus.[1,31] CT scan is usually necessary to define these fractures fully. All patients with orbital margin or floor fractures require referral. Complications of surgical treatment of orbital floor fractures include persistent diplopia, hypoaesthesia/ hyperaesthesia or paraesthesia, ectropion and epiphora.[32]

Maxillary fractures

Fractures of the maxilla include fractures of the alveolar ridge of the maxilla, fracture of the anterolateral wall of the maxillary sinus, and the Le Fort fractures. Isolated maxillary fractures are rare.

Le Fort described a classification of patterns of mid face fractures, following cadaveric experiments, in Paris in 1901:[33] Le Fort I (horizontal maxillary fracture) involves only the maxilla at the level of the nasal fossae; Le Fort II (pyramidal fracture) is the most common midface fracture[34] and involves the maxilla, nasal bones and medial aspect of the orbit; Le Fort III (craniofacial dysjunction) separates the midfacial skeleton from the base of the cranium, with the fracture extending through the base of the nose and ethmoid region and across the orbits and zygomatic arches bilaterally.

Most midface fractures are combination injuries, with different Le Fort classifications on each side of the face.[1] Airway compromise is more common with Le Fort II and III fractures, and may require urgent reduction in the emergency department. Le Fort II and III fractures may demonstrate midface mobility and are associated with skull-base fractures, leading to CSF rhinorrhoea. All patients require a complete eye examination, and these injuries necessitate referral.

Nasal fractures

These are the most common facial fractures. Diagnosis is largely clinical, plain X-rays are unreliable and usually unnecessary, and the major concerns for the emergency physician are control of epistaxis and examination for a septal haematoma. Displaced fractures should be reduced within 7–10 days.

Nasoethmoidal fractures are more complicated and are caused by trauma to the bridge of the nose.[1,35] This may produce an increase in the intercanthal distance; disruption of the medial canthal ligaments may produce rounding of the palpebral fissures or widening of the inter-canthal distance (telecanthus).[36] Persistent epistaxis and CSF rhinorrhoea may also be evident. Referral is necessary for these patients.

Temporomandibular joint dislocation

Dislocation of the temporomandibular joint may follow trauma to the face or may occur as a result of simply opening the mouth widely. Patients complain of inability to close the mouth and moderate discomfort. X-rays should be performed to confirm that no fracture is present, and dislocation will be evidenced by the appearance of the condyle anterior to the articular eminence of the fossa. A directed history will exclude extrapyramidal dystonia mimicking a dislocation. Reassurance, sedation and firm downward pressure of the physician's thumbs on the patient's posterior teeth, with upward tilting of the symphysis, is usually successful in relocating the mandibular condyles.[1] Postreduction X-rays are necessary. Analgesia and a soft diet should be prescribed and the patient warned to avoid wide opening of the mouth in the short term.

PENETRATING INJURIES TO THE FACE

Penetrating trauma of the face from gunshot, shotgun and stab wounds, and impaling foreign bodies is often dramatic at the time of presentation. It is rarely fatal, but may result in significant morbidity. The wounding capability of penetrating projectiles (bullets and pellets) is proportional to the energy imparted to the tissue;[37-39] thus, the mass of the slug, its velocity and design, and the density of the body tissue penetrated determine the amount of tissue destruction.[40,41]

Early aggressive airway management is necessary in patients with gunshot wounds to the face, as respiratory decompensation may be rapid: approximately one-third of patients will require emergency airway intervention.[42] Shotgun and stab wounds are less likely to require an emergency airway, although the presence of a significant vascular injury or oedema remains a universal indication for airway intervention, and patients with mandible entry sites are more likely to require an emergency airway than those with midface entry sites.[41] Orotracheal intubation can usually be achieved,[42,43] with cricothyroidotomy the preferred alternative if necessary. Central nervous system injuries are common, and CT scan of the head and/ or cervical spine should be performed if indicated on neurological examination, or when the bullet entry site is above the lower face,[42] especially when the trajectory passes along or across the base of the skull.[43]

Arterial injury is suggested by evidence of active bleeding and an expanding haematoma; angiography (carotid and vertebral arteries), which is required in approximately 35–40% of cases,[42,43] should be performed when the bullet trajectory suggests proximity to major vessels or the skull base,[41,43-45] or where the knife or foreign body is in close proximity to a major vascular structure.[41]

Peripheral nerve injuries, especially of the facial nerve and mandibular branch of the trigeminal nerve, are also frequently present.[43] Careful eye examination is necessary because ocular trauma is the most common overall complication of penetrating facial trauma.[41]

Antibiotics and tetanus prophylaxis are indicated, and wounds are managed with

CONTROVERSIES

❶ Consideration of an immediate surgical airway, rather than attempted oral intubation, in a patient with significant facial trauma and a compromised or deteriorating airway.

❷ The role of angiography and selective embolization in the management of patients with significant haemorrhage from blunt and penetrating trauma.

conservative debridement, closed reduction of facial fractures, and early repair of palate injuries. Open facial fracture reduction is usually delayed.[42]

CONCLUSION

Facial trauma in the emergency department is common, encompasses many types of injury, and after rapid exclusion of life-threatening complications, requires thorough patient evaluation to exclude other more urgent injuries. The aim of management of isolated facial injuries is the maintenance of normal function and appearance.

REFERENCES

1. Cantrill SV 1992 Facial trauma. In: Rosen P, Barkin RM (eds) Emergency Medicine – Concepts and Clinical Practice, 3rd edn. Mosby Year Book, St Louis, pp 355–70
2. Dolan KD, Jacoby CG 1978 Facial fractures. Seminars in Roentgenology 13: 37–51
3. Murray JF, Hall HC Fractures of the mandible in motor vehicle accidents. Clinics in Plastic Surgery 2: 131–41
4. Davidoff G, Jakubowski M, Thomas D, Alpert M 1988 The spectrum of closed-head injury in facial trauma victims: incidence and impact. Annals of Emergency Medicine 17: 6–9
5. Schultz RC, Oldham RJ 1977 An overview of facial injuries. Surgical Clinics of North America 57: 987–1010
6. Robson MC, Smith DJ 1990 Maxillofacial area. In: Moore EE (ed.) Early Care of the Injured Patient, 4th edn. BC Decker, Toronto, pp 138–48
7. Carithers JS, Koch BB 1997 Evaluation and management of facial fractures. American Family Physician 55: 2675–82
8. Shepherd SM, Lippe MS 1987 Maxillofacial trauma - evaluation and management by the emergency physician. Emergency Medicine Clinics of North America 5: 371–92
9. Dutton GN, al-Qurainy I, Stassen LFA, Titterington DM, Moos KF, el-Attar A 1992 Ophthalmic consequences of mid-facial trauma. Eye 6(1): 86–9
10. Joseph E, Zak R, Smith S, Best WR, Gamelli RL, Dries DJ 1992 Predictors of blinding or serious eye injury in blunt injury. Journal of Trauma 33: 19–24
11. Hunter JG 1992 Paediatric maxillofacial trauma. Pediatric Clinics of North America 39: 1127–43
12. Hendler BH 1996 Maxillofacial trauma. In: Tintinalli JE (ed.) Emergency Medicine: A Comprehensive Study Guide, 4th edn. McGraw-Hill, pp 1093–103
13. Goubran GF 1989 Maxillofacial injuries. In: Westaby S (ed.) Trauma: Pathogenesis and Treatment. Heinemann Medical, Oxford, pp 230–45
14. Finkle DR, Ringler SL, Lutterton CR, et al 1985 Comparison of the diagnostic methods used in maxillofacial trauma. Plastic and Reconstructive Surgery 75: 32–41
15. Russel JL, Davidson MJ, Daly BD, Corrigan AM 1990 Computed tomography in the diagnosis of maxillofacial trauma. British Journal of Oral and Maxillofacial Surgery 28: 287–91
16. Davidson JS, Birdsell DC 1989 Cervical spine injury in patients with facial skeletal trauma. Journal of Trauma 29: 1276–8
17. Hills MW, Deanne SA 1993 Head injury and facial injury: is there an increased risk of cervical spine injury. Journal of Trauma 34: 549–53
18. Williams J, Jehle D, Cottington E, Shuffleberger C 1992 Head, facial, and clavicular trauma as a predictor of cervical spine injury. Annals of Emergency Medicine 21: 719–22
19. Sinclair D, Schwartz M, Gruss J, McLellan B 1988 A retrospective review of the relationship between facial fractures, head injuries, and cervical spine injuries. Journal of Emergency Medicine 6: 109–12
20. Joynt GM, Oh TE 1997 Faciomaxillary and upper airway injuries. In: Oh TE (ed.) Intensive Care Manual, 4th edn. Butterworth-Heinemann, Oxford, pp 582–9
21. Ardekian L, Samet N, Shoshani Y, Taicher S 1993 Life-threatening bleeding following maxillofacial trauma. Journal of Craniomaxillofacial Surgery 21: 336–8
22. Murakami WT, Davidson TM, Marshall LF 1983 Fatal epistaxis in craniofacial trauma. Journal of Trauma 23: 57–61
23. Slupchynskyj OS, Berkower AS, Byrne DW, Cayten CG 1992 Association of skull base and facial fractures. Laryngoscope 102: 1247–50
24. Geronemus RG, Mertz PM, Eaglstein WH 1979 Wound healing: the effects of topical antimicrobial agents. Archives of Dermatology 115: 1311
25. Yarington CT Jr 1977 Managing soft tissue injuries. American Family Physician 16: 109
26. Hussain K, Wijetunge DB, Grubnic S, Jackson IT 1994 A comprehensive analysis of craniofacial trauma. Journal of Trauma 36: 34–47
27. Luce EA, Tubb TD, Moore AM 1979 Review of 1000 major facial fractures and associated injuries. Plastic and Reconstructive Surgery 63: 26
28. Halazonetis JA 1968 The 'weak' regions of the mandible. British Journal of Oral Surgery 6: 37–48
29. Chu L, Gussack GS, Muller T 1994 A treatment protocol for mandible fractures. Journal of Trauma 36: 48–52
30. Winstanley RP 1984 The management of fractures of the mandible. British Journal of Oral and Maxillofacial Surgery 22: 170–7
31. Pathria MN, Blaser SI 1989 Diagnostic imaging of craniofacial fractures. Radiology Clinics of North America 27: 839–53
32. Whitaker LA, Yaremchuk MJ 1990 Secondary reconstruction of posttraumatic orbital deformities. Annals of Plastic Surgery 25: 440–9
33. Le Fort R 1972 Experimental study of fractures of the upper jaw. Revue Chirurgie Paris 1901; 23: 208–27, 360–79 (reprinted in Plastic and Reconstructive Surgery 50: 497–506)
34. Manson PN, Hoopes JE, Su CT 1980 Structural pillars of the facial skeleton: an approach to the management of Le Fort fractures. Plastic and Reconstructive Surgery 66: 54–61
35. Curtin JW 1973 Basic plastic surgical techniques in repair of facial lacerations. Surgical Clinics of North America 53: 33
36. Stranc MF, Robertson GA 1979 A classification of injuries of the nasal skeleton. Annals of Plastic Surgery 2: 468–74
37. Khalil AF 1980 Civilian gunshot injuries to the face and jaws. British Journal of Oral Surgery 18: 205–11
38. Cole RD, Browne JD, Phipps CD 1994 Gunshot wounds to the mandible and midface: evaluation, treatment, and avoidance of complications. Otolaryngology Head and Neck Surgery 111: 739–45
39. Stiernberg CM, Jahrsdoerfer RA, Gillenwater A, Joe SA, Alcalen SV 1992 Gunshot wounds to the head and neck. Archives of Otolaryngology Head and Neck Surgery 118: 592–7
40. Jahrsdoerfer RA, Johns ME, Cantrell RW 1979 Penetrating wounds of the head and neck. Archives of Otolaryngology Head and Neck Surgery 105: 721–5
41. Chen AY, Stewart MG, Raup G 1996 Penetrating injuries of the face. Otolaryngology, Head and Neck Surgery 115: 464–70
42. Kihitir T, Ivatury RR, Simon RJ, Nassoura Z, Leban S 1993 Early management of civilian gunshot wounds to the face. Journal of Trauma 35: 569–75
43. Dolin J, Scalea T, Mannor L, Sclafani S, Trooskin S 1992 The management of gunshot wounds to the face. Journal of Trauma 33: 508–14
44. Stanley RB, Canalis RF, Colman MF 1981 Gunshot wounds to the mandible with secondary neck injuries. Archives of Otolaryngology Head and Neck Surgery 107: 565–7
45. Kreutz RW, Bear SH 1985 Selective emergency arteriography in cases of penetrating maxillofacial trauma. Oral Surgery, Oral Medicine, Oral Pathology 60: 18–22

2.5 ABDOMINAL TRAUMA

GARRY J. WILKES

ESSENTIALS

1 Abdominal trauma is an important cause of morbidity and mortality.

2 The abdominal cavity has a large capacity to accommodate haemorrhage with no external sign, and this can easily be overlooked if a high index of suspicion is not maintained.

3 Investigations of value include focused trauma ultrasound (FAST), computer tomography and diagnostic peritoneal lavage. The use of these investigations, along with repeated clinical assessments, will detect injuries early and reduce morbidity and preventable mortality in trauma patients.

INTRODUCTION

One in 10 deaths from trauma is due to abdominal injuries. These may be difficult to detect initially, as the abdominal cavity cannot be viewed with the naked eye, plain radiography is insensitive to intra-abdominal bleeding and solid organ injury, and signs and symptoms of blood loss may be attributed to more obvious injuries. It is, therefore, not surprising that missed abdominal injuries are a major cause of preventable death in trauma patients. A high index of suspicion should be maintained for this important cause of morbidity and mortality.

A stepwise approach to the management of the multiply injured patient will address the possibility of significant intra-abdominal injury. The principles of initial management are to identify the presence or otherwise of such injury and to determine the need for surgery and the most appropriate timing of interventions. This process requires the presence of an experienced clinician at the earliest possible stage to direct and coordinate the trauma team. Ideally, the trauma surgeon should be present at the initial resuscitation.

The initial resuscitation, history, examination and specific investigations will be reviewed in turn.

PRIMARY AND SECONDARY SURVEYS

The abdomen does not normally form part of the primary survey. The unstable patient requiring continued fluid resuscitation without other sources of haemorrhage must be considered to have ongoing intra-abdominal bleeding. Specific points to remember are to expose the patient fully, including an examination of the back as well as the rectum and vagina.

History

The history will provide vital clues to the increased likelihood of significant intra-abdominal trauma (Table 2.5.1). Ambulance personnel will be able to provide valuable details of the incident. It is important to remember that trauma does not skip body regions and that significant intra-abdominal injuries frequently occur in the absence of external signs of abdominal trauma. Other aspects of history that should be sought are known adverse

Table 2.5.1 Risk factors for intra-abdominal injury in trauma patients

High-speed vehicular collisions
Pedestrian struck by vehicle
Fall from greater than standing height
Hypotension or history of hypotension (systolic BP <100 mmHg) at any time
Presence of significant chest or pelvic injuries
Significant injuries on physically opposing sides of the abdomen.

drug reactions, the medical history and medications of the patient, and when they last ate and drank.

Abdominal examination

Penetrating injuries are overt and dramatic, whereas blunt trauma is more common and more difficult to assess on clinical grounds. Bruising and abrasions are associated with intra-abdominal pathology. The spleen and liver are the most commonly injured organs, with different patterns of injury seen in blunt and penetrating injuries (Table 2.5.2)[1] Marks from lap-type seatbelts carry a high association with Chance fractures (T12/L1), small bowel injury and pancreatic injury. Palpation of the abdomen may reveal local/generalized tenderness and evidence of peritonism but is less reliable in detecting retroperitoneal injury and in the presence of altered sensorium. Auscultation is rarely useful; however, the absence of bowel sounds should increase the suspicion of intra-abdominal injury.

Rectal examination may demonstrate frank blood from injured bowel, a high-riding or mobile prostate from urethral rupture, and may allow direct palpation of fractures or breaches of bowel wall integrity. Vaginal examination is important for similar reasons, and may detect an unrecognized gravid uterus. The examination of the abdomen is not complete until the back, buttocks and perineum have been fully exposed.

Although unexplained hypotension suggests intra-abdominal haemorrhage, not all patients with significant blood loss will display the typical pattern of hypotension and tachycardia.[2] This is especially true of the younger patient. Less than one-third of patients with significant blood loss will have both hypotension and tachycardia.[3] More important are changes in pulse and blood pressure with time and in response to fluid resuscitation. Continuing falls in blood pressure and rises in pulse rate indicate ongoing

Table 2.5.2 Organ injuries associated with blunt and penetrating trauma[1]

	Blunt trauma (%)	Stabbing (%)	Gunshot (%)
Spleen	40–55	–	–
Liver	35–45	40	30
Retroperitoneal haematoma	15	–	–
Small bowel	–	30	50
Diaphragm	–	20	–
Colon	–	15	40
Abdominal vascular structures	–	–	25

Table 2.5.3 Indications for laparotomy

Immediate
Evisceration
Gunshot wound
Stab wound with peritoneum breached
Haemodynamic instability despite correction of estimated blood loss from extra-abdominal sites
Frank peritonism (initially or on repeat examination)
Free gas on plain radiography
Ruptured diaphragm

Emergent
Positive trauma ultrasound
Positive DPL

haemorrhage which, if no other source is identified, must be assumed to be intra-abdominal. Abdominal distension does not occur until several litres of blood have been sequestered, and can initially be confused with obesity.

Once the patient has been examined a urinary catheter should be inserted, unless there is suspicion of a urethral injury. Blood at the urethral meatus, scrotal haematoma and a high-riding or mobile prostate are suggestive of urethral injury, and a urological opinion should be sought before attempting to insert a catheter. In these circumstances a suprapubic catheter may be preferable. Patients with a suspicion of abdominal injury also require a gastric catheter. Nasogastric catheterization is more comfortable for the patient than the oral route, but is contraindicated by evidence of basilar skull fracture. Gastric decompression may be both diagnostic and therapeutic. Penetration of the stomach or proximal small bowel will produce a bloodied aspiration. Aspiration of air will relieve gastric tamponade, which is occasionally an unrecognized cause of hypotension from impaired venous return. Urinary and gastric catheterization are mandatory prior to diagnostic peritoneal lavage (DPL).

A penetrating object, such as a knife protruding from the abdomen, should be left in situ unless it is an immediate threat to life. It is tempting to remove such objects when the patient appears stable in order to examine the patient and the wound tract, but following this impulse can lead to disastrous consequences if the object is adjacent to or penetrates vascular structures. The sudden release of a tamponade may kill the patient in a very short time. The only place to remove a knife or other penetrating object is in an operating theatre, with staff on hand capable of dealing with all possible complications.

Investigations

In the initial resuscitation of all trauma patients blood is drawn for full blood count, urea and electrolytes, blood sugar determination, cross-matching, arterial blood gases (if available) and a trauma radiology series. There is little place for plain radiology of the abdomen.

The indications for immediate laparotomy are listed in Table 2.5.3. Gunshot wounds can produce secondary missiles, are unpredictable in their path, and all require laparotomy. Stab wounds that have penetrated the peritoneum may also require laparotomy and need immediate assessment by an experienced trauma surgeon. In cases where immediate laparotomy is indicated the patient should be escorted to theatre with no further investigations. If other operations are required the order is determined by the surgeons concerned. If laparotomy is to be delayed by other, more urgent procedures, further investigations such as trauma ultrasound or DPL may be performed in theatre, allowing the timing of laparotomy to be planned.

Unstable patients require surgical intervention as soon as possible. Stable patients can be investigated further, allowing better planning of further management. The difficulty arises in the common situation where there are multiple injuries and only a suspicion – not confirmation – of significant intra-abdominal pathology. Some patients are at risk of abdominal injury but cannot be assessed on clinical grounds. These include those with head, chest and spinal injuries, intoxicated or sedated patients, and those who will be inaccessible while undergoing lengthy operations on other body regions. For these patients it is important to make a further assessment of the presence or otherwise of intra-abdominal injury. Additional investigations of benefit are DPL, computer tomography (CT) and ultrasound. Each has advantages and disadvantages (Table 2.5.4). They may also be consecutive and complementary, thereby minimizing the disadvantages of each individually. Areas poorly imaged by all modalities are hollow organ injury, such as small bowel rupture and vascular compromise. Serial clinical examination is essential to detect these injuries, even if investigation results are normal.

DPL was first described by Root et al in 1965.[4] Several modifications of the technique have been described, including open, semiopen and closed techniques, with and without pressure infusion of lavage fluid. Experienced operators can complete lavage in less than 4 minutes.[5] A positive lavage is indicated by aspiration of frank blood, exit of lavage fluid out of other catheters (e.g. intercostal),

Table 2.5.4 Comparison of abdominal CT, DPL and ultrasound for investigation of abdominal trauma

Abdominal CT	DPL	Ultrasound
Advantages		
Anatomical information	Rapid, cheap, sensitive	Rapid, portable, repeatable
Non-invasive	Minimal training	Non-invasive
Visualizes retroperitoneum	Ideal in unstable patients	Ideal in unstable patients
Also views chest, pelvis	Can be done in resusc. room	Can be done in resusc. room
		Also views chest, pelvis
Disadvantages		
Not suitable for unstable patients	Not organ specific	Requires specific training
Requires transport from resus room	False negative	Operator dependent
	Retroperitoneal injuries	False negative
Patient safety	Hollow viscus injury	Retroperitoneal injuries
Inaccessible while scanning	Diaphragm injury	Hollow viscus injury
Time	Iatrogenic injury	Diaphragm injury
Cost		False positive
False negative		Ascites
Hollow viscus injuries		
IV contrast reactions		

drainage of intestinal material or bile, or sufficient bloodstaining of the lavage fluid to prevent the reading of standard newspaper print. Additional tests on lavage fluid, such as red cell count, white cell count and amylase levels, have been suggested. The time taken to obtain these results, as well as deciding what constitutes a significant result, limit these other investigations.[6] For example, the most widely accepted cut-off point for significance in red cell count is 100 000 mm^{-3}.[1] Others have suggested a lower level of 10 000 mm^{-3} for penetrating trauma, and levels as low as 1000 mm^{-3} have been suggested in the presence of other injuries.[7] Despite these limitations, a specificity of 99% and accuracy of 95% have been achieved for intra-abdominal haemorrhage, which, when combined with clinical assessment, reduce the non-therapeutic laparotomy rate to below 5% in the presence of systolic hypotension.[8] DPL can also be performed in the operating theatre if desired. DPL does not exclude retroperitoneal injury. The final disadvantage is the lack of organ specificity. Only the presence of an intraperitoneal injury is determined, not its location.

Abdominal CT

Abdominal CT is non-invasive and provides precise anatomical details of intra-abdominal pathology. The major disadvantages are associated with the use of intravenous contrast and the need for the patient to be transported from the resuscitation area to the CT scanner, where they are not accessible during the procedure. Intravenous contrast may rarely produce allergic reactions and can precipitate or exacerbate renal impairment, particularly in higher doses and in the presence of renal hypoperfusion and hypofunction. Although modern machines complete scans in a single breath-hold, time is still required to load and unload the patient. Transport and transfer are times of maximum patient risk and minimum monitoring. Only stable patients are, therefore, suitable for transfer for CT scanning. Unstable patients require further resuscitation or operative intervention if this is unsuccessful. The definition of stable is not agreed. The final decision can only be made by the most experienced physician available, although a systolic pressure of at least 90 mmHg and no requirement for additional fluids after correction of estimated losses would be minimum requirements.

Focused trauma ultrasound

Focused ultrasound is a relatively new technique in acute trauma management. Abdominal ultrasound is non-invasive, may be done at the bedside, and can be repeated as needed. The technique of focused assessment by sonography in trauma (FAST) can be easily learnt by clinicians and completed in less than 5 minutes without interfering with the function of a trauma resuscitation team.[9–12] Ultrasound combines the advantages of being rapid, accurate and non-invasive, and can be performed at the bedside without interfering with the resuscitation. Ultrasound is at least as accurate as DPL, and in experienced hands has similar results to CT in determining the presence of intraperitoneal injury. As a decision making tool for identifying the need for laparotomy in hypotensive patients (systolic BP <90), FAST has a sensitivity of 100%, specificity of 96% and negative predictive value of 100% (NPV).[13] Interest and experience in this technique continue to grow with ACEP and ACEM established credentialling.[14, 15] It is the bedside investigation of choice if an experienced operator is available.

Laparoscopy

Laparoscopy has been investigated in some centres, but the skills required and the time taken for a thorough examination limit the widespread usefulness of this modality in acute blunt trauma. However, it is useful in excluding peritoneal penetration in abdominal stab wounds.

PENETRATING INJURIES

Penetrating injuries produce a different pattern of injury (see Table 2.5.2) and are managed in a different manner from blunt injuries (Figs 2.5.1 and 2.5.2). The potential for gunshot wounds to produce secondary missiles and cause widespread injury mandates formal laparotomy in all cases. Stab wounds with haemodynamic compromise or other indications should also proceed to laparotomy without delay for other investigations. Local exploration of stab wounds by experienced surgeons in patients without evidence of internal injury may be useful, as up to one-third

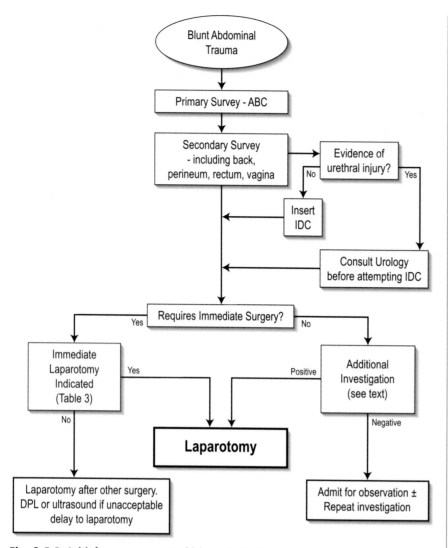

Fig. 2.5.1 Initial management of blunt abdominal trauma.

mation at the bedside in the resuscitation area rapidly, without the need for invasive techniques. The other area of development will be in non-operative management of injuries using radiological or minimally invasive surgical techniques, thereby decreasing the need for laparotomy.

of wounds do not breach the peritoneum. Selected patients may then be managed conservatively.

DISPOSITION

Disposition decisions may be difficult in the less seriously injured patient or those with suspected injury. Every patient suspected or at significant risk of intra-abdominal injury should be admitted for observation and serial examinations, ideally by the same individual. Injuries to the bowel wall or intestinal blood supply may not be evident on initial clinical examination or investigation, and may take 24 hours to declare themselves.

A higher index of suspicion is required for patients who cannot be assessed clinically. Unconscious, intubated, head-injured and spinal-injured patients are all at increased risk of abdominal injuries and less able to declare them. Serial investigations and clinical vigilance are vital.

FUTURE DIRECTIONS

The difficulty in managing abdominal trauma is determining the presence, location and details of intra-abdominal injury. Current imaging techniques have their disadvantages and limitations. The refinement of modalities such as ultrasound will provide more detailed infor-

REFERENCES

1. American College of Surgeons Committee on Trauma 1997 Advanced Trauma Life Support Student Manual, 6th edn. ACS, Chicago
2. Wilkes GJ, McSweeney PA 1996 The diagnosis of traumatic intra-abdominal haemorrhage in patients with normal vital signs. Emergency Medicine 8: 19–23
3. Grant RT, Reeve EB 1941 Clinical observations on air-raid casualties. British Medical Journal 2: 293–7
4. Root HD, Hauser CW, La Fave JW, Mendiola RP 1965 Diagnostic peritoneal lavage. Surgery 57: 633–7
5. Sugrue M, Seger M, Gunning K, Sloane D, Deane S 1995 A modified combination technique for performing diagnostic peritoneal lavage. Australian and New Zealand Journal of Surgery 65(8): 604–6
6. Feliciano DV, Bitondo Dyer CG 1994 Vagaries of the lavage white blood cell count in evaluating abdominal stab wounds. American Journal of Surgery 168(6): 680–3; discussion 683–4
7. Feliciano DV, Rozycki GS 1995 The management of penetrating abdominal trauma. Advances in Surgery 28: 1–39
8. Day AC, Rankin N, Charlesworth P 1992

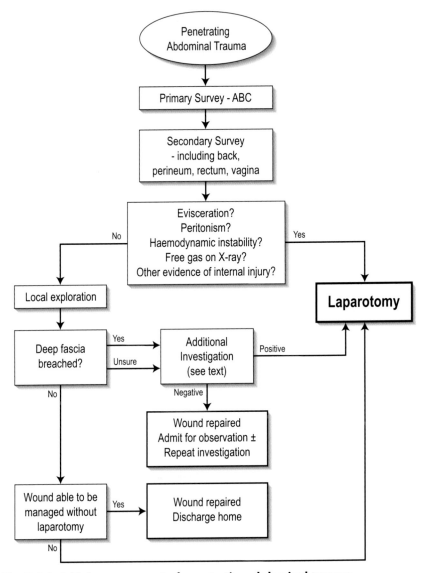

Fig. 2.5.2 Initial management of penetrating abdominal trauma.

Diagnostic peritoneal lavage: integration with clinical information to improve diagnostic performance. Journal of Trauma 32(1): 52–7

9. Rozycki GS, Feliciano DV, Davis TP 1998 Ultrasound as used in thoracoabdominal trauma. Surgical Clinics of North America 78(2): 295–310

10. Shackford SR 1993 Focused ultrasound examinations by surgeons: the time is now. Journal of Trauma 35(2): 181–2

11. McGahan JP, Rose J, Coates TL, Wisner DH, Newberry P 1997 Use of ultrasonography in the patient with acute abdominal trauma. Journal of Ultrasound Medicine 16(10): 653–62; quiz 663–4

12. Shackford SR, Rogers FB, Osler TM, et al 1999 Focused abdominal sonogram for trauma: the learning curve of nonradiologist clinicians in detecting hemoperitoneum. Journal of Trauma 46: 553–62

13. http://www.trauma.org/radiology/FASThowgood.html Accessed May 2002

14. http://www.trauma.org/radiology/FASTintro.html Accessed May 2002.

15. http://www.acem.org.au/open/documents/ultrasonography.htm Updated July 2000. Accessed May 2002

2.6 CHEST TRAUMA

MARK C. FITZGERALD • ROBERT GOCENTAS

ESSENTIALS

1 Less than 10% of blunt chest trauma patients require thoracic operations.

2 Radiographs do not reliably exclude rib fracture or other complications.

3 Adequate analgesia is essential to prevent complications from chest-wall injury.

4 Resuscitative thoracotomy should be restricted to those patients likely to benefit.

INTRODUCTION

Thoracic trauma is responsible for 25% of all trauma deaths and contributes to a further 25%. In Australasia and the UK 90–95% of chest trauma is secondary to blunt injury.

The majority of chest trauma patients may be managed non-operatively. Only 10% of blunt thoracic trauma patients will require thoracotomy, the remainder requiring supportive care including chest decompression and drainage.

Supportive care, in particular resuscitation, is often suboptimal. Delayed or inadequate ventilatory resuscitation, inadequate shock management, insufficient monitoring of arterial blood gases, and delay or failure to perform intercostal catheterization remain identifiable problems that contribute to preventable morbidity and mortality.[1,2] Recently controversy has developed regarding the place of aggressive fluid resuscitation in chest trauma with penetrating trauma, which may exacerbate uncontrolled intrathoracic bleeding. It is certainly not a substitute for early operative intervention.[3]

Flail chest, pulmonary contusion, thoracic aortic transection, pneumothorax, haemothorax and ruptured hemidiaphragm are life-threatening injuries that may not be apparent on initial presentation. These diagnoses need to be pursued and actively excluded.

Patients with underlying airway disease and the elderly with diminished compliance are at particular risk.

Anatomically the thorax may be divided into:

- Chest wall and diaphragm
- Pleura
- Lung parenchyma
- Bronchi and trachea
- Mediastinum, including heart, great vessels and oesophagus
- Vertebral column and spinal cord.

When dealing with chest trauma a systematic approach should consider injury in each of these anatomical areas.

CHEST WALL INJURY

Fractured ribs

Fractured ribs are common sequelae of focal trauma. Fractured ribs cause pain, which may then interfere with ventilation and coughing, causing ventilatory impairment and atelectasis. This impairment may not be manifest for hours and occasionally days post injury.

Underlying structures are often injured concomitantly, particularly the lungs, pleura and intercostal vessels. Fractures of the lower left ribs are associated with splenic injury, the lower right with hepatic injury, and the lower posterior ribs with renal injury. The first and second ribs are stronger and less easily injured, and when fractured are usually indicative of significant force to the upper mediastinum. Although first and second rib fractures have been traditionally associated with thoracic aortic injury, the positive predictive value of this association has been questioned.[4]

Rib fracture is essentially a diagnosis based on the clinical findings of local rib tenderness with or without deformity and crepitus. Up to 50% of fractured ribs are not apparent on the initial chest X-ray. A follow-up film is recommended to improve sensitivity.[5] Reliance on the X-ray to diagnose fractured ribs inevitably results in underdiagnosis. This may lead to delays in diagnosis and therapy and an adverse outcome, particularly with elderly patients and those with coexisting airways disease.

The management of rib fractures centres on pain relief, minimizing pulmonary sequelae and actively excluding associated injury. Oral analgesics usually provide adequate pain relief for single rib fractures. Local anaesthetic intercostal blocks, epidural analgesia and narcotic infusions improve ventilation when impaired by pain and are often required for multiple rib fractures, particularly in the elderly patient. Breathing exercises, coughing and incentive spirometry minimize subsequent atelectasis.

Fractured sternum

This is a clinical diagnosis confirmed on lateral chest X-ray. As with rib fractures, concern centres on associated intrathoracic injuries, specifically myocardial and other mediastinal injuries.

The possibility of underlying injury has been related to the mechanism of injury. For example, in North America it is reported that up to 66% of patients with sternal fractures have associated injuries. It is believed that low seatbelt usage results in sternal fractures secondary to impact against the steering wheel. In Australasia, where seatbelt usage is high, sternal fracture is more often caused by the restraining belt. Therefore, comparatively lower deceleration forces are evident, resulting in a decreased association with underlying injury.[5–7]

For isolated sternal fractures admission for analgesia is usually required, although this may be only necessary for 1–2 days. Monitoring is not required unless the mechanism or subsequent investigations suggest underlying mediastinal injury.

Flail chest

Flail chest may occur where the continuity of the bony skeleton of the chest wall is disrupted in two places. It is characterized by paradoxical movement of the associated unanchored chest wall segment. Because of muscular spasms and splinting this segment may not be apparent initially, and may flail some time after the accident. Elderly patients have a less compliant chest wall and are at greater risk of developing a flail segment.

Flail chest is often associated with ventilatory insufficiency. Ventilatory disturbance is caused by hypoventilation of the affected hemithorax due to the mechanical disruption and associated pain, compounded by the underlying pulmonary contusion. Therapy centres on maintaining oxygenation, ventilation and euvolaemia. Adequate analgesia should be supplemented with intercostal nerve blocks or epidural analgesia. In general, patients with a significant flail, which impairs ventilation, will require intubation and positive-pressure ventilation or pressure support.

Ruptured hemidiaphragm

Diaphragmatic rupture may be difficult to diagnose. High-velocity injuries with lateral torso trauma or thoracoabdominal crush injuries should alert the clinician to the possibility of underlying diaphragmatic injury. Associated injuries, such as lateral rib fractures, penetrating left upper quadrant wounds and fractured pelvis, are associated with an increased incidence of diaphragmatic disruption. There may be respiratory compromise, with diminished air entry in the involved hemithorax. Placement of a radio-opaque nasogastric tube will facilitate the diagnosis of left hemidiaphragmatic disruption on chest X-ray. Although gross rupture may be apparent initially, the classic radiological findings of viscera in the thoracic cavity, the nasogastric tube coiled in the thoracic cavity, or marked hemidiaphragm elevation are present only 50% of the time, with no intra-thoracic pathology seen on 15% of occasions.[8] Thus many diaphragmatic injuries present late, with complications of diaphragmatic hernias. Spiral CT scan will display gross disruption but may miss small defects. Occult diaphragmatic lacerations are associated with penetrating injuries of the thoracoabdominal region, and should be actively excluded by laparoscopy, thoracoscopy or open operation.

The treatment of diaphragmatic disruption is operative repair.

PLEURAL INJURY

Open pneumothorax

Open pneumothorax presents an immediate threat to life. An open chest wall defect disrupts the generation of a negative inspiratory pressure. If the opening is approximately two-thirds the diameter of the trachea, air will pass preferentially through the defect (a 'sucking' chest wound) and respiratory failure will occur.[9]

Initial management includes covering the defect with a sterile dressing and taping it on three sides to achieve a flutter-valve effect, prior to placement of an intercostal catheter and sealing of the defect. Definitive surgical closure is required.

Pneumothorax

Simple pneumothorax is characterized by a visceral pleural rent and pleural air preventing expansion of the associated lung. Although small (<20%) pneumothoraces may be managed conservatively, larger ones mandate intercostal catheter insertion and underwater seal or flutter-valve drainage. Intercostal catheters should also be inserted for all pneumothoraces if positive-pressure ventilation is anticipated or has been commenced. If small traumatic pneumothoraces are not drained, the patient should be followed closely with repeat chest X-rays. Intercostal catheters should be placed if the patient is to be air-transported to another facility.

Thoracic CT scanning will demonstrate pneumothoraces that may not be apparent on plain radiology.[10] This also mandates intercostal catheter placement in ventilated patients.

Tension pneumothorax

Tension pneumothorax occurs with the formation of a 'one-way valve' from the lung through disrupted visceral pleura. Air collects under tension in the hemithorax, collapsing the lung and displacing the mediastinum, impairing ventilation and obstructing venous return. Tension pneumothorax is more commonly associated with positive-pressure ventilation. It is essentially a clinical diagnosis, characterized by tachypnoea, tracheal deviation away from the affected hemithorax, diminished ipsilateral breath sounds, diminished compliance, oxygen desaturation and hypotension.

If clinically suspected, the affected hemithorax should be immediately decompressed and an intercostal catheter subsequently inserted. Needle thoracentesis using a 14G needle inserted anteriorly in the second intercostal space, in the midclavicular line, is the currently recommended initial approach.[11] There should be no attempt to delay chest decompression in favour of a chest X-ray.

Some thoracic trauma patients, after intubation and ventilation, demonstrate air under tension subcutaneous emphysema on initial chest X-ray, without a pneumothorax being visible. This should mandate immediate chest-tube placement, as this is a precursor of ipsilateral tension pneumothorax. The subcutaneous tissues in communication with the air leak offer less initial resistance and display air under pressure, prior to tension developing within the pleural space.

Haemothorax

Blood may accumulate within the pleural space after lung laceration or laceration of a chest-wall vessel and, less commonly, after mediastinal injury. It is indicated by diffuse opacification of a hemithorax on supine chest X-ray, or blunting of the costophrenic angle on an upright film. The haemothorax is best drained via placement of a 32Fr or larger intercostal catheter, positioned in the fifth intercostal space just anterior to the midaxillary line on the affected side. The use of suction (20 cmH$_2$O) facilitates chest drainage. If haemorrhage is ongoing the blood can be collected in a suitable closed system and may then be autotransfused.

Bleeding is usually self-limiting following drainage. Drainage of more than 1500 mL following initial intercostal catheter insertion, or a sustained loss of more than 200 mL per hour for more than 2 hours, are indications for thoracotomy.[12] Large blood losses frequently come from intercostal arteries.

Clamping the intercostal catheter in an attempt to tamponade bleeding and 'buy time' for an intubated and ventilated, unstable patient with a massive and ongoing hemithorax could be considered if delays to thoracotomy arise. However, this technique is yet to be validated in a controlled trial.

LUNG INJURY

Pulmonary contusion

Pulmonary contusion follows focal pulmonary trauma and is characterized by the leakage of blood into the alveoli and pulmonary interstitium, culminating in consolidation and atelectasis. Associated hypoxia may be profound and is evident on arterial blood gases. Tachypnoea with rales is a common clinical finding. The initial chest X-ray may not demonstrate the severity of injury. Pulmonary contusion may take some time to be radiologically apparent, with 21% of experimentally incurred contusions still not visible on chest X-ray 6 hours post injury.[13]

CT scans provide the most sensitive test for gauging the extent of pulmonary contusion, although arterial blood gases provide the best measure of physiological derangement requiring intervention. Therapy is based on ensuring adequate oxygenation, ventilatory support and fluid restriction. Ventilation should involve low-volume, low-pressure techniques to reduce barotrauma and secondary injury. Steroids have not been shown to improve outcome.[11]

TRACHEOBRONCHIAL INJURY

Injuries to the trachea and bronchi are rare, accounting for less than 1% of injuries after blunt chest trauma.[14] Eighty per cent of injuries occur near the carina, with mediastinal and cervical emphysema resulting. A persistent air leak should alert the clinician to the possibility of a tracheobronchial injury. Fibreoptic bronchoscopy is the investigative modality of choice. Persistent air leaks often require operative repair.

MEDIASTINAL INJURY

Myocardial contusion

Although myocardial contusion occurs commonly, significant sequelae are rare. Cardiac failure and hypotension are uncommonly associated with myocardial contusion. Although the ECG is used as a predictor of myocardial contusion, it is non-specific and poorly portrays the right ventricle – the area most commonly injured. Cardiac enzyme elevation does occur but is non-predictive and unhelpful. Echocardiography may demonstrate dyskinesis of the ventricular wall. Patients with hyperacute ECG changes or conduction defects should be admitted and monitored for dysrhythmias.

Myocardial laceration and cardiac tamponade

Precordial penetrating injury is associated with myocardial laceration. Bedside echocardiography is useful in demonstrating myocardial injury and pericardial collections. Patients presenting with signs of pericardial tamponade (hypotension, diminished heart sounds, jugular venous distension) require urgent surgical intervention.

Patients who acutely deteriorate into cardiac arrest yet who had signs of life en route to hospital or on arrival require a resuscitative thoracotomy in the emergency department.[15] Outcome for blunt trauma patients without initial signs is very poor (<2%), but penetrating injury has a higher survival rate.[15] This procedure should only be undertaken judiciously because of the infection risks to personnel. Prolonged (>9 minutes) external cardiac massage is futile in these patients.[15]

Tension pneumopericardium

Tension pneumopericardium, although much less common than tension pneumothorax, is thought to arise via a similar 'one-way valve' mechanism, particularly after the institution of positive-pressure ventilation. It is characterized by raised jugular/central venous pressure and hypotension, and requires urgent pericardiocentesis.[16]

Thoracic aortic transection

Eighty-five per cent of patients with transection of the thoracic aorta die before reaching hospital. Of the survivors, 50% die within the next 48 hours if not operated upon. Sixty-five per cent of injuries are to the proximal descending aorta.

A mechanism of injury involving violent/high deceleration forces should alert the physician to the possibility of thoracic aortic injury. Lateral-impact, as well as frontal-impact, motor vehicle crashes contribute to aortic transection.[17]

Clinical signs, such as pulse deficits, upper body hypertension, unequal blood pressures bilaterally or dysphonia, are uncommon findings. The initial chest X-ray may demonstrate mediastinal widening, loss of the aortic knuckle, loss of the paraspinal stripe, massive haemothorax, and tracheal or oesophageal deviation from the midline.

When blunt thoracic aortic injury was studied prospectively, mediastinal widening was demonstrated in 85% of cases.[18] Mediastinal widening on chest X-ray is 90% sensitive and 10% specific for aortic transection. This means that approximately 10% of patients with aortic transection have a normal mediastinum on the initial chest X-ray. Associated fractures of the thoracic spine also cause mediastinal widening and make interpretation difficult. There is no thoracic skeletal injury that is a clinically useful predictor of acute thoracic aortic transection.[5]

At present, angiography remains the imaging gold standard. CT has been shown to be diagnostic in 75% of cases and transoesophageal echocardiography (TOE) in 80%.[18] CT will reliably demonstrate mediastinal haematoma and is, therefore, a useful screening test. If aortic injury is not apparent and mediastinal haematoma is evident on CT, the patient should undergo angiography. However, better definition with new multi-slice CT scans is increasing the diagnosis of intimal injury (see Chapter 2.8 Radiology in Major Trauma).

TOE accuracy is operator dependent. It has been used as a screening tool for aortic tears[19] and is useful for patients in theatre or those unable to be moved to angiography.[20,21]

Multicentre studies of aortic transection demonstrate that three patient populations exist: those in extremis, unstable patients, and one-third more 'stable' group.[22] Patients in extremis from aortic transection rarely survive. In unstable patients (systolic BP <90 mmHg) surgical repair is indicated, although overall mortality is greater than 85%. Recent research suggests that in 'stable' patients (systolic BP >90 mmHg) blood pressure control with β-blockade is indicated prior to surgical repair. Blood pressure control reduces shearing forces at the site of aortic transection, increasing the likelihood of containment within the mediastinal haematoma prior to operative repair. 'Stable' patients with coronary artery disease and 'stable' patients aged over 55 may fare worse with immediate operative repair, and non-operative management or endoluminal graft placement should be considered.[22]

Oesophageal perforation

Oesophageal rupture after blunt chest trauma is rare. The lower third of the oesophagus is the commonest site of rupture, presumably secondary to a forced Valsalva manoeuvre. Mediastinitis is a subsequent development. Retrosternal pain is common and mediastinal air may be seen on chest X-ray.

Gastrografin is the study of choice. Mortality is directly related to time to operative repair.[23]

Gunshot injuries across the truncal midline more commonly involve mediastinal and spinal structures and, therefore, have a much greater mortality than unilateral injuries.[24] It is important to exclude oesophageal injury early with penetrating and transmediastinal wounds, as it

constitutes significant morbidity and mortality in those patients who survive to hospital.

VERTEBRAL COLUMN AND SPINAL CORD INJURY

Exclusion of thoracic spine fractures and spinal-cord injury forms part of the routine work-up of the chest trauma patient. Occult injuries are common, and unstable injuries in ventilated patients require skilled nursing. Such injuries are easily overlooked.

OPERATIVE INTERVENTION

The majority of thoracic trauma in Australasia is due to blunt injury. The Alfred Emergency and Trauma Centre in Melbourne has the largest, adult major trauma workload (defined as ISS > 15, death or >24 hours ventilation) in Australasia. From July 2001 to June 2002, 729 major trauma patients were received: 95.3% were blunt trauma patients, 67.4 % sustained some form of thoracic injury and 25% required intercostal catheter insertion.

Emergency operative procedures are uncommon and amongst this group included 32 (4.4%) emergency thoracotomies and 7 (1%) resuscitative thoracotomies.

INDICATIONS FOR EMERGENCY THORACOTOMY[25]

Although more than 90% of chest-trauma patients may be managed non-operatively, the following categories warrant surgical intervention:

- Cardiac tamponade
- Acute deterioration – cardiac arrest in patients with penetrating truncal trauma
- Vascular injury at the thoracic outlet
- Traumatic thoracotomy (loss of chest-wall substance)

- Massive air leak from chest tube
- Massive or continuing haemothorax
- Mediastinal traversing penetrating injury
- Endoscopic or radiographic demonstration of oesophageal injury
- Endoscopic or radiographic demonstration of tracheal or bronchial injury
- Radiographic evidence of great vessel injury
- Thoracic penetration with industrial liquids (especially coaltar products).

RESUSCITATIVE THORACOTOMY

Left antero-lateral thoracotomy as a rescucitative manoeuvre allows direct access to the heart and pericardial decompression for patients who have lost output following penetrating injury to the heart. Myocardial wounds can then be directly controlled. Right atrial catheterization facilitating IV fluid adminstration, pulmonary hilar clamping, descending aorta cross-clamping and open cardiac massage are adjunctive procedures performed if indicated.

Survival rates of better than 40% have been reported in some subgroups of penetrating trauma arrest – specifically precordial stab wounds. Survival was dependent on resuscitative thoracotomy performed within 10 minutes of arrest secondary to penetrating chest trauma and an organized cardiac electrical rhythm being present.[26,27,28,29]

The role or resuscitative thoracotomy in blunt trauma arrest is more controversial. The rationale is to relieve rare cases of tamponade, initiate open cardiac massage, provide a route for IV fluid, clamp the descending aorta to control infra-diphragmatic haemorrhage and clamp pulmonary hilar injuries. Only a few survivors (<3%) are reported.[30]

CONCLUSION

Less than 10% of blunt thoracic trauma patients will require thoracotomy, the remainder requiring supportive care, including chest decompression and drainage. The significance and severity of chest trauma may not be obvious on initial examination. Patients with underlying airway disease and the elderly with diminished compliance are at particular risk. Delayed or inadequate ventilatory resuscitation, inadequate shock management, insufficient monitoring of arterial blood gases, and delay or failure to perform intercostal catheterization remain identifiable problems in emergency departments.

REFERENCES

1. McDermott F 1994 Severe chest injuries: problems in Victoria. Issues and controversies in the early management of major trauma. Alfred Hospital and Monash University Department of Surgery, Melbourne
2. Danne P, Brazenor G, Cade R, et al 1998 The Major Trauma Management Study: an analysis of the efficacy of current trauma care. Australian and New Zealand Journal of Surgery 68: 50–7
3. Civil I 1993 Resuscitation following injury: an end or a means? Australian and New Zealand Journal of Surgery 63: 5–10
4. Lee J, Harris JH, Duke JD, Williams JS 1997 Noncorrelation between thoracic skeleton injuries and traumatic aortic tear. Journal of Trauma 43: 400–4
5. Hehir MD, Hollands MJ, Deane SA 1990 The accuracy of the first chest X-ray in the trauma patient. Australian and New Zealand Journal of Surgery 60: 529–32
6. Brookes JG, Dunn RJ, Rogers IR 1993 Sternal fractures: A retrospective analysis of 272 cases. Journal of Trauma 35: 46–54
7. Hills MW, Delprado AM, Deane SA 1993 Sternal fractures: associated injuries and management. Journal of Trauma 35: 55–60
8. Brasel KJ, Borgstrom DC, Meyer P, Weigelt JA 1996 Predictors of outcome in blunt diaphragm rupture. Journal of Trauma 41: 484–7
9. American College of Surgeons Committee on Trauma 1997 Advanced trauma life support student manual. American College of Surgeons, p. 127
10. Blostein P, Hodgman CG 1997 Computed tomography of the chest in blunt thoracic trauma: results of a prospective study. Journal of Trauma 43: 3–18
11. American College of Surgeons Committee on Trauma 1997 Advanced trauma life support student manual. American College of Surgeons, p. 153
12. American College of Surgeons Committee on Trauma 1997 Advanced trauma life support student manual. American College of Surgeons, p. 134
13. Cohn S 1997 Pulmonary contusion: review of the clinical entity. Journal of Trauma 42: 973–9
14. Mulder DS, Barkun JS 1991 Injuries to the trachea, bronchus and oesophagus. In: Moore EE, Mattox KL, Feliciano DV (eds) Trauma. Appleton & Lange, Norwalk, pp 345–55
15. Jorden RC 1993 Penetrating chest trauma. Emergency Medicine Clinics of North America 11: 97–106
16. Fitzgerald MC, Foord K 1993 Tension pneumopericardium following blunt trauma. Emergency Medicine 5: 74–7
17. Katyal D, McLellan B, Brenneman F, Boulanger B, Sharkey P, Waddell J 1997 Lateral impact motor vehicle collisions: a significant cause of traumatic rupture of the thoracic aorta. Journal of Trauma 45: 769–72
18. Fabian T et al 1997 Prospective study of blunt aortic injury: multicenter trial of the American Association for the Surgery of Trauma. Journal of Trauma 42: 374–83
19. Cohn SM, Burns, GA, Jaffe C, Milner KA 1995 Exclusion of aortic tear in the unstable trauma patient: the utility of transosophageal echocardiography. Journal of Trauma 39: 1087–90
20. Ben-Menachem Y 1997 Assessment of blunt aortic-brachiocephalic trauma: should angiography be supplanted by transosophageal echocardiography? Journal of Trauma 42: 969–72
21. Mattox K 1997 Red River anthology. Journal of Trauma 3: 353–68
22. Camp PC, Shackford SR and the Western Trauma Association Multicenter Study Group 1997 Outcome after blunt thoracic aortic laceration: identification of a high-risk cohort. Journal of Trauma 43: 413–22
23. Jackimczyk K 1993 Blunt chest trauma. Emergency Medicine Clinics of North America 11: 81–96
24. Hirshberg A, Or J, Stein M, Walker R 1996 Transaxial gunshot injuries. Journal of Trauma 41: 460–1
25. Pickard LR, Mattox KL 1988 Thoracic trauma and indications for thoracotomy In: Mattox KL, Moore EE, Feliciano DV (eds) Trauma. Appleton & Lange, Norwalk, pp 315–20
26. Tyburski, JG, Astra, L, Wilson, RF, Dente, C, Steffes, C 2000 Factors affecting prognosis with penetrating wounds of the heart. Journal of Trauma-Injury Infection & Critical Care 48(4): 587–91
27. Battistella, FD, Nugent, W, Owings, JT, Anderson, J T 1999 Field triage of the pulseless trauma patient. Archives of Surgery 134(7): 742–6
28. Renz BM, Stout MJ 1994 Rapid right atrial cannulation for fluid infusion during resuscitative emergency department thoracotomy. Am Surg 60(12): 946–9
29. Mattox KL, Feliciano DV 1982 Role of external cardiac compression in truncal trauma. Journal of Trauma 22(11): 934–6
30. Aihara, R, Millham, FH, Blansfield, J, Hirsch EF 2001 Emergency room thoracotomy for penetrating chest injury: effect of an institutional protocol. Journal of Trauma – Injury Infection & Critical Care 50: 1027–30

2.7 LIMB TRAUMA

RICHARD HARROD

ESSENTIALS

1 The aim of treatment is pain-free return of normal function with acceptable cosmesis.

2 Limb trauma assessment is a part of the secondary survey and involves look, feel, movement, and neurovascular and functional assessment.

3 Management of fractures and dislocations consists of reduction, immobilization and rehabilitation.

4 Optimal emergency management will decrease the incidence of life- and limb-threatening complications.

INTRODUCTION

Limb trauma may be an isolated injury or part of the injury complex involved in a multitrauma presentation. In the multitrauma patient it is important not to be distracted by the limb injury and to undertake initially the primary survey and resuscitation, with limb injury management being restricted to replacement and control of revealed and concealed haemorrhage.

Hypovolaemic shock is the only acute life-threatening complication of limb trauma. Correct initial management decreases the incidence of delayed life-threatening problems such as sepsis, crush syndrome and fat embolism. Only when resuscitation is under control can the secondary survey commence, which includes limb examination and management of injuries, with the initial emphasis on limb salvage, the overall goal of treatment being the return of full, pain-free normal function and an acceptable cosmetic result. Although not strictly part of emergency care, it is vital to emphasize the importance of rehabilitation in the healing process, and this must be taken into consideration from the outset.

PRESENTATION

History and examination

The key to history taking is obtaining a good description of the mechanism of injury. This will allow determination of a pattern of injury as well as focused examination and investigation, in conjunction with a meticulous secondary survey. Problems arise when the history and examination are difficult or incomplete, due to factors such as head injury, intoxication, distracting injuries, language or extremes of age. The history should also include:

- Prehospital scene history from EMS personnel and other observers, including blood loss at scene
- Whether patient is left- or right-handed, and his or her occupation
- Tetanus prophylaxis
- Assessment of anaesthetic suitability, including allergies.

The key points of the secondary survey of limb trauma are:

- Look, feel and move – then assess the neurovascular state and limb function and compare with the opposite side.
- Examine for swelling, bruising and deformity, and check for any open wounds (potentially compound injuries).

- Feel for areas of pain, tenderness, deformity or crepitus.
- There is no need to elicit crepitus and abnormal movement at fracture sites as this increases bleeding and local acute inflammatory response, as well as causing unnecessary pain.
- Movement should be both active (patient controlled) and passive (physician controlled) to assess function, range of movement and joint stability.
- The neurovascular examination is based on an anatomical knowledge of vascular and nerve distribution. Peripheral nerve examination includes an assessment of motor and sensory components.
- The most accurate indicator of sensory function is two-point discrimination.
- Vascular injury is particularly important in penetrating injuries. The limb may be obviously ischaemic or there may be signs of vascular injury, such as absent or decreased distal pulses, ongoing bleeding from the wound, or an expanding haematoma. Occasionally a bruit may be heard. Vascular injury is *not* excluded if these findings are absent.

If the skin and soft tissue overlying the fracture site are intact then the fracture is simple or closed. Any exposure to the external environment means the fracture is an open or compound one. Compound fractures are classified as follows:

- Grade 1: Wound less than 1 cm long punctured from below (by tip of fracture fragment).
- Grade 2: Wound up to 5 cm long without contamination or crush or excessive skin loss or tissue necrosis.
- Grade 3: Large laceration with associated contamination or crush (may be closed after debridement). Periosteal stripping of bone (will require a skin flap for closure). Associated major vascular injury.
- Grade 4: Total or subtotal amputation.

INVESTIGATIONS
Plain radiographs

- This is the investigation of choice in the diagnosis of fractures and dislocations.
- At least two views of an injury site, including the joint above and below, are required to diagnose fractures. An emergency physician needs to be aware when special views are required, e.g. a skyline view of the patella.
- If there is doubt then comparison views of the opposite limb can be taken.
- Look for other indicators of injury, such as soft tissue swelling, air or foreign bodies in soft tissue or joints, and evidence of joint injury, such as effusion or lipohaemarthrosis, which suggests an intra-articular fracture is present.
- If a clinical suspicion persists then symptomatic treatment should be undertaken and reassessment and repeat X-ray organized as a part of the follow-up. New bone produced beneath the periosteum at the fracture site will become apparent radiographically.
- Interpretation of X-rays needs to be meticulous, with a viewing box and a hot light available.

Angiography

Angiography should be performed if vascular injury is obviously present or suspected. This can be done in the emergency department or in the operating theatre as part of life- or limb-saving surgery. Angiography should always be considered in penetrating limb injury and in injuries such as knee joint disruption, where the mechanism suggests blood vessel injury.

Computerized tomography scan

Computerized tomography (CT) does not have a major role in the emergency management of limb injuries but may be used to assess injuries that are difficult on plain radiology, such as carpus and tarsus injuries, and to better define alignment or fragmentation.

Magentic resonance imaging

This modality has a role in assessment of soft tissue injuries but is usually not available during the emergency department phase of care.

Ultrasound

Ultrasound is becoming more available in the emergency department setting and has a role especially in the diagnosis of non-radio-opaque foreign bodies.

MANAGEMENT

The primary survey and resuscitation always take precedence and limb injuries must not distract from this initial management. The control of external haemorrhage by pressure, the sterile dressing of open wounds and the splinting of fractures are indicated in the initial phase of care. Distal limb swelling should be anticipated, therefore, all rings and other constricting items of clothing and jewellery must be removed as early as practicable. Early tetanus prophylaxis and appropriate antibiotics for compound injuries need to be instituted. Current antibiotic guidelines for the management of muscular, skeletal and soft tissue trauma, crush injuries and stab wounds suggest the likely pathogens are *Staphylococcus aureus*, *Streptococcus pyogenes*, *Clostridium perfringens* and aerobic Gram-negative bacilli. The recommendations include a combination of flucloxacillin, gentamicin and metronidazole, or a combination of cephalothin and metronidazole.[1] The guidelines for compound fractures suggest treatment be aimed against *Staphylococcus aureus*, with flucloxacillin or cephalothin. If wound soiling, severe tissue damage or devitalized tissue is present, then gentamicin to cover Gram-negative organisms and benzylpenicillin to cover *Clostridium perfringens* are indicated.

Compound injuries should be protected from further contamination by gentle normal saline washing and coverage with a moist sterile dressing.

Ideally, a polaroid photograph can be taken of the wound and placed on the dressing to prevent future disturbance until definitive care is performed.

Decontamination of wounds

There has been little work published on the best wound management prior to definitive care in theatre. Certainly time to theatre is critical, as this reduces the incidence of wound colonization ($>10^6$ colonies per gram of tissue). Most published work on wound-cleansing solutions has been done on long-term wounds. It is known that bacteria cause local inflammation, delay wound contraction, reduce wound tensile strength and are leucocytotoxic. However, many antiseptics are also cytotoxic and a balance needs to be reached. Povidone-iodine has been shown to delay wound healing in chronic wounds and to increase infection rate. There is no evidence to suggest it has a role in the acute management of contaminated wounds. If povidone-iodine is used it should be diluted to less than 1%. Shaving should also be avoided as this causes increased infection rates due to damage of the infundibulum of hair follicles.

The most appropriate emergency management is to remove gross contamination and irrigate with normal saline. This can remove up to 90% of contaminating bacteria, and its efficacy is related to the irrigation pressure. Pulsatile pressure delivered at 7–10 psi (48–69 kPa) effectively removes debris and bacteria without disseminating micro-organisms into the deeper tissue. This pressure can be produced with a 20 mL syringe and a 19 gauge needle (and splash guard). Higher pressure can also cause tissue damage (see Wound management). There is no value in taking preoperative wound swabs unless pus is present.

Analgesia

Relief of pain should be considered early, including the use of such simple measures as fracture reduction and splinting. Narcotic analgesia should be given early unless contraindicated. Narcotics are best titrated in small aliquots i.v. until adequate analgesia is achieved without side effects. Local nerve block

and regional anaesthesia can be used if local neurological damage is not evident. A femoral nerve block is particularly useful for a fractured shaft of femur (see Chapter 21.1 Pain Relief in Emergency Medicine). Pain makes assessment of other injuries difficult and may distract both patient and clinician from less evident injuries.

Reduction

The definitive management of fractures and dislocations is reduction, immobilization and rehabilitation. Early reduction helps relieve pain and reduce progressive soft tissue damage. It also reduces damage to the overlying skin and traction pressure on nerves and arteries. Increased initial haematoma and obligate oedema lead to increased scar tissue formation and consequent increased problems with rehabilitation. If there is a suspicion of penetrating joint injury then the joint should be lavaged in the operating theatre.

Immobilization

Immobilization in the emergency department may be temporary or permanent. If a fracture is adequately reduced then a plaster cast may be sufficient. All patients who are discharged after reduction of a dislocation or the application of a plaster cast must have a radiograph after reduction to ensure correct positioning. If anatomical reduction cannot be obtained then temporary immobilization should be undertaken.

Splints that have been applied correctly by prehospital personnel need not be removed as long as a neurovascular examination can be performed. The limb should be totally exposed during the initial examination. Most injuries are splinted in an anatomical position by simple board splints or air splints: their correct use prevents further tissue damage and assists in transport, as well as providing pain relief. The joints above and below the injury need to be immobilized, and the limb is then elevated. Fractures of the femoral shaft need immobilization with a traction splint because of associated muscle spasm. There are several devices (e.g. Thomas, Donway) that operate on the principle of a proximal ring engaging the ischial tuberosity and then longitudinal traction being applied through an attachment to the ankle. The circulation needs to be checked after application.

Rehabilitation with the goal of pain-free return of normal function begins in the emergency department. Early mobilization of non-involved joints must be encouraged to prevent limb disuse syndromes.

Early orthopaedic and other specialist consultation is vital, as these units will be responsible for further management and follow-up.

DISPOSITION

Admission may be required for the definitive management of limb injuries or because of other injuries.

If the limb injury has been definitively managed in the emergency department and the patient has adequate support to cope at home, then discharge can be organized with specific discharge instructions. If a plaster has been applied then advice about signs and symptoms of tightness should be given to the patient and carers verbally, and written instructions should also be issued. This should be noted on the history. It is particularly important to emphasize that pain un-relieved by simple analgesia and elevation, or increasing pain under a plaster, demands urgent review and splitting of the plaster and underlying padding.

Strict instruction to rest and elevate the injured part to reduce swelling particularly in the first 48 hours, is important. Analgesia should be given and written advice about the mobilization of un-involved joints provided. A plaster should be reviewed within 24 hours (advising an earlier return if there are problems), and an outpatient appointment with an appropriate specialist must be arranged.

COMPLICATIONS OF LIMB TRAUMA

Arterial injury

Arterial injury is both a life-threatening and a limb-threatening complication that must be diagnosed quickly and dealt with urgently. An ischaemic time of 4–6 hours results in permanent damage to nerves and muscles. The initial assessment of limb trauma always involves an assessment of distal circulation. Peripheral pulses should be assessed and sides compared. It is important to exclude hypovolaemic shock and consequent generalized inadequate tissue perfusion as a cause of diminished pulses. If there is evidence of decreased peripheral circulation then limb deformity should be corrected and any tight splints, dressings or plasters loosened.

Arterial injury, if it occurs, may be partial or complete. Complete transection, from either penetrating trauma or bony fragments, leads to initial brisk bleeding. This is often followed by vessel wall contraction and clotting and, if associated with a decrease in mean arterial pressure, will often cease. This is the basis of the argument for hypotensive resuscitation in patients with penetrating injury. A large fluid load will often distend the contracted vessel and cause vigorous bleeding to recommence. Partial vessel wall laceration may lead to more prolonged bleeding, as the vessel wall is unable to retract.

Arterial injury is diagnosed by distal signs or local signs at the injury site. These include decreased or absent pulses, or evidence of limb ischaemia (pallor or cyanosis) without systemic evidence of hypovolaemia to explain this finding. Local signs include evidence of brisk, bright blood loss from an open wound, or expanding haematoma in a closed wound. A bruit may be detected. Delayed signs include false aneurysm formation or arteriovenous fistulae. If pulses cannot be palpated then a Doppler stethoscope should be used to listen for flow. Palpable pulses may be misleading. In up to 15% of significant arterial injuries the distal pulses may initially be normal: this may be due to an intimal flap and progressive thrombosis.

There are also specific sites where arteries are at particular risk and angiography may need to be considered, even if there is no evidence of vascular compromise. These include:

- The brachial artery at the proximal humeral shaft
- The brachial artery in the supracondylar area of the humerus
- The deep femoral artery at the subtrochanteric level of the femur
- The popliteal artery at the level of the adductor canal in the supracondylar area of the femur
- The popliteal artery at the level of trifurcation adjacent to the metaphyseal area of the tibia (particularly associated with a dislocated knee)
- The anterior tibial artery in the middle third of the tibia.

Angiography is the investigation of choice.

Nerve injury

Nerve injury results from direct laceration in penetrating trauma, from a fractured bone fragment, or indirectly from contusion or stretching. It is important to exclude ischaemia as a cause of neurological symptoms and signs.

Nerve injuries can be classified as follows:

- **Neuropraxia.** A transient alteration in conduction, usually as a result of mild contusion. There is usually an early return of function within days, and complete return of function within 8 weeks.
- **Axonotmesis.** Complete denervation with an intact nerve sheath, usually as a result of blunt trauma causing severe contusion or stretching. The nerve reinnervates over months, with axonal regeneration along the intact nerve sheath.
- **Neurotmesis.** Results from complete division of a nerve and its sheath. There is no spontaneous resolution and surgical repair is required.

Any evidence of nerve injury associated with penetrating trauma will require exploration and repair in theatre, allowing optimal operating conditions. With blunt trauma it is vital to reduce all fractures and dislocations and to ensure adequate arterial supply if there is evidence of neurological dysfunction. It is vital always to reassess neurovascular status after manipulations and immobilization, to ensure that no damage has occurred during the procedure. It is rare in blunt trauma to require exploration for nerve injury. Some common nerve injuries that do occur are:

- Axillary nerve injury with fractures and dislocations of the shoulder
- Radial nerve injury with fractures of the distal third of the humerus
- Ulnar nerve injury with fracture of the medial epicondyle of the humerus
- Median nerve injury in the carpal tunnel associated with displaced wrist fractures (may require urgent carpal tunnel decompression)
- Sciatic nerve injury with fractures and posterior dislocation of the hip
- Peroneal nerve injury with fracture of the neck of the fibula.

It is possible with nerve injury to delay repair if complete disruption is thought unlikely, and to follow progress with serial EMG.

FAT EMBOLISM

Fat embolism may follow the fracture of a single long bone or, more usually, in the patient with multiple fractures, associated with prolonged hypovolaemia. It occurs between 6 and 24 hours after injury and presents as adult respiratory distress syndrome.

The clinical signs are tachypnoea, tachycardia, increasing confusion, and the appearance of petechial haemorrhage on the upper part of the body, including the conjunctivae. The emboli result from direct embolism of fat from the bone marrow into the venous plexus of long bones, and also from alterations in lipid solubility in trauma, causing embolism to the brain and lungs and other parts of the body.

There is no diagnostic test and, in patients with hypoxaemia after trauma, fat embolism needs to be considered along with pulmonary contusion, post-traumatic shock lung (ARDS), and overhydration.

There is no specific treatment and management is optimal control of oxygenation, including mechanical ventilatory support if required. The condition is self-limiting but may be exacerbated during manipulation of long-bone fractures, particularly if internal fixation is required.

COMPARTMENT SYNDROME

Compartment syndrome is caused by increased pressure in a limb compartment due to bleeding and oedema. Compartments are anatomical regions bound by bone, interosseous membrane and fascia, and are relatively inexpansile. Increasing compartment pressure decreases vascular flow, particularly in the small vessels supplying muscle and nerves initially. Presentation usually consists of a combination of ischaemic muscle pain (difficult to control pain in excess of that expected of the injury) and distal neurological signs due to nerve ischaemia and direct pressure effects. However, increased compartment pressure may not be greater than mean arterial pressure, and so distal pulses will be palpable even with significant compartment syndrome. The syndrome can be exacerbated by external pressure on the compartment from tight casts or dressings.

Causes of compartment syndrome include fractures, crush or wringer injuries, injection into compartments, snakebite, electric shock, burns, muscle trauma and exercise. An awareness of the possibility needs always to be borne in mind, and further elevation of pressure must be avoided. Thus splinting to prevent further bleeding and the avoidance of tight casts and dressings is essential.

Compartment syndrome most commonly occurs in the leg (anterior, lateral, deep posterior and superficial posterior compartments) (Fig. 2.7.1) and in the forearm (volar and dorsal compartments). Less commonly it can occur in the hand (interosseous), thigh (quadriceps), arm (deltoid and biceps) and buttock (gluteal).

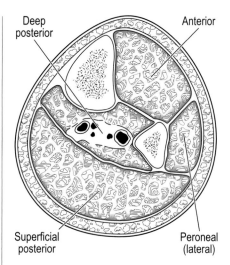

Fig. 2.7.1 Compartments of the leg.

The diagnosis is made by a combination of clinical symptoms and signs, and by direct compartment pressure measurement. The key symptom is pain out of proportion to that expected of the injury, exacerbated by passive stretching of the muscles in that compartment. There may be associated muscle weakness but this is difficult to assess because of the pain. Hyperaesthesia or paraesthesia may also be present. On palpation the compartment often feels tense. Sides must always be compared. There will also be marked tenderness. If suspected, then pressure monitoring is essential. Pressure monitoring may also be required if the patient is unconscious, intoxicated, or has distracting injuries. Some units continuously monitor compartment pressures in such patients.

The normal resting muscle pressure is about 4 mmHg. A tissue pressure greater than 40 mmHg impairs local circulation, whereas a pressure less than 30 mmHg usually does not. An initial pressure greater than 50 mmHg is an absolute indication for compartment pressure release. The intracompartmental tissue pressure is best measured using a commercial product (e.g. Stryker intracompartmental pressure monitor), although pressures can be measured by inserting an intra-arterial pressure monitor into the compartment using a saline-filled intravenous set.

If compartment syndrome is diagnosed the management is surgical decompression of the affected compartment with fasciotomy.

CRUSH SYNDROME

Crush syndrome is a systemic manifestation of an injury to a limb by a compressive force of sufficient duration and severity to cause significant muscle crush injury and cell death. It is a time- and pressure-dependent phenomenon. The compressive force is usually external, e.g. a wooden beam or brick wall, but the compressive force may be generated by the patient's own weight, e.g. coma from stroke or overdose.

The muscle is damaged by a combination of factors, leading to rhabdomyolysis:

- Vascular compression due to external pressure preventing arterial flow. This leads to initial anaerobic cell metabolism, cell death and cell wall breakdown.
- Direct compressive forces due to external pressure and raised compartment pressure, causing disruption of cell membrane integrity directly.
- Extreme compression force may cause immediate mechanical cell disruption and death.

Substances released during rhabdomyolysis, especially after ischaemia and anaerobic metabolism, include lactic acid, potassium, myoglobin, uric acid, phosphate, lysosomes, muscle enzymes (especially creatine kinase, which is useful as a biochemical marker), superoxide and other free radicals, histamine, leukotrienes and peroxides. There is also damage to blood vessels, leading to a capillary leakage syndrome and local bleeding. This disintegrating local environment, however, is usually completely insolated from the rest of the systemic circulation as venous return is impeded. The major systemic problems occur with the release of compressive force and reperfusion. Damaged vessels start to bleed, capillaries leak and cause third space loss, and oedema develops. The products of anaerobic metabolism and cell-wall breakdown return to the central circulation, causing hyperkalaemic acidosis and myoglobinuria. Sudden cardiac arrhythmias can occur, and the longer-term problems of myoglobinuria cause acute renal failure, particularly if associated with hypovolaemia and an acidic urine.

Diagnosis is based on the history of a crush injury. Examination may reveal tender, swollen muscles and often the overlying skin is blistered as a result of ischaemic pressure. The urine will be dark red-brown (machinery oil) and will test positive for blood, but no red blood cells will be seen under the microscope. Biochemical rests will reflect the cellular breakdown, with elevated CK being the major biochemical indicator.

The key to treatment is to anticipate the problem and resuscitate adequately, with fluid replacement to maintain a high urine output. Alkalinization of the patient with sodium bicarbonate prior to extrication is helpful. ECG monitoring should be used to look for evidence of arrhythmias secondary to acid-base and electrolyte flux. Hyperkalaemia is most frequent. Local management of associated limb injuries, including splinting and a careful check for compartment syndrome, is required. Ongoing fluid resuscitation matched to a urine output of 2 mL/kg/h is vital. CVP monitoring may be required, and mannitol may be used to maintain urine output. Mannitol also theoretically helps by binding oxygen free radicals. If, despite adequate filling, the urine output is inadequate, then dopamine is required. The urinary pH needs to be checked regularly, as an acidic urine increases myoglobin toxicity. Bicarbonate at 50 mmol/h will generally maintain an alkaline urine. Haemodialysis will be required if the patient is anuric.

CONTROVERSIES

❶ Emergency department management of wounds associated with compound limb injuries. Currently, the most appropriate management involves irrigation with saline to reduce contamination. There is no evidence for the use of antiseptic agents.

❷ The role of angiography in limb injuries associated with arterial injury, with no arterial compromise clinically. It may be better to plan angiography on the basis of associated injury and mechanism.

❸ Which patients should receive limb compartment pressure monitoring. Currently, many units are reluctant to monitor compartment pressures without clinical evidence of compartment syndrome.

REFERENCES

1. Victorian Drug Usage Advisory Committee 1999 Antibiotic Guidelines, 10th edn.
2. Driscoll P, Skinner D 1999 ABC of Major Trauma, 3rd edn. British Medical Journal Publishing
3. Rosen Barkin (eds) 1997 Emergency Medicine: Concepts and Clinical Practice. Mosby Year Book
4. McCrae R 1994 Practical Fracture Treatment, 3rd edn. Churchill Livingstone, London

2.8 RADIOLOGY IN MAJOR TRAUMA

TONY JOSEPH • ROGER HARRIS • KAREN FALK

ESSENTIALS

1 Trauma team leader should supervise the primary and secondary survey and the initial trauma series X-rays.

2 The trauma team should be mindful of the risks of irradiation and wear adequate protection.

3 The full 'trauma series' X-rays should be done unless there is a good reason for not doing so.

4 Evaluation of facial trauma requires an adequate clinical and radiological examination.

5 Correct evaluation of the cervical spine X-rays will exclude most bony cervical spine abnormalities.

6 Injuries to the thoracolumbar spine should be actively sought in the multi-trauma patient.

7 Chest computerized tomography (CT) has become a useful screening test for mediastinal or large vessel injury.

8 CT pelvis is invaluable for the classification of pelvic fractures.

EMERGENCY DEPARTMENT RECEPTION

The reception of the major trauma patient requires planning and organization.

This involves adequate communication by the ambulance officers preferably directly from the scene to the hospital resuscitation area to allow time to assemble the trauma team. Membership of the trauma team will vary from place to place and will include medical, nursing and radiology staff.

The information that should be available from the ambulance personnel to the trauma team leader on arrival will include mechanism of injury, injuries, treatment given and vital signs (MITV).

The team leader will supervise the completion of the primary and secondary surveys as well as coordinate the initial trauma X-ray series which are usually taken at the completion of the primary survey. There is no place for any radiological investigation until the primary survey and initial resuscitation are complete.

The initial trauma X-rays (lateral cervical spine, chest and pelvic X-rays) are best done by use of an overhead X-ray tube rather than a bulky mobile X-ray unit. X-rays taken by portable equipment are usually inferior in quality to fixed equipment in the radiology department. The reasons for this include the lower power of the portable machines and less effective grids for the portable films resulting in more photon scatter reaching the film. In order to reduce magnification distortion the tube-film distance for the chest X-ray (CXR) and lateral cervical (Cx) spine should ideally be 1.8 metres (72 inches)[1] and the X-ray plate should be as close as possible to the area being imaged. The reality of achieving 1.8 m target-film distance in the trauma room is difficult to achieve.

The film processing unit should be as close as possible to the resuscitation area to enable rapid viewing of the films by the trauma clinicians before a formal report by a radiology specialist. If possible there should be a joint review of the X-rays by the senior trauma clinician and the radiologist.

HAZARDS OF RADIATION

Exposure of both trauma team members and patients to ionizing radiation should be minimized by the wearing of protective lead gowns and thyroid shields. The number of X-rays in the resuscitation area should be kept to a minimum and the use of permanent lead barriers should be considered.

Radiation exposure decreases inversely with the square of the distance from the source.

The absorbed dose (mGy) (typical skin radiation dose) in the primary beam has been estimated in the 'trauma series' to be a total of 7.2 mGy. This breaks down to 0.2 mGy for the AP chest X-ray, 4.0 mGy for the AP pelvic X-ray and 3.0 mGy for the lateral cervical spine.[2] Note that 1 mGy = 0.1 rad. Adverse effects to a developing foetus from a dose of irradiation have been calculated to occur at a dose of 50 to 100 mGy. The dose for adverse event to occur in a trauma team member is unknown but estimated to be much higher.

Radiation dose may also be calculated in 'whole body effective doses' in microSieverts (µSv). Table 2.8.1 gives calculated doses for selected radiological procedures as well as some 'naturally occurring' sources.[3,4]

Table 2.8.1 Whole body effective doses (µSv)	
Examination	Radiation dose (µSv)
CXR	40
Pelvis X-ray	1100
SXR	100
Chest CT	7800
Abdo CT	7600
Pelvis CT	7100
Head CT	1800
Natural sources	
Background (1 year)	2400
1 week skiing	15
Round trip transcontinental US Flight	60

THE TRAUMA SERIES

The initial 'trauma series' X-rays should consist of the lateral cervical (Cx) spine, AP chest (CXR) and AP pelvic X-rays. The lateral Cx spine X-ray should be taken with a team member exerting gentle traction on the arms in order to pull down the shoulders and expose the lower Cx spine to the C7-T1 junction. Traction on the arms is contraindicated in the presence of known cervical spine or cord pathology.

Systematic examination of this film which includes assessment of alignment, bony structures, cartilage and soft tissue (ABCS) will detect 80–90 % of bony Cx spine injuries[5] (Fig. 2.8.1).

The CXR performed is usually a supine antero-posterior (AP) rather than erect (PA) film due to the inability to clear the spine both clinically and radiologically. This film should include both clavicles, all ribs, lung fields, mediastinum and diaphragm. If there is adequate penetration, the thoracic spine may be

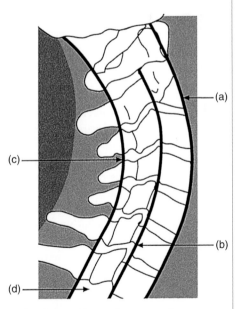

Fig. 2.8.1 Normal structural relationships of the lateral cervical spine.
(a) Anterior vertebral line
(b) Posterior vertebral line
(c) Spinolaminar line
(d) Spinal canal.
(From Rosen P, Doris PE, Barkin RM, Barkin SZ, Markovchick VJ (eds) 1992 Diagnostic Radiology in Emergency Medicine. Mosby-Year Book Inc., St Louis)

seen. The mediastinum is often magnified due to the frontal nature of the film and this should be taken into account. This X-ray film will exclude life-threatening injuries such as haemo-pneumothorax and may show signs of major vessel injury indicated by a widening of the mediastinum.

The pelvic X-ray will include all the bony pelvic components and the hip joints. The object of this view is to provide information regarding the integrity of the bony pelvic structures and the pelvic contents

SPECIFIC REGIONAL RADIOLOGY

Head

Head trauma is responsible for 50-70% of the mortality associated with major trauma. The spectrum of head injury ranges from mild concussion to major open head injury not compatible with life.

A computerized tomography (CT) brain scan is the investigation of choice for all but minor head injuries. See Table 2.8.2 for CT indications in serious head injury. A non-contrast CT brain scan is adequate for the detection of intracranial haematoma or cerebral oedema with or without mid-line shift. Bone windows should be performed if there is a suspicion of a skull fracture (Table 2.8.2).

In a recent large prospective study of over 2000 patients with minor head trauma as defined by a history of any loss of consciousness, or amnesia and a GCS of 15, Miller et al[6] concluded that in the presence of one or more of: severe headache, nausea, vomiting and a depressed fracture on physical examination, there was a significantly increased risk of the presence of an intracranial lesion, which would require neurosurgical intervention. However, they found that of the patients with none of the above risk factors for a significant intracranial lesion, there was a 3.7% incidence of abnormal CT scans. These abnormalities included cerebral contusions, subdural haematomas and skull fractures, but did not require neurosurgical intervention. The significance

Table 2.8.2 Indications for a CT brain in significant head injury

Glasgow Coma Score (GCS) <9 after resuscitation
Neurological deterioration of 2 or more points on the GCS
Drowsiness or confusion (GCS 9-13 that persists for longer than 2 hours)
Persistent headache or vomiting
Focal neurological signs (e.g pupillary abnormalities or focal neurological signs)
Skull fracture known or suspected
Penetrating injury known or suspected
Age over 50 years with a suspicious mechanism of injury
Any head injury in a patient on anticoagulation therapy

of an abnormal CT in these patients is unclear as there is little evidence to support its predictive value for neurological outcomes.

The Canadian CT Head Rule[7] for patients with minor head injury does much to answer the question as to which patients with minor head injury, as characterized by GCS 13–15, will require CT scan of the brain. The authors found that the presence of any of the high-risk factors (Table 2.8.2) was 100% sensitive for predicting the need for neurological intervention. They also found that the presence of medium-risk factors was 98.4% sensitive for detecting clinically important brain injury.

They postulated that patient care would be standardized and improved, and that the accuracy of this rule would lead to large savings in health-care expenditure.

Skull X-Ray (SXR)

There are very few indications for a SXR in the presence of neurotrauma if a CT scanner is available. If a fracture is visible on a SXR, this will raise the likelihood of the presence of an intracranial haematoma and the need for a CT brain scan.

A SXR may be of value in the presence of a penetrating metallic injury to the head, e.g. a bullet, as this will cause significant artefact on the CT scan. The SXR will demonstrate that the skull table has been penetrated and will delineate the position of the bullet. If a compound depressed fracture of the skull is suspected clinically, a CT brain scan should be performed. This complicated fracture is considered a neurosurgical emergency because the underlying dura is lacerated and this significantly increases the risk of infection, such as meningitis or brain abscess. A depressed fracture increases the likelihood of post-traumatic epilepsy.

Cerebral angiography

Angiography will be required if there is a clinical suspicion of a traumatic dissection of either the carotid or vertebral arteries.

If a CT brain scan demonstrates a cerebral aneurysm or an arterio-venous malformation, angiography will be required to delineate the lesion.

Some trauma centres use carotid Doppler instead of cerebral angiography for the demostration of vascular injuries in the presence of penetrating head or neck trauma. Although Doppler is less invasive it is more user dependant than cerebral angiography which is considered the gold standard.

Magnetic resonance imaging

There is no indication for magnetic resonance imaging (MRI) scanning of the brain in acute neurotrauma due to the technical difficulties associated with the presence of patient monitoring and life-support equipment which interferes with the MRI scanning process.

FACE

Facial trauma may range from the relatively trivial undisplaced nasal bone fractures to the life-threatening problems of airway protection and haemorrhage associated with mid-face (Le Fort) fractures. There may also be underlying cerebral injury associated with frontal bone fractures.

The commonest injury to the mid-face is the blow-out fracture (Fig. 2.8.2) caused by a direct blow to the orbit which

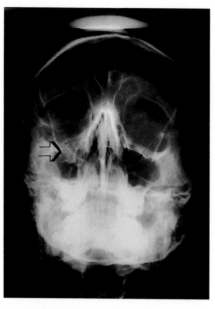

Fig. 2.8.2 Waters view. Blow out fracture right orbit (arrow) with fluid in right maxillary sinus.

results in a fracture of the orbital floor or the medial wall of the orbit. There may be tenderness over the fractured bone associated with diplopia due to entrapment of orbital contents or (less commonly) visual disturbance due to globe or optic nerve injury. These fractures are best seen on both the Waters (Fig. 2.8.3) view and the Caldwell views. There is often blood or soft tissue shadows in the maxillary antrum, but the fractures are difficult to see on plain X-rays and require plain tomography or a CT scan for clearer definition of displacement of bony segments. Providing there is no visual impairment, entrapment of orbital contents is treated less urgently with elevation of the depressed fracture at 10–14 days if diplopia persists once the initial swelling settles.

Mandibular fractures are usually obvious clinically due to pain, malocclusion and drooling. PA and oblique X-rays may be used to show mandibular fractures, but a panoramic view in the form of an ortho-pantomogram (OPG) provides optimal demonstration of the ramus, body and angle of the mandible as well as good visualization of the mandibular neck and condyle. The patient is required to remain vertically upright for an OPG and, hence, this form of imaging cannot

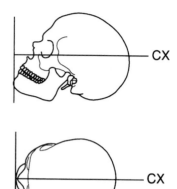
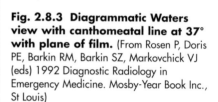

Fig. 2.8.3 Diagrammatic Waters view with canthomeatal line at 37° with plane of film. (From Rosen P, Doris PE, Barkin RM, Barkin SZ, Markovchick VJ (eds) 1992 Diagnostic Radiology in Emergency Medicine. Mosby-Year Book Inc., St Louis)

be performed until a cervical spine injury has been excluded. Some information may be obtained from a Towne projection of the skull that may show fractures of the condyle and neck of the mandible (Fig. 2.8.4). Tomography and CT scan of the temporo-mandibular joint are further means of assessing the mandible.

Fractures of the zygoma are classified as (a) tripod fractures and (b) isolated fractures of the zygomatic arch.

Tripod fractures (Fig. 2.8.5) are usually caused by a significant force to the body of the zygoma or the malar eminence. The three fractures that constitute the tripod fracture are located in the inferior orbital margin, the lateral orbital margin or zygomatico-frontal suture and the zygomatic arch. The zygomatic arch may also be visualized by a submento-vertical X-ray (Fig. 2.8.6) or tangential views. In addition, the lateral wall of the maxillary sinus is often fractured. The presence of one of the fractures in the tripod series should raise the suspicion of other possible fractures and is an indication for further plain radiology or CT evaluation.

The Le Fort fractures (Fig. 2.8.7) are due to direct trauma to the mid-face. The Le Fort 1 fracture involves the maxilla at the level of the nasal floor and will allow mobility of the palate. The Le Fort 2 fracture passes through the nasal bones, as well as medial, inferior and lateral walls

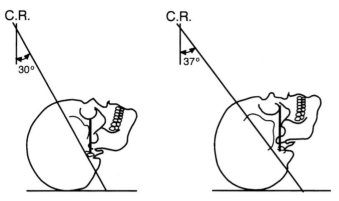

Fig. 2.8.4 Diagrammatic representation of Towne view. (From Rosen P, Doris PE, Barkin RM, Barkin SZ, Markovchick VJ (eds) 1992 Diagnostic Radiology in Emergency Medicine. Mosby-Year Book Inc., St Louis)

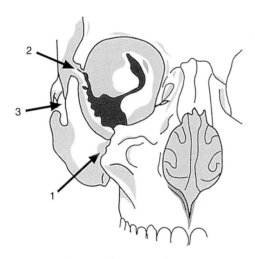

**Fig. 2.8.5 Tripod fracture showing fracture of
(1) Inferior orbital margin
(2) Lateral orbital margin
(3) Zygomatic arch.**
(From Rosen P, Doris PE, Barkin RM, Barkin SZ, Markovchick VJ (eds) 1992 Diagnostic Radiology in Emergency Medicine. Mosby-Year Book Inc., St Louis)

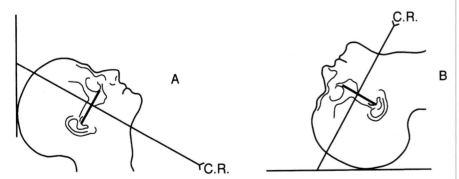

Fig. 2.8.6 Diagrammatic representation of submento-vertical (axial) projection will give good views of the zygomatic arch. (From Rosen P, Doris PE, Barkin RM, Barkin SZ, Markovchick VJ (eds) 1992 Diagnostic Radiology in Emergency Medicine. Mosby-Year Book Inc., St Louis)

Table 2.8.3 Minor head injury indications for CT scan
Canadian CT Head Rule Risk Factors
High risk
Failure to reach Glasgow Coma Score =15 within 2 hours
Suspected open skull fracture
Any sign of fracture in base of skull
>2 episodes of vomiting
Age >65
Medium risk
Amnesia prior to impact >30 minutes
Dangerous mechanism of injury

of the maxillary antrum, The Le Fort 3 fracture involves the nasal bones, the medial and lateral orbital walls, and zygomatic arch.

Some facial fractures are unable to be classified due to marked fragmentation of the bones and are termed as 'central facial smash'. Plain X-rays are often unhelpful in making the diagnosis and the best information is obtained from coronal CT scans with 3-D reformatting.

Frontal sinus fractures occur commonly due to direct force and are often compound with the risk of associated intracranial infection. There may be an associated intracranial haematoma or cerebral contusion. These fractures are best demonstrated on the Towne, Caldwell and lateral skull X-rays, but may also require CT scan to determine the involvement of posterior sinus wall fracture that often requires surgical exploration for debridement and repair.

SPINE

Cervical spine

Cervical spine injuries can be classified into those with fractures and no neurological deficit, and those with fractures associated with neurological deficit. There is a small group of cord injuries classified as spinal cord injury without radiological abnormality (SCIWORA) that occur mainly in children.

The cervical spinal column is the most frequently injured part of the spinal canal (60%)[8] due to its flexibility and exposure. Any patient with significant blunt trauma and some patients who have penetrating

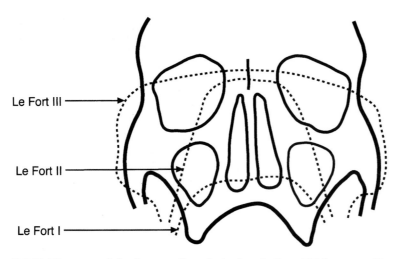

Fig. 2.8.7 Diagram of the fracture lines in Le Fort I, II and III fractures (Courtesy of Dr K Falk)

Le Fort III

Le Fort II

Le Fort I

injuries are at risk for cervical spine fracture.[9]

Patients who sustain blunt trauma injury have an estimated overall incidence of cervical spine fracture of 3–8%.[9] It has been estimated that up to 30% of patients with cervical spine fractures have an additional injury above the clavicles[9]. Despite this, meta-analysis of multiple publications cannot demonstrate a definite association between any single injury above the clavicles and cervical spine injury. There is considerable evidence to confirm that patients with an altered level of consciousness are at increased risk for cervical spine fracture[10].

Ryan et al[11] found, however, that if there was a fracture of C1-C2, there was a 9% chance of a cervical fracture below C3; hence the importance of imaging the entire cervical spine to the cervico-thoracic junction. Unconscious patients with a significant mechanism of injury should have full spinal precautions until there is the opportunity for clinical and radiological evaluation of the spinal column and its contents.

Absolute indications for radiology of the cervical spine include patients who present with signs of cord injury and those with an altered level of consciousness. Other indications for imaging of the cervical spine in victims of trauma are stated in Table 2.8.4 as derived from the NEXUS Study (National Emergency X-Radiography Utilization Study)[12].

The NEXUS study was a very large validation study that included over 34 000 patients and was 99.6% sensitive for clinically important cervical spine injuries. However, the specificity was only 12.9%, which led to some concern that cervical X-rays may actually increase. Moreover, there was no inter-rater reliability assessed for assessment of 'intoxication' and the presence of 'distracting injuries'.

The Canadian C-Spine Rule for radiography in alert and stable trauma patients[13] may be more clinically useful in that it comprises three main questions in a prospective cohort study.

❶ Is there a presence of any high risk factor which requires radiography? e.g. age >65, dangerous mechanism, limb paraesthesias.
❷ Is there any low risk factor which allows assessment of range of motion? e.g. simple rear end collision, sitting position in the emergency

department, able to walk at any time after injury, delayed onset of neck pain, absence of midline Cx spine tenderness.
❸ Can the patient rotate the neck 45° to left and right.

If 2. and 3. were positive, then no imaging was required.

This rule demonstrated 100% sensitivity and 42.5% specificity for clinically important cervical spine injuries. There was good interobserver agreement for each variable with κ value >0.6 and strong association with outcome (spinal injury) P < 0.05.

The presence or absence of a cervical spine or cord injury is determined on both clinical and radiological grounds.

Children who are less than 2 years of age and with a suggestive mechanism of injury should have plain radiology of the cervical spine to exclude cervical bone injury. If the plain X-rays require further clarification, a CT of the cervical spine should be performed. Similarly, the above criteria do not apply to the elderly who, due to the relative immobility of the cervical spine or due to pre-existing spinal disease, may sustain cervical spine fractures even in the presence of a seemingly trivial injury.[9]

Alignment

Inspection of alignment (Fig. 2.8.1) should include the four lordotic lines that are: anterior and posterior vertebral lines, as well as the spinolaminar line and tips of the spinous processes. In adults up to 1.0 mm of anterior subluxation (and up to 3 mm in children) may be normal in a true lateral film taken at 1.8 m. This variant of normal may be confirmed by normal alignment of the spinolaminar line and careful flexion/extension films if

Table 2.8.4 Indications for X-ray views of the cervical spine in a multi-trauma patient
Disturbed conscious state e.g. head injury, intoxication for any reason
Any neurological motor or sensory signs
Neck pain or midline cervical tenderness
Other major distracting injuries in a multi-trauma patient

Table 2.8.5 Radiological examination of the lateral cervical spine	
A	Alignment
B	Bony Structures
C	Cartilage spaces
S	Soft Tissue

the patient is alert and neurologically intact. Indications for flexion/extension films are ongoing pain or tenderness of the cervical spine in a patient who is neurologically intact and fully alert. The patient must be able to flex and extend his or her neck voluntarily and these X-rays should be supervised by the medical officer who ordered the investigation.

True pseudosubluxation is commonest in children up to the age of 8 years, but may be seen up to age 18 years.[5] It commonly occurs between C2-3 and, less commonly, at the C3-4 and C4-5 levels. The key radiological feature in determining pathological from non-pathological subluxation is the preservation of the spinolaminar line in all lateral views including the cross-table lateral and careful flexion/extension views [5].

Angulation between adjacent vertebrae up to 11° may be normal.[14] The sagittal (AP) diameter of the spinal canal should be measured. At the C2 level the lower limit radiographic measurement of the A-P diameter of the spinal canal is 14 mm and the upper limit of the cord AP measurement is 11 mm. At the C7 level the lower limit of the AP canal diameter is 12 mm and the upper limit of the cord measurement is 9 mm.[15]

Bony canal

All the cervical vertebrae should be systematically examined including vertebral body, pedicles, facet joints, laminae and spinous processes and the interspinous distance (Table 2.8.5).

In the upper cervical spine a line drawn along the clivus to the tip of the odontoid should point to the junction of the anterior and middle thirds of the odontoid peg. A line drawn tangentially to the lamina of C1 should intersect the posterior margin of the foramen magnum. The space between the odontoid and the anterior ring of C1 measured at its most inferior margin should not exceed 2.5 mm in adults and may be up to 4.5 mm in children. If this distance is exceeded there may be a rupture of the transverse ligament of the odontoid peg (Fig. 2.8.8).

The 'ring' of increased radio-density formed by the odontoid process and the

facet joints of C1-C2 is known as 'Harris ring'. This ring should be intact anteriorly, superiorly and posteriorly indicating an intact odontoid process and facet joints of C1-2. A type-2 fracture of the odontoid process may be visible on the lateral Cx spine X-ray.

Cartilage

All the spaces between adjacent vertebrae should be inspected for equality.

Soft tissue

The pre-vertebral soft tissue should be inspected. A distance greater than 7 mm at C2 and 22 mm at C6 in the adult indicates the presence of a pre-vertebral haematoma[16]. If this is present, then a fracture or ligamentous disruption must be excluded. In children the upper pre-vertebral space may be larger than in adults due to increased nasopharyngeal lymphoid tissue and it may also increase in infants when crying. When the soft tissues are abnormal, further radiological investigation is indicated to exclude a bony or (more rarely) a ligamentous injury.

Atlanto-occipital and atlantoaxial bony injuries

Occipital condyle[17] and C1-C2 fractures are often missed on the lateral cervical spine X-ray with the only indication of a fracture being an increase in soft tissue

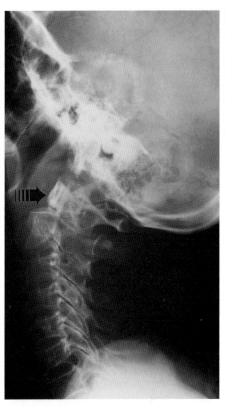

Fig. 2.8.8 Lateral cervical spine X-ray showing Type 2 fracture of the odontoid peg (arrow).

swelling in this area. The initial lateral cervical spine X-ray should be accompanied by an open mouth (odontoid process) and an A-P view. The three films will exclude up to 95% of bony cervical

Table 2.8.6 Examination of the lateral Cx spine X-ray
Upper Cx Spine (occipital condyles to C2)
Clivoodontoid relationship
C1-odontoid measurement
2.0 to 2.5 mm in adults
4.0 to 4.5 mm in children
Retropharyngeal space
Posterior pharyngeal wall to anteroinferior body of C2 (7 mm in adults and children)
Lower Cx Spine (C3-7)
Anteroinferior margin of C3 to pharyngeal airway (4 to 5 mm)
Prevertebral fat stripe
Retrotracheal spaces (posterior tracheal wall to anteroinferior body of C6)
Normal in adults, ≤22 mm
Normal in children, ≤14 mm
Anterior spinal line
Posterior spinal line
Spinolaminar line
Disc spaces
Facet joints
Spinous processes and interspinous distance

Source: Reprinted from *Imaging of Orthopedic Trauma* ed 2 by TH Berquist, 1991, Raven Press, © Mayo Foundation.

spine injuries.[5] The open mouth (odontoid) view should be inspected for alignment of the lateral masses of C1-C2, which is abnormal in the Jefferson fracture, fracture of the odontoid process (Types 1–3) and rotatory subluxation of C1 on C2. Rotation of the head can simulate pathological malalignment in this region. The A-P view of the cervical spine should be checked for alignment of the articular pillars and vertebral bodies. The spinous processes should be centred and deviation of these from the midline may indicate a unilateral facet dislocation. Widening of the interspinous distance may indicate subluxation or dislocation. Fractures and dislocations may cause malalignment or compression of the vertebral bodies. Conventional tomography may be utilized in the patient with a suspected odontoid fracture, but a CT scan with sagittal and coronal reconstruction is preferable.

Many centres routinely perform a CT scan of the occipital condyles and the C1-C2 area at the same time as a CT brain scan in order to exclude such fractures. If there is a difficulty in visualizing the C7-T1 junction, a swimmer's view or oblique views of the lower cervical spine may be useful. If the above are inconclusive, a CT scan of the lower cervical spine is indicated.

If no fracture is seen on the three-view films in a patient with continuing pain or midline cervical tenderness without neurological deficit, careful flexion/extension lateral X-rays of the cervical spine are indicated as described above.

Any fracture of the cervical spine, which involves the vertebral foramina, may involve the vertebral artery and consideration should be given to assessing the vertebral artery for acute dissection by angiography. Vertebral artery dissection may result in brainstem ischaemia or infarction.

MRI (Table 2.8.6)

Indications MRI of the cervical spine include:

- Patients with complete or incomplete neurological deficit
- Deteriorating neurological status

Table 2.8.7 Spinal abnormalities seen on the MRI scan
Spinal-cord injury
Disc herniation
Epidural haematoma
Epidural abscess
Bone fracture/dislocation
Ligamentous rupture

Table 2.8.8 Conditions unsuitable for MRI scan
Metallic components, e.g bullets, aneurysm clips
Haemodynamically unstable patients
Patients requiring ventilation and **extensive** physiological monitoring

- Suspected ligamentous or intervertebral disc injury.

MRI has largely superceded CT myelography in spinal trauma due to the ability to provide clear and concise pictures of all structures particularly the spinal cord, intervertebral discs and soft tissues. Bony structures are also demonstrated but fine bony detail is best seen on a CT scan. An MRI scan may show abnormalities in different planes and will highlight solid/fluid structures depending on the weighting of the images.

An MRI scan also provides information regarding spinal cord injury patterns, such as central cord syndrome, which have been previously unavailable with other imaging modalities.

Spinal cord oedema has a much better prognosis than spinal cord haemorrhage, while contusion of the cord has an intermediate prognosis.[16]

Thoracolumbar spine

The second most frequently injured area of the spinal column after the cervical spine is the thoracolumbar junction (T11–L2). Cord injuries in this region comprise about 20% of all spinal cord injuries.[8] The main reasons for the susceptibility of this region are the abrupt transition from the rigidly fixed thoracic spine to the more mobile lumbar spine and that the spinal canal in the thoracic region is more circular and smaller in diameter than the cervical or lumbar spinal canals resulting in increased risk to the cord.

It is also of note that injuries in the T1–T10 region comprise 16% of cord injuries and lumbosacral injuries such as cauda equina lesions comprise approximately 4% of spinal neurological injuries.[8]

Classification of thoracolumbar spine injuries are as follows:

- **Minor** (stable) fractures, which include transverse process fractures, spinous process fractures and pars interarticularis fractures
- **Major** (unstable) fracture/dislocations, which include compression fractures, the 'chance' fracture, the burst fracture and the flexion/distraction injuries.

Although there is a lack of evidence-based guidelines that provide indications for plain X-rays of the thoracolumbar spine, the criteria for radiography of this region may be reasonably applied from those criteria for the cervical spine (see above). In particular, the patient with a decreased level of consciousness is at risk for spinal column/cord injury at any level and victims of multiple trauma may have spinal injuries at more than one level. Radiography of the thoracolumbar spine includes a lateral and an anteroposterior (AP) view. The alignment, both anterior and posterior, of the vertebral bodies as well as the anterior and posterior height of the body should be checked. Wedge compression fractures which occur commonly in the elderly from T12–L2 are generally stable, but if the anterior border has lost more than 50% of the height compared to the posterior margin, there is a potential for instability of the posterior ligaments. In the upper thoracic spine the anterior height of the vertebral body is usually 1.5 mm less than the posterior height.

On the lateral view one should also check the integrity of posterior bony elements and the interspinous distance that may indicate rupture of the

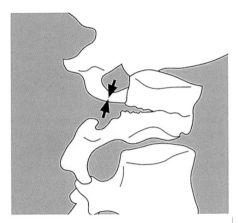

Fig. 2.8.9 Representation of the Chance fracture showing a horizontal fracture through the posterior vertebral elements of the lumbar spine. (From Rosen P, Doris PE, Barkin RM, Barkin SZ, Markovchick VJ (eds) 1992 Diagnostic Radiology in Emergency Medicine. Mosby-Year Book Inc., St Louis)

posterior ligaments. The anteroposterior view should be checked for the height of the vertebral bodies, interpedicular distance and/or disruption of the pedicles (e.g. chance fracture) and the alignment of the vertebral bodies and the spinous processes. A paravertebral shadow, which may represent a haematoma may alert the clinician as to the presence of a thoracolumbar spinal fracture.

The Chance fracture (Fig. 2.8.9) is an example of the distraction or seatbelt injury with the lap belt as the axis of rotation and failure of the spinal column in its posterior ligamentous and bony elements. This fracture is horizontal through the entire bony column including vertebral body, pedicles, laminae and spinous processes and is, by definition, unstable. This fracture may also be associated with injuries to the abdominal contents, e.g. pancreas or duodenum.

It is often difficult to obtain satisfactory images of the upper thoracic spine particularly the T1–T4 region and, in these circumstances, further imaging should be performed by CT scan or MRI.

Patients with unexplained neurological deficit or a major fracture/dislocation on plain X-ray should proceed to CT scan of the relevant area followed by sagittal reconstruction as directed by the clinical examination.

Standard axial CT scans are adequate to demonstrate most injuries of the thoracolumbar spine, however, Chance fractures are an exception and often require sagittal reconstruction for more accurate delineation.

MRI scanning is often of value for defining injury to the spinal cord itself (see above) and for excluding the presence of a spinal epidural haematoma or abscess.

MRI scan is the investigation of choice in the uncommon SCIWORA, which is seen in children. This injury is associated with ligamentous rupture and/or cord ischaemia, contusion or haematoma.

Fractures of the lower lumbar spine and sacrum may involve the cauda equina and associated sacral nerve roots. There may be bladder, bowel or sexual dysfunction as well as variable motor and sensory deficit in the lower limbs. There is often significant neuralgia that is disabling and difficult to treat. Plain X-rays will give some indication of the severity of the bony injury, but CT scan is required for definitive information if surgical fixation is required.

Coccygeal fractures are due to direct blows and are treated and diagnosed clinically. Radiological diagnosis is not usually necessary. There may be an associated rectal injury which may require repair and otherwise analgesia only is required.

CHEST TRAUMA

The chest X-ray has a key role in the investigation in multi-trauma involving the thorax. There remains controversy, however, regarding the roles of CT chest scans, aortography and transoesophageal echo (TOE). Investigations other than CXR may be decided to some extent by the availability of the above modalities at different institutions. The CT chest scan has become more accessible in recent years, whereas the use of TOE and angiography remains confined to the major centres. It is important that the trauma team leader has a clear understanding of the advantages, disadvantages and limitations of each investigation so

that he can carefully choose the most appropriate investigation available at his institution.

The trauma room chest X-ray (CXR) should ideally be performed in the erect position with a nasogastric tube in situ. However, since it is often impossible to clear the cervical or thoraco-lumbar spine in the trauma room, the CXR is frequently taken in the supine position. This can create a number of difficulties in the interpretation of the X-ray results. The AP projection of the X-ray beam will magnify the mediastinal structures and, when the patient is supine, the thoracic veins will passively distend and add to this appearance of mediastinal widening. Small pneumothoraces and haemothoraces are also difficult to detect on the supine CXR because the air distributes as a thin film anteriorly[18] and blood as a thin homogenous layer posteriorly. A haemothorax of 200–300 mL will normally be visible on a good quality erect CXR whereas it will usually require 800–1000 mL to produce the 'fuzzy' appearance of a haemothorax seen on the supine CXR[18]. In some trauma centres these problems are overcome with the use of trauma beds that are capable of a reverse-Trendelenburg position. This allows the patient to remain flat on the bed with the spine immobilized, while the bed is tilted 30° to 40° head-up and thus providing a semi-erect CXR.

Examination of the CXR will often begin with a review of the bones and soft-tissues. The CXR is a poor diagnostic aid for rib fractures as it will miss up to 50% of anterior and lateral fractures.[18] The CXR assessment should be more directed towards the complications of rib fractures such as pneumothorax or haemothorax, and oblique rib views will better delineate rib fractures. It is also important to remember that the clavicles and scapulae are often visible on the CXR. Fractures of these bones, along with fractures of the first and second ribs, are indicators of significant blunt thoracic trauma and should prompt a careful examination for underlying visceral and vascular injuries.

Sternal fractures are not evident on the AP or PA CXR but may be seen on a lateral or oblique sternal view X-ray. The significance of sternal fractures will largely direct the examination towards underlying mediastinal injuries. Brookes et al in a retrospective study[19] found a 2% incidence of sternal fractures associated with motor vehicle accidents. These patients had a very low incidence (1.5%) of cardiac arrhythmias requiring treatment and a mortality rate of less than 1%. The authors found that those at risk of cardiac arrhythmias requiring treatment were over 65 years of age and either had pre-existing ischaemic cardiac disease or were on digoxin treatment. They recommended that cardiac monitoring was not required unless the patient fulfilled the above criteria and there was no other specific indication. They also found that the 12-lead ECG was not predictive for the development of arrhythmias requiring treatment.

In cases of penetrating chest trauma, a foreign body may be evident on the CXR. An AP and lateral projection with appropriate skin markers will normally be required to aid in locating the position of the foreign object. In cases where the foreign object is embedded close to or in a pulsatile thoracic structure, the object may appear blurred on the CXR indicat-ing the proximity of the foreign body to the vessel.

Subcutaneous emphysema (Fig. 2.8.10) may be seen on the CXR and may result from injury to the lung, the tracheo-bronchial tree, the larynx, pharynx and oesophagus. Subcutaneous emphysema should prompt a careful examination for evidence of a pneumothorax and pneumo-mediastinum. Subcutaneous emphysema and pneumothorax are common findings in traumatic injury to the lung and also occur in tracheobrochial injury.

In cases of suspected tracheal lacera-tion, where the patient has been intu-bated, the appearance of the endotracheal tube on the CXR should be carefully examined (Table 2.8.9).

The normal appearance of the balloon is 2.5 cm proximal to the tip of the endotracheal tube.

If a pneumothorax is suspected but not visible on the supine CXR, an erect CXR should be performed and films obtained in both inspiration and expira-tion. If an erect CXR cannot be performed, a shoot-through lateral CXR with the patient supine may show an anterior pneumothorax. A CT chest is the defini-tive investigation when a pneumothorax cannot be excluded.

Table 2.8.9 Chest X-ray signs of tracheal laceration
Subcutaneous emphysema
Mediastinal emphysema
Pneumothorax
Deviation of the endotracheal tube tip to the right relative to the tracheal lumen
Distension of the endotracheal tube balloon
Migration of the endotracheal tube balloon distally towards the tube tip

In cases of penetrating chest trauma, the development of a detectable pneu-mothorax may be delayed and so it is recommended that check X-rays be performed at 6 and 12 hours.[18]

The lung fields may become opacified by contusion, aspiration, pulmonary fat embolism and either cardiogenic or non-cardiogenic pulmonary oedema. Lung contusions will usually develop rapidly within 6 hours of an injury whereas the changes of aspiration and pulmonary infarction are often delayed for 12 to 24 hours. Rib fractures are frequently associated with pulmonary contusions, although in paediatric patients and young adults the ribs are more compliant and may bend-in causing a contusion without fracture.

Diaphragmatic injuries are more fre-quent in penetrating than blunt trauma. In blunt trauma however, 80% of diaph-ragmatic injuries occur on the left side because the liver and its ligamentous attachments protect the right side (see Table 2.8.10).

If a nasogastric tube is in situ, it may be seen to pass down into the abdomen and back up into the chest contained within the herniated stomach. Lower rib fractures are often seen in association with injuries to the diaphragm.

Thoracic aortic injury

Ninety per cent of injuries occur in the region of the aortic isthmus that is that part of the proximal descending aorta between the origin of the left subclavian artery and the site of attachment of the

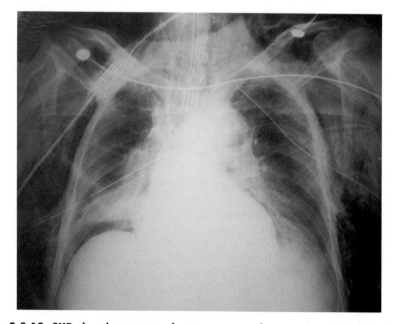

Fig. 2.8.10 CXR showing gross subcutaneous emphysema in an intubated patient with a tracheal laceration. Note bilateral thoracostomy tubes.

Table 2.8.10 Signs of diaphragmatic injury on CXR

Elevated hemi-diaphragm

Abnormal or indistinct contour of the diaphragm

Collapse of the lower lung fields

Inhomogenous mass in the relevant hemi-thorax

Displacement of the mediastinum away from the injury.

Table 2.8.11 Chest X-ray signs of aortic disruption[20]

Widened mediastinum
  >6 cm in erect PA film
  >8 cm in supine AP film

Deviation of the oesophagus / NG tube to the right of T4 spinous process

Obliteration of aortic knob

Opacification of the aortopulmonary window

Deviation of the trachea to the right of the T4 spinous process

Depression of the left main bronchus to below 40o from the horizontal.

Increased right paratracheal stripe (>4 mm)

Increased left paravertebral stripe (>5 mm)

Left apical cap

ligamentum arteriosum (1.5 cm in length). The ascending aorta is involved in only 5% of cases.[20]

As previously described, the supine AP CXR magnifies the mediastinal silhouette. Superior mediastinal widening is a common finding in cases of both penetrating and blunt trauma to the great thoracic vessels. The mediastinal width is measured at the top of the aortic knob. A width greater than 8.0–8.5 cm in a supine film or 6 cm in an erect CXR is suggestive of a mediastinal haematoma[18] (Fig. 2.8.11).

The sensitivity of a widened mediastinum on a CXR for the detection of thoracic aortic injuries has been estimated at 67% and the specificity 45%.[21]

Deviation of a nasogastric tube more than 1–2 cm to the right of the spinous process of T4 in a non-rotated film is highly suggestive of a para-aortic haematoma[20] (Table 2.8.11).

The paravertebral stripes are lines of opacification that lie between the thoracic spines and the pleura reflection. The left paravertebral line is distinguished from the descending thoracic aorta because it is not continuous with the aortic knob.

The right paratracheal stripe lies between the right margin of the trachea and the pleural reflections. It is normally less than 4-5 mm in diameter.

Injuries to the oesophagus may occur in association with both blunt and penetrating chest trauma. The predominant X-ray finding in oesophageal injury is pneumomediastinum and this may be associated with subcutaneous emphysema, pneumothorax, a left pleural effusion or a widened mediastinum.

Thoracic CT scan

Thoracic CT has become a common diagnostic aid in investigating the multi-trauma patient with chest injuries. The increasing speed and greater clarity of the helical CT scanner gives a reliable and rapid means of screening for most intrathoracic injuries. The CT scan of the chest is a sensitive test for detecting pneumothorax, pneumomediastinum, pulmonary contusion, haemothorax and/or mediastinal haematoma.

Mediastinal haematoma is an indirect sign of aortic injury and appears as soft tissue attenuation around mediastinal structures[21] (Fig. 2.8.11).

Some controversy has surrounded the role of CT chest versus arch angiography for investigating the widened mediastinum to exclude a possible aortic disruption. The arch aortogram remains the gold standard against which the other investigations are measured, but the helical CT scan has become more reliable as a screening test for mediastinal haematoma which, if present, will mandate an arch aortogram in patients considered low-to-moderate risk of traumatic aortic disruption.[21]

Aortography should be done if there is obvious mediastinal widening on CXR and a high clinical suspicion of aortic injury. Alternatively, if the chest X-ray is equivocal and the patient is stable, a dynamic contrast-enhanced helical CT scan with 5 mm cuts through the mediastinum is recommended. A helical CT scan of the chest with contrast may overlook an intimal flap in the thoracic aorta. Three-dimensional CT angiography with 2–3 mm slices may be reconstructed to produce detailed images of the aorta.

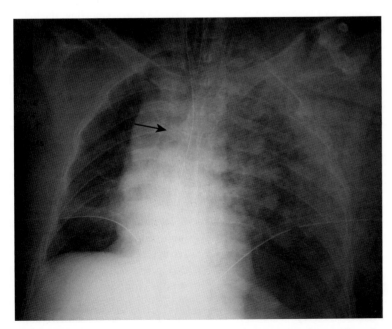

Fig. 2.8.11 CXR showing a widened mediastinum in a patient with a thoracic aortic dissection. Note deviation of the trachea to the right (arrow)

Aortography

Transfemoral angiography remains the investigation of choice for the diagnosis of major thoracic vascular injuries, in particular those involving the aorta and great vessels.[20] This investigation is not free from complications, although the morbidity and mortality are low. Significant complications such as rupture at the site of injury during contrast injection are rare, but have been reported.[20] At least two projections must be obtained usually the left anterior oblique and the antero-posterior views. Arch angiography is more expensive than CT chest scan especially when used as a screening tool for the exclusion of aortic injury, while the CT scan is less invasive and will show other traumatic chest injuries. Hunink[21] calculated that the cost per life saved was $2 million when CXR and angiography alone were used compared to $500 000 per life saved when CT was introduced into the screening algorithm for low-to-moderate risk of aortic rupture.

Digital subtraction angiography (DSA)[22] offers some advantages over conventional angiography with shorter examination times and smaller amounts of contrast required. This may be of use in those with renal impairment or known contrast allergy, but the CT scan is less invasive, cheaper and will often show other traumatic injuries such as rib fractures, pneumothorax, haemothorax and pulmonary contusion.

The aortogram remains the key investigation for the stable patient with penetrating injury to the thorax and lower neck. However, in one small study[23] aortography displayed a sensitivity of 67% and a specificy of 98%, while transoesophageal echocardiography (TOE) was accurate in predicting the presence or absence of an aortic injury with both a sensitivity and specificity of 100%.

Transoesophageal echocardiography (TOE)

In the investigation of a suspected mediastinal haematoma, the TOE has many proponents of its value both as a screening and diagnostic test. Some authors[23,24] suggest that the TOE is more accurate than aortography in detecting aortic injuries, although it is acknowledged that interpretation is operator-dependent.

Advantages of TOE are: that it can be performed quickly in the resuscitation area, it is minimally invasive and has a low complication rate such as aspiration and oesophageal perforation. It can demonstrate myocardial, pericardial and valvular injuries. Disadvantages are that it may require sedation and intubation in the trauma patient and may be of limited value in providing information about the distal ascending aorta, the aortic arch and the arch vessels.[24] Although the incidence of injury to the arch and major branch vessels is rare, aortography is required when injury to these vessels is suspected The role of intravascular ultrasound is limited, but it may be of use to confirm subtle angiographic changes in the vertical descending aorta[25]. MRI for the diagnosis of traumatic aortic rupture is generally not practical in the trauma victim.

Gastograffin/barium studies

Oral contrast provides useful information in the investigation and diagnosis of oesophageal and diaphragmatic injuries. In cases of oesophageal perforation, gastrograffin is the preferred contrast media as it is less irritant than barium should there be a leak into the surrounding mediastinal tissues. However, there is a 25% incidence of false negatives[18] with the use of gastrograffin and this incidence decreases if barium is used. A gastrograffin swallow is mandatory in the evaluation of suspected penetrating injuries of the oesophagus. If there is a risk of aspiration, gastrograffin should not be used as it produces a severe pneumonitis. In these circumstances contrast designed for intravenous use can be administered orally in order to demonstrate oesophageal perforation.

Flexible or rigid oesophagoscopy may also be utilized to exclude oesophageal perforation.

ABDOMEN/PELVIS

Abdominal X-ray

The role of the plain abdominal X-ray (AXR) in the investigation of abdominal trauma is limited. In cases of penetrating injuries, it may be useful in detection of foreign bodies. Free intra-abdominal gas may also be seen with perforation of a hollow viscus. An erect CXR may show 'free-gas' under the left hemidiaphragm more commonly than on the right. The free-gas is distinguished from normal intra-gastric air because it appears directly beneath the diaphragm highlighting the thin diaphragmatic silhouette and it does not conform to the contained appearance of air in the fundus of the stomach. If the patient's condition precludes an erect CXR, a left lateral decubitus X-ray may be performed to demonstrate free intra-abdominal gas. In cases of duodenal perforation, free retroperitoneal air may be seen as pockets of gas along the right psoas-line (shadow) on a supine AXR. Both blunt and penetrating abdominal trauma may result in an ileus that is seen as dilated bowel loops containing fluid levels on both the erect and lateral decubitus X-rays. Dilated small bowel can form a 'step-ladder' like appearance of the small intestine as it forms multiple loops lying one on top of the other.

Abdominal CT scan (Abdo CT)

Abdo CT is usually performed with both oral and intravenous contrast. However, as most multi-trauma patients have delayed gastric emptying, the bulk of oral contrast tends to remain in the stomach and upper GIT. This phenomenon has led some authors to suggest that oral contrast is of little use in this setting.[26] The increased speed of the helical CT scanner has resulted in excellent resolution for the detection of vascular injuries involving the liver, spleen and kidneys after intravenous contrast. In stable patients with possible intra-abdominal injuries, the abdo CT has become the investigation of choice because, as well as being non-invasive, it reliably identifies intraperitoneal fluid, solid organ injury, retroperitoneal injuries as well as spine and pelvic fractures. The use of intravenous contrast will also give some indication of both renal perfusion and function as contrast is excreted into the ureters and bladder. This has largely negated the use of the one-shot intravenous pyelogram (IVP) as a marker of renal perfusion and function. One of the main limitations of the abdo CT is that the investigation must be done in the radiology department and, as a result, is inappropriate for any unstable patient. Injuries that may be missed on abdo CT include upper intestinal perforation as well as injury to the diaphragm, pancreas and bladder. [26]

In a review of prospective studies of haemodynamically stable patients with blunt abdominal trauma and equivocal findings on physical examination, Catre[27] found the mean sensitivity and specificity of DPL was 98% and 92% respectively, while he found the mean sensitivity and specificity of abdo CT was 60% and 98% respectively. He concluded that the two investigations were complimentary rather than equivalent.

Focused assessment by sonography for trauma (FAST)

Since the introduction of the focused ultrasound examination for trauma in the early 1990s in North America and in the late 1990s in Australasia, there has been some debate regarding the sensitivity, specificity and accuracy of the examination compared to diagnostic peritoneal lavage (DPL). In those centres that use the FAST exam on a regular basis, there has been a markedly decreased requirement for DPL. One of the criticisms of DPL has been its low specificity resulting in an excessive non-therapeutic laparotomy rate of up to 30% in some centres.[28,29] The main utility of the FAST exam has been shown in the unstable trauma patient with intra-abdominal haemorrhage who requires urgent surgery.

The FAST exam requires the examination of four areas (Table 2.8.12).

The limitations of the FAST exam include:

- Requires training
- Cannot differentiate fluids (blood v ascites v urine)
- Poor quality images in obesity, subcutaneous emphysema and dilated loops of bowel.[30]

The FAST exam can be completed in 2–5 minutes, is non-invasive and is repeatable. The focused examination is very poor in detecting specific intra-abdominal injuries, but if abdominal haemorrhage is ruled out and the patient is haemodynamically stable, then abdominal CT is indicated.

Tiling et al[31] reported that the FAST exam could consistently detect 200–250 mL of blood. Many studies have consistently reported for the detection of intraperitoneal blood a sensitivity of 80–100% and a specificity of 88–100%.[30] It has also been consistently reported that FAST will not detect hollow viscus injuries, lacerations in the intra-abdominal solid organs, retroperitoneal or diaphragmatic injuries.

There is also some evidence that FAST is of value in penetrating trauma. Boulanger et al[32] found that the routine use of FAST in penetrating trauma was useful with regard to the detection of pericardial and peritoneal fluid. However, they cautioned that a negative FAST did not exclude hollow viscus or diaphragmatic injuries.

Many centres have introduced FAST into the algorithm for the routine assessment of victims of trauma. Boulanger et al[33] have demonstrated in a prospective study that a FAST-based algorithm for blunt abdominal injury was more rapid, less expensive, and as accurate as an algorithm that used CT or DPL only. Hence there is a growing body of evidence that shows that the indications for DPL are probably only for suspected perforated bowel and the diagnosis for this condition is usually made clinically or by CT.

There is also ample evidence in the literature that both emergency physicians[34] and surgeons[35] can learn to perform the FAST exam with clinically acceptable sensitivity, specificity and accuracy after a relatively short introductory course and hands-on practical supervision combined with a supervised period of clinical scanning.

Radiology in pelvic trauma

In addition to plain radiology, pelvic CT scan and angiography are becoming increasingly important in the diagnostic and therapeutic work-up of pelvic trauma.

Table 2.8.12 The FAST Examination
1. The right upper quadrant (Morison's pouch)
2. The left upper quadrant (splenorenal recess)
3. The subxiphoid area (pericardium)
4. The suprapubic area (pouch of Douglas/rectovesical pouch)

The trauma room antero-posterior (AP) X-ray of pelvis should include all the bony pelvic components as well as both hip joints and proximal femora, including greater and lesser trochanters.

Most anterior pelvic fractures are able to be seen on the A-P film but up to 30% of posterior fractures involving the sacrum and sacro-iliac joints will not be seen on the plain radiology. These fractures will be best seen on a 2-dimensional or re-formatted 3D CT scan of the pelvis. Acetabular fractures are often difficult to visualise on the A-P film and oblique (Judet) films or a CT scan of the pelvis may be required. Inlet and outlet films have now been largely superceded by CT scan.

There are a number of radiological classifications of pelvic fractures that must be interpreted in association with the clinical impression of the fracture and associated complications. The greater the A-P disruption of the pelvic ring and, as a result, the greater the pelvic cavity volume, the more the potential for severe haemorrhagic shock and visceral damage.

The key considerations in any assessment of pelvic fractures are:

- Major or minor?
- Open or closed?
- Haemodynamic compromise or hollow viscus injury?
- Bony stability or instability?

A useful current classification is that by Young and Resnik,[36] which is a modification of the Pennel and Tile classification of pelvic fractures. This classifies fractures by mechanism of injury into AP compression, lateral compression, vertical shear and a combination; and takes into consideration rotational and/or vertical instability of the pelvic ring. If the pelvic ring is fractured anteriorly and posteriorly, stability is usually lost with disruption of the posterior ligaments (the sacro-iliac, sacro-tuberous and sacro-spinous ligaments) and there will be widening of the sacro-iliac joint(s) on the AP view. The classification provides a graded probability of bleeding related to the fracture, development of haemorrhagic shock and associated organ damage.

The Young and Resnik classification

AP compression

- Type 1: Disruption of the symphysis pubis with less than 2.5 cm diastasis; no significant posterior pelvic injury
- Type 2: Disruption of the symphysis pubis of more that 2.5 cm with tearing of the anterior sacroiliac, sacrospinous and sacrotuberous ligaments
- Type 3: Complete disruption of the pubic symphysis and posterior ligament complexes, with hemipelvic displacement.

Lateral compression

- Type 1: Posterior compression of the sacroiliac joint without ligament disruption; oblique pubic ramus fracture
- Type 2: Rupture of the posterior sacroiliac ligament; pivotal internal rotation of the hemipelvis on the anterior SI joint with a crush injury of the sacrum and an oblique pubic ramus fracture. (Fig. 2.8.12)
- Type 3: Findings as in Type 2 injury with evidence of an AP compression injury to the contralateral hemipelvis.

Vertical shear Complete ligament or bony disruption of a hemipelvis associated with hemipelvis displacement.

This classification does not take into consideration isolated fractures outside the bony pelvic ring or acetabular fractures.

CT scan of the pelvis

CT and plain X-rays are complementary modalities in the evaluation of pelvic fractures. Patients with pelvic fractures associated with haemodynamic instability are not suitable for placement in the CT scanner. CT scan is useful for demonstrating posterior fractures involving the sacrum and sacro-iliac joints, as well as sacro-iliac joint diastasis. Reformatted 3-D images are particularly useful for the assessment acetabular and pubic bone fractures.

Angiography

Pelvic fractures that disrupt the posterior aspect of the pelvic ring have the potential to cause considerable arterial and venous injury. 'Open-book' or AP compression pelvic ring fractures are more likely to have venous rather than arterial bleeding and compression of the pelvic ring by external fixation should help to minimize this blood loss, although this practice has not been validated by prospective, randomized controlled trials. Angiography will detect only arterial bleeding which occurs in approximately 15% of pelvic fractures. In patients with ongoing blood loss and pelvic fractures not amenable to acute compressive treatment, angiography and embolization is recommended. The femoral artery is catheterized and angiography of both internal iliac arteries is performed. If arterial bleeding is identified, then the vessels can be selectively embolized or the entire internal iliac vessels may be occluded. There is a rich vascular supply to the pelvic viscera and major ischaemic complications are rare following pelvic embolization, however, other problems such as impotence may occur.

Contrast studies

The main contrast studies used in pelvic fractures are the urethrogram and cystogram. Rupture of the membranous urethra may occur in association with pelvic fractures, particularly those involving distraction of the pubic symphysis or 'butterfly' fractures involving both superior and inferior pubic rami. If there is clinical and radiological suspicion of potential urethral damage, a urethrogram should be performed. This is done by inserting a soft catheter into the urethral meatus and injecting contrast (urograffin) while screening with an image intensifier. The urethral passage, if patent, will be visualized and it may be possible to catheterize the urethra. If there is obstruction to the passage of dye or a false track is identified, a suprapubic

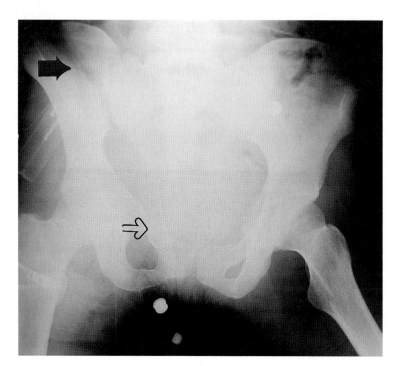

Fig. 2.8.12 AP X-ray of pelvis showing a lateral compression Type 2 fracture.
Note fractures of pubic rami (open arrow) and right iliac crest (solid arrow)

catheter will be required. Further contrast is then injected into the bladder and PA and oblique views taken to assess for extravasation of contrast suggesting bladder rupture.

EXTREMITIES

Missed injuries occur in the order of 2–6% of blunt trauma patients. One retrospective study[37] found that musculoskeletal injuries and spinal fractures featured highly (6%) amongst the injuries not found after the initial primary and secondary surveys. The musculoskeletal injuries comprised mainly fractures and a small number of soft tissue injuries. Amongst the factors contributing to the missed injuries were the presence of closed head injury and intoxication. In comparison, one study[38] found the rate of abdominal missed injuries to be 2%.

A careful clinical examination of all joints and limbs looking for swelling, deformity and crepitus must be made to direct radiological investigation. Fractures, dislocations and ligamentous instability are more likely to be missed in the smaller, peripheral bones. As these injuries may be a source of ongoing incapacitiation due to late diagnosis,there may also be a potential source of litigation. Joint dislocations such as anterior shoulder and elbow should be readily obvious, but less so are posterior shoulder and lunate/perilunate dislocation in the wrist. AP and lateral X-rays should be taken of any joint considered abnormal on examination during the secondary survey. In the lower limb, posterior dislocation of the hip and knee joints may cause serious sciatic nerve and popliteal artery damage respectively and require urgent reduction. If the viability of the limb or skin is threatened, a dislocation (e.g. knee or ankle) should be immediately reduced on clinical grounds, and X-ray performed post-reduction to check for position and bony fractures.

Bony fractures in the upper limb which are commonly missed include medial or lateral epicondyle fractures, and supracondylar fractures of the elbow in children. In the adult, fractures of the carpal bones, in particular the scaphoid and triquetrum, may be missed unless carefully looked for and these injuries may result in significant disability. Fractures and dislocations involving the metacarpals and phalanges are also easily missed in the multi-trauma patient. The skier's (or gamekeeper's thumb)[39] is an acute sprain or rupture of the ulnar collateral ligament at the metacarpophalangeal joint caused by forceful abduction of the thumb. This injury may be missed unless the joint is specifically examined for stability and stress views taken if indicated.

In the lower limb, fractures of the tibial plateau and calcaneus, which may occur as a result of a fall, may be missed unless sought clinically and radiologically. Appropriate AP and lateral X-rays should be taken of these areas. In the foot, loss of Boehler's angle (normal 25–40°) may indicate a depressed fracture of the subtalar part of the calcaneus.

Falls, in general, and calcaneal fractures, in particular, may be associated with fractures of the upper lumbar spine, especially L2.

Other imaging modalities in extremity injury

CT scans of complex fractures and dislocations may assist the orthopaedic surgeon in planning appropriate fixation. Joints where this may be helpful include large joints such as shoulder, hip and knee, e.g. tibial plateau fractures. Calcaneal fractures are often not clearly seen on plain X-rays and require a CT scan for a more accurate view of these complex fractures.

Angiography is required when there is suspected or clinically obvious vascular compromise to either upper or lower limb. The axillary or brachial arteries may be damaged or transected in blunt or penetrating injuries to the upper limb. The commonest serious vascular injury to the lower limb may be associated with posterior dislocation of the knee and intimal disruption of the popliteal artery. Angiography will give accurate information regarding the degree of arterial damage and the state of the collateral flow.

CONCLUSION

Radiology in the multitrauma patient requires judicious decision making and interpretation of X-rays and other specialized modalities such as CT scans, MRI and ultrasonography. Much information can be gleaned from the initial trauma series of X-rays. Further information can be obtained from plain X-rays in the radiology department as well as more specialized imaging provided the patient remains haemodynamically stable. Missed injuries that are not diagnosed in the first 24–48 hours often contribute significantly to patient morbidity and mortality. These often involve the musculoskeletal system in the form of limb or spinal fractures and must be actively sought and excluded by appropriate clinical and radiological examination.

REFERENCES

1. Harris J H, Edeiken-Monroe B 1987 Radiographic examination. In: The Radiology of Acute Cervical Spine Trauma, 2nd edn. William and Wilkins, Baltimore pp 45–64
2. International Commission on Radiological Protection 1982 Publication 34. Protection of the patient in diagnostic radiology. Annals of the ICRP 9: 2–3
3. International Commission on Radiological Protection.1991 Publication 62. Radiological protection in biomedical research. Annals of the ICRP 22: 3
4. International Commission on Radiological Protection 1990 Publication 60. Recommendations of the international commission on radiological protection. Annals of the ICRP 21: 1–3
5. Berquist TH 1992 Cervical spine trauma. In: Kricum ME (ed.) Imaging of Sports Injuries. Aspen Publications, pp 31–64
6. Miller EC, Holmes JF, Derlet RW 1997 Utilising clinical factors to reduce head CT scan ordering for minor trauma patients. Journal of Emergency Medicine 15: 453–7
7. Stiel IG, Wells GA, Vandemheen K, et al 2001 The Canadian CT Head Rule for patients with minor head injury. Lancet: 357(9266): 1391–6
8. Satisky E, Votey S 1997 Emergency department approach to acute thoracolumbar spine injury. Journal Emergency Medicine 15: 49–59
9. Bell RM Clearing the cervical spine. Personal communication
10. Williams J, Jehle D, Cottington E, et al 1992 Head, facial and clavicular trauma as a predictor of cervical-spine injury. Annals of Emergency Medicine 21: 719–22
11. Ryan MD, Henderson J 1992 Injury 23: 38–40
12. Hoffman JR, Mower WR, Wolfson AB, et al 2000 Validity of a set of clinical criteria to rule out injury to the cervical spine in patients with blunt trauma. National Emergency X-Radiography Utilisation Study Group. New England Journal of Medicine 343 (2): 94–9
13. Stiell IG, Wells, GA, Vandemheen K et al.2001 The Canadian C-Spine Rule for Radiography in

CONTROVERSIES

❶ The skull X-ray (SXR). There are very few indications for a SXR in the evaluation of head trauma provided a CT scan is readily available. The only current indication for a SXR is for the detection of a metallic foreign body associated with a penetrating head injury.

❷ Cervical spine clearance in the unconscious patient. There is general agreement that there is a need for both clinical and radiological clearance of the cervical spine in the obtunded or unconscious patient on whom a neurological examination is unable to be performed. This becomes particularly problematic in the patient with severe head injury who remains unconscious, or sedated and ventilated for a prolonged period of time. Bell[9] suggests from an extensive review of the literature that the absolute risk of missing an unstable cervical spine injury when there is an adequate screening examination, which is said to be normal by an experienced person, is much less than 1%. He further suggests that it may be reasonable to remove the hard collar and place the patient in a soft collar until alert or have dynamic fluoroscopy[40] performed by an experienced examiner. The usefulness of dynamic fluoroscopy is yet to be conclusively validated. The East Group[41] make more definitive recommendations in this group of patients after consideration of all the available published evidence. They conclude that the safest approach to this group is a screening cervical spine X-rays (three -views with axial CT through suspicious or poorly visualized areas). They also suggested that during the inital or follow-up head CT, the upper two cervical vertebrae should be visualized with thin axial cuts. If all these studies are adequate and correctly interpreted, the cervical spine should be considered stable and immobilization deviced removed. There may be an argument for simply performing a CT of the entire cervical spine from occiput to T 2-3 with sagittal reconstructions as a means of achieving radiological clearance. These recommendations are based on opinion only and are not supported by good quality data from randomized controlled trials. This approach will not detect the rare isolated spinal ligamentous injury.

❸ Clearing the cervical spine in the alert, asymptomatic blunt trauma victim. Bell[9], Hoffman et al[12], Stiel et al[13] and Velmahos[42] provide good evidence that clinical examination alone can reliably assess the victims of blunt trauma who are alert, not intoxicated, do no have neck pain or tenderness, are neurologically intact and do not have a major distracting injury. The evidence provided by Stiel et al appears to be best validated and the risk of 'occult' injury in these patients approaches zero. The exceptions, as previously stated, are children under the age of 2 years with a suggestive mechanism of injury and the elderly.

❹ Indications for radiology of the thoracolumbar spine in multiple trauma. Terregino et al[43] found that, in blunt trauma victims who could not be evaluated for symptoms and signs of spinal injury due to a depressed level of consciousness or had cervical spine neurological deficit, there was a 5% incidence of thoracolumbar spine fractures.

In patients who could be evaluated clinically, they found that in the absence of pain, tenderness, thoracic or lumbar neurological deficit, or a major distracting injury (including a cervical spine fracture) there was no need for imaging of the thoracolumbar spine. Pain and tenderness, in particular, had a high correlation with the presence of a thoracolumbar fracture. More importantly, they found that if there was a spinal fracture at any level, there was an 11% chance of a spinal fracture elsewhere that correlates with other studies.

The current recommendations for thoracolumbar radiology are that it should be performed in those patients with a suggestive or unknown mechanism of injury who:

– are unable to be examined clinically due to decreased level of consciousness, intoxication or a cervical spine injury;
– are able to be examined clinically and have one or more of: pain or tenderness in the area, a major distracting injury, other spinal fractures and thoracic or lumbar neurological deficit.

❺ The investigation of choice for the assessment of traumatic aortic injury (TAI) secondary to blunt trauma. There is general agreement that patients, who are hypotensive after blunt or penetrating trauma and who have clinical or radiological evidence of mediastinal injury, should proceed immediately to the operating theatre for a thoracotomy. There remains considerable debate about which investigation is most suitable for the otherwise stable patient who has a significant mechanism of injury, an equivocal or widened mediastinum on CXR, or concern that there may be significant extrathoracic injuries (e.g. head, abdominal). Morgan et al[44] suggest that a dynamic, contrast-enhanced CT scan of the chest can accurately detect mediastinal haematoma and recommend arch aortography only on those patients with a positive CT scan. Chan,[45] however, advocates the use of transoesophageal echocardiography (TOE) on the grounds that it can be used in the resuscitation room, it is reliable, non-invasive, and has a low complication rate. There are, however, conflicting studies where the sensitivity and specificity for TOE range from 63–100% and 45–63%, respectively. It seems from the current literature that further evaluation is required to determine the efficacy of the TOE and it may be very operator-dependent.[46, 47]

From the evidence available to date, it would seem reasonable that a patient with a significant mechanism of injury, a clinical examination suggestive of TAI and a definite widened mediastinum on CXR should go directly to the operating theatre for thoracotomy if haemodynamically unstable or via the angiography suite if stable.

❻ The stable patient with a suspicious mediastinal appearance should have a dynamic, contrast-enhanced CT scan of the chest looking for mediastinal haematoma and then proceed to the angiography suite if positive. There is insufficient evidence to date to make a recommendation for the place of TOE in the evaluation of these patients.

alert and stable trauma patients. Journal of the American Medical Association 286(15): 1841–8

14. Murphy MD, Batnizsky MD, Bramble JM 1989 Diagnostic imaging of spinal trauma. In: Sartoris DJ (ed.) Musculoskeletal trauma. The radiological clinics of North America. W B Saunders Co, Philadelphia PA 27: 855–72

15. Lusted LB, Keats TE 1967 The spine. In: Atlas of Roentgenographic Measurement, 2nd edn. Yearbook Medical Publications Inc., Chicago pp 101–3

16. Keene JG, Daffner RH 1992 Spinal trauma. In: Rosen P, Doris PE, Barkin RM, Barkin SZ, Markovchick VJ (eds) Diagnostic Radiology in Emergency Medicine. Mosby-Year Book, St Louis

17. Noble EF, Smoker WRK 1996 The forgottern condyle: The appearance, morphology, and classification of occipital condyle fractures. AJNR 17: 507–13

18. Wilson RF 1996 Thoracic trauma. In:Tintinalli JE, Ruiz E, Krone RC (eds) Emergency Medicine. A Comprehensive Study Guide. American College of Emergency Physicians, 4th edn. McGraw-Hill pp 1156–82

19. Brookes JG, Dunn RJ, Roger IR 1993 Sternal fractures: A retrospective analysis of 272 cases. Journal of Trauma 35: 46

20. Creasy JD, Chiles C, Routh WD, et al 1997 Overview of traumatic injury of the thoracic aorta. Radiographics 17: 27–45

21. Hunink MGM, Bos JJ 1995 Triage of patients to angiography for detection of aortic rupture after blunt chest trauma: cost-effectiveness analysis of using CT. AJNR. 165: 27–36

22. Mirvis SE, Pais SO, Gens DR 1986 Thoracic aortic rupture: advantages of intra-arterial digital subtraction angiography. AJR. 146: 987–91

23. Keaney PA, Wesley Smith D, Johnson SB, et al 1993 Use of transoesophageal echocardiography in the evaluation of traumatic aortic injury. Journal of Trauma 34: 696–703

24. Smith MD, Cassidy JM, Souther S, et al 1995 Transoesophageal echocardiography in the diagnosis of traumatic rupture of the aorta. New England Journal of Medicine 332: 356–62

25. Williams DM, Dale MD, Bolling SF, et al 1993

The role of intravascular ultrasound in acute traumatic aortic rupture. Seminar Ultrasound, CT, MRI 14: 85–90

26. Tsang BD, Panacek EA, Brant WE, et al 1997 Effect of oral contrast administration for abdominal computed tomography in the evaluation of acute blunt trauma. Annals Emergency Medicine 30: 7–13

27. Catre MG 1995 Diagnostic peritoneal lavage versus abdominal computed tomography in blunt abdominal trauma: a review of prospective studies. Canadian Journal of Surgery 38: 117–22

28. Ross SE, Dragor GM, O'Malley KF, et al 1995 Morbidity of negative celiotomy in trauma. Injury 26: 393–4

29. Henneman PL, Marx JA, Moore EE, et al 1990 Diagnostic peritoneal lavage: Accuracy in predicting necessary laparotomy following blunt and penetrating trauma. Journal of Trauma 30: 1345

30. Melanson SW, Heller M 1998 The emerging role of bedside ultrasonography in trauma cases. Emergency Medical Clinics of North America 16: 165–89

31. Tiling T, Bouillon B, Schmid A, et al 1990 Ultrasound in blunt abdomino-thoracic trauma. In Border JR. Allgoewer M, Hansen ST, et al (eds): Blunt multiple trauma: comprehensive pathophysiology and care. Marcel Dekker, New York pp 415–33

32. Boulanger BR, Kearney PA, Tsuei B, et al 2001 The routine use of sonography in penetrating torso injury is beneficial. Journal of Trauma (2): 320–5

33. Boulanger BR, McLellan BA, Brenneman FD et al 1999 Prospective evidence of the superiority of a sonography-based algorithm in the assessment of blunt abdominal injury. Journal of Trauma 47(4): 632–7

34. Mandevia DP, Aragona J, Chan L, et al 2000 Ultrasound training for emergency physicians – a prospective study. Academic Emergency Medicine 7(9): 1008–14

35. Shackford SR, Rogers FB, Osler TM, et al 1999 Focused abdominal sonogram for trauma: the learning curve of nonradiologist clinicians in detecting haemoperitoneum. Journal of Trauma 46(4): 553–64

36. Gill Cryer H, Johnson E 1996 Pelvic fractures. In: Feliciano DV, Moore EE, Mattox KJ (eds). Trauma, 3rd edn. Appleton and Lange, Stamford pp 635–59

37. Kremli MK 1996 Missed musculoskeletal injuries in a University Hospital in Riyadh: types of missed injuries and responsible factors. Injury 27: 503–6

38. Sung C, Kim KH 1996 Missed injuries in abdominal trauma. Journal of Trauma 41: 276–8

39. Musharafieh RS, Bassim YR, Atiyeh BS 1997 Ulnar collateral ligament injury in the emergency department. Journal of Emergency Medicine 15: 193–6

40. Davis JW, Parkes SN, Detlefs CL, et al 1995 Clearing the cervical spine in obtunded patients: the use of dynamic fluroscopy. Journal of Trauma 39: 435–8

41. East Practice Parameter Workgroup for cervical spine clearance 1998 Practice Management guidelines for identifying cervical spine injuries following trauma. Eastern Association for the Surgery of Trauma. www.east.org

42. Velmahos GC, Theodorou D, Tatevossion R, et al 1996 Radiographic cervical spine evaluation in the alert asymptomatic blunt trauma victim: Much ado about nothing? Journal of Trauma 40: 768–74

43. Terregino CA, Ross SE, Lipinski MF, et al 1995 Selective indications for thoracic and lumbar radiography in blunt trauma. Annals of Emergency Medicine 26: 126–9

44. Morgan PW, Goodman LR, Aprahamian C, et al. 1992 Evaluation of traumatic aortic injury: does dynamic contrast-enhanced CT play a role? Radiology 182: 661–6

45. Chan D 1998 Echocardiography in thoracic trauma. Emergency of Clinics North America 16: 191–207

46. Kearney PA, Smith N, Johnson SB, et al 1993 Use of transoesophageal echocardiography in the evaluation of traumatic aortic injury. Journal of Trauma 34: 696–701

47. Saletta S, Lederman E, Fein S, et al 1995 Transoesophageal echocardiography for the initial evaluation of the widened mediastinum in trauma patients. Journal of Trauma 39: 137–41

2.9 TRAUMA IN PREGNANCY
STEVEN TROUPAKIS

ESSENTIALS

1 Trauma in pregnancy is the most common cause of non-obstetric maternal death, with most of the mortality due to head injury and haemorrhagic shock.

2 Fetal death occurs far more often than maternal death and is dependent on the severity of the maternal injuries. Placental abruption and direct fetal trauma cause most deaths.

3 Common causes of trauma are motor vehicle accidents, falls and assaults.

4 Important sequelae are bruising, fractures, premature labour, placental abruption, disseminated intravascular coagulation, fetomaternal haemorrhage, intra-abdominal injuries, uterine rupture and haemorrhagic shock.

5 The physiological changes that occur with pregnancy, such as the relative hypervolaemia and the gravid uterus, may make clinical assessment of the patient difficult.

6 Continuous cardiotocographic monitoring for at least 4 hours is the best predictor for placental abruption and fetal distress. Ultrasound and CT are also useful, especially in assessing intra-abdominal organs and for intraperitoneal fluid.

7 Maternal resuscitation remains the best method of fetal resuscitation.

INTRODUCTION

Trauma during pregnancy presents a unique set of challenges for the emergency department, as the anatomical and physiological changes that occur during pregnancy will influence the evaluation of the patient. An appreciation of these changes is important. Aggressive resuscitation of the mother remains the best treatment for the fetus. Early obstetric consultation will help improve the outcome of these patients.

ANATOMICAL AND PHYSIOLOGICAL CHANGES IN PREGNANCY

Cardiovascular
Blood volume increases by about 45% by the end of the third trimester.[1] With relative hypervolaemia the patient may lose up to 35% of her blood volume before signs of haemorrhagic shock appear. Maternal cardiac output increases by 1–1.5 L/min in the first 10 weeks. The resting heart rate increases by 15–20 beats/min by the end of the third trimester. Systolic and diastolic blood pressure fall by 10–15 mmHg during the second trimester, but rise again towards the end of the pregnancy. ECG changes may occur with the cephalic displacement of the heart, such as left axis deviation by 15°, T-wave inversion or flattening in leads III, V1 and V2 and Q waves in III and AVF.[2] After 20 weeks' gestation, supine positioning may cause inferior vena cava (IVC) obstruction by the gravid uterus, leading to a fall in cardiac output.

Haematological
A dilutional anaemia occurs with a fall in the haematocrit (31–35% by the end of pregnancy). Pregnancy induces a leucocytosis, with levels up to 18000/mm³ in the third trimester. The ESR is elevated by the third trimester (average 78 mm/h). Coagulation factors increase (fibrinogen, factors VII, VIII, IX, X), increasing the risk of venous thrombosis. The buffering capacity of the blood is decreased.[3]

Respiratory
The diaphragm is elevated by about 4 cm. Tidal volume increases by 40% and the residual volume falls by about 25%. A respiratory alkalosis results, with a fall in PCO_2 to 30 mmHg. The anteroposterior diameter of the chest is increased, and the mediastinum is widened on chest X-ray.

Gastrointestinal
Cephalic displacement of intra-abdominal structures and delayed gastric motility increase the risk of aspiration. The intestines are displaced to the upper part of the abdomen and may be shielded by the uterus. The peritoneum is stretched by the gravid uterus, which may make signs of peritonism less reliable.[3] Alkaline phosphatase levels may triple because of placental production.

Urinary
Dilatation of the renal pelvis and ureters occurs from the 10th week of gestation. The bladder becomes hyperaemic and is displaced into the abdomen from the 12th week, making it more susceptible to trauma.

Uterine
There is a massive increase in uterine size. Blood flow to the uterus increases from 60 to 600 mL/min by the end of pregnancy.

EPIDEMIOLOGY

The incidence of trauma during pregnancy is approximately 7%,[4] the causes being similar to those in the general population. Blunt trauma is the commonest injury, with motor vehicle accidents, falls and assaults being the other common causes in that order. Penetrating injuries are less common and usually the result of domestic violence. Stab wounds have a better prognosis for the fetus than do projectile wounds. Most trauma is of a minor nature, resulting in bruising, minor fractures and threatened premature labour. Maternal death from trauma is rare, but is the leading non-obstetric cause of death, with most fatalities due to head injuries and haemorrhage from internal injuries. Fetal death occurs in about 1–2% of cases and is dependent on the gestational age and the pattern and severity of maternal injury. Most fetal deaths are due to placental abruption or direct trauma. High-speed (>80 km/h) and broadside motor vehicle accidents have a higher incidence of placental abruption and fetal and maternal death than do frontal collisions.[5] Similarly, ejection from a vehicle, motorcycle and pedestrian collisions are associated with poor fetal outcome.[6] Maternal hypotension and vaginal bleeding are associated with increased fetal loss.[7] In one pregnant trauma series, patients with an Injury Severity Score (ISS) greater than or equal to 12 had a fetal death rate of 65%; those with an ISS <12 had no fetal deaths.[8] Other studies have shown pregnancy loss with low ISS.[7]

SPECIFIC INJURIES

Pelvic fracture

Pelvic fracture is often the result of a high-speed motor vehicle accident. Massive haemorrhage can occur from the uterus, as well as bladder, urethral and ureteric lacerations. Retroperitoneal haemorrhage occurs and may be difficult to diagnose. Direct fetal skull fractures can lead to fetal death. The most common type of pelvic fracture involves the pubic rami of one half of the pelvic rim.[9] The majority of patients with a pelvic fracture can be delivered vaginally.

Placental abruption

Placental abruption complicates 1–5% of patients with minor trauma and between 20 and 50% of cases with major trauma.[10] The placenta separates from the underlying decidua because of shearing forces between the relatively inelastic placenta and the more elastic uterus. It leads to fetal hypoxia and death. Thromboplastin release may lead to the development of disseminated intravascular coagulopathy (DIC).

Uterine rupture

Uterine rupture is rare but leads to considerable haemorrhage and almost 100% fetal mortality. It should be suspected when there is maternal shock, fetal death, difficulty defining a uterus, easily palpable fetal parts and a positive peritoneal lavage.[11]

Fetomaternal haemorrhage

Fetomaternal haemorrhage is the transplacental spread of fetal blood into the maternal circulation. It occurs in approximately 8–30% of trauma cases, and may lead to Rhesus sensitization of the mother, neonatal anaemia, fetal cardiac arrhythmias and fetal death.[3] The Kleihauer-Betke test is used to identify and quantify fetomaternal haemorrhage. This test relies on the principle that fetal cells are stable in acid (pH 3.2), whereas adult haemoglobin is eluted from maternal red cells. Microscopy will identify fetal red blood cells on blood smear.

PRESENTATION

History

Questions should be directed to determining the severity and type of trauma, as well as an obstetric history. In a motor vehicle accident, high speed, side collisions, ejection from the vehicle, and improper use of seatbelts and lap belts alone are associated with a greater likelihood of serious injuries.[5] Direct trauma to the abdomen is more likely to cause fractures, splenic and liver injuries, whereas indirect trauma via shearing forces is more likely to cause placental abruption. Pelvic pain, uterine contractions and vaginal bleeding may indicate placental abruption. An obstetric history is essential. The gestational age (>22 weeks) is the main determinant for fetal viability. Lack of fetal movements may indicate fetal death.

Primary survey

The airway should be assessed and cleared. Intubation may be difficult because of the aspiration risk, breast enlargement and cervical trauma. Breathing should be assessed and the patient given supplemental oxygen to improve both maternal and fetal oxygenation. If the patient is more than 20 weeks pregnant she should be placed on her side – preferably the left – to relieve any caval compression. If spinal immobilization is necessary, wedges can be placed underneath a spinal board, or alternatively the uterus pushed to the left manually. The blood pressure and circulation can then be assessed, remembering that signs of shock may present late because of relative hypervolaemia.

A quick assessment of conscious level and any major neurological deficits should be made. The patient should be adequately exposed for a thorough examination, but protected from a drop in temperature.

Secondary survey

The sequence of the secondary survey is the same as in the non-pregnant patient, but with an obstetric examination included in the abdominal examination. The uterus should be assessed for fundal height, tenderness, contractions, fetal heart tone, fetal movements and position. A Doppler ultrasound, stethoscope or fetoscope should be used to assess the fetal heart rate. An obstetrician should perform the pelvic examination, looking for trauma to the genital tract, cervical dilatation, fetal presentation and station relative to the ischial spines. Nitrazine paper can be used to test for the presence of amniotic fluid: it turns blue in the presence of the alkaline fluid. Rectal examination and urinalysis are essential.

INVESTIGATIONS

Blood tests

Routine blood tests, such as full blood examination, electrolytes, coagulation studies, group and hold, should be performed looking for evidence of anaemia and DIC.[2] A Kleihauer-Betke test will indicate the necessary dose of Rhesus immunoglobulin in Rh-negative patients, but has proved unreliable in predicting fetal outcome.[4]

X-rays

In severe trauma it is necessary to take cervical spine, chest and pelvic films. The abdomen should be shielded and repetition of films avoided. There has been no increased risk to the fetus when radiation exposure has been limited to less than 0.1Gy, and after 20 weeks' gestation radiation is unlikely to cause abnormalities.[2,12] A standard pelvic film delivers less than 0.01Gy.

Ultrasonography

Ultrasonography is useful in determining gestational age, placental position and fetal well-being, and estimating amniotic fluid volume.[13] It can be used to diagnose placental abruption and uterine rupture, but this is dependent on the expertise of the operator. Rapid ultrasonography in the emergency department can indicate the presence of intraabdominal fluid, especially in patients too unstable for CT.[14] Ultrasonography will detect only 40–50% of placental abruptions.[15] Cardiotocography (CTG) has proved more sensitive in diagnosing placental abruption.[8,16]

Cardiotocography

CTG monitoring beyond the 20th week of pregnancy has proved a sensitive way of diagnosing placental abruption early. It should be instituted early and continuously for at least 4 hours.[3,17] Frequent uterine contractions and fetal distress are suggestive of placental abruption. In one study no placental abruptions were missed if CTG monitoring remained normal for the first 4 hours.[10]

Computerized tomography

Computerized tomography (CT) is an accurate and non-invasive way of assessing uterine and retroperitoneal structures, but it is time-consuming and involves a higher radiation dose than normal X-rays, with exposure generally between 0.05 and 0.1Gy.[2]

Diagnostic peritoneal lavage

Diagnostic peritoneal lavage (DPL) is highly sensitive in indicating significant intra-abdominal trauma.[9] However, it does not indicate which organ is involved or if there is a retroperitoneal injury. It is safe and accurate in pregnancy as long as the operator is experienced in using an open technique, with the incision above the fundus.[2]

MANAGEMENT

Maternal resuscitation is the best method of fetal resuscitation. If the injuries are severe the patient should be in a resuscitation area, with a team approach to management and early surgical and obstetrical consultation. Attention to adequate oxygenation, proper positioning and aggressive fluid replacement is important. Oximetry, ECG, blood pressure monitoring and cardiotocography should be started early. A nasogastric tube should be inserted to reduce the risk of aspiration, as should an indwelling catheter for urinalysis and to allow better assessment of the uterus. X-rays as indicated should be performed as well as CT, DPL and ultrasound as necessary, to evaluate abdominal injuries. The choice between the three depends on the injuries suspected, the experience of the staff and the stability of the patient. If the patient remains unstable with hypotension or continued bleeding, laparotomy is indicated.[1]

The presence of vaginal bleeding, abdominal tenderness or pain, hypotension, absent fetal heart sound, fetal distress on CTG and amniotic fluid leakage requires an urgent obstetric opinion and possibly caesarean section.

Premature labour can be treated with tocolytic agents such as intravenous salbutamol. However, salbutamol causes maternal and fetal tachycardia, which may mask symptoms of hypovolaemia. Magnesium sulphate is recommended as alternative tocolytic in abdominal trauma.[15,18]

Disseminated intravascular coagulation (DIC) may develop from placental abruption, amniotic fluid embolism and fetal death. Clotting factors may need to be replaced.

In general, penetrating injuries should be explored by laparotomy, especially if they involve the upper abdomen, where there is a high possibility of bowel perforation. Some authors argue that stab wounds over the uterus with no evidence of visceral injury, and missile wounds where the entrance wound is below the fundus, the patient is stable and the missile is within the uterine cavity, can be treated conservatively.[11]

Postmortem caesarean section should be considered within the first 4 minutes of the mother arresting. There have been many cases of fetal survival up to 20 minutes after maternal death. The fetuses who have the best chance of surviving neurologically intact are those delivered within 5 minutes of the maternal arrest, who weigh more than 1000 g and are of more than 28 weeks' gestation.[2,9]

DISPOSITION

Patients who are haemodynamically unstable and who have extensive head or chest injuries will require surgical intervention and intensive-care support. Patients who are stable but show signs of fetal distress should undergo caesarean section. All patients with minor injuries who are more than 20 weeks pregnant should have CTG monitoring for at least 4 hours, preferably in a labour ward.

PROGNOSIS

Most authors agree that pregnancy does not increase maternal morbidity from trauma.[9,19] There is greater maternal and fetal mortality in pregnant women with higher Injury Severity Scores. Placental abruption can still occur from minor trauma 24–48 hours after the accident, but 4 hours of CTG monitoring should detect this group of patients.[3]

PREVENTION

Properly worn seatbelts reduce both maternal and fetal mortality. In one study of serious motor vehicle accidents maternal mortality following ejection from the vehicle was 33%, compared to only 5% in those who were not ejected: fetal mortality was 47% and 11%, respectively.[11] A three-point seat bar system should be used, with the lap portion as low as possible, preferably over the thighs, and with the shoulder portion passing between the breasts and above the gravid uterus.

In a small series it appears that side airbags do not increase the risk of injury to pregnant women as long as other three-point restraints are used as well.[20]

CONTROVERSIES

❶ The length of CTG monitoring: most authors agree 4 hours should be enough to predict placental abruption, although some argue that 24-48 hours may be needed.

❷ Exploration of penetrating wounds to the abdomen: some authors argue a conservative approach to a wound below the uterine fundus, whereas others argue that all such wounds should be explored.

REFERENCES

1. American College of Surgeons 1993 Advanced Trauma Life Support. ACS, Chicago
2. Esposito TJ 1994 Trauma during pregnancy. Emergency Medicine Clinics of North America 12: 167–99
3. Pearlman MD, Tintinalli JE, Lorenz RP 1990 Blunt trauma during pregnancy. New England Journal of Medicine 323: 1609–13
4. Connolly A, Katz VL, Bash KL, McMahon MJ, Hansen WF 1997 Trauma and pregnancy. American Journal of Perinatology 14: 331–6
5. Aitokallio-Tallberg A, Halmesmaki E 1997 Motor vehicle accident during the second or third trimester of pregnancy. Acta Obstetrica Gynecologica Scandinavica 76: 313–7
6. Curet MJ, Schermer CR, Demarest GB, Bienek EJ, Curet LB 2000 Predictors of outcome in trauma during pregnancy: Identification of patients who can be monitered for less than 6 hours. Journal of Trauma 49: 18–25
7. Baerga-Varella Y, Zietlow SP, Bannon MP, Harmsen WS, Ilstrup DM 2000 Trauma in pregnancy. Mayo Clinic Proceedings 75: 1243–8
8. Ali J, Yeo A, Gana TJ, McLellan BA 1997 Predictors of fetal mortality in pregnant trauma patients. Journal of Trauma 42: 782–5
9. Kuhlmann RS, Cruikshank DP 1994 Maternal trauma during pregnancy. Clinical Obstetrics and Gynaecology 37: 274–93
10. Pearlman MD, Tintinalli JE, Lorenz RP 1990 A prospective controlled study of outcome after trauma during pregnancy. American Journal of Obstetrics and Gynecology 162: 1502–10
11. Vaizey CJ, Jacobson MJ, Cross FW 1994 Trauma in pregnancy. British Journal of Surgery 81: 1406–15
12. Goldman SM, Wagner LK 1996 Radiological management of abdominal trauma in pregnancy. American Journal of Roentgenology 166: 763–7
13. Bode PJ, Niezen RA, Van Vugt AB, Schipper J 1993 Abdominal ultrasound as a reliable indicator for conclusive laparotomy in blunt abdominal trauma. Journal of Trauma 34: 27–31
14. Stone IK 1999 Trauma in the obstetric patient. Obstetric and Gynaecology Clinics of North America 26: 459–67
15. Henderson SO, Mallon WK 1998 Trauma in pregnancy. Emergency Medicine Clinics of North America 16: 209–28
16. Goodwin TM, Breen MT 1990 Pregnancy outcomes and foetomaternal haemorrhage after noncatastrophic trauma. American Journal of Obstetrics and Gynecology 162: 665–71
17. Connolly A, Katz VL, Bash KL, McMahon MJ, Hansen WF 1997 Trauma in pregnancy. American Journal of Perinatology 14: 331–6
18. Pak LL, Reece EA, Chan L 1998 Is adverse pregnancy outcome predictable after blunt abdominal trauma? American Journal of Obstetrics and Gynaecology 179: 1140–4
19. Shah KH, Simons RK, Holbrook T, Fortlage D, Winchell RJ, Hoyt DB 1998 Trauma in pregnancy: maternal and fetal outcomes. Journal of Trauma Injury Infectious Critical Care 45: 83–68
20. Asterita DC, Feldman B 1997 Seat belt placement resulting in uterine rupture. Journal of Trauma 42: 738–40

2.10 TRAUMA IN THE ELDERLY

PETER RITCHIE

ESSENTIALS

1 The elderly patient has less physiological reserve due to the degenerative effects of ageing, comorbidity and drug therapy.

2 Early invasive monitoring to guide resuscitation in severely injured elderly patients results in better outcomes.

3 Adherence to basic principles of resuscitation of trauma patients and an organized team approach to management are as essential in the elderly as in the young.

4 Elderly patients with an initial Glasgow Coma Score of 8 or less due to head injury frequently die or survive to live in a persistent vegetative or dependent functional state.

5 Return to functional independence should be the ultimate goal in elderly trauma patients.

INTRODUCTION

Elderly patients are generally defined as those over 65 years with injured patients over 80 having significantly poorer outcomes. Physiological age may be greater than chronological age in some (e.g. those with disease in the major organ systems, or accelerated degenerative processes).[1]

Elderly patients comprise 15–20% of major trauma victims[2], with blunt trauma accounting for more than 95% of this group. The mean inpatient length of stay for elderly trauma victims is significantly longer than the average of 16 days and intensive care usage is high (>25%). Thus, despite the small number compared with other admission diagnoses, trauma patients consume a disproportionate amount of resources. Considering the rising proportion of the population that is elderly (i.e. over 65 years) this resource utilization is likely to increase.

The elderly are predisposed to injury by degenerative processes associated with ageing and the prevalence of disease processes (comorbidity). Deterioration of hearing, vision, joint position sense, the vestibular system, coordination, motor strength and the common problem of postural hypotension (iatrogenic or otherwise) all lead to an increased incidence of injury. Osteoporosis is a major contributing factor to fractures, which consequently may be caused by minimal trauma in the elderly. Advances in the treatment of chronic disease, such as arthritis and cardiovascular disease, allow people to remain more physically active into their later years, thus predisposing them to injury. Falls are the most common mechanism. Injuries of similar severity to those from which the young may rapidly recover often lead to greater morbidity and mortality in the elderly, and mortality increases directly with age. Complications after trauma are common in the elderly, including infections (14.5%), and complications involving the pulmonary (10.7%), cardiac (5.5%) and renal (3.7%) systems.[3,4]

AETIOLOGY

Falls

Over the age of 80, falls are the most common mechanism of injury leading to death.[5] Most falls occur on level surfaces or stairs. Each year 3.8% of the elderly have a significant fall,[6] mostly in the home. Risk factors for falls include increasing age, sensory impairment, neuromuscular disorders, unstable gait, dementia, acute illness, lower limb weakness, postural hypotension, cerebrovascular disease and drugs, including benzodiazepines, phenothiazines, antidepressants and diuretics. About 25% of falls in the elderly are caused by an underlying medical problem;[7] thus investigation of the cause of the fall is important, as well as treatment of injuries. Up to 50% of the elderly hospitalized for falls die within a year.[8]

Motor vehicle accidents

Most fatalities from trauma in the 65–80-year age group are due to motor vehicle accidents (25% of fatalities from all injuries).[5,9] When standardized for distance driven, the elderly have a high crash rate, particularly those over 85. The elderly are also more commonly involved as pedestrians struck by vehicles than any other age group.

Violence

Elderly people are easy targets for violent crime. Elder/parent abuse has recently been recognized and requires vigilance similar to that for child abuse. Victims may be poorly nourished, unkempt, or have multiple bruises and injuries in varying stages of repair. The involvement of emergency department care coordinators or social workers and appropriate community service agencies is necessary in such cases.

Burns

The elderly form a small percentage of the population with burn injuries but have the highest case fatality of any age group. Mortality from burns is directly related to the percentage of body surface area burnt, and age. Those who survive to hospital discharge do not subsequently have an accelerated death rate compared to the non-burned population.[3]

PATHOPHYSIOLOGY

'Physiological reserve' is reduced in the elderly. There is a reduction in cardiac index, pulmonary compliance, renal function and ability to respond physiologically to fluid loss or gain. Pathophysiological states such as chronic renal impairment, chronic liver disease, chronic respiratory disease and ischaemic heart disease are more common in the elderly, and also impair the response to hypovolaemia (and also to hypervolaemia from over-enthusiastic resuscitation). Many elderly patients are taking diuretics, which may deplete intravascular volume and potassium; and other drugs with cardiovascular actions, such as β-blockers and calcium channel blockers, which impair the cardiovascular response to trauma, including volume loss. Early use of invasive haemodynamic monitoring (arterial blood pressure monitoring, pulmonary artery catheterization) in conjunction with pulse oximetry, cardiac monitoring and measurement of urine output is recommended in the elderly multiple-trauma patient in order to optimize oxygen delivery, which is the ultimate goal of initial treatment.

GENERAL MANAGEMENT OF RESUSCITATION

Early attention to an accurate history of the event and of previous medical conditions is important, and relatives, the general practitioner or paramedics may be useful to this end if the patient is not able to give an accurate account.

General principles of assessment and resuscitation should follow standard guidelines, such as advanced trauma life support (ATLS).[10] However, elderly trauma patients may have an occult shock state despite apparently unremarkable clinical examination and vital signs.[1] This may be partly cardiogenic in origin. The early use of invasive monitoring, as outlined above, is recommended in the elderly patient with multiple injuries. In one study, severely injured geriatric patients who had early (2.2 hours) invasive monitoring, which included Swan-Ganz catheterization and intra-arterial blood pressure monitoring, had a much higher survival rate (53%, compared to 7%) than patients in whom invasive monitoring was started later (5.5 hours).[11]

Early initial radiography of multiple-trauma patients is as vital in the elderly as in the young, and should include chest, pelvis and cross-table cervical spine imaging without interruption of resuscitation.

MANAGEMENT OF SPECIFIC INJURIES

Head

Elderly patients with severe head injury have much poorer neurological recovery and higher mortality than younger patients. Falls are the most common mechanism, and are often precipitated by physical illness or alcohol. Subdural haematoma is common due to fragile bridging veins, which are firmly adherent to the dura and the cerebral hemispheres and increased mobility of the brain due to cerebral atrophy in the elderly. Extradural haematoma is uncommon because the dura becomes more adherent to the skull as the brain ages.

In a study published in 1996,[12] all patients over 65 with an admission Glasgow Coma Score (GCS) of 3 died in hospital, and all with an admission GCS of 4–7 either died, or lived in persistent vegetative or dependent functional states. In another study[13] practically all patients with a GCS <9 with intracranial space-occupying lesions (mostly subdural haematomata) died, and 80% with non-surgical lesions and a GCS <9 also died. This led the authors to suggest limited or no treatment of those with GCS <9 with a 'surgical' lesion, and 24 hours of aggressive treatment of those with a 'non-surgical' lesion, limiting of further 'maximal' therapy to those with a significant improvement over that time. A more recent study in Australia[14] found poor outcomes in all elderly patients with GCS<11 on arrival in the emergency department. Patients over the age of 51 with coma due to head injury of longer than 5.5 days have no chance of recovery.[15]

The management of head injury in the elderly is similar to that in younger patients, with maintenance of cerebral perfusion and early CT scanning to diagnose specific injuries. Early use of invasive haemodynamic monitoring and of intracranial pressure monitoring are specific considerations in the elderly. Medical and ethical decisions about the continuation of aggressive treatment should be made in light of the above evidence, and in consultation with the patient's family whenever possible.

Thoracic and abdominal injuries

Management of thoracic trauma in the elderly follows similar guidelines to that in the young but there should be a lower threshold for admission to hospital for the elderly patient. Osteoporosis results in a greater propensity for rib fractures, and cardiorespiratory reserve is lower in the elderly. Blunt chest trauma is common after falls and may go unrecognized, unless all elderly patients who fall are fully examined. Blunt chest trauma is also common in motor vehicle accidents (vehicle versus pedestrian and vehicle versus vehicle). Arterial blood gases should be measured in all cases of chest trauma. Good pain management is an essential component of the successful management of rib fractures, and may include epidural anaesthesia/analgesia or

narcotic infusions with careful monitoring of respiratory status.

Abdominal trauma management is the same as for younger patients except that the elderly tolerate shock less well, and thus the need for rapid diagnosis and intervention when necessary is paramount. The elderly may have less clinically obvious signs of intra-abdominal injury than a younger patient. Double-contrast CT scan is the radiological investigation of choice in the stable patient with abdominal injury, and there should be a lower threshold for this in the elderly. Bedside focused abdominal ultrasound should be considered an extension of the clinical examination of the abdomen in trauma and will be increasingly utilized in the emergency department. Peritoneal lavage may have a small place in the assessment of patients with combined abdominal and pelvic injuries. Unstable patients, those with abdominal signs consistent with hollow organ perforation or those with a positive ultrasound, should have urgent surgery.

Pelvis

Early and aggressive control of major haemorrhage, with early stabilization by external fixation and/or arterial embolization by a radiologist, is potentially life saving.

Spinal injuries

Elderly patients are more likely to sustain spinal trauma from falls, whereas younger patients are more likely to sustain such trauma in a motor vehicle accident. Elderly patients with spinal cord injury are more likely to develop the complications of bed rest. Functional recovery also tends to be worse in the elderly.

Cervical spine injury tends to involve the upper vertebrae of the neck (C1, C2). Pre-existing spinal disease makes bony and spinal cord injury more likely due to rigidity and a narrowed spinal canal. Evaluation may include plain radiography, CT and MRI imaging. (see Radiology in Major Trauma Chapter 2.8)

Fractures

Shock may occur with multiple fractures as a result of haemorrhage from bone, periosteum and surrounding soft tissues. Osteoporosis is common in the elderly, and a fractured neck of femur is the most common admission diagnosis for trauma. All patients with hip pain after a fall must be X-rayed regardless of their ability to walk afterwards, as it is sometimes possible to walk with an impacted subcapital fracture which is in danger of becoming displaced without internal fixation, thereby increasing the propensity for avascular necrosis. Early surgery and mobilization lead to lower morbidity and mortality from the complications of bed rest in the elderly: pneumonia, venous thromboembolism, decubitus ulcers, gastrointestinal haemorrhage (gastro-oesophageal reflux, peptic ulceration) and urinary sepsis from catheterization. Colles' fracture and fractured neck of humerus are common in the elderly, and may lead to significant social problems in those who may already be barely coping at home alone. Discharge of such patients from the emergency department must include a thorough social assessment.

Penetrating injuries

These are rare in the elderly but may result from suicide attempts or interpersonal violence. Specific management should be the same as in the young patient.

Burns

Management should include careful attention to fluid balance and respiratory state because of the lack of cardiorespiratory reserve and decreased renal function in the elderly.

DISPOSITION

There should be a low threshold for admission of the elderly injured patient to hospital, and the multiply injured elderly patient to the intensive care unit.

Identification of precipitating causes, such as neurological or cardiac events or postural hypotension, is especially important in the elderly prior to discharge from hospital, to prevent recurrent falls.

OUTCOMES

In 1984, Oreskovich et al[15] found an 85% overall survival rate in elderly trauma patients, but 88% did not return to their previous level of independence and only 8% were fully independent 1 year post discharge; 17% required home assistance and 72% were still in nursing homes. Mean ISS score in the study group was 19.

More recent studies have had more promising results. An Australian study by Day et al[16] of 118 patients over 60 with ISS scores >15 found a mortality of 30% in hospital (severe head injury being the main cause of death); of those surviving to hospital discharge, followed for an average of 3 years, 31% died, but of the long-term survivors 43 of 53 (i.e. 36% of the original 118) lived independently, and 41 of 54 scored maximum points in activities of daily living assessment. The authors assert that, although age is an important factor in survival after major trauma, those who do survive generally return to full activity and independence. Similar results were found in patients 75 years and over by Battistella et al[17] (47% mortality overall but 77 of 93 survivors living independently). In a study by DeMaria et al[18] of multiple-trauma patients over 65 with a mean ISS score of 15.8, there was a 21% mortality (which included patients who died in the study period after discharge), and of the survivors 89% returned home, 57% returned to independent living and 11% remained in nursing homes. Nursing home admission was more likely in the older patient, in those with a higher ISS, and those with more severe head and neck trauma. A subsequent study by the same authors[19] found that mortality was related to these same factors, and also to ventilator dependence for 5 or more days, cardiac complications and pneumonia. Two-thirds of survivors aged 80 or older also returned home. Carillo et al[20] found an 87% hospital survival rate and 87% of survivors were ultimately able to live independently at home. Broos et al[21] reported high survival and functional independence rates. Results such as these suggest that an aggressive approach to

trauma care in the elderly multiple-trauma patient is justified, with the caveat that elderly patients with head injury and a presenting Glasgow Coma Score of 8 or less have a very poor prognosis. Resuscitation using early invasive monitoring of blood pressure, cardiac output, central venous and pulmonary capillary wedge pressures in an intensive care unit has been shown to improve survival, and this approach is, therefore, recommended.[11]

Comorbidity is common in the elderly and has the potential to influence outcome adversely. Early identification may influence management.

PREVENTION

Prevention has greater potential to reduce trauma morbidity and mortality than treatment after the event. Legislative factors (e.g. seatbelt legislation, random breath testing, compulsory retesting of elderly drivers, reporting and delicensing of unfit drivers such as unstable epileptics) and community education programmes have great potential to improve the prevention of trauma. Technological advances (e.g. air bags and ABS braking systems in cars) may reduce injury severity. Improvement of the stabilization, resuscitation, surgical and inpatient care phases has been the traditional role of the emergency physician and surgeon, but there is great scope for medical practitioners involved in trauma care in promoting and participating in research into injury causation and prevention, and to influence government policy and the public in prevention.

REFERENCES

1. Mandavia D, Newton N 1998 Geriatric trauma. Emergency medicine. Clinics of North America 16(1): 257–75
2. Cameron P, Dziukas L, Hadj A, et al 1995 Major trauma in Australia: a regional analysis. Journal of Trauma 39(3): 545–52
3. Santora TA, Schinco MA, Trooskin SZ 1994 Management of trauma in the elderly patient. Surgical Clinics of North America 74(1): 163–86
4. Smith DP, Enderson BL, Maull KI, et al 1990 Trauma in the elderly: determinants of outcome. Southern Medical Journal 83: 171–7
5. Schwab CW, Kauder DR 1992 Trauma in the geriatric patient. Archives of Surgery 127: 701–6
6. Ryynanen OP, Kivela S, Honkanen R, et al 1991 Incidence of falling injuries leading to medical

treatment in the elderly. Public Health 105: 373–86
7. Duthie EH 1989 Falls. Medical Clinics of North America 73: 1321–36
8. Nelson RC, Murlidhar AA 1990 Falls in the elderly. Emergency Medical Clinics of North America 8: 309
9. McCoy GF, Johnstone RA, Duthie RB 1989 Injury to the elderly in road traffic accidents. Journal of Trauma 29(4): 494–7
10. American Committee on Trauma 1997 Advanced Trauma Life Support. Student Manual, American College of Surgeons
11. Scalea TM, Simon HW, Duncan AO, et al 1990 Geriatric blunt multiple trauma: improved survival with early invasive monitoring. Journal of Trauma 30: 129–36
12. Kilaru, S, Garb J, Emhoff T, et al 1996 Long-term functional status and mortality of elderly patients with severe closed head injuries. Journal of Trauma 41(6): 957–63
13. Kotwica Z, Jakubowski JK 1992 Acute head injuries in the elderly. An analysis of 136 consecutive patients. Acta Neurochirurgica 118: 98–102
14. Ritchie PD, Cameron PA, Ugoni AM, et al 2000 A study of the functional outcome and mortality in elderly patients with head injuries. Journal of Clinical Neuroscience 7: 301–4
15. Oreskovich MR, Howard J, Copass MK, et al 1984 Geriatric trauma: injury patterns and outcome. Journal of Trauma 24: 565–72
16. Day RJ, Vinen J, Hewitt-Falls E 1994 Major trauma outcomes in the elderly. Medical Journal of Australia 160: 675–8
17. Battistella FD, Din AM, Perez L 1998 Trauma patients 75 years and older: long-term follow-up results justify aggressive management. Journal of Trauma 44: 618–23
18. DeMaria EJ, Pardon R, Merrim MA, et al 1987 Aggressive trauma care benefits the elderly. Journal of Trauma 27(11): 1200–6
19. DeMaria EJ, Pardon R, Merrim MA, et al 1987 Survival after trauma in geriatric patients. Annals of Surgery 206(6): 738–43
20. Carrillo EH, Richardson J, Malias MA, et al 1993 Long-term outcome of blunt trauma care in the elderly. Surgery, Gynecology and Obstetrics 176: 559–64
21. Broos PLO, D'Hoore A, Vanderschot P, et al 1993 Multiple trauma in elderly patients. Factors influencing outcome: importance of aggressive care. Injury 24: 365–8

2.11 WOUND CARE AND REPAIR

RICHARD WALLER

ESSENTIALS

1 Good cosmesis can be achieved in the emergency department with conservative but thorough debridement and accurate apposition of everted skin edges.

2 Choose a suture that is monofilament, causes little tissue reactivity, and retains tensile strength until the healing wound strength has equalled that of the suture.

3 Dirty, contaminated, open wounds should generally be cleaned, debrided and closed within 6 hours to minimize the chance of wound infection.

4 Suspected tendon injuries require examination of the full range of movement of joints distal to the wound while observing the tendon in the base of the wound for breaches.

5 The success of a tendon repair (as measured by function) relates in large part to the postoperative care and therapy, not simply to the suture and wound closure.

6 Appropriate splinting and elevation of limb wounds at risk of infection takes precedence over antibiotics in the postoperative prevention of infection.

7 If prophylactic antibiotics are used, they should be given intravenously prior to wound closure to achieve adequate concentrations in the tissues and haematomas that may collect.

8 Wounds breaching body cavities, such as the peritoneum and joints, or involving flexor tendons, nerves and named arteries, should be referred to a surgeon for consideration of repair.

9 Foreign bodies such as clay directly chemically impair wound healing.

10 Puncture wounds such as bites may be managed by either second-intention healing after thorough lavage, or better still by excisional debridement, lavage, antibiotics and atraumatic closure, if less than 24 hours old (preferably less than 6 hours).

INTRODUCTION

Open wound injury comprises a significant component of emergency department (ED) workload. Data from the Victorian Injury Surveillance System databank (1998, personal communication), which records 80% of Victorian Emergency Department presentations, show that more than 8% of all recorded principal injuries are open wounds. In addition, open wounds may accompany other injuries such as fractures. More than a quarter of open wound injury types are in the paediatric age group (0–14 years), more than 60% occur in people under 30, and less than 10% in the over 60s age group. Overall 70% of patients are male.

Location data show that more than 40% of these wounds occur in the home, mostly during activity described as leisure. The three major causes are falls up to 1 metre; contact with cutting or piercing objects; or having been struck or collided with. Most are accidental and only 3.7% are due to an assault. Injuries to the face and head comprise one-third, and the hand is involved in another one-third. The rest are scattered over the remainder of the body. The majority are repaired in the emergency department and the patient discharged home (87%). Almost half are referred to GPs and specialists for review. It is those wounds that are suitable for emergency department repair that will be further discussed.

CLINICAL PRESENTATION

An initial general assessment of the patient is important as it defines the likely mode of repair and the injured structures, and identifies factors for complications. The assessment includes the traditional history, examination and investigation of the patient.

It is important in the history to identify the time and mechanism of injury, the likely presence of foreign bodies, and the tetanus immunization status. Past medical history; allergies to agents such as local anaesthetics, antibiotics, preparation solutions and tapes; and current medications such as warfarin or cytotoxics all have a bearing on the management. For example, there is a greater risk of infection and poor wound healing in diabetic patients with extremity wounds of the lower limbs sustained in a crush injury. Other relevant general conditions, particularly in the setting of dirty wounds such as bites, include prior mastectomy, and other causes of chronic oedema of the affected region, prior splenectomy, liver dysfunction, immunosuppression, or autoimmune disease such as SLE. Smokers have impaired collagen production in healing wounds.[1]

The general examination comprises a search for all injuries sustained and concurrent medical illness that may have a bearing on the results of repair, such as poor circulation in patients with peripheral vascular disease. The patient needs to be recumbent (beware of syncope) and any clothing that may obstruct a thorough examination removed. A general examination is performed, followed by a local preliminary screening examination of the wound coupled with initial cleansing. This is designed to assess the need to perform additional investigations.

Investigations include radiographs for fractures or ultrasound for foreign bodies, and precede a detailed examination of the depth of the wound, which usually requires good anaesthesia. A surface wound caused by the entrance of a foreign body does not necessarily mean that the foreign body has remained in the vicinity.

An injury to a tendon in the base of the wound may only be apparent when the joints over which it acts are in a particular position, reflecting the position of the limb at the time of injury. At other positions the tendon injury may slide out of view. Marked pain with use may be a clue to a partial tendon injury.

The initial assessment may suggest factors such as nerve damage, indicating the need for referral to a plastic surgeon. Having completed the preliminary investigations the wound depths are explored with good anaesthesia to identify any additional structural damage, and further cleansing is carried out before repair is commenced.

WOUND CLEANSING

To provide optimum conditions to heal without infection it is essential to remove all contaminants, foreign bodies and devitalized tissue prior to wound closure.

Universal precautions, including eye protection (goggles or similar), clothing protection (gown) and gloves, must be taken for all wound care and repair. Gloves should be powder free to avoid adding starch foreign body to the wound, which will delay healing and produce granulomas.[2] One must be aware of the risk of latex allergy to both the glove wearer and the patient.[2]

There is a wide variety of cleansing solutions available (Table 2.11.1), with differing attributes.

The surrounding skin surface is prepared with chlorhexidine or povidone-iodine using caution near the eyes and mucous membranes, particularly if the solution is surgical scrub strength. Despite their bactericidal nature, bottles of povidone-iodine may become contaminated by bacteria as a result of multiple usage.[3] Thus fresh sterile solution should be used whenever possible. Concentrations of more than 1% have proved toxic to tissues.[4] If there is to be a delay in closure, the wound may be kept moist with either 0.5% povodine-iodine or 0.05–0.1% chlorhexidine, or saline-soaked gauze. Alcoholic solutions should not be used in open wounds.

Anaesthesia is necessary for wounds to be cleansed adequately. Extensive wounds or particularly heavily contaminated wounds that need vigorous scrubbing, such as road metal tattooing, may require general anaesthesia. Local anaesthetic may be given by local infiltration or as a regional nerve blockade. Needles introduced through the wound cause less pain, but may theoretically track bacteria into the tissues, although this has not been demonstrated to be a problem clinically. After anaesthesia, irrigation with a pressure of at least 8 psi (55 kPa)[5,6] is required to dislodge bacteria and reduce the incidence of infection. This can be achieved with a 19G needle, a 25–50 mL syringe, a three-way tap and a flask of fluid such as sterile saline (Fig. 2.11.1).[7] High-pressure irrigation (>20 psi, 138 kPa) may cause tissue damage.[8]

Radio-opaque foreign bodies, such as gravel, metal, pencil lead and glass may be identified using portable fluoroscopy and removed. This is not sensitive for plastic or wood, however,[9] which may be detectable with ultrasound.

Adequate debridement of devitalized tissue has always been a tenet of surgical practice. More recently, there has been a change in emphasis from radical to meticulous debridement. If the skin is devitalized it should be removed using a scalpel blade. Viable tissue will bleed when cut, and viable muscle will contract when stimulated. If viability is in doubt it may be better to wait for demarcation over the following days, with regular close observation. Fat and fascia are relatively avascular and, if semiviable, in contamin-

Table 2.11.1 Preparation solutions and their properties				
Solution	Properties	Mechanism of action	Uses	Disadvantages
N. Saline	Isotonic, nontoxic	Simply washing action	In wound for irrigation	No antiseptic action
Chlorhexidine 0.1% w/v – aqueous	Bacteriostatic	Antibacterial and washing action	Cleanse skin surrounding wound	Not near eyes (causes keratitis), perf. ear drum or meninges
Chlorhexidine 0.1% w/v + cetrimide 1% w/v	Bacteriostatic	Antibacterial and soap action, removes sebum, 'wetting' the skin	Cleanse skin surrounding wound	Not near mucous membranes, eyes (causes keratitis), perf. ear drum or meninges
H_2O_2 3%	Bacteriocidal to anaerobes	Forms superoxide radicals	Severely contaminated wounds with anaerobic type pathogens	Obstruction of wound surface capillaries and subsequent necrosis
Povidone-iodine 10% w/v	Bacteriocidal fungicidal viricidal sporicidal	Releases free iodine	On surrounding skin, or in severely contaminated wounds (dilute 1% w/v)	Use on/in large wounds may cause acidosis due to iodine absorption[28]

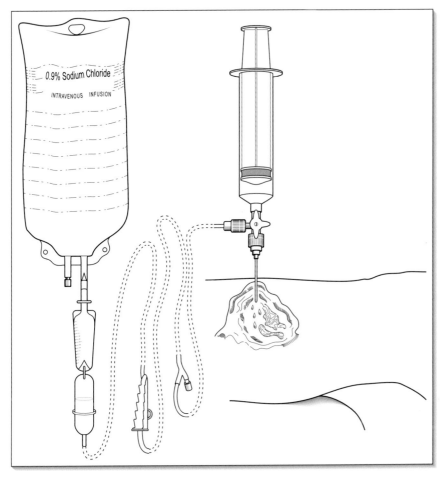

Fig. 2.11.1 Wound irrigation set-up comprising flask of fluid, IV tubing, three-way tap, syringe and 19 G needle designed to deliver fluid at at least 8 psi (55 kPa). (From an original drawing by Elaine Wheildon)

ated wounds, should be removed. Semi-viable muscle can usually be preserved when well drained.[10] Nerves, major vessels and tendons should not be debrided in the emergency department. Lavage and debridement should be continued until the wound is clean. Organic material and anionic soils such as clay pose the greatest risk of infection if not removed. The highly charged clay particles directly affect leucocytes, preventing phagocytosis of bacteria. They also react chemically with antibiotics, limiting their action.

Once the wound is clean the decision to close immediately or later is made.

Guidelines for delayed closure may include:

- Puncture wounds, such as with a tooth or a knife;
- Wounds unable to be adequately debrided;

- Contaminated wounds more than 6 hours old;
- Too much tension in the wound, particularly with crush injury.

In some cases, such as thoroughly lavaged puncture wounds, it may be prudent to allow healing by secondary intention. If in doubt, consult with a plastic surgeon. When repair in the emergency department may be delayed, it is prudent to have nursing staff perform a preliminary preparation of the wound along the lines shown in Table 2.11.2.

TETANUS PROPHYLAXIS

The risk of tetanus is greatest in the very young and the very old, with an overall death rate of 1 in 10 in Australia,[11] so prevention is all important. An average

of 10 cases per year occur in Australia,[10] usually in older adults who have not been immunized or who have allowed it to lapse. The anaerobic bacterium *Clostridium tetani* is present in soil and animal faeces. After incubation of 3–21 days post innoculation into a wound, the toxin produced by the bacteria causes severe muscle spasm and convulsions. Death occurs commonly from respiratory failure. The types of wounds at risk are listed in Table 2.11.3, but tetanus may occur after apparently trivial wounds.

Tetanus immunoglobulin is given into the opposite limb to the tetanus toxoid for patients with inadequate protection against tetanus (Table 2.11.4), providing passive protection.

WOUND-HEALING MECHANISMS

Wounds never gain more than 80% of the strength of intact skin.[12] There are three phases of wound healing. Days 1–5 are the initial lag phase (inflammatory), where there is no gain in the strength of the wound. Days 5–14 are a period of rapid increase in wound strength, associated with fibroplasia and epithelialization. The wound has only 7% of its final strength at day 5. Wound maturation progresses from day 14 onwards, with production, cross-linking and remodelling of collagen.

The surgical maxim that wounds heal from side to side is only partly true: if left to heal by itself the entire wound will contract around its margin prior to epithelialization. This has been termed secondary closure or healing by second intention. Allowing the wound to close without intervention relies on healing up from the base and from the edges, and often results in unsightly scars. Primary closure involves the apposition of wound edges, preferably within 6 hours of injury, with sutures, staples, tissue adhesive glue, etc. After a delay of 6 hours or more the chance of a wound infection increases. Delayed primary closure is performed 4–5 days after injury, when it is clear there is no infection. This may be used for contaminated wounds that present more than 6 hours post injury.

Table 2.11.2 Preliminary wound preparation procedure instructions for nurses

Explain the procedure to the patient

Identify any allergies, especially to iodine-like products and adhesive tapes

Medicate the patient prior to the irrigation, as needed for pain control

Protect patient clothing from soiling by the irrigation solution or wound drainage

Position the patient so that irrigating solution can be collected in a basin, depending on the wound's location

Maintain a sterile field during the irrigation procedure as appropriate

Irrigate wound with appropriate solution, using a large irrigating syringe and set-up (see Fig. 2.11.1)

Instil the irrigation solution at 8 psi (55 kPa), reaching all areas

Avoid aspirating the solution back into the syringe

Cleanse from cleanest to dirtiest areas of the wound

Continue irrigating the wound until the prescribed volume is used or the solution returns clear

Position the patient after the irrigation to facilitate drainage

Cleanse and dry the area around the wound after the procedure

Dispose of soiled dressing and supplies appropriately

Lightly pack the wound with well wrung out, saline soaked lint-free sterile gauze, or an alginate dressing

Apply a sterile dressing as appropriate until repair is performed

Table 2.11.3 Wounds that are prone to tetanus

Compound fractures

Deep penetrating wounds

Wounds containing foreign bodies, e.g. wood splinters, thorns

Crush injuries or wounds with extensive tissue damage, e.g. burns

Wounds contaminated with soil or horse manure

Wound cleansing delayed more than 3–6 hours

SUTURE TYPES

Wounds may be closed with tape, staples, sutures or tissue adhesive.

Purpose-made commercial tapes reinforced with rayon provide an excellent means of closure. The adherence of tapes (Fig. 2.11.2) may be improved with the application of adhesive adjuncts, such as tincture of benzoin, or gum mastic paint.[13] These adhesives must not be allowed to enter the wound[14] as they potentiate infection and cause intense pain. The rates of infection with tapes and staples are lower than with conventional sutures.[15]

Staples have the advantage of rapid insertion and wound closure, particularly for extensive wounds. They are applied using a staple gun and must be removed using the appropriate removal device, which may be a problem with follow-up arrangements.

From horsehair in World War Two[16] to today's soluble monofilament plastics with prolonged tensile strength, necessity has seen the development of many different suture materials (Fig. 2.11.3) of different grades and with different types of needles. The ideal suture is monofilament, causes no tissue reaction, does not promote infection, is completely absorbed, and yet has a tensile strength and secure knots that last until tissue strength has equalled that of the suture. It should stretch to accommodate wound oedema, recoil to its original length, and be inexpensive. However, as yet no such suture exists.

Table 2.11.4 Tetanus vaccination schedule for acute wound management

History of tetanus vaccination	(CDT) Td	Type of wound	DTP, DT (ADT)* or tetanus toxide as appropriate	Tetanus immunoglobulin
3 doses or more	If less than 5 years since last dose	All wounds	no	no
	If 5–10 years since last dose	Clean minor wounds	no	no
		All other wounds	yes	no
	If more than 10 years since last dose	All wounds	yes	no
Uncertain, or less than 3 doses		Clean minor wounds	yes	no
		All other wounds	yes	yes

*DTP, diphtheria tetanus pertussis for children before 8th birthday
DT, Child diphtheria tetanus (CDT) if pertussis is contraindicated
Td, adult diphtheria tetanus (ADT) for children after their 8th birthday
Adapted from.[11]

Factors that affect the rate of wound healing include:

- Technical factors of the repair
- Anatomic factors (intrinsic blood supply, etc.)
- Drugs (steroids, cytotoxics, etc.)
- Associated conditions and diseases (diabetes, vitamin C, zinc deficiency, etc.)
- The general nutritional state of the patient.

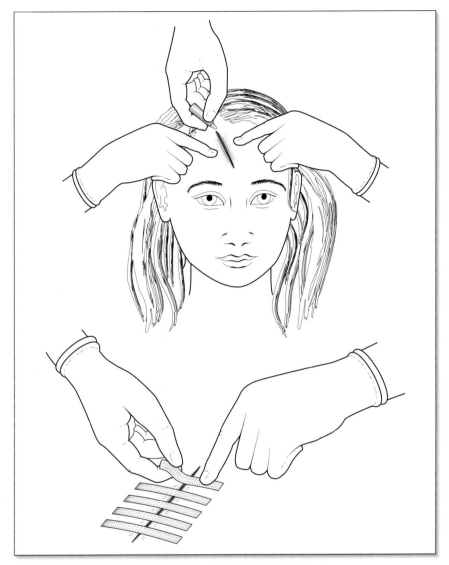

Fig. 2.11.2 Steristrips and glue are typically used for children in most simple split lacerations, thereby avoiding the use of needles. (From an original drawing by Elaine Wheildon)

In the future, biological tissue adhesive agents such as fibrin sealant[16] for use in the wound may replace sutures as the means of wound closure. As yet these are experimental in sterile, surgically created wounds.

NEEDLES

Early surgical needles had eyes like traditional sewing needles and caused tissue trauma as the bulk of folded-back thread and needle passed through the tissues. The first swaged needles were invented over 100 years ago, and modern disposable swaged needles have largely replaced the reusable eye needles. There are three parts to a needle: the swage, the body and the point (Fig. 2.11.4).

Advances in metallurgy have allowed the production of nickel maraged stainless steel wire, from which needles are cut. They may be straight, or curved in arcs of varying degrees to produce portions of a circle, such as 90°, 135°, 180° and 225° parts. A compound curved needle comprises two different arcs, limiting the amount of supination necessary to pass it through tissue. Skin repair requires usually either or half circle needles. The points of surgical needles may be tapered, cutting, or a combination. Taper-point needles are generally round or oval bodied and are not suitable for skin as they are difficult to pass through the tightly bundled collagen fibres of the dermis. Their role is in repair of soft tissues such as fascia, blood vessels and bowel, etc. Cutting needles are for skin, and have a triangular point with sharp cutting edges to facilitate tissue penetration. Conventional cutting needles have the apex of the triangle towards the concavity of the curved needle (see Fig. 2.11.4). Reverse cutting needles have the apex on the convexity of the needle. This style of needle and suture will not cut out when the needle is passed through tissue, or once the knotted suture is resting against a block of tissue rather than a cut. Such needles are structurally stronger.[19] Combination cutting at the point and taper for the remainder of the body are for slightly denser tissues such as tendon or aponeu-

A key factor in choosing absorbable suture is the length of time over which it retains adequate strength. The inflammatory phase of healing lasts for 7 days. Catgut prolongs this phase and is removed by enzymatic action, whereas absorbable plastics simply hydrolyse. Braided sutures produce greater tissue reaction than monofilaments. Braided and catgut sutures should be avoided in contaminated wounds,[17] as the interstices provide a haven for bacteria from phagocytes. Traditional absorbable sutures have included Vicryl® and Dexon®, both braided multifilament. Extensive studies have shown new monofilament absorb-able sutures to have superior strength both initially and at 4 weeks; less interference with bacterial clearance; more secure knots with fewer throws; and lower drag forces through tissue, compared to the braided absorbable types.[18]

Tissue adhesive agents such as Histo-acryl (enbucrilate; B. Braun Surgical GmbH) - 'superglue' - have been developed particularly with the minor superficial paediatric wound in mind. The results can be excellent, provided good wound edge apposition is achieved prior to application of the glue on the surface (see Fig. 2.11.2).

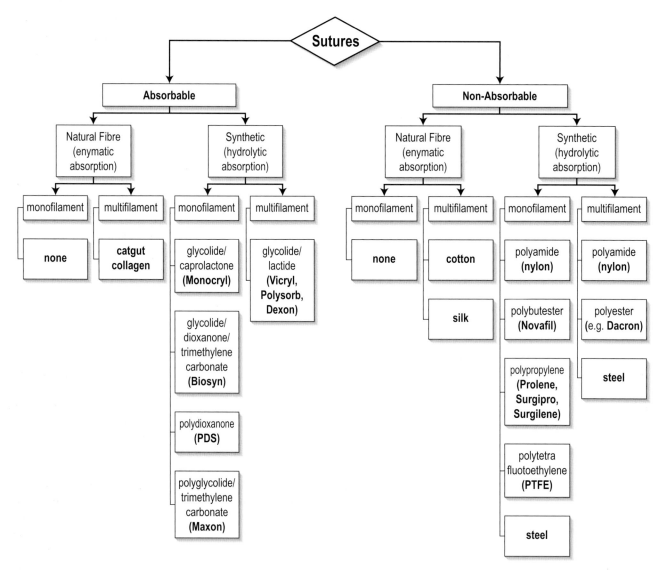

Fig. 2.11.3 A simple classification of suture types in current usage, adapted from[17].

rosis. Needle holders are generally used with curved needles, and straight needles are hand held. The risk of needle-stick injuries with handheld needles makes their use hazardous.

BASIC SUTURE TECHNIQUE

Prior to closure, prophylactic antibiotics (see Chapter 8.10) should be given intravenously if required. This ensures that any haematoma that collects in the wound after or during closure will contain antibiotic.

Having prepared a sterile field with the contents of a suture tray (Table 2.11.5)

laid out, the wound anaesthetized and cleaned, and the sterile drapes placed around the wound, repair can begin. A very contaminated wound should be anaesthetized, lavaged and cleansed before repreparing with antiseptic and draping for formal debridement, further lavage and repair.

One should choose the thinnest possible suture that will tolerate the tissue tensions and provide adequate strength. The needle holder must grasp the needle in the body, usually two-thirds of the length from the tip of the needle, rather than over the swage where the metal is relatively weak. Stretching the suture in the hands, supporting it at the needle swage, will remove its

'memory', making handling easier. The needle holder should be held in the palm of the hand and controlled with the index finger, using a supination/pronation action in the arc of the needle (Fig. 2.11.5). The placement of the first suture varies with the wound: in a small linear wound it may be convenient to simply suture from one end to the other. In longer wounds without good corresponding landmarks on either side it is helpful to subdivide the wound serially, to ensure one does not finish up with a 'dog ear'. If an assistant is available, stretching the wound is helpful (see Fig. 2.11.5). In more irregular complex wounds it is helpful to approximate corresponding landmarks first. For example,

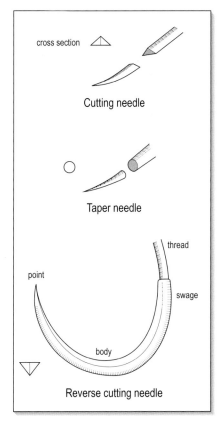

cross section

Cutting needle

Taper needle

thread

point

swage

body

Reverse cutting needle

Fig. 2.11.4 Surgical needle characteristics and types. (From an original drawing by Elaine Wheildon)

Table 2.11.5 Surgical instruments required for wound repair	
Contents of a typical simple suture tray	*Contents of a typical 'plastics' suture tray*
1× Nelson Hegar needle holder 6 1/2 in 1× Curved artery forceps 1× Gillies dissectors 1× McIndoe dissectors 2× Small bowls 1× Kidney dish autoplas 255 mm 1× Fenestrated drape 1× Huck towel	2× Mosquito forceps curved 2× Mosquito forceps straight 1× Hegar needle holder 5 1/2" 1× Gillies needle holder 1× Straight Mayo scissors 1× Curved Mayo scissors 1× Vein straight scissors 1× Vein curved scissors 1× McIndoe dissectors 1× Adson dissectors 1× Gillies toothed dissectors 2× Skin hooks 2× Catspaw refractors 1× Bard–Parker handle no. 3 1× Bard–Parker handle no. 4 1× Vein hook Alcot 1× Rampley sponge holder 3× Gallipots 1× Kidney dish 3× Towel clips 4× Huck towel

the apex of a flap is best stitched first (Fig. 2.11.6).

After wound contraction has occurred the wound edge has a natural tendency to inversion, resulting in a shallow crater. To prevent this the edges must be everted at closure. To do this the skin near the wound edge is depressed (Fig. 2.11.7) or lifted with a skin hook or forceps, such that the needle enters and exits perpendicularly to the skin in both running and interrupted sutures. The sutures so placed may be interrupted with separate tied closed loops or continuous loops passing through tissue, tied at either end. Vertical mattress sutures (Fig. 2.11.8) and horizontal mattress sutures (Fig. 2.11.9) are designed to evert wound edges that are difficult to maintain in eversion with simple sutures.

Knots are the weakest link in the suture, particularly for continuous sutures, where the failure of a knot will release the whole suture along the length of the wound. The knots may be tied with

instruments or by hand. One must be careful, when using instrument ties, not to damage the suture by either crushing with the serrated jaws of a needle holder or tearing on the edges of the jaws. A reef knot with a snug third throw produces the best results for nylon or polypropylene. Synthetic monofilament sutures require several twists in the first and second throws to prevent unknotting (see Fig. 2.11.5). It is important that the wound closure be achieved without excessive tension on the sutures.

Interrupted sutures have the advantage of individual removal to allow drainage of an infected wound, or for cosmetic reasons to limit the time a suture stays in while retaining some sutures for wound strength; however, there is a trade-off in the time it takes to close a wound using multiple knots. Sutures tied too tightly, exacerbated by oedema in the wound and from the trauma created by the needle's passage, will cause suture marks due to local ischaemia on the skin surface. An individual suture strangling tissue will continue to do so until it is cut. One way to avoid tissue strangulation is to use a loop throw in an interrupted suture[12] (Fig. 2.11.10).

Studies have shown no increase in wound infection or decrease in wound strength with the use of continuous sutures,[20] which may be placed rapidly in

long linear wounds, distributing tension evenly. However, if one knot fails or the stitch is cut they will loosen along the length of the wound. Continuous sutures may be percutaneous or intradermal (subcuticular). If intradermal they should surface every 3 cm to facilitate removal.[21]

Intradermal sutures are most appropriate for surgical wounds. Monofilament polypropylene has a very low surface coefficient of friction and is thus easiest to remove in the setting of continuous percutaneous or subcuticular closure.[22] One should ensure that the suture glides easily through each segment and is not looped, otherwise removal may become very difficult. Recently, absorbable monofilament such as glycolide caprolactone - Monocryl (Ethicon Inc.) - has supplanted polypropylene for continuous subcuticular suture as it does not have to be removed.

Historically, Halstead[23] considered it important to 'obliterate with the greatest care all of the dead spaces of a wound'. In 1974 it was demonstrated that suture closure of dead space increases the incidence of infection secondary to the foreign body (the suture) in the wound, thereby eliminating the benefits of dead space closure.[24] Some authors[12] stress the importance of using buried sutures to obtain wound edge eversion and dead space closure. Modern hydrolysable

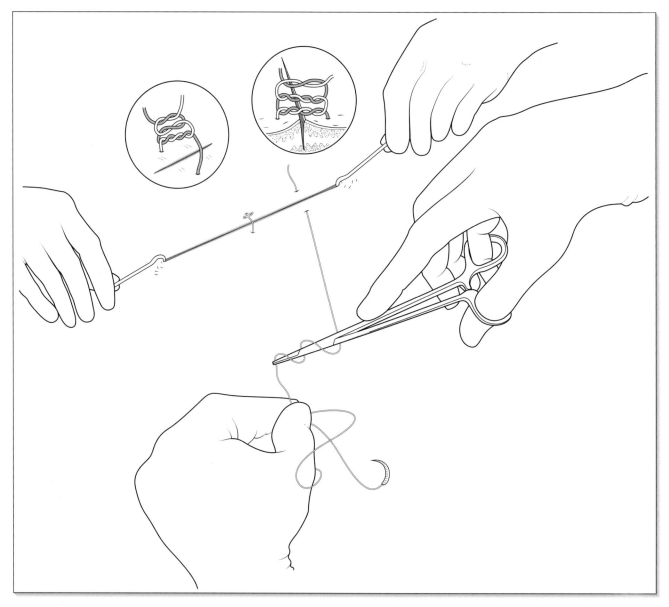

Fig. 2.11.5 The basic technique of how to hold a needle driver, put the wound on the stretch, and suture a long wound in halves using surgical knots. For synthetic sutures the reef knot with the third throw requires several twists, as illustrated, to prevent loosening. (From an original drawing by Elaine Wheildon)

monofilament sutures allow this. The long-term maintenance of dermal edge apposition, either with or without deep sutures, is the key to obtaining the narrowest possible scar. Techniques have been developed to encourage this and to avoid leaving buried sutures, with their attendant risk of wound infection. To allow the removal of a deep space-obliterating suture without disrupting the wound some creative methods have been devised (Fig. 2.11.11).[25]

Wounds that slice obliquely through thick skin, such as on the back, can be trimmed with a scalpel blade perpendicular to the skin or sutured with a vertical mattress to prevent one bevelled edge sliding over the other. If necessary to prevent a wound edge step, adjustments in the height of the wound edges can be achieved by exiting the needle superficially on the high side and deeper on the low side, using either continuous or interrupted sutures.[12]

SPECIAL SITES AND SITUATIONS

The face, particularly with dirty wounds such as bites, requires early repair to achieve good cosmesis. Delay for up to 24 hours is acceptable, prior to definitive debridement and repair in the operating theatre, provided interim wound care is of a good standard. To enable adequate cleansing, local nerve blocks should be used.

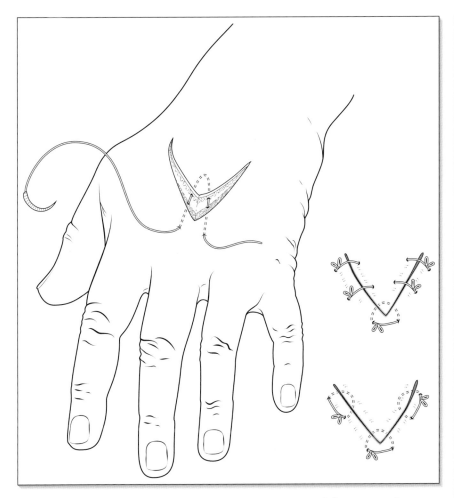

Fig. 2.11.6 Closure of a flap requires an initial suture of the apex, after which either simple or horizontal mattress sutures may be used. (From an original drawing by Elaine Wheildon)

A field block is generally required for ears. Ear cartilage must be aligned and skin coverage achieved to prevent perichondritis.

Injuries involving the eyelid need a good examination of the underlying globe to exclude scleral and conjunctival lacerations; also, canaliculi may be torn. A lacerated canaliculus should be microsurgically repaired and stented within 24 hours. Accurate apposition of eyebrows and vermilion border is essential. Never shave an eyebrow.

Damaged facial muscle must be repaired in the interests of facial symmetry. In cheek injuries, the facial nerve and parotid duct must be checked for intactness. The nerves are generally deep in the cheek. Terminal repair of nerves medial to the midpupillary line is unnecessary.

Tattooing should be removed within 12 hours to avoid tissue fixation. Use a sterile brush and magnification and be meticulous. It is useful to have sterile toothbrushes available in the emergency department for this. After 12 hours a formal dermabrasion and/or debridement may be needed.

Complications of facial wounds are numerous and provide some special problems (Table 2.11.6).

SPECIAL SUTURE TECHNIQUES

Techniques for relieving the tension in a wound include limited undermining, and the use of horizontal mattress sutures (see Fig. 2.11.9). Very rarely should skin flaps be raised in acute trauma. These may be advancement (e.g. V-Y advancement), rotation or transposition in design. It is usually better to apply a split skin graft to heal the wound primarily and perform later scar revision or reconstruction. In some settings V-Y flaps can be advanced or retreated, depending on the direction of tension (Fig. 2.11.12).

THE 'DOG EAR'

The term 'dog ear' refers to a conical pucker of redundant skin that may collect at the end of a wound towards the end of closure (Fig. 2.11.13), particularly in wounds with an eliptical area of skin defect. In order to avoid a 'dog ear' the wound should be sutured in halves, placing each new stitch between the previous ones (see Fig. 2.11.5). There are several ways to remove a dog ear.[26]

- The direct overlap excision technique involves drawing the redundant skin from one side across the wound and excising along the line of the wound. Any remaining redundant skin is drawn across the wound from the other side, and excised along the line of the wound (see Fig. 2.11.13).
- Unilateral dog ears are best removed by elevating the redundant skin with a skin hook in the centre, followed by incising along the edge of the fold and then allowing the created flap to fall back along the line of the sutures, where it is trimmed off. This results in a J-shaped repair (see Fig. 2.11.13).
- An elliptical excision of the dog ear in line with the closure can excise the defect (see Fig. 2.11.13), but this also lengthens the wound.
- In very large dog ears a V-Y excision and closure will provide good closure.
- Thick dog ears that are aligned perpendicularly to the original closure can be excised and closed in a T repair (see Fig. 2.11.13).

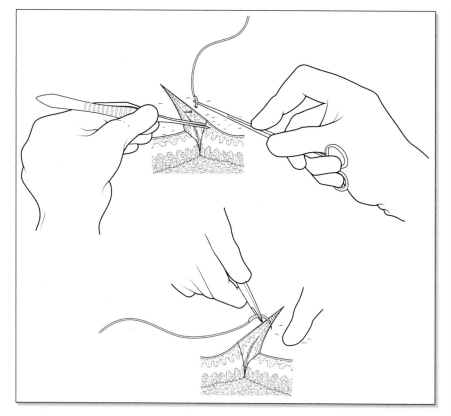

Fig. 2.11.7 Everting the wound edge using Gillies tissue forceps or digital pressure when placing a suture improves the cosmetic result. (From an original drawing by Elaine Wheildon)

WOUND DRAINAGE

Fluid trapped within the closed wound predisposes to infection by:

- Progressively losing opsonins
- Interfering with access of phagocytes to bacteria
- Providing a nutrient medium for bacterial growth
- Putting pressure on adjacent vasculature, compromising blood supply.

Fluid also prevents the apposition of healing tissues. The build-up of fluid can be prevented by immobilization, preventing shearing forces between tissue planes; firm but not tight dressings; and drainage. The indications for drainage are:

- Dead-space elimination to prevent fluid accumulation (with an active suction drain or a compressive dressing with a passive drain)
- Removal of established fluid collections.

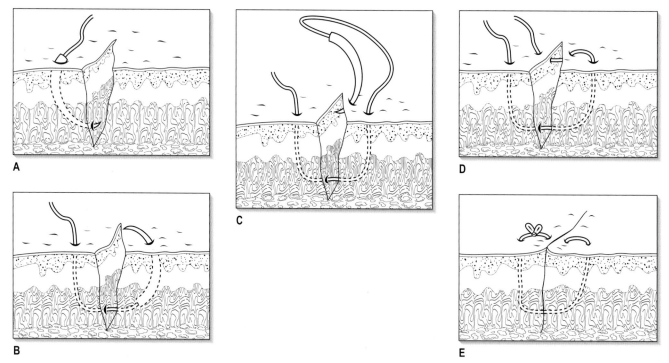

Fig. 2.11.8 The vertical mattress suture technique is useful to evert wound edges with a natural tendency to roll inward despite correctly placed simple sutures. (From an original drawing by Elaine Wheildon)

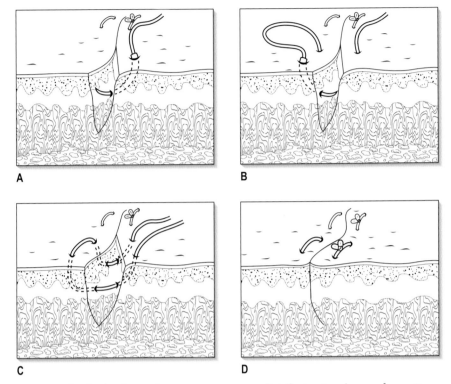

A

B

C

D

Fig. 2.11.9 The horizontal mattress suture redistributes tension and everts wound edges. (From an original drawing by Elaine Wheildon)

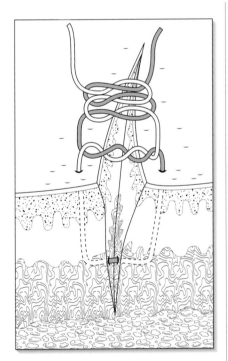

Fig. 2.11.10 The loop suture method of avoiding excessive tension on a stitch.[12] (From an original drawing by Elaine Wheildon)

Suction drains are superior to passive drains, which rely on gravity; however, blockage of drain holes and of the drain tube lumen can be a problem. There are many commercial closed suction systems on the market. A simple suction drain can be constructed from a 'butterfly' cannula and a vacuum blood specimen tube (Fig. 2.11.14)[6] by cutting off the syringe adapter and fenestrating the tubing prior to placement through a stab incision into the wound. The vacuum tube can be changed as necessary. Clamp the tubing before changing the tube to prevent the ingress of contaminants into the wound via the drain. Patients with drains will need regular review, either in the emergency department or by the local doctor. Drains are generally removed at 48 hours unless draining copiously.

DRESSINGS

It has long been recognized that the dressing and subsequent wound care are as important as the operative technique.[27] The depths of the wound must be moist for healing, but the skin surface must not become macerated.

The appropriate style of dressing for abrasions is still debated. The 'moist' versus 'dry' debate revolves around saline packs, sterile paraffin, solugel, seaweed preparations, occlusive plastic film dressings and various foam preparations.

In covering the sutured wound, the dressing aims to keep the primarily apposed skin edges dry, wicking away any ooze, haemorrhage or exudate. It should only be changed if its capacity to absorb fluid is exceeded, and ideally it should stay on until the time of suture removal. Where this is not possible, the wound may be bathed or showered 24 hours after closure, provided it is thoroughly dabbed dry and not immersed and soaked in water. In the case of scalp wounds this allows showering and hair washing, and avoids the problem of fixing a dressing to hairy skin. Plastic spray such as OpSite® may be useful in this setting. Wounds that are contaminated and at high risk of infection need review and redressing at 48 hours.

IMMOBILIZATION

Wounds that traverse joints or which occur on highly mobile skin, such as in the hand, require immobilization. Splinting with plaster slabs is a cheap, traditional and reliable method. Apart from protecting and stabilizing the wound to allow healing, the splint also reduces the likelihood of infection. If practicable, potentially infected wounds of the upper limbs should be in a sling, elevated to reduce oedema. Lower limbs may be rested using crutches, and elevated whenever possible.

DISPOSAL/REMOVAL

Despite an apparently good cosmetic result at the time (Table 2.11.7) of suture removal (5–14 days) in head and neck wounds, there is evidence of a poor correlation with wound appearance 6–9

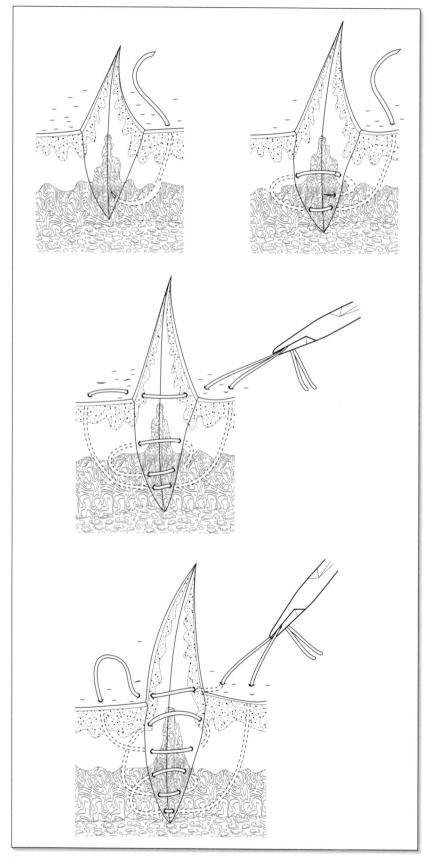

Fig. 2.11.11 A deep closure method utilizing a variable number of loops, adapted from a Mayo Clinic stitch.[25] (From an original drawing by Elaine Wheildon)

Table 2.11.6 Complications of facial wounds

Complication	Notes
Infection	Potentially fatal owing to the valveless venous communication with the brain
AV fistulae	Due to profuse vascularity – uncommon
Scarring	Producing facial asymmetry and cosmetic implications
Deformity	Due to unrecognized fractures, such as of the nose or malar bone
Facial palsy	Due to damaged facial nerves
Epiphora	With tissue loss or scarring everting the lower lid, or canaliculus damage
Salivary fistula	After disruption of the parotid duct
Drooling	With tissue loss, scar contracture or local nerve damage
Corneal exposure	With tissue loss, scar contracture or local nerve damage

Table 2.11.7 Guide to time for removal of sutures

Location	Days to removal
Scalp	6–8
Face (incl. ear)	4–5
Chest/abdomen	8–10
Back	12–14
Arm/leg*	8–10
Hand*	8–10
Fingertip	10–12
Foot	12–14

*Add 2–3 days for lacerations crossing extensor surfaces of joints and if early motion is required for rehabilitation, e.g. post flexor tendon repair. Adapted from[30]

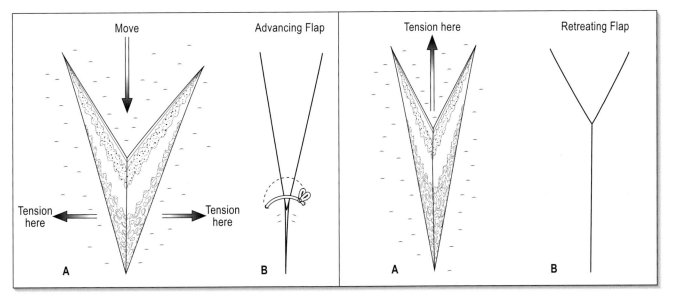

Fig. 2.11.12 The V-Y flap advancement or retreat is useful to redistribute and reduce tension across a wound. (From an original drawing by Elaine Wheildon)

months later.[28] The degree to which different factors, such as wounding mechanism, wound repair technique and patient host factors, have a role remains to be determined. Keloid or hypertrophic scarring is more common in negroid and Asian races, and in wounds located over the deltoid muscle or sternum.

All percutaneous stitches will cause needle marks if left in situ longer than 8 days, as epithelium migrates down the needle track. Removal too early predisposes to wound dehiscence (see Fig. 2.11.15); however, the wound may be supported by skin tapes. If tapes were the primary method of closure they may be left on for at least 10 days, or until they fall off, providing the skin is not sensitive to the adhesive, as evidenced by erythema or bulla formation.

Suture removal technique is also important. To avoid tissue trauma and additional scarring stitches should be cut at the knots with iris scissors after gentle washing with saline to remove the eschar, and the suture gently pulled through. So-called suture scissors are actually too big for the task. 'Stitch cutters', requiring a sawing motion to cut through the suture, put traction on the underlying tissue and risk causing trauma.

Inelastic paper tape can be used to support a wound and help stop the scar from stretching until such time as the collagen is near maturation, beyond 3 months. Paper tape is also useful in the setting of keloid scar in an attempt to provide pressure and encourage remodelling. In some cases silicone gel pads and even pressure garments are required to control keloid scarring.

If the wound suppurates then the sutures will need to be removed, either partly or in total, to allow the egress of pus.

CONTROVERSIES

❶ Drainage will remove fluid and haematoma that potentiates infection, but the drain itself may predispose to infection; this is less the case with suction drains.

❷ Subcutaneous sutures will close dead space, thereby reducing haematoma and wound infection, yet of themselves may potentiate wound infection.

❸ The degree of debridement required for a dirty wound has moved from radical to conservative but meticulous, with an emphasis on preservation of viable skin to improve cosmesis.

❹ Povidone-iodine packs, which are tissue toxic, may be used by some surgeons in the setting of open wounds over compound fractures while the patient awaits transfer to the operating theatre for definitive repair.

❺ Opinion as to the appropriate dressings for abrasions range from moist, such as plastic film, to dry, such as mercurochrome paint and dry gauze.

REFERENCES

1. Jorgensen LN Kallenhave F, Christensen E, Siana JE 1998 Less collagen production in smokers. Surgery 123(4): 450–5
2. Ellis H 1997 Hazards from surgical gloves. Annals of the Royal College of Surgeons of England 79(3): 161–3
3. Birnbach DJ Stein DJ, Murray O, Thys DM, Sordillo EM 1988 Povidone iodine and skin disinfection before initiation of epidural anesthesia. Anesthesiology 88(3): 668–72
4. Keating JP, Neill M, Hill GL 1997 Sclerosing encapsulating peritonitis after intraperitoneal use of povidone iodine. Australian and New Zealand Journal of Surgery 67(10): 742–4
5. Rodeheaver GT Pettry D, Thacker JG et al 1975 Wound cleansing by high pressure irrigation.

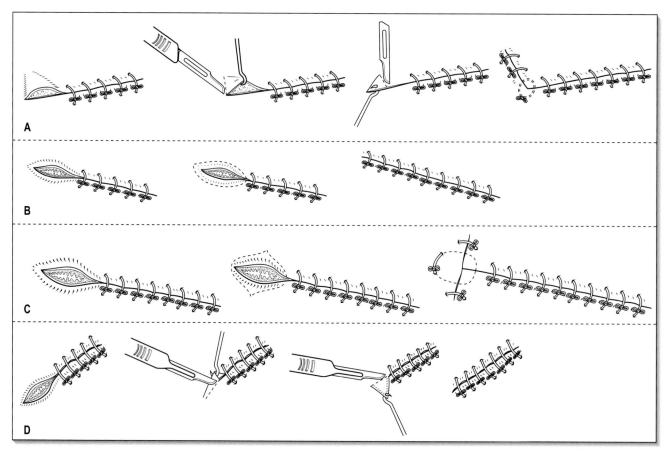

Fig. 2.11.13 Various methods of dealing with a dog ear. (a) Hockey-stick or back-cut technique; (b) Double elliptical incision technique; (c) Perpendicular elliptical T-repair technique; (d) Direct overlap excision technique. (From an original drawing by Elaine Wheildon)

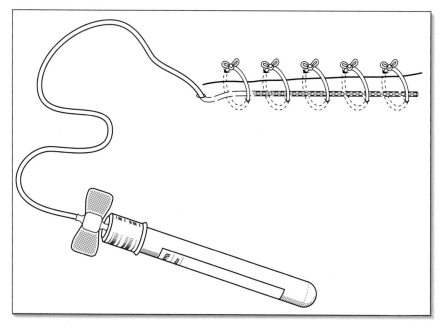

Fig. 2.11.14 A simple suction drain. (From an original drawing by Elaine Wheildon.)

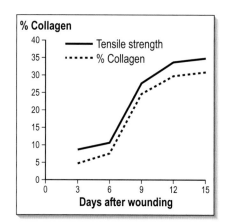

Fig. 2.11.15 The relationship between tensile strength and collagen deposition. (From an original drawing by Elaine Wheildon)

Surgery, Gynecology and Obstetrics 141: 357–62

6. Brown LL 1978 Evaluation of wound irrigation by pulsatile jet and conventional methods. Annals of Surgery 187: 170

7. Gfeller RW, Crow DT 1994 The emergency care of traumatic wounds: current recommendations. Veterinary Clinics of North America 24(6): 1249–74

8. Wheeler CB, Rodeheaver GT, Tracker JG, et al 1976 Side-effects of high pressure irrigation. Surgery, Gynecology and Obstetrics 143: 775–8

9. Wyn T, et al 1995 Bedside fluoroscopy for the detection of foreign bodies. Academic Emergency Medicine 2(11): 979–82

10. Fackler MI, et al 1989 Open wound drainage versus wound excision in treating the modern assault rifle wound. Surgery 105: 576–84

11. National Health and Medical Research Council 1977 The Australian Immunisation Handbook, 6th edn.

12. Moy RL, Lee A, Zalka A 1991 Commonly used suturing techniques in skin surgery. American Family Physician 44(5): 1625–34

13. Moy RL, Quan MB 1990 An evaluation of wound closure tapes. Journal of Dermatology, Surgery and Oncology 16(8): 721–3

14. Panek P, Prusak MP, Bolt D 1972 Potentiation of wound infection by adhesive adjuncts. American Surgeon 38: 343–5

15. Edlich RF, Becker DG, Thacker JG, Rodheaver GT 1990 Scientific basis for selecting staple and tape skin closures. Clinics in Plastic Surgery 17(3): 571–8

16. Spotnitz WD, Falstrom MA, Rodeheaver GT 1997 The role of sutures and fibrin sealant in wound healing. Surgical Clinics of North America 77(3): 651–69

17. Van Winkle W Jnr, et al 1972 Considerations in the choice of suture material for various tissues. Surgery, Gynecology and Obstetrics 135: 113–26

18. Rodeheaver GT, et al 1996 Biomechanical and clinical performance of a new synthetic monofilament absorbable suture. Journal of Long-Term Effects of Medical Implants 6: 181–98

19. Bendel LP, Trozzo LP 1993 Tensile and bend relationships of several surgical needle materials. Journal of Applied Biomaterials 4(2): 161–7

20. Mclean NR, et al 1980 Comparison of skin closure using continuous and interrupted nylon sutures. British Journal of Surgery 67: 633–5

21. Drake DB, Gear AL, Mazzarese PM, Faulkner BC, Woods JA, Edlich RF 1997 Search for a scientific basis for continuous suture closure: a 30 year odyssey. Journal of Emergency Medicine 15(4): 495–504

22. Pham S, Rodeheaver GT, Dang MC, Foresman PA, Hwang JC, Edlich RF, et al 1990 Ease of continuous dermal suture removal. Journal of Emergency Medicine 8: 539–43

23. Halstead WS 1990–91 The treatment of wounds with especial reference to the value of blood clot in the management of dead spaces. Bulletin of the Johns Hopkins Hospital 2: 255

24. De Holl D 1974 Potentiation of infection by suture closure of dead space. American Journal of Surgery 127: 716–20

25. Arnold PG 1997 Space obliterating skin suture. Plastic and Reconstructive Surgery 100(6): 1506–8

26. Gusman D 1995 Wound closure and special suture techniques. Journal of the American Podiatric Medical Association 85(1): 2–10

27. Ivy RH, et al (eds) 1943 Manual of Standard Practice of Plastic and Maxillofacial Surgery. WB Saunders, Philadelphia

28. Hollander JE, Blasko B 1995 Poor correlation of short and long-term cosmetic appearance of lacerations. Academic Emergency Medicine 2: 983–7

29. Pietsch J, Meakins JL 1976 Complications of povidone-iodine absorption in topically treated burns patients. Lancet 1: 280–2

30. Trott AT 1997 Wounds and Lacerations: Emergency Care and Closure, 2nd edn. Mosby Year Book, St Louis

2.12 BURNS

TIM GRAY

ESSENTIALS

1 Advances in treatment of severely burned patients including fluid resuscitation, control of sepsis, early excision and use of skin substitutes has made previously lethal burns survivable.

2 Airway burns account for most deaths from burn injury and signs of laryngeal oedema should prompt early intubation.

3 Burn resuscitation formulas should be considered as a guide only. Fluid administration must be based on haemodynamic response. Hartmanns solution should be used as the initial resuscitation fluid.

4 Meta-analysis suggests that resuscitation with colloid, as opposed to crystalloid, does not improve survival.

5 Extensive or complicated burns should be managed in a specialized burns unit.

6 Chemical burns, after decontamination and specific antidotes, are treated in a similar fashion to thermal burns.

INTRODUCTION

Advances in burn management over the last three decades have significantly reduced mortality and improved quality of life for burns victims. In the past, inadequate fluid administration resulted in high death rates, however, with the advent of vigorous fluid resuscitation, sepsis has replaced hypovolaemia as the major cause of death in the burned patient.

PATHOPHYSIOLOGY

The skin is the largest organ of the body. Its most important functions are:

- To act as a vapour barrier to prevent water loss from the body
- To present the body's major barrier against infection
- Temperature regulation.

The skin consists of two main layers. The epidermis is stratified squamous epithelium that acts as the major barrier to passive water loss from the body. The dermis contains the adnexal structures, namely sweat glands, hair follicles and sebaceous glands, as well as pain and pressure receptors, and the cutaneous blood vessels, which play a major role in temperature regulation by controlling radiant heat loss (Fig. 2.12.1)

The adnexae are embryologic downgrowths of the epidermis. Following burn injury, the epithelial cells of these structures undergo metaplastic change to stratified squamous epithelium, proliferate and gradually cover the wound.

Thus burns that partially or completely

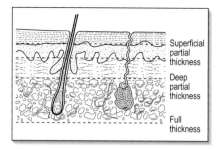

Fig. 2.12.1 Diagram of skin layers.

spare these structures will usually heal without scarring. Deeper burns involve greater loss of adnexal cells, resulting in poorer epithelial coverage and hence greater scarring.

Burned skin undergoes coagulative necrosis with three distinct zones of injury. A central zone of coagulation, in which irreversible cell death occurs, is surrounded by a zone of stasis, in which vasoconstriction and intravascular coagulation contribute to local ischaemia. A zone of hyperaemia surrounds the wound. In the early stages of the burn, evolution of these zones results in a progressive deepening of the wound, which may be minimized by appropriate early treatment.[1]

CLASSIFICATION

Burns may be classified according to their depth as superficial, partial thickness or full thickness.

Superficial burns involve only the epidermis. Pain and swelling usually subside within 48 hours and the superficial epidermis peels off within a few days. Healing occurs by proliferation of undamaged cells of the germinal layer of the epidermis and is usually complete within 7 days.

Partial thickness burns involve destruction of the epidermis and superficial dermis. They are characterized by blister formation and may be further classified into superficial and deep partial thickness. Healing is dependent on the amount of intact epithelium in the adnexae.

Superficial partial thickness burns are typically bright red with a moist surface, are exquisitely sensitive to stimulus and heal in 2–3 weeks, generally with minimal

scarring. Deep partial thickness burns are typically dark red or yellow-white and take longer than 3 weeks to heal as few epithelial elements survive. Hypertrophic scarring usually occurs.

Full thickness burns involve the epidermis and dermis including the epidermal appendages. Clinically they appear charred or pearly white in appearance and are usually insensate. Because loss of epidermal adnexae is complete, full thickness burns only heal by scarring or skin graft.

THERMAL BURNS

PRESENTATION

History

History may be obtained from the patient, from witnesses and from fire or ambulance personnel. Details of the nature of the injury are important, especially the nature of the burning materials, duration of exposure, whether the patient was trapped in an enclosed space or lost consciousness, or whether there was an associated fall, vehicular accident or blast injury.

A history of altered consciousness or confinement in a burning environment suggests the likelihood of carbon-monoxide poisoning.

Past medical history, current medications, allergies, and tetanus status should also be obtained.

Examination

Initial examination should be directed to identification of signs suggestive of airway burns as well as the presence of other injuries. Early haemodymamic compromise is rarely due to burn injury alone and should prompt a search for other causes.

Facial and oral burns, singed nasal hairs, carbonaceous sputum, tachypnoea and wheeze are clinical signs suggesting an increased risk of inhalation injury, however, in the absence of laryngeal oedema, inhalation injury may not become clinically evident for 12–24 hours.[2,3]

Signs of laryngeal oedema, namely hoarseness, brassy cough or stridor

indicate the need for early endotracheal intubation as oedema formation may rapidly distort the anatomy, necessitating a surgical airway.

The adequacy of peripheral circulation should be assessed, particularly in the setting of circumferential limb burns.

Evaluation of burn area

The extent and depth of the burn wound must be assessed as accurately as possible. Representation of the burn area diagrammatically on a body chart aids assessment. The simplest method is the 'Rule of nines' where the adult body is divided into anatomical regions that represent 9% of the total body surface area.

In infants and young children the Lund and Browder chart is used to correct for proportional variation at different ages, for instance an infants head is approximately 18% of the total body surface area compared to 9% in an adult (Fig. 2.12.2).

INVESTIGATIONS

Blood should be taken for baseline full blood examination, serum electrolytes and creatinine, createnine kinase as well as blood group and crossmatch.

There is no test to quantitate the severity of inhalational injury. Chest X-ray and blood gases should be obtained to assess alveolar function, however, these may be normal initially.

Carboxyhaemoglobin levels extrapolated to the time of injury may give an estimate of the severity of exposure. An admission carboxyhaemoglobin level greater than 15% suggests significant smoke inhalation. If the diagnosis remains in doubt, fibreoptic laryngoscopy is indicated.[1]

Urine myoglobin should be measured in extensive burns, particularly those resulting from electrical injury.

MANAGEMENT

Prehospital

Prehospital care of the burned patient should be directed at stopping the

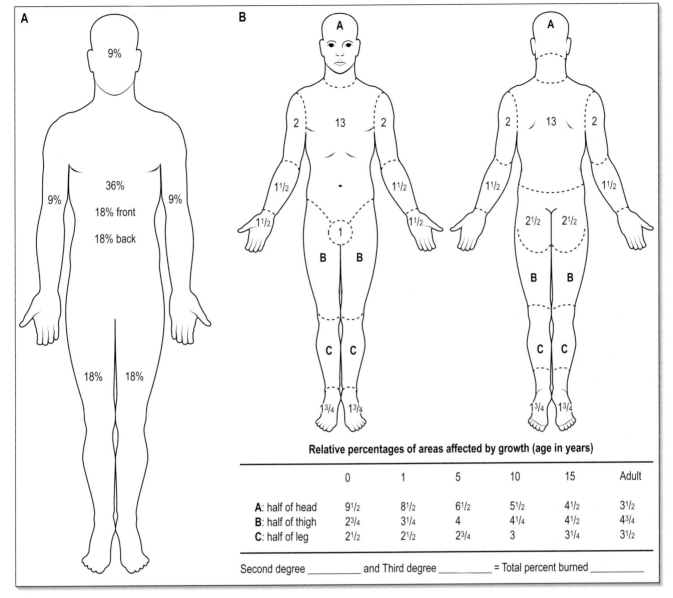

Fig. 2.12.2 (A) 'Rule of nines' diagram and (B) Lund and Browder chart.

Relative percentages of areas affected by growth (age in years)

	0	1	5	10	15	Adult
A: half of head	$9^1/_2$	$8^1/_2$	$6^1/_2$	$5^1/_2$	$4^1/_2$	$3^1/_2$
B: half of thigh	$2^3/_4$	$3^1/_4$	4	$4^1/_4$	$4^1/_2$	$4^3/_4$
C: half of leg	$2^1/_2$	$2^1/_2$	$2^3/_4$	3	$3^1/_4$	$3^1/_2$

Second degree _____ and Third degree _____ = Total percent burned _____

burning process, assessing and stabilizing the airway, breathing and circulation, and rapidly transferring the patient to hospital.

Where possible, major burns should be triaged to a burn centre (Table 2.12.1).

Recent burns should be covered with a clean cloth soaked in cool water so as to limit the depth of burn by dissipation of heat. After this cooling process, or if not required, the burns should be covered with a clean, preferably sterile sheet or dressing. Prolonged exposure to cool water should be avoided and ice should

Table 2.12.1 Patients who fulfil the following criteria should be considered for transfer to a specialist burns unit

Partial thickness burns of greater than 20% in all age groups or greater than 10% in the under 10 and over 50 age groups

Full thickness burns of greater than 5% in any age group

Burns involving face, eyes, ears, hands, feet, genitalia, perineum or a major joint

Inhalation burns

Electrical burns including lightning injury

Burns associated with other significant injuries

Smaller burns in patients with pre-existing disease that could complicate management never be applied directly to the wound as it may increase the depth of burn.

The patient should be kept warm, supplemental oxygen administered and where prolonged transport times are anticipated, intravenous fluid therapy should be instituted.

Emergency department

Initial management

Supplemental oxygen should be administered, cardiac and oxygen saturation monitoring instituted.

Stabilization of the airway and treatment of life-threatening injuries take priority over management of the burn wound itself. As previously discussed, signs of laryngeal oedema indicate the need for early endotracheal intubation, particularly if the patient is to be transferred. Fluid resuscitation with Hartmann's solution as outlined below should be commenced in any patient with burns of more than 20% total body surface area (TBSA). Peripheral venous access, even if through burned skin is preferable to central venous access in the initial phase of resuscitation. A urinary catheter should be inserted to assess the adequacy of fluid resuscitation.

Subsequent management

Having stabilized the patient and initiated fluid resuscitation, a careful secondary survey should be performed looking for associated injuries.

All burn wounds are painful, thus adequate analgesia is an important facet of management.

Small burns may be managed with a combination of cool compresses and oral analgesia, however, larger burns require opiate analgesia.

As a general guide, haemodynamically stable patients should be given morphine in an intravenous loading dose of 0.1 mg/kg followed by an infusion of 0.05 mg/kg/h. Higher doses may be required to adequately control pain. Hypovolemic patients should receive small incremental doses of intravenous morphine (0.02 mg/kg) to achieve adequate analgesia. The intramuscular route should be avoided because of erratic absorption.[4]

Tetanus immunoglobulin should be given if the burn is grossly contaminated or more than 6 hours old, or if the patient has not had a tetanus booster within the preceding 5 years.

A nasogastric tube should be inserted in patients with major burns to avoid gastric dilatation.

Escharotomy may occasionally be necessary in the setting of circumferential limb burns with circulatory compromise, or circumferential chest burns with respiratory compromise.

Extensively burned limbs should be elevated early and frequent observations of pulse strength, capillary return and sensation – particularly two point discrimination – must be performed. Escharotomy may be necessary even when pulses are present, however, the receiving unit should be consulted before escharotomies are performed.[1]

Fluid resuscitation[3,4]

Many formulae exist for the fluid resuscitation of burns victims. While considerable debate continues, the general principles of fluid resuscitation are:

- In the first 24 hours, isotonic salt solution should be used to replace the large volumes lost to tissue oedema with about half the fluid given in the first 8 hours after injury, coincident with the period of most rapid oedema formation.
- The administration of colloid is unnecessary for patients with burns of less than 40% TBSA and during the first 8 hours. Meta-analysis suggests that resuscitation with colloid does not result in improved survival.[5]
- Fluid resuscitation formula are a guide only, and the patients haemodynamic status must be monitored by cardiovascular parameters and hourly urine volume measurement. Increased resuscitation fluid volume is required in children less than 30 kg, in high voltage electrical injuries, if resuscitation is delayed and in the presence of inhalation injury.

Most burn formulae use between 2 to 4 mL of crystalloid per kg body weight

per per cent TBSA burned. It is felt that the latter rate allows a more rapid correction of shock.

The Parkland formula allows for 4 mL/kg/% TBSA burned over 24 hours, with half the total fluid requirement to be given in the first 8 hours. In children under 30 kg, the above fluid should be given in addition to calculated maintenance fluid.[1]

Haemodynamic status may be difficult to evaluate in the severely burned patient. Parameters that indicate adequacy of resuscitation are urinary output of 50 mL per hour in adults and 1 mL/kg/h in children, normalization of haemodynamic parameters and correction of metabolic acidosis.

Strategies to reduce the total volume of resuscitation fluid including the use of colloid and hypertonic salt solutions are somewhat controversial.

The generalized increase in capillary permeability that occurs with major burns results in the loss of plasma protein, particularly albumin, from the circulation. There is a coincident decrease in hepatic albumin production post burn. Colloid administration helps maintain oncotic pressure, but does not reduce tissue oedema in the first 8 hours and has not been shown to improve clinical outcome.[1]

Hypertonic saline solution may be useful in patients with limited cardiopulmonary reserve, however, there is considerable debate over the safety of this technique.[2,3]

Management of the burn injury

The development of effective topical antimicrobial agents has minimized the incidence of early burn wound infection.

Infecting organisms are most likely to originate from the patient's own gastrointestinal tract. The most important primary infecting agents are the Gram-negative bacteria, particularly *Pseudomonas aeruginosa*, *Proteus*, *Klebsiella* and *E. coli* species. β-haemolytic streptococci, *Staphylococcus aureus* and *Candida* are also important pathogens.[1]

Silver sulfadiazine (SSD) cream is the agent most commonly used and is relatively free from side effects, apart from rashes, transient leucopenia and occasionally serum hyperosmolarity.

Other agents used include silver nitrate solution, which may cause hyponatremia, and mafenide acetate cream, which has the advantage of rapidly penetrating the burn eschar, making it useful in treating invasive burn-wound infections. Mafenide is associated with metabolic acidosis when used continuously on large burns.

BURN SHOCK

The pathophysiology of burn shock is complex and involves a combination of haemodynamic and local tissue factors.

The early post-burn period, i.e. within the first 8 hours, is marked by rapid formation of tissue oedema, predominantly in the wound itself, but also in non-burned tissue. Factors contributing to this fluid accumulation are not fully understood but include local release of inflammatory mediators, particularly prostaglandins and leukotrienes. These increase capillary permeability locally and systemically, as well as increasing regional blood flow. Increased interstitial osmotic pressure in burned tissue due to the release of osmotically active cellular components and partial degradation of collagen also contributes to tissue oedema.[1,3]

Major evaporative loss from burned skin due to loss of epithelial integrity significantly adds to fluid losses. In addition to the fluid shifts, cardiac output may fall by 30–50% in major burns, possibly due to a circulating myocardial depressant factor.[1]

INHALATION INJURY

Respiratory complications account for most deaths from burn injury.

Direct thermal trauma below the larynx is rare except in the case of steam inhalation.

Pulmonary complications are largely due to inhalation of toxic products of combustion, particularly in house or vehicular fires. Smoke consists of a particulate fraction – predominantly carbon – and a gaseous fraction, which may include carbon dioxide, carbon monoxide, oxides of nitrogen and sulfur, hydrogen cyanide and PVC, depending on the materials being burnt. These agents adhere to the moist respiratory mucosa, forming corrosive compounds that cause inflammation, hypersecretion and mucosal sloughing resulting in airway obstruction and atelectasis. Smoke inhalation also triggers the release of thromboxane, resulting in increased pulmonary artery pressures.[2]

DISPOSITION

Patients with major burns as outlined in Table 2.12.1 should be managed in a specialist burns unit. The patient should be discussed with the receiving unit prior to transfer so that appropriate measures may be undertaken to stabilize them. Such burns should be covering with a sterile towel or burn dressing. Plastic cling wrap applied directly over the burn wound provides a good non-adherent dressing that will reduce heat and fluid loss. SSD cream should not be applied to these burns as it interferes with subsequent evaluation.

Current management of full and deep partial thickness burns involves early excision and autologous skin grafting. In extensive burns, excision and autologous grafting can be staged, allowing sufficient skin to regenerate. Alternatively, complete early excision with a combination of autologous and cadaveric skin grafts or skin substitute membranes may be used.[2,3]

Less extensive burns may be admitted to a general or plastic surgery service. These burns may be gently cleansed with a non-irritant antiseptic solution. Blisters are best left intact, however, loose skin and broken blisters should be debrided. SSD cream with an overlying non-adherent dressing should be applied to areas of epithelial loss.

Superficial or partial thickness burns involving less than 10% TBSA may be suitable for outpatient management subject to the criteria in Table 2.12.1 and depending on the social and psycholo-gical status of the patient. The choice of dressings for outpatient management depends on the depth of the burn, the extent and size of blisters and the amount of exudate from the burn surface.[1]

Superficial burns simply require protection from mechanical trauma. Self adhesive semipermeable film dressings such as Op-site® or Tegaderm® provide ideal protection.

Burns with multiple small-surface blisters pose a low infection risk. Such burns are best treated with a hydro-colloid dressing such as Duoderm® that allows some evaporation of exudate.

Superficial partial thickness burns involve loss of epithelium with considerable exudate and hence are prone to infection. After gentle cleansing and debridement of loose tissue, SSD cream should be applied. A secondary non-adherent dressing such as Melolin® should be used to cover the cream. The dressing should be changed daily to maximize the effectiveness of the SSD cream and to minimize crusting and dressing adherence. Epithelialization commences at 7–10 days, by which time the burn surface should be drying out. At this stage the more convenient hydrocolloid or film dressings may be used until epithelialization is complete.

If healing is not well established by 10–14 days, then the patient should be referred for specialist opinion, as excision and grafting may be required.[5]

CHEMICAL BURNS

A wide range of products available in both the industrial and domestic environments can lead to burns. Although the mechanism is different, chemical burns demonstrate a similar spectrum of injury to thermal burns. Superficial burns are associated with itching, burning or pain; partial thickness burns are associated with tissue oedema and formation of bullae; and full thickness burns are associated with damage extending through the dermis. The extent of tissue damage in chemical burns is determined by the nature and concentration of the chemical, as well as the extent and duration of contact.

In addition to the burn itself, toxicity may occur due to systemic absorption.

The majority of chemical burns are caused by acids and alkalis. Acids cause coagulation, with formation of a tough eschar that may limit further tissue damage. Alkalis cause liquifactive necrosis, allowing deeper penetration. Many other types of chemicals cause burns, however, disinguishing them by mechanism of action is not relevant to the clinician as management, apart from a few exceptions, is similar.

GENERAL PRINCIPLES

Chemical agents continue to damage tissue until they are removed or inactivated. Therapy then is directed to decontamination and where appropriate use of specific antidotes as well as recognition and treatment of systemic toxicity.

Adequate protection of medical personnel to prevent secondary contamination is essential. Copious irrigation is the cornerstone of therapy, however, contaminated garments should be removed and dry chemical particles brushed away before irrigation commences. Adherent or oily compounds may need to be removed with mild soap and scrubbing brush and nails, hair and intertriginous areas should be carefully checked.

The duration of irrigation depends on the agent. Alkali in particular may require prolonged lavage due to its tissue penetration. The use of litmus paper to determine wound pH may guide the duration of irrigation in acid and alkali burns.

Other than decontamination and treatment of systemic toxicity, management is similar to that for thermal burns.[7]

DISPOSITION

Most patients with chemical burns can be treated on an outpatient basis.

Indications for admission include:

- Partial thickness burns of greater than 15% TBSA
- All full thickness burns
- Burns involving hands, feet, eyes, ears or perineum
- Evidence of or potential for systemic toxicity
- Significant associated injuries or complicating medical conditions.

Specific chemicals

Hydrofluoric acid

Hydrofluoric acid is a relatively weak acid used in glass etching, electronics and oil refining industries. It is also a component of many industrial and domestic rust removers. In strong solution, it causes corrosion of tissue due to release of hydrogen ions, however, its major toxicity is caused by the dissociated fluoride ion that complexes calcium and magnesium to form insoluble salts. Cell destruction associated with severe pain results. In severe burns, hyopcalcaemia and hypomagnesemia may occur.

Contact with strong solution (greater than 50%) causes immediate pain and tissue destruction, however, exposure to weaker solutions, particularly less than 20%, may cause little or no pain initially. Thus it may take from several to 24 hours for the burn to become apparent.

Once apparent the burn causes excruciating pain that is difficult to control even with parenteral narcotic.

After irrigation, specific therapy is aimed at precipitation and hence neutralization of free fluoride ions. Methods depend on the severity and location of the burn. Calcium gluconate gel, made by mixing calcium gluconate with a water soluble lubricant to make a 2.5–10% solution, should be applied directly to the affected area.

Relief of pain is the marker of adequate treatment. If pain is not relived, or recurs, parenteral therapy is required. Generally this consists of subcutaneous injection of calcium gluconate, aiming for 0.5 mL of 10% solution per square centimetre.

Hand and digital burns pose a problem as vascular compromise may occur if too much fluid is injected. Alternatives include intra-arterial injection of calcium gluconate, or regional perfusion using Bier's technique.[7,8]

Metals

Burns due to molten metal are treated as thermal burns. Some elemental metals such as sodium, lithium, potassium, magnesium, calcium and aluminium spontaneously ignite on exposure to air. Water should not be used to extinguish burning metal fragments as an intensive exothermic reaction may occur. Burning metal embedded in skin should be covered with mineral oil or sand.

White phosphorous

White phosphorous is used in munitions as an incendiary as well as some insecticides and rodenticides. Like elemental metals, it may ignite spontaneously on exposure to air, however, treatment is by copious irrigation with water. Brief irrigation with dilute copper sulphate solution may colour the phosphorous particles black, aiding removal and reducing the rate of oxidation.

Care must be taken to avoid systemic copper toxicity.[7]

REFERENCES

1. Shaw A, Anderson J, Hayward A, Parkhouse N 1994 Pathophysiological basis of burn management. British Journal of Hospital Medicine 52(11): 583–7
2. Nguyen TT, Gilpin DA, Meyer NA, Herndon DN 1996 Current treatment of severely burned patients. Annals of Surgery 233(1): 14–25
3. Monafo WW 1996 Initial management of burns. New England Journal of Medicine 335(21): 1581–6
4. Finkelstein JL, Schwartz SB, Madden MR, Marano MA, Goodwin CW 1992 Paediatric burns: An overview. Paediatric Clinics of North America 39(5): 1145–63
5. Alderson P, Schierhout G, Roberts I, Bunn F 2002 Colloids versus crystalloids for fluid resuscitation in critically ill patients (Cochrane Review). In: The Cochrane Library, Issue 2, Oxford
6. Judson R 1997 Minor burns: modern management techniques. Australian Family Physician 26(9): 1023–6
7. Benda B 1992 Chemical injuries. In: Rosen P, Barkin R, et al (eds) Emergecy Medicine: Concepts and Clinical Practice. Mosby, St Louis pp 965–8
8. Bretolini JC 1992 Hydrofluoric acid: A review of toxicity. Journal of Emergency Medicine 10: 163–8

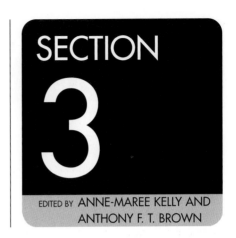

ORTHOPAEDIC EMERGENCIES

3.1 Upper limb: injuries of the shoulder girdle 130

3.2 Fractures of the humerus 132

3.3 Dislocations of the elbow 136

3.4 Fractures of the forearm 138

3.5 Hand injuries 142

3.6 Pelvic injuries 148

3.7 Hip injuries 152

3.8 Femur injuries 157

3.9 Knee injuries 159

3.10 Tibia and fibula injuries 165

3.11 Ankle joint injuries 168

3.12 Foot injuries 171

3.1 INJURIES OF THE SHOULDER GIRDLE

ANNE-MAREE KELLY

ESSENTIALS

1 Most clavicular fractures heal despite displacement, thus reduction is not necessary.

2 Injuries to the shoulder region may also involve injury to local neurovascular structures.

3 Acromioclavicular joint injuries and fractures of the scapula are usually treated conservatively.

4 Posterior sternoclavicular dislocations require reduction.

5 In dislocation of the shoulder, careful examination of the axillary (circumflex) nerve, brachial plexus and axillary artery is mandatory pre and post reduction.

6 In anterior dislocation of the shoulder, surgical repair of the capsule is recommended for recurrent dislocators and first-time dislocators who are young and engaged in high-risk sports.

FRACTURES OF THE CLAVICLE

Fractures of the clavicle usually result from a direct blow on the point of the shoulder but may also be due to a fall on the outstretched hand or a direct blow. The most common site of fracture is the junction of the middle and outer thirds of the clavicle. There are varying degrees of displacement of the fracture ends, with overlapping fragments and shortening being common. Due to its strategic location, injury to the pleura, axillary vessels and/or brachial plexus is possible, but fortunately these complications are rare.

The clinical signs of clavicular fractures are that of a patient supporting the weight of their arm at the elbow and local pain and tenderness, often accompanying by deformity.

In most cases, treatment consists of an elbow-supporting sling (e.g. broad arm sling) for 2–3 weeks. For comfort, this may be worn under clothes for the first few days. The sling may be discarded when local tenderness has subsided. Note, clinical union precedes radiological union by weeks. Early shoulder movement should be encouraged within the limits of pain. Even in the presence of off-ending, reduction of most clavicular fractures is not necessary as healing is rapid and remodelling, even in an adult, produces an acceptable result. Fractures of the outer third of the clavicle may involve the coracoclavicular ligaments. If displaced, non-union is not uncommon and surgical management should be considered.

Late complications include shoulder stiffness and a local lump at the site of fracture healing, which is rarely of cosmetic significance.

ACROMIOCLAVICULAR JOINT INJURIES

Acromioclavicular (AC) joint injuries usually result from a fall where the patient rolls onto his shoulder. The degree of the injury relates to the number of ligaments damaged. The clavicle is attached to the scapula by acromioclavicular, trapezoid and conoid ligaments. In sprains and subluxations, only the AC ligament is damaged; in dislocations, the conoid and trapezoid ligaments are also ruptured and displacement may be severe.

On clinical examination of the standing patient, the outer end of the effected clavicle will be prominent and there will be local tenderness over the AC joint. The degree of damage can be ascertained by taking standing X-rays of both shoulders with the patient holding weights in both hands. ('Routine' shoulder X-rays may fail to show the injury, as spontaneous reduction tends to occur when the patient is lying down – the usual position for shoulder X-rays.)

Treatment is with a broad arm sling. For minor sprains 1–2 weeks is usually sufficient; dislocations may require 4–6 weeks of immobilization. If there is gross instability and there are strong occupational reasons for optimal stability, surgery may be considered.

STERNOCLAVICULAR SUBLUXATION AND DISLOCATION

Sternoclavicular injury is usually due to a fall on the outstretched hand or a blow to the front of the shoulder. Subluxation is more common, with the effected medial end of the clavicle displaced forwards and downwards. Dislocations may be anterior or, rarely, posterior. In the latter case, the great vessels or trachea may be damaged.

Clinical features include local tenderness and assymetry of the medial ends of the clavicles. The diagnosis is essentially clinical. X-rays are difficult to interpret. They are not necessary for subluxations but may be helpful to confirm major dislocations.

Subluxations should be treated in a broad arm sling for 2 to 3 weeks. Gross displacements and dislocations, especially posterior location, should be reduced under general anaesthesia, then supported by a clavicular brace and sling for 4 to 6 weeks.

FRACTURES OF THE SCAPULA

Fractures of the blade of the scapula are usually due to direct violence. Clinical features are local tenderness, sometimes with marked swelling. Healing is usually rapid, even in the presence of comminution and displacement, with an excellent outcome. Treatment is a broad arm sling with early mobilization.

Fractures of the scapula neck are often comminuted and may involve the glenoid. Swelling and bruising of the shoulder may be marked. Clinical examination and X-rays should ensure that the humeral head is enlocated. Computerized tomography (CT) scans may be useful in defining the degree of involvement of the glenoid and any steps in the articular surface. If there is no significant damage to the articular surface, treatment is with a broad arm sling with mobilization as early as possible to prevent shoulder stiffness. In these cases, a good outcome is the rule. Surgery should be considered if there are significant steps in the articular surface.

ROTATOR CUFF INJURIES

Rotator cuff injuries may follow minor trauma in older patients in whom degeneration has weakened the cuff or there is sudden application of traction to the arm. The clinical features of a strain include a painful arc of abduction centred at 90° of abduction and tenderness under the acromion. If the tear is complete, no abduction at the gleno-humeral joint will occur, although some abduction to 45–60% is possible by scapular rotation. In both cases, there is full passive range of abduction. Treatment of both injuries is aggressive physiotherapy after acute symptoms have begun to settle. Local injection of hydrocortisone may be useful if symptoms persist. Surgery is rarely required, with the indication being prolonged, persistent pain.

DISLOCATION OF THE SHOULDER

Dislocation of the shoulder results in the humeral head lying anterior, posterior or inferior to the glenoid. Of these, anterior dislocation is the most common.

Anterior dislocation

Anterior dislocation of the shoulder is most often due to a fall resulting in external rotation of the shoulder, for example the body rotating internally over a fixed arm. It is most common in young adults, often being related to sports. There is inevitable damage to the capsule of the joint (stretching or tearing) and there may be associated damage to subscapularis and the greater trocanter of the humerus. Complications may include damage to the axillary (circumflex) nerve (resulting in inability to contract deltoid and numbness over the insertion of deltoid) and rarely the axillary vessels and the brachial plexus.

Clinical features include severe pain, reluctance to move the shoulder and the effected arm supported at the elbow often in slight abduction. The contour of the shoulder is 'flattened off' and there is a palpable gap just under the acromion where the humeral head usually lies. The displaced humeral head may be palpable anteriorly in the hollow behind the pectoral muscles. Dislocation is confirmed by X-ray. The dislocation may be evident on the AP film but cannot be ruled out on a single view. Additional views (e.g. an axial lateral, translateral, tangential lateral) are required. These may reveal an associated fracture of the greater trocanter, but this does not influence initial management.

The principles of management are the provision of adequate analgesia as soon as possible (ideally, this should take the form of titrated intravenous opioid), reduction of the dislocation, immobilization followed by physiotherapy. There are several effective methods for reduction of anterior dislocations. These include the Spaso technique,[1] modified Kocher's manoeuvre[2] and scapular rotation.[3,4] The Hippocratic method is not recommended as the traction involved may damage neurovascular structures. Gravitational traction, having the patient lie face down with a weight strapped to the limb, is occasionally successful and may be worthwhile if there will be a delay to reduction by another method. All reduction methods require adequate analgesia. Sedation, in an appropriately

controlled environment, may be of assistance in augmenting analgesia and providing a degree of muscle relaxation and amnesia. Failure of reduction under analgesia/sedation is rare and mandates reduction under general anaesthesia.

Spaso technique[1]

The patient is placed in the supine position. The affected arm is held by the forearm or wrist and gently lifted vertically, applying slight traction. While maintaining vertical traction, the shoulder is externally rotated, resulting in reduction.

Modified Kocher's manoeuvre[2]

Applying traction to the arm by holding it at the elbow, the shoulder is slowly externally rotated, pausing if there is muscle spasm or resistance. External rotation to about 90° should be possible and reduction often occurs during this process. The elbow is then adducted until it starts to cross the chest and then internally rotated until the hand lies near the opposite shoulder.

Scapular rotation[3]

This technique is traditionally performed with the patient prone but can be performed in a seated patient.[4] For both variations, the scapula is manipulated by adducting (medially displacing) the inferior tip using thumb pressure while stabilizing the superior aspect with the other hand.

Post reduction X-rays confirm reduction and neurovascular status must be rechecked. The arm should be immobilized in a sling under clothes for several days and the patient advised not to abduct or externally rotate the arm. This should be followed by an external broad arm sling for 2–6 weeks and physiotherapy. The duration of immobilization and the timing of physiotherapy are controversial.

If there is an associated fracture of the greater trochanter, it usually reduces when the shoulder is reduced. If it remains displaced, open reduction and internal fixation may be required.

Primary surgical repair of the capsule, usually by arthroscopic techniques, is recommended for patients having suffered recurrent dislocations and for first-time dislocators who are young and engaged in high-risk sports.

Recurrence is rare in the elderly but approaches 50% in younger patients.

Posterior dislocation

Posterior dislocation is frequently mentioned in medicolegal reports as it is easy to miss, especially in the unconscious. It may result from a fall on the outstretched or internally rotated hand, or from a blow from the front. It is also associated with seizures and electrocution injuries where it is not uncommonly bilateral. The dislocation is usually not apparent on an AP film so additional views are required (see above). Reduction is performed by traction on the limb in the position of 90° abduction followed by external rotation. Aftercare is the same as

for anterior dislocation. Posterior dislocation is prone to recurrence.

Inferior dislocation

This type of dislocation is rare and usually obvious as the arm is held in abduction. Neurovascular compromise is a significant risk requiring careful examination and prompt reduction. Reduction is by traction in abduction followed by swinging the arm into adduction. Aftercare is the same as for anterior dislocation.

REFERENCES

1. Miljesic S, Kelly AM 1998 Reduction of anterior dislocation of the shoulder: the Spaso technique. Emergency Medicine 10: 173–5
2. McRae R, Esser M 2002 Practical Fracture Treatment, 13th edn. Churchill Livingstone, Edinburgh

CONTROVERSIES

❶ The place of clavicular braces.

❷ Timing of mobilization after dislocation of the shoulder.

❸ The best technique for reduction of anterior dislocation of the shoulder.

❹ The role of surgery in acromioclavicular joint dislocations.

3. Anderson D, Zvirbulis R, Ciullo J 1982 Sacpular manipulation for reductions of anterior shoulder dislocations. Clinical Orthopedics Related Research 164: 181–3
4. McNamara RM 1993 Reduction of anterior shoulder dislocations by scapular manipulation. Annals of Emergency Medicine 21:1140–4
5. Solomom L, Warwick D, Nayagam S 2001 Apley's System of Orthopaedics and Fractures, 8th edn. Arnold, London

3.2 FRACTURES OF THE HUMERUS

TIMOTHY HUDSON RAINER

ESSENTIALS

1 Fractures of the proximal humerus occur primarily in the elderly.

2 Falls producing fractures in elderly patients are often precipitated by an underlying medical problem that should be sought and managed.

3 Most proximal humeral fractures do not require surgical intervention.

4 The aim of treatment is to minimize pain, to maximize the return of normal function as soon as possible and to achieve acceptable cosmesis.

5 Humeral shaft fractures, displaced distal humeral fractures and fractures associated with neurovascular compromise require early orthopaedic review.

INTRODUCTION

The function of the upper limb is dependent upon an intact shoulder girdle that, in turn, is affected by the integrity of muscles, tendons and ligaments, bones, joints, blood vessels and nerves. Fractures of the humerus severely limit efficient function of the upper limb and may be divided into proximal (neck), middle

(shaft) and distal (supracondylar) segments.

FRACTURES OF THE PROXIMAL HUMERUS

Patterns of injury

Fractures of the proximal humerus represent 5% of all fractures presenting to emergency departments and typically

occur as a result of an indirect mechanism in elderly, osteoporotic patients who fall on their outstretched hand with an extended elbow. These injuries are important to understand as the majority do not require surgical intervention and may be initially treated by emergency physicians. A subset, require early surgical intervention and, therefore, it is important not to misdiagnose or fail to refer this group. Fractures of the humerus may also occur in patients with multiple injuries or in the elderly with fractures of the neck of femur.[1]

Clinical assessment

History and examination

Patients typically present soon after injury holding their arm close to the chest wall. They complain of pain and exhibit swelling and tenderness of the shoulder and upper arm. Although crepitus and bruising may occur, the former is not usually illicited because it causes excessive and unnecessary pain.

Bruising is usually delayed, occuring several days after injury. It appears around the lower arm rather than at the fracture site as a result of gravity and blood tracking distally.

A neurovascular examination is essential as both the brachial plexus and axillary artery may be damaged. The axillary nerve is the most commonly injured nerve and presents with altered sensation over the badge area (insertion of the deltoid) and reduced deltoid muscle contraction (which may be hard to assess because of pain). The axillary artery is the commonest vessel to be injured and may present with any combination of limb pain, pallor, paraesthesia, pulselessness, a cool limb and paralysis.

As these injuries frequently occur in elderly patients, careful attention must be paid to the reason for the fall, as an underlying acute medical condition may have precipitated the event and require management in its own right.

Investigations
Three radiographic views - anteroposterior, lateral and axillary - will allow most proximal humeral fractures to be correctly diagnosed.

Fracture classification and management
Although the majority of these fractures are easily managed by emergency physicians, the challenge is to differentiate these from the minority that require orthopaedic intervention.

Neer classification system
In this sytem, fractures are classified first, according to four anatomical sites (anatomical and surgical necks, greater and lesser tuberosities), second, according to the number of fragments (one to four part), and third, according to the degree of fracture displacement, defined as 1 cm separation or >45° angulation (see Figs 3.2.1 & 3.2.2).

One-part fracture   One-part fractures account for 80% of proximal humeral fractures. Any number of fracture lines may exist but none are significantly displaced. Treatment includes a collar and cuff, adequate analgesia and follow-up. Early mobilization is important and the prognosis is good.

Two-part fracture   Two-part fractures account for 10% of proximal humeral fractures, and usually one fragment is significantly displaced. Initial treatment includes a collar and cuff, adequate analgesia and immediate orthopaedic advice. Definitive management may include open (intra-operative) or closed reduction depending upon neurovascular injury, rotator cuff integrity, associated dislocations, likelihood of union and function.

Two-part fractures of the humerus may involve the anatomical neck (see Fig. 3.2.1a), the surgical neck (see Fig. 3.2.1b), the greater tuberosity (see Fig. 3.2.1c). or the lesser tuberosity (see Fig. 3.2.1d).

Three- and four-part fracture   Three- and four-part fractures account for the remaining 10% of proximal humeral fractures, with two or three significantly displaced fragments (see Figure 3.2.2a-c). Management is similar to that of two-part fractures, with early orthopaedic input.

The surgical management of displaced proximal humeral fractures remains varied and controversial.[2] Small, randomized controlled trials suggest that external fixation may confer some benefit over closed manipulation[3] and that conservative treatment is better than tension band osteosynthesis,[4] but no large scale studies provide any definitive answers. Other small-scale studies suggest that some bandaging styles may be better than others,[5] that early physiotherapy may improve functional outcome but that pulsed high frequency electromagnetic energy adds no additional benefit.[6]

Anatomical neck and articular surface fractures
Fractures at these sites are uncommon, but are important to recognize as they may compromise the blood supply to the

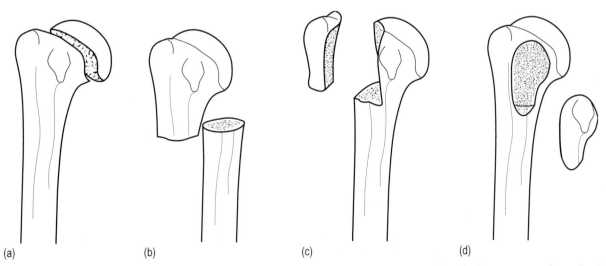

Fig. 3.2.1 Neer classification with two part fractures of anatomical neck (a), surgical neck (b), greater tuberosity (c) and lesser tuberosity (d).

(a)   (b)   (c)   (d)

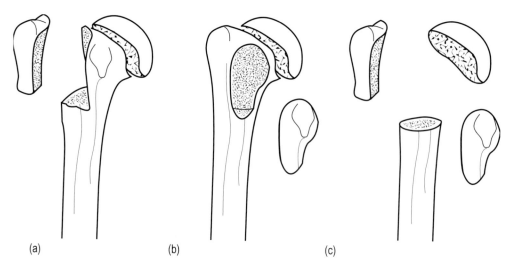

Fig. 3.2.2 Neer classification with three part fractures of greater tuberosity and anatomical neck (a), of lesser tuberosity and anatomical neck (b), and four part fracture involving anatomical neck, greater tuberosity and lesser tuberosity (c)

articular segment, may result in avascular necrosis and may require a humeral head prosthesis.

Fracture dislocations

Fractures of the greater tuberosity accompany 15% anterior glenohumeral dislocations and may be associated with rotator cuff tears. Although the fracture may be grossly displaced, reduction of the dislocated shoulder usually also reduces the fracture. In patients who require the full range of movement of their shoulders, surgical repair of the cuff may be required.

Fractures of the lesser tuberosity are associated with posterior glenohumeral dislocations.

Disposal

Most patients may be discharged from the emergency department with a collar and cuff sling, analgesia, and appropriate follow-up. High-risk patients require orthopaedic consultation and admission pending surgical intervention, as do those with medical problems requiring investigation or treatment.

FRACTURES OF THE SHAFT OF HUMERUS

Patterns of injury

Fractures of the humeral shaft commonly occur in the third decade (active young men) and in the seventh decade of life

(osteoporotic elderly women). The commonest site is the middle third. The close proximity of the fracture to the radial nerve and brachial artery commonly produces neurovascular deficits.

Direct blows tend to produce transverse fractures, while falls on the outstretched hand produce torsion forces and consequent spiral fractures. Combinations of the two mechanisms may produce a butterfly segment. Pathological fractures are also common resulting from metastatic breast cancer.

The angle and degree of displacement of the fracture depends on the site of injury and its relationship to the action and attachment of muscles either side of the injury (Fig. 3.2.3).

Clinical assessment

History and examination

Patients typically present complaining of pain and supporting the forearm of the injured limb, flexed at the elbow, held close to the chest wall. Examination of the limb reveals tenderness, swelling and possibly deformity. The skin should be assessed for tension or disruption, and particular attention should be paid to the shoulder and elbow for associated fractures or dislocations. Initial and post-reduction assessments of the brachial artery and vein, and ulnar, median and radial nerves must be performed.

The commonest complication is radial nerve injury resulting either from injury or reduction of the fracture, and evidenced by wrist drop and altered sensation in the first dorsal web space.

Investigations

Two radiographic views – anteroposterior and lateral – will allow the correct diagnosis in most cases.

Fracture management and disposal

Uncomplicated, closed fractures account for the majority of injuries and may be treated by immobilization, analgesia, a hanging or U-shaped cast (see Fig. 3.2.3), and a broad arm or collar and cuff sling. Most patients should be referred for orthopaedic review . Some departments may prefer a humeral brace rather than U-shaped plaster immobilization, as the former may permit greater functional use without affecting fracture healing or alignment.[7] Complications affecting the vessels require surgical repair, but the majority of radial nerve injuries recover without surgical intervention.

FRACTURES OF THE DISTAL HUMERUS

Classification and patterns of injury

Unlike children, fractures of the distal humerus in adults are very uncommon

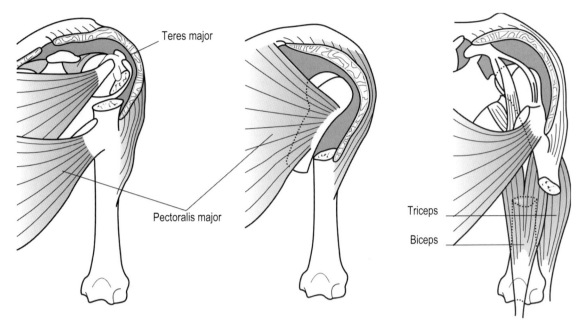

Fig. 3.2.3 Relationships between humeral fracture site and the actions of inserting muscles determine bony angulation and displacement.

and patterns of injury tend to reflect the anatomical two-column construction (condyles) of the humerus. These fractures may be classified into supracondylar, intercondylar and other types. Supracondylar fractures lie transversely, whilst intercondylar T or Y fractures include an additional vertical extension between the condyles.

Mechanisms of injury usually involve a direct blow to the flexed or extended elbow. In the former, the olecranon is driven upwards thus either splitting the condyles apart producing a T or Y pattern, or shearing off one condyle.

Clinical assessment

History and examination

Patients typically present with a swollen, tender, deformed elbow. As very little subcutaneous or other tissue separates the bone from skin, any disruption of the skin should be carefully examined for the possibility of a compound fracture. Although distal neurological and vascular injury must be assessed carefully, neurovascular injury is uncommon.

Investigations

Two radiographic views – anteroposterior and lateral – should be requested but pain and inability to extend the elbow often result in poor quality radiographs. Although high-quality radiographs are essential for operative planning, repeat films should not be attempted in the emergency department as they rarely provide the desired result. They should be delayed until after the patient is anaesthetized.

Undisplaced fractures may not be visible on radiography but may be suggested by posterior or anterior fat pad signs which result from fat displaced by an underlying haemarthrosis.

Ultrasonography, computerized tomography and magnetic resonance imaging may all improve diagnostic precision, but whether such findings alter management and improve outcome is unknown.

Fracture management and disposal

Uncomplicated, undisplaced, closed fractures with minimal swelling should be immobilized at 90° flexion with an above elbow cast and a broad arm sling for 3 weeks followed by active mobilization.

Patients with severe swelling, compound fractures, displaced fractures or neurovascular compromise should be referred for orthopaedic consultation.

CONTROVERSIES

❶ Guidance for management is based primarily on experience rather than rigorous research evidence.

❷ For humeral shaft fractures, it is unclear whether hanging plasters are better than U-shaped plasters for pain relief, and fracture healing and position.

❸ Small-scale studies suggest that fracture bracing may yield better functional results than U-shaped plaster immobilization for fractures of the shaft of humerus.

❹ Low-intensity pulsed ultrasound may be useful in the treatment of non-union.[8] Whether it may enhance normal fracture healing is not known.

❺ The role of magnetic resonance imaging in the diagnosis of bone bruising and humeral fracture has not been studied.

REFERENCES

1. Mulhall KJ, Ahmed A, Khan Y, Masterson E 2002 Simultaneous hip and upper limb fracture in the elderly: incidence, features and management considerations. Injury 33: 29-31

2. Weber E, Matter P 1998 Surgical treatment of proximal humerus fractures - an international multicenter study [In German]. Swiss Surgery 4: 95–100

3. Kristiansen B, Kofoed H 1988 Transcutaneous reduction and external fixation of displaced fractures of the proximal humerus. A controlled clinical trial. Journal of Bone and Joint Surgery British Volume 70: 821–4

4. Zyto K, Ahrengart L, Sperber A, Tornkvist H 1999 Treatment of displaced proximal humeral fractures in elderly patients. Journal of Bone and Joint Surgery British Volume 79: 412–7

5. Rommens PM, Heyvaert G 1993 Conservative treatment of subcapital humerus fractures. A comparative study of the classical Desault bandage and the new Gilchrist bandage. Unfallchirurgie 19: 114–8

6. Livesley PJ, Mugglestone A, Whitton J 1992 Electrotherapy and the management of minimally displaced fracture of the neck of the humerus. Injury 23: 323–7

7. Camden P, Nade S 1992 Fracture bracing the humerus. Injury 23: 245–8

8. Nolte PA, van der Krans A, Patka P, Janssen IM, Ryaby JP, Albers GH 2001 Low-intensity pulsed ultrasound in the treatment of nonunions. Journal of Trauma 51: 693–702

FURTHER READING

McRae R (ed.) 1994 Practical Fracture Treatment. Churchill Livingstone, Edinburgh, UK, pp 99–127

Uehara DT, Rudzinski JP 2000 Injuries to the shoulder complex and humerus. In: Tintinalli JE, Kelen GD, Stapczynski JS (eds) Emergency Medicine. A Comprehensive Study Guide. American College of Emergency Physicians and McGraw-Hill Companies Inc, US, pp 1783–91

Willet K 1997 Upper limb injuries. In: Skinner D, Swain A, Peyton R, Robertson C (eds) Cambridge Textbook of Accident and Emergency Medicine. Cambridge University Press, Cambridge, UK, pp 601–17

3.3 DISLOCATIONS OF THE ELBOW

TIMOTHY HUDSON RAINER

ESSENTIALS

1 Elbow dislocations are the third most common large joint dislocation.

2 Surgical intervention is rarely required for simple elbow dislocations.

3 Surgical intervention may be required when fractures of the radius, ulnar and humerus are associated with elbow dislocations or when neurovascular injury occurs.

4 The commonest neurovascular complication involves the ulnar nerve.

5 After reducing elbow dislocations, it is important to reassess for joint stability and for neurovascular complications.

INTRODUCTION

Elbow dislocation, along with glenohumeral and patellofemoral joint dislocations, is one of the three most common large joint dislocations.[1] The elbow joint is a hingelike articulation involving the distal humerus and proximal radius and ulna. Due to strong muscular and ligamentous supports, the joint is normally quite stable, and rarely requires operative intervention even for acute instability after dislocation.

Elbow dislocations usually involve a fall on the outstretched hand with some degree of flexion or hyperextension at the elbow. The radius and ulna commonly dislocate together and the injury, in relation to the distal humerus, may be described as posterolateral, posterior, medial, anterior or lateral. Of these, posterolateral dislocations are the most common.

Less commonly, the radius or ulna alone may dislocate at the elbow. In such cases there is always a fracture of the other bone. One common example is in Monteggia fractures where anterior or posterior radiohumeral dislocation occurs alongside a fracture of the ulna shaft (see Fig. 3.3.1). A rarer example is a posterior ulnahumeral dislocation with fracture of the radial shaft. Therefore, although elbow dislocations may appear to be isolated, it is important to look for associated intraarticular or shaft fractures.

CLINICAL ASSESSMENT

History and examination

Patients typically present holding the lower arm at 45° to the upper arm and with swelling, tenderness and deformity of the elbow joint. The three-point anatomical triangle of olecranon, medial and lateral epicondyles should be assessed for abnormal alignment as this strongly suggests dislocation.

The commonest neurovascular injury involves the ulnar nerve, but the median and radial nerves, and the brachial artery may also be affected.

The differential diagnosis is a complex distal humerus fracture, which in a swollen elbow may be hard to differentiate from an elbow dislocation.

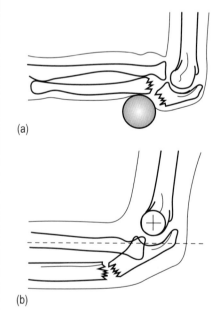

(a)

(b)

Fig. 3.3.1 Monteggia fracture dislocation. Fracture of the ulna shaft may be associated with anterior radiohumeral dislocation (a) or posterior radiohumeral dislocation (b).

INVESTIGATIONS

Anteroposterior and lateral radiographic views should be requested and scrutinized for associated fractures of the coronoid process, radial head, capitellum and olecranon.

Magnetic resonance imaging characterizes bony injury more accurately than radiography in children with elbow injuries, but its potential role for diagnosis and guiding management in adults has not been well evaluated.[2]

MANAGEMENT

Dislocation of the stable elbow joint produces severe soft tissue injury and resultant instability. One consequence is that, with adequate sedation, gentle traction and countertraction, the joint relocates quite easily. Medial and posterolateral dislocations may also require sideways correction.

There is little evidence that surgical intervention improves outcome in patients with medial or lateral elbow instability after dislocation. One small randomized controlled trial showed no evidence that surgical ligamentous repair produced better results than conservative management.[3] Another small study, a case-series of patients with humeral medial condyle fracture, suggested good results after surgical management using absorbable implants compared with removal of the bony fragment.[4] Current practice is to treat all Monteggia fractures by open reduction and internal fixation. However, about 45% these cases are associated with complications and poor long-term functional outcome.[5]

Reassessment

After reduction, the limb should be assessed for elbow stability, range of motion and neurovascular complications. Inability to fully flex or extend the elbow suggests a loose bone or cartilagenous fragment, or capsular tear. Therefore, post-reduction films should be assessed, not only for correct joint relocation, but also for associated fractures.

The elbow should be placed in a posterior plaster cast at 90° of flexion after reduction. Cylinder casts are contraindicated because of the likelihood of severe soft-tissue swelling. Thus, the limb should be reassessed for neurovascular injury both after reduction and several hours later.

DISPOSAL

Current practice is that most patients may be discharged from the emergency department with analgesia, plaster cast and broad arm sling with appropriate follow-up. However, a recent prospective, randomized, French study suggested that early mobilization is superior to plaster immobilization in terms of functional recovery, without any increased instability or a recurrence of dislocation for patients with uncomplicated posterior dislocations.[6] Patients with irreducible dislocations, neurovascular complications, associated fractures or open dislocations require orthopaedic intervention.

REFERENCES

1. Uehara DT, Chin HW 2000 Injuries to the elbow and forearm. In: Tintinalli JE, Kelen GD, Stapczynski JS (eds) Emergency Medicine. A Comprehensive Study Guide. American College of Emergency Physicians and McGraw-Hill Companies Inc, US, pp. 1763–72
2. Griffiths JF, Roebuck DJ, Cheng JCY, Chan YL, Ng BKW, Rainer TH, Metreweli C 2001 Comparison of radiography and magnetic resonance imaging in the detection of injuries after paediatric elbow trauma. American Journal of Roentgenology 176: 53–60
3. Josefsson PO, Gentz CF, Johnell O, Wendeberg B 1987 Surgical versus non-surgical treatment of ligamentous injuries following dislocation of the elbow joint. A prospective randomized study. Journal of Bone and Joint Surgery – American Volume 69: 605–8
4. Partio EK, Hirvensalo E, Bostman O, Rokkanen P 1996 A prospective controlled trial of the fracture of the humeral medial epicondyle-how to treat? Annales Chirurgiae et Gynaecologiae 85: 67–71

CONTROVERSIES

❶ There are no large-scale randomized studies comparing operative and non-operative management of elbow dislocation. It is, therefore, unclear whether one method may produce better outcomes than the other.

❷ Early mobilization may be superior to plaster immobilization after reduction of uncomplicated posterior dislocations.

❸ The epidemiology of elbow injury including dislocation in patients presenting to emergency departments has not been well described and, therefore, requires further studies.

❹ Roles for ultrasound, computerized tomography and magnetic resonance imaging in evaluating elbow injury and influencing management require further study.

5. Reynders P, De Groote W, Rondia J, Govaerts K, Stoffelen D, Broos PL 1996 Monteggia lesions in adults. A multicenter Bota study. Acta Orthopaedica Belgica 62 Suppl 1: 78–83
6. Rafai M, Largab A, Cohen D, Trafeh M 1999 Pure posterior luxation of the elbow in adults: immobilization or early mobilization. A randomized propsective study of 50 cases. Chirurgie de la Main 18: 272–8

FURTHER READING

McRae R 1994 Practical Fracture Treatment. Churchill Livingstone, Edinburgh, UK, pp 129–54
Uehara DT, Chin HW 2000 Injuries to the elbow and forearm. In: Tintinalli JE, Kelen GD, Stapczynski JS (eds) Emergency Medicine. A Comprehensive Study Guide. American College of Emergency Physicians and McGraw-Hill Companies Inc, US, pp. 1763–72
Willet K 1997 Upper limb injuries. In: Skinner D, Swain A, Peyton R, Robertson C (eds) Cambridge Textbook of Accident and Emergency Medicine. Cambridge University Press, Cambridge, UK, pp 601–17

3.4 FRACTURES OF THE FOREARM

PETER WRIGHT

ESSENTIALS

1 Most fractures of the radial head and neck can be managed conservatively.

2 Fractures involving both radius and ulna are commonly open and often displaced. Most of these fractures require open reduction and internal fixation.

3 Monteggia fracture-dislocation is fracture of the proximal ulna with dislocation of the radial head. The dislocation is easily missed. All cases require open reduction and internal fixation.

4 Galeazzi fracture dislocation involves fracture of the distal radius and dislocation/subluxation at the distal radio-ulnar joint. All cases require surgical intervention.

5 Median nerve injury may complicate fractures of the distal radius.

6 Significant or persistent symptoms with the absence of a visible fracture on plain X-ray may be due to an undetected fracture or significant soft-tissue injury. A computerized tomography scan and review by a sports physician or orthopaedic surgeon should be considered.

7 According to the World Health Organization, fractures of the distal radius in post-menopausal women are indications for evaluation of bone-mineral density.[1]

RADIAL HEAD AND NECK FRACTURES

History

Patients have usually had a fall onto their outstretched hand or received a direct blow to the lateral side of their elbow. They present with pain and restricted movement at the elbow.[2,3,4]

Examination

Usually there is swelling and tenderness over the radial head. Sometimes, with more subtle injuries, rotating the forearm while palpating the radial head may be necessary to elicit tenderness. Elbow extension and forearm rotation are limited.[3,5] Severely comminuted fractures may have proximal displacement of the radius, which can be associated with disruption of the interosseous membrane and subluxation of the distal radioulnar joint (Essex-Lopresti fracture-dislocation).[3,4]

Imaging

Anteroposterior (AP) and lateral X-rays of the elbow are needed. A radiocapitellar view may be necessary if the fracture is subtle.[3,4] The presence of an anterior fat pad sign alone on X-ray is associated with an underlying radial head or neck fracture in up to 50% of patients.[6,7] In this case a fracture should be assumed to be present if there is an appropriate mechanism and local signs. A follow-up X-ray or computerized tomography (CT) scan is indicated only in the presence of persistent pain, stiffness or locking.[3,4,8]

Classification

Radial head fractures may be described as hairline, marginal (displaced and undisplaced), segmental (displaced and undisplaced) or comminuted.[3] They may also be classified into 4 types (Fig. 3.4.1).

Fractures of the radial neck may be undisplaced or have various degrees of lateral tilting.[3]

Management

Type I and minor type II radial head fractures without mechanical block may be managed with a bandage and sling.[2-5,9,10] If there is severe pain, aspiration of the fracture haematoma, intra-articular bupivacaine, or a backslab may be useful. Mobilization can occur after 1–2 days depending on symptoms.[2] Prognosis is good, but full extension may not be possible for many months.

All type III and those type II fractures with the presence of a mechanical block to movement require surgical intervention. Mechanical block can be difficult to assess acutely. Intra-articular injection of bupivacaine may assist early assessment or assessment may be deferred. Surgical options include open reduction and internal fixation, and excision of the radial head plus or minus implantation of a prothesis.[5,9]

Radial neck fractures with up to 20° tilts can be managed conservatively. More severe tilt can be reduced using intra-articular bupivacaine. The forearm is pronated until the most prominent part of the radial head is felt. Then traction is applied to the forearm and pressure applied to the radial head. Open reduction is indicated if closed methods fail or displacement is gross.[3]

Complications

Neurovascular complications and compartment syndrome are uncommon. Most complications relate to disturbance of the relationships of the proximal radioulnar and radiocapitallar articular surfaces causing limitation of movement. This is uncommon with minor fractures and often responds to radial head excision.[5]

SHAFT FRACTURES

Fracture of both radius and ulna

History

This type of injury requires great force, typically from a motor-vehicle accident, fall from a height or a direct blow. These fractures are commonly open and nearly always displaced.

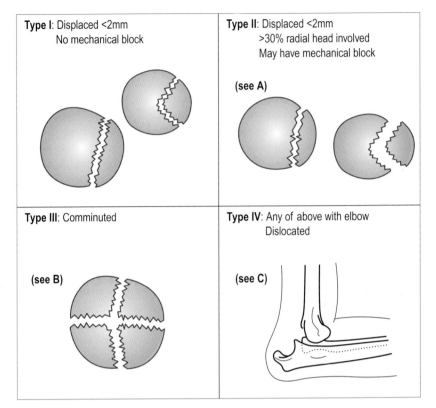

Type I: Displaced <2mm
No mechanical block

Type II: Displaced <2mm
>30% radial head involved
May have mechanical block

(see A)

Type III: Comminuted

(see B)

Type IV: Any of above with elbow
Dislocated

(see C)

Fig. 3.4.1 Mason-Hotchkiss classification of radial head fractures.[2,5,9]

Examination

The forearm is swollen and tender and may be angulated and rotated. Examination looking for an open wound, local neurovascular compromise, compartment syndrome, or musculotendinous injury is required. Given the mechanism of injury, other injuries should also be sought.

Imaging

AP and lateral X-rays of the forearm, including the wrist and elbow joints, are needed. Displacement and angulation are easily determined, but torsional deformity may be subtle. Because the ulna and radius are rectangular in cross-section rather than circular, a change in bone width at the fracture sight indicates rotation. The radial and ulnar styloid processes normally point in opposite directions to the bicipital tuberosity and coronoid process respectively. A change in this alignment also suggests torsion.

Management

Adult forearm fractures are less stable than those in children and limited remodelling limits tolerance to incomplete reduction. Undisplaced fractures may be managed with an above elbow cast, but must be reviewed at 1 week for displacement and angulation. Most fractures, however, are displaced and require open reduction and internal fixation.

Complications

Early complications include wound infection, osteomyelitis, neurovascular injury and compartment syndrome. Later, non-union, malunion, reduced forearm rotation and reflex sympathetic dystrophy are possible complications.[2,4,11]

Isolated ulnar shaft fracture

These fractures are due to a direct blow to the ulna, often when raised in defence; hence they are also known as 'nightstick' fractures. Patients present with localized pain and swelling. AP and lateral X-rays delineate the location of the fracture and degree of angulation. Look for associated dislocation of the radial head if displacement is present (Monteggia fracture-dislocation).

Fractures displaced less than 50% of the ulna width heal well with a non-union rate 0–4%. Traditional treatment involves fixing the forearm in mid-pronation with a plaster cast, extended above elbow if the middle or proximal thirds of the ulna are fractured. The cast is removed once union occurs, usually in 6–8 weeks. Other proven options include below elbow plaster (BEPOP) for proximal fractures, early mobilization with bandage after 1–2 weeks in BEPOP, and functional bracing.[12]

Fractures with greater than 10° of angulation or displaced more than 50% of the diameter of the ulna require surgical intervention.[2,4,11,12]

Monteggia fracture-dislocation

This is a rare fracture of the proximal ulna with dislocation of the radial head. It occurs either through a fall onto the outstretched hand with hyperpronation or through a force applied to the posterior aspect of the proximal ulna. Patients present with pain, swelling and reduced elbow movement. The forearm may appear shortened and the radial head may be palpable in the antecubital fossa. Associated posterior interosseous nerve injury is common.

On X-ray the fracture is obvious, but the dislocation is commonly missed. Check that a line through the radial shaft bisects the capitellum on both views. Dislocation is anterior in 60%, but may be anterolateral or posterolateral.

All Monteggia fractures require open reduction and internal fixation. Common complications include malunion and non-union of the ulna fracture and an unstable radial head.[2,4,11]

Isolated radial shaft fracture

Isolated fractures of the proximal two-thirds of the radial shaft are uncommon and are usually displaced. The rare undisplaced fractures can be treated similarly to isolated ulna shaft fractures. Displaced fractures require open reduction and internal fixation.

Galeazzi fracture-dislocation

Fractures of the distal third of the radial shaft occur through a fall onto the outstretched hand or a direct blow. There may be an associated subluxation or dislocation of the distal radioulnar joint (DRUJ) known as the Galeazzi fracture-dislocation. Patients have pain and swelling at the radial fracture site. Those with a Galeazzi injury will also have pain and swelling at the DRUJ with a prominent ulnar head.

X-rays show the radial fracture, which is tilted ventrolaterally. Widening of the DRUJ space on the AP and dorsal displacement of the ulnar head on the lateral are seen with the Galeazzi fracture (Fig. 3.4.2). An ulnar styloid fracture is seen in 60% of cases.

All Galeazzi fracture-dislocations require surgical management. Complications include malunion or non-union of the radial fracture with subsequent instability of the DRUJ.[2,4,11]

DISTAL RADIUS AND ULNA

Colles' fracture

First described in 1814, the Colles' fracture is the most common adult wrist fracture. As osteoporosis is often contributory, this fracture is most prevalent among post-menopausal women. Patients

AP view wrist

(see A)

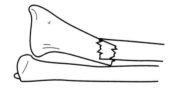

(see B)

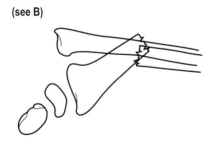

Fig. 3.4.2 The Galeazzi fracture-dislocation.

usually describe a fall on the outstretched hand and present with pain and deformity of the wrist.[13-15]

Examination

The wrist has a classic 'dinner-fork' appearance, with swelling and tenderness. Associated median nerve injury and vascular compromise may occur. Associated injuries may include the scaphoid, elbow and shoulder.[13-15]

Imaging

Anteroposterior (AP) and lateral X-rays of the wrist demonstrate the injury (Fig. 3.4.3). Damage to the radioulnar fibrocartilage is often associated. There may be comminution, commonly dorsally, which can extend into the radiocarpal or radioulnar joints.[13-15]

AP view wrist

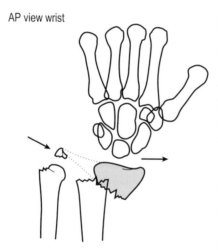

Lateral view wrist

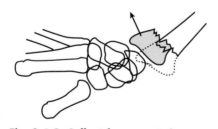

Fig. 3.4.3 Colles' fracture. A fracture of the distal radial metaphysis with 6 classic deformities. The lateral view shows anterior angulation, dorsal displacement and impaction. The AP view reveals radial displacement, ulnar angulation and an ulnar styloid fracture.

Management

Prompt attention to analgesia, splinting and elevation is essential while awaiting X-rays. Reduction is necessary if there is visible deformity of the wrist, if there is loss of volar tilt of the distal radial articular surface beyond neutral, if the ulnar styloid is displaced, or if there is ulnar angulation. Greater deformity can be accepted in elderly, frail patients.[13,16] Anaesthetic options in the ED include intravenous regional anaesthesia (Bier's block), haematoma block and conscious sedation. In some institutions, general anaesthesia is preferred and the patient admitted from the ED or booked to return for the next operating list.

The aim of reduction is to restore radial length, volar tilt, and radial angulation. A minimum of zero degrees tilt is acceptable if full reduction is not possible.[15] Reduction is achieved by first disimpacting the fracture with traction in the line of the forearm. If this fails traction in the line of the deformity should be tried. Then volar tilt is restored with volar pressure over the dorsum of the distal fragment while traction is maintained. Lastly, correct ulnar angulation and radial displacement with ulnar pressure over the radial side of the distal fragment. In order to maintain reduction, cast immobilization must fix the wrist joint in 10° flexion, full ulnar deviation and pronation, and be carefully moulded over the dorsum of the distal fragment and the anteromedial forearm.[13,16] Peripheral neurovascular function must again be documented.[14] Patients with more comminuted or displaced injuries or marked swelling should be considered for non-encircling casts or admission for limb observation.

An orthopaedic surgeon should review all fractures within 7 days. This should be done early for fractures with marked dorsal comminution or displacement or intra-articular extension as loss of reduction often occurs.[14] Discharged patients must first be instructed regarding plaster care and complications.

Immediate surgical intervention is indicated in the presence of neurovascular compromise, the presence of an open injury or if reduction fails.[13-15]

Complications

Median nerve injury may occur acutely due to the injury, as a result of reduction, or later due to pressure effects from the plaster. Loss of reduction may require delayed surgical intervention. Malunion with chronic wrist pain, arthritis, secondary radioulnar and radiocarpal instability are associated with intra-articular extension of the fracture.[14–16] Delayed ruptures of the extensor pollicus longus can occur.[13]

Smith fracture

Clinical features

This fracture of the distal radius occurs through a direct blow or fall onto the back of the hand or a fall backward onto the outstretched hand in supination. Swelling and fullness is seen anteriorly in the wrist.

Imaging

AP and lateral X-rays of the wrist show a 'reverse Colles' fracture' with a similar AP appearance, but with volar displacement and dorsal angulation on the lateral view.

Management

Management issues are similar to those seen with Colles' fractures. Closed reduction to achieve anatomical radial length and volar tilt should be attempted. Traction is first applied to restore length, followed by dorsal pressure over the volar surface of the distal radius to reverse displacement and angulation. A full above-elbow cast is applied with the wrist in supination and fully dorsiflexed to prevent loss of reduction.

Surgical intervention is needed for open injuries or if reduction is inadequate. Early follow-up as for Colles' fractures is required.

Complications

Complications are similar to those seen with Colles fractures.[13-16]

Barton fracture

Barton fractures are dorsal or volar intra-articular fractures of the distal radial rim (Fig. 3.4.4). The mechanisms of injury are similar to those seen with Colles' and Smith fractures respectively. There is often significant soft-tissue injury and

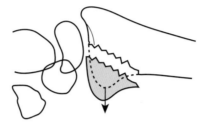

Dorsal Barton's

Volar Barton's

Fig. 3.4.4 Barton fractures demonstrated on lateral views of the wrist.

the carpus is usually dislocated or subluxed along with the distal fragment. These fractures are complicated by arthritis of the radiocarpal joints and carpal instability.

Minimally displaced fractures involving less than 50% of the joint surface and without carpal displacement may be reduced along the lines of a Colles' or Smith fracture. However, most fractures are unstable and potentially disabling, requiring early operative management, especially for younger patients.[13–15] Early orthopaedic follow-up is mandatory.

Radial styloid (Hutchison or Chauffeur) fracture

This oblique intra-articular fracture of the radial styloid is caused by a direct blow or fall onto the hand. Displacement is associated with carpal instability and long-term arthritis. The fracture is seen best on AP X-rays of the wrist (Fig. 3.4.5). Undisplaced fractures can be treated with a cast for 4-6 weeks. Displaced fractures should be referred to an orthopaedic surgeon for anatomical reduction and fixation.[13–15]

Ulnar styloid fracture

An isolated fracture can occur through forced radial deviation, dorsiflexion, rotation, or a direct blow. If displaced

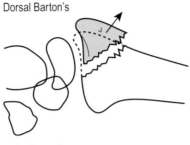

AP view wrist

(see A)

Fig. 3.4.5 Radial styloid (Hutchison or Chauffeur) fracture.

CONTROVERSIES

1 The role of backslab versus encircling cast in Colles' fracture that have undergone reduction.

2 Relative merits of intravenous arm block, haematoma block and general anaesthesia for reduction of fractures of the distal radius.

3 Many alternatives exist to the traditional methods of conservative fracture management. Debates in the literature exist regarding the optimal position of wrist fixation for distal radial fractures; the relative benefits of splints, functional braces and encircling casts; the duration of immobilization for undisplaced fractures and the need for above-elbow plaster for isolated proximal ulnar shaft fractures.

there may be associated damage to the triangular radioulnar fibrocartilage with subsequent DRUJ instability. Fractures should be treated with a splint or cast with the wrist in ulnar deviation and referred to an orthopaedic surgeon to assess DRUJ stability.[15]

REFERENCES

1. Hanel DP, et al Wrist Fractures. Orthopaedic Clinics of North America 2002; 33(1): 35–57
2. Geiderman JM, Magnusson AR. Humerus and Elbow. In: Rosen P, Barker R, et al (eds) 1998 Emergency Medicine, 4th edn. Mosby-Year Books Inc., St. Louis
3. McRae R 1994 Injuries about the elbow. In: McRae R Practical Fracture Treatment, 3rd edn. Churchill Livingstone, London

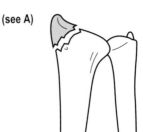

ORTHOPAEDIC EMERGENCIES

3

4. Uehara DT, Chin HW 2000 Injuries to the elbow and forearm. In: Tintinalli JE, et al (eds) Emergency Medicine, 5th edn. McGraw Hill, New York
5. Kuntz DG Jr, Bararz ME 1999 Fractures of the elbow. Orthopaedic Clinics of North America 30(1): 37–61
6. Irshad F, Shaw NJ, Gregory RJ 1997 Reliability of fat-pad sign in radial head/neck fractures of the elbow. Injury 28(7): 433–5
7. de Beaux AC, Beattie T, Gilbert F 1992 Elbow fat-pad sign: implications for clinical management. Journal of the Royal College of Surgeons of Edinburgh 37(3): 205–6
8. Miller TT 1999 Imaging of elbow disorders.

Orthopaedic Clinics of North America 30(1): 21–36
9. Van Glabbeek F, Van Riet R, Verstreken J 2001 Current concepts in the treatment of radial head fractures in adults. A clinical and biomechanical approach. Acta Orthopaedica Belgica 67(5): 430–41
10. Villarin LA Jr, Belk KE, Freid R 1999 Emergency department evaluation and treatment of elbow and forearm injuries. Emergency Medicine Clinics of North America 17(4): 843–58
11. McRae R 1994 Injuries to the forearm bones. In: McRae R Practical Fracture Treatment, 3rd edn. Churchill Livingstone, London
12. Mackay D, Wood L, Rangan A 2000 The

treatment of isolated ulnar fractures in adults: a systematic review. Injury 31: 565–70
13. McRae R 1994 The wrist and hand. In: McRae R Practical Fracture Treatment, 3rd edn. Churchill Livingstone, London
14. Eisenhauer MA 1998 Wrist and forearm. In: Rosen P, Barker R, et al (eds) Emergency Medicine, 4th edn. Mosby-Year Books Inc., St. Louis
15. Uehara DT, Chin HW 2000 Wrist injuries. In: Tintinalli JE, et al (eds) Emergency Medicine, 5th edn. McGraw Hill, New York
16. Szabo RM 1993 Extra-articular fractures of the distal radius. Orthopaedic Clinics of North America 24(2): 229–37

3.5 HAND INJURIES

PETER FREEMAN

ESSENTIALS

1 A thorough knowledge of hand anatomy and function is essential for proper management of the injured hand.

2 Most hand injuries carry a good prognosis if treated early and appropriately.

3 Aftercare and rehabilitation are vital.

INTRODUCTION

The effect of hand injury on an individual cannot be overestimated. Apart from the initial pain and trauma, occupational and psychological concerns play a major role in the aftermath of the injury. Even a relatively minor fingertip injury can result in an individual being away from work for several days, with the resulting loss in earnings and concerns for long-term function and appearance. It is, therefore, essential that assessment and management are appropriate.

PRESENTATION

History

Time taken eliciting an accurate history of the mechanism of injury is never more important than in the case of hand injury. When did the injury occur and what was the position of the hand at the time? Was the hand injured with a sharp implement such as glass or was it crushed in a machine? Incised wounds tend to damage structures such as nerves and tendons, whereas crush injuries will fracture bones and cause soft tissue damage. Was there brisk bleeding and does any part of the hand feel numb? These features are important as in the fingers the digital arteries lie adjacent to the nerves. What was the environment of the injury and is it likely that the wound is contaminated or contains foreign bodies? All glass is radio-opaque to a varying degree and, if there is any doubt, it is best to assume the wound contains glass.

The hand is very well supplied with nerve endings and has an extensive cortical sensory representation. Hand injuries are, therefore, painful, although the initial trauma may have been felt as no more than a 'knock'. The patient is likely to require analgesia, so routine questioning about medication and allergies is required. It is also essential to inquire about the tetanus prophylaxis status of the patient. Hand dominance, occupation and leisure activities are all important.

Examination

The injured hand must be examined in a well-lit cubicle with the patient comfortably reclined. Temporary dressings may need to be soaked off if they have been allowed to dry out and become adherent. An initial saline-soaked gauze dressing is ideal, with firm pressure and elevation if there is significant haemorrhage.

Hand and finger injuries are painful and suitable analgesia must be given to allow full examination. Local infiltration of lidocaine without adrenaline (epinephrine) around a wound or as a digital nerve block will allow examination of all except sensation, which must be tested and recorded prior to anaesthesia. Adrenaline (epinephrine) should not be injected around digital arteries. Inadvertent injection of adrenaline (epinephrine) with local anaesthetic in a digital nerve block can be treated by rapid infiltration of phentolamine (α-blocker) into the ischaemic area.

Testing sensation is achieved by light touch or two-point discrimination in the distribution of the three main nerves that supply the hand. The median nerve supplies the palmar aspect of the thumb, index, middle and half of the ring finger extending to supply the fingertip and nailbed. The ulnar nerve supplies both palmar and dorsal aspects of the other half of the ring finger and the little finger. The radial nerve supplies the radial dorsum of the hand, thumb, index, middle and radial aspect of the ring finger (Fig. 3.5.1). It is inadvisable to use a hypodermic needle to test cutaneous sensation. If the patient is unable to describe sensation because they are too young or unconscious, it is useful to remember

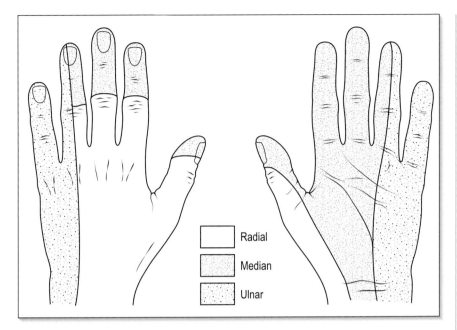

Fig. 3.5.1 Nerve supply to the hand.

INVESTIGATIONS

Most information will be obtained from a full history and examination. Radiology of the hand and fingers will be necessary if bone or joint deformity or tenderness is elicited. Dislocations should always be radiographed prior to manipulation, however trivial they may seem. Radiography can reveal radio-opaque glass in a wound. Organic foreign bodies can often be detected by ultrasound imaging using a small parts soft tissue probe.

Blood investigations are rarely of use in the injured hand.

Magnetic resonance imaging (MRI) is useful (when available) as it shows the soft tissues of the hand well, but it is expensive and should be reserved for conditions where clinical examination requires supplementary information about the integrity of the soft structures in the hand, e.g. tendon injury and tissue tumours.

CLASSIFICATION

There are many ways of cataloguing hand injuries and conditions are often grouped by tissue, e.g. tendon injuries. However, a more *practical* approach is to describe injuries by anatomical site.

FINGERTIP INJURIES

The fingertips have an excellent blood supply and will usually heal if given the correct environment. Fingertip avulsions are classified as type A when the skin loss is oblique dorsal, type B when the loss is transverse, and type C when the loss is oblique volar[1] (Fig. 3.5.2).

The most complex to manage is type C, as there is loss of palmar skin. When there is a type A or B injury involving less than 50% of the nailbed, conservative treatment is often the best option. Care of the finger initially is likely to require a haemostatic dressing, which may be followed by an occlusive silver sulphadiazine dressing. There is good evidence that this kind of dressing promotes healing by being non-adherent and

that the digital nerves also carry the sympathetic supply to the fingers and that division will cause a dry finger in the distribution of the digital nerve.

The examination should be comprehensive and not just concentrate on the obvious injury. Inspection of the hand will provide information about the colour of the tissues, local swelling and position of wounds. The resting position of the hand may be a clue to tendon injury, as the normal uninjured position is with the fingers in increasing flexion from the index to the little finger. A 'pointing finger' may indicate a flexor tendon injury. Obvious bone or joint deformity should be recorded. It is important to remember that glass injuries can cause division of structures distant from the wound entry point.

Palpation of the hand will elicit any local tenderness, and the metacarpals and phalanges are all easily palpable subcutaneously.

Functional testing should be a routine for all injured hands. Tendon function is tested by asking the patient to perform specific movements. Some tendon injuries may be obvious, such as mallet finger injuries and the pointing finger. However, two flexor tendons supply each finger, and simply asking the patient to flex the finger will not exclude a divided flexor digitorum superficialis tendon. The profundus tendon flexes the distal interphalangeal joint and is tested by asking the patient to flex the tip of each finger in turn while the examiner holds the proximal interphalangeal joint immobilized. The superficialis tendon is tested by asking the patient to flex each finger individually, while the examiner holds the other fingers straight. The extensor tendons to the fingers are tested by asking the patient to hyperextend the fingers. It is important to remember that the interconnections between the extensor tendons make it possible to extend to near neutral in the presence of a divided tendon. Partial tendon injuries may still exist despite normal functioning of the fingers. The functioning hand should allow full extension of all fingers and comfortable flexion of the fingers into the palm.

Displaced fractures may be apparent as a deformity. The tips of the flexed fingers should point to the scaphoid bone, and rotational deformity will be detected by a finger crossing its neighbour when flexed.

Rings should be removed from injured fingers to prevent subsequent compromise of circulation as the finger swells.

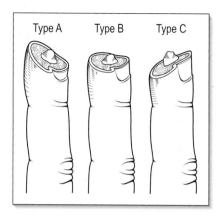

Fig. 3.5.2 Classification of fingertip amputations.

allowing fast re-epithelialization of the fingertip.[2] The dressing is quick to apply, easily removed and comfortable for the patient. The finger has a macerated appearance after a few days but this quickly returns to normal, leaving a fingertip which has pulled good-quality skin to cover the deficit. Most other dressings adhere to the wound and pull epithelial cells off when removed. Alternatives to conservative dressings include skin grafts to the fingertips, advancement flaps and cross-finger flaps. These should be performed by surgeons trained in the specialist techniques, and should be reserved for injuries involving large areas of skin loss.

Major amputations of the fingertip or crush injuries may require terminalization of the finger, and this should be fully discussed with the patient, who may be prepared to forgo finger length in exchange for early healing. Small tuft fractures of the underlying terminal phalanx are stable and will be supported by the dressing.

Fingertip injuries are very painful and digital block local anaesthesia is the preferred technique for analgesia. Occasionally patients will bring amputated pieces of the injured fingertip with them into the emergency department. This tissue may be useful for harvesting full-thickness skin and should be thoroughly defatted before use. No attempt should ever be made to resuture avascular tissue. If there is any doubt of the viability of fingertip tissue the patient should be referred to a specialized hand service.

Nerve repairs distal to the distal interphalangeal joint are rarely rewarding. Digital nerves proximal to the distal interphalangeal joint may be repaired using magnification. Salvage of the digital nerve will depend on the extent of local tissue damage.[3] Good results are achieved with early repair of digital nerves when the ends can be approximated without tension using a fine (8/0) suture. The return of protective sensation depends on the level of repair and axon regeneration.

NAILBED INJURIES

These injuries are frequently under-estimated, often because of a reluctance to remove the nail. An underlying fracture or growth-plate slip of the terminal phalanx will often be associated with nailbed disruption. A subungual haematoma larger than 25% of the area of the nail mandates removal of the nail itself. Small painful subungual haematomas can be released using a hot paperclip or trephine burr. Often damage to the nailbed results in separation of the nail spontaneously, preceded by new nail growth which pushes the damaged nail off. Assuming the nail root is intact a new nail will grow back at a rate of 1 mm per week; full growth of a new nail takes approximately 80 days. Removal of the damaged nail is achieved under digital nerve block using blunt dissection with a pair of fine forceps or scissors. The nail should be retained for use as a dressing later. Underlying fractures should be reduced with pressure, and fracture haematoma irrigated away to achieve anatomical approximation of the bone ends. Fractures distal to the insertion of the profundus tendon are stable. Repair of the fragmented nailbed should be performed with fine (6/0 or 7/0) absorbable suture on an atraumatic needle. Care needs to be taken not to cut out with the needle as the nailbed is fiable. Haemostasis can be achieved with the prior application of a finger tourniquet or firm pressure. The nail is, ideally, trimmed and reapplied as an organic splint and dressing.

TERMINALIZATION

Terminalization of a finger is sometimes necessary when fingertip damage excludes reconstruction. Full discussion with the patient must ensure acceptance of the loss of the fingertip. Occupation and leisure activities must be considered before embarking on finger terminalization. This procedure can be performed under digital nerve/ring block anaesthesia. The fingertip is supplied by the palmar digital nerves, which are best approached from the palmar surface of the finger at the proximal skin crease (Fig. 3.5.3). A rubber tourniquet around the base of the finger provides a bloodless field, but this should be removed to ensure haemostasis prior to skin closure.

Terminalization of a finger requires a level of surgical skill as removal of the nail root and fashioning of the stump are vital for a good cosmetic result. The terminal phalanx should be nibbled down short enough to allow loose closure. Ideally, the insertion of the profundus tendon into the base of the terminal phalanx should be preserved, but often this needs to be sacrificed to achieve skin closure. Terminal vessels and digital nerves should be cauterized with bipolar diathermy. Loose closure of the skin should be performed with 5/0 or 6/0 non-absorbable monofilament suture, being careful to avoid dog ears. The skin flaps must be observed to ensure capillary refill. Postoperatively the hand should be elevated and analgesia provided.

DISTAL INTERPHALANGEAL JOINT INJURIES

Acute flexion injuries of the terminal phalanx may either rupture the extensor tendon at the level of the distal interphalangeal joint or avulse the insertion into the terminal phalanx. This produces an acute flexion deformity of the distal interphalangeal joint, known as a mallet finger. An X-ray of the finger should be taken as an intra-articular fracture involving more than one-third of the joint surface may require internal fixation.

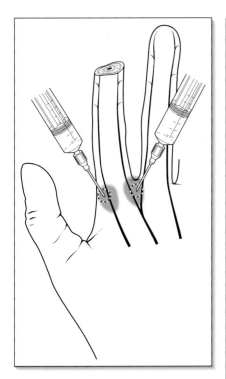

Fig. 3.5.3 Digital nerve block - palmar approach.

Small avulsion fractures and tendon ruptures are best treated by the application of a correctly fitting mallet splint, which should not be removed for 8 weeks. Persisting mallet finger deformity after treatment or late presentations are often best ignored as the finger is still functional despite the deformity. Avulsion fractures resulting from hyperextension of the fingertip are unstable owing to the attachment of the profundus tendon and require internal fixation. Simple dislocations of the distal interphalangeal joint are easily reduced and rarely cause long-term instability. However, prior radiography should be performed to differentiate dislocation from the more complicated intra-articular fractures.

MIDDLE PHALANGEAL INJURIES

The middle phalanx takes the insertion of the superficialis tendon slips through, which passes the profundus tendon. Fracture of the middle phalanx can disrupt the fibrous tunnel of the profundus tendon and cause adhesions. These

fractures need to be accurately reduced and may require internal fixation. They are usually unstable owing to the pull of the tendons. Palmar wounds at this level are likely to divide the profundus tendon or digital nerves and should be explored by a specialized hand service if these injuries are suspected on clinical grounds.

PROXIMAL INTERPHALANGEAL JOINT INJURIES

This is the joint that causes most long-term complications, as a result of stiffness and joint contracture. The proximal interphalangeal joint is mechanically complex and is supported dorsally by the extensor apparatus; on the palmar aspect is the strong fibrous volar plate. Rupture of either structure will result in joint instability and potential long-term disability. Dislocations of the proximal interphalangeal joint invariably displace both structures. Occasionally, the central slip of the extensor tendon or the volar plate avulses a small fragment from the middle phalanx, and this will be visible on X-ray. Reduction of dislocations should be followed by extension splintage and appropriate follow-up. The boutonnière deformity is a hand surgeon's nightmare and should, ideally, be prevented, as long-term results from reconstructive surgery are poor. Tears in the extensor apparatus may result from relatively minor trauma. A high index of suspicion and early splintage should be adopted. These injuries should not be underestimated, and recently ultrasound has been used to aid with early diagnosis.

PROXIMAL PHALANGEAL INJURIES

Both flexor tendons pass along the palmar aspect of the proximal phalanx, and, therefore, fractures of this bone tend to be unstable. Rotational deformity is particularly disabling and may not be noticeable with the finger held straight. These fractures usually require internal

fixation. The lateral X-ray will often be the most useful in determining the degree of angulation or displacement. Wounds may damage digital nerves or either flexor tendons on the palmar aspect. Examination of the finger should detect these injuries, and referral to a specialized hand service will be required.

MCPJ INJURIES

Subluxation of the metacarpophalangeal joint may occur in the older patient after relatively minor trauma. The clinical appearances are subtle and the injury is easy to miss on X-ray. The clue is the inability of the finger to extend fully. Reduction is achieved in recent injury with traction of the finger, although once the displacement is established reduction becomes difficult even with open procedures.

Fist-tooth injuries involving the metacarpophalangeal joint are common and should be assumed to be infected. The extensor tendon may be divided and X-ray may show fracture of the metacarpal head. These injuries should be treated aggressively by joint irrigation, splintage and antibiotics.

The ulnar collateral ligament (gamekeeper's thumb) rupture results from an abduction injury of the thumb and, when complete, results in metacarpophalangeal joint instability. The ligament when completely ruptured may become folded back outside the adductor aponeurosis. X-rays must be taken to identify avulsion fractures of the base of the proximal phalanx. Stress X-ray views will confirm joint instability. Early repair gives superior results to conservative splintage when complete rupture is diagnosed.

METACARPAL INJURIES

These injuries are caused by punching, crush injury, or falls on to the closed fist. The commonest injury is the fifth metacarpal neck fracture, which is usually best treated conservatively. Correction of significant angulation will only be achieved by open reduction and internal fixation. Spiral fractures of the shaft of a metacarpal will result in shortening of the bone and loss of the contour of the knuckle. Conservative management of these fractures should involve resting the hand in a volar splint with the metacarpophalangeal joint flexed to at least 70%. The fingers must be splinted straight, with support to the fingertip. Abduction injuries of the thumb may cause a Bennett fracture, which is an intra-articular fracture, of the base of the thumb metacarpal. The Bennett fracture when displaced should be referred for internal fixation.

DORSAL HAND INJURIES

Wounds on the dorsum of the hand may divide the extensor tendons, which are relatively superficial. Division may be apparent by loss of full extension, but the extensor tendons have extensive cross-insertions and, therefore, visualization of the intact tendon throughout its range of movement is the only safe way to exclude damage. Repair of these tendons is

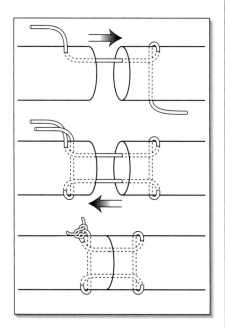

Fig. 3.5.4 Kessler technique of tendon repair. An alternative technique is to begin the suture between the tendon ends and tie, and bury the knot within the tendon.

relatively straightforward, if there are suitable facilities and equipment. Good exposure of the tendon is required, and haemostasis may be achieved using an ischaemic arm block. Good approximation of the tendon ends is required, using the Kessler technique (Fig. 3.5.4) and non-absorbable sutures. Splintage of the hand in extension will be required for 3 weeks, followed by guarded active flexion. Aftercare must be provided, with access to occupational therapy or physiotherapy during rehabilitation.

PALMAR HAND INJURIES

Penetrating wounds on the palm of the hand are likely to divide flexor tendons or main digital nerves. These injuries should be detected by examination. Briskly bleeding wounds proximal to an area of anaesthesia are a clue to digital nerve injury because of coexisting damage to both neurovascular structures. Tendon damage will require referral for specialist repair.

Foreign bodies in the hand can be notoriously difficult to find and damage to other structures can result from injudicious exploration. The best results are achieved in a bloodless field with full anaesthesia. Nailgun injuries require an X-ray prior to removal of the nail to establish its location in respect to bone, and to see whether the nail has barbs that will make removal difficult. High-pressure grease- or paint-gun injuries result in extensive tissue penetration and should never be underestimated. Wide exposure and decompression of the tract will require the care of a specialist hand services.

DISPOSITION

Many hand injuries can be appropriately managed in a well-equipped emergency department. Initial inspection of the injury should take place in a well-illuminated room with the hand resting comfortably. Procedures should only be performed with the patient supine. No attempt should be made to operate surgically on

a hand without good instruments and fine sutures, and the operator must have a good knowledge of anatomy and confidence in his or her abilities. After surgery the hand should be elevated and suitable analgesia provided. Some injuries will require access to a specialized plastic or orthopaedic hand service.

PROGNOSIS

Hand injuries do best with early definitive treatment, as badly managed injuries can be notoriously difficult to salvage at a later date. Stiffness and loss of function can be avoided if good surgical principles of wound management are adhered to. Appropriate splintage and early mobilization are the cornerstones of rehabilitation. The injured hand recovers best when splintage has been in a functional position (extrinsic plus). Whenever possible, the hand should be immobilized with the fingers straight and the metacarpophalangeal joints flexed to at least 70°. This can be achieved in even the most swollen hand by careful application of a volar plaster cast. Grooving of the plaster will give strength without the need for extra layers. Early referral for definitive surgery and subsequent rehabilitation will be essential for severe injuries. An explanation to the patient of the need to prevent joint stiffness will be important when the finger requires dressings for more than 3 weeks. A finger that is kept bandaged and protected for excessive periods after injury will become stiff and sensitive. The fingertips become sensitive after injury and gradual desensitization of the skin can be achieved by gentle percussion of the finger.

PREVENTION

Hand and finger injuries should be prevented, and it is the responsibility of the emergency physician to become actively involved in injury prevention. Unfortunately, fingertips are all too frequently injured. Study of occupational injury – in butchers, for instance, shows that the commonest fingers injured are

ORTHOPAEDIC EMERGENCIES

CONTROVERSIES

❶ **Fingertip dressings** Clinicians should keep an open mind to new products and techniques. There is good evidence that a sterile moist environment for wound healing is beneficial and promotes re-epithelialization. There is no doubt that dressings that adhere to wounds are uncomfortable to remove and damage new epithelial cells.

❷ **Hand splintage** There is often a conflict between the need for appropriate splintage and the desire for early mobilization. The volar plaster splint allows for adequate rest for a wide range of hand and finger injuries without contributing to major joint contraction. The old boxing glove bandage tends to leave the hand clawed and is not a good dressing for an acutely injured and swollen hand.

❸ **Fifth metacarpal fractures** It is tempting to attempt manipulation of displaced neck of fifth metacarpal fractures. Experience shows that these fractures rarely remain reduced even if the position is initially improved. Grossly angulated fractures may warrant internal fixation in selected cases. Functional results are surprisingly good despite angulation.

❹ **Foreign bodies** Foreign body removal from the hand can range from being entirely straightforward to being excessively difficult and damaging. A judgement needs to be made on the likely ease of removal and the facilities available. The first attempt is the easiest. Wood and glass can be very difficult to find in the tissues without a bloodless field. Fish-hooks in the skin can be removed by pushing through the barb and then cutting off the shank.

❺ **To suture or not?** Injudicious suture of an acutely injured finger can compromise circulation and confer a secondary injury. Steristrips may be used to bring the skin edges together or, where there is gross swelling, tulle gauze may be used to maintain the anatomy of the finger. This can be achieved using steristrip skin closures, but these need to be kept dry to adhere and should not be removed until the wound margins have become adherent. When the finger is grossly swollen and fragmented, dressing with a tulle gauze mould can maintain the anatomy of the finger without further adding to the injury.

❻ **Antibiotics** Antibiotics have no role in the initial management of hand injuries. The exception to this is the grossly contaminated injury and those known to be caused by bites. Open fractures of the hand bones will need to be admitted for surgical debridement.

the left index finger and the left thumb, resulting from holding a knife in the right hand and meat in the left hand. Simple measures such as chain-mail gloves can prevent these injuries. Slow door closures and patio door guards will help prevent toddlers getting their fingers caught in the door jamb. Strategies for prevention involve providing data for public awareness and lobbying officials to legislate for sensible measures to prevent injury.

REFERENCES

1. Rob C, Smith R, Birch R, Brooks D 1984 Rob and Smith's Operative Surgery: The Hand, 4th edn. Butterworths, London
2. de Boer P, Collinson PO 1981 The use of silver sulphadiazine occlusive dressings for finger tip injuries. Journal of Bone and Joint Surgery 63B(4)
3. Jabaley M 1984 Technical aspects of peripheral nerve repair. Journal of Hand Surgery 9: 9–14

FURTHER READING

Atasoy E, Lokamidis E, Kasdan M, et al 1970 Reconstruction of the amputated finger tip with a triangular volar flap. Journal of Bone and Joint Surgery 52A(5): 921–6
Davies D, Smith R 1985 The hand 1 & 11. British Medical Journal 290: 1729–34
Hart RG, Kleinert HE 1993 The hand in emergency medicine. Emergency Medicine Clinics of North America 11(3): 755–6
Henderson HP 1984 The best dressing for a nail bed is the nail itself. Journal of Hand Surgery 9B(2): 197–8
Scott JE 1974 Amputation of the finger. British Journal of Surgery 61: 574–6
Stewart C 1997 Hand injuries. Emergency Medicine Reports 18(22): 223–34

3.6 PELVIC INJURIES

MICHAEL CADOGAN

ESSENTIALS

1 Pelvic fractures constitute 3% of skeletal fractures.

2 They are either stable or unstable.

3 Unstable fractures are often associated with considerable mechanical forces, concomitant injuries and a resultant high mortality.

4 Understanding the mechanism of injury and observing the pelvic fracture pattern will provide insight into the potential complicating factors of associated neurovascular or urogenital injuries.

5 Isolated stable pelvic fractures are usually treated conservatively.

ANATOMY

The pelvic ring is formed by two innominate bones and the sacrum. The innominate bones are made up of the ilium, ischium and pubis and are joined anteriorly at the symphysis pubis and posteriorly at the left and right sacroiliac joints. The lateral surface of the innominate bone forms a socket, the acetabulum, to which the ilium, ischium and pubis all contribute. Stability of the pelvic ring is dependent on the strong posterior sacroiliac, sacrotuberous and sacrospinous ligaments.

Disruption of the ring can result in significant trauma to the neurovascular and soft tissue structures it protects

CLASSIFICATION OF PELVIC FRACTURES

Pelvic fractures are stable or unstable, dependent on the degree of ring disruption. They may be open or closed; major or minor and may be associated with haemodynamic compromise and hollow viscus injury.

The Young and Resnik classification scheme is outlined in the chapter on 'Radiology in Major Trauma' and classifies pelvic fractures by mechanism of injury and direction of the causative force. It does not include isolated fractures out with the pelvic ring, or acetabular fractures. These will be detailed later in the chapter.

Young and Resnik classification

Most pelvic fractures result from lateral compression, anteroposterior compression or vertical shear forces. These injuries may be suggested by the history and are confirmed radiographically.

Lateral compression injuries

Lateral compression of the pelvis accounts for 50% of pelvic fractures. They commonly occur when a pedestrian or motor vehicle is struck from the side. Most of these injuries are stable, but as a result of the considerable forces involved, the potential for associated injuries is high. This mechanism of injury can produce several fracture patterns and involves anterior and posterior pathology.

Anteriorly there is always a transverse fracture of at least one set of pubic rami. These fractures may be unilateral or bilateral and may include pubic symphysis disruption. The posterior element of lateral compression fractures is important. This component may be overlooked by the emergency physician concentrating on the anterior findings, but is critical in determining the functional stability of the pelvic ring and defining associated injuries.

Type 1 fractures are the commonest. They involve a compression injury to the sacrum posteriorly and oblique pubic rami fractures anteriorly. These injuries are observed on the side of impact and are usually stable involving impaction of the cancellous bone of the sacrum without ligamentous disruption. X-rays confirm discontinuity of the sacral foramina posteriorly.

Type 2 fractures result from greater lateral compressive forces. The iliac wing is fractured posteriorly and the fracture line often extends to involve part of the sacroiliac joint. This leaves part of the ilium firmly attached to the scarum. Anteriorly the obligatory pubic rami fractures are observed. Stability is determined by the degree of sacroiliac joint disruption and mobility of the involved anterior hemipelvis. These fractures are usually stable to external rotation and vertical movement but are more mobile to internal rotation.

Type 3 injuries usually occur when one hemipelvis is trapped against the ground and a lateral force rolls over the mobile hemipelvis, producing a lateral compression injury to the side of primary impact and an unstable anteroposterior compressive injury to the contralateral sacroiliac joint.

Anteroposterior compression injuries

Anteroposterior compression of the pelvis accounts for 25% of pelvic fractures.

These injuries result from anteriorly directed forces applied directly to the pelvis or indirectly via the lower extremities to produce open-book type injuries.

Type 1 injuries result from low energy forces that stretch the ligamentous constraints of the pelvic ring. The pubic symphysis is disrupted anteriorly with less than 2.5 cm diastasis observed radiographically. These fractures are stable and there is usually no significant posterior pelvic injury.

Type 2 injuries are classically open-book fractures. They involve rupture of the anterior sacroiliac, sacrospinous and sacrotuberous ligaments posteriorly with disruption of the pubic symphysis anteriorly. Radiographically there is widening of the anterior sacroiliac joint, diastasis of the pubic symphysis more than 2.5 cm and occasionally avulsion of the lateral border of the lower sacral segments. Considerable force is involved to disrupt these ligaments and neurovascular injuries and complications are common. The pelvis is unstable to external rotation and external compression will 'spring' the pelvis.

Type 3 injuries occur when even greater forces are applied and involve disruption of all the pelvic ligaments on the affected side. Rupture of the posterior sacroiliac ligaments leads to lateral displacement and disconnection of the affected hemipelvis from the sacrum. They are completely unstable and are associated with the highest rate of neurovascular injury and haemorrhage.

Vertical shear injuries (Malgaigne fracture)

These injuries account for only 5% of pelvic fractures. They usually occur following a fall from a height or during a motor vehicle accident when the victim reflexly extends their leg against the break pedal before impact. These mechanisms force the hemipelvis in a vertical direction and result in complete ligamentous or bony disruption with cephaloposterior hemipelvic displacement.

Anterior disruption occurs through the pubic symphysis or pubic rami. Posteriorly, dissociation usually occurs through the sacroiliac joint, but may occur vertically through the sacrum. They are usually unilateral, but may be bilateral and may be associated with significant intra-abdominal injuries.

CLINICAL ASSESSMENT

In the multi-trauma patient, it is essential that standard trauma protocols are adhered to with attention being paid first to the airway, breathing and circulation in the primary survey and resuscitation phases of initial care.

The pelvis is examined within the secondary survey. The suprapubic, pelvic and urogenital regions are examined for signs of bruising, abrasions, open wounds and obvious deformity. In males the urethral meatus is inspected for the presence of frank blood and the scrotum inspected for bruising. Flank bruising may indicate retroperitoneal haemorrhage.

Palpation of the pelvis commences at the anterior superior iliac spines. Evidence of internal rotation is assessed by compressing the spines towards each other and external rotation is tested by pushing both the spines outwards. The pelvic compression test does not always correlate with the significance of the injury. In the haemo-dynamically unstable patient this examination should only be performed once, to avoid exacerbating haemorrhage by dislodging any clots.

The back is examined with attention to the lumbar spine, sacroiliac regions and the coccyx. Abdominal, rectal, vaginal and perineal examinations are required.

The rectal examination includes observation for fresh blood, assessment of anal sphincter tone and the position and tenderness of the prostate. A thorough neurovascular examination must be performed.

The AP pelvis X-ray will usually reveal anterior fractures, but posterior fractures are often difficult to visualize. If clinically indicated further X-rays or a CT scan are warranted.

INJURIES ASSOCIATED WITH PELVIC FRACTURES

Haemorrhage

Haemorrhage is the most significant complication of pelvis fractures. It may result from bleeding at fracture sites, local venous and arterial tears and disruption of major vessels. Catastrophic bleeding may result from disruption of the internal iliac arteries, their tributaries and accompanying veins as they pass over the anterior aspect of the sacroiliac joint. Severe hypovolemia following persistent haemorrhage without major vessel disruption is a significant cause of mortality. Up to 4 L of blood can be lost into the retroperitoneal space before tamponade occurs.

Anteroposterior type 3 injuries and vertical shear injuries disrupt the sacroiliac joint and are associated with significant haemorrhage. Treatment to minimize or cease haemorrhage associated with pelvic fractures includes angiography and embolization, external fixation and open reduction with internal fixation.

Genitourinary and bladder injuries

Pelvic fractures have an associated injury to the lower urinary tract in up to 16% of cases. They are more prevalent in males who sustain a much higher level of urethral injury. Pelvic trauma may also result in bladder rupture. The bladder is normally protected by the pelvis and rupture is usually indicative of significant disruption of the pelvic ring. Blunt trauma victims with bladder rupture have an associated pelvic fracture in nearly 90% of cases. Patients usually present hypotensive with frank haematuria. However, gross haematuria is a general sign of genitourinary trauma and is not specific for bladder rupture. A retrograde urethrogram is, therefore, performed to delineate any urethral trauma prior to performing retrograde cystography.

Urethral and genital injuries

Urethral rupture is mainly associated with males and is rare in females. Rupture of the urethra secondary to blunt trauma commonly occurs in the anterior bulbous urethra just distal to the urogenital diaphragm. It is associated with bilateral pubic rami fractures, pubic symphysis disruption and vertical shear injuries.

Clinically, a urethral rupture must be suspected in the male adult with a pelvic fracture, blood at the urethral meatus, a high-riding prostate, perineal haematoma and urinary retention. However, these 'classic' signs may not be present. A retrograde urethrogram is diagnostic and may be performed prior to Foley catheterization if clinically indicated.

Injury to the female genitalia is often overlooked. Vaginal lacerations are associated with pelvic fractures in 4% of cases. They normally present with bleeding, but may be occult. A bimanual pelvic examination is required in all women with pelvic fractures. This may necessitate anaesthesia as a result of patient discomfort.

Complications of these uncommon injuries, such as abscess formation and sepsis may be severe.

MANAGEMENT OF UNSTABLE PELVIC FRACTURES

The mainstay of pelvic fracture management within the emergency department is to identify and assess the degree of pelvic injury; provide adequate fluid resuscitation and analgesia and to minimize life-threatening haemorrhage. Early identification of pelvic trauma and mobilization of specialists including the orthopaedic surgeon, vascular surgeon and radiologist is essential.

Fluid resuscitation

Fluid resuscitation of hypotensive patients with pelvic trauma commences with intravenous crystalloid through two large bore peripheral cannulae. Blood products are used if the patient remains hypotensive despite intravenous fluids. The average blood transfusion requirements for anteroposterior compression fractures is 15 units, vertical shear injuries 9 units and lateral compression injuries 3.5 units.

Pelvis immobilization

Immobilization of the pelvis and re-approximation of the bony fragments creates a tamponade effect and reduces the risk of continuing haemorrhage prior to definitive treatment. This may be achieved initially by simply bracing the pelvis in a sheet and supporting it laterally with sandbags. The efficacy of pneumatic anti-shock garments (PASG) within the emergency department is controversial. They may be useful in the pre-hospital setting and have provided stabilization and immobilization during transport. PASG reduce haemorrhage from anteroposterior compression fractures, but conversely may increase fracture displacement with lateral compression injuries. Other complications with their use include catastrophic hypotension on injudicious sudden removal, compart-

ment syndrome and reduced access to the lower limbs.

External fixation is a rapid and simple emergency department procedure designed to stabilize and immobilize the pelvis and reduce pelvic haemorrhage prior to definitive treatment. Three pins are placed through each iliac crest and then clamped to an external frame to reduce the displaced pelvic ring injury. Advantages of external fixation are that it is quick, effective and can proceed within the emergency department without delaying the continued management of the multiply injured patient. The disadvantages include the lack of support for the posterior component of pelvic ring fractures and difficulty in placement in the obese patient.

Embolization

Angiography with embolization is used as an adjunct to external or internal fixation and may also be used to primarily control haemorrhage. It is operator-dependent, time consuming, is performed outside the emergency department and does not address the venous blood loss.

OPEN PELVIC FRACTURES

These fractures are rare and associated with an increased morbidity and mortality. Open fractures with pelvic ring disruption lose the tamponade effect offered by a closed space and can result in massive and fatal haemorrhage. Control of haemorrhage is a priority in open pelvic injury. Sterile gauze packed into the wounds applies a direct pressure tamponade. Urgent operation to repair associated open bowel and bladder injuries and debride bleeding wounds is paramount and stabilization of the pelvic fracture is the last step in treatment.

STABLE FRACTURES OF THE PELVIS

Isolated avulsion fractures

These are often sustained by young adults following stress of the muscular

and ligamentous insertions onto the bony pelvis. They include:

Anterior superior iliac spine fracture

The anterior superior iliac spine may be fractured by powerful contraction of the sartorius muscle and occurs in jumping activities. Such injuries usually involve pain on weight bearing with local tenderness and swelling at the fracture site. Active flexion and abduction of the thigh will reproduce the pain. There is usually minimal displacement of the avulsed fracture on the AP film of the pelvis.

Anterior inferior iliac spine fracture

Forceful contraction of the rectus femoris muscle may avulse the anterior inferior iliac spine, which usually occurs in sports that involve kicking. These patients complain of a sharp pain in the groin and are unable to actively flex the hip. The fracture is usually evident on plain AP pelvis views with the fragment displaced distally.

Ischial tuberosity fractures

Fractures of the ischial tuberosity are rare and occur with forceful contraction of the hamstrings. They occur in young adults whose apophyses are not fully united and are associated with hurdling and other jumping activities. Pain may be reproduced by local palpation and active flexion of the hip with the knee extended. Plain X-rays of the pelvis reveal minimal displacement of the apophysis from the ischium.

Isolated pubic ramus fractures

These injuries are commonly seen in the elderly with direct trauma following a fall. The patient has difficulty in weight bearing and local pain and tenderness in the groin.

Pain is usually reproduced with the *FABER* test. The ipsilateral foot is placed on the contralateral knee forcing the ipsilateral hip to be Flexed, ABducted and Externally Rotated. Pelvic radiographs confirm non-displaced isolated pubic rami fractures.

Iliac wing fractures (Duverney fracture)

Direct lateral trauma may result in an isolated iliac wing fracture. Patients complain of severe pain on weight bearing and walk with a waddling gait. Localized tenderness and bruising are usually apparent over the site of injury. Abdominal guarding, ileus and lower quadrant tenderness are associated features. These fractures are generally minimally displaced, rarely comminuted and easily visualized on AP pelvis X-rays.

Coccyx fractures

These fractures are more frequent in women and are caused by a falls onto the buttocks with both hips flexed. Patients have extreme difficulty in mobilizing and have local pain, swelling, bruising and tenderness over the lower sacral region.

Radiographic confirmation is not necessary if physical examination confirms an isolated injury.

MANAGEMENT OF ISOLATED STABLE FRACTURES

Avulsion fractures, pubic ramus fractures and iliac wing fractures are treated conservatively with non-steroidal anti-inflammatory drugs and non-weight bearing crutches for 10 days. Slow mobilization and physiotherapy will allow resumption of normal activities in 3–4 weeks. Coccygeal fractures require bed rest, analgesia and stool softeners. Sitting is often very painful and a donut-ring cushion is helpful.

ACETABULAR FRACTURES

Acetabular fractures account for 20% of pelvic fractures. They are usually associated with lateral compression forces but also occur with posterior forces applied distally through the femur. They are often associated with other pelvic injuries, knee injuries, hip fractures and dislocations.

Acetabular fractures are caused by direct impaction of the femoral head and are usually associated with hip dislocations. Their classification is complex. These fractures are associated with sciatic and femoral nerve injury depending on the position of the hip dislocation. A thorough neurovascular examination is mandatory.

Standard radiographs of the hip and pelvis are useful in defining the fracture, but CT scans are essential to show the anterior and posterior fragments and the involvement of ilioischial and iliopubic columns.

FURTHER READING

Burgess AR, Eastridge BJ, Young JW, Ellison TS 1990 Pelvic ring disruptions: effective classification system and treatment protocols. Journal of Trauma 30: 848

CONTROVERSIES

❶ The use of the PASG in transport and pre-hospital has been fully evaluated, but its efficacy within the emergency department requires further research.

❷ The placement of external fixation devices within the emergency department has been shown to reduce mortality and should be implemented.

❸ The optimum timing of embolization to control primary haemorrhage in the multi-trauma victim is unclear.

Dalal SA, Burgess AR, Siegel JH, et al 1989 Pelvic fracture in multiple trauma: classification by mechanism is key to pattern of organ injury, resuscitative requirements, and outcome. Journal of Trauma 29: 981–1002

Fallon B, Wendt JC, Hawtrey CE 1984 Urological injury and assessment in patients with fractured pelvis. Journal of Urology 131: 712–4

Gokcen EC, Burgess AR, Siegel JH, Mason-Gonzalez, Dischinger PC, Ho SM 1994 Pelvic fracture mechanism of injury in vehicular trauma patients. Journal of Trauma 36: 789–96

Kellam JF 1989 The Role of external fixation in pelvic disruptions. Clinical Orthopedics 241(Apr): 66–82

Mattox KL, Bickell W, Pepe PE, Mangelsdorff AD 1986 Prospective randomized evaluation of antishock MAST in post-traumatic hypotension. Journal of Trauma 26: 779–86

Pennal GF, Tile M, Waddell JP 1980 Garside pelvic. Disruption: assessment and classification. Clinical Orthopedics 151(Sep): 12–21

Rothenberger DA, Velasco R, Strate R, Fischer RP, Perry JF Jr 1978 Open pelvic fracture: a lethal injury. Journal of Trauma 18: 184–7

ORTHOPAEDIC EMERGENCIES

3

3.7 HIP INJURIES

MICHAEL CADOGAN

ESSENTIALS

1 Trauma to the hip is a major cause of morbidity and mortality and has a huge impact on health care and resources.

2 Hip injuries are usually pathological and a disease of the elderly, however, there has been an increased incidence of hip fractures and dislocations in young people sustaining high-energy trauma.

3 Femoral head avascular necrosis is a complication of intracapsular femoral-neck fractures.

4 Extracapsular neck of femur fractures may be associated with significant haemorrhage necessitating early recognition and treatment.

5 The hip joint is least stable when flexed and adducted and prone to dislocation.

6 Posterior hip dislocations are associated with sciatic nerve injury and avascular necrosis and are an orthopaedic emergency.

7 Anterior hip dislocations are associated with femoral neurovascular injury and occult hip joint fractures.

ANATOMY

The hip joint is a large ball and socket articulation encompassing the acetabulum and proximal femur. The hip joint provides a high degree of stability and mobility.

Blood supply

The head and intracapsular portion of the femoral neck receive the majority of their blood supply from the extracapsular arterial ring (trochanteric anastomosis), with a minor supply arising from the obturator artery via the ligamentum teres (foveal artery). Retinacular arteries from the extracapsular ring pass under the reflection of the hip capsule to supply the femoral neck and head in a retrograde manner. Intracapsular fractures will disrupt this 'distal to proximal flow' and so may result in avascular necrosis of the femoral head.

Avascular necrosis (AVN)

In the context of hip injuries, avascular necrosis is ischaemic bone death that occurs within the femoral head following compromise to its blood supply. In neck of femur fractures, AVN results primarily from the disruption of the trochanteric anastomosis, and is the commonest early complication of these fractures. Traumatic haemarthrosis, with or without a fracture, may result in intracapsular tamponade. If the intracapsular pressure exceeds the diastolic blood pressure, AVN can occur.

The risk of AVN with posterior dislocations is related to the degree of trauma and the duration of time the femoral head is out of the joint. Their management is an orthopaedic emergency.

Chronic pancreatitis, alcohol abuse, sickle cell anaemia, vasculitis, irradiation, decompression illness and the prolonged use of corticosteroids may all result in AVN. Increased bone density of the femoral head is a radiographic feature of AVN, but may take up to 6 months to become manifest.

CLASSIFICATION OF HIP FRACTURES

Hip fractures are either intracapsular or extracapsular. Intracapsular fractures involve the femoral neck or head. Extracapsular fractures include intertrochanteric, trochanteric and subtrochanteric fractures and are four times more common than intracapsular fractures.

The incidence of hip fractures increases exponentially with age as the fracture rate doubles for every decade over 50 years. Hip fractures occur most frequently in white postmenopausal females with 50% of 65-year-old females, and 100% of females over the age of 85 have a bone mineral content below fracture threshold level.

Intracapsular fractures

Femoral head

Femoral head fractures are uncommon and are usually associated with dislocations of the hip. They often occur in younger patients, and 75% of cases are associated with motor vehicle accidents.

Classification Fractures of the superior aspect of the femoral head are usually associated with anterior dislocations, and inferior femoral head fractures occur with posterior dislocations. Fractures may involve a single fragment (type 1) or comminution (type 2).

Clinical evaluation The symptoms and signs of femoral head injuries are usually those of the associated dislocation rather than the fracture itself. The femoral head fractures are not always picked up on initial X-rays. Further radiological imaging should be sought in the presence of persistent pain post reduction of a hip dislocation, in the absence of abnormality on plain radiographs.

Management Orthopaedic consultation is important as prompt reduction of the dislocation and appropriate stabilization of the fracture reduce the risk of AVN and increase the chance of full return of mobility. The prognosis is related to the severity of the initial trauma, time to definitive reduction and number of failed closed relocation attempts.

Complications AVN occurs in 15–20% of cases, posttraumatic arthritis in 40% and myositis ossificans in 2%.

Femoral-neck fractures

Intracapsular fractures are four times more common in females than males.

There are four main causes of this type of injury:

❶ Elderly, with minimal trauma following a fall onto the greater trochanter (pathological fracture).

❷ Elderly, with torsion or twisting injury prior to fall (pathological fracture).

❸ Young persons involved in high energy trauma (excessive loading).

❹ Repetitive stress or cyclical loading injuries (stress fracture).

Classification The Garden classification system is commonly used to describe intracapsular neck of femur fractures.

Garden I   Incomplete, impacted or stress fractures that are stable. Trabeculae of the inferior neck are still intact and, although they may be angulated, they are still congruous.

Garden II   Undisplaced fracture across the entire femoral neck. The weight-bearing trabeculae are interrupted without displacement. These fractures are inherently unstable and must be fixed.

Garden III   Complete femoral neck fracture with partial displacement. There is associated rotation of the femoral head with non-congruity of the head and acetabular trabeculae.

Garden IV   Complete subcapital fracture with total displacement of fracture fragments. There is no congruity between proximal and distal fragments but the femoral head maintains a normal relationship with acetabulum.

Fractures may be further simplified into non-displaced (Garden I and II) and displaced (Garden III and IV).

Clinical assessment and management

Non-displaced fractures Non-displaced fractures include stress fractures, Garden I and Garden II fractures. Stress fractures are usually the result of repetitive abnormal forces on normal bone in fit and active young people such as military recruits or marathon runners, but may occur with repetitive normal stresses on abnormal bones such as in rheumatoid arthritis or patients taking long-term steroids.

They present with pain that is of gradual onset, worse after activity that radiates from the groin to the medial aspect of the knee. Patients walk with a limp and often present late. Physical examination reveals no obvious deformity; although there is mild discomfort on passive movement at the extremities of motion and percussion tenderness over the greater trochanter.

Additional radiological examination with a bone scan and/or MRI is indicated in the high probability patient with initially normal X-rays but persistent pain. MRI is the investigation of choice. It is not time-dependent and is more sensitive than bone scans in the first 24 hours. It is of similar accuracy as bone scans in fracture assessment at 72 hours.

Stress fractures and Garden I impacted fractures are considered stable and may be treated conservatively under close orthopaedic supervision. Garden II fractures, although non-displaced, are inherently unstable and must be internally fixed.

Displaced fractures Elderly patients with displaced fractures usually present with pain in the hip area and markedly reduced hip movement. The lower limb is shortened, abducted and externally rotated (though less than with intertrochanteric fractures) distal to the fracture. XR reveals the fracture and the degree of posterior comminution of the proximal fragment. Adequate systemic analgesia and a femoral nerve block reduce discomfort. Skin traction will also reduce pain and attempt to preserve femoral head vascularity.

Traumatic femoral neck fractures in the young adult are uncommon injuries and usually involve normal bone. These fractures are outside of the Garden classification. They require a large degree of force and have a high risk of AVN in up to 35% and non-union in up to 57%.

Complications

Mortality Femoral-neck fractures are associated with a mortality of 14–36% in the first year after injury. The rate returns to the pre-fracture level after the first year. Mortality is increased threefold in those patients who were institutionalized prior to the fracture, with concomitant factors of male sex, increased age, malnutrition, multiple medical problems and end-stage renal failure also increasing the mortality.

Morbidity AVN is the most common complication despite optimal treatment. Non-union, post-operative infection and osteomyelitis are also common.

Extracapsular femur fractures

Intertrochanteric femur fractures

Fractures of the proximal femur that occur along a line between the greater and lesser trochanters are referred to as intertrochanteric. They are usually pathological, occur in the elderly and have a female predominance.

Mechanism In the elderly population, a simple fall with a direct force applied to the greater trochanter is enough to cause an intertrochanteric femur fracture. In young adults they are associated with high-speed motor-vehicle accidents or falls from a height.

Clinical assessment Patients sustaining an intertrochanteric fracture are unable to weight bear and have significant pain on hip movement. There is often a large haematoma overlying the greater trochanter due to the highly vascular bone that has been fractured without any intracapsular containment.

Examination reveals a markedly shortened, abducted, significantly externally rotated lower limb.

In most cases, X-ray confirms the fracture, however, internal rotation of the hip on the AP view prevents rotation of the greater trochanter and this may obscure of the fracture. The lateral view radiograph depicts size, location and degree of comminution of the fracture fragments and determines stability.

Classification Numerous classification systems are available for intertrochanteric fractures, the simplest of which was postulated by Evans, which divides intertrochanteric fractures into stable and unstable.

However, for the emergency physician an anatomical description of the fracture detailing the degree of comminution, subtrochanteric extension and presence of displaced posterior fragments is adequate (see Fig. 3.7.1).

Management A complete patient evaluation is critical in formulating any treatment plan, as intertrochanteric fractures occur most frequently in the elderly. Patients may lose up to 1.5 litres of blood from comminuted fractures and are often dehydrated, malnourished and in significant pain on arrival in the emergency department. Systemic analgesia and fluid resuscitation are essential preparation for theatre.

Skin traction or immobilization with sandbags prevents further soft tissue damage and bony comminution and reduces blood loss. Full pre-operative evaluation includes a search for associated injuries such as rib fractures, radial fractures and spinal compression at the level of T12 and L1. ECG, bloods, and CXR to elucidate the cause of the fall and treatment of associated medical problems are essential.

Treatment aims to return the patient to their pre-fracture status. Open reduction with internal fixation (ORIF) produces better anatomical alignment, shorter hospital stay, and improved function with a decreased mortality than conservative management.

Complications There is a mortality rate of 10–30% in the first year, which returns to that of the general population after the first year. Survival is directly related to the patient's age and pre-existing medical factors.

Greater trochanteric fracture

Mechanism
Isolated greater trochanter fractures are uncommon. They usually occur between 7 and 17 years of age and involve true epiphyseal separation secondary to indirect trauma. Forceful muscular contraction by gluteus medius causes avulsion of the apophysis. The displaced, non-comminuted fragment may be separated by up to 6 cm.

Greater trochanteric fractures in adults are rare and usually result from direct trauma causing a comminuted fracture whose fragments are rarely displaced and usually involves only part of the trochanter.

Clinical assessment
Patients with a greater trochanter injury are tender to palpate over the area of avulsion or comminution, but bruising is uncommon. There is often an associated flexion deformity of the hip as a result of pain and muscle spasm and weight bearing produces a limp.

Management
The prognosis after these fractures is good. Most are treated with bed rest for 3 days followed by non-weight-bearing crutches for 4 weeks. Open reduction and internal fixation is required when there is marked separation of the bony fragment.

Lesser trochanteric fracture
Isolated fractures of the lesser trochanter usually occur in children and young athletes with 85% occurring before the age of 20.

Mechanism
Lesser trochanter fractures are usually an apophyseal avulsion secondary to the forceful contraction of iliopsoas.

Clinical assessment
Patients complain of pain on flexion and internal rotation of the hip. Examination reveals tenderness in the femoral triangle. The patient is unable to flex the hip and raise the foot off the ground in a seated position (Ludloff sign).

Radiology is often inconclusive as there may not be complete separation of the bony fragment and comparison views may be required.

Management
Ten days of bed rest and slow mobilization will result in a full recovery. Open reduction and internal fixation is

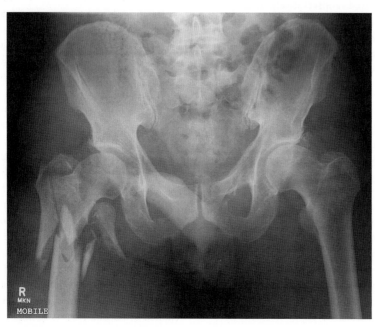

Fig. 3.7.1 Unstable comminuted intertrochanteric fracture with subtrochanteric extension

unnecessary, even in wide apophyseal separation.

Subtrochanteric femur fractures

The subtrochanteric region of the femur lies between the lesser trochanter and a point 5 cm distally. Fractures arising within this region are termed subtrochanteric fractures.

They account for 11% of hip fractures and occur in the elderly with osteoporosis, bone metastases or end-stage renal failure. High-energy injuries in young adults with normal bone are less common.

Mechanism

Ninety per cent of these fractures are as a result of blunt trauma, either from a simple fall in the elderly or following a high speed MVA or fall from a height in young adults, with up to 10% due to high-energy gunshot wounds in the USA.

Classification

A variety of classification systems are available but none widely used. As with intertrochanteric fractures it is best to describe the location, presence of comminution and the position of the lesser trochanter proximal or distal to the fracture line.

Clinical assessment

In the elderly, subtrochanteric fractures are usually isolated. However, substantial force is required in young adults, and the presence of other injuries must be actively sought. The limb distal to the fracture is usually held in abduction, flexion and external rotation. Haemorrhage from a comminuted subtrochanteric fracture may be up to 2 litres. The patient's circulatory status must be assessed and fluid resuscitation commenced to prevent hypovolaemic shock.

Management

Following the administration of analgesia, the affected limb should be immobilized in a splint such as a Donway or Thomas splint, and fluid resuscitation commenced as required. Orthopaedic referral is necessary for open reduction and internal fixation of these fractures.

Complications

There is around a 20% mortality associated with these fractures in the first year, mainly in the elderly. Subtrochanteric bone is cortical, unlike the cancellous bone involved in intertrochanteric fractures. These fractures often lack the vascularity for adequate new bone growth and repair and are associated with a higher rate of non-union and implant failure. Of note, the further down the shaft of femur the fracture line is located, the greater the degree of non-union and implant failure.

Hip dislocation

The hip joint is inherently stable and, as considerable force is required to produce a dislocation, associated injuries must always be sought.

Hip dislocations are classified anatomically into anterior and posterior dislocations dependent on the final position of the femoral head relative to the acetabular rim.

As a result of the femoral head's precarious blood supply and the proximity of the sciatic nerve, non-prosthetic dislocations are an orthopaedic emergency. Failure to reduce a dislocation within 6 hours dramatically increases the risk of AVN and sciatic nerve ischaemia.

Posterior dislocation

Mechanism Posterior dislocations represent 85-90% of traumatic hip dislocations. Classically a direct distal force applied to the flexed knee, with the hip in varying degrees of flexion causes a posterior dislocation of the hip. When seated in the front of a car, the hip and knee are usually flexed to 90° and the hip adducted, which is the least stable position for the hip to be in. The force applied by the dashboard in a head on collision to a seated individual may produce a simple posterior dislocation.

The abducted and partially flexed hip in the same scenario is more stable and if the force of impact is great enough will result in a posterior dislocation with displaced acetabular fracture.

Clinical assessment Examination of the affected limb will reveal shortening, adduction, internal rotation and some degree of flexion. A single AP pelvis radiograph is usually adequate to confirm a posterior dislocation. However, with up to half of these dislocations being associated with an acetabular, femoral head or femur fracture, further radiological imaging is essential. Judet views, AP hip with internal rotation and AP and lateral femur will reveal these associated fractures.

Neurological examination is important in posterior dislocations, as those particularly with marked internal rotation may compress the sciatic nerve and its branches, resulting in deficits especially in the peroneal nerve distribution. It is important to be aware of associated injuries such as ipsilateral knee ligament disruption especially a posterior cruciate rupture.

Management The orthopaedic team must be consulted early. Adequate imaging, a thorough search for associated peri-articular and distal limb injuries and neurological evaluation are essential in the emergency department.

Closed reduction of posterior hip dislocations may be performed within the emergency department under conscious sedation, unless there is immediate access to an operating theatre.

There are numerous methods of relocation, many requiring significant physical force.

The most commonly used procedure is the Allis manoeuvre, whereby the patient lies supine with an assistant stabilizing the pelvis with downward pressure on the anterior superior iliac spines. The operator forcefully distracts the lower leg with the hip and knee at 90° of flexion. Other techniques include the lateral traction-countertraction method or the Whistler technique.

Complications The risk of developing AVN is directly proportional to the length of time the hip remains dislocated, and increases dramatically if the dislocation is not reduced within 6 hours of injury. Sciatic nerve neurapraxia may occur in 15% of cases but is usually relieved by reduction. Permanent ischaemic changes with neurological deficit secondary to pressure necrosis have been reported in up to 3% of cases usually in the peroneal nerve distribution. Missed knee injuries occur in up to 15% of cases, as well as patella, tibial plateau and posterior cruciate injuries.

Anterior dislocation

Anterior dislocations account for 10–15% of traumatic hip dislocations, and are associated with femoral neurovascular injury and occult hip joint fractures. They usually result from a direct blow to the abducted and externally rotated hip. When the hip is in abduction, the femoral neck or greater trochanter impinges on the rim of the acetabulum. A direct force applied distally can lever the head out of the acetabulum and tear the anterior capsule of the hip.

Classification Anterior dislocations may be superior or inferior. Type I or superior dislocations occur when the hip is extended at the time of injury. These are also known as iliac dislocations. Type II or inferior dislocations occur when the hip is flexed at the time of injury. These are also known as obturator dislocations. They may be further sub classified as a) simple dislocation; b) associated femoral neck fracture or c) associated acetabular fracture.

Clinical assessment The superior-type of injury causes an extended, externally rotated and slightly abducted distal limb. The distal limb in the inferior-type dislocation is externally rotated, abducted and in flexion. The femoral head may be palpated around the anterior superior iliac spine in superior types and in the obturator foramen in inferior.

A neurovascular examination is essential in anterior dislocations, particularly the superior-type, where trauma to the femoral artery, vein and nerve is common. Hip and pelvis radiographs must be carefully studied for associated fractures of the acetabulum and femoral head. Further imaging with CT scanning may be indicated for persistent post reduction pain.

Management These injuries are usually associated with high energy trauma and a thorough multi-system examination looking for associated life-threatening injuries is essential. Orthopaedic consultation is mandatory due to the high probability of vascular injury and the requirement for closed reduction under general anaesthesia.

Complications

Early Superior-type dislocations produce direct pressure on the femoral vessels with the potential for distal neurovascular compromise.

Late Post traumatic arthritis and AVN may occur. Recurrence is common when anterior capsular healing is incomplete following inadequate immobilization post reduction.

FURTHER READING

Dahners LE, Hundley JD 1999 Reduction of posterior hip dislocations in the lateral position using traction-countertraction: safer for the surgeon? Journal of Orthopaedic Trauma 13: 373–4

Garden RS 1961 The structure and function of the proximal end of the femur. Journal of Bone and Joint Surgery 43B: 576–89

Hirasawa Y, Oda R, Nakatani K 1977 Sciatic nerve paralysis in posterior dislocation of the hip. Clinical Orthopedics, 126: 172–5

Holmberg S, Conradi P, Kalen R, Thorgren KG 1986 Mortality after cervical hip fracture; three thousand two patients followed for six years. Acta Orthopaedica Scandinavica 57: 8–11

Jazayeri M 1978 Posterior fracture dislocations of the hip joint with emphasis on the importance of hip tomography in their management. Orthopedic Review 7: 59–64

Keller CS, Laros GS 1980 Indications for open reduction of femoral neck fractures. Clinical Orthopedics 152: 131–7

Walden PD, Hamer JR. 1999 Whistler technique used to reduce traumatic dislocation of the hip in the emergency department setting. Journal of Emergency Medicine 17: 441–4

CONTROVERSIES

❶ The application of skin traction and immobilization for extracapsular femur fractures within the emergency department to reduce mortality warrants further investigation.

❷ Further research into the use of CT and MRI to evaluate the acutely reduced non-prosthetic hip may reduce associated morbidity.

❸ Although it is essential to treat hip dislocations early, it remains contentious as to whether the reduction should occur within the emergency department or in the operating theatre.

3.8 FEMUR INJURIES

MICHAEL CADOGAN

ESSENTIALS

1 The femur is the longest and strongest bone in the body.

2 Early fracture reduction and immobilization in traction reduces mortality.

3 Haemorrhagic shock is a major complication with an average blood loss from a closed femoral fracture of 1200 mL.

4 Femoral shaft fractures are often associated with other significant injuries which should be sought.

FEMORAL SHAFT FRACTURE

Mechanism

Considerable force is required to break the adult femur in the absence of a pathological process such as osteoporosis or metastatic disease. The majority of injuries occur in young adults following road traffic accidents, falls from a height or gun shot wounds.

Clinical evaluation

The clinical diagnosis of femoral shaft fractures is usually readily apparent. The thigh is shortened and externally rotated, with the hip held in slight abduction.

Palpation reveals tenderness over the fracture site and on attempted movement. Neurovascular injuries are rare, but thorough examination of the distal pulses, capillary refill and distal sensation must be performed.

In closed fractures, vascular damage is usually limited to rupture of the profunda femoris perforating branches. The resultant tense, swollen haematoma is limited to the thigh and is not associated with distal circulatory compromise. Penetrating trauma and open fractures may cause femoral artery disruption and

repeated vascular evaluations are important. Any evidence of diminished distal pulses, or an expanding haematoma should prompt further investigation with Doppler imaging or arteriography.

Commonly associated injuries include fractures of the pelvis, femoral head and neck, dislocation of the hip and soft tissue disruption of the knee. Up to 50% of closed femur injuries are associated with knee meniscal and collateral injuries; however, it is often impossible to reliably evaluate for these injuries in the acute setting.

Up to 1.5 litres of blood may extravasate into the surrounding soft tissues. Frequent examination for signs of hypovolemia such as hypotension and tachycardia is essential.

Management

In the setting of multi-trauma, the treatment of associated head, neck, thoracic and pelvic injuries must take priority. Fracture reduction and immobilization, fluid resuscitation and the administration of analgesia are performed before X-ray of the lower limb.

Analgesia

Pain relief is important in the emergency department. Intravenous opioid analgesia is the first line of treatment, titrated to effect. A femoral nerve block is an important adjunct that should be considered prior to fracture reduction.

Reduction and immobilization

Early fracture reduction and immobilization in traction reduces mortality. With appropriate analgesia, and the knee in extension, fractures are reduced to near anatomic alignment using longitudinal traction. This limits blood loss, reduces pain and decreases the risk of fat embolus. Hare, Buck and Thomas splints have been the mainstay of skin traction within the emergency department. However, the pneumatic Donway splint is becoming increasingly popular. It provides

smooth and gentle traction with minimal discomfort to the patient, and has the additional benefit of reducing blood loss by direct pressure and tamponade of haematoma formation. Traction is applied through a padded wrap around the foot and heel with cushioned countertraction in the groin. Limb rotation is controlled by multiple straps that encompass the thigh.

Traction cannot maintain a constant force of sufficient magnitude to maintain the length and alignment of adult femur fractures and is only an interim procedure prior to definitive management.

Fluid resuscitation

Haemorrhagic shock is a major complication with an average blood loss from a closed femoral fracture of 1200 mL. In addition to maintenance fluids, patients with suspected significant blood loss should be resuscitated with crystalloids, and all patients must be cross matched for blood, kept fasted and an indwelling catheter inserted to monitor fluid balance.

Orthopaedic management

Adults are best treated with immediate operative fixation, typically intramedullary nailing. Open fractures require immediate operative debridement followed by delayed intramedullary nailing with antibiotic coverage.

Classification

The description of a femoral shaft fracture is important but no universally accepted classification system exists. An adequate description of femoral shaft fractures provides the surgeon with an indication of potential blood loss and the urgency of definitive fixation. Femoral fractures are either open or closed and may be transverse, oblique, spiral or segmental. Their location is within the proximal third, midshaft or distal third of the femur. The degree of fracture comminution, soft tissue involvement

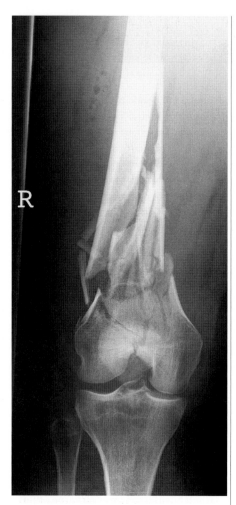

Fig. 3.8.1 Comminuted femur fracture.

and neurovascular status should also be described.

The majority of fractures occur in young adults with healthy bones and result in transverse fractures. Larger mechanical forces usually result in severe comminution (see Fig. 3.8.1). Minimal force with pathological bone tends to produce metaphyseal fractures with propagation into the shaft. Stress fractures of the femoral shaft are becoming increasingly common. They occur when repetitive mechanical stress is applied to the femur such as in marathon running or as a military recruit. They are associated with pain in the mid thigh and usually normal X-rays, although a bone scan will detect the fracture and low impact training such as cycling is used in rehabilitation. They are rarely displaced.

Complications

Complications include fat embolus syndrome, haemorrhagic shock and adult respiratory distress syndrome, with a higher incidence in comminuted fractures.

Long term complications of shortening, malalignment and non-union may eventuate in post-traumatic arthritis. Early mobilization following intramedullary nailing greatly reduces those complications associated with prolonged immobilization. Patients older than 60 years with closed fractures of femur have a mortality rate of 17% and a complication rate of 54%.

FURTHER READING

Provost R, Morris J 1969 Fatigue fracture of the femoral shaft. Journal of Bone and Joint Surgery 51A: 487–98

Russell RH 1987 Fracture of the femur. A clinical study (Abridged by Peltier LF). Clinical Orthopedics 224: 4–11

Taylor M, Banerjee B, Alpar E 1994 Injuries associated with a fractured shaft of the femur. Injury 25: 185–7

Vanganess C, DeCampos J, Merritt P, Wiss D 1993 Meniscal injury associated with femoral shaft fractures. An arthroscopic evaluation of incidence. Journal of Bone and Joint Surgery 75: 207–9

West H, Turkovich G, Donnell C, Luterman A 1989 Immediate prediction of blood requirements in trauma victims. Southern Medical Journal 82: 186–9

3.9 KNEE INJURIES

MICHAEL CADOGAN

ESSENTIALS

1 The knee bears the entire weight of the body, is essential to ambulation, and is the most commonly injured joint in the body.

2 Knee injuries often occur in the young and are usually associated with sport.

3 The history must always include the mechanism of injury and examination must include the hip and ankle joint.

4 Lateral tibial plateau fractures are associated with anterior cruciate and medial collateral ligament disruption whilst medial plateau fractures are associated with posterior cruciate and lateral collateral ligament disruption.

5 Anterior cruciate ligament disruption is associated with meniscal and collateral ligament injuries in 50% of cases.

6 Knee dislocations are orthopaedic emergencies that require emergent reduction and post reduction angiography.

ANATOMY

The knee is the largest and most complicated joint in the body. It is a synovial complex-hinge joint comprising of the patellofemoral and tibiofemoral joints. Movement ranges form 10° of extension to 140° of hyperflexion with up to 12° of rotation present through the full arc.

The ligaments of the knee may be classified as extracapsular or intracapsular.

The main extracapsular ligaments are the medial and lateral collaterals (MCL and LCL). The main intracapsular ligaments are extra-synovial and are the anterior and posterior cruciate ligaments (ACL and PCL). Collateral ligaments provide lateral stability and stability in extension, whilst the cruciate ligaments are essential to knee stability in flexion.

Muscular extensions enhance knee stability such as the vastus medialis in patella stability. The fibrous extension of vastus lateralis and medialis (the patellar retinaculum) strengthens the knee anteriorly and the iliotibial tract strengthens the knee in slight flexion.

CLINICAL ASSESSMENT

The history of the injury, degree of force, presence of immediate swelling and the ability to weight bear immediately post injury are important in diagnosing soft tissue injuries, which may involve valgus or varus stresses and may be due to direct or indirect trauma.

Physical examination

Both legs must always be examined with the patient undressed lying supine. Visual inspection may reveal bruising, swelling, erythema, deformity and associated wounds. Palpation detects warmth, swelling, crepitus, muscle mass and neurovascular status, and is started away from the point of trauma, then used to localize the areas of maximal tenderness to help define the underlying pathology. As well as the bony structures of the knee joint, it is important to assess the insertion points of the quadriceps tendon, patella tendon, collateral ligaments and the medial and lateral joint lines.

Swelling observed within the first few hours after trauma is usually associated with a vascular response to subchondral, bone or synovial injury causing a *haemarthrosis*. Swelling developing gradually over several hours to days is an *effusion* as a result of synovial reaction. Active and passive movements of the knee joint are assessed with the degree of flexion, extension, internal and external rotation noted. The ability to straight leg raise whilst supine is observed for potential damage to the extensor mechanism of the knee.

The basic knee examination is then completed with an assessment of the knees functional stability. Ligamentous laxity decreases with age and comparison with the opposite knee is more important than absolute laxity. The stability of the anterior and posterior cruciate ligaments may be crudely determined with the anterior and posterior drawer tests. The patient must be supine with the hip flexed at 45° and the knee flexed at 90°. The examiner sits on the patient's foot to stabilize the procedure and promotes firm forward movement of the tibia on the femoral condyles in the anterior drawer test and backwards in the posterior drawer test.

Posterior displacement of the tibia by more than 5 mm is indicative of PCL ruptures. The posterior drawer test remains the best test of PCL instability with a sensitivity of 85%. However, the accuracy of the anterior drawer test, as defined by subsequent arthroscopy, is only 56% for rupture of the ACL.

In the acute setting, Lachman's test is the most sensitive manoeuvre for testing ACL integrity especially in the presence of haemarthrosis. With the knee in 20–30° of flexion, the operator supports the distal femur with one hand and uses the other hand to draw the tibia forwards on the femoral condyles. Increased anterior displacement of the proximal tibia compared to the unaffected limb indicates a positive test.

The collateral ligaments are assessed with the application of varus and valgus stresses to the knee at zero and 30° of flexion. The degree of ligamentous laxity is determined by the amount of movement produced between the tibia and fibula in comparison to the normal side.

McMurray's test may demonstrate a meniscal injury. The patient lies supine and the knee is passively flexed and extended. One hand is placed over the knee to feel for crepitus whilst the other hand rotates the tibia on the femur. Internal rotation tests the lateral meniscus and external rotation assesses the medial meniscus. A positive test reveals pain and crepitus at the extremes of movement.

Apley's test involves the patient lying prone with the knee flexed to 90°. The tibia is rotated on the femur with downward pressure on the heel. Meniscal tears are associated with pain on downward pressure in the extremes of movement, relieved by release of pressure.

Radiology

Clinical decision rules to determine the requirement of knee radiography have been published, that aim to reduce emergency department radiographs, waiting times and costs. At present, with none having gained wide acceptance, all knee injuries associated with significant pain, haemarthrosis or joint line tenderness should be X-rayed.

Standard knee X-ray evaluation includes AP and lateral views. AP views assess integrity of the medial and lateral joint spaces and the femoral tibial angle. They also show the size, position and integrity of the patella. Lateral views may identify lipohaemarthrosis and various fractures. Oblique X-rays are particularly useful in elucidating tibial plateau fractures. The tunnel view enhances imaging of the intercondylar region. Skyline X-rays may be taken to further evaluate the patella and patellofemoral joint. They can identify undisplaced vertical fractures of the patella and subtle subluxation not seen on the conventional views.

Computerized tomography (CT) is a useful adjunct in defining certain fractures such as those of the tibial plateau, and magnetic resonance imaging (MRI) is reserved for evaluation of complex soft tissue knee injuries.

FRACTURES AROUND THE KNEE JOINT

Distal femur

Distal femoral fractures account for 4% of femoral fractures. They are usually associated with high-energy injuries secondary to a fall or a direct blow to the femur as in motor vehicle accidents.

Classification

Distal femur fractures may be divided anatomically into supracondylar, inter-condylar and isolated condylar fractures. Supracondylar fractures are extra-articular and occur immediately above the femoral condyles. Intercondylar fractures involve separation of the femoral condyles, although the fracture line may extend through the supracondylar region but in general they are treated as intra-articular fractures. Isolated condylar fractures are uncommon and occur when a varus or valgus force is applied to the weight-bearing, extended knee. The tibial eminence is thus driven into the femoral intercondylar notch creating an intra-articular fracture with severe ligamentous disruption.

Clinical assessment

Patients with injuries to the distal femur are in significant pain and are unable to weight bear. Examination may reveal swelling, deformity, rotation and short-ening. The joint is tender to palpate along the medial or lateral joint line and an acute haemarthrosis secondary to associated ligamentous injury or intra-articular involvement is common.

The whole lower limb must be examined to exclude ipsilateral hip dislocation, associated tibial fractures and quadriceps damage. Neurovascular deficit is assessed including sensation in the web space between first and second toe for deep peroneal nerve function.

Anteroposterior and lateral X-rays of the femur and knee will reveal the fracture and its degree of displacement or com-minution. A pelvis X-ray is necessary to exclude an associated proximal femur fracture or hip dislocation.

Management

Adequate analgesia is administered and a splint is applied in the emergency depart-ment to prevent excessive motion at the fracture site. Early orthopaedic con-sultation is required.

Cast immobilization is usually enough for undisplaced or impacted fractures without joint involvement. Those frac-tures with joint incongruity usually require open reduction and internal fixation. Distal femur fractures are a complex orthopaedic problem and long-term complications of malunion, quadriceps adhesion and osteoarthritis are common.

Tibial plateau

The tibial plateaus are the superior articulating surfaces of the medial and lateral condyles. Hyaline cartilage and a fibrocartilaginous meniscus cover them and their integrity is vital for knee alignment, articulation and stability.

Mechanism

Tibial plateau fractures account for 1% of all skeletal fractures and are commonest in the elderly. They occur when a valgus or varus deforming force is applied to the weight-bearing knee. Lateral tibial plateau fractures are twice as common as medial injuries and both plateaus are involved in 10–30% of cases. Anterior fractures occur when the knee is in extension and posterior fractures when the knee is flexed.

Classification

Fracture classification is complex due to the varying degrees of comminution, displacement and compression of the plateaus. The most widely used system was proposed by Schatzker, which divides the factures into six different types. Fracture types 1, 2 and 3 involve the lateral tibial plateau with increasing articular depression (see Fig. 3.9.1). Type 4 in-volves the medial plateau. Fracture types 5 and 6 involve both tibial plateaus and demonstrate increasing comminution and joint instability.

Tibial plateau avulsion fractures at the site of lateral capsular ligament insertion are called Segond fractures. They are asso-ciated with excessive internal rotation and varus stress to the flexed knee, and are usually associated with sporting injuries. Segond fractures are important markers of ACL disruption and rotatory instability.

Clinical assessment

Pain and haemarthrosis limit active and passive movements of the knee. Patients

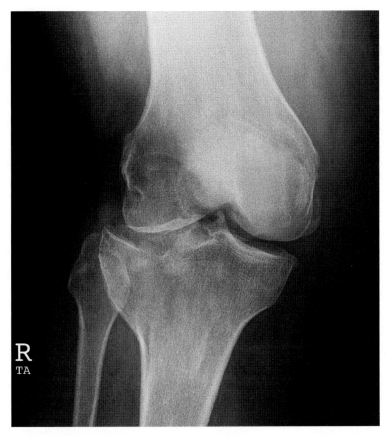

Fig. 3.9.1 Schatzker type 3 tibial plateau fracture.

are usually unable to weight-bear and present with a painful swollen knee. Focal tenderness may be palpated at the fracture site and over any associated collateral ligament tears. Distal circulatory compromise may be present secondary to the compression of the popliteal artery by comminuted subcondylar fragments.

Peroneal nerve neurapraxia and paralysis may complicate displaced lateral condylar fractures. Soft-tissue injuries are associated with up to 35% of injuries. In general, lateral plateau fractures are associated with ACL and MCL disruption whilst medial plateau fractures are associated with PCL and LCL disruption.

Radiology

Most plateau fractures are evident on standard knee X-rays, although oblique views may be required to elucidate subtle fractures and further classify obvious fractures. CT is used to further evaluate non-displaced and comminuted fractures, whereas MRI helps quantify the degree of associated ligamentous damage.

Management

Orthopaedic consultation is essential for further management. Many fractures may be treated conservatively with closed reduction and casting, however comminuted fractures with articular surface disruption require open reduction and internal fixation.

Common complications include undiagnosed neurovascular injuries, compartment syndrome and osteoarthritis.

Fractures of the tibial spine and intercondylar eminence

The tibial spine separates the medial and lateral tibial condyles and is divided into anterior and posterior areas by the intercondylar eminence. These areas provide flat surfaces for the attachment of the ACL and PCL respectively. The intercondylar eminence is divided into a medial and lateral tubercle visible on anteroposterior X-rays. Nothing is attached to these tubercles.

Mechanism

Most tibial spine and intercondylar eminence fractures occur in children, as the cruciate ligaments are stronger than the skeletal physeal plates. Considerable force is required for these fractures to occur in adults. In both cases the tibial spine is usually fractured during violent twisting knee movements with anterior tibial spine fractures occurring ten times more frequently than posterior. Intercondylar eminence fractures are associated with severe hyperextension or hyperflexion injuries.

Clinical assessment

The patient usually complains of severe pain, inability to weight-bear and immediate swelling of the knee. Examination confirms the presence of an acute haemarthrosis and limited knee movement. The knee is usually held in slight flexion and cannot be fully extended. An associated ACL disruption may be confirmed with a positive Lachman's or anterior drawer test.

Radiology

Tunnel or oblique views are used in addition to AP and lateral X-rays to confirm the diagnosis. MRI best demonstrates the associated ligamentous injuries.

Management

Most injuries are treated conservatively but displaced fractures with marked ligamentous injury require open reduction and internal fixation.

Patella fracture

The patella is the largest sesamoid bone in the body and lies within the quadriceps tendon. It provides protection to the femur and improves the stability and strength of the extensor mechanism.

Mechanism

Patella fractures account for 1% of skeletal injuries and occur predominantly in males between the ages of 20 and 50 years by direct or indirect trauma. Direct trauma to the anterior aspect of the patella results in incomplete, stellate, comminuted or vertical patella fractures, which commonly occur in motor vehicle accidents when the knee strikes the dashboard. There is usually little or no separation of the bony fragments as the medial and lateral quadriceps expansions remain intact.

Indirect trauma usually occurs when stumbling or falling forwards. The combination of powerful quadriceps contraction proximally and the strong distal patellar insertion overcomes the intrinsic strength of the patella and a transverse fracture ensues. Transverse fractures account for up to 80% of patellar fractures and mainly occur in the central and lower third of the patella. The extent of the fragment separation is dependent on the degree of quadriceps expansion tearing.

Clinical assessment

Physical examination reveals pain, swelling and bruising over the patella. The ability to walk and actively extend the knee is dependent on the type of fracture, and is important when considering surgical repair such as the ability to perform a straight leg raise whilst in a supine position, which confirms the integrity of the knees extensor mechanism. Patients with undisplaced fractures may be ambulatory and able to demonstrate active knee extension against gravity. Patients with displaced transverse patella fractures are unable to extend the knee actively.

Management

Non-displaced patella fractures with an intact extensor mechanism are treated conservatively with a long cast in full extension for 6 weeks. Fractures with fragment displacement of more than 3 mm are associated with disruption of the extensor mechanism. They require open reduction and internal fixation with tension band wiring.

DISLOCATION AROUND THE KNEE JOINT

Proximal tibiofibular joint dislocation

Mechanism

The proximal tibiofibular joint is supported by a capsule anteriorly, the popliteus muscle posteriorly and the LCL superiorly. Dislocation is rare and only possible when the LCL support is relaxed with the knee in flexion. Thus they occur mainly in violent athletic twisting injuries such as the shot put.

Clinical assessment

The patient is able to weight bear with difficulty, holds the knee flexed at 20–30° and has point tenderness over the fibula head. Common peroneal nerve neurapraxia is unusual.

Radiology

AP and lateral comparison views reveal the dislocation, which is usually anterolateral.

Management

Reduction requires adequate analgesia. Firm pressure is applied over the fibula head towards the centre of the knee. Reduction is associated with a satisfying click and surgical intervention is rarely required.

Patella dislocation

Traumatic patellar dislocation is common and may become recurrent with further patellar subluxation or dislocation. The majority of dislocations occur in the setting of patellofemoral dysplasia and malalignment syndromes secondary to hypoplastic vastus medialis, a shallow trochlear groove or genu valgum. Lateral dislocations are the most common and are usually caused by a direct blow to the anterior or medial surface of the patella. In all cases the medial retinaculum is disrupted either being stretched in subluxations or torn in dislocations.

Clinical assessment

Patients complain of the knee suddenly giving way accompanied by immediate pain and swelling. They are unable to weight bear or extend the knee. Palpation reveals an anterior defect, a laterally deviated patella, swelling and medial joint line tenderness.

Standard AP and lateral X-rays confirm the diagnosis, and are important to exclude an associated osteochondral fracture.

Management

Many dislocations spontaneously reduce or are reduced prior to arrival at the emergency department. Closed reduction is performed with analgesia or sedation. Anteromedial pressure is applied to the lateral aspect of the patella with gentle leg extension. Following post reduction X-rays, the knee should be immobilized in extension for 3–6 weeks to allow the medial retinaculum time to heal.

Complications

Recurrent dislocation occurs in 15% of cases and may necessitate surgical intervention. Up to 50% of patients following traumatic dislocation suffer symptoms of instability or anterior knee pain.

Dislocation of the knee

Knee dislocations are rare and usually occur in males in their third decade. They are orthopaedic emergencies associated with vascular damage that require urgent reduction.

Mechanism

Tibial femoral knee dislocation usually requires the rupture of both cruciate ligaments and one collateral ligament. Such injuries are, therefore, associated with high velocity accidents such as from a motorcycle. They are described with respect to the displacement of the tibia in relation to the femur. Anterior dislocations are the most common.

Evaluation

Initial examination usually reveals gross distortion of the knee with the clinical deformity being easily palpable. Knee dislocations are associated with a high rate of peroneal nerve and popliteal artery injury. A thorough neurovascular assessment is essential. Compression and distortion of the posteriorly placed popliteal artery and vein may cause distal vascular compromise, although 10% of vascular injuries are associated with normal pedal pulses. Peroneal nerve dysfunction is present in up to 50% of patients suffering knee dislocation.

Radiology

Radiological confirmation of the dislocation is ideal prior to reduction but must never delay this procedure.

Management

Early reduction under conscious sedation in the ED and prompt consultation with the orthopaedic and vascular teams is essential. If reduction is not performed within 6 hours, the risk of compartment syndrome and amputation is increased considerably. Failed reduction secondary to buttonholing of the femoral condyle is uncommon and requires open reduction in theatre. An angiogram is required following all reductions to assess the extent of any vascular injury.

SOFT TISSUE INJURIES

Collateral ligaments

Medial collateral ligament

The medial collateral ligament (MCL) complex comprises a long superficial ligament with a distal point of insertion and a short deep ligament attached to, and stabilizing, the medial meniscus. In conjunction with the capsule and semimembranosus, the MCL provides medial stabilization to the knee joint, resisting valgus laxity and medial rotational instability.

MCL injuries are the most common isolated knee ligament injury. They occur when an excessive valgus force is applied to the knee, usually by a direct blow to the lateral aspect. The magnitude of the valgus deforming force determines the risk of associated ACL disruption.

Lateral collateral ligament

The lateral collateral ligament (LCL) is the phylogenetically degenerate part of peroneus longus. It is a cord-like ligament running from the lateral epicondyle of the femur to the head of the fibula. It is separated from the lateral meniscus by the tendon of popliteus. The LCL is the major lateral stabilizer of the knee. It provides the main resistance to varus deforming forces, especially when the knee is extended.

LCL injuries are less common but more debilitating than MCL injuries. The lower incidence of LCL injuries is a result of the lateral ligament's mobility and the protective effect of the opposite leg. They result from a direct blow to the medial aspect of the knee. Associated injuries to the biceps femoris at its insertion and common peroneal nerve at the fibula head must also be excluded.

Clinical evaluation of the collateral ligaments

Medial and lateral ligament damage is usually a significant injury and often associated with sporting events. Examination for point tenderness at the site of injury, demonstrable laxity and haemarthrosis is essential. Stressing the affected ligament complex especially with partial tears can duplicate pain. Complete rupture of the ligament complex is associated with instability and stress testing causes the joint line to open up on the affected side.

The MCL is tested at 0 and 30° of flexion. Pressure is applied to the lateral joint line with one hand whilst the other hand creates a valgus stress by gently pushing the medial malleolus laterally. At 0° the medial complex is reinforced by the ACL, but at 30° the testing is specific for the MCL. Lateral instability is assessed when pressure is applied to the medial joint line with one hand and a varus stress administered with a hand moving the lateral malleolus medially.

Radiology Standard X-rays will only reveal collateral ligament injury if there has been a bony avulsion. Calcification at the origin of the MCL occurs in chronic injuries (Pellegrini-Stieda). MRI helps delineate the degree of ligamentous disruption and highlights associated injuries in complex cases.

Management All isolated collateral ligament injuries are treated conservatively providing damage to the ACL and PCL complexes has been excluded. Discomfort is reduced by knee immobilization in a splint such as a Richards splint, or elastic knee support, ice massage and anti-inflammatory drugs. Recovery is aided by quadriceps strengthening exercises and early return to movement using a hinged splint.

Cruciate ligaments

The cruciate ligaments are the primary stabilisers of the knee in flexion and extension.

Anterior cruciate ligament

The anterior cruciate ligament (ACL) extends from the medial aspect of the lateral femoral condyle to the anterior intercondylar area of the tibia. It prevents backward displacement of the femur on the tibial plateau and limits extension of the lateral condyle of the femur. It helps control the rotation of the knee in twisting and turning activities and is much more commonly injured than the PCL.

Mechanism The ACL is commonly injured during sporting activities such as skiing and rugby with patients readily able to define the causative mechanism. The injury may result from direct trauma as the tibia is forcefully displaced anteriorly on the femur or the femur posteriorly on the tibia. Indirect injury may occur when the flexed knee suffers a sudden twisting movement, with the foot firmly planted on the ground.

Clinical assessment ACL injuries are classically associated with sudden severe pain, an audible 'pop', an acute haemarthrosis and inability to weight-bear. Immediate significant swelling of the knee is indicative of the serious intra-articular pathology. The anterior drawer test or Lachman's test is used to clinically assess ACL integrity. ACL disruption is associated with meniscal and collateral ligament injuries in 50% of cases. The most common combination involves the triad of ACL and MCL disruption with a lateral meniscal tear.

Radiology X-rays may reveal avulsion of the anterior tibial spine although an MRI scan is the most accurate in determining ACL rupture with over 90% sensitivity and specificity.

ORTHOPAEDIC EMERGENCIES

3

Management Arthroscopy is still the gold standard in assessing the integrity of the ACL and has the advantage of allowing simultaneous debridement and repair. Arthroscopic repair or reconstruction is usually performed on young, active patients after 2–3 weeks to allow the initial swelling to subside.

Posterior cruciate ligament

The posterior cruciate ligament (PCL) extends from the lateral aspect of the medial femoral condyle to the posterior intercondylar area of the tibia. It prevents excessive forward displacement of the femur on the tibia and as the only stabilizing structure in the flexed, weight-bearing knee, is essential in providing mechanical support when walking downhill or down stairs.

Mechanism PCL disruption is normally caused by a posteriorly directed force on the proximal tibia such as with falls onto the tibial tubercle, knee dislocations and dashboard injuries and is less commonly associated with sporting injuries.

Clinical assessment Immediate pain and swelling are common with PCL rupture, which unlike with the ACL, are rarely associated with popping or tearing sensations and stability is usually enough to allow partial weight bearing. Associated MCL and ACL disruptions are common and must be actively sought. Isolated PCL ruptures may result in posterior 'sag' of the tibia in comparison with the unaffected limb. The posterior drawer test is performed to asses PCL integrity.

Radiology X-rays may reveal avulsion of the posterior tibial spine, but as with ACL injuries, MRI is over 90% specific and sensitive for PCL rupture. Arthroscopic PCL examination is less reliable.

Management The treatment of isolated PCL rupture is largely non-operative and focuses initially on pain management and non-weight bearing immobilization. When PCL injuries are combined with other ligamentous injuries, operative intervention within 2 weeks is more usual.

Patella tendon rupture

The patella tendon is the final connection of the extensor mechanism from the inferior pole of the patella to the tibial tuberosity. Rupture usually occurs under the age of 40 years often associated with a previous history of patella tendinitis or steroid injections. Injury is usually associated with stressful sporting activity and occurs with forceful quadriceps contraction. It is associated with significant pain.

Examination reveals a palpable defect, which may be masked by significant swelling. Comparison lateral X-ray views of both knees may reveal a high riding patella with an MRI differentiating partial and complete tears in complex cases. Partial tears may be treated non-operatively with cast immobilization in extension for 6 weeks. Complete tears of the patella tendon require surgical intervention.

Quadriceps tendon injury

The quadriceps tendon is a trilaminar junction of the quadriceps muscle. Rupture is commonest in older age groups with the decline in tendinous blood supply. Young persons usually suffer a muscular disruption. It occurs three times more commonly than patella tendon rupture and is usually by a direct blow to the knee or a hyperextension injury. It is associated with intense pain, and the patient is unable to walk without assistance.

Examination reveals a tender, palpable defect more apparent on attempted knee extension. Swelling secondary to a haemarthrosis and bruising are usually present.

Straight leg raise is impossible in a complete rupture whereas extension of the knee from a flexed position cannot be performed in a partial tear. Comparison lateral knee X-rays may demonstrate a low lying patella in the affected knee. MRI scans can distinguish between a partial and complete rupture.

Management

Partial tears can be treated non-operatively, but a complete rupture requires early surgical intervention for the best results.

Patella and quadriceps tendinitis (jumper's knee)

Both these extensor tendons are susceptible to tendinitis secondary to repetitive overloading. Patella tendinitis is commoner than quadriceps tendinitis. Patients present with anterior knee pain with point tenderness over the inferior or superior pole of the patella. It is common in athletes participating in running and jumping activities.

In patella tendinitis, inflammation at the insertion point of the patella tendon into the patella is six times commoner than at the insertion to the tibial tuberosity. It may be associated radiologically with fragmentation of the inferior pole of the patella.

Initial treatment involves rest, ice and anti-inflammatory medication. Longer term recovery and prevention requires conditioning and training of the extensor musculature.

Meniscal injury

The menisci are semilunar fibrocartilaginous structures found on the medial and lateral sides of the superior aspect of the tibia. They enhance the fluidity of articulation between the femoral and tibial condyles and increase the stability of the tibiofemoral articulation. The medial meniscus is immobile, being firmly attached to the deep portion of the medial collateral ligament and joint capsule. The lateral meniscus has a uniform thickness and a larger tibial area than the medial. It has no attachment to the LCL and is more mobile than the medial meniscus, making it more prone to injury.

Mechanism

Meniscal injuries are uncommon in isolation and are usually associated with collateral or cruciate ligament injury, which should be sought when examining the acutely injured knee. The menisci are injured commonly by a single traumatic process. Chronic degenerative processes account for only a small percentage of injuries. An isolated meniscal injury should be suspected in the young athlete sustaining a violent twisting or rotational injury to the weight-bearing knee.

Clinical assessment

Following meniscal injury, the patient is able to partially weight bear and usually complains of medial or lateral joint line pain. Delayed swelling, intermittent locking and a sensation of the knee 'giving way' are also clues to meniscal damage.

Examination usually confirms the presence of an effusion and joint line tenderness, especially in the extremes of flexion and extension. McMurray's test may be positive, however it is not pathognomonic, and in the acute setting pain often prevents adequate hyper-flexion for the test to be accurate.

The 'locked' knee is usually held in 30° of flexion and examination reveals a springy block to extension with associated pain. Bucket-handle meniscal tears are classically associated with a true 'locked knee'. They are longitudinal tears, usually of the medial meniscus, and frequently associated with ACL disruption.

Radiology

Routine X-rays do not reveal direct evidence of meniscal damage. However, they should be obtained to exclude commonly associated bony injuries. An MRI may determine both meniscal and ligamentous injuries in complex cases.

Management

Arthroscopy is used in evaluation and treatment of meniscal injuries. It can reveal the extent of meniscal damage and determine whether resection of the torn cartilage or meniscectomy is required.

FURTHER READING

Bandyk DF 1995 Vascular injury associated with extremity trauma. Clinical Orthopedics 318: 117–24

Kendall NS, Hsu SY, Chan KM 1992 Fracture of the tibial spine in adults and children. Journal of Bone and Joint Surgery Br 74: 848

Kode L, et al 1994 Evaluation of tibial plateau fractures: Efficacy of MR imaging compared with CT. American Journal of Roentgenology 163: 141

CONTROVERSIES

❶ Further studies to evaluate a clinical decision tool for the use of radiographs in acute knee injuries are required.

❷ Current research is evaluating replacing cylindrical plaster cast treatment of patella fractures and some soft tissue injuries with Richards's splints and hinged supports.

Roberts DM, Stallard TC 2000 Emergency department evaluation and treatment of knee and leg injuries. Emergency Medical Clinics of North America 18: 67–84

Schatzker J 1987 Fractures of the tibial plateau. In: Schatzker J, Tile M (eds.) Rationale of operative fracture care. Springer, New York, p 279

Seaburg DC, et al 1999 Multicenter comparison of two clinical decisions rules for the use of radiography in acute, high-risk knee injuries. Annals of Emergency Medicine 32: 8–13

Wascher DC, et al 1997 Knee dislocation: initial assessment and implications for treatment. Journal of Orthopedic Trauma 11: 525–9

3.10 TIBIA AND FIBULA INJURIES

MICHAEL CADOGAN

ESSENTIALS

1 Tibial shaft fractures are the commonest long bone fracture.

2 The subcutaneous nature of the tibia leaves it vulnerable to open fractures.

3 Emergency department documentation of the lower legs neurovascular status is vital, as compartment syndrome is a real risk in tibial shaft fractures.

4 Proximal fibula fractures may be associated with common peroneal nerve injury.

5 Tibial tubercle injury ranges from apophysitis to acute fracture.

ANATOMY

The tibia is the weight-bearing structure of the lower leg. Proximally, the tibia articulates with the femoral condyles and distally it provides the bony extension to allow medial stability to the ankle joint. Its shaft is triangular in cross section and is subcutaneous anteromedially. The fibula head is proximal and connects to the shaft by the fibula neck. Distally it is palpable subcutaneously as the lateral malleolus. The tibia and fibula are connected by superior and inferior tibiofibular joints and a dense interosseus membrane. Distally the union is strengthened by the syndesmosis, which enhances the stability of the ankle mortice.

Compartments

The lower leg is divided by bone and fascia into four compartments. Each compartment contains a sensory nerve and muscles with specific functions. Increased pressure within a compartment may be readily evaluated clinically if the functional anatomy is understood.

The anterior compartment contains the tibialis anterior and the long toe extensor muscles that dorsiflex the ankle and foot. The deep peroneal nerve supplies these muscles and the first web space of the foot. The anterior tibial artery is constrained within the compartment up to the ankle, where it becomes the dorsalis pedis.

The lateral compartment contains peroneus longus and brevis that evert the foot, and the superficial peroneal nerve that supplies sensation to the dorsum of the foot. The superficial posterior compartment contains gastrocnemius, plantaris

Table 3.10.1 Compartments of the lower leg

Compartment	Muscles	Muscle action	Artery	Nerve
Anterior	Tibialis anterior Long toe extensors	Dorsiflex ankle and foot	Anterior tibial	Deep peroneal
Lateral	Peroneus longus Peroneus brevis	Evert foot		Superficial peroneal
Superficial posterior	Gastrocnemius Soleus Plantaris	Plantarflex ankle		Sural
Deep posterior	Tibialis posterior Long toe flexors	Plantarflex toes	Posterior tibial Peroneal	Tibial

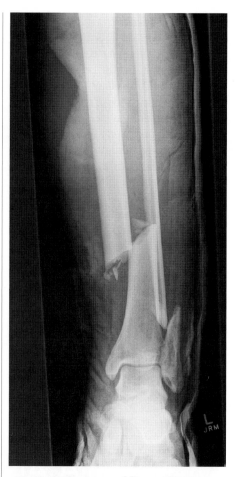

Fig. 3.10.1 Open, oblique, distal third tibia fracture with displaced varus deformation and fibula involvement.

and soleus muscles that plantarflex the ankle. The sural nerve lies in this compartment before piercing the fascia to supply the lateral side of the foot and distal calf.

The deep posterior compartment contains the tibialis posterior and long toe flexor muscles that plantarflex the toes. The tibial nerve is incorporated in the compartment and supplies sensory function to the sole of the foot. The posterior tibial and peroneal arteries also lie in this compartment (Table 3.10.1).

FRACTURES OF THE TIBIA AND FIBULA

Tibia

Tibial shaft fracture

Tibial shaft fractures are the commonest long bone fracture. They are also the commonest open fracture, due to the subcutaneous nature of the tibial shaft.

Mechanism A considerable amount of energy must be applied in a direct or indirect manner for the tibial shaft to fracture. Indirect torsional forces applied to the tibia produce spiral fractures as the body rotates about a fixed foot. Such injuries are common in skiing accidents and have increasing degrees of comminution dependent on the amount of energy applied.

Direct injuries may occur secondary to bending forces or a direct blow. Direct violence in motor vehicle and pedestrian accidents causes deformation at the site

of contact resulting in transverse or comminuted fractures. High-energy injuries have an increased degree of displacement, comminution, soft tissue injury and fibula involvement. They are associated with marked vascular, interosseus and bony involvement and are unstable, with a high risk of compartment syndrome.

Clinical assessment Pain is usually severe at the site of the fracture. The patient is unable to weight bear and inspection reveals swelling and deformity of the leg. The skin must be checked for its integrity and to identify areas of pressure caused by displaced fragments. The neurovascular status of the lower leg and foot must also be assessed as a matter of urgency. Skin colour, capillary refill and the distal dorsalis pedis and posterior tibial pulses are assessed.

Although direct nerve trauma is rare in closed tibial shaft fractures, contusion of the peroneal nerve may occur in high energy injuries with proximal fibula fractures. The motor function of the deep peroneal nerve is tested with active ankle and toe dorsiflexion. Active foot eversion assesses the motor component of the superficial peroneal nerve. The sensory function of the deep peroneal nerve is tested in the first dorsal web space. The superficial peroneal nerve supplies sensory function to the dorsal lateral aspect of the foot.

Associated injuries of the ipsilateral femur, hip, knee, foot and pelvis must be excluded.

Radiology AP and lateral views of the lower leg should include the entire tibia and fibula from the knee to the ankle. These views are designed to document tibial shaft fractures, the fracture pattern, degree of comminution and displacement and to identify associated fibula fractures (see Fig. 3.10.1).

Classification The description of the fracture must be clear and concise in relation to the following:

❶ Skin integrity: open or closed
❷ Anatomical site: proximal, middle or distal third.
❸ Fracture type: transverse, oblique, spiral or comminuted.
❹ Angulation of the distal fragment in relation to the proximal fragment

expressed in degrees and direction (anterior, posterior, varus or valgus).

❺ Degree of displacement and rotation.

❻ Involvement of the fibula.

Management Open wounds must be assessed for depth and associated soft-tissue damage, then dressed to avoid further contamination. Tetanus status is checked and empiric antibiotics administered such as intravenous cephalexin 1 g.

Emergency department documentation of the lower legs neurovascular status is vital, as compartment syndrome is a real risk in tibial shaft fractures. This baseline evaluation may be compared with any deterioration in function that may occur later with increasing compartmental pressures.

Pain is managed with intravenous opiates and the lower leg is immobilized as early as possible in a cast or splint. Reduction of displaced, rotated and angulated fractures may be performed within the emergency department under appropriate conscious sedation.

Reduction aims to arrest local swelling, release the tension of skin tented over a displaced fracture and reduce associated soft-tissue damage.

Following reduction, a posterior long leg cast, with 20° of knee flexion is applied and post reduction films taken to confirm the position. Circumferential casts should *never* be applied in the acute setting because of the inherent risk of compartment syndrome.

Fibula fractures

Proximal fibula fractures may occur in isolation or in association with tibial and ankle injuries.

Associated tibial shaft fracture

Most fibula fractures are associated with fractures of the tibial shaft and are managed in the same manner as for tibial fractures. The pattern of the associated fibular fracture indicates the degree of energy imparted. Severe comminution of the fibula or tibia-fibula diastasis implies disruption of the interosseus membrane and indicates an unstable fracture. The fibula usually heals well, whatever treat-

ment is selected for the tibia, and with a better rate of union. Complications of fibula fractures associated with tibial shaft fractures are rare.

Isolated proximal fibula fractures

Isolated proximal fibula and fibula shaft fractures are less common. They are usually associated with a direct blow to the lateral aspect of the leg with typical symptoms of local tenderness, swelling, bruising, and difficulty walking. A neurovascular assessment is important, as the common peroneal nerve wraps around the proximal neck of the fibula and may be contused or disrupted in these isolated injuries. Rarely, thrombosis of the anterior tibial artery may occur.

Full length AP and lateral X-rays of the tibia and fibula, including the ankle and knee joints will confirm the fracture pattern.

Non-displaced fractures may be associated with little pain and are treated with ice, compression bandage, analgesia and non-weight-bearing crutches for 3 weeks. Weight bearing is advanced progressively as tolerated. Mildly displaced fractures or those with significant pain may require a long leg cast for up to 6 weeks. Severely displaced fractures, or those associated with peroneal nerve deficit such as foot drop, require orthopaedic consultation and consideration for fixation.

Maisonneuve fractures

A proximal fibula fracture with an associated medial malleolus or distal tibial fracture is termed a Maisonneuve fracture. These fractures occur when an external rotatory force is applied to the ankle resulting in partial or complete syndesmotic disruption and are unstable. Palpation of the proximal fibula following ankle injuries is thus essential to assess for this fracture. All such fractures must be referred to the orthopaedic team for operative fixation.

Tibial tubercle fracture

The tibial tubercle lies proximally on the anterior border of the shaft of the tibia.

It is readily palpable beneath the infrapatellar bursa, and receives the insertion

of the patella tendon. Fractures of the tubercle are uncommon and usually occur in adolescents typically from indirect injury. Avulsion fractures of the tubercle are usually the result of violent flexion of the knee against tightly contracted quadriceps muscle.

Watson-Jones described three grades of injury. In type I injuries the tubercle is hinged upwards without displacement. Type II injuries involve avulsion of a small portion of the tubercle proximally. Type III injuries are intra-articular. The fragment is displaced and may be comminuted.

Examination reveals pain and tenderness over the anterior aspect of the knee and proximal tibia. There may be a haemarthrosis and loss of active extension depending on the severity of the injury.

Plain X-rays confirm the diagnosis. The lateral tibial view reveals the avulsion fragment, its degree of displacement and comminution.

Management is dependent on the degree of displacement and the presence of joint involvement. Type I and II injuries are treated with cylindrical long leg casts until healed. Type III injuries require open reduction and internal fixation with tension band wiring and fixation screw.

The differential diagnosis of Osgood-Schlatter disease should be considered. This condition is an apophysitis of the tibial tubercle caused by repeated micro-trauma to the growing tubercle during adolescence. It is chronic and associated with repetitive activity. Unlike tubercle fractures, it is never accompanied by a haemarthrosis and, active knee extension though painful, is possible. Treatment is conservative with rest, ice and compression. A return to full mobilization requires rehabilitation and strengthening of the quadriceps complex.

> ## CONTROVERSIES
>
> **❶** The use of compartment pressure monitors is becoming more widespread and their placement should be considered an emergency department procedure.

FURTHER READING

Balmat P, Vichard P, Pem R 1990 The treatment of avulsion fractures of the tibial tuberosity in adolescent athletes. Sports Medicine 9: 311

McQueen MM, Christie J, Court-Brown CM 1990 Compartment pressures after intramedullary nailing of the tibia. Journal of Bone and Joint Surgery 72B: 395–7

Nicoll EA 1964 Fractures of the tibial shaft: A survey of 705 cases. Journal of Bone and Joint Surgery 46B: 373–87

3.11 ANKLE JOINT INJURIES

MICHAEL CADOGAN

ESSENTIALS

1 Ankle injuries are a common emergency department presentation. They occur as isolated injuries or as adjunctive findings in high-energy multi-trauma.

2 In adults with isolated acute ankle injuries, the requirement for imaging of the ankle or foot may be determined using the Ottawa Ankle Rules (OAR).

3 The Henderson classification is the simplest system for describing ankle fractures.

4 Lateral malleolar fractures are the commonest ankle fracture.

5 The Simmonds's test can confirm the diagnosis of squeeze tendon rupture.

ANATOMY

The ankle joint is a complex hinge joint providing a stable but mobile support for the weight of the body that permits articulation between the tibia, fibula and talus. It helps to absorb the forces of ambulation, maintain an upright posture and allow accommodation for uneven terrain.

The stability of the ankle joint arises from a combination of the bony architecture, joint capsule and the ligaments. The bones and ligaments, which provide the stability, are best visualized as a ring structure centring on the talus. This ring of stability is made up of the tibial plafond, medial malleolus (MM), deltoid ligaments, calcaneus, lateral collateral ligaments, lateral malleolus (LM) and syndesmotic ligaments. When more than one element of this structure is disrupted, the joint becomes unstable.

The distal fibula (LM), distal tibia (MM) and distal tibial plafond form the mortice of the joint. This constrains the wedge-shaped talus distally, providing intrinsic bony stability. Most injuries to the ankle joint are as a result of abnormal movement of the talus within the mortice. This movement causes stress to the encompassing ring of structures of the ankle joint. Instability arises when disruption of malleoli or their associated ligaments results in distraction of the talus within the mortice.

CLINICAL ASSESSMENT

History

Inability to weight bear and the presence of swelling immediately following an injury implies significant pathological disruption. Further essential information includes the circumstances surrounding the injury, the position of the foot at the time of the injury and the magnitude and direction of loading forces applied, particularly rotational.

Examination

The patient should be given appropriate analgesia and the affected limb is iced and elevated. It is important to note that examination of the ankle includes the entire lower leg, and commences with a comparison between the injured and non-injured limb. In particular, the integrity of the skin and the presence of bruising, swelling or deformity should be noted. The range of active and passive movement at the ankle joint is then assessed including inversion, eversion, plantar and dorsiflexion. If there is a significant difference between the active and passive ranges of movement a soft tissue injury is likely.

Palpation for point tenderness may localize ligament, bone or tendon injury and should commence at a site away from the area of obvious injury. The entire length of the tibia and fibula, as well as the base of the fifth metatarsal, calcaneus and Achilles tendon must be examined. Palpation of the posterior aspects of the malleoli should commence 6–10 cm proximally and include both ends of the collateral ligament attachments. The anterior plafond and the medial and lateral aspects of the talar dome are then palpated in plantar flexion.

The foot should always be checked for motor or sensory impairment, capillary return, the presence of dorsalis pedis and posterior tibial pulses and injury to the base of the fifth metatarsal.

In the acutely injured ankle, stress tests for ligamentous stability, and an evaluation of weight-bearing ability should only proceed if clinical suspicion of a fracture is low.

Radiology

The standard radiographic evaluation of the acutely injured ankle includes anteroposterior, lateral and mortice views. In adults with isolated acute ankle injuries, the requirement for imaging of the ankle or foot may be determined using the Ottawa Ankle Rules (OAR). These have determined that an ankle X-ray series is only required if there is any pain in the malleolar region and:

❶ bone tenderness over the posterior aspect of the distal 6 cm of the lateral malleolus
 or
❷ bone tenderness over the posterior aspect of the distal 6 cm of the medial malleolus
 or
❸ inability to bear weight for at least 4 steps both immediately after the injury and at the time of evaluation.

A foot X-ray is required if there is pain in the mid-foot region and:

❶ bone tenderness at the navicular
 or
❷ bone tenderness at the base of the fifth metatarsal
 or
❸ inability to bear weight for at least 4 steps both immediately after the injury and at the time of evaluation in ED.

The OAR only apply to patients over the age of 18 years and have a sensitivity of over 98% for detecting clinically significant malleolar zone ankle fractures. In addition, they only apply to acute ankle injuries in a competent historian.

Further imaging

Stress X-rays are used to confirm suspected ligamentous instability compared to the opposite ankle. Computerized tomography (CT) may be used to further evaluate complex fractures and ligamentous injuries. Bone scans may delineate osteochondral and stress fractures. Some highlight ligamentous disruption but are usually used in subacute conditions.

FRACTURE CLASSIFICATION

Multiple classification systems are used to describe ankle fractures and dislocations.

These allow appreciation of the ankle's stability following an injury, and may indicate the need for orthopaedic intervention.

Lauge-Hansen

The Lauge-Hansen classification is based on experimental, clinical and radiographic observations. In this system, the position of the foot at the time of the injury is described first and the direction of the deforming force second. It is useful as it characterizes the mechanism and sequence of injury and emphasizes the associated ligamentous injuries.

Danis-Weber

The Danis-Weber classification system divides ankle fractures into three types based on the level at which the fibula fractures. The more proximal the fibula fracture, the greater the associated syndesmosis disruption and potential for ankle instability:

Type A fractures involve the distal fibula below the level of the tibial plafond and occur in supination-adduction injuries.
Type B fractures involve an oblique or spiral fracture at the level of the syndesmosis and are associated with supination-eversion injuries.
Type C fractures occur with pronation-abduction injuries when the fibula is fractured above the level of the syndesmosis. These injuries are universally associated with syndesmosis disruption, making the ankle unstable.

AO system

The AO classification system adds three subdivisions to each Danis-Weber fracture type to enhance the description of associated medial injuries and further defines potential ankle stability.

Henderson system

The Henderson classification is a simple system based on radiographic findings.

❶ Unimalleolar fractures include lateral malleolar fractures where the stability is dependant on the level of fracture in relation to syndesmosis (Danis-Weber). Medial malleolar fractures associated with external rotation. Posterior malleolar fractures are rare and associated with posterior tibiofibular, medial and

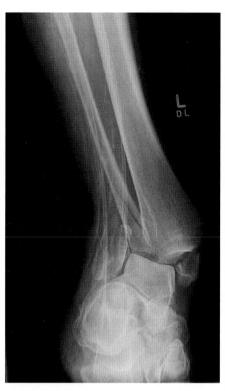

Fig. 3.11.1 Unstable bimalleolar ankle fracture.

lateral ligament disruption. Finally, the anterior malleolar fracture is uncommon and often results from vertical loading and is associated with calcaneal fractures.
❷ Bimalleolar fractures involve disruption of at least two elements of the ankle ring and are unstable. They are usually associated with abduction injuries.
❸ Trimalleolar fractures involve medial, lateral and posterior fractures, are unstable and require ORIF.

INCIDENCE

Ankle fractures are commonest in males under 50 years and in females over 50 years. The commonest fracture is that of the lateral malleolus (15%).

Management

Minimally displaced avulsion fractures of the distal fibula less than 3 mm in diameter, which are not associated with medial ligament disruption are treated as sprains.

Extra-articular or non-displaced fractures with an intact mortice joint on X-ray may be treated non-operatively in a below knee cast, with the ankle at 90°, to maintain the correct anatomical position of the talus. They should be referred for follow-up in the orthopaedic fracture clinic in the event operative intervention is required.

Displaced and potentially unstable fractures require immediate orthopaedic consultation, including all bimalleolar and trimalleolar fractures and those unimalleolar fractures with contralateral ligamentous injuries.

Complications

Early operative complications include osteomyelitis, pin-site infection and skin necrosis. Late complications include non-union, chronic instability, traumatic arthritis and reflex sympathetic dystrophy.

PILON FRACTURES

These fractures involve the distal tibial metaphysis and result from high-energy injuries directed through the talus into the distal tibia with tibial plafond disruption. Their frequency has increased with the greater numbers of motor vehicle accidents and falls from heights. They are rarely isolated and are usually associated with multiple other injuries. They are also often open, comminuted and associated with massive soft tissue deformity.

The fracture is reduced and splinted under sedation to lessen the potential for massive soft tissue swelling and conversion of a closed fracture to an open one from overlying skin necrosis. Treatment usually then requires open reduction and internal fixation, or external fixation with gross soft tissue changes.

DISLOCATIONS

Ankle dislocations are frequently associated with a fracture, but do occur in isolation. They require considerable force and may be open or closed occurring when an external force is directed against the plantar flexed foot, squeezing the talus out of the mortice. The direction of the initial loading force determines the final position of the dislocation. Posterior dislocations are the most common.

Closed dislocations are associated with marked soft-tissue disruption and skin tethering, although neurovascular compromise is uncommon. They should be reduced promptly with gentle manipulation under sedation in the emergency department to minimize any associated soft-tissue injury. Despite the potential for ligamentous disruption, they usually have an excellent outcome following immobilization for 8 weeks.

Open dislocations are often associated with disruption of the dorsalis pedis and posterior tibial vessels. They require surgical debridement in theatre, but again should initially be reduced and splinted in the emergency department. Open injuries are associated with more long-term complications than closed, in particular traumatic arthritis and reduced mobility.

SOFT TISSUE INJURIES

Ligamentous injuries

Ankle sprains are one of the commonest presentations to the emergency department.

Most of the sprains involve the lateral ligament complex. Medial ligament disruption is more frequently associated with lateral malleolar fractures or Maisonneuve type injuries involving the proximal fibula and syndesmosis disruption.

Lateral ligamentous injuries are graded according to severity and are then treated as either stable or unstable:

Grade I   Microscopic tearing within the ligament substance. Patients are able to weight bear, with minimal swelling and normal stress testing.

Grade II   Partial tear of the ligament. Patients have difficulty weight bearing, significant localized swelling and moderate joint instability.

Grade III   Complete ligament rupture. Patients are unable to weight bear, there is gross swelling, bruising and joint instability.

All Grade I, and some Grade II injuries are stable. These patients are able to weight bear and have normal ankle stress testing. They are treated conservatively with rest, ice, compression bandage, elevation and non steroidal anti-inflammatory drugs for 24 hours. Physiotherapy to promote early mobilization results in a quicker return to normal activities.

Patients with unstable and potentially unstable sprains include all Grade III and some Grade II injuries. These patients are unable to weight bear and have demonstrable joint instability or are unable to have stress testing performed as a result of the pain and swelling. Operative intervention is controversial, although direct repair is usual for athletes. Conservative treatment involving cast immobilization for 6–8 weeks with orthopaedic follow-up is appropriate in the others.

Delayed surgical repair or reconstruction has similar results to early intervention.

Achilles tendon injuries

Achilles tendon rupture is associated with sedentary middle-aged individuals during a burst of unaccustomed strenuous physical activity. Predisposing medical conditions include rheumatoid arthritis, SLE, chronic renal failure, gout, hyperparathyroidism and long-term steroid use.

Rupture usually occurs whilst pushing off with the weight-bearing foot, but may occur with sudden dorsiflexion or direct trauma. An audible 'pop' and the sensation of a direct blow to the back of the ankle are followed by difficulty in walking. The segment of the Achilles tendon particularly prone to rupture lies 2–6 cm proximal to the tendon's insertion into the calcaneus. The blood vessels that supply this area are prone to atrophy and the resultant reduction in collagen cross-linking leads to a reduced tendon tensile strength.

Examination may reveal a visible and palpable deficit in the tendon, but swelling around the tendon sheath may rapidly mask these signs. The calf-squeeze test or Simmonds's test confirms the diagnosis. This is best performed with the patient kneeling on a chair with the feet hanging free over the edge. Initially, the unaffected calf is gently squeezed just distal to its maximal girth and normal plantar flexion demonstrated. Absence of plantar flexion in the affected limb confirms Achilles rupture.

The choice of operative or non-operative treatment is controversial. Non-operative management includes applying a cast to the ankle placed in the equinus position to bring the two ends of the ruptured tendon into apposition. One regimen involves a cast for 4 weeks in equinus, 4 weeks in partial plantar flexion and then 2 weeks in the neutral position. Complications of non-operative management include a higher re-rupture rate requiring surgical intervention.

Operative risks include fistula formation, skin necrosis, and infection. However, the procedure has a lower rate of

CONTROVERSIES

❶ Physiotherapy and early mobilization are considered the treatment of choice for low grade sprains but lengthy periods of immobilization and crutches are still employed.

❷ Operative intervention for grade III sprained ankles is currently reserved for elite athletes but should the enhanced stability and early return to mobilization be offered to all patients?

❸ Operative versus conservative management of Achilles tendon ruptures remains contentious.

muscle atrophy, lower re-rupture rate and allows an earlier resumption of physical activity.

FURTHER READING

Brennan MJ 1990 Tibial pilon fractures. In: Greene WB (ed.) Instructional course lectures, vol 39. American Academy of Orthopaedic Surgeons

Cetti R, et al 1993 Operative versus non-operative treatment of Achilles tendon rupture: a prospective randomized study and review of the literature. American Journal of Sports Medicine 21: 791

Karlsson J, Eriksson BI, Sward L 1996 Early functional treatment for acute ligament injuries of the ankle joint. Scandinavian Journal of Medicine & Science in Sports 6: 341

Muller ME, Nazarian S, Koch P 1988 The AO Classification of Fractures. New York, Springer-Verlag

Oloff-Solomon J, Solomon MA 1988 Computed tomographic scanning of the foot and ankle. Clinics in Podiatric Medicine & Surgery 5: 931

Plint AC et al 1999 Validation of the Ottawa ankle rules in children with ankle injuries. Academic Emergency Medicine 6: 1005

Wedmore IS, Charette J 2000 Emergency department evaluation and treatment of ankle and foot injuries. Emergency Medical Clinics of North America 18: 85

3.12 FOOT INJURIES

MICHAEL CADOGAN

ESSENTIALS

1 Standard radiological imaging includes AP, lateral and 45° internal oblique projections.

2 Major talar fractures have a significant risk of subsequent avascular necrosis.

3 The majority of calcaneal fractures are intra-articular and associated with a Boehler's angle of less than 20°.

4 Navicular body fractures may require internal fixation.

5 Fractures of the base of the second metatarsal are pathognomic of Lisfranc injury (Fleck sign).

ANATOMY

The foot is composed of 28 bones and 57 articulating surfaces. It can be divided into three anatomical regions including the hindfoot containing the talus and calcaneum; the midfoot containing the navicular, cuboid and cuneiforms and the forefoot containing the metatarsals and phalanges.

The subtalar joint collectively describes the three articulations of the inferior aspect of the talus with the calcaneus and allows inversion and eversion of the hindfoot. The midtarsal joints incorporate the talonavicular and calcaneocuboid joints. They join the hindfoot and midfoot and allow abduction and adduction of the forefoot. The five tarsometatarsal joints (Lisfranc joints) join the midfoot and forefoot. They form an arch, which lends stability to the foot.

CLINICAL ASSESSMENT

History

Injury to the foot occurs due to direct or indirect trauma. Indirect trauma from a twisting injury usually results in minor avulsion-type injuries. Direct trauma is often associated with considerable soft tissue swelling and fractures. A record of any pain, swelling, loss of function, decreased sensation and deformity or associated ankle injuries is made.

Examination

Inspection commences with the patient lying on a bed with both lower limbs exposed. Comparison with the unaffected limb helps identify bruising, swelling, deformity, skin wounds, pallor or cyanosis. Gentle and careful palpation over the entire foot commences at a site away form the area of maximal pain. This may elicit point tenderness or crepitus at the site of fracture. Specific sites, which must be palpated, include the Achilles tendon, calcaneus, base of the fifth metatarsal and the area under the head of the second metatarsal.

The patient is then asked to demonstrate active foot movements before the examiner performs gentle passive movements of the foot. Comparison is made with the other foot. Subtalar motion is evaluated with the foot in a neutral position, with one hand on the lower leg and the other holding the heel. The heel is inverted and everted and should attain 25° of motion. Midtarsal motion is assessed with one hand stabilizing the heel whilst the other hand grasps the forefoot at the bases of the metatarsals. The forefoot is pronated, supinated, adducted and abducted. Finally forefoot motion is evaluated by individually flexing and extending the metatarsophalangeal (MTP) and interphalangeal (IP) joints.

If no obvious focus of the pain is found during the initial examination, the patient is asked to stand and walk to assess gait and the ability to weight bear. The circulation of the foot is then assessed by observing capillary refill, skin colour and the presence of dorsalis pedis and the posterior tibial pulses. The posterior tibial pulse is palpable behind the medial malleolus unless there is excessive swelling or damage to the artery. The dorsalis pedis is more variable, being too small or absent in 12% of the population. Doppler may be used to determine the presence of flow if there is doubt.

Neurological assessment includes motor and sensory function.

Radiology

Standard radiological imaging includes AP, lateral and 45° internal oblique projections. The lateral view visualises the hindfoot and soft tissues, whilst oblique and AP projections provide the best imaging of the midfoot and forefoot. An axial calcaneal view is best to visualize the hindfoot if there is pain around the heel or there is a history of a fall from a height.

Bone scans are indicated when a stress fracture is suspected and may be positive 2–3 weeks before conventional radiographs demonstrate a fracture. Computerized tomography (CT) is an excellent modality for imaging the calcaneum, subtalar joint and Lisfranc joint complex in more difficult injuries.

FOOT FRACTURES

Hindfoot

Talar fractures

The talus is one of the most vital bones in the foot. It provides support for the body when standing and bears more weight per surface area than any others. It has no muscular attachments and is held in place by the malleoli and ligaments. It is composed of a head, neck and body. The head has articulations with the navicular and calcaneus, whilst the body articulates with the tibia, fibula and calcaneus. The neck joins the head and body and is extra-articular. The blood supply to the talus arises from an anastomotic ring involving the peroneal, posterior and anterior tibial arteries and is tenuous and easily disrupted leading to avascular necrosis.

Mechanism and classification Talar fractures are the second commonest tarsal fracture. They are either major or minor. Minor fractures are caused by inversion injuries to the plantar or dorsiflexed foot often from minimal trauma and may present as an apparent ankle sprain.

Major talar fractures require significant force such as motor vehicle accidents or involve axial loading in a fall from a height when they are associated with calcaneal fractures. Talar neck fractures account for 50% of major talar injuries and are associated with extreme dorsiflexion injuries. Hawkins' classification of talar fractures is commonly used. Type 1 fractures are undisplaced; type 2 fractures have associated subtalar subluxation and type 3 fractures involve dislocation of the talar body and are usually open. Commonly associated injuries include vertebral compression, calcaneal and medial malleolar fractures.

Talar head fractures are uncommon and result from a compressive force applied to the plantar-flexed foot. They are associated with disruption of the talonavicular joint, navicular fractures and anterior malleolar fractures. Talar body fractures are usually of the minor avulsion type.

Clinical evaluation Minor talar fractures are usually subtle. The patient presents following an inversion injury with mild swelling around the ankle joint and are able to partially weight bear. Active plantar and dorsiflexion are possible but inversion and eversion at the subtalar joint is painful. Major talar fractures are associated with large compressive forces and cause considerable swelling and tenderness dorsally.

Radiology Standard X-rays of the foot will reveal all but the most subtle avulsion fractures, which may require stress views of the ankle mortice or CT for further evaluation.

Management Major talar fractures have a significant risk of subsequent avascular necrosis. Displaced fractures, especially if associated with neurovascular or cutaneous compromise, should be reduced in the emergency department. Closed reduction is performed under conscious sedation by grasping the hindfoot and midfoot and applying longitudinal traction in plantarflexion. A posterior slab is applied with the ankle at 90°. Emergency closed reduction is used to improve fracture alignment and to reduce the risk of vascular compromise. Most fractures require orthopaedic referral for consideration of open reduction and internal fixation. Minor talar fractures are treated with a below knee, non-weight-bearing posterior cast with orthopaedic follow-up.

Subtalar dislocation

Subtalar dislocations are rare and are associated with considerable deforming forces. Such injuries involve the simultaneous dislocation of the talonavicular and talocalcaneal joints with preservation of the tibiotalar joint.

Mechanism and classification Subtalar dislocations are often associated with motor vehicle accidents, but a significant number are incurred during sport, particularly basketball. They are described in terms of the final position of the foot in relation to the talus following dislocation. Medial dislocations account for 85% of these injuries and are caused by forceful foot inversion in plantarflexion. Ten per cent of subtalar dislocations are open and 50% are associated with proximally located injuries.

Clinical assessment Subtalar dislocations are associated with obvious deformity, swelling and tension of the skin over the opposing joint margin. Neurovascular status must be examined but is rarely compromised. Standard X-rays are difficult to interpret due to the distortion of the foot. The most helpful is the AP view, which confirms disruption of the talonavicular joint.

Management All closed subtalar dislocations should be reduced in the emergency department under conscious sedation to minimize the chance of the skin tented over the head of the talus becoming necrotic. Closed reduction of a medial subtalar dislocation requires firm longitudinal traction applied to the foot with countertraction on the leg. The assistant providing countertraction must flex the knee to relax the tension of the Achilles tendon on the calcaneum increasing the mobility of the hindfoot. The foot is initially inverted to accentuate the deformity, and then everted with digital pressure over the head of the talus to reverse the deformity. Eighty per cent of dislocations may be reduced nonoperatively. Following reduction, the ankle is placed in a posterior slab at 90°. Orthopaedic consultation is required.

Calcaneal fractures

The calcaneus is the largest bone of the foot and is the most commonly fractured tarsal bone. The calcaneus forms the heel of the foot and provides vertical support for the body weight and functions as a springboard for locomotion.

Mechanism Fractures of the calcaneus occur with direct axial compression during falls from a height and 7% are bilateral. Lower extremity injuries are present in 25% of cases and vertebral compression fractures are found in 10%.

Classification Twenty five per cent of calcaneal fractures are extra-articular and 75% intra-articular. Fractures may be non-displaced, displaced or frequently comminuted due to the cancellous nature of the calcaneal bone, and the magnitude of force associated with these fractures (see Fig. 3.12.1).

Clinical assessment Patients usually present following a fall, involving direct trauma to the heel. The patient may be able to walk, but weight bearing on the heel is usually impossible. Examination reveals pain, swelling and tenderness over the heel with bruising that may extend over the sole of the foot. Associated fractures are common and examination of the vertebral column, affected lower extremity and opposing calcaneus is important.

Radiology Standard X-rays are usually sufficient to reveal most comminuted calcaneal fractures.

The AP view highlights the anterosuperior calcaneus and calcaneocuboid joint. The lateral view may reveal compression fractures of the body and posterior facet. Boehler's angle normally ranges from 20 to 40° measured on the lateral X-ray. If the angle is less than 20°, a compression fracture is likely. An additional Harris or axial view demonstrates the more subtle fractures seen poorly on a lateral view. CT scan is important in defining complex fractures and is useful in pre-operative planning.

Management Intra-articular, displaced and comminuted fractures are prone to gross swelling of the foot and have an increased incidence of compartment syndrome. They should be referred to the orthopaedic team for consideration of admission for operative intervention. They have a poor long-term prognosis with up to 50% suffering chronic pain

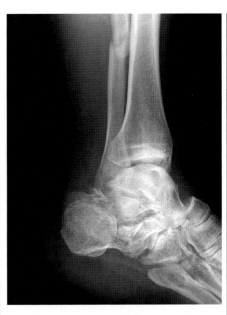

Fig. 3.12.1 Intra-articular comminuted calcaneal fracture.

and functional disability. Extra-articular fractures are usually undisplaced and are treated conservatively in a posterior non-weight bearing cast for 6 weeks. Displaced fractures require orthopaedic consultation and CT analysis.

Midfoot

The midfoot comprises the navicular, cuboid and cuneiform bones. It is an inherently stable portion of the foot and is rarely injured. However, midfoot fractures are often associated with a delay in diagnosis due to the difficulty in X-ray interpretation and poorly localized pain.

Navicular fractures

The navicular is a curved bone with extensive articulations. It has a tenuous blood supply and like the talus is susceptible to avascular necrosis.

Mechanism and classification The navicular is the most commonly injured of the midfoot bones, although the overall incidence is rare. Fractures may involve the dorsal surface, tuberosity or the body. Dorsal avulsion fractures are commonest. They occur in eversion injuries and are associated with deltoid ligament or talonavicular capsular injury. Tuberosity fractures also result from eversion injuries with avulsion of the posterior tibial tendon insertion. Body fractures from axial loading are rare and are frequently comminuted.

Clinical evaluation Point tenderness may be elicited over the dorsum and medial aspect of the midfoot. Passive eversion and active inversion reproduce the pain. Standard X-rays usually reveal the fracture, but bone or CT scans may be required.

Management All intra-articular, displaced and comminuted fractures require orthopaedic review in the emergency department. These are frequently complicated by subsequent avascular necrosis. Dorsal avulsion and tuberosity fractures are treated conservatively in a walking cast for 6 weeks. Navicular body fractures may require internal fixation.

Cuboid fractures

Isolated cuboid fractures are rare. They are most commonly associated with Lisfranc-type injuries with lateral subluxation of the midtarsal joint, the 'nutcracker' fracture, and fractures of the posterior malleolus. They are best visualized with an oblique foot X-ray.

Management Treatment ranges from weight bearing casts for undisplaced fractures to operative fixation for displaced and comminuted fractures. All cuboid fractures require orthopaedic consultation.

Cuneiform fractures

These fractures are extremely rare. They usually occur with direct trauma and an associated Lisfranc injury should be excluded. Displaced fractures require orthopaedic intervention whilst non-displaced fractures are treated conservatively in a cast.

Lisfranc fractures and dislocations

The Lisfranc joint involves the articulation of the first three metatarsal bases with their respective cuneiforms, and the fourth and fifth metatarsal bases with the cuboid. The second metatarsal is the most important structure within this complex holding the key to its stability.

Mechanism and classification Injury results from rotational forces applied to the fixed forefoot, axial loads and crush injuries. Although commonly associated with vehicular accidents, Lisfranc injuries may also occur in sports that involve fixation of the forefoot, such as horse-riding and rowing. They are classified by the direction of dislocation in the horizontal plane. Divergent dislocations usually involve medial and lateral splaying of the first and second metatarsals. In homolateral injuries all five metatarsals are displaced in the same direction, either medially or laterally. In isolated dislocations, one or more of the metatarsals are displaced away from the others.

Lisfranc dislocations are usually associated with fractures of the metatarsals, especially the second metatarsal base, and with fractures of the midfoot in 40% of cases. Although vascular compromise is uncommon, significant haemorrhage may occur with disruption of the dorsalis pedis branch to the plantar arch as it passes between the first and second metatarsal bases.

Clinical assessment Lisfranc injuries should be suspected when mid-foot fractures are present. They are associated with severe midfoot pain and an inability to bear weight on the toes. Examination may reveal deformity, swelling and bruising over the dorsum of the foot. Point tenderness over the joint, with pain on passive abduction and pronation may also be present.

Radiology Standard X-rays are sufficient to visualize most Lisfranc injuries. AP views identify Lisfranc fractures and oblique views determine their alignment. Lateral views demonstrate the soft tissues and identify the presence of dorsal or plantar displacement. Fractures of the base of the second metatarsal are pathognomic of Lisfranc injury (Fleck sign). Stress radiographs may be helpful if spontaneous reduction of the dislocation has occurred.

Management All Lisfranc injuries require orthopaedic consultation. Most are treated with closed reduction and K-wire

fixation followed by non-weight bearing for 12 weeks. Despite aggressive management chronic pain, reflex sympathetic dystrophy and degenerative arthritis are common complications.

Forefoot

Metatarsal fractures

Metatarsal fractures account for 35% of foot fractures.

Metatarsal shaft fractures

Metatarsal shaft fractures occur as a result of direct trauma or a rotational injury to the fixed forefoot. They are associated with difficulty in weight bearing and ill-defined tenderness and bruising over the plantar aspect of the foot. The third metatarsal is most commonly affected. They are also commonly associated with Lisfranc injuries and phalangeal fractures. Standard X-ray views will detect nearly all these fractures and determine their alignment, angulation and displacement.

Management Undisplaced shaft fractures of the second to fifth metatarsals are treated in a below knee walking cast for 3–4 weeks. If these fractures have more than 3 mm of displacement or 10° of angulation they require closed reduction and application of a non-weight-bearing cast for 6 weeks. The great toe metatarsal requires more aggressive treatment due its load-bearing function. Non-displaced fractures require 4–6 weeks in a non-weight-bearing cast, whereas displaced fractures require operative treatment. Orthopaedic consultation is therefore required for multiple or displaced fractures and all fractures of the great toe metatarsal.

Metatarsal head and neck fractures

These fractures are usually the result of direct trauma and are often multiple. Non-displaced fractures are treated with a walking cast for 4–6 weeks, and displaced fractures require closed reduction to maintain the transverse arch integrity.

Base of fifth metatarsal fractures

These are the most common of the metatarsal fractures. Two distinct types exist. The most common fracture is that of the fifth metatarsal tuberosity, which occurs when the plantarflexed foot undergoes sudden inversion. It is caused by avulsion of the lateral band of the plantar aponeurosis and is usually extra-articular. The second type of fracture is known as the Jones fracture, and is defined as a transverse fracture through the base of the fifth metatarsal from 15 to 31 mm distal to the proximal end of the bone. This fracture is intra-articular as it involves the intermetatarsal articulation of the fourth and fifth metatarsals. Jones fractures occur when a load is applied to the lateral aspect of the foot without inversion. Activities such as jumping and dancing are typically associated with such injuries, which may also occur as 'stress-type' injuries from repetitive strains.

In both types of fracture the patient has difficulty weight bearing and there is point tenderness over the fifth metatarsal tuberosity and passive inversion is painful. Extra-articular tuberosity fractures heal well regardless of size or degree of displacement. They are treated symptomatically in either a walking cast for 3 weeks or a compression bandage. Intra-articular fractures, which involve more than 30% of the articular surface or with more than 2 mm of displacement may require surgical fixation. Non-displaced fractures are treated in non-weight bearing cast for 6 weeks.

Metatarsophalangeal dislocations

MTP dislocations are uncommon. The fifth MTP joint is most commonly dislocated laterally when the little toe is caught on an object. First or hallux MTP joint dislocations are usually dorsal and follow violent hyperextension injuries. They are usually obvious with the metatarsal head palpable on the plantar surface. Other dislocations are usually more subtle.

Management Most MTP joint dislocations are easily reduced with longitudinal traction under local anaesthesia. Post-reduction they are managed in a buddy strap. First MTP joint dislocations are more difficult to reduce and may require open reduction. They should be treated in a walking cast with a toe-plate extension for 3 weeks.

Phalangeal fractures and dislocations

Phalangeal fractures are common and usually occur with direct trauma most often involving the proximal phalange. They are associated with pain, deformity and difficulty walking.

Management Non-displaced fractures heal well and are 'buddy strapped' to reduce pain and prevent displacement. Gauze should be placed between the splinted toes to prevent skin maceration. Pain may be expected for up to 3 weeks until stabilized by callus.

Displaced fractures are reduced with traction under digital nerve anaesthesia. Operative fixation may be indicated if the fracture is unstable, especially if the fracture is intra-articular or involves the hallux.

Interphalangeal dislocations are uncommon and usually involve the hallux.

They are reduced with longitudinal traction under digital nerve anaesthesia. Those, which involve the great toe, require a toe plated walking cast for 3 weeks post reduction. All other interphalangeal dislocations are treated with a buddy strap once reduced.

CONTROVERSIES

❶ Optimal use of nurse-initiated X-ray in lower limb injuries.

❷ Imaging of osteochondral talar dome fractures.

❸ Role of the bone scan, CT and MRI in other limb injuries.

FURTHER READING

Chen MY, Bohrer SP, Kelley TF 1991 Boehler's angle: a reappraisal. Annals of Emergency Medicine 20: 122

Heckman JD 1991 Fractures and dislocations of the foot. In: Rockwood CA, Green DP, Bucholz RW (eds) Rockwood and Green's Fractures in Adults, 3rd edn. JB Lippincott, Philadelphia

Lawrence SJ, Botte MJ 1993 Jones' fractures and related fractures of the proximal fifth metatarsal. Foot and Ankle International 14: 358

Merchan EC 1992 Subtalar dislocations: Long-term follow-up of 39 cases. Injury 23 :97–100

Vuori J, Aro HT 1993 Lisfranc joint injuries: Trauma mechanisms and associated injuries. Journal of Trauma 35: 40

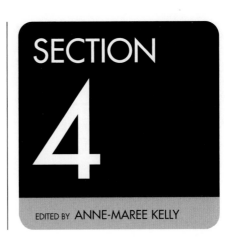

CARDIOVASCULAR

4.1 Chest pain 178

4.2 Ischaemic heart disease: acute coronary syndromes 182

4.3 Assessment and management of acute pulmonary oedema 193

4.4 Arrhythmias 197

4.5 Pulmonary embolism 210

4.6 Pericarditis, cardiac tamponade and myocarditis 215

4.7 Heart valve emergencies 223

4.8 Peripheral vascular disease 231

4.9 Hypertension 237

4.10 Aortic dissection 242

4.11 Aneurysms 248

4.1 CHEST PAIN

MICHAEL BRYANT

ESSENTIALS

1 In the absence of a clear alternative diagnosis an acute coronary syndrome cannot be excluded on initial testing in the emergency department.

2 Exclusion of acute myocardial infarction (AMI) requires at least 12 hours.

3 Troponin I detects a subset of unstable angina patients likely to have further episodes of angina or an AMI, but requires at least 12 hours of testing to do so.

4 Normal troponin levels do not guarantee the absence of complications including death.

5 Acute coronary syndromes such as unstable angina require further investigation, including provocative testing, for diagnosis.

INTRODUCTION

Correctly diagnosing patients with the symptom of chest pain is a major challenge. Missing the diagnoses of acute myocardial infarction (AMI) or ischaemia may have serious consequences for the patient.

CLINICAL FEATURES

History

The importance of obtaining a detailed history cannot be overemphasized. Examination findings and investigation results may not enable one to make a firm diagnosis: the management of the patient then depends upon the clinical impression of the aetiology of the pain. Unless a clear alternative diagnosis is present, an acute coronary syndrome cannot be excluded. Where pain is clearly pleuritic or musculoskeletal in nature an acute coronary syndrome can usually be excluded. The parietal pleura is richly innervated by somatic afferents via the intercostal nerves. Inflammation causes localized pain, which is referred to the shoulder or neck via the phrenic nerve (C3–C5) if the central diaphragm is involved, or the epigastric area if the peripheral diaphragm is involved. The visceral pleura is innervated by visceral afferents and does not cause readily localized pain when inflamed.

Cardiac pain is visceral - classically crushing and dull in nature, although patients with myocardial ischaemia sometimes describe burning or sharp pains. Care must be exercised, particularly in patients of non-English-speaking background, as some patients may use the adjective 'sharp' to describe the severity of the pain rather than its nature. Also some patients with asthma may complain of chest tightness. Gastrointestinal pathology may be indicated by a relationship to meals. The presence of pain radiation to the neck, jaw and arms is associated with cardiac ischaemic pain as are the associated symptoms of breathlessness, nausea, vomiting and diaphoresis.

Details of past medical history and medication usage are essential. For example, erythromycin may be the cause of epigastric/chest pain. Although a family history of coronary artery disease and a personal history of hypertension, diabetes, cigarette smoking and hypercholesterolaemia are predictive epidemiologically in assessing an individual's lifetime risk of coronary-artery disease, they are of no predictive help in the instance of an acute presentation.[3]

Examination

Patients with cardiac pain are often quiet rather than restless. They may have sweating, pallor, and can look extremely unwell. Clinical examination findings are often lacking. Examination contributes to diagnosis by identification of alternative pathologies. A blood-pressure differential between arms may be indicative of aortic dissection, but also sometimes occurs as a result of atherosclerosis involving the great vessels. The presence of chest-wall tenderness may indicate a local musculoskeletal cause. A pericardial rub may be present, indicating pericarditis.

In a quarter of patients with anterior AMI an abnormal systolic pulsation develops in the periapical area in the first days, and then may resolve. It sometimes occurs in patients experiencing angina. A third heart sound (S3) may be heard. This low-pitched ventricular sound occurs at the termination of rapid filling. It is frequent in children, and also in adults with high cardiac output. In patients aged over 40 years, it is indicative of ventricular decompensation. An audible fourth heart sound (S4) is common in patients in sinus rhythm with an AMI. It is associated with effective atrial contraction and its presence indicates decreased ventricular compliance. A transient apical systolic murmur due to mitral regurgitation can occur secondary to papillary muscle dysfunction during AMI. It may be mid or late systolic in timing. Pericardial friction rubs are heard in many patients with transmural AMI at some time during their course.

Abdominal examination may reveal right-upper-quadrant tenderness consistent with biliary disease, or left hypochondrial tenderness with pancreatitis. Epigastric tenderness may indicate peptic ulcer disease. However, it is dangerous to assume that these findings exclude cardiac pain, particularly if the pain is not exactly reproduced.

Examination of the lower limbs may reveal the presence of deep venous thrombosis and make the diagnosis of pulmonary embolism more likely.

Response to therapeutic challenge

The 'gastrointestinal cocktail', consisting of mylanta with or without lidocaine, is not a good diagnostic test, as it has been demonstrated to be almost as effective an analgesic for myocardial ischaemia as for gastrointestinal pain.[4]

It is also important to remember that, although anginine (GTN) is effective when used for angina, it may also reduce oesophageal spasm and diminish chest-wall pain. It too, is not reliable as a 'diagnostic test'.

INVESTIGATIONS

ECG

This is the quickest and most useful test, but it cannot be used as a single definitive test to 'rule out MI' as it may initially be normal, with changes evolving over time. Patients with ongoing pain or hyper-acute changes should have repeat ECGs performed at 15–30 minutely intervals. The initial ECG can be used to stratify the risk of adverse events occurring and enables one to decide where patients should be admitted – to the CCU, tele-metry, or a general ward. Patients with normal ECGs and a suspicion of acute coronary ischaemia or unstable angina are at low risk unless pain recurs, and may go to an unmonitored bed. Should pain recur the patient should be trans-ferred to the CCU. Clear AMIs should be monitored closely in the CCU, and those with abnormal but non-diagnostic ECGs should be on telemetry as a minimum.

Chest X-ray

The chest X-ray is often unhelpful but may exclude alternative diagnoses, such as hiatus hernia, aortic dissection, pneumonia or malignancy. Complica-tions such as congestive cardiac failure (CCF) may be detected.

Laboratory

Cardiac markers require serial measure-ment over 12–24 hours to exclude AMI. They cannot be used to diagnose unstable angina. There are a variety of different tests, including CK, CKMB, CKMB subforms, troponin T and tropo-nin I.[5] The recommended laboratory investigation for the detection of myo-cardial injury is now troponin.[6] Elevated troponin levels are predictive of further episodes of angina or AMI in patients with unstable angina. Elevations of troponin are thought to indicate the presence of a microinfarct. Repeat test-ing for troponin T or I is required for 12 hours for 95% sensitivity for AMI. The role of troponins appears to be to stratify the risk of complications of cardiac ischae-mia, rather than to accurately diagnose AMI (see Chapter 4.2). Recent research has shown that elevations of troponin during sequential testing over 24 hours are predictive of complications. The con-verse is not true – a negative troponin does not rule out the development of complications, including death.[7,8,9]

Myoglobin is also used occasionally, although its exact role is uncertain. It has a high sensitivity at a very early stage, but a low specificity. Liver function tests and amylase may be useful in some patients in whom it is difficult to discern whether the pain is in the lower chest or the epigastrium.

Arterial blood gases (ABGs) may be helpful in the diagnosis of pulmonary embolism if hypoxia or an increased A-a gradient is present. A normal ABG result cannot be used to exclude the diagnosis of pulmonary embolism.

Full blood examination may indicate a leucocytosis suggestive of infection. The presence of anaemia may indicate the presence of peptic ulcer disease, but may also be responsible for myocardial ischaemia.

Other

V/Q scans are helpful in confirming the diagnosis of pulmonary embolism, but are less reliable in the presence of pre-existing lung disease.[10] Delays in the performance of V/Q scan produce less definitive results because of the break-up of the embolus into smaller fragments and the opening of collateral channels. Helical CT is increasingly being used in some centres to diagnose pulmonary emboli. (see Chapter 4.5).

Thallium scans reflect regional coronary blood flow. Uptake in patients with acute pain is proportional to myocardial blood flow. Images at 2–24 hours reflect the presence of viable or non-viable myocardium. Reversible defects indicate unstable angina. This test may be logistically difficult. Images must be obtained shortly after injection, when the patient may not be stable enough for transfer.

Technetium-99m (^{99m}Tc) sestamibi scans can be used to detect areas of recently ischaemic myocardium up to 8 hours later (if tracer is injected at the time of pain). Technetium is taken up by myocardial cells in proportion to blood flow and cellular metabolism. Saturation of the myocardium occurs within 50 minutes, and little change in distribution occurs for 4 hours afterwards. The test has a sensitivity of 96–100% and a specificity of 88–100% for the detection of AMI. In the absence of previous AMI it shows promise in the early detection of AMI. Resting sestamibi scans are not a reliable test for angina or ischaemia.[11]

Echocardiography can be used to demonstrate acute wall motion abnormalities in patients with AMI or myocardial ischaemia. It shows decreased myocardial wall motion in areas with occluded arteries, but is highly operator dependent. It is most useful in those with no prior cardiac history. It cannot detect unstable angina. Transoesophageal echocardiography is better than transthoracic for detection of aortic dissection, pulmonary embolism and pericarditis.

Exercise testing may be performed after AMI has been excluded. The testing interval from when the patient is pain free is controversial, and varies from 1 to 24 hours.

Dobutamine stress nuclear myocardial perfusion imaging is a technique available for those patients with limited exercise capacity.

DIFFERENTIAL DIAGNOSES

Cardiovascular

- Myocardial infarction
- Unstable angina
- Pericarditis
- Pulmonary embolism
- Aortic dissection
- Aortic stenosis
- Hypertrophic obstructive cardiomyopathy
- Pulmonary hypertension
- Right ventricular strain.

Gastrointestinal

- Peptic ulcer disease
- Oesophageal reflux and spasm
- Biliary disease
- Pancreatitis.

Musculoskeletal

- Arthritis of shoulder or spine
- Costochondritis
- Radicular pain from cervical or thoracic roots.

Respiratory

- Pneumonia
- Pneumothorax
- Pleurisy
- Tumour.

Other

- Breast disorders
- Chest wall tumours
- Herpes zoster.

SPECIFIC DISEASES

Breast

Important causes of mastalgia are inflammatory breast disease, benign and malignant tumours, mastitis and breast abscess. Local breast abnormalities are usually found.

Costochondritis

This is a condition that is most frequently found in women over the age of 40. It most commonly affects the third, fourth or fifth ribs.[12]

In contrast, Tietze syndrome is commoner in those under 40 years of age and affects both sexes equally. It manifests as a painful swelling of one joint.

Herpes zoster

Pain precedes the development of an eruption by 48–72 hours. A vesicular eruption occurs along a dermatome, most commonly the dermatomes between T3 and L3. Up to 4 weeks may be required before the skin returns to its normal appearance. The incidence of herpes zoster infection increases with age. It is treated with aciclovir 800 mg five times per day for 7 days.

Mediastinal emphysema

Pneumomediastinum may occur spontaneously or secondary to blunt or penetrating trauma. It occurs primarily in young adults and is caused by yelling, shouting or active exercise, vigorous vomiting and asthma. It has been reported after pulmonary barotrauma from scuba diving, smoking crack cocaine and the use of ecstasy, with puncture wounds and lacerations of the hypopharynx, dental procedures, airway instrumentation and colonoscopy.[13-20]

Retrosternal pain and dyspnoea are the most common symptoms. On examination subcutaneous emphysema may be found. Auscultation may reveal Hamman's crunch sign.

The diagnosis is made on chest X-ray and is often best seen on the lateral view.

Symptomatic treatment and reassurance are all that is required. Rarely air from a pneumomediastinum may rupture into the pleural space, resulting in a pneumothorax, or extend up into the neck and on to the chest. Haemodynamic compromise and cardiovascular collapse have been reported, but are rare.

Musculoskeletal

A clear history of exertion or injury, with appropriately tender muscle on examination, is quite straightforward. However, patients with reproducible chest-wall pain on palpation can have an AMI. It may be that rubbing on the chest after the onset of pain creates a tender area that can be found on palpation.

Oesophageal reflux and spasm

Diffuse oesophageal spasm is a motor disorder of the oesophageal smooth muscle characterized by multiple spontaneous contractions and by swallowing-induced contractions of simultaneous onset.[21] Cholinergic stimulation, distension, acid reflux and hyperventilation may provoke it. Patients with symptomatic oesophageal spasm present with chest pain, dysphagia or both. The pain is retrosternal and may radiate to the back, the sides of the chest, both arms and the jaw. It lasts for seconds or minutes and may mimic the pain of myocardial ischaemia. The presence of odynophagia may be a clue that the oesophagus is the site of disease. The diagnosis of oesophageal spasm is confirmed by oesophageal manometry.

Smooth muscle relaxants, such as sublingual GTN, isosorbide dinitrate or nifedipine, are helpful in some cases.

Pleurisy

Pleurisy implies pleural inflammation without effusion. The aetiology is often viral, although pulmonary embolism needs to be excluded. Bornholm disease (epidemic myalgia) is usually due to a Coxsackie B virus (sometimes A) and echo virus. It most frequently affects children and young adults. In this condition fever, sore throat and myalgias follow a 3–5-day incubation period. Table 4.1.1 lists the differential diagnoses.

Rib fractures

Clinical features are local tenderness, bony crepitus, pain at the fracture site on springing, and rarely ecchymosis. In elderly patients with osteoporosis, rib fractures may occur with minimal trauma. A chest X-ray is indicated to detect complications, particularly pneumothorax, and also to detect the presence of suspected pathological fractures.

MANAGEMENT

All patients should receive supplemental oxygen and have IV access created. Ideally, the ECG should be obtained

Table 4.1.1 Pleurisy: differential diagnoses

Underlying pulmonary disease	No apparent underlying pulmonary disease
Pneumonia	Infection – viral, Bornholm disease
Bronchiectasis	Connective tissue disease (SLE, RA)
Tuberculosis	Pulmonary embolism
Pulmonary infarction	Asbestosis exposure
Neoplasm	Chest-wall pain Familial Mediterranean fever Uraemia Sickle cell crisis Dressler syndrome

while the history and examination are being performed. Aspirin should be given to all those in whom a diagnosis of myocardial ischaemia is considered, and the patient made painfree with titrated doses of IV narcotics.

Management thereafter depends on the provisional diagnosis. Detailed management of myocardial ischaemia and AMI is given in Chapter 4.2.

Large numbers of patients attend emergency departments with chest pain. In response, several centres have developed models for the rapid rule-out of myocardial ischaemia. Some of these models are housed in units known as chest pain centres or chest pain emergency departments. In those patients where the likelihood of ischaemic heart disease is low, the patient is kept in the chest pain emergency department until the diagnosis has been either confirmed or excluded using a testing protocol. Algorithms such as the Goldman algorithm[22] for MI are used in some centres to define this low-risk group. Patients in this group undergo testing over a variable time period, generally 9–12 hours to exclude AMI, usually using cardiac markers. Once AMI is excluded they have a provocative test such as an exercise test. If the test is positive they are admitted for further investigation. If the test is negative they are discharged for further follow-up. Numerous centres have shown this approach to be safe.[23, 24,25]

Patients with unstable angina and AMI are admitted at the time the diagnosis is made.

DISPOSITION

The aim should be to make a positive diagnosis of patients with chest pain and treat accordingly. If this cannot be done the patient should be admitted for observation, as acute myocardial infarction cannot be excluded for 12–24 hours. Unstable angina cannot be excluded until further tests, such as an exercise test, have been performed.

CONTROVERSIES

❶ The Braunwald subclassification of unstable angina patients may identify a group who can be discharged with early follow-up.

❷ Sestamibi scans do not detect all patients with unstable angina.

❸ Troponin levels are more specific than CKMB, but still require repeated measurements over at least 12 hours.

❹ The sensitivity of troponin for complications is low and normal levels cannot be relied upon to guarantee safety.

❺ The development of chest pain centres has followed the identification of a clinical pathway that encourages the early identification of patients with acute coronary syndromes. The best interval to exclude AMI prior to exercise testing is yet to be determined.

REFERENCES

1. Braunwald E 1989 Unstable angina. A classification. Circulation 80: 410–14
2. van Milztenburg-van Zijl AJM, Simoons ML, Veerhoek RJ, Bossuyt PMM 1995 Incidence and follow-up of Braunwald subgroups in unstable angina pectoris. Journal of the American College of Cardiologists 25: 1286–92
3. Green LA, Yates FJ 1995 Influence of pseudodiagnostic information on the evaluation of ischemic heart disease. Annals of Emergency Medicine 25: 451–7
4. Wrenn K, Slovis CM, Gongaware J 1995 Using the "GI cocktail": a descriptive study. Annals of Emergency Medicine 26: 687
5. Sarko J, Pollack CV Jr 1997 Beyond the twelve-lead electrocardiogram: diagnostic tests in the evaluation of suspected acute myocardial infarction in the emergency department. Journal of Emergency Medicine 15: 839–47
6. Jaffe AS, The World Health Organization, The European Society of Cardiology, The American College of Cardiology 2001 New standard for the diagnosis of acute myocardial infarction. Cardiology in Review 9(6): 318–22
7. Polanczyk CA, Lee TH, Cook F, et al 1998 Cardiac troponin I as a predictor of major cardiac events in emergency department patients with acute chest pain. Journal of the American College of Cardiology 32: 8–14
8. Kontos MC, Anderson FP, Alimard R, Ornato JP, Tatum JL, Jesse RL 2000 Ability of troponin I to predict cardiac events in patients admitted from the emergency department. Journal of the American College of Cardiology. 36: 1818–23
9. Limkakeng A Jr, Gibler WB, Pollack C, et al 2001 Combination of Goldman risk and initial cardiac troponin I for emergency department chest pain patient risk stratification. Academic Emergency Medicine 8(7): 752–3
10. The PIOPED Investigators 1990 Value of the ventilation/perfusion scan in acute pulmonary embolism: results of the prospective investigation of pulmonary embolism diagnosis (PIOPED). Journal of the American Medical Association 263(20): 2753–9
11. Kontos MC, Jesse RL, Schmidt KL, Ornato JP, Tatum JL 1997 Value of acute rest sestamibi perfusion imating for evaluation of patients admitted to the emergency department with chest pain. Journal of the American College of Cardiologists 30: 976–82
12. Disla E, Rhim HR, Reddy A, Karten I, Taranta A 1994 Costochondritis: a prospective analysis in an emergency department setting. Archives of Internal Medicine 154: 2466–9
13. Rezvani K, Kurbaan AS, Brenton D 1996 Ecstasy induced pneumomediastinum. Thorax 51: 960–1
14. McHugh TP 1997 Pneumomediastinum following penetrating oral trauma. Paediatric Emergency Care 13: 211–3
15. Mirzayan R, Cepkinian V, Asensio JA 1996 Subcutaneous emphysema, pneumomediastinum, pneumothorax, pneumopericardium, and pneumoperitoneum after rectal trauma. Journal of Trauma 41: 1073–5
16. Mumford AD, Ashkan K, Elborn S 1996 Clinically significant pulmonary barotrauma after inflation of party balloons. British Medical Journal 313: 1619
17. Sullivan TP, Pierson DJ 1997 Pneumomediastinum after freebase cocaine use. American Journal of Roentgenology 168: 84
18. Tetzlaff K, Reuter M, Leplow B, Heller M, Bettinghausen E 1997 Risk factors for pulmonary barotrauma in divers. Chest 112: 654–9
19. Stack AM, Caputo GL 1996 Pneumomediastinum in childhood asthma. Paediatric Emergency Care 12: 98–101
20. Uva JL 1997 Spontaneous pneumothoraces, pneumomediastinum, and pneumoperitoneum:

consequences of smoking crack cocaine. Paediatric Emergency Care 13: 24–6
21. Cooke FA, Wang AA, Chambers JB, Owen M 1996 Hyperventilation and esophageal dysmotility in patients with noncardiac chest pain. American Journal of Gastroenterology 91: 480–4
22. Lee TH, Juarez G, Cook EF, Weisberg MC, Rouan GW, Brand DA, Goldman L 1991 Ruling out acute myocardial infarction: A prospective

multicenter validation of a 12-hour strategy for patients at low risk. New England Journal of Medicine 324: 1239–46
23. Lewis WR and Amsterdam EA 1994 Utility and safety of immediate exercise testing of low-risk patients admitted to the hospital for suspected acute myocardial infarction. American Journal of Cardiology 74: 987–90
24. Gibler WB, Runyon JP, Levy RC, et al 1995 A

rapid diagnostic and treatment center for patients with chest pain in the emergency department. Annals of Emergency Medicine 25: 1–8
25. Fiebach NH, Cook EF, Lee TH, Brand DA, Rouan GW, Weisberg M, Goldman L 1990 Outcomes in patients with myocardial infarction who are initially admitted to stepdown units: Data from the multicenter chest pain study. American Journal of Medicine 89: 15–20

4.2 ISCHAEMIC HEART DISEASE: ACUTE CORONARY SYNDROMES

CORINNE GINIFER

ESSENTIALS

1 Ischaemic heart disease (IHD) remains the major cause of death for men and women in the developed world.

2 Myocardial ischaemia results from an imbalance between myocardial oxygen supply and demand.

3 The initial electrocardiograph (ECG) in acute myocardial infarction (AMI) may be normal.

4 10–30% of patients with AMI will have an 'atypical presentation'.

5 Cardiac markers do not help initial decision making.

6 Early thrombolysis/reperfusion has become the standard of care for AMI.

7 Aspirin alone saves as many lives as thrombolysis alone; together they have an additive benefit.

8 Urgent angioplasty is the only intervention to demonstrate benefit for patients with cardiogenic shock following AMI.

9 Primary and secondary prevention strategies are at the forefront of modern management of IHD.

INTRODUCTION

Myocardial ischaemia results when coronary arterial flow is insufficient to meet myocardial oxygen needs. This deficiency is manifested clinically by anginal pain, cardiac failure and conduction disturbances.

EPIDEMIOLOGY

According to the World Health Report 1997, ischaemic heart disease is still the leading cause of global mortality. There were 7.2 million deaths worldwide in 1996 attributable to IHD compared to 6.3 million in 1990, despite advances in treatments and the implementation of earlier detection and prevention programmes.[1]

Patients who survive AMI face a significant increase in morbidity compared to the general population. Thirty per cent will subsequently develop non-trivial angina pectoris, whilst the annual re-infarction rate is 6%. In addition, they have a markedly increased risk of heart failure and sudden death.[2]

There has been a significant decline in mortality from IHD over the last 25 years. The reasons for this decline are multifactorial including primary prevention strategies directed at reduction in coronary risk factors through life-style change, improved prehospital and inpatient medical care and advances in surgical and angioplasty techniques. Reduced dietary fat intake, lowering of blood cholesterol levels, reduced cigarette smoking, increased exercise and better management of hypertension are the main primary prevention strategies, but these account only partly for the observed decline in mortality.

PATHOPHYSIOLOGY

Coronary blood flow is tightly coupled to variations in myocardial oxygen demand through autoregulation. Failure to ensure adequate oxygen delivery results in ischaemia.

Occlusion of coronary arteries by atherosclerosis is the primary cause of IHD. Haemorrhage and rupture of an atheromatous plaque with subsequent formation of intravascular thrombus results in artery-specific ischaemia. Increased vascular tone resulting in coronary artery spasm is believed to be responsible for a significant proportion of IHD. Such vasomotor changes may result in complete spastic occlusion, increasing the likelihood of subsequent thrombus formation. Other less common causes of occlusive vascular disease include coronary embolus, coronary arteritis and hypercoagulable states.

There is an increasing body of evidence to suggest that atherosclerosis is a

CARDIOVASCULAR

chronic inflammatory condition that develops in response to sustained insults such as hypercholesterolaemia, hypertension or cigarette smoking.[3,4] Autopsies of patients with unstable angina (UA) have revealed infiltration of the coronary arteries by inflammatory cells. In addition, recent research shows that inflammatory markers, such as C-reactive protein and serum amyloid A protein, are elevated in patients with unstable angina.[5,6] Local inflammation of coronary arteries may precipitate thrombus formation with subsequent occlusion. Such an underlying inflammatory process may explain the observed phenomenon in some studies of regression of coronary atherosclerosis following aggressive treatment with lipid lowering drugs. [7]

Myocardial ischaemia is accompanied by a variety of physiological changes. The increase in myocardial wall stiffness leads to a reduction in compliance, an increase in left ventricular end-diastolic pressure (LVEDP) and a reduction in ejection fraction and thus cardiac output. This leads to activation of neuroendocrine and baroreceptor reflexes. The resultant increases in afterload and heart rate only serve to increase myocardial oxygen demand at a time of failing supply.

The ischaemic process may be transient and reversible (angina), or prolonged, resulting in myocardial infarction with its attendant mechanical and electrical dysfunction.

RISK FACTORS

Years of research have identified and stratified a number of risk factors for the development of IHD. These include a family history of coronary artery disease, hypercholesterolaemia, hypertension, diabetes mellitus and cigarette smoking. In addition, other life style factors such as obesity and lack of exercise may play a contributory role. When assessing a patient with chest pain, the presence of risk factors places the patient in a higher risk group for IHD, but the absence of risk factors cannot be used to exclude the diagnosis of cardiac ischaemia. Previous

history of IHD obviates the need for risk factor assessment.

Clinical manifestations of IHD include:

- angina
- acute myocardial infarction
- dysrhythmias
- sudden cardiac death
- left ventricular failure and cardiogenic shock
- thromboembolism
- pericarditis
- syncope.

ANGINA SYNDROMES

Clinical features

The diagnosis of angina is made on history rather than by examination or special investigations. A description of 'typical' ischaemic chest pain (see Chapter 4.1 Chest Pain) that is related to exertion and promptly relieved by rest or nitrates is characteristic of stable angina.

Unstable angina

In a patient with a previously stable pattern of angina, an increase in frequency or intensity of angina, angina occurring in response to lesser degree of exertion or not promptly relieved by rest indicates that angina has become unstable. Unstable angina may be the first presentation of IHD.

Unstable angina may be due to a number of causes. Extra-cardiac factors include uncontrolled hypertension, tachycardia and anaemia. Local causes include intermittent coronary artery thrombosis, coronary artery spasm or an acute complication of an atheromatous plaque.

Variant angina (Prinzmetal)

Although most cases of angina occur in patients with structural heart disease, a significant proportion have no identifiable coronary atheroma on angiography or post-mortem examination. Spasm of coronary arteries has been demonstrated angiographically during episodes of chest pain in association with ST-segment depression. This phenomenon was first

described in 1959.[8] Since that time it has been increasingly recognized as a cause of ventricular dysrhythmia and sudden death.[9]

Silent ischaemia

Silent ischaemia appears to play a much greater role than previously realized. Considerable evidence for the concept of mixed anginal syndromes has been gathering over recent years. Previously it was assumed that myocardial ischaemia only occurred in the presence of anginal pain. With the greater application of continuous ambulatory ST-segment monitoring, it has become clear that even in patients with stable angina, frequent episodes of silent ischaemia occur throughout the entire 24-hour period.[10] Research has shown that both silent and painful ischaemia are major prognostic factors in patients with coronary disease. Such silent episodes are thought to contribute to the overall ischaemic burden, although this is difficult to quantify in the individual patient.

Management

The purpose of treating angina is not only to prevent AMI and long-term complications such as heart failure,[11] but also to improve quality of life. Anti-anginal medication lessens the frequency and severity of episodes of angina through several mechanisms, ultimately altering the balance of oxygen supply and demand. Anginal symptoms alone are not a reliable guide to the extent of patients' ischaemic heart disease and silent episodes of ischaemia are associated with increased morbidity and mortality.[12] It has become apparent that effective treatment of ischaemia will have to target the pattern of ischaemic events seen in patients' daily lives and treatment strategies must aim to eliminate both silent and symptomatic episodes of ischaemia. The complementary effects of combination therapy with nitrates, beta-blockers and calcium channel antagonists have been demonstrated in this regard. A detailed review of their pharmacology is beyond the scope of this chapter and readers are referred to a comprehensive review by Cohn.[13] In addition, recent evidence suggests that some of these newer agents may also halt or even reverse the underlying pathophysiological processes.[14]

The standard of care for unstable angina proceeds along the same lines as for AMI (see below) including the early administration of aspirin. The patient should be commenced on heparin therapy, either intravenous unfractionated heparin or subcutaneous low-molecular-weight heparin. If IV heparin is used, the aim is to achieve an activated partial thromboplastin time of 1.5–2.5 times control. This has been shown to be even more effective than aspirin at reducing the risk of death or myocardial infarction.[15] Low-molecular-weight heparins (LMWH) have improved pharmacologic and pharmacokinetic properties over standard heparin that may result in greater efficacy and safety. LMWH may be given in fixed, weight-based doses subcutaneously without monitoring, resulting in greater clinical utility and cost-effectiveness compared with standard heparin.

Research by Blomberg has shown that in patients with unstable angina, high level thoracic epidural anaesthesia (TEA) reduces ST-segment depression during exercise stress testing, presumably through a favourable change in the ratio of oxygen supply and demand. TEA may have application in patients with recurrent angina who cannot be weaned from nitrate infusions and perhaps for the long-term treatment of anginal pain.[16] Some patients with refractory unstable angina may require treatment with intra-aortic balloon counter pulsation to relieve their symptoms. Counter pulsation improves coronary blood flow during diastole when the balloon inflates and reduces afterload during cardiac systole (balloon deflation).

Persistent angina despite optimum combination medical therapy indicates a poor prognosis. Such patients should be considered for urgent revascularization.

For further information on the diagnosis and management of unstable angina, the consensus paper by Braunwald et al is recommended.[17]

MYOCARDIAL INFARCTION

Pathophysiology

ST-segment elevation myocardial infarction (STEMI)

Anterior AMI This is the most common site of infarction, usually due to occlusion of the left anterior descending coronary artery (LAD) or one of its branches and is evidenced by ST-segment elevation in the precordial leads of the ECG. Some patients present with marked sympathetic stimulation (compared with inferior AMI - see below) and control of heart rate may be essential to relieve symptoms of ischaemia. Large anterior infarctions result in left ventricular dysfunction and are prone to mural thrombus formation. There may be associated inferior infarction.

Inferior AMI Acute inferior infarction is diagnosed by elevation of ST segments or the development of Q waves in the inferior ECG leads (II, III and aVF). Inferior infarction is generally associated with less impairment of the left ventricle than anterior infarction. When there is associated ST-segment depression in leads V_{1-4}, there is likely to be additional LAD disease with poor left ventricular function. These patients may present clinically with epigastric pain, nausea and vomiting (a picture suggestive of vagal over-activity) and are at increased risk of early complications including arrhythmias, heart block and cardiogenic shock.

Right-ventricular AMI[23] Isolated right ventricular (RV) infarction accounts for less than 3% of all cases of infarction. More commonly it occurs in association with almost half of inferior AMIs. RV infarction results from occlusion of the right coronary artery (RCA) proximal to the marginal branches or less commonly with occlusion of the circumflex artery in patients with dominance of the left coronary circulation.

The presence of RV infarction may be diagnosed on ECG RV leads (RV_{4-6}). These will show ST-segment elevation in the presence of AMI. All patients with inferior infarction who show clinical signs of right-heart failure (hypotension, clear lung fields, elevated jugular venous pressure) should have RV leads performed to exclude RV infarction as the management is significantly different in this group of patients. RV infarction may be complicated by shock, heart block (usually in association with inferior infarction), atrial fibrillation, pulmonary embolism from RV thrombus formation, tricuspid incompetence and a high incidence of pericarditis.

The pathophysiology of RV infarction is quite distinct from that of left ventricular infarction. Right ventricular preload must be maintained through adequate filling, maintenance of sinus rhythm and avoidance of drugs that reduce preload (e.g. nitrates and diuretics). Inotropic support with dobutamine is indicated for inadequate cardiac output despite aggressive fluid management. When associated with left ventricular dysfunction, intra-aortic balloon counterpulsation or arteriodilators (e.g. sodium nitroprusside) may help to reduce the afterload of both ventricles. Although there has been little systematic study of RV infarction, the recommendations for thrombolysis and acute angioplasty are the same as for infarctions in other regions of myocardium.

Posterior AMI The presence of a posterior AMI should be suspected when ST-segment depression in leads V_1 and V_2 are seen on the ECG of patients with ischaemic chest pain. Posterior ECG leads (V_{7-9}) should be performed and elevation of the ST segments in these leads confirms the diagnosis of posterior AMI.

Non ST-segment elevation myocardial infarction

Subendocardial or non-ST-segment elevation myocardial infarction (NSTEMI) accounts for up to 40% of AMIs. They tend to be smaller than transmural infarctions, with better left ventricular ejection fractions and are less likely to produce new onset congestive cardiac failure. They have a lower in-hospital mortality. However, they carry a higher risk of post-infarct angina and recurrent infarction.

Clinical features

The diagnosis of AMI is frequently difficult to make and easy to miss. Certain subgroups of patients are more at risk of being misdiagnosed than others. The majority of patients with AMI who are inappropriately discharged home are either young patients with unsuspected AMI or elderly patients with 'atypical' symptoms such as acute weakness, syncope, confusion or cerebrovascular accident (CVA). The incidence of 'painless' AMI increases with age and is reported to be 60–70% of patients over the age of 85.[18] Furthermore, 2–6% of AMIs occur in patients younger than 40, a group previously regarded as being 'too young' to have a heart attack. Patients with left bundle branch block (LBBB), those presenting with altered conscious state and diabetic patients with autonomic neuropathy can also present a diagnostic challenge.

In order to make a diagnosis of STEMI, at least two of the following must be present:

- Typical ischaemic chest pain present for at least 30 minutes.
- ECG changes – ST-segment elevation of at least 2 mm in two or more consecutive chest leads, or 1 mm in two limb leads, or a new LBBB. (NB The ECG can be normal initially).
- Elevation of the serum levels of the cardiac markers.

Whilst the primary aim of the emergency department assessment of the patient with chest pain is to exclude acute ischaemic syndromes and thus avoid inappropriate discharge, it is just as important to identify those patients who do not have an ischaemic cause for their pain. Some of these patients will have other equally life-threatening conditions, such as pulmonary embolism, which require prompt recognition and intervention.

Investigations

ECG

The ECG is essential in the assessment of patients with potential IHD. Acute ischaemic changes on the ECG may indicate the need for urgent thrombolytic therapy, whilst continuous cardiac monitoring allows rhythm analysis and early intervention for serious dysrhythmias.

As aggressive reperfusion therapy with either thrombolysis or percutaneous coronary intervention (PCI) is most effective within 60–90 minutes of symptom onset, the selection of patients for reperfusion therapy still relies on ECG criteria as specified above. However, 25–50% of patients with AMI have a normal initial ECG on presentation to the ED. This contributes to the finding that 2–8% of ED patients with AMI are undiagnosed.[19] Where clinical suspicion is high and the initial ECG does not confirm AMI, then serial ECGs at 15–30 minute intervals are recommended until either the patient's symptoms resolve with anti-anginal therapy/analgesia or ECG changes meeting criteria for thrombolysis appear.

The use of additional ECG leads may assist in the diagnosis of right ventricular or posterior infarction, and certainly has been shown to help define the full extent of myocardial injury in patients with myocardial infarction. However, performing routine 15-lead ECGs has not been shown to alter the diagnosis, therapy, rate of thrombolysis or disposition of patients.[20]

Cardiac markers

Despite the ongoing search for better serum markers to aid early identification of patients with myocardial infarction, none of the available tests are useful in this regard as they all require serial sampling over a period of at least 12 hours. Much research has revolved around serum markers such as myoglobin, cardiac troponin T and I, and CKMB.

Myoglobin is the smallest of these markers and is, therefore, measurable in the serum earliest. However, the assay cannot distinguish between myoglobin of skeletal muscle origin and that of cardiac muscle origin – so while it remains a very sensitive test, its specificity is very low.

Assays for cardiac troponins have recently been improved and are becoming more widely available. However, they have failed to fulfil the need for an early, accurate serum marker of myocardial infarction. Cardiac troponin has been shown in clinical trials to offer no advantage over the more traditional CKMB in either sensitivity or specificity shortly after onset of symptoms. Within 6 hours of symptom onset, each test has 40% sensitivity and 98% specificity for the diagnosis of AMI. However, troponin remains elevated much longer than CKMB and thus is a more useful marker of recent infarction in patients who present late. At 24 hours after symptom onset, troponin-I is 100% sensitive compared to CKMB at 57% sensitive.[21]

Neither test is useful as a marker of AMI among patients with chest pain of less than 6 hours duration. In addition, measurement of serum cardiac markers does not detect unstable angina and certainly should not be used as a tool to rule out an acute coronary syndrome (ACS), especially when making decisions about which patients may be discharged. Recent studies have demonstrated that elevated levels of troponin I in patients with unstable angina places these patients at higher risk for subsequent AMI.[21]

Chest X-ray

The chest X-ray is only useful in the acute phase if aortic dissection is suspected on clinical grounds. Certainly the initiation of thrombolysis should not be delayed in order to first obtain a chest X-ray. The X-ray will also provide information regarding cardiac size and the degree of pulmonary congestion.

Echocardiography

There is no evidence to support the routine use of echocardiography to assess patients with AMI. Echocardiography provides useful information in patients with evidence of ventricular dysfunction. The presence of akinetic/dyskinetic segments of ventricular wall, their size and the presence of aneurysmal dilatation and mural thrombus may be detected and quantified. In addition, acute valvular dysfunction (especially mitral regurgitation) can be assessed.

Differential diagnosis

See Chapter 4.1.

Management

Patients with potentially ischaemic chest pain should be assessed promptly and have treatment initiated without delay. This includes continuous ECG and vital sign monitoring, ongoing reassessment of cardiac rhythm and response to therapeutic interventions and serial ECGs if indicated. All patients should have intravenous access established and receive supplemental oxygen. Aspirin should be routinely administered unless a contraindication exists.

Early mortality in patients with ischaemic heart disease is mainly due to acute dysrhythmias or left ventricular failure. Continuous ECG monitoring allows early recognition and treatment of dysrrhythmias, whilst aggressive treatment of heart failure increases the likelihood of recovery.

Management of acute AMI is aimed primarily at the preservation of myocardium and the reduction of morbidity and mortality. The standard of care has been outlined in the ACC/AHA Guidelines (last issued in 2000). These guidelines are comprehensive and outline the evidence available at the time for each intervention.[22]

Thrombolysis

Early reperfusion of infarcting myocardium has become the standard of care. Many large multi-centre trials have now validated the use of thrombolytic therapy. As it is often more readily available than angioplasty, it has become the most commonly used reperfusion technique.

Thrombolytic therapy should be initiated as soon as possible after the diagnosis of STEMI. The aim of thrombolysis is to prevent extension of thrombus, preserve ventricular function and reduce morbidity and mortality. Ideally, patients should receive treatment within an hour of onset of symptoms to gain maximal benefit. Clearly for a number of reasons (late presentation, initially normal ECG, silent infarction, etc.) this will not

be the case for the majority of patients. Patients treated after 6 hours of symptoms will still gain some benefit, but initiation of thrombolysis after 12 hours is of little benefit.[24] It is important for emergency departments to have processes in place aimed at keeping 'door-to-needle' time for these patients to a minimum and to audit their performance in this area.

Streptokinase (SK) and plasminogen activators are the most often used and best investigated thrombolytic agents. A number of plasminogen activators are now commercially available including, alteplase, reteplase, tenecteplase and lanoteplase. The newer plasminogen activators differ from alteplase with respect to their fibrin specificity, plasma half-life and resistance to plasminogen activator inhibitor type 1.[25] Numerous large multi-centre trials have attempted to define the best thrombolytic agent, the optimal dose and administration regime and the best combination of adjuvant therapies in order to achieve the lowest mortality rates whilst minimizing the complications of therapy. Little difference has been shown between streptokinase and front-loaded tissue plasminogen activator (tPA) when given with heparin, except in the subgroup of patients less than 75 years old with anterior-wall infarcts who present within 4 hours of onset of pain. In this group the 30-day mortality rate was significantly lower and the 90-minute patency rate significantly higher in the tPA group compared to the streptokinase group.[26]

The newer plasminogen activators are replacing front loaded tPA because their longer plasma half lives allow for easier administration regimens whilst maintaining the safety and effectiveness profiles of older agents.[25]

Indications for thrombolytic therapy

Typical ischaemic chest pain of greater than 30 minutes and less than 6 hours duration, plus one of: ST-segment elevation of at least 1 mm in two or more consecutive limb leads; or ST-segment elevation of at least 2 mm in two or more consecutive chest leads; or new-onset LBBB and the absence of absolute contraindications to thrombolysis.

Contraindications to thrombolysis

Absolute

- Uncontrolled hypertension (>180/120 mmHg)
- Bleeding diathesis
- Recent gastrointestinal bleeding
- Haemorrhagic stroke (<6 months)
- Trauma, surgery, organ biopsy (<6 weeks)
- Pregnancy to 1 week post-partum
- Aortic dissection
- Acute pericarditis
- Acute pancreatitis
- Neurosurgery (<6 months).

Relative contraindications to thrombolysis

- Non-compressible vessel puncture site
- History of cerebrovascular disease
- Controlled hypertension
- Acute ventricular thrombus
- Endocarditis
- Non-traumatic cardio-pulmonary resuscitation.

If relative contraindications are present it is necessary to individually balance the potential advantages of thrombolysis and possible disadvantages due to side effects.

Complications of thrombolytic therapy

Bleeding complications The cerebral haemorrhage rate in AMI trials is remarkably constant at 0.5–1.5%.[24] The risk of cerebral haemorrhage is greater when the systolic blood pressure is greater than 150 mmHg, the patient's age is over 65 years, the patient has a low body weight and tPA is the thrombolytic agent.[27] Most bleeding complications are relatively minor.

Allergy and anaphylaxis SK is a bacterial protein and induces an antigenic response. Patients with high antibody titres (after streptococcal infection or previous exposure to SK) are less likely to achieve thrombolytic efficacy when treated with SK and in addition are more likely to experience an allergic reaction. Therefore, reuse of SK should be avoided.[28] Anaphylaxis is very rare with any of the thrombolytic agents (<0.5%).

A serum sickness-like illness may develop late after the use of SK and should be treated in the standard way.

Hypotension Hypotension due to kinin release may be seen during the administration of SK and is related to the rate of administration of the drug. It will respond to fluid loading and slowing the rate of infusion.

Reperfusion arrhythmias Arrhythmias following thrombolytic therapy are usually self-terminating and seldom require specific therapy. Their occurrence often signals reperfusion of the ischaemic and irritable myocardium.

Revascularization

Revascularization techniques aim to restore myocardial oxygen supply by either relieving or circumventing the atherosclerotic obstruction responsible for ischaemic symptoms. However, initially successful coronary artery bypass grafting (CABG) and PCI may be followed by recurrence of angina due to graft or stent occlusion, restenosis post angioplasty or the progression of coronary artery disease.

Large multicentre trials have provided no evidence that surgical treatment is superior to medical treatment in increasing long-term survival in patients with mild angina and lesser degrees of coronary atherosclerosis. Such patients are best treated medically.[13] However, surgery has been shown to be superior to medical therapy in increasing longevity in patients with significant stenosis of the left main coronary artery.[29] Surgical management may also be preferable to medical therapy in patients with triple vessel disease regardless of symptoms, especially in those with continuing ischaemia and impaired left-ventricular function. In addition, surgery is recommended for patients with angina that fails to respond to medical therapy. Comparison of coronary angioplasty with bypass surgery has shown no clear-cut advantage in terms of morbidity and mortality,[30] however, PCI remains an alternative for patients with medically refractory angina who are high-risk candidates for surgery.

Angioplasty

Although balloon angioplasty has been associated with lesion success rates approximating to 89%[31], not all lesions lend themselves anatomically to this approach. In addition, restenosis and stent occlusion remain significant problems. Approximately 50% of patients treated with percutaneous transluminal coronary angioplasty (PTCA) following myocardial infarction will require another revascularisation procedure (either PTCA or CABG) over the subsequent 2–3 years.[32]

Newer interventional modalities such as directional atherectomy, rotablation, transluminal extraction catheterization, laser coronary angioplasty and coronary stenting all have the potential to offer reduced rates of restenosis in certain patients.

Cardiac bypass surgery

Coronary artery bypass surgery is still the most widely used treatment for patients with multi-vessel coronary artery disease.[33] Bypass surgery is the preferred revascularization technique for patients with LAD disease and three-vessel disease. In contrast, PTCA is the preferred technique for patients with a previous history of PTCA or coronary bypass surgery, for NSTEMI and if there is a possibility of placing a coronary stent.[33]

Operative management continues to improve and the use of arterial grafts may have a survival advantage, however, the long-term results of surgery lie with the secondary prevention of cardiac risk factors.[32]

Newer surgical techniques of minimally invasive coronary artery surgery are becoming increasingly popular. The two principal techniques involve surgery on the beating heart without cardiopulmonary bypass and thoracoscopic or small incision surgery with the use of an endoluminal aortic cross clamp. These techniques are not yet suitable for acutely ill patients and the long-term benefits are yet to be assessed.

Medical therapy

Aspirin

Since thrombosis is responsible for most acute manifestations of coronary artery disease, including unstable angina and NSTEMI, antiplatelet therapy has played a major role in reducing the risk of ischaemic events. Aspirin has been shown to significantly reduce the incidence of death or MI in patients with unstable angina or NSTEMI.[34] Aspirin also significantly reduces mortality following STEMI,[26] but this benefit is limited to patients where aspirin is administered early.[34] Importantly, however, this early benefit is preserved for several years following infarction. In addition, ISIS-2 (1988)[35] demonstrated that the combination of aspirin with streptokinase is more effective in reducing mortality following AMI than either therapy alone. As a consequence, aspirin is recommended in all patients with unstable angina and acute myocardial infarction. What remains unresolved is the minimum effective dose and optimal formulation of aspirin that should be used for inhibition of platelet function. It should be noted that aspirin does not confer any benefit to patients whose symptoms are due to coronary artery spasm.[34]

Beta blockers

Randomized trials have demonstrated that beta-blockers improve survival after AMI. Not only do they have antiarrhythmic properties but they also decrease infarct size and reduce reinfarction rates. Early therapy is more effective.[33] Sympathetic stimulation increases myocardial metabolic requirements. Beta-blockers blunt the cardiovascular responses to adrenergic stimulation, and are effective in reducing both symptomatic and silent ischaemia, thus conferring protection to the myocardium after infarction.[13] However, they also have negative chronotropic and inotropic properties and are contraindicated in patients with advanced heart block, symptomatic bradycardia, low cardiac output and severe left ventricular impairment. In addition, beta-blockers can precipitate coronary spasm, and for this reason a nitrate or calcium channel blocker is preferred over a beta-blocker for the treatment of patients in whom coronary artery spasm is believed to play a causative role.

The use of beta-blockers in unstable angina is based upon data from studies involving patients with AMI. In patients with stable angina, beta-blockers have been shown to reduce the frequency of symptoms and to increase the anginal threshold. This effect is most pronounced during exercise or in the presence of increased sympathetic activity. However, there is no evidence to date that shows that beta-blocker therapy in patients with unstable angina reduces the incidence of mortality or AMI.[36]

Angiotensin converting enzyme inhibitors

The efficacy of angiotensin converting enzyme inhibitors (ACE inhibitors) used early after AMI has been established in meta-analyses of large randomized trials.[37,38] These demonstrated a 6.5% reduction in early mortality.

Nitrates

Nitrates exert their anti-anginal activity by a number of mechanisms. Reduction in venous return and LVEDP lowers myocardial oxygen demand and at the same time enhances blood flow to the sub-endocardium. They also directly increase myocardial oxygen supply by dilating the epicardial coronary arteries. In particular, organic nitrates have been shown to dilate stenotic segments and increase collateral blood flow. More recent data suggest that nitrates may also have anti-platelet and antithrombotic properties.[39] Both the vasodilatory action of nitrates and the proposed anti-platelet effect of these drugs are believed to involve nitric oxide.

Following acute AMI, nitrates reduce ventricular dilatation and by doing so reduce pulmonary congestion and mitral regurgitation. Early short-term use (4–6 weeks) may reduce mortality in the absence of hypotension.[37,38] Despite their well-documented benefit in angina and congestive heart failure, their longer term impact on the morbidity and mortality of survivors of AMI has yet to be determined.[40]

Calcium-channel blockers

Despite their vasodilatory properties and efficacy in relieving angina, calcium-channel blockers do not reduce mortality

during or after AMI.[41] They are useful for patients who cannot tolerate beta-blockers for relief of ongoing ischaemic pain and as antiarrhythmics.[22]

Glycoprotein IIb/IIIa receptor inhibitors

Despite adjunctive therapy with heparin and aspirin, patients undergoing PCI have a significantly high re-occlusion rate. In an attempt to improve patency rates, more potent agents have been developed, including direct thrombin inhibitors and the glycoprotein (GP) IIb/IIIa receptor inhibitors. The GP IIb/IIIa receptor is the major platelet surface receptor involved in the final common pathway of platelet aggregation. The inhibitors work by preventing fibrinogen from binding to GP IIb/IIIa receptor sites on activated platelets. The goal of treatment is to block 80% of receptors. This class of drug includes abciximab, tirofiban, eptifibatide and lamifiban.

The overall efficacy of GP IIb/IIIa inhibitors in unstable angina and NSTEMI is still unclear. Studies thus far do not consistently show a decrease in mortality or long-term benefit.[42] Both eptifibatide and tirofiban have been shown to have benefits in patients with UA/NSTEMI who do not undergo PCI.[43,44] The rates of death and AMI were reduced with each agent during medical management. This reduction is further magnified with intervention.[44,45] In patients with UA who do undergo PCI, the GP IIb/IIIa inhibitors have been shown to be effective in preventing complications associated with PCI. The GUSTO IV ACS trial demonstrated the important contribution of invasive management in attaining the optimal benefits from GP IIb/IIIa inhibition.[46]

In summary, the GP IIb/IIIa receptor inhibitors have been shown to produce a modest reduction in combined endpoints of death, AMI and urgent revascularization, conferring additional benefit over aspirin/heparin. Increased benefit is seen in those patients with elevated troponin and when PCI is performed early. Improved outcomes have been demonstrated when these agents are used in the hours preceding PCI.

In the management of STEMI, improved patency and a reduction in re-occlusion rates (when used in conjunction with tPA, aspirin and heparin) suggest that these agents may be as efficacious as primary angioplasty. However, their use has also been associated with an increase in bleeding complications.[30,47,48] Trials to date suggest that reduced-dosage thrombolytic plus full-dosage GP IIb/IIIa blocker enhance efficacy compared with full-dosage thrombolytic alone; however, none have been large enough to confirm safety.

Until there is further evidence from clinical trials, reversible GP IIb/IIIa inhibitors should be considered for medical management of ACS in addition to therapy with aspirin and heparin in the following situations:

- NSTEMI or unstable angina at high risk for AMI.
- STEMI when fibrinolytic therapy is contraindicated.
- Patients who are not able to undergo emergency PCI due to unavailability of a 24-hour service or who are treated more than12 hours after symptom onset.
- Patients with ECG changes that do not meet criteria for thrombolysis.

Adenosine diphosphate inhibitors

The adenosine diphosphate inhibitors (ADP) inhibitors prevent ADP-mediated platelet aggregation by selectively binding to adenylate cyclase-coupled ADP receptors on the surface of platelets. This results in inhibition of platelet aggregation and binding of fibrinogen to the GP IIb/IIIa receptor on activated platelets. Clopidogrel and ticlopidine have been studied with regards to their role in the management of acute coronary syndromes, in particular as adjuvant therapy in patients undergoing PCI with stent placement. In this regard their safety and efficacy has been established.[48]

ADP inhibitors may also be considered an alternative in patients with a contraindication to aspirin therapy. They may also be used for recurrent ischaemia despite treatment with aspirin. There are no data to suggest that they are equivalent to aspirin in the primary or secondary prevention of AMI.

Heparin

Thrombus formation is central in the pathogenesis of AMI, unstable angina and re-occlusion following angioplasty. Heparin is the mainstay of antithrombin therapy and works indirectly requiring antithrombin III as co-factor. Heparin is indicated in unstable angina in addition to aspirin. Many studies have shown that its use reduces the incidence of non-fatal AMI and recurrent ischaemia.[36] In addition, its role as adjuvant therapy to thrombolysis has been clearly established. However, the routine administration of heparin in addition to aspirin following STEMI does not confer any survival benefit and may increase the incidence of haemorrhagic complications.[49, 50] Recent studies have compared the low molecular weight heparins (LMWH) (dalteparin and enoxaparin) with unfractionated heparin (UFH) in patients with unstable angina and NSTEMI.[48] They appear to offer greater efficacy and the advantage that monitoring of the aPTT is not required. They are, however, associated with an increased risk of minor bleeding complications. Their role in the management of STEMI and following PCI has not been established.

Direct thrombin inhibitors

Hirudins are polypeptides derived from the leech *Hirudo medicinalis*. Recent studies have compared UFH with hirudin in the management of acute ischaemia. Hirudin appears to be associated with improved measures of coronary reperfusion and vessel patency compared to UFH[51] and may decrease the risk of non-fatal AMI.[52] Although these compounds have to-date, not been compared with LMWH, they should be considered as alternatives for patients who are unable to tolerate UFH or LMWH due to heparin induced thrombocytopenia.[48]

Magnesium

The role of magnesium in the setting of AMI is still unclear as clinical studies have produced conflicting results.[53,54] The early administration of magnesium may reduce reperfusion-related injury, but it has no effect on mortality following AMI.[41] At this time the routine administration of magnesium is not recommended.

COMPLICATIONS

Arrhythmias and conduction disturbances

See Chapter 4.4.

Acute left ventricular failure and cardiogenic shock

AMI is invariably accompanied by some degree of left ventricular dysfunction. The degree of left ventricular failure can be correlated with acute in-hospital mortality. The Killip classification has been commonly used in cardiac trials.

Class	Clinical manifestations	Approx. mortality (%)
I	Asymptomatic	5
II	Mild LVF, bibasal crepitations	20
III	Pulmonary oedema	40
IV	Cardiogenic shock	80

Cardiogenic shock is associated with loss of more than 40% of left ventricular myocardium and carries a grave prognosis. General management includes adequate oxygenation and ventilation, correction of electrolyte disturbances, ensuring adequate filling pressures and the early institution of inotropes for hypotension, inadequate perfusion and oliguria in the face of adequate intravascular volume. No large trials have demonstrated that thrombolysis improves the survival of patients with cardiogenic shock and the intervention of choice in these critically ill patients is urgent angioplasty.[55] Intra-aortic balloon counterpulsation produces only temporary clinical and haemodynamic improvement in patients with cardiogenic shock. Clinical trials are lacking, but its utility appears to be limited to those patients who subsequently undergo urgent revascularization.[55]

Treatment of cardiac failure

See Chapter 4.3.

Beta-blockers improve functional capacity, ventricular function and decrease mortality in patients with heart failure due to ischaemic heart disease.[56] This mortality risk reduction may be as great as 20% in subgroups of patients with heart failure following AMI.[57]

Several studies indicate that patients with left ventricular dysfunction after an AMI should receive long-term treatment with an ACE inhibitor.[58,59,60] This may improve survival, reduce the incidence of overt heart failure and reduce the risk of reinfarction.[61]

Mechanical defects

Large anterior AMIs will result in ventricular wall motion abnormalities most readily visualized with echocardiography. This is the underlying mechanism of acute left ventricular failure. In addition, hypokinesis predisposes to mural thrombus formation with attendant risks of systemic or pulmonary embolism (depending upon which ventricle is involved).

Acute mitral insufficiency may develop secondary to papillary muscle rupture or dysfunction, most commonly in the setting of inferior infarction. Such an event will be manifested clinically by cardiogenic shock and a new pansystolic murmur. Emergency therapy is required in the form of afterload reduction with sodium nitroprusside or intra-aortic balloon counterpulsation whilst the diagnosis is confirmed and the patient prepared for urgent valve replacement surgery.

Ventricular septal defect can occur in the setting of anterior AMI and can be difficult to distinguish clinically from acute mitral insufficiency. Emergency treatment is the same for both conditions.

Cardiac rupture is an uncommon complication that presents clinically as acute pericardial tamponade. Immediate management comprises aggressive fluid resuscitation, pericardiocentesis in unstable patients and surgical repair. The prognosis is grim.

Thromboembolism

Thrombus forms in hypokinetic areas of ischaemic myocardium. Inflammatory changes of the myocardial muscle in these areas together with a relative stasis of blood flow predispose to thrombus formation. Presence of intracardiac thrombus can be confirmed with echocardiography. These patients require systemic anticoagulation to prevent embolic complications.

Pericarditis

Inflammation of the overlying pericardium may accompany transmural infarction and is manifest by pain and a friction rub in the first week following AMI. An immune mediated form of pericarditis known as Dressler syndrome may occur later. Management is with non-steroidal anti-inflammatory medications.

DISPOSITION

All patients with unstable coronary syndromes require further evaluation and management as inpatients. A diagnosis of unstable angina, NSTEMI or STEMI is based on initial evaluation. Further management is determined by risk stratification dependent on duration of ischaemic pain, ECG changes and elevation of cardiac markers as well as clinical evidence of cardiac dysfunction.[62,63,64,65] Patients at low risk (including those with stable angina) should undergo further evaluation and ongoing management on an outpatient basis. High-risk patients should be admitted to an intensive care or coronary care unit. Intermediate-risk patients may be admitted to an intermediate acuity unit or telemetry bed.[62] Patients at low risk for ischaemic heart disease who are being admitted for the investigation of atypical chest pain may be admitted to general ward beds.

PROGNOSIS

The major determinants of prognosis are age, left ventricular function, effort tolerance and the clinical stability or instability of angina.[66] Measures that improve survival after AMI include treatment with thrombolytic agents, aspirin and beta-adrenergic blockers and smoking cessation. Lowering serum lipid concen-

trations in patients with IHD and hypercholesterolaemia has been shown to reduce the risk of subsequent cardiovascular death.[67] Concerns have been raised that the cardiovascular benefits of lowering cholesterol concentrations might be outweighed by the increased risk of other causes of death, however, this concern has not been validated in recent trials.[68]

LONG-TERM MANAGEMENT

Cardiac rehabilitation

The aim of cardiac rehabilitation is to restore patients as nearly as possible to their pre-infarct level of functioning in terms of both physical and emotional health. By ensuring that they are well adjusted, well educated and fit, they are best able to cope with the long-term consequences of ischaemic heart disease. Patient education is paramount for a successful rehabilitation programme. The majority of patients enrolled in exercise programmes are medically stable and relatively symptom-free. Programmes include not only exercise regimes usually supervised by physiotherapists, but also devote time to patient education, risk factor modification and individual counselling. There is increasing evidence that those with extensive myocardial damage, left ventricular dysfunction or failure and ongoing myocardial ischaemia may also benefit.[69]

Such rehabilitation programs have been shown to be cost-effective in terms of productivity and return to active employment, as well as reduced incidence of depression, anxiety and cardiac events including hospital admission.[70] Despite this, however, follow-up and ongoing preventive care in the community following discharge is often less than ideal with only 30–40% of patients eligible to attend a structured rehabilitation programme actually doing so.[71]

Primary prevention

The importance of primary prevention is highlighted by the fact that about 25% of new cases of ischaemic heart disease

present as sudden death. Over recent years there has been substantial investment of time and money by government bodies in many countries to promote healthy life-style programmes aimed at public education and the primary prevention of disease including life-style and risk factor modification. A reduction in preventable ischaemic heart disease would mean substantial cost savings worldwide.

Primary prevention strategies include cessation of cigarette smoking and avoidance of obesity through regular exercise and reduction of dietary fat intake. In individuals with a strong family history of IHD, early detection and treatment of risk factors such as hypertension, hypercholesterolaemia and diabetes may substantially reduce their risk.

Studies have shown that small daily amounts of alcohol have a beneficial effect in reducing the risk of IHD.[72] This protective effect does not appear to depend on the type of alcohol consumed and may be related to antithrombotic effects of alcohol.[73] High levels of intake, however, are associated with an increased risk of IHD in addition to other medical and social burdens associated with heavy alcohol consumption.

The role of low dose aspirin in the secondary prevention of AMI, stroke and death from cardiovascular causes has been well established. Its role in the primary prevention of IHD has been less well studied. One trial demonstrated a reduction of 33% in the incidence of first AMI in men taking low doses of aspirin.[74] Despite such promising results, more research is need before recommending prophylactic low-dose aspirin to everyone. Current recommendations for its use in primary prevention of AMI is in men over 40 years of age who have risk factors for the development of IHD that outweigh the risks of complications from long-term aspirin therapy.[75]

Of unique importance to women is the role that hormone replacement therapy plays in the primary prevention of IHD. It has been recognized for some time that following menopause, the incidence of IHD in women starts to approach that for men. This difference has been attributed to the protective effect of ovarian hormones in the premenopausal woman. The effectiveness of hormone-replacement therapy in primary prevention of IHD has been confirmed.[76] Oestrogen therapy alone has been estimated to reduce the risk of IHD by up to 44%.[73] Data also suggest a reduction in risk with combined therapy. In addition, the newer low-dose oral contraceptive pills do not carry the same increased risk for IHD as the older formulations.

Secondary prevention

Secondary prevention should be considered just as important as primary prevention because morbidity and mortality from IHD carry a considerable social and financial burden for individuals as well as communities.

Lipid-lowering regimens are effective as both primary and secondary preventive measures. Available evidence suggests that aggressive lipid lowering treatment is clinically indicated for both men and women who have proven ischaemic heart disease across a wide range of LDL cholesterol concentrations. In addition, treatment with lipid lowering drugs is effective in reducing major coronary events even in people with IHD who have cholesterol concentrations in the 'normal' range.[67]

The role of daily low-dose aspirin has been well established as has long-term beta-blockade in survivors of myocardial infarction.[22]

FUTURE DIRECTIONS

As more evidence is coming to light regarding the role of inflammation in the pathogenesis of IHD, research is now concentrating on the identification of the causative agents and the modification of cellular and physiologic response to these agents. To this end, primary and secondary prevention strategies are gaining more recognition as being central to efforts to curb the steady increase in IHD worldwide. Research continues in the areas of risk stratification and the role of newer drugs (particularly the antiplatelet agents) in the conservative management of acute coronary syndromes.

CONTROVERSIES

❶ Are plasminogen activators superior to streptokinase, and does any additional benefit justify the cost?

❷ Should thrombolysis or primary angioplasty be the treatment of choice in AMI?

❸ The role and cost-benefit of chest pain units.

❹ Pre-hospital thrombolysis.

❺ The emerging role of newer antiplatelet agents (doses and combination with standard therapy) in the management of acute coronary syndromes.

REFERENCES

1. World Health Report 1997 Conquering suffering, enriching humanity. Geneva: WHO
2. Kannel WB 1976 Some lessons in cardiovascular epidemiology from Kramingham. American Journal of Cardiology 37: 269
3. Munro JM, Cotran RS 1988 The pathogenesis of atherosclerosis: atherogenesis and inflammation. Laboratory Investments 58: 249–61
4. Alexander RW 1994 Inflammation and coronary artery disease. New England Journal of Medicine 331: 468–9
5. Liuzzo G, Biasucci LM, Gallimore JR, et al 1994 The prognostic value of C-reactive protein and serum amyloid A protein in severe unstable angina. New England Journal of Medicine 331: 417–24
6. Mendall MA, Patel P, Ballam L, Strachan D, Northfield TC 1996 C-reactive protein and its relation to cardiovascular risk factors. British Medical Jouranl 312: 1061–5
7. Brown G, Albers JJ, Fisher LD, et al 1990 Regression of coronary artery disease as a result of intensive lipid-lowering therapy in men with high levels of apolipoprotein B. New England Journal of Medicine 323: 1289
8. Prinzmetal M, Kennamer R, et al 1959 Angina pectoris. I. A variant form of angina pectoris: Preliminary report. American Journal of Medicine 27: 375–88
9. Myerburg RJ, Kessler KM, et al 1992 Life-threatening ventricular arrhythmias in patients with silent myocardial ischaemia due to coronary artery spasm. New England Journal of Medicine 326: 1451–5
10. Taylor SH 1992 Therapeutic targets in ischaemic heart disease. Drugs 43(1): 1–8
11. Pepine CJ, Cohn PF, et al 1994 For the ASIST Study Group: Effects of treatment on outcome in mildly symptomatic patients with ischaemia during daily life: The Atenolol Silent Ischaemia Study (ASIST). Circulation 90: 762–8
12. Deanfield J 1996 Treatment effects on the total ischaemic burden and prognostic implications. European Heart Journal 17(G): 64–8
13. Cohn PF 1997 Pharmacological treatment of ischaemic heart disease. Monotherapy vs combination therapy. European Heart Journal 18(B): B27–B34
14. Simons LA 1991 Is regression of human atherosclerosis a clinical reality? Medical Journal of Australia 160: 531–2
15. Turpie AG 1997 Low-molecular-weight-heparins and unstable angina: current perspectives. Haemostasis. 27(1): 19-24
16. Blomberg S, Curelaru I, Emanuelsson H et al 1989 thoracic epidural anaesthesia in patients with unstable angina pectoris. European Heart Journal 10: 437–44
17. Braunwald E, et al 1994 Diagnosing and managing unstable angina. Circulation 90: 613–22
18. Brady WJ 1997 Missing the diagnosis of AMI. Emergency Medicine Reports
19. Sirois J 1995 Acute Myocardial Infarction. Emergency Clinics of North America 13(4): 759–69
20. Brady WJ, Hwang V, et al 2000 A Comparison of 12- and 15-Lead ECGs in ED Chest Pain Patients: Impact on Diagnosis, Therapy and Disposition. American Journal of Emergency Medicine 18(3): 239–43
21. Brogan GX, et al 1997 Evaluation of a new assay for cardiac troponin I vs creatine kinase-MB for the diagnosis of acute myocardial infarction. Academy of Emergency Medicine 4: 6–12
22. Braunwald E, Antman EM, Beasley JW, et al 2000 ACC/AHA guidelines for the management of patients with unstable angina and non-ST segment elevation myocardial infarction: executive summary and recommendations. A report of the American College of Cardiology/American Heart Association task force on practice guidelines (committee on the management of patients with unstable angina). Circulation 102(10): 1193–209
23. Kinch JW, Ryan TJ 1994 Current concepts - right ventricular infarction. New England Journal of Medicine 330: 1211–6
24. Cairns JA, et al 1995 Fourth ACCP consensus conference on antithrombotic therapy: Coronary thrombolysis. Chest 108(4) (suppl): 401S–423S
25. Spinler SA, Inverso SM 2001 Update on strategies to improve thrombolysis for acute myocardial infarction. Pharmacotherapy 21(6): 691–716
26. The GUSTO Angiographic Investigators 1993 The effects of tissue plasminogen activator, streptokinase, or both on coronary artery patency, ventricular function, and survival after acute myocardial infarction. New England Journal of Medicine 329: 1615–22
27. Huber K, Runge MS, Bode C, Gulba D 1996 Thrombolytic therapy in acute myocardial infarction – update 1996. Annals Hematology 73(suppl I): S29–S38
28. Cross D 1994 Should streptokinase be readministered? Medical Journal of Australia 161: 100–1
29. Taylor HA, Deumite NJ, Chaitman BR, Davis KB, Killip T, Rogers WJ 1989 Asymptomatic left main coronary artery disease in the Coronary Artery Surgery study (CASS) Registry. Circulation 79: 1171–9
30. RITA Trial Participants 1993 Coronary angioplasty versus coronary artery bypass surgery: the Randomised Intervention treatment of Angina (RITA) trial. Lancet 341: 573–80
31. Konstam MA 1997 New trends in the interventional treatment of Ischaemic heart disease. European Heart Journal 18 (B): B16–20
32. Anderson JR, Parker DJ 1997 Long-term results of coronary artery surgery. Coronary Heart Disease 8(3-4): 205–12
33. De-Servi S, et al 1997 Factors affecting the therapeutic choice in patients with multivessel coronary artery disease. The Studio Lombardo Angiografia Multivasali (SLAM) study group. Heart 77(5): 443–8
34. Kerins DM, Fitzgerald GA 1991 The current role of platelet-active drugs in ischaemic heart disease. Drugs 41(5): 665–71
35. ISIS-2 collaborative group 1988 Randomised trial of intravenous streptokinase, oral aspirin, both, or

neither among 17187 cases of suspected acute myocardial infarction: ISIS-2 (Second International Study of Infarct Survival) Collaborative Group. Lancet II: 349–60

36. Chai AU, Crawford MH. 1999 "Traditional" medical therapy for unstable angina. Cardiology Clinics 17(2): 359–72

37. ISIS-4 (Fourth International Study of Infarct Survival) Collaborative Group 1995 ISIS-4: a randomised factorial trial assessing early captopril, oral mononitrate and intravenous magnesium sulphate in 58,050 patients with suspected acute myocardial infarction. Lancet 87: 38–52

38. GISSI 3 study protocol on the effects of lisinopril, of nitrates, and of their association in patients with acute myocardial infarction. American Journal of Cardiology 70: 62C

39. Loscalzo J 1992 Antiplatelet and antithrombotic effects of organic nitrates. American Journal of Cardiology 70: 18B–22B

40. Thadani U 1996 Secondary preventive potential of nitrates in ischaemic heart disease. European Heart Journal 17(F): 30–6

41. Wood A 1996 Adjuvant drug therapy of acute myocardial infarction – evidence from clinical trials. New England Journal of Medicine 335: 1660–7

42. Harrington RA 1999 Overview of clinical trials of glycoprotein IIb-IIIa inhibitors in acute coronary syndromes. American Heart Journal 138(4): S276–S286.

43. PRISM Study Investigators 1998 A comparison of aspirin plus tirofiban versus aspirin plus heparin for unstable angina. New England Journal of Medicine 338: 1498–505

44. The PURSUIT Trial Investigators 1998 Inhibition of platelet glycoprotein IIb/IIIa with eptifibatide in patients with acute coronary syndromes. New England Journal of Medicine 339: 436–43

45. The PRISM-PLUS Study Investigators 1998 Inhibition of the platelet glycoprotein IIb/IIIa receptor with tirofiban in unstable angina and non-Q-wave myocardial infarction. New England Journal of Medicine 338: 1488–97

46. Simoons ML 2001 Effect of glycoprotein IIb/IIIa receptor blocker abciximab on outcome in patients with acute coronary syndromes without early coronary revascularisation: the GUSTO IV-ACS randomised trial. Lancet 357(9272): 1915–24

47. Adgey AA 1996 Haemostasis 26(5): 237–46

48. Wiggins BS, Wittkowsky AK, Nappi JM 2001 Clinical use of new antithrombotic therapies for medical management of acute coronary syndromes. Pharmacotherapy 21(3): 320–37

49. Julian DG, Chamberlain DA, Pocock SJ 1996 A comparison of aspirin and anticoagulation following thrombolysis for myocardial infarction (the AFTER study): a multicentre unblinded randomised clinical trial. British Medical Journal 313: 1429–31

50. Collins R, et al 1996 Clinical effects of anticoagulant therapy in suspected acute myocardial infarction; systematic overview of randomised trial. British Medical Journal 313: 652–9

51. Cannon CP, Braunwald E 1995 Hirudin: Initial results in acute myocardial infarction, unstable angina and angioplasty. Journal of the American College of Cardiology 25(suppl): 30S–7S

52. GUSTO IIb Investigators 1996 A comparison of recombinant hirudin with heparin for the treatment of acute coronary syndromes. New England Journal of Medicine 335: 775–82

53. Woods KL, Fletcher S, Roffe C, et al 1992 Intravenous magnesium sulphate in suspected acute myocardial infarction: Results of the second Leicester Intravenous magnesium Intervention Trial (LIMIT-II). Lancet 339ii :1553–8

54. Woods KL, Fletcher S 1994 Long term outcome after intravenous magnesium sulphate in suspected acute myocardial infarction: The second Leicester Intravenous Magnesium Intervention Trial (LIMIT-2). Lancet 343: 816–9

55. Califf RM, Bengtson JR 1994 Cardiogenic shock. New England Journal of Medicine 330: 1724–9

56. Kelly DT 1996 Beta-blocker therapy in heart failure: myths or realities. Journal of Cardiovascular Failure 2(4): S239-S242

57. Sharpe N 1996 Beta-blockers in heart failure. Future directions. European Heart Journal 17(B): 39–42

58. Pfeffer MA, Braumwald E, et al 1992 Effect of captopril on mortality and morbidity in patients with left ventricular dysfunction after myocardial infarction – results of the survival and ventricular enlargement (SAVE) trial. New England Journal of Medicine 327: 669–77

59. The Acute Infarction Ramipril Efficacy (AIRE) Study Investigators 1993 Effect of ramipril on mortality and morbidity of survivors of acute myocardial infarction with clinical evidence of heart failure. Lancet 57: 84–95

60. The TRACE Study Group 1994 The Trandolapril Cardiac Evaluation (TRACE) study. American Journal of Cardiology 73

61. Sigurdsson A, Swedberg K 1995 Prevention of congestive heart failure by ACE inhibition in patients with acute myocardial infarction. Journal of Cardiovascular Risk 2(5): 406–12

62. Antman EM, Fox KM 2000 Guidelines for the diagnosis and management of unstable angina and non-Q-wave myocardial infarction: Proposed revisions. American Heart Journal 139(3): 461–75

63. Aroney C, Boyden AN, Jelinek MV, et al 2001 Current guidelines for the management of unstable angina: A new diagnostic and management paradigm. Internal Medicine Journal 31: 104–11

64. Pollack CV, Gibler WB 2000 ACC/AHA guidelines for the management of patients with unstable angina and non-ST-segment elevation myocardial infarction: A practical summary for emergency physicians. Annals of Emergency Medicine 38(3): 229–40

65. O'Rourke RA, Hochman JS, Cohen MC, et al 2001 New approaches to diagnosis and management of unstable angina and non-ST-segment elevation myocardial infarction. Archives of Internal Medicine 161: 674–82

66. Maseri A, Pasceri V, Giordano A, Trani C, et al 1996 Expanding concepts in ischaemic heart disease: implications for clinical practice and research. Queensland Journal of Nuclear Medicine 40(1): 4–8

67. Byrne CD, Wild SH 1996 Lipids and secondary prevention of ischaemic heart disease. British Medical Journal 313(23): 1273–4

68. Scandinavian Simvastatin survival study group. 1994 Randomised trial of cholesterol lowering in 4444 patients with coronary heart disease: the Scandinavian simvastatin survival study (4S). Lancet 344: 1383–9

69. Todd IC, Wosornu D, Stewart I, Wild T 1992 Cardiac rehabilitation following myocardial infarction. A practical approach. Sports Medicine 14(4): 243–59

70. Chua TP, Lipkin DP 1993 Cardiac Rehabilitation. British Medical Journal 306: 731–2

71. Bradley F, Morgan S, Smith H, Mant D 1997 Preventive care for patients following myocardial infarction. Family Practice 14(3): 220–6

72. Kemm J 1993 Alcohol and heart disease; the implications of the U-shaped curve. British Medical Journal 307: 1373–4

73. Rich-Edwards JW, Manson JE, Hennekens CH, Buring JE 1995 The primary prevention of coronary heart disease in women. New England Journal of Medicine 332: 1758–66

74. Antiplatelet Trialists' Collaboration 1994 Collaborative overview of randomised trials of antiplatelet therapy – I; prevention of death, myocardial infarction, and stroke by prolonged antiplatelet therapy in various categories of patients. British Medical Journal 308: 81–106

75. Aspirin prophylaxis 1989 In: Guide to clinical preventive services; report of the U.S. Preventive Services Task Force. Baltimore; Williams & Wilkins, pp 258–60

76. Grodstein F, et al 1996 Postmenopausal estrogen and progestin use and the risk of cardiovascular disease. New England Journal of Medicine 335: 453–61

FURTHER READING

American College of Emergency Physicians 1994 Prehospital use of thrombolytic agents. Annals of Emergency Medicine 23: 1146

Bahr RD (ed.) 1997 The strategy of chest pain units (in emergency departments) in the war against heart attacks. Supplement to the Maryland Medical Journal

Harrington RA 1999 Overview of clinical trials of glycoprotein IIb-IIIa inhibitors in acute coronary syndromes. American Heart Journal 138(4): S276–S286

Ohman EM 1999 Troponin and other cardiac markers: role in management of acute coronary syndromes. Australian and New Zealand Journal of Medicine 29: 436–43

Pollack CV, Gibler WB 2000 ACC/AHA guidelines for the management of patients with unstable angina and non-ST-segment elevation myocardial infarction: a practical summary for emergency physicians. Annals of Emergency Medicine 38(3): 229–40

Roberts R (ed.) 1996 La difference: long-term benefit of one thrombolytic over another. Circulation 94: 1203–4

Solomon DH, Stone PH, Glynn RJ Ganz DA, et al 2001 Use of risk stratification to identify patients with unstable angina likeliest to benefit from an invasive versus conservative management strategy. Journal of the American College of Cardiology 38(4): 969–76

Spinler SA, Inverso SM 2001 Update on strategies to improve thrombolysis for acute myocardial infarction. Pharmacotherapy 21(6): 691–716

Storrow AB, Gibler WB 2000 Chest Pain Centres: Diagnosis of Acute Coronary Syndromes. Annals of Emergency Medicine 35(5): 449–61

Wiggins BS, Wittkowsky AK, Nappi JM 2001 Clinical use of new antithrombotic therapies for medical management of acute coronary syndromes. Pharmacotherapy 21(3): 320–37

4.3 ASSESSMENT AND MANAGEMENT OF ACUTE PULMONARY OEDEMA

DAVID LIGHTFOOT

ESSENTIALS

1 Severe APO is associated with high morbidity and mortality.

2 APO is a pathophysiological state characterized by a maldistribution of fluid; most patients do not have fluid overload.

3 Therapy is aimed at maintaining oxygenation and cardiac output. Reversible causes should be sought and corrected.

4 Hypotensive patients require ventilatory and inotropic support.

5 For most patients, the mainstays of therapy are high-flow oxygen, nitrates and CPAP.

6 CPAP is safe and effective in APO. It has been shown to decrease rates of intubation and ICU admission.

INTRODUCTION

Acute pulmonary oedema (APO) occurs mainly in elderly patients and is associated with a very poor long-term prognosis if severe (1-year mortality approaching 40%).[1] It is a pathophysiologic state characterized by fluid-filled alveolar spaces, with resultant impaired alveolar gas exchange and decreased lung compliance. Acute dyspnoea, hypoxia, and increased work of breathing are the resultant symptoms and signs. APO occurs when increased pulmonary capillary pressure, decreased plasma oncotic pressure or pulmonary capillary permeability changes lead to plasma leaving the capillaries and building up in the pulmonary interstitium. When this occurs at such a rate that lymphatic drainage from

the lung cannot keep up, flooding of the alveoli results.

PATHOPHYSIOLOGY

The causes of APO can be divided into cardiogenic (the commonest cause in emergency department patients) and non-cardiogenic. In cardiogenic APO, an acute reduction in cardiac output associated with an increase in systemic vascular resistance, leads to back pressure on the pulmonary vasculature with resultant increased pulmonary capillary pressure. Once established APO can lead to a downward spiral where decreasing oxygenation and increasing pulmonary vascular resistance (with its resultant increased right ventricular end-diastolic pressure) worsens left ventricular dysfunction and worsens pulmonary oedema.[2] In most cases the patient has a maldistribution of fluid rather than being fluid overloaded. They may, in fact, have a whole body fluid deficit. This understanding has lead to a change in the management of this condition from the use of large doses of diuretics, to a focus on vasodilators and non-invasive ventilation. Some of the causes of cardiogenic pulmonary oedema are listed in Table 4.3.1.

In non-cardiogenic APO, the mechanism is thought to be changes in pulmonary vascular permeability, brought about by the causative insult. (This may also play some role in cardiogenic APO.) Some of the causes of non-cardiogenic pulmonary oedema are listed in Table 4.3.2.

CLINICAL ASSESSMENT

History

As with all emergencies, the clinical assessment and management should occur in parallel. There is usually a history of sudden onset, severe dyspnoea. A focused

Table 4.3.1 Causes of cardiogenic pulmonary oedema
Acute valvular dysfunction
Anaemia
Arrhythmias
Dietary, physical or emotional excess
Fluid overload- may be iatrogenic
Medication adverse effect
Medication non-compliance
Myocardial ischaemia/infarction
Myocarditis
Post cardioversion
Pulmonary embolus
Worsening congestive cardiac failure

history concentrating on the recent occurrence of chest pain, a past history of ischaemic heart disease or congestive heart failure, or other causative factor is sought. Details of current medication and compliance are also important.

Examination

Patients are pale or cyanosed, sweaty (sometimes profusely) and frightened. They strive to maintain an upright position at all costs, and may be unable to sit still. They may cough up pink or white frothy sputum, adding to their feeling of drowning. The respiratory rate is high, with use of the accessory muscles of respiration, and breathing is often noisy. Oxygen saturation is severely reduced indicating hypoxia. Most patients are hypertensive or normotensive. Hypotension indicates cardiogenic shock and a very poor prognosis. There may also be a raised JVP, third heart sound or gallop rhythm, and signs of right heart strain. Signs of chronic heart failure should also

Table 4.3.2 Causes of non-cardiogenic pulmonary oedema

Airway obstruction
Asthma
DIC
Eclampsia
Head injury, intracerebral haemorrhage
Hyperbaric oxygen treatment
Inhalation injury
Lung re-expansion, e.g. after treatment of a pneumothorax
Near drowning/cold water immersion
Opiates and opiate antagonists (naloxone and naltrexone)
Pancreatitis
Pulmonary embolism (thrombus, fat, amniotic fluid, other)
Rapid ascent to high altitude
Renal/hepatic failure
SCUBA diving
Sepsis
Shock
Toxins

be sought, as well as murmurs that may hint at the cause. The chest may be dull to percussion and fine crepitations, which are often extensive, will be heard on auscultation. Importantly, there may be other adventitial lung sounds including wheeze, so-called 'cardiac asthma'.

INVESTIGATION

ECG is required looking for ischaemia and chest X-ray will show cardiac size and help differentiate APO from airways disease. The chest X-ray findings of pulmonary oedema reflect the changes in fluid distribution. Initially blood is diverted to the upper lobe veins, which become more prominent than normal. As the oedema worsens, interstitial oedema results in basilar and hilar infiltrates, which are hazy and more confluent than patchy, and interlobular oedema is seen as Kerley B lines. There is loss of vascular delineation. In severe APO widespread changes representing alveolar oedema appear. There may also be changes associated with the underlying cause, e.g. cardiomegaly and pleural effusions in cardiogenic APO.

Blood tests include haemoglobin, electrolytes, cardiac markers or other cause specific bloods as indicated eg amylase. Oximetry (in some cases supplemented with arterial blood gases) will reflect severity, and help guide and monitor the patient's response to therapy. Rarely, in some more severe cases invasive monitoring including pulmonary artery catheterization may be useful.

MANAGEMENT

In all patients with APO, management strategies should provide supportive care to maximize cardiac output and oxygenation, followed by treatment of the underlying cause.

Treatment of the patient with non-cardiogenic pulmonary oedema consists of removing the patient from a causative environment, supportive therapies aimed at maintaining oxygenation, including non-invasive ventilation, and treating the underlying cause.

Most patients with APO in the ED have a cardiogenic aetiology. Therapy varies according to haemodynamic parameters.

Normotensive or hypertensive patients

The mainstays of treatment are preload and afterload reduction with nitrates, and optimizing oxygenation, often with non-invasive ventilatory support. The patient should be managed sitting up.

Nitrates

Nitrates act to increase cyclic guanosine monophoshate (cGMP) in smooth muscle cells, leading to relaxation. In lower doses this predominantly causes venodilation and preload reduction. At higher doses the arterioles are also affected leading to afterload and blood pressure reduction. In addition coronary artery dilatation leads to increased coronary blood flow. Myocardial work and oxygen demands are reduced whilst oxygen delivery is improved. Nitrates are, therefore, the ideal agents for treating APO by reversing the pathophysiological process. Their use is limited by their hypotensive effect and by tachyphylaxis that occurs with prolonged use. Therefore, they should be titrated against the patient's haemodynamics and if used intravenously require careful monitoring. Nitrates may be used topically, sublingually or by intravenous (IV) infusion. In the patient with APO the IV route is preferred as dosing can be titrated to effect and therapy ceased promptly if the patient becomes hypotensive. Topical or sublingual therapy is often used as a temporizing measure until IV access can be secured. Peak effect of IV nitrates occurs after 5 minutes,[3] which compares well with furosemide, which causes venodilatation after about 15 minutes.[4]

The usual dosing regime is to begin the infusion at 5 µg/minute and increase the rate by 5 µg/minute every 3 minutes titrated to clinical effect and limited by falling blood pressure. A reasonable blood pressure target is a systolic pressure of 110 to 120 mmHg. Recent studies[5,6] have looked at using higher dose bolus IV nitrates and have shown good efficacy and safety, with improved results over low dose nitrates, furosemide and non-invasive ventilation. Patient numbers, however, have been small and these dosing regimes are not currently widely used.

Furosemide

Furosemide has been the first line treatment for patients with APO for many years. Its usefulness is due to venodilatory properties that lead to decreased preload as well as to its diuretic properties. The venodilation occurs before diuresis begins.[3] It can, however, lead to increased peripheral vascular resistance via reflex sympathetic and renin-angiotensin system actions.[7] As mentioned above, fluid overload is not usually a contributing factor in acute heart failure and thus diuresis is not a necessary endpoint of therapy. The obvious exception is in patients with APO of iatrogenic aetiology after IV fluid therapy.

Although it is an established therapy, there are no controlled studies that show benefit from the use of furosemide in APO. At least two studies have shown that nitrates are more beneficial than frusemide in relation to haemodynamic and clinical outcomes.[4,8] Nevertheless, a single dose of furosemide at 1–1.5 mg/kg is still commonly recommended in the initial management of this illness.

Morphine

Morphine's main role is in the relief of chest pain that is resistant to nitrate therapy. Its other effects in APO result from central sympatholysis and anxiolysis. The resultant vasodilation with reduced heart rate, blood pressure, and cardiac contractility causes decreased preload and myocardial oxygen demand. In addition, it may help alleviate some of the terror felt by patients with APO, but at the risk of reduced respiratory effort. Other negative aspects include its respiratory and central nervous system depressant effects, thus there must be close observation for any signs of narcosis. Patients with hypotension, altered conscious state or with respiratory depression should not be given morphine.

There have been no controlled studies looking at the role of morphine in the emergency department management of APO and one retrospective analysis linked its use to increased rates on intubation and ICU admission[9].

Morphine has been one of the major drugs used in the treatment of APO but its use is now controversial. If it is used, it should be in small titrated IV doses with close observation.

Ventilatory support

All patients with APO should be given high flow supplemental oxygen using an oxygen delivery system that can meet their minute volume needs, such as a venturi system. They are hypoxic and uncorrected this will worsen APO through direct pulmonary vascular constriction and reduced myocardial oxygen delivery.

Patients with severely decreased level of consciousness, agonal respirations, or respiratory arrest require endotracheal intubation and mechanical ventilatory support. This should be accomplished using rapid sequence induction.

In recent years, non-invasive ventilation, using continuous positive airway pressure (CPAP), or bi-level positive airway pressure (Bi-PAP), has allowed many patients to avoid endotracheal intubation. CPAP pressures of 5–10 cm H_2O are used. When using Bi-PAP expiratory pressures are usually begun at 3–5 cmH_2O with the inspiratory pressure 5–8 cm higher. The benefits of these therapies result from a number of effects. Oxygen concentration can be accurately controlled and higher percentages can be delivered than via a facemask. By using CPAP, functional capacity is increased by alveolar recruitment with a resultant increase in gas exchange area, improved pulmonary compliance and decreased work of breathing. The addition of inspiratory pressure support with Bi-PAP further decreases the work of breathing. Cardiovascular effects result from positive intrathoracic pressures, with decreased venous return and decreased left ventricular transmural pressures. These preload and afterload effects improve cardiac output without increasing myocardial oxygen demand. In general these therapies have had few complications and are considered safe. Complications that have been reported include nasal bridge abrasions, patient intolerance, gastric distension and aspiration, pneumothorax, and air embolism. The last two potentially serious adverse events are extremely rare and appear to occur in selected populations with other underlying disease processes (e.g. pneumothorax in patients with *Pneumocystis carinii* pneumonia).[10]

A number of studies have compared CPAP to conventional therapy in APO. They have been reviewed by Kosowsky et al,[11] Pang[12] and Cross.[10] There were significant improvements in oxygenation, ventilation, respiratory rate and distress, and heart rates, without significant adverse events. There were also decreased rates of endotracheal intubation and intensive care lengths of stay, without benefit being shown in terms of total length of hospital stay or mortality. The evidence for Bi-PAP is controversial. When compared to conventional therapy in the only randomized trial[13] it showed benefits in terms of more rapid resolution of symptoms, improved oxygenation, and decreased intubation rates. There was no difference in mortality or length of stay. However, this was a very small study and there were differences in underlying morbidity between the control and study groups. There has been one trial comparing Bi-PAP to CPAP in APO[14] that showed more rapid improvements in the Bi-PAP arm, without any medium-term benefit. This study was terminated early, however, because of a high rate of myocardial infarction in the Bi-PAP group. In another study comparing Bi-PAP to high dose nitrate therapy[6] the study was also terminated due to high rates of AMI, intubation and death in the Bi-PAP arm. As there is no convincing evidence of benefit of Bi-PAP over CPAP, and there is evidence of increased morbidity, Bi-PAP cannot be recommended for use in the treatment of APO at this time.

New agents

Nesiritide This drug is currently available in the USA. It is a recombinant brain natriuretic peptide. Its actions are to cause arterial (including coronary) and venous vasodilation, increase sodium excretion and to suppress the renin-angiotensin-aldosterone and sympathetic nervous systems.[15] It has been shown to increase cardiac index and to reduce pulmonary capillary wedge pressure, vascular resistance, and dyspnoea in patients with decompensated heart failure. Adverse events include dose-related hypotension and bradycardia.

This drug has recently been compared with IV nitrates and placebo in patients with decompensated heart failure and dyspnoea at rest. There were early improvements in pulmonary capillary wedge pressure and cardiac index with nesiritide, with equivalence by nitrates at 3 hours. There were equivalent improvements in dyspnoea by nesiritide and nitrates over placebo. Adverse events were similar, although hypotension was of longer duration with nesiritide.[16] Overall its therapeutic efficacy was equivalent to nitrates. There are no studies using the drug only in APO and thus its cannot be recommended as first line therapy at this time.

Endothelin antagonists Drugs from this class act to reduce systemic and pulmonary vascular resistance, increase cardiac output and decrease pulmonary capillary wedge pressure.[17] They have not yet been studied in the treatment of APO but may in the future be shown to be of benefit.

Hypotensive patients

In general patients with APO who are hypotensive are at the most severe end of the disease spectrum, having cardiogenic shock. They requirement both ventilatory and haemodynamic support. Endotracheal intubation, using rapid sequence induction, and ventilation maximize oxygen delivery and minimize oxygen utilization. Positive end expiratory pressure of 5–10 cm H_2O may be useful. These patients may have a fluid deficit and therefore cautious fluid bolus resuscitation should be titrated against haemodynamics and clinical effect. Inotropic support is also required with adrenaline (epinephrine) or dopamine being the first-line agents. These drugs will increase cardiac output but do so at the expense of increased myocardial oxygen demand and increased arrhythmogenicity. Invasive monitoring may be most useful in this group, as it helps guide fluid and inotropic management. Some time may be bought with

---

CONTROVERSIES

❶ The use of standard dose infusions versus high dose bolus nitrates.

❷ The use of Bi-PAP.

❸ The use and dosage of furosemide and morphine.

❹ The role of new agents such as nesiritide.

---

the use of invasive therapeutic manoeuvres such as an intra-aortic balloon pump. This device decreases myocardial oxygen demand via afterload reduction and increases coronary flow through diastolic augmentation. Reversible causes should be treated, e.g. PTCA for acute myocardial infarction, surgical correction of acute valvular dysfunction.

REFERENCES

1. Adnet F, Le Toumelin P, Leberre A, et al 2001 In-hospital and long-term prognosis of elderly patients requiring endotracheal intubation for life-threatening presentation of cardiogenic pulmonary edema. Critical Care Medicine 19: 891–5
2. Cotter G, Kaluski E, Moshkovitz Y, et al 2001 Pulmonary edema: new insight on pathogenesis and treatment. Current Opinion in Cardiology 16: 159–63
3. Morrison RA, Wiegand UW, Janchen E, et al 1983 Isosorbide dinitrate kinetics and dynamics after intravenous, sublingual and percutaneous dosing in angina. Clinical Pharmacology Therapy 33: 747–56
4. Dikshit K, Vyden JK, Forrester JS, et al 1973 Renal and extrarenal hemodynamic effects of furosemide in congestive heart failure after acute myocardial infarction. New England Journal of Medicine 288: 1087–90
5. Cotter G, Metzkor E, Kaluski E, et al 1998 Randomised trial of high-dose isosorbide dinitrate plus low-dose furosemide versus high-dose furosemide plus low-dose isosorbide dinitrate in severe pulmonary oedema. Lancet 351: 389–93
6. Sharon A, Shpirer I, Kaluski E, et al 2000 High-dose intravenous isosorbide dinitrate is safer and better than Bi-PAP ventilation combined with conventional treatment for severe pulmonary oedema. Journal of the American College of Cardiology 36: 832–7
7. Francis GS, Siegel RM, Goldsmith SR, et al 1985 Acute vasoconstrictor response to intravenous furosemide in patients with congestive heart failure. Annals of Internal Medicine 103: 1–6
8. Nelson GIC, Silke B, Ahuja RC, et al 1983 Haemodynamic advantages of isosorbide dinitrate over frusemide in acute heart failure following myocardial infarction. Lancet 1: 730–3
9. Sacchetti A, Ramoska E, Noakes ME, et al 1999 Effect of ED Management on ICU use in Acute Pulmonary Edema. American Journal of Emergency Medicine 17: 571–4
10. Cross AM 2000 Review of the role of non-invasive ventilation in the emergency department. Journal of Accident Emergency Medicine 17: 79–85
11. Kosowsky J, et al 2000 Continuous and bilevel positive airway pressure in the treatment of acute cardiogenic pulmonary edema. American Journal of Emergency Medicine 18: 91–5
12. Pang D, Keenan SP, Cook DJ, et al 1998 The effect of positive pressure airway support on mortality and the need for intubation in cardiogenic pulmonary edema. A Systematic review. Chest 114: 1185–92
13. Masip J, Betbesé AJ, Póez J, et al 2000 Non-invasive pressure support ventilation versus conventional oxygen therapy in acute cardiogenic pulmonary oedema: a randomised trial. Lancet 356: 2126–32
14. Mehta S, Jay GD, Woolard RH, et al 1997 Randomized, prospective trial of bilevel vs continuous positive airway pressure in acute pulmonary edema. Critical Care Medicine 25: 620–8
15. Colucci W, Elkayam U, Horton DP, et al 2000 Intravenous Nesiritide, a natriuretic peptide, in the treatment of decompensated congestive heart failure. New England Journal of Medicine 343: 246–53
16. Young JB, Abraham WT, Stevenson LW, et al 2002 Intravenous Nesiritide vs nitroglycerin for treatment of decompensated congestive heart failure. A randomized controlled trial Journal of American Medical Association 287: 1531–40
17. Spieker L, Mitrovic V, Noll G, et al 2000 Acute hemodynamic and neurohumeral effects of selective ET(A) receptor blockade in patients with congestive heart failure. ET 003 Investigators. Journal of the American College of Cardiology 35: 1745–52

4.4 ARRHYTHMIAS

ALASTAIR D. McR. MEYER

ESSENTIALS

1 The assessment of cardiac arrhythmias requires an understanding of the normal conducting system of the heart.

2 Tachyarrhythmias are generated by three fundamental mechanisms: re-entry; enhanced automaticity; after polarizations.

3 Bradyarrhythmias arise as a result of depression of sinus node activity or conduction system block.

4 Manage the patient, not just the ECG.

5 Haemodynamically stable patients with arrhythmias may not require urgent treatment.

6 Patients who are hypotensive, confused, have ischaemic chest pain or left ventricular failure with arrhythmias require urgent treatment.

7 A broad complex tachycardia should be considered VT until clear evidence is found to prove otherwise.

INTRODUCTION

Management of cardiac arrhythmias in the emergency department should be directed towards the patient and not the specific arrhythmia. In general, patients who are haemodynamically stable do not require immediate therapy. The key objective in a patient with abnormal haemodynamic parameters is the restoration of adequate cardiac output to maintain cerebral perfusion as well as a stable rhythm, using interventions least likely to cause harm.

Normal conducting system

The heartbeat originates in pacemaker cells that undergo spontaneous depolarization and initiate an electrical impulse.

This impulse is spread via conducting cells that form a specialized conducting system throughout the heart (Fig. 4.4.1).

The sinoatrial (SA) node, the internodal atrial pathways, the atrioventricular (AV) node, the bundle of His and its branches and the Purkinje system are anatomically and physiologically identifiable parts of this conducting system. The conducting system rapidly propagates an electrical impulse throughout the heart. The various parts of the conducting system are also capable of spontaneous discharge under abnormal conditions. The SA node is normally the dominant cardiac pacemaker and is located near the junction of the superior vena cava (SVC) and the right atrium (see Fig. 4.4.1). The rapidly propagated electrical impulse depolarizes the contractile cells of the heart, converting electrical energy into mechanical energy and causing myocardial contraction.

The blood supply of the sinoatrial (SA) node is from its own artery, which arises from the proximal right coronary artery in 55% of individuals and from the left circumflex in the remaining 45%. The SA node is innervated by both sympathetic and parasympathetic nerve endings. The intrinsic SA node discharge rate is between 90 and 100 beats per minute; however, because of the predominant resting parasympathetic tone, a healthy individual's heart rate is usually lower than this at rest.

The electrical conduction speed is different in the various parts of the conducting system (Table 4.4.1). Depolarization initiated in the SA node spreads rapidly through atrial tissue and converges on the AV node. The atria and ventricles are electrically isolated from each other by the annulus fibrosis. Under normal conditions the electrical impulses from the atria reach the ventricles by passing through the AV node and then the infra-

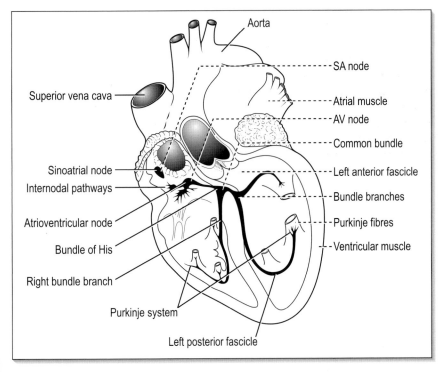

Fig. 4.4.1 Conducting system of the heart. (Reproduced with permission from Ganong WF 1995 A review of medical physiology, 17th edn. Appleton & Lange, Connecticut)

Table 4.4.1 Conduction speeds in cardiac tissue. (Reproduced with permission from Ganong WF 1995 A review of medical physiology, 17th edn. Appleton & Lange)

Tissue	Conduction rate (m/s)
SA node	0.05
Atrial pathways	1
AV node	0.05
Bundle of His	1
Purkinje system	4
Ventricular muscle	1

nodal conducting system. The AV node is located in the right atrial endocardium, near the insertion of the septal leaflet of the tricuspid valve. It receives its blood supply via a branch from the right coronary artery in 90% of people. In the remaining 10% the AV node receives its blood supply from the left circumflex artery.

Conduction velocity in the AV node is slow to allow time for atrial contraction to be completed, thus ensuring adequate ventricular filling. The delay of electrical conduction is shortened by stimulation of the sympathetic nerves to the heart, and lengthened by parasympathetic (vagal) discharge. This delay also serves to protect the ventricles from excessively rapid stimulation.

After leaving the AV node the electrical impulse travels along the bundle of His, which traverses the posterior margin of the membranous portion of the interventricular septum to reach the top of the ventricular muscle mass. The bundle is 1–2 cm long and divides at the crest of the muscular interventricular septum into the right and left bundle branches, the left having two distinct pathways to the base of the papillary muscles, the left anterior fascicle and the left posterior fascicle. These intraventricular conduction pathways are composed of specialized cells known as Purkinje cells, which have the ability to rapidly conduct electrical impulses as well as possessing a pacemaker ability. The electrical impulse travels to the endocardium via networks of Purkinje

cells that extend just beneath the surface of the right and left endocardia. The impulses then proceed slowly from endocardium to epicardium throughout the right and left ventricles. The right bundle branch and the left anterior fascicle receive blood from the AV nodal artery in 50% of people, and from the left anterior descending artery in the remaining 50%. The left posterior inferior fascicle receives blood supply from the AV nodal artery alone in 50% of people, and from both the AV nodal artery and left anterior descending artery in the remaining 50%.

Embryonic remnants of myocardium persist as accessory tracts. These are most commonly found about the AV node and are capable of conducting electrical activity between the atria and ventricles, thus bypassing the AV node. These bypass tracts are the anatomical basis for certain supraventricular tachyarrhythmias.

PATHOGENESIS OF ARRHYTHMIAS

Tachyarrhythmias

There are three fundamental mechanisms for the generation of tachyarrhythmias:

❶ Re-entry.
❷ Enhanced automaticity.
❸ After polarizations (triggered arrhythmias).

Re-entry

Re-entry occurs when a closed loop of conducting tissue transmits an electrical impulse around the loop and stimulates atrial or ventricular electrical activity with each pass around the circuit. Re-entry may occur on a large (macro) or small (micro) scale. Atrial and ventricular flutter and fibrillation are examples of micro re-entry; paroxysmal supraventricular tachycardia (PSVT) is an example of macro re-entry.

The features of a re-entry circuit are a conduction pathway that forms a closed loop and part of the closed loop exhibits unidirectional blockade of conduction. The area of unidirectional block allows an impulse to traverse the loop in one direction only, returning to its starting

point via the area of unidirectional block, allowing another circuit to commence. Re-entry can occur around anatomically defined circuits, resulting in a regular rapid rhythm such as paroxysmal supraventricular tachycardia (PSVT). Conversely, re-entry can also occur in a disorganized and chaotic fashion through a syncytium of myocardial tissue, as in atrial fibrillation or ventricular fibrillation.

Enhanced automaticity

Abnormal or ectopic impulse formation may be the result of enhanced automaticity. The primary pacemaker cells of the SA and AV nodes may generate slow response action potentials, and have the ability to spontaneously depolarize, thus demonstrating automaticity. The cells of the conducting system generate fast action potentials and may also spontaneously depolarize. These cells are, however, normally overridden by the dominant SA node. Under adverse physiological conditions of hypokalaemia, hypoxaemia or catecholamine activity the threshold potential of conducting and contracting cells may be altered, thereby creating a situation of enhanced automaticity and secondary ectopic pacemakers. An example of enhanced automaticity is multifocal atrial tachycardia, which is due to multiple secondary ectopic atrial pacemakers associated with hypoxaemia.

After polarizations (triggered arrhythmias)

Abnormal impulse formation is often due to oscillations of the transmembrane potential during or after repolarization. These oscillations may reach the threshold membrane potential and trigger a second complete depolarization. This process may be self-perpetuating. Torsades de pointes is the classic example of a triggered arrhythmia.

Bradyarrhythmias

Two mechanisms are responsible for bradyarrhythmias:

❶ Depression of sinus node activity.
❷ Conduction system block.

In spite of these, a subsidiary pacemaker may take over and pace the heart.

GENERAL PRINCIPLES FOR THE MANAGEMENT OF ARRHYTHMIAS

Patients presenting to the emergency department with an arrhythmia should be managed in an area where they can be closly monitored. Such patients commonly show evidence of hypoperfusion, and, therefore, a team approach to find the cause and treat the arrhythmia may be required.

Attention is first directed to management of the patient's ABCs, as described in Chapter 1.2.[1-4] Intravenous access is gained and blood drawn for routine tests and specific biochemistry, as indicated by the history. A 12-lead ECG is essential and a chest X-ray should be performed. Routine blood biochemistry includes full blood examination, electrolytes, urea and creatinine level, magnesium and calcium levels. Cardiac markers should also be measured.

Specific investigations may also be clinically indicated, e.g. thyroid function tests, digoxin level and theophylline level.

The key objective in an unstable patient is the restoration of adequate cerebral perfusion and a stable rhythm. Haemodynamically stable patients generally do not require immediate treatment, despite the arrhythmia. The objective in these patients is to establish a diagnosis and to determine whether cardioversion is low risk and the resultant rhythm, once reverted, is likely to be sustained.

Bradyarrhythmias

The need to treat bradyarrhythmias is dictated primarily by the clinical state of the patient. If there is evidence of hypoperfusion, most bradyarrhythmias will respond initially to atropine.[5]

Sinus bradycardia

Sinus rhythm with a ventricular rate of less than 60 beats per minute is termed sinus bradycardia, the clinical significance of which is determined by a thorough history and a clinical examination. Physiological sinus bradycardia is associated with young adults and athletes. Patients on beta-blocker therapy and some calcium channel antagonists may also present with sinus bradycardia.

Sinus bradycardia may also be caused by acute inferior myocardial ischaemia and infarction, raised intracranial pressure (Cushing's reflex), bradycardia-tachycardia syndrome, hypothermia and hypothyroidism. Special investigations are directed to these causes.

Clinical features   Often no signs or symptoms are evident. Dizziness, light-headedness and syncope are the most common symptoms.

ECG features
- Normal P-wave morphology
- Normal PR interval
- 1:1 AV conduction
- Atrial rate less than 60 beats per minute.

Management   Special management is not usually required. If the patient has evidence of hypoperfusion, 0.4–0.6 mg of atropine IV is indicated as a temporizing measure while the cause is investigated.

Disposition   This is very much dependent on the cause of the sinus bradycardia. Pharmacological agents responsible should be ceased, and the patient's response monitored. If it can be established that myocardial pathology is not the cause of the problem, the patient may be safely discharged home.

Bradycardia-tachycardia syndrome (sick sinus syndrome)

The bradycardia-tachycardia syndrome is most commonly found in the elderly as a result of fibrosis around the sinus node. It may also occur with ischaemia and congenital heart disease. There is often an association with more widespread conduction pathway disease. The bradycardia-tachycardia syndrome is caused by sinus bradycardia and intermittent failure of sinus node function. P-wave activity is ceased and a prolonged pause is seen, interrupted by a temporary escape rhythm. The episode may be exacerbated by pharmacological agents (beta-blockers, digoxin), and these should be ceased.

Clinical features   Typical features are syncope, light-headedness and/or collapse.

ECG features
- Sinus bradycardia
- Intermittent cessation of P-wave activity
- Long pause, interrupted by escape rhythm
- Resumption of sinus node activity, often tachycardiac.

Management   Emergency department management is indicated for haemodynamically compromised patients. Management consists of atropine 0.4–0.6 mg IV as a temporizing measure prior to pacing. A transcutaneous or temporary transvenous pacemaker should be considered if atropine is ineffective.

Disposition   All patients have the potential to degenerate into ventricular standstill. Consequently, referral to the cardiology team and admission is essential. Permanent pacing will be required.

Heart block

First-degree AV block

In first-degree AV block atrial activity is conducted to the ventricles but there is a delay in the conduction. A P wave precedes each QRS complex, but the PR interval is greater than 0.2 seconds. This represents a delay in the conduction in the AV node (Fig. 4.4.2). First-degree AV

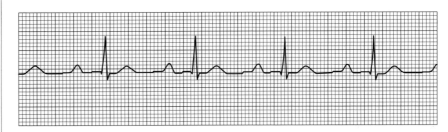

Fig. 4.4.2 Rhythm strip of first-degree AV block.

block is found in normal hearts as a result of increased vagal tone, digoxin toxicity, inferior myocardial infarction, idiopathic fibrosis and aortic valve disease.

Clinical features

There are no specific clinical features.

ECG features

- Sinus rhythm
- PR interval greater than 0.2 seconds, constant.

Management

No treatment is required unless associated with acute ischaemia, where monitoring with a view to pacing is required. There are no accepted indications for pacing in isolated first-degree block.

Disposition

Unless associated with acute ischaemia, first-degree AV block is not, in itself, an indication for hospital admission.

Second-degree AV block: Mobitz I (Wenckebach)

This is exemplified by progressive prolongation of the PR interval before an atrial impulse fails to stimulate the ventricle, resulting in a 'missed' or 'dropped' QRS complex. The block is anatomically above the bundle of His in the AV node. The pathogenesis is believed to be due to prolongation of the refractory period of the AV node (Fig. 4.4.3).

Second-degree Mobitz I is often transiently associated with inferior myocardial infarction, digoxin toxicity and high vagal tone. This condition is nearly always benign and asymptomatic; however, in the setting of an acute myocardial infarction it may progress to complete heart block.

Clinical features

Usually there are no specific clinical features. Patients may complain of palpitations, missed beats or a thumping heart.

ECG features

Progressive lengthening of the PR interval until an atrial impulse is completely blocked. This is often a cyclical pattern.

Management

The stable patient requires no therapy, and management is aimed at excluding myocardial ischaemia. If the patient's cardiac output is poor, 0.4–0.6 mg of IV atropine may be used. Cardiac pacing may be indicated in selected cases.

Disposition

This is nearly always a benign condition. If it occurs in association with ischaemia, admission is recommended.

Second-degree AV block: Mobitz II

In second-degree AV block (Mobitz II), the PR interval remains constant, with regular intermittent failure of P-wave conduction. Mobitz II blocks usually occur in the infranodal conducting system (the bundle of His) and are frequently associated with bundle branch blocks or fascicular blocks. Advanced second-degree block is the block of two or more consecutive P waves (Fig. 4.4.4).

Clinical features

There are usually no specific clinical features, but some patients may experience syncope.

ECG features

- Constant PR interval
- Intermittent omission of QRS complex.

Management

Intravenous atropine, 0.4–0.6 mg IV, prior to pacing.

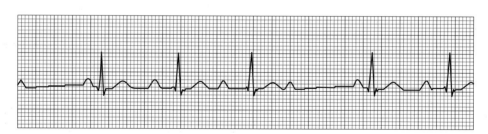

Fig. 4.4.3 Rhythm strip of second-degree AV block, Mobitz I.

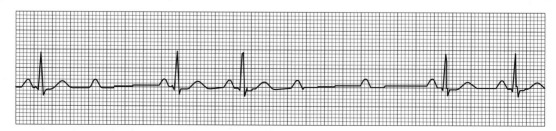

Fig. 4.4.4 Rhythm strip of second-degree AV block, Mobitz II.

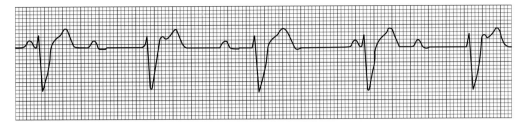

Fig. 4.4.5 Rhythm strip of third-degree heart block.

Disposition

Patients with this condition must be admitted, as second-degree AV block can deteriorate to complete heart block.

Third-degree heart block (complete heart block)

Third-degree heart block is complete dissociation of the atrial and ventricular rhythms (Fig. 4.4.5). The ventricles are paced by an escape pacemaker at a rate slower than the atrial rate. Anatomically, the block can occur either at the AV node or at the infranodal level. The width of the QRS complex and the rate of the ventricular rhythm may help to decide at which level the block is occurring. A narrow QRS with a junctional escape rhythm of 40–60 beats per minute implies a nodal block, whereas a widened QRS with a ventricular escape rhythm of less than 40 beats per minute implies an infranodal block.

The commonest cause of complete heart block is myocardial fibrosis; however, in the emergency department complete heart block is seen in up to 8% of acute inferior myocardial infarctions. In the latter setting it is often transient. Complete heart block is also associated with sick sinus syndrome, Mobitz II, and transient second-degree block with a new bundle branch or fascicular block.

Clinical features

The patient may be asymptomatic. Syncope is common. Cannon 'a' waves may be seen in the neck veins, and there is varying loudness of the first heart sound.

ECG features

• Complete dissociation of P waves and QRS complex

• Ventricular escape pacemaker at 20–50 bpm
• QRS complexes may be wide or narrow.

Management

Treatment of complete heart block is similar to that for Mobitz II. Temporary pacing is required for patients who are haemodynamically compromised. Again, temporizing measures may be taken, with cautious use of intravenous atropine (0.4–0.6 mg). Isoprenaline infusion titrated to effect may be used as a temporizing agent only. It may worsen the patient's condition as a result of vasodilatation of skeletal muscle vascular beds and resultant coronary hypoperfusion. In the setting of myocardial ischaemia and complete heart block it is, therefore, preferable to use external cardiac pacing prior to placement of a pacing wire. Adrenaline (epinephrine) infusion, titrated to effect, is preferable in ischaemic tissue as coronary perfusion is better maintained.

Disposition

Admission to a monitored bed is usually indicated. Sometimes patients present with a history over days to weeks, in which case a permanent pacing wire may be inserted electively.

Bundle branch blocks

Bundle branch blocks are caused by abnormal conduction of the electrical impulse through the conducting network of the heart.

Right bundle branch block

Clinical features

Right bundle branch block (RBBB) can be a normal variant. It may also be seen

in massive pulmonary embolus, right ventricular hypertrophy, ischaemic heart disease, congenital heart disease and cor pulmonale.

ECG features

Incomplete RBBB shows a QRS complex which has an rSR pattern, most noted in right ventricular leads V_1 and V_2. Left ventricular leads show a broad S wave. Complete RBBB shows a widened QRS of more than 120 ms duration, rSR pattern and broad S wave in the left ventricular leads (Fig. 4.4.6).

Management

If RBBB is new, the cause should be determined. Monitoring is advised to document progression, especially in the setting of myocardial ischaemia.

Disposition

If new, consider admission and monitoring.

Left bundle branch block

Left bundle branch block (LBBB) is due to the interventricular septum being activated from right to left, rather than the normal left to right. In the presence of LBBB, myocardial ischaemia and infarction can be difficult to diagnose. It is noted in Chapter 4.2 that a new LBBB with clinical features of myocardial ischaemia must be considered as evidence of an infarct.[6]

Clinical features

LBBB may present with no clinical abnormality. It is associated with congenital heart disease, left ventricular hypertrophy, left ventricular strain and left ventricular ischaemia.

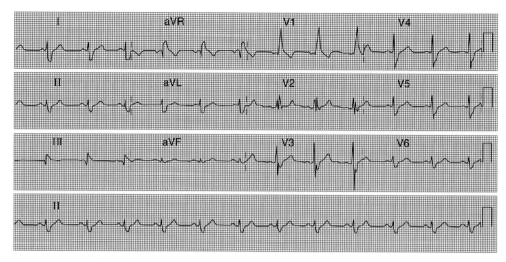

Fig. 4.4.6 Right bundle branch block.

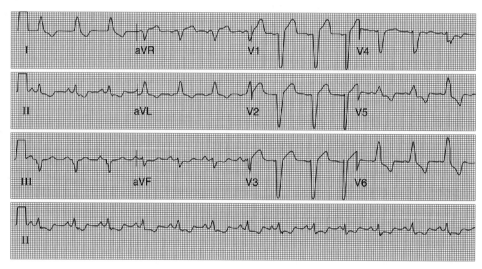

Fig. 4.4.7 Left bundle branch block.

ECG features
- Wide QRS (>120 ms)
- RR pattern, best seen in left ventricular leads (V₅, V₆) (Fig. 4.4.7).

Management

Usually no treatment is required, unless a new LBBB is found in the setting of features of myocardial ischaemia (see Chapter 4.2).

Disposition

If new myocardial ischaemia cannot be excluded, the patient should be admitted and monitored.

Fascicular blocks

Block of the infranodal conduction pathway is seen in RBBB, left anterior fascicular block (LAFB) and left posterior fascicular block (LPFB). Blockade of electrical conduction through any of these pathways can be caused by ischaemia, cardiomyopathy, valvular heart disease, myocarditis, cardiac surgery and congenital heart disease.

LAFB

Clinical features

There are usually no specific clinical features.

ECG features
- Normal QRS duration, left axis deviation.

Management and disposition

Emergency department management is directed at determining the cause for the conduction block. Ischaemic heart disease is the most common cause, and if clinical features indicate this, the patient should be admitted and monitored.

LPFB

Clinical features

There are usually no specific clinical features.

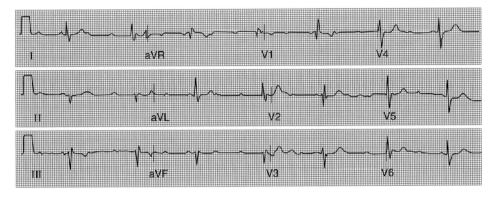

Fig. 4.4.8 Incomplete RBBB and LAFB.

ECG features
- Right axis deviation, normal QRS duration.

Management and disposition
Aimed at determining the cause of the conduction block.

Combination blocks (Fig. 4.4.8)
Bifascicular block refers to conduction blocks of two fascicles:

- RBB and LAFB
- RBB and LPFB
- LBBB.

Clinical features
There are usually no specific clinical features.

Management and disposition
Aim to identify and treat ischaemia. In the setting of acute ischaemia, prophylactic pacemaker insertion may be indicated.

Trifascicular block is a combination of conduction blocks in all three fascicles. It may be permanent or a transient abnormality.

- RBBB and LAFB with 1° AVB
- RBBB and LPFB with 1° AVB
- LBBB and 1° AVB
- Alternating RBBB and LBBB.

In the setting of AMI, both bi- and trifascicular blocks may degenerate to complete heart block. Consequently, admission to a monitored bed is essential, and prophylactic pacemaker insertion is advised.

Tachyarrhythmias

There is a wide range of tachyarrhythmias. Immediate diagnosis and management may be considered on the basis of the width of the QRS complex. Broad complex tachyarrhythmias have a QRS complex greater than 120 ms; narrow complex tachyarrhythmias have a QRS complex less than 120 ms. Broad complex tachyarrhythmias should be considered to be ventricular in origin.[1,7]

Broad complex tachycardia

The differential diagnosis for a regular broad complex tachycardia includes ventricular tachycardia (VT), or a supraventricular tachycardia (SVT) with aberrant conduction.[8] Considerable research has been undertaken in an attempt to define 12-lead ECG criteria that can reliably distinguish VT from SVT. Sensitivities and specificities of greater than 90% have been reported for some criteria (Brugada[9] and Wellens[10]); however, the high prevalence of VT in the emergency department (approximately 80% of all broad complex tachycardias) lowers the predictive value of even the best criteria[11] (Table 4.4.2).

Ventricular tachycardia is the occurrence of three or more beats from a ventricular ectopic pacemaker. It is usually secondary to ischaemic heart disease, acute myocardial infarction or dilated cardiomyopathy. Any disease of the myocardium that results in fibrosis can also lead to VT in the younger patient.

Ventricular tachycardia

Clinical features
The patient may have no symptoms, or palpitations. Dizziness and/or angina may be described. Cannon '*a*' waves may

Table 4.4.2 Features that increase the chance of broad complex tachycardia being diagnosed as VT[6–8]		
History	*Clinical features*	*ECG features*
Age >35 years	Cannon '*a*' wave in JVP	AV dissociation
Smoker	Variable intensity of S1	Fusion beats
Ischaemic heart disease	Unchanged intensity of S2	Capture beats
Previous VT		QRS with >140 ms (<120 ms SVT)
Active angina		Concordance of QRS vectors in pericardial leads
		Left axis variation >30° favours VT
		QRS morphology in V1
N: If any doubt, treat as VT!		

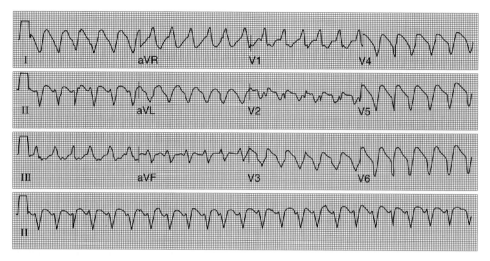

Fig. 4.4.9 Ventricular tachycardia (VT).

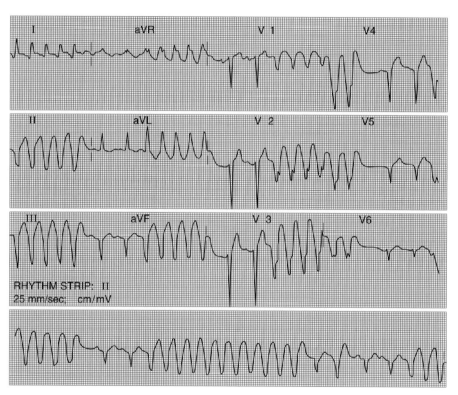

Fig. 4.4.10 Non-sustained VT.

be seen in the neck veins. The patient may also lose consciousness.

ECG features
- Wide QRS greater than 140 ms
- Rate greater than 100 bpm (commonly 150–200 bpm)
- Rhythm regular, although some beat-to-beat variability

- QRS axis constant (Figs 4.4.9 and 4.4.10).

Management
VT should be managed in accordance with AHA ECC guidelines[8] (Fig. 4.4.11). An unstable patient must be treated with cardioversion. Shock resistant VT may respond after the administration of IV amiodarone. Lidocaine, magnesium and procainamide are considered second-line adjunct to cardioversion, but have less evidence for their efficacy.[8,12] A patient who has a cardiac output sufficient to provide adequate cerebral perfusion may be treated with cardioversion, amiodarone (2–3 mg/kg IV) or procainamide (1 mg/kg IV) in the first instance.

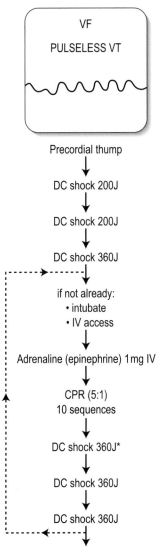

Fig. 4.4.11 VF/VT protocol.

Notes
- *the interval between these two shocks should be less than 2 min
- adrenaline (epinephrine) should be given every 2–3 min
- after three loops consider alkalinizing agents and/or antiarrhythmic drugs

PROLONGED RESUSCITATION:
Consider alkalinizing agents
e.g. 50 mmol sodium bicarbonate
(50 ml of 8.4%)
or according to blood gas analysis

POST RESUSCITATION CARE CHECK:
- arterial blood gases
- electrolytes
- chest X-ray
Observe, monitor and treat
in an intensive care area

Lidocaine may also be used, however this agent is relatively ineffective for termination of haemodynamically stable VT of unknown aetiology.[8] Lidocaine may suppress ventricular tachyarrythmias associated with acute myocardial ischaemia and infarction. Sotalol (1 mg/kg) may be considered as a second line agent.

Misdiagnosis of broad complex is common. More than 50% of broad complex tachycardias in adults are misdiagnosed by initial care providers and patients subsequently receive inappropriate treatment. Verapamil, a calcium channel blocker often used for the treatment of SVT, may cause hypotension if administered to patients with VT.

Torsades de pointes

Torsades de pointes (from the French, meaning 'twisting of the points') was first described in 1966 by Dessertenne (Fig. 4.4.12).[13] This is a polymorphic VT that rotates around the isoelectric line of the ECG, thereby continually changing its axis. This arrhythmia may be self-limiting and recurrent, and may degenerate rapidly into ventricular fibrillation (VF).

It is thought that the basic prerequisite for this condition is a prolonged QT interval, which is usually the result of the use of antiarrhythmic drugs, especially class I antiarrhythmics and amiodarone and sotalol. Tricyclic antidepressants, which have class I activity, are also associated with prolongation of the QT interval, as are phenothiazines. Congenital long QT syndrome is a rare familial disorder. Torsades de pointes is occasionally secondary to ischaemia (Table 4.4.3).

Clinical features
Syncope is the usual presenting symptom.

ECG features
- Regular or irregular fast, wide QRS complexes
- Variable, twisting axis.

Management
Torsades de pointes is very sensitive to magnesium.[14] A 2 g bolus given over 1 minute, followed by an infusion, will usually cause reversion. Defibrillation is

Table 4.4.3 Causes of torsades de pointes
Hypomagnesaemia
Hypocalcaemia
Class I and class II antiarrhythmic drugs
Phenothiazines
Tricyclic antidepressants
Congenital prolonged QT syndrome
Organophosphates
Complete heart block
Drug interaction of terfenidine with erythromycin

recommended if the patient is haemodynamically compromised; however, torsades de pointes can be resistant to defibrillation. Accelerating the heart rate, thereby shortening ventricular repolarization, may be successful. This may be precipitated by overdrive pacing to a heart rate of 90–120 beats per minute, isoprenaline infusion (titrated to effect) and/or transcutaneous pacing can be tried to accelerate the heart rate.

Attention to the underlying cause is essential, as torsades de pointes is very difficult to control.

Disposition
Admission to CCU for monitoring and investigation.

Narrow complex tachyarrhythmias

Sinus tachycardia
This is defined as a heart rate greater than 100 beats per minute. Sinus tachycardia is not an arrhythmia but is usually a marker of an underlying disorder. Assessment is directed towards identifying the underlying cause, and management is of the identified disorder. The diagnosis is established by the presence of P waves of normal morphology in the normal relationship to the QRS complex. Common causes include shock, cardiac failure, anaemia, drug intoxication, fever, pain, anxiety, thyrotoxicosis and pregnancy.

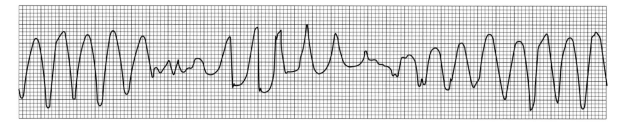

Fig. 4.4.12 Torsades de pointes.

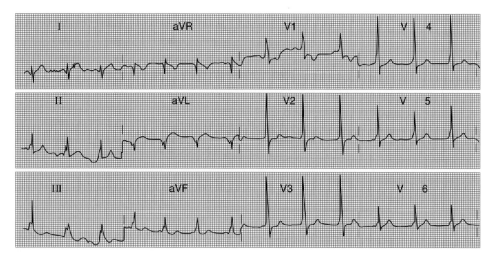

Fig. 4.4.13 Wolff-Parkinson-White syndrome: 12-lead ECG showing d waves.

Paroxysmal supraventricular tachycardia

Paroxysmal supraventricular tachycardia (PSVT) is a broad and rather confusing label that encompasses arrhythmias of varied aetiologies. Strictly, the term PSVT is applied to those arrhythmias that incorporate the atrium in the tachycardia circuit. Atrial tachycardias, atrial fibrillation (AF), atrial flutter and AV re-entry tachycardia are included in this group. AF and atrial flutter will be considered separately.

PSVT originates from either an ectopic atrial focus or a re-entry circuit. An ectopic focus discharges at a rate of 100–250 beats per minute, and can be seen in acute myocardial ischaemia, lung disease, alcohol intoxication and digoxin toxicity. Re-entry circuits are responsible for pre-excitation, which exists when the whole or part of the ventricular muscle is activated earlier than anticipated. The majority of these re-entry circuits involve the AV node. Re-entry SVT within the AV node is usually initiated when an ectopic atrial impulse encounters the AV node during the partial refractory period. There are two functionally different parallel conducting limbs within the AV node, connected above at the atrial end and below at the ventricular end of the node.

Retrograde conduction may also involve an AV bypass tract. Wolff-Parkinson-White syndrome is the most common of these, with an incidence of 1–3 per 1000; 40–80% of whom experience PSVT. The features of Wolff-Parkinson-White syndrome were described in 1930 and are characterized by an electrically conductive muscle bridge (bundle of Kent) connecting atria and ventricle, bypassing the AV node. During sinus rhythm the ECG shows a PR interval less than 0.12 seconds, slurred upstroke (the delta wave) and a wide QRS >0.10 seconds (Fig. 4.4.13).

Clinical features

Patients experience palpitations, chest pain and syncope, with tachycardia paroxysms.

ECG features

Narrow complex tachycardia (Fig. 4.4.14).

Management

The initial management of PSVT in the patient with abnormal haemodynamic parameters is DC reversion.[1-4,15] Sedation is usually required and energy levels of 100–360J should be used.

If the patient is asymptomatic and has a blood pressure higher than 100 mmHg, non-invasive vagal manoeuvres may be of benefit.

Adenosine, administered in a large proximal vein with a 20 mL flush in increasing doses, will terminate most PSVT. Intravenous bolus doses of 6 mg, 12 mg and 18 mg should be tried sequentially, prior to consideration of second-line drugs. Patients experience a transient sense of anxiety, impending doom, chest discomfort and shortness of breath with adenosine, this can be quite distressing for some and may be tempered with pre-treatment of midazolam.[16]

Verapamil 5–15 mgIV slowly over a

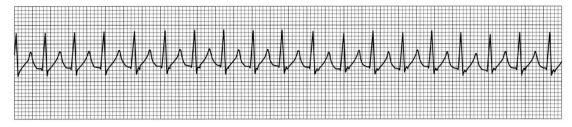

Fig. 4.4.14 Paroxysmal supraventricular tachycardia (PSVT).

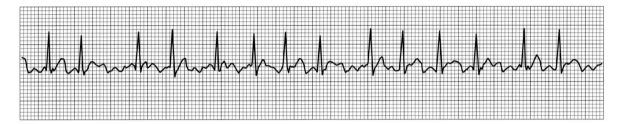

Fig. 4.4.15 Rhythm strip of atrial fibrillation.

2–5-minute period may be used with caution, as a precipitant drop in blood pressure may occur. Concurrent use of beta-blockers may add to the negative inotropic effects of verapamil in these patients.[17]

Flecainide in a dose of 2 mg/kg over 15–45 minutes may be considered as a third-line agent in the treatment of PSVT. Haemodynamically normal patients, who are resistant to chemical reversion, may be cardioverted.

Disposition

If myocardial ischaemia is not suspected the patient may be discharged from the emergency department once sinus rhythm is restored. Outpatient followup is essential.

Atrial fibrillation

Atrial fibrillation (AF) is the result of chaotic atrial depolarization from multiple areas of re-entry within the atria. It is the commonest sustained disorder of cardiac rhythm. There is an absence of coordinated atrial activity. AF is characterized by the absence of discrete P waves, and a narrow complex ventricular rate, which is irregularly irregular.[18]

Clinical features

Paroxysmal AF is typically fast and symptomatic. Irregular palpitations, dyspnoea

and dizziness are experienced; angina may also occur.

Patients with chronic AF usually experience no specific features, especially if the ventricular rate is less than 100 beats per minute. If the ventricular rate becomes rapid (130–180 beats per minute) dyspnoea, angina and syncope may be evident.

Causes of rapid AF seen in the emergency department

Cardiac

- Ischaemic heart disease
- Pericarditis
- Hypertension
- Rheumatic heart disease
- Pre-excitation syndromes
- Cardiomyopathy
- Atrial septal defect
- Atrial myxoma
- Postoperative (especially thoracotomy).

Non-cardiac

- Electrolyte disturbances
- Sepsis
- Pulmonary embolus
- Drug and alcohol intoxication
- Chronic obstructive airways disease
- Thyrotoxicosis
- Lung carcinoma
- Intrathoracic pathology.

ECG features

- Fibrillatory waves of atrial activity may be seen in V_1, V_2, V_3 and aVF
- Ventricular response rate is irregularly irregular (Fig. 4.4.15).

Management

Emergency department management depends on the chronicity of the arrhythmia, the ventricular response rate, the presence or absence of underlying structural heart disease, and the presence of associated or underlying disorders.

The aim of treatment in those with chronic AF is to control ventricular rate by slowing AV node conduction. In those with paroxysmal AF the aim is not only to control ventricular rate, but to effect cardioversion to sinus rhythm.[19]

Investigations for patients with paroxysmal AF include full blood examination, electrolytes, magnesium and thyroid function tests. A 12-lead ECG and chest X-ray are also necessary. The purpose of these tests is to identify a cause of AF.

An otherwise well patient with paroxysmal atrial fibrillation in the absence of structural heart disease or another underlying disorder has at least a 90% chance of spontaneously reverting to sinus rhythm without specific treatment, within 48 hours. These patients are said to have 'idiopathic' or 'lone' atrial fibrillation; this is a diagnosis of exclusion. It may be paroxysmal or persistent, and is present in 3–11% of all patients with AF. Such patients may be simply observed, or given an agent to control the ventricular response rate if this is greater than 100 beats per minute.[18]

Ventricular rate control can be achieved by slowing AV node conduction. Beta-blockers and calcium channel blockers are effective AV nodal blocking agents and may be used for this purpose, however, such agents must be used with caution if there is evidence of CCF. Metoprolol (5–10 mg IV over 2 minutes), propranolol (1 mg over 2 minutes, repeat up to 5 mg) and verapamil (5–10 mg over 2 minutes) are in common use. Digoxin is also used in the acute setting; however, digoxin is a weak AV nodal-blocking agent and ventricular rate control is mainly through its vagal tonic effect. It may take several hours to have an effect on ventricular rate, and some studies have implied that the use of digoxin may actually prolong the duration of AF. Amiodarone alone or in conjunction with digoxin is effective for rate control.[20]

High sympathetic tone will increase AV node conduction. Consequently, associated features such as pain, hypoxia and hypovolaemia should be corrected. Electrolyte disturbances should also be corrected.

The second aim of treatment, that of cardioversion, may be achieved electrically or pharmacologically. Synchronized DC reversion is the treatment of choice if there is haemodynamic compromise. Sixty per cent of patients can be cardioverted with 100J, 80% with 200J.[2,18,19]

Pharmacological cardioversion can be achieved with flecainide (2 mg/kg IV over 20–30 minutes), amiodarone (2–3 mg/kg IV over 5 minutes, repeated if unsuccessful) or sotalol (1 mg/kg over 30 minutes). Flecainide should not be used if there is evidence of ischaemic heart disease or cardiac failure. In patients with Wolf-Parkinson-White syndrome extremely rapid ventricular responses may occur during episodes of AF. In such cases, the use of adenosine, calcium channel blockers, beta-blockers or digoxin may adversely accelerate the ventricular response. Amiodarone or procainamide are the preferred agents to use.

Cardioversion (electrical or pharmacological) carries a risk of left atrial embolization if the arrhythmia has been present for longer than 24 hours. Cardioversion to sinus rhythm has an increased chance of success if the AF has been of short duration (less than 72 hours) and the left atrium is not dilated.[18,19]

Disposition

Patients with paroxysmal AF which does not revert should be admitted. Those with chronic AF who present with uncontrolled ventricular rate should also be admitted. Most patients can be discharged if they have been successfully cardioverted and there is no evidence of myocardial ischaemia. Outpatient review is essential.

Atrial flutter

Atrial flutter rarely occurs in the absence of underlying heart disease. It is a rhythm that originates from a small area within the atria. The exact mechanism, re-entry or triggered, is not clear.

Causes of atrial flutter

- Ischaemic heart disease
- AMI (2% of all AMI)
- Congestive cardiac failure
- Pulmonary embolus
- Myocarditis
- Chest trauma
- Rarely digoxin toxicity.

Clinical features

Commonly asymptomatic. Palpitations are the most common complaint. Importantly, flutter is associated with ischaemia.

ECG features

- Atrial flutter is characterized by a sawtooth-type pattern of atrial activity, best seen in leads II, III and aVF
- Atrial rate of 300 beats per minute
- Commonest AV block is 2:1, resulting in a ventricular rate of 150 beats per minute (Fig. 4.4.16).

Management

Atrial flutter is an unstable rhythm and usually responds to low-energy cardioversion. In the haemodynamically unstable patient 90% of cases revert to sinus rhythm with 25–50J of energy. Flecainide may be used to revert atrial flutter. Verapamil will control ventricular rate, but reversion is rare. Spontaneous reversion is also commonly seen during treatment for the underlying illness. In the haemodynamically stable patient treating the underlying cause is best, with no specific management of the arrhythmia required.

Atrial ectopic beats

Atrial ectopic beats appear on the ECG as an early P wave, often with an abnormal morphology. They may be followed by a QRS complex and are less common than ventricular ectopics. Up to 60% of adults have atrial ectopics on a 24-hour ECG recording, and they are mostly asymptomatic. Treatment in the

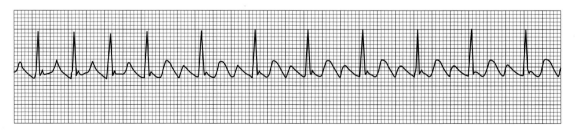

Fig. 4.4.16 Rhythm strip of atrial flutter.

ED is not indicated, other than advice in regard to modification of risk factors. Atrial ectopics can be precipitated by nicotine, alcohol and caffeine.

Multifocal atrial tachycardia

Multifocal atrial tachycardia (MFAT) is a rare atrial arrhythmia is characterized by three or more atrial foci, a ventricular rate of more than 100 beats per minute, and variable PP, PR and RR intervals. It is seen in patients with electrolyte disturbances, especially hypocalcaemia and hypomagnesaemia, hypoxia (especially COAD and pulmonary embolus), and is a feature of digoxin toxicity. Treatment is directed at improving the underlying condition. Treatment of the arrhythmia specifically with antiarrhythmic agents is rarely required and often not helpful.

PRETERMINAL ARRHYTHMIAS

Pulseless electrical activity

Pulseless electrical activity (PEA) or electromechanical dissociation is the presence of ventricular electrical activity with no evidence of cardiac output. The aetiology can be considered as either mechanical or metabolic (Table 4.4.4).

PEA results in circulatory collapse. The observed rhythm rapidly degenerates into VF or asystole. Management is directed at the presumed cause and in accordance with ALS protocols. The prognosis for PEA is very poor.

Asystole

Asystole is demonstrated by a complete absence of electrical activity. It is impor-

Table 4.4.4 Causes of PEA	
Mechanical	Metabolic
Pericardial tamponade	Acidosis
Tension pneumothorax imbalance leading to excitation contraction coupling discruption	Electrolyte
Massive pulmonary embolism	Hypothermia
Severe hypovolaemia	

CONTROVERSIES

❶ Asystole: has a very poor outcome. Does ALS improve survival once diagnosis has been confirmed?

❷ High-dose adrenaline (epinephrine): is there any value in its use? Initial enthusiasm following reports of increased return of circulation has been tempered by a lack of survivors leaving hospital.

❸ Post resuscitation care: routine use of lidocaine infusions post VF/VT. It is unclear whether these infusions alter outcome.

❹ Second-line antiarrhythmics: poor evidence for the use of many second-line agents, e.g. amiodarone in AF, bretylium in VF.

tant to exclude lead displacement, fine VF and extreme bradycardia. Asystole may be secondary to hyperkalaemia, acidosis, digoxin toxicity or pacemaker failure.

The outcome from this rhythm is invariably poor, but it is best to treat as fine VF. Standard ALS protocols should be followed.[1] In the pre-hospital arena, once the diagnosis of asystole has been reached, no further action is indicated.[21,22]

REFERENCES

1. American Heart Association ECC Guidelines 2000 Circulation 102: I-1-I-171
2. Adult advanced life support 1993 The Australian Resuscitation Council Guidelines. Medical Journal of Australia 159: 616–21
3. Advanced Life Support Working Party of the European Resuscitation Council Guidelines for advanced life support 1992 Resuscitation 24: 111–21
4. Colquhoun MC, Handley AJ, Evans TR (eds) 1996 ABC of resuscitation. BMJ Publishing, London
5. Brady WJ Jr, Harrigan RA 1998 Evaluation and management of bradyarrhythmias in the emergency department. Emergency Clinics of North America 162: 361–87
6. Sgarbossa EB, Pinski SL, Barbagelata A, et al 1996 Electrocardiographic diagnosis of evolving acute myocardial infarction in the presence of left bundle branch block. New England Journal of Medicine 34: 481–7
7. Shah CP, Thakur RK, Xie B, Hoon VK 1998 Clinical approach to wide QRS complex

tachycardias. Emergency Clinics of North America 16(2): 331–59
8. Atkins DC, Dorian P, Gonzalez ER, et al 2001 Treatment of Tachyarythmias. Annals of Emergency Medicine 37(4): S91–S110
9. Brugada P, Brugada J, Mont L, et al 1991 A new approach to the differential diagnosis of regular tachycardia with a wide QRS complex. Circulation 83: 1649–59
10. Wellen HJJ, Frits WHM, Lie KI 1978 The value of the electrocardiogram in the differential diagnosis of a tachycardia with a widened QRS complex. American Journal of Medicine 64: 27
11. Herbert ME, Votey SR, Morgan MT, Cameron PA, Dziukas L 1996 Failure to agree on the electrocardiographic diagnosis of ventricular tachycardia. Annals of Emergency Medicine 27(1): 35–8
12. Doriamp, Cass D, Schwartz B, et al 2002 Amiodarone as compared with Lidocaine for shock-resistant ventricular fibrillation. New England Journal of Medicine 346(12): 884–90
13. Dessertenne F 1996 La tachycardie ventriculaire a deux foyers opposés variables. Archives de Mal de Coeur 59: 263–72
14. Tzivoni D, Banai S, Schuger C, et al 1998 Treatment of torsades de pointes with magnesium sulphate. Circulation 77: 392–7
15. Dreifus LS, Hessen SE 1990 Supraventricular tachycardia: diagnosis and treatment. Cardiology 77: 259–68
16. Meyer ADMcRM 2000 Pre-medication with midazolon for patients in P(SVT) receiving adenosine. Emergency Medicine 13: A9
17. Marsden CD, Pointer JE, Lynch TG 1995 A comparison of adenosine and verapamil in treatment of supraventricular tachycardia in the prehospital setting. Annals of Emergency Medicine 25(5): 649–55
18. Lip GY (ed.) 1996 ABC of atrial fibrillation. BMJ Publishing, London
19. Li H, Easley A, Bennington W, Windle J 1998 Evaluation and management of atrial fibrillation in the emergency department. Emergency Clinics of North America 16(2): 389–403
20. Cotter G, Blatt A, Karluslei E, et al 1999 Conversion of recent onset paroxysmal atrial fibrillation to normal sinus rhythm and the effect of no treatment and high dose amiodarone: a randomized placebo-controlled study. European Heart Journal 20: 1833–42
21. Meyer ADMcRM, Bernard S, Smith KC, McNeil JJ, Cameron PC 2001 Aysystolic cardiac arrest in Melbourne, Australia. Emergency Medicine 13: 186–9
22. Meyer ADMcRM, Cameron PA, Smith KC, McNeil JJ 2000 Out-of-hospital cardiac arrest. Medical Journal of Australia 172: 2–5

FURTHER READING

ACLS Committee of the ERC 1994 Management of peri-arrest arrhythmias. Resuscitation 28: 151–9
Ganong WF 1995 Review of Medical Physiology, 17th edn. Appleton and Lange, Connecticut
Guidelines for cardiopulmonary resuscitation and emergency cardiac care 1992. Journal of the American Medical Association 268: 16
Proceedings of the guidelines 2000 Conference for cardiopulmonary resuscitation and emergency cardiovascular care: an international consensus on science. The American Heart Association in Collaboration with the International Liaision Committee on Resuscitation (ILCOR)
Xie B, Thakur RK, Shah CP, Hoon VK 1998 Clinical differentiation of narrow QRS complex tachycardias. Emergency Clinics of North America 16(2): 295–327

4.5 PULMONARY EMBOLISM

PETER CAMERON

ESSENTIALS

1 Patients with a diagnosis of pulmonary embolus left untreated, have a high mortality rate. This is significantly reduced by anticoagulation.

2 The decision to treat is based on the probability of serious morbidity and mortality after history, examination and investigation.

3 The investigative algorithm involves ECG and X-ray to exclude other causes. The use of D-dimer, lower limb ultrasound, V/Q scan and CT angiogram to refine probability will depend on local resources.

4 In massive embolism transoesophageal echocardiography is a useful investigative modality.

5 The gold standard test of pulmonary angiography should be reserved for the small group of patients where the probability of thromboembolic disease is high, less invasive tests have failed to rule out the disease and there is significant risk of an adverse event if undiagnosed.

6 Thrombolysis is indicated for massive embolus, but improvement in mortality has not been conclusively demonstrated.

7 Low molecular weight heparin is now recommended for treatment of deep-vein thrombosis and pulmonary embolus. It can safely be used on an outpatient basis in selected patients.

8 Thromboembolic disease should be considered as a continuum from deep-vein thrombosis to pulmonary embolism. Investigation should be considered in terms of risk stratification, rather than aiming for a definitive diagnosis.

INTRODUCTION

Pulmonary embolus (PE) is the third most common cardiovascular disease, and historical data suggest that if it is left untreated it is associated with a high hospital mortality. Treating PE with anticoagulation reduces the overall hospital mortality to about 10%, however most of these patients die of a comorbidity and only 2.5% of PE.

Most PEs are either idiopathic (40%) or secondary to surgery/trauma (43%); heart disease (12%), neoplasms (4%) and systemic disease (1%). Many risk factors have been proposed for PE. The most important appear to be trauma, surgery, heart disease, and other factors causing stasis of blood flow as well as coagulation disorders such as antithrombin 111 deficiency, antiphospholipid syndrome and deficiency of protein C and S. Other proven risk factors include age, male sex, oral contraceptive pill, neoplasm, obesity and a past history of DVT/PE.

The diagnosis and management of PE is difficult and relies on the estimation of probabilities rather than any definitive test. The probability is based on history, examination and investigations, which may include chest X-ray, aerterial blood gas analysis, ECG, ventilation/perfusion (V/Q) scan and angiography where necessary. More recently, D-dimer assay, CT angiography, ultrasound and MRI have been included in the diagnostic algorithm (Fig. 4.5.1).

HISTORY

The history is the most important screen. Virtually all patients with PE will present with a recent onset of dyspnoea, chest pain or both (sensitivity 97%, specificity 10%).[1] Other symptoms are less important in the diagnosis of PE, but help to exclude other causes. Associated risk factors increase the probability of PE and should be documented. No single symptom or sign has the sensitivity or specificity to either establish or exclude the diagnosis.

EXAMINATION

Physical signs are most useful in excluding other pathology, but a mild fever (less than 38°C), tachycardia, tachypnoea, elevated JVP, loud S2 and pulmonary systolic murmur are all associated with a diagnosis of PE.

INVESTIGATIONS

The initial screening tests for PE are:

- **CXR** This is reportedly abnormal in 80% of patients diagnosed with PE. However, the signs are subtle and non-specific. Pleural effusion, plate atelectasis, enlarged descending pulmonary artery, enlarged heart shadow and 'Hampton's hump' (a semicircular opacity with the base abutting the pleural surface) are all suggestive of PE.[2] The main role of CXR is in the identification of alternative causes for symptoms.

- **ECG** At least 21 potential signs have been postulated, but these are all non-specific. The most significant are RBBB, right axis deviation, T-wave inversion (especially V_1, V_2) right ventricular hypertrophy, p pulmonale and $S_1Q_3T_3$.[2]

- **Arterial blood gas (ABG)** In recent years the role of ABG in the diagnosis of PE has been challenged. A P_aO_2 less than 80 mmHg in the absence of another cause makes PE likely; however, 12% of patients with PE have P_aO_2 higher than 80 mmHg. An abnormal A-a gradient increases the likelihood of PE, but 20% of patients with PE will have a normal A-a gradient.[3] If there is coexisting pulmonary disease then a previous ABG is essential to interpret

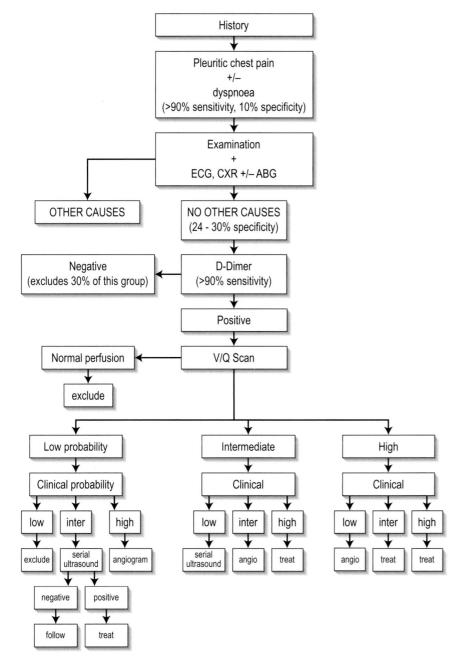

Fig. 4.5.1 Investigation algorithm for pulmonary embolism.

Table 4.5.1 Wells clinical criteria for PE	
Clinical signs of DVT	3.0
Pulse rate >100	1.5
Immobilized ≥ 3 days	1.5
Surgery < 4 weeks	1.5
Past history PE/DVT	1.5
Haemoptysis	1.0
Current/recent Neoplasm	1.0
PE likely clinically including ECG, ABG	3.0
Score	
Low	<2
Moderate	2-6
High	>6

and would only be useful in excluding a diagnosis in patients assessed as low or moderate probability on clinical assessment.[4] More recent studies have cast doubt on the sensitivity of rapid D-dimer tests (such as Simpli-Red®) and have suggested they should not be used independent of clinical probability. So that a negative D-dimer should only be used to rule out PE or DVT if there is a low clinical probability or negative V/Q scan.[5] Wells has validated this approach using a clinical risk scoring system (see Table 4.5.1), to detect clinically low-risk patients. This is followed by D-dimer to exclude the need for further investigation[6].

Following screening tests, more definitive investigations including V/Q scan, pulmonary angiography, CT, MRI and TOE, should be performed. The choice of test will depend on the clinical state of the patient, the estimated risk of PE, the presence of co-exisiting pulmonary disease and availability of modalities.

V/Q scan

V/Q scanning is the usual next step, because it is readily available and has a low complication rate. Unfortunately, it is an imprecise tool that can only give clinicians a range of probabilities. Two major studies (PIOPED[7] and McMaster[8]) have helped to define these probabilities. Scans were defined as normal, near-normal or low, intermediate, and high probability, according to the number and size of lung segments not perfused, and

the result. In current clinical practice an oxygen saturation measurement is sufficient to exclude significant hypoxaemia (<90%). There is little to be gained in using an ABG for routine screening for PE.

- **D-dimer** This investigation has been used clinically since the early 1980s, but problems with sensitivity, specificity and process have limited its utility. D-dimer is a fibrin degradation product which can be

measured using enzyme-linked immunosorbent assay (ELISA), latex agglutination techniques or rapid D-dimer assays. The latex test is easy to use but lacks sensitivity. The ELISA test is sufficiently sensitive but is too complex for routine use and not available at all hospitals. Newer techniques using rapid D-dimer assays have been reported to be as sensitive as the ELISA and quick to process. They still lack specificity, whether perfusion defects were matched to ventilation defects. Although variations on the definitions have occurred, the basic concept has remained. There are also variations in the technique used. The initial investigations used xenon for ventilation scans, whereas Australian centres now mostly use technetium, which allows better views. More recently it has been suggested that the number of segments may be less open to interpretation errors and just as accurate in predicting the probability of PE as the number and size of the segments.[9] The interobserver variability in the intermediate and low-probability scan interpretations was as high as 70% in the PIOPED study.

V/Q scanning is often of doubtful benefit in patients with known preexistent lung disease because of the difficulty in interpreting the significance of abnormalities.

Normal/near-normal scan

A normal/near-normal perfusion scan excludes a PE, however, only 14% had a normal/near-normal scan.

High probability

A high-probability scan was associated with a greater than 85% chance of PE, but only 13% had a high-probability scan. Also, 15% of patients treated on the basis of a high-probability scan would be anticoagulated, or even thrombolysed unnecessarily.

Low/intermediate

The low- and intermediate-probability groups had a 15–30% and greater than 30% chance, respectively, of having PE.[10]

Combination with clinical probability

The predictive value of VQ scans may be greatly refined by combining clinical and scanning probabilities. If patients without previous PE and significant cardiopulmonary disease are excluded, then a low-probability scan and a low clinical probability makes PE unlikely (less than 5%). For those patients with intermediate-probability scans with low clinical suspicion, the risk of PE is also low. In this group it has been shown that

exclusion of proximal vein thrombosis by serial impedance plethysmography (IPG) (or more recently by compression ultrasonography, which has equivalent accuracy) will reduce the risk of PE to less than 3%.[10] This approach is based on the premise that the pathology of venous thromboembolism (VTE) is a continuum. Forty per cent of patients with diagnosed DVT have asymptomatic PE. However, 30% of patients with PE will have no clot in proximal leg veins.[11]

The combination of high-probability V/Q scan with high clinical suspicion raises the chance of PE to more than 95%. This means that more aggressive therapy, such as thrombolysis, can be given in appropriate cases.

The group with low/intermediate probability and high clinical suspicion ± cardiopulmonary disease ± previous PE has a wide range of probabilities, from 15–75%. This comprises a relatively large group and, although pulmonary angiography has been advocated in US centres to further refine the probabilities in this group, in the Australian setting this is rarely done. In the lower-probability patients in this group it may be reasonable to follow clinically with serial ultrasound and clinical assessment. An alternative would be to further reduce the probability by using D-dimer and/or CT angiogram (see below).

However, the risk of missing a PE should be acknowledged. The risk of serial clinical assessment in this group, as opposed to treatment, has not been assessed. There is some evidence that patients with no evidence of central PE or proximal leg vein clot and low/ntermediate clinical probability are at low risk of recurrent PE.[12] This approach acknowledges that the aim of investigation is risk stratification, rather than diagnosis. Treatment is based on the risk of an adverse event, rather than ultimate diagnosis. At all times the risk of investigation and treatment must be balanced with the risk of the untreated disease.

Computerized tomography

Computerized tomography (CT) angiogram is becoming increasingly available in most centres and after hours avail-

ability is frequently higher than V/Q scanning. CT is preferable to V/Q in patients with preexistent lung disease. CT appears to be accurate in diagnosing main, lobar and segmental vessel emboli. Sensitivity for subsegmental emboli is low, however, the prevalance (6–30% reported) and clinical significance of this group of PEs is not known. Many centres are now using CT and lower limb ultrasound to exclude significant PE. Their belief is that risk of recurrent PE and death is minimal if both tests are negative. A further advantage, apart from availability, is that other thoracic causes of chest pain can be imaged. If this approach is adopted, then careful follow-up is advised[13] (Fig. 4.5.2.).

Pulmonary angiography

Pulmonary angiography is promoted as the 'gold standard' in diagnosing PE; however, there are significant technical difficulties in interpretation. It has a mortality of 0.3% and a complication rate of 3%. Experts disagree on the presence of PE in 8% of cases and its absence in 17%.[7,14] Digital subtraction angiography may decrease complication rates and allow adequate images with improvements in technique. Pulmonary angiography should be directed to the segments suspected of being involved on the basis of the V/Q scan.

Magnetic resonance imaging

Magnetic resonance imaging (MRI) techniques are improving rapidly. Sensitivity for central emboli is already greater than 90%, with high specificity. However, there is little place at this stage for MRI in the acute setting because of access, cost and availability. The advantage of both MRI and CT is that they allow simultaneous imaging of other thoracic structures.

Transoesophageal echocardiography

A further advance in the diagnosis of massive PE has been the development of transoesophageal echocardiography (TOE). This provides a rapid and relatively accurate diagnosis in the haemodynamically unstable patient. TOE will

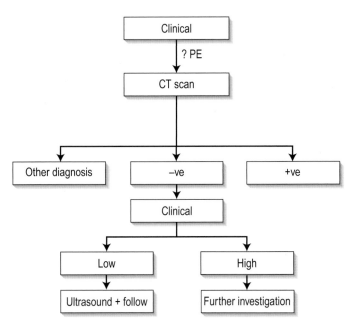

Fig. 4.5.2 Alternative algorithm.

exclude other causes of hypotension and raised venous pressure (such as tamponade, valve or myocardial dysfunction), and in most cases of massive PE will demonstrate the pulmonary artery clot and right heart dysfunction. Importantly, it can be performed in the resuscitation room. TOE is not sensitive for peripheral emboli.

MANAGEMENT

General measures

The management of PE begins with prevention. Thromboembolic disease should be considered a continuum from DVT to PE. The greatest single preventable cause of DVT is surgery. Low-dose anticoagulation should be routine, and the introduction of low molecular weight heparin has made this safer and more effective for some groups. Venous stasis as a result of bed rest, cardiopulmonary disease and travel is a further important cause of PE. Mobilization techniques are important and low dose anticoagulation has been demonstrated to improve outcomes for medical patients admitted for bed rest.

Most patients presenting with PE have significant ventilation/perfusion [V/Q] mismatch and require supplemental oxygen. Severe hypoxaemia may require endotracheal intubation and ventilation. Haemodynamic instability occurs late and indicates a massive PE. Initially intravascular fluid loading may be sufficient to maintain blood pressure. However, persistent hypotension will require inotropic support. There is little evidence to support the use of noradrenaline (norepinephrine) over adrenaline (epinephrine) as the inotrope of choice.[15] Patients requiring inotropes should not be treated with isoprenaline. This results in vasodilatation, decreased peripheral resistance and increased cardiac output, without an improvement in coronary perfusion.

SPECIFIC TREATMENTS

Anticoagulation

Unfractionated heparin treatment for PE has been standard for 30 years. LMW heparin has been shown to be as effective, for example enoxaparin subcutaneously 1 mg bd or 1.5 mg daily. This raises the potential for outpatient management of small PEs.[16] The duration of warfarin treatment should be 3 months for nonsurgical DVT and 1 month for surgical DVT. There is increasing interest in antiphospholipid antibodies and their role in recurrent DVT and PE. Those patients without obvious cause for VTE (e.g. surgery, heart failure) should have an antibody screen. If antibodies are detected then patients should be anticoagulated for life and at a higher INR level (3.5–4.5 vs 2–3).

Thrombolysis

The widespread use of thrombolytic therapy for coronary disease has led to a reappraisal of thrombolytics in PE. Although no controlled, randomized studies have convincingly shown improvement in mortality with their use, there is definite evidence of decreased pulmonary artery pressures and improved right ventricular function, which seem to persist following the acute episode.[17] Very few clinicians would withhold thrombolytics for massive PE. There is widespread use of thrombolytics in Europe for moderate-sized PE, with some evidence of improved mortality[18] but there seems to be less acceptance in the USA and Australia for this indication. Tissue plasminogen activator (TPA) appears to be the most effective and to have the fewest side effects when compared to urokinase and streptokinase. TPA has been used as an infusion of 100 mg over 2 hours.[17] Bolus reteplase (10 u/s + 10 u/s separated by half an hour) may be just as effective and easier to use.

The risk of anticoagulation is approximately 14–22 bleeding episodes per 1000 treatment months. Thrombolysis is associated with a major bleeding episode in up to 4% of patients. Although the overall in-hospital mortality from untreated PE approaches 30%, the risk of not treating low-probability scans (and, therefore, small PEs) and following clinically may be much lower.

Surgery

Patients with persistent haemodynamic instability or hypoxia should be considered for thoracotomy and embolectomy. Patients in this category are not necessarily at hospitals with facilities for cardiopulmonary bypass, and, therefore, alternative therapies have been developed. The use of mechanical clot disruption for massive PE has been reported in case studies, but controlled studies are difficult to design because of the infrequency of the event and the emergent nature of massive PE. By passing a standard pulmonary artery catheter J wire past the clot, sliding the catheter over this and withdrawing the catheter, the clot can be fragmented. Unlike other surgical techniques, the expertise and equipment for this procedure are readily available in most large hospitals. Pulmonary embolectomy without cardiac bypass has been used as a last resort for haemodynamically unstable patients, with a reported survival of greater than 50%.[19] Following cardiac arrest, survival rates are much lower, although survivors have been reported.

There is no evidence that mechanical removal of clot results in better outcome than does thrombolysis.

The use of caval interruption techniques should be considered in cases of recurrent PE despite coagulation, or where there is bleeding. It has also been recommended for massive PE. Fatal PE usually occurs as a result of further clot progressing along the inferior vena cava (IVC). Percutaneous IVC umbrellas may be inserted relatively easily and prevent further deterioration.

PROGNOSIS

The prognosis is largely dependent on coexistent illness. With anticoagulation, hospital mortality is still high (10%). Recurrent PE occurs in 25% of patients by 8 years.[11]

DISPOSITION

Patients with haemodynamic instability or significant hypoxia should be admitted

---

CONTROVERSIES

❶ The role of pulmonary angiography: the risk of anticoagulation, and the lack of 'definitive' diagnosis, versus the benefit of angiography.

❷ Whether helical CT should replace V/Q scanning as the first imaging technique in PE.

❸ The role of thrombolysis: it is generally accepted for use in large PEs. European countries have advocated thrombolysis for medium PEs and DVT to prevent long-term complications.

❹ Outpatient treatment of PE with LMW heparin.

---

to an ICU. Surgical referral should be considered for ongoing instability. Most patients with PE can be admitted directly to the ward, although early discharge with LMW heparin should be considered for small PEs.

CONCLUSION

The diagnosis and management of PE is based on an estimate of the probability of diagnosis versus the risk of treatment. Nowhere else in medicine is the 'art' of medicine more in evidence.

REFERENCES

1. Palla A, Putruzelli S, Donnamaria V, Giuntini C 1995 The role of suspicion in the diagnosis of pulmonary embolism. Chest 107(Suppl): 21–4
2. Manganelli D, Palla A, Donnamaria V, Giuntini C 1995 Clinical features of pulmonary embolism: doubts and certainties. Chest 107(Suppl): 25–32
3. Stein PD, Goldhaber SZ, Henry JW 1995 Alveolar-arterial oxygen gradient in the assessment of acute pulmonary embolism. Chest 107: 139–43
4. Mountain D, Brown AFT 1996 A review of the usefulness of D-dimer in the diagnosis of pulmonary embolism. Emergency Medicine 8: 253–9
5. Ginsberg JS, Wells PS, Kearon C, et al 1998 Sensitivity and specificity of a rapid whole-blood assay for D-Dimer in the diagnosis of pulmonary embolism. Annals of Internal Medicine 129(12): 1006–11
6. Wells PS, Anderson DR, Rodger M, et al 2001 Excluding pulmonary embolism at the bedside without diagnostic imaging: management of patients with suspected pulmonary embolism presenting to the emergency department by using a simple clinical model and d-dimer. Annals of Internal Medicine 135: 98–107
7. The PIOPED Investigators 1990 Value of the ventilation/perfusion scan in acute pulmonary embolism. Journal of the American Medical Association 263: 2753–9
8. Hull RD, Hirsh J, Carter CJ, et al 1985 Diagnostic value of ventilation-perfusion lung scanning in patients with suspected pulmonary embolism. Chest 88: 819–28
9. Stein PD, Henry JW, Gottschalk A 1993 The addition of clinical assessment to stratification according to prior cardiopulmonary disease further optimises the interpretation of ventilation/ perfusion lung scans in pulmonary embolism. Chest 104: 1472–6
10. Kelley M, Carson J, Palevsky H, Schwartz J 1991 Diagnosing pulmonary embolism: new facts and strategies. Annals of Internal Medicine 114: 300–6
11. Hirsch J, Hoak J 1996 Management of deep vein thrombosis and pulmonary embolism (AHA medical/scientific statement). Circulation 93: 2212–45
12. Myers TM 1995 Diagnosis of pulmonary embolism. Thorax 50: 930–2
13. Ginsberg JS, Bates SM 2000 Helical computed tomography and the diagnosis of pulmonary embolism. Annals of Internal Medicine 132: 240–2
14. Matsumoto A, Tegfmeyer C 1995 Contemporary diagnostic approaches to acute pulmonary emboli. Radiologic Clinics of North America 33: 167–83
15. Tapson VF, Witty LA 1995 Massive pulmonary embolism. Clinics in Chest Medicine 16(2): 329–40
16. Simonneau G, Sors H, Charbonnier B, et al 1997 A comparison of LMW heparin with unfractionated heparin for acute pulmonary embolism. New England Journal of Medicine 337: 663–9
17. Goldhaber SZ, Haire WB, Feldstein MI, et al 1993 Altephase vs heparin in acute PE: randomised trial assessing right-ventricular function and pulmonary perfusion. Lancet 341: 507–11
18. Konstantinides S, Geibel A, Olschewski M, et al 1997 Association between thrombyltic treatment and the prognosis of hemodynamically stable patients with major pulmonary embolism: results of a multicenter registry. Circ 96:882–8
19. Clarke DB, Abrams LD 1986 Pulmonary embolectomy: 25 years' experience. Journal of Thoracic and Cardiovascular Surgery 92: 442–5

4.6 PERICARDITIS, CARDIAC TAMPONADE AND MYOCARDITIS

JAMES HAYES

PERICARDITIS

ESSENTIALS

1 Myocarditis is often associated with the clinical condition pericarditis. This has important clinical implications.

2 Pericarditis is most commonly diagnosed on ECG findings, but may ultimately be a purely clinical diagnosis.

3 The majority of cases of pericarditis have a presumed viral aetiology and most run a benign course.

4 The correct distinction of pericarditis from AMI is essential, as the administration of thrombolytics in cases of pericarditis may result in life-threatening complications.

5 Longer-term follow-up is essential as a subacute or chronic course can develop, with further complications such as chronic constrictive pericarditis.

INTRODUCTION

Pericarditis is defined as inflammation of the pericardium. It should be noted, however, that the condition is better described as perimyocarditis. In the majority of cases there are variable degrees of associated 'epimyocarditis', which has important clinical implications. The causes of pericarditis are listed in Table 4.6.1.

CLINICAL FEATURES

History

Idiopathic or viral types may have a history of a recent viral illness, and the history should be directed towards the known causative pathologies. The pain is usually retrosternal, sometimes with radiation to the trapezius muscle ridges but not generally the arms. It may also be pleuritic in nature, worse with movement and respiration, typically worse lying supine, and better sitting up and leaning forward. True dyspnoea is not a feature, but respiration may be shallow because of pain.

Examination

With viral or idiopathic types fever may be present. Sinus tachycardia is common.

A pericardial friction rub may be heard, caused by rubbing between parietal and visceral pericardial layers or between parietal pericardium and lung pleura. The rub may, therefore, be heard despite the presence of a large effusion. It may be audible anywhere over the precordium, but is best heard with the diaphragm over the lower left sternal edge, where the least amount of lung tissue intervenes, and while the patient holds his or her breath after full exhalation and leans forward. The rub has a superficial scratching or 'velcro-like' quality, most commonly triphasic, but may be biphasic or rarely monophasic. The triphasic components correlate to atrial systole, ventricular systole and ventricular diastole. Rubs may be difficult to detect, as they can be transient and migratory. The patient should be examined for any signs of a complicating cardiac tamponade. A search should also be made for any signs of an underlying causative condition.

INVESTIGATIONS

Blood tests
- FBE
- ESR provides confirmatory evidence of an inflammatory process, and can be used to follow treatment.

Table 4.6.1 Causes of pericarditis	
Idiopathic	Many of these cases are probably due to viral infection
Infective	Viral, e.g. Coxsackie B, mumps, EBV, influenza, HIV Bacterial, e.g. staphylococcal, streptococcal, G-ves and TB Mycotic, e.g. histoplasmosis
Autoimmune/connective tissue diseases	*Especially rheumatoid arthritis and SLE*
Radiation injury	
Trauma	Penetrating Blunt Post pericardiotomy syndrome
Malignancy	Primary, e.g. sarcoma and mesotheliomas Secondary, e.g. haematological, breast, lung and melanoma
Myocardial infarction associated	Acute: days to weeks following *transmural* AMI Dressler's syndrome: weeks to months following AMI
Drugs	SLE-type syndromes, e.g. hydralazine Hypersensitivity syndromes, e.g. penicillin
Systemic diseases	Renal failure, uraemia Myxoedema

- Cardiac enzymes may be elevated because of the associated myocarditis.

Chest X-ray

Chest X-ray (CXR) does not confirm the diagnosis of pericarditis but will rule out other causes of pleuritic chest pain, find evidence of a complicating pericardial effusion, or evidence of causative pathology such as malignancy.

ECG

ECG changes are the result of the associated epimyocarditis. The pericardium is electrically neutral and of itself does not produce ECG changes. Therefore, in the occasional 'pure' case of pericarditis the ECG will be normal. The ECG is the most important investigation in making the diagnosis of pericarditis, but it has limitations. It may follow the typical evolution of changes but in a sizeable minority will not.

The typical pattern follows four stages:

- Stage 1: hours to days
  - diffuse concave upwards ST elevation; this may occur in all leads apart from AVR and often VI.
  - PR-segment depression(reflecting sub-epicardial atrial injury); this may occur in all leads apart from AVR and V1. These two leads may in fact show PR-segment elevation.
- Stage 2: the PR and ST segments normalize, which can lead to a transiently normal ECG
- Stage 3: days to weeks, T-wave inversion occurs
- Stage 4: normalization of the ECG; over a period of up to 3 months, however, in some cases the T-wave changes may be permanent.

Atypical ECGs may include the following:[1]

- A normal ECG in cases of 'pure' pericarditis (remembering that during stage 2 the ECG may also be transiently normal during a typical evolution)
- The PR-segment depression may occur in isolation, without any ST segment elevation

- Stages 1 and 2 without progression to stage 3
- Localized as opposed to diffuse ECG changes.

Echocardiography

This may give indirect evidence for pericarditis by showing the presence of an effusion or a thickened pericardium. High-quality echocardiograms are able to distinguish bloody from serous effsions. TOE is better at measuring thickness of the pericardium than TTE. A normal echocardiogram does not rule out a diagnosis of pericarditis.

CT scan

CT scan may show effusions and and pericardial thickening. It may be useful in those patients who do not have a good echocardiographic 'window', (COAD, thoracic skeletal deformities).

Nuclear medicine scanning

This is not currently a useful investigation for the diagnosis of pericarditis. It may detect associated myocarditis.

MAKING THE DIAGNOSIS

Stage 1 ST-segment deviations are virtually diagnostic of acute pericarditis when typically distributed among limb and precordial leads. However, a sizeable minority of ECGs will be atypical, and, indeed, in some cases may be normal. The diagnosis of pericarditis may, therefore, ultimately be a clinical one based on the presence of typical pain and a rub heard on auscultation or presence of an effusion on echocardiogram. Cases where pain is typical but a rub is not heard present more difficulty, and should be followed closely. If clinical suspicion is high, again an echcardiogram finding of an effusion in the presence of typical pain would be highly suggestive. Convenient diagnoses, such as 'muscular', 'fibrositis', 'costochondritis' and 'viral' should be avoided until more important conditions, such as pericarditis, pulmonary embolus and pneumothorax, are excluded. The most difficult clinical decision in the

emergency department is differentiating between pericarditis, benign early repolarization (BER) and AMI. This is especially so when the decision to use thrombolytics is being considered. Thrombolytic therapy may result in life threatening hemmorhagic cardiac tamponade in patients who have pericarditis.

Pericarditis versus BER

To help distinguish pericarditis from BER (a normal variant generally seen in patients under 45):

- Look at the ST/T-wave segment ratio in lead V_6. If this is less than 0.25 then BER is more likely to be the diagnosis than pericarditis.
- If available, examine old ECGs: BER changes tend to be permanent, at least over years, whereas ST elevation of pericarditis is never permanent.

ST changes in BER are seen in the precordial leads and not the limb leads.

Pericarditis versus AMI

- The descriptive nature of the pain, that is, pleuritic versus crushing
- Distinguishing features on the ECG (Table 4.6.2)
- Cardiac enzymes: these may be elevated in perimyocarditis, but only to a modest degree compared to AMI, where they may be greatly elevated
- Echocardiography may provide useful information. Pericarditis may show effusion without myocardial wall motion abnormalities, whereas AMI or ischaemia will show regional wall motion abnormalities.

MANAGEMENT

The symptoms of pericarditis are generally well controlled with non-steroidal anti-inflammatory agents. Occasionally more severe symptoms of pain will require steroids. Rest is essential, as exercise may exacerbate an associated myocarditis. Complications such as arrhythmias are treated along conventional lines. If a significant effusion is suspected this should be confirmed on echocardiogra-

Table 4.6.2 Pericarditis vs AMI vs BER

ECG feature	Acute pericarditis	AMI	BER
ST segment morphology	Concave upwards ST elevation	Convex upwards ST elevation	Concave upwards ST elevation
ST segment elevation	Usually <5 mm	May be >5 mm, more suspicious the greater the elevation	<5 mm
ST segment changes distribution	Diffuse	Anatomic	Precordial only
Reciprocal changes	No, mild depressions only in AVR, V$_1$	Deep reciprocal changes opposite ST elevated segments	No
Q waves	No (unless associated with infarction)	Yes	No
PR segments	PR-segment depressions (may be elevated in AVR and V1)	No	No
T wave inversion	T-wave inversion after ST segments normalize	T waves may invert concurrently with elevation of ST segments	No
ST/T ratio	>0.25	N/A	<0.25
Usual pattern of evolution of changes	Days to weeks	Minutes to days	Stable over many years

phy and signs of early cardiac tamponade looked for. An underlying cause for the pericarditis should be sought and treatment directed at this, though the majority will be viral. In high-risk patients HIV should also be considered as a possible underlying aetiology.

DISPOSITION

The clinical course really depends on the underlying pathology. The majority of cases fall into the viral and idiopathic groups, and these most commonly follow a benign and self-limiting course over 10–14 days.

Patients with severe symptoms should be admitted; some may require narcotic analgesia. Those with evidence of a significant associated myocarditis, such as elevation of cardiac enzymes, arrhythmias or significant ST elevation, should be admitted to a coronary care unit. Those with evidence of effusion causing tamponade should be admitted to an intensive care unit. Patients in whom the diagnosis remains uncertain, especially when other serious conditions such as AMI cannot be ruled out, should be admitted. Patients with presumed viral causation who are otherwise well are often

treated as outpatients, but close follow-up is essential. Longer-term follow-up is also essential to look for the development of chronicity and constrictive pericarditis.

CONTROVERSIES

❶ Whether all patients with pericarditis should be admitted. Although patients with usual pericarditis are at low risk of adverse events, clinical diagnosis is not always accurate.

NON-TRAUMATIC CARDIAC TAMPONADE

ESSENTIALS

1 Cardiac tamponade is a life-threatening condition.

2 The signs and symptoms of cardiac tamponade are non-specific and often not present, or at least difficult to elicit. A high index of suspicion is, therefore, essential to ensure that the condition is not missed.

3 The 'gold standard' investigation is echocardiography. It is the most sensitive and the most specific.

4 The urgency and type of treatment will depend on the rapidity of, as well as the degree of, accumulation of pericardial contents. It will also depend on the aetiology.

5 Needle pericardiocentesis is best reserved as a drainage procedure of last resort. The preferred method should be subxiphoid pericardiotomy if the clinical situation allows. In cases of myocardial rupture and aortic dissection, thoracotomy with drainage and definitive repair is the method of choice, rather than attempts at pericardiocentesis.

INTRODUCTION

Pericardial effusion is the accumulation of fluid (exudate, transudate, blood and chylus) within the pericardial cavity. Normally this cavity contains up to 35 mL of fluid. More than this can be accommodated in the short term to about 200 mL, and then in the longer term up to 2 liters, with little clinical consequence. However, above these values the process of cardiac tamponade will occur, with lethal consequences if unrecognized.

Cardiac tamponade can be defined as an accumulation of pericardial contents that inhibits the diastolic filling of the atria and ventricles and, if left unchecked, will lead to a clinical state of shock. It may be recognized by the clinical signs in the late stages, but the diagnosis should be confirmed by echocardiography as these signs are non-specific. It is now recognized that the process of cardiac tamponade may occur before significant clinical signs develop.[2] Echocardiography can diagnose this early 'compensated' stage of the process, whereas in the late 'decompensated' stages a clinical picture of shock will be apparent.

The best classification for cardiac tamponade is traumatic (dealt with elsewhere in this book) and non-traumatic (Fig. 4.6.1), as not only the aetiology but the clinical course and approach to management are very different.

CLINICAL FEATURES

History
The symptoms and signs of cardiac tamponade are non-specific and occur relatively late, in the gradual-onset group. They are also inconsistent and sometimes difficult to elicit. A high index of suspicion for the condition must

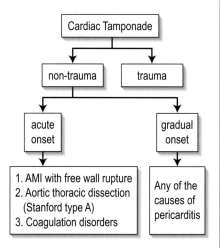

Fig. 4.6.1 Causes of pericardial effusion and cardiac tamponade.

therefore be maintained, which requires thorough knowledge of the clinical settings in which it can occur.

The commonest symptom of cardiac tamponade is dyspnoea. Most other symptoms will relate to those of diminished cardiac output (e.g. dizziness, apprehension) or to the underlying disease process (e.g. pain of pericarditis).

Examination
Loss of the apical impulse or, if present, an area of cardiac dullness extending beyond the apical impulse, may give a clinical clue to the presence of an effusion but not cardiac tamponade. These signs are difficult to elicit and very non-specific. In the later stages of cardiac tamponade, tachycardia and tachypnoea are common. The classically described 'Beck's triad' may be present in part or in whole (i.e. hypotension, diminished heart sounds and elevated jugular venous pressure). It should be noted that cardiac tamponade may be present in the absence of an elevated JVP in conditions of significant hypovolaemia, and that diminished heart sounds is a very non-specific and subjective finding. Furthermore, the absence of hypotension does not rule out cardiac tamponade: indeed, in some cases hypertension may be present.[3]

Pulsus paradoxus is a good indicator of cardiac tamponade but may be difficult to detect, especially in a hypotensive patient, and again is non-specific. Its presence is more readily appreciated on an arterial pressure line tracing. A degree of 'peripheral cyanosis', often more of the upper body, head, neck, chest and upper limbs, may also be present. If cardiac function is otherwise normal the lung fields are typically 'clear'. There may be associated pleural effusions and signs of pericarditis (e.g. fever, pericardial rub). Pleuropericardial rubs may still be heard even in the presence of a large effusion. The differential diagnosis of cardiac tamponade is given in Table 4.6.3.

INVESTIGATIONS

CXR
This may provide clues to the presence of an effusion, such as 'globular' cardio-

Table 4.6.3 The differential diagnosis of cardiac tamponade
Massive pulmonary embolism
Tension pneumothorax
Superior vena cava obstruction
Chronic constrictive pericarditis
Air embolism
Right ventricular infarct
Severe congestive cardiac failure/ cardiogenic shock
Extrapericardial compression: haematoma tumour

megaly and an increased epicardial fat pad, together with clear lung fields; however, these signs will not indicate whether tamponade is occurring. It should be remembered that in cases of acute tamponade, the cardiac silhouette may appear entirely normal. At least 250 mL of fluid must be present within the pericardial cavity before an increase in the cardiac silhouette can be appreciated.

ECG
This may provide clues to the presence of an effusion, with low voltages and electrical alternans, but again will not indicate whether tamponade is occurring. It has been claimed that total electrical alternans indicates tamponade, but the evidence for this is tenuous at best and should not be relied on to make the diagnosis.

Echocardiography
Echocardiography is the current 'gold standard' investigation for the diagnosis of cardiac tamponade. It is the most specific and sensitive investigation for the detection of effusion and of the process of tamponade. It can be performed rapidly and non-invasively (in the case of transthoracic echocardiography) in the emergency department. In patients in whom a transthoracic study (TTE) is difficult to perform or in whom the result is equivocal, then a transoesophageal (TOE) study may be performed. This technique may detect occult

loculated effusions missed by TTE and may even be performed in the intubated patient during CPR. Echocardiography can provide valuable information about associated cardiac function and abnormalities. It may also detect the process of tamponade before significant clinical signs develop.

Computerized tomography and magentic resonance imaging

Computerized tomography (CT) and magentic resonance imaging (MRI) are sensitive and specific for the detection of pericardial fluid and are good alternatives if echocardiography is not available. They are much less reliable in determining whether tamponade is occurring, giving only indirect clues. Neither is suitable in the critically ill patient.

Haemodynamic monitoring

In the ICU setting, the pulmonary artery catheter findings of 'equalization' of the right heart diastolic pressures (i.e., right atrial, right ventricular end-diastolic, diastolic pulmonary artery and pulmonary artery wedge pressures) suggests the diagnosis of cardiac tamponade.

TREATMENT

General measures

Attention to airway, breathing and circulation is the first priority. Fluid loading may provide some minor 'temporizing' support of the cardiac output. Inotropes may similarly provide some temporary benefit; however, attempts at fluid loading and inotropic support should never be allowed to delay the definitive measure of a drainage procedure.

Definitive measures

Drainage procedures

Needle pericardiocentesis should be considered a method of last resort. It is best reserved for the prearrest or just arrested patient, as it can be technically difficult and has significant complications, especially when smaller volumes of fluid are involved. If it is to be carried

out it is best followed up with the insertion of an indwelling 'pigtail'-type catheter for ready aspiration should the patient's condition again deteriorate. The safety of the procedure is enhanced if done under echocardiographic guidance. It must be remembered that CPR in the arrested patient will not be effective in cases of cardiac tamponade, when immediate needle drainage followed by thoracotomy will be required.

Subxiphoid pericardiotomy is the preferred method of drainage, provided an operator skilled in this technique is readily available. Here the pericardium is opened and a drain tube placed under direct vision, thereby avoiding many of the complications of needle pericardiocentesis.[4,5] This procedure may also be done under local anaesthesia, thus avoiding the significant risks of general anaesthesia under these conditions. Again, a pigtail catheter should be left in situ for further easy drainage should tamponade recur, until a more definitive procedure can be performed. The subxiphoid approach offers an additional advantage in that a biopsy specimen may be readily obtained, which will increase the diagnostic yield over pericardial fluid analysis alone.

Thoracotomy without attempts at drainage should be performed when definitive surgical repair of the causative pathology is necessary. Examples in this category include trauma, rupture of the myocardium, and dissecting thoracic aneurysm causing cardiac tamponade. Indeed, attempts at drainage before definitive repair in the case of dissecting aortic aneurysm may be positively detrimental.[6]

Treatment must also be directed at the underlying pathology.

DISPOSITION

Pericardial effusion may with time lead to cardiac tamponade. All cases of cardiac tamponade will lead to shock and death if left untreated, the rapidity of which will depend on the amount of fluid present, the rate at which it accumulated, and the compliance of the pericardium.

Cases of 'compensated' non-traumatic cardiac tamponade should be admitted to ICU for close observation while a definitive drainage procedure is planned and organized. In cases of decompensated tamponade, management will depend on the aetiology, clinical urgency and expertise available.

CONTROVERSIES

❶ The distinction between clinical and echocardiographic tamponade with the advent of more sensitive imaging.

❷ The type and timing of drainage procedures in the critically ill.

MYOCARDITIS

ESSENTIALS

1 Myocarditis is most commonly caused by viral infection; the majority of cases run a benign course, with full recovery.

2 Occasionally acute fulminating episodes occur, giving rise to arrhythmias, cardiac failure and death. Survivors of these episodes may, however, make a full recovery with supportive treatment.

3 Diagnosis is difficult and is usually made on clinical grounds. The definitive investigation is endomyocardial biopsy, although false negative results can occur.

4 Myocarditis may present in a similar manner to AMI , including similar chest pain, ECG changes and elevation of cardiac enzymes.

5 Long-term follow-up is important in patients who have had myocarditis, as some cases may progress to a chronic form with the development of dilated cardiomyopathy.

INTRODUCTION

The best working definition of myocarditis is myocardial inflammation and injury in the absence of ischaemia.[7] The condition is frequently associated with pericarditis, resulting in a myopericarditis.

Pathophysiolgy

The exact mechanism by which viral myocarditis and its longer term complications develop is unknown. It probably involves the interplay of three factors. These are direct damage due to the virus itself, damage in the acute and long term by the host's immune responses and finally a genetic predisposition in an individual. The relative contributions of these three factors in causing disease is unknown.

CLINICAL FEATURES

The clinical spectrum of myocarditis is variable. It may manifest as any of the following:

❶ Asymptomatic/subclinical.
❷ Fever with 'viral' illness, with minimal cardiac features.
❸ Acute myopericarditis.
❹ Unexplained arrythmias, including conduction delays.
❺ Unexplained cardiac failure, ranging from mild to to frank cardiogenic shock.
❻ Sudden, unexpected cardiac death.
❼ May present years later as dilated cardiomyopathy.

History

Many cases are asymptomatic. There may be a history of an antecedent viral illness. Ten to 14 days following this illness, symptoms relating to cardiac involvement develop, such as arrhythmias causing palpitations or dizziness, or cardiac failure causing shortness of breath. Pleuritic-type pain may be a feature owing to an associated pericarditis. Occasionally a non-pleuritic type chest pain of a nature indistinguishable from AMI may occur.[8]

Examination

On examination a fever may be present; however, patients are often afebrile.

Sinus tachycardia is often found and is said to be 'out of proportion' to the degree of fever. Other arrhythmias may be found. A pericardial rub due to an associated pericarditis may also be present. There may be signs of heart failure, ranging from mild pulmonary edema to frank cardiogenic shock.

INVESTIGATIONS

Blood

A number of blood tests can give support to a diagnosis of myocarditis, but none is specific. These include elevation of the white cell count, elevation of the ESR and elevation of the CRP. Cardiac enzymes may also be elevated. These parameters may be used to assess response to treatment.

CXR

This may show cardiomegaly with changes of congestive failure in severe cases, but again is non-specific. The chest X-ray may also be normal.

ECG

In most cases the ECG will be abnormal; however, the changes are not specific for myocarditis. Sinus tachycardia is usually seen. The most common finding is non-specific ST-T-wave changes. Rhythm disturbances of any type may occur, including a significant proportion with conduction delays. Occasionally ST elevation may occur that is indistinguishable from AMI.[9]

Echocardiography

This can give supportive evidence but is not diagnostic. Global wall motion abnormalities are a characteristic finding, but in some cases more regional abnormalities will be seen. An associated effusion may be found. Evidence of myocardial failure can be found with ventricular cavity dilation and reduced ejection fractions.

Nuclear medicine scanning

Radiolabelled (^{111}I) antimyosin Fab is currently the most specific marker for myocyte membrane damage. It is non-specific for myocarditis but is a useful screening tool to select patients for biopsy, as a normal scan makes myocarditis unlikely. In myocarditis there will be a generalized uptake of tracer, as opposed to the localized uptake pattern seen in cases of ischaemia, spasm or embolus.[10]

Endomyocardial biopsy

This is currently the only way to make a definitive diagnosis, according to the standardized 'Dallas criteria'.[7] The investigation is still not a gold standard, as the following problems may be encountered:

- Acute myocarditis may be patchy and diagnosis may be missed on a single specimen.
- False-positive results are possible.
- May underestimate more minor cases of myocarditis.

Although not included in the Dallas criteria, the detection of viral material within biopsy specimens gives further support to a diagnosis of viral myocarditis. The Dallas criteria have been critisized as underestimating the true incidence of myocarditis. Molecular biological techniques, such as PCR tesing for viral material are evolving rapidly. It is likely that further refinement of diagostic these criteria will occur.

MAKING THE DIAGNOSIS

A definitive diagnosis of acute viral myocarditis cannot be made in the emergency department and must in the first instance be presumptive. The commonest scenario will be the young patient who presents with cardiac failure, shock or arrhythmias for which there is no obvious aetiology.

A small number of cases of myocarditis may present with a history and ECG findings indistinguishable from AMI. This situation poses a real dilemma in the emergency department, especially when thrombolytics are being considered. The only clinical clue to the possibility of myocarditis in this setting may be extreme young age (a child or adolescent),

Table 4.6.4 Causes of myocarditis

Bacterial	e.g. Lyme disease via arthropod inoculation of the spirochaete *Borrelia burgdorferi*
Bacterial toxins	Diphtheria Clostridia
Protozoal agents	Toxoplasmosis South American trypanosomiasis (Chagas' disease)
Rickettsial agents	Typhus Q fever
Drugs and toxins	
Ionizing radiation	
Systemic diseases/autoimmune	SLE Sarcoidosis Kawasaki's disease Rheumatic fever

Viral infection is the commonest cause of myocarditis and most cases occur in younger age groups, such as neonates, children and young adolescents. Causative agents include Coxsackie B, influenza A and B, varicella, HIV, adenovirus, EBV and CMV. Many other viruses have been implicated. The other causes of myocarditis are rare.

Table 4.6.5 Some distinguishing features: myocarditis vs AMI

	Myocarditis Child/young	AMI Adult
	Age	
Pain	Recurrent/intractable despite treatment	Resolves with treatment
ECG	Does not follow the normal evolution of ischaemic changes	Follows typical evolution of ischaemic changes
Echocardiography	Global wall motion abnormalities	Wall motion abnormalities confined to a vascular distribution
Nuclear scan	Diffuse uptake	Localized uptake confined to a vascular distribution
Coronary angiography	Normal	Vascular occlusion/angiographic narrowing

perhaps with a clear history of a recent viral illness (Table 4.6.4). In older patients the diagnosis will usually not even be considered until angiography demonstrates normal coronary arteries, including no abnormality on ergonovine challenge for spasm (Table 4.6.5).

TREATMENT AND DISPOSITION

Treatment is supportive, with attention directed firstly to the airway, breathing and circulation. Oxygenation is important, and in cases of pulmonary oedema CPAP may be necessary. Analgesia will be required if pain is a significant feature. Strict bed rest is advised, as exercise has been shown to increase the degree of myocyte necrosis. Complicating arrhythmias and cardiac failure are treated along conventional lines. In patients who develop cardiogenic shock, intervention should be early and aggressive. The use of inotropes, ECMO, intraaortic balloon pumps or ventricualr assist devices is strongly justified as with aggressive

intervention survival, either by bridge to transplant or recovery approaches 70%.[11] Cardiac transplantation may ultimately be required in severe refractory cases. Immunosuppressive treatment has been advocated for myocarditis, but the myocarditis treatment trial did not show any benefit.[12] Survivors of myocarditis must be followed up carefully for the possible future development of dilated cardiomyopathy. Patients should not undergo any competitive sport for 6 months following the onset of clinical myocarditis.[13]

All patients with suspected acute myocarditis should be admitted to CCU/ICU.

NATURAL HISTORY OF MYOCARDITIS

Complications at presentation are usually the result of arrhythmias and heart failure; however, the majority of these will run a benign course with a full recovery. Arrhythmias may include conduction delays with a potential for sudden death. Occasionally an acute fulminant course may occur, with intractable arrhythmias or, more often, with acute heart failure rapidly progressing to cardiogenic shock and death. Survivors of this fulminant course will often make a complete recovery. The whole spectrum of asymptomatic through to fulminant cases may progress to a chronic course. Myocarditis is currently thought to be the cause of a significant percentage of cases of dilated cardiomyopathies. It may also explain some instances of recurrent unexplained

CONTROVERSIES

❶ The role of immunosuppressive agents in the management of myocarditis.

❷ The role of antiviral drugs and vaccines.

❸ The indications for endomyocardial biopsy in patients suspected of having viral myocarditis.

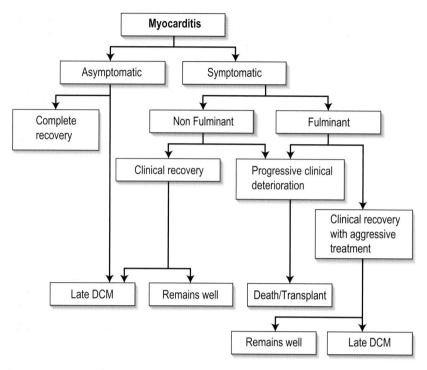

Fig 4.6.2 Natural history of myocarditis.

arrhythmias and sudden unexpected cardiac death, especially in younger age groups.

See Figure 4.6.2 for a summary of the natural history of myocarditis.

REFERENCES

1. Bruce MA, Spodick DH 1980 Atypical electrocardiogram in acute pericarditis: characteristics and prevalence. Journal of Electrocardiology 13: 61–6

2. Fowler NO 1993 Cardiac tamponade: a clinical or echocardiographic diagnosis? Circulation 87: 1738–41

3. Brown J, MacKinnon D, King A, Vanderbush E 1992 Elevated arterial blood pressure in cardiac tamponade. New England Journal of Medicine 327: 463–6

4. Alcan KE, Zabetakis PM, Marino ND, Franzone AJ, Michelis MF, Bruno MS 1982 Management of acute cardiac tamponade by subxiphoid pericardiotomy. Journal of the American Medical Association 247: 1143–8

5. Allen KB, Faber LP, et al 1999 Pericardial Effusion: Pericardiostomy Versus Percutaneous Catheter Drainage. Annals of Thoracic Surgery 67: 437–40

6. Coplan NL, Goldman B, Mechanic G, et al 1986 Sudden haemodynamic collapse following relief of cardiac tamponade in aortic dissection. American Heart Journal 111: 406

7. Aretz HT, Billingham ME, Edwards WD, et al 1987 Myocarditis: a histopathologic definition and classification. American Journal of Cardiovascular Pathology 1: 3–14

8. Narula J, Khaw BA, Dec GW, et al 1993 Brief report: recognition of acute myocarditis masquerading as acute myocardial infarction. New England Journal of Medicine 328: 100–4

9. Spodick DH, Greene TO, Saperia G 1995 Acute myocarditis masquerading as acute myocardial infarction. Circulation 91: 1886–7

10. Morguet AJ, Munz DL, Kreuzer H, Emrich D 1994 Scintigraphic detection of inflammatory heart disease. European Journal of Nuclear Medicine 21: 666–74

11. Acker MA 2001 Mechanical circulatory support for patients with acute fulminant myocarditis annals of thoracic surgery. 71 S73–S76

12. Mason JW, OConnell JB, Herskowitz A, et al 1995 A clinical trial of immunosuppressive therapy for myocarditis. New England Journal of Medicine 333: 269–75

13. Maron BJ, Isner JM, McKenna WJ 1994 Taskforce three: cardiomyopathy, myocarditis, and other myopericardial diseases and mitral valve prolapse. Journal of the American Cardiology Clinics 24: 845–99

FURTHER READING

Feldman AM, McNamarra D 2000 Myocarditis: New England Journal of Emergency Medicine 343 (19): 1388–98

Hancock EW 1994 Cardiac tamponade. Heart Disease and Stroke 3: 155–8

Hayes JE 1997 Cardiac tamponade. Emergency Medicine 9: 123–35

Raftos JR 1996 Acute fulminant viral myocarditis. Emergency Medicine 8: 235–8

4.7 HEART VALVE EMERGENCIES

MARIAN LEE

ESSENTIALS

1 Infective endocarditis is an often missed diagnosis.

2 Infective endocarditis is effectively a multi-organ disease.

3 Degenerative heart disease and prosthetic valve endocarditis are currently the high-risk factors in infective endocarditis in developed countries.

4 Antibiotic prophylaxis in patients with valvular or congenital heart disease is an important consideration in the appropriate clinical context.

5 Surgical intervention must be considered in valvular emergencies. Medical treatment may only be a temporizing measure. Early surgical consultation should be sought.

6 The causes of acute deterioration in chronic valve lesions must be recognized and treated expediently to prevent life-threatening haemodynamic instability.

INTRODUCTION

Heart valve emergencies are a cause of sudden deterioration in cardiac function. The underlying cause depends on the valve involved. The emergency physician has a crucial role in the diagnosis and management of these conditions.

INEFECTIVE ENDOCARDITIS

This is a commonly missed diagnosis. A high index of suspicion must be maintained as delay in diagnosis will increase the mortality and morbidity.

EPIDEMIOLOGY

The incidence in the developed world in the 1980s was between 1.7 and 2.0 cases per 100 000 population.[1] The median age has increased from 30–40 years to 50–55 years.[1-3] Previously, the major predisposing factor was rheumatic heart disease. Mitral valve prolapse, degenerative heart disease and prosthetic valve endocarditis are now the prominent pathologies.[1,3] Intravenous drug use (IVDU) is a major predisposing behaviour in younger patients. The incidence of infective endocarditis (IE) in this group is 150–2000 cases per 100 000 person-years.[4]

PATHOLOGY

In the developing countries, rheumatic heart disease is the commonest risk factor for infective endocarditis. In the developed world the risk factors are:

- Host related factors[4,5]
  - poor oral hygiene
  - severe renal disease on haemodialysis
  - diabetes mellitus
  - mitral valve prolapse – particularly in the presence of valve incompetence or thickening of the leaflets.
- Procedure related factors[4]
  - infected intravascular device
  - post genitourinary procedure
  - post gastrointestinal procedure
  - surgical wound infection.

Pathogens of native valve endocarditis (NVE)[4]

In adults (15 years of age or above) the ranking of the responsible organisms is the same across age groups, with some difference in the magnitude of the percentages in those above the age of 60 years (Table 4.7.1).

In 15–60 year-olds, *Streptococcus viridans* accounts for up to two-thirds, with

Table 4.7.1 Pathogens of NVE		
Organism	15–60 years	60+ years
Streptococcus species	45–65%	30–45%
Staphylococcus aureus	30–40%	25–30%
Coagulase-negative	4–8%	3–5%
Staphylococcus aureus		
Enterococci	5–8%	14–17%
Gram-negative bacillus	4–10%	1–2%
Culture-negative	3–10%	5%
Fungi	1–3%	1–2%
Polymicrobial	1–2%	1–3%

Staphylococcus aureus being responsible for up to 30%.[1-3] Over 60 years, the major pathogens are similar, however, enterococci are more highly featured than in any other age group.[1] Resistant infective endocarditis is frequently caused by by enterococci. Enterococci also commonly causes nosocomial bacteraemia. The incidence of infective endocarditis in enterococcal bacteraemia is of the order of 10%.[4] *S. bovis* is also peculiar to this age and is associated with colonic polyps and gastrointestinal malignancy.[1,2]

In intravenous drug users (IVDU), *Staph. aureus* accounts for at least 50% of the pathogens. It is responsible for up to 77% of right-sided endocarditis.[1] Unusual organisms can be found, including fungus species. Notably, polymicrobial endocarditis is found only in this group and in neonates.

Pathogens of prosthetic valve endocarditis (PVE)[4]

The risk of infection at 12 months is 1% and this rises to 2–3% at 60 months.[4]

The patients can be divided into three groups according to the time the infection occurs post-surgery (Table 4.7.2). Early prosthetic endocarditis occurs in less than 2 months. The infection is

Table 4.7.2 Pathogens of PVE. The organisms are ranked in order of likelihood

Early	Intermediate	Late
Coagulase - negative	Staphylococcus aureus	Coagulase-negative
Staphylococcus aureus	Streptococcus species	
Staphylococcus aureus	Staphylococcus aureus/enterococci	Staphylococcus aureus
Gram- negative bacillus	Streptococcus species	Coagulase-negative Staphylococcus aureus
Enterococci	Culture-negative/polymicrobial	Enterococci

acquired in hospital. Late prosthetic endocarditis occurs after 12 months. The infection is community-acquired. Between 2 to 12 months, the organisms responsible are a combination of nosocomial and community acquired.

PATHOGENESIS

In IE, the interactions between host and organism are complex. Platelet-fibrin deposits form at sites of endothelial damage and are called non-bacterial thrombotic endocarditis (NBTE).[1] Invasion and multiplication of the virulent microbe in these cases lead to enlargement of these vegetations, which become infected. The consequences are the basis of the clinical complications of IE. The vegetations can fragment and embolize, leading to distal foci of infection. Obstruction of vessels by these fragments can result in tissue ischaemia and infarction. Seeding from the fragments perpetuates the bacteraemia. Local destruction of the valve may extend to its supporting structures and surrounding tissue, hence the conducting tissue and myocardium may be involved.

CLINICAL FEATURES

IE should be considered a multisystem disease. The symptoms and signs are non-specific, compounding the difficulty of diagnosis. Symptoms usually occur within two months of the event responsible for the initiation of bacteraemia,[1] although this may be difficult to identify.

The two most frequent systemic features are fever and malaise. Fever is present in 80–85% of cases.[1,2] It can be absent in the severely debilitated, the elderly and those with cardiac failure, chronic renal failure, liver failure, recent antibiotic use and if the infection is by an organism with low virulence.[1,4] The height of the fever is rarely above 39.4°C.[1]

Malaise is reported in up to 95% of cases.[1,2] Other symptoms are variable and non-specific, and may include headache, confusion, cough, chest pain (more common in IVDU with IE), dyspnoea, abdominal pain, anorexia, weight loss and myalgia.

With respect to cardiac features, a new or changed incompetent murmur may be found. However, in 70–95% of cases a murmur is pre-existent, hence the discovery of an acute murmur is an uncommon but highly significant finding. The absence of a murmur does not exclude the diagnosis of IE. A new or a change of murmur is more likely in patients with a prosthetic valve or congestive cardiac failure.

Congestive cardiac failure is one of the complications of IE. It is usually a result of infection-induced valvular damage. Involvement of the aortic valve is more likely to cause congestive cardiac failure than mitral valve damage. The other cause is extension of the infective process beyond the valvular annulus. Involvement of the septum produces atrioventricular, fascicular and bundle branch blocks.

Pericarditis can result from extension into the sinus of Valsalva. Haemopericardium and tamponade may occur. Myocardial infarction as a result of infective embolism to the coronary arteries can also occur, but is rare.

Neurological manifestations are present in 30 to 40% of patients and are more likely if the pathogen is *Staph. aureus*. Sixty-five per cent of all embolic events occur in the central nervous system (CNS). These include meningoencephalitis, focal deficits, transient ischaemic attacks and stroke. Embolic stroke is the most frequent event, but intracranial haemorrhage may occur as a result of rupture or leak of a mycotic aneurysm, septic arteritis or bleeding into an infarct. The mortality is high.[1,2]

Systemic embolization occurs in 40% of cases and gives rise to the peripheral manifestations of infective endocarditis. The embolization usually antedates the diagnosis. Its incidence falls with the administration of appropriate antibiotics. Notably, systemic emboli are absent in IE of the tricuspid valve.[1]

Petechiae are commonly found in the palpebral conjunctivae and are also present in the mucosal membranes. Splinter haemorrhages under the fingernails, Osler's nodes (painful tender swellings of the fingertips or toe pads), Janeway lesions (small haemorrhages with a slightly nodular character on the palms and soles) and Roth's spots (oval retinal haemorrhages with a clear pale centre) are uncommon.[1,2]

Renal dysfunction may be due to altered renal haemodynamics, immune complex-mediated glomerulonephritis or nephrotoxicity from medications.

Splenomegaly is present in 30% of cases. This is due to splenic abscesses arising from direct seeding from the bacteraemia or from an infective embolus. It leads to persistent fever, abdominal pain and diaphragmatic irritation. Tender hepatomegaly may also be present. Anaemia is common.

DIAGNOSIS

The diagnosis of IE requires an integration of data from various sources. This is due to the non-specific nature of the clinical manifestations. The Duke criteria for IE are a useful diagnostic tool that has good specificity and a negative predictive value above 92%.[4] These combine patient risk factors, isolates from blood cultures, the persistence of bacteraemia, echocardiographic findings and other clinical and laboratory data.

When fever is persistent and unexplained, infective endocarditis must be considered:

- In patients with acquired or congenital valvular heart disease, pre-existing prosthetic valve, hypertrophic cardiomyopathy, congenital heart disease (PDA, VSD, coarctation of the aorta), intracardiac pacemakers, central venous lines or intra-arterial lines or a new or changed cardiac murmur.
- Known bacteraemia. In *Staph. aureus* bacteraemia, the risk of IE is higher if: it is community acquired; there is no primary focus of infection; there is a metastatic complication; in the context of an intravascular catheter being a possible focus of infection, if fever or bacteraemia is present for greater than 3 days, despite removal of the catheter
- Recent procedures likely to cause a bacteraemia – dental, bronchoscopy, gastrointestinal and genitourinary procedures.
- There are features of an embolic event, especially if recurrent.
- In young patients with unexpected stroke or subarachnoid haemorrhage.
- In patients with a history of IVDU, especially if there are pulmonary features such as cough and pleuritc chest pain.
- When there is persistent bacteraemia despite treatment, persistent fever despite treatment, congestive cardiac failure or new ECG features of atrioventricular heart block, fascicular block and bundle branch block.

INVESTIGATIONS

Blood cultures are crucial to the diagnosis of IE. If no prior antibiotics have been given, blood cultures are positive in 95–100% of cases, often in the first two sets.[1] The major causes of culture-negative IE are prior use of antibiotics and fastidious organisms. In the stable patient without evidence of complications, three sets of blood cultures should be collected over 24 hours prior to the start of empirical antibiotics. An aerobic and an anaerobic medium is used in each set. Bacteraemia in IE is continuous and hence there is no need to collect cultures in relationship to fever.[1]

Arterial and venous blood are equally likely to be infected.

Anaemia is demonstrated in most patients. It is usually normochromic and normocytic. There is a leucocytosis in acute IE but this is absent in subacute IE. Thrombocytopenia is rare. The ESR is a non-specific test; however, it is raised in almost all patients to a magnitude of greater than 55 mm/h. A normal ESR makes IE less likely.[1] The exceptions are patients with congestive cardiac failure, renal failure and disseminated intravascular dissemination.

The urinalysis is abnormal in 50% of patients,[1] with proteinuria and microscopic haematuria. Normal renal function may be maintained.

Echocardiography provides morphological confirmation of the diagnosis. Two modes of echocardiography are used. Both are useful in imaging the valve and perivalvular lesions. Transthoracic echocardiography (TTE) has a specificity for vegetations of 98%, but a sensitivity of less than 60–70%. The reason for the low sensitivity is the technical problems in those with chest-wall deformity, chronic airway limitation and obesity. However, it has the benefit of being non-invasive. Transoesophageal echocardiography (TOE) is invasive and more difficult to obtain. It has a specificity of 85–98% and the sensitivity is 75–95% for vegetations. In particular, it will detect perivalvular lesions and abscesses. The indication for TTE in IE is suspected native valve IE with no technical hindrance to imaging. If the result is negative and coupled with a low clinical suspicion, a subsequent TOE is not warranted. The indications for TOE in IE are:

- Prosthetic valves
- Suspected myocardial involvement
- Unexplained gram-negative coccus bacteraemia
- Catheter related *Staph. aureus* bacteraemia
- Current intravenous drug use
- Suspected perivalvular extension of disease.

Despite the virtues of TOE, a negative study does not exclude the diagnosis or the need to start treatment if clinical suspicion is high. The false-negative range is 6–18%, which decreases to 4–13% with a repeat study.[1] There are a number of limitations of echocardiography: infectious vegetations cannot be distinguished from marantic lesions on native valves or thrombus on prosthetic valves and healed lesions cannot be easily separated from active ones. Entities that may mimic vegetations are thickened valves, ruptured chordae or valves, calcifications and nodules.

MANAGEMENT

Management involves the use of antibiotics to eradicate the pathogen and other interventions to deal with the intracardiac and distal complications of the infections. Surgery may be required for the latter.

Antibiotic therapy

In the emergency department, a microbiological diagnosis is not possible. Toxic patients must start empirical antibiotics after the collection of three sets of cultures at three separate venepuncture sites. These do not need to be separated in time in the septic patient.[6] *Staph. aureus* is commonly the pathogen in fulminant IE. There are different regimens available, but all recommend intravenous therapy for a period of 4–6 weeks.

Microbiological consultation should be made and the appropriate antibiotic used when the sensitivities are available. The organism must be retained until a cure is confirmed. This is due to frequent adverse reactions necessitating a change in antibiotic. The principle of the therapy is to use a synergistic bactericidal combination of a cell-wall active agent (penicillin, ampicillin or vancomycin) together with an aminoglycoside. The following empirical regimens are derived from the *Therapeutic Guidelines*.[6]

❶ General regimen: benzylpenicillin 1.8 g, 4 hourly AND flucloxacillin 2 g, 4 hourly AND gentamicin 4–6 mg/day intravenously

❷ Patients with nosocomial infection, prosthetic valves or penicillin hypersensitivity: vancomycin 1 g, intravenously 12 hourly AND gentamicin 4–6 mg/kg daily intravenously.

Prophylactic antibiotics[1,6]

Prophylaxis is widely accepted but unproven. The effectiveness is based on animal models and empirical observations and not on placebo-controlled trials. The two factors that requires consideration are the cardiac condition and the procedure being performed in that patient. The risk of adverse effect from the antibiotic must be weighed against the risk of endocarditis. The publication *Therapeutic Guidelines*[6] is a useful guide. Microbiological consultation can be sought.

Anticoagulation[4]

The use of anticoagulants to prevent embolic events have not been proven. It increases the risk of intracranial haemorrhage. Aspirin has also not be shown to be effective. In native valve endocarditis, use of antocoagulants is indicated only if the need is separate from the IE. If an intracranial haemorrhage or a mycotic aneurysm is present, anticoagulation must be stopped. In prosthetic valve endocarditis, anticoagulants should be used with caution and ceased if any of the above complications are present. The risk of intracranial haemorrhage in patients on anticoagulants is high if the organism responsible is *Staph. aureus*.

Surgery

Surgical intervention has been shown to improve mortality under certain circumstances:

- Congestive cardiac failure. Moderate to severe congestive cardiac failure is the strongest indication for surgery. The mortality drops from a range of 56–86% to 11–35%. The haemodynamic status at surgery determines the mortality.
- Uncontrolled infection despite appropriate medical therapy. Medical therapy is not adequate if the causative organisms are *Pseudomonas aeruginosa*, brucella species, *Coxiella burnetti*, enterococcus or fungus.
- *Staph. aureus* infections. Survival requires a combination of medical and surgical treatment.
- Perivascular infection.
- In prosthetic valve endocarditis, if there is relapse after therapy or instability of the prosthesis.

Contraindications to surgery are relative. The risk of post-operative neurological deterioration is present after surgery. Surgery should be delayed by at least 4 weeks in those with an intracranial haemorrhage. In patients with an embolic event, the delay should be at least 2–3 weeks.

Mortality and prognosis

The overall mortality for native and prosthetic valve endocarditis is 20–25%.[4] In right sided lesions in intravenous drug users, the mortality is 10%. The most important determinant of mortality is congestive cardiac failure. Mortality is also related to the organism isolated. It is greater than 50% in *Pseudomonas aeruginosa*, enterobacteriacae or fungal infection. *Staph. aureus* infection has a mortality of 25–47%. The major causes of death are haemodynamic deterioration and embolic complications of the CNS.

Relapse occurs usually within 2 months of stopping antibiotics. The rate of relapse in native valve endocarditis is <2% for penicillin sensitive organisms and 8–10% for enterococci. In prosthetic valve endocarditis the relapse rate is 10–15%. Primary treatment failure can occur even with combined medical and surgical treatment if the organism is *Staph. aureus*, enterobacteriacae or fungi.

PATHOPHYSIOLOGY

An acute and progressive volume overload within a left ventricle that has not had time to compensate is the essence of the haemodynamic problem. The consequence is an elevated left ventricular end-diastolic pressure (LVEDP). Transmission of this pressure elevation to the left atrium and pulmonary venous bed leads to pulmonary oedema. The cardiac output is diminished as the stroke volume is shared between forward and regurgitant flow into the left atrium. The compensatory mechanisms via the sympathetic nervous system (SNS) result in positive inotropy and chronotropy. However, the rise in the systemic peripheral vascular resistance (SVR) impedes left ventricular outflow and worsens the regurgitation. Ventricular oxygen demand is also increased and myocardial ischaemia is a real risk even if coronary artery disease is not present.

The causes, in order of frequency, are infective endocarditis, proximal aortic dissection, blunt chest trauma, and spontaneous rupture of an abnormal valve.[1,6]

CLINICAL FEATURES

Acute aortic incompetence is poorly tolerated. Severe congestive cardiac failure and hypotension are typical. Hence the patients essentially present with pulmonary oedema and cardiogenic shock. The diastolic murmur is soft and extends only to mid-diastole. The pulse pressure is large.

INVESTIGATION

The CXR may reveal the underlying cause. Pulmonary congestion is often present without cardiac enlargement. Echocardiography is diagnostic and provides useful data especially in the selection of timing for surgery. A TOE is required if aortic root dissection is thought to be the cause. Cardiac catheterization precedes surgery except under dire circumstances.[6]

MANAGEMENT[7]

Valve replacement is crucial to survival, as severe left ventricular failure (LVF) is the commonest cause of death. Medical treatment with a positive inotrope (dopamine or dobutamine) and concurrent vasodilatation (with nitroprusside) are used, but only serve as preoperative measures.

Inra-aortic balloon counterpulsatoin is contraindicated. Beta-blockers should be used with caution as the compensatory tachycardia will be prevented. In patients with infective endocarditis with stable haemodynamics, surgery may be deferred;[1] however, early surgical consultation is needed.[1,6,8]

ACUTE DETERIORATION IN CHRONIC AORTIC INCOMPETENCE

PATHOPHYSIOLOGY

In chronic aortic valve (AV) incompetence the pathophysiology is dictated by the combination of pressure and volume overload. The initial stage of compensation is achieved by hypertrophy of the left ventricle. The LVEF is never in the normal range even in the compensated stage. However, the patient can be asymptomatic for decades. This is followed by the uncompensated stage where there is a significant reduction of the left ventricular ejection fraction, defined as a LVEF of 50% or less at rest. This results predominantly from volume overload. It is reversible initially, with full recovery of left ventricular function if AV replacement is performed.

The uncompensated phase becomes irreversible with enlargement of the left ventricle. The symptoms become severe and reversal by surgery is then not possible.

Apart from abnormalities intrinsic to the aortic valve, aortic root dilatation from various causes must be considered.

CLINICAL FEATURES

The patient may be asymptomatic. As the left ventricular dysfunction deteriorates, clinical features of cardiac failure are present. The patients are usually hypertensive.

INVESTIGATION

The aim of investigations is to identify those who will need surgery. Serial investigations are usually performed. The most important is the assessment of LVEF and LV systolic and diastolic volumes by echocardiogram.

MANAGEMENT

Medical management

The objective is to improve forward stroke volume and to reduce the regurgitant load on the left ventricle and therefore preservation of LV systolic function and reduction of LV mass. This is achieved by using vasodilators. The dose is titrated to the blood pressure, aiming to reduce it to a level tolerated by the patient. Decreasing the BP to a normal range is rarely possible. This therapy is contraindicated in patients with normal blood pressure. In patients with normal BP who has mild AV incompetence and normal LV size, no treatment is required. Nifedipine and hydralazine have been used with good effect on the LV. Angiotensin converting enzyme inhibitors (ACE) have provided less consistent results.

Surgical management

Indications for AV replacement are :

- Symptomatic patients
- Asymptomatic patients with LVEF ≤50%
- Asymptomatic patients with severe LV dilatation with LV end systolic volume (LVESV) of >55 mm or LV end-diastolic volume (LVEDV) >75 mm.

ACUTE MITRAL INCOMPETENCE

PATHOPHYSIOLOGY

Acute volume overload into the left atrium by the regurgitant stream is the crucial factor in acute mitral incompetence. The left atrium has limited capacity to accommodate this insult, and pulmonary oedema occurs. There is an associated rise in the pulmonary vascular resistance. Right ventricular failure may result. Cardiac output is reduced owing to a low stroke volume. The consequent elevation in the SVR impedes cardiac output. Tachycardia occurs but confers no benefit as the diastolic filling time is reduced.[8]

CAUSES

- Papillary muscle disorder
  - ischaemia or infarction
  - trauma
  - infiltrative disease.
- Rupture of the chordae tendinae
  - acute rheumatic fever
  - infective endocarditis
  - chest trauma
  - balloon valvotomy
  - myxomatous degeneration
  - spontaneous rupture.
- Mitral leaflet disorder
  - infective endocarditis
  - myxomatous degeneration
  - atrial myxoma
  - systemic lupus erythematosus
  - trauma.

CLINICAL FEATURES

Acute mitral valve imcompetence (MVI) is poorly tolerated and patients are always symptomatic. The patient looks extremely unwell with poor forward output and acute dyspnoea from pulmonary congestion. The blood pressure is variable and can be normal or low. The precordial findings do not correlate with the severity of the pathology. A normal

CARDIOVASCULAR

LV will not produce a hyperdynamic apical impulse. The third heart sound may be the only finding, although a fourth heart sound is common. The apical mitral murmur is soft and occurs in early systole and does not become pansystolic. It radiates to the axilla and is commonly accompanied by a short apical diastolic murmur.

INVESTIGATION

The CXR will show pulmonary oedema but not cardiomegaly. The ECG may show a recent infarct. Echocardiography is diagnostic and provides valuable information on left ventricular function. A TTE may underestimate the severity of the lesion due to inadequate imaging. If the information is insufficient for assessment, a TOE should be used.

MANAGEMENT

Mitral valve replacement is urgently required. Medical treatment is usually only a temporizing step.

Surgical treatment

Left heart studies and consideration for surgical treatment should be carried out prior to the development of severe LVF. If the patient can be stabilized by medical treatment, then surgery can be deferred.

Medical treatment

The mortality in patients with severe left-ventricular failure (LVF) is high. Medical treatment is directed at the reduction of the regurgitant volume and hence diminishing the pulmonary congestion. It also aims to improve the forward output of the left ventricle. The modalities used depend on the blood pressure.

In normotensive patients, sodium nitroprusside (SNP) may achieve all of the above objectives. In hypotensive patients, a combination of SNP and an inotrope such as dobutamine is required. Aortic ballon counterpulsation may be required to improve LV ejection volume

and further assists in the reduction of the regurgitant volume. This may be the only method of stabilization prior to emergency surgery.

ACUTE DETERIORATION IN CHRONIC MITRAL INCOMPETENCE

PATHOPHYSIOLOGY

In chronic MVI the increased LVEDV leads to an increased LV stroke volume and hence forward flow is preserved. The other factors that enable this are the increased preload on the LV and the ability of the LV to reduce afterload by backfilling into the left atrium. The result is enlargement of the left atrium and ventricle. In this compensated phase the patient is asymptomatic and this may last for years.

In the phase of decompensation, LV systolic dysfunction occurs due to contractile failure. This causes a rise in the LVESV leading to further LV dilatation and LV preload. A fall in forward LV outflow and pulmonary congestion may result. However, the factors are often still in favour of the LV and the LVEF may be in the lower range of normal, i.e. 0.5–0.6.

The cause may be ischaemic or non-ischaemic (mitral valve prolapse, degenerative). Ischaemic causes have the worst prognosis as myocardial dysfunction is often coexistent.

CLINICAL FEATURES

The role of the emergency physician is to identify the patient who now presents in the decompensated phase of their mitral-valve disease. This will require records of previous clinical assessment as the onset of symptoms can be subtle. Notably, in the examination, the displacement of the apical impulse is an indication of the dilatation of the LV. A third heart sound is commonly found and is not necessarily evidence of left-ventricular failure.

INVESTIGATIONS

Serial CXR and ECG are important. The most important test is the ECG. The size of the LV and left atrium should be documented. Data on the LVEF and the severity on the MVI are collected. The integrity of the tricuspid valve is also important.

MANAGEMENT

The emergency department management often requires the initiation of treatment and/or cardiology consultation. This depends on the clincial presentation.

Medical treatment

Atrial fibrillation (AF) is a common morbidity in chronic MVI. The ventricular rate requires control. Anticoagulation is used as prophylaxis for embolic complications. AF is also an independent predictor of poor outcome after surgery. It is more likely to remain post surgery if it has been present for greater than 1 year or the left atrial size is greater than 50 mm.

In the presence of systemic hypertension, vasodilators can be used, although there are no studies supporting long-term benefit. In patients with no systemic hypertension, there is no indication for the use of vasodilators if the left ventricular function is preserved. In some centres, asymptomatic patients with normal left ventricular function are offered surgery (see below).

Surgical treatment

Surgery is indicated in symptomatic patients with preserved LV function as defined by a LVEF >0.6 or a ESV <45 mm. In these patients surgery, whether this is repair or valve replacement, improves symptoms of cardiac failure and preserves LVF. It is also indicated if there is LV dysfunction. Surgery should also be considered in asymptomatic patients with a recent or chronic atrial fibrillation.

ACUTE DETERIORATION IN CRITICAL AORTIC STENOSIS

The patient with a severely stenosed aortic valve can remain asymptomatic for many years. Medical treatment can achieve a 5-year survival of 40% and a 10-year survival of 20%.[1] The risk of sudden death in the asymptomatic patient is 2%, even when critical stenosis is present.[1] With the development of syncope and angina, the survival falls to 2–3 years. When cardiac failure is present the survival is 1.5 years;[1] 50% will die within 18 months with no surgical intervention.

PATHOPHYSIOLOGY

Aortic valve stenosis restricts left ventricular outflow and imposes a pressure load on the left ventricle. The latter is hypertrophied, with consequent poor compliance, and it is at risk of ischaemia and dysrhythmia. Cardiac function is delicately balanced between preload and afterload. Preload on the hypertrophied ventricle is elevated to support the stroke volume, but not high enough to lead to pulmonary congestion. The SVR is elevated but does not cause an increase in the oxygen demand that will not be met. The reserve margin is slim. A small and sudden alteration in any of these factors will precipitate pump failure.

CAUSES OF ACUTE DETERIORATION

- **Acute fall in preload:** hypovolaemia, excessive diuresis and vasodilatation.
- **Atrial flutter or fibrillation.** These are both uncommon and should raise suspicion of associated mitral valve disease. Unfortunately, in these patients atrial systole contributes 40% (normal is 25%) to the left ventricular preload and may result in hypotension.[1,8]

- **Acute afterload reduction.** This leads to a reduction in coronary artery perfusion and places the hypertrophied LV at risk of ischaemia. It does not improve the LV stroke volume as the problem lies in the stenotic valve and not the SVR.

CLINICAL FEATURES

The patient presents with acute pump failure: shock and pulmonary oedema. The murmur will not be impressive as the cardiac output is poor.

MANAGEMENT

Rapid reversal of the precipitant is essential. Medical therapy may allow cardiac catheterization to be performed prior to surgery. Expedient treatment of atrial dysrhythmias may necessitate cardioversion. Definitive treatment is valve replacement. Sudden death is common.[8]

ACUTE DETERIORATION IN MITRAL STENOSIS

PATHOPHYSIOLOGY

The adult mitral orifice is 4–6 cm². Critical stenosis occurs when this is reduced to 1 cm² but the patient may remain asymptomatic for many years. A pressure load is imposed on the left atrium; pulmonary congestion and pulmonary hypertension are the consequences. The major damage is incurred by the lungs and right ventricle.

CAUSES OF ACUTE DETERIORATION

Acute deterioration can be precipitated in two ways. When the heart rate is increased, the ventricular filling time in diastole is reduced. The atrial pressure rises and is transmitted retrogradely to the pulmonary bed, leading to acute dyspnoea and pulmonary oedema. Atrial fibrillation with a rapid ventricular response is a common example of this. In addition, loss of atrial systole in atrial fibrillation leads to a 20% decrease in cardiac output.[1] Therefore, major haemodynamic instability can occur.

The second cause of acute deterioration is related to flow across the stenosed valve. When the flow is increased, the transvalvular pressure gradient is increased by a factor equal to the square of the flow rate.[1] The left atrial pressure rises and can precipitate pulmonary congestion. The common clinical contexts in which the transvalvular flow is increased are exercise, pregnancy, hypervolaemia and hyperthyroidism.

CLINICAL FEATURES

Patients may be asymptomatic for many years. The commonest symptom is dyspnoea, which may be accompanied by wheezing and coughing. In severe cases orthopnoea is present, with dyspnoea at rest. Precipitant pulmonary oedema may occur under the circumstances mentioned previously.

Signs of critical stenosis are small pulse pressure, soft first heart sound, early opening snap, long diastolic murmur, diastolic thrill and evidence of pulmonary hypertension. Acute pulmonary oedema may be present. Atrial fibrillation with a rapid ventricular rate is frequently the cause. Evidence of systemic embolization of a left atrial thrombus should be sought.

INVESTIGATIONS

The CXR features are those of an enlarged left atrium, pulmonary congestion and pulmonary hypertension. The heart size is usually normal. Left atrial enlargement on the ECG is found in 90% of patients in sinus rhythm.[1] A detailed echocardiograph assessment is required to develop a management plan.

MANAGEMENT

In acute pulmonary oedema the underlying cause must be treated as well as the pulmonary congestion. Rapid ventricular response in atrial fibrillation may require cardioversion in the unstable patient. Surgical considerations should be pursued after the resolution of the acute deterioration.

PROSTHETIC VALVE COMPLICATIONS

Prosthetic valve complications are common. As discussed previously they are prone to IE so antibiotic prophylaxis is essential in the preventation of this.

ANTITHROMBOTIC THERAPY[7]

This is given to prevent embolic complications. The risk is greater in mitral than aortic prosthesis regardless of the type.It is also highest in the first few months as the prothesis has not been fully endothelialized. Warfarin is the anti-coagulant of choice.

Target INR values for mechanical valves

Position	Valve	INR range
Aortic	bileaflet of Medtronic Hall	2.0–3.0
	Starr-Edward or other discs	2.5–3.5
Mitral	Any	2.5–3.5

Aspirin in the dose range of 80–100 mg/day may be used in addition to warfarin in patients with an embolic event with the INR in the therapeutic range, known vascular disease or a susceptibility to hypercoagulability. This has been shown to reduce the risk of thromboembolism and cardiovascular mortality. The data only refer to aspirin doses within this range.

Biological valves

The increased risk of thromboembolism is in the first 3 months. The incidence is

at its height during the initial few days. Heparin therapy is started as soon as surgical bleeding is reduced. After the 3-month period, the biological prosthetic valve can be regarded as a native valve. Warfarin is ceased in two-thirds of the patients. The remaining one-third stay on a lifetime treatment with an INR in the range of 2.0–3.0. Patients requiring lifetime warfarin therapy include those with atrial fibrillation, a past history of thromboembolism, a risk of hypercoagulability and those with severe left ventricular dysfunction with a LVEF <0.3.

Complications of antithrombotic therapy

These are not uncommon findings in the emergency department:

Embolic episode

The treatment depends on the anti-thrombotic regime used. There are several options:

- INR 2.0–3.0 – increase dose to achieve an INR of 3.5
- INR 2.5–3.5 – increase dose to achieve an INR of 3.5–4.5
- Add aspirin – 80–100 mg/d
- Increase aspirin – up to a dose of 325 mg/d
- Add warfarin if on aspirin alone.

Excessive anticoagulation

Most institutions will have guidelines for this, based on the presence of absence of haemorrhage and the level of anticoagulation. In general, in the aymptomatic patients, the INR should be reduced gently and vigilance for overshooting the therapeutic range must be kept.

Management when surgery is required

The risk of stopping anticoagulation must be weighed against the risk of intraoperative bleeding. Those patients requiring heparin until warfarin can be used again are:

- Those with an episode of thromboembolism within the last 12 months
- Those with thromboembolic episode whilst off warfarin

- Patients with a Bjork-Shiley valve
- Those with greater than or equal to three of the following: atrial fibrillation; hypercoagulable syndrome; past history of thromboembolis, mechanical prosthesis and left-ventricular dysfunction
- Patients with mitral valve prosthesis, any one of the above risk factors is sufficient.

OBSTRUCTION OF PROSTHETIC VALVES

The mechanical and porcine xenograft prostheses used, have a smaller orifice than a normal native valve. Endothelialization after implantation reduces the orifice further. Hence they are essentially stenotic, but this is not functionally important.

In general, a grade 1–2 systolic murmur is acceptable. Additionally,most prostheses have a degree of incompetence. However, audible diastolic murmurs should be followed up.

MANAGEMENT

Significant obstruction of the prosthetic valve may occur as a result of thrombosis or pannus infiltration or both. If the obstruction is due to pannus infiltration, thrombolytic therapy is ineffective and surgery is required.

The indication for surgery is a large obstructive clot associated with a NYHA Class III or IV symptoms. In general, thrombolytic therapy is ineffective in 16–18% of patients. The mortality is high at 6%. The risk of complications is also insubstantial with a risk of a disabling haemorrhage of 5% and the likelihood of rethrombosis of 11%. Hence it can only be indicated in patients with contra-indications to surgery or where the latter carries a high mortality. Streptokinase and urokinase are used. The duration depends on the resolution of the pressure gradient across the valve and the recovery of the valvular area. Therapy is ceased if no improvement is present after 24 hours. The maximum duration is 72 hours. If the treatment is successful, heparin is given until an INR of 3–4 is achieved in aortic prosthesis and an INR of 3.5–4.5 for mitral prosthesis. In partial success, subcutaneous heparin (APTT 55–80 seconds) and warfarin (INR 2.5–3.5) is given for 3 months.

When the thrombus is smaller and the clinical features are consistent with a NYHA Class I and II, short-term intravenous heparin can be given and followed by thrombolysis, reoperation or an expectant regime as an outpatient. The latter uses a combination of subcutaneous heparin and warfarin.

SUMMARY

The spectrum of heart valve emergencies is broad. Acute emergencies may involve an acute valve lesion, but frequently the problem is an acute deterioration of a chronic lesion. Good management in the emergency department must centre on early diagnosis, expedient stabilization of haemodynamic problems, and timely surgical consultation.

REFERENCES

1. Karchmer AW 1997 Infective endocarditis. In: Braunwald E (ed.) Heart Disease. A Textbook of Cardiovascular Medicine, 5th edn. WB Saunders, Philadelphia
2. Dunmire SM, Ahrens B 1992 Endocarditis and acquired valvular heart disease. In: Rosen P, Barkin R (eds) Emergency Medicine: Concepts and Clinical Practice, 3rd edn. Mosby Year Book, USA
3. Bansal RC 1995 Infective endocarditis. Medical Clinics of North America 79(5): 1205–40
4. Mylonakis E, Calderwood SB 2001 Medical progress: infective endocarditis in adults. The New England Journal of Medicine 345(18): 1318–30
5. Strom BL, et al 2000 Risk factors for infective endocarditis – oral hygiene and nondental exposures. Circulation 102(23): 2842
6. Therapeutic Guidelines: Antibiotic 2000 Version 11. Therapeutic Guidelines Limited. Melbourne
7. Bonow RO, et al 1998 Guidelines for the Management of Patients with Valvular Heart Disease. Circulation Vol 98: pp 1949–84.
8. Simpson PC, Bristow JD 1979 Recognition and management of emergencies in valvular heart disease. Medical Clinics of North America 63(1): 155–71
9. Talley T, O'Connor S 1989 Clinical Examination: A Guide to Physical Diagnosis. MacLennan & Petty Pty Ltd, Artamon, New South Wales

4.8 PERIPHERAL VASCULAR DISEASE

TAJEK B. HASSAN • JACK BERGMAN

ESSENTIALS

1 The incidence of peripheral arterial and venous disease in the developed world continues to increase significantly with the continuing rise in the elderly population.

2 Claudication is the single most important symptom of arterial occlusive disease in an extremity, although a well developed collateral circulation will delay the onset of symptomatic extremity ischaemia.

3 Acute arterial occlusion is usually associated with a number of classical symptoms and signs. It is a time critical emergency requiring urgent access to an experienced vascular team.

4 Irreversible changes begin to occur within 4–6 hours after acute arterial occlusion.

5 If venous thrombosis is suspected, detailed assessment is essential. Unfortunately the presence or absence of signs and symptoms of deep venous thrombosis (DVT) does not correlate at all well with the presence or absence of actual venous clot. Homan's sign is very non-specific and unreliable.

6 Optimal assessment for DVT should consist of defining a pre-test probability of disease and then performing appropriate non-invasive investigations in the first instance.

7 Non-invasive ultrasound scanning is the investigation of choice for diagnosis of DVT depending upon expertise and availability. Alternatives include impedance plethsmography or venography.

8 Anticoagulation is the recommended treatment for DVT above the level of the popliteal vein. Treatment of below-knee DVT remains controversial but evidence suggests that these patients should also receive anti-coagulation treatment to prevent complications.

9 Extensive ileo-femoral thrombus or thrombus of the upper limb may require early surgical and or thrombolytic treatment to minimize the risk of post thrombotic syndrome.

ARTERIAL DISEASE

INTRODUCTION

Extremity ischaemia may be acute, chronic or acute on chronic. The onset and severity of symptoms may be modified by the development of collateral circulation.

CHRONIC ARTERIAL ISCHAEMIA

The prevalence of peripheral arterial disease increases with age (most symptomatic patients being aged over 60 years) and is twice as high in men as in women between age 50 and 70 years, but almost identical after the age of 70.[1]

Peripheral arterial disease is usually due to atherosclerosis of lower abdominal aorta, iliac femoral and/or politeal arteries. The common disease processes that exacerbates arterial disease include diabetes mellitus, hypertension, smoking, cholesterol abnormalities, ischaemic heart disease, and previous limb surgery or trauma. Good collateral circulation is made up of pre-existing pathways arising from the distributing branches of large and medium-sized arteries. It develops over time when there is an increase in the velocity of flow through them secondary to arterial occlusion developing in a main vascular pathway. Collateral flow can usually provide adequate needs to the resting limb, and sufficient additional needs to sustain moderate exercise. The effects of acute total occlusion may be dire should the collateral circulation not be sufficiently established.

PRESENTATION

Presentation may be acute or chronic. Symptoms consist of pain, ulceration or changes in appearance with swelling or discolouration. Lower limb ischaemia manifests usually as claudication – the most important symptom of extremity arterial occlusive disease. Chronic critical lower limb ischaemia is defined by either of the following two criteria:

❶ Recurring ischaemic rest pain persisting for more than 2 weeks and requiring regular analgesics. There should be an ankle systolic pressure of less than or equal to 50 mmHg, a toe systolic pressure of less than or equal to 30 mmHg, or both.

❷ Ulceration or gangrene of the foot or toes, with similar haemodynamic parameters.[2]

The classical description of of claudication is of pain in a functional muscle unit that occurs as a result of a consistent amount of exercise and is promptly relieved by rest. Limp may also be pronounced. The commonest site of occlusion leading to claudication is the superficial femoral artery leading to pain in one or both calves. This occurs on walking upstairs or slopes and relieved by rest. Less common aorto-iliac disease produces symptoms of pain in the thigh or buttock. Night pain experienced in the foot, relieved by either dependency or, paradoxically, by walking around, implies a reduction in blood flow to a level below that required for normal resting tissue metabolism. Typically the rest pain tends to be distal to the metatarsals, severe, persistent and worsened by elevation.

A detailed examination of the peripheral vascular system is essential. Abnormalities tend to be related to changes in the peripheral arteries and tissue ischaemia. Superficial arteries may feel thick and hardened. Distal pulses may be absent or diminished in amplitude, and bruits (commonly femoral) may be present. Capillary return is usually reduced, atrophic changes are present and the foot is cool to touch. Pallor may be apparent on exercise, usually associated with pain. There may also be pallor on elevation of the foot. The less the elevation resulting in pallor, the greater the degree of stenosis. As the ischaemia becomes more advanced the skin becomes shiny and scaly with associated atrophy of the subcutaneous tissues and muscle. There may be red discoloration in advanced stages of stenosis, caused by capillary blood stasis and a high oxygen extraction. There may

also be tissue necrosis and non-healing wounds or ulcers secondary to trauma, which may progress to gangrene.

INVESTIGATIONS

Standard biochemical blood tests should be carried out to derive baselines for renal and hepatic function as well as to exclude anaemia, polycythaemia, hyperglycaemia, thrombocythaemia and hyperlipidaemia. If there is any doubt about the diagnosis, the ankle-brachial pressure index (ABPI) should be measured. This is calculated (for each leg) by dividing the highest systolic pressure recorded at the respective ankle by the highest systolic brachial pressure obtained in recordings from both arms. Resting ABPI is normally >1, and figures of <0.92 indicate arterial disease. Values >0.5 but <0.9 may be associated with claudication and <0.5 with rest pain. Normal ABPI may be recorded in diabetic patients even though they have claudication due to the presence of medial arterial calcification.

MANAGEMENT

In those patients with a chronic stable disease process, treatment is focused mainly around preventing progression of the disease process. This is usually co-ordinated by the patient's primary physician and consists of regular exercise, control of associated medical diseases and cessation of smoking. In more advanced progressive disease, strategies to minimize other complications including lower limb ulcers and gangrene should also be considered. Patients presenting to the emergency department at this stage or with debilitating symptoms that have not been previously investigated merit early referral for vascular surgical assessment with view to operative intervention.

ACUTE LIMB ISCHAEMIA

Acute limb ischaemia, or 'limb-threatening' ischaemia is associated with significant morbidity and mortality. Early recognition of the signs and symptoms is critical. The arterial occlusion will cause symptoms most obviously when there is inadequate collateral circulation. Causes may be embolic, thrombotic, traumatic, or iatrogenic/self-inflicted in nature. Most (85%) arterial emboli originate in thrombus formation from the heart. Left ventricular thrombus from myocardial infarction accounts for 60% to 70% of arterial emboli, the remainder being from the left atrium. Other causes such as arterial thrombosis are due to endothelial injury or alterations in the blood flow to the limb. Iatrogenic causes may be secondary to intra-arterial cannulation or ischaemic limb anaesthesia.

PRESENTATION

Sudden occlusion of a previously patent artery is a dramatic event. Unfortunately recognition can be difficult particularly in elderly people with chronic confusional states and careful examination is therefore essential. Occlusion may be portrayed by one or more of the classical signs of pulselessness, pain, pallor, paraesthesia and later of paralysis (the '5Ps'). However, none of the above, either alone or in combination, is sufficient to definitely establish or exclude the diagnosis of an acute ischaemic limb. Loss of a palpable pulse in the symptomatic limb as compared to the other side should raise significant concern.

Pain is a severe, constant ache which requires intravenous opiates for relief. The ischaemic periphery is pale, white or cadaveric in appearance, and feels cold to touch. Progression occurs with blotchy areas of cyanosis and further discoloration. Pain, tense swelling and acute tenderness of a muscle belly are late findings. If these findings persist for longer than 12 hours, irreversible ischaemia with gangrene is highly likely.

INVESTIGATION

Doppler ultrasound should be used in all patients where there is concern about the arterial circulation of a limb. A handheld Doppler probe will confirm the presence or absence of a pulse and give some quantification of flow. Other investigations, including basic haematology and biochemical profiles as well as electrocardiography help to rule out other diagnostic possibilities, e.g. low cardiac output state, polycythaemia, identify other contributing factors and establish fitness for surgical intervention.

DIFFERENTIAL DIAGNOSIS

It is important to differentiate between an embolic event and acute progression of a thrombus. The embolic event will tend to be sudden in onset and exhibit some combination of the '5Ps'. In situ progression of thrombus will occur in patients who have longstanding significant peripheral atherosclerosis and well developed collateral circulation. Other diagnoses that must be considered include aortic dissection and phlegmasia cerulea dolens. The latter is a condition of massive ileo-femoral deep venous thrombosis. The initial symptom may be of an acutely swollen and painful leg. As the swelling continues there may be secondary arterial insufficiency. Acute embolus, however, tends to produce pallor and a sharp demarcation, whereas with phlegmasia cerula dolens there is a large cyanotic appearing limb.

It is important to consider other medical causes that can mimic acute embolism of the upper or lower limb. These include neurological disorders (spinal subarachnoid haemorrhage) and low-output states such as sepsis, myocardial infarction or pulmonary embolus.

MANAGEMENT

Key to management for these patients is rapid diagnosis and access to definitive care. Irreversible changes begin to occur within 4–6 hours of onset of symptoms and revascularization is reported to be less effective after 8–12 hours of ischaemia.

Immediate heparinization should be commenced and other correctable aggravating factors (dehydration, sepsis, arrhythmias, myocardial infarction) should be considered and addressed appropriately. Urgent surgical intervention is critical. Embolectomy using a Fogarty catheter, with or without a more definitive revascularization procedure, is the preferred procedure. Angiography is not usually necessary in such circumstances as it tends to introduce unnecessary delay. Ultrasound may be used to rapidly establish a level of occlusion. Intra-arterial thrombolytic therapy has been used in selected cases. Unfortunately, complications can include partial clot lysis, further distal embolization and it can be time-consuming. In general, the risks will outweigh the benefits in many cases.[3]

UPPER LIMB ISCHAEMIA

Symptomatic vascular disease of the upper limb is relatively rare as compared to the lower limb. Presentation to the emergency department is usually due to coldness or colour change in the upper limb or digits.

Acute arterial obstruction may arise secondary to emboli, or from penetrating, blunt or iatrogenic trauma. In rare circumstances, acute occlusion may be associated with thoracic aortic dissection. Diagnosis may be obvious (e.g. trauma) or suggestive by virtue of the presenting history and clinical findings. Thoracic outlet syndrome has a number of mechanical causes leading to brachial plexus or vascular compromise. Arterial complications constitute approximately 1% of such cases.

Examination of the limb, comparing with the other side, palpation of the pulses and delayed capillary return, as well as detailed examination of the neck may help localize the level of occlusion. Use of the handheld Doppler and ultrasound may negate the need for preoperative angiography. In the presence of acute ischaemic symptoms of the forearm and hand due to trauma, urgent operative repair is mandatory. In the case of injuries to the radial or ulnar arteries, if only one vessel is damaged and the collateral flow is satisfactory, the vessel may be ligated.

Emboli to the upper limb most frequently involve the brachial artery. Radial and ulnar artery embolization tends to arise from atherosclerotic plaques, aneurysms of subclavian and axillary arteries, and from complications of thoracic outlet syndrome, rather than from a cardiac source. Embolectomy is the treatment of choice, although in some cases thrombolysis may be considered.

Acute occlusion of a digital artery results in profound ischaemia of the involved digit. Diagnosis is again on clinical grounds with sudden onset of pain, cyanosis, coldness and numbness in the affected digit. A chest X-ray may identify a cervical rib. Referral to a vascular surgeon is again indicated for further investigation as to the exact cause.

VENOUS DISEASE: LOWER LIMB

INTRODUCTION

In contrast to arterial disease, peripheral venous disease most commonly causes cosmetic concerns (varicose veins) only. However, thrombosis in the deep venous system is a life threatening emergency requiring urgent treatment.

It is important to understand that the the venous drainage of the lower limb comprises superficial and deep systems connected by means of perforating veins. A complex framework of valves and muscle pumps ensure that blood is carried up from the feet back to the heart. Venous pathology such as valvular destruction results in directional flow change and venous pooling.

VARICOSE VEINS

Primary varicose veins develop in the absence of deep venous thromboses (DVT). The main underlying physiolo-gical defect in varicose veins is a venous valvular incompetence. Varicose veins may also arise secondary to venous outflow obstruction plus valvular incompetence, or there may even be a primary venous outflow obstruction only. Acute presentation of complications of varicose veins is uncommon. However, the skin overlying varices can become thin and erosion can occur spontaneously or with minor trauma alone, resulting in bleeding. The essentials of treatment include elevation of the limb and gentle digital pressure on the site. Ligation of the offending vein may be necessary. Surgical treatment or injection of the varicosities is required as a later procedure.

SUPERFICIAL VENOUS THROMBOSIS

This is a benign self-limiting disease in most cases. Exclusion of DVT is usually required, although on occasions the diagnosis is obvious. Patients usually present with pain, tenderness and induration along the course of the vein, which may feel firm, cord like and have associated erythema. There are usually no signs of impaired venous return. Underlying causes include varicose veins, surrounding cellulitis or a history of preceding trauma. In the upper limb, the commonest cause is intraveous cannulation.

Treatment depends on the extent, aetiology and symptoms. Superficial, mildly tender and well-localized thrombophlebitis may be treated with mild analgesics, elastic supports and continued daily activity. More severe thrombophlebitis with marked pain, tenderness and erythema may require a period of rest and elevation of the limb. Antibiotics are not indicated. Anticoagulation is necessary only if the process extends into the deep venous system or approaches the sapheno-femoral junction. The prognosis is usually good and there is not an associated tendency for the development of deep venous thrombosis. The process may take 3–4 weeks to resolve. If associated with a varicose vein, superficial thrombophlebitis may recur unless the varix is excised.

DEEP VENOUS THROMBOSIS

Deep venous thrombosis (DVT) is a condition characterized by active thrombosis in the deep venous system of one or both lower limbs. Depending upon the thrombus load and the level of extension of the thrombotic process, embolism proximally into the central pulmonary circulation can lead to sudden collapse and death. Early recognition and treatment is, therefore, essential. The diagnosis and management of acute DVT has changed in recent years with a move towards structured assessment, non invasive investigations and more aggressive treatment for patients with distal clots.

Clinical assessment

Symptoms and signs vary, with one-third having no clinical signs at all. A small number may have classical manifestations. Pain may be located in the calf and/or the thigh, ranging from a dull ache to a tight sensation and is sometimes related to exercise. Examination findings include calf swelling, calf tenderness, tenderness over popliteal or femoral veins, and oedema, but may occasionally be entirely normal. Circumferential limb measurements may be helpful, but up to 1 cm difference occurs naturally. Homan's sign is very non-specific and unreliable.[4] In addition, it is important to incorporate an assessment of risk factors for DVT. These include, a period of acute immobilization, trauma to the lower limbs (especially fractures in cast), hereditary coagulation disorders, previous DVT, pregnancy and the postpartum period (6 weeks) and cancer in an active phase.

One validated method for assessment resulting in the generation of a pre-test probablility[5] of DVT is summarized in Table 4.8.1. Following this initial assessment, radiological investigations are directed by the clinical probability of DVT using either ultrasound, plethysmography or venography according to local protocols and expertise. In some institutions a D dimer assay is used as an addi-

Table 4.8.1 Clinical prediction rule to rank DVT assessment[5]

Ask about:

Score	
Active cancer (on-going treatment, diagnosed within the last 6 months or having palliative care)	+1
Paralysis, paresis or plaster immobilization of a leg	+1
Recently bedridden >3 days or major surgery within past 4 weeks	+1

Look for:

Localized tenderness over distribution of the deep veins	+1
Entire leg swollen	+1
Calf circumference 10 cm below tibial tuberosity is >3 cm greater than other calf	+1
Pitting oedema only in the symptomatic leg	+1
Collateral dilated (but not varicose) veins	+1
An alternative diagnosis as or more likely than DVT	−2

Match the patient's score to the risk:

Score	*Risk of DVT*
3 or more	High
1–2	Moderate
0 or less	Low

CARDIOVASCULAR

tional aid for those defined as low clinical probability.

Investigations

Being non-invasive, cheap and easy to perform at the bedside, ultrasound is currently the most commonly used and readily available test in most institutions.[6] For high clinical probability patients, a negative scan should continue to raise enough concern to proceed to venography at the first visit if clinically warranted. A negative ultrasound result in the setting of intermediate clinical probability for DVT warrants repeat serial ultrasound testing at 5–7 days. If this remains negative, and clinical suspicion becomes strong for DVT, venography should be considered. In most circumstances, an alternative diagnosis is more likely at this stage. Few patients will have a positive second scan. In a study that rescanned all patients with a first negative scan, only 0.9% had a positive second scan and 0.06% developed further symptoms in the intervening week.[7] A positive ultrasound result in the setting of an intermediate to high clinical probability of DVT requires treatment.

However, if there is a low clinical probability for DVT but a positive ultrasound, the scan should be discussed with the radiologist and a venogram should be considered. The overall sensi-

tivity of ultrasound for any lower limb DVT is in the range of 95%, with 96% specificity. In the setting of a low clinical suspicion for DVT, the negative predictive value of the ultrasound is of the order of 99%.[6,8] Failing a satisfactory result with ultrasound, venography would be the next definitive investigative step. Venography has been considered to be the gold standard against which other investigations are rated, but it has the disadvantages of being invasive, painful, expensive, inconvenient to perform, and associated with potential phlebitis, anaphylaxis and other complications.[6] Both ultrasound and venography are operator dependent, and reporting accuracy will be influenced by the skills and experience of the radiologist.

A number of studies have suggested that markers of intravascular thrombosis such as D-dimer assays could be a used as an adjunct in patients with a low clinical risk for DVT.[9] However, D-dimer test characteristics vary greatly depending upon whether the method used is an enzyme-linked immunosorbent assay (ELISA) or a variant of a whole blood latex agglutination study. In some centres, patients with a negative D dimer and low clinical risk for DVT are discharged from the ED with no further follow-up. Local expertise in the interpretation of these markers is essential in

such circumstances. It does, however, reduce the workload of the ultrasonographers for those patients with a low clinical risk for DVT. Despite this, by virtue of its ease and non-invasive nature, venous ultrasound in conjunction with clinical assessment has become the first-line investigation for possible DVT.

Differential diagnosis

The prevalence of DVT for in patients with suggestive symptoms attending the emergency department ranges from 16–30%.[10] Other alternative diagnoses to consider include cellulitis, superficial thrombophlebitis, a ruptured Baker's cyst, chronic leg oedema, chronic venous insufficiency, post operative swelling and arthritis. Rare causes not to miss include pelvic tumours.

Management

Treatment for acute DVT consists of adherence to a number of basic principles and specific treatment strategies according to location and duration of the thrombus. The standard treatment for established DVT is anticoagulation. If clinical suspicion is high and there is a delay in confirming the diagnosis, anticoagulation should be commenced provided there are no contraindications, such as active bleeding. Otherwise, anticoagulation should await confirmation of the diagnosis. Controversy exists as to whether all DVTs require anticoagulation, the role of low-molecular-weight heparins and the potential for outpatient treatment of this condition.[10,11]

Treatment can usually be carried out either as ambulatory care in the home or be hospital based. Hospital-based treatment is certainly indicated if there is severe oedema of the whole of the lower limb or there is thrombus above the groin. Treatment at home is possible as long as there is adequate follow-up of the anti-coagulation regimen and potential complications are explained to the patient.

For patients with a high and large ileofemoral thrombus, consideration should be given to thrombolysis especially if there is haemodynamic changes suggestive of multiple pulmonary emboli.

Thrombectomy may be indicated if the vital functions of the lower limb are threatened. The aim is to reduce the risk of post thrombotic syndrome. Occlusive lower extremity venous thrombi respond poorly to systemic thrombolysis, and the risks of bleeding may outweigh the justification of its use. Catheter-directed thrombolytic therapy, however, has been used to treat large symptomatic iliofemoral thrombi with some success.[12] Alternatively, heparin or low-molecular-weight heparin (e.g. dalteparin 200 iu/kg/day) can be given for 5–7 days with warfarin being started concomitantly.

There is agreement that when a DVT is evident in the popliteal vein and above, anticoagulation is indicated. In these circumstances, low-molecular-weight heparin can again be administered on an outpatient basis.[13] Recent studies suggest the latter approach to be efficacious, safe and cost-effective. Irrespective of the initial anticoagulation regimen employed, all patients require ongoing anticoagulation with warfarin for 3–6 months.

A dilemma arises when there is an isolated DVT below the level of the popliteal vein, or when there is an equivocal finding in the infrapopliteal area and negative findings above. Options include withholding anticoagulation and following the patient with serial ultrasound studies; performing a venogram in equivocal cases where there is a strongly suggestive history; or implementation of anticoagulation. In the setting of an infrapopliteal or calf-vein clot where anticoagulation is not commenced, repeat ultrasound at 3–5 days and again at 7–14 days will determine whether the clot has propagated above the knee with a high degree of sensitivity. Given the risk of pulmonary embolism from calf DVT of the order of 5% and the safety of low-molecular-weight heparin treatment, it is probably prudent to treat confirmed below-knee DVT and to further investigate equivocal cases with venography or serial ultrasound studies.[11,14]

Those patients with recurrent emboli, or who have contraindications for anticoagulation, should be referred for insertion of an inferior vena caval filter.

VENOUS DISEASE: UPPER LIMB

AXILLARY SUBCLAVIAN VEIN THROMBOSIS

Thrombosis of the subclavian and axillary veins is much less common than thrombosis of the lower extremity veins. This occurs predominately in males and often follows upper extremity exertion – 'effort thrombosis'. It may also occur in association with heart failure, metastatic tumours of the mediastinum, trauma and central line placement particularly in chemotherapy patients.

Patients present with swelling of the extremity, either rapidly or slowly over a period of weeks. Severe pain is uncommon, with the usual symptoms being arm heaviness and discomfort exacerbated by activity and relieved by rest.

Clinical findings may include an increased prominence of hand and forearm veins, venous patterning over the shoulder and hemithorax, skin mottling or cyanosis, and non-pitting oedema. There may be tenderness to palpation of the axillary vein within the axilla. The ipsilateral internal jugular vein is not usually enlarged. If it is, the possibility of a superior vena caval obstruction should be considered. Diagnosis may be made by Doppler assessment or ultrasound scanning.

Treatment

Standard treatment consists of anticoagulation with heparin to prevent progression of thrombosis. Symptomatic relief will be attained with elevation of the arm in a sling. A more multidisciplinary approach incorporating catheter-directed thrombolytic therapy, anticoagulation and possibly transluminal balloon angioplasty may be more effective in restoring vein patency and reducing the risk of rethrombosis. Consideration of thoracic outlet decompression should also be considered if appropriate.

The use of long-term anticoagulation may be justified in cases of late diagnosis.

CONTROVERSIES

❶ The role of catheter-directed thrombolytic agents in the treatment of acute arterial ischaemia.

❷ The role of new D-dimer assays in the assessment of patients with a low clinical risk for DVT.

❸ Risk-to-benefit ratios for the treatment or non-treatment of below-knee DVT.

❹ The role of thrombolytic agents in the treatment of extensive ileofemoral DVT.

❺ The management of superficial thrombophlebitis extending above the knee.

However, because of the risk of persistent symptoms that may arise with vigorous upper extremity activity, an aggressive approach to therapy as discussed above may be more beneficial.[2] Axillary vein thrombosis secondary to local trauma associated with central venous cannulation may be treated conservatively, provided the patient is asymptomatic and there are no clinical signs of propagation.

REFERENCES

1. Dormandy JA, Ray S 1996 The natural history of peipheral arterial disease. In: Tooke JE, Lowe GDO (eds). Textbook of Vascular Medicine. Arnold, London
2. Rutherford RB (ed.) 2000 Vascular Surgery, 5th ed., Vols 1 & 2. WB Saunders, London
3. Ricotta JJ, Green RM, DeWeese JA 1987 Use and limitations of thrombolytic therapy in the treatment of peripheral arterial ischaemia: results of a multi-institutional questionnaire. Journal of Vascular Surgery 6: 45–50
4. Banerjee A 1997 The assessment of acute calf pain. Postgraduate Medical Journal 73: 86–8
5. Wells PS, et al 1997 Value of assessment of pre-test probability of deep venous thrombosis in clinical management. Lancet 350: 1795–8
6. Haines ST, Bussey HI 1997 Diagnosis of deep vein thrombosis. American Journal of Health-System Pharmaceuticals 54: 66–74
7. Cogo, et al 1998 Compression ultrasonography for diagnostic management of patients with clinically suspected deep venous thrombosis: prospective chort study. British Medical Journal 316: 17–20
8. Hirsch J, Hoak J 1996 Management of deep vein thrombosis and pulmonary embolus. American Heart Association Scientific Council 93: 2212–45

9. Becher, et al 1996 D-dimer testing and acute venous thromboembolism: a shortcut to accurate diagnosis? Archives of Internal Medicine 156: 939–46
10. Anand SS, et al 1998 The rational clinical exam: does this patient have deep venous thrombosis Journal of the American Medical Association 279: 1094–9
11. Ginsberg JS 1996 Management of venous thromboembolism. New England Journal of Medicine 335: 1816–28
12. Ouriel K 1996 Thrombolytic therapy in peripheral vascular disease. Advances in Surgery 29: 191–206
13. Schulman S 1996 Anticoagulation in venous thrombosis. Journal of the Royal Society of Medicine 89: 624–30
14. Pearson SD, Polak JL, Cartwright S, et al 1995 A critical pathway to evaluate suspected deep vein thrombosis. Archives of Internal Medicine 155: 1773–8
15. Cooke JP, Ma AO 1995 Medical therapy of peripheral arterial occlusive disease. Surgical Clinics of North America 75: 569–79
16. Comerota AJ 1995 Modern day treatment of acute deep venous thrombosis. Australian and New Zealand Journal of Surgery 65: 773–9
17. Turkstra F, Koopman MMW, Büller R 1997 The treatment of deep vein thrombosis and pulmonary embolism. Thrombosis and Haemostasis 78(1): 489–96

4.9 HYPERTENSION

MARIAN LEE

ESSENTIALS

1 Hypertension is defined as a systolic blood pressure (sBP) greater than or equal to 140 mmHg and/or a diastolic blood pressure (dBP) greater than or equal to 90 mmHg.

2 A hypertensive crisis is present when diastolic blood pressure is greater than 120 mmHg.

3 The exact mechanism for the acute rise in blood pressure in hypertensive crisis is not well understood.

4 The pathophysiological consequences of hypertensive crisis are fibrinoid necrosis in arteries, followed by endothelial damage, platelet and fibrin deposition, loss of autoregulatory function and microangiopathic haemolytic anaemia.

5 Management depends on the clinical syndrome, the presence of complications or coexisting conditions, and the risks of intervention.

6 Hypertensive encephalopathy and pre-eclampsia are emergencies that mandate urgent control of the blood pressure.

INTRODUCTION

Hypertension is defined as a systolic blood pressure (sBP) greater than or equal to 140 mmHg and/or a diastolic blood pressure (dBP) greater than or equal to 90 mmHg. It is present in 31% of men and 26% of women over the age of 25 years in Australia. In the period 1999–2000 surveyed, more than 3.6 million Australians in this age group had hypertension. (Australian Bureau of Statistics.)

A hypertensive crisis is uncommon and occurs in less than 1% of the hypertensive population. It is defined by a dBP that is greater than 120 mmHg[2,3] However, some have argued that the absolute magnitude of the blood pressure is not important. Rather, it is the presence of end-organ dysfunction that is the defining factor. End-organ dysfunction is uncommon when the dBP is less than 130 mmHg.[4]

Hypertensive crisis can be divided into 2 distinct clinical entities. Where the sudden rise in the systolic and diastolic BP is associated with end-organ dysfunction, a hypertensive emergency is present. A hypertensive urgency is when there is no evidence of end-organ dysfunction. When a hypertensive crisis is present, it is crucial to the outcome of the patient that this entity is recognized early and appropriate management is rendered.

PATHOPHYSIOLOGY

The pathophysiology of hypertensive crisis remains incompletely deciphered. Any cause of hypertension can lead to a hypertensive crisis. The actual magnitude of the blood pressure is not a dependable guide to the likelihood of end-organ damage. The majority of hypertensive crises occur in patients with pre-existing hypertension. The chronicity of the pathology means that adaptive vascular mechanisms are present. Hence end-organ damage occurs at a higher pressure than in the novice.[4,5] For instance, a previously well patient with an acute rise in the blood pressure as a result of acute glomerulonephritis, will have end-organ dysfunction at a lower blood pressure then a patient a patient with longstanding hypertension.

The actual precipitant of an acute increase in vascular tone is unknown. Activation of the renin-angiotensin-aldosterone (RAS) system is thought to be an important contributor. This may be via the release of vasoconstrictors such as angiotensin II and noradrenaline (nor-epinephrine).[4] Relative hypovolaemia may also precipitate vasoconstriction.[2] The initial rise in the blood pressure leads to vascular compensation through the release of vasodilatory substances that reside in the endothelium. These have been identified as nitric oxide and prostacyclin.[4] If the hypertension is severe and/or sustained, local homeostatic mechanisms are overwhelmed. Consequently, there is endothelial damage. At the histological level, fibrinoid necrosis has been identified as the main pathology with a resultant increase in vascular permeability, inhibition of the local endothelial fibrinolysis and activation of the coagulation cascade. Platelet aggregation and degranulation occur at the damaged endothelium. This promotes local inflammatory changes of the endothelium, thrombosis and further vasoconstriction. Hence a cycle of progressive endothelial damage and increase in vascular resistance occurs.[4,5] This results in end-organ dysfunction from ischaemia and microangiopathic haemolytic anaemia from vascular injury.

CLINICAL ASSESSMENT

The immediate aim in the emergency department is to distinguish between a hypertensive emergency and a hypertensive urgency, by determining the presence or absence of end-organ dysfunction. A secondary objective is to identify the precipitant of the acute rise in blood pressure.

The clinical presentation of the patient with a hypertensive emergency is varied, being dependent on the organ that has dysfunctioned. The hypertensive emergencies are:

- Hypertensive encephalopathy
- Acute pulmonary oedema
- Acute myocardial infarction/unstable angina
- Acute aortic dissection
- Acute deterioration in renal function (in end-stage renal disease)
- Preeclampsia and eclampsia
- Microangiopathic haemolytic anaemia.

Hypertensive encephalopathy

This is an acute organic brain syndrome resulting from a failure of cerebral vascular autoregulation. Autoregulation occurs between a mean arterial pressure (MAP) of 60–120 mmHg and cerebral

blood flow is constant between this range. As the mBP rises, there is compensatory vasoconstriction to prevent hyperperfusion. The upper limit of the compensatory mechanism is a MAP of 180 mmHg. When this point is reached, vasodilatation occurs resulting in cerebral oedema. The magnitude of the MAP at which hypertensive encephalopthy is manifested depends on the chronicity of the hypertension. In previously normotensive patients, this can occur at a BP of 160/100, i.e. MAP of 120 mmHg. In patients with known hypertension, encephalopathy may not occur until much higher blood pressures.[4]

The pathological changes of oedema and micro-haemorrhage are due to the increased permeability of the endothelium. On MRI, changes are predominantly found in the white matter of the parietal and occipital lobes. These findings are symmetrical and due to vasogenic and not cytotoxic oedema. When timely and appropriate management is rendered, the vasogenic oedema is reversible. The MRI findings are recognized as reversible posterior leucoencephalopathy syndrome. It can be found in all age groups and not specific to hypertensive encephalopathy. [4]

Hypertensive encephalopathy presents as an altered level of consciousness associated with an elevation blood pressure. Generalized or focal seizures may occur. Visual abnormalities may also be present. New onset of proteinuria and acute retinopathy may or may not be present and is not required for the diagnosis. If unrecognized, cerebral haemorrhage, oedema and death result. Patients at higher risk include those with untreated or inadequately controlled hypertension, renal disease, thrombotic thrombocytopaenic purpura, preeclampsia and eclampsia and those on medications such as erythropoietin and certain immunotherapy treatments.

Acute pulmonary oedema: myocardial ischemia/unstable angina

An acute and severe rise in the blood pressure can cause an acute myocardial ischaemia syndrome and acute pulmonary

oedema without obstructive coronary arteries disease. However, in patients who have pre-existing hypertension, coronary artery disease may already be present and the risk of myocardial dysfunction is increased. An acute blood pressure rise leads to increased mechanical stress on the left-ventricular wall and consequently, a rise in the myocardial oxygen demand

In patients presenting with symptoms and signs consistent with acute pulmonary oedema and myocardial ischaemia, the magnitude of the blood pressure will identify those with a hypertensive emergency.

Acute aortic dissection

This is the most rapidly deteriorating hypertensive emergency. It is also the most devastating and the mortality remains high. The crucial role of the emergency department is to diagnose and treat this condition expediently. This is discussed in detail in Chapter 4.10.

Acute deterioration in renal function

Acute and severe elevation in the blood pressure may lead to deterioration in the renal function. This manifestation of a hypertensive emergency is difficult to recognize initially. The hypertension will be evident on arrival to the emergency department, but the renal dysfunction may not be recognized for a period of time until oliguria or anuria is present. Biochemical evidence of renal failure is rarely at hand in the emergency department.

Additionally, renal insufficiency may itself be the cause of the hypertensive emergency. This creates a vicious cycle of deterioration in renal function leading to an elevation of the blood pressure, which in turn, compounds the renal dysfunction. Risk groups include patients with chronic renal failure, especially those requiring dialysis and patients who have had a renal transplant, especially if taking corticosteroids and ciclosporin.[4,5]

Preeclampsia

Preeclampsis is a hypertensive emergency, although it is often not thought of as such. It is a syndrome that is present after 20 weeks of gestation. It is comprised of pregnancy-induced hypertension with proteinuria or oedema. Hypertension in pregnancy is defined by sBP ≥140 mmHg or a dBP of ≥90 mmHg. Usually, blood pressure falls in the second trimester of pregnancy. Therefore, a better criteria to use is a change from baseline of sBP by 30 mmHg and dBP of 15 mmHg. The quantitative criteria for proteinuria is 300 mg or more during a 24 hour urine collection. A qualitative correlation using a urine dipstick is a reading of 1+, in the absence of concomitant urinary tract infection.

Preeclampsia is a multisystem disease. The cause is unclear. The HELLP syndrome is a variation of preeclampsia that illustrates the multisystem involvement. HELLP is the acronym for haemolysis, elevated liver enzymes and low platelets. The most severe complication of this syndrome is liver rupture with significant maternal and fetal mortality. The course of preeclampsia is difficult to predict. The hypertension and the proteinura may be mild and yet, progression to eclampsia occurs.

The women at risk of preeclampsia are those with a previous history of preeclampsia, at the extremes of maternal age, with multiple gestations, a family history of preeclampsia, trophoblastic disease, chronic hypertension, diabetes mellitus, connective tissue disease and renal disease.

The course of preeclampsia is difficult to predict. The hypertension and the proteinura may be mild and yet, progression to eclampsia can occur.

Severity markers in preeclampsia include:

- Systolic BP ≥160 mmHg on more than one reading
- Diastolic BP ≥110 mmHg on more than one reading
- Proteinura in the nephrotic range, i.e. 3.5 g/24 hours or more
- Renal insufficiency with a serum creatinine > 0.11 mmol/L
- Thrombocytopaenia <100 × 10⁹/L
- Evidence of neurological dysfunction, pulmonary oedema, hepatocellular injury or microangiopathic haemolytic anaemia.[7,8]

Microangiopathic haemolytic anaemia

Microangiopathic haemolytic anaemia is a result of vascular damage. It is not specific to hypertensive emergencies but in this context, it is an indicator of vascular damage resulting from a rise in blood pressure. It can involve macrovessels. Schistocytes on the blood film are markers of this non-immune haemolytic anaemia.

Phaeochromocytoma

This is a catecholamine-secreting tumour of the adrenal medulla. Hypertension is initially episodic and associated with headache, anxiety, palpitations, diaphoresis, nausea and vomiting.

INVESTIGATIONS

The objectives of the investigations are to detect the presence of end-organ dysfunction as well as to identify the underlying cause of the hypertension.

Essential investigations include:

- Full blood count (FBC) and film to detect microangiopathic haemolytic anaemia and thrombocytopaenia
- Electrolytes – to assess renal function and hyperkalaemia due to secondary hyperaldosteronism from pressure induced natriuresis (present in 50% of patients with hypertensive emergencies)
- Urinalysis for casts and cells
- CXR for evidence of cardiac failure
- ECG for evidence of iscahemia.

Special investigations will be guided by clinical assessment and potential differential diagnoses but may include:

- Imaging : CT, Doppler studies, echocardiogram, MRA
- Blood tests: plasma levels of aldosterone and renin. In the pregnant patient suspected of preeclampsia, serum transaminases, serum albumin, lactate dehydrogenase and serum uric acid should be added.
- Urine collection for metanephrine levels.

MANAGEMENT

General

Management depends on the clinical syndrome, the presence of complications or coexisting conditions and the potential risks of intervention. If the BP is to be manipulated pharmacologically this should take place in a resuscitation area with intra-arterial BP monitoring.

Reduction of the BP carries significant risks, in particular, iatrogenic ischaemia or infarction of tissues may occur as a result of hypoperfusion. The patient is extremely vulnerable to any pressure manipulation because of the loss of autoregulation, and so both the magnitude and the rate of the pressure reduction must be tempered by this consideration. For extra-cerebral emergencies, a decrease in mean arterial pressure (MAP) by 20–25% is generally safe. In hypertensive emergencies the aim is to achieve this within 1–2 hours in order to halt progressive damage.[3,4,5] Another guide is a drop in dBP to 100–110 mmHg. This target level is then maintained for several days prior to further reduction to the normal level. The latter is achieved over the ensuing weeks. It must be emphasized, however, that any evidence of further end-organ compromise during treatment must be heeded as iatrogenic. Further BP reduction must be ceased until the ischaemia resolves and recommenced on a slower and smaller scale.

It should be recognized that large clinical trials looking at the optimum therapy in hypertensive emergencies are not available. The design and interpretation will be confounded by the heterogeneity of the clinical manifestations.[4] Hence the specific treatment discussed below are largely not evidence based but supported by consensus.

Specific conditions

Hypertensive encepalopathy

The divide between the risk and benefit of treatment in hypertensive encephalopathy is small. The clinical manifestation may be reversible, however, the risks of treatment are ischaemia and infarction from too rapid a fall in the MAP. The consensus is a drop of the MAP to 20–25% or a diastolic blood pressure of 100–110 mmHg, whichever value is greater, over 2–4 hours.[2,4,6,10] Vigilant monitoring is essential as any deterioration of clinical status must be followed by a reduction or cessation of the drug used. This is irrespective of the magnitude of the decrease in the mBP. Therefore the agent used must be rapidly titratable.

Centrally acting drugs that can affect the mental status are not used. Suitable agents are sodium nitroprusside (SNP), intravenous labetalol and nitroglycerin (GTN). SNP is considered the first-line therapy. The dose range is 0.5 mcg/kg/minute to 10 mcg/kg/minute. SNP requires normal hepatic and renal function for its metabolism and excretion and hence cannot be used in patients with renal or hepatic impairment. Labetolol, an α and β adrenergic blocker, is given as an infusion of 1–2 mg/minute.

Management of hypertension in stroke syndromes

Hypertension is frequently associated with stroke syndromes. It is not the immediate cause of the stroke but a physiological response to maintain cerebral perfusion to the surrounding ischaemic but not infarcted area. This ischaemic penumbrum is dependent on the MAP for adequate cerebral perfusion, as the autoregulation is no longer functional.

In embolic and ischaemic strokes, the hypertension is not substantial and treatment of the hypertension is not required. Greater than 80% of patients have hypertension on admission. There is a gradual fall over the subsequent 10 days after which only one-third remains hypertensive. The risk of treatment, especially in patients with chronic hypertension, is ischaemia in the vascular watershed areas. There is no evidence that treatment of the hypertension will improve outcome. Untreated hypertension in this context has not been shown to cause deterioration.[4] The indication for pharmacotherapy is a dBP greater than 140 mmHg. The latter is rare.[6] The titration point is a reduction of the MAP by 20% over the first 24 hours.

Intracranial haemorrhage from a variety of causes commonly leads to profound hypertension. The cause is intracranial hypertension and stimulation of the autonomic nervous system. Notably, this hypertension is transitory. The management of hypertension in this context remains controversial. Treatment of this hypertension has not been shown to reduce the risk of rebleeding or vasogenic oedema.[5] The accepted indication for pharmacotherpay is a sBP of >200 mmHg or a dBP of >120 mmHg.

Rapid reduction in blood pressure in the first 24 hours has been shown to increase mortality.[5] The optimal antihypertensive should be intravenous and have a short half life. SNP is commonly used but it has a narrow therapeutic index. Intravenous labetalol is also useful. Nicardipine and fenoldopam are also alternatives but they are not currently available in Australia. Intravenous ACE inhibitors and hydralazine, and oral or sublingual nifedipine are not recommended as they are not as accurately titratable and predictable.

Aortic dissection

See Chapter 4.10.

Acute pulmonary oedema and myocardial ischaemia

Reduction of blood pressure relieves ventricular wall tension and, hence, decreases the myocardial oxygen demand. Intravenous nitrates improve coronary perfusion, reduce left-ventricular preload and, hence, are well suited for use in this context. Pure vasodilators should be avoided because of reflex tachycardia (see Chapter 4.3).

Acute renal insuffiency

In patients with CRF, hypertension is commonly due to an increase in the extracellular fluid volume secondary to sodium retention by the diseased kidneys. This is frequently associated with vasoconstriction from hyperactivity of the renin-angiotensin system. Hypertension leads to further deterioration of renal function. The appropriate antihypertensive is one that will preserve the residual renal blood flow and calcium channel

antagonists are the preferred agents. Second-line therapy is SNP, hydralazine and fenoldapam. Diuretic use should be judicious as use in the absence of hypervolaemia may be deleterious. Emergency ultrafiltration may be required in cases refractory to medical treatment.

Preeclampsia

The objectives in the management of preeclampsia are to reduce maternal and fetal morbidity and mortality. No specific treatment is available as the precipitant and the pathogenesis is largely unknown. The definitive cure is termination of the pregnancy, however, other options may need to be considered if the fetus is immature.

The majority of these patients will primarily be under the care of the obstetricians. The involvement of the emergency department may be in the diagnosis or in the management of the complications. Preeclamptic and eclamptic patients are treated in the same manner.

Magnesium sulphate (Mg So4) is given as a prophylaxis for eclampsia and also to prevent further seizures in an eclamptic patient. From 4 to 6 g are given intravenously over 15 minutes, followed by an infusion of 1–2 g/hour. Monitoring is via regular assessment of deep tendon reflexes and serum magnesium. MgSo4 can cause neuromuscular depression.

With respect to anti-hypertensive agents, there is no evidence that one drug is better than another. The use depends on the experience of the clinician.[11] All drugs used cross the placenta. It is important to note that the maternal adverse effects are not the same as in the non-pregnant patient. $MgSO_4$ in the dose described above is used. Hydralazine 2.5 mg IV followed by 5–10 mg IV 20-minutely until a maximum dose of 40 mg has been reached is an alternative. Labetalol 20 mg IV followed by an infusion of 1–2 mg/minute or IV boluses of 40–80 mg every 10 minutes until a maximum of 300 mg is also commonly utilized. Contraindicated agents include ACE inhibitors because of deleterious fetal effects and diazoxide that can cause severe hypotension.

HYPERTENSIVE URGENCY

The appropriate management of hypertensive urgency is reliant on an accurate assessment of the presence or absence of end-organ dysfunction. In the asymptomatic patient it can be difficult to determine whether the dysfunction is acute or pre-existing. Past history and laboratory results are extremely useful to provide a comparison. It may be that this decision cannot be made and treatment is started without a clear distinction between an emergency or an urgency. The importance of the clinical assessment in hypertensive urgency is to identify the subset that is most likely to progress to hypertensive emergencies. The features suggestive of this are first presentation of severe hypertension, a history of poorly controlled hypertension, ischaemic heart disease or cerebrovascular disease.[7]

The treatment goal in this group is a reduction of the blood pressure over 24 to 48 hours using an oral antihypertensive. The aim is to reduce the mAP by 20% over this period of time. The patient should be admitted and an oral antihypertensive is started if the dBP remains above 120 mmHg 30–60 minutes after resting.

A wide range of oral antihypertensives is available. Angiotensin-converting enzyme inhibitors are a reasonable first line in most patients. Note, the majority of patients are hypertensive due to poor or non-compliance with medications. In general, the disposition of the patient depends on the presence of significant co-morbidities, response to treatment and the availability and accessibility for out-patient follow-up within 24 hours of discharge.

DISPOSITION

All patients with hypertensive emergencies should be admitted to an intensive care unit. The high-risk patient with hypertensive urgency requires hospital admission for observation and BP stabilization.

CONTROVERSIES

❶ Reduction of the elevated BP in the acute phase of a stroke remains controversial. There is no consensus on the indication to treat or the timing of intervention. Each case should be considered individually, with careful consideration given to the risks and benefits of lowering the BP.

❷ Choice of antihypertensive in preeclampsia and eclampsia.

FURTHER READING

1. Cardiovascular Health - High Blood Pressure. Australian Bureau of Statistics
2. Calhoun DA, Oparil S 1990 Treatment of hypertensive crisis. New England Journal of Medicine. 323(17): 1177–83
3. Bales A 1999 Hypertensive crisis. Postgraduate Medicine 105(5)
4. Vaughan C, Delanty N 2000 Hypertensive emergencies. Lancet 356(9227): 411–7
5. Varon J, Marik Paul E 2000 Chest 118(1): 214–27
6. Wu Melissa M, Chanmuyam A 2000 Hypertension. In: Tintinalli, et al (eds) Emergency Medicine. A Comprehensive Study Guide, 5th edn. McGraw Hill, Australia
7. Garoric Vesna D 2000 Hypertension in pregnancy: diagnosis and treatment. Mayo Clinic Proceedings 75(10): 1071–6
8. Branch DW, Porter TF 1999 Hypertensive disorders of pregnancy. In: Scott, et al (eds) Danforth's Obstetrics and Gynaecology, 8th edn. Lippincott Williams and Wilkins, Maryland, USA
9. Johnson Gary A 2000 Aortic dissection and aneurysms. In: Tintinalli, et al (eds) Emergency Medicine. A Comprehensive Study Guide, 5th edn. McGraw Hill, Australia
10. Murphy C 1995 Hypertensive emergencies. Emergency Clinics of North America 13(4): 1249–65
11. Duley L, Henderson-Smart DJ 2002 Drugs for rapid treatment of very high blood pressure during pregnancy. The Cochrane Database of Systematic Review Issue 1
12. Thach AM, Schultz PJ 1995 Nonemergent hypertension: new perspectives for the emergency medicine physician. Emergency Medicine Clinics of North America 13(4): 1009–36

4.10 AORTIC DISSECTION

MICHAEL COMAN • DALE HANSON

ESSENTIALS

1 Untreated aortic dissection has a mortality rate of approximately 1% per hour for the first 48 hours and 90% at 3 months. Early diagnosis and aggressive management improve mortality rates to 20–40%.

2 Aortic dissection is a clinical diagnosis confirmed through focused investigation. A high index of suspicion is required.

3 Both false-negative and false-positive diagnoses of aortic dissection result in increased morbidity and mortality. This is particularly true in patients with a clinical diagnosis of myocardial infarction. Only 0.26% of these patients have dissection. Routine chest X-ray to exclude dissection in this group may delay thrombolysis, resulting in a worse outcome for patients with AMI.

4 If available, transoesophageal echocardiography in the unstable patient and CT aortography or magnetic resonance imaging in the stable patient are excellent imaging modalities for patients suspected of suffering aortic dissection.

5 Therapy aimed at reducing blood pressure and the force of ventricular contraction should commence as soon as the diagnosis is suspected.

6 Proximal dissections require emergency surgery, whereas distal dissections are generally treated medically, surgery offering no improvement in outcome for the majority of patients.

INTRODUCTION

Aortic dissection (AD) is an uncommon yet potentially lethal condition. A high index of suspicion is required due to the broad range of presenting signs and symptoms of AD. Investigations must be carefully chosen and rapidly performed to confirm the diagnosis. It is imperative to institute emergency therapy as soon as the diagnosis is suspected, as untreated, the mortality rate for AD is approximately 1% per hour for the first 48 hours.[1]

EPIDEMIOLOGY

The annual incidence of AD is 5–10 patients/million/year.[1,2] One third to one half of all cases are diagnosed at autopsy.[3] Although the overall incidence is low, AD is the most common catastrophe of the aorta, 2–3 times more common than rupture of the abdominal aorta.[1]

Most cases occur in males, particularly between the ages of 50–70. Proximal dissections have a peak incidence 10 years earlier than distal dissections.[3] Risk factors for AD are shown in Table 4.10.1. Of note, hypertension is the single most important risk factor. Any

Table 4.10.1 Predisposing factors for aortic dissection

Major associations
Hypertension
Congenital cardiovascular disorders
  Aortic stenosis
  Bicuspid aortic valve
  Coarctation of the aorta
Connective tissue disorders
  Marfan's syndrome
Ehlers-Danlos syndrome.

Other associations
Iatrogenic (post cardiac surgery or balloon angioplasty for coarctation)
Cocaine
Pregnancy
Inflammatory diseases
  Giant-cell arteritis.

patient with a history of hypertension who presents with sudden severe chest, back or abdominal pain must have the diagnosis of AD considered.

PATHOPHYSIOLOGY

Arterial hypertension and degeneration of the aortic media are the two key elements of AD. Dissection occurs when blood is forced along a low resistance pathway created by the diseased and weakened media. Two pathophysiological processes have been proposed. The traditional explanation for AD requires a breach in the intima (the intimal tear) to initiate the dissection process. The tear occurs at sites where hydrodynamic and torsional forces on the aorta are greatest, most commonly a few centimetres above the aortic valve (60–65%) or just beyond the insertion of the ligamentum arteriosum (30–35%).[1,4] A column of high-pressure aortic blood gains access to the media and, under pressure, dissects through the weakened tissue plane creating a false lumen. The dissecting column of blood can extend in an antegrade or retrograde direction. The alternative proposed mechanism suggests that diseased or unsupported vasa vasorum within the media rupture as a result of medial degeneration, initiating AD.[4] A haematoma develops, which dissects through the media as it expands. The intima loses its support as dissection progresses, and is subjected to increased shearing forces during diastolic recoil of the aorta. Eventually, but not necessarily, this may lead to a tear in the intima. In this scenario, an intimal tear is a consequence of the dissection, not an initiating factor. An intimal tear is not identified in 12% of autopsies, suggesting that the intimal tear is not a mandatory precursor for AD.[4,5]

Regardless of the primary process producing dissection, the sequelae are identical. As the dissection extends, any structures caught in its path may be affected. Branch vessels of the aorta may be distorted or occluded resulting in signs and symptoms of ischaemia to the organs they supply. Proximal dissection may produce acute aortic valve incompetence and continued proximal extension may enter the pericardial sac, tamponading the heart. The false lumen created by the dissection may also partially or completely obstruct the true lumen. It may end in a blind sac or rupture back into the true lumen at any point. The false lumen may also rupture outwards through the adventitia. If this occurs, rapid exsanguination will occur if the haematoma is not contained. Common sites of external rupture are into the left pleural cavity or mediastinum.

Once the dissection begins, its propagation is dependent on the blood pressure and the gradient of the arterial blood pressure wave ($\Delta p/\Delta t$), which is a function of the velocity of left ventricular contraction. Hence urgent pharmacological treatment is aimed at lowering arterial blood pressure and decreasing ventricular contractile force.

CLASSIFICATION

AD may be classified anatomically or pathophysiologically. The Stanford and De Bakey systems are the two anatomically based classification systems in use. Both systems describe the site of the dissection, providing information that is pivotal in determining patient management.

The Stanford system divides AD into two types (Fig. 4.10.1). Type A (65–70%) involves the ascending aorta, with or without involvement of the descending aorta. The presence or absence of an intimal tear, the site of the intimal tear, and the extent of distal extension are not considered in this classification. Type B (30–35%) dissections involve the descending aorta only,[6] which by definition, begins distal to the origin of the left subclavian artery. The Stanford system is simple, easy to remember, and reflects the two major management pathways of AD. Type A generally requires surgical repair while type B is generally managed medically.

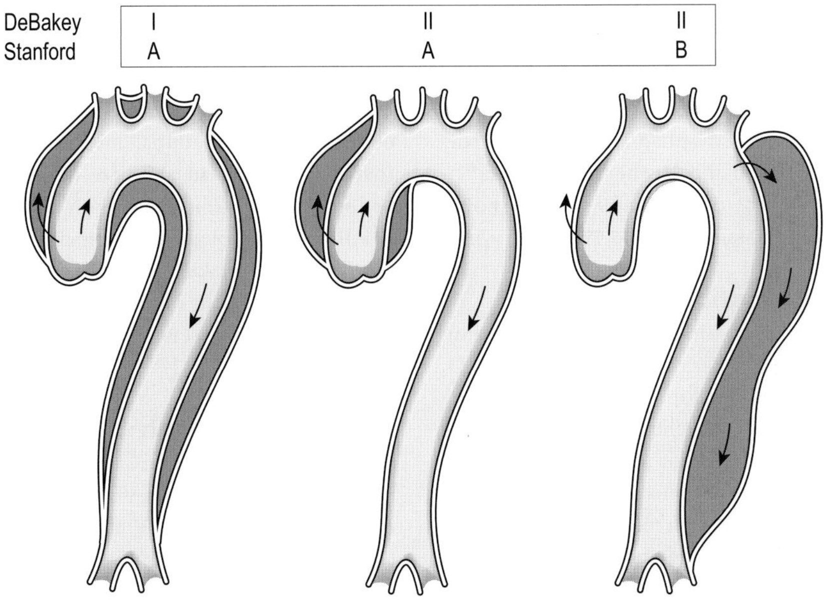

The DeBakey classification system divides AD into three types (Fig. 4.10.1). Type I involves both the ascending and descending aorta. Type II involves the ascending aorta only. Type III involves the descending aorta only, and is subdivided into type IIIa, which is confined to the thoracic aorta, and type IIIb, which extends into the abdominal aorta.

A new pathophysiological classification system has been proposed.[5] This system divides the causes of AD into five classes (Fig. 4.10.2):

Class 1: classical aortic dissection with an intimal flap between the true and false lumen.
Class 2: medial disruption with formation of intramural haematoma.
Class 3: subtle-discreet AD. A partial tear or structural weakness of the aortic wall can either lead to clinically inapparent disease or minor forms of AD.
Class 4: plaque rupture leading to aortic ulceration, followed by AD or aortic perforation.
Class 5: iatrogenic or traumatic AD, often due to catheter-induced intimal separation.

It is unknown whether this more comprehensive but complicated pathophysiological classification system will gain widespread acceptance, and whether the use of this system will lead to improvements in the diagnosis and emergency management of AD.

AD is classified as acute if symptoms are present for less than 14 days, chronic if longer than 14 days. Note, the term 'dissecting thoracic aneurysm' is confusing and should be avoided, as dissections can and usually do occur in the absence of aneurysmal dilatation of the aorta.

CLINICAL FEATURES

History

Pain is the most common presenting symptom occurring in 74–95% of patients.[1,3] Pain is classically described as severe, unremitting, tearing or ripping in nature, and maximal at onset.[1] The pain is often migratory, reflecting proximal or

Fig. 4.10.1 Anatomical classification of AD. (Reproduced with permission Erbel R, Alfonso F, Boileau C, et al 2001 Diagnosis and management of aortic dissection. European Heart Journal 22: 1642–81)

| DeBakey | I | II | II |
| Stanford | A | A | B |

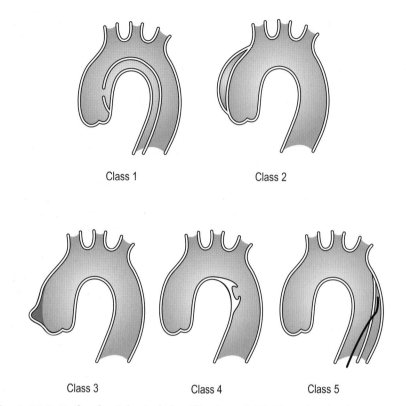

Fig. 4.10.2 Pathophysiological classification of AD. (Reproduced with permission Erbel R, Alfonso F, Boileau C, et al 2001 Diagnosis and management of aortic dissection. European Heart Journal 22: 1642–81

distal extension of the tear. The site of the pain may reflect the site of the dissection, with involvement of the ascending aorta typically producing anterior chest pain, while neck and jaw pain may suggest aortic arch dissection. Interscapular pain can occur with involvement of the descending aorta, and as distal dissection continues, pain may migrate to the lower back or abdomen.[1] In a minority of patients, a history of pain may not be forthcoming (4–15%). This is more common in those with severe neurological impairment.[6]

Other symptoms of AD are related to the effects of major aortic side branch occlusion. Almost 20% of dissections present with coma, confusion or stroke.[1,6] This may signify carotid artery involvement, or may reflect end organ hypoperfusion from hypovolaemic shock from external rupture of the aorta, or cardiogenic shock caused by pericardial tamponade. Neurological symptoms may often fluctuate. Lower limb paraplegia or paraesthesia (2–8%) may occur as spinal

arteries are separated from the aortic lumen.[3] Syncope (18% type A and 3% type B) may suggest rupture into the pericardial sac.[3,6]

Symptoms may also be due to local compression from a contained rupture. These are uncommon but may include superior vena cava syndrome, hoarseness, dyspnoea, dysphagia, upper airway obstruction and Horner's syndrome.[3]

A history of risk factors for AD should also be obtained (Table 4.10.1).

Examination

There is no single examination finding that will confirm the diagnosis of AD. It is common for patients to be acutely distressed, apprehensive and for their pain to be resistant to narcotic analgesia.

Patients are generally tachycardic due to a combination of pain, anxiety and possibly shock. Hypertension is seen in 50–78% of patients, especially those suffering from type-B dissection. This may reflect an underlying history of hypertension or an acute response to pain and

anxiety. Hypotension is an ominous sign, suggesting free rupture of the aorta or pericardial tamponade. Evidence of side branch occlusion may include stroke, limb ischaemia or neurological dysfunction, pulse deficits or a difference of 15 mmHg or more in manually taken blood pressures between the upper limbs.

Evidence of proximal extension to involve the aortic valve or pericardium may produce acute aortic incompetence possibly with signs of acute left ventricular failure. A diastolic murmur indicative of acute aortic incompetence is a common finding in proximal dissection (50–68%). Pericardial tamponade may manifest with hypotension, muffled heart sounds, a raised jugular venous pressure, pulsus paradoxus or pericardial friction rub. Involvement of the renal arteries may result in oliguria or anuria.

Aortic rupture may present with shock or clinical signs of a pleural effusion, usually left sided. Frank haemoptysis or haematemesis also suggests aortic rupture. Compression of local structures by a contained haematoma, particularly within the mediastinum may be evident.

Serial examination is very important, as signs may change as the dissection progresses.

INVESTIGATION

Specific investigations are required to confirm or exclude AD. There are, however, a number of initial investigations that may identify an alternate diagnosis or increase the clinical suspicion of AD. Routine haematological or biochemical investigations are of little value in the immediate diagnosis of AD, and at best, provide baseline renal function and haemoglobin.

Electrocardiograph

An electrocardiograph (ECG) should be performed on all patients with suspected AD, as acute myocardial infarction (AMI) is a major differential diagnosis. However, 10–40% of patients with AD have ECG evidence suggestive of acute ischaemia.[7] Seven per cent of dissections involve the coronary arteries, yet only

0.9–2.4% of patients will have ECG changes in keeping with AMI.[3,6] Total coronary occlusion is less common than partial occlusion, and the right coronary is more commonly involved than the left. The ECG may display voltage criteria for left ventricular hypertrophy, reflecting a longstanding history of hypertension.

Chest X-ray

A number of chest X-ray (CXR) abnormalities have been described in patients with AD (Table 4.10.2). The sensitivity and specificity of each individual finding is poor, and for this reason, no single finding should be used in isolation for predictive purposes. Many findings are subtle and are best seen on a good quality erect PA film. In reality, the clinical condition of the patient may only allow a supine, mobile, AP film. Retrospective audits of plain radiographs of patients known to have dissection reveals abnormalities suggesting AD in 72–90% of cases, however, attempts to prospectively identify AD in blinded studies yield less reliable results (sensitivity of 81% and specificity of 82–89%).[8] Up to 20% of radiographs are normal in patients suffering dissection. At best, the CXR may increase the clinical suspicion of AD or identify alternate pathology. A normal appearing CXR must never be used to exclude AD.

Specific investigations

All patients in whom AD is suspected must have a diagnostic test performed. Options include computerized tomography (CT), echocardiography, aortography and magnetic resonance imaging (MRI). The aim of the diagnostic test is to determine whether a dissection is present, its site, the structures involved and the presence of complications. Unfortunately no test is ideal, and the most appropriate investigation may differ between individual patients and individual institutions. Factors such as patient stability, test availability, operator availability and expertise, the physical location of the diagnostic equipment, and the variable institutional sensitivity and specificity of each test need to be taken into account. Each emergency department should have a pre-arranged imaging strategy for the diagnosis of suspected AD factoring in the above variables.

Computerized tomography

Technological advances over the past decade have revolutionized the amount and rate of information that can be acquired by CT. Spiral CT with rapid administration of intravenous contrast can be timed to acquire data during peak contrast opacification of the aorta, effectively creating a CT aortogram. Images can be reconstructed in multiple planes, and motion artefact, once a problem with older and slower scanners has been greatly reduced as data acquisition takes place during a single breath hold. Increased availability, after hours reporting via teleradiology, and the trend to position scanners in close proximity to emergency departments have made CT a good option for those patients who are able to be transported. It is the preferred study, particularly in stable patients with a low-to-moderate index of suspicion for AD as it is effective in identifying alternate pathology. Diagnosis is based on the demonstration of an intimal flap, shown as a low attenuation linear structure within the aortic lumen. Secondary findings of AD include internal displacement of luminal calcification, and delayed contrast enhancement of the false lumen. Sensitivity and specificity for diagnosing arch vessel involvement are high (93 and 98% respectively).[5] CT can identify complications of AD including pericardial, mediastinal and pleural blood. Disadvantages of CT include the requirement for intravenous contrast and patient transport. CT cannot provide a functional assessment of the aortic valve.

Echocardiography

Transthoracic echocardiography (TTE) is no longer considered a useful screening test in view of its low sensitivity and specificity (Table 4.10.3). TTE is parti-

Table 4.10.2 Radiographic features suggesting dissection
Widening of the superior mediastinum (52–75%)
Dilatation of the aortic arch (31–47%)
Change in the configuration of the aorta on successive CXR (47%)
Obliteration of the aortic knob
Double density of the aorta (suggesting true and false lumina)
Localized prominence along aortic contour (38%)
Disparity of calibre between descending and ascending aorta (34–67%)
Displacement of the trachea or nasogastric tube to the right
Distortion of the left mainstem bronchus
Calcium sign (more than 6 mm between the intimal calcium and the shadow of the outer aortic wall: 7–17%)
Pleural effusion, more common on the left (15–20%)
Cardiomegaly (21%).

Table 4.10.3 Sensitivity and specificity of diagnostic investigations		
Investigation	Sensitivity (%)	Specificity (%)
CT	83–100[6]	90–100[6]
TTE	78–100[6]: type a 31–55[6]: type b 59–85[6]: all	63–96[6]
TOE	97–99[4]	97–100[4]
Aortography	81–91[6]	94[6,15]
MRI	95–100[16]	95–100[16]

cularly poor at imaging the transverse arch and the descending aorta, owing to interference from the airways.

Transoesophageal echocardiography (TOE) has emerged as an excellent diagnostic investigation for AD in centres where this facility is available. Ideal for critically ill patients, TOE can be rapidly and safely performed at the bedside and is highly sensitive and specific[8,9] (Table 4.10.3). In addition, TOE can give a functional assessment of the aortic valve and the left ventricle, and can identify other complications of AD including the involvement of coronary arteries and the presence of pericardial blood. Disadvantages of TOE include the limited availability outside major centres and the requirement for a skilled and available operator. TOE is invasive and patients may require sedation and airway protection to perform the test. It is contraindicated in patients with known oesophageal pathology including varices, strictures or tumours. The diagnosis is confirmed by demonstrating the intimal flap separating the true and false lumens. The true lumen can be distinguished from the false lumen as it is usually smaller, expands during systole (compared to compression of the false lumen during systole) and is less commonly thrombosed.[10] Central displacement of luminal calcium may confirm the presence of AD in situations where the false lumen has thrombosed.

Aortography

Formerly the gold standard investigation for AD, aortography is now less commonly performed due to the development and refinement of less invasive, more sensitive and rapid alternatives. Aortography is able to identify branch vessel involvement and aortic incompetence, however, involvement of surrounding structures cannot be assessed as only the endoluminal contour of the vessels is displayed.

Aortography is an invasive, lengthy and expensive procedure, requiring the assembly of a specialized team and transport to an angiography suite. In addition, intraarterial contrast must be given. Diagnosis is made by the visualization of the intimal flap or the recognition

of two separate lumens. The diagnosis may be missed if the false lumen has thrombosed.

Magnetic resonance imaging

MRI is highly sensitive and specific, providing excellent visualization of the site and extent of the dissection, and the complications of dissection including side branch involvement. The availability of MRI is improving, and data acquisition is becoming more rapid. The major disadvantages of MRI relate to patient safety. Studies are still lengthy, patient accessibility is poor during the study, and patient monitoring is problematic due to the requirement of equipment that is compatible with the magnetic field. MRI equipment is frequently located at a distance from resuscitation facilities. For these reasons, MRI is unsafe for unstable or potentially unstable patients despite the comprehensive information that it can provide.

DIFFERENTIAL DIAGNOSIS

The diagnosis of AD is rarely straightforward, and there is a long list of differential diagnoses (Table 4.10.4), due to the wide range of presenting symptoms and signs. The fear of misdiagnosing AD for acute myocardial infarction and the subsequent administration of a thrombolytic agent is a concern of many clinicians. The facts show this to be a rare occurrence. AMI is approximately 1000 times more common than AD[11] and only a small percentage of patients suffering AD (0.9–2.4%)[3,6] have ECG changes suggesting AMI. Despite the widespread use of thrombolysis for AMI, only 21 cases of inappropriate administration of thrombolysis were reported by 1994. Sixteen of 21 patients died, giving a mortality rate of 71%, similar to that of AD in the presurgical era.[11] Clearly, only a minority of patients with a presentation suggesting AMI with ST elevation on ECG will ultimately prove to have AD. CXR is sometimes advocated as a screening test to exclude dissection in this circumstance. However, based on the reported sensiti-

Table 4.10.4 Differential diagnosis of aortic dissection

Cardiovascular
  Acute coronary syndrome with or without ST segment elevation
  Shock
  Acute pulmonary oedema
  Acute valvular dysfunction
  Pericarditis
  Acute extremity ischaemia

Pulmonary
  Pulmonary embolus
  Pneumothorax

Gastrointestinal
  Pancreatitis
  Peptic ulcer disease (including perforation)
  Oesophageal spasm/reflux
  Ischaemic bowel

Neurological
  Stroke/transient ischaemic attack
  Spinal cord compression

Renal
  Renal colic

vity of 81%, specificity of 89%[8] and an AD incidence of 0.26% in patients with a clinical diagnosis of AMI,[12] the positive predictive value of CXR is 1.9%. That is, 49 patients suffering AMI would be falsely labelled as potentially suffering an AD for every true case identified. Delay in thrombolysis while a definitive investigation is performed may result in an adverse outcome for these patients. Unless the clinical presentation suggests AD, routine CXR is an ineffective screening tool in patients with a clinical presentation suggesting AMI.

MANAGEMENT

Treatment must be started as soon as the diagnosis is suspected. Unstable patients require immediate resuscitation. Diagnostic investigations and management of life-threatening complications may need to take place simultaneously. Measures to minimize progression of the dissection need to be instituted rapidly, and early surgical referral is mandatory. Early diagnosis, control of blood pressure and heart rate, and early surgical repair are all associated with improved survival.

Patients with AD are usually in severe pain and require large doses of titrated IV narcotic analgesia, which should not be delayed or withheld. A secondary benefit from the relief of pain is a reduction in blood pressure and heart rate.

Pharmacological treatment is aimed at decreasing the pulsatile load ($\Delta p/\Delta t$) delivered by the left ventricle to the column of blood within the false lumen. This minimizes the likelihood of ongoing dissection.[5] The pulsatile load is determined by the systolic blood pressure and the velocity of blood ejected from the heart. Importantly, blood pressure must be lowered without increasing the velocity of ventricular contraction, which can occur if afterload is reduced prior to blocking the reflex tachycardia and increased contractile velocity of the heart that afterload reduction produces.

If there is no contraindication, beta blockade is the ideal first-line agent due to its negative inotropic and chronotropic effects on the heart. Esmolol, a short acting beta-blocker (half-life 9 minutes), which can be given by peripheral intravenous infusion and titrated to heart rate and blood pressure, is effective. A loading infusion of 0.5 mg/kg may be given by hand-held syringe over 1 minute. Following this, a maintenance infusion ranging from 50 to 200 mcg/kg/minute is commenced. If esmolol is unavailable, or experience in its use is limited, titrated intravenous boluses of atenolol or metoprolol are equally effective. A heart rate of 60–80 beats per minute and a systolic blood pressure (BP) of 100–120 mmHg are commonly quoted target ranges,[5] but these figures are not absolute. Blood pressure must be titrated to the clinical condition of the patient, being modified if signs of end organ hypoperfusion, or signs and symptoms of ongoing dissection become evident. Intraarterial blood pressure monitoring is necessary for optimal BP management.

If further BP reduction is required following beta blockade, a vasodilator may be added. Sodium nitroprusside reduces afterload via systemic vasodilatation. Delivered by intravenous infusion, it is effective, has a rapid onset and short duration of action and can be readily titrated to effect. The usual infusion range is 0.5–10 mcg/kg/minute. Due to the possibility of cyanide toxicity, the infusion should not continue beyond 24 hours. An alternative agent to reduce BP is glyceryl trinitrate (GTN), a drug more commonly and confidently used by most clinicians. Delivered by peripheral IV infusion, GTN reduces both preload and afterload by relaxing vascular smooth muscle. Reflex tachycardia is a common side effect, and must be prevented by prior beta blockade. The infusion range is 5–50 mcg/minute, and can be rapidly titrated to clinical effect.

Surgical intervention

Immediate surgery is the treatment of choice for acute proximal (type A) AD. The aim of surgery is to prevent rupture of the false lumen, re-establish blood flow to regions affected by occluded side branches, correct any associated acute aortic valve incompetence, and prevent pericardial tamponade. Usual practice is to excise the section of the aorta containing the intimal tear and replace this section with a prosthetic interposition graft. Operative mortality ranges from 5–21%.[13] Without surgery, up to 90% of patients with acute type A dissection will die within 3 months.[13] With surgery, there is a 56–87% 5-year survival.[13]

The traditional treatment for type B dissections has been medical management, with survival rates approaching 80%. Surgical intervention in these cases is complicated by tissue friability, coagulopathy, the risk of spinal cord ischaemia and resulting paraplegia, renal failure, distal arterial embolization and infection. Despite these risks, there are circumstances where surgical management for type B dissections is indicated, usually when life-threatening complications develop or medical management has failed. These are listed in Table 4.10.5.

Recent advances in endovascular stent grafting have challenged the traditional management of type B dissections.[14] Expandable metal stents covered by a prosthetic fabric graft material are deployed percutaneously through the femoral artery. These stents may be seated over the intimal flap to occlude flow between the true and false lumena. In addition, stenting of occluded side branches of the aorta including visceral and renal arteries has been successfully performed, avoiding the need for high-risk surgery. Studies have reported success in restoring flow to side branches of the aorta occluded by AD in excess of 90%, with average 30-day mortality rates of 10%.[5]

All patients are discharged on lifelong beta-blockers, regardless of initial medical or surgical treatment, or whether the patient is hypertensive or normotensive.[5] Serial MRI examinations are necessary for long-term surveillance of the aorta.

Table 4.10.5 Indications for surgical repair of type B aortic dissection
Leaking or ruptured aorta
Ischaemic compromise of vital organs
Marfan's syndrome
Extension of dissection despite appropriate medical therapy
Intractable pain
Intractable hypertension
Aortic dilatation (greater than 5 cm).

PROGNOSIS

A dramatic improvement in survival has been observed over the past 30 years due to advances in medical and surgical management of AD. One-year survival rates of 52–69% for type A and 70% for type B have been reported.[5] Eighty-six per cent of deaths from AD are from aortic rupture, 70% of those rupturing into the pericardial sac.[6] Multiorgan failure is another major cause of death following medical or surgical therapy.

DISPOSITION

Those patients not eligible or stable enough for emergency surgery require admission to an intensive care area for monitoring and aggressive therapy aimed at minimizing propagation of their dissection. Patients in peripheral or regional centres will require transfer to a specialist cardiothoracic unit after their condition has been stabilized.

REFERENCES

1. Zappa MJ, Harwood-Nuss A 1993 Recognition and management of acuta aortic dissection and thoracic aortic aneurysm. Emergency Medicine Reports 14: 1–8
2. Chen K, Varon J, Wenker OC 1997 Acute aortic dissection and its variants. Journal of Emergency Medicine 15: 859–67
3. Spittel PC, Spittel JA, Joyce JW, et al 1993 Clinical features and differential diagnosis of aortic dissection: experience with 236 cases. Mayo Clinic Proceedings 68: 642–51
4. O'Gara PT, DeSanctis RW 1995 Acute aortic dissection and its variants. Circulation 92: 1376–8
5. Erbel R, Alfonso F, Boileau C, et al 2001 Diagnosis and management of aortic dissection. European Heart Journal 22: 1642–81
6. Richards KA 1995 Emergency department recognition and management of dissecting thoracic aneurysm. Emergency Medicine 7: 99–105
7. Bourland MD In: Rosen P, Barkin RM, et al (eds) 1992 Emergency Medicine: Concepts and Clinical Practice. Mosby, Chicago, pp 1384–90
8. Jagannah AS, Sos TA, Lockart SH, Saddenki S, Sniderman KW 1986 Aortic dissection: a statistical analysis of the usefulness of chest pain radiographic findings. American Journal of Radiology 147: 1123–6
9. Weintraub AR, Erbel R, Gorge G, et al 1994 Intravascular ultrasound imaging in acute aortic dissection. Journal of the American College of Cardiologists 24: 495
10. Erbel R, Zamorano J 1996 The aorta. Critical Care Clinics 12: 733–66
11. Kamp TJ, Goldschmidt-Clermont PJ, Brinker, JA, Resar JR 1994 Myocardial infarction, aortic dissection, and thrombolytic therapy. American Heart Journal 128: 1234–7
12. Wilcox RG, Olssen CG, Von der Lippe G, et al 1988 Trial of tissue plasminogen activator for mortality reduction in acute myocardial infarction. Anglo-Scandenavian study of early thrombolysis (ASSET). Lancet 2: 525–30
13. Kouchoukos NT, Dougenis D 1997 Medical progress: surgery of the thoracic aorta. The New England Journal of Medicine 336(26): 1876–88
14. Vlahakes GJ 2000 Concise Review: Endovascular stent-graft placement in the treatment of aortic dissection. In: Braunwald E, Fauci AS, Isselbacher DL, et al (eds) Harrisons Online
15. Erbel R, Daniel W, Visser C, Engberding R, Roelandt, J Rennollet H 1989 Echocardiography in the diagnosis of aortic dissection. Lancet i: 457–61
16. Sarasin FP, Louis-Simonet M, Gaspoz JM, Jonod AF 1996 Detecting acute thoracic aortic dissection in the emergency department: time constraints and choice of the optimal diagnostic test. Annals of Emergency Medicine 28: 278–88

4.11 ANEURYSMS

ROGER SWIFT

ESSENTIALS

1 Mortality from the rupture of an abdominal aortic aneurysm (AAA) is over 90%, including approximately 50% mortality for those reaching the operating theatre. Mortality from elective repair is generally less than 10%.

2 Ruptured AAA mimics other conditions. Therefore, a high degree of suspicion is required in the patient over the age of 65 presenting with abdominal or back pain, and/or unexplained hypotension.

3 Treatment of ruptured or symptomatic AAA is emergency surgical repair which, when clinically indicated, should not be delayed for further investigation.

4 Percutaneous endovascular aortic stenting may become a treatment option for the urgent management of symptomatic AAA as experience with this procedure grows.

5 Management for ruptured or symptomatic AAA in the emergency department is oxygen, two large-bore peripheral intravenous cannulae, analgesia, blood cross-match and baseline tests and expedited emergency surgery.

6 Large-volume fluid resuscitation for patients with ruptured AAA should be delayed until aortic cross-clamping unless the patient is severely hypotensive or in hypovolaemic arrest. Rapid expansion of the intravascular space or hypertension may result in loss of stabilizing tamponade and worsen outcome.

INTRODUCTION

This chapter deals with non-cerebral 'true' arterial aneurysms. A true aneurysm is an 'aberrant, localized and irreversible dilatation of an artery of a minimum of 1.5 times its normal diameter'.[1] A true aneurysm contains all three layers of the arterial wall. By far the most common site of aneurysm is the infrarenal abdominal aorta (>95%).

Atherosclerosis was thought to be the main cause of aneurysm formation but this relationship is now questioned.[1] Rather, there may be a defect in connective tissue metabolism, with loss of elastin and collagen in the arterial wall. Aneurysms are commonly associated with generalized arteriomegaly. There is a 12–33% incidence of abdominal aortic aneurysm (AAA) in first-degree relatives of affected patients. This association is higher if the affected relative is female and relatively young.[2] Atherosclerosis is common in both non-aneurysmal arterial disease and aneurysm.

INFRARENAL AORTIC ABDOMINAL ANEURYSM

The distal aorta is subject to the greatest arterial pressure changes.[3] Although an AAA is usually distal, approximately 2% involve the renal arteries or other visceral branches. They may also involve either of the common iliac arteries. The diameter of the infrarenal aorta is normally less than 2 cm, and may be considered aneurysmal if the diameter is 3 cm or more.

Estimates of prevalence vary and are usually based on records of clinical referral or autopsy studies. An increase has been reported in population studies in several countries.[4] In Western Australia the prevalence in men aged over 55 years is reported to have increased from 74.8 per 100 000 to 117.2 per 100 000 between 1971 and 1981.[5] The cause of this increase is unclear. AAA is uncommon before 55 years of age, and rupture uncommon before 65 years.[6] The peak incidence occurs in men between 70 and 74 years of age.

Risks factors for AAA include male gender (male preponderance of between 3 and 8:1),[4] age greater than 55 years, hypertension, tobacco use, peripheral vascular disease, chronic obstructive airways disease, Marfan's and Ehlers-Danlos syndromes, and a first-degree relative with AAA.[1,6]

AAA is usually asymptomatic until complicated. The most frequent complications are rupture (usually into the left retroperitoneum), symptomatic expansion, thrombosis and embolism. Rupture may be contained in the retroperitoneal space, resulting in tamponade. Intraperitoneal rupture may occur primarily, or follow retroperitoneal rupture. Rarely AAA may be complicated by chronic rupture, with false aneurysm, inflammatory aneurysm, aortovenous fistula, aortoenteric fistula (often causing a minor 'herald bleed' before major GI haemorrhage), atheroembolism ('trash foot syndrome'), small bowel obstruction, or ureteric obstruction.

The risk of rupture is proportional to aneurysm diameter, hypertension, chronic obstructive airways disease and, probably, rapid expansion of the aneurysm (more than 0.5–1 cm per year).[1,7]

AAAs are often estimated to expand at an average rate of 4–5 mm per year,[6] although reports vary.[7] They may rupture without evidence of expansion in the prior 6 to 12 months. Although they can rupture at any size, the risk increases mildly when the diameter is more than 4 cm, and increases substantially if the diameter is greater than 5 cm.

CLINICAL ASSESSMENT

History

The patient is more often male and usually over the age of 65 years. A non-ruptured AAA is initially asymptomatic and may be found coincidentally on abdominal examination or imaging. Rupture may present with a varied combination of pain (in the abdomen, back, flank or leg), syncope due to hypotension and occasionally neurological deficit due to spinal cord ischaemia (usually T10–T12). That said, the classical combination of flank pain, hypotension and a pulsatile abdominal mass is found in less than 50% of patients with ruptured AAA.[1] Pain may be due to rupture, symptomatic expansion, arterial branch occlusion or embolus, or irritation of adjacent structures (e.g. the sciatic nerve).

Symptomatic expansion or rupture may mimic other conditions, such as musculoskeletal back pain, perforated viscus, intra-abdominal sepsis, myocardial ischaemia, and renal colic; 9.5% of presentations of ruptured AAA have flank pain radiating to the groin and haematuria.[1] Therefore, a high degree of suspicion of AAA is advocated for patients over the age of 65 years with undifferentiated abdominal or back pain, syncope, or hypotension.

Examination

Classically an AAA is felt as a pulsatile mass in the epigastrium below the costal margin and above the umbilicus. A left-sided pulsatile swelling that does not cross the midline is more likely a tortuous non-aneurysmal abdominal aorta, but this finding alone cannot be relied on to rule out AAA. Abdominal examination may be insensitive in the detection of AAA, particularly with obesity, abdominal distension, and when the aneurysm is 5 cm or less.

Findings with ruptured AAA may include tachycardia, hypotension, pulsatile abdominal mass (77%[8]), abdominal bruit, peripheral arterial insufficiency, and peritonism. A patient with a contained rupture may have an unremarkable examination. The finding of a tender AAA is usually considered an indication for urgent surgery, even in a stable and otherwise asymptomatic patient.

INVESTIGATION

Patients who present with hypotension and a suspected AAA should not have surgery delayed by further imaging. Blood should be taken for full blood picture, serum electrolytes, urea, creatinine, glucose, coagulation profile, and cross-match of 6–10 units of blood.

Twelve-lead ECG and chest X-ray should be performed if time permits as pre-operative investigations.

Imaging

A cross-table lateral abdominal X-ray may show the presence of a calcified AAA in 60% of patients with acute rupture.[8] This is not sensitive and is not recommended as a routine investigation for suspected ruptured AAA. Bedside abdominal ultrasound may have over 90% sensitivity to detect AAA[9] but cannot distinguish rupture from non-rupture. Ultrasound may be useful when the diagnosis is in doubt and the patient unstable. The sensitivity of ultrasound is dependent on the operator and is reduced with abdominal distension from ileus secondary to retroperitoneal or intraperitoneal blood. Computerized tomography (CT) may detect rupture as well as the presence of AAA or other intra-abdominal pathology in the *stable* patient when the diagnosis is uncertain. CT angiography is a precursor to endovascular stenting but its role in the unstable patient with symptomatic AAA prior to stenting has not yet been clarified. CT should be avoided in the unstable patient.

MANAGEMENT

Patients with suspected ruptured AAA require full cardiovascular monitoring in an area equipped for resuscitation. They require high-flow oxygen and two proximal wide-bore intravenous cannulae. Narcotic analgesia should be given intravenously in small increments, titrated to response. A nasogastric tube and urethral catheter should be inserted if time allows before surgery. The patient should be kept warm.

Intravenous fluid resuscitation should be performed cautiously. Rapid volume expansion may cause loss of retroperitoneal tamponade and accelerated bleeding. Therefore, volume resuscitation should be delayed in patients who have adequate perfusion to vital organs until emergency surgery is under way and the

aorta cross-clamped. However, fluid resuscitation may be required en route to surgery for those in hypovolaemic arrest, in whom arrest appears imminent, who are severely hypotensive or have evidence of inadequate vital organ perfusion. Although there is a lack of evidence to guide the setting of an optimal blood pressure target, a systolic pressure of the order of 80 mmHg to 100 mmHg would seem reasonable.

Specific treatments

Standard management is currently the surgical replacement of the affected aorta with a synthetic graft, usually Dacron.

Endovascular aortic stenting can be inserted under local anesthetic via the femoral arteries. Stenting would be advantageous in ruptured AAA because it does not require opening of the peritoneal cavity and potential release of tamponade, or cross-clamping of the aorta. However it requires on table arteriography and preferably preoperative imaging of the aneurysm by CT angiography. Its regional availablity may be limited to a few centres. Its use in symptomatic AAA is currently under study.

PROGNOSIS

Annually between 1 and 2% of people over 65 die of a ruptured aorta;[4] 27–50% die before reaching hospital, 24–58% die after reaching hospital but before reaching theatre, and 42 to 80% of those reaching theatre die. The usual cause of death in theatre is uncontrollable haemorrhage and cardiovascular failure. Postoperatively death is most commonly due to hypotension-induced multiorgan failure and less commonly to myocardial infarction. The overall mortality of rupture is 78–94%. In comparison, mortality for elective AAA repair is between 4 and 11%. Long-term survival is significantly improved with elective repair and life expectancy afterwards is equivalent to that of the age-matched population.[8]

THORACIC AORTIC ANEURYSM (see Chapter 4.10)

VISCERAL ANEURYSMS[1,10,11]

The incidence of visceral aneurysm is 0.01 to 0.2% at autopsy. Aetiology includes atheroma, trauma, inflammation, arterial fibrodysplasia (e.g. polyarteritis nodosa), and mycotic (e.g. from bacterial endocarditis associated with illicit intravenous drug use). They are usually sacular. Angiography is most useful in the stable patient but CT and ultrasound may also image the aneurysm.

Splenic artery

Splenic artery aneurysms account for 60% of visceral arterial aneurysms. Risk factors include female gender (female:male 4:1), portal hypertension and pregnancy (probably owing to the influence of oestrogen on the arterial wall). These aneurysms tend to present in either young women or the elderly. The aneurysm is usually less than 2 cm. Two per cent go on to life-threatening rupture, often in pregnant women in the third trimester. Mortality from rupture is reported as 35–70%, with 95% fetal mortality. Rupture presents with epigastric or right upper quadrant pain, sweating, and hypotension. X-ray may show characteristic signet-ring or eggshell calcification, particularly in the older age group.

Hepatic artery aneurysm

Hepatic artery aneurysms account for 20% of visceral arterial aneurysms. They usually occur in those aged over 60, and are commonly asymptomatic. Rupture may mimic biliary colic and pancreatitis. It may rupture into bile duct (triad of biliary colic, GI bleed and jaundice), bowel or peritoneum. X-ray shows characteristic calcification.

Superior mesenteric aneurysm

Superior mesenteric artery aneurysms account for 8% of visceral arterial aneurysms They present with symptoms of thrombosis and ischaemia. The patient may complain of postprandial pain that resolves over several hours. Rupture is rare.

Renal artery aneurysm

These are very rare – accounting for less than 0.1% of visceral aneurysms. They are bilateral in 20% of cases and present with hypertension, often coexisting with renal artery stenosis and ischaemia. Haematuria is commonly associated.

PERIPHERAL ARTERIES

Peripheral artery aneurysms tend to present with thrombosis, embolism and distal ischaemia rather than rupture. The aetiology is similar to aneurysms elsewhere, although peripheral sites are more commonly due to trauma.

Popliteal artery aneurysm

This aneurysm is the most common peripheral site, although it may not be evident symptomatically or clinically. It may present with distal ischaemia or as a coincidental finding. Rupture is uncommon. It is often bilateral and associated with aneurysms in other arteries. Investigation looking for a coexisting AAA should be considered. Elective repair may prevent ischaemic complications.

Femoral artery aneurysms

These aneurysms are less common and more prone to rupture than popliteal aneurysms.

Upper limb

The subclavian, axillary and brachial arteries rarely form aneurysms. If present they may lead to a palable pulsatile mass, compression of local structures and distal ischaemia.

CONTROVERSIES

❶ The most controversial issue is withholding surgery for those with ruptured AAA and a very high risk of death despite treatment. This high-risk group includes female gender, age over 80, persistent preoperative hypotension, cardiac arrest, admission haematocrit less than 25%, and those requiring more than 15 units of blood.[12–14] Operative mortality is over 90% in this group.

❷ Some patients may decline or be advised against elective repair because of coexisting medical illness. However, they may subsequently opt for life-saving emergency repair after rupture.[12]

❸ Endovascular aortic stents are likely to have a growing role in the management of selected patients with ruptured AAA, however, experience to date is limited. It requires angiographic imaging of the arterial system during stenting and preferably prior to the procedure.

Carotid artery aneurysm

This aneurysm is rare and may be mistaken for a tortuous carotid artery. Emboli present a much greater risk than rupture. Trauma may cause false aneurysms.

REFERENCES

1. Walker D 1996 Vascular abdominal emergencies. Emergency Medicine Clinics of North America 14(3): 584–91
2. Norman PE, Castleden WM, et al 1992 Screening for abdominal aortic aneurysms. Australian and New Zealand Journal of Surgery 62(5): 333–7
3. Dobrin PB 1989 Pathophysiology and pathogenesis of aortic aneurysms. Surgical Clinics of North America 69(4): 687–703
4. Reilly JR, Tilson MD 1989 Incidence and etiology of abdominal aortic aneurysms. Surgical Clinics of North America 69(4): 705–71
5. Castleden WM, Mercer JC 1985Abdominal aortic aneurysm in Western Australia: descriptive epidemiology and patterns of rupture. British Journal of Surgery 72(2): 109–12
6. Vliert JAVD, Boll APM 1997 Abdominal aortic aneurysm. Lancet 349: 863–6
7. Ernst CB 1993 Abdominal aortic aneurysm. New England Journal of Medicine 328(16): 1167–72
8. Rutherford RB, McCroskey BL 1989 Ruptured abdominal aortic aneurysm. Surgical Clinics of North America 69(4): 859–68
9. Rowland J, Kuhn M, Bonnin RL, Davey Mj, Langlois SL 2001 Accuracy of emergency department bedside ultrasonography. Emergency Medicine (Fremantle) 13: 305–13
10. Panayiotopoulus YP, Taylor PR, et al 1996 Aneurysms of the visceral and renal arteries. Annals of the Royal College of Surgeons of England 78: 412–9
11. Rokke O, Sondenaa K, et al 1996 The diagnosis and management of splanchnic artery aneurysms. Scandinavian Journal of Gastroenterology 31(8): 737–43
12. Glovickzki P, et al 1992 Aggressive management of ruptured abdominal aortic aneurysm. Journal of Vascular Surgery 15(5): 851–9
13. Johansen K 1993 Ruptured abdominal aortic aneurysm: should repair ever be denied? Journal of Vascular Surgery 17(2): 446–7
14. Robinson D, Englund R, et al 1997 Treatment of abdominal aortic aneurysm disease in the 9th and 10th decades of life. Australian and New Zealand Journal of Surgery 67: 640–2

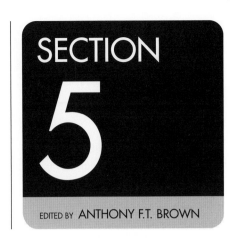
RESPIRATORY

5.1 Oxygen therapy 254

5.2 Upper respiratory tract 265

5.3 Asthma 271

5.4 Community-acquired pneumonia 275

5.5 Chronic obstructive airways disease 286

5.6 Pneumothorax 291

5.7 Pleural effusion 296

5.8 Haemoptysis 300

5.1 OXYGEN THERAPY

DAVID R. SMART

ESSENTIALS

1 Oxygen is the most commonly used drug in emergency medicine.

2 Oxygen-delivery systems may be divided into variable performance (delivering a variable concentration of oxygen), and fixed performance (delivering a fixed concentration of oxygen, including systems that deliver 100% oxygen).

3 Fixed-performance systems are essential where precise titration of oxygen dose is required, such as with chronic obstructive pulmonary disease, or where 100% oxygen is required.

4 In attempting to deliver 100% oxygen, free flowing circuits are least efficient. A reservoir or demand system improves efficiency, and a closed circuit delivery system is most efficient.

5 Pulse oximetry provides valuable feedback regarding the appropriateness of oxygen dose provided to individual patients.

6 Oxygen should never be abruptly withdrawn from patients in circumstances of suspected CO_2 narcosis.

INTRODUCTION

Oxygen (O_2) constitutes 21% of dry air by volume. It is essential to life. Cellular hypoxia results from a deficiency of oxygen regardless of aetiology. Hypoxaemia is a state of reduced oxygen carriage in the blood. Hypoxia leads to an anaerobic metabolism that is inefficient, and may lead to death if not corrected. A major priority in acute medical management is correction of hypoxia, hence oxygen is the most frequently admin-

istered and important drug in emergency medicine. There are sound physiological reasons for the use of supplemental oxygen in the management of acutely ill and injured patients to:

- Correct defects in delivery of inspired gas to the lungs. A clear airway is essential.
- Supplement oxygen in circumstances where there is inadequate oxygenation of blood due to defects in pulmonary gas exchange.
- Maximize oxygen saturation of the arterial blood (SaO_2) where there is inadequate oxygen transport by the cardiovascular system.
- Maximize oxygen partial pressure and content in the blood in circumstances of increased or inefficient tissue oxygen demand.
- Provide 100% oxygen where clinically indicated.
- Titrate oxygen dose in patients with impaired ventilatory response to carbon dioxide.

Oxygen was first discovered by Priestley in 1772 and was first used therapeutically by Beddoes in 1794. It now forms one of the cornerstones of medical therapy.

PHYSIOLOGY OF OXYGEN

Oxygen proceeds from inspired air to the mitochondria via a number of steps known as the oxygen transport chain. These steps include:

❶ Ventilation
❷ Pulmonary gas exchange
❸ Oxygen carriage in the blood
❹ Local tissue perfusion
❺ Diffusion at tissue level
❻ Tissue utilization of oxygen.

Ventilation

Normal inspired air oxygen partial pressure (P_IO_2) is approximately 20 kPa (150 mmHg) at sea level. Hypoxia results

if there is a reduction in the fraction of inspired oxygen (F_IO_2) as occurs at altitude. This is relevant in the transport of patients at 2400 m altitude in commercial 'pressurized' aircraft where ambient cabin pressures of 74.8 kPa (562 mmHg), result in a P_IO_2 of 14.4 kPa (108 mmHg).

Hypoxia can result from inadequate delivery of inspired gas to the lung. The many causes include airway obstruction, respiratory muscle weakness, neurological disorders interfering with respiratory drive (seizures, head injury), disruption to chest mechanics (chest injury) or extrinsic disease interfering with ventilation (intra abdominal pathology). These processes interfere with maintenance of an adequate alveolar oxygen partial pressure (P_AO_2), which is approximately 13.7 kPa (103 mmHg) in a healthy individual. An approximation of the alveolar gas equation permits rapid calculation of the alveolar oxygen partial pressures:

$$P_AO_2 = F_IO_2 \times (\text{Barometric pressure} - 47) - P_aCO_2 / 0.8$$

Pulmonary gas exchange

Oxygen diffuses across the alveoli and into pulmonary capillaries and carbon dioxide diffuses in the opposite direction. The process is passive occurring down concentration gradients. Ficks law summarizes the process of diffusion of gases through tissues:

$$\dot{V}O_2 \propto \frac{A}{T} \times \frac{Sol}{\sqrt{MW}} \times (P_AO_2 - P_{pa}O_2)$$

where $\dot{V}O_2$ = rate of gas (oxygen) transfer, $\propto$ = proportional to, A = Area of tissue, T = tissue thickness, Sol = solubility of the gas, MW = molecular weight, P_A = alveolar partial pressure, P_{pa} = pulmonary artery partial pressure.

In healthy patients, oxygen passes rapidly from the alveoli to the blood and after 0.25 seconds, pulmonary capillary blood is almost fully saturated with oxygen resulting in a systemic arterial oxygen partial pressure (P_aO_2) of approximately 13.3 kPa (100 mmHg). The difference between the P_AO_2 and the P_aO_2 is known as the alveolar to arterial oxygen gradient (A - a gradient). It is usually small and increases with age. The *expected* A - a gradient breathing air approximates to: age ÷ 4 + 4.

An approximation of the *actual* value can be calculated:

Aa O_2 gradient = 140 − (PO_2 + PCO_2)

If the calculated value exceeds the expected value then there is a defect in pulmonary gas exchange. The Aa O_2 gradient is increased if there is a barrier to diffusion (such as pulmonary fibrosis or oedema) or a deficit in perfusion such as pulmonary embolism. An increased Aa gradient also reflects widespread ventilation-perfusion inequality. In circumstances of impaired diffusion in the lung, raising the F_IO_2 assists oxygen transfer by creating a greater pressure gradient from the alveoli to the pulmonary capillary. The increase in F_IO_2 may not be as helpful when lung perfusion is impaired due to increased intra-pulmonary shunting.

Oxygen carriage in the blood

Three steps are required to deliver oxygen to the periphery:

❶ Uptake of oxygen by haemoglobin (Hb).
❷ Generation of a cardiac output to carry the oxygenated haemoglobin to the peripheral tissues.
❸ Dissociation of oxygen from haemoglobin to allow diffusion from blood to cell.

The haemoglobin-oxygen (Hb-O_2) dissociation curve is depicted in Figure 5.1.1, which also summarizes the factors which influence the position of the curve. If the curve is shifted to the left, this favours the affinity of haemoglobin for oxygen. These conditions are encountered when deoxygenated blood returns to the lung. A shift of the curve to the right favours unloading of oxygen, and subsequent delivery to the tissues.

A number of advantages are conferred by the shape of the Hb-O_2 dissociation

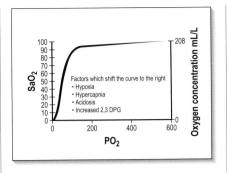

Fig. 5.1.1 Haemoglobin oxygen dissociation curve.

curve that favour uptake of oxygen in the lung and delivery to the tissues:[1]

- A flat upper portion of the curve allows some reserve in the P_AO_2 required to keep the haemoglobin fully saturated; P_AO_2 reduction of 20% will have minimal effect on O_2 loading of Hb.
- The flat upper portion of the curve also ensures that a large difference remains between P_AO_2 and the pulmonary capillary O_2 partial pressure ($P_{pc}O_2$) even when much of the haemoglobin has been loaded with oxygen. This pressure difference favours maximal Hb-O_2 loading.
- The lower part of the curve is steeper, which favours offloading of oxygen in peripheral tissues with only small falls in capillary PO_2. This maintains a higher driving pressure of oxygen facilitating diffusion into cells.
- The right shift of the Hb-O_2 dissociation curve in circumstances of increased temperature, fall in pH, increased PCO_2 and increased erythrocyte 2, 3 DPG assists in further off-loading of oxygen even when the driving pressure has fallen and PO_2 has reached 5.3 kPa (40 mmHg); i.e. venous blood, which is still 75% saturated with oxygen.

Oxygen is carried in the blood as dissolved gas and in combination with haemoglobin. At sea level (101.3 kPa), breathing air (F_IO_2 = 0.21), the amount of oxygen dissolved in plasma is very small (0.03 mL O_2 per litre of blood for each mmHg P_aO_2). This dissolved component assumes greater significance in a hyperbaric situation, where at 284 kPa, and F_IO_2 = 1.0, up to 60 mL oxygen can be carried in the dissolved form per litre of blood.

Haemoglobin carries 1.34–1.39 mL O_2 per gram when fully saturated. Blood with a haemoglobin concentration of 15 g/L carries approximately 200 mL O_2 per litre. The total amount of oxygen delivered to the body per minute is known as oxygen flux.[1]

Oxygen flux = (oxyhaemoglobin + dissolved O_2) × cardiac output = (1.39 ×

$$Hb \times \frac{S_aO_2}{100} + 0.03 \times P_aO_2) \times Q$$

where: Hb = haemoglobin concentration g/L; S_aO_2 = arterial oxygen saturation (percentage); P_aO_2 = partial pressure of arterial oxygen (mmHg); Q = cardiac output (L/min).

A healthy individual breathing air transports approximately 1000 mL O_2 per minute to the tissues with a cardiac output of 5 L/minute. Thirty per cent or 300 mL/minute of this oxygen is not available because at least 2.7 kPa (20 mmHg) driving pressure is required to allow oxygen to enter the mitochondria, and, therefore, approximately 700 mL/minute is available for utilization by peripheral tissues. This provides considerable reserve above the 250 mL/minute consumed by a healthy resting adult. In illness or injury this reserve may be eroded considerably. Factors which reduce oxygen flux include falls in cardiac output of any aetiology (including shock states), anaemia or a reduction in functional haemoglobin (carbon monoxide poisoning) and a drop in the S_aO_2. These situations are frequently encountered in emergency medicine; supplemental oxygen is required in addition to specific therapy such as volume replacement, transfusion, and measures to improve cardiac output.

Local tissue perfusion and diffusion

Cellular hypoxia results if there is impairment of perfusion to local tissues.

Oedema associated with medical illness or local injury increases the diffusion distance between blood and cell thus mandating a higher P_aO_2 to ensure adequate tissue oxygen delivery.

Tissue utilization of oxygen

Increased oxygen flux is required if:

- Tissue demands for oxygen are higher than normal
  or
- Tissue utilization of oxygen is impaired.

Elevation of cardiac output increases oxygen flux in these circumstances but frequently this too is significantly impaired by the disease state.

Tissue demands for oxygen increase by 7% for each degree Celsius elevation in body temperature, and considerably greater increases in demand occur in seizures, sepsis, severe dyspnoea, restlessness and shivering.[2] Tissue extraction of oxygen is impaired in sepsis, and by poisons such as CO or cyanide. In all cases, oxygen therapy must be combined with general measures (such as reduction of fever), and specific treatment of the primary disease process.

OXYGEN DELIVERY SYSTEMS

Oxygen delivery systems can be classified into three groups (Table 5.1.1):

Table 5.1.1 Oxygen delivery systems
Variable performance systems
Nasal cannulae
Hudson mask +/- reservoir
T pieces and Y connectors
Fixed performance systems:
Venturi mask
Oxygen blenders
100% oxygen systems
Non rebreathing circuits
– Free flowing circuits
– Self refilling circuits
– Soft reservoir bags
– Oxygen powered resuscitators
Partial rebreathing circuits
Closed circuit systems

❶ Variable-performance systems
❷ Fixed-performance systems
❸ One hundred per cent oxygen systems

Definitions

Variable-performance oxygen delivery systems

These systems deliver a variable F_IO_2 to the patient that is altered by the inspiratory flow rate, the minute volume of the patient, and the physical characteristics of the delivery system.

Fixed-performance oxygen delivery systems

These systems deliver a specificied F_IO_2 to the patient that is not altered by changes in ventilatory pattern, volume or inspiratory flow rate.

100% oxygen systems

This is a subgroup of 2 wherein 100% oxygen is delivered to the patient.

General principles

The oxygen source in most Australasian emergency departments consists of a wall-mounted flow meter that is capable of delivering oxygen up to 15 L/minute. Most available oxygen delivery systems connect to this apparatus. The 15 L/minute flow rate limits the delivery of high F_IO_2 to adults for the following reasons:

- A quietly breathing adult has a peak inspiratory flow rate (PIFR) of approximately 30–40 L/min which exceeds the oxygen supply. Hence a free flowing system such as a Hudson Mask must entrain air into the system in order to match the patient's PIFR, with a resultant reduction in F_IO_2 to a maximum of 0.6.[3]
- A quietly breathing adult has a respiratory minute volume of 4–8 litres and in a child this value is approximately 150 mL/kg. By incorporating a reservoir into the circuit, oxygen is stored during expiration for use during inspiration with a considerable improvement in economy of oxygen use. This system is limited by the patient's minute

volume. If the minute volume exceeds 15 litres there is danger of the patient asphyxiating due to insufficient gas supply, or if safety valves allow air into the system, the F_IO_2 falls.

Multiple port oxygen supply outlets can overcome the above limitations of inspiratory flow rate and minute volume. The use of 'Y' connectors and 'T' pieces enables 30, 45 or 60 litres per minute to be delivered to the patient, to achieve F_IO_2 of very nearly 1.0. Extra source oxygen flow may cause variable performance systems such as the Hudson mask to become fixed performance systems. Hence the terms 'variable performance' and 'fixed performance' are loosely applied and are largely dependent on whether or not the flow of gas delivered to the patient is sufficient to match their ventilatory requirements. A fine example of this is in paediatric oxygen delivery. A high F_IO_2 can be delivered using standard 15 L/minute oxygen source because the child's ventilatory requirements are smaller in proportion to the available oxygen supply.

The oxygen delivery systems available for use in emergency medicine are broadly summarized in Table 5.1.1. They can be further subdivided according to economy of oxygen use and whether or not the system can be used to manually ventilate the patient. Figures depicting the various systems have been published elsewhere.[3]

VARIABLE PERFORMANCE SYSTEMS

The F_IO_2 delivered by these systems is summarized in Table 5.1.2.

Options available for use in emergency medicine include:

- Nasal cannulae
- Face masks with air inlets
- T pieces and Y connectors.

Nasal cannulae

The system must be used at flow rates 4 L/minute or less to avoid painful drying of the nasal mucosa. A flow rate

Table 5.1.2 Variable performance oxygen delivery systems

Apparatus	Oxygen flow L/min	Oxygen concentration (%)
Nasal catheters	1–4	24–40
Semi-rigid mask	6–15	35–60
Semi-rigid mask with double O_2 supply	15–30	Up to 80
Semi-rigid mask with reservoir bag	12–15	60–90

of 2 L/minute or less is insufficient to create a nasopharyngeal reservoir during the expiration pause, for inspiration with the next breath. The inspired oxygen concentration is a function of the patient's inspiratory flow rate, and is usually in the vicinity of 22–28%. At flow rates of 2–4 L/minute, the nasopharynx acts as a partial reservoir during the expiratory pause resulting in an increased F_1O_2. The delivered F_1O_2 is then influenced by the pattern of breathing (mouth or nose), and the positioning of the nasal cannula.[4]

Nasal cannulae provide a higher F_1O_2 in paediatric patients and nose breathers. They are less effective in dyspnoeic patients because of greater amounts of air inspired through the mouth. They are frequently used in patients with stable COPD due to absence of dead space that prevents CO_2 rebreathing. However, fluctuations in F_1O_2 make nasal cannulae less than ideal in management of patients who rely on hypoxic respiratory drive and they are second choice after venturi masks in emergency management of these patients. Advantages for home therapy include the ability to eat and drink, less noise than masks, and economy of oxygen use.

Face masks (Hudson, Edinburgh, Medishield)

A small reservoir of oxygen is provided by these masks but this has little effect on F_1O_2. The small increase in dead space created by the mask necessitates a flow rate of greater than 6 L/minute to prevent rebreathing of CO_2. Two factors influence the F_1O_2 provided by this system:

❶ The patient's inspiratory flow rate
❷ The source oxygen supply flow rate.

At O_2 flow rates of 6–14 L/minute, the delivered F_1O_2 varies from 0.35–0.6. The F_1O_2 will be less in a dyspnoeic patient due to higher inspiratory flow rate, and greater in a paediatric patient because the converse applies. If the PIFR increases, greater amounts of air will be entrained into the mask, diluting the oxygen. During expiration, the exhaled gas and excess oxygen is vented through the side perforations. Attaching a reservoir bag to this mask improves the economy of oxygen use by storing this vented gas during the expiratory phase. This increases the delivered F_1O_2 but it may be at the expense of increased CO_2 rebreathing. Commercially available reservoir bags have a volume of 750 mL–1 L, which is inadequate for a dyspnoeic patient. The authors recommend a minimum flow rate of 12 L/minute to avoid CO_2 retention.

Using a source oxygen supply of 15 L/min the maximum F_1O_2 delivered via Hudson mask to a quietly breathing adult is 0.6.[3] By attaching another source oxygen using a 'T' piece or 'Y' connector, the resultant flow rate of 30 L/minute can deliver F_1O_2 up to 0.8. With even greater flow rates the mask may be converted into a fixed performance system delivering almost $F_1O_2 = 1.0$; the ability to deliver 100% oxygen is limited by the mask 'fit'.

The Medishield mask is stated to be more efficient than the Hudson mask because dead space is reduced by bringing the oxygen supply closer to the mouth, and more effective entrainment of oxygen occurs during inspiration. A

$F_1O_2 = 0.75$ may be obtained with a gas flow rate of 15 L/minute.

T pieces and Y connectors

The term 'T piece' has been used to describe a number of different oxygen delivery systems including the 'T piece' for supplying humidified oxygen to patients with a tracheostomy and the Ayre's T piece which is the Mapleson E circuit. The use of 'T pieces' or 'Y connectors' in emergency medicine is to supplement an existing oxygen supply with 1) extra oxygen, 2) nebulized medication or 3) humidification. The disadvantage of the system is that multiple oxygen ports are necessary, which is untidy and may restrict the patient's mobility. There is loss of economy of O_2 use because of higher flow rates. T pieces allow a higher F_1O_2 to be delivered to severely dyspnoeic patients.

FIXED-PERFORMANCE SYSTEMS

Two systems are available for use in emergency departments:

❶ High-flow venturi masks
❷ Oxygen blenders.

Venturi mask

Oxygen flow through a venturi system results in air entrainment with delivery of a fixed concentration of oxygen to the patient. The masks deliver F_1O_2 values of 0.24, 0.28, 0.35, 0.40, 0.50 and 0.60 using different adaptors that are colour coded.

Many studies have assessed their accuracy.[5,6,7,8] It is generally considered that the patient receives the stated F_1O_2 provided the total flow rate exceeds 60 L/minute or is 30% higher than the patient's PIFR.[9,10] As the patient's PIFR increases the system functions with variable performance. In supplying $F_1O_2 = 0.24$ using 6 L/minute oxygen flow rate, the total flow rate delivered to the patient is 120 L/minute. This falls to 30 L/minute total flow for $F_1O_2 = 0.6$ using 15 L/minute oxygen supply.[3] This latter total flow rate is just equal to the PIFR of a quietly breathing adult, and unlikely to be sufficient to provide consistent performance in delivery of the stated F_IO_2. In severe dyspnoea these masks may not deliver the stated F_IO_2.[6] Increasing the oxygen flow rate above the manufacturers recommendations will increase the total gas flow to the mask whilst maintaining the stipulated F_IO_2.[8] At very high flow rates, however, turbulence is likely to reduce the performance of the system.

Venturi masks provide the best means of managing patients with chronic obstructive airways disease in the emergency department because they provide a predictable F_IO_2 and the air entrained is more humid than fresh oxygen. The entrained gas mixture can be further heated and humidified to assist with sputum clearance. High gas flows minimize rebreathing of CO_2 and claustrophobia, but cause problems with sleeping due to noise.

Oxygen blenders

Air is blended with oxygen from a number of inlet ports to supply a fixed F_IO_2 to the patient. It is a high-flow system and fine tuning of F_IO_2 from 0.21 to 1.0 is possible. The resultant mixture can then be channelled to the patient through systems such as continuous positive airways pressure, or humidifiers. Lack of portability and high cost are disadvantages, and oxygen blenders are best suited to the resuscitation room and critical-care settings.

100% OXYGEN DELIVERY SYSTEMS

These systems vary in their economy of oxygen use, and are summarized in Table 5.1.3. The least economical is the free-flowing system, because this system can only deliver 100% oxygen if the flow rate exceeds the patient's PIFR. Incorporating a reservoir and unidirectional valves into the circuit enables greater economy of oxygen use by storing oxygen during expiration ready for the inspiratory phase.

Devices incorporating a reservoir into the circuit are capable of delivering 100% oxygen only if total oxygen flow equals or exceeds the patient's respiratory minute volume (RMV) and there are no leaks in the system. The reservoir volume must exceed the patient's tidal volume, otherwise storage of oxygen is inefficient, fresh gas loss occurs when the reservoir is full, and there is a risk of asphyxia during inspiration.

A demand valve system delivers precisely the patient's minute volume without the added bulk and problems of a reservoir. It is able to cope with changes in RMV, provided fresh gas flow always exceeds the patients PIFR. Closed-circuit systems are the most economical in O_2 consumption. Carbon dioxide is absorbed by sodalime and low flow fresh oxygen replaces the O_2 consumed during metabolism - approximately 250–1000 mL/minute; which is considerably less than the patient's minute volume.

Classification

One hundred per cent oxygen-delivery systems available for use in emergency medicine are summarized in Table 5.1.3.

Free-flowing circuits

In order to provide 100% oxygen using a free-flowing system, flow rates in excess of the patient's PIFR are required. This necessitates the use of multiple oxygen ports. The system may not deliver 100% oxygen, is wasteful of oxygen and may be untidy, restricting patient mobility for investigations. Sophisticated free-flowing systems using oxygen blenders and humidification are available, but restrict the ability to move the patient.

Table 5.1.3 Classification of 100% oxygen systems				
System	Rebreathing of gases	Fresh gas flow to deliver 100% O_2	Use for spontaneous and fo manual ventillations	Comments
Free flowing systems	Non-rebreathing	45–90 L/min	Spontaneous	High fresh gas flow prevents CO_2 rebreathing
Soft reservoir bag circuit (Laerdal, Air viva)	Non-rebreathing	7–15 L/min	Spontaneous	Can increase to 15–30 L/min with Y connectors to maintain F_IO_2=1.0 If minute volume exceeds O_2 flow, then F_IO_2<1.0
Demand valve system	Non-rebreathing	Delivers up to 120 L/min Usual RMV = 7–15 L/min	Spontaneous/ manual during inspiration only	Actual delivered volume of O_2 equals minute volume Requires 'trigger' pressure
Mapleson circuits	Partial rebreathing	15–40 L/min	Spontaneous/manual	Fresh gas flow must be at least double minute volume to avoid CO_2 build up
Oxy resuscitator	Closed circuit rebreathing	0.5–2 L/min	Spontaneous/manual	Requires intermittent purging of reservoir to remove exhaled nitrogen from functional residual capacity

Soft reservoir circuits

These are non rebreathing systems incorporating unidirectional valves to channel fresh oxygen to the patient and exhaled gas to the atmosphere. With one oxygen supply port the system delivers 100% oxygen provided the patient's minute volume is less than 15 L/minute. Two O_2 supply ports enable delivery of up to 30 L/minute. Fresh gas flow is titrated to the patient's minute volume by watching the reservoir bag – it should be fully distended at the start of inspiration and more than one-third full when inspiration is complete. The reservoir bag has a minimum volume of 3 litres and for optimal performance the patient's tidal volume should not exceed 2 litres. A soft silicone mask is strapped to the head to ensure a firm but comfortable fit without leaks. The system cannot be used to manually ventilate patients and may be hazardous if the patient has impaired conscious state because of the risk of aspiration if they vomit, and asphyxiation if there is a fall in fresh gas flow or a sudden rise in minute volume. Complications can be avoided with careful clinical vigilance, and the use of safety valves to entrain air, if the oxygen supply ceases.

Self-refilling, non-rebreathing resuscitators (Air viva® and Laerdal® systems)

Most Australasian emergency departments possess at least one type of these self-refilling systems. The systems can be used to manually ventilate patients as well as allow spontaneous ventilation. The Laerdal system has three sizes for adults, children and infants, whereas the Air viva system has one size for adults only (Table 5.1.4).

Advantages of these systems include:

- Self inflation and hence the ability to ventilate patients with air if oxygen supply is exhausted.
- Low resistance unidirectional valves prevent rebreathing of CO_2.
- Can be used in spontaneously ventilating patients and for manual ventilation.
- Provided fresh gas flow exceeds minute volume and the reservoir bag is attached the system is capable of delivering $F_IO_2 = 1.0$. Without the reservoir bag, maximum $F_IO_2 = 0.6$ is obtainable.
- If there is a sudden rise in minute volume, a safety valve entrains air into the system to prevent asphyxiation. This is at the expense of F_IO_2.
- Over pressure valves are incorporated into the Laerdal paediatric and infant apparatus to prevent barotrauma in these patients.
- Positive end-expiratory pressure (PEEP) can be added to the system by attaching a PEEP valve to the expiratory limb. Close apposition of the mask to the face, or endotracheal intubation is required for this to be effective.

The disadvantages include:

- A reduction in F_IO_2 occurs when minute volume exceeds fresh gas flow. Dual oxygen supply ports can minimize this problem, especially in very dyspnoeic patients.
- The unit is bulky and disconnections sometimes occur.
- There is less 'feel' during manual ventilation than with soft bag circuits and inflation of the stomach is more likely during bag/mask ventilation especially if there is airway obstruction or decreased pulmonary compliance.

Oxygen-powered resuscitators

Examples of this system include the Oxy viva®, Laerdal®, and DAN demand valve system. High pressure oxygen is fed to a demand valve which delivers high flow oxygen to the patient. The system can be used in spontaneously breathing patients and for manual ventilation by depressing a manual override button. Spontaneously ventilating patients initiate oxygen flow of up to 120 L/minute by generating a negative pressure of 0.3 kPa (2.25 mmHg) at the start of inspiration. Fresh gas flow is delivered at a pressure of up to 5.3 kPa (40 mmHg).

Advantages of the system include:

- Portability - it is easy to attach to an oxygen cylinder and take to the field. There are no bulky reservoir bags attached.
- Economy of oxygen use - the patient's minute volume is precisely delivered at sufficient flow rates to match the PIFR. Provided there are no leaks the system delivers $F_IO_2 = 1.0$.

Disadvantages include:

- Increased work of breathing for spontaneous ventilation because negative pressure must be generated to initiate O_2 flow.
- When fresh gas supply is exhausted the system cannot function.
- During manual ventilation it is almost impossible to judge ventilatory volume except by observing the patient's chest. The safety over-pressure valve may not prevent barotrauma, especially in children. Lack of 'feel' during manual ventilation may lead to over inflation of the stomach if there is airway obstruction or reduced pulmonary compliance.

Mapleson circuits

A detailed description of these circuits has been previously published.[11] Partial rebreathing of gases occurs with all of

Table 5.1.4 Self-refilling, non rebreathing resuscitators		
	Self-refilling bag volume	O_2 reservoir bag volume
1. Air viva	1700 mL	2300 mL
2. Laerdal (Adult)	1600 mL	2600 mL
3. Laerdal (Child)	500 mL	2600 mL
4. Laerdal (Infant)	240 mL	600 mL

the circuits and CO_2 retention can be avoided if fresh gas flow exceeds minute volume by a ratio of 2–2.5 to 1.

The circuits are still used in some emergency departments. The most commonly used versions are the Mapleson B and the Mapleson F, which are covered under paediatric considerations. Mapleson A, C, D and E circuits will not be discussed.

Advantages of the Mapleson B circuit for oxygen delivery include:

- It can be used for both spontaneous and manual ventilation, and its performance is similar in both circumstances.
- The soft bag has excellent 'feel' for manual ventilation, and it is easy to monitor spontaneous ventilation by observing the filling and emptying of the reservoir bag.

Disadvantages include:

- Carbon dioxide build up with lower O_2 supply flow rates. This can be avoided with higher flow rates, or intermittently purging the reservoir bag.
- The system cannot function without fresh gas supply.
- It may be difficult to use when manually ventilating patients using a mask.
- The valve assembly may occasionally 'stick'.

Closed-circuit systems

An example is the M.D. oxyresuscitator. The circuit is the same as the Boyle's anaesthetic circle system. A sodalime canister absorbs exhaled CO_2, and a low flow oxygen supply replaces O_2 consumed by metabolism; approximately 0.5–2 L/minute. Considerable economy of oxygen use is achieved by rebreathing from the circuit.

Advantages of this system include:

- Economy of oxygen use. More than 6 hours O_2 can be provided by a 'C' sized oxygen cylinder at 1 L/minute. This markedly exceeds the endurance of the cylinder using other systems.
- It can be used for spontaneous or manual ventilation. A soft reservoir

bag provides excellent 'feel' to ventilation.
- The pressure on the system is controlled by the operator during manual ventilation. This minimizes gastric distension.
- It is portable and can easily be taken to the field.

Disadvantages are as follows:

- The circuit ceases to function when fresh gas flow is exhausted.
- Exhaled nitrogen from the patients early breaths may enter the circuit and reduce F_1O_2 below 1.0. This can be prevented by intermittent purging of the reservoir.
- CO_2 accumulation may occur if the sodalime canister is old or stops functioning.
- Incorrect packing of the sodalime canister may result in sodalime dust inhalation (this is extremely rare).
- The reservoir bag is remote from the patient mask and the system may be cumbersome to operate.

MEASUREMENT OF OXYGENATION

Clinical assessment of oxygenation is unreliable, and the time-honoured sign of cyanosis varies with the level of haemo-globin, skin pigmentation, perfusion and external light.[1,12,13] Arterial blood gases and pulse oximetry provide objective measurement of oxygenation and enable precise titration of oxygen therapy to the clinical situation.

As it is non-invasive, pulse oximetry has become the most frequently used indicator of oxygenation in emergency medicine.[14,15] It is colloquially known as the 'fifth vital sign', and provides continuous real time assessment of a patient's oxygenation and response to therapy. It has a proven role in emergency medicine and is an excellent clinical tool provided the limitations are understood. The principles behind pulse oximetry have been described elsewhere.[16,17]

A detailed knowledge of the haemoglobin-oxygen dissociation curve is required to interpret pulse oximetry as well as the factors that influence readings obtained by this equipment. These factors are summarized in Table 5.1.5.

PAEDIATRIC CONSIDERATIONS IN OXYGEN THERAPY

The general principles of oxygen therapy and its indications apply equally well in children as for adults. There are a

Table 5.1.5 Factors which influence pulse oximetry readings[12,13,16,17]

Factor	Cause
Signal interference	High intensity external light source Diathermy Shivering/movement of digit
Reduced light transmission	Dark coloured nail polish Dirt (melanin pigment/jaundice - no effect)
Reduction in plethysmographic volume	Peripheral vasoconstriction (shock, hypothermia)
Inaccurate readings due to abnormal haemoglobin	COHb causes over estimation because not distinguished from O_2Hb Methaemoglobin >10% reads 85% saturation regardless of O_2 saturation Profound anaemia - insufficient hamoglobin for accurate signal
Falsely low readings	Intravenous dyes with absorption spectra near 660 nm, e.g. methylene blue Stagnation of blood flow

number of important differences in relation to body size, psychology and oxygen toxicity.

Body size

Anatomical and physiological parameters are smaller in children. Any increases in equipment dead space will significantly increase CO_2 retention. Children are less able to tolerate increased resistance to ventilation; particularly if negative pressure must be generated to open valves in the apparatus. Peak inspiratory flow rate and respiratory minute volume are lower; hence a given oxygen supply flow rate will produce a higher F_IO_2 for a child than an adult. A Hudson mask at 8 L/minute may supply a F_IO_2 of 0.8 in a young child.[2] Reservoir bags are not required to deliver F_IO_2 values near 1.0 to children weighing less than 15 kg because available supply flow rates (maximum 15 L/minute) exceed the child's PIFR.

Appropriately sized equipment is essential; multiple sized oxygen masks, oximeter probes, laryngoscopes and endotracheal tubes must be available to manage children of different ages. Serious barotrauma may result from the use of excessive volume during manual ventilation. Resuscitator bags are available with paediatric sized reservoirs. The Laerdal system has paediatric and infant sizes. These units also have a pressure relief valve designed to prevent barotrauma. Pressure rapidly rises as the child's lung reaches full inflation. A smaller Mapleson circuit is available to ventilate children; the Jackson-Rees (or Mapleson F) circuit. It can be used for spontaneous ventilation and to manually ventilate children. Rebreathing of carbon dioxide does not occur provided fresh gas flow is 2–3 times minute volume, and the bag is separated from the patient by a tube of internal volume greater than the patients tidal volume. The overall relationship between fresh gas flow, minute volume and P_aCO_2 is complex.[11] The principal advantages over the Laerdal system are that the operator can observe bag movement in spontaneous respiration and has a better 'feel' for airway obstruction in manual ventilation.

However, considerable skill and experience is required to use the system safely.

Psychological considerations

Gaining the trust and confidence of an ill child is an art to be learnt with experience. They frequently respond with fear when oxygen therapy is administered. It is helpful to obtain assistance by asking their parents to nurse the child during treatment. A tight fitting mask is less important in a child because source flow rate more closely approximates PIFR. Parents may assist by holding the oxygen mask close to the child's face, or by directing high flow oxygen straight at the child's mouth using a tube only. A cupped hand with the oxygen tube held between middle and ring fingers can serve as a useful oxygen 'mask'.

Oxygen toxicity

Prolonged administration of oxygen at $F_IO_2 > 0.6$ for longer than 24 hours may be toxic to infants. This toxicity may not become apparent during their acute stay in the emergency department, however, the oxygen dose received there contributes to cumulative toxicity. Appropriate monitoring using pulse oximetry ensures administration of the correct oxygen dose and minimizes the risk of toxicity. Supplemental oxygen should *never* be withheld because of fear of toxicity.

TRANSFER OF PATIENTS ON OXYGEN THERAPY

Supplemental oxygen therapy is a vital part of transporting the ill patient, and is especially important for air travel where lower ambient P_IO_2 may exacerbate hypoxia already present due to the patient's disease process. The partial pressures of oxygen at various altitudes have been summarized elsewhere.[18] Patients with decompression illness or arterial gas embolism should not be transported at cabin pressures lower than 101.3kPa (1 atmosphere absolute, ATA) because lower ambient pressure exacerbates their disease process by increasing bubble size. A number of factors must be considered for successful oxygen therapy during transport of a patient.[19]

Knowledge of the oxygen delivery apparatus and its maximum rate of oxygen delivery is essential for estimating transport oxygen requirements. These estimates take into account: current oxygen consumption, duration of transport (including delays), oxygen required in the event of deterioration, and adding a safety factor of at least 50%. The sizes of oxygen cylinders available in Australasia, their filling pressures and approximate endurances are summarized in Table 5.1.6. The most economical circuit for a prolonged transport with $F_IO_2 = 1.0$ is a closed circuit with a CO_2 absorber and the least economical is a free-flowing circuit.

Monitoring during transport should be of the same standard initiated in the emergency department. Pulse oximetry provides an essential monitoring tool to detect hypoxia during transport, and should include audible and visual alarms. Oxygen therapy can be titrated against SaO_2, and this is particularly important in air travel where P_IO_2 varies with ascent and descent. All the usual clinical parameters must also be monitored.

Table 5.1.6 Oxygen cylinder sizes

Cylinder size	Water capacity	Volume at 15000 kPa 15°C	Approximate endurance		
			8 L/min	15 L/min	30 L/min
C	2.8 kg	420 L	52 min	28 min	14 min
D	9.5 kg	1387 L	173 min	92 min	46 min
E	23.8 kg	3570 L	446 min	238 min	119 min
G	48 kg	7200 L	900 min	480 min	240 min

OXYGEN THERAPY IN SPECIFIC CIRCUMSTANCES

Asthma

Hypoxia in asthma results from ventilation – perfusion inequality created by bronchospasm, secretions and airway inflammation and oedema. Supplemental oxygen should be titrated to provide a SaO_2 greater than 90%, preferably 94%, and must be continued during the interval between doses of inhaled bronchodilators.

Initial management should include a Hudson mask at 8 L/minute O_2 flow rate. SaO_2 should be monitored continuously by pulse oximetry. The oxygen dose should be rapidly increased up to 100% if the patient remains hypoxic. Bronchodilator therapy should be administered proportionate to the severity of the attack, using oxygen to drive the nebulizer. Oxygen should not be withheld or administered in low doses because of fear of respiratory depression. Hypercapnia is an indication of extreme airway obstruction and its presence mandates aggressive therapy and/or mechanical ventilation.

Occasionally patients with asthma become hypoxic during nebulizer therapy because O_2 flow rates driving the nebulizer (6–8 L/minute) are lower than the flow rate required to maintain $SaO_2 >90\%$. In these circumstances, extra oxygen may be supplied to maintain SaO_2 via a T piece or Y connector, during the nebulizer therapy.

Chronic obstructive pulmonary disease

Most patients with chronic obstructive pulmonary disease (COPD) possess a degree of *acute* respiratory failure that has caused their emergency presentation. This may be due to infection, bronchospasm, retention of secretions, coexistent left ventricular failure, worsening right heart failure, pulmonary embolism, pneumothorax, or sedation. The vast majority will have normal ventilatory response to CO_2 and if these patients develop hypercapnia, there is danger of impending respiratory arrest because their disease is severe and progressive. Any patient with impaired consciousness due to respiratory failure should be manually ventilated, whilst they are clinically assessed and treated.

It is useful in terms of management, to divide patients with COPD into two groups, although this simple classification is still a source of debate.[20,21,22]

- Patients with normal ventilatory response to CO_2 ('can't breathe' = most common). Gas exchange and air flow into the lungs is impaired but ventilatory drive is normal.
- Patients with impaired ventilatory response to CO_2 ('won't breathe' = uncommon). Ventilation does not increase in response to hypercapnia and acidosis.

There is overlap between the advanced stages of illness. The aims of oxygen therapy are to ensure SaO_2 of greater than 90% in the first group, and to identify the second group of patients so that oxygen dose can be titrated to achieve an acceptable clinical response without excessive elevation of P_aCO_2. Serial arterial blood gas analysis is an essential tool in the management of these patients.

It is reasonable to use a consistent initial approach to oxygen therapy for conscious patients with advanced COPD because at the time of presentation their ventilatory response to CO_2 is unknown. These patients should be treated with controlled supplemental oxygen therapy commencing with $F_IO_2 = 0.28$. Oxygen dose should be adjusted as information is gathered concerning the patients ventilatory response to CO_2. Clues may be obtained from the patients history, past clinical records, emergency department blood gases and their response to initial oxygen therapy. Clinical indicators of patients at risk of CO_2 retention include a housebound patient, a FEV_1 <1 litre, polycythaemia, a warm vasodilated periphery and cor pulmonale. Arterial blood gas (ABG) samples taken during the initial assessment of these patients (with or without supplemental O_2) will assist management. If the bicarbonate level is >30 mmol/L or elevated by more than 4 mmol/L for each 1.3 kPa (10 mmHg) rise in $PaCO_2$ above normal (5.3 kPa, 40 mmHg) this provides strong evidence of chronic hypercapnia provided there is no other cause of metabolic alkalosis.[23]

The patient's response to initial oxygen therapy ($F_IO_2 = 0.28$) will direct further oxygen dose changes and identify any patients not already known to be suffering chronic hypercapnia. A repeat ABG sample should be taken after 10 minutes of breathing $F_IO_2 = 0.28$. The P_aCO_2 may rise slightly because of the 'Haldane effect'.[1,21] If this rise is excessive (greater than 1–1.3 kPa [8–10 mmHg]), it is consistent with an impaired ventilatory response to CO_2. The F_IO_2 should then be adjusted downwards in steps to achieve a satisfactory pulse oximetry reading that is compatible with acceptable CO_2 levels. Arterial blood gases should be checked at regular intervals during titration of the oxygen dose.

If the patient becomes progressively more hypoxic and the elevation of P_aCO_2 persists or worsens, or their conscious state deteriorates, they require non-invasive, or mechanical ventilation. Supplemental oxygen should never be withdrawn abruptly from these patients because a catastrophic fall in P_aO_2 will occur. In the majority of cases an acceptable balance between P_aO_2 and P_aCO_2 can be achieved while both hypoxia and hypercarbia are reversed by specific therapy. A lower SaO_2 in the range of 85–90% may be accepted if the patient's clinical staus and conscious state is stable. Administration of bronchodilators using oxygen driven nebulizers in the acute management of chronically hypercapnic patients has been shown to be safe in a pilot study.[24]

Patients with normal ventilatory response to CO_2 will not exhibit significant elevation of P_aCO_2 in response to oxygen therapy. They constitute the majority of patients, especially those with early disease. Oxygen dose should commence with $F_IO_2 = 0.28$, then be progressively increased until a satisfactory $S_aO_2 > 90\%$ is achieved (monitored by continuous pulse oximetry). Specific therapy should be initiated, aiming to reverse the cause of the acute deterioration. If at any stage the patient becomes agitated or confused, hypoxia or CO_2 narcosis should be suspected, and the patient fully re-evaluated.

Oxygen therapy for shock, sepsis and myocardial infarction

Supplemental oxygen therapy is provided in order to overcome inefficiencies in the oxygen transport chain created by these conditions. A Hudson mask delivering oxygen at 6–8 L/minute is usually sufficient, however, the O_2 dose should be titrated to provide a SaO_2 >90% if there is respiratory compromise. Treatment must also be directed at reducing oxygen consumption (antibiotics, antipyretics and analgesia) and at repairing the specific deficits in the oxygen transport chain (volume and blood replacement for shock, vasodilators and thrombolytics for myocardial infarction). If there is concern about the extent of coexisting chronic obstructive airway disease, a venturi mask delivering 28% oxygen is satisfactory for initial management, then careful titration of oxygen dose using ABG measurements.

Pulmonary oedema

Increased diffusion gradients and intrapulmonary shunting contribute to hypoxia in the oedematous lung, which in turn exacerbates the disease process. Supplemental oxygen is one of the definitive modes of therapy for pulmonary oedema. Oxygen dose should initially commence with a Hudson mask at 6–15 L/minute and be titrated to achieve a SaO_2 of 90%, preferably 94%. It may be necessary to use a 100% O_2 delivery system if higher flows (15–30 L/minute) via a Hudson mask do not elevate SaO_2 sufficiently.

Continuous positive airways pressure (CPAP) coupled with 100% oxygen is now an essential component of treatment; reducing the need for endotracheal intubation and ventilation in severe cardiogenic pulmonary oedema.[25] This is covered in more detail under the section on CPAP.

COMPLICATIONS OF OXYGEN THERAPY

These can be classified into three categories:

❶ Equipment-related complications
❷ Carbon-dioxide narcosis
❸ Oxygen toxicity.

Equipment-related complications

These are entirely preventable with careful monitoring and many have been dealt with in the discussion of each individual apparatus. Tight-fitting masks may cause asphyxia if there is insufficient O_2 reservoir or flow, and aspiration of vomitus may occur if the patient has depressed airway reflexes. Use of appropriate O_2 flow rates with rebreathing circuits prevents CO_2 accumulation. During mechanical ventilation, barotrauma can be prevented by use of appropriate volumes and pressures, although it may be difficult to avoid when there is reduced lung compliance as in the moribund asthmatic. Knowledge of potential complications due to equipment enables prompt intervention should they arise. When investigating a sudden deterioration in the patient's condition, a thorough check of the equipment in use is mandatory.

Carbon-dioxide narcosis

This can be prevented by controlled oxygen therapy, titrating the F_1O_2 against SaO_2, arterial blood gases and conscious state. Unconscious patients should be intubated and manually ventilated using high F_1O_2, preferably 100% O_2. Patients with deteriorating conscious state and respiration due to CO_2 narcosis need to be vigorously stimulated and encouraged to breathe, whilst F_1O_2 is reduced in a step-wise manner. Oxygen should never be suddenly withdrawn because this precipitates severe hypoxia. Reversible causes of respiratory failure should be treated. Doxapram may be useful as a respiratory stimulant in the 'won't breathe' group, but a recent review suggests that non-invasive ventilation is more effective.[26]

Oxygen toxicity

Oxygen is toxic in higher doses and this toxicity is a function of P_1O_2 and duration of exposure. The toxicity is thought to occur by formation of 'free radicals' and toxic lipid peroxides, inhibition of enzyme systems and direct toxic effect on cerebral metabolism.[27] Toxicity is mainly restricted to the respiratory system and central nervous system (CNS), although it may affect other regions such as the eye; premature infants develop retrolental fibroplasia after prolonged exposure to high F_1O_2. CNS oxygen toxicity manifested by neuromuscular irritability and seizures (Paul Bert effect) is restricted to hyperbaric exposures.

Pulmonary oxygen toxicity (Lorraine-Smith effect) is of greatest relevance to emergency medicine, although exposures of 0.6–1 ATA for greater than 24 hours are required to produce it.[27] Acute changes such as oedema, haemorrhages and proteinaceous exudates are reversible on withdrawal of O_2. Longer durations of high P_1O_2 may lead to permanent fibrosis and emphysema. Physicians should be alert to acute symptoms of cough, dyspnoea and retrosternal pain; these are non-specific symptoms of oxygen toxicity. A progressive reduction in vital capacity may be demonstrated. As with all drugs, oxygen dose should be monitored and carefully titrated against SaO_2 and clinical effect; however, oxygen therapy should never be withheld acutely because of fear of toxicity.

SPECIAL DELIVERY SYSTEMS

Humidification of oxygen

This may be desirable when prolonged use (>6 hours) of supplemental oxygen is required because oxygen is totally dry, possessing no water vapour. Humidification is particularly necessary where patients are intubated because the natural humidification that occurs in the nose, mouth and nasopharynx is bypassed. Patients with COPD and retained secretions benefit from humidification.

Additional heat is required to provide effective humidification by vaporization of water. Various systems are available to humidify inspired gas and, ideally, they should be able to deliver inspired gas to the trachea at 32–36 °C with low resistance and at greater than 90% humidity. The devices should be simple to use, and able to maintain temperature and humidity at varying gas flows and F_IO_2. There should also be safety alarms monitoring temperature and humidity.[23] Humidification of warmed inspired gas also enables heat transfer to hypothermic patients, and is essential in treating the pulmonary complications of near drowning. Dry oxygen will exacerbate hypothermia. The Fischer and Paykel apparatus provides more effective humidification by using a heating coil with a large surface area for contact with inspired gas.

Continuous positive airways pressure

This topic has been reviewed in detail by Duncan, Oh and Hillman.[28] Continuous positive airways pressure (CPAP) has a role in the management of pulmonary oedema, pneumonia, bronchiolitis, respiratory tract burns and acute respiratory failure.[25,29,30,31,32] Benefit to the patient is achieved as a result of increasing functional residual capacity and reduced pulmonary compliance. Hypoxaemia is reversed by reduction in intrapulmonary shunting, and work of breathing is reduced.[28]

Circuit designs generally consist of a reservoir based on the Mapleson D circuit, or a high flow turbine system.[25] Humidification can be added to the system, and is considered essential for long-term use (>6 hours). Use of an oxygen blender enables valuable F_IO_2 to be administered. In emergency medicine, CPAP has a proven role in the acute management of cardiogenic pulmonary oedema. Reduced requirements for endotracheal intubation have been demonstrated when CPAP is used for severely ill patients.[25] Complications of CPAP include aspiration, and pulmonary barotrauma. It may elevate intracranial pressure, and precipitate hypotension by reducing venous return to the thorax.

Hyperbaric oxygen treatment

Hyperbaric oxygen (HBO) treatment consists of administering oxygen at pressures greater than 1 ATA, usually in the range of 1.5–2.8 ATA. This requires a hyperbaric chamber that is pressurized with air whilst the patient breathes F_IO_2 = 1.0 from various delivery systems for periods of 2–7 hours. The high P_IO_2 results in P_aO_2 of up to 267 kPa (2000 mmHg) if 2.8 ATA treatment pressure is used. This is beneficial because there is increased dissolved O_2 in the plasma (up to 300 mL O_2 may be carried to the periphery each minute in the dissolved form), which maintains O_2 flux even if Hb is non functional (CO poisoning). Increased P_IO_2 enables more rapid elimination of toxic gases from the body, for example CO or H_2S. The increased PO_2 creates a greater driving pressure of oxygen into ischaemic tissues (problem wounds), and reduces swelling by vaso-constriction (crush injuries). HBO treatment has a number of benefits in treating gas embolism and decompression illness. It provides extra oxygen to tissues rendered ischaemic by nitrogen bubbles, increased pressure reduces bubble size and enhanced nitrogen removal from the body. HBO treatment is also of benefit in anaerobic infections by being bacterio-static to anaerobes, inhibiting clostridial α toxin, and stimulating host defences (granulocyte function). Recognized indications for acute referral to a hyperbaric facility for HBO treatment are summarized in Table 5.1.7.[27]

Table 5.1.7 Indications for acute treatment with hyperbaric oxygen[27]

1. Decompression illness
2. Air or gas embolism
3. Carbon monoxide poisoning
4. Gas gangrene and anaerobic fasciitis
5. Necrotizing soft tissue infections
6. Acute crush injury with compartment syndrome
7. Acutely compromised skin flaps or grafts due to injury or post surgery

---

REFERENCES

1. West JB 1999 Respiratory physiology - the essentials, 6th edn. Lippincott, Williams and Wilkins. Baltimore USA
2. Oh TE, Duncan AW 1988 Oxygen therapy. Medical Journal of Australia 149: 141–6
3. Smart DR, Mark PD 1992 Oxygen therapy in emergency medicine. Part 1. Physiology and delivery systems. Emergency Medicine 4(3): 163–78
4. Bethune DW, Collins JM 1967 An evaluation of oxygen therapy equipment. Thorax 22: 221–5
5. Campbell EJM 1960 A method of controlled oxygen administration which reduces the risk of carbon dioxide retention. Lancet 2: 10–1
6. Hill SL, Barnes PK, Hollway T, Tennant R 1984 Fixed performance oxygen masks: an evaluation. British Medical Journal 288: 1261–3
7. Fracchia G, Torda TA 1980 Performance of venturi oxygen delivery devices. Anaesthesia and Intensive Care 8: 426–30
8. Friedman SA, Weber B, Briscoe WA, Smith JP, King TKC 1974 Oxygen therapy. Evaluation of various air-entraining masks. Journal of the American Medical Association 228(4): 474–8
9. Goldstein RS, Young J, Rebuck AS 1982 Effect of breathing pattern on oxygen concentration received from standard face masks. Lancet 27(2): 1188–90
10. Woolner DF, Larkin J 1980 An analysis of the performance of a variable Venturi-type oxygen mask. Anaesthesia and Intensive Care 8: 44–51
11. Dorsch JA, Dorsch SE 1984 The breathing system. II. The Mapleson systems. In: Dorsch JA, Dorsch SE (eds) Understanding anaesthesia equipment. Construction, care and complications, 2nd edn. Williams and Wilkins, Baltimore
12. Morgan-Hughes J O 1968 Lighting and cyanosis. British Journal of Anaesthesia 40: 503–7
13. Hanning CD 1985 "He looks a little blue down this end". Monitoring oxygenation during anaesthesia. British Journal of Anaesthesia 57: 359–60
14. Jones J, Heiselman D, Cannon L, Gradisek R 1988 Continuous Emergency Department monitoring of arterial saturation in adult patients with respiratory distress. Annals of Emergency Medicine 17: 463–8
15. Lambert MA, Crinnon J 1989 The role of pulse oximetry in the Accident and Emergency Department. Arch Emerg Med 6: 211–5
16. Adams AP 1989 Capnography and pulse oximetry. In: Atkinson RS, Adams AP (eds) Recent Advances in Anaesthesia and Analgesia. Churchill Livingstone, Edinburgh, pp 155–75
17. Phillips GD, Runciman WB, Ilsley AH 1989 Monitoring in Emergency Medicine. Resuscitation 18 Suppl: 21–35
18. Hackett PH, Roach RC, Sutton JR 1989 High altitude medicine. In: Auerbach PS, Geehr EC (eds). Management of wilderness and environmental emergencies, 2nd edn. CV Mosby, Missouri USA, pp 1–34
19. Saunders CE 1989 Aeromedical transport. In: Auerbach PS, Geehr EC (eds) Management of wilderness and environmental emergencies, 2nd edn. CV Mosby, Missouri USA, pp 359–88
20. Stradling JR 1986 Hypercapnia during oxygen therapy in airways obstruction: a reappraisal. Thorax 41: 897–902
21. Aubier M, Murciano D, Milic-Emili J, et al 1980 Effects of the administration of oxygen on ventilation and blood gases in patients with chronic obstructive pulmonary disease during acute respiratory failure. Am Rev Resp Dis 122: 747–54
22. Sassoon CSH, Hassell KT, Mahutte CK 1987 Hyperoxic induced hypercapnia in stable chronic obstructive pulmonary disease. American Review of Respiratory Disease 135: 907–11

23. Tuxen DV 1990 Acute respiratory failure in chronic obstructive airways disease. In: Oh TE (ed.) Intensive Care Manual, 3rd edn. Butterworths, Sydney

24. Cameron P, Coleridge J, Epstein J, Teichtahl H 1992 The safety of oxygen driven nebulisers in patients with chronic hypoxaemia and hypercapnia. Emergency Medicine 4 (3): 159–62

25. Bersten AD, Holt AW, Vedig AE, Skowronski GA, Baggoley CJ 1991 Treatment of severe cardiogenic pulmonary oedema with continuous positive airway pressure delivered by face mask. New England Journal of Medicine 325(26): 1825–30

26. Greenstone M 2000 Doxapram for ventilatory failure due to exacerbations of chronic obstructive pulmonary disease. Cochrane Database Systematic Reviews 2:CD 000223

27. Hampson NB 1999 Hyperbaric Oxygen Therapy: 1999 Committee Report. Undersea and Hyperbaric Medicine Society, Kensington, Maryland USA

28. Duncan AW, Oh TE, Hillman DR 1986 PEEP and CPAP. Anaesthesia and Intensive Care 14: 236–50

29. Taylor GJ, Brenner W, Summer WR 1976 Severe viral pneumonia in young adults. Therapy with continuous airway pressure. Chest 69: 722–8

30. Beasley JM, Jones SEF 1981 Continuous positive airways pressure in bronchiolitis. British Medical Journal 283: 1506–8

31. Venus B, Matsuda T, Copiozo JB, Mathru M 1981 Prophylactic intubation and continuous positive airways pressure in the management of inhalation injury in burn victims. Critical Care Medicine 9: 519–23

32. Katz JA, Marks JD 1985 Inspiratory work with and without continuous positive airway pressure in patients with acute respiratory failure. Anaesthesiology 63: 598–607

5.2 UPPER RESPIRATORY TRACT

KEN OOI

ESSENTIALS

1 Airway management and the ABCs take precedence over the history, examination and specific treatment of upper airway obstruction.

2 Direct laryngoscopy is both an important investigation and management technique in upper airway obstruction.

3 The Heimlich manoeuvre (abdominal thrust) is a useful first aid technique in foreign body upper airway obstruction, though unproven.

4 Acute viral respiratory infections are a frequent reason for seeking medical attention. Over-prescribing of antibiotics is an increasing problem.

5 Bacterial infections and collections are uncommon but may compromise the upper airway.

6 A high index of suspicion is needed to diagnose blunt trauma injuries to the larynx and trachea.

7 Cervical spine injuries frequently accompany significant blunt laryngeal injuries.

Table 5.2.1 Causes of upper airway obstruction

Altered conscious state
Head injury
CVA
Drugs and toxins
Metabolic – hypoglycaemia, hyponatraemia, etc.

Foreign bodies

Infections
Tonsillitis
Peritonsillar abscess (quinsy)
Epiglottitis
Ludwig's angina
Other abscesses and infections

Trauma
Blunt or penetrating trauma resulting in oedema or haematoma formation
Uncontrolled haemorrhage
Thermal injuries
Inhalation burns

Neoplasms
Larynx, trachea, thyroid

Allergic reactions
Anaphylaxis
Angioedema

Anatomical
Tracheomalacia – congenital or acquired (secondary to prolonged intubation)
Other congenital malformations.

INTRODUCTION

The upper respiratory tract extends from the mouth and nose to the carina. It comprises a relatively small area anatomically, but is of vital importance. Presenting conditions may be acute and potentially life threatening requiring immediate evaluation or treatment, although the majority of presentations to most general emergency departments are not life threatening.

Urgent conditions requiring immediate attention or intervention are those likely to compromise the airway. Protection and maintenance of airway, breathing and circulation (the ABCs) take precedence over history taking, detailed examination or investigations. Possible causes of airway obstruction are listed in Table 5.2.1.

Non urgent presentations include rash or facial swelling not involving the airway, sore throat in a non-toxic patient and complaints that have been present for days or weeks with no recent deterioration. Pharyngitis and tonsillitis are common causes for presentation in both paediatric and adult emergency practice.

TRIAGE AND INITIAL EVALUATION

Initial evaluation should be aimed at differentiating those patients needing urgent management to prevent significant morbidity and mortality, from those needing less immediate intervention.

Triage must be based on the chief complaint and on vital signs since the same clinical presentation may result from a range of pathophysiologies e.g. stridor can be due to trauma, infection, drug reactions or anatomical abnormalities such as tracheomalacia.[1]

Symptoms and signs of airway obstruction include dyspnoea, stridor, altered voice, dysphonia and dysphagia. Evidence of the increased work of breathing includes subcostal, intercostal and suprasternal retraction, flaring of the nasal alar as well as exhaustion and altered mental state. The presence of these signs may vary with age and accompanying conditions. Cyanosis is a late sign.

Further examination will be directed by the presenting complaint and initial findings and includes:

- General appearance – facial symmetry, demeanour
- Vital signs – temperature, heart rate, respiratory rate, BP, pulse oximetry
- Head and face – rash, swelling, mucous membranes, lymphadenopathy
- Oropharynx – mucous membranes, dental hygiene, tongue, tonsils, uvula.

UPPER-AIRWAY OBSTRUCTION

Upper-airway obstruction may be acute and life threatening or may have a more gradual onset. It is essential that the adequacy of the airway is assessed first. Any emergency interventions that are required to maintain the airway should be instituted before obtaining a detailed history and examination. This may range from relieving the obstruction to providing an alternative airway.

Obstruction may be physiological with the patient unable to maintain and protect an adequate airway due to a decreased conscious state. Despite the plethora of possible causes the initial treatment of securing the airway is the same regardless of the cause. Mechanical obstruction may be due to pathology within the lumen (aspirated foreign body), in the wall (angioedema, tracheomalacia) or by extrinsic compression (Ludwig's angina, haematoma, external burns). Obstruction may be due to a combination of physiological and mechanical causes. A summary of potential causes of upper airway obstruction is provided in Table 5.2.1.

INVESTIGATION

Investigations are secondary to the assessment of and/or provision of an adequate airway. Once the airway has been assessed as secure the choice of investigations is directed by the history and examination.

Endoscopy

Direct laryngoscopy in experienced hands is the single most important manoeuvre in patients with acute upper airway obstruction. It may concurrently form part of the assessment, investigation or treatment. By visualizing the laryngopharynx and upper larynx the cause of the obstruction is seen. Any foreign bodies may be removed or if necessary a definitive airway such as an endotracheal tube introduced. In the case of the stable patient with an incomplete obstruction this should only be attempted when there are full facilities available for intubation and provision of a surgical airway and may be more appropriately deferred until expert airway assistance is available.

Bronchoscopy may be required to assess the trachea and distal upper airway but it is not part of the initial resuscitation. In the stable patient it is more appropriate to transfer the patient to the operating suite or ICU for this procedure.

Pathology

Some tests may be useful in guiding further management. These include full blood count, arterial blood gases, and throat swab and blood cultures. Initial treatment in the emergency department should not await their results.

Neck X-rays

A lateral soft tissue X-ray of the neck is sometimes helpful once the patient has been stabilized. Metallic or bony foreign bodies, food boluses or soft tissue masses may be seen. A number of subtle radiological signs have been described in epiglottitis (Table 5.2.2)

Computerized tomography

In the patient with a mechanical obstruction, a computerized tomography (CT) scan of the neck and upper thorax may be helpful in diagnosing the cause of the obstruction as well as the extent of any local involvement. It may aid in planning further management, especially if surgical intervention is indicated, for example for a retrothyroid goitre or head and neck neoplasm.

Table 5.2.2 Radiological findings in adult epiglottitis	
The 'thumb' sign	Oedema of the normally leaf-like epiglottis resulting in a round shadow resembling an adult thumb. The width of the epiglottis should be less than 1/3 the antero-posterior width of C4.
The vallecula sign	Progressive epiglottic oedema resulting in narrowing of the vallecula. This normally well defined air pocket between the base of the tongue and the epiglottis may be partially or completely obliterated.
Swelling of the aryepiglottic folds	
Swelling of the arytenoids	
Prevertebral soft tissue swelling	The width of the pre-vertebral soft tissue should be less than half the antero-posterior width of C4.
Hypopharyngeal airway widening	The ratio of the width of the hypopharyngeal airway to the antero-posterior width of C4 should be less than 1.5.

MANAGEMENT

Management initially consists of securing the airway. This is discussed in more detail elsewhere (advanced airway management), but simple interventions include chin lift or jaw thrust and the oropharyngeal airway, to more sophisticated items such as the laryngeal mask, endotracheal tube or surgical airway. A surgical airway is rarely necessary in the emergency department, although it is important that equipment is always available and that the technique has been practised, such as needle insufflation and cricothyrostomy. A number of commercial kits such as the 'Mini-trach® II' and the Melker Emergency Cricothyroidotomy Catheter Set are available. Further management will depend on the underlying cause.

TRAUMA

Trauma to the upper airway may involve obstruction by a foreign body, blunt or penetrating trauma or thermal injury.

FOREIGN BODY AIRWAY OBSTRUCTION

Foreign body aspiration is often associated with an altered conscious state including from alcohol or drug intoxication as well as cerebrovascular accident (CVA) or dementia. Elderly patients with dentures are at increased risk. Laryngeal foreign bodies are almost always symptomatic and are more likely to cause complete obstruction than foreign bodies below the epiglottis. If the obstruction is incomplete and adequate air exchange continues, care should be taken not to convert partial obstruction into a complete block by over zealous interference.

Management

The Heimlich manoeuvre or abdominal thrusts is one recommended technique whereby the rescuer stands behind the patient placing clenched fists over the patient's upper abdomen well clear of the xiphisternum. A short sharp upward thrust is made to force the diaphragm up and expel the foreign body.[2] There is a risk of injury to internal organs and thus should only be done by rescuers who have been trained in the technique.

Chest thrusts are a similar technique that may be used in children or in pregnant women and back blows can be used in small children. Patients who are asymptomatic after uncomplicated removal of a foreign body should be observed for a time in the emergency department and if they remain well may be discharged home.

In the unconscious patient direct laryngoscopy may be performed with removal of the foreign body under direct vision with Magill forceps or suction.

BLUNT TRAUMA

The upper airway is relatively protected against trauma since the larynx is mobile and the trachea compressible and because the head and mandible act as shields. Blunt trauma may be difficult to diagnose as external examination may be normal and there may be distracting head or chest injuries.

Mechanism

'Clothesline injuries' involve cyclists or other riders hitting fences or cables. Direct trauma from assaults, sporting equipment or industrial accidents also occur. Suicide attempts by hanging may cause traumatic injuries to the neck as well as airway obstruction due to the ligature. 'Dashboard injures' occur when seatbelts are not worn, with sudden deceleration resulting in hyperextension of the neck and compression of the larynx between the dashboard and cervical spine.

Pathology

The most common laryngeal injury is a vertical fracture through the thyroid cartilage. Fractures of the hyoid bone and cricoid cartilage also occur and may be found in cases of manual or ligature strangulation. The cricothyroid ligament and the vocal cords may be ruptured and the arytenoids dislocated. Complete cricotracheal transection may occur. Mortality rates depend on the location of the injury, ranging from 11% for isolated fractures of the thyroid cartilage to 50% for injuries involving the cricoid cartilage, bronchi or intrathoracic trachea.[3] Up to 50% of patients sustaining significant blunt airway trauma have a concurrent cervical spine injury.[4]

Clinical

Tracheal or laryngeal injury should be suspected if aphonia, hoarseness, stridor, dysphagia or dyspnoea occur. Patients may present with complete obstruction or may deteriorate rapidly after arrival. There may be minimal external evidence of injury or the larynx may be deformed or tender and there may be subcutaneous emphysema. It is important to check for associated head, chest and cervical spine injuries.

PENETRATING TRAUMA

Mechanism

Penetrating injuries may by secondary to assault or to sporting or industrial accidents. A focused history is mandatory.

Clinical

Penetration of the airway should be suspected if there is difficulty breathing, change in voice, pain on speaking, subcutaneous emphysema or bubbling from the wound. This is often associated with great vessel or pulmonary injuries and the patient may require an emergency airway procedure. Uncontrolled haemorrhage is a potentially life-threatening condition. Other causes include head and neck malignancies eroding vascular structures or post radiotherapy. Uncontrolled haemorrhage may lead to exsanguination as well as compromising the airway and requires prompt surgical intervention.

Management

Airway management with protection of the cervical spine is essential. Fibre-optic bronchoscopic intubation is preferable to minimize complications such as laryngeal disruption, laryngo-tracheal separation or creating a false tracheal lumen. Crico-thyrostomy is relatively contraindicated due to the altered anatomy. Emergency tracheostomy may even be required, ideally performed in the operating theatre.

THERMAL INJURY

Pathology

Burns may affect the airway because of facial and perioral swelling, laryngeal oedema or constricting circumferential neck burns. Smoke inhalation occurs in about 25% of burn victims and may cause bronchospasm, retrosternal pain and impaired gas exchange.

Clinical

External examination may show evidence of burns. Carbonaceous material in the mouth, nares or pharynx suggests the possibility of upper airway thermal injury. If the patient presents with stridor or hoarseness, early intubation is essential because of the danger of increasing airway oedema. Smoke inhalation may be associated with carbon-monoxide poisoning, and in the setting of domestic or industrial fires cyanide poisoning should also be considered.

INVESTIGATIONS

Plain X-ray

X-rays should only be considered if the patient is stable with adequate ventilation. Lateral soft tissue X-rays of the neck may provide information about airway patency, subcutaneous or soft tissue emphysema, and fractures of the hyoid and larynx. They may also confirm the presence of a foreign body. Cervical spine X-rays should be considered due to the association between upper airway injuries and cervical spine injuries. Chest X-rays may show signs of trauma and subcutaneous or mediastinal emphysema.

Endoscopy

Endoscopy includes both laryngoscopy and bronchoscopy, performed in the

Table 5.2.3 Grading of blunt laryngeal injury[5]

Grade	Endoscopic and radiological findings
I	Minor laryngeal haematoma without detectable fracture
II	Oedema, haematoma or minor mucosal disruption without exposed cartilage, or non-displaced fractures on CT
III	Massive oedema, tears, exposed cartilage, immobile cords

operating theatre, as urgent surgical intervention may be required. Fuhrman et al[5] suggested a classification system for severity of blunt upper airway injury based on endoscopic and radiological findings (see Table 5.2.3).

CT

CT of the neck is useful in assessing the extent of injuries to larynx, oesophagus, cervical spine and adjacent structures but should only be considered in the stable patient.

INFECTIONS

Infections may involve the upper respiratory tract directly or affect adjacent structures. They range from the common and trivial to the rare and potentially life threatening. Croup and epiglottitis usually occur in children, but may be seen in adults. Acute respiratory infections are the most frequent reason for seeking medical attention in the USA and are associated with up to 75% of total antibiotic prescriptions there each year.[6] Unnecessary antibiotic use can cause a number of adverse effects for the individual including allergic reactions, GIT upset, yeast infections, drug interactions, an increased risk of subsequent infection with drug resistant *S. pneumoniae* and added costs of over-treating.

Non-specific upper-airway infections

Upper-airway infections are generally diagnosed clinically. Symptom com-

plexes where the predominant complaint is of sore throat are labelled pharyngitis or tonsillitis and where the predominant symptom is cough bronchitis. Acute respiratory symptoms in the absence of a predominant sign are typically diagnosed as 'upper-respiratory-tract infections'.[7] Each of these syndromes may be caused by a multitude of different viruses and only occasionally by bacteria. Most cases resolve spontaneously within 1–2 weeks. Bacterial rhino-sinusitis complicates about 2% of cases and should be suspected when symptoms have lasted at least 7 days and include purulent nasal discharge and other localising features. High-risk patients for developing bacterial rhino-sinusitis or bacterial pneumonia include infants, the elderly and the chronically ill. A recent American survey revealed an antibiotic prescription rate for uncomplicated URTIs of 52%[8] despite the fact that they are typically viral in origin and that antibiotic treatment does not enhance illness resolution nor alter the rates of these complications. Treatment should be symptomatic only.

Pharyngitis/tonsillitis

Sore throat is one of the top ten presenting complaints to emergency departments in the USA.[9] The differential diagnosis is large and includes a number of important conditions (Table 5.2.4). Pharyngitis has a wide range of causative bacterial and viral agents most of which produce a self-limited infection with no significant sequelae. The major role for antibiotics in treating pharyngitis is for suspected Group A beta-haemolytic streptococcal infection (GABHS) or *Strep. pyogenes*. Antibiotic use in this setting decreases the duration of both symptoms and infectivity and the incidence of suppurative complications such as quinsy and retropharyngeal abscess. Also if given in the first 9 days they prevent the development of acute rheumatic fever.[9] Antibiotics have not been shown to decrease the incidence of post-streptococcal glomerulonephritis, which is related to the subtype of streptococcus.[10] Antibiotic therapy is also recommended for patients from the following groups: patients with scarlet

Table 5.2.4 Differential diagnosis of sore throat in the adult

Infective pharyngitis
  Bacterial: Group A beta haemolytic streptococcus most common pathogen. Diphtheria should be considered in patients with membranous pharyngitis
  Viral: including EBV

Traumatic pharyngitis (exposure to irritant gases)

Non-specific upper respiratory tract infection

Quinsy (peritonsillar abscess)

Epiglottitis

Ludwig's angina

Parapharyngeal and retropharyngeal abscesses

Gastro-oesophageal reflux

Oro-pharyngeal or laryngeal tumour.

fever, with known rheumatic heart disease or from populations with high incidence of acute rheumatic fever including some Aboriginal populations in Central and Northern Australia.[11]

Up to 50% of pharyngitis in children is caused by GABHS, but only between 5 and 15% of adult cases. The most reliable clinical predictors for GABHS are Centor's criteria.[12] These include tonsillar exudates, tender anterior cervical lymphadenopathy or lymphadenitis, absence of cough and history of fever. The presence of three or more criteria has a positive predictive value of 40–60% while the absence of three or more has a negative predictive value of approximately 80%.

Rapid antigen tests are available which have sensitivities ranging between 65 and 97% but are not widely used in emergency departments in Australia. They may have a future role in deciding the need for antibiotics. Throat cultures take 2–3 days and may give false positive results from asymptomatic carriers with a concurrent non-GABHS pharyngitis. The American Heart Association recommends cultures for patients with appropriate clinical criteria but negative rapid antigen testing. Serological testing is not useful in the acute treatment of pharyngitis.

Most patients with pharyngitis are managed as outpatients. Airway compromise is rare as the nasal passages provide an adequate airway. Some patients who are toxic or dehydrated may need admission for IV hydration and antibiotics. High-dose penicillin remains the drug of choice. The role of oral, IM or IV steroids remains controversial but they may be useful in relieving airway obstruction and decreasing the duration of symptoms.

Quinsy/peritonsillar abscess

Peritonsillar infections occur between the palatine tonsil and its capsule. Peritonsillar cellulitis may form pus and progress to abscess formation. Cellulitis responds to antibiotics alone, but differentiating between the two and identifying those that require drainage may be difficult clinically. Peritonsillar abscesses occur most commonly in males between 20 and 40 years of age. Symptoms include progressively worsening sore throat, fever and dysphagia. On examination the patient may have a muffled 'hot potato' voice, trismus, drooling, a swollen red tonsil with or without purulent exudate and contralateral deviation of the uvula. GABHS is the most common organism associated with quinsy but other organisms include *S. aureus, H. influenzae* and anaerobic species such as fusobacterium, peptostreptococcus and bacteroides.[14] Treatment requires admission for IV penicillin and metronidazole. Clindamycin may be used as an alternative. Needle aspiration in experienced hands can be useful but has a 12% false-negative rate and carries the risk of damaging the carotid artery.[15] Formal surgical drainage may be necessary.

Ludwig's angina

Cellulitis of the submandibular space is the most common neck space infection. It was first described by Wilhelm Fredrick von Ludwig in 1836 and at that time was usually fatal because of rapid compromise to the airway. With prompt treatment including IV antibiotics the mortality rate has declined to less than 5%. Clinical features include toothache, halitosis, neck pain, swelling, fever, dysphagia and trismus. Infection may spread rapidly into adjacent spaces including the pharyngomaxillary and retropharyngeal areas and the mediastinum. Ludwig's angina is related to dental caries involving the mandibular molars, or it may be associated with peritonsillar abscess, trauma to the floor of the mouth or mandible and recent dental work. Cultures are usually polymicrobial and include viridans streptococci (40.9%), *S. aureus* (27.3%), *S. epidermidis* (22.7%) and anaerobes (40%) such as bacteroides species. Treatment necessitates admission and careful airway management. This may include endotracheal intubation as abrupt obstruction can occur. Surgical drainage is indicated if the infection is suppurative or fluctuant. The IV antibiotics of choice are high dose penicillin plus metronidazole or clindamycin.[16]

Other abscesses

Parapharyngeal abscesses involve the lateral or pharyngomaxillary space. Presentation and treatment are similar to Ludwig's angina, from which they may develop. As well as the complications of Ludwig's angina including airway obstruction and spread to contiguous areas, there is the added risk of internal jugular vein thrombosis and erosion of the carotid artery.

Retropharyngeal abscesses are more common in children below 5 years of age. In adults they often result from foreign bodies or trauma. Presenting symptoms and signs include fever, odynophagia, neck swelling, drooling, torticollis, cervical lymphadenopathy, dyspnoea and stridor. Lateral neck X-rays show widening of the prevertebral soft tissues and sometimes a fluid level. CT of the neck may help in determining the extent and in differentiating abscess from cellulitis. Treatment requires admission, airway management, IV antibiotics and may include surgical drainage.

Epiglottitis

Epiglottitis is becoming an adult disease although in adults there is significantly less risk to the airway than in children.[17]

The incidence of adult epiglottitis has remained relatively stable at 1–4 cases per 100 000 per year with a mortality of 7%, but this may change over the next 10–20 years as vaccinated children grow into adolescents and adults.[18] Acute adult epiglottitis is often referred to as supraglottitis because inflammation is not confined to the epiglottis, but also affects other structures such as the pharynx, uvula, base of tongue, aryepiglottic folds and false vocal cords. *H. influenzae* has been isolated in 12–17% of cases and the high rate of negative blood cultures may reflect viral infections or prior treatment with antibiotics in cases that present late. *Strep. pneumoniae, H. parainfluenzae* and herpes simplex have also been isolated. Epiglottitis may also occur following mechanical injury such as ingestion of caustic material, smoke inhalation and following illicit drug use (smoking heroin).

Sore throat and odynophagia are the most common presenting symptoms. Drooling and stridor are infrequent. Factors shown to be associated with an increased risk of airway obstruction include stridor, dyspnoea, sitting upright and short duration of symptoms. A number of X-ray changes have been described in epiglottitis which are listed in Table 5.2.2.[19,20] Management requires admission and IV ceftriaxone or cefotaxime. The role of steroids and nebulized or parenteral adrenaline (epinephrine) is controversial. Chloramphenicol may be used in patients with cephalosporin

CONTROVERSIES

❶ The role of steroids in acute pharyngitis/tonsillitis and quinsy.

❷ The role of rapid antigen testing in diagnosing Group A beta haemolytic streptococcal infections.

❸ The role of intubation, steroids and nebulized or parenteral adrenaline (epinephrine) in adult epiglottitis.

sensitivity. Most adults can be treated conservatively without the need for an artificial airway.[21]

REFERENCES

1. Howes DS, Dowling PJ 2000 Triage and initial evaluation of the oral facial emergency. Emergency Medicine Clinics of North America1: Oral-Facial Emergencies 8(3): 371–8
2. American Heart Association 1992 Guidelines for cardiopulmonary resuscitation and emergency cardiac care. Journal of the Australian Medical Association 268(16): 2171–302
3. Thierbach AR, Lipp MDW 1999 Airway management in trauma patients. Anesthesiology Clinics of North America 17(1): 63–82
4. Cicala RS 1996 The traumatized airway. In: Benumof JE (ed) Airway Management: Principles and Practice. St. Louis, Mosby-Year Book, p. 736
5. Fuhrman GM, Stieg FH, Buerk CA 1990 Blunt laryngeal trauma: Classification and management protocol. Journal of Trauma 30(1): 87–92
6. Gonzales R, Bartlett JG, Besseer RE, Cooper RJ, Hickner JM, Hoffman GR, Sande MA 2001 Principles of appropriate antibiotic use for treatment of acute respiratory tract infections in adults: Background, specific aims, and methods. Annals of Emergency Medicine 37: 690–7
7. Gonzales R, Bartlett JG, Besser, RE, Hickner JM, Hoffman JR, Sande MA 2001 Principles of appropriate antibiotic use for treatment of nonspecific upper respiratory tract infections in adults: Background. Annals of Emergency Medicine 37: 698–702
8. Gonzales R, Steiner JF, Sande MA 1997 Antibiotic prescribing for adults with colds, upper respiratory tract infections and bronchitis by ambulatory care physicians. Journal of the American Medical Association 278: 901–4
9. Stewart MH, Siff JE, Cydulka RK 1999 Evaluation of the patient with sore throat, earache, and sinusitis: an evidence based approach. Emergency Medicine Clinics of North America: Evidence Based Emergency Medicine 17(1): 153–88
10. Richardson MA 1999 Sore throat, tonsillitis, and adenoiditis. Medical Clinics of North America: Otolaryngology for the Internist 83(1): 75–84
11. Victorian Medical Postgraduate Foundation 2000 Therapeutic Guidelines: Antibiotic Version 11: 129–31
12. Centor RM, Witherspoon JM, Dalton HP, Brody CE, Link K 1981 The diagnosis of strep throat in adults in the emergency room. Med Decis Making 1: 239–46
13. Cooper RJ, Hoffman JR, Bartlett JG, Besser RE, Gonzales R, Hickner JM, Sande MA 2001 Principles of appropriate antibiotic use for acute pharyngitis in adults: Background. Annals of Internal Medicine 134: 509–17
14. Steyer TE 2002 Peritonsillar abscess: diagnosis and treatment. Am Fam Phys 65(1): 93–6
15. Scott PMJ, Loftus WK, Kew J, Ahuja A, Yue V, Van Hasselt CA 1999 Diagnosis of peritonsillar infections: a prospective study of ultrasound, computerized tomography and clinical diagnosis. J Laryngol Otol 113: 229–32
16. Harpavat M 2001 Index of suspicion: Case 2. Pediatric Review 22(7): 245–50
17. McCollough M 1999 Update on emerging infections from the centers for disease control and prevention: commentary. Annals of Emergency Medicine 34(1): 110–1
18. Ames WA, Ward WMM, Tranter RMD, Street M 2000 Adult epiglottitis: an under-recognized, life-threatening condition. B J Anaes 85(5): 795–7
19. Schamp S, Pokieser P, Danzer M, Marks B, Denk D-M 1999 Radiological findings in acute adult epiglottitis. Eur Radiol 9(8): 1629–31
20. Nemzek WR, Katzberg RW, Van Slyke MA, Bickley LS 1995 A reappraisal of the radiologic findings of acute inflammation of the epiglottis and supraglottic structures in adults. Am Jour Neuro Radiol 16(3): 495–502
21. Frantz TD, Rasgon BM, Quesenberry CP 1994 Acute epiglottitis in adults. Journal of the American Medical Association 272(17): 1358–60

5.3 ASTHMA

ANNE-MAREE KELLY

ESSENTIALS

1 Asthma is a major health problem worldwide, resulting in significant morbidity and mortality.

2 Asthma is characterized by episodic bronchoconstriction and wheeze in response to a variety of stimuli.

3 Features suggesting an increased risk of life-threatening asthma include a previous life-threatening attack, previous intensive care admission with ventilation, and having required a course of oral corticosteroids within the previous 6 months.

4 Attacks vary in severity from mild to life threatening, and may develop over minutes.

5 Clinical features supported by bedside pulmonary function tests and pulse oximetry are reliable guides to the severity of attacks.

6 Oxygen, β-adrenergic agents and corticosteroids are the mainstay of therapy.

7 Hospital admission is essential if pretreatment PEFR or FEV_1 is less than 25% of predicted, or post-treatment levels are less than 40% of predicted.

INTRODUCTION

The prevalance of asthma varies significantly between regions across the world. In Australasia, New Zealand and the United Kingdom it is thought to affect about 20% of children and 10% of adults. Sufferers tend to present to emergency departments when their usual treatment plan fails to adequately control symptoms. The respiratory compromise caused can range from mild to severe and life-threatening. For these patients the main role of the emergency physician is therapeutic. Other reasons for patients with asthma to attend emergency departments include having run out of medication, having symptoms after a period of being symptom and medication free, and a desire for a 'second opinion' about the management of their asthma. For this smaller group the primary role is one of educating about the disease, of planning an approach to the current state of the asthma, and of referral to appropriate health professionals, e.g. respiratory physicians or general practitioners.

Asthma is a major health problem in many countries resulting in significant morbidity and mortality. The cost in terms of long-term medications and lost school and work days is difficult to quantify, but would run to millions of US dollars annually. Australasia, United Kingdom and North America have a greater prevalence of asthma than the Middle East and some Asian countries. There is also considerable geographic variation in severity with Australasia reporting the highest proportion of severe disease. The reason for this geographical variation is unclear, but may relate in part to ethnicity, rural versus metropolitan environment and air pollution. A number of epidemiological studies suggest that the prevalence and severity of asthma is slowly increasing worldwide.

PATHOPHYSIOLOGY

Asthma is characterized by hyper-reactive airways and inflammation leading to episodic, reversible bronchoconstriction in response to a variety of stimuli. Traditionally, it has been divided into extrinsic (allergic) and intrinsic (idiosyncratic) types.

Extrinsic asthma is initiated by a type I hypersensitivity reaction induced by an extrinsic allergen. IgE-mediated activation of mucosal mast cells results in the release of primary mediators (histamine and eosinophilic and neutrophilic chemotactic factors) and secondary mediators including leukotrienes, prostaglandin D_2, platelet-activating factor and cytokines. These result in bronchoconstriction by direct and cholinergic reflex actions, increased vascular permeability and increased mucous secretions.

In contrast, intrinsic asthma is initiated by diverse non-immune mechanisms, including respiratory infections (in particular viruses), drugs such as aspirin and β-blockers, pollutants and occupational exposure, emotion and exercise.

The morphological changes in asthma are overinflation of the lungs, bronchoconstriction, and the presence of thick mucous plugs in the airways. Histologically there is thickening of the basement membrane of the bronchial epithelium, oedema and an inflammatory infiltrate in the bronchial walls, increased numbers of submucosal glands and hypertrophy of bronchial wall muscle.

Pathophysiologically the effects of acute asthma are:

- Respiratory muscle fatigue
- Increased physiological dead space
- Intrinsic positive end-expiratory pressure secondary to hyperventilation with air trapping.

There is increasing evidence that there are different phenotypes of both acute and chronic asthma. For acute asthma, a rapid onset may be closer to anaphylaxis in pathology with minimal inflammation and may respond more quickly to treatment.

CLINICAL ASSESSMENT

History

Asthma is characterized by episodic shortness of breath, often accompanied by wheeze, chest tightness and cough.

Symptoms may be worse at night, which is thought to be due to variation in bronchomotor tone and bronchial reactivity. Attacks may progress slowly over days or rapidly over minutes.

Features in the history indicating a significant risk of life-threatening asthma include a previous life-threatening attack, previous intensive care admission with ventilation and having required a course of oral corticosteroids within the previous 6 months.

Examination

Physical findings vary with the severity of the attack and may range from mild wheeze and dyspnoea to respiratory failure. Findings indicative of more severe disease include an inability to speak normally, use of the accessory muscles of respiration, a quiet or silent chest on auscultation, restlessness or altered level of consciousness, and cyanosis. Clinical features are a good guide to the severity of attacks. Features of the major severity categories are summarized in Table 5.3.1.

INVESTIGATION

For mild and moderate asthma investigations should be limited to pulmonary function tests (PEFR or FEV_1) and pulse oximetry. A chest X-ray is only indicated if examination of the chest suggests pneumothorax or pneumonia. Arterial blood gases are not useful in this group of patients.

For severe asthma, a chest X-ray is necessary as localizing signs in the chest may be hard to detect. Arterial blood gas analysis is useful if the O_2 saturation is less than 92% on room air at presentation, if improvement is not occurring as expected, and if the patient appears to be tiring. For those with severe asthma, blood gases may show respiratory alkalosis and mild-to-moderate hypoxia (reflecting an increase in respiratory rate in an attempt to maintain oxygenation) or hypoxia and respiratory acidosis as the $PaCO_2$ rises with fatigue and air trapping. Blood gases may also be helpful if intubation is being considered. Otherwise, their impact taken early in management is minimal. They must never be considered 'routine'.

Full blood examination is usually not useful as a mild to moderate leucocytosis may be present in the absence of infection. Electrolyte measurements may show a mild hypokalaemia, particularly if frequent doses of β-agonists have been taken, but this is rarely of clinical significance.

MANAGEMENT

The emergency management of acute asthma varies according to severity, as defined by the clinical parameters above. The principles are ensuring adequate oxygenation, reversing bronchospasm and minimizing the inflammatory response.

Mild asthma

Mild attacks are managed using inhaled β-adrenergic agonists such as salbutamol by metered dose inhaler (MDI) or spacer, the commencement of inhaled corticosteroids if the patient is not already taking them, and education about the disease and the proposed management and follow-up plan.

Moderate asthma

Patients with moderate attacks may require oxygen therapy titrated to achieve oxygen saturation in excess of 92%. The mainstays of therapy are inhaled β-adrenergic agents (by metered dose inhaler [MDI] with a spacer or nebulizer) and systemic corticosteroids. The dosage of salbutamol is 5–10 mg by nebulizer or eight puffs by MDI and spacer, every 15 minutes for three doses. Corticosteroids are equally effective given by the oral or intravenous routes. The usual dose is 50 mg prednisolone orally or 250 mg hydrocortisone intravenously. Reassessment, including repeat pulmonary function tests, should occur at least 1 hour after the last dose of β-agonist, with a view to the need for further therapy and decision on hospital admission.

Severe asthma

Severe attacks require supplemental oxygen to achieve oxygen saturation in excess of 92%. Because of high respiratory rates it is important to ensure adequate gas flow by the use of either a reservoir-type

Table 5.3.1 Categorization of asthma severity based on clinical features*

Severity category	Features	Respiratory function
Near death	Exhaustion, confusion Cyanotic, sweating Silent chest Reduced respiratory effort Unable to speak	FEV_1, PEFR not appropriate O_2 saturation <90% despite supplemental O_2
Severe	Laboured respirations Sweating, restless Difficulty speaking: words or phrases only Tachycardia	FEV1, PEFR not able or less than 40% predicted/best PEFR <200L/min O_2 saturation <90% on air
Moderate	Dyspnoea at rest Able to speak short sentences Chest tightness Wheeze Partial/short-lived relief from usual therapy Nocturnal symptoms	FEV_1 PEFR 40%–60% predicted/best PEFR 200–300 L/min
Mild	Exertional symptoms Able to speak normally Good response to usual therapy	FEV_1, PEFR >60% predicted/best PEFR >300 L/min

* Modified after Guidelines for Emergency Management of Adult Asthma, Canadian Association of Emergency Physicians[1]

mask or a Venturi system. High oxygen concentrations may be necessary. Patients should have continuous cardiac and oximetric monitoring and should receive continuous β-agonist by nebulizer at the doses described above, plus oral or intravenous corticosteroids. The addition of nebulized ipratropium and/or intravenous magnesium may be beneficial (see below). If patients fail to respond, intravenous β-agonist (e.g. salbutamol as a bolus of 5 μg/kg followed by an infusion at 1-20 μg/min) and/or ventilation should be considered.

For patients with an acceptable conscious state and airway protective mechanisms, non-invasive ventilation may be suitable. Continuous intensive monitoring is mandatory. Otherwise, endotracheal intubation and ventilation will be needed. Ketamine, which has been shown to be an effective bronchodilator, is the induction agent of choice.[2] Care must be taken with ventilation, as severe air trapping results in markedly raised intrathoracic pressure with cardiovascular compromise. A slow ventilation rate of 6–8/min with prolonged expiratory periods is recommended.

A number of other therapeutic modalities are outlined below.

Adrenaline (epinephrine)

Small studies have suggested that adrenaline (epinephrine) administered by nebuliser and subcutaneously has a similar effect to nebulised salbutamol. These studies are limited by small sample size and the inclusion of patients with mild and moderate asthma.

Adrenaline (epinephrine) may have advantages over salbutamol as a parenteral agent. This is based on the theoretical reduction of bronchial mucosal oedema by α–adrenergic mechanisms and inhibition of cholinergic neurotransmission. Anecdotes and a small case series[3] indicate that adrenaline (epinephrine) is safe and effective, but no studies comparing adrenaline (epinephrine) to more selective agents have been published.

Aminophylline

One randomized, controlled trial in children admitted to hospital with asthma who were unresponsive to nebulized salbutamol and ipratropium and intravenous steroids showed a greater improvement in spirometry at 6 hours and a lower intubation rate.[4] This is supported by a Cochrane review of the use of aminophylline in children with acute severe asthma.[5] A number of other studies have failed to demonstrate a benefit from the use of aminophylline when optimal doses of β-agonists and corticosteroids are used.[6-9] A recent Cochrane review of the use of aminophylline in adults with asthma concluded that the use of aminophylline did not result in additional bronchodilation compared with the use of beta-agonists and was associated with more adverse events.[10] Concerns have also been raised about the potential for serious side effects from its use, in particular cardiac arrhythmias and death.[11]

Bicarbonate

The postulated mechanism of action of bicarbonate in severe asthma is the facilitation of adrenergic effects and the countering of acidosis, thus improving respiratory muscle function. To date only small case series support this view, and the quality of evidence is poor.[12,13]

Non-invasive ventilation (NIV: CPAP and BIPAP)

In acute asthma, CPAP has been shown to reduce airways resistance, result in bronchodilation, counter atelectasis, reduce the work of respiration and reduce the cardiovascular impact of changes in intrapleural and intrathoracic pressures caused by asthma. It does not, when used alone, improve gas exchange. An unrandomized study of CPAP in combination with pressure support ventilation for patients with severe asthma found rapid correction of pH and improvement in ventilation at lower pressures than were necessary with mechanical ventilation.[14] Other small studies also suggest that NIV may reduce the need for intubation in selected patients with severe asthma[15,16]. NIV also appears to be associated with a lower risk of adverse events.

Heliox

Heliox is a blend of 70% helium and 30% oxygen. It may have advantages in asthma because of better gas flow dynamics. Small studies have had conflicting results. A recent Cochrane review concluded that the existing evidence did not support the use of heliox in patients with acute severe asthma in the emergency department.[17]

Ipratropium

β-agonists have been shown to be more effective bronchodilators than ipratropium when these agents are used alone, but evidence about the impact of combined therapy is contradictory. A meta-analysis concluded that combination therapy resulted in a statistically significant additional improvement in FEV_1, but doubted the clinical significance of this difference.[18] Prospective trials have conflicting results, however, there is little if any benefit from the addition of ipratropium to nebulized salbutamol in mild or moderate asthma. Subgroup analysis suggests that there may be benefit from combination nebulized therapy in severe asthma (PEFR <200 L/min).

Ketamine

A potential benefit from cautious subinduction doses of ketamine in severe asthma has been suggested. The postulated mechanisms of action of ketamine in asthma are sympathomimetic effects, direct relaxant effects on bronchial smooth muscle, antagonism of histamine and acetylcholine and a membrane-stabilizing effect. There is only one randomized trial investigating the role of ketamine in acute asthma. It showed that in doses with an acceptable incidence of dysphoria, ketamine did not confer benefit.[19]

Magnesium

The postulated mechanisms for the action of magnesium in acute asthma are a bronchodilator effect by impeding the uptake of calcium ions into smooth muscle cells, and an anti-inflammatory effect by attenuation of the neutrophil respiratory burst associated with asthma. A Cochrane review suggests that there is no benefit from the use of magnesium (in addition to standard therapy) in mild or moderate asthma, but that for severe asthma (FEV_1 less than 25% predicted) the addition of magnesium resulted in highly significant increases in FEV_1 and reduced admission rates. No serious adverse reactions were noted in any of the studies.[20] Similar results were found in a recent randomized controlled trial.[21]

High-dose parenteral salbutamol

Some centres, particularly in New Zealand, advocate the use of high doses of salbutamol intravenously. Doses as high as a 2000 µg (2 mg) bolus with total doses in the first 1-2 hours of treatment up to 10000 µg (10 mg) have been suggested. There is no published evidence to support this approach, which carries a risk (based on animal studies) of myocardial toxicity. At present, this approach cannot be recommended.

Racemic salbutamol

The salbutamol in common use comprises a racemic mixture of (R) and (S) isomers. The (R) isomer is responsible for the therapeutic effects. The (R) isomer has been shown to oppose the bronchodilatory effects of the (S) isomer and to be proinflammatory.[22] It is also metabolized slower than the (R) isomer. The single isomer salbutamol preparation ((R) isomer, levalbuterol) is more potent with fewer side effects but is much more expensive. The place of single isomer salbutamol in routine clinical practice is yet to be established.

Leukotriene inhibitors

Leukotriene receptor antagonists (e.g. montelukast) were developed in response to finding that leukotrienes exhibit biological activity that mimics some of the clinical features of asthma and are found in increased amounts in patients with asthma, especially during exacerbations. They may have a role in the management of chronic asthma. There have been no emergency department-based studies of acute asthma investigating the potential role of these agents.

DISPOSITION

Patients with severe or life-threatening asthma require admission to an intensive care unit or respiratory high-dependency unit. Patients with mild disease can usually be discharged after treatment and the formulation of a treatment plan. Those for whom the admission or discharge may be in question is the moderate group. Bedside pulmonary function tests can be useful to guide these decisions. Hospital admission is mandated if pretreatment PEFR or FEV_1 is less than 25% of predicted, or post-treatment less than 40% of predicted.

For those with post-treatment pulmonary function tests in the 40–60% of predicted range, discharge may be possible if improvement is maintained over a number of hours. In addition, other factors should be considered in estimating the safety of discharge. These include history of a previous near-death episode, recent emergency department visits, frequent admissions to hospital, current or recent steroid use, sudden attacks, poor understanding or compliance, poor home circumstances, and limited access to transport back to hospital in case of deterioration.

All discharged patients should have an Asthma Action Plan to cover the

following 24–48 hours with particular emphasis on what to do if their condition worsens. They should also have scheduled review within that time. A short course of oral steroids (e.g. 50 mg/day for 5–7 days) is usual.

CONTROVERSIES

❶ The relative efficacy and safety of intravenous adrenaline (epinephrine) compared to high- and standard-dose intravenous salbutamol.

❷ The role of intravenous magnesium in severe asthma.

❸ The role of non-invasive continuous positive airway pressure as an alternative to intubation and mechanical ventilation.

❹ The role of (R)-isomer salbutamol.

❺ The role of leukotriene inhibitors.

REFERENCES

1. Beveridge RC, Grunfeld AF, Hodder RV, Verbeek PR 1996 Guidelines for the emergency management of asthma in adults. CAEP/CTS Asthma Advisory Committee. Canadian Medical Association Journal 155: 25–37
2. L'Hommedieu CS, Arens JJ 1987 The use of ketamine for the emergency intubation of patients with status asthmaticus. Annals of Emergency Medicine 16: 568–71
3. Tirot P, Bouacher G, Varache N, et al 1992 [Use of intravenous adrenaline in severe acute asthma]. Revue des Maladies Respiratoires 9: 319–23
4. Yung M, South M 1998 Randomised controlled trial of aminophylline for severe acute asthma. Archives of Diseases in Childhood 79: 405–10
5. Coleridge J, Cameron P, Epstein J, Teichtahl H 1993 Intravenous aminophylline confers no benefit in acute asthma treated with intravenous steroids and inhaled bronchodilators. Australia and New Zealand Journal of Medicine 23: 348–54
6. Mitra A, Bassler D, Ducharme FM 2001 Intravenous aminophylline for acute severe asthma in children over 2 years using inhaled bronchodilators. Cochrane Database Systematic Reviews (4) CD 001276
7. Needleman JP, Kaifer MC, Nold JT, Shuster PE, Redding MM, Gladstein J 1995 Theophylline does not shorten hospital stay for children admitted for asthma. Archives of Paediatric and Adolescent Medicine 149: 206–9
8. Strauss RE, Wertheim DL, Bonagura VR, Valacer DJ 1994 Aminophylline therapy does not improve outcome and increases adverse effects in children hospitalised with acute asthmatic exacerbations. Pediatrics 93: 205–10
9. DiGiulio GA, Kercsmar CM, Krug SE, Alpert SE, Marx CM 1993 Hospital treatment of asthma: lack of benefit from theophylline given in addition to nebulised albuterol and intravenously administered corticosteroids. Journal of Paediatrics 122: 464–9
10. Parameswaran K, Belda J, Rowe BH 2000 Addition of intravenous aminophylline to beta2-agonists in adults with acute asthma. Cochrane Database Systematic Reviews (4) CD 002742
11. Rodrigo C, Rodrigo G 1994 Treatment of asthma: lack of therapeutic benefit and increase of the toxicity from aminophylline given in addition to high doses of salbutamol delivered by metered dose inhaler with a spacer. Chest 106: 1071–6
12. Bouacher G, Tirot P, Varache N, Harry P, Alquier P 1992 [Metabolic acidosis in severe asthma: effect of alkaline therapy]. Revue de Pneumologie Clinique 48: 115–9
13. Mansmann HC, Abboud EM, McGready SJ 1997 Treatment of severe respiratory failure during status asthmaticus in children and adults using high flow oxygen and sodium bicarbonate. Annals of Allergy and Asthma Immunology 78: 69–73
14. Shivaram U, Miro AM, Cash ME, Finch PJ, Heurich AE, Kamholz SL 1993 Cardiopulmonary responses to continuous positive airway pressure in acute asthma. Journal of Critical Care 8: 87–92
15. Fernandez MM, Villagra A, Blanch L, Fernandez R 2001 Non-invasive mechanical ventilation in status asthmaticus. Intensive Care Medicine 27: 486–92

16. Holley MT, Morrissey TK, Seaberg DC, Afessa B, Wears RL 2001 Ethical dilemmas in a randomized trial of asthma treatment: can Bayesian statistical analysis explain the results? Academy Emergency Medicine 8: 1128–35
17. Rodrigo G, Rodrigo C, Pollack C, Travers A 2001 Helium-oxygen mixture for nonintubated acute asthma patients. Cochrane Database Systematic Reviews (1): CD002884
18. Osmond MH, Klassen TP 1995 Efficacy of ipratropium bromide in acute childhood asthma: a meta-analysis. Academy of Emergency Medicine 2: 651–8
19. Howton JC, Rose J, Duffy S, Zoltanski T, Levitt MA 1996 Randomised, double blind, placebo controlled trial of intravenous ketamine in acute asthma. Annals of Emergency Medicine 27: 170–5
20. Rowe BH, Bretzlaff JA, Bourdon C, Bota GW, Camargo CA Jr 2000 Magnesium sulfate for treating exacerbations of acute asthma in the emergency department. Cochrane Database Systematic Reviews (2) CD 001490
21. Silverman RA, Osborn H, Runge J, et al 2002 IV magnesium sulfate in the treatment of acute severe asthma: a multicenter randomized controlled trial. Chest 122: 489–97
22. Handley D 1999 The asthma-like pharmacology and toxicology of (S)-isomers of beta agonists. Journal of Allergy and Clinical Immunology 104: S69–S76

5.4 COMMUNITY-ACQUIRED PNEUMONIA

GARRY J. WILKES

ESSENTIALS

1 Community-acquired pneumonia is a common infection that, despite recent advances in diagnosis and treatment, still has an in-hospital mortality rate of approximately 10%.

2 The initial antibiotic treatment of community-acquired pneumonia is almost always empirical, as early investigations rarely identify the responsible pathogen. Factors guiding the initial antibiotic treatment include the local epidemiology of pneumonia, the patient's medical history, clinical findings, and chest X-ray results.

3 Rational, consistent prescribing of antibiotics will help to limit the spread of drug-resistant organisms.

4 Different types of pathogens are responsible for hospital-acquired pneumonia, aspiration pneumonia and pneumonia in the immunocompromised host. Different antibiotic regimens will, therefore, be required in these patients.

INTRODUCTION

Pneumonia has been documented from the beginning of recorded time. The term is derived from 'Peripneumonia' as described by Hippocrates in the 4th century BC. Laennec (who also introduced the stethoscope to clinical assessment in 1806) first described the classic stages of lobar pneumonia in 1834. The first stage of engorgement is associated with a congested and oedematous lung parenchyma. Auscultatory findings are minimal with reduced air entry and crackles. In the second stage of red hepatization the lung becomes dry, solid and red and resembles a normal liver on gross examination. Bronchial breathing and whispering pectoriloquy coincide with the onset of this stage. In the third stage, grey hepatization occurs with organization of the inflammatory exudate. Healing follows with break-down of the alveolar debris and expectoration of the purulent material. Respiratory crackles return in the final stage of resolution.

In 1881 Frieländer first found bacteria in the lungs during post mortem examinations using the newly developed staining technique of Gram. Fraenkel isolated an organism from a dying man in 1884 and named it 'pneumoniemikroccus'. This settled the debate as to the cause of the condition with evidence of an infectious agent rather than atmospheric conditions being the sole cause of pneumonia.

PATHOPHYSIOLOGY

The lower respiratory tract has a formidable array of protective barriers. Almost all of the defence mechanisms of the body are represented. These will be reviewed with respect to the route of potential infection.

Inhalation

Infection may result from inhalation of aerosols containing infective micro-organisms. Large droplets (>10 μm diameter) impact on the nasal and oropharyngeal mucosa and are either expectorated, swallowed, or must compete for survival against the normal, protective flora. Organisms contained in smaller droplets can be successfully transported to the smaller airways and alveoli where they meet further barriers. Mucous cells secrete a protective bilayer on the lower airways. The outer viscous layer traps inhaled particles while cilia beating 1000 times per minute in coordinated waves in the less viscous inner layer carry them from the lower respiratory tract. The cilia-driven 'escalator' is effective against particles 2–10 μm in size and returns particles to the oropharynx within hours.

Immunoglobulins protect against viruses and bacteria. IgA is predominantly in the upper respiratory tract with IgG and smaller amounts of IgA in the lower respiratory tract. Direct actions of the immunoglobulins include reduced attachment of bacteria to the respiratory mucosa, neutralization of bacterial toxins, agglutination of bacteria and bacterial lysis. Indirect actions include activation of complement, opsonization of bacteria, and promotion of chemotaxis of macrophages and granulocytes.

Alveolar macrophages are present in alveoli and represent the final barrier to tissue penetration. Organisms able to reach the tissue are then subject to the humoral and cell-mediated immunity of the body. Systemically produced antibodies, complement factors, phagocytic macrophages and granulocytes continue the defence of the body against the invading microorganisms.

Aspiration

The most common route of infection for pneumonia is aspiration of oropharyngeal flora. Many potential respiratory pathogens such as *S. pneumoniae*, *H. influenzae*, and *S. aureus* can be isolated from the oropharynx of normal individuals. The respiratory tract below the vocal cords remains relatively sterile and protected from disease by the mechanisms listed above and the airway reflexes of glottic closure and cough. Aspiration of small volumes of oropharyngeal material may occur in normal individuals during sleep, but this does not result in colonization or infection.

Other routes of infection

Pneumonia may develop via haematogenous seeding from remote foci. Sources of infection include generalized septicemia, infected intravascular devices and organisms introduced through intravenous drug abuse. The lungs may become secondarily involved from adjacent areas of infection such as subphrenic or mediastinal abscesses. Traumatic inoculation of organisms directly through the chest wall is a less common mechanism of infection.

Effect of disease processes

The normal protective mechanisms can be interfered with by a variety of disease processes.

Coliforms are uncommon in the oropharynx of normal individuals but are found in greater numbers in smokers, alcoholics, institutionalized and hospitalized patients. Diabetes mellitus, glucocorticoid therapy and immunosuppression are also associated with alterations in the normal flora. Gram negative infection is more likely in these groups of patients.

Normal individuals have minimal aspiration of oropharyngeal and/or gastric contents during waking hours but may aspirate larger volumes whilst asleep. Impairment of consciousness and/or

protective reflexes occurs with general debility, neurological disease and alcohol and drug abuse. Significant aspiration may occur under these circumstances.

The acid environment of the stomach provides protection against transmission of coliforms to the upper airway. Gastric acidity is reduced by a variety of pharmacological agents. Patients who are unwell from any cause also have a reduction in gastric acid production. In association with the increase in gastric pH, there is an increased incidence of Gram negatives in the oropharyngeal flora of these individuals.

Mucociliary transport is reduced by smoking and by viral infection. Chronic bronchitis and cystic fibrosis are associated with an increase in the volume and viscosity of mucus, which may be difficult to clear.

Immunosuppression from malignancy (particularly haematogenous malignancies), chemotherapeutic agents or conditions such as HIV infection are associated with infection from opportunistic organisms in addition to the usual pathogenic organisms.

CLINICAL FEATURES

The presentation of community-acquired pneumonia (CAP) may be classified as 'typical' or 'atypical.' The 'atypical' presentation refers to both clinical and radiological features.

In the pre-antibiotic era the principle organism causing pneumonia was *S. pneumoniae*. The 'typical' pattern of disease produced by this pathogen was as follows: Prior to the illness the patient is usually well or has only a minor respiratory infection. The patient becomes unwell abruptly with a sudden onset of fever, rigors, pleuritic chest pain and a cough, which quickly progresses from dry to productive of mucopurulent sputum. The majority of patients with pneumococcal pneumonia have a single rigor only. Repeated rigors make another etiological agent likely. Constitutional symptoms are usually present but mild and overwhelmed by the pulmonary features. The patient remains unwell as

the disease progresses. Spontaneous recovery in survivors of untreated pneumococcal pneumonia typically occurs after 7 to 10 days. Resolution of illness occurs by 'crisis' with a dramatic onset of sweats, sudden resolution of fever, and return to health.

A 'typical' presentation is most likely to be due to *S. pneumoniae*, and is also characteristic of other bacterial pneumonias such as *H. influenzae* and *S. aureus* (more commonly seen post-influenza or in intravenous drug users).

Although other organisms have subsequently been isolated from patients with the 'atypical' symptom complex (Table 5.4.1), *M. pneumoniae* remains the most common isolate.

The history taken from patients with pneumonia should include details of recent travel and contact with others suffering from similar illnesses. Some diseases are more common following contact with specific sources: farm animals (Q fever: *C. burnetii*); rabbits and ticks (tularaemia); birds (psittacosis); and rats (plague, leptospirosis). A careful inquiry as to the patient's occupation and exposure to animals is essential.

Knowledge of local disease patterns is of benefit at times of epidemics. Viral infections including influenza are more common in winter months and are associated with an increase in secondary bacterial pneumonias. *S. aureus* in particular is more common following infection due to influenza viruses. Legionellosis occurs in sporadic outbreaks with multiple cases infected from exposure to a single source (often associated with air-conditioning units). Endemics of *M. pneumoniae* tend to occur every 3-4 years.

Table 5.4.1 Likely pathogens causing 'atypical' pneumonia
Mycoplasma pneumoniae
Legionella pneumophilia
Viral infections
Chlamydia pneumoniae
Atypical presentation of 'typical' agents

Physical examination findings in patients with pneumonia usually include fever, tachypnoea and tachycardia. Examination of the chest may reveal evidence of consolidation with dullness to percussion, decreased breath sounds, bronchial breathing and whispering pectoriloquy. Classic signs of consolidation are present in less than 30% of patients with CAP. Physical findings in the chest may be limited to crackles only. Infections limited to the lingula or medial segment of the right middle lobe may have no abnormalities on chest examination.

General examination may give additional clues to the type of pneumonia. Herpes labialis is characteristic of pneumococcal infection. Herpes zoster pneumonitis is likely in the presence of a thoracic zoster rash.

Elderly patients and those with depressed immune function may have less prominent symptoms and signs of pulmonary infection.

INVESTIGATION

Radiographic features

The single most useful investigation in patients with suspected pneumonia is a chest X-ray demonstrating the presence and extent of any pulmonary infiltrate. Pulmonary opacities may also be due to other causes such as non-infectious inflammatory conditions, atelectasis, malignancy, industrial and chemical exposure or drug reactions.

The extent of the radiographic involvement does not always match the severity of the clinical status. The radiological changes associated with infection due to 'atypical' agents are often more extensive than the clinical examination suggests. Pneumonia can be present without obvious pulmonary infiltrates in the early stages of the disease and in patients who are dehydrated. Radiographic changes may be delayed or absent if the patient is unable to mount an inflammatory response due to other disease or immunosuppressive therapy.

The chest X-ray may demonstrate other relevant pathology such as hilar lymphadenopathy, pulmonary metastases, Ghon lesions or complexes of TB, apical fibrosis, or the presence of cavitating lesions. Pleural effusions are present in 30–50% of patients with CAP.

Pneumococcal pneumonia was originally classified on anatomical grounds as lobar or bronchopneumonia. *S. pneumoniae* remains the most common cause of lobar pneumonia. Consolidation of a single segment or lobe may also be secondary to obstruction of the associated bronchus. Malignancy or foreign body causing obstruction must be suspected if there is a failure to respond to treatment or if the disease is progressive.

The infecting agent can not be inferred reliably from the radiological appearances alone, although some features are more commonly seen in association with particular pathogens:

Infection due to *Klebsiella* spp. most commonly produces bulging of involved segments with downward displacement of the horizontal fissure. However, this finding is neither specific nor sensitive for *Klebsiella* infections.

Features of pulmonary anatomy and physiology predispose to particular patterns of disease. The right main bronchus is longer and more vertical than the left favouring aspiration of material into the dependent portions of the right lung. The dependent portions of the lungs also have the lowest ventilation-perfusion ratio. The reduced PaO_2 favours the growth of anaerobic organisms. Aspiration of oropharyngeal anaerobes typically produces foci of infection more in the dependent portions of the lungs and more often on the right hand side. In contrast, secondary infection from the obligate aerobe, *M. tuberculosis*, is seen almost exclusively in the oxygen-enriched apices where the ventilation-perfusion ratio is highest.

Pulmonary infiltrates should be examined closely for the presence of cavitation, which implies unusual pathology. This is discussed in more detail below (see 'Notes on specific conditions').

Computerized tomography (CT) displays greater anatomical detail than plain radiography and identifies multi-focal disease more accurately. CT is more sensitive for detecting interstitial disease, cavitation, and adenopathy and is a useful adjunct for the investigation of complicated cases.

Sputum analysis

The relative value of sputum microscopy and culture is debated. Analysis of the initial Gram's stain of sputum may give some important clues as to the identity of the etiological agent. The results of a correctly collected and processed sample of sputum provide a useful guide to initial therapy. Unfortunately, this analysis is neither specific nor sensitive for correct identification of the true pathogenic agent.

Collection of an adequate sample, use of correct transportation media and expert and expedient laboratory processing of these samples are crucial to the relevance of the information obtained from this procedure. An adequate sample of sputum is indicated by the presence of greater than 25 leucocytes and less than 10 epithelial cells per high power field. Difficulties in collecting adequate sputum include that 10–30% of patients have a non-productive cough and other patients are unable to expectorate sputum adequately. Often, induced sputum may be successfully obtained with the aid of physiotherapy and inhalation of nebulized saline.

The absence of identifiable pathogens in an adequately collected sample does not exclude their presence. *S. pneumoniae* is isolated from sputum in only 50% of patients with bacteraemic pneumococcal pneumonia. Mycobacteria and many of the 'atypical' organisms may not be evident on initial microscopy and require special staining techniques or the use of immunoflourescent antibodies to reveal their presence (e.g. acid-fast stains for mycobacteria, Giemsa stain for pneumocystis). The predominance of one microbial agent does not always indicate its pathological significance as *S. pneumoniae* and *H. influenzae* can be isolated from a small percentage of normal individuals in the absence of clinical disease. These findings are greatly increased in patients with chronic bronchitis from whom *H.*

influenzae and *S. pneumoniae* can be isolated from the sputum of up to 80% and 40% of individuals respectively who have stable disease and are clinically well.

The sputum Gram's stain result acts as a useful adjunct to guide initial therapy when considered in conjunction with the clinical and radiological patterns. In experienced hands, sputum analysis indicates the likely pathogenic agent in 50% of cases with a 90% correlation between organisms identified on initial Gram's staining and those in subsequent culture. Culture results and antibiotic sensitivity profiles are only of additional value when positive. This process takes at least 2 days and prior use of antibiotics may prevent growth of organisms identified on initial sputum microscopy.

Further investigations

In an otherwise well patient with community-acquired pneumonia who is suitable for outpatient management, no further investigations are required. In this group of patients a thorough clinical assessment (including pulse oximetry when available), examination of the chest radiograph and analysis of an adequate sputum sample (if possible) is sufficient.

Additional information is useful when deciding on the need for hospital admission or intensive care therapy (see 'Disposition'). The results of further investigations may give clues as to the etiological agent or may indicate the severity of the disease (Table 5.4.2). The results of these investigations should be viewed as an adjunct to and not a substitute for a thorough clinical assessment.

Blood should be sent for culture in all hospitalised patients. At least two cultures taken from different sites are necessary to avoid confusion from growth of contaminants. The yield from blood cultures is directly related to the magnitude of bacteraemia. Cultures taken during febrile periods (>38°C) have a higher positive culture rate. Positive blood cultures have been reported in 11% of hospitalized patients, with *S. pneumoniae* comprising 67% of all bacteraemia.

Samples of fluid can be collected from associated pleural effusions. Diagnostic needle thoracentesis is indicated when a

Table 5.4.2 Features indicating more severe pneumonia

History
Confusion
Syncopal episodes
*Inability to clear secretions
Debilitating coexistent disease
Previous splenectomy
Failure of oral therapy
*Rapidly progressive disease
Inability to cope at home

Examination
Confusion
Temperature >38.5°C or <37°C
*Shock
*Systolic blood pressure <90 mmHg
*Diastolic blood pressure <60 mmHg
*Respiratory rate >30/min
Extrapulmonary disease

Radiological features
*Multilobe involvement
*Bilateral infiltrates
*Increase in size of infiltrate ≥50% in 48 hours

Laboratory findings
*PaO_2 <60 mmHg (8 kPa) or SaO_2 < 90%
*$PaCO_2$ >50 mmHg (6.7 kPa)
White cell count >30 or <4 × 10^9/L
Neutrophil count <1 × 10^9/L
Haemoglobin <90 g/L
Impaired or deteriorating renal function

Intensive care unit admission should be considered

*, Intensive care

Table 5.4.3 Mortality from community-acquired pneumonia

Factor	Mortality odds ratio
Hypothermia	5.0
Systolic hypotension	4.8
Neurological disease	4.6
Multi-lobar infiltrates on CXR	3.1
Tachypnoea	2.9
Neoplastic disease	2.8
Bacteraemia	2.8
Leucopoenia	2.5
Diabetes mellitus	1.3
Male sex	1.3
Pleuritic chest pain	0.5

microbiological diagnosis is required and cannot be obtained by non-invasive methods. Pleural fluid should be examined for organisms and sent for culture. Cultures from these sources are highly specific for the causative agent. Biochemical examination of aspirated fluid is also of value. A low glucose indicates bacterial infection but is not organism specific. The pH of pleural fluid is predictive of the need for subsequent drainage of the effusion. If the pH is above 7.3 antibiotic treatment is likely to be successful. If the pH is lower, drainage is usually required. Therapeutic aspiration/drainage of large effusions is indicated when there is evidence of respiratory compromise.

In bacterial pneumonia the total white cell count (WCC) is raised with a predominance of neutrophils and a shift to the left ('toxic granulation'). The WCC is usually greater than 15 × 10^9/L.

Infections due to the atypical agents are usually associated with a normal or only mildly elevated WCC (10–12 × 10^9/L). Viral disease is also associated with a normal or slightly raised WCC and more commonly induces a lymphocytosis. Pneumonia may be predisposed to by leucopoenia. A neutrophil count of less than 1 × 10^9/L is associated with immunosuppression or may result from overwhelming sepsis. Severe pneumonia can be associated with a high or low WCC. The prognosis is significantly worse if the total WCC is >30 or <4 × 10^9/L or if the neutrophil count is <1 × 10^9/L (Table 5.4.2).

Subclinical haemolysis from IgM directed anti-I cold agglutinins is a feature of infection with *Mycoplasma* and can be pronounced enough to induce haematuria or a mild anaemia. Anaemia may also result from chronic disease or severe pneumonia of any cause.

Non-invasive pulse oximetry quickly and accurately identifies hypoxaemia and monitors response to supplementary oxygen delivery. The major draw-back of pulse oximeters is the inability to distinguish between oxy- and carboxy-haemoglobin (CO-Hb). The SaO_2 calculated by pulse oximetry will, therefore, be falsely elevated in the presence of significant CO-Hb levels. The most common cause of a raised CO-Hb is cigarette smoking. Heavy smokers may have a CO-Hb of up to 15%. The true SaO_2 can be calculated by subtracting the measured CO-Hb from the SaO_2 obtained from pulse oximetry.

A relative hypoxaemia and respiratory alkalosis are typical arterial blood gas (ABG) analysis findings in CAP. ABG determinations are indicated for patients with severe disease and in those patients in whom CO_2 retention is suspected. There is no indication for ABG in patients with a normal SaO_2 who appear well. Patients who are cyanosed, have an abnormal mental status, and those who have a low SaO_2 reading on pulse oximetry should never have oxygen withheld solely for the purpose of obtaining an ABG 'on air'. A SaO_2 of 90% is equivalent to a PaO_2 of 60 mmHg and is the level at which hospital admission is standard and ICU admission should be considered.

Abnormal liver function tests are seen in up to 50% of patients with bacterial pneumonia and are not organism specific. Hyponatraemia is most frequently associated with Legionella infection but this finding is neither sensitive nor specific. Impaired or deteriorating renal function is seen with severe pneumonia of any cause.

Abnormalities of serum glucose may occur as a consequence of the infection or provide a clue to the presence of associated diabetes. Pneumonia is more common in diabetics. There is a higher incidence of infection due to *H. influenzae* and mortality is increased.

All patients with an abnormal mental status should have the serum glucose determined in order to detect hypoglycaemia. Hypoglycaemia may result from severe infection or as a consequence of inadequate food intake in diabetic patients who are unwell from any cause. Confused patients may not volunteer a diagnosis of diabetes. Hypoglycaemia may also be the cause of a depressed mental status precipitating pulmonary aspiration. Hyperglycaemia may result from poor compliance with medications or from increased requirements with intercurrent disease.

Table 5.4.4 Guide to the interpretation of sputum gram's stain

Sputum Gram's stain	Likely organism
Gram-positive diplococci or short chains	S. pneumoniae
Gram-positive cocci in clusters	S. aureus
Gram-negative coccobacilli or pleomorphic forms	H. influenzae
Small gram-negative bacilli	Coliforms
Polymorphonuclear cells without organisms	M. pneumoniae and other 'atypical' agents
Polymorphonuclear cells with mixed organisms (often abundant, foul smelling sputum)	Anaerobic agents

On occasions it may be necessary to obtain respiratory secretions by more invasive techniques in complex patients unable to expectorate an adequate sputum sample. Various techniques are available including tracheal puncture and aspiration, bronchoscopic washings with double sheathed brushes, and transthoracic needle aspiration. The decision to use these techniques should only be made by experienced specialists familiar with the appropriate investigation.

TREATMENT

Treatment is both general and specific. General measures such as bed rest, adequate nutrition and fluid intake, analgesics, antipyretics, and prevention of exposure to excessive heat or cold are as important as antimicrobial therapy. Coughing and expectoration of secretions aids pulmonary clearance and should be encouraged. Cough suppressants may be necessary to reduce the disturbance to sleep. Patients who are hypoxic, hypotensive, or who are unwell require specific treatment in hospital and may require intensive care admission (see Disposition).

Antibiotics

Mortality from untreated pneumonia is high and increases to over 80% in the presence of bacteraemia. Treatment with antibiotics has been associated with a dramatic reduction in mortality.

Unfortunately, the etiological agent is usually unknown when patients first present. Sputum Gram's stain (when available) may indicate a likely etiological agent and aids the choice of initial antibiotic therapy (Table 5.4.4). Initial therapy is often commenced before a firm bacteriological diagnosis is made. Treatment may be modified if laboratory results suggest the presence of an agent unresponsive to this initial therapy. This process takes at least 24–48 hours and may not provide any useful information if these results are inconclusive. Patients are initially treated in relation to the clinical presentation prior to the availability of these results. Treatment guidelines based on a bacteriological diagnosis are, therefore, of little value in the emergency department when a patient first presents.

The most practical guidelines are based on dividing patients into broad groups with respect to the clinical scenario. The likely etiological agents and initial therapy can be based on this classification. Clinically based guidelines have been developed in Australia, the USA, the UK, and Canada.

Treatment guidelines cannot cover every possible clinical presentation and do not represent a comprehensive treatment plan. Treatment should always be individualized with guidelines providing a practical framework on which to base therapy. The emerging spectrum of antimicrobial resistance necessitates the updating of guidelines every few years and pocket-sized versions (such as the *Therapeutic Guidelines Antibiotic* 2000) are particularly useful to the clinician.

Table 5.4.5 classifies CAP into five clinical groups. Group 1 is the most

Table 5.4.5 Pathogens and therapy associated with community acquired pneumonia in adults

Classification	Most common pathogens	Less common pathogens	Oral therapy	Parenteral therapy
Group 1 Mild to moderate age < 60 years. No coexistent illness	S. pneumoniae M. pneumoniae	H. influenzae C. pneumoniae Legionella spp. S. aureus	Macrolide or amoxycillin or doxycycline	Macrolide plus either benzylpenicillin or procaine penicillin or cephalothin or cephazolin
Group 2 Mild to moderate pneumonia age > 60 years and/or coexisting illness	S. pneumoniae H. influenzae	M. catarrhalis aerobic Gram-negative bacilli Legionella spp. S. aureus	Amoxycillin or amoxycillin/ potassium clavulanate or ceflacor or roxithromycin or doxycycline	Benzylpenicillin or procaine penicillin or cephalothin or cephazolin (for resistant organism or slow response, treat as for severe pneumonia)
Group 3 Severe pneumonia and/or a condition predisposing to Pseudomonas infection, e.g. bronchiectasis, cystic fibrosis	S. pneumoniae Legionella spp H. influenzae aerobic Gram-negative bacilli P. aeruginosa	M. pneumoniae C. pneumoniae S. aureus		Erythromycin plus either cefotaxime or ceftriaxone Erythromycin plus gentamicin plus either ceftazidime or ticarcillin/potassium clavulanate
Group 4 Aspiration pneumonia and lung abscess	Anaerobes S. anginosus	Gram-negative bacilli		Benzylpenicillin plus metronidazole or clindamycin as single agent
Group 5 Staphlococcal pneumonia	S. aureus		Flucloxacillin or (for MRSA) vancomycin	

Refer to Therapeutic Guidelines Antibiotic (Version 12, 2003) for latest antibiotic recommendations.

commonly encountered group. *S. pneumoniae* usually produces a classical bacterial pneumonia whereas *M. pneumoniae* is more likely to cause an atypical pneumonia. Macrolides (erythromycin or roxithromycin) are effective against both common pathogens and are preferred as the initial therapy. If there are no atypical features suggesting mycoplasma infection, and local resistance to *S. pneumoniae* is low, amoxycillin is an alternative initial therapy.

S. pneumoniae is also the most common pathogen for Group 2 patients. Elderly patients and those with coexisting illness are less likely to have mycoplasma infection and more likely to be affected by *H. influenzae*. Macrolides are less effective against *H. influenzae* and penicillins or cephalosporins are the preferred initial treatment.

Features indicating severe pneumonia (Group 3) are listed in Table 5.4.2. Patients in this group can deteriorate suddenly and initial therapy is designed to cover all of the common pathogens. These patients require treatment with intravenous, broad-spectrum antibiotics.

Therapy can be altered with the substitution of more narrow spectrum antibiotics once the results of cultures and antibiotic sensitivities are available.

Group 4 patients are those with aspiration syndromes and lung abscesses. The most common pathogens are oral anaerobes and, less frequently, Gram-negative bacilli. Monotherapy with benzylpenicillin has been the traditional treatment for this group of patients but is not effective against all anaerobes. Combination therapy with metronidazole or the use of clindamycin as a sole agent has been shown to be superior to monotherapy with benzylpenicillin (see also 'Lung Abscess').

Infection due to *S. aureus* (Group 5) is more frequent following influenza infection and is a common blood-borne pathogen complicating intravenous drug abuse. *S. aureus* is an infrequent cause of pneumonia and carries a high mortality (Table 5.4.6). Treatment is with intravenous flucloxacillin or vancomycin if methicillin resistant *S. aureus* (MRSA) is present.

Monitoring of antibiotic levels is

recommended for gentamicin and vancomycin in particular to avoid nephrotoxicity and ototoxicity. Both the dose and dose interval may require alteration in the presence of renal impairment for a variety of other antibiotics including the penicillins, the cephalosporins (with the exception of ceftriaxone), and pentamidine.

Doxycycline causes staining of teeth and may be associated with bone-marrow suppression. It is, therefore, contraindicated in children under 12 years of age and in pregnant and breast-feeding mothers. Intravenous erythromycin should be infused slowly over at least an hour. Rapid infusion produces pain, phlebitis, QT prolongation and has been associated with a variety of cardiac arrhythmias including Torsades de pointes and ventricular fibrillation. Clindamycin has also been associated with serious cardiovascular side effects when infused rapidly and should also be administered over at least 1 hour.

The optimal duration of therapy is not clearly delineated in the literature. For patients admitted to hospital, IV therapy

Table 5.4.6 Community acquired pneumonia

Aetiological agent	Frequency (%)*	Mortality (%)#
S. pneumoniae	63	17
H. influenzae	12	7.4
M. pneumoniae	7.2	1.4
Mixed bacterial species	4.3	24
Legionella spp.	3.9	15
Coxiella burnetii	2.6	0.5
S. aureus	2.2	32
Gram-negative bacteria	1.5	37
Chlamydia pneumoniae	0.6	10
Viruses	2.8	6.1
P. aeruginosa	0.25	61.1
Klebsiella spp.	0.79	35.7
E. coli	0.24	35.3
Proteus spp.	0.17	8.3
Streptococci spp.	0.08	16.7
Influenza A virus	1.42	9.0
Parainfluenza virus	0.42	6.7
Influenza B virus	0.40	0
Respiratory syncytial virus	0.28	5.0
Adenovirus	0.27	0
Cause unknown	61	12.8

*percentage of identified isolates
#percentage mortality for each etiological agent

is preferred to obtain higher tissue levels of antibiotics. IV therapy should be continued until the patient has been afebrile for 24 hours and the SaO_2 remains above 95%. Oral therapy should be continued for 5–10 days for uncomplicated cases. Ten to 14 days is recommended if mycoplasma or chlamydia infection is suspected or proven, and 14–21 days for Legionella, S. aureus, and when infection occurs in an immunocompromised host.

Response to therapy

Response to therapy may be delayed and therapy should not be changed within the first 72 hours unless there is a marked clinical deterioration. For normal individuals fever may persist for 2–4 days, leucocytosis for 4 days, and pulmonary crackles remain in one-third of patients after 1 week of treatment. The rapidity of resolution varies with the etiological agent. Fever resolves more rapidly with S. pneumoniae infection than other agents.

Radiological changes are usually delayed compared to the clinical response. It is common for the chest radiograph to show some deterioration in the first few days of treatment. If the patient is improving or has only mild disease, the radiographic changes are not of clinical significance. In contrast, the presence of increasing pulmonary infiltrates in

patients with severe CAP is a poor prognostic feature. Radiographic clearance is related to the etiological agent and the presence of significant comorbid disease. In otherwise healthy patients less than 50 years of age with S. pneumoniae pneumonia, radiographic clearance will be complete in 4 weeks in 60% of cases. Only one-quarter of patients who are older, bacteraemic, or have associated chronic disease will have radiographic clearance by 4 weeks. Infection due to M. pneumoniae clears more rapidly and infection due to Legionella spp. slower than pneumococcal pneumonia. Radiological features other than consolidation (such as volume loss, pleural changes) resolve much slower than pulmonary infiltrates and may become permanent.

Failure to improve can be for a variety of reasons and each must be considered in turn in the patient who is deteriorating or not improving. Firstly the diagnosis must be reconsidered. Conditions such as pulmonary embolism and infarction, congestive cardiac failure, inflammatory lung disease, and malignancy can all mimic pneumonia. Further imaging including thoracic CT, lung scanning, and pulmonary angiography may establish the presence of an alternative diagnostic condition. Thoracic CT may also demonstrate previously undetected collections or effusions that are amenable to diagnostic sampling. Bronchoscopy may reveal information on local anatomical detail and can provide material for microscopic examination and culture.

If patients are not responding to treatment, the history should be repeated with an emphasis on risk factors for immunosuppression and potential exposure to tuberculosis and other unusual agents. Non-prescribed medications may contain significant amounts of corticosteroids and can be a less obvious cause of immunosuppression. Further investigation for the presence of unusual agents may be indicated, (see also Clinical Features and Notes on Specific Conditions).

Prior treatment with antibiotics increases the false negative rate of sputum analysis and blood culture and increases the likelihood of a resistant organism if the patient is not responding to the initial therapy. If antibiotic resistance is suspected, an alternative antibiotic regime should be considered in consultation with the local infectious disease unit.

Resistance to antimicrobial therapy is an increasing problem. The first clinically significant penicillin resistant *S. pneumoniae* isolate was reported in Australia by Hansman and Bullen in 1967. Despite the origination from Australia, this country has remained relatively protected. Resistance rates to penicillin have risen to 50% in Spain, 25% in parts of the USA, and are rising in Australia. Results from an Australian review showed higher rates of resistance for most other antibiotics (chloramphenicol, 6%; erythromycin, 11%; tetracycline, 15%; co-trimoxazole, 42%). Resistance to the cephalosporins is also an area of concern. Approximately 10% of strains resistant to penicillin are also resistant to cephalosporins and multiple drug resistance is common with this combination.

Overall mortality from pneumococcal pneumonia is higher in the presence of penicillin resistance. However, exclusion of patients with polymicrobial pneumonia and adjustment for other predictors of mortality produces the same mortality for penicillin sensitive and penicillin-resistant strains.

DISPOSITION

The majority of patients with pulmonary infections are well and managed on an out-patient basis. As few as 20% of patients with pneumonia are admitted to hospital. The decision to admit a patient to hospital is made on individual clinical and laboratory or radiological assessment.

Hospitalization should be considered if any features of more severe disease are present (Table 5.4.2). Intensive care admission may be necessary in the presence of rapidly progressive disease and/or the inability to maintain normal physiological parameters. Early consultation with specialty units is an integral part of the management of patients with more severe disease.

Hospital admission may be necessary on social grounds if the patient is not able to be cared for adequately at home. If there is any doubt about the ability of the patient to cope at home or if there are unusual features in the history a short period (1–2 days) of observation in hospital will usually delineate any unclear issues. Patients who remain stable during this observation period can then be discharged and managed on an outpatient basis.

PROGNOSIS

The majority of patients with pneumonia do not have comorbid disease, are treated on an out-patient basis and have a complete resolution and return to health. In contrast, two-thirds of review articles on community-acquired pneumonia in the last 30 years deal with hospitalized patients only and 10% are restricted to ICU patients. Overall mortality rates are approximately 10% for hospitalized patients and 35% for ICU patients.

Mortality is intimately related to the underlying etiological agent and to a variety of patient characteristics.

Mortality rises with increasing age, extent of disease, presence of malignancy, comorbid disease, and abnormalities of vital signs. The factor most significantly associated with outcome is hypothermia with a five-fold increase in mortality. Pleuritic chest pain is the only characteristic consistently associated with a reduction in mortality (Table 5.4.3).

The agent most frequently associated with death is *S. pneumoniae*. Gram-negative pneumonia is more commonly associated with debility and significant comorbid disease and carries a worse prognosis. Mortality rates are greater than 30% for *Klebsiella* spp. and *E. coli* and more than 60% for *P. aeruginosa*. Collectively these three agents only account for just over 1% of all pneumonias and, therefore, contribute little to overall mortality. Infection due to *S. aureus* is also infrequent but associated with a mortality twice that of *S. pneumoniae*.

Infection due to atypical agents is generally associated with a favourable outcome. *M. pneumoniae* is the most common of the atypical agents and is associated with a mortality of less than 2%. Viral infections account for less than 3% of all isolates. Mortality from viral infections overall is 6%. Influenza A virus is the most frequent viral isolate (1.4% of all isolates) with a mortality of 9%. Death from Influenza B virus or adenovirus is rare.

DIFFERENTIAL DIAGNOSIS

Pneumonia may be present with minimal or no respiratory complaints. Infection with the atypical agents, in particular, may have prominent extra-pulmonary symptoms, which may overwhelm and obscure the respiratory component of the illness. Abdominal pain or back pain may be the primary complaint with lower lobe and atypical pneumonias. Elderly patients and those with depressed immune function may have less prominent symptoms. Pneumonia should, therefore, be included in the differential diagnosis of every febrile illness of indeterminate origin.

Infiltrates on a chest X-ray in the setting of a febrile patient are not always due to pneumonia. Opacities may be due to previous illness or disease and the febrile illness due to a non-respiratory cause. Comparison with previous radiographs is important. Pulmonary infiltrates may also be due to malignancy, radiation, drugs, chemical exposure, or hypersensitivity pneumonitis. These conditions must all be considered if the patient is not responding to therapy for pneumonia.

NOTES ON SPECIFIC CONDITIONS

Streptococcal pneumonia

S. pneumoniae is responsible for the majority of cases of community-acquired pneumonia and remains the most common single isolate in almost every subgroup of patients. The current reported incidence is highly variable (20–75%) and appears to be largely related to publication bias.

Published studies are mostly from academic institutions and do not reflect the full community perspective. Patients with other pathology, particularly immune deficiency conditions, constitute a disproportionately high percentage of the population seen at academic institutions. Infection due to uncommon agents (principally *Pneumocystis carinii*) is more frequent in this subgroup even though *S. pneumoniae* is still the most common isolate. The vast majority of community-acquired pneumonias are due to *S. pneumoniae*, treated on an out-patient basis and are not reported.

The mortality from pneumonia in which no agent is identified is almost identical to that from *S. pneumoniae*. After discriminant functional analysis of data on patients in whom no pathogen was identified, the conclusion of the British Thoracic Society's Pneumonia Research Committee was that most cases were probably due to *S. pneumoniae*. It is likely that the frequency of infection due to *S. pneumoniae* is under-represented in the literature.

The typical presentation is described in 'Clinical features'. Less commonly, infection due to *S. pneumoniae* presents with an atypical pneumonic pattern. Hyperbilirubinaemia, jaundice, and rhabdomyolysis with myoglobinuria and renal failure have been described, but are rare.

Pneumococcal pneumonia usually produces a lobar infection of a single lobe. Up to one-quarter of patients have involvement of two lobes. The classic stages of lobar pneumonia were originally described in relation to pneumococcal pneumonia. Bronchopneumonia is seen more commonly in young children and elderly patients.

Patients at increased risk of pneumococcal sepsis may be immunized with a polyvalent vaccine. Identification and prophylactic treatment of these patient is discussed further in 'Prevention'.

Legionella

Legionnaires' disease derives its name from an American Legion Convention in Philadelphia in 1976 at which 200 people fell ill from an unknown illness. A Gram-negative bacillus was determined to be the causative agent and named *Legionella pneumophilia*. Retrospective analysis has discovered *Legionella* bacterium in specimens from as early as 1943. It is likely that the same organism was responsible for 'Pontiac fever' in Pontiac, Michigan, in 1968 and for an outbreak of pneumonia in Washington DC, in 1965.

Transmission of disease is usually from inhalation of contaminated droplets. Multiple cases are infected from a single aerosol source (mostly cooling towers, air-conditioning units, and whirlpool spa units) resulting in outbreaks of the condition. There is little or no person-to-person transmission. The increased use of evaporative cooling and air-conditioning in summer explains the greater incidence of epidemics during that season.

The clinical presentation is initially 'atypical' with prominent extra-pulmonary symptoms. The deterioration may be rapid as the classic features of bacterial pneumonia develop.

Sputum Gram stain demonstrating few polymorphonuclear cells and no bacteria is suggestive of legionella infection. Hyponatraemia is seen more commonly in association with legionella than any other cause of pneumonia.

Confirmation of diagnosis from culture of sputum will take at least 2 days. Antigen testing of sputum is highly specific for *L. pneumophilia* (which is responsible for over 90% of clinical infections) but is negative for other serotypes. Serological diagnosis of legionella infection requires a rise in titre of at least 1:128. Titres may rise within one week but more commonly take 3 to 6 weeks for the diagnosis to be confirmed. This delay makes the results of serologic titre testing of value for epidemiological purposes only.

Following confirmation of infection, the history must be carefully examined to identify the contact which would have occurred at the beginning of the 2–10 day incubation period. Other people infected from the same source may be unaware of the cause of their illness.

Penicillins are ineffective against legionella. Macrolides are the preferred initial therapy.

Table 5.4.7 Differential diagnosis of cavitating lesions on chest X-ray
S. aureus pneumonia
Anaerobic abscess
Fungi
Gram-negative bacteria
M. tuberculosis
S. pneumoniae serotype III
Malignancy
Infected cyst/bullae
Pulmonary infarction

Cavitating lesions

Cavitation within an area of consolidation is unusual for the common causes of pneumonia (Table 5.4.7). The presence of such lesions should raise the suspicion of infection due to *S. aureus*, fungi, or anaerobes with the production of an abscess. Anaerobes are aspirated from infective foci in teeth so edentulous patients are protected from this complication. Cavitation is also seen more commonly in Gram-negative infection and as a complication of tuberculosis. *S. pneumoniae* serotype III may cause cavities whereas the other serotypes of *S. pneumoniae* and infection due to *H. influenzae*, *M. pneumoniae* and viruses almost never produce cavities.

Cavitation within a pulmonary lesion may also indicate the presence of a malignancy, secondary infection of a pre-existent cyst or bullae, pulmonary infarction or necrosis in an inflammatory lesion. These conditions may mimic pneumonia and must be included in the differential diagnosis.

All cavitating lesions require further investigation. Comparison with previous chest films is desirable before commencing invasive investigations. Thoracic CT provides more detailed information about the lesion, the presence and location of hilar lymph nodes, and can be used to guide needle aspiration and/or biopsy of lesions. Bronchoscopy delineates the presence of disease in the local airways and can provide brushings or biopsy samples for analysis. As bronchoscopy may lead to inadvertent intrapulmonary spread of infection, it should be delayed until antibiotics have been commenced.

Nosocomial pneumonia

Nosocomial pneumonia refers to the development of a new episode of pneumonia more than 2 days after a patient has been admitted to hospital. Such illnesses are the third most common nosocomial infections (after urinary tract and wound infections) and occur in 0.5 to 5% of hospitalized patients. The source of infection is most commonly aspiration of the patients own oropharyngeal flora. Less common sources of infection are transfer from patient to patient on equipment or directly by staff contact. Outbreaks of legionella have been reported from hospital heating and water systems.

Pneumonia developing in patients already admitted to hospital is usually more severe and associated with a worse prognosis than CAP. Hospitalized patients have more significant comorbid disease and are frequently on antibiotic therapy (increasing the false-negative rate of bacteriological diagnosis). Pulmonary infiltrates may pre-exist due to other conditions. As a result of these factors, the presence of superimposed pneumonia may not be apparent until disease is advanced.

Patients and staff in hospitals and institutions have a higher incidence of Gram-negative oropharyngeal colonization. Infection with Gram-negative bacilli occurs in half of all isolates of nosocomial pneumonia and is associated with a poorer prognosis. Normal gastric acidity is reduced in patients who are unwell from any source and in patients on therapy aimed at increasing gastric pH. The normal protective barrier to spread of coliforms is reduced in these patients. The combination of reduced host defences and more virulent organisms increases the incidence of and mortality from nosocomial pneumonia compared to community-acquired pneumonia. Mortality ranges from 25–50% and survivors have a prolongation of hospital stay.

Table 5.4.8 provides a clinically based classification of nosocomial pneumonia, indicates the likely etiological agent and lists suggested initial therapy for each group. Parenteral therapy is preferred in order to achieve higher tissue levels of antibiotics. Initial therapy is commenced with the broad-spectrum third-generation cephalosporins until the result of culture and sensitivities are available. Potential infection with resistant Gram-negative infections is more common is patients with severe pneumonia and patients with multiple risk factors for nosocomial pneumonia (Groups 3 and 2d). Initial therapy for these patients must also include an aminoglycoside for effective Gram-negative cover.

Empyema

Collections of purulent material in the interpleural space may result as an extension of pneumonia, spread from adjacent foci of infection, direct inoculation through the thoracic wall, or as a result of haematogenous seeding from a distal focus. In the pre-antibiotic era, empyema occurred in 5–8% of patients with pneumococcal pneumonia. Empyema is now uncommonly seen in association with pneumococcal pneumonia.

Table 5.4.8 Pathogens and therapy associated with nosocomial pneumonia

Pneumonia classification	Most common organisms	Other organisms to consider	Parenteral therapy
Group 1 Mild to moderate No specific risk factors	S. pneumoniae H. influenzae	Klebsiella spp. and other Gram-negative rods	Cefotaxime or ceftriaxone
Group 2 Mild to moderate Specific risk factors a) aspiration, thoraco-abdominal surgery	As above	As above Anaerobes	As for Group 1 plus either metronidazole or clindamycin
b) diabetes, coma, head injury	As above	As above S. aureus	As for Group 1 plus flucloxacillin or (if MRSA suspected) vancomycin
c) high dose corticosteroids	As above Klebsiella spp. and other Gram-negative rods	Legionella spp.	As for Group 1 plus erythromycin
d) multiple risk factors ICU, antibiotics, prolonged hospitalization	As above	P. aeruginosa Multiresistant Gram-negative rods	See Group 3 below
Group 3 Severe pneumonia	As above	P. aeruginosa Legionella spp.	Aminoglycoside plus erythromycin together with either ceftazidime or ticarcillin/potassium clavulanate

Refer to Therapeutic Guidelines Antibiotic (Version 12, 2003) for latest antibiotic recommendations.

An empyema may be obscured by pneumonia and should be considered in patients who remain febrile or do not respond to antibiotic therapy. Small collections may be difficult to detect on clinical examination. Larger collections can be further delineated by ultrasound examination or thoracic CT. Needle thoracentesis returning purulent material confirms the diagnosis and provides samples for microbiological analysis. In the early stages of infection the aspirated material may not be frankly purulent on gross examination. Microscopic analysis reveals organisms and leucocytes.

Adequate treatment requires drainage of the empyema and emptying of the infected interpleural space by tube thoracentesis. Thoracic surgical consultation is needed if tube thoracostomy does not achieve adequate drainage.

CONCLUSION

The initial management of the patient with community-acquired pneumonia requires a sound knowledge of pathophysiology, microbiology and epidemiology, in addition to a thorough clinical assessment. Emergency physicians should be able to determine the most likely pathogen in cases of pneumonia, so that decisions regarding early antibiotic treatment are both rational and effective.

CONTROVERSIES AND FUTURE DIRECTIONS

❶ Prospective clinical trials are required to validate the efficacy and assess the cost-effectiveness of current clinical practice guidelines for pneumonia.

❷ Research is currently being conducted to develop tests that measure specific microbial antigens for a number of the pathogens responsible for community-acquired pneumonia. If successful, these tests may provide the clinician with a more timely microbiological diagnosis, and assist in guiding early antibiotic therapy.

REFERENCES

1. Ashbourne JF, Downey PM 1992 Pneumonia. In: Rosen P, Barkin RM (eds) Emergency Medicine - Concepts and Clinical Practice, 3rd edn. Mosby Year Book, St. Louis, pp 1162–77
2. Bartlett JG, Mundy LM 1995 Community-acquired pneumonia. New England Journal of Medicine 333: 1618–23
3. British Thoracic Society 1993 Guidelines for the management of community-acquired pneumonia in adults admitted to hospital. British Journal of Hospital Medicine 49: 346–50
4. Currie B, Howard D, Nguyen VT, et al 1993 The 1990-1991 outbreak of melioidosis in the Northern Territory of Australia: clinical aspects. Southeast Asian Journal of Tropical Medicine and Public Health 24: 436–43
5. Fang GD, Fine M, Orloff J, et al 1990 New and emerging etiologies for community-acquired pneumonia with implications for therapy. A prospective multicenter study of 359 cases. Medicine (Baltimore) 69: 307–16
6. Fein AM, Niederman MS 1995 Guidelines for the initial management of community-acquired pneumonia: savory recipe or cookbook for disaster? American Review of Respiratory Critical Care 152: 1149–53
7. Fine MJ, Smith DN, Singer DE 1990 Hospitalization decision in patients with community-acquired pneumonia: a prospective cohort study. American Journal of Medicine 89: 713–21
8. Gleason PP, Kapoor WN, Stone RA, et al 1997 Medical outcomes and antimicrobial costs with the use of the American Thoracic Society guidelines for outpatients with community-acquired pneumonia. Journal of the American Medical Association 278: 32–9
9. Jernigan DB, Cetron MS, Breiman RF 1996 Minimizing the impact of drug-resistant Streptococcus pneumonia (DRSP). Journal of the American Medical Association 275: 206–9
10. Karalus NC, Cursons RT, Leng RA, et al. 1991 Community acquired pneumonia: aetiology and prognostic index evaluation. Thorax 46: 413–8
11. Lim I, Shaw DR, Stanley DP, et al 1989 A prospective hospital study of the etiology of community-acquired pneumonia. Medical Journal of Australia 151: 87–91
12. Neill AM, Martin IR, Weir R, et al 1996 Community acquired pneumonia: aetiology and usefulness of severity criteria on admission. Thorax 51: 1010–6
13. Niederman MS, Bass JB, Campbell GD, et al 1993 Guidelines for the initial management of adults with community-acquired pneumonia: diagnosis, assessment of severity, and initial antibiotic therapy. American Review of Respiratory Disease 148: 1418–26
14. Schuller D 1995 Pulmonary diseases. In: Ewald GA, McKenzie CR (eds) Manual of Medical Therapeutics, 28th edn. Little, Brown, Boston, pp 236–61
15. Thompson JE 1997 Community acquired pneumonia in northeastern Australia – a hospital based study of Aboriginal and non-Aboriginal patients. Australian and New Zealand Journal of Medicine 27: 59–61

5.5 CHRONIC OBSTRUCTIVE AIRWAYS DISEASE

MARTIN DUFFY

ESSENTIALS

1 Chronic obstructive airways disease (COAD) is a common medical condition.

2 The majority of exacerbations of COAD are due to infection, but other important precipitants need to be excluded.

3 Therapeutic options are limited because of the essentially irreversible nature of the disease.

4 Clinically significant carbon dioxide retention is a much feared but uncommon complication of oxygen therapy.

5 Support for the widespread use of steroids is limited.

6 Non-invasive ventilatory assistance has an important role in the management of acute respiratory failure.

INTRODUCTION

The term chronic obstructive airways disease (COAD) can be applied to any respiratory condition characterized by chronic reduced expiratory airflow. In clinical practice most emergency physicians use the term more specifically for the conditions of emphysema and chronic bronchitis, tending to view patients with conditions such as asthma, bronchiectasis and cystic fibrosis as different entities, even though the clinical margins are often blurred and treatment options overlap considerably.

COAD is a major public health problem and commonly quoted figures are probably significant underestimates.

It affects approximately 5% of the population[1] and is the fourth leading cause of death in the world.[2] Projections from the Global Burden of Disease Study suggest COAD will be the fifth leading cause of disability-adjusted-life-years lost worldwide by the year 2020.[3] Despite the enormity of the problem there is a shortage of well-conducted research to guide present management.

For emergency physicians COAD is important for two reasons. First, it may present as life-threatening respiratory failure; second, it is a common co-morbidity that may impact on the management of other illnesses.

DEFINITIONS

Chronic bronchitis is a clinical diagnosis characterized by the presence of chronic cough with sputum production for at least 3 months per year for at least 2 consecutive years. Histological features include inflammatory cell infiltration of the bronchial mucosa, goblet cell metaplasia, mucosal oedema and increased mucus secretions.

Emphysema is a pathological diagnosis characterized by the destruction of lung units distal to the terminal bronchioles, leading to abnormal permanent airspace enlargement.

An acute exacerbation is a clinical state characterised by worsening of dyspnoea, increase in sputum purulence, and increase in sputum volume. However, there are no standardized, validated grading systems for the severity of an acute exacerbation.[4]

AETIOLOGY

By far the most important factor leading to the development of COAD is cigarette smoking. Less common factors include genetic disorders such as α_1-antitrypsin deficiency, occupational exposure and exposure to air pollution.

Why one patient with the above risk factors develops COAD and another patient with similar risk factors does not, remains unclear. For instance, only 10–15% of smokers develop clinically significant emphysema, and almost two-thirds of those homozygous for α_1-antitrypsin deficiency have well preserved pulmonary function.[5] These discrepancies continue to stimulate research into the pathophysiology of COAD and question the roles of such factors as cytokines, eicosanoids, neurogenic mechanisms and respiratory muscle dysfunction.

HISTORY

Most patients with COAD experience a slow, steady deterioration in their respiratory function. The majority of presentations to the emergency department are the result of a superimposed acute exacerbation.

It is important to have a good understanding of the patient's baseline function. Questioning to determine this should include the following:

Background

- When did the patient first develop symptoms
- When was the diagnosis first made (from the time of initial diagnosis the 10-year mortality rate exceeds 50%)[6]
- The presence of risk factors
- Is the patient a smoker – past or present
- Maintenance therapy
- Use of oral steroids
- Normal level of activity
- Home monitoring, e.g. PEFRs
- Use of home oxygen therapy

- Record of hospitalizations, including ICU admissions.

Acute deterioration

- Fever
- Increased cough and sputum production
- Chest pain suggestive of a pulmonary embolus or pneumothorax
- Coexisting illnesses
- Inhaler technique
- Intercurrent use of inappropriate medications, e.g. β-blockers, sedatives.

EXAMINATION

Classically, patients with COAD have been described as 'pink puffers' (predominantly emphysema) and 'blue bloaters' (predominantly chronic bronchitis). In clinical practice there is usually a variety of presentations between the two extremes. The 'pink puffer' is typically described as a thin, barrel-chested patient with obvious dyspnoea and tachypnoea, but no cyanosis. Use of the accessory muscles of respiration is evidenced by the classic tripod posture, with both elbows resting on the patient's knees or other surfaces, as well as sternomastoid muscle hypertrophy. Pursed-lip breathing completes the picture. The 'blue bloater' is typically described as an overweight, oedematous, cyanosed patient suffering from chronic cough and sputum production. Despite evidence of hypoxaemia they are not usually dyspnoeic. Features of cor pulmonale may be present in the later stages.

Clinical features strongly suggestive of airflow obstruction, with specificities of 98–99%, are the presence of wheezes, a barrel chest, decreased cardiac dullness, and a subxiphoid cardiac impulse. Unfortunately, the sensitivities of these features are extremely poor (8–15%), limiting their clinical usefulness.[7]

Noting the classic features above, the goal of the initial evaluation of a patient presenting with an exacerbation of COAD is to determine the severity of the attack, as well as to search for and treat any precipitating factors and complications. The patient with flushed, cyanosed warm peripheries, a bounding pulse, diaphoresis and an altered level of consciousness obviously needs urgent resuscitation. The patient who is awake, alert and able to talk in sentences despite their respiratory distress, can be assessed at a less urgent pace.

Important precipitants and complications to search for include:

Precipitants of acute respiratory failure

- Infection
  - Acute bronchitis
  - Pneumonia
- Bronchospasm
- Sputum retention
- Pneumothoraces and bullae
- Pulmonary embolism
- Decreased respiratory drive, e.g. inappropriate sedative use
- Decreased respiratory muscle strength, e.g. metabolic or neuromuscular cause
- Increased metabolic demands
  - Sepsis
  - Fever
- Left ventricular failure.

Complications of COAD

- Pulmonary hypertension
- Right ventricular failure
- Secondary polycythaemia
- Loss of weight
- Complications secondary to long-term steroid use.

INVESTIGATIONS

The following investigations may be used during the evaluation of a patient with COAD. Not all will be necessary in every patient in every situation: it is important to choose wisely and use tests that will have an impact on management decisions.

Tests performed at the bedside include:

- Pulse oximetry: provides invaluable 'real-time' non-invasive evaluation of oxygenation, helping with the initial assessment of the patient and allowing observation of trends in response to therapy; typical goal is a saturation of >90%.
- Spirometry: provides confirmation of obstruction – FEV_1 <80% of predicted and FEV_1/FVC <0.7. In the acute situation spirometry often cannot be performed by the patient, and it has little role in management decisions such as intubation. Clinical practice guidelines from the American College of Physicians-American Society of Internal Medicine and the American College of Chest Physicians (ACP-ASIM/ACCP) state that for patients being hospitalized with an acute exacerbation of COAD spirometry should not be used to diagnose an exacerbation nor to assess its severity.[8]
- Electrocardiography: along with continuous ECG monitoring, is used to detect associated dysrhythmias and may also detect intercurrent ischaemic heart disease. ECG evidence of pulmonary hypertension and right ventricular hypertrophy may be present, but is often insensitive and non-specific.

Tests that have results available within minutes include:

- Arterial blood gases: provide information regarding acute versus chronic respiratory failure and monitor improvement or deterioration with several measurements. An acute rise in P_aCO_2 by 10 mmHg leads to an increase in HCO_3 levels by 1 mmol/L, up to a HCO_3 value of 30 mmol/L; a chronic rise in P_aCO_2 by 10 mmHg leads to an increase in HCO_3 levels by 4 mmol/L up to a HCO_3 value of 36 mmol/L.[9] In the acute setting an acidotic pH value in a patient with chronic carbon dioxide retention signifies superimposed acute decompensation. Although this information is useful, ABGs play little part in *clinical* decisions such as intubation.

- Chest radiograph: in the acute setting provides valuable information regarding the presence of coexisting illnesses which may be life-threatening and require specific interventions, e.g. pneumothorax, pneumonia, pleural effusions, heart failure. Studies have demonstrated that up to 23% of admitted patients may have a change in their management related to their chest X-ray (CXR) findings.[8] Classic features of the predominantly emphysematous patient include hyperinflation, flattened diaphragms, bullae, increased retrosternal airspace, decreased vascular markings and a small heart.

Other tests that may be useful, although with limited or no role in the acute setting, include:

- Sputum culture: up to 80% of exacerbations secondary to acute bronchitis may be due to bacteria, with *H. influenzae*, *S. pneumoniae* and *Moraxella catarrhalis* the predominant pathogens. The remaining 20% are due to viruses, such as influenzae, rhinoviruses, parainfluenzae and coronaviruses;[5] exacerbations complicated by pneumonia have similar bacterial pathogens. Colonization of the respiratory tract can make interpretation of results difficult.
- Full blood examination: may reveal evidence of secondary polycythaemia. A raised white cell count may be due to an infection, but the contribution of long-term steroid use to any neutrophilia must be considered, as too should the hyperadrenergic stress response of the acutely ill patient.
- Electrolytes: with particular note of potassium levels.
- Theophylline level: as required, noting that a patient may be toxic despite having a measured level within the therapeutic range.
- Respiratory function tests: demonstrate largely irreversible airflow obstruction with elevated lung volumes; reduced carbon monoxide uptake implies emphysema.
- High-resolution chest CT: demonstrates air trapping, hence useful in the diagnosis of emphysema,[10] but of questionable value given limited availability, high cost, and as yet undetermined advance on other diagnostic modalities available for the assessment of most patients with COAD.
- Cardiac studies: such as echocardiography and gated nuclear scans may be required to determine the role of ventricular dysfunction in the clinical picture; the utility of brain natriuretic peptide (BNP) measurements in differentiating dyspnoea due to heart failure from COAD is yet to be fully determined.

MANAGEMENT

The management of a patient with COAD is difficult because of the predominantly irreversible nature of the disease process, thereby limiting therapeutic options. However, seemingly small improvements often lead to substantial symptomatic relief. As with all patients presenting to the emergency department, the timing and level of intervention depends on the severity at the time of presentation. It is important to remember that management decisions for the patient in extremis are solely clinical: no further investigation is necessary to determine whether immediate intubation is required.

The following is a summary of the therapeutic modalities typically used to treat an acute exacerbation of COAD.

Oxygen therapy

Hypoxemia must be corrected. Oxygen therapy for most patients with COAD will not produce clinically significant carbon dioxide retention, a multifactorial condition caused by changes in pulmonary blood flow and V/Q mismatching, not simply hypoventilation.[11] The minimal acceptable oxygen saturation in most cases is approximately 90%. For the mildly unwell patient this may be achieved with the use of nasal prongs at 2L/min. For patients with more severe disease the use of a ventimask with an appropriate fractional inspired oxygen concentration is more appropriate. In most cases these devices are of the fixed-performance type, i.e. the FiO_2 is independent of patient factors. However, beware of the severely dyspnoeic patient whose peak inspiratory flow rate may exceed the peak flow rate of the device, leading to fluctuations in the FiO_2. To avoid this a circuit with a large reservoir will be necessary. Persisting hypoxia (SpO_2 <85%) necessitates a search for complicating factors such as pneumonia, pulmonary oedema, pulmonary embolus or pneumothorax,[12] as well as consideration for ventilatory assistance.

Ventilatory assistance

Ventilatory assistance may be non-invasive (NIV) or invasive. One of the critical factors in deciding which form is most appropriate is determining whether the patient can protect their own airway - if not, intubation is required.

The role of NIV in the management of acute respiratory failure in patients with COAD continues to grow. A common feature of acute deterioration is the presence of dynamic hyperinflation and the development of intrinsic positive end expiratory pressure (PEEPi) leading to an increased work of breathing. The application of CPAP or external PEEP at levels to overcome PEEPi, has been shown to reduce respiratory work.[13,14,15] This has resulted in patients reporting less dyspnoea and laboratory evidence of better gas exchange.[16,17] The use of inspiratory pressure support ventilation, either on its own or in combination with CPAP (i.e. BiPAP), has also proved an effective form of NIV in acute respiratory failure. Initiation of ventilation triggers the inspiratory positive airway pressure response, which is limited to a predetermined level, usually 10–20 cmH_2O. Expiratory positive airway pressure of approximately 5 cmH_2O, is predetermined and persists throughout expiration. The whole process thus decreases the work of breathing. Numerous studies, using either a face mask or nasal mask and varying combinations of the above airway pressure manipulations, have shown significant reductions in the need for intubation.[18-22] Brochard et al's prospective randomized study demonstrated that NIV in selected patients not only reduced the need for intubation, but also reduced length of hospital stay, complications and in-hospital mortality.[22] A subsequent meta-analysis of five randomized-controlled trials concluded that the addition of NIV to standard therapy in patients with an acute exacerbation of COAD complicated by acute respiratory failure improves survival and decreases the need for endotracheal intubation.[23] Clinical practice guidelines from ACP-ASIM/ACCP and evidenced-based management guidelines from the Global Initiative for Chronic Obstructive Lung Disease (GOLD) support these findings.[8,2] Although the above is very promising it is important to note that NIV is not uniformly effective, with success rates ranging from 50 to 92%, raising the question of which patients are most likely to benefit from the intervention.[24] Factors that may predict success or failure remain unclear. A decrease in P_aCO_2 of >10 mmHg or improvement in pH of >0.05 after 30 minutes of nasal mechanical ventilation can be used to predict successful nasal ventilation.[24] Whether these guidelines can be extrapolated to other forms of NIV remains to be determined. The concurrent delivery of nebulized β_2- agonists with NIV is an important therapeutic issue. Theoretical concerns of reduced drug delivery because of the rates of fresh gas flow required to effectively run CPAP circuits have been confirmed. However, these concerns were not of clinical significance in a group of stable asthmatic patients.[25] Extrapolation to COAD patients with acute respiratory failure should be made with caution, but may be appropriate given the favourable effects of CPAP on respiratory mechanics and subsequent drug delivery.[25]

Endotracheal intubation with positive-pressure ventilation is used in patients who fail non-invasive ventilatory assistance or who have indications for intubation present at the outset, e.g. unprotected airway, respiratory arrest. The major problems with positive-pressure ventilation in this patient population are the risk of barotrauma and the production of PEEPi. Commonly recommended ventilation strategies include using tidal volumes of approximately 8 mL/kg, using a reduced respiratory rate, and using an inspiratory:expiratory ratio of 1:3. Most patients also usually require a bolus of intravenous fluids to counter the effects of positive-pressure ventilation on venous return and cardiac output.

Concerns about subsequent ventilator dependence are often unfounded, with premorbid level of activity and FEV_1 being the best predictors of successful weaning. In a retrospective analysis by Menzies et al, 100% of patients with good premorbid function and an FEV_1 >40% of predicted were successfully weaned.[26] It is important to note that for the purposes of the study successful weaning was defined as 72 hours survival post-extubation without the need for ventilatory assistance. Those with poor premorbid function and an FEV_1 <25% of predicted had an almost 50% chance of weaning within 4 months. Menzies et al further noted that the albumin level, an indicator of nutritional status, also predicted successful weaning.

Bronchodilators

Bronchodilators are used in the management of acute exacerbations because of the possibility of a small reversible component to the airflow obstruction. In the emergency department setting these drugs are usually given via a nebuliser, though there is little evidence to support this route over metered-dose inhalers, particularly when used in conjunction with a spacer device.[4,27] It is common practice to use the drugs below in combination. Although there are at present few studies to support this approach, addition of a second bronchodilating drug once the maximal dose of the initial drug has been reached may be of some additional benefit.[8]

Anticholinergic agents

The effectiveness of anticholinergic agents compared to β_2-agonists has been confirmed[4,28] and, because of their lower adverse effect profile, recommendations for their use as first line agents have been made.[8] The most commonly used agent in Australia is ipratropium bromide. The usual dose is 500 µg via nebulizer, with doses as frequent as every 20 minutes being used in clinical practice, though with little supporting evidence.

Tiotropium bromide is a new long-acting anticholinergic agent currently not yet available in Australia. A number of studies have now confirmed its efficacy, both in terms of improvements in spirometry and in health-related quality of life.[29-32]

β_2-agonists

Salbutamol is commonly used as a first-line agent in Australia. The usual dose is 5 mg via nebulizer, repeated as necessary, often continuously in the severely ill patient. Occasionally in the patient with a severe exacerbation the intravenous route may be required, though evidence for or against this practice is lacking.[33] Common side effects include tachycardia and tremor. A decrease in potassium levels is seen.

Theophylline

Rarely used in the acute setting because of significant side effects and questionable efficacy.

Corticosteroids

Data supporting the use of oral or intravenous steroids in the treatment of acute exacerbations of COAD are limited. Corticosteroids can be useful if there is an asthmatic component in the disease process, according to the American Thoracic Society's consensus document of 1995.[34] ACP-ASIM/ACCP and GOLD guidelines currently recommend the use of steroids.[8,2] Prednisolone, starting at 50 mg per day, is commonly prescribed. Evidence suggests that oral administration is just as effective as parenteral administration of steroids, exceptions being conditions that preclude the oral route, e.g. vomiting.[35] Short courses have minimal side effects, whereas the complications of long-term use are myriad. The potential role of hypothalamic-pituitary-adrenal axis suppression complicating patient presentations needs to be remembered.

Antibiotics

The role of bacteria, and hence antibiotics, in acute exacerbations of COAD is more controversial than previously believed, although they are still the most common cause of an exacerbation. In 30% of patients no clear cause for their exacerbation may be found.[2] In general, the more severe the exacerbation the more likely antibiotics will provide some benefit.[8] The increased production of purulent sputum is a reasonable trigger for the commencement of antibiotic therapy.[2] Drugs should cover *H. influenzae*, *S. pneumoniae* and *Moraxella catarrhalis*: depending on local sensitivities, a β lactamase-resistant drug (e.g. ampicillin with clavulanic acid) is often required. Third-generation cephalosporins (e.g. ceftriaxone) are commonly used for intravenous therapy.

Chest physiotherapy

Chest physiotherapy, in the form of mechanical percussion in an attempt to improve mucus clearance, has been shown to be ineffective and is currently not recommended.[8]

OTHER THERAPIES

- Nutritional support
- Correction of electrolyte abnormalities
- Longer-term measures
  – Smoking cessation
  – Vaccinations
    – pneumococcal
    – influenza
  – Home oxygen therapy
  – Lung volume reduction surgery
  – Transplantation.

DISPOSITION

At the heart of all decisions regarding the disposition of patients with COAD is the knowledge that one is dealing with a predominantly irreversible disease process.

CONTROVERSIES

❶ The role of heliox in the management of acute exacerbations.

❷ Criteria for admission and discharge of moderately severe exacerbations.

❸ The role of novel agents such as immunomodulators.

Most presentations are due to a superimposed acute deterioration in lung function, precipitated by any one or more of a number of previously outlined factors. Whether the patient requires admission will depend on the severity of the present exacerbation, how easily correctable is the precipitating factor, and how well the patient responds to therapy in the emergency department. In clinical practice this translates into a stay in hospital for 1, 2 or more days for most patients. A decision to discharge the patient from the emergency department requires the physician to ensure the presence of good home conditions, social supports and the organization of appropriate follow-up.

REFERENCES

1. Higgins MW 1989 Chronic airways disease in the United States: trends and determinants. Chest 96: 328S
2. Global Initiative for Chronic Obstructive Lung Disease. www.goldcopd.com
3. Murray CJL, Lopez AD (eds) 1996 The global burden of disease: a comprehensive assessment of mortality and disability from diseases, injuries and risk factors in 1990 and projected to 2020. Harvard University Press, Cambridge, MA
4. McCrory DC, Brown C, Gelfand S, Bach PB 2001 Management of acute exacerbations of COPD: a summary and appraisal of published evidence [special report]. Annals of Internal Medicine 134: 600–20
5. Morris DG, Szekely LA, Thompson BT 1997 Chronic obstructive pulmonary disease. In: Lee BW, Hsu SI, Stasiar DS (eds) Quick Consult Manual of Evidence-based Medicine. Lippincott-Raven, Haggerson, USA
6. Ferguson GT, Cherniack RM 1993 Management of chronic obstructive pulmonary disease. New England Journal of Medicine 328(14): 1017
7. Holleman DR Jr, Simel DL 1995 Does the clinical examination predict airflow limitation? Journal of the Australian Medical Association 273(4): 313
8. Snow V, Lascher S, Mottur-Pilson C for the Joint Expert Panel on COPD of the American College of Chest Physicians and the American College of Physicians-American Society of Internal Medicine

2001 The evidence base for management of acute exacerbations of COPD: Clinical Practice Guideline, Part 1 [special report]. Annals of Internal Medicine 134: 595–9
9. Worthley LIG 1996 Handbook of emergency laboratory tests. Churchill Livingstone, Edinburgh
10. Miniati M, Filippi E, Falaschi F, et al 1995 Radiologic evaluation of emphysema in patients with chronic obstructive pulmonary disease - chest radiography versus high resolution computed tomography. American Journal of Respiratory and Critical Care Medicine 151: 1359
11. Aubier M, Murciano D, Fournier M, et al 1980 Central respiratory drive in acute respiratory failure of patients with chronic obstructive pulmonary disease. American Review of Respiratory Disorders 122: 191
12. Tuxen DV 1997 Acute respiratory failure in chronic obstructive airways disease. In: Oh TE (ed) Intensive Care Manual. Butterworth-Heinemann, Oxford
13. Van den Berg B, Aerts JG, Boyaard JM 1995 Effect of continuous positive airway pressure (CPAP) in patients with chronic obstructive pulmonary disease (COPD) depending on intrinsic PEEP levels. Acta Anaesthesiologica Scandinavica 39(8): 1097
14. Goldberg P, Reissmann H, Maltais F, Ranieri M, Gottfried SB 1995 Efficacy of noninvasive CPAP in COPD with acute respiratory failure. European Respiratory Journal 8(11): 1894
15. Ranieri VM, Dambrosio M, Brienza N 1996 Intrinsic PEEP and cardiopulmonary acute ventilatory failure. European Respiratory Journal 9(6): 1283
16. de Lucas P, Tarancon C, Peuente L, Rodriguez C, Tayay E, Monturiol J 1993 Nasal continuous positive airway pressure in patients with COPD in acute respiratory failure. Chest 104(6): 1694
17. Miro A, Shivaram U, Hertig I 1993 Continuous positive airway pressure in COPD patients in acute hypercapnic respiratory failure. Chest 103(1): 266
18. Brochard L, Isabey D, Piquet J, et al 1990 Reversal of acute exacerbations of chronic obstructive lung disease by inspiratory assistance with a face mask. New England Journal of Medicine 323: 1523
19. Meduri G, Abou-Shala N, Fox R, Jones C, Leeper K, Wunderink R 1991 Non-invasive face mask mechanical ventilation in patients with acute hypercapnic respiratory failure. Chest 100: 445
20. Fernandez R, Blanch L, Valles J, Baigorri A, Artigas A 1993 Pressure support ventilation via face mask in acute respiratory failure in hypercapnic COPD patients. Intensive Care Medicine 19: 456
21. Kramer N, Meyer T, Meharg J, Ace R, Hill N 1995 Randomized prospective trial of non-invasive positive pressure ventilation in acute respiratory failure. American Journal of Respiratory Critical Care Medicine 157: 1799
22. Brochard L, Mancebo J, Wysocki M, Lefaso P, Centi G 1995 Non-invasive ventilation for acute exacerbations of chronic obstructive pulmonary disease. New England Journal of Medicine 333: 817
23. Keenan SP, Kernerman PD, Cook DJ, Martin CM, McCormack D, Sibbald WJ 1997 Effect of non-invasive positive pressure ventilation on mortality in patients admitted with acute respiratory failure: a meta-analysis. Critical Care Medicine 25(10): 1685–92
24. Soo Hoo G, Santiago S, Williams A 1994 Nasal mechanical ventilation for hypercapnic respiratory failure in chronic obstructive pulmonary disease. Determinants of success and failure. Critical Care Medicine 22: 1253
25. Parkes S, Bersten A 1997 Aerosol kinetics and bronchodilator efficacy during continuous positive airway pressure delivered by face mask. Thorax 52: 171
26. Menzies R, Gibbons W, Goldberg P 1989 Determinants of weaning and survival among

patients with COPD who require mechanical ventilation for acute respiratory failure. Chest 95: 398

27. Turner MO, Patel A, Ginsburg S, et al 1997 Bronchodilator delivery in acute airflow obstruction: a meta-analysis. Archives of Internal Medicine 157: 1736–44

28. Karpel JP, Pesin J, Greenberg D, Gentry E 1990 A comparison of the effects of ipratropium bromide and metaproterenol sulfate in acute exacerbations of COPD. Chest 98: 835

29. Casaburi R, Mahler DA, Jones PW, et al. 2002 A long-term evaluation of once-daily inhaled tiotropium in chronic obstructive pulmonary

disease. European Respiratory Journal 19(2): 217–24

30. Vincken W, van Noord JA, Greefhorst AP, Bantje TA, Kesten S, Korducki L, Cornelissen PJ Dutch/Belgian Tiotropium Study Group 2002 Improved health outcomes in patients with COPD during 1 yr's treatment with tiotropium. European Respiratory Journal. 19(2): 209–16

31. Rees PJ 2002 Tiotropium in the management of chronic obstructive pulmonary disease. European Respiratory Journal 19(2): 205–6

32. Donohue JF, van Noord JA, Bateman ED, et al 2002 A 6-month, placebo-controlled study comparing lung function and health status changes

in COPD patients treated with tiotropium or salmeterol. Chest 122(1): 47–55

33. Travers A, Jones AP, Kelly K, Barker SJ, Camargo CA Jr, Rowe BH 2002 Intravenous beta2-agonists for acute asthma in the emergency department. (Cochrane Review) In: The Cochrane Library Issue 3. Oxford, Update Software

34. Celli BR 1995 Standards for the diagnosis and care of patients with chronic obstructive pulmonary disease. American Journal of Respiratory Critical Care Medicine 152: S77

35. Gibson PG 1996 Corticosteroids - clinical applications. Exacerbations of asthma in adults. Australian Prescriber 19: 44

5.6 PNEUMOTHORAX

JANET TALBOT-STERN

ESSENTIALS

1 Pneumothorax can occur spontaneously, as a result of trauma, or iatrogenically. Common presenting symptoms are chest pain and dyspnoea.

2 The diagnostic test of choice is a chest X-ray, the expiratory view being the most sensitive.

3 Treatment options include observation, aspiration, thoracostomy and surgery. Video-assisted thoracoscopy has recently become an alternative to thoracotomy for patients with recurrent pneumothoraces or those who have failed conventional therapy.

4 Tension pneumothorax is rarely seen after spontaneous pneumothorax. It is, however, a life-threatening problem and must be managed immediately. It is a clinical, not a radiological, diagnosis.

INTRODUCTION

Pneumothorax is the presence of free air in the interpleural space. Normally the visceral and parietal pleura are in close apposition, with only a potential space between them.

The most common form of pneumothorax is spontaneous. The incidence varies from 2.5 to 18 per 100 000 patients. It has a bimodal distribution with peaks for the young (20–40 years) and those more than 50 years. Primary spontaneous pneumothorax occurs in patients with no obvious pulmonary parenchymal disease. An asymptomatic pulmonary or subpleural bleb (usually apical) ruptures into the pleural space, air leaks from the alveoli, and increased intrapleural pressure collapses the lung. Tall thin males aged 20–40 years who smoke are more likely to develop this form of pneumothorax.

Secondary spontaneous pneumothorax occurs as the result of underlying lung disease with a peak incidence of 60–65 years. Chronic airway limitation, chronic bronchitis and asthma are responsible for the majority of secondary spontaneous pneumothoraces. Less common associated diseases include bacterial or tuberculous pneumonia, cancer, honeycomb lung disorders and cystic fibrosis. Chronic obstruction and bronchospasm cause increased intra-bronchial and intra- alveolar pressures which disrupt weakened and dilated alveolar walls.

Some women with pelvic endometriosis may develop pneumothoraces (predominantly right sided) within 72 hours of menstruation, possibly caused by endometrial metastases to the lungs. HIV patients with active pneumocystis pneumonia, particularly if it is apical, can develop pneumothoraces. There is rupture of necrotic diseased lung tissue, destruction of the alveolar septae, and rupture of bullae which have formed. The incidence has decreased, however, with improvement in prophylaxis and early steroid use. Secondary pneumothorax has also been seen in association those who abuse amphetamine, cocaine, ecstasy, marijuana and nitrous oxide.

Iatrogenic pneumothorax results from central line placement, intercostal blocks, thoracocentesis, lung biopsy, bronchoscopy and high pressures from artificial ventilation. It may occur more commonly with apical procedures, as airflow is greater there than in the bases. Traumatic pneumothorax occurs in up to 15–20% of patients who sustain blunt chest trauma, and is usually secondary to fractured ribs. It may also be the result of penetrating wounds or barotrauma.

In most cases the air leak seals spontaneously, but in some the air continues to leak, and in a subset of these a ball-valve effect can occur, with the development of tension pneumothorax. The trachea and mediastinal structures are pushed away from the collapsed lung, the inferior vena cava may become kinked, and venous return is decreased. The patient develops severe respiratory distress and hypotension. Tension is rare as a complication of spontaneous primary pneumothorax.

CLINICAL FEATURES

History

Symptoms of primary spontaneous pneumothorax often begin suddenly when the patient is at rest, but can be associated with deep inspiration, hyperventilation or coughing. It may also be precipitated by changes in atmospheric pressure that occur with flying and diving. Chest pain on the side of the pneumothorax is the most common presenting symptom (90% of cases). It can be sharp and pleuritic or dull, and may radiate to the back or neck. Dyspnoea occurs in up to 80% of patients but is generally not severe. Some patients, however, may be relatively asymptomatic or become asymptomatic after 24 hours.

Chest pain is less common with secondary pneumothorax and dyspnoea, the predominant presenting complaint, may be severe as patients have less respiratory reserve. Patients are more likely to be hypoxic. In this group the other symptoms include tachycardia, cough and blood-streaked sputum.

Examination

The classic signs of pneumothorax are decreased breath sounds and hyperresonance to percussion; however, at times the chest examination is unremarkable. Less common findings include unilateral enlargement of the chest, decreased excursion of the hemithorax with respirations, inferior liver displacement, Hamman's crunch (a noise heard with each heartbeat from mediastinal emphysema) and subcutaneous emphysema. If the chest is scratched anteriorly on both sides with the stethoscope in the middle, the side with the louder noise represents the pneumothorax. Those with pneumothorax and pneumomediastinum post drug abuse may also have neck pain, sore throat and dysphagia.

Patients who develop tension pneumothorax have evidence of air hunger, distended neck veins, tachycardia, hypo-tension and, classically as a late sign, a deviated trachea.

DIFFERENTIAL DIAGNOSIS

The differential diagnosis of this type of presentation includes costochondritis, pneumonia, pleurisy, pulmonary embolus, exacerbation of bronchospastic disease and myocardial ischaemia.

INVESTIGATIONS

No investigations are indicated for patients with suspected tension pneumothorax and cardiorespiratory compromise. It is a clinical, not a radiologic diagnosis, and requires immediate treatment.

In stable patients with a suspected pneumothorax the investigation of choice is chest X-ray. If there is any doubt an expiratory view, which increases the relative size of the pneumothorax, may be helpful. Findings include hyperlucency, lack of markings at the periphery and a fine line which represents the retraction of the visceral from the parietal pleura. There may also be blunting of the costophrenic angle. If the findings are not convincing, a lateral decubitus view may better reveal air. Large bullae or lung cysts may mimic a pneumothorax, and again a lateral decubitus view may be helpful or a computerized tomography (CT) scan of the chest may be diagnostic.[1]

If a supine X-ray is taken the only clue to a pneumothorax may be a deep sulcus sign on the affected side, an unusually distinct cardiac apex or increased hyperlucency of the upper abdominal quadrants.[2] A cross-table lateral view should confirm the diagnosis. Thoracic ultrasound has recently been advocated if X-ray is delayed.[3] Associated pneumomediastinum is seen in 1.5% of pneumothoraces.

Pneumothoraces are graded as small (<15% or a small rim of air around the lung), moderate (15–60% or collapse halfway towards the heart border) and complete (>60% or an airless lung).

Several methods have been suggested to more accurately estimate the extent of collapse. Clinically useful in the emergency department are the following: the average of the interpleural distance in centimetres at the apex, the upper zone and the lower zone of the frontal chest X-ray approximates the pneumothorax[4] (Fig. 5.5.1). Alternatively the percentage of pneumothorax may be estimated by the formula:

$$100 - \text{average lung diameter/average hemithorax diameter} \times 100.[5]$$

The patient's oxygenation should be assessed as initially there may be a decrease in P_aO_2 from arterial shunting past non-ventilated areas. Pulse oximetry is acceptable in most patients, but arterial blood gases may be necessary in sicker patients.

An ECG will often be part of the assessment, particularly if myocardial ischaemia is a differential diagnosis. Findings may include anterior non-Q wave changes, right axis deviation, decreased R waves or T-wave inversion in the precordial leads, and decreased QRS amplitude.

MANAGEMENT

General measures

All patients should initially receive supplemental oxygen, particularly if hypoxic. This increases the rate of pleural air absorption by at least four times, by decreasing the partial pressure of nitrogen and increasing the gradient for nitrogen absorption. It is useful for both pneumothorax and pneumomediastinum.

Specific treatments

Patients who present in severe respiratory insufficiency or shock should be treated with immediate decompression as a temporizing measure. This involves the placement of a large (e.g. 14 gauge) cannula in the second intercostal space, midclavicular line (or the fifth intercostal space midaxillary line). Definitive therapy is then required.

Present management options for those without a tension pneumothorax include

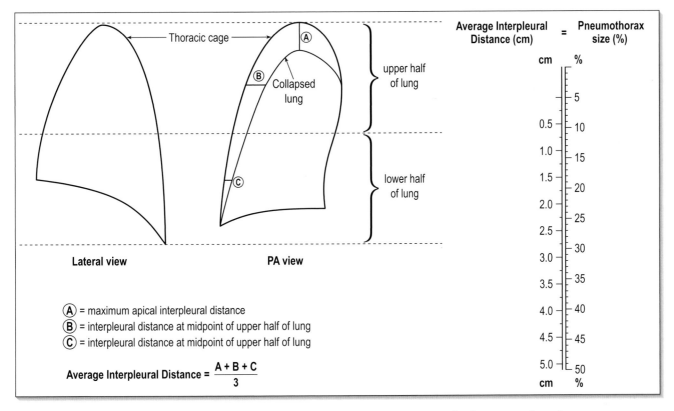

Fig. 5.6.1 Determining the size of pneumothorax in the upright patient. (Reprinted with permission from Rhea JT, De Luca SA, Green RE 1982 Determining the size of pneumothorax in the upright patient. Radiology 144: 727–36).

observation, aspiration, small-lumen catheter drainage, thoracostomy tubes, thoracoscopy and thoracotomy. These treatments, however, are not founded on evidence based medicine, being more individual and institution specific. Fifty years ago much experience of pneumothoraces was in the treatment of tuberculosis, with the creation of unilateral or bilateral pneumothoraces. Patients were managed at home, with spontaneous resolution of the intrapleural air. When healthy patients developed pneumothoraces they were treated by simple aspiration using the same equipment employed to create a pneumothorax in the tuberculous patients.

Subsequently aspiration was abandoned in favour of thoracostomy tubes, with the idea that there would be more rapid lung expansion and better outcome.

Until recently the management of pneumothoraces greater than 15–20% was with wide-bore thoracostomy tubes. Currently, more conservative approaches

are now advocated by most authors. The British Thoracic Society, in response to concerns about the liberal use of intercostal catheters by inexperienced doctors, developed a protocol in 1993.[6] This advocated a more conservative approach that included observation, aspiration for all stable patients, and thoracostomy tubes only if aspiration failed.

Observation

Even without treatment pneumothoraces should resolve. The mean rate of re-expansion of the lung is 1.25% per day, so a 15% pneumothorax could take up to 12 days to dissipate. Generally patients with a primary spontaneous pneumothorax of less than 20% who are without respiratory compromise do not require admission.

Those with underlying lung pathology should be admitted for observation in case there is sudden deterioration or the development of tension pneumothorax. Others have a period of observation in

the emergency department, a repeat X-ray and discharge home if no change has occurred. A subsequent film is taken 24 hours later. Another approach is to X-ray the following day and every 3–5 days afterwards until the lung is fully expanded.[7]

Simple aspiration

The concept of aspiration re-emerged in the 1980s. Up to 80% success has been seen for iatrogenic pneumothoraces, 70% for primary pneumothoraces and 30% for secondary pneumothoraces. It is not indicated for traumatic pneumothoraces or associated haemo- or hydrothorax. There may be a correlation between success and the size of the pneumothorax.[8] Advantages of this method include less pain, ease of procedure, fewer complications and an ability to discharge patients home if successful.

The method involves the placement of a 14 or 16 gauge cannula into the pleural space in the second intercostal space, midclavicular line. The air is aspirated with a 50 mL syringe and a three-way stopcock until the patient feels discomfort, coughs, or no more air is aspirated. It is considered unsuccessful if there is excessive coughing, more than 3 litres is aspirated, or the lung remains unexpanded. An X-ray is done after the procedure and repeated in the ED in 4–6 hours. If the lung remains expanded the patient may be discharged home, with close follow-up and repeat X-ray in 24–48 hours. A method to predict successful outcome using marker gas has been developed. Its presence is predictive of aspiration failure or early recollapse, requiring patients to be admitted for observation even if aspiration was successful. Its absence allowed immediate discharge.[9] The British Thoracic Society (BTS) protocol recommends admission for patients with underlying lung disease after successful aspiration. If immediately unsuccessful or the pneumothorax recurs at 6 hours, alternative therapy is indicated.[6]

However, a recent consensus statement from the American College of Chest Physicians (ACCP) recommends small bore catheters less than 14 Fr or 16–22 thoracostomy tubes rather than aspiration for moderate to large pneumothoraces, because of the perceived high failure rate with aspiration.[10] Additionally, studies looking at the compliance with the BTS guidelines showed that they were not being adhered to. In one case review only 73% of patients had aspiration[11] and a questionnaire in Wales found only 44% would discharge patients with small asymptomatic primary pneumothoraces, 72% would aspirate larger primary pneumothoraces and only 20% would aspirate secondary pneumothoraces.[12]

Small-lumen catheters

These were developed to extend the role of the 16 gauge cannula. They may be placed in the same position as for aspiration, or in the fourth intercostal space, midaxillary line. The operator must be sure there is no lung underlying, as it is placed by the Seldinger technique. They can be used for aspiration but can also be connected to underwater seal

drains or Heimlich valves to manage the pneumothorax if aspiration fails. The most common problem of tube blockage with these small catheters can be prevented by a daily flush with a small volume of saline or a specific pigtail catheter design that decreases blockage. If this method fails after 3 days surgery may be indicated, rather than switching to a thoracostomy tube.[13]

One author feels that these small lumen catheters may replace aspiration. However, all patients would then require admission.[14]

Thoracostomy

Thoracostomy tubes were traditionally placed for all pneumothoraces greater than 15–20% until the re-emergence of aspiration and small lumen catheters. They are still necessary for haemopneumothorax, tension pneumothorax after decompression, traumatic pneumothorax, and when positive-pressure ventilation is planned. In other forms of pneumothorax in stable patients they should only be considered after failure of observation or aspiration. The ACCP recommends them for all secondary pneumothoraces: 16–22 Fr in stable patients, or 24–28 Fr if unstable.[10] Patients should be pretreated with a combination of aliquots of a narcotic and benzodiazepine.

The arm should be raised above the shoulder to open up the rib spaces. After local anaesthesia to the area over the rib at the level of the fourth or fifth intercostal space, anterior axillary line, a 2–3 cm incision is made along the rib. Blunt dissection by tunnelling over the rib with large artery forceps allows access to the pleura. A gush of air confirms release of the pneumothorax. A finger-sweep inside the pleural cavity is essential to check for adhesions, and the thoracostomy tube can then be placed. Connection to an underwater seal prevents the pneumothorax from recurring.

Patients require admission until the lung is fully expanded and no bubbling occurs in expiration. The tube remains in place for an additional 24 hours. Recurrence after thoracostomy tube placement is greater than 25%, and is higher with secondary pneumothorax than

with primary pneumothorax. In some institutions, a chemical pleurodesis agent such as talc, silver nitrate, tetracycline or minocycline is injected via the chest tube to prevent recurrence. Recurrence is then reduced to about 16%.[16] This is often used for AIDS patients even without a demonstrated air leak as the rate of recurrence is high.[1] One institution uses CT to look for bullous disease. If fit for surgery patients undergo pleural abrasion and bullectomy via thoracoscopy; those unfit for surgery undergo only chemical pleurodesis.[2]

Thoracotomy

Axillary thoracotomy with bullectomy, pleural abrasion and partial pleurectomy was, in the past, the routine surgical approach for recurrent pneumothoraces or failure of more conservative treatment. The immediate problem is corrected and an attempt made to prevent recurrence by obliterating the pleural space. It has a low recurrence rate but is associated with morbidity secondary to sputum retention and chest infection.

Thoracoscopy

In the 1990s video assisted thoracoscopy was increasingly used for the treatment of primary pneumothoraces. This involves general anaesthesia with double-lumen endotracheal intubation. It has been recommended for all patients with pneumothoraces,[15] but this is felt by others to be too aggressive for potentially benign disease. Most authors recommend it for patients who continue to have an air leak after 3–7 days, recurrent pneumothoraces, airline pilots, frequent plane travellers and divers, contralateral or bilateral pneumothoraces, and failure of sclerosant through the chest tube.[15–19]

A range of techniques are used according to the findings, including pleurodesis with talc or scarification, blebectomy and/or bullectomy with electrocautery and stapling. It is not used routinely for secondary pneumothoraces and patients need to be carefully selected.[20] An alternative more controversial treatment involves thoracoscopy under local anaesthesia and nitrous oxide/oxygen inhalation with insufflation of talc.

PROGNOSIS

Recurrence after the first pneumothorax is up to 50% for primary and secondary pneumothoraces, half of which occur within 4 months.[17] This increases to 60-70% for subsequent recurrences.

DISPOSITION

Patients with small, asymptomatic primary pneumothoraces and those with primary pneumothoraces successfully treated with simple aspiration may be discharged home, with close follow-up. All other patients require admission for either observation or definitive management.

CONCLUSION

Spontaneous primary pneumothorax is an essentially benign condition and intervention should be kept to a minimum. Patients with a pneumothorax less than 20% can be observed as outpatients, with careful follow-up. Simple aspiration may still be considered as initial treatment for these patients followed by small-lumen catheter drainage rather than wide-bore thoracostomy tubes if unsuccessful. Although spontaneous secondary pneumothorax can be associated with greater respiratory distress, an initial conservative management may be indicated in the absence of tension pneumothorax. If that

CONTROVERSIES

❶ Is aspiration still the appropriate first treatment for stable primary pneumothoraxes or should they all now be treated with small lumen catheters?

❷ Could stable patients with small lumen catheters be safely discharged home with heimlich flutter valves?

❸ If patients fail conservative therapy, should they have a thoracostomy tube placed or be referred for thoracoscopy?

❹ Should all patients with pneumothoraces, regardless of aetiology, be referred for surgical evaluation now that thoracoscopy is available, rather than thoracotomy with its attendant risks?

is unsuccessful more aggressive treatment in the form of tube thoracostomy or thoracoscopy should be initiated.

REFERENCES

1. Sahn S, Heffner JE 2000 Spontaneous pneumothorax. New England Journal of Medicine 343(12): 868–74
2. Karnik AM. 2001 Management of pneumothorax and barotrauma: Current concepts. Com Ther 27(4): 311–21
3. Dulchavsky SA. Schwarz KL, et al 2001 Prospective evaluation of Thoracic ultrasound in the detection of pneumothorax. Journal of Trauma 50: 201–5
4. Rhea JJ, Deluca SA, Green RE 1980 Determining the size of pneumothorax in the upright patient. Radiology 130: 25
5. Noppen M, Alexander P, et al 2001 Quantification of the size of primary spontaneous pneumothorax: accuracy of the light index.Respiration 68: 396–9
6. Miller AC, Harvey JE Guidelines for the management of spontaneous pneumothorax. British Medical Journal 307: 114–6
7. Kelly AM 1993 Options in the management of spontaneous pneumothorax. Emergency Medicine 5: 201–8
8. Aplin P 1996 Size does make a difference in the management of pneumothorax. Emergency Medicine 8: 221–5
9. Kiely DG, Ansari S, et al 2001 Bedside tracer gas technique accurately predicts outcome in aspiration of spontaneous pneumothorax. Thorax 56: 617–21
10. Baumann Mh. Strange C, et al 2001 Management of Spontaneous Pneumothorax. An American College of Chest Physicians Delphi Consensus Statement. Chest 119: 590–602
11. Mendia, El-Shanawany T, et al 2002 Management of spontaneous pneumothorax: are British Thoracic Society guidelines being followed. Postgraduate Medicine J 78: 80–4
12. Yeoh JH, Ansare S, et al 2000 Management of spontaneous pneumothorax – a Welsh survey. Postgrad Med J 76: 496–500
13. Martin T, Fontana G, Olak J, et al 1996 Use of a pleural catheter for the management of simple pneumothorax. 110(5): 1169–72
14. Hart SP 2001 Management of spontaneous pneumothorax.Letters to the editor. Postgraduate Medicine 77: 215–6
15. Schramel FM, Sutedja TG, et al 1996 Cost-effectiveness of video-assisted thoracoscopic surgery versus conservative treatment for first time or recurrent spontaneous pneumothorax. European Respiratory Journal 9: 1821–5
16. Yim AP, Ho JK, et al 1995 Primary spontaneous pneumothorax treated by video assisted thoracoscopic surgery – results of intermediate follow up. Australian and New Zealand Journal of Medicine 25: 146–50
17. Light RW 1993 Management of spontaneous pneumothorax. American Review of Respiratory Disease 148: 245–8
18. Frexinet J, Canalis E, et al 1997 Surgical treatment of primary spontaneous pneumothorax with video-assisted thoracic surgery. European Respiratory Journal 10: 409–11
19. Waller DA 1997 Video assisted thoracoscopic surgery (VATS) in the management of spontaneous pneumothorax. Thorax 52: 307–8
20. Yim AP, Ng CSH 2001 Thoracoscopy in the management of Pneumothorax. Current Opinion in Pulmonary Medicine 7: 210–4

5.7 PLEURAL EFFUSION

SUZANNE MASON

ESSENTIALS

1 In the vast majority of patients a posteroanterior and lateral chest X-ray will confirm and localize an effusion. Lateral decubitus films, ultrasound and CT scanning are more sensitive in diagnosing and localizing small effusions.

2 Pleural fluid analysis is the principal investigation to determine the underlying cause of the effusion. The key to management is the differentiation of transudates from exudates.

3 Pleural biopsy improves the diagnostic yield in the presence of TB and malignancy to 80% and 90%, respectively, when combined with pleural fluid analysis.

4 Treatment is dependent on the underlying disease. Large pleural effusions with cardiorespiratory compromise should be aspirated to provide symptomatic relief.

5 Transudates respond to treatment of the underlying condition. Exudates usually require further investigative procedures and specific local treatments.

INTRODUCTION

A pleural effusion is an accumulation of fluid in the pleural space as a result of a disruption of the homeostatic forces that control normal flow. Massive pleural effusions may produce significant cardio-respiratory compromise requiring urgent attention in the emergency department. However, many are asymptomatic or produce minimal disturbance. In this latter group the role of the emergency physician is to ascertain the aetiology of the effusion, as this dictates the most appropriate treatment.

Much information regarding the likely cause can be obtained by a thorough history and physical examination. Important adjuvant investigations include the chest X-ray, the examination of pleural fluid and biopsies obtained during thoracocentesis. Bronchoscopy and thoracoscopy have a role to play in the small group of patients in whom the above procedures fail to establish a cause, but their use is beyond the scope of initial emergency department assessment and stabilization.

PATHOPHYSIOLOGY

The pleural cavity in health is a small space bordered by the visceral and parietal pleura. It contains between 1 mL and 15 mL of clear fluid.[1] The pleura act as semipermeable membranes and fluid movement is determined principally by capillary pressure and plasma oncotic pressures and capillary permeability, governed by Starling's Law. Net flow is from parietal pleura to visceral pleura via the pleural cavity. Additional pleural fluid drainage occurs via pleurolymphatic communications or stomas augmented by an active muscle pump. Overall absorptive capacity exceeds production by a factor of 10–20. Pleural effusions occur in one of the following:

- Disturbances in the hydrostatic-osmotic pressure gradients, resulting in a transudate.
- Pleural inflammation with loss of semipermeable membrane function, resulting in a protein-rich exudate.
- Lymphatic obstruction (usually producing a transudate).

Transudates are ultrafiltrates of plasma and arise as a result of a relatively small number of conditions. Exudates are produced by a wider variety of inflammatory conditions and often require more extensive investigation.

AETIOLOGY

Tables 5.7.1 and 5.7.2 list the causes of transudative and exudative pleural effusions. The commonest causes are congestive cardiac failure, pneumonia and malignancy.[2]

CLASSIFICATION

Pleural effusions are classified according to their aetiology as transudates or exudates. Light first proposed the criteria to differentiate the two. This involved measurement of both serum and pleural markers[3]. An exudate is present if one or more of the following three are present:

1 Ratio of pleural-fluid LDH level to serum LDH level >0.6

2 Pleural-fluid LDH level > two-thirds upper limit of normal for serum LDH level

3 Ratio of pleural-fluid protein level to serum protein level >0.5.

If the fluid is found to be an exudate, then further tests are required to determine the underlying cause of disease.

CLINICAL FEATURES

History

The history will often identify the cause of a pleural effusion. Features suggestive of the common causes (congestive heart failure, pneumonia, malignancy and pulmonary embolism) should be sought. Specific questioning regarding previous occupational exposures, drug treatments,

Table 5.7.1 Causes of exudative pleural effusions

Infectious
Bacterial pneumonia
Tuberculosis
Parasites
Fungal disease
Atypical pneumonia
Nocardia, actinomyces
Subphrenic abscess
Hepatic abscess
Splenic abscess
Hepatitis
Spontaneous oesophageal rupture

Iatrogenic
Drug-induced (nitrofurantion, dantrolene, methysergide, procarbazine, methotrexate, medications causing drug-induced lupus syndrome such as procainamide, hydralazine, quinidine)
Oesophageal perforation
Oesophageal sclerotherpay
Central venous catheterization
Enteral feeding

Malignancy
Carcinoma
Lymphoma
Mesothelioma
Leukemia
Chylothorax

Other inflammatory disorders
Pancreatitis
Benign asbestos pleural effusion
Pulmonary embolism
Radiation therapy
Uraemic pleurisy
Sarcoidosis
Postcardiac injury syndrome
Haemothorax
ARDS

Increased negative intrapleural pressure
Atelectasis
Cholesterol effusion

Connective tissue disease
Lupus pleuritis
Rheumatoid pleurisy
Mixed connective tissue disease
Churg-Strauss syndrome
Wegener granulomatosis
Familial Mediterranean fever

Endocrine dysfunction
Hypothyroidism
Ovarian hyperstimulation syndrome

Lymphatic abnormalities
Malignancy
Yellow nail syndrome
Lymphangiomyomatosis

Movement of fluid from the abdomen to pleural space
Pancreatitis
Pancreatic pseudocyst
Meigs syndrome
Carcinoma
Chylous ascites

Table 5.7.2 Causes of transudative pleural effusions

Effusion always transudative
Congestive cardiac failure
Cirrhosis
Nephrotic syndrome
Peritonael dialysis
Hypoalbuminaemia
Urinothorax
Atelectasis
Constrictive pericarditis
Superior vena caval obstruction

'Classic' exudates that can be transudates
Malignancy
Pulmonary embolism
Sarcoidosis
Hypothyroidism

radiation therapy, trauma, tuberculosis exposure and collagen vascular disease may be rewarding. Pleural effusions rarely cause symptoms other than dyspnoea, although a mild non-productive cough is sometimes described. A more severe or productive cough suggests underlying pulmonary pathology. Chest pain in association with an effusion may indicate malignancy, pulmonary embolus or pleural inflammation. More unusually a chest wall swelling may be due to metastatic cancer or an expanding empyema.

Patients may have myriad associated systemic symptoms due to the underlying pathological process such as fever, weight loss, abdominal and joint pain.

Physical examination

Small effusions may be undetectable clinically. However, mild hypoxemia is common in patients, often associated with dyspnoea which can be due to distortions of the diaphragm or chest wall during respiration. The classic signs of pleural effusion are reduced chest-wall expansion, stony dullness to percussion, diminished or absent vocal resonance and tactile fremitus on the affected side and absent breath sounds. In large unilateral effusions, tracheal displacement toward the unaffected side may be detected. In addition, signs of underlying disease should be sought.

INVESTIGATIONS

Chest X-ray

In the majority of patients a postero-anterior and lateral chest X-ray will provide the required information to confirm and localize an effusion. The classic radiological features of effusion are of a gravity-dependent homogenous opacity within the pleural cavity with a concave lateral air-fluid interface (meniscus sign). Effusions greater than 150 mL are seen as blunting of costophrenic angles on erect films. Very small and/or isolated effusions may not be seen on standard views.

Occasionally the collection may be subpulmonary. Signs suggestive of this include apparent elevation of the diaphragm, abnormal diaphragmatic contour (lateral displacement of the apex on PA film, sharp angulation of apparent anterior diaphragm on lateral film), and more than a 2 cm space between the gastric bubble and apparent left diaphragm.

Lateral decubitus films are often helpful where a fluid level at least 1 cm deep indicates that the effusion is accessible by thoracocentesis. If the fluid does not form a uniform level, this may indicate the presence of a loculated effusion that requires more careful management. Chest ultrasound and computerized tomography (CT) are more sensitive in diagnosing and localizing small effusions. CT can also be helpful in examining the lung parenchyma and mediastinum for associated pathology.

The chest X-ray can also provide other diagnostic clues to the aetiology of the effusion. Large effusions with lack of mediastinal shift indicate a bronchial obstruction, infiltration of the lung with tumour, mesothelioma or a fixed mediastinum (due to tumour or fibrosis). Bilateral effusions with an enlarged heart shadow are usually due to congestive cardiac failure. Pleural plaques and calcification indicate asbsetos exposure and findings consistent with pneumonia or malignancy may indicate a cause for the associated effusion.

Thoracocentesis

If the diagnosis is known (e.g. congestive heart failure with recurrent effusions) further investigations need only be performed to aid management of the underlying problem. When the diagnosis is still uncertain the most useful investigation is diagnostic thoracocentesis. A variety of techniques have been reported, but the common underlying principle is the advancement of a needle, trocar or cannula into the pleural space under strict aseptic conditions, and the withdrawal of a volume of fluid for analysis. Fluid should be procured for biochemical, microbiological and cytological analysis in order to classify the effusion as outlined above and indicate an underlying cause.

The gross apperance of the pleural fluid can be helpful in diagnosis. Table 5.7.3 outlines the common differentials according to gross findings. With respect to exudates, microscopy, Gram stain and cytology should be performed. The diagnostic yield in malignant disease ranges from 50 to 80%[4] and is improved with larger-volume collections and repeated sampling. Pleural fluid pH may be helpful in diagnosis. In parapneumonic effusions, a pH < 7.2 indicates the need for urgent drainage of the effusion whereas a pH >7.3 suggests that treatment with systemic antibiotics should be sufficient management.[5] In malignant effusions, a pleural pH <7.3 indicates more extensive pleural involvement and shorter survival times.[6] A low pleural fluid pH also correlates well with glucose levels. Glucose <0.5 times serum is suggestive of bacterial infection, malignancy or rheumatoid arthritis. An elevated amylase in the pleural fluid suggests oesophageal rupture, effusion associated with pancreatitis, or malignancy. Pleural fluid antinuclear antibody and rheumatoid factor tests should be ordered when collagen vascular diseases are suspected.

There are no absolute contraindications to thoracocentesis, but relative contraindications include bleeding diathesis or anticoagulation, small fluid volumes, mechanical ventilation and cutaneous disease over the proposed puncture site.[7,8] The puncture location is chosen based on clinical examination and chest X-ray findings. Smaller effusions can often be located with ultrasound guidance.

Additional techniques

Two other procedures may be considered when thoracocentesis is not diagnostic. Percutaneous pleural biopsy involves obtaining a closed biopsy of the parietal pleura using either an Abrams or Cope needle. It is relatively easy to perform and improves the diagnostic yield in the presence of tuberculosis and malignancy to 80% and 90% respectively, when combined with pleural fluid analysis. The second is thoracoscopy, which involves pleural biopsy under direct visualization through a thoracoscope. Thoracoscopy has a very high yield for diagnosing both benign and malignant pleural disease, however, it requires general anesthesia and is usually employed only after other procedures are non-diagnostic.

Table 5.7.3 Gross appearance of pleural fluid[2]		
Appearance of fluid	Test indicated	Interpretation of result
Bloody	Haematocrit	<1% non-sigificant 1–20% malignancy, pulmonary embolus, trauma >50% haemothorax
Cloudy or turbid	Centrifugation Triglyceride level	Turbid supernatant – high lipid levels >110mg/dL chylothorax >50mg/dL need lipoprotein analysis Chylomicrons chylothorax <50 mg/dL and cholsterol>250mg/dL pseudochylothorax
Putrid odour	Gram stain and culture	Possible anaerobic infetion

MANAGEMENT

If a pleural effusion is causing respiratory distress it should be drained regardless of whether it is a transudate or an exudate. Drainage of a relatively small volume of fluid can cause significant relief from symptoms. All patients undergoing this procedure should be well oxygenated with oxygen saturations monitored and kept above 90% since thoracocentesis may increase ventilation-perfusion mismatches.[9] Removal of large volumes (usually more than 1500 mL) may produce reexpansion pulmonary oedema, so large effusions should be drained in stages, with at least 12 hours between procedures.

All transudates should be managed by treating the underlying disease. Large-bore tube thoracostomy should be employed for empyema and traumatic haemothorax. Empyemas tend to loculate early, in which case 250 000 units of streptokinase may be instilled to dissolve the fibrin membranes. Should this fail, surgical drainage or decortication should be performed. Systemic organism-specific antibiotic therapy should also be instituted.

Malignant effusions can be managed by thoracostomy and tetracycline pleurodesis, thoracoscopy and talc poudrage, or pleuroperitoneal shunt. Chylothoraces should be treated by pleuroperitoneal shunting, as long-term drainage may result in malnutrition and altered immunocompetence.

COMPLICATIONS

Pleural effusions can produce significant respiratory distress alleviated only through drainage. Other complications are those of the underlying pathological process such as fever and toxicity in the case of parapneumonic effusions.

There are recognized complications associated with thoracocentesis such as pain at the puncture site, cutaneous or internal bleeding, pneumothorax, empyema and splenic or hepatic puncture.[7] Pneumothorax complicates around 12% of thoracocenteses. Those at increased risk of complication include patients with chronic obstructive or fibrotic pulmonary disease previous chest irradiation, using larger thoracocentesis needles, multiple passes to obtain fluid and aspiration of air during the procedure.[10,11]

DISPOSITION

The requirement for inpatient investigation and management will depend on the degree of respiratory compromise, the presence of coexisting or underlying disease, and the patient's wishes. In many cases chronic relapsing effusions in the otherwise stable patient may be managed on an outpatient basis.

SUMMARY

Pleural effusion complicates many local and systemic illnesses. The vast majority can be detected with a good history, physical examination and a chest X-ray. The key to management is the differentiation of transudates from exudates. In general transudates respond to treatment of the underlying condition. Exudates usually require further investigative procedures and specific local treatments.

REFERENCES

1. Light RW 1995 Diseases of the pleura, mediastinum, chest wall and diaphragm. In: George RB, et al (eds) Chest Medicine: Essentials of Pulmonary and Critical Care Medicine, 3rd edn. Williams & Wilkins, Baltimore
2. Light RW 2002 Pleural Effusion. New England Journal of Medicine 346(25): 1971–7
3. Light RW, Macgregor MI, Luchsinger PC, Ball WC Jr 1972 Plerual Effusions: the diagnostic separation of transudates and exudates. Annals of Internal Medicine 77: 507–13
4. Health and Public Policy Committee 1985 American College of Physicians. Diagnostic thoracocentesis and pleural biopsy. Position paper. Annals of Internal Medicine 103: 799–802
5. Good JT Jr, Taryle DA, Maulitz RM, Kaplan RL, Sahn SA 1980 The diagnostic value of pleural fluid pH. Chest 78(1): 55–9
6. Sahn SA, Good JT Jr 1988 Pleural fluid pH in malignant effusions: diagnostic, prognostic, and therapeutic implications. Annals of Internal Medicine 108(3): 345–9
7. Sahn SA 1988 State of the art: the pleura. American Review of Respiratory Disease 138(1): 184–234
8. Bartter T, Santarelli R, Akers SM, Pratter MR 1994 The evaluation of pleural effusion. Chest 106(4): 1209–14 [Erratum, Chest 1995;107(2): 592]
9. Estenne M, Yernault JC, De Troyer A 1983 Mechanism of relief of dyspnoea after thoracocentesis in patients with large pleural effusions. American Journal of Medicine 74(5): 813–9
10. Doyle JJ, Hnatiuk OW, Torrington KG 1996 Necessity of routine chest roentgenography after thoracocentesis. Annals of Internal Medicine 124(9): 816–20
11. Raptopoulos V, Davis LM, Lee G 1991 Factors affecting the development of pneumothorax aasociated with thoracocentesis. Americal Journal of Roentgenology 156(5): 917–20

FURTHER READING

Boutin C, et al 1990 The role of thoracoscopy in the evaluation and management of pleural effusions. Lung (Suppl): 113–21
Burgess KR 1997 MJA practice essential 3. The chest wall and pleural space. Medical Journal of Australia 166: 604–9
Pleural disease. In: Rosen P, et al 1992 Emergency Medicine Concepts and Clinical Practice, 3rd edn. Mosby, St Louis

5.8 HAEMOPTYSIS

STUART DILLEY

ESSENTIALS

1 The majority of patients are stable and can be managed as outpatients.

2 Patients may have difficulty differentiating between haemoptysis and haematemesis.

3 Chest X-ray is normal in 20–30% of patients with haemoptysis.

4 Bronchoscopy is the specific investigation of choice if haemoptysis is thought to be due to a lesion in the bronchial tree.

5 In 30% of cases, no cause for haemopytysis will be found.

6 The priorities in massive haemoptysis are the maintenance of ventilation, circulatory support and the identification of the source of bleeding.

INTRODUCTION

Most patients who present with haemoptysis describe small amounts of blood mixed with sputum or saliva. The majority of patients are stable and can be managed as outpatients. Rarely, patients present with massive haemoptysis where respiratory and circulatory systems are severely compromised and death by asphyxiation can be quite rapid. These patients require urgent skillful management of airway and circulatory systems. Nonetheless, by obstructing an airway, a small blood clot may compromise ventilation just as effectively as a massive bleed that floods an entire lung.

AETIOLOGY

The causes of haemoptysis are summarized below. In approximately 30% of cases no cause will be found (see Table 5.8.1).

CLINICAL ASSESSMENT

The relative importance of resuscitation, history, examination, and investigation in patients presenting with haemoptysis depends very much on the degree of bleeding and respiratory compromise. Most patients do not have compromised respiratory or circulatory systems, so the emphasis is on clinical assessment.

Patients may have difficulty in differentiating between haemoptysis and haematemesis. Bronchial blood is usually bright red, frothy and alkaline, while gastrointestinal blood is usually darker, may be mixed with food particles, and is acidic. History and examination should be tailored to elicit information relevant to the common causes of haemoptysis as listed above.

INVESTIGATIONS

Imaging

Chest X-ray

Between 20 and 30% of patients with haemoptysis will have a normal chest X-ray. 'Abnormal' X-rays tend to reflect pre-existing chronic lung disease rather than identifying a definitive cause for the bleeding. Evidence of infection, abscess formation, tuberculosis, bronchiectasis or tumours may be seen.

Computerized tomography

Computerized tomography (CT) of the chest may occasionally provide additional information not evident on chest X-ray, and is particularly useful in cases of bronchocarcinoma and bronchiectasis to further delineate anatomy.

Other

Ventilation-perfusion scan, CT angiography and other investigations may be indicated if the diagnosis is thought to be pulmonary embolism.

Pulmonary and bronchial angiography may be indicated if bleeding is ongoing and no source is found by other means.

Bronchoscopy

Bronchoscopy allows direct visualization of the bronchial tree and the source of bleeding, and is the specific investigation of choice in cases of haemoptysis thought to be due to abnormalities of the bronchial tree. In the case of massive haemoptysis, bronchoscopy should be performed early. It should also be performed on those patients diagnosed with pneumonia or bronchitis who continue to bleed or who do not respond to antibiotic therapy. In addition to direct

Table 5.8.1	
Pulmonary	*Extra-pulmonary*
Pneumonia	Pulmonary embolism
Neoplasm	Coagulopathies
Bronchitis	Mitral stenosis
Lung abscess	Oral or pharyngeal blood
Bronchiectasis	Heart failure
Tuberculosis	Thoracic aortic aneurysm
Connective tissue disorder	Oesophageal carcinoma
Arterio-venous malformation	

visualization of the bronchial tree, bronchoscopy facilitates the gathering of sputum and cytological samples for further analysis.

Rigid bronchoscopy allows for more complete removal of blood and better ventilation in the case of massive haemoptysis, although upper lobe airways are not well visualized. The fibreoptic bronchoscope (FOB) is more flexible and thinner and can be used to visualize areas of the bronchial tree not seen by the rigid bronchoscope. It cannot cope with the large volumes of blood that need suctioning in massive haemoptysis, but can be passed down the lumen of the rigid bronchoscope once the majority of blood has been removed.

Sputum

When the origin of haemoptysis is thought to be infective or neoplastic, sputum should be collected for bacteriological and cytological assessment, including Zeihl-Neelsen staining for acid-fast bacilli.

Other

Haemoglobin, platelet count, and clotting studies will usually be normal in an otherwise healthy individual. A raised white cell count may indicate the presence of infection. Arterial blood gases and/or pulse oximetry are useful for the patient with respiratory distress and massive bleeding, or when pulmonary embolism is being considered. Blood cross-matching may be needed in the case of massive haemoptysis.

DISPOSITION

In most cases haemoptysis is mild and transient and is usually due to an infective process. If so, patients can be discharged on appropriate antibiotics for outpatient or general practitioner follow-up of sputum studies, repeat chest X-rays, CT scans and bronchoscopy, as indicated. Those with respiratory compromise, pulmonary emboli or carcinoma should be managed accordingly.

MASSIVE HAEMOPTYSIS

Massive haemoptysis is rare, accounting for less than 2 % of all cases of haemoptysis. It is not only frightening to the patient, but can also test the skill of the emergency physician. Usually originating from the high-pressure bronchial arteries, massive haemoptysis has been arbitrarily defined by various authors as being as little as 100 mL to as much as 1000 mL of blood loss in 24 hours.[1] Exsanguinating haemoptysis of more than 150 mL per hour and a loss of more than 1000 mL per day has a mortality of 75%.[2]

The general principles of 'ABCs' apply as in all serious illness. The immediate threat to the patient is asphyxia. Patients may rapidly become severely hypoxic, restless and uncooperative, and immediate intubation may be necessary. The airway should be vigorously suctioned and supplemental oxygen administered. Blood should be collected for full blood count, cross-matching and arterial blood gases, and intravenous fluids or blood infused through one or more large bore IV cannulae. Although it is customary to nurse the patient with the suspected bleeding lung dependant to prevent aspiration into the normal lung,[1,3] some have argued that this may increase the rate of bleeding.[4] The Trendelenburg position is also recommended to aid drainage of blood from the thorax.

The need to secure an airway provides a dilemma for the emergency physician. A large bore endotracheal tube (ETT) will permit ventilation but may not protect the lungs. However, it will allow the passage of an FOB and large bore suction catheter to both visualize the bronchial tree and remove blood. In extreme circumstances, the ETT may be advanced into the right main-stem bronchus to protect the right lung if bleeding appears to be left sided, but may lead to occlusion of the right upper lobe bronchus. The ETT can be used to guide a balloon occlusion catheter into the right main-stem bronchus to tampo-

nade the right lung if bleeding appears to be right sided, although the ETT will then need to be replaced so that circuit connections can still be made. Blindly advancing the ETT into the left main bronchus is a more difficult procedure. Balloon catheters may be more accurately placed under bronchosopic guidance.[1]

Double lumen tubes, such as the Robertshaw or Carlen tubes, provide protection for the normal lung and a chance to suction or tamponade the bleeding lung. However, they may not be readily available in the emergency department and take considerably more skill to insert than a standard single-lumen ETT. High rates of misplacement have been reported.[3] They are also too narrow to allow the passage of a FOB, and hence limit further assessment of the bleeding source. They are perhaps best reserved for use after bronchoscopy has been performed.[5]

In a survey of 227 delegates at the American College of Chest Physicians meeting in 1998,[6] 85% agreed that early endotracheal intubation was desirable for life-threatening haemoptysis. Fifty-seven per cent favoured a large bore single lumen tube. While 43% preferred a double lumen tube, only 29% of respondents felt they were proficient in its use, deferring to their anaesthesia colleagues for insertion.

Urgent bronchoscopy should be performed early in unstable patients with massive haemoptysis.[1] Bronchoscopy can help to localize the source of bleeding and may facilitate the passage of a balloon-tip catheter into the bleeding bronchus for tamponade of the bleeding source.

Based on several retrospective studies quoting mortality rates of 78–85% for 'operable patients' treated conservatively, surgical resection of the bleeding site and adjacent lung has traditionally been the treatment of choice for massive haemoptysis. It may be difficult to identify the source of the bleeding, however, and most surgeons prefer to operate on a stable patient whose bleeding has ceased. Some patients will not have the pulmonary reserve to cope with a partial or full lobectomy.

Some authors have suggested a more conservative approach.[7] Conservative management, including airway management, suction, endobronchial balloon tamponade, antibiotics, iced saline lavage, topical adrenaline (epinephrine) and bronchial artery embolization resulted in mortality rates of 0–25% in these studies. In their opinion, surgery should be reserved for patients who continue to suffer massive haemoptysis despite these measures.

Radiologically guided bronchial artery embolization is a useful procedure, halting bleeding in most patients. Twenty per cent of patients will re-bleed within 6 months, and 50 % will have significant bleeds in the longer term.[8] However, this procedure may buy some time to allow thoracotomy to be performed semi-electively. Significant complications such as spinal cord injury and arterial dissection, although rare, have been reported.

CONTROVERSIES

❶ What is the appropriate positioning for the patient with massive haemoptysis?

❷ Should CT scan or bronchoscopy be the investigation of choice following CXR?

❸ What method of endotracheal or endobronchial intubation is most appropriate for acute massive haemoptysis in the emergency department?

❹ Should rigid or flexible bronchoscopy be used to assess massive haemoptysis?

❺ Conservative versus operative management of massive haemoptysis.

REFERENCES

1. Dweik R, Stoller J, 1999 Role of bronchoscopy in massive hemoptysis. Clinics in Chest Medicine 20: 89–105
2. Rudzinski JP, delCastillo J 1987 Massive Hemoptysis. Annals of Emergency Medicine 16(5): 561–4
3. Jean-Baptiste E. 2000. Clinical assessment and management of massive haemoptysis. Critical Care Medicine 28: 1642–7
4. Patel U, Pattison CW, Raphael M 1994 Management of massive haemoptysis. British Journal of Hospital Medicine 52: 74–8
5. Goldman J 1989 Hemoptysis: Emergency assessment and management. Emergency Medicine Clinics of North America 7(2): 325–38
6. Haponik E, Fein A, Chin R 2000 Managing life-threatening hemoptysis. Has anything really changed? Chest 118: 1431–5
7. Jones D, Davies R 1990 Massive haemoptysis: Medical management will usually arrest the bleeding. British Medical Journal 300: 889–90
8. Marshall T, Flower C, Jackson J 1996 Review: The role of radiology in the investigation and management of patients with haemoptysis. Clinical Radiology 51: 391–400

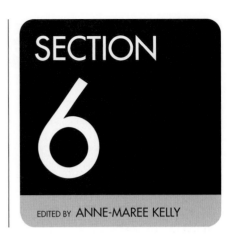

SECTION 6

EDITED BY ANNE-MAREE KELLY

DIGESTIVE

6.1 Dysphagia 304

6.2 Bowel obstruction 306

6.3 Hernia 309

6.4 Gastroenteritis 311

6.5 Haematemesis and melaena 316

6.6 Peptic ulcer disease and gastritis 322

6.7 Biliary tract disease 326

6.8 Pancreatitis 329

6.9 Acute appendicitis 332

6.10 Inflammatory bowel disease 335

6.11 Acute liver failure 338

6.12 Rectal bleeding 341

6.13 Perianal conditions 344

6.1 DYSPHAGIA

GRAEME THOMSON

ESSENTIALS

1 Dysphagia presents emergency physicians with diagnostic challenges and a broad differential diagnosis should be considered. A carefully taken history will reveal the likely cause in most cases.

2 A patient with dysphagia may be at risk of aspiration, particularly if it is the result of neurological dysfunction. An assessment of that risk should be made prior to allowing the patient to take oral fluids or food.

3 A patient with moderate to long-term dysphagia may have significant fluid and electrolyte abnormalities and may have severe nutritional disturbances.

4 Emergency-department investigations should be directed to the detection of high-grade obstructions and lesions causing significant risks from airway compromise, haemorrhage or sepsis. Most other investigations to detect abnormalities of function or inflammation are non-urgent.

5 Dysphagia is very rarely caused by a psychological disorder. There is nearly always a physical cause to be found.

INTRODUCTION

Dysphagia is a broad term encompassing the many forms of difficulty with deglutition (swallowing). The main issues are to determine the likely causes, to identify those patients at risk of significant complications, to treat those causes that are amenable to acute intervention and to refer appropriately for further investigations and treatment.

Dysphagia may be associated with odynophagia (pain on swallowing). Globus is a related term that means the sensation of a lump in the throat. This is rarely of psychological origin. Since the advent of sophisticated investigative techniques it has been recognized that in the great majority of cases there is an identifiable physical cause.

CLINICAL FEATURES

Symptoms may appear suddenly or develop insidiously. If insidious there may be an acute precipitating event leading to presentation, often complete or partial obstruction due to impaction of a food bolus in the oesophagus. This may present as pain, a feeling of a lump in the neck or central chest, severe retching or drooling with inability to swallow saliva. Patients may report increasing difficulty swallowing solids and then fluids but in some cases there may be no previous history of dysphagia. Several drugs are recognized to induce odynophagia or dysphagia. They include antibiotics such as tetracyclines, nonsteroidal anti-inflammatory drugs, ascorbic acid, quinidine, ferrous sulphate and potassium chloride.

Where a neurological disorder is causing difficulty initiating swallowing there may be other neurological deficits and the patient may not be able to give a history. Regurgitation of food from the mouth or nose, coughing or frank aspiration may be evident when the patient eats. It should be assumed that patients with recent cerebrovascular events or bulbar dysfunction are dysphagic until formal assessment of swallowing and airway protection can be undertaken.

Examination is often unrewarding but should focus on careful examination of cranial nerve function and examination of the neck, chest and abdomen.

INVESTIGATION

Investigations are directed by the history and likely aetiology.

For oropharyngeal and upper oesophageal lesions a lateral X-ray of the soft tissues of the neck may reveal a lesion impinging on the oesophagus. An impacted dense bone or other solid foreign body may also be seen. Video oesophagoscopy is the best semi-elective investigation. It will reveal structural abnormalities as well as disorders of muscular coordination. Endoscopy may also be indicated. Manometric studies are less reliable.

Table 6.1.1 Causes of dysphagia

Oropharyngeal dysphagia
Abnormalites of neurological function
Cerebrovascular accidents
Motor neurone disease
Parkinson's disease
Cerebral tumours
Cerebral palsy
Other degenerative diseases

Abnormalities of muscular function
Muscular dystrophies
Various types of myositis
Upper oesophageal sphincter dysfunction

Local structural abnormalities
Dental diseases
Infections and inflammatory lesions
Tumours
Trauma
Pharyngeal diverticulae
Cervical masses

Oesophageal dysphagia
Abnormalities of muscular function
Scleroderma
Achalasia
Lower oesophageal sphincter dysfunction

Abnormalities of luminal structure
Tumours
Foreign bodies
Strictures
Oesophageal webs

Abnormalities of adjacent structures
Retrosternal thyroid
Mediastinal tumours
Thoracic aortic aneurysms and other enlarged vessels

For suspected mid and lower oesophageal lesions, frontal and lateral chest radiographs may reveal a mediastinal tumour, tuberculous lesions or an aneurysm of the thoracic aorta. Oesophageal perforation may also be detected. A formal gastrograffin swallow or computerized tomography (CT) scan may be indicated, but in most cases can be deferred and performed on a semi-elective basis. Endoscopy is usually indicated as part of the investigation of this region.

Electrolytes and full blood examination are usually indicated to detect electrolyte disturbances and anaemia.

MANAGEMENT

Definitive treatment varies with the underlying cause and will rarely be completed in the emergency department. The degree of oesophageal obstruction, the acuity of onset and the presence of complications dictate the need for emergency treatment. Patients with high-grade obstruction should have oral fluids and food withheld and should be given intravenous fluids if the obstruction persists for more than a few hours. For food bolus obstruction endoscopic removal will be required in many cases, although this is usually attempted after a period of expectant treatment.

Intramuscular or intravenous glucagon may relax oesophageal muscles enough to allow a bolus to pass through. An initial dose of 1 mg may be followed by a 2 mg dose if necessary. Complications are rare but include allergy, nausea and hypotension. Phaeochromocytoma is a contraindication to use of glucagon.

Sublingual glyceryl trinitrate may be used as an alternative to glucagon but hypotension may occur. A gas-producing substance may be given in an attempt to distend the oesophagus and allow the bolus to pass. Aerated drinks are adequate for this purpose. This technique should be used very cautiously as a patient with upper oesophageal obstruction will be at risk of aspiration if given a foaming substance. It should also be avoided if there is any suspicion of perforation.

Odynophagia may be relieved by parenteral or topical analgesia. Oral administration of a viscous preparation of lidocaine will relieve the pain caused by luminal inflammatory disorders. The maximum recommended dose is 300 mg and should be reduced in the elderly who may be more affected by systemic absorption.

Bones or similar foreign bodies impacted in the pharynx can often be removed in the emergency department. Topical anaesthetic sprays may suppress the pharyngeal reflexes adequately to allow direct or indirect laryngoscopy and removal with forceps. Removal may immediately relieve the dysphagia however symptoms may persist owing to local oedema or abrasions.

DISPOSITION

Appropriate disposition will depend on the likely aetiology and the presence of complications. Admission will be indicated for patients at risk of airway compromise, severe haemorrhage, sepsis or who have high-grade oesophageal obstruction. It will also be indicated

CONTROVERSIES

❶ There is argument about which specialists are best able to treat oesophageal food bolus obstruction, particularly of the upper oesophagus. Gastroenterologists, otorhinolaryngologists, thoracic surgeons and others have provided endoscopy services and there appear to be no strong arguments to favour any single specialty. Flexible endoscopy has a lower complication rate than rigid endoscopy so the choice of specialist should be made on the basis of skills in flexible endoscopy.

❷ Proteolytic enzymes have been used to dissolve impacted food boluses but complications have included oesophageal perforation and pneumonitis. Their use cannot be recommended.

when dysphagia is part of a broader disease process.

FURTHER READING

Braunwald E, Fauci AS, Kasper, et al 2001 Harrison's Principles of Internal Medicine, McGraw-Hill Inc, Australia, pp 233–6

Haubrich WS, Schaffner F, Berk JE 1995 Bockus Gastroenterology. WB Saunders Company, Pennsylvania, pp 35–8

Rosen P, Barkin RM, Danzi DF, et al 1998 Emergency medicine - concepts and clinical practice. Mosby Year Book Inc, St Louis, pp 1964–9

Taylor MB, Gollan JC, Steer ML, Wolfe MM 1997 Gastrointestinal emergencies. Williams and Wilkins, Hagerstown, USA, pp 65–75

Tintinalli JE, Kelen GD, Stapczynski JS 2000 Emergency Medicine - A Comprehensive Study Guide. McGraw Hill Inc, Australia, pp 523–9

6.2 BOWEL OBSTRUCTION

KIM YATES

ESSENTIALS

1 Obstruction of the small bowel is most often caused by adhesions, whereas obstruction of the large bowel more commonly results from neoplasms.

2 Paralytic ileus may be caused by other intra-abdominal conditions, serious systemic illnesses, metabolic disturbances or drugs.

3 The common clinical features of bowel obstruction are colicky, poorly localized abdominal pain, constipation/obstipation, abdominal distension and hyperactive or high-pitched bowel sounds.

4 Examination for hernias is essential.

5 The presence of dilated loops of bowel with multiple air-fluid levels on abdominal X-ray (supine and erect or decubitus) is diagnostic of bowel obstruction.

6 Initial treatment consists of correction of dehydration and electrolyte abnormalities, decompression, analgesia and assessment particularly to identify strangulating bowel obstruction.

7 Strangulating bowel obstruction is an indication for urgent surgery.

INTRODUCTION

Bowel obstruction is the interruption of the normal peristaltic progression of intestinal contents in either the small or the large bowel. Mechanical bowel obstruction can be caused by lesions outside or within the bowel wall, or within the lumen itself. It may be partial or complete, strangulating or non-strangulating.[1] Ileus, either adynamic/ paralytic, spastic or ischaemic, is obstruction without a mechanical cause, associated with abnormal propulsive motility.[1] Pseudo-obstruction is also associated with abnormal neuromuscular activity but refers to more chronic processes.[1]

In the emergency situation trying to differentiate the type of bowel obstruction is important, as the management of paralytic ileus or pseudo-obstruction focuses on diagnosing and treating the underlying cause, whereas surgical treatment may be required for mechanical bowel obstruction. Recognition of the potential complications, such as perforation or bowel strangulation, and hence the need for urgent surgery, is also important.

CAUSES AND PATHOPHYSIOLOGY (see Tables 6.2.1 and 6.2.2)

Adhesions and herniae rarely cause large bowel obstruction.

Paralytic ileus or pseudo-obstruction can be caused by a wide range of conditions including endocrine, cardiovascular, post-traumatic, postoperative, inflammatory, infectious, respiratory, metabolic, neurologic, vasculitic and pharmacologic disorders.[1, 6] Metabolic causes include hypokalaemia (most common), hyponatraemia, hypomagnesaemia, and hypoalbuminaemia.[1, 6] Drugs such as tricyclic antidepressants, opiates, antihistamines, beta-adrenergic agonists, and quinidine have also been implicated.[1]

The pathophysiology of mechanical bowel obstruction relates to changes in bowel function seen with rising intraluminal pressure. The bowel proximal to the obstruction gradually distends, initially with gas, fluid and electrolytes. As intraluminal pressure rises, hypersecretion escalates while the bowel absorptive ability decreases, causing large and progressive systemic volume losses. Initially, peristalsis increases proximal to the

Table 6.2.1 Causes of small bowel obstruction[1,2,3,4,5]
Adhesions (43–75%, usually postoperative)
Hernias (7–44%, inguinal most common)
Neoplasms (7–14%)
Inflammatory bowel disease
Gallstones
Bezoars
Foreign bodies
Strictures
Radiation
Diverticulitis
Endometriosis
Abscesses
Haematomas
Intussusception, volvulus and congenital lesions, which are more common causes of small bowel obstruction in children, are very rare in adults.[1]

Table 6.2.2 Causes of large bowel obstruction[3, 6-8]
Neoplasm (55–65%) particularly colorectal carcinoma
Diverticulitis (12–20%)
Volvulus (5% in Europe and North America but 50% in India, Africa, Eastern Europe [sigmoid volvulus is more common than caecal])
Faecal impaction (uncommon)
Inflammatory bowel disease
Tuberculosis
Ischaemic or radiation strictures
Extraintestinal tumours.

obstruction, in an attempt to overcome the blockage. Continuous peristalsis transforms into bursts of peristaltic activity, where frequency of bursts depends on location of obstruction – every 3–5 minutes if in the proximal small intestine, longer if more distal – giving rise to cyclic abdominal pain and high-pitched peristaltic rushes. As the obstruction persists and intraluminal pressure rises further, the proximal bowel is less able to contract vigorously, and bowel sounds become infrequent and quiet. Eventually, vomiting may ensue, worsening dehydration and electrolyte disturbances, with possible progression to haemoconcentration, hypovolaemia, renal insufficiency or shock. Increasing intraluminal pressures and distension can also lead to vascular compromise, especially venous stasis. The bowel wall becomes oedematous and bacterial translocation to the bloodstream may occur. Toxins produced by proliferating bacteria can have local or systemic effects. As pressures rise and/or blood flow diminishes, strangulation, hemorrhagic necrosis and/or gangrene may follow, with consequent perforation and sepsis. A closed-loop obstruction implies both proximal and distal obstruction, as is seen in a strangulating hernia or volvulus, and is likely to cause vascular compromise sooner, thus speeding the progression to gangrenous bowel.[1, 5, 7, 8]

CLINICAL FEATURES

History

In early bowel obstruction abdominal pain is poorly localized and colicky in nature, but as the obstruction progresses it may become more constant, and if severe suggests ischaemia or peritonitis. Pain from small bowel obstruction tends to be more severe earlier, and cramps tend to be more frequent compared to the pain pattern of large bowel obstruction where dull, lower abdominal cramps are more common. Vomiting is more common in small bowel obstruction and is a late symptom in large bowel obstruction. Faeculent vomiting suggests a more distal bowel obstruction. Decreased or absent flatus or stool is typical. Distension suggests a more distal obstruction.[1,2, 4–7]

A thorough gastrointestinal and surgical history helps in differentiating the possible mechanical causes of bowel obstruction, and drug history and systems enquiry may identify potential causes of non-mechanical obstruction.

Examination

Fever, tachycardia and abdominal tenderness or mass are more common in strangulating obstruction, however, variable signs and vascular compromise can occur in their absence.[1, 2, 9] Signs of dehydration are often present.[4] Abdominal distension and hyperresonance are present more commonly in large or distal small bowel obstruction.[1,4,5,7] Guarding or peritoneal irritation, suggests a strangulating obstruction, however, tenderness is a variable sign and vascular compromise is still possible in its absence.[2,4,6] Auscultation may reveal the rushes or gurgles of increased peristalsis, or high-pitched tinkles, but bowel sounds are not an absolute indicator of obstruction.[1,4,5,7] Surgical scars suggest adhesions as a possible cause of obstruction and examination for hernias is essential.[4] Rectal examination may be normal in small bowel obstruction, but the presence of faecal impaction, blood or a mass may assist with diagnosis.[4–7] Pelvic examination may be useful if abscesses or inflammation are suspected.

A focused medical examination should also be performed to exclude causes of paralytic ileus and pseudo-obstruction, and to assess anaesthetic risk.

INVESTIGATIONS

Blood and urine tests

Laboratory tests are of limited value for making the diagnosis of bowel obstruction[4,5] but may assist in assessment of severity and be a useful guide to resuscitation. Leukocytosis on a full blood count suggests ischaemia or strangulation,[4–6,10] but occurs in only 38–50% of strangulating obstructions, compared to 27–44% of non-strangulating obstructions.[9] Hematocrit may be raised if dehydration is present.[1,4,5] Electrolyte abnormalities, such as hyponatraemia, hypokalaemia, and impaired renal function, commonly occur[1,4,5] and abnormal serum calcium, phosphate and magnesium occur occasionally.[5,11,12] Serum amylase may be mildly raised in small bowel obstruction.[5] Arterial blood gases may be disturbed, with metabolic alkalosis if vomiting is severe, metabolic acidosis if shock, dehydration, or ketosis is present, or hypoxia/hypercapnia if distension impairs breathing.[1] Recent studies suggest that raised levels of serum lactate and interleukin-6 are associated with the presence of ischaemic bowel.[13] A blood or urine pregnancy test where appropriate, and urine microscopy are important in excluding other causes of abdominal pain, although sterile pyuria may be seen.[2]

Imaging

The presence of dilated loops of bowel with multiple air-fluid levels on abdominal X-rays (supine and erect or decubitus) is diagnostic of bowel obstruction,[4,5,7] although up to five air-fluid levels may be normal.[14] Plain film radiography has a sensitivity of only 66% in small bowel obstruction[15] and 84% in large bowel obstruction.[6] The dilated bowel loops may give a clue to the level of the obstruction, as the presence of dilated colon, identified by haustral sacculation, suggests large bowel obstruction.[16] The dilated single loop of colon ('bent inner tube') in the left abdomen suggests sigmoid volvulus or, in the midabdomen or epigastrium, caecal volvulus.[6] Perforation risk is higher when caecal dilatation exceeds 12 cm.[17] Dilated small bowel, identified by valvulae conniventes that extend across the bowel, may be present in either small or large bowel obstruction.[16] Absence of bowel gas distal to the obstruction may be seen as obstruction progresses.[16] Abdominal X-rays have not been shown to help distinguish strangulating from non-strangulating bowel obstruction,[2,18] however, the presence of a single loop of dilated small bowel in the presence of acute, severe pain suggests a strangulated closed-loop obstruction.[4]

An erect chest X-ray or left lateral decubitus X-ray should be checked, looking for free gas indicating perforation.[1, 5, 16]

Although many patients with suspected mechanical large bowel obstruction will eventually require a barium enema for diagnostic purposes, the role of contrast studies in acute bowel obstruction is controversial.[1,6,15] Abdominal ultrasound appeared less sensitive (88% vs 96%), but more specific (96% vs 65%) than plain radiography in the diagnosis of bowel obstruction in one study,[19] and superior to plain radiography in the diagnosis of strangulation (91% vs 30%).[18]

Abdominal computerized tomography (CT) is being used more commonly in small bowel obstruction to identify patients with complete obstruction, and is useful in large bowel obstruction if abscesses or malignancy are suspected.[4,16] Fast magnetic resonance imaging had a sensitivity of 90% and specificity of 86% in diagnosing small bowel obstruction in one study,[20] compared to 100% sensitivity for CT.[4]

Endoscopy

Careful sigmoidoscopy is safe in large bowel obstruction, and therapeutic in sigmoid volvulus when used to place a flatus tube.[6,8] In some centres, endoscopy is performed acutely to diagnose the nature, level and severity of a large bowel obstruction, then to decompress the obstruction by inserting drainage tubes or metallic stents using guidewire techniques.[21-23]

MANAGEMENT

Resuscitation and general measures

Measurement of vital signs and a survey for dehydration, toxicity and shock, are important initially so that appropriate resuscitation can be instigated.

As most patients with bowel obstruction are dehydrated, intravenous fluid therapy with crystalloid should be commenced according to the degree of dehydration. Electrolyte disturbances should be corrected. The response to therapy, by monitoring vital signs and urine output, should determine further fluid therapy. Analgesia is often required, with titrated intravenous increments of opioid being prompt and effective. Nasogastric decompression is customary.[1,4,5,7]

Conservative therapy

Ongoing intravenous fluid therapy and decompression are indicated in partial bowel obstruction and in those awaiting surgery.[1,4,5,7] Decompression via nasogastric tube is usual.[1,4,5,7] Nasogastric and nasointestinal tubes have been tried but the evidence for both is limited.[1,2,4,12] Monitoring of vital signs, urine output and clinical state should continue, and deterioration or failure to improve are indications for surgical therapy.[1,2,4,10,12] In patients with acute colonic pseudo-obstruction unresponsive to conservative therapy, intravenous neostigmine 2 mg has initiated rapid colonic decompression.[17] A non-strangulating sigmoid volvulus can be temporarily decompressed by a rectal tube passed through a sigmoidoscope.[8]

Endoscopic placement of a transanal drainage tube or a self-expanding metallic stent has been used in some cases. It allows decompression and cleansing in acute colonic obstruction due to malignancy prior to elective surgical resection and can be used as definitive palliative therapy in others. Reported complications of metallic stent use include perforation (0–16% of patients), stent migration (0–40%), restenosis (0–25%), pain, and bleeding.[21-23]

Surgical therapy

Strangulating bowel obstruction is an indication for urgent surgery. This might be suspected in the presence of severe pain, localized tenderness, a mass, fever, acidosis, marked leucocytosis, hernia, shock, sepsis, or ultrasound findings.[1,2,5,10,18] It can, however, occur without these features.[1,2,4] Raised lactate and/or interleukin-6 levels may be useful, if available, however, their sensitivity and specificity for detecting strangulation are not yet determined.[13] Parenteral antibiotics (e.g. cefoxitin, or ceftazidime/metronidazole or equivalent) are indicated preoperatively and if sepsis is suspected.[24]

Mortality escalates dramatically the longer surgery is delayed in strangulating bowel obstruction or perforation (~30% compared to 3–5% in non-strangulating bowel obstruction),[9] so prompt surgery is vital. The surgical approach adopted will depend on the suspected pathology and operative findings.[1,2,4,6,25,26] In small bowel obstruction laparotomy is usual, although a groin incision may be used in the presence of herniae. Adhesions can be lysed and any gangrenous bowel or tumour resected, followed by primary anastomosis, or bypass if this is not possible.[1,2,4,25,26] Some centres use laparoscopy in the treatment of acute small bowel obstruction with success rates that vary between 33 and 87%, and this seems more successful in patients

CONTROVERSIES

❶ Diagnosis of strangulating bowel obstruction. Clinical features and plain radiography may not be helpful.[1,2,4,5,9] Ultrasound may be a more sensitive test.[18,19] Serum lactate and interleukin-6 levels may prove useful, but further studies are required to determine sensitivity and specificity.[13]

❷ Tube decompression therapy in small bowel obstruction. Both short nasogastric and long nasointestinal tubes have been used in adhesive small bowel obstruction. Non-operative therapy may be more successful, with a long tube placed (often by fluoroscope) in the small bowel.[4,11,12]

❸ The role of self-expanding metallic stents in acute colonic obstruction caused by malignancy. Endoscopic placement of a stent may preclude the need for surgery when used as palliative therapy, or allow a one-stage surgical procedure when used for decompression and cleansing but complications are common.[6,21-23]

❹ Non-operative therapy. Some surgeons prefer early surgery because of the difficulty in diagnosing strangulating bowel obstruction. In adhesive small bowel obstruction, without signs of strangulation, a 48-hour trial of non-operative therapy with frequent reassessment appears safe.[10]

with a history of appendicectomy only, or in those with band adhesions.[27]

In large bowel obstruction there are a number of options, determined by the nature and site of the obstructing lesion, the patient's condition and surgical preference. Decompressive stomas followed by a definitive operation at a later date are sometimes useful in very sick patients; however, right-sided lesions can often be resected at laparotomy with a primary anastomosis, avoiding a stoma completely. One-stage resection/anastomosis is possible with left-sided lesions, but there is a higher risk of contamination in the unprepared bowel of emergency procedures and higher mortality rates.[6,25,26]

DISPOSITION

Patients with bowel obstruction and haemodynamic compromise, shock or sepsis, require combined ongoing management by surgical and intensive-care teams. Patients with suspected strangulating bowel obstruction or perforation should have urgent surgery. Patients with partial bowel obstruction can be commenced on conservative therapy and monitored closely as surgical inpatients for signs of deterioration.

REFERENCES

1. Fischer JE, Nussbaum MS, Chance NT, Luchette F, et al 1999 Manifestations of Gastrointestinal Disease. In: Schwartz SI (ed.) Principles of Surgery, 7th edn. McGraw-Hill, Australia 1033–61
2. Deutsch AA, Eviator E, Gutman H, Reiss R, et al 1989 Small bowel obstruction: a review of 264 cases and suggestions for management. Postgraduate Medical Journal 65: 463–7
3. McKellar DP, Reiling RB, Eiseman B 1999 Prognosis and outcomes in surgical disease: Quality Medical Publishing, St Louis, Missouri
4. Hodin RA, Matthews JB 2001 Small intestine. In: Norton JA BR, Chang AE, Lowry SF, Mulvihill SJ, Pass HI, Thompson RW (eds) Surgery: Basic Science and Clinical Evidence. Springer-Verlag, New York, pp 617–42
5. Rohovsky S, Bleday R 2000 Small bowel obstruction. In: Morris PJ WW (ed.) Oxford Textbook of Surgery, 2nd edn. Oxford University Press, Oxford 1345–9
6. Lopez-Kostner F, Hool GR, Lavery IC 1997 Management and causes of acute large bowel obstruction. Surgical Clinics of North America 77(6): 1265–90
7. Welch JP 2000 Large-bowel obstruction. In: Morris PJ WW (ed.) Oxford Textbook of Surgery, 2nd edn. Oxford University Press, Oxford 1511–14
8. Berry AR 2000 Volvulus of the colon. In: Morris PJ WW (ed.) Oxford Textbook of Surgery, 2nd edn. Oxford University Press, Oxford 1515–19
9. Ellis H 1997 The clinical significance of adhesions: focus on intestinal obstruction. European Journal of Surgery 577(Suppl): 5–9
10. Cox MR, Gunn IF, Eastman MC, et al 1993 The safety and duration of non-operative treatment for adhesive small bowel obstruction. ANZ Journal of Surgery 63(5): 367–71
11. Gowen GF 1997 Decompression is essential in the management of small bowel obstruction. American Journal of Surgery 173: 459–60
12. Fleshner PR, Siegman MG, Slater GI, et al 1995 A prospective randomized trial of short versus long tubes in adhesive small-bowel obstruction. American Journal of Surgery 170(4): 66–370
13. Firoozmand E, Fairman N, Klar J, Vaxman K, et al 2001 Intravenous interleukin-6 levels predict need for laparotomy in patients with bowel obstruction.

14. Billittier AJ, et al 1996 Radiographic imaging modalities for the patient in the emergency department with abdominal complaints. Emergency Medical Clinics of North America 14(4): 889–51
15. Gupta H, Dupuy DE 1997 Advances in imaging of the acute abdomen. Surgical Clinics of North America 77(6): 1245–63
16. Nicholson, DA Driscoll PA 1995 ABC of Emergency Radiology. BMJ Publishing Group, London
17. Ponec RJ, Saunders MD, Kimmey MB 1999 Neostigmine for the treatment of acute colonic pseudo-obstruction. New England Journal of Medicine 341(3): 137–41
18. Czechowski J 1996 Conventional radiography and ultrasonography in the diagnosis of small bowel obstruction and strangulation. Acta Radiologica 37(2): 86–218
19. Ogata M, Mateer JR, Condon RE 1996 Prospective evaluation of abdominal sonography for the diagnosis of bowel obstruction. Annals of Surgery 223(3): 37–241
20. Regan F, Beall DP, Bohlman ME, et al 1998 Fast MR imaging and the detection of small-bowel obstruction. AJR 170: 1465–69
21. Mauro MA, Koehler RE, Baron TH 2000 Advances in Gastrointestinal intervention: the treatment of gastroduodenal and colorectal obstructions with metallic stents. Radiology 215: 659–69
22. Law WL, Chu KW, Ho JW, et al 2000 Self-expanding metallic stent in the teatment of colonic obstruction caused by advanced malignancies. Diseases of the Colon and Rectum 43: 1522–7
23. Tanaka T, Furukawa A, Murata K, Sakamoto T, et al 2001 Endoscopic transanal decompression with a drainage tube for acute colonic obstruction. Diseases of the Colon and Rectum 44: 418–22
24. Farber MS, Abrams JH 1997 Antibiotics for the acute abdomen. Surgical Clinics of North America 77(6): 395–417
25. Isbister WH, Prasad J 1996 The management of left-sided large bowel obstruction: an audit. ANZ Journal of Surgery 66: 602–4
26. McLeish A 1996 The management of large bowel obstruction. ANZ Journal of Surgery 66: 584
27. Levard H, Boudet MJ, Msika S, et al 2001 Laparoscopic treatment of acute small bowel obstruction: a multicentre retrospective study. ANZ Journal of Surgery 71: 641–6

American Surgeon 67(12): 1145–9

6.3 HERNIA

ANDREW DENT

ESSENTIALS

1 A diagnosis of symptomatic hernia mandates early surgical repair to avoid life-threatening complications.

2 Hernia may present as a reducible lump, or may incarcerate, strangulate and/or present as bowel obstruction.

3 Femoral herniae are often misdiagnosed and are associated with high morbidity when complicated.

4 All herniae presenting with a complication should undergo surgical repair promptly.

INTRODUCTION

A hernia is defined as a protrusion of a viscus or part of a viscus through a weakness in the wall of the containing cavity. It has an aperture, coverings (usually peritoneum and abdominal wall layers) and contents, which may be any intra-abdominal organ but are usually omentum or small bowel. Surgical treatment requires reduction of the contents and closure of the aperture, with reinforcement to prevent recurrence.

There are a number of described sites for herniae. This chapter will focus on the more common, but the principles of assessment and treatment apply in general to herniae at other sites.

INGUINAL HERNIA

Inguinal herniae are extremely common, with a lifetime risk of occurrence of 27% for men and 3% for women, and an annual incidence of 130 per 100 000 population. Up to 9% of hernia repairs are performed urgently. Emergency repairs are more common in the elderly and carry greater morbidity than elective repair.[1]

Direct inguinal herniae bulge directly through the posterior wall of the inguinal canal. They are caused by weak abdominal musculature, are common in the elderly and frequently bilateral. They have a large neck and hence seldom become irreducible or strangulate until they are of considerable size.

For indirect inguinal herniae the hernial sac comes through the internal inguinal ring, travels the length of the inguinal canal and emerges from the external inguinal ring. Thus it usually lies above and medial to the symphysis pubis. Later the internal inguinal ring may stretch and the hernial sac and its contents may descend to and fill the scrotum, occasionally becoming very large. As the internal inguinal ring is usually narrow, irreducibility is common. Indirect inguinal herniae occur throughout life.

Direct and indirect inguinal herniae may be distinguishable by simple clinical tests. When an indirect hernia is reduced, finger pressure over the site of the internal ring may hold it reduced; however, a direct inguinal hernia will flop out again unless several fingers or the side of the hand props up the entire length of the inguinal canal.

FEMORAL HERNIA

Femoral herniae appear lateral and inferior to the symphysis pubis. They are formed by the peritoneal sac and contents, which enlarge the potential space of the femoral canal, medial to the femoral vein. They are proportionately more common in women and rarely large. Symptoms usually occur early and complications are common.

The femoral canals should be closely examined in any patient presenting with abdominal pain or signs of bowel obstruction, as femoral herniae are frequently overlooked, especially in patients who are elderly and obese.[2] Diagnosis of a femoral hernia mandates early surgery. Morbidity from emergency femoral hernia repair increases with the presence of small bowel obstruction, and mortality with emergency surgery can be as high as 5%.[3]

UMBILICAL HERNIA

Umbilical and periumbilical herniae protrude through and around the umbilicus. They are very common in the newborn, but most resolve by 4 years of age. As they have a broad neck, emergency complications are uncommon. They can be difficult to diagnose in very obese people. If complicated, they can present resembling abdominal wall cellulitis.

EPIGASTRIC HERNIA

Epigastric herniae appear in the midline above the umbilicus. A small extraperitoneal piece of fat may be stuck in this hernia, causing pain.

OTHER HERNIA
Obturator hernia
Rarely viscera may pass through a defect in the obturator foramen and present as a small bowel obstruction. This occurs most commonly in elderly emaciated women with chronic disease.[4] Diagnosis of this internal hernia, and the hernia of the foramen of Winslow, is seldom made preoperatively.

Spigelian hernia
These are rare and are due to a defect in the anterolateral abdominal wall musculature. They usually present as a reducible lump in the elderly male, lateral to the rectus muscle in the lower half of the abdomen.[5] Complications are rare.

Incisional hernia
These may occur at any previous abdominal wound, such as appendicectomy or laparotomy. The wound area becomes weak, allowing the protrusion of a viscus or part of a viscus.

Sportsman's hernia
This is a term used for those who present with the painful symptoms of a hernia in the groin following exertion, but without a demonstrable lump.[6] Although some progress over time to full-blown herniae, an alternative diagnosis for the pain will often be found, such as nerve entrapment or visceral pain.[7]

COMPLICATIONS

In the early stages herniae are usually reducible, only producing intermittent pain in the groin. Reducible herniae may become irreducible (incarcerated). Incarcerated herniae may lead to a bowel obstruction. Strangulation, interruption of the blood supply to the contents of the hernia (usually small bowel) may supervene. In this case there will be increasing, local pain and tenderness, warmth and overlying erythema accompanied by signs of bowel obstruction, and leucocytosis.

Rarely only part of the bowel wall is caught in a hernial constricting ring. Bowel wall necrosis ensues that is not circumferential; this is termed a Richter's hernia. In this case, there may be signs of strangulation, i.e. without signs of obstruction.

Very rarely, neglected herniae can fistulate, with bowel contents appearing at the abdominal wall or through the hernial orifices.

TREATMENT
Reduction
It may be possible to reduce a hernia that initially appears irreducible in the emergency department, but caution must be

exercised. If the skin over the herniae is already inflamed and pain is severe, the contents may be compromised and urgent surgical exploration is required. Reduction of the contents in this circumstance can be dangerous, as false reassurance can occur followed by the later development of peritonitis due to intra-abdominal perforation of the contents.

As a general rule, if the hernia has been irreducible for less than 4 hours, vital signs are normal and there are no symptoms of bowel obstruction, reduction of an incarcerated hernia may be attempted. This is achieved by giving adequate analgesia to relax the patient and applying gentle pressure manipulating the hernia site for several minutes. Elevating the foot of the bed may be helpful. Successful reduction relieves pain, may prevent strangulation and reduces the urgency for surgical intervention. Notwithstanding, all herniae that have undergone a complication require surgical consultation at the time of presentation.

Surgical repair

Timely repair of herniae decreases the incidence of complications and avoids the greater risk associated with emergency surgery.[8] Laparoscopic transabdominal preperitoneal hernia repair takes longer than open surgery, but is being increasingly performed as it reduces post operative pain and significantly reduces time off work.[9]

Patients requiring emergency surgery for bowel obstruction or strangulation should be prepared with adequate fluid resuscitation and analgesia.

REFERENCES

1. Primatesta P, Goldacre MJ 1996 Inguinal hernia repair: incidence of elective and emergency surgery, readmission and mortality. International Journal of Epidemiology 25(4): 835–9
2. Camary VL 1993 Femoral hernia: intestinal obstruction is an unrecognized source of morbidity and mortality. British Journal of Surgery 80(2): 230–2
3. Brittenden J, Heys SD, Eremerin O 1991 Femoral hernia: mortality and morbidity following elective and emergency repair. Journal of the Royal College of Surgeons of Edinburgh 36(2): 86–8
4. Lo CY, Lorentz TG, Lau PW Obturator hernia presenting as small bowel obstruction. American Journal of Surgery 167(4): 396–8
5. Spangen L 1989 Spigelian hernia. World Journal of Surgery 13(5): 573–80
6. Fredberg U, Kissmeyer-Nielsen P 1996 The Sportsman's hernia - fact or fiction? Scandinavian Journal of Medicine and Science in Sports 6(4): 201–4
7. Gallegos NC, Hobsley M 1990 Abdominal wall pain: an alternative diagnosis. British Journal of Surgery 77(10): 1167–70
8. Devsine M, Grimson R, Soroff HS 1987 Benefits of a clinic for the treatment of external abdominal wall hernias. American Journal of Surgery 153(4): 387–91
9. McCormack K, Scott NW, Go PM, Ross S 2002 Laparoscopic techniques versus open techniques for inguinal hernia repair. Cochrane Database of Systematic Reviews. Issue 2

CONTROVERSIES

❶ The diagnosis and management of the 'sportsman's hernia'.

❷ The role of laparoscopy in hernia repair.

6.4 GASTROENTERITIS

CORINNE GINIFER • SIMON YOUNG

ESSENTIALS

1 Gastroenteritis is usually a benign, self-limiting disease that can be diagnosed clinically, warrants no specific investigation and settles spontaneously with symptomatic treatment and oral fluid therapy.

2 The cardinal clinical feature of gastroenteritis is diarrhoea, which may be accompanied by varying degrees of nausea and vomiting, abdominal cramping and pain, lethargy and fever.

3 The clinical examination is directed at confirming the diagnosis of gastroenteritis, excluding alternative diagnoses and determining the degree of dehydration.

4 A wide variety of viruses, bacteria and protozoa may cause gastroenteritis. Common viral agents include rotavirus and Norwalk virus. Common bacteria include *Campylobacter jejuni*, *Staphylococcus aureus*, *Escherichia coli*, *Shigella dysenteriae* and *Salmonella enteriditis*. Common protozoa include *Giardia lamblia*.

5 The principles of treatment of gastroenteritis are to replace the fluid losses orally or intravenously, minimize the patient's symptoms by use of antiemetic or antidiarrhoeal therapy, and in some circumstances administer specific antimicrobial agents.

INTRODUCTION

Gastroenteritis is a common clinical syndrome. Globally it poses one of the world's major clinical and public health problems. In developing countries with poor-quality drinking water and low levels of sanitation it is a major cause of morbidity and mortality, especially among children and the elderly.

Gastroenteritis is caused by infection of the gastrointestinal tract by various viruses, bacteria and protozoa, which have most commonly been transmitted by the faecal-oral route. The syndrome consists of diarrhoea, abdominal cramping or pain, nausea and vomiting, lethargy, malaise and fever. Each of these features may be present to a varying degree, and may last from 1 day to more than 3 weeks.

In developed countries, even though serious morbidity and mortality are low, gastroenteritis may be an extremely painful and unpleasant event causing disruption to daily living routines and significant loss of working and school days. Patients often seek emergency medical care because of the acuteness of onset or the frequency of the diarrhoea, the severity of abdominal pain and cramps, and because of concerns regarding dehydration.

Gastroenteritis may occur in many settings. It may be a sporadic isolated event, a small outbreak either within a family or other close living group, or part of a larger community epidemic. The latter can place extreme strain upon emergency department resources. It may occur in a traveller, either while still overseas or on their return home. It is important to be aware of the circumstances and context in which the illness occurs, as these will often dictate the course of investigation or management undertaken.

PATHOPHYSIOLOGY AND MICROBIOLOGY

Micro-organisms of all descriptions are constantly entering the gastrointestinal tract through the mouth. Extremely few of these progress to cause clinical illness. The natural defences of the gastrointestinal tract against infection include gastric acid secretion, normal bowel flora, bile salt production, bowel motility, mucosal lymphoid tissue and secreted immunoglobulin A. People with disturbances in any of these defences are more prone to a clinical infection. For example, patients with achlorhydria, bowel stasis or blind loops, immunodeficiency states or recent antibiotic therapy that has disturbed bowel flora are prone to gastroenteritis. Some organisms such as rotavirus occur principally in children, as previous infection confers immunity.

A wide variety of viruses, bacteria and protozoa may cause gastroenteritis, and the list is continually growing. Viral agents include rotavirus, enteric adenovirus, astrovirus, calicivirus, Norwalk virus, coronavirus and cytomegalovirus.

Bacteria include *Campylobacter jejuni*, *Staphylococcus aureus*, *Bacillus cereus*, *Escherichia coli*, *Vibrio cholerae*, *Shigella dysenteriae*, *Salmonella enteriditis*, *Yersinia enterocolitica* and *Clostridium perfringens* and *difficile*. Protozoa include *Giardia lamblia*, *Cryptosporidium parvum* and *Entamoeba histolytica*. These micro-organisms cause gastroenteritis by a number of mechanisms. They may release preformed toxins prior to ingestion; multiply and produce toxins within the gastrointestinal lumen; directly invade the bowel wall; or utilize a combination of toxins and invasion. *Staphylococcus aureus* and *Bacillus cereus* produce a variety of toxins in stored food that are subsequently ingested. These toxins are absorbed and act within hours on the central nervous system to produce an illness characterized predominantly by vomiting and mild diarrhoea.

Invasive bacteria are characterized by *Salmonella*, which invades the mucosa, primarily of the distal ilium mucosa, producing cell damage and excessive secretion. *Shigella* likewise invades the mucosa but also produces toxins that have cytotoxic, neurotoxic and enterotoxic effects.

The many strains of *E. coli* have been divided into five groups, depending upon the pathology of the diseases they cause. These are enteropathogenic, enterotoxigenic, enteroinvasive, enteroaggregative and enterohaemorrhagic. Enterohaemorrhagic *E. coli* is associated with haemorrhagic colitis and the haemolytic uraemic syndrome, whereas enterotoxigenic *E. coli* is associated with traveller's diarrhoea. The protozoan *Giardia lamblia* adheres to the jejunum and upper ileum, causing mucosal inflammation, inhibition of disaccharidase activity and overgrowth of luminal bacteria.

CLINICAL PRESENTATION

The clinical history and examination is directed at confirming the diagnosis of gastroenteritis, excluding other diagnoses, and determining the degree of dehydration present.

The principal clinical manifestation of gastroenteritis is diarrhoea. This is often watery and profuse in the early stages of the illness, and may last for up to 3 weeks. It is essential to determine as far as possible the frequency, volume and characteristics of the stool. Some organisms, such as enterohaemorrhagic *E. coli*, *Shigella*, *Salmonella*, *Campylobacter* and *Entamoeba histolytica*, may cause acute and bloody diarrhoea, whereas others such as *Giardia* may cause loose, pale and greasy stools.

Abdominal pain is common and is most often described as a diffuse intermittent colicky pain situated centrally in the abdomen. It may occur just prior to, and be partially relieved by, a bowel action. Severe pain is often caused by *Campylobacter*, *Yersinia* and *E. coli*. Abdominal pain is also the hallmark of many other forms of intra- and extra-abdominal pathology. Diagnoses other than gastroenteritis should be seriously considered if the pain is well localized, constant and severe, or radiates to the back or shoulder. Vomiting may be present, often early in the illness, and can be of variable severity and persistence. The amount of vomiting and the ability to keep down clear fluids should be determined, as this will dictate the management of dehydration. Severe vomiting often occurs with organisms that produce preformed toxin, although it does not usually persist for longer than 24 hours. Anorexia, nausea and lethargy are common. Fever and systemic symptoms such as headache are prominent with organisms that invade the bowel wall and enter the systemic circulation, such as *Yersinia*. Lethargy may be related to the dehydration or merely the strain of constant and persistent diarrhoea from any aetiology.

Specific inquiry regarding fluid status is essential. The aim should be to determine the amount of fluids that have been taken orally and kept down over the course of the illness, along with the estimated urine output. A recent weight may also be useful in children. It is also important to ensure that the patient does not have any pre-existing or intercurrent illness, such as diabetes or immunosuppression, which may alter management.

CLINICAL EXAMINATION

Suitable infection control procedures should be instituted prior to the examination to prevent spread to the examining doctor and hence to other patients. Handwashing before and after the consultation, the use of gloves and prompt disposal of soiled clothing and linen are important.

A careful clinical examination should be performed, concentrating on the abdomen and the circulatory state of the patient. The vital signs, temperature and urinalysis should be obtained.

In mild to moderate gastroenteritis the clinical examination is often unremarkable. There may be some general abdominal tenderness, active bowel sounds and facial pallor, but little else. In more severe disease the abdominal tenderness may be pronounced and signs of dehydration present. Of note, uncomplicated gastroenteritis is extremely unlikely if the abdominal examination reveals localized tenderness or signs of peritoneal irritation.

Fluid losses through diarrhoea, vomiting and fever, together with poor oral fluid intake, can lead to clinically apparent dehydration. This may be manifest as tachycardia, tachypnoea, decreased tissue turgor, delayed capillary return, decreased urine output and, in its more severe stages, hypotension, impaired conscious state and death.

Extra-abdominal signs of a primary gastroenteritis can occur. *Campylobacter* has been associated with reactive arthritis and Guillain-Barré syndrome. The clinical features, course and complications for various causative agents are summarized in Table 6.4.1.

Table 6.4.1 Pathogen-specific syndromes

Causative agent	Incubation period	Duration of illness	Predominant symptoms	Foods commonly implicated
Bacteria				
Campylobacter jejuni	3–5 days	2–5 days occ. >10 days	Sudden onset of diarrhoea, abdominal pain, nausea, vomiting	Raw or undercooked poultry, raw milk, meat, untreated water
Escherichia coli enteropathogenic, enterotoxigenic, enteroinvasive, enterohaemorrhagic	12–72 hours (enterotoxigenic) longer in others	3–14 days	Severe colicky abdominal pain, watery to profuse diarrhoea, sometimes bloody. May cause haemolytic uraemic syndrome	Many raw foods, unpasteurized milk, contaminated water, minced beef
Salmonella serovars	6–72 hours	3–5 days	Abdominal pain, diarrhoea, chills, fever, malaise	Meat, chicken, eggs and egg products
Shigella species	12–96 hours	4–7 days	Malaise, fever, vomiting, diarrhoea commonly with blood mucus	Any contaminated food or water
Yersinia enterocolitica	3–7 days	1–21 days	Acute diarrhoea sometimes bloody, fever, vomiting	Raw meat and poultry, milk and milk products
Vibrio cholerae	Few hours to 5 days	3–4 days	Asymptomatic to profuse dehydrating diarrhoea	Raw seafood, contaminated water
Vibrio parahaemolyticus	12–24 hours	1–7 days	Abdominal pain, moderate diarrhoea/ vomiting of moderate severity	Raw and cooked fish, shellfish, other seafoods
Viruses				
Small round structured viruses (SRSVs) such as astrovirus, adenovirus, calicivirus,	24–48 hours	12–48 hours	Severe vomiting, diarrhoea	Oysters, clams, other food contaminated by human Norwalk virus, excreta
Rotaviruses	24–72 hours	3–7 days	Malaise, headache, fever, vomiting, diarrhoea	Contaminated water
Parasites				
Cryptosporidium	1–12 days	4–21 days	Profuse watery diarrhoea	Contaminated water and food
Giardia lamblia	1–3 weeks	1–2 weeks to months	Loose pale greasy stools, abdominal pain	Contaminated water, food contaminated by infected food handlers
Entamoeba histolytica	2–4 weeks	Weeks–months	Colic, mucous or bloody diarrhoea	Contaminated water and food
Toxin-producing bacteria				
Bacillus cereus (toxin in food)	1–6 hours	<24 hours	Nausea, vomiting, diarrhoea, cramps	Cereals, rice, meat products, soups, vegetables
Clostridium perfringens (toxin in gut)	8–20 hours	24 hours	Sudden-onset colic, diarrhoea	Meats, poultry, stews, gravies, (often reheated)
Staphylococcus aureus (toxin in food)	30 mins–8 hours	24 hours	Acute vomiting, purging, may lead to collapse	Cold foods (much handled during preparation), milk products, salted meats

Adapted from Guidelines for the Control of Infectious Diseases – The Blue Book. Infectious Diseases Unit, Public Health Division, Victorian Government Department of Human Services, 1997 (Reproduced with the kind permission of the Infectious Diseases Unit, Public Health Division, Victorian Government Department of Human Services)

DIARRHOEA IN CERTAIN CIRCUMSTANCES

Traveller's diarrhoea

Millions of travellers each year are affected by diarrhoea. Southeast Asia, the Middle East, the Mediterranean basin, Central and South America are areas of frequent occurrence. The incidence of diarrhoea in travellers to these areas is as high as 30–50%.[1] Several pathogens including *Salmonella, Shigella, Campylobacter, Giardia, Entamoeda histolytica* and rotavirus are responsible. However, the most common cause is enterotoxigenic *E.coli*. Many cases do not become symptomatic until after return home. A history of recent travel to one of these areas should be sought. Antibiotic prophylaxis for traveller's diarrhoea, although effective, is not usually recommended as in most instances the illness will be self-limiting.

The immunocompromized patient

Patients with impaired immunity (AIDS, IgA deficiency, immunosuppressive therapy following organ transplantation and long-term corticosteroid usage) are not only more susceptible to the common causes of gastroenteritis, but are also vulnerable to the less common organisms such as *Cryptosporidium, Microsporidium, Isopora* and *Cytomegalovirus*. Infections are often more severe, have a higher incidence of complications and may be more resistant to conventional therapy. Isolation of the causative organism and determination of antibiotic sensitivity is essential to guide management.

Hospital-acquired diarrhoea

Antibiotic-associated diarrhoea as a result of *Clostridium difficile* infection is the most common cause of acute diarrhoea in hospitalised patients.[1] It may range from a mild disease to life-threatening pseudomembranous colitis and can follow treatment with almost any antibiotic but particularly cephalosporins and clindamycin. Tissue culture cytotoxicity and ELISA tests for toxins A and B should be performed to establish the diagnosis. Patients should be treated with oral metronidazole or oral vancomycin.

DIFFERENTIAL DIAGNOSIS

Many pathological conditions, especially early in their course, may present with a clinical picture similar to that of gastroenteritis. Appendicitis, mesenteric adenitis, small bowel ischaemia and inflammatory bowel disease can all present in a similar fashion. Conversely, *Campylobacter* may cause severe abdominal pain with little diarrhoea, and may be misdiagnosed as appendicitis or inflammatory bowel disease. Medical conditions such as toxic ingestions, diabetic ketoacidosis, hepatitis and pancreatitis can present with vomiting, abdominal pain and tenderness and 'loose' stools.

Although a meticulous history and examination, combined with judicious use of investigations, should be able to differentiate many of these at the time of presentation, careful observation over a period of time looking for a change in signs and symptoms may be necessary.

INVESTIGATIONS

In most circumstances no investigations are necessary in order to make the diagnosis of gastroenteritis or to manage the patient effectively.

Identification of the infective agent may be useful when there is an outbreak of gastroenteritis to ensure that adequate public health measures are instituted, in an attempt to limit spread of the disease. Additionally, in a patient who has a persistent illness or clinical features of a specific illness, such as *Campylobacter, Giardia* or *Salmonella*, identification of the organism may be helpful in directing antimicrobial therapy or identifying a carrier state. Although the history and examination may give clues as to the aetiological agent, they are unreliable as many similarities exist between the clinical syndromes produced by each organism. Laboratory identification is the only accurate method.

The infective agent may be identified by microscopy and culture of faeces, looking specifically for pathogenic bacteria, cysts, ova or parasites. A fresh specimen of faeces will assist in detection. Occasionally multiple specimens are required, especially for organisms which may shed into the faeces only sporadically. Once collected, the specimen must be kept cool (4°C) and transported promptly to the laboratory.

Rotavirus infection is detected by looking for rotavirus antigen in the stool by electron microscopy, ELISA or latex agglutination.

If a patient is dehydrated or systemically unwell, a full blood examination, serum electrolyte determination and serum glucose are warranted. In rare cases where there are signs suggestive of septicaemia or severe systemic illness, blood cultures and liver function tests may be indicated.

Abdominal X-rays are only of assistance if it is necessary to exclude a bowel obstruction or free intra-abdominal gas.

TREATMENT

The principles of treatment of gastroenteritis are to replace fluid and electrolyte losses, minimize symptoms if possible and, in selected cases, administer specific antimicrobial therapy. Clear fluids for 24 hours are often recommended, with the rationale that keeping the stomach empty will minimize vomiting. If the patient wishes to eat it is allowable. Strictly withholding feeding, especially from children, is not necessary.

Replacement of fluid losses may be achieved enterally, either by mouth or via a nasogastric tube, or intravenously. The method of rehydration selected will depend on the cooperation of the patient, the degree of dehydration, the rate at which rehydration is desired, and the presence of other diseases such as diabetes.

Specific oral rehydration solutions are the most appropriate fluid for oral or nasogastric use. There are a number of commercially available preparations available through pharmacies without prescription. These consist of a balanced formula of glucose, sodium and potassium salts, and in worldwide trials have been shown to be extremely effective and safe, even when used in the most primitive of conditions.[2] Although many commonly available fluids may be used and will probably be effective in mild disease, fluids that contain large amounts of glucose, such as degassed lemonade or undiluted fruit juice, should not be encouraged in adults and are contraindicated in children. These fluids are hyperosmolar and deficient in electrolytes, thus promoting further fluid losses. Glucose-containing electrolyte solutions utilize the gut's co-transport system for glucose and sodium thereby facilitating the absorption of water as well. Milk and other lactose-containing products should be avoided during the acute phase of the illness as viral or bacterial enteropathogens often result in transient lactose malabsorption. Caffeine-containing products should also be avoided.[1] Caffeine increases cyclic AMP levels, thus promoting secretion of fluid and worsening diarrhoea.

Intravenous rehydration is necessary in patients who are shocked or who are becoming progressively more dehydrated despite oral or nasogastric fluids. Resuscitation should be commenced with normal saline at a rate which accounts for ongoing losses, as well as replaces the estimated fluid deficit. In severely dehydrated patients one or two 20 mL/kg boluses of normal saline may be necessary. Patients should also be encouraged to take oral fluids, unless vomiting is prohibitive. As soon as an adequate intake is achieved the intravenous fluids can be scaled back and ceased.

Close monitoring of the serum electrolytes is necessary during intravenous rehydration. In particular it is important to monitor serum sodium, as the exclusive use of normal saline for rehydration can lead to hypernatraemia. Potassium should be added to the fluid as determined by the serum potassium, remembering that a low serum potassium in this circumstance is indicative of a low total body potassium.

In adults, parenterally administered antiemetic drugs such as metoclopramide or prochlorperazine may be useful in the management of severe vomiting. In children, however, an unacceptably high incidence of dystonic reactions precludes their use. Antimotility agents such as loperamide or diphenoxylate plus atropine may be used, and have been shown to decrease the number of diarrhoeal stools and the duration of the illness. Both these agents have significant side-effects and should only be used if it is essential. Anticholinergic agents are ineffective for controlling symptoms and have significant adverse side effects.

Even though many bacteria that cause gastroenteritis respond to antibiotics they are rarely indicated. Recent antibiotic guidelines suggest that most infections with *Campylobacter, Salmonella, Shigella, Yersinia* and *E. coli* do not need antibiotics. In the majority of these cases the illness will be short-lived and mild. Because of the previous widespread use of antibiotics to treat gastroenteritis from any cause, and the current use of antibiotics in animals bred for food, many isolates of *C. jejuni, Shigella* and *Salmonella* are resistant to many antibiotics.[1] Choice of antibiotics should be based on antibiotic sensitivity patterns. Antibiotics may be indicated in *Giardia* infections, *Shigella* causing severe disease, *Salmonella* in infants, the immunosuppressed or the elderly, *Campylobacter* in food handlers, and in traveller's diarrhoea. Antibiotics are contraindicated in uncomplicated *Salmonella* infections as they may prolong the carrier state. Recommended antibiotic regimens are summarized in Table 6.4.2.

Table 6.4.2 Antibiotic treatment regimens

Giardia lamblia
Tinidazole 2 g orally as a single dose. Children: 50 mg/kg/day up to adult dose
OR
Metronidazole 400 mg orally, 8 hourly for 7 days
Amoebiasis
Metronidazole 600 mg orally, 6 hourly for 6–10 days. Children: 45 mg/kg/day up to adult dose in three divided doses
PLUS
Diloxanide furonate 500 mg orally 8 hourly for 10 days. Children: 20 mg/kg/day up to adult dose in three divided doses (to prevent relapse)

Shigellosis
Norfloxacin 400 mg orally, 12 hourly for 7–10 days (not in children)
OR
Ampicillin 1 g orally, 6 hourly for 7–10 days. Children: 100 mg/kg/day up to adult dose in four divided doses
OR
Co-trimoxazole 160/800 mg orally, 12 hourly for 7–10 days. Children: 8/40 mg/kg/day up to adult dose in two divided doses
Campylobacter
Erythromycin 500 mg orally, 6 hourly for 7–10 days. Children: 40 mg/kg/day up to adult dose in four divided doses
Traveller's diarrhoea
Norfloxacin 800 mg orally as a single dose or 400 mg orally 12 hourly for 3 days (not in children)
OR
Co-trimoxazole 320/1600 mg orally, as a single dose or 160/800 mg orally, 12 hourly for 3 days
IN CHILDREN GIVE
Co-trimoxazole 8/40 mg/kg/day up to a maximum of 160/800 mg/day in two divided doses orally for 3 days
Clostridium difficile
Metronidazole 400 mg orally 8 hourly for 7–10 days. Children: 30 mg/kg/day up to adult dose in three divided doses
If unresponsive or severe disease:
Vancomycin 125 mg orally 6 hourly for 1–2 weeks. Children: 5 mg/kg up to adult dose.

Reference: Therapeutic Guidelines: Antibiotic. Version 11, 2000. Therapeutic Guidelines Limited. VMPF Therapeutics Committee, Melbourne

CONTROVERSIES

❶ The role of faecal microscopy and culture.

❷ The public health role of emergency departments in monitoring and reporting the prevalence of gastroenteritis in the community.

❸ When is it appropriate to prescibe antiemetic or antidiarrhoeal therapy, given that this is most commonly a benign and self-limiting disease?

❹ The reliability of clinical examination in determining the degree of dehydration.

❺ The circumstances in which the empirical use of antibiotics may be appropriate.

REFERENCES

1. Aranda-Michel J, Giannella RA 1999 Acute diarrhea: a practical review. American Journal of Medicine 106: 670–6
2. Guerrant RL, Van Gilder T, Steiner S, et al 2001 Practice guidelines for the management of infectious diarrhea. Clinical Infectious Diseases 32: 331–50

6.5 HAEMATEMESIS AND MELAENA

PETER WYLLIE • SUE IERACI

ESSENTIALS

1 Assessment and stabilization of intravascular volume is the first priority.

2 Identifying the most likely source of bleeding is crucial: it guides specific therapy and further investigations, and predicts prognosis.

3 Disposition must be individualized in order to minimize further morbidity and mortality.

INTRODUCTION

Gastrointestinal bleeding (GIB) is a common medical emergency with significant morbidity and mortality. Over the last decade there have been advances in pharmacotherapy for peptic ulcer disease and varices, improvements in endoscopic techniques, interventional radiology and surgical management, in addition to advances in resuscitation and supportive care in the emergency department and the ICU. Despite these advances, mortality for patients presenting with upper gastrointestinal haemorrhage remains around 5–10%, with approximately 16% requiring emergency surgery.[1-4]

HISTORY AND EXAMINATION

The aim of the history is to establish:
- The likely site of the bleeding
- The acuity of the bleed
- Pre-existing conditions/ comorbidities.

Determining the site of bleeding

First it is necessary to determine whether the blood loss is from a gastrointestinal source. Blood from the nose or oropharynx can be swallowed, resulting in haematemesis and/or melaena.

The next step is to distinguish upper GIB from lower GIB. Haematemesis and/or positive nasogastric aspirates indicate bleeding in the upper GI tract. Bright blood per rectum, although usually associated with lower GIB, may also be associated with brisk upper GIB bleeding. Melaena (black, tarry stools as a result of bacterial degradation of haemoglobin), although more commonly associated with upper GIB, may also be seen with lower GIB bleeds bacterial degradation of haemoglobin. Development of melaena requires a period of at least 4–8 hours for as little as 50–100 mL of blood to be degraded in the gut. It generally implies slow blood loss and does not always result in haemodynamic instability or anaemia. It is not associated with any increase in mortality, complications, or the need for surgery when compared with brown stools. Red stools, however, are generally associated with accelerated bleeding and do correlate with increased mortality, complications and surgery.

Role of nasogastric aspiration

When upper GI bleeding is strongly suspected, early endoscopy is the investigation treatment of choice. When this is not readily available, nasogastric aspiration may assist in confirming the site of bleeding and prioritizing the need for endoscopy. Table 6.5.1 shows the correlation of nasogastric findings with bleeding status at endoscopy in 1498 patients. Furthermore, it has been demonstrated that mortality increases from 6% with clear aspirates, to 10% if 'coffee grounds' were found, and 18% when bright blood was aspirated.

There are limitations to the use of the nasogastric tube as a diagnostic tool. Multiple factors, including pylorospasm, incorrect localization of the NGT and tube blockage limit the sensitivity of the nasogastric aspirate in detecting active bleeding to 79%. However, if the nasogastric aspirate is clear it is unlikely

Table 6.5.1 Nasogastric aspirate and bleeding status at endoscopy (1498 patients)

| Nasogastric aspirate | No. of patients | Bleeding status at endoscopy | |
		No blood or clot (%)	Oozing or pumping (%)
Clear	214	180 (84.1)	34 (15.9)
Coffee grounds	599	420 (70.1)	179 (29.9)
Red blood	685	355 (51.8)	350 (48.2)

(Reproduced with permission from Silverstein FE, et al 1981 The National ASGE survey on upper gastrointestinal bleeding. Gastrointestinal Endoscopy 27: 73–79, Mosby Inc., St Louis)

Table 6.5.2 Causes of upper gastrointestinal bleeding at endoscopy

Disease	% total
Erosive gastritis	29.6
Duodenal ulcer	22.8
Gastric ulcer	21.9
Varices	15.4
Oesophagitis	12.8
Erosive duodenitis	9.1
Mallory–Weiss tear	8.0
Neoplasm	3.7
Oesophageal ulcer	2.2
Stomach ulcer	1.9
Osler–Rendu–Weber	0.5
Other	7.3

(Reproduced from Gilbert DA, et al 1981 The National ASGE survey on upper gastrointestinal bleeding. Endoscopy in upper gastrointestinal bleeding. Gastrointestinal Endoscopy 27: 94–102, Mosby Inc., St Louis)

that a bleeding site is present in the oesophagus or stomach. The specificity for detecting active bleeding is also poor. In a study by Cuellar et al,[5] only 53% of patients with a positive aspirate were found to be actively bleeding at endoscopy. Nasal trauma secondary to the NGT may also result in false positives. However, there is no evidence that NGT placement aggravates bleeding from Mallory–Weiss tears or varices.

Upper GI bleeding

If bleeding is thought to be from the upper GI tract, then a number of diagnoses need to be considered. The most common causes are shown in Table 6.5.2.

Some historical clues and caveats must be considered:

- A history of epigastric pain or dyspepsia suggests peptic ulcer disease. However, peptic ulcer disease may be painless, particularly in the elderly.
- A positive history of gastric or duodenal ulcer disease or reflux oesophagitis is associated with an approximately 50% chance of finding the same diagnosis at endoscopy.
- The risk of GI bleeding in patients taking NSAIDs is double that of patients not taking NSAIDs.
- The classic history of nausea and vomiting prior to bleeding occurs in approximately one-third of cases of Mallory–Weiss tears.
- GI bleeding with a history of alcohol abuse and the stigmata of portal hypertension is suggestive of varices. However, up to 40% of patients with cirrhosis who present with GI bleeding are bleeding from causes other than varices (commonly from gastric erosions).
- Conditions associated with stress ulcers include burns, major trauma, head injury, sepsis and hypotension.
- Patients with chronic renal failure have a high incidence of angiodysplasia, peptic ulcer disease and oesophagitis.
- A history of aortic surgery and GI bleeding should alert the clinician to the possibility of an aortoenteric fistula, even if the initial bleeding episode is not significant.
- Clinical evidence of a coagulopathy should also be sought, as this will influence subsequent investigation, treatment and prognosis.
- A rectal examination is essential. As described above, stool colour has prognostic significance. Testing for occult blood further increases the sensitivity of this examination, as kits such as Hematest™ are able to detect as little as 6 mg of haemoglobin per gram of stool. A positive test is dependent on the time of onset of bleeding in relation to gastrointestinal transit time. False-positives may be produced by certain bacterial and vegetable peroxidases, such as bananas and horseradish. False-negatives may result from ferrous salts.

Acuity of the bleed

Clues to the speed or acuity of blood loss include:

- The most likely diagnosis, especially varices or aortoenteric fistulae
- The character of the vomitus: haematemesis, altered blood or clear fluid
- The colour of the stool: brown/black or red
- Signs of haemodynamic instability and response to resuscitation
- The nasogastric aspirate
- Initial haemoglobin.

Comorbidities

Patients with upper GI bleeding do not usually die from exsanguination but rather from decompensation of other organ systems. Therefore, comorbidities should be sought in order to predict potential morbidity and mortality. The presence of pre-existing cardiac, central nervous system, hepatic, pulmonary or renal disease is known to increase mortality in GI bleeding, and should, therefore, increase the urgency of investigations and the aggressiveness of therapy.

INVESTIGATIONS

Blood tests

Blood should be drawn for full blood count, coagulation studies (APTT and INR/PT), electrolytes, urea, creatinine, glucose level and cross-matching. Liver function tests should be performed if liver disease is suspected. Note that the initial haemoglobin is of limited value, as 24–48 hours are required for the intravascular volume to equilibrate. Thrombocytopenia and leucocytosis are associated with increasing morbidity and mortality. Upper GI bleeding may also result in an elevation of the urea level (relative to the creatinine), as there is a combination of an increased protein load in the gut and intravascular hypovolaemia.

Imaging

A chest X-ray may be indicated where aspiration is suspected, in the elderly, or in patients with cardiopulmonary comorbidities requiring anaesthesia. It should also be performed if perforation is suspected, however perforation associated with GIB is very rare. It must be noted that in one-third of patients with perforation no free gas is seen.

Endoscopy

Although clinical and historical features are helpful in indicating the most likely diagnosis, they are not specific. Furthermore, there is no empirical therapy that effectively treats all causes of upper GI bleeding. As a result, a specific diagnosis needs to be made.

Most centres rely on endoscopy to:

- provide information on the source of bleeding with a high degree of specificity (90–95%)
- allow prediction of the likelihood of rebleeding and mortality, according to the nature and location of the lesion and evidence of recent haemorrhage (Table 6.5.3). These factors help in deciding how closely the patient needs to be monitored or whether they may be treated as an outpatient
- provide therapy. Endoscopy facilitates haemostasis through sclerotherapy, coagulation techniques and banding of varices, and allows histological or microbiological diagnosis. In high-risk peptic ulcers endoscopic therapy has been shown to decrease rebleeding by 75% and mortality by 40%

Table 6.5.3 The prevalence and outcomes of bleeding ulcers, based on endoscopic appearance (without endoscopic therapy)

Endoscopic appearance	Prevalence	Percentages		
		Rebleeding	Surgery	Mortality
Clean base	42	5	0.5	2
Flat spots	20	10	6	3
Adherent clot	17	22	10	7
Non-bleeding visible vessel	17	43	34	11
Active bleeding	18	55	35	11

(Adapted with permission from Laine L, Peterson WL[18] 1994 Medical progress: bleeding peptic ulcer. New England Journal of Medicine 331: 717–727. © 1994 Massachusetts Medical Society. All rights reserved)

- diagnose with safety (morbidity less than 0.01%). Safety is further maximized if endoscopy is delayed until the patient is haemodynamically stable and the airway patent and protected.

The sensitivity of endoscopy is optimized if performed within 12–24 hours of presentation. Urgent endoscopy should be performed in patients with active or recurrent bleeding, bright red blood on NG aspirate, haematemesis, large bleeds (>2 units blood required), and when variceal bleeding is suspected. Early endoscopy facilitates management and results in earlier discharge.

INITIAL ASSESSMENT AND STABILIZATION

Oxygen should be administered to all patients. The intravascular volume should then be assessed. The presence of shock places the patient at high risk for rebleeding, surgery and mortality. Note that in the elderly, patients with autonomic neuropathies or those taking beta-blockers or calcium channel antagonists, vital signs (including postural hypotension) may not be a reliable indicator of the degree of blood loss.

Intravascular volume should initially be replaced with isotonic crystalloid (saline or Hartmann's) or colloid (e.g. Haemaccel®). Blood should be given if there is persistent haemodynamic instability despite 2 litres of crystalloid or colloid, if the initial haemoglobin level is less than 8 mg/dL, if there is significant risk of rebleeding, and in those patients with comorbidities making them unable to tolerate periods of hypoperfusion or anaemia. Aggressive resuscitation with early blood transfusion is indicated in the elderly patient. However, overhydration of patients with suspected varices should be avoided with careful monitoring.

Monitoring

Continuous ECG monitoring, non-invasive blood pressure monitoring and pulse oximetry should be instituted, with repeated measurements made in conjunction with frequent clinical reassessment. Urine output should be monitored. CVP monitoring may be necessary in massive bleeds and those with comorbidities.

Coagulation

Fresh frozen plasma should be given when the prothrombin time is 3 seconds greater than the control or when large transfusions are required. Platelets are rarely required unless the platelet count is less than 50×10^9/L or the platelets are dysfunctional.

ACUTE SPECIFIC THERAPY

Peptic ulcer disease

Peptic ulceration is the most common cause of upper GI haemorrhage, accounting for approximately 50% of cases. As bleeding ceases spontaneously in 80% of cases, the mortality rate is approximately 5–6%, significantly less than with variceal bleeding.

Pharmacotherapy

As in vitro studies have shown haemostasis to be a pH dependent process, it is hypothesized that medications which inhibit acid secretion will also reduce the three main end points of the studies: rebleeding, the need for surgery and mortality. The two main drug classes are the H_2-antagonists and the proton pump inhibitors (PPIs).

H_2-antagonists Most data relating to the benefit of H_2-antagonists in acute upper GI bleeds are unconvincing. Most trials are too small to assess reliably the effect of treatment on end-points such as mortality. A large trial by Walt et al,[6] involving 1005 patients, found no benefits in terms of mortality, rebleeding or surgery with IV famotidine.

Proton pump inhibitors The PPIs are becoming the most commonly used drug in peptic disease based on more profound and persistent acid suppression. However, the many trials of PPIs have yielded conflicting results, as they involve different treatment and placebo arms, with varying inclusion and exclusion criteria. In summary, the available data suggests that:

- When all causes of upper GI bleeding are included, there are no significant benefits (rebleeding, need for surgery or mortality) with PPIs.
- When all groups of non-variceal/peptic bleeding are included, there are no significant benefits (rebleeding, need for surgery or mortality).
- When only patients with high risk peptic ulcers are included (Forrest Class 1 and 2 with and without endoscopic treatment), some studies showed reduced need for surgery and rebleeding but no change in mortality. Note that these benefits were not found in all studies, were only found in patients with specific high risk endoscopic features (as shown in Table 6.5.3) and the

treatment arms most commonly used omeprazole in large doses of 80 mg IV followed by infusions of 8 mg/h.

Therefore high dose therapy should be restricted to those patients found to have high risk lesions at endoscopy.

For patients with peptic ulcer disease, the aim should be to eliminate reversible risk factors such as *H. pylori* and NSAIDs, and aim for long-term healing. As PPIs have been shown to be provide better rates of healing, they are thus drugs of first choice for this purpose. It is reasonable to initiate oral therapy when feeding is recommened, or intravenous therapy when feeding is delayed.

Somatostatin/octreotide Conflicting results have been found in studies of the use of somatostatin and octreotide in peptic ulcer disease. One small study noted the successful use of somatostatin in controlling severe upper GI bleeding in patients in whom surgery was hazardous.[8] However, other trials have not shown either agent to conclusively influence rebleeding, surgery or mortality,[9,10] and, therefore, these agents cannot be routinely recommended. Further studies are required to establish the role of somatostatin or octreotide in non-variceal bleeding.

Endoscopy

Endoscopic therapy has been shown to achieve haemostasis in approximately 90% of cases, reduce rebleeding by 62%, reduce emergency surgery by 64% and mortality by 45%. The incidence of bleeding and perforation associated with endoscopic therapy was 0.38% and 0.61%, respectively.[11] The ongoing development of new endoscopic techniques for coagulation of bleeding sites means that endoscopy is continuing to supplant surgery as definitive therapy.

Surgery

Surgery is required in approximately 15% of patients. It is indicated for continuous or recurrent active bleeding, especially in patients over 60, in whom early elective surgery produces significant benefits in terms of mortality. Other indications include blood transfusion exceeding 5

units, refractory shock, and failure to respond to endoscopic therapy. Early elective surgery in selected cases is preferable to emergency surgery because of the significant mortality associated with the latter.

Surgical consultation should be considered early in patients aged over 60, those with significant comorbidities, those with active bleeding (haematemesis, bright red blood on aspirate), when there is a significant risk of rebleeding, or when there is haemodynamic instability at any stage.

Embolization

This is a therapeutic alternative in high-risk patients with recurrent or severe bleeding.

Gastro-oesophageal varices

Although haemorrhage from gastro-oesophageal varices accounts for 2–15% of all upper GI bleeding, it is a significant therapeutic challenge to the physician. Bleeding ceases spontaneously in only 20–30%, yet as bleeding is often more severe and recurrent, mortality approaches 25–40% for each episode of variceal haemorrhage. Factors influencing mortality include the stage and rate of deterioration of the underlying liver disease, the presence of comorbidities, variceal size, and specific endoscopic criteria.

Pharmacotherapy

Drugs should be used when endoscopic expertise is not available, if massive bleeding prevents immediate sclerotherapy, or as an adjunct to further treatment if continued variceal haemorrhage is suspected. However, sclerotherapy or other surgical procedures are still required after drug therapy.

Somatostatin/octreotide This therapy produces dramatic decreases in splanchnic arterial blood flow and portal venous pressure, while preserving cardiac output and systemic blood pressure. It is the pharmacological method of choice as it is comparable to injection sclerotherapy, vasopressin and balloon tamponade in terms of bleeding control and survival, with the advantage of fewer side effects.

Treatment results in the control of bleeding in 74–92% of cases, with endoscopic evidence of cessation of bleeding in 68% of patients within 15 minutes. The suggested rate of administration of somatostatin is 250 mg/hour after an initial bolus of 250 mg. Octreotide is administered at 50 mg/hour after an initial bolus of 50 mg. There may be additional benefits from daily boluses.

Vasopressin This drug increases peripheral vascular resistance and mean arterial pressure, with reduced cardiac output and coronary blood flow. It is, therefore, contraindicated in patients with coronary artery disease, and is associated with complications necessitating withdrawal of treatment in up to 25% of patients. This makes vasopressin the second choice of pharmacotherapy. However, combination with IV nitroglycerin (if tolerated) reduces the incidence of complications with no effect on efficacy. Vasopressin results in the control of bleeding in 50–75% of cases. The recommended infusion rate is 0.2–0.4 U/min to a maximum of 0.8 U/min with nitroglycerin if tolerated (40 mg/minute increasing to 400 mg/minute, titrated to blood pressure).

Endoscopic sclerotherapy

Endoscopy is essential to confirm the diagnosis of variceal haemorrhage, as in patients with known varices an alternative bleeding site was noted up to 81% of cases. Endoscopy may also have therapeutic benefits as endoscopic sclerotherapy (EST) can be performed at the time of the initial endoscopy. Control of bleeding can be achieved subsequently in up to 95% of cases,[12] with a reduction in the risk of rebleeding. Therefore, EST is considered first-line therapy in the control of bleeding from oesophageal varices.

However, complications are noted in up to 41% of patients. These include perforation, aspiration, pyrexia, chest pain, tachycardia, oesophageal ulcers and strictures. Because recurrence rates are 20–30%, patients need repeated treatments.

EST is not recommended for gastric varices owing to the high complication rate and poor efficacy. Two possible alternative therapeutic strategies of benefit are tissue adhesives or thrombin.

Endoscopic variceal ligation

Although technically more difficult, endoscopic variceal ligation (EVL) has been shown to be as effective as EST in the control of variceal haemorrhage, with significantly fewer complications, rebleeding and mortality. It requires fewer treatment sessions than EST. Additional benefits (more effective control of variceal bleeding) may be gained by combining sclerotherapy with octreotide.

Balloon tamponade

Compression of fundal and distal oesophageal varices by balloon tamponade results in control of bleeding in 70–90% of cases. Balloon tamponade may be used as a temporary means of controlling bleeding which is refractory to medical or endoscopic treatment, or when it is too massive for endoscopy to be performed successfully.

Because of the problems of pooling of secretions in the oesophagus (thereby increasing the risk of pulmonary aspiration), the standard Sengstaken-Blakemore tube has been modified to the form of the Minnesota tube to incorporate an oesophageal aspiration port. Alternatively, an NGT may be placed to drain the oesophagus. Further modifications have been made with the Linton-Nachlas tube, which incorporates a single large gastric balloon (600 mL) for the tamponade of gastric varices.

There are number of problems with balloon tamponade:

- It can only be used for a maximum of 48–72 hours. As up to 50% of patients rebleed when the tube is deflated, further definitive procedures need to be performed (EVL, EST, surgery).
- There is a significant (25–30%) risk of complications, particularly pulmonary aspiration and oesophageal perforation.
- Balloon tamponade requires skilled staff and monitoring in an intensive-care setting for the initial insertion and maintenance of balloon position and function.
- Owing to the risks of pulmonary aspiration, endotracheal intubation should be considered in all patients requiring balloon tamponade.

Transjugular intrahepatic portosystemic stent

Transjugular intrahepatic portosystemic stent-shunt (TIPS) involves the insertion of a stent under radiological guidance via the jugular vein, forming a portosystemic shunt between the hepatic and portal veins. This technique is effective, achieving control of bleeding in up to 90% of patients, and is less invasive and faster to perform (range 30 minutes to 3 hours) than other surgical shunt procedures. However, it requires an experienced operator and often results in complications similar to those seen after other portosystemic shunts, particularly encephalopathy and deteriorating liver function.

The main role of TIPS, therefore, appears to be in patients who continue to bleed in spite of sclerotherapy or ligation therapy, and who do not have hepatic encephalopathy, preterminal liver failure, portal vein thrombosis, intrahepatic sepsis or significant cardiac disease. TIPS then acts as a bridging procedure until other definitive surgical procedures can be performed (such as liver transplantation, shunt surgery or oesophageal transection).

Surgery

Since the advent of EST, the role of surgery in the control of acute bleeding has decreased and it is now largely confined to patients who continue to bleed despite endoscopic intervention. Shunt surgery and oesophageal transection have been shown to reduce bleeding. However, these techniques have not been shown to improve survival, and provide no cost advantage compared to EST.

Radiologic embolization

Radiologic embolization via a transhepatic or minilaparotomy approach is another non-operative option for control of bleeding varices. It is effective, controlling bleeding in 70–90% of patients, yet there is a significant rebleeding rate over the next 2–6 months. The role of embolization has largely been superseded by interventions such as TIPS.

DISPOSITION

The primary decision in most cases is whether the patient is to be admitted to the ward or to an intensive care (ICU) or high-dependency unit (HDU).

The main indications for ICU/IDU admission include:

- Known or suspected variceal bleeding
- Haemodynamic instability
- Significant comorbidities, including cardiac, renal, pulmonary or hepatic dysfunction
- Endoscopic features suggesting recent haemorrhage (arterial bleeding, adherent clot or visible vessel).

It is also suggested that the threshold for ICU/HDU admission be lowered in patients over 60 years of age, owing to the high incidence of comorbidities and poor physiological compensatory reserve.

Other low-risk patients may be admitted to the general ward for approximately 3 days, as the major risk of rebleeding is during the first 48–72 hours.

The guidelines for outpatient management of upper GI bleeding are less clear. Most cases cease spontaneously and most patients compensate well, not requiring transfusion or surgery. As a result, some authors advocate outpatient management of approximately 20% of patients presenting with upper GI bleeding.[13] To minimize the risk of adverse events if the patient is managed as an outpatient, early endoscopy is advocated. Early discharge is then suggested for those who were noted to have clean-based ulcers or non-bleeding Mallory–Weiss tears. In this group, with no stigmata of recent haemorrhage, the risks of rebleeding and need for emergency surgery are between 0 and 5% and death is rare.[14] This subgroup of patients may be discharged after a 6-hour observation period if they also satisfy all of the criteria listed in Table 6.5.4.[14,15]

Table 6.5.4 Criteria for the selection of patients for outpatient management of upper gastrointestinal haemorrhage

Absolute
No high-risk endoscopic features, varices or portal hypertensive gastropathy

Not absolute
No debilitation and age less than 60
Haemoglobin levels >10 g/dL
Lack of significant comorbidities (cirrhosis, coronary or peripheral vascular disease, anticoagulation/coagulopathy, aortic prosthesis, renal disease or irreversible lung disease
No fresh voluminous haematemesis or multiple episodes of melaena on the day of presentation
No orthostatic vital sign changes
Adequate support at home/reliable and compliant
Lack of syncopal symptoms or signs
No medications likely to cloud assessment, such as calcium channel blockers or β-blockers

(Adapted with permission from Longstreth GF, Feitelberg SP[14] 1995 Outpatient care of selected patients with acute non-variceal upper gastrointestinal haemorrhage. Lancet 354: 108–111)

CONTROVERSIES

❶ Nasogastric aspiration is an important diagnostic tool; however, a range of factors limit its sensitivity.

❷ Although the early use of H₂-antagonists is widespread, the evidence of benefit in acute gastrointestinal haemorrhage is not convincing and is limited to gastric ulceration.

❸ There are many therapeutic modalities available for the treatment of oesophageal varices. Octreotide and transjugular intrahepatic portosystemic stent-shunt (TIPS) are becoming more established, the high complication rate of balloon tamponade makes it a less desirable option.

❹ A case is now being made for the outpatient management of selected low-risk cases of gastrointestinal bleeding.

REFERENCES

1. Dronfield M 1987 Specialised units for acute upper gastrointestinal bleeding. British Medical Journal 294: 1308–9
2. Gostout CJ, Wang KK, Ahlquist DA, et al 1992 Acute gastrointestinal bleeding: experience of a specialised management team. Journal of Clinical Gastroenterology 14: 260–7
3. Duggan JM 1986 Haematemesis patients should be managed in special units. Medical Journal of Australia 144: 247–50
4. Hunt PS, Hansky J, Korman MG 1979 Mortality in patients with haematemesis and melaena: a prospective study. British Medical Journal 1: 1238–40
5. Cuellar RE, Gavaler JS, Alexander JA, et al 1990 Gastrointestinal hemorrhage: the value of the nasogastric aspirate. Archives of Internal Medicine 150: 1381–4
6. Walt RP, Cottrell J, Mann SG, Freemantle NP, Langman MJS 1992 Continuous intravenous famotidine for haemorrhage from peptic ulcer. Lancet 340: 1058–62
7. Collins R, Langman M 1985 Treatment with histamine H2 antagonists in upper gastrointestinal haemorrhage: implications of randomised trials. New England Journal of Medicine 313: 660–6
8. Jenkins SA, Taylor BA, Nott DM, Ellenbogen S, Haggie J, Shields R 1992 Management of upper gastrointestinal haemorrhage from multiple sites of peptic ulceration with somatostatin and octreotide - a report of five cases. Gut 33: 404–7
9. Sommerville KW, Davies JG, Hawkey CJ, Henry DA, Hine KR, Langman MJS 1985 Somatostatin in the treatment of haematemesis and melaena. Lancet i: 130–2
10. Christiansen J, Ottenjann R, Von Arx F 1989 Placebo-controlled trial with the somatostatin analogue SMS 201–995 in peptic ulcer bleeding. Gastroenterology 97: 568–74
11. Cook DJ, Guyatt GH, Salena BJ, Laine LA 1992 Endoscopic therapy for acute nonvariceal upper gastrointestinal hemorrhage: a met-analysis. Gastroenterology 102: 139–48
12. Westaby D, Hayes P, Grimson AE, Polson RJ, Williams R 1989 Controlled trial of injection sclerotherapy for active variceal bleeding. Hepatology 9: 274–7
13. Packham CJ, Rockall TA, Logan RFA 1995 Outpatient care for selected patients with acute upper gastrointestinal bleeding (letter). Lancet 345: 659–60
14. Longstreth GF, Feitelberg SP 1995 Outpatient care of selected patients with acute non-variceal upper gastrointestinal haemorrhage. Lancet 345: 108–11
15. Rockall TA, Logan RFA, Devlin HB, Northfield TC 1996 Selection of patients for early discharge or outpatient care after acute upper gastrointestinal haemorrhage. Lancet 347: 1138–40
16. Silverstein FE, Gilbert DA, Tedesco FJ, et al 1981 The national ASGE survey on upper gastrointestinal bleeding III endoscopy in upper gastrointestinal bleeding. Gastrointestinal Endoscopy 27: 94–102
17. Gilbert DA, Silverstein FE, Tedesco FJ, et al 1981 The national ASGE survey on upper gastrointestinal bleeding. Gastrointestinal Endoscopy 27: 73–9
18. Laine L, Peterson WL 1994 Bleeding peptic ulcer. New England Journal of Medicine 331: 717–27

FURTHER READING

Besson I, Ingrand P, Person B, et al 1995 Sclerotherapy with or without octreotide for acute variceal bleeding. New England Journal of Medicine 333: 555–60

DIGESTIVE

Brewer TG 1993 Treatment of acute variceal hemorrhage. Medical Clinics of North America 77: 993–1010

Cello JP, Chan MF 1993 Octreotide therapy for variceal hemorrhage. Digestion 54(1): 20–6

Daneshmend TK, Hawkey CJ, Langman MJS, Logan RFA, Long RG, Walt RP 1992 Omeprazole versus placebo for acute upper gastrointestinal bleeding: randomised double blind controlled trial. British Medical Journal 304: 143–7

Goff JS 1993 Gastroesophageal varices: pathogenesis and therapy of acute bleeding. Gastroenterology Clinics of North America 22: 779–800

Harland R, Neilson D 1992 Criteria for selective admission of patients with haematemesis. Journal of the Royal Society of Medicine 85: 26–8

Jenkins SA, Taylor BA, Nott DM, Ellenbogen S, Haggie J, Shields R 1992 Management of upper gastrointestinal haemorrhage from multiple sites of peptic ulceration with somatostatin and octreotide - a report of five cases. Gut 33: 404–7

Kolkman JJ, Meuwissen SGM 1996 A review on the treatment of bleeding peptic ulcer: a collaborative task of gastroenterologist and surgeon. Scandinavian Journal of Gastroenterology 31(218): 16–25

Liebermann D 1993 Gastrointestinal bleeding: initial management. Gastroenterology Clinics of North America 22: 723–36

Luk GD, Bynum TE, Hendrix TR 1979 Gastric aspiration for localisation of gastrointestinal haemorrhage. Journal of the American Medical Association 241: 576–8

Navarro VJ, Garcia-Tsao G 1995 Variceal hemorrhage. Critical Care Clinics 11: 391–414

Roberts SK, Dudley FJ 1997 Management of haematemesis and melaena. Medical Journal of Australia 166: 549–53

Rockall TA, Logan RFA, Devlin HB, Northfield TC 1996 Selection of patients for early discharge or outpatient care after acute upper gastrointestinal haemorrhage. Lancet 347: 1138–40

Sandford NL, Kerlin P 1995 Current management of oesophageal varices. Australian New Zealand Journal of Medicine 25: 528–34

Silverstein FE, Gilbert DA, Tedesco FJ, et al 1981 The national ASGE survey on upper gastrointestinal bleeding. II Clinical prognostic factors. Gastrointestinal Endoscopy 27: 80–93

Williams SGJ, Westaby D 1994 Management of variceal haemorrhage. British Medical Journal 308: 1213–7

Wrenn KD, Brindley Thompson L 1991 Hemodynamically stable upper gastrointestinal bleeding. American Journal of Emergency Medicine 9: 309–12

Yung JJY, Chung S, Lai CW, et al 1993 Octreotide infusion or emergency sclerotherapy for variceal haemorrhage. Lancet 342: 637–41

6.6 PEPTIC ULCER DISEASE AND GASTRITIS

STUART DILLEY

ESSENTIALS

1 *Helicobacter pylori* is responsible for 70–90% of peptic ulcers, with non-steroidal anti-inflammatory drugs accounting for most of the remainder.

2 Emergency presentations of peptic ulcer disease vary from mild indigestion to severe life-threatening complications.

3 Endoscopy is the investigation of choice for definitive diagnosis.

4 Most patients can be managed medically with a combination of antisecretory drugs and antibiotics as indicated.

5 Surgical treatment may be indicated for complications such as haemorrhage, perforation and obstruction.

6 A 'negative' erect chest X-ray does not exclude ulcer perforation.

INTRODUCTION

In recent years the discovery of the organism *Helicobacter pylori* has resulted in a dramatic change in our understanding of the aetiology and pathophysiology of peptic ulcer disease. What was once a chronic disease prone to relapse and recurrence has now become eminently treatable and curable.

Patients presenting to emergency departments may do so with 'classic' ulcer symptoms, undifferentiated abdominal or chest pains, or more dramatically with life-threatening complications such as perforation or haemorrhage.

PATHOPHYSIOLOGY

Although the vast majority of patients harbouring *H. pylori* are asymptomatic, it is now accepted that *H. pylori* is the major cause of peptic ulceration, or at least a major cofactor in the development of peptic ulcer disease. *H. pylori* has been isolated from 20–50% of patients with dyspeptic symptoms. More importantly, 90–95% of patients with duodenal ulcers and 70% of those with gastric ulcers are infected with the organism. Eradication of *H. pylori* has been shown to markedly reduce the recurrence rate for ulceration.[1,2]

Non-steroidal anti-inflammatory drugs (NSAIDs), including low-dose aspirin, are the second most common cause of peptic ulceration and account for most ulcers not due to *H. pylori*. NSAIDs cause ulcers by inhibiting the production of prostaglandins in the stomach and duodenum (a vital part of the stomach's mucosal defence mechanisms), and hence may also cause ulceration when given by non-oral routes. NSAIDs are more commonly associated with gastric ulceration. At least 50% of patients taking NSAIDs will have endoscopic evidence of erythema, erosions or ulcers, even if asymptomatic.[1,3]

Some NSAIDS are more likely to produce ulcers than others. In general, shorter acting agents such as ibuprofen and diclofenac are less likely to lead to ulcers than longer acting agents.[4]

Acid is an important ingredient in the pathogenesis of both NSAID- and *H. pylori*-induced ulceration. Traditional risk factors such as smoking, alcohol and stress may increase the risk of ulceration and delay healing, but their relative importance as aetiological agents has fallen considerably with the discovery of *H. pylori*.[1] Other causes of peptic ulceration, such as Zollinger-Ellison syndrome, are rare.

CLINICAL FEATURES

History

'Indigestion' is the most common symptom in patients found to have peptic ulcer disease. Patients describe a burning or gnawing pain in the epigastrium that may radiate into the chest or straight through to the back. Food may either exacerbate or relieve the pain. The pain is classically both fluctuating and periodic, with bouts of discomfort of variable severity interspersed with symptom-free periods.

However, 'indigestion' or 'dyspepsia' has a relatively poor sensitivity and specificity for diagnosing the various peptic syndromes. Less than 25% of patients with dyspepsia have peptic ulcer disease proven by gastroscopy, and between 20 and 60% of patients presenting with complications of ulcer disease report no antecedent symptoms.[5]

Emergency patients may present or be referred with this classic symptom complex. Others present with chest or abdominal pains which need to be differentiated from conditions such as myocardial ischaemia, biliary tract disease, pancreatitis and other abdominal emergencies.

Patients also present frequently with the two most common complications of ulcer disease, namely acute gastrointestinal haemorrhage or acute perforation.

Examination

In uncomplicated peptic ulcer disease abdominal findings may be limited to epigastric tenderness without peritoneal signs.

INVESTIGATIONS

The extent of investigations performed in the emergency department depends greatly on the patient's presentation and the degree of severity of symptoms. Most will be referred for definitive diagnosis.

Haematology and biochemistry

Pathology investigations relevant to the emergency management of these patients are aimed primarily at eliminating alternative diagnoses or identifying the complications of peptic ulceration.

Full blood examination

Anaemia is most likely to represent chronic rather than acute blood loss, unless bleeding is particularly heavy and hence clinically obvious. A microcytic, hypochromic anaemia suggests chronic blood loss with iron deficiency, and can be confirmed with iron studies.

Blood cross-match

Patients with active bleeding will need replacement with blood products. Several units of blood may be required.

Clotting studies

These are indicated in patients taking warfarin and those with massive bleeding and/or a history of liver disease and/or alcoholism.

Liver function tests/amylase

Biliary tract disease and pancreatitis are common differential diagnoses in patients presenting with non-specific epigastric or upper abdominal pain. Pancreatitis may also be the consequence of ulcer penetration through the posterior wall of the stomach.

Radiology

Radiological imaging has a very limited place in the diagnosis of uncomplicated peptic ulcer disease. However, an erect chest X-ray (CXR) is an important investigation when ulcer perforation is being considered. Gas is usually visible under the diaphragm, but its absence does not rule out perforation. Several studies have quoted the sensitivity of erect CXR for detection of pneumoperitoneum as ranging from 70–80%.[6,7] Lateral chest X-ray in addition to the PA view may increase the sensitivity.[7] Lateral decubitus abdominal X-rays may be needed to demonstrate free gas in those unable to sit erect. CT scan of the abdomen may be more sensitive in detecting small pneumoperitoneums.

Contrast studies are no longer considered first-line investigations in the assessment of patients with dyspeptic symptoms. Abdominal X-ray and ultrasound studies are useful to exclude alternative diagnoses, as indicated.

Endoscopy

Endoscopy is the investigation of choice for patients with dyspeptic symptoms, allowing direct visualization of the mucosa of the oesophagus, stomach and proximal duodenum. It provides a definitive diagnosis, which forms the basis of rational drug use, and allows biopsies to be taken to exclude malignant disease and to isolate *H. pylori*. Endoscopy may also be therapeutic in some cases of upper gastrointestinal haemorrhage.

H. pylori status

The discovery of *H. pylori* was quickly followed by the development of tests to identify its presence. Currently there are a number of tests available, both invasive and non-invasive[8] though their exact role in the emergency-department setting have not been defined. It should be remembered that the majority of patients infected with *H. pylori* do not in fact have peptic ulcer disease, and that the identification of *H. pylori* infection often has little relationship to presenting symptoms. In particular, neither of the non-invasive tests can make a diagnosis of peptic ulcer disease, only of *H. pylori* infection. However, a negative test in a patient not taking NSAIDs makes the likelihood of peptic ulcer low.[1]

The invasive tests for *H. pylori* include haematoxylin and eosin staining of mucosal biopsies and rapid urease tests (e.g. CLOtest). The latter are performed on biopsy specimens. Positive tests rely on the organism's ability to produce ammonia from urea. For both tests sensitivity is reliant on the number of organisms present, and hence may be affected by pretreatment.[2,8]

The non-invasive tests include urease breath tests and IgG serology. Regarding breath tests, the high urease activity of *H. pylori* is used to cleave ingested ^{13}C- or ^{14}C-labelled urea, with the resultant labelled carbon dioxide measured on exhalation. Urea breath tests are highly sensitive and specific for the presence of *H. pylori*.[9] At present, they are most useful in assessing H. *pylori* eradication without the need for further gastroscopy. A number of IgG serology tests are available with varying specificities and sensitivities. Most are qualitative tests that remain positive for some time after treatment, and may not be useful to confirm eradication.[1,8]

MANAGEMENT

Emergency department management of patients with dyspeptic symptoms requires the exclusion of other diseases, the removal of known precipitants such as NSAIDs, alcohol and cigrattes, the institution of simple treatment measures aimed at symptomatic relief, and referral for further investigation and management.

There is debate about the merits of starting specific antiulcer therapy and *H. pylori* eradication in patients with dyspeptic symptoms before a formal diagnosis has been made on gastroscopy and biopsy.

For patients with mild symptoms of recent onset, empirical treatment with antacids and/or histamine receptor antagonists aimed at symptomatic relief is reasonable. Given the poor correlation between dyspeptic symptoms and gastro-oesophageal disease, early gastroscopy should be considered for most cases, particularly if symptoms are not controlled or promptly recur.

A recent review of the literature concluded that for patients with non-ulcer dyspepsia, H_2-receptor blockers were significantly more effective at reducing symptoms than placebo whereas proton pump inhibitors and bismuth salts were only marginally so.[10] Antacids and sucralfate were not statistically superior to placebo.

Early treatment prior to endoscopy may cure some patients without the need for expensive invasive procedures.

However, this plan of action may hinder subsequent *H. pylori* isolation and delay definitive diagnosis, including the diagnosis of malignant disease.[1] Endoscopy and biopsy should precede the institution of eradication therapy and proton pump inhibitors.

In reality, proton pump inhibitors and the *Helicobacter* eradication triple packs are currently only available in Australia on authority or restricted prescription after definitive diagnosis of ulceration and *H. pylori* infection has been made.

Antacids

'Antacids', containing combinations of calcium, magnesium, local anaesthetics and alginates, are useful in providing symptomatic relief for patients with relatively mild symptoms. In many instances, patients have already tried these agents prior to presentation.

Histamine-receptor antagonists

The H_2-receptor antagonists such as cimetidine, ranitidine, famotidine and nizatidine all have similar efficacies with regard to ulcer healing. All are well absorbed orally, however, their absorption may be reduced when used with antacids.[11] Eighty to 90% of duodenal ulcers will be healed in 4–8 weeks, and 70% of gastric ulcers within 8 weeks. Relapse rates of 80% over the course of 1 year are to be expected if *H. pylori* eradication is not also undertaken.[5,12]

Proton pump inhibitors

Omeprazole, lansoprazole and pantoprazole are currently available in Australia. They act by binding to $H^+/K^+ATPase$ in gastric parietal cells, inhibiting the cells' proton pump. Compared to H_2-receptor antagonists, these agents result in more rapid ulcer healing and pain relief over 2–4 weeks, although differences at 8 weeks are not significant. Again, relapse rates are high, particularly if *H. pylori* is present and eradication therapy is not used.[12]

Cytoprotectants

Cytoprotective agents include colloidal bismuth subcitrate (De-Nol®) and sucralfate. Both act by binding to or chelating with proteins in the base of the ulcer. Bismuth compounds also suppress *H. pylori*. A 6–8-week course is recommended and relapse rates are still high. Bismuth compounds lead to the formation of black stools that may be confused for melaena by the unwary clinician. Sucralfate should not be taken with antacids as it requires an acid environment to achieve its optimal effects.[12]

Prostaglandin analogues

Misoprostol, a synthetic analogue of PGE_1, interferes with histamine-dependent gastric acid secretion as well as being cytoprotective for the gastric mucosa. It is particularly useful in the prevention of NSAID-induced ulcers, although it is probably no better than the other agents in actually treating such ulcers.[12]

H. pylori eradication

A number of eradication therapies have been postulated, all with very high eradication (>80%) and low relapse rates (<5%). The development of resistance to metronidazole has resulted in amoxycillin and clarithromycin being recommended as the antibiotics of choice. These are usually combined with a proton pump inhibitor or colloidal bismuth subcitrate for a 1-week course. Several single prescription packages are now available.[9] It is generally accepted that acid suppresion therapy be continued for 4–8 weeks after cessation of antibiotic therapy.

H. pylori eradication therapy in patients with non-ulcer dyspepsia may have a small, yet statistically significant effect on symptoms.[13]

Prevention of NSAID-induced ulcers

The best protection against the development of NSAID induced ulcers is to avoid their unnecessary use. However, there are many patients who need to take NSAID, putting them at risk of peptic ulceration and its associated complications. For these patients, co-therapy may be beneficial.

H_2-receptor antagonists appear to offer little protection against NSAIDs. However, misoprostol and the proton pump inhibitors have been shown to protect against NSAID-induced ulceration.[4]

Misoprostol significantly reduced the risk of endoscopic ulcers.[14] Standard doses of H_2-blockers were effective at reducing the risk of duodenal but not gastric ulcers. Double dose H_2-blockers and proton pump inhibitors were effective at reducing the risk of both duodenal and gastric ulcers, and were better tolerated than misoprostol.[14]

Treatment of NSAID-induced ulcers

NSAIDs, including aspirin should be ceased if at all possible. Treatment should consist of a 4–8 week course of H_2-receptor antagonist or proton pump inhibitor.

SURGICAL MANAGEMENT

With the newfound success of medical treatment of peptic ulcer disease, surgical intervention has been restricted to the management of complications rather than of the primary disease.

COMPLICATIONS

Haemorrhage

Peptic ulceration is a common cause of upper GI bleeding, occurring in 10–20% of ulcer patients and accounting for approximately 50% of all upper GI bleeds. Urgent endoscopy is usually indicated and surgical intervention may be required. A recent meta-analysis concluded that the use of acid-reducing agents was associated with a statistically significant decrease in rebleeding, but not mortality.[15] Assessment and management of these patients is discussed in detail elsewhere in this book (Chapter 6.5).

Perforation

Perforation occurs in approximately 5% of ulcers, usually those on the anterior wall of stomach and duodenum. Chemical peritonitis develops suddenly, with acute severe generalized abdominal pain. Examination reveals a 'sick patient' with a rigid, quiet abdomen and rebound tenderness. Delay in presentation and treatment, which may occur in the elderly and debilitated, sees the rapid development of bacterial peritonitis and subsequent sepsis and shock. The overall mortality rate is about 5%.

Diagnosis should be confirmed with an erect chest X-ray, bearing in mind a sensitivity of 70–80%,[6,7] and vigorous fluid resuscitation instituted. Renal function (via urine output) should be closely monitored. Ampicillin, gentamicin and metronidazole should be given, along with adequate analgesia. Cardiac and respiratory support may be needed in some cases.

The majority of patients with perforation should undergo surgery for decontamination and repair. It may be possible to observe the stable patient who presents late, and in whom there is no evidence of an ongoing leak. Contrast studies may be useful in this setting.

Penetration

Posterior ulcers may perforate the gastric or duodenal wall and continue to erode into adjacent structures, most commonly the pancreas. Patients may describe their pain as becoming more severe and constant, radiating to the back and no longer eased by antacids. The serum amylase level may be mildly raised. Endoscopy may reveal ulceration, but 'penetration' is difficult to confirm.

Gastric outlet obstruction

Obstruction may occur in up to 2% of patients with ulcer disease. It may arise acutely secondary to inflammation and oedema of the pylorus or duodenal bulb, or more commonly as a consequence of scarring due to chronic disease.

CONTROVERSIES

❶ Should specific H_2-blockers, proton pump inhibitors or *H. pylori* eradication therapy be instituted prior to formal diagnosis via gastroscopy?

❷ Conservative versus surgical management of perforated ulcer.

REFERENCES

1. Katelaris P 1996 Peptic ulcer disease: clinical implications of current thinking. Current Therapeutics 37(7): 41–6
2. NIH consensus development panel on *Helicobacter pylori* in peptic ulcer disease 1994 *Helicobacter pylori* in peptic ulcer disease. Journal of the American Medical Association 1994; 272(1): 65–9
3. Yeomans N 1997 How do we treat NSAID-induced ulcers? Current Therapeutics 38(4): 45–51
4. Yeomans N 2001 Approaches to healing and prophylaxis of nonsteroidal anti-inflammatory drug-associated ulcers. American Journal of Medicine 110: 24S–28S
5. Tierney L, McPhee S, Papadikis A (eds) 1994 Current Medical Diagnosis and Treatment, 33rd edn. Prentice Hall, New Jersey
6. Svanes C, Salvesen H, Bjerke Larssen T, Svanes K, Soreide O 1990 Trends in and value and consequences of radiologic imaging of perforated gastroduodenal ulcer. Scandanavian Journal of Gastroenterology 25(3): 257–62
7. Woodring J, Heiser M 1995 Detection of pneumoperitoneum on chest radiographs: Comparison of upright lateral and posteroanteiror projections. American Journal of Roentgenology 165(1): 45–7
8. Cutler A 1996 Testing for *Helicobacter pylori* in clinical practice. American Journal of Medicine 100: 35S–41S
9. Madge S, Yeomans N 2001 Stomach and duodenal ulcers. Diagnosis and treatment. Current Therapeutics 42: 69–73
10. Soo S, Moayyedi P, Deeks J, Delaney B, Innes M, Forman D 2001 Pharmacological interventions for non-ulcer dyspepsia. Cochrane Database of Systematic Reviews Issue 4.
11. ETG 1998 Gastrointestinal, 2nd edn. Therpeutic Guidelines Limited, Version 1.1.990701
12. Katelaris P 1996 Disease management guide: recommended regimens for peptic ulcer treatment: guide chart. Current Therapeutics 37(6): 24
13. Moayyedi P, Soo S, Deeks J, et al 2001 Eradication of *Helicobacter pylori* for non-ulcer dyspepsia. Cochrane Database of Systematic Reviews Issue 4.
14. Rostom A, Wells G, Tugwekk P, Welch V, Dube C, McGowan J 2001 Prevention of NSAID induced gastroduodenal ulcers. Cochrane Database of Systematic Reviews Issue 4.
15. Selby N, Kubba A, Hawkey C 2000 Acid supression in peptic ulcer haemorrhage: A meta analysis. Alimentary Pharmacology and Therapeutics 14(9) 1119–26

6.7 BILIARY TRACT DISEASE

ANDREW WALBY • MICHAEL BRYANT

ESSENTIALS

1 Greater than 95% of biliary tract disease is attributable to gallstones.

2 Most patients with gallbladder disease present with abdominal pain.

3 Investigations are directed to confirming the diagnosis and detecting the presence of complications.

4 The management of acute biliary pain is supportive and discharge is often possible.

5 The management of cholecystitis and other complications of gallbladder disease is both supportive and surgical.

6 Acalculus cholecystitis occurs in the absence of gallstones.

7 Antibiotics are indicated for treatment of cholecystitis and ascending cholangitis.

7 Ultrasound is the imaging test of choice for most biliary tract disease.

INTRODUCTION

The most frequent cause of gallbladder disease is gallstones (95%). It is more common in women than men and incidence increases with age. Recurring episodes of symptoms are characteristic. It is diagnosed by a combination of clinical features, laboratory investigations, and organ imaging. Patients present with biliary pain due to obstruction of the biliary tree by a calculus. Cholecystitis and ascending cholangitis develop when secondary infection occurs. Calculus disease is the most frequent cause of pancreatitis. Acalculus cholecystitis occurs in the absence of gallstones and may complicate major illness.

CLINICAL FEATURES

History

Patients usually present with abdominal pain that may be midline and visceral or somatic and right upper quadrant. The pain is usually constant and may be severe. Nausea and vomiting are often present. Complaints of fevers and chills may be indicative of either cholecystitis or ascending cholangitis. Rigors suggest cholangitis.

Examination

Right upper quadrant tenderness is the most common examination finding. Fever and tachycardia are usually present in acute cholecystitis although, at presentation, they may be absent in 59–90% of cases. Local peritonism and Murphy's sign also suggest acute cholecystitis. Jaundice is usually absent in biliary colic and acute cholecystitis. The presence of pain, jaundice, high fever and shaking chills (Charcot's triad) are indicative of ascending cholangitis.

DIFFERENTIAL DIAGNOSIS

The differential diagnoses of right upper quadrant pain include:

- Peptic ulcer disease, including perforation
- Acute pancreatitis
- Coronary ischaemia, especially involving the inferior myocardial surface
- Appendicitis, especially retrocaecal or in pregnancy
- Renal disease, including renal colic and pyelonephritis
- Colonic conditions
- Hepatic pathology, especially hepatitis
- Right lower lobe pneumonia.

INVESTIGATIONS

Investigations of biliary pain are aimed at confirming the diagnosis, establishing the presence of gallstones and detection of complications.

Imaging

Ultrasound is the investigation of choice to confirm the diagnosis, measure the thickness of the gallbladder wall and CBD. It can also detect the presence of calculi in the CBD and the presence of any local fluid collection. It has high sensitivity and specificity, is non-invasive and requires little preparation of the patient.

In the majority of cases, plain radiographs are not helpful in the diagnosis of gallbladder disease. On occasion, they may be useful to rule out other potential diagnoses. Rare X-ray findings include radiopaque calculi (only 10–15% of biliary calculi are radio-opaque), the presence of gas in the biliary tree in a biliary-gastrointestinal fistula, gas or an air fluid level in emphysematous cholecystitis or a localized ileus in the right upper quadrant.

Blood

Blood tests are fairly non-specific. Bilirubin and alkaline phosphatase levels are mildly elevated in uncomplicated biliary colic and cholecystitis. Amylase is elevated if pancreatitis is also present. Full blood examination shows a leucocytosis and left shift in the majority of cases of cholecystitis and cholangitis, however, 32–40% do not have a leucocytosis.

COMPLICATIONS

Complications of biliary disease include:

- Cholecystitis
- Obstructive jaundice
- Ascending cholangitis and Gram-negative septicaemia

- Gall stone ileus
- Perforation: the elderly and diabetics are at particular risk of rapid necrosis and perforation.
- Pancreatitis.

MANAGEMENT

The management of biliary pain depends on the presence or absence of complications. In the emergency department phase, patients should receive analgesia in the form of titrated intravenous opioids and intravenous fluids. In the absence of cholecystitis or complications like biliary obstruction, ascending cholangitis or pancreatitis they may be discharged for outpatient surgical follow-up if pain settles.

Antibiotics are indicated for the treatment of cholecystitis or ascending cholangitis. The appropriate antibiotics for cholecystitis in which Gram-negative organisms are most frequently implicated is ampicillin and gentamicin, or cefotaxime if the patient is penicillin allergic. Ascending cholangitis should be treated with cefotaxime or ceftriaxone.

ERCP is indicated for the treatment of biliary obstruction. Surgery for removal of gallstones is indicated for all patients who are fit for the procedure. The timing of surgery is a matter of surgeon's preference and theatre time availability.

DISPOSITION

Many patients with biliary colic can be discharged. Most patients with complications such as acute cholecystitis, ascending cholangitis or pancreatitis require hospital admission. Admission may also be indicated in some cases because of recurrent severe pain.

CHOLELITHIASIS

Epidemiology

Gallstones are present in 10–20% of adult population in developed countries, but more than 80% are 'silent'. The prevalence increases throughout life. In young adults, more females are affected than males, but the disparity narrows with age. Predisposing factors include older age, female gender, obesity, weight loss (especially if rapid), drugs including clofibrate, oral contraceptives and other exogenous oestrogens and ceftriaxone, genetic predisposition, diseases of the terminal ileum and abnormal lipid profile. Pregnancy is also a predisposing condition. Gallstone precipitation is common, especially in late pregnancy (but most remain asymptomatic at least until delivery). Symptomatic cholelithiasis can complicates the puerperium and each first postnatal year. Forceful gallbladder contraction postpartum increases the potential for cystic or common bile duct obstruction.

Clinical features and investigation

Many gallstones are present for decades before symptoms develop and 70–80% remain asymptomatic throughout their lives. Asymptomatic patients convert to symptomatic at a rate of 1–3% per year (risk decreases with time). The most common presentations are biliary colic, cholecystitis, obstructive pancreatitis and ascending cholangitis. Less common presentations are empyema, perforation, fistula formation, gallstone ileus, hydrops or mucocoele of the gallbladder and carcinoma of the gallbladder.

The investigation of choice is ultrasound, which has a sensitivity of 84–97% and a specificity of 95–100%.

Treatment

Cholecystectomy is the definitive treatment of choice for symptomatic cholelithiasis. It provides symptomatic relief in up to 99% of patients. Laparoscopic cholecystectomy is the technique of choice. Dissolution methods and lithotripsy are of limited utility due to restricted indications for their use and gallstone recurrence in approximately 50% of cases at 5 years.

ACUTE CHOLECYSTITIS

Epidemiology

Distribution parallels that of cholelithiasis.

Pathology

Cholelithiasis is present in most acute cases; a single large calculus being the most common finding. Bacteria are present in approximately 50% of cases, but bacterial infection is not thought to cause acute cholecystitis. Rather, it results from chemical irritation and inflammation of the obstructed gallbladder.

Clinical features

Right upper quadrant pain and fever are the most common features. Usually, but not always, patients have experienced previous episodes of biliary pain. A distended, tender gallbladder is not usually evident. The right upper quadrant mass palpated in approximately 20% of patients represents omentum overlying the inflamed gallbladder. Only approximately 20% of patients are jaundiced. The presence of hyperbilirubinaemia suggests common bile duct obstruction. Neutrophilia may be present.

Ultrasound

Findings on ultrasound are often diagnostic showing cholelithiasis, an increase in transverse gallbladder diameter greater than 4–5 cm in up to 87% of cases and gallbladder wall thickening greater than 5 mm. Ultrasonic Murphy's sign is a sensitive indicator of cholecystitis if positive.

Complications

Complications include bacterial superinfection leading to ascending cholangitis or sepsis, gallbladder perforation leading to local abscess formation or diffuse peritonitis, biliary enteric (cholecystenteric) fistula, with a risk of gallstone-induced intestinal obstruction (gallstone ileus) and deterioration in pre-existing medical illness.

Treatment

Treatment is with antibiotics, hospital admission and cholecystectomy. (Amoxy)ampicillin 1 g IV, 6 hourly, plus gentamic at 4–6 mg/kg IV, daily are recommended. If these are contraindicated and alternatives are cefotaxime 1 g IV, 8 hourly or ceftriaxone 1 g IV, daily. It is important to note that cephalosporins are not active against enterococci. Cholecystectomy is required to prevent recurrence or other complications. The timing of cholecystectomy will be determined by the treating surgical unit.

Acute acalculous cholecystitis is acute inflammation of the gallbladder in the absence of gallstones, generally in the severely ill patient and accounts for 10% of cases of acute cholecystitis. Predisposing factors include post-operative state after major, non-biliary surgery, severe trauma or burns, multi-system organ failure, sepsis, prolonged intravenous hyperalimentation and being post-partum. It is thought to be ischaemic in pathogenesis. Contributing factors include dehydration, multiple blood transfusions, gallbladder stasis, accumulation of biliary sludge, viscous bile and gallbladder mucus and bacterial contamination. Compared with acute calculous cholecystitis, there is a much higher incidence of empyema, gangrene and perforation of the gallbladder.

CHOLEDOCHOLITHIASIS

Features

Gallstones are present within the biliary tree, almost all derived from the gallbladder. Approximately 10% of patients with cholelithiasis have choledocholithiasis, which may be asymptomatic, intermittently or permanently obstructive. Choledocholithiasis is the second most common cause of CBD obstruction after neoplasms.

Symptomatic cases present due to obstruction (resulting in jaundice), pancreatitis, cholangitis, hepatic abscess, secondary biliary cirrhosis or acute acalculous cholecystitis.

Imaging

Ultrasound is less reliable in choledocholithiasis. Common bile duct measurement may yield false-positive or false-negative results, but is more accurate in jaundiced patients, approaching 80% accuracy. In addition, the precise level and cause of obstruction is sometimes difficult to identify, especially if it lies near the pancreatic head. ERCP is more accurate and often therapeutic. Interval cholecystectomy to prevent recurrence is recommended.

CHOLANGITIS

Aetiology

Cholangitis is a purulent bacterial infection of the biliary tree, including the intrahepatic ducts related to obstruction to bile flow (e.g. choledocholithiasis, stents, tumours, acute pancreatitis, strictures and rarely parasites). Bacteria are usually Gram-negatives such as *E.coli*, *Klebsiella*, *Clostridia*, *Bacteroides* and *Enterobacter* or group D streptococci. They are thought to enter the biliary tree via the sphincter of Oddi.

Charcot's biliary triad (fluctuating jaundice, recurrent abdominal pain and intermittent fever with rigors) is present in 70% of patients.

Treatment

The principles of treatment are antibiotics and prompt drainage of the biliary obstruction. For the latter, the method will depend on the underlying cause, surgical preference and the state of the patient. The recommended antibiotics are (amoxy)ampicillin 1 g IV, 6 hourly, plus gentamicin 4–6 mg/kg IV, daily and metronidazole 500 mg IV, 12 hourly in patients with a history of previous biliary tract surgery.

FURTHER READING

Cotran RS, Kumar V, Collins T 1999 Robbins Pathologic Basis of Disease, 6th edn. W.B.Saunders Company, Pennsylvania

Epstein FB 1994 Acute abdominal pain in pregnancy. Emergency Medical Clinics of North America 12(1): 151–65

Feldman M, et al 1998 Sleisenger & Fordtran's Gastrointestinal and Liver Disease, 6th edn. W.B.Saunders Company, Pennsylania

Gruber PJ, et al 1996 Presence of fever and leukocytosis in acute cholecystitis. Annals of Emergency Medicine 28: 273–7

Hudson PA, Promes SB 1997 Abdominal ultrasonography. Emergency Medical Clinics of North America 15(4): 825–48

Moscati RM 1996 Cholelithiasis, cholecystitis and pancreatitis. Emergency Medical Clinics of North America 14(4): 719–37

Singer AJ, et al 1996 Correlation among clinical, laboratory and hepatobiliary scanning findings with acute cholecystitis. Annals of Emergency Medicine 28: 267–72

Therapeutic Guidelines: Antibiotic. Version 11. Therapeutic Guidelines Limited, 2000

6.8 PANCREATITIS

MICHAEL BRYANT

ESSENTIALS

1 The incidence of acute pancreatitis is increasing and the in-hospital mortality is 5–10%.

2 Investigations are directed to measuring the severity of illness and identifying the underlying aetiology.

3 The management of acute pancreatitis is supportive.

4 The use of antibiotics has been shown to reduce the development of pancreatic sepsis in those with necrotizing pancreatitis and to reduce the mortality rate.

5 The management of chronic pancreatitis is often the same as for a chronic pain syndrome. Additional problems for patients who suffer chronic pancreatitis are malabsorption states, impaired glucose tolerance and gastrointestinal bleeding secondary to peptic ulceration or gastritis.

6 Narcotic addiction and the development of a chronic pain syndrome is not uncommon in patients with chronic pancreatitis.

ACUTE PANCREATITIS

INTRODUCTION

The incidence of acute pancreatitis is increasing and the in-hospital mortality is 5–10%. It is diagnosed by a combination of clinical features, laboratory investigations and organ imaging. The most frequent causes of pancreatitis are alcohol (35–66%) and choledocholithiasis (45%). In males alcohol is most frequently the cause; in females calculus disease is more likely. Miscellaneous and idiopathic causes account for 10% each.

CLINICAL FEATURES

History

The sudden onset of constant abdominal pain radiating through to the back is the most typical presention of acute pancreatitis. Sitting up and leaning forward may relieve the pain. Nausea, vomiting and abdominal distension are also commonly present. If present, symptoms of dyspnoea or circulatory compromise are indicative of severe disease.

After the diagnosis of acute pancreatitis has been established, questioning should be directed to identifying its underlying cause. Excluding the two most common causes of alcohol and calculus disease, other causes are listed in Table 6.8.1.

Examination

Low-grade fever is common. Manifestations of severe disease are the presence of tachycardia, hypotension, and the respiratory findings of crepitations and pleural effusions. Tenderness in the epigastrium without guarding or rigidity is the most frequent examination finding. Uncommon examination findings are the presence of a pseudocyst, Cullen's sign (a blue periumbilical discoloration secondary to haemoperitoneum) or Turner's sign (flank discoloration due to haemoglobin catabolism). These usually occur some time after the initial insult and are not usually seen in the emergency department.

INVESTIGATIONS

Biochemical

Amylase

The degree of elevation of serum amylase does not correlate with prognosis. Serum amylase level returns to normal quickly and is not as highly elevated in alcoholic forms of pancreatitis as in other forms. Amylase usually rises within hours of onset of symptoms. Levels usually peak within 24 hours and return to normal within 48 to 72 hours.

Elevations of amylase may occur in the absence of pancreatitis. Other causes of raised serum amylase are summarized in Table 6.8.2. Using amylase levels three times the upper limit of normal as a cutoff for diagnosing pancreatitis is said to be more specific, although this reduces sensitivity.[1]

Table 6.8.1 Causes of acute pancreatitis, other than alcohol and choledocholithiasis

Obstructive	Infections
Ascaris	HIV, as the result of both the disease and the treatments
Choledochal cysts	Viral: mumps, rubella, viral hepatitis, Epstein–Barr virus; cytomegalovirus and coxsackie B virus infections
Carcinoma of the pancreas	Bacterial: *Mycoplasma, Campylobacter, Mycobacteria* and *Legionella*
Toxins and drugs	
Organophosphate insecticides	
Azathioprine, mercaptopurine, valproic acid, didanosine, pentamidine, cotrimoxazole	
Trauma	**Vascular**
Blunt abdominal	Hypoperfusion
Postoperative	Vasculitis: systemic lupus erythematosus, polyarteritis
ERCP, sphincterotomy	Nodosa
Metabolic	**Miscellaneous**
Hypertriglyceridaemia	Penetrating peptic ulcer
Hyperlipidaemia	Crohn's disease
Hypercalcaemia	Reye syndrome
	Hypothermia

Table 6.8.2 Causes of elevated serum amylase other than pancreatitis

Pancreatic	Non-pancreatic
Perforated viscus	Pregnancy
Intestinal obstruction and infarction	Renal transplantation and renal insufficiency
Ruptured ectopic pregnancy	Salivary gland lesions: mumps, calculus
Peritonitis	Tumours of lung, oesophagus, breast, ovary
Aortic aneurysm	Macroamylasaemia
Chronic liver disease	Burns
	Diabetic ketoacidosis
	Cerebral tumours

COMPLICATIONS

Local

Pancreatic necrosis is present when a non-perfused area on contrast-enhanced CT scan measures either more than 3 cm or more than 30% of the gland. Pancreatic necrosis may be found in severe disease, and differentiation cannot be made clinically between sterile and infected necrotic areas. CT-guided needle aspiration is used to diagnose the presence of infection. If infection is present surgery is indicated.

Acute fluid collections occur early in 30–50% of cases and are located in or near the pancreas. Pseudocyst and pancreatic abscess formation may be identified on CT scan.

Systemic

The morbidity and mortality of acute pancreatitis are directly related to the presence or absence of systemic complications. The development of pulmonary complications, such as pleural effusions, pneumonitis or adult respiratory distress syndrome (ARDS), and renal failure with oliguria and azotaemia, are markers of severe disease.

Cardiovascular complications include pericardial effusion. Gastrointestinal manifestations of erosive gastritis and peptic ulceration may also occur as may disseminated intravascular coagulation, hyperglycaemia, hypocalcaemia and encephalopathy.

Lipase

Serum lipase levels remain elevated longer than amylase levels. Lipase levels are elevated to the same extent in both forms of pancreatitis. Current literature suggests that lipase levels are more sensitive and specific for pancreatitis than amylase and that lipase measurement should replace amylase as the initial test of choice.[1]

Other blood tests

- Clotting profile: coagulation may be abnormal.
- As up to 25% of patients with acute pancreatitis have been shown to be hypoxic on arterial blood gases, all patients should as a minimum have pulse oximetry and, if this is less than 96% arterial blood gases should be taken.

Imaging

- Plain radiographs are of very limited use in the diagnosis of acute pancreatitis. Erect chest X-ray may, however, be useful to distinguish acute pancreatitis from perforated peptic ulcer. Uncommonly, abdominal films may reveal the presence of gallstones or an ileus. The presence of calcification may indicate chronic pancreatitis. Chest X-ray may also demonstrate complications such as atelectasis or pleural effusions.
- Contrast-enhanced computerized tomography (CT) scan is normal in 15–30% of those with mild disease, but is nearly always abnormal in those with moderate-to-severe disease.

Severity markers

The Ranson criteria[2] can be used to predict the severity of disease. This entails measurement of serum electrolytes, glucose, LDH and AST, calcium, arterial blood gases and full blood count. Intended for use for inpatients, some of these parameters are measured at admission and others 'within 48 hours'. The criteria and the level that constitutes a risk factor are summarized in Table 6.8.3.

In the presence of one or two risk factors the mortality is <1%. An increase to three or four risk factors increases the mortality to 15%. A mortality of 100% is found with six or seven risk factors.

Obesity is an independent risk factor for severe acute pancreatitis, with a 36% mortality rate compared to 6% in non-obese patients.[3]

Table 6.8.3 Ranson criteria

Initial	Within 48 hours
Age over 55 years	Haematocrit fall >10%
WCC >16 000	Urea rise >1.8 mmol/L
Glucose >11 mmol/L	Ca^{2+} <1.9 mmol/L
LDH >400 IU/L	Arterial PO_2 <60 mmHg
AST >250 IU/L	Base deficit >4 mEq/L
	Estimated fluid sequestration >4000 mL

MANAGEMENT

The diagnosis and management of acute pancreatitis involves the detection of the underlying aetiology, the alleviation of pain and the early detection of complications. Management may require aggressive resuscitation, with care in an ICU.

General measures

For the majority of patients the initial management of acute pancreatitis is supportive. In the emergency department, patients should receive supplemental oxygen, analgesia in the form of titrated intravenous opioids, and intravenous fluids. Anti-emetics are also often required. Sphincter of Oddi spasm is frequently cited as a reason to avoid the use of morphine in this setting. All narcotics increase pressure in the sphincter of Oddi. There has been no trial comparing the effects of pethidine and morphine on sphincter of Oddi spasm.[4] The use of nasogastric tubes has not been shown to improve pain relief or to reduce the length of hospital stay.[5] They are, however, appropriate for symptomatic relief of ileus or severe vomiting.

Urinary catheterization, arterial lines and central venous lines may be required, depending on the patient's condition.

Specific treatments

If biliary tract calculus is the cause of acute pancreatitis, endoscopic stone removal reduces biliary sepsis and mortality. Patients with acute necrotizing pancreatitis are at greatest risk of developing infection from the translocation of enteric Gram-negative or Gram-positive bacteria from the bowel lumen into the necrotic pancreatic tissue.[5] Several trials of antibiotic prophylaxis have shown a reduction in the development of pancreatic and non-pancreatic sepsis (imipenem; ceftazidime, amikacin and metronidazole), with some (cefuroxime) showing a reduction in mortality.[6,7] Pseudocysts that do not resolve spontaneously may require surgical drainage.

DISPOSITION

Many patients with acute pancreatitis can be managed on a general ward. Patients with hypoxia and haemodynamic instability should be admitted to an intensive care unit.

CHRONIC PANCREATITIS

CLINICAL FEATURES

The symptoms of chronic pancreatitis are identical to those of acute pancreatitis, but patients may also present with persistent abdominal pain with or without steatorrhoea and weight loss. The cause of pain is multifactorial and includes intraductal pressure resulting from ductal stricture, interstitial hypertension, pancreatic ischaemia, neuronal inflammation and extra-pancreatic complications.[8] Chronic pancreatitis is notable for the progressive loss of exocrine and endocrine pancreatic function.

INVESTIGATION

In contrast to acute pancreatitis, the amylase is often not elevated. Serum lipase levels still rise in patients with an episode of acute on chronic pancreatitis. Elevations of bilirubin and alkaline phosphatase may indicate cholestasis secondary to chronic inflammation around the common bile duct. The abdominal X-ray is of limited clinical use in guiding management, but may show pancreatic calcification.

COMPLICATIONS

Approximately 40% of patients with chronic pancreatitis have B_{12} malabsorption. There may also be impaired glucose tolerance or diabetes mellitus, or gastrointestinal bleeding secondary to peptic ulceration or gastritis. Icterus may occur secondary to oedema of the head of the pancreas or secondary to chronic inflam-

CONTROVERSIES

❶ Cytokines and other non-cytokine mediators are produced rapidly during acute pancreatitis and may be responsible for the majority of systemic manifestations. Blocking these has been shown to be of benefit in animals.[10]

❷ Antibiotic usage has been shown to reduce morbidity and mortality in patients with necrotizing pancreatitis.

❸ The use of octreotide and antioxidants may be of benefit in severe acute pancreatitis.[11]

❹ There is no evidence to support the use of pethidine in preference to morphine.

mation around the common bile duct. Fat necrosis can occur in subcutaneous tissues, and intramedullary fat necrosis can cause bone pain. Although rarely present, pleural, pericardial and peritoneal effusions contain elevated amylase levels.

Narcotic addiction and a chronic pain syndrome are well-recognized problems in patients with chronic pancreatitis, and may pose a significant management challenge.

Other complications include pseudocysts, venous thromboses, duodenal obstruction, biliary cirrhosis and pancreatic cancer.[9]

MANAGEMENT

Management is difficult and requires a multidisciplinary approach. Involvement of pain management services and drug and alcohol services are frequently necessary.

REFERENCES

1. Vissers RJ, Abu-Laban RB, McHugh DF 1999 Amylase and lipase in the emergency department evaluation of acute pancreatitis. The Journal of Emergency Medicine. 17: 1027–37
2. Ranson J 1985 Risk factors in acute pancreatitis. Hospital Practice 20: 69

3. Funnell IC, Bornman PC, Weakley SP, Terblanche J, Marks IN 1993 Obesity: an important prognostic factor in acute pancreatitis. British Journal of Surgery 80: 484–6
4. Thompson DR. 2001 Narcotic analgesic effects on the sphincter of Oddi: a review of the data and therapeutic implicaitons in treating pancreatitis. American Journal of Gastroenterology 96: 1266–72
5. Steinberg W, Tenner S 1994 Acute pancreatitis.

New England Journal of Medicine 330: 1198–210
6. Foxx-Orenstein A, Orenstein R 1997 Antibiotics and pancreatitis. Gastroenterologist 5: 157–64
7. Kramer KM, Levy H. 1999 Prophylactic antibiotics for severe acute pancreatitis: the beginning of an era. Pharmacotherapy 19: 592–602
8. Pitchumoni CS 1998 Chronic pancreatitis: pathogenesis and management of pain. Journal of Clinical Gastroenterology 27: 101–7

9. Apte MV, Keogh GW, Wilson JS 1999. Chronic pancreatitis: complicaitons and management. Journal of Clinical Gastroenterology 29: 225–40
10. Norman J 1998 The role of cytokines in the pathogenesis of acute pancreatitis. American Journal of Surgery 175: 76–83
11. Haber PS, Pirola RC, Wilson JS 1997 Clinical update: management of acute pancreatitis. Journal of Gastroenterology and Hepatology 12: 189–97

6.9 ACUTE APPENDICITIS

ANDREW DENT

ESSENTIALS

1 Appendicitis is the most common acute abdominal surgical condition.

2 In the majority of patients appendicitis is a clinical diagnosis based on history and findings on clinical examination.

3 Investigations are of limited use in the confirmation of clinical appendicitis, although ultrasound may be useful in cases of doubt, particularly in women.

4 The management of appendicitis is surgery.

INTRODUCTION

Appendicitis is the most common acute abdominal surgical condition. Although the incidence appears to be declining: 100 new cases per 100 000 population per year occur in developed countries. It is more common in males, but in females poses a significant diagnostic challenge. Pathologically there appear to be two types: those that perforate early (19%; more common in the very young and very old) and those that progress far more slowly.[1,2]

PRESENTATION

The diagnosis of appendicitis remains clinical despite the advent of multiple investigative procedures to assist the clinician.

History

Pain is the hallmark of appendicitis. The presence of continuous abdominal pain is typical of an acute inflammatory abdominal condition. Classically, pain is initially located in the central region of the abdomen, owing to visceral irritation. Visceral pain is poorly localized and while appendicitis is developing, takes on the small bowel pain pattern. Systemic symptoms may commence soon after pain, with the onset of anorexia and possibly vomiting. Vomiting is, however, not usually a dominant early symptom and its occurrence prior to the onset of pain makes the diagnosis of appendicitis unlikely.[3]

After a variable period of time (2–18 hours) the pain usually migrates to the right lower quadrant and becomes constant. In most cases symptoms of peritoneal inflammation, such as pain on movement, deep breathing and coughing, are present at this time. If the appendix is located away from the parietal peritoneum (e.g. retrocaecal or retroileal, or high and subhepatic with a non-descended caecum) the migration of pain may be late, atypically located and symptoms of peritoneal irritation may be minimal. Should there be a delay in diagnosis or presentation, perforation of the appendix may occur, with the onset of generalized peritonitis and constant severe generalized pain.

Nausea and anorexia are common early, and may be followed by vomiting. The retention of good appetite is strongly against the diagnosis of appendicitis. Diarrhoea is an unusual symptom in adults and, if prominent, appendicitis is unlikely. Fever is usually low grade but present, typically 37.5–38.0°C in the early stages. High fever can occur in frank peritonitis or appendiceal abscess.

Examination

Examination findings vary according to stage and severity. Often patients lie still, as movement exacerbates pain. Vital signs may be normal, but a mild tachycardia is usual along with low-grade fever. There may be some halitosis, associated with anorexia-induced starvation ketosis or recent vomiting, and the tongue may be dry or coated.

The most useful abdominal findings are local tenderness in the right iliac fossa. The presence of guarding is a sensitive sign, as is rebound tenderness. Other findings might include decreased movement with respiration, with the abdomen held still to minimize pain. Asking the patient to suck their abdomen in or to blow it out to touch the examining hand held a few centimetres above the abdominal wall may bring on pain or assist in localizing pain. Asking the patient to cough may elicit a weak or interrupted cough and a protective clutch over the right lower abdomen. In the obese or in early and doubtful cases, Rovsing's sign may be useful. Gentle slow pressure from the lateral aspect of the left side of the abdomen compresses and displaces abdominal contents towards the right. On release, pain is felt in the right iliac fossa, often to the patient's surprise.

In most cases, rectal examination in patients with suspected appendicitis is of little value and does not alter management.[4] It may be helpful when the diagnosis is in doubt, particularly in the elderly. It may elicit tenderness indicative of pelvic appendicitis or an intra-abdominal abscess.

DIFFERENTIAL DIAGNOSIS

Appendicitis can mimic most acute abdominal conditions and should be considered in any patient with symptoms referable to the abdomen.

Occasionally another condition causes symptoms and signs typical of appendicitis. The list of differential diagnoses is very long (Table 6.9.1). As far as the emergency physician is concerned, it is important to recognize the presence of a condition requiring surgical intervention and to initiate appropriate investigation, treatment and consultation simultaneously, so as to minimize preoperative time. On occasion, the diagnosis can only be confirmed at surgery or laparoscopy.

INVESTIGATION

Acute-phase reactants

A white cell count (WCC) is not usually helpful as 70% of patients with appendicitis with free pus or an abscess have a WCC of less than 15 000.[5] Although frequently requested, research has shown that knowledge of a normal WCC did not significantly influence surgical decision-making in suspected appendicitis.[6]

C-reactive protein has been advanced as an exclusion test for appendicitis, but has a low specificity.[7]

Imaging

Plain abdominal radiography rarely provides helpful information in the work-up of clinical appendicitis.[8]

Ultrasound is not necessary when clinical signs are straightforward. On meta-analysis, ultrasound has a sensitivity of about 85%.[9] A false positive rate of up to 20% in patients with few clinical signs suggests it is not a good tool for screening non specific abdominal pain. It has the advantage of picking up alternative causes for pain, especially in women.

Debate continues on the precise role of CT in the diagnosis of acute appendicitis. Sensitivity of the test has been reported as high as 98%, but in settings of an adult acute emergency department may be as lower than 90%, with a positive predictive value of 78%, and a negative predictive value of 96%.[10] Particular concern has been expressed at the increase in negative CTs requested (up to 70% in some series) with little benefit demonstrated by decreased negative laparotomy rate.[11]

Clinical decision tools

Several tools have been described to assist clinical diagnosis. The best known of these is the ten point Alvarado score for acute appendicitis, also known as MANTRELS criteria (migration of pain, anorexia, nausea and vomitting, tenderness in right lower quadrant, rebound tenderness, elevated temperature and leucocytosis with a left shift).[12]

Two points are given each for right iliac fossa tenderness and a total white cell count of more than 10 000. One point each is awarded for pain migration, anorexia, nausea and vomiting, percussion or rebound pain, temperature above 37.5°C, and a neutrophil differential count of more than 75%.

Alvarado recommended surgery for scores of seven or more, and observation for scores of 5 and 6. It has proved of some use with a positive predictive value of 77% above for scores above 7, and negative predictive value of 97% when the score is below 4. More recently, it has been suggested as a tool to determine which cases should be further investigated. Thus those patients with an Alvarado score between 4 and 8 could benefit from ultrasound or CT.[13] CT and clinical assessment with the MANTRELS model had similar sensitivity (90–92%) in one study, but clinical assessment had less specificity (85% vs 94%). Combining the two increased sensivity to 98% and and specificity to 96%.[14]

Other

Neutrophil scanning with ^{99m}Tc-HMPAO-labelled white cells has a 92% specificity and sensitivity and has been recommended for diagnosing appendicitis in the elderly patient with equivocal physical signs.[15]

Table 6.9.1 Differential diagnosis of right iliac fossa pain
In general
Gastroenteritis, including amoebiasis and *Yersinia enterocolitica*
Infestations, including *Enterobius vermicularis, Ascaris lumbricoides*
Mesenteric adenitis
Non-specific abdominal pain
Diverticulitis: Meckel's, caecal, sigmoid
Crohn's disease and other inflammatory bowel disease involving terminal ileitis
Cholecystitis; cholelithiasis pancreatitis
Renal colic and urinary-tract infections
Testicular conditions, hernia
Perforated peptic ulcer
Medical causes: pneumonia diabetes, Addison's disease, familial Mediterranean fever, porphyria
In women
Salpingitis/pelvic inflammatory disease
Complication of an ovarian cyst
Ectopic pregnancy
In the elderly
Caecal carcinoma (complicated)
Acute retention of urine
Abdominal aortic aneurysm
Ischaemic bowel.

TREATMENT

The treatment for appendicitis remains appendicectomy, which may be open or laparoscopic. Laparoscopy is being increasingly preferred. There is an increase in operative time but a reduction in postoperative analgesia requirements and inpatient stay and a more rapid return to work.[16,17] Preoperative preparation will include analgesia (small doses of intravenous narcotic) and intravenous hydration. Antibiotics, commonly metronidazole and ampicillin, when given preoperatively or intraoperatively reduce the incidence of postoperative wound infection and intra-abdominal abscess.[18]

When the indication for surgery is in doubt, a period of observation in or out of hospital can be helpful. In this way non-specific abdominal pain can be managed conservatively. Great caution needs to be exhibited in the very young and the very old, who may have atypical signs and symptoms, and in patients with diabetes whose signs may be masked.

ACUTE APPENDICITIS IN PREGNANCY

Acute appendicitis is the commonest cause for non-obstetric laparotomy in the pregnant, occurring in about 1 in

CONTROVERSIES

❶ The usefulness of WCC in the diagnosis of appendicitis. It is neither highly sensitive nor specific.

❷ What is the acceptable negative laparotomy rate?

❸ The role of laparoscopy in diagnosis and treatment.

1100 deliveries. Symptoms of appendicitis are similar, but in late pregnancy the site of tenderness and other signs may be masked or altered. Fetal loss as a result of appendicitis and laparotomy may be as high as 20%.

REFERENCES

1. Anderson R, et al 1994 Indications for operation in suspected appendicitis and incidence of perforation. British Medical Journal 308: 107–10
2. McCahy P 1994 Continuing fall in the incidence of acute appendicitis. Annals of the Royal College of Surgeons of England 76: 282–3
3. Wagner JM, McKinney WP, Carpenter JL 1996 Does this patient have appendicitis? Journal of the American Medical Association 276: 1589–94
4. Dunning PG, Goldman MD 1991 The incidence and value of rectal examination in children with suspected appendicitis. Annals of the Royal College of Surgeons of England 73: 233–4
5. Blennerhassett L, Hall JL, Hall JC 1996 White blood cell counts in patients undergoing abdominal surgery. Australian and New Zealand Journal of Surgery 66: 369–71
6. Vermeulen B, Morabia A, Unger PF 1995 Influence of white cell count on surgical decision making in patients with abdominal pain in the right lower quadrant. European Journal of Surgery 161: 483–6
7. Hallan s, Asberg A 1997 The accuracy of C-Reactive protein in diagnosing acute appendicitis. Scandinavian Journal of Clinical and Laboratory Investigation 57: 373–80
8. Rothrock et al 1991 Plain abdominal radiography in the detection of acute medical and surgical disease in children: a retrospective analysis. Pediatric Emergency Care 7: 281–5
9. Orr RK, Porter D, Hartman D 1995 Ultrasonography to evaluate adults for appendictis: decion making based on a meta-analysis and probablistic reasoning. Academic Emergency Medicine 2: 644–50
10. Ujiki MB, Murayama KM, Cribbins AL, et al 2002 CT in the management of acute appendicitis. Journal of Surgical Research 105: 119–22
11. Weyant MJ, Barie PS, Eachempati SR 2002 Clinical role of noncontrast helical computerised tomography in diagnosis of acute appendicitis. American Journal of Surgery 183: 97–8
12. Alvarado A 1986 A practical score for the early diagnosis of acute appendicitis. Annals of Emergency Medicine 15: 1557–64
13. Douglas CD, MacPherson NE, Davidson PM, Gani JS 2000 Randomised controlled trial of ultrasonography in diagnosis of acute appendicitis, incorporating the Alvarado score. British Medical Journal 321: 919–92
14. Gwynn LK 2001 The diagnosis of acute appendicitis: Clinical assessment versus computerised tomography evaluation. Journal of Emergency Medicine 21: 119–23
15. Lin WY, et al 1997 99Tcm-HMPAO-labelled white blood cell scans to detect acute appendicitis in older patients with an atypical clinical presentation. Nuclear Medicine Communications 18: 75–8
16. Sauerland S, Lefering R, Neugebauer EAM 2002 Laparoscopic versus open surgery for suspected appendicitis. Cochrane Database for Systematic Reviews. Issue 2
17. Garbutt JM, Sopper NJ, Shannon WD, et al 1999 Meta-analysis of randomized controlled trials comparing laparoscopic and open appendicectomy. Surgical Laparoscopy and Endoscopy 9: 17–26
18. Anderson BR, Kallehave FL, Andersen HK 2002 Antibiotics versus placebo for prevention of postoperative infection after appendicectomy. Cochrane Database of Systematic Reviews. Issue 2

6.10 INFLAMMATORY BOWEL DISEASE

KIM YATES

ESSENTIALS

1 The two major forms of inflammatory bowel disease (IBD) are Crohn's disease and ulcerative colitis.

2 The basis of the lesions of IBD is immunological; however, the cause of this response remains unclear.

3 IBD is chronic and relapsing. Patients may present with increased disease activity or with complications of the disease process or treatments.

4 Gastrointestinal complications may include dehydration, bleeding, strictures, obstruction, fistulae, sepsis, perforation, neoplasia and toxic megacolon.

5 Acute arthropathy is the most common extra-intestinal manifestation of disease in IBD.

6 The principal clinical features of IBD are diarrhoea and/or abdominal pain.

7 Patients with moderate or severe IBD require admission to hospital. Emergency surgery is required for a small group of patients with intra-abdominal sepsis, perforation, obstruction or toxic megacolon, the remainder being managed initially with medical therapy.

INTRODUCTION

Inflammatory bowel disease (IBD) classically refers to Crohn's disease and ulcerative colitis (UC), which are chronic inflammatory diseases of the gastrointestinal tract of uncertain aetiology.

Patients with IBD may present as an emergency with problems related to increased disease activity, or with complications of the disease process or its treatments.

EPIDEMIOLOGY AND PATHOGENESIS

Incidence rates of IBD vary with both geography and age. It is more common in cooler latitudes and the age incidence is bimodal, with the larger peak at 15–30 years and a smaller one at 60–80 years.[1] Incidence rates in Australasia are thought to be in the range of 0.8–6/100 000 of population.[2,3] Crohn's disease is more common in women.[1]

A genetic predisposition to developing IBD has been observed,[1,4,5] with positive family history being the strongest risk factor for developing IBD.[6] Current thought is that IBD is a heterogenous group of diseases that have mucosal inflammation as a common final manifestation, where several genetic and environmental factors contribute to pathogenesis.[7,8] It is theorized that genetic susceptibility leads to abnormal T-cell activation and cytokine-mediated tissue damage/inflammation with exposure to luminal bacteria and environmental antigens.[4,5,7,8] Infectious and non-infectious initiators are under investigation (see Controversies). Whatever the initiator, an immune response against gut constituents appears a critical feature of the pathogenesis.[8]

Pathologically the two major forms of IBD differ considerably. Crohn's disease is a discontinuous transmural inflammation characterized by transmural lesions, skip lesions, aphthoid ulcers, granulomas, and giant cells, and associated with fistulas, abscesses, strictures and obstruction.[9,10] It can affect any part of the GI tract, from mouth to anus, with ileocolonic disease being the most common.[1] On the other hand, UC is a continuous colonic mucosal inflammation, often associated with bleeding.[10] The majority of UC patients have disease limited to the rectum, rectosigmoid or left colon.[1]

Rarer atypical forms of IBD have been described. These include collagenous, lymphocytic and diversion colitis.[11]

COURSE AND COMPLICATIONS

Patients with IBD may present acutely at any stage of the illness, as IBD is chronic and relapsing. Anatomic location and extent of the disease, particularly on initial diagnosis, can help to predict the course of both forms to some extent.[1,3] Gastrointestinal complications may include dehydration, bleeding, strictures, obstruction, fistulae, sepsis, perforation, neoplasia and toxic megacolon.[1,10,12] Toxic megacolon (colonic dilatation with severe colitis, fever, abdominal distention and tachycardia) occurs in 1.6–18% of UC patients, and 1–7.8% of those with Crohn's disease.[1,9,10,13] In Crohn's disease patients with small bowel disease are more likely to develop obstructive disease.[1,3] Those with colonic involvement may develop bleeding or toxic megacolon. Most patients with Crohn's disease require surgical treatment at some time, with up to 74% requiring bowel resections; however, this is rarely curative as recurrence is frequent.[1,3,12,14]

In UC an initial diagnosis of pancolitis (which occurs in 14–36.7% of cases) is associated with more complications and a higher requirement for surgery.[1,10] Conversely, initial proctitis is less likely to be associated with complications, extra-intestinal manifestations or cancer.[1,15] Patients with fulminant colitis are most at risk of toxic megacolon and perforation.[16] Medical treatment reduces relapses in both major forms of IBD.[17–19]

Extraintestinal complications of IBD can be rheumatological, ocular (episcleritis, uveitis), dermatologic (erythema nodosum, pyoderma gangrenosum) or hepatobiliary. The most common is acute arthropathy (10–20%).[1,10,12] Sclerosing cholangitis occurs in 2–7.6% of UC patients, whereas cholelithiasis and nephrolithiasis are more frequent in Crohn's disease.[1] Patients with IBD have an increased risk of developing bowel cancer, which in UC is proportional to the degree of colonic involvement, but is smaller and less well-defined in Crohn's disease.[1,15]

CLINICAL FEATURES

Clinical features vary depending on the form and anatomic distribution of the disease.[1,10] In an acute presentation, although a diagnosis and assessment of disease activity should be made, the emphasis should be on identifying potentially serious complications of the disease and its treatments.

To determine severity, the Truelove and Witts criteria for UC use stool frequency, the presence of blood, fever, tachycardia, anaemia, raised ESR, colonic X-ray features and abdominal signs.[10,20] The Crohn's Disease Activity Index is more subjective, using abdominal pain, general well-being and opiate use, as well as stool frequency, presence of complications, abdominal masses, anaemia and weight loss.[10,20]

History

Diarrhoea is a frequent complaint, and the duration, number and type of motions per day are useful in assessing the activity and form of IBD.[1,10,20]

In UC more than 10 motions per day suggests fulminant disease, whereas fewer than four suggests mild disease.[20] Bloody diarrhoea, mucus, tenesmus and rectal complaints are more common in UC.[9,10] In Crohn's disease anal complaints and fissures, along with diarrhoea without blood, are more common.[10,20]

Abdominal pain in Crohn's disease is commonly right-sided, postprandial and associated with vomiting.[21] In UC, pain is less frequent and usually crampy, lower abdominal, and relieved by passing a motion.[21] If pain is more severe it may herald the onset of fulminant colitis or other complications.[21] Weight loss is more common in Crohn's than in UC.[21] Fever may occur in either form and is a marker of disease severity.[10,20,21]

Further enquiry should include a search for extraintestinal manifestations and evidence of past surgical procedures. A careful drug history is essential, as treatments such as steroids and immuno-suppressants are possible causes of complications in their own right.

Examination

Anaemia, fever higher than 37.5°C, pulse greater than 90 per minute and abdominal tenderness are markers of more severe disease, particularly in UC.[10,20] The presence of fever, abdominal tenderness, peritoneal irritation, distention and absent bowel sounds suggests fulminant colitis.[9] An abdominal mass is more common in Crohn's disease and is associated with increased disease severity.[20,21] The presence of abdominal distension raises the question of fulminant colitis, toxic megacolon or obstruction.[9,13,16,21] Rectal examination may show anal fissures, abscesses or fistulae (more common in Crohn's disease). In patients taking immunosuppressants, a specific search for sepsis should be made. A survey of joints, eyes, skin and vasculature may help identify extraintestinal complications.

INVESTIGATIONS

Blood tests

A full blood count to quantify anaemia and determine the need for transfusion is usually important.[10,16,20,21] Leucocytosis may be present in acute disease,[21] but leucopenia may be seen if the patient is on immunosuppressants.[20–22] The ESR is usually greater than 30mm/hour in severe UC.[20] Electrolytes and renal function may be abnormal in dehydration.[9] Iron and folate deficiencies, and hypoalbuminaemia are common in IBD, and hypomagnesaemia and hypocalcaemia may occur in Crohn's disease.[23] Disturbed liver function tests suggests hepatobiliary complications.[24]

Microbiology

Infective diarrhoea may cause presentations similar to IBD, and so faeces culture may be helpful in diagnosis.[10]

Radiology

On acute presentation abdominal X-rays (supine and erect/decubitus) are useful where complications are suspected, looking for free gas with perforation; dilated bowel loops and air-fluid levels with obstruction or dilated transverse colon (>6 cm) with toxic megacolon.[9, 25] Computerized tomography (CT) will identify an intra-abdominal abscess or fistula.[26] Barium studies will diagnose and differentiate between Crohn's (skip lesions, fistulae, deep ulcers, cobblestoning) and UC (granularity, ulceration more super ficial and continuous, confined to colon), but are contraindicated in acutely unwell patients because of the risks of perforation or obstruction.[21,26]

Endoscopy

Endoscopic findings and biopsies are useful in differentiating IBD from infective or ischaemic processes, as well as determining the form of IBD, staging activity, and screening for strictures or cancer.[15,21,26] Cautious rigid proctosigmoidoscopy is safe in the acutely unwell patient, but colonoscopy, although performed acutely in some centres, carries a risk of perforation.[21,26] Upper gastrointestinal endoscopy is being used more commonly to diagnose upper gastrointestinal Crohn's disease.[21]

MANAGEMENT

General measures

Initial assessment should focus on the detection and treatment of life-threatening conditions such as septic or hypovolaemic shock, severe anaemia or dehydration. Thereafter, assessment focuses on disease activity/severity and the presence of complications. Intravenous fluid therapy may be necessary if dehydration or shock are present. Electrolyte disturbances and anaemia should be corrected. For abdominal pain, analgesia with opiates can be used, but with caution in severe colitis as toxic megacolon may be precipitated. If toxic megacolon is suspected, nasogastric drainage should be started and intravenous steroids and broad-spectrum antibiotics are indicated, as discussed below. Complications requiring surgery, such as bowel obstruction, intra-abdominal sepsis or perforation, should be ruled out early.

Medical therapy

Corticosteroids induce remission of IBD but are not useful as maintenance therapy.[17–19] Rectal steroids are used in mild-to-moderate distal IBD, and prednisone 40–60 mg/day or equivalent is used for moderate or more proximal IBD.[17–19] High-dose parenteral steroids (≥60 mg prednisone equivalent/day) are reserved for severe or fulminant disease.[16] Budesonide which has low bioavailability but high potency appears effective both topically and orally in IBD with fewer systemic side effects.[16–19]

Aminosalicylates (sulfasalazine, 5ASA/mesalamine) are used to treat mild-to-moderate IBD and to maintain remission.[17–19] Mesalamine (5ASA) is better tolerated but more expensive than sulfasalazine, and is used topically/rectally in distal disease, and orally in more proximal disease.[18,20]

Immunomodulators such as azathioprine and 6-mercaptopurine are used as steroid-sparing agents or in steroid resistant disease, but pancreatitis and bone-marrow suppression can be problems.[17–19] Trials of infliximab (anti Tumour Necrosis Factor a) have shown clinical response rates of 65–81% in moderate-to-severe Crohn's with a marked steroid-sparing effect.[17,18] Initial studies also suggest good response rates to infliximab in refractory UC.[27] Other immunosuppressants have been trialled (see Controversies).

Antibiotic therapy with metronidazole is effective in treating perianal disease in Crohn's disease and has been shown to prevent relapses when used as long-term therapy postoperatively, but peripheral neuropathy can complicate prolonged use.[17,18] Ciprofloxacin is an alternative.[17,18] Apart from treating pouchitis after resection with anastomosis, benefit from antibiotics is not proven in UC.[17]

Nutritional support, such as elemental diets and parenteral nutrition, is more helpful in Crohn's disease than in UC.[17] Vitamin and trace element supplements are required in patients on steroid therapy.[17] Loperamide or cholestyramine may be useful in reducing diarrhoea in mild Crohn's ileitis.[17]

Surgical therapy

Intra-abdominal abscesses, seen more commonly in Crohn's disease, can be drained percutaneously using CT or ultrasound guidance but may require laparotomy.[21] If toxic megacolon fails to respond to medical therapy, or if perforation occurs, then urgent surgery is indicated.[9] Intractable gastrointestinal bleeding may also require urgent surgery.[21]

In Crohn's disease, intestinal obstruction is the commonest indication for surgery.[13] Indications for elective surgery in IBD include intractable disease, stricture with obstruction, fistulae or cancer.[13] In UC, total proctocolectomy with ileostomy is considered 'curative'; however, subtotal procedures and anastomoses are often performed when disease is limited or when patients wish to avoid a stoma.[13] In Crohn's, because surgical 'cure' is not possible, resection with anastomosis is most commonly performed.[13] As Crohn's has a high recurrence rate, patients often have multiple operations and risk short bowel syndrome.[13, 21]

DISPOSITION

Patients with moderate or severe IBD require admission, usually for a trial of medical therapy. Surgical admission is indicated for perforation, obstruction, intra-abdominal sepsis or toxic megacolon. Patients with mild IBD and no complications can be managed as outpatients, with gastroenterology follow-up.

REFERENCES

1. Andres PG Friedman LS 1999 Epidemiology and the natural course of IBD. Gastroenterology Clinics of North America 28(2): 255–81
2. Isbister WH 1997 The surgical management of nonspecific IBD: a small personal experience. New Zealand Medical Journal 110: 56–8
3. Anseline PF 1995 Crohn's disease in the Hunter Valley region of Australia. ANZ Journal of Surgery 65(8): 564–9
4. Farrell RJ Peppercorn MA 2002 Ulcerative colitis. Lancet 359: 331–40
5. Shanahan F 2002 Crohn's disease. Lancet 359: 62–9

CONTROVERSIES

❶ Causes of IBD. Numerous infectious agents have been postulated as causative or initiative, including *Mycobacteria* (particularly *M. paratuberculosis*), paramyxovirus (measles), and *Listeria*; however, there is no definitive evidence to date.[1] A cohort study implicating childhood measles vaccination has not been substantiated by later case-control studies.[28] Non-infectious agents under investigation include non-steroidal anti-inflammatory drugs, toxic food additives, smoking, oral contraceptive agents and antibiotic-related changes in gut flora.[1]

❷ Medical therapies. Aminosalicylates are widely used but their anti-inflammatory actions are poorly understood.[17] Methotrexate has been trialled in severe Crohn's disease with mixed results.[17,18] Cyclosporin A is sometimes used cautiously in severe refractory IBD where surgery is not possible, but has significant adverse effects, including renal dysfunction.[17, 18]

❸ Smoking and IBD. Epidemiologically the risk of developing UC is higher in non-smokers than in smokers, and trials with transdermal nicotine or nicotine gum have shown some improvement in patients with active disease; however, this remains controversial.[1] In contrast to UC, smoking is associated with increased risk of Crohn's disease, or Crohn's disease flares.

❹ Cancer and IBD. Patients with UC are more at risk of colorectal cancer than those with Crohn's, but the effectiveness of colonoscopic surveillance programmes is controversial.[12,15] Genetic or biochemical markers predicting cancer risk are currently being researched.[15]

6. Annese V Andreoli A, et al 2001 Clinical features in familial cases of Crohn's disease and ulcerative colitis in Italy: A GISC study. American Journal of Gastroenterology 96: 2939–45

7. Papadakis KA Targan SR 1999 Current theories on the causes of IBD. Gastroenterology Clinics of North America 28(2): 283–96

8. Panes J 2001 IBD: pathogenesis and targets for therapeutic interventions. Acta Physiologica Scandinavica 173: 159–65

9. Roy MA 1997 IBD. Surgical Clinics of North America 77(6): 1419–31

10. Moses PL, et al 1998 IBD: origins, presentation and course. Postgraduate Medicine 103(5): 77–102

11. Giardiello FM Lazenby AJ 1999 The atypical colitides. Gastroenterology Clinics of North America 28(2): 479–90

12. Andrews J Norton I, Dent O, Goulston K 1995 IBD: a retrospective review of a specialist-based cohort. Medical Journal of Australia 163: 133–6

13. Becker JM 1999 Surgical therapy for UC and Crohn's disease. Gastroenterology Clinics of North America 28(2): 371–90

14. Wolff BD 1998 Factors determining recurrence following surgery for Crohn's Disease. World Journal of Surgery 22: 364–9

15. Solomon MJ Schnitzler M 1998 Cancer and IBD: bias, epidemiology, surveillance and treatment. World Journal of Surgery 22: 352–8

16. Michetti P Peppercorn MA 1999 Medical therapy of specific clinical presentations. Gastroenterology Clinics of North America 28(2): 352–70

17. Stein RB Hanauer SB 1999 Medical therapy for IBD. Gastroenterology Clinics of North America 28(2): 297–321

18. Sands B 2000 Therapy of IBD. Gastroenterology 118: S68–S82

19. Kho YH, Oudkerk-Pool M, et al 2001 Pharmacotherapeutic options in IBD: an update. Pharmacy World & Science 23(1): 17–21

20. Hannauer SB 1996 IBD. New England Journal of Medicine 334(13): 841–8

21. Katz J (ed.) IBD. Medical Clinics of North America 78(6): 1207–493

22. Lofberg R 1997 Medical treatment for IBD - refinements and new modalities (editorial). Journal of Intensive Care Medicine 241: 1–4

23. Han PD Burke A, Baldesanno R, et al 1999 Nutrition and IBD. Gastroenterology Clinics of North America 28(2): 423–43

24. Raj V Lichtenstein DR 1999 Hepatobiliary manifestations of IBD. Gastroenterology Clinics of North America 28(2): 491–513

25. Nicholson DA Driscoll PA 1995 ABC of Emergency Radiology. BMJ Publishing Group, London

26. Scotiniotis I Rubesin SE, Geinsberg GG 1999 Imaging modalities in IBD. Gastroenterology Clinics of North America 28(2): 391–421

27. Chey WY 2001 Infliximab for patients with refractory ulcerative colitis. Inflammatory Bowel Disease 7(Suppl 1): S30–S33

28. Feeney M Clegg, Winwood, Snook J 1997 A case-control study of measles vaccination and IBD. Lancet 350: 764–6

6.11 ACUTE LIVER FAILURE

JOHN M. RYAN

ESSENTIALS

1 The diagnosis of acute liver failure is based on the presence of increasing coagulopathy, hepatic encephalopathy and deepening jaundice.

2 The aetiology is varied and related to a number of geographical and social factors. Viral hepatitis remains the commonest cause worldwide, but paracetamol toxicity is an increasingly common cause in the Western world.

3 Early diagnosis is important because of the therapeutic option of using antidotes in the presence of a reversible cause.

4 Patients should be transferred to an intensive care unit or a specialized liver unit once the diagnosis of acute liver failure has been made.

5 Management involves optimizing the patient's haemodynamic, renal, pulmonary and cerebral status, in addition to preventing bacterial and fungal infections. Orthotopic liver transplantation may improve survival rates.

INTRODUCTION

Acute liver failure (ALF) is an umbrella term covering a spectrum of disease from subacute to hyperacute. The fundamental components are altered mental status and coagulopathy occurring in the setting of an acute hepatic disease.[1] Acute hepatic encephalopathy can be graded according to clinical signs:[2]

Grade 1: Confused or altered mood

Grade 2: Inappropriate behaviour or drowsiness

Grade 3: Stuporous but rousable, markedly confused behaviour

Grade 4: Coma unresponsive to painful stimuli.

Hyperacute liver failure implies encephalopathy coming on within 1 week of jaundice, and is often associated with paracetamol toxicity. Subacute failure results in encephalopathy coming on within 1 and 24 weeks of jaundice, and is may be the result of non-A non-B hepatitis where no virus is detected.[3]

Although the causative agent of ALF is usually detectable, the pathogenesis of organ failure is not well understood. The common factors shared by all causes are cerebral oedema and a shock-like state, with failure to perfuse vital organs. Tumour necrosis factor, disturbed prostaglandin metabolism and group-specific component protein are frequently present, but are not universal.

AETIOLOGY

Although uncommon, ALF is nevertheless a devastating illness resulting in multisystem failure with a mortality of up to 80%, depending on the cause. The aetiology is geographically and socially linked. In the Western world paracetamol is the single most frequently indicted agent. Although paracetamol is the causative agent in only 3% of fatal overdoses, it is responsible for 50–60% of cases of ALF.[4] Fatalities have also been reported with therapeutic amounts of paracetamol when ingested by chronic alcoholics or by patients taking phenytoin and other enzyme-inducing agents.[5]

In France and California, mushrooms (*Amanita phalloides*) have also been implicated.[6] Halothane and other drugs, such as antituberculous medications, are uncommon causes.[7] More recently, the statins including lovastatin have been incriminated as have Cox-2 inhibitors and antiretroviral HIV medication.

On a worldwide basis, however, viral hepatitis remains the commonest cause of ALF, constituting in excess of 70% of cases. Significant geographical variations exist, however. For instance, hepatitis C is a major cause of ALF in Japan and the Far East, though rarely seen in Europe.[8] Hepatitis A rarely leads to ALF and has a relatively good survival rate of 60%. Hepatitis B is the commonest cause of viral-associated ALF and is particularly prevalent in the Far East. Hepatitis D is usually only implicated on a background of previous or coincidental hepatitis B infection and, although uncommon in the USA, it is the cause of 50% of cases of ALF in patients who are hepatitis B positive. Hepatitis E is seen in subtropical areas, particularly in pregnancy, when it is often fatal.[9]

Other rarer causes of ALF include lymphoma, ischaemia, Budd-Chiari syndrome, ecstasy poisoning, and other viruses such as coxsackie B and herpes simplex. In Australia some rare causes of ALF have been described, including chronic copper toxicosis.

Herbal hepatotoxicity as a cause of ALF, most notably kava kava an antidepressant, is a reminder of the importance of taking a detailed drug history. Acute fatty liver of pregnancy as a cause of ALF is usually self-evident.

PRESENTATION

The diagnostic hallmark of ALF is the clinical presentation of hepatic encephalopathy, severe coagulopathy and worsening jaundice. As the disease progresses features of shock and multiorgan failure develop, including adult respiratory distress syndrome, renal failure and superinfection with bacteria and fungi.

Hypotension and hypoxia lead to a worsening cycle as further damage to the injured liver occurs.

The mode of presentation may give some clue to the aetiology. Patients with paracetamol toxicity may present with severe coagulopathy and encephalopathy, with jaundice being a late feature. Conversely, patients with non-A non-B hepatitis are more likely to present with deep jaundice prior to the onset of confusion.

INVESTIGATIONS

The clinical scenario of coagulopathy, altered mental status and jaundice strongly suggests the diagnosis. However, determining the aetiology is important because of the availability of antidotes. Extensive investigations should be performed to determine both the aetiology and the severity of the condition. Laboratory testing should include a full blood count, coagulation screen, liver enzymes, renal function and arterial blood gases. A prothrombin time exceeding 4 seconds in the presence of altered mental status confirms the clinical diagnosis. Viral studies, caeruloplasmin levels and drug screens should be sent at an early stage, as the assays are not always available immediately. Recently it has been suggested that arterial blood lactate measurement rapidly and accurately identifies patients who will die from paracetamol-induced acute liver failure. It is thought that its use may increase the speed and selection of patients suitable for liver transplantation.[10]

MANAGEMENT

A number of therapeutic options exist in the management of ALF in the emergency department and are dependent on the aetiology. In some cases, specific antidotes such as silibinin (milk thistle extract), penicillin or *N*-acetylcysteine (NAC) may be available to treat ALF or impending ALF. Generally, however, the treatment centres on good intensive care, addressing pulmonary complications,

haemodynamic factors, adequate tissue oxygenation and cerebral perfusion, and prevention of infection. Liver transplantation has been a major factor in improving survival in recent years.

Antidotes

Patients with acute liver failure as a result of paracetamol toxicity should be treated with NAC.[11] Research has shown that even when given up to 36 hours after ingestion, NAC reduces mortality from paracetamol poisoning.[12]

Other antidotes available include penicillin and silibinin (milk thistle extract) for *Amanita phalloides* poisoning. Antidotes should be commenced at the earliest opportunity, but do not reduce the importance of the management of complications and preventing and managing multiorgan failure.

General measures

Fundamental to the management of patients with ALF is management in a specialized or intensive care unit. Aggressive monitoring is required to detect respiratory and haemodynamic complications, neurological changes, infections and gastrointestinal haemorrhage. Central venous access and invasive and non-invasive arterial blood pressure monitoring are useful for monitoring vascular status. Swan-Ganz pulmonary artery pressure monitoring gives helpful information about cardiac output. All patients should have a urinary catheter placed to monitor urine output. Volume resuscitation should be with colloids and can be titrated to a pulmonary wedge pressure of 12–14 mmHg. Intravenous dopamine may be required to encourage renal perfusion, and noradrenaline (norepinephrine) may be required for systemic hypotension. Patients should be monitored with pulse oximetry and assisted ventilation may be required for deteriorating pulmonary function. Metabolic derangements such as hypoglycaemia should be sought and treated aggressively. Hypokalaemia is common and should be managed with intravenous supplements. Intravenous phosphate and magnesium supplements may also be required. Platelets may be required if the count falls below 20000/mL. H_2-receptor blockers are given for prophylaxis against gastrointestinal bleeding. Dialysis may be required for deteriorating renal function and worsening acidosis.

Maintaining adequate cerebral perfusion is paramount and the patient should be nursed in a quiet environment with 10° head-up tilt. Intracranial pressure monitoring may be helpful in some patients for directing therapy to prevent brain-stem herniation. Dietary protein withdrawal is commonly recommended to treat acute hepatic encephalopathy, although the traditional use of lactulose for enteral decontamination is now more controversial. Instead, other agents such as metronidazole and neomycin have been recommended to treat acute hepatic encephalopathy, although early introduction of systemic antibiotics is the most important intervention. Systemic antimicrobial therapy with or without enteral decontamination reduces infection rate in patients with acute liver failure.[13]

Recent developments in tissue engineering have included the development of flat membrane bioreactor utilizing hepatocytes for the creation of a bioartificial liver.[14] These extracorporeal liver assist devices have been seen as providing a potential bridge to definitive liver transplantation.

Some experimental work has suggested that mild hypothermia may prevent encephalopathy and brain oedema in ALF.[15]

DISPOSITION

Patients with ALF should be managed in a specialized liver unit or an intensive care unit. Any patient with altered mental status or evidence of significant coagulopathy requires intensive care and close monitoring for deteriorating renal function, shock and cerebral oedema.

PROGNOSIS

Survival rates for patients with ALF have improved with the advent of specialized liver and intensive care units. Survival for all-cause acute liver failure is now in excess of 50%. Aetiology, however, remains the most important independent predictor of outcome. Survival from paracetamol toxicity in patients with grades 3–4 hepatic encephalopathy is now as high as 64% in one specialized unit.[16] The prognosis is best for acute fatty liver of pregnancy, followed by the viral causes, with hepatitis A having the best outcome, hepatitis B an intermediate outcome and non-A non-B viruses having the worst prognosis. Patients with slow progression of failure tend to do worse than those with a rapid downhill course to encephalopathy. Other factors associated with a poor prognosis include the presence of a metabolic acidosis and, in cases of paracetamol toxicity, a continuing rise in the prothrombin time at days 3–4, which may rise to 180 seconds. Orthotopic liver transplantation is one of the most important advances in the treatment of acute liver failure and has improved survival rates to 60–80%.[17]

CONTROVERSIES

❶ Lactulose, although still advocated in some centres for the treatment of hepatic enecephalopathy, has been withdrawn in others because of the fear of fluid overload. H_2 blockers have been used since 1977 for stress ulceration, although lately sucralfate has been considered of more benefit than acid-suppressing drugs for the prevention of stress ulceration.

❷ The addition of vasodilators such as epoprostenol (prostacyclin) or NAC to increase oxygenation remains controversial. NAC is available intravenously in the UK, Australia and many other countries but only the oral form is available in the USA.[18]

❸ Extracorporeal liver-assist devices may be the latest development, but await further controlled studies before they are widely applied in cases of acute liver failure.[19]

PREVENTION

The prevention of acute liver failure, worldwide, is dependent on improvements in public health and hygiene as viral hepatitis is the commonest cause. In Western society paracetamol toxicity is becoming an increasingly common problem. The incidence, although rising, is not as high in France as in other countries. One reason for this may be the lack of availability of paracetamol tablets in more than 8 g packages, and there may be a case for advocating such practice worldwide, although there is conflicting evidence of the effect of introducing legislative change regarding its availability. One suggestion, of adding methionine to paracetamol, is unlikely to be adopted because of financial implications. Avoiding other toxic substances, such as the newer recreational drugs, might also decrease the incidence.

REFERENCES

1. Trey C, Davidson CS 1970 The management of fulminant hepatic failure. In: Popper H, Schaffer F (eds) Progress in Liver Failure. Grune and Stratton, New York, pp 292–8
2. Caraceni P, Van Theil DV 1995 Acute liver failure. Lancet 345: 163–9
3. Grady JG, Schalm, Williams R 1993 Acute liver failure: redefining the syndromes. Lancet 342: 273–5
4. Spooner JB, Harvey JG 1993 Paracetamol overdose - facts not misconceptions. Pharmaceutical Journal 252: 706–7
5. Zimmerman HJ, Maddrey WC 1995 Acetaminophen (paracetamol) hepatotoxicity with regular intake of alcohol: analysis of instances of therapeutic misadventure. Hepatology 22: 767–73
6. Klein AS, Hart J, Brems JJ, Goldstein L, Lewin K, Busuttil RW 1989 *Amanita* poisoning: treatment and the role of liver transplantation. American Journal of Medicine 86: 187–93
7. Mitchell I, Wendon J, Fitt S, Williams R 1995 Anti-tuberculous therapy and acute liver failure. Lancet 345: 555–6
8. Yoshiba M, Seikiyama K, Inoue K, et al 1994 Contribution of hepatitis C virus to non-A, non-B fulminant hepatitis in Japan. Hepatology 19: 829–35
9. Asher LVS, Innis BL, Shrestha MP, Ticehurst J, Baze WB 1990 Virus-like particles in the liver of a patient with fulminant hepatitis and antibody to hepatitis E virus. Journal of Medical Virology 31: 229–33
10. Bernal W, Donaldson N, Wyncoll D, Wendon J 2002 Blood lactate as an early predictor of outcome in paracetamol-induced acute liver failure: a cohort study. Lancet 359: 558–63
11. Prescott IF, Illingworth RN, Critchley JAJH, Stewart MJ, Adam RD, Proudfoot AT 1979 Intravenous *N*-acetylcysteine: the treatment of choice for paracetamol poisoning. British Medical Journal ii: 1097–100

12. Harrison PM, Keays R, Bray GP, Alexander GJM, Williams R 1990 Improved outcome of paracetamol induced fulminant hepatic failure by late administration of acetylcysteine. Lancet 335: 1572–3

13. Rolando N, Grimson A, Wade J, et al 1993 Prospective study comparing prophylactic parenteral antimicrobials, with or without enteral decontamination, in patients with acute liver failure. Hepatology 17: 196–201

14. O'Grady JG, Alexander G, Hayllar K, Williams R 1988 Early indicators of prognosis in fulminant hepatic failure. Gastroenterology 94: 1186–92

15. Boudjema K, Bachellier P, Wolf P, Tempe JD, Jaeck D 2002 Auxiliary liver transplantation and bioartificial bridging procedures in treatment of acute liver failure. World Journal of Surgery 26(2): 264–74

16. Chatauret N, Rose C, Therrien G, Butterworth RF 2001 Mild hypothermia prevents cerebral edema and CSF lactate accumulation in acute liver failure. Metabolic Brain Disease 16(1–2): 95–102

17. O'Grady JG, Alexander GJM, Thick M, Potter D, Calne RY, Williams R 1988 Outcome of orthoptic liver transplantation in the etiological and clinical variants of acute liver failure. Journal of Medicine 69: 817–24

18. Harrison PM, Wendon JA, Gimson AES, Alexander GJM, Williams R 1991 Improvement by acetylcysteine of haemodynamics and oxygen transport in fulminant hepatic failure. New England Journal of Medicine 324: 1852–7

19. Butler A, Friend PJ 1997 Novel strategies for liver support in acute liver failure. British Medicine Bulletin 4: 719–29

FURTHER READING

Caraceni P, Van Theil DV 1995 Acute liver failure. Lancet 345: 163–9

Lee WM Medical progress: acute liver failure. New England Journal of Medicine 329: 1862–74

Williams R 1996 Classification, etiology and considerations of outcome in acute liver failure. Seminars in Liver Disease 16: 4

6.12 RECTAL BLEEDING

SCOTT J. PEARSON • PETER J. AITKEN

ESSENTIALS

1 All patients over 50 years with rectal bleeding should have complete investigation of their large bowel regardless of the presence of anorectal disease.

2 Mortality from significant lower gastrointestinal bleeding has decreased to 5–10% with early resuscitation and improved diagnostic techniques.

3 Eighty to 90% of lower gastrointestinal haemorrhages will stop spontaneously.

4 Colonoscopy is the investigation of choice in both elective and acute situations, but is controversial in the acute setting. There is wide institutional variation in the use of colonoscopy, angiography and red blood cell scans owing to availability, access and local expertise.

5 Treatment options consist of colonoscopic, angiographic and surgical techniques. Surgery is occasionally necessary in the acute situation. Results of surgery are optimized by prior haemodynamic stabilization.

INTRODUCTION

Rectal bleeding is a common problem in most Western societies, with over 20% affected at some stage in their lives. Patients may present with minor self-limiting episodes, evidence of occult blood loss with anaemia, or more severe bleeding with haemodynamic instability.

Per rectal blood loss usually originates distal to the ligament of Trietz (duodenal suspensory ligament at the junction of the duodenum and the jejunum) in the distal duodenum. However, in 10–15% of cases the cause of the bleeding may be proximal in the duodenum, stomach or distal oesophagus.[1,2]

The primary pathology causing bleeding varies with age. Appropriate investigation and management is dictated by the severity of the presentation and the age of the patient. Those with minor bleeds can often be investigated and managed as an outpatient. Moderate and severe bleeding, although frequently ceasing spontaneously, requires inpatient investigation. In some cases immediate resuscitation may be necessary. Mortality from acute lower gastrointestinal bleeding has declined to 5–10%.[1] The risk of mortality is increased by increased age, concomitant medical problems, difficulty in locating a bleeding source, and surgery in the unstable patient.

AETIOLOGY

In patients under 50 haemorrhoids are by far the most common cause of rectal bleeding, with anal fissures, benign polyps and inflammatory bowel disease being much less common.[3] Other causes, such as colitis and diverticulosis, feature sporadically in this age group. Over the age of 40 the risk of sporadic colonic neoplasms increases with every year of age.[4] This should be borne in mind in investigating this age group.

Diverticulosis and angiodysplasia are the most common causes in patients over 50, with carcinoma, polyps, haemorrhoids and colitis also featuring. The presence of disease in the rectum or anus in this age group should not discourage a more thorough investigation of the gastrointestinal tract,[5] as dual pathology exists in as many as 25% of cases. Despite thorough investigation, about 10% of people suffering rectal bleeding will remain undiagnosed.[6] As better techniques become available for imaging the gastrointestinal tract, this number should gradually decrease.

Diverticulosis

Colonic diverticula are acquired defects in the bowel wall occurring at the point of entry of nutrient vessels. The incidence increases with age and they are present in

341

>50% of people over 60 years of age.[1,7] Diverticula are far more common distally, with only 15% of patients having involvement of the caecum and ascending colon. Significant diverticular bleeding occurs in only 3–5%[6] of patients with diverticulosis, and 50–70% of this occurs in the right colon despite the lower incidence of right-sided disease.[1] There is usually no association with diverticulitis.

Bleeding is arterial and usually from a single diverticulum. It is acute, painless, and can be alarming in its volume. Intermittent minor bleeding is not characteristic. Bleeding stops spontaneously in 80–90% of cases. Rebleeding will occur in as many as 25%.[8]

Angiodysplasia

Angiodysplastic lesions are acquired submucosal vascular ectasia, which occur as part of the degenerative process of ageing. Their exact aetiology is unclear. They can affect up to 25% of the population of over 60 year olds, and involve mainly the right colon and caecum. They are usually small (<5 mm) and multiple in 25%.[1] The majority do not cause problems and diagnosis is often incidental. Bleeding is usually chronic, although a minority can present with acute haemorrhage. These will settle spontaneously in 90%, but almost all will rebleed.[6] Other, rarer vascular anomalies may include true arteriovenous malformation, haemangiomas, and those associated with syndromes such as hereditary haemorrhagic telangiectasia (Osler–Rendu–Weber syndrome).

Neoplasia

Neoplasms arising from any portion of the bowel usually cause occult or minor bleeding. Significant haemorrhage occurs in less than 20%.[6] There may be associated symptoms such as weight loss, altered bowel habit, abdominal pain or symptoms of obstruction. Isolated rectal bleeding without associated symptoms is a very uncommon presentation of bowel malignancy.[9]

Inflammatory bowel disease

Inflammatory bowel disease (IBD) is usually associated with small to moderate amounts of bright blood mixed in with the stool. Significant bleeding only occurs in 1–2% of individuals. These patients are usually young (25–30 years) with widespread disease.

Colitis

Radiation colitis may occur early in treatment (acute) or months to years afterwards (chronic), and bleeding may be severe. A variety of parasitic and bacterial infections can cause colitis, but bleeding is rarely severe. Bleeding may also occur with ischaemia.

Anorectal disorders

Haemorrhoids are generally the most common cause of rectal bleeding, usually causing intermittent painless bleeding associated with defecation. Significant haemorrhage may occur following haemorrhoidectomy. It may also occur when prolapsed internal haemorrhoids are mistaken for thrombosed external haemorrhoids and an attempt is made at incision and drainage. Rectal varices may occur in association with portal hypertension.

Aortoenteric fistula

This complication occurs in 0.5–2.5% of abdominal aortic aneurysm repairs. In 75% of cases, it involves the third part of the duodenum in association with graft material. It is rare in the absence of previous vascular surgery. There may be a 'herald bleed' prior to catastrophic exsanguinating haemorrhage. High levels of suspicion should be maintained for all patients with gastrointestinal bleeding and previous abdominal aortic aneurysm repair.

Miscellaneous

Rectal ulcers may result from pressure necrosis of bowel mucosa. Local trauma may result from unusual sexual practices or the insertion of foreign bodies. Non-steroidal anti-inflammatories are also thought to predispose to lower gastrointestinal bleeding, but the area is controversial. Inherited or acquired bleeding disorders may exacerbate gastrointestinal bleeding. Nocturnal epistaxis and swallowed blood from oral or nasal sources may result in erroneous investigation of lower or upper gastrointestinal tracts. Massive rectal bleeding is a rare complication of prostatic biopsy. More unusual causes, often infective, also need to be considered in association with HIV.

HISTORY

Important features in the history are an estimate of the severity of the bleeding, localization of the source and information offered by the patient. Although patient estimates of the amount of bleeding are unreliable, the number and frequency of motions and symptoms of volume depletion (syncope, dizziness, dyspnoea) are more helpful.

The diagnosis of neoplasia may be suggested by altered bowel habit or abdominal pain and constitutional symptoms such as weight loss and lethargy. Pain is unusual with bleeding from diverticular disease or angiodysplasia.

A history of haematemesis is useful in directing initial investigation to the upper tract. Routine questioning should also include past medical history (especially any cardiorespiratory disease), anticoagulation, non-steroidal anti-inflammatory use and alcohol intake.

EXAMINATION

Initial evaluation should focus on haemodynamic stability. Vital signs should include systolic blood pressure and pulse rate. A postural blood pressure drop indicates a significant blood volume loss (also caused by drugs and autonomic functions). Respiratory rate is an important early indicator of shock. Both mental status and urine output are also important. Examination should look for abdominal signs and evidence of chronic liver disease and coagulopathy. Digital rectal examination is essential to confirm rectal bleeding and detect local pathology.

INVESTIGATIONS

Proctoscopy

This procedure takes minimal time and should be the initial investigation in almost all patients. It offers the highest detection rate for haemorrhoids and anal fissures.

Rigid or flexible sigmoidoscopy

This procedure enables inspection of the mucosa of the rectum, sigmoid colon and distal descending colon.

Double-contrast barium enema

Barium studies have no place in the acute setting largely because of practical difficulties and inadequately prepared bowel. It also lacks sensitivity in detecting smaller dysplastic lesions and cannot provide a tissue diagnosis. Barium studies may complement colonoscopy if a source is not found, or may be used in conjunction with sigmoidoscopy in the younger patient.[3,10]

Colonoscopy

This offers the most complete view of the colonic mucosa with the added ability to establish tissue diagnosis by biopsy and perform therapeutic interventions. It is the investigation of choice in the stable patient with adequate bowel preparation.[11] The role of colonoscopy in acute lower gastrointestinal bleeding is more controversial. Care should be taken to ensure the procedure is performed in an appropriate area of the hospital where resuscitation can be continued.

Technetium-labelled red blood cell (^{99m}Tc RBC) scans

Serial scans can be obtained up to 36 hours after injection of the tracer, which may be useful in intermittent bleeding. Localization of bleeding sources is often imprecise, however.[6]

Angiography

Where available this involves contrast injection of the superior mesenteric artery, inferior mesenteric artery and coeliac trunk, in that order. Sensitivity varies widely.

Other investigations

If investigation of the colon has failed to identify a cause of bleeding then investigation of the upper gastrointestinal tract, including gastroscopy and a small bowel contrast series of X-rays should be considered. Abdominal CT scanning may very occasionally be helpful. Plain abdominal X-rays are of little use, but may be considered if there is clinical suspicion of bowel obstruction or possibly bowel ischaemia.

TREATMENT

The approach to the patient with rectal bleeding will differ depending on the severity of bleeding.

Minor intermittent bleeding

After initial assessment these patients may be investigated on an outpatient basis. Even in the presence of anorectal pathology, further imaging of the colon is necessary in the over-50 age group. The extent of further imaging in the younger age group is controversial, but many would extend the age range down to those over 40 years and anyone with significant risk factors for colonic carcinoma.[10] These people should proceed to either colonoscopy or double-contrast barium enema, as local resources permit. Anoscopy and rigid sigmoidoscopy can potentially be performed in the emergency department, although there are issues of performer experience and adequate bowel preparation that need to be considered. Those discharged home should have adequate arrangements for outpatient follow-up with either surgical or gastroenterology services.

Major and/or persistent rectal bleeding

Immediate assessment should follow the standard ABC approach, with care to ensure adequate fluid resuscitation with crystalloid/colloid, followed by blood products if necessary. A haemodynamically stable, resuscitated patient has less morbidity, with improved tolerance of further procedures. The usual care with fluid resuscitation should be exercised in the elderly. Most severe bleeding will cease spontaneously,[1,6] and further investigation can proceed when the bowel has been properly prepared. In a minority of instances bleeding continues and further management should occur as an emergency. Again controversy exists and local practice varies. Early colonoscopy with the aid of saline/polyethylene glycol purge results in improved diagnostic and treatment rates.[11] Technetium-labelled red blood cell scanning and angiography are available in some institutions.

As most lower gastrointestinal bleeding ceases spontaneously, the majority of patients will need no treatment other than initial resuscitation. Definitive therapy may then be performed on an elective basis if needed. Treatment options include the investigative modalities of colonoscopy and angiography, as well as surgery.

Colonoscopic therapy

Treatment options include electrocoagulation, laser and polypectomy. Most success has been achieved with angiodysplasia, and occasionally with diverticulosis. Endoscopic control of bleeding is achieved in 50–86% of cases.[12,13] Risks are rebleeding and perforation. In addition to proven efficacy, emergency colonoscopy may be the most cost-effective management approach.[14]

Angiographic treatment

Vasopressin may give temporary control of bleeding. Transcatheter embolization of angiodysplastic lesions has been reported but has a significant risk of intestinal ischaemia and infarction.[6]

Surgery

Surgery is most useful as an interval procedure in a resuscitated stable patient for definitive treatment of established diagnoses. Emergency surgery has a high morbidity and mortality, as patients are usually elderly and haemodynamically unstable.

Laparotomy is performed as a final option. Every effort should be made to locate a bleeding source prior to any planned bowel resection. Right hemicolectomy is often performed, and has a lower morbidity and mortality than subtotal colectomy.[6]

CONCLUSION

Rectal bleeding is a common problem but rarely acutely life threatening. Care needs to be exercised to ensure that all patients are adequately investigated, otherwise disease progression may occur and result in increased morbidity. Uncommonly, large-volume rectal bleeding will occur and cause shock, usually in the older patient. Resuscitation should include active intravascular volume replacement with appropriate fluids and blood products. Care should be taken in view of the high incidence of coexisting medical illness. Surgical colleagues should be involved early so that plans can be made regarding appropriate investigation.

CONTROVERSIES

❶ The use of colonoscopy, red cell scanning and angiography. Much of this is dictated by local resource availability, including expertise.

❷ The extent of investigation in the younger (under 40 years) age group.

REFERENCES

1. Demarkles MP, Murphy JR 1993 Acute lower gastrointestinal bleeding. Medical Clinics of North America 77: 1085–99
2. Lichtiger S, Kornbluth A, Saloman P, et al 1992 Lower gastrointestinal bleeding. In: Taylor MB, Gollan JL, Peppercorn MA, et al (eds) Gastrointestinal Emergencies. Williams and Wilkins, Baltimore
3. Korkis AM, McDougall CJ 1995 Rectal bleeding in patients less than 50 years of age. Digestive Diseases and Sciences 1520–23
4. Fleischer DE, Goldberg S, Browning T, et al 1992 Detection and surveillance of colorectal cancer. Journal of the American Medical Association 61(4): 580–5
5. Helfaud M, Marton KI, et al 1997 History of visible rectal bleeding in a primary care population. Initial assessment and 10 year follow-up. Journal of the American Medical Association 1277: 44–8
6. Ellis DJ, Reinus JF 1995 Lower intestinal haemorrhage. Critical Care Clinics 11: 369–87
7. Katkov WN 1992 Case records of the Massachusetts General Hospital. Case 14–1992. New England Journal of Medicine 326: 936
8. Zuckerman DA, Bocchini TP, Birnbaum EH 1993 Massive haemorrhage in the lower gastrointestinal tract in adults: diagnostic imaging and intervention. American Journal of Roentgenology 161: 703–11
9. Richter JM, Christensen MR, Kaplan LM, et al 1995 Effectiveness of current technology in the diagnosis and management of lower gastrointestinal haemorrhage. Gastrointestinal Endoscopy 41(2): 93–8
10. Douek M, Wickramasinghe M, Clifton MA 1999 Does isolated rectal bleeding suggest colorectal cancer? Lancet 354: 393
11. Gane EJ, Lane MR 1992 Colonoscopy in unexplained lower gastrointestinal bleeding. New Zealand Medical Journal 105: 31–3
12. Jenson DM, Machicado GA 1988 Diagnosis and treatment of severe hematochezia: the role of urgent colonoscopy after purge. Gastroenterology 95: 1569–74
13. Santos JC Jr, Aprilli F, Guimaraes AS, et al 1998 Angiodysplasia of the colon: endoscopic diagnosis and treatment. British Journal of Surgery 75: 256–8
14. Machicado GA, Jensen DM 1997 Acute and chronic management of lower GI bleeding:Cost effective approaches. Gastroenterologist 5: 189–201

6.13 PERIANAL CONDITIONS

ANDREW DENT

ESSENTIALS

1 Perianal and pilonidal abscesses require incision and drainage. In some cases this can be done safely in the emergency department but some surgeons prefer that all anorectal abscesses are drained in theatre.

2 Incision and drainage of cutaneous abscesses is not associated with bacteraemia in afebrile adults, and so routine antibiotic cover is not required.

3 Supralevator, intersphincteric and ischiorectal abscesses require formal surgical exploration and drainage in theatre.

4 Irreducible haemorrhoids require urgent reduction and surgery.

PILONIDAL ABSCESS/SINUS

Pilonidal abscess/sinus is a recurrent disease of young adults, affecting men twice as often as women. It is more common in obese and sedentary patients.[1] The natural history of the disease is for spontaneous regression in the fourth decade of life.[2] The pathological basis of the condition is the migration of hair ends into the natal cleft, where they become embedded, cause irritation, and an abscess forms around them.

The patient presents with a painful lump over the sacrum. Systemic symptoms are uncommon. Examination shows an abscess usually slightly to one side of the midline. One or more midline pits are often present, and occasionally hair is seen protruding.

Treatment is drainage. Simple drainage, under local anaesthesia, leaving the wound open, relieves symptoms and allows immediate return to work. Healing is very slow, occurring in 58% of cases by 10 weeks, and in 76% by 18 months.[3]

Prevention of recurrence by careful attention to hair control with natal cleft shaving and improved perineal hygiene is recommended. More aggressive excisional procedures are not favoured as they produces similar results at greater cost and more loss of working days.[4]

ANORECTAL ABSCESSES

Anorectal abscesses can be classified into one of four groups. Depending on local practice, some may be able to be treated in the emergency department. The concern for the emergency physician is to identify those that can be safely drained in the emergency department without harming continence, causing seeding infection, or missing another diagnosis.

Perianal abscess

This presents as a painful lump around the anal verge, usually lateral and posterior to the anus. It may result from an infected anal gland or, more rarely, be a presentation of Crohn's disease. Systemic symptoms are uncommon. On examination most will be pointing, with an indurated red area which may be fluctuant.

Such abscesses can be drained under local anaesthesia, with the assistance of sedation or inhalation analgesia. Incision should be stab-like, circumferential to the anal ring but long enough to allow complete evacuation of pus. The drainage site can be opened a little more widely with artery forceps. It is often best to leave it to drain freely for a few minutes, and then insert a small wick of gauze into the cavity to prevent early closure. A dressing will usually prevent soiling of clothes. Regular review and dressing change should continue until healing is confirmed.

Ischiorectal abscess

This abscess usually has more systemic symptoms. Patients are often febrile and look toxic. The area of induration is likely to be large and more lateral. Pointing may not occur until late, and it may seem more like a 'buttock cellulitis'. Treatment should be exploration and drainage under general anaesthesia, usually with proctosigmoidoscopy and possibly biopsy at the same time.

Supralevator abscess

This may be the cause of a pyrexia of unknown origin. The patient may present with pain on defecation and an altered bowel habit. In reality, this is a pelvic abscess and is often secondary to an intra-abdominal condition such as diverticular or Crohn's disease. Inspection of the perineum may be normal, but rectal examination will reveal a firm, spongy, tender mass. Treatment is exploration and drainage under general anaesthesia by a surgeon with a colorectal interest.

Intersphincteric or submucous abscess

These abscesses are within the anal canal, so no external swelling may be visible. They point within the anal canal and may rupture spontaneously. Traditionally the search for a fistulous internal opening followed by fistulotomy has been the standard treatment for perianal suppuration. Recently simple drainage under general anaesthesia has been advocated, as this will be the only treatment required in most cases. The risk of recurrence is low.[5]

Complex and recurrent anorectal abscesses may be well delineated by intrarectal ultrasound.[6]

Fistula formation and recurrence following the first presentation of an anorectal abscess occurs in up to 50% of cases, and is more common with bowel-derived organisms such as *E. coli* and *Bacterioides fragilis*.[7]

FISTULAE

Anal fistula rarely present as an emergency de novo, but rather as recurrent perianal suppuration. A fistula is a connection between two epithelial surfaces, and in this setting, between rectal lumen and perianal skin. They may be secondary to a complicated anorectal abscess, Crohn's disease, diverticular disease or carcinoma. Diagnosis is suspected on a history of recurrent perianal suppuration and is confirmed by the delineation of fistulous tracks during surgery under anaesthesia. Fistula surgery can be difficult and complex, and recurrence is common.

HAEMORRHOIDS

Haemorrhoids are dilatations of the internal venous plexuses of the anus, usually located in the 3, 7 and 11 o'clock positions as viewed through a proctoscope with the patient in the lithotomy position.

First-degree haemorrhoids are never visible, but they cause symptoms by bleeding. Second-degree haemorrhoids prolapse, usually after straining at stool, but are immediately reducible. Third-degree haemorrhoids are permanently prolapsed to some degree.

Bleeding from otherwise uncomplicated haemorrhoids is typically painless and bright red. It is often described as a splash in the pan or streaks on toilet paper. Bleeding between bowel actions or blood mixed with the stool should raise the suspicion of other pathology, such as diverticular disease or carcinoma. In any patient with rectal bleeding, it is important to rule out carcinoma.

Examination involves observing the perineum with the patient straining. Redundant skin tags may be present. Grape-like structures may be seen to bulge around the classic 3, 7 and 11 o'clock positions. Proctosigmoidoscopy, looking particularly on withdrawal of the scope, may reveal one or more haemorrhoids.

For first-, second- and reducible third-degree haemorrhoids, treatment consists of stool softeners and a high-fibre diet to prevent straining. The use of locally soothing suppositories and creams such as Anusol may be symptomatically helpful if there is associated irritation or pain.

Irreducible haemorrhoids

These will require early surgery. Discomfort can be reduced and, on occasion, reduction achieved by the use of systemic analgesia, a foot-up tilted trolley, the application of ice, local anaesthetic gel, and firm slow pressure applied digitally. This can change the requirement for surgery from emergency to urgent elective.

Thrombosed external haemorrhoid, or perianal haematoma

This is quite a different condition from internal haemorrhoids and lends itself to simple, effective treatment in the emergency department. After straining at stool the patient describes a sensation of pain and a lump. Examination reveals a bluish, exquisitely tender skin-covered lump sited lateral to the anus.

Treatment is incision under local anaesthetic. A small amount of lidocaine with adrenaline (epinephrine) is injected extremely slowly until the skin bleb blanches. A small longitudinal incision is made over the crest of the thin skin, and a broad-bean-sized blood clot is shelled out. Local pressure with a piece of gauze, taped in place for a short period, will prevent bleeding. No other follow-up treatment is required. Pain relief is immediate and permanent. If the condition is left untreated it will usually improve spontaneously within 5 days.

FISSURE IN ANO

Fissure in ano, a vertical crack in the anal mucosa with associated spasm of the anal sphincter, can usually be suspected on history. Typically, the patient has noticed some pain on defecation, often following a period of constipation. A feeling of being 'split open' with the passage of hard stool is described. Following the passage of stool there may be a burning sensation for a few minutes followed by some relief, until the next attempt at defecation when there is recurrence of pain. It may be accompanied by a smear of blood on the toilet paper. Pain induces a fear of passing stool and some people may even resort to codeine compound analgesics, which hardens the stool even further. A vicious cycle is set up, with further constipation, hard stool and pain. In this way the fissure may become chronic.

Inspection of the perineum may reveal tightening of the corrugator cutis ani, an almost diagnostic sign of anospasm which is usually secondary to a fissure. If a small midline 'sentinel' pile is seen, the diagnosis is confirmed. Rectal examination and proctosigmoidoscopy should be deferred until acute pain has subsided.

Treatment is aimed at reducing pain and spasm around the acute fissure. This can be achieved by the use of local anaesthetic jelly, such as that usually used for the insertion of urinary catheters. This is most accurately applied by the patient, who knows where it hurts. Once pain is eased, a glycerine or Anusol suppository can be inserted. Combining

this treatment with stool softeners and a high-fibre diet brings resolution of symptoms over a few days. More recently, nitrate pastes, such as isosorbide dinitrate and nitroglycerin, have gained popularity.[8] Local application reduces anal pressure and improves anodermal blood flow. Twice-daily application of 0.25% glyceryl trinitrate ointment to the fissure may be successful in up to 88% of cases after 6 weeks. Injection with botulinum toxin A maybe even more effective.[9,10] Recurrence of symptoms after initial success withconservative treatment is not uncommon.[10]

Although most acute fissures can be dealt with conservatively as described, a small group do not respond and require surgical referral for sphincterotomy.

Anal fissure is sometimes complicated by abscess formation in the sentinel pile. This is suspected by a very swollen oedematous tag and will require surgical drainage. Anal fissure can also be associated with systemic illnesses such as Crohn's disease.

PRURITUS ANI

Persistent itchiness in the anal region can be a difficult condition to treat. It may be due to any generalized skin condition, such as eczema, psoriasis, scabies or pediculosis, or a more specific condition such as threadworm or pinworm. In most cases it is difficult to identify a specific cause. Occasionally pruritus ani is due to excessive attempts at hygiene, causing local irritation. Other generalized skin conditions or important local conditions to exclude are condylomata lata, condylomata acuminata, chancre, lymphoma, Kaposi's sarcoma and squamous cell carcinoma.

PROCTALGIA FUGAX

Proctalgia fugax is the sudden and unpredictable onset of shearing or knife-like pain in the anus and rectum. It is

usually of short duration and is most common in males. It is thought to be due to dysfunction of the internal anal sphincter.[12] Apart from reassurance no specific therapy is usually required. Salbutamol inhalation is recommended for severe episodes, but the mechanism of action is uncertain.[12]

INJURIES TO THE PERIANAL REGION

History is paramount and abuse needs to be excluded. Examination should focus on the function of the sphincter and be alert to the possibility of intra-abdominal extension of penetrating injuries.

REFERENCES

1. Sondenaa K, et al 1995 Patient characteristics and symptoms in chronic pilonidal sinus disease. International Journal of Colorectal Disease 10(1): 39–42
2. Clothier PR, Haywood IR 1984 The natural history of the post anal (pilonidal) sinus. Annals of the Royal College of Surgeons of England 66(3): 201–3
3. Jensen SL, Harling H 1988 Prognosis after simple incision and drainage for a first episode acute pilonidal abscess. British Journal of Surgery 75(1): 60–1
4. Armstrong JH, Barcia PJ 1994 Pilonidal sinus disease. The conservative approach. Archives of Surgery 129(9): 914–9
5. Tang CL, Chew SP, Seow-Choen F 1996 Prospective randomized trial of drainage alone vs. drainage and fistulotomy for acute perianal abscesses with proven internal opening. Diseases of the Colon and Rectum 139: 1415–7
6. Cataldo PA, Senagore A, Luchtefeld MA 1993 Intrarectal ultrasound in the evaluation of perirectal abscesses. Disease of the Colon and Rectum 36(6): 554–8
7. Janicke DM, Pundt MR Anorectal disorders. Emergency Clinics of North America 14(4): 757–88
8. Lund JN, Armitage NC, Schofield JH 1996 Use of glyceryl trinitrate ointment in the treatment of anal fissure. British Journal of Surgery 83(6): 776–7
9. Watson J, Kamm MA, Nicholls RJ, Phillips RK, et al 1996 Topical glyceryl trinate in the treatment of chronic anal fissure. British Journal of Surgery 83(6): 771–5
10. Hananel N, Gordon PH 1997 Reexamination of clinical manifestations and response to therapy of fissure in ano. Diseases of the Colon and Rectum 40(2): 229–33
11. Babb RR 1996 Proctalgia fugax, would you recognise it? Postgraduate Medicine 99(4): 263–4
12. Eckardt VF 1996 Treatment of proctalgia fugax with salbutamol inhalation. American Journal of Gastroenterology 91(4): 686–9

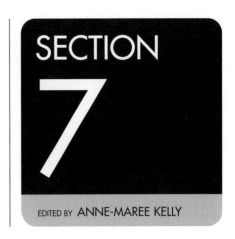

SECTION
7

EDITED BY ANNE-MAREE KELLY

NEUROLOGY

7.1 **Headache** 348

7.2 **Stroke and transient ischaemic attacks** 352

7.3 **Subarachnoid haemorrhage** 361

7.4 **Altered conscious state** 365

7.5 **Seizures** 371

7.1 HEADACHE

ANNE-MAREE KELLY

ESSENTIALS

1 The pathophysiological basis of headache is traction or inflammation of extracranial structures, the basal dura or the large intracranial arteries and veins, or dilatation/distension of cranial vascular structures.

2 Severity of headache is not a reliable indicator of the underlying pathology.

3 History is of paramount importance in the assessment of headache.

4 Sudden, severe headache or chronic, unremitting headache is more likely to have a serious cause and should be investigated accordingly.

5 NSAIDs are the most effective treatment for tension headache.

6 As most patients have tried oral medications prior to attending emergency departments, parenterally administered agents are usually indicated for emergency department treatment of migraine.

7 Typical characteristics of migraine are unilateral location, pulsating quality, moderate or severe intensity, aggravation by routine physical activity and association with nausea, photophobia and phonophobia. An aura (neurological symptoms localizable to the cerebral cortex or brain stem) may precede the headache.

8 Based on current evidence, the most effective agents for treating migraine are sumatriptan and chlorpromazine. Pethidine is not indicated because it is less effective than other agents, has a high rebound headache rate, and carries the potential for the development of dependence.

INTRODUCTION

Headache is a common ailment that is often due to a combination of physical and psychological causative factors. The vast majority are benign and self-limiting and are managed by patients in the community. Only a very small proportion of patients experiencing headache attend emergency departments for treatment. The challenges for emergency physicians are to distinguish potentially life-threatening causes from the more benign, and to effectively manage the pain of headache.

PATHOPHYSIOLOGY

The structures in the head capable of producing headache are limited. They include:

- Extracranial structures, including skin and mucosae, blood vessels, nerves, muscles and fascial planes.
- The main arteries at the base of the skull (as arteries branch they progressively lose the ability to produce painful stimuli).
- The great venous sinuses and their branches.
- The basal dura and dural arteries, but to a lesser extent than the other structures.

The bulk of the intracranial contents, including the parenchyma of the brain, the subarachnoid and pia mater and most of the dura mater, are incapable of producing painful stimuli.

The pathological processes that may cause headache are:

- Tension. This usually refers to contraction of muscles of the head and/or neck, and is thought to be the major factor in the so-called 'tension headache'.
- Traction. Traction is caused by stretching of intracranial structures from a mass effect, as with a tumour. Pain caused by this mechanism is characteristically constant, but may vary in severity.
- Vascular processes. These include dilatation or distension of vascular structures, and usually result in pain that is throbbing in nature.
- Inflammation. This may involve the dura at the base of the skull or the nerves or soft tissues of the head and neck. This mechanism is responsible for the initial pain of subarachnoid haemorrhage and meningitis, and for sinusitis.

The pathophysiological causes of headache are summarized in Table 7.1.1.

Table 7.1.1 A pathophysiological classification of headache		
	Extracranial	*Intracranial*
Tension/traction	Muscular headache 'Tension headache'	Intracranial tumour Cerebral abscess Intracranial haematoma
Vascular	Migraine	Severe hypertension
Inflammatory	Temporal arteritis Sinusitis Otitis media/mastoiditis Tooth abscess Neuralgia	Meningitis Subarachnoid haemorrhage

ASSESSMENT

In the assessment of a patient with headache, history is of prime importance. Specific information should be sought about the timing of the headache (in terms of both overall duration and speed of onset), the site and quality of the pain, relieving factors, the presence of associated features such as nausea and vomiting, photophobia and alteration in mental state, medical and occupational history and drug use.

Intensity of the pain is important from the viewpoint of management but is not a reliable indicator of the nature of underlying pathology. This said, sudden, severe headache and chronic, unremitting or progressive headache are more likely to have a serious cause.

Physical examination should include temperature, pulse rate and blood pressure measurements, assessment of conscious state and neck stiffness, and neurological examination, including fundoscopy. Abnormal physical signs are uncommon, but the presence of neurological findings makes a serious cause probable. In addition, a search for sinus, ear, mouth and neck pathology and muscular or superficial artery tenderness should be made.

Headache patterns

Some headaches have 'classic' clinical features: these are listed in Table 7.1.2. It must be remembered that, as with all disease, there is a spectrum of presenting features and the absence of the classic features does not rule out a particular diagnosis. Every patient must be assessed on their merits and, if symptoms persist without reasonable explanation, further investigation should be undertaken.

INVESTIGATION

For the vast majority of patients with headache no investigation is required. The investigation of suspected subarachnoid haemorrhage and meningitis is discussed elsewhere in this book. If tumour is suspected, the investigations of choice are magentic resonance imaging (MRI) or a contrast computerized tomo-graphy (CT) scan. An elevated ESR may be supporting evidence for a diagnosis of temporal arteritis. With respect to sinusitis, facial X-rays are of very limited value.

TENSION HEADACHE

The pathological basis of tension headaches remains unclear, however, increased muscular tension of the neck or cranial muscles is a prominent feature. A family history of headaches is common and there is an association with an injury in childhood or adolescence. The most common precipitants are stress and alteration in sleep patterns.

Aspirin, non-steroidal anti-inflammatory agents and paracetamol have all been shown to be effective in the treatment of tension headaches with success rates between 50–70%. Ibuprofen 400 mg or ketoprofen 25–50 mg appear to be the most effective, followed by aspirin 600–1000 mg and paracetamol 1000 mg.

MIGRAINE

INTRODUCTION

Migraine can be a disabling condition for the sufferer. Most migraine headaches are successfully managed by the patient and their general practitioner, but a small number fail to respond or become 'fixed', and sufferers may present for treatment at emergency departments. As most patients have tried oral medications

Table 7.1.2 Classic clinical complexes and cause of headache

Preceded by an aura Throbbing unilateral headache, nausea Family history	Migraine
Sudden onset Severe occipital headache; 'like a blow' Worst headache ever	Subarachnoid haemorrhage
Throbbing/constant frontal headache Worse with cough, leaning forward Recent URTI Pain on percussion of sinuses	Sinusitis
Paroxysmal, fleeting pain Distribution of a nerve Trigger manoeuvres cause pain Hyperalgesia of nerve distribution	Neuralgia
Unilateral with superimposed stabbing Claudication on chewing Associated malaise, myalgia Tender artery with reduced pulsation	Temporal arteritis
Persistent, deep-seated headache Increasing duration and intensity Worse in morning Aching in character	Tumour: primary or secondary
Acute, generalized headache Fever, nausea and vomiting Altered level of consciousness Neck stiffness +/− rash	Meningitis
Unilateral, aching, related to eye Nausea and vomiting Raised intraocular pressure	Glaucoma
Aching, facial region Worse at night Tooth sensitive to heat, pressure	Dental cause

prior to attending, parenterally administered agents are usually indicated for emergency department treatment.

Migraine is a clinical diagnosis and, in the emergency department setting, a diagnosis of exclusion. Other causes of severe headache, such as subarachnoid haemorrhage and meningitis, must be ruled out before this diagnosis is made. In particular, the response of the headache to antimigraine therapy should not be used to assume that the cause was migraine. There have been reports that the headaches associated with subarachnoid haemorrhage and meningitis have, on occasion, responded to these agents.

PATHOPHYSIOLOGY

The pathophysiology of migraine is complex and not completely understood. It is probably the result of interaction between the brain and the cranial circulation in susceptible individuals.

The phenomenon of 'cortical spreading depression' is probably the event underlying the occurrence of an aura in migraine. This is a short-lasting depolarization wave that moves across the cerebral cortex. A brief phase of excitation is followed by prolonged depression of nerve cells. At the same time there is failure of brain ion homeostasis, an efflux of excitatory amino acids from nerve cells, and increased energy metabolism. This phenomenon appears to be dependent on the activation of an N-methyl-D-aspartate receptor, which is a subtype of the glutamate receptor.

The headache pain of migraine seems to result from the activation of the trigeminovascular system. The trigeminal nerve transmits headache pain from both the dura and the pia mater. The triggers for the development of migraine headache are probably chemical and are thought to originate in the brain, blood vessel walls and the blood itself. These triggers stimulate trigeminovascular axons, causing pain and the release of vasoactive neuropeptides from perivascular axons. These neuropeptides act on mast cells, endothelial cells and platelets, resulting in increased extracellular levels of arachi-

donate metabolites, amines, peptides and ions. These mediators and the resultant tissue injury lead to a prolongation of pain and hyperalgesia.

Serotonin has been specifically implicated in migraine. By activation of afferents, it causes a retrograde release of substance P. This, in turn, increases capillary permeability and oedema.

CLASSIFICATION AND CLINICAL FEATURES

Migraine is defined as an idiopathic recurring headache disorder with attacks that last 4–72 hours. Typical characteristics are unilateral location, pulsating quality, moderate or severe intensity, and aggravation by routine physical activity. There is also usually nausea, photophobia and phonophobia.

In some patients migraine is preceded by an 'aura' of neurological symptoms localizable to the cerebral cortex or brain stem, such as visual disturbance, paraesthesia, diplopia or limb weakness. These develop gradually over 5–20 minutes and last less than 60 minutes. Headache, nausea and/or photophobia usually follow after an interval of less than an hour. The headache usually lasts less than 72 hours.

Several variant forms of migraine have been defined, including ophthalmoplegic, abdominal and retinal migraine, but all are uncommon. In ophthalmoplegic migraine the headache is associated with paralysis of one or more of the nerves supplying the ocular muscles. Horner syndrome may also occur. Abdominal migraine manifests as recurrent episodes of abdominal pain for which no other cause is found. Retinal migraine, which is fortunately very rare, involves recurrent attacks of retinal ischaemia, which may lead to bilateral optic atrophy.

TREATMENT

The complexity of the mechanisms involved in the genesis of migraine suggests that there are a number of ways

to interrupt the processes to provide effective relief from symptoms.

A number of pharmacological agents and combinations of agents for the relief of migraine have been studied, with varying results. A review of the published literature[1] reached the following conclusions:

Ketorolac and lidocaine fail to reach acceptable effectiveness and, as such, are not recommended for use in acute migraine. Metoclopramide and pethidine perform a little better, but each has been shown to be inferior to other treatments. The potential for dependence and abuse must also be considered with pethidine. The data on dihydroergotamine are difficult to interpret because it is often used in combination with other agents, e.g. metoclopramide; however, it has also been shown to be less effective than chlorpromazine and sumatriptan in acute treatment, and to have a high rate of unpleasant side effects. Prochlorperazine and haloperidol have both been reported to be highly effective,[2,3] but numbers in these studies were small and further studies are needed to determine their performance in comparison to other agents.

Recently, there have been several small studies of other agents. Civamide, a vanilloid receptor agonist and neuronal calcium channel blocker that inhibits the neuronal release of excitatory neurotransmitters, showed moderate efficacy[4] as did intravenous valproate sodium (300 mg).[5] The efficacy of intravenous magnesium sulphate (1 or 2 mg) remains unclear. It has been shown in a small placebo-controlled trail to be effective,[6] however, in another study the combination of magnesium with metoclopramide was less effective than metoclopramide and placebo.[7] Intramuscular droperidol 2.5 mg has been shown to be moderately effective, but with a 13% rate of akasthisia.[8] Further research would be required before these agents could be recommended.

At present the most effective agents seem to be chlorpromazine and the triptans, each of which has achieved greater than 70% efficacy in a number of studies.[9-13]

Chlorpromazine

The mechanism by which chlorpromazine acts in migraine is uncertain. It is possibly the result of a combination of actions: anti-5HT effect, antidopamine effect in the chemoreceptor trigger zone, vascular effects via its α-blocking action, and modulation of serotonin receptors.

The usual dosing regimen is 12.5 mg intravenously, repeated every 20 minutes as needed to a maximum dose of 37.5 mg. Because of the significant incidence of postural hypotension associated with this treatment, an infusion of 1 litre of normal saline over 1 hour is strongly recommended. Side effects include postural hypotension and dystonic reaction, which is idiosyncratic but rare.

Sumatriptan

Sumatriptan is a specific and selective serotonin (subtype 1D) agonist that has no effect on other serotonin receptor subtypes. The antimigraine effect of sumatriptan is thought to be due to its effect on the 5HT subtype 1D receptors in cranial blood vessels. It blocks neurogenic inflammation by acting at prejunctional serotonin receptors on trigeminovascular fibres.

Sumatriptan may be administered intranasally, orally or by subcutaneous injection. The recommended dose is 6 mg subcutaneously, 20 mg intranasally or 50 mg orally. Clinical response begins within 10–15 minutes of subcutaneous injection and within 30 minutes of oral administration. Adverse effects include drowsiness, weakness, dizziness, flushing,

rash, pruritus, elevation of blood pressure, chest pain or chest tightness. Sumatriptan is contraindicated in patients with a history of ischaemic heart disease, uncontrolled hypertension or the concomitant use of ergot preparations. There are also a significant number of non-responders (up to 18%),[14] for which no clinical, pharmacokinetic or genetic explanation has been found.

A range of 'triptan' agents are now available (including rizatriptan, zolmitripan and eletriptan). Efficacy seems to be similar but some (e.g. naratriptan) report less reduction in coronary blood flow.

The choice between chlorpromazine and the triptans will depend on issues of cost, convenience and resource utilization.

CONTROVERSIES

❶ Choice of drug therapy.

❷ Role and timing of investigations in atypical migraine. CT or MRI may be indicated acutely to rule out other intracranial pathology.

❸ Role and timing of investigations, in particular neuroimaging, for persistent or atypical headache.

REFERENCES

1. Kelly AM, Bryant M, Zebic S 1995 The emergency department management of migraine. Emergency Medicine 7: 162
2. Jones J, Sklar D, Dougherty J, White W 1989 Randomized double-blind trial of intravenous prochlorperazine for the treatment of acute headache. Journal of the American Medical Association 261: 1174–6
3. Fisher H 1995 A new approach to emergency department therapy of migraine headache with intravenous haloperidol: a case series. Journal of Emergency Medicine 13: 119–22
4. Diamond S, Freitag F, Phillips SB, Bernstein JE, Saper JR. 2000 Intranasal civamide for the acute treatment of migraine headache. Cephalalgia 20: 597-602
5. Mathew NT, Kailasam J, Maedors L, Chernyschev O, Gentry P 2000 Intravenous valporate sodium (depacon) aborts migraine rapidly: a preliminary report. Headache 40: 720–3
6. Demirkaya S, Vural O, Dora B, Topcuoglu MA 2001 Efficacy of intravenous magnesium sulphate in the treatmnent of acute migraine attacks. Headache 41: 171–7
7. Corbo J, Esses D, Bijur PE, Iannaccone R, Gallagher EJ 2001 Randomised clinical trial of intravenous magnesium sulphate as an adjunctive medication in the emergency department treatment of migraine. Annals of Emergency Medicine 38: 621–7
8. Richman PB, Allegra J, Eskin B, Doran J, Reischel U, Kaiafas C, Nashed AH 2002 A randomised clinical trial to assess the efficacy of intramusculalr droperidol for the treatment of acute migraine headache. American Journal of Emergency Medicine 20: 39–42
9. Bell R, Montoya D, Shuaib A, Lee MA 1990 A comparative trial of three agents in the treatment of acute migraine headache. Annals of Emergency Medicine 19: 1079–82
10. Cady RK, Wendt JK, Kirchner JR, Sargent JD, Rothrock JF, Skaggs H Jr 1991 Treatment of acute migraine with subcutaneous sumatriptan. Journal of the American Medical Association 265: 2831–5
11. McEwen JI, O'Connor HM, Dinsdale HB 1987 Treatment of migraine with intramuscular chlorpromazine. Annals of Emergency Medicine 16: 758–63
12. The Subcutaneous Sumatriptan International Study Group 1991 Treatment of migraine attacks with sumatriptan. New England Journal of Medicine 325: 316–21
13. Akpunonu BE, Mutgi AB, Federman DJ, et al 1995 Subcutaneous sumatriptan for the treatment of acute migraine in patients admitted to the emergency department. Annals of Emergency Medicine 25: 464–9
14. Moschiano F, D'Amico D, Grazzi L, Leone M, Bussone G 1997 Sumatriptan in the acute treatment of migraine without aura: efficacy of 50 mg dose. Headache 37: 421–3

7.2 STROKE AND TRANSIENT ISCHAEMIC ATTACKS

PHILIP APLIN

ESSENTIALS

1 Ischaemic strokes and transient ischaemic attacks (TIAs) are most commonly due to atherosclerotic thromboembolism from the cerebral vasculature or emboli from the heart. Other causes should be considered in younger patients, those presenting with atypical features, or when evaluation is negative for the more common aetiologies.

2 Haemorrhagic and ischaemic strokes cannot be reliably differentiated on clinical grounds alone, therefore, computerized tomography (CT) scanning is required prior to the commencement of anticoagulant or thrombolytic therapy.

3 A carotid bruit in a patient with an ipsilateral ischaemic event may predict a moderate-to-severe internal carotid artery stenosis. On the other hand, the absence of a bruit in such patients does not exclude a significant underlying stenotic lesion.

4 Differentiating strokes from other acute neurological presentations may be difficult in the emergency department. This issue has implications for the use of high-risk therapies in the emergency department, such as thrombolysis.

5 The early phase of stroke management concentrates on airway and breathing, rapid neurological assessment of conscious level, pupil size and lateralizing signs, and blood sugar measurement. Hyperglycaemia may worsen neurological outcome in stroke, and so glucose should not be given in likely stroke patients unless a low blood sugar level is objectively demonstrated.

6 TIAs and non-disabling strokes should be evaluated in a similar way to detect an underlying treatable cause that may lead to a subsequent major stroke.

7 Echocardiography is not a high-priority investigation in a patient with a TIA or non-disabling stroke in the absence of cardiac disease on clinical evaluation and a normal ECG.

INTRODUCTION

Cerebrovascular disease is the third largest cause of death in developed countries, after heart disease and cancer. A stroke is an acute neurological injury secondary to cerebrovascular disease, either by infarction (80%) or by haemorrhage (20%). The incidence of stroke is steady, and, although mortality is decreasing, it is still a leading cause of long-term disability. Transient ischaemic attacks (TIAs) are defined as a focal loss of brain function attributed to cerebral ischaemia that lasts less than 24 hours, although most last less than 1 hour. Causes are similar to those of ischaemic stroke, particularly atherosclerotic thromboembolism related to the carotid and cerebral artery circulation, and cardioembolism. Diagnosis of the cause with appropriate management is important in order to prevent stroke.

PATHOPHYSIOLOGY

Brain tissue is very sensitive to the effects of oxygen deprivation. The effect of occlusion of any part of the cerebral vasculature depends on the vessel involved, the collateral blood supply and the duration of occlusion. Modification of the ischaemic injury to potentially salvage tissue surrounding the infarcted area of the brain following acute vascular occlusion is the subject of intensive research. These studies focus on improving blood supply to the ischaemic area using thrombolytic, anticoagulant and antiplatelet agents, or amelioration of the metabolic effects of ischaemia and reperfusion through glutamate receptor antagonists, calcium channel blockers and antioxidants.

Ischaemic strokes

These are the result of several possible pathological processes (Table 7.2.1).

- Most commonly due to thromboembolism originating from the cerebral vasculature, the heart, or occasionally the aorta. Thrombosis usually occurs at the site of an atherosclerotic plaque secondary to a combination of shear-induced injury on the vessel wall, turbulence and flow obstruction. It may also be the site of emboli that dislodge and subsequently occlude more distal parts of the cerebral circulation. Atherosclerotic plaques develop at sites of vessel bifurcation. Lesions affecting the origin of the internal carotid artery (ICA) are the most important source of thromboembolic events. The more distal intracerebral branches of the ICA and vertebrobasilar system are also significant sites.

- Approximately 20% of cerebrovascular events are due to emboli originating from the heart. Rarely, emboli may arise from peripheral circulation, the latter being carried to the cerebral circulation via a patent foramen ovale.

Table 7.2.1 Causes of stroke

Ischaemic stroke
Arterial thromboembolism
  Carotid and vertebral artery atheroma
  Intracranial vessel atheroma
  Small vessel disease – lacunar infarction
  Haematological disorders –
  hypercoagulable states

Cardioembolism
  Aortic and mitral valve disease
  Atrial fibrillation
  Mural thrombus
  Atrial myxoma
  Paradoxical emboli

Hypoperfusion
  Severe vascular stenosis } or a
  Hypotension   combination
  Vasoconstriction – drug   of these factors
  induced, post SAH,
  pre-eclampsia

Other vascular disorders
  Arterial dissection
  Gas embolism syndromes
  Moyamoya disease
  Arteritis

Intracerebral haemorrhage
Hypertensive vascular disease –
Lipohyalinosis and microaneurysms

Aneurysms
  Saccular
  Mycotic

Arteriovenous malformations

Amyloid angiopathy

Bleeding diathesis
  Anticoagulation
  Thrombolytics
  Thrombocytopenia/disseminated
  Intravascular coagulation
  Haemophilia

Secondary haemorrhage into a lesion –
tumour or infarction

- Hypertension-induced lipohyalinosis and microatheroma affecting the small penetrating vessels of the brain are the postulated causes of lacunar infarcts.
- Haemodynamic reduction in cerebral blood flow may occur as a result of systemic hypotension or severe carotid stenosis. In these cases cerebral infarction typically occurs in a vascular watershed area.
- Vasoconstriction, as seen in subarachnoid haemorrhage (SAH), migraine and pre-eclampsia, and with drugs such as sympathomimetics and cocaine.
- Less common vascular disorders such as arterial dissection, arteritis, venous

thrombosis, sickle cell disease and moyamoya disease.

Haemorrhagic stroke

This is the result of vessel rupture into the surrounding intracerebral tissue or subarachnoid space. Subarachnoid haemorrhage is the subject of a separate chapter in this book. The neurologic defect associated with an intracerebral haemorrhage may be the effect of direct brain injury, secondary occlusion of nearby vessels, and reduced cerebral perfusion caused by associated raised intracranial pressure and cerebral herniation.

The causes of intracerebral haemorrhage (ICH) include:

- Aneurysmal vessel dilatation. Vascular dilatation occurs at a site of weakness in the arterial wall, resulting in an aneurysm that expands until it ruptures into the subarachnoid space and, in some cases, the brain tissue as well.
- Arteriovenous malformation (AVM). A collection of weakened vessels exists as a result of abnormal development of the arteriovenous connections. AVMs may rupture to cause haemorrhagic stroke or, more rarely, cerebral ischaemia from steal.
- Hypertensive vascular disease. Lipohyalinosis may be the underlying cause of microaneurysms of small penetrating vessels, which rupture, causing haemorrhage in characteristic locations: in the putamen, thalamus, upper brain stem and cerebellum.
- Amyloid angiopathy. Postmortem pathologic examination has found these changes, principally in elderly patients with lobar haemorrhages.
- Haemorrhage into an underlying lesion, e.g. tumour or infarction.
- Drug toxicity from sympathomimetics and cocaine.
- Anticoagulation and bleeding diatheses.

RISK FACTORS FOR STROKE/TIA

Non-modifiable risks

These include:

- Increasing age: stroke rate more than doubles for each 10 years above age 55
- Gender: male slightly more common than female
- Family history.

Modifiable risks

Hypertension is the most important modifiable risk factor. The efficacy of anti-hypertensive treatment in stroke reduction has been well shown.[2] The other major risk factors for atherosclerosis and its complications – diabetes, smoking and hypercholesterolaemia – also contribute to increased stroke risk.

Atrial fibrillation, both chronic and paroxysmal, is the most important cardiac risk factor. Warfarin is recommended to prevent cardioembolism except in patients under 75 years with no history of hypertension, diabetes, TIA or stroke, and with a normal echocardiogram, and in those with a contraindication to warfarin. These patients should initially receive aspirin.

Other major cardiac risk factors include endocarditis, mitral stenosis, prosthetic heart valves, recent myocardial infarction and left ventricular aneurysm. Less common factors include complicated mitral valve prolapse (i.e. with associated atrial fibrillation or endocarditis), atrial myxoma, a patent foramen ovale and atrial septal aneurysm.

Procedures such as cardiac catheterization and cardiac surgery increase the stroke risk.

A carotid bruit or carotid stenosis found in an otherwise asymptomatic patient is associated with an increased stroke risk. However, the role of carotid endarterectomy in these patients is very controversial. In a highly selected patient group, the Asymptomatic Carotid Atherosclerosis Study (ACAS)[1] showed a small but significant benefit in reduction of stroke or death at 5 years following surgery for angiographically proven carotid stenoses >60%, compared to medical therapy. This benefit was much lower than that achieved in symptomatic carotid stenoses >70% shown in the North American Symptomatic Carotid Endarterectomy Study (NASCET)[2] study and can only be achieved with extremely low perioperative mortality and stroke rates.

ISCHAEMIC STROKE SYNDROMES

The symptoms and signs of stroke or TIA obviously correspond to the area of the brain affected by ischaemia or haemorrhage (Table 7.2.2).

In ischaemic brain injury the history and pattern of physical signs may correspond to a characteristic clinical syndrome according to the underlying cause and the vessel occluded. This has an important bearing on the direction of further investigation and treatment decisions. Differentiating between anterior and posterior circulation ischaemia/infarction is important in this respect, but is not always possible on clinical grounds alone. Determining the cause of the event is the next step. Once again, clues may be present on clinical evaluation. For accurate delineation of the site of the lesion, exclusion of haemorrhage and assessment of the underlying cause it is usually necessary to undertake imaging studies.

Anterior circulation ischaemia

The anterior circulation supplies blood to 80% of the brain and consists of the ICA and its branches, principally the ophthalmic, middle cerebral and anterior cerebral arteries. Hence this system supplies the optic nerve, retina, frontoparietal and most of the temporal lobes. Ischaemic injury involving the anterior cerebral circulation commonly has its origin in atherothrombotic disease of the internal carotid artery. Atherosclerosis of this artery usually affects the proximal 2 cm, just distal to the division of the common carotid. Advanced lesions may be the source of embolism to other parts of the anterior circulation, or cause severe stenosis and subsequent hypoperfusion distally if there is inadequate collateral supply via the Circle of Willis. This is usually manifested by signs and symptoms in the middle cerebral artery (MCA) territory. Less commonly, stenosing lesions of the intracranial ICA and MCA cause similar clinical features.

Embolism to the ophthalmic artery or its branches causes monocular visual symptoms of blurring, loss of vision and field defects that, when transient, are referred to as amaurosis fugax, or transient monocular blindness.

Symptoms and signs of MCA involvement include homonymous hemianopia or quadrantanopsia, with more distal branch occlusion. Contralateral motor and cortical sensory changes affect the face and hands more than the legs. Higher brain dysfunction can be a feature. Dominant parietal hemispheric lesions may cause disturbances of speech (dysphasia), writing (agraphia), calculation (acalculia), left–right orientation and finger recognition (agnosia), the latter four characterizing Gerstman syndrome. Non-dominant parietal lobe lesions are manifested by unilateral spatial neglect (left-sided in 90%) and constructional and dressing difficulties (dyspraxias).

The anterior cerebral artery is least commonly affected because of its collateral supply via the anterior communicating artery. If embolism occurs distally, or the collateral supply is inadequate, then ischaemic injury may occur. This characteristically gives rise to sensory and motor changes, in the leg more so than the arm. More subtle changes of personality may occur with frontal lobe lesions, as may disturbances of micturition and conjugate gaze.

Major alterations of consciousness, as in coma or with Glasgow Coma Scores of less than 8, imply bilateral hemispheric or brain-stem dysfunction. The brain stem may be primarily involved by a stroke or secondarily affected due to compression by supra- or infratentorial ischaemic or haemorrhagic lesions.

Posterior circulation ischaemia

Ischaemic injury in the posterior circulation involves the vertebrobasilar arteries and their major branches, which supply the cerebellum, brain stem, thalamus,

Table 7.2.2 Location of TIA

Symptom	Carotid	Arterial territory Either	Vertebrobasilar
Dysphasia	+		
Monocular visual loss	+		
Unilateral weakness*		+	
Unilateral sensory disturbance*		+	
Dysarthria+		+	
Homonymous hemianopia		+	
Dysphagia+		+	
Diplopia+			+
Vertigo+			+
Bilateral simultaneous visual loss			+
Bilateral simultaneous weakness			+
Bilateral simultaneous sensory disturbance			+
Crossed sensory/motor loss			+

*Usually regarded as carotid distribution; +Not necessarily a transient ischemic attack if an isolated symptom. (Reproduced with permission from Hankey GJ 2001 Management of first time transient ischaemic attack. Emergency Medicine 13: 70–81)

medial temporal and occipital lobes. Posterior cerebral artery occlusion is manifested by visual changes of homonymous hemianopia, typically with macular sparing if the MCA supplies this part of the occipital cortex. Cortical blindness, of which the patient may be unaware, occurs with bilateral posterior cerebral artery infarction.

Brain-stem and cerebellar involvement manifests as a combination of motor and sensory abnormalities, which may be uni- or bilateral, cerebellar signs of ataxia, vertigo and nystagmus and gaze and cranial nerve palsies, producing dysarthria, diplopia and vertigo. Ipsilateral cranial nerve/cerebellar signs with crossed long tract signs are the classic presentation of a brain-stem stroke. Major alterations in consciousness occur with involvement of the reticular activating system (RAS) in the pons or upper midbrain due to primary ischaemic injury, or from secondary compression by posterior fossa or herniating supratentorial lesions. The locked-in syndrome, in which the patient is unable to move the limbs but has retained consciousness and is only able to look up, may be caused by a stroke affecting the ventral pontine motor tracts.

Lacunar infarction
Lacunar infarcts are primarily associated with hypertension and diabetes. They occur in small penetrating arteries affecting the internal capsule, thalamus and upper brain stem. Isolated motor or sensory deficits are most commonly seen.

INTRACEREBRAL HAEMORRHAGE

Intracerebral haemorrhage (ICH) is most commonly associated with hypertension, with haemorrhage characteristically affecting the internal capsule, thalamus, pons and cerebellum. However, the basic differentiation between an ischaemic and a haemorrhagic stroke cannot be reliably made on clinical grounds alone. A history of prolonged hypertension is usual in hypertensive

ICH. Other clues to a haemorrhagic cause include sudden onset in the awake state, associated headaches, vomiting and collapse, and a history of anticoagulant use or a bleeding diathesis. Hypertension is often present and rapid progression to coma may ensue as a result of brain-stem compression by herniating supratentorial contents or a posterior fossa mass. Pontine haemorrhage will cause deep coma and quadriplegia from the outset. Amyloid angiopathy is an increasingly recognized cause of ICH, particularly of lobar haemorrhages in the elderly. Other causes of ICH include rupture of a Circle of Willis aneurysm into brain substance, AVMs, and haemorrhage into a tumour. Ischaemic strokes may undergo haemorrhagic transformation either spontaneously or subsequent to the administration of anticoagulant and thrombolytic therapy, often with associated clinical deterioration.

HISTORY

This includes particularly the circumstances, time course and progression of signs and symptoms. The possibility of trauma or drug abuse should be remembered, along with past medical, family and medication history to look for risk factors for cardio/cerebrovascular disease, cardiac embolism and increased bleeding risk. A past history of similar events should be carefully sought. In young patients with an acute neurologic deficit, dissection of the carotid or vertebral arteries should be considered. This is often associated with neck pain and headache/retro- orbital pain and a history of neck trauma, which can be minor, as in a twisting or hyperextension/flexion injury sustained in a motor accident or playing contact sports.

Cardioembolism tends to produce ischaemic injury in different parts of the brain, resulting in non-stereotypic recurrent TIAs, whereas atherothrombotic disease of the cerebral vessels may cause recurrent TIAs of similar nature, particularly in stenosing lesions of the internal carotid or vertebrobasilar arteries.

EXAMINATION
Central nervous system
This includes assessing the level of consciousness, pupil size and reactivity, extent of the neurologic deficit, presence of neck stiffness, and fundoscopy for signs of papilloedema and retinal haemorrhage. The gag reflex should be assessed both as part of the neurologic assessment and for aspiration risk.

All signs may have resolved in the case of TIAs. The average TIA lasts less than 15 minutes.

Cardiovascular examination
This includes carotid auscultation and is directed toward findings that are associated with a cardioembolic source. An ECG is part of this assessment. A carotid bruit in a symptomatic patient may predict a moderate-to-severe carotid stenosis. Conversely, the absence of a carotid bruit does not exclude carotid artery disease as the cause of a TIA or stroke.

Major risk factors for cardioembolism that can be identified in the emergency department include atrial fibrillation, mitral stenosis, prosthetic heart valves, infective endocarditis, recent myocardial infarction, left ventricular aneurysm and cardiomyopathies.

UNCOMMON CAUSES OF STROKE AND TIA

There are many uncommon causes of stroke and TIAs. Those that should be considered in the emergency department evaluation include arterial dissection, antiphospholipid antibody syndrome, hypercoagulable states, gas embolism syndromes and vasculitis.

DIFFERENTIAL DIAGNOSIS (Table 7.2.3)

The acute onset of stroke and TIA is characteristic; however, misdiagnosis is common in the emergency department, even by experienced clinicians.[3] The

Table 7.2.3 Differential diagnosis of stroke

Intracranial space-occupying lesion
Subdural haematoma
Brain tumour
Brain abscess
Postictal neurological deficit – Todd's paresis
Head injury
Encephalitis
Metabolic or drug-induced encephalopathy
Hypoglycaemia, hyponatraemia etc.
Wernicke–Korsakoff syndrome
Drug toxicity
Hypertensive encephalopathy
Multiple sclerosis
Migraine
Peripheral nerve lesions
Functional

most common include seizures, systemic infection, brain tumour and toxic-metabolic. Others include subdural haematoma, encephalitis, multiple sclerosis, migraine and conversion disorder. This has implications when considering more aggressive stroke interventions, such as thrombolysis.

COMPLICATIONS OF STROKE

CNS complications include cerebral oedema and raised intracranial pressure (ICP). This is rarely an acute problem in the first 24 hours following ischaemic stroke, compared to ICH, where acutely raised ICP may lead to herniation and brain-stem compression in the first few hours. Haemorrhagic transformation may occur either spontaneously or associated with treatment. Seizures can also occur and should be treated in the standard way. Seizure prophylaxis is not generally recommended.

Non-CNS complications include aspiration/pneumonia, hypoventilation, deep vein thrombosis and pulmonary embolism, urinary tract infections and pressure ulcers.

INVESTIGATIONS

Standard investigations that may identify contributing factors to stroke/TIA or guide therapy include a complete blood picture, ESR, blood glucose, coagulation profile, electrolytes and liver function tests. Oxygen saturation should be monitored and arterial blood gases performed if the adequacy of ventilation is in doubt. An ECG should be performed to identify dysrhythmias and signs of pre-existing cardiac disease.

Further investigation depends on the nature of the neurological deficit and other risk factors for stroke identified in the prior evaluation, but usually involves a combination of brain and vascular imaging.

Imaging in TIAs

TIAs and non-disabling strokes should be evaluated similarly in order to promptly diagnose and manage a potentially treatable process that may lead to a subsequent major stroke. This should be done expeditiously and may require hospital admission. Certain patients are at increased risk of stroke, such as those with multiple frequent TIAs and hemispheric TIAs, each of which may indicate underlying severe carotid stenosis. Also those with a probable or proven cardioembolic source should be considered high risk.

Imaging vessels

Ultrasound If the aetiology of a TIA is likely to be carotid disease, e.g. a history of amaurosis fugax or hemispheric TIAs, with or without a carotid bruit, then a carotid duplex ultrasound is the initial investigation of choice to investigate the presence and degree of carotid stenosis if the patient would be suitable for surgery if severe carotid stenosis was demonstrated. In some cases it is difficult or impossible to determine clinically whether the aetiology of the event is due to carotid or vertebrobasilar disease. In these cases a carotid ultrasound is also indicated.

Magnetic resonance imaging (MRI) and magnetic resonance angiography (MRA) provide non-invasive imaging of the brain and major cerebral vasculature. MRA can show features suggestive of a vascular aetiology for TIAs, such as absence of the normal flow void in the ICA and vertebrobasilar arteries, or vascular ectasia, stenosis, dissection and venous thrombosis. MRI/MRA is not routine in TIA work-up but may be indicated in patients in whom an uncommon cause is suspected, or there is absence of a more obvious cause and in young patients.

Angiography Formal angiography is reserved for cases where the carotid ultrasound reveals a stenosis of >50%. If angiography or MRA demonstrates >70% stenosis, the findings of the NASCET study suggest that this group should be considered for endarterectomy. It should also be done to confirm or exclude complete carotid occlusion shown on ultrasound. Angiography and MRI/MRA may be performed to detect intracranial carotid disease or vertebrobasilar disease, although surgical options in such cases are controversial, difficult, and generally reserved for patients with failed medical therapy.

Cardiac imaging

If the clinical evaluation indicates that a cardioembolic source is the most likely cause of TIA, such as a patient with atrial fibrillation or a recent myocardial infarction, then echocardiography is a priority. However, if there is no evidence of cardiac disease on clinical evaluation and the ECG is normal, then echocardiography should be reserved for patients in whom no other cause can be found by other investigations. A transthoracic echocardiogram (TTE) is the first-line investigation in cardiac imaging. A trans-oesophageal echocardiogram (TOE) is more sensitive in detecting potential cardiac sources of emboli, such as mitral valve vegetations, atrial thrombi, and mural thrombi than the transthoracic approach, and should be considered in patients with a likely cardioembolic source on clinical grounds but inconclusive or normal transthoracic echo, and in patients with persistent diagnostic uncertainty with a normal TTE. This particularly applies to patients under 45 years with no history of cardiac disease and unexplained TIAs, or non-disabling stroke in order to detect causes such as atrial myxoma, patent foramen ovale, which may transmit a paradoxical embolus, and atheromatous plaque affecting the aortic arch.

Brain imaging

A non-contrast CT scan is indicated in most patients with a TIA to exclude lesions that occasionally mimic TIAs, such as subdural haematoma and brain tumours. CT may also show areas of infarction which match the symptoms of a TIA that have completely resolved. It is less reliable in showing posterior territory ischaemic events than MRI, particularly in the brain stem. CT, to exclude haemorrhage, is recommended to precede full anticoagulation, such as in the setting of multiple, frequent or cardioembolic TIAs.

Imaging in stroke

Brain imaging

CT In the setting of completed stroke the principal investigation is the non-contrast CT scan. Clinical evaluation cannot reliably exclude ICH. A current-generation CT scanner is extremely sensitive in detecting ICH at onset and will detect up to 90–95% of SAH in the first 2 days post bleed. The scan is often normal in the first hours following ischaemic stroke. In 60% of cases there will be changes at 24 hours and in 100% at a week. The earliest sign of ischaemic stroke is loss of the cortical grey/white matter distinction in the affected arterial distribution. Early signs of cerebral oedema, such as effacement of the cortical sulci or compression of the ventricular system, are indicative of large infarcts. Occasionally a hyperdense clot will be seen in the region of the MCA. A

CT scan must be performed before considering full anticoagulation or thrombolytic therapy to exclude ICH. However, one recent study revealed an inability of emergency physicians, neurologists and radiologists to detect difficult intracerebral haemorrhage on CT scan.[4]

The location of an ICH can indicate the likely cause. Haemorrhage in the basal ganglion region suggests hypertensive ICH. Lobar haemorrhage is associated with AVM in younger patients and amyloid angiopathy in the elderly. Haemorrhage located at the base of the frontal lobe suggests aneurysmal rupture.

MRI Standard MRI is superior to CT in showing early signs of infarction, with 90% showing changes at 24 hours on the T2 weighted images. However, it is inferior in diagnosing ICH and SAH, therefore CT is the first-line investigation. In cases of diagnostic doubt, or where further information is required, MRI in combination with MRA/MRV can be useful, particularly in suspected stroke caused by vasculitis, venous thrombosis or arterial dissection. This is particularly the case in young patients. It is also indicated in strokes involving the braistem and posterior fossa where CT has poor accuracy, particularly if basilar artery thrombosis is suspected. Diagnosis is important in these cases as it may alter management. Anticoagulation therapy may be indicated where venous thrombosis or arterial dissection is demonstrated and the use of intrarterial thrombolysis in case series of basilar artery thrombosis appears to improve outcome, even when therapy is delayed for up to 10–12 hours.

Recent advances in MR technology are likely to have a major role in acute stroke imaging. Diffusion MR scans show areas of reduced water diffusion in the parts of the brain that are ischaemic and likely to be irreversbly injured. This occurs rapidly after vessel occlusion and manifests as an area of high scan signal in the core ischaemic area less than an hour after stroke onset and is detectable much earlier than abnormalities on standard T2 weighted MRI or CT images. Perfusion scans indicate the area of brain

with reduced or delayed bood flow. This is the area likely to become infarcted if flow is not restored.

The areas of diffusion and perfusion abnormality can then be compared. A significantly larger perfusion than diffusion abnormality is a marker of potentially salvagable brain; the ischaemic penumbra. It is in those acute stroke patients with this pattern that are most likely to benefit from vessel opening strategies such as thrombolysis. Large areas of diffusion abnormality may also be a marker for increased risk of ICH with thrombolysis. An MRA can be performed at the same time to identify a major vessel occlusion.

Other

Other investigations may be indicated, particularly in young people in whom the cause of a stroke/TIA may be obscure, and include tests to detect prothrombolic states and uncommon vascular disorders. The list is potentially long and includes antithrombin III, protein C and S levels, antiphospholipid antibodies, a vasculitic and luetic screen, echocardiography and angiography.

TREATMENT

The treatment of cerebrovascular events must be individualized as determined by the nature and site of the lesion and the underlying cause, but then incorporated into assessment of the whole patient and the benefits and risks of any treatment contemplated. This is particularly so with the use of more aggressive therapies, such as anticoagulation, thrombolysis and surgery.

General

Emergency department management of TIA and stroke requires the usual priorities of initially stabilizing the airway and ensuring adequate ventilation and oxygenation. Airway intervention may be necessary in the setting of severely depressed level of consciousness, neurological deterioration or signs of raised intracranial pressure and cerebral herniation. Vital signs should be monitored and blood sugar assessed early to exclude hypoglycaemia. Hyperglycaemia should be avoided as it may worsen the outcome. Hypotension is very uncommon except in the terminal phase of brainstem failure. Hypertension is much more likely to be associated with stroke because of the associated pain, vomiting and raised intracranial pressure, and/or pre-existing hypertension, but rarely requires treatment in the stroke patient. It may be due to cerebral hypoxia and raised intracranial pressure as the physiologic response to maintain cerebral perfusion pressure. The use of antihypertensives in this situation may aggravate the neurologic deficit.

Guidelines[5] recommend cautious and controlled lowering of a persistently raised blood pressure higher than 220/140 mmHg or a mean arterial pressure greater than 130, using rapidly titratable IV drugs such as sodium nitroprusside, esmoloc or glycerin trinitrate at low initial doses, and with continuous haemodynamic monitoring in a critical-care setting. However, there is a paucity of scientific data to support such an approach in the ischaemic stroke patient. Oral or sublingual nifedipine is contra-indicated as it may cause a rapid un-controlled fall in blood pressure, causing or aggravating cerebral ischaemia. The threshold blood pressure for initiation of antihypertensive therapy is often lowered in ICA in consultation with the inpatient specialist. Analgesia is appropriate if pain is thought to be contributory, and urinary retention should be excluded. An elevated temperature can occur in stroke but should raise suspicion of other causes for the neurologic findings or an associated infective focus.

After stabilization of vital functions, the clinical evaluation must focus on determining the nature and cause of the neurologic lesion through a focused history and examination, then selecting appropriate investigations that will assist in guiding therapy.

TIAs

The main aim of therapy in TIAs and minor strokes is to prevent a major subsequent cerebrovascular event. Following a TIA the risk of stroke is 4–8% in the first month and 12–13% during the first year. The risk of stroke is not uniform for all types of TIAs: for example, hemispheric TIAs with an associated >70% carotid stenosis have a 2-year stroke rate of about 40%.

Antiplatelet therapy

Aspirin should be commenced at a dose of 300 mg and maintained at 75–150 mg/d in patients with TIAs or minor ischaemic strokes as it has been shown to be effective in preventing further ischaemic events. The antiplatelet agent clopidogrel may be substituted for aspirin if the patient does not respond or is intolerant of aspirin. Clopidogrel is possibly more effective than aspirin in stroke prevention, but is often more expensive.

Dipyridamole alone has no advantage over aspirin, but may have a modest additional benefit in combination with aspirin. Studies are being undertaken to evaluate the optimal antiplatelet regime for secondary prevention.

Warfarin anticoagulation has not been shown to be superior to aspirin except in TIA/minor stroke due to cardio-embolism. It can be considered in other cases if antiplatelet treatment fails.[6]

Anticoagulant therapy

Patients with a cardioembolic source of TIA should be fully anticoagulated with heparin and warfarin following a normal CT scan, except those with endocarditis. In endocarditis the risk of haemorrhagic complications is increased.

Heparinization in TIA is controversial (other than with a cardioembolic source). This should be considered for patients with crescendo TIAs, i.e. frequent, multiple or progressing events, and is also used in some patients with high-risk TIAs, i.e. anterior circulation TIA and >70% carotid stenosis, while they are awaiting surgical evaluation.

Surgery

The NASCET trial demonstrated a beneficial outcome of surgery for symptomatic carotid stenosis in patients with anterior circulation TIAs and an angiographically demonstrated carotid stenosis of >70–99%, as long as the operational perioperative mortality/stroke morbidity is low.

Surgery for TIA and vertebrobasilar disease and intracranial carotid stenosis is occasionally considered in cases of continued symptoms despite maximal medical therapy. Studies have failed to show a benefit from ECA/ICA bypass surgery in patients with occlusion of the ICA, with continued symptoms, compared to medical therapy.

Advances in surgical treatment of cerebrovascular disease, such as carotid angioplasty and vascular stenting, continue to evolve and are undergoing study.

Ischaemic stroke

A more active approach to the acute management of ischaemic stroke is seen as having the potential to improve neurological outcome. The emergency department is the place where these important treatment decisions will largely be made. Most patients with a stroke will require hospital admission for further evaluation and treatment, observation, and possibly rehabilitation. Studies of stroke units show that these patients will benefit from being under the care of physicians with an active interest in stroke management.

Aspirin

In the large International Stroke Trial (IST)[7] and Chinese Acute Stroke Trial (CAST)[8] aspirin administered within 48 hours of onset was found to improve the outcome of early death or recurrent stroke when given to acute stroke patients rather than placebo. A CT scan should be performed to exclude ICH prior to commencing aspirin.

Thrombolysis

Thrombolytic agents are increasingly being seen as having a place in the management of acute ischaemic stroke, although their use is still controversial.[9] Only one large randomized controlled trial, the National Institute of Neurological Diseases Study (NINDS),[10] has shown a significant improvement in long-term neurological outcome when patients with an ischaemic stroke were given a thrombolytic agent. In the NINDS study, patients with a stroke of well-defined onset with a CT scan showing no signs of ICH and satisfying other strict inclusion criteria, were randomized to receive tissue plasminogen activator (tPA) at a dose of 0.9 mg/kg (maximum 90 mg) or placebo. For inclusion, treatment must have commenced within 3 hours of stroke onset. Patients were excluded if they were on anticoagulants but not if taking aspirin. In the thrombolysis group there was a significant increase in intracerebral haemorrhage rate(6.4% in tPA vs 0.6% in placebo group), of which half were fatal, although there was no overall excess mortality. Hence, the significant overall clinical benefit of little or no neurological deficit at 3 months was gained at an appreciable risk. It is currently unclear in which patients this risk can be reduced, although factors such as increased age, increased severity of stroke and early CT scan changes of a large ischaemic stroke may be important in increasing the risk of intracerebral haemorrhage with thrombolysis. Since the publication of the NINDS study, the ECASS 2 [11]and ATLANTIS [12] trials of tPA use up to 6 hours post onset of acute stroke have been published. Both were negative for the primary endpoint of favourable neurologic outcome. Studies evaluating the use of tPA in United States hospitals since the approval of IV tPA for stroke by the FDA, have yielded conflicting results.[13,14] The 2000 American Heart Association guidelines [15] gave IV tPA, in acute stroke up to 3 hours, a grade 1 rating (definetely recommended) despite concerns expressed by members of the emergency medicine community.[16]

Intra-arterial thrombolysis has been evaluated in the PROACT 2 study.[17] Two hundred patients with angiographically demonstrated MCA occlusion were randomized to intra-arterial urokinase and low-dose heparin or low-dose heparin alone, up to 6 hours post stroke onset. A significant improvement was found in the number of patients with independent neuologic outcomes in the urokinase group. The lack of availability of the interventional expertise required to perform this therapy makes it unlikely to have a significant impact on stroke therapy for the vast majority of patients within the foreseeable future.

Future trials of thrombolysis in acute stroke will be aimed at identifying those patients most likely to benefit from revascularization therapy, lessening the risk of ICH and extending the time window for treatment, particularly through the use of advanced imaging techniques. Specifically diffusion/perfusion MRI holds great promise in achieving these goals and clinical trials are underway.

Heparin

Heparin is used in some ischaemic stroke syndromes but evidence is lacking regarding indications, timing, dosing, efficacy and safety. In the IST trial high-dose heparin (12 500 units bd s.c.) was associated with a significantly worse outcome. Heparin anticoagulation can be considered in patients at high risk of recurrent embolism, such as those in AF and associated mitral stenosis, or with mechanical heart valves, where intracardiac thrombus is established. This depends on the severity of the existing neurologic deficit and overall clinical state. A CT scan to exclude ICH and neurological consultaion should be obtained prior to considering anticoagulation in any patient with a stroke of likely cardioembolic origin.

Neuroprotection

Neuroprotective therapies include calcium antagonists; drugs that decrease glutamate release or mode of action, such as N-methyl-D-aspartate (NMDA) receptor antagonists, anticonvulsants and opioids; and antioxidant drugs such as the 21-aminosteroids, which inhibit lipid peroxidation. These and other therapies are undergoing study, particularly to follow thrombolytic therapy, but at this stage none is recommended for the treatment of stroke.

Surgery

There are limited data on the indications, efficacy and safety of surgical procedures in acute stroke. Emergency carotid endarterectomy is occasionally performed, and endovascular techniques are being developed and studied.

Intracerebral haemorrhage

Surgery

Surgical management of ICH depends on the location, cause, neurologic deficit and the overall clinical state. Early neurosurgical consultation should be obtained to consider haematoma evacuation and/ or cerebrospinal fluid drainage if acute hydrocephalus develops. Evidence for improved outcomes following drainage of supratentorial haematomas is lacking, but the procedure may be indicated in selected patients.[18] The presence of a cerebellar haematoma is a particular indication for surgery, with the potential for neurologic recovery.

Medical

Hyperventilation and diuretics may transiently reduce intracranial pressures in cases of cerebral herniation while neurosurgical review is awaited. The calcium antagonist nimodipine is used in selected cases of SAH. Steroids are not indicated. Anticonvulsant prophylaxis is common practice.

CONCLUSION

The emergency physician is involved not only in the diagnosis of stroke and TIA, but also increasingly in important decisions regarding the investigation, treatment and disposition of such patients, with the potential for improved survival and reduced disability.

REFERENCES

1. Executive Committee of the Asymptomatic Carotid Atherosclerosis Study 1995 Endarterectomy for asymptomatic carotid artery stenosis. Journal of the American Medical Association 273: 1421–8
2. North American Symptomatic Carotid Endarterectomy Trial Collaborators (NASCET) 1991 Beneficial effects of carotid endarterectomy in symptomatic patients with high grade carotid stenosis. New England Journal of Medicine 325: 445–53
3. Libman RB, Wirkowski E, Alvir J, Rao TH 1995 Conditions that mimic stroke in the emergency department. Archives of Neurology 52: 1119–22
4. Schriger DL, Kalafut M, Starkman S, et al 1998 Cranial computer tomography interpretation in

CONTROVERSIES

❶ Thrombolysis is a high-risk therapy which may improve neurological outcome in patients with ischaemic stroke when given within 3 hours of onset. Only one study has so far demonstrated such a significant improvement without excess overall mortality. Problematic issues for thrombolytic therapy in stroke include the small number of patients who currently present within the time window for treatment, identification in the emergency department of subgroups with higher risks of haemorrhagic complications or less treatment benefit; the significant rate of stroke misdiagnosis, with subsequent potential for unnecessary exposure to a high-risk therapy and the requirement and availability of neuroradiologic expertise to exclude subtle intracerebral haemorrhage prior to thrombolysis. Advances in neuro-imaging, particularly diffusion/perfusion MRI hold great promise for improved selection of patients likely to benefit from thrombolytic therapy.

❷ Selection of the most approriate anti-platelet agent for the treatment of TIAs is debated. Aspirin is cost effective. Clopidogrel and aspirin/dipyridamole combinations are usually reserved for those with aspirin contra indications/intolerance or ongoing TIAs on aspirin.

❸ Anticoagulation is indicated in TIAs and minor ischaemic strokes from a proven cardioembolic source, except in endocarditis and after CT exclusion of haemorrhage. There are little data to support the use of heparin in stroke or TIA outside this group, but it is commonly given in the clinical setting of 'crescendo TIAs', particularly while awaiting further investigation or surgery.

❹ Antihypertensive therapy is rarely necessary in the acute management of stroke. An elevated blood pressure may be a physiologic response to maintain cerebral perfusion pressure. Rapid uncontrolled BP reduction can occur with agents such as oral or sublingual nifedipine, thereby aggravating cerebral ischaemia.

acute stroke. Physician accuracy in determining eligibility for thrombolytic therapy. Journal of the American Medical Association 279: 1293–7
5. Adams HP Jr, Brott TG, Crowell RM, et al 1994 Guidelines for the management of acute ischaemic stroke. Stroke 25: 1901–14
6. Frienberg WM, Albers GW, Barnett HJM, et al 1994 Guidelines for the management of transient ischaemic attacks. Stroke 25: 1320–35
7. International Stroke Trial Collaborative Group 1997 The International Stroke Trial (IST): a randomised trial of aspirin, subcutaneous heparin, both, or neither among 19435 patients with acute ischaemic stroke. Lancet 349: 1569–81
8. CAST (Chinese Acute Stroke Trial) Collaborative Group 1997 CAST: randomised placebo controlled trial of early aspirin use in 20000 patients with acute ischaemic stroke. Lancet 349: 1641–9
9. Wardlaw JM, Warlow CP, Counsell C 1997 Systematic review of evidence on thrombolytic therapy for acute ischaemic stroke. Lancet 350: 607–14
10. The National Institute of Neurological Disorders and Stroke rt-PA Stroke Study Group 1995 Tissue plasminogen activator for acute ischaemic stroke. New England Journal of Medicine 333(24): 1581–7
11. European Cooperative Acute Stroke Study(ECASS) 1995 Intravenous thrombolysis with recombinant tissue plasminogen activator for acute hemispheric stroke. Journal of the American Medical Association 274: 1017–125
12. Clark WM, Albers GW, et al 2000 for the Thrombolytic Therapy in Acute Ischaemic Stroke Study Investigators. The rtPA 0 to 6 hour acute stroke trial par A. Stroke 31: 811–6
13. Albers GW 2000 Intravenous tissue-type plasminogen activator for treatment of acute stroke: the Standard Treatment with Alteplase to Reverse Stroke (STARS) study. Journal of the American Medical Association 83: 1145–50
14. Katzan IL, Furlan AJ, Lloyd LE, et al 2000 Use of tissue type plasminogen activator for acute ischaemic stroke: the Cleveland Area Experience. Journal of the American Medical Association 283: 1151–8
15. American Heart Association in Collaboration with the international Liasion Committee on Resuscitation Guidelines 2000 for cardiopulmonary resuscitation and emergency cardiovascular care. Part 7 : The era of reperfusion: Section 2 : acute stroke. Circulation 102(8suppl I): 204–16
16. Hoffman JR 2000 Should physicians give tPA to patients with acute ischaemic stroke? Against: and just what is the emperor of stroke wearing? West J Med 173: 149–50
17. Furlan A, Higashida R, Wechsler L, et al 1999 Intra-arterial prourokinase for acute ischaemic strike. The PROACT II study: arandomised trial. PRolyse in Acute Cerebral Thromboembolism. Journal of the American Medical Association 282: 2003–11
18. Hankey GJ, Hon C 1997 Surgery for primary intracerebral haemorrhage: is it safe and effectivefi A systematic review of case series and randomised controlled trials. Stroke 28: 2126–32

7.3 SUBARACHNOID HAEMORRHAGE

PAMELA ROSENGARTEN

ESSENTIALS

1 The diagnosis of subarachnoid haemorrhage (SAH) demands a high index of suspicion for the condition.

2 Up to 50% of patients with SAH experience a warning leak, the sentinel haemorrhage, in the hours to days prior to the major bleed.[1]

3 Brain CT scan without contrast is the initial investigation of choice.

4 A negative CT scan for SAH must be followed by lumbar puncture and examination of the CSF.

5 The patient with SAH requires urgent neurosurgical referral and management.

6 Early definitive surgery to repair the aneurysm reduces early complications and improves outcome.[2]

INTRODUCTION

Patients with headache account for approximately 1% of all emergency department visits and of these 1 to 4% have been demonstrated to have subarachnoid haemorrhage.[2] Early accurate diagnosis of aneurysmal subarachnoid haemorrhage is imperative as early definitive surgery has been shown to reduce early complications of re-bleeding and vasospasm and improve outcome.[2]

SAH is the presence of extravasated blood within the subarachnoid space. Excluding head trauma, which remains the most common cause, non-traumatic or spontaneous SAH results from rupture of a cerebral aneurysm in approximately 85% of cases.

Aneurysmal SAH occurs most commonly in the 40–60-year age group.[3] Risk factors include cigarette smoking, a family history of first-degree relatives with SAH, hypertension, heritable connective tissue disorders, particularly polycystic kidney disease and neurofibromatosis, sickle cell disease and α-1 antitrypsin deficiency.[1,2,4]

The following discussion refers to aneurysmal SAH.

HISTORY

The history is critical to the diagnosis of SAH:

- Headache is the principal presenting symptom, being present in up to 95% of patients with SAH. It is typically of sudden onset and severe, being the worst headache ever experienced by the patient. Up to 50% of patients experience a warning leak (sentinel haemorrhage) in the hours to days before the major bleed.[1] This headache may be less severe, generalized or localized, resolve spontaneously or respond to analgesic therapy. It does, however, tend to develop abruptly and differ in quality to other headaches that the patient may have previously experienced.[2]
- Upper neck pain is common.
- One-third of patients will develop SAH during strenuous exercise, e.g. bending or lifting, whereas in the remaining two-thirds it will occur during sleep or routine daily activities.[2,3]
- Nausea and vomiting are present in 75% of patients.[1]
- Brief or permanent loss of consciousness occurs in the majority of patients. Severe headache is usually experienced when the patient regains consciousness, although a brief episode of excruciating headache may occur prior to losing consciousness.
- Seizures occur in 15% of patients.
- Prodromal symptoms such as cranial neuropathy (particularly third cranial

nerve with pupillary dilatation and sixth cranial nerve palsies), seizures, mass effect or cerebral ischaemia due to clot passing distal to the aneurysm, may suggest the presence and location of a progressively enlarging unruptured aneurysm.[2]

EXAMINATION

There is a wide spectrum of clinical presentation with the level of consciousness and clinical signs being dependent upon the site and extent of the haemorrhage:

- Conscious state may vary from normal to drowsy to coma.
- Signs of meningism, including fever, photophobia and neck stiffness, are present in 75% of patients but may take several hours to develop.
- Focal neurological signs may be present in up to 25% of patients and are secondary to associated intracranial haemorrhage, cerebral vasospasm, local compression of a cranial nerve by the aneurysm (e.g. oculomotor nerve palsy by posterior communicating aneurysm) or raised intracranial pressure (sixth-nerve palsy).[1]
- Ophthalmologic examination may reveal unilateral or bilateral subhyaloid haemorrhages or papilloedema.
- Patients are categorized into clinical grades from I to V, according to their conscious state and neurological deficit. Two grading schemes, that of Hunt and Hess and that of the World Federation of Neurosurgeons, are depicted in Table 7.3.1.[1]

INVESTIGATIONS

Investigations specific for the diagnosis of SAH are as follows:

Table 7.3.1 Clinical grading schemes for patients with SAH

Grade	Grading scheme of Hunt and Hess	Grading scheme of WFNS GCS	Motor deficit
1	No symptoms or minimal headache, slight nuchal rigidity	15	No
2	Moderate to severe headache, no neurological deficit other than cranial nerve palsy	13–14	No
3	Drowsy, confused, mild focal deficit	13–14	Yes
4	Stupor, moderate to severe hemiparesis, vegetative posturing	7–12	Yes or no
5	Deep coma, decerebration, moribund	3–6	Yes or no

WFNS = World Federation of Neurosurgeons, GCS = Glasgow Coma Score
(Reproduced with permission from Sawin PD, Loftus CM 1997 Diagnosis of spontaneous subarachnoid hemorrhage. American Family Physician 55(1): 145–156)

- Brain CT scan without contrast is the initial investigation of choice. In the first 24 hours following haemorrhage it can demonstrate the presence of subarachnoid blood in 90–95% of cases.[4] The sensitivity, however, decreases with time, with only 80% of scans positive at 3 days and 50% positive at 1 week.[4] CT scan will also demonstrate the site and extent of the haemorrhage, indicate the possible location of the aneurysm, and demonstrate the presence of hydrocephalus and other pathological changes.
- Lumbar puncture is necessary when there is clinical suspicion of SAH, the CT scan is negative, equivocal or technically inadequate and no mass lesion or signs of raised intracranial pressure are found. In at least 5–10% of patients with SAH the CT scan will be normal.

Measuring the opening pressure when performing a lumbar puncture is important as CSF pressure may be elevated in SAH or in other conditions such as cerebral venous sinus thrombosis or pseudotumor cerebri.

Diagnosis of SAH is then dependent upon the finding of red blood cells not due to traumatic tap, or red blood cell breakdown products within the CSF. Differentiation of a traumatic tap, which can occur in up to 20% of lumbar punctures, from SAH may be difficult.[2]

Examination of the red cell count in three sequentially collected tubes of CSF implies SAH when the red cell count is constant in all three tubes, and traumatic tap when there is a decrease in the red cell count across the three tubes. This test, although suggestive of SAH, is, however, unreliable.[5,6.]

Xanthochromia, the yellow discolouration of CSF due to haemoglobin breakdown products, oxyhaemoglobin and bilirubin, is generally agreed to be the primary criterion for diagnosis of SAH and to differentiate between SAH and traumatic tap.[2 6] Xanthochromia requires lysis of red blood cells and metabolism of haemoglobin and is usually present within 6 hours of SAH and has been demonstrated in all patients with SAH between 12 hours and 2 weeks following the haemorrhage.[5] Xanthochromia is not reliably detected by visual examination of centrifuged CSF. Spectrophotometric analysis of CSF is considered the most sensitive means of detecting xanthochromia and should be undertaken to detect its presence when visual examination is negative.[5,6] In a small number of patients with SAH xanthochromia may not be present until 12 hours following headache onset, and controversy exists as to the optimal timing of lumbar puncture. Early lumbar puncture within 12 hours may have negative or equivocal CSF findings whereas delayed lumbar puncture may result in an increased risk of early re-bleeding as well as having

practical implications for the emergency department. In general at least 6 to 12 hours should have elapsed between headache onset and lumbar puncture, however, when lumbar puncture is performed within 12 hours of headache onset and CSF result is equivocal, blood stained and negative for xanthochromia or where spectrophotometric analysis of the CSF is not possible, then neurosurgical consultation and vascular imaging should be performed.

Although detection of xanthochromia is indicative of SAH it does not entirely rule out traumatic lumbar puncture and can occur in extremely bloody taps (>12 000 RBC/mL) or where the lumbar punture has been repeated after an initial traumatic tap.[14]

Other studies of the CSF such as D-dimer assay and detection of erythrophages have been found to be inconsistent in differentiating SAH from traumatic tap.[2] Although the presence of erythrophages confirms SAH they are found inconsistently and may take several days to be positive.[4]

- MRI with FLAIR (fluid attenuated inversion recovery) is reliable in demonstrating early SAH and is superior to CT in detecting extravastaed blood in days (up to 40) post haemorrhage. Availability and logistical considerations make MRI impractical for use in the initial diagnostic work up of SAH but it may be considered in patients who present 1 to 2 weeks post symptom onset.[15]
- Four-vessel cerebral angiography has been the gold standard for confirming the presence of an aneurysm, its location and the presence of vasospasm. It should be performed as soon as possible following the diagnosis of SAH.
- CT angiography has a sensitivity of 85 to 95% when compared with catheter angiography for detecting aneurysms and may evolve as an alternative imaging modality to conventional angiography.[15]
- MR angiography is currently useful as a screening tool for the diagnosis

of intracranial aneurysms in patients at increased risk. It does not reliably detect small aneurysms, nor does it provide sufficient information for surgical planning.

General investigations to be performed include full blood examination, erythrocyte sedimentation rate, urea, electrolytes, blood glucose, clotting profile and ECG.

ECG changes are frequently present and include ST and T-wave changes which may mimic ischaemia, QRS and QT prolongation and arrhythmias.

COMPLICATIONS

- Rebleeding: 4% of patients rebleed within the first 48 hours after the initial haemorrhage, and overall 20% of patients rebleed within the first 2 weeks.[3,4] It is associated with a 60% mortality and poor outcome which is eliminated by early treatment.[2]
- Subdural haematoma can be life threatening and require immedicate drainage. Similarly a large intracerebral haematoma may be contributing to the poor clinical condition and warrant drainage simultaneously with clipping of the aneurysm.
- Global cerebral ischaemia: irreversible brain damage resulting from haemorrhage at the time of aneurysm rupture. Probably seconday to a marked rise in incranial pressure resulting in inadequate cerebral perfusion.
- Cerebral vasospasm: clinically significant vasospasm occurs in approximately 20% of patients with SAH and is a major cause of death and morbidity.[3] It tends to occur between day 3 and day 15 after SAH, with a peak incidence at days 6–8.[3] Vasospasm causes ischaemia or infarction and should be suspected in any patient who suffers a deterioration in their neurological status or develops neurological deficits.
- Hydrocephalus: occurs in approximately 15% of patients with SAH. It can occur within 24 hours

of haemorrhage and should be suspected in any patient who suffers a deterioration in mentation or conscious state pariticularly if associated with slowed pupillary responses.
- Seizures.
- Fluid and electrolyte disturbances: patients with SAH may develop hyponatraemia and hypovolaemia secondary to excessive natriuresis (cerebral salt wasting), or alternatively may develop a syndrome of inappropriate ADH (SIADH).

MANAGEMENT

The management of SAH requires general supportive measures particularly airway protection and blood pressure control as well as specific management of the ruptured aneurysm and the complications of aneurysmal haemorrhage.

General measures

- Stabilization of the unconscious patient, with particular attention to the airway. Endotracheal intubation with oxygenation and ventilation will be required in patients with higher grade (4 to 5) SAH.
- In all patients maintain oxygenation and circulation ensuring adequate blood volume.
- Analgesia, sedation and antiemetics as required. Ensure bed rest with minimal stimulation.
- Blood pressure control: blood pressure levels are often in the order of 150/90 immediately following SAH, and in most patients can be adequately controlled by sedation and analgesia. Normotensive levels extending to mild to moderately hypertensive levels especially in patients with pre-existing hypertension are acceptable. Antihypertensive therapy should be reserved for patients with severe or complicated hypertension and short acting antihypertensive agents (e.g. esmolol or nitroprusside) and intensive haemodynamic monitoring be used.

- Seizures should be treated as they occur. The use of prophylactic phenytoin is controversial.
- Correct electrolyte imbalances. Hyponatraemia of excessive natriuresis must be differentiated from that of SIADH. Hypovolaemia should be avoided.
- Treatment of vasospasm: nimodipine, a calcium channel antagonist, when given orally, has been shown to decrease the proportion of patients with poor outcome and ischaemic neurological deficits after aneurysmal SAH.[11] It is worthy to note that this efficacy and the recommended dosage are based upon the results of a single large trial. [11] Nimodipine, 60 mg orally 4–6-hourly, should be commenced within 48 hours of haemorrhage.[8]

Vasospasm has also been treated with induced hypervolaemia and hypertension. This therapy aims for a systolic blood pressure of 180–220 mmHg but requires definitive treatment of the aneurysm with exclusion from the circulation and intensive haemodynamic monitoring.[8] Athough hypervolaemia and hypertension is widely practiced there is litle evidence from clinical trials to support its use.[15]

- Antifibrinolytic agents, including e-aminocaproic acid, which inhibit clot lysis, reduce the incidence of rebleeding after initial aneurysmal rupture.[1,5] Their use has, however, been associated with an increase in neurological deficits and failed to improve outcome. [12] They are not advocated for routine use in SAH.
- Intracranial pressure monitoring and medical management is beneficial in patients with raised intracranial pressure.
- Treatment of hydrocephalus by ventricular drainage may be required.

Specific treatment

Surgical clipping of the neck of the aneurysm remains the definitive treatment of choice for ruptured cerebral aneurysm. Early surgery within 72 hours secures the aneurysm, prevents rebleeding and removes the clot. It is technically more difficult than delayed surgery but is the option most neurosurgeons prefer for good grade (I-III) patients as it reduces the incidence of early complications and improve outcomes.[2] Delayed surgery at 10–14 days post haemorrhage is generally reserved for poor-grade (IV-V) patients.[1,4]

Endovascular treatment, in which metallic coils are placed in the aneurysm under radiological guidance, has been used in selected cases, but long-term effectiveness and its exact role are yet to be determined.[4]

PROGNOSIS

SAH has a 40–60% mortality rate from the initial haemorrhage, with up to one-third of survivors having a significant neurological deficit.[3,4] The most important prognostic factor is the clinical condition at time of presentation, with coma and major neurological deficits generally associated with a poor prognosis.[4] Survival rates have been reported at 70% for grade I, 60% for grade II, 50% for grade III, 40% for grade IV and 10% for grade V.[9]

It is worthy to note, however, that survival without brain damage is possible even after respiratory arrest.[15] In these circumstances outcome and persistence of neurological dysfunction usually become evident in the hours following resuscitation.

OTHER CAUSES FOR SAH

Nonaneurysmal perimesencephalic haemorrhage accounts for approximately 10% of all occurences of SAH. It is defined by the distribution of extravasated blood on CT scan (confined to the cisterns around the midbrain with centre of bleeding immediately anterior to the midbrain) and the absence of an aneurysm. The prognosis in this group of patients is excellent – rebleeds and delayed cerebral ischaemia do not occur.[15]

Other causes of SAH are less common accounting for approximately 5% of cases and include arterial dissection, AV malformations, septic aneuryms, pituitary apoplexy, cocaine abuse, sickle cell disease, neoplasms, medical conditions including infections, collagen vascular disorders, blood dyscrasias, bleeding diatheses and anticoagulant therapy.[1,2] Congenital vascular malformations account for the majority of bleeds occurring in children and young adults.

In patients where SAH is present and no cause is found, then the distribution of extravasated blood on the CT scan should be reviewed. If this confoms to the peri mesencephalic distribution of non aneurysmal haemorrhage, then no repeat investigations are warranted. If, however, an aneurysmal pattern of haemorrhage is present, then a second angiogram is recommended as occasionally an aneurysm may have gone undetected on the original test.[15]

CONCLUSION

Clinical suspicion of the diagnosis of SAH gained from a history of sudden, severe or atypical headache demands a full investigation, including brain CT scan and, if necessary, lumbar puncture. Once SAH has been diagnosed then urgent neurosurgical referral and management are required.

REFERENCES

1. Sawin PD, Loftus CM 1997 Diagnosis of spontaneous subarachnoid hemorrhage. American Family Physician 55(1): 145–56
2. Edlow JA, Caplan LR. 2000 Primary care: Avoiding pitfalls in the diagnosis of subarachnoid hemorrhage. The New England Journal of Medicine 342(1): 29–36
3. Kopitnik T, Horowitz M, Samson D 1997 Management of subarachnoid haemorrhage. In: Hughes RAC (ed.) Neurological emergencies, 2nd edn. BMJ publishing, London, pp 188–244
4. Schievink WI 1997 Intracranial aneurysms. The New England Journal of Medicine 336: 28–40
5. Vermeulen M 1996 Subarachnoid haemorrhage: diagnosis and treatment. Journal of Neurology 243: 496–501
6. Vermeulen M, van Gijn J 1990 The diagnosis of subarachnoid haemorrhage. Journal of Neurology, Neurosurgery and Psychiatry 53(5): 365–72
8. Lang DT 1990 Rapid differentiation of subarachnoid haemorrhage from traumatic lumbar puncture using the D-dimer assay. American Journal of Clinical Pathology 93: 403–5
9. Thompson WR 1997 Acute cerebrovascular complications. In: Oh TE (ed.) Intensive Care Manual, 4th edn. Butterworth-Heinemann, Oxford, pp 386–94
10. Barson WG, Kothari R 1998 Stroke. In: Rosen P (ed.) Emergency Medicine: Concepts and Clinical Practice, 4th edn. Mosby, Chicago, pp 2184–98
11. Feigin VL, Rinkel GJE, Algra A, Vermeulen M, Ginjn J 2002 Calcium antagonists for aneurysmal subarachnoid haemorrhage (Cochrane Review). The Cochrane Library, Issue 2
12. Roos YBWEM, Rinkel GJE, Vermeulen M, Algra A, Gijn J 2002 Antifibrinolytic therapy for aneurysmal subarachnoid haemorrhage. The Cochrane Database of Systematic Reviews, Issue 2
13. de Gans K, Nieuwkamp DJ, Rinkel GJ, Algra A 2002 Timing of aneurysmal surgery in subarachnoid hemorrhage: a systematic review of the literature. Neurosurgery 50(2): 336–40
14. Holdgate A, Cuthbert K 2001 Perils and ptfalls of lumbar puncture in the emergency department. Emergency Medicine 13: 351–8
15. van Gijn J, Rinkel GJE 2001 Subarachnoid haemorrhage: diagnosis, causes and management. Brain 124: 249–78

CONTROVERSIES

❶ The timing of lumbar puncture following haemorrhage. Diagnostic CSF xanthochromia has not been reliably demonstrated to be present until 12 hours post SAH, although most are positive by 6 hours. Recommendations to delay the lumbar puncture until 12 hours after the onset of headache may be associated with an increased risk of early rebleeding. The timing of lumbar puncture should probably be at least 6 hours after onset of headache following a non-diagnostic CT scan. If the CSF result is inconclusive, neurosursurgical consultation and vascular imaging should be performed.[2]

❷ Vascular imaging for patients with negative CT scan and negative CSF is indicated in patients with ambiguous test results, those at high risk for SAH and patients presenting greater 2 weeks.[2]

❸ Timing of surgery: early or delayed. Generally early surgery for good clinical grade patients and delayed for poor grade patients, although evidence is still lacking for the best timing of surgery.[13]

❹ Prophylactic anticonvulsant therapy for patients with SAH.

7.4 ALTERED CONSCIOUS STATE

RUTH HEW

ESSENTIALS

1 For clinical purposes, the ability of the individual to respond appropriately to environmental stimuli provides a quantifiable definition of consciousness.

2 The Glasgow Coma Scale can be used to quantify conscious state and monitor progress.

3 The causes of altered conscious state can be divided pathophysiologically into structural insults and metabolic insults.

4 As in all life-threatening conditions, assessment and management proceed concurrently with the focus on assessment of the consequences of the coma, commencement of resuscitation and identification and management of the cause.

5 Bedside blood glucose measurement is essential and can be life-saving.

INTRODUCTION

Consciousness can be defined as a state of awareness of self and environment. This presumes subjectivity, unity and intentionality implying that each individual's perception is unique, consisting of a moulding of various sensory modalities over time and interpreted within the full range of that individual's experiences. It is clear even from this limited description that the definition of consciousness is metaphysical and difficult to quantify. It would also include what is clinically described as mental state but psychiatric disease and its differentiation from medical pathology is excluded from this discussion as it is addressed elsewhere.

For clinical purposes, the ability of the individual to respond appropriately to environmental stimuli provides a quantifiable definition of consciousness. Pragmatically, consciousness equals responsiveness.

PATHOPHYSIOLOGY

The level of consciousness describes the arousability of the individual while the content of consciousness may be assessed in terms of the appropriateness of the individual's response. Broadly speaking the first is a brainstem function while the second is an attribute of the forebrain.

The physical portions of the brain involved in consciousness consist of the ascending arousal system that begins with monoaminergic cell groups in the brainstem and culminates in extensive diffuse cortical projections throughout the cerebrum. En route there is input and modulation from both thalamic and hypothalamic nuclei, as well as basal forebrain cell groups.

The integration of the brainstem and the forebrain is illustrated by individuals who have an isolated pontine injury. They remain awake but the intact forebrain is unable to interact with the external world, hence the aptly named 'locked-in syndrome'. At the other end of the spectrum are individuals in a persistent vegetative state who, in spite of extensive forebrain impairment, appear awake but totally lack the content of consciousness. These clinical extremes underscore the important role of the brainstem in modulating motor and sensory systems through its descending pathways and regulating the wakefulness of the forebrain through its ascending pathways.

Impairment of conscious state implies dysfunction of the ascending arousal system in the paramedian portion of the upper pons and midbrain, its targets in the thalamus of hypothalamus, or both

cerebral hemispheres. The resultant changes in the conscious state range from awakeness through lethargy and stupor to coma with a progressively depressed response to various stimuli.

There are a myriad of scales that have attempted to define consciousness but the one that has found universal acceptance is the Glasgow Coma (or Responsiveness) Scale (GCS) (Table 7.4.1). Initially described in 1974,[1] for the assessment of traumatic head injuries, 25 years of experience has shown that the scale can also be used in non-traumatic situations to provide a structured assessment of an individual's conscious state at various points in time and also to monitor progress. In quantifying and standardizing the various responses, the GCS has enabled clinicians worldwide to compare data and therapies.

In the spectrum from full awareness to unrousability, coma or unconsciousness has been arbitrarily defined as a GCS less than or equal to 8.[2]

Table 7.4.1 Glasgow Coma Scale

The GCS is scored between 3 and 15, 3 being the worst, and 15 the best. It is composed of three parameters: Best Eye Response, Best Verbal Response, Best Motor Response, as given below:

Best Eye Response (score out of 4):
1 – No eye opening.
2 – Eye opening to pain.
3 – Eye opening to verbal command.
4 – Eyes open spontaneously.

Best Verbal Response (score out of 5):
1 – No verbal response.
2 – Incomprehensible sounds.
3 – Inappropriate words.
4 – Confused
5 – Orientated

Best Motor Response (score out of 6):
1 – No motor response.
2 – Extension to pain.
3 – Flexion to pain.
4 – Withdrawal from pain.
5 – Localizing pain.
6 – Obeys commands

DIFFERENTIAL DIAGNOSES

As the main diagnostic challenge in a patient with an altered conscious state is to identify the cause, it is reasonable to approach the assessment of the patient armed with a knowledge of the possible differential diagnoses.

There are several well-known mnemonics to assist in remembering the rather diverse list. Some are listed below:

T	Trauma	**A**	Alcohol and other toxins
I	Infection	**E**	Endocrinopathy Encephalopathy Electrolyte disturbances
P	Psychogenic	**I**	Insulin - Diabetes
(P)	(Porphyria)	**O**	Oxygen: Hypoxia of any cause Opiates
S	Seizure Syncope Space-occupying lesion	**U**	Uraemia including Hypertension

Or if you prefer,

C erebral
O verdose
M etabolic
A sphyxia and other **A** ssociations

However, the long list of apparently disparate causes can be divided pathophysiologically into structural insults and metabolic insults (Table 7.4.2).

Structural insults are usually focal intracranial lesions that exert direct or indirect pressure on the brainstem and the more caudal portions of the ascending arousal system. They tend to produce lateralising neurological signs that can assist in pinpointing the level of the lesion. As there is little space in and around the brainstem, any extrinsic or intrinsic compression will rapidly progress through coma to death unless the pressure on the brainstem is relieved surgically or pharmacologically.

Metabolic insults are usually due to systemic pathology affecting primarily the forebrain, although direct depression of the brainstem may also occur. There are seldom lateralising signs. The solution to the problem is the correction of the underlying metabolic impairment. Naturally, as in all clinical practice, there are no absolute distinctions. Any of the metabolic causes can, uncorrected, eventually cause cerebral oedema and herniation leading thence to brainstem compression with lateralizing signs and death.

Table 7.4.2 lists the more common and important causes of an altered conscious state.

CLINICAL ASSESSMENT

As in all life threatening conditions, assessment and management proceed concurrently. There are two primary considerations, neither of which is mutually exclusive - assessment of the consequences of the coma and commencement of resuscitation and identification and management of the cause.

As in other time critical situations, the primary survey and secondary survey approach often proves useful.

Primary survey

This focuses on attention to the airway, breathing and circulation. It commences the identification of life-threatening problems and allows immediate therapeutic measures such as airway support to be implemented. Supplemental oxygen is indicated, as is frequent monitoring of vital signs and GCS. Endotracheal intubation is required at this stage if the patient is unable to maintain a safe airway. This usually corresponds with a GCS of 8 or less. Mild hyperventilation to a $pCO2$ of 30–35 mm Hg will correct underlying acidosis and reduce intracranial pressure. Cervical spine precautions are imperative if trauma is suspected until clearance of the spine can be obtained.

A bedside glucose determination may identify clinical or biochemical hypoglycaemia, which should be treated with glucose. These is no evidence that 50 mL of intravenous 50% dextrose will cause harm even in an already hyperglycaemic patient and a case could be made for

Table 7.4.2 Causes of alteration in conscious state

STRUCTURAL INSULTS
Supratentorial
Haematoma
– epidural
– subdural
Cerebral tumour
Cerebral aneurysm
Haemorrhagic CVA
Infratentorial
Cerebellar AVM
Pontine haemorrhage
Brainstem tumour

METABOLIC INSULTS
Loss of substrate
Hypoxia
Hypoglycaemia
Global ischaemia
Shock
– hypovolaemia
– cardiogenic
Focal ischaemia
– TIA/CVA
– vasculitis

Derangement of normal physiology
Hypo or hypernatraemia
Hyperglycaemia/hyperosmolarity
Hypercalcaemia
Hypermagnesaemia
Addisonian crisis
Seizures
– status epilepticus
– post-ictal
Post-concussive
Hypo or hyperthyroidism
Cofactor deficiency
Metastatic malignancy
Psychiatric illness
Toxins
Drugs
– alcohol
– illicit
– prescription
Endotoxins
– subarachnoid blood
– liver failure
– renal failure
Sepsis
– systemic
Focal
– meningitis
– encephalitis
Environmental
– hypothermia/heat exhaustion
– altitude illness/decompression
– envenomations.

routinely administering glucose to any patient with an altered conscious state if bedside glucose estimation is not readily available.[3]

A history of opiate usage combined with the clinical signs of pinpoint pupils and hypoventilation may make the administration of naloxone both diagnostic and therapeutic. Parenterally, 0.2–0.4 mg aliquots can be given to a maximum of 10 mg. The likelihood of serious adverse reactions such as pulmonary oedema is very low.[4] However, in combination overdoses, the negation of the opiate effect may unmask the effects of other toxins including those with pro-convulsant or pro-arrhythmic tendencies. Parenteral administration in uncontrolled situations with a flailing patient is not without its risks to both patient and staff. In particular, there is a risk to staff from needlestick injuries and blood-borne infections. Research is underway into the effectiveness of intranasal administration via atomizer which would eliminate this risk.[5]

The administration of thiamine, 100 mg, is advocated in patients suspected of having hepatic encephalopathy but its effect is rarely immediate and delayed administration will not change the course of the initial resuscitation.[6] The old dogma that thiamine should be withheld until hypoglycaemia is corrected to avoid precipitating Wernicke's encephalopathy is unfounded. The absorption of thiamine is so much slower than that of glucose, timing is irrelevant.

Concern that there might be delay in the recognition of hypoglycaemia, opiate toxicity and hepatic encephalopathy led to the promotion of the routine administration of a so-called 'coma cocktail' to unconscious patients. This consisted of intravenous 50% dextrose, thiamine and naloxone. Its routine use is no longer advocated.[6]

Secondary survey

After initial resuscitation of the patient, it is important to complete the assessment by obtaining a full history, conducting a full examination and performing adjunctive investigations. This will assist in identifying the cause of the condition and planning further management.

History

Obtaining a full history can be difficult as the patient may be confused or obtunded. Details have to be garnered from supplemental sources such as ambulance or police officers, relatives or carers and primary care physicians. Medical records, when obtainable, may provide clues and patients will occasionally carry cards or wear bracelets that alert you to particular conditions.

It is crucial to establish the events leading up to the presentation with specific questioning about prodromal events, ingestions, IV drug usage, trauma, underlying illness, medications, allergies, and associated seizures and abnormal movements. For example, the presence or absence of a headache and its onset and duration would aid in the clinical diagnosis of a subarachnoid haemorrhage and a history of head injury with loss of consciousness would increase the likelihood of an extra-axial intracranial collection. Patients who are taking anticoagulants also have an increased risk of intracranial haemorrhage with minimal trauma.

Examination

A general physical examination, bearing in mind the various differential diagnoses, is the next step. Vital signs may suggest sepsis or other causes of shock. A keen sense of smell might detect fetor hepaticus or the sweet breath of ketosis. Bitter almonds scent is pathognomonic of cyanide poisoning. Of note, alteration of consciousness can be attributed to alcoholic intoxication only by the process of exclusion. Thus, the characteristic odour of alcoholic liquor is indicative but cannot be presumed to be diagnostic.

Neurological examination clearly must be as comprehensive as possible. There are several obstacles to this goal. Initial resuscitation measures such as endotracheal intubation will reduce the ability of the patient to cooperate with the examination and language difficulties will be accentuated as the neurological examination is strongly language oriented. Thus patients who do not share a common language and those with dysphasia may be disadvantaged. Also sensory modalities are difficult to assess in patients with impaired mentation, although deficits are often paralleled by deficits in the motor system.

The primary aims of the neurological examination is to differentiate structural and non-structural causes and to identify groups of signs that may indicate specific diagnoses such as meningitis and to pinpoint the precise location of a structural lesion. Therefore, emphasis needs to be given to signs of trauma, tone, reflexes, papillary findings and eye signs as well as serial estimations of the GCS.

Signs of trauma need to be documented and spinal precautions taken as indicated. Palpation of the soft tissues and bones of the skull may detect deformity or bruising and a haemotympanum may herald a fracture of the base of the skull.

Hypotonia is common in acute neurological deficits. Specific examination of anal sphincter tone will uncover spinal cord compromise and is crucial in trauma patients. An upgoing Babinski response is indicative of pyramidal pathology and asymmetry of the peripheral limb reflexes may help to 'side' a lesion. Conversely, heightened tone in the neck muscles (neck stiffness) may indicate meningitis or subarachnoid haemorrhage.

Pupillary findings and eye signs may also be useful to differentiate metabolic and structural insults and more importantly detect incipient uncal herniation. Intact oculocephalic reflexes and preservation of the 'doll's eyes response' indicates an intact medial longitudinal fasciculus and by default an intact brain stem suggesting a metabolic cause for coma (see Table 7.4.3). There are four pairs of nuclei governing ocular movements and they are spread between the superior and inferior midbrain and the pons. The pattern of ocular movement dysfunction can be used to pinpoint the site of a brainstem lesion (see Table 7.4.4). Likewise, specific testing of the oculovestibular reflex and the cranial nerve examination can be used to precisely locate a brainstem lesion but is of limited use in the emergent setting except as a predictor of herniation (see Table 7.4.3).

More generally, skin examination may reveal needle tracks suggestive of drug use. Mucosal changes such as cyanosis or the cherry red glow of carbon monoxide poisoning can be diagnostic. Cardiac

Table 7.4.3 Ocular responses to cold caloric testing of the oculovestibular reflex

Response	Cerebrum	Medial longitudinal fasciculus	Brainstem
Bilateral nystagmus	Intact	Intact	Intact
Bilateral conjugate deviation towards the stimulus	Metabolic dysfunction	Intact	Intact
No response			Structural or metabolic dysfunction
Ipsilateral dysconjugate deviation			Structural dysfunction

monitoring and cardiovascular examination should identify rhythm disturbances, the murmurs of endocarditis and valvular disease or evidence of shock from myocardial ischaemia or infarction. Respiratory patterns may aid in identifying the site of the lesion (see Table 7.4.4). Abdominal examination may detect organomegaly, ascites, bruits or pulsatile masses.

INVESTIGATIONS

Specific laboratory and radiological investigations must be guided by the history and examination and their timing determined by the priorities of resuscitation.

Haematology

A full blood examination may reveal anaemia, immunocompromise, thrombocytopaenia, inflammation or infection but is rarely specific. CRP and ESR are nonspecific acute phase reactants and single determinants are not initially useful, although they may later be followed to monitor regression of the illness or response to therapy. Coagulation profiles are particularly useful in haematological and liver disease or if patients are taking anticoagulants such as warfarin.

Biochemistry

Serum electrolyte levels aid in the differentiation of the various hypo and hyper-elemental causes of coma. Electrolyte imbalances may also be secondary to the causative insult and may not need specific correction. In hypotensive patients, a high to normal sodium and a low potassium suggests primary or secondary Addisonian crisis.

Liver, renal and thyroid function tests may confirm focal organ dysfunction. The last may not always be readily available but hypothyroidism should be considered in the hypothermic patient and hyperthyroidism in the presence of tremor and tachyarrhythmias.

A serum glucose provides confirmation of bedside testing. Serum lactate determinations may reveal a metabolic acidosis and reflect the degree of tissue hypoxia which may again be primary or secondary. Creatinine kinase and myoglobinuria are useful to determine the presence and extent of rhabdomyolosis and to predict the likelihood of requiring dialysis. Serum and urine osmolarity may be useful in toxic ingestions such as ethylene glycol.

Blood gas analysis may give important information regarding acid-base balance and along with the anion gap and the serum electrolytes can help distinguish between the various types and causes of acidosis and alkalosis. Knowledge of the oxygen and carbon dioxide partial pressures is vital to resuscitative efforts.

Microbiology

Sepsis is a major metabolic cause of conscious state alteration and may present with no localizing symptoms or signs, especially in the elderly. In this case, blood cultures, preferably multiple sets obtained before antibiotic therapy, may be the only means of isolating the causative organism. Naturally system specific specimens such as sputum, urine and cerebrospinal fluid should be collected when clinically indicated. Although as a rule specimens should be

Table 7.4.4 Patterns of dysfunction in various parameters determined by the site of the structural or metabolic insult

	Respirations	Motor response	Pupillary light response	Eye movements
Forebrain	Cheyne-Stokes – waxing and waning	Localizing to pain	Symmetrical, small, reactive Pretectal-symmetrical, large, fixed	
Midbrain	Hyper-ventilation	Decorticate	Fixed	Upper midbrain – CN III palsy Lower midbrain – CN IV deficit – loss of ipsilateral adduction
Pons	Apneusis – halts briefly in full inspiration	Decerebrate	Symmetrical, pinpoint, reactive. Uncal – ipsilateral, fixed, dilated	CN VI deficit – loss of ipsilateral abduction
Medulla	Ataxic irregular rate and uneven depth Apnoeic Bilateral ventrolateral medulla lesions			

obtained prior to therapy, in suspected meningitis or encephalitis, the administration of antibiotics or antiviral agents should not be delayed while a lumbar puncture/computerized tomography (CT) scan is performed.

Specific laboratory testing

Based on information from the history and examination, specific drug assays and urine screens may be indicated. These may include prescribed medications such as lithium or theophylline or drugs of addiction such as amphetamine or opiates. Routine urine drug screens are, however, of very limited value.

Venom detection kits can be utilized in specific clinical situations and evidence of systemic envenomation can be screened for with other tests such as coagulation profiles and creatinine kinase.

Imaging

A chest X-ray may reveal primary infection or malignancy. In a patient with an altered conscious state and any suspicion of trauma, a full cervical spine series is mandatory. Imaging of the rest of the spine and the pelvis should be guided by clinical assessment.

Intracranial imaging is best achieved with a plain CT of the head, which, if normal, may be followed by a contrast enhanced scan or magnetic resonance imaging (MRI). The latter has a higher sensitivity for encephalitis and cerebral vasculitis although it may not always be easily accessible from the emergency department. Also the technical constraints of MRI require a stable patient. Emergent angiography has a role in the delineation of cerebral aneurysms and can provide therapeutic options particularly in a patient who is progressing towards herniation.

Other tests

The 12 lead ECG can highlight tachycardia as well as arrhythmias. Specific changes such as the U wave of hypokalaemia, the J wave of hypothermia and focal infarction and ischaemic patterns may offer pointers to the cause of the coma.

MANAGEMENT

Management is necessarily governed by the assessment and likely diagnoses. Usually assessment and management simultaneously. The algorithm in Figure 7.4.1 is aimed at correcting immediate life-threatening pathology and then identifying and treating reversible structural and metabolic causes.

Following initial resuscitation, it is important to identify patients in whom trauma is known or suspected. These have a higher risk of skull fractures and focal intracranial pathology and are more likely to have increased intracranial pressure requiring urgent imaging and subsequent neurosurgical consultation and definitive management. The same

pathway is required for patients who have a non-traumatic cause for coma but who have lateralizing signs suggesting a focal intracranial lesion. Evidence of brain-stem herniation is a neurosurgical emergency. A CT scan is helpful in diagnosing the cause of cerebral herniation and should be obtained expeditiously. Neurosurgical consultation can be arranged concurrently so as not to impede smooth transit to theatre for those requiring urgent craniotomy. Cerebral resuscitation is continued concurrently, with relative hyperventilation to maintain a $pCO2$ of 30–35 mm Hg. The role of mannitol is still controversial but may be used in consultation with the neurosurgical team. The diuretic effect may, however, add to haemodynamic

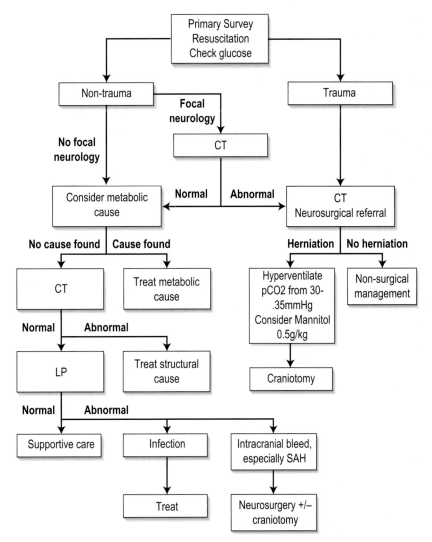

Fig. 7.4.1

compromise and secondary neurological embarrassment.

Should there be no lateralising signs then a metabolic cause needs to be sought. A metabolic screen and, if indicated, a toxicological screen is performed. If a cause is found, it is further specifically investigated and definitively managed. If no cause is identified or suggested on initial or other first-line specific investigation, a CT brain scan is performed. Thereafter, patients with identified causes are stabilized and referred for appropriate continuing care, for example, neurology in the case of cerebravascular incidents, neurosurgery for tumours and extra-axial haemorrhages and medical units for endocrinopathies and infections. Depending on the pathology, prophylactic anticonvulsants and corticosteroids may be considered.

A normal CT scan does not exclude treatable intracranial infection or subarachnoid haemorrhage. Therefore, depending upon the patient's conscious state and the level of clinical suspicion, a lumbar puncture may further assist with diagnosis. However, it must be emphasized that, in suspected intracranial infection, an obtunded patient should be treated empirically with appropriate antiviral agents or antibiotics and the lumbar puncture defered until the risk of herniation is minimized.[7] In the absence of any identifiable cause, supportive care is provided until specific investigation or the natural evolution of the disease process points to the diagnosis.

DISPOSITION

Patients with continuing altered consciousness should be admitted to an inpatient bed in a hospital with the range of services and clinical disciplines to manage the primary diagnosis. The level of care required would depend on the state of the patient on presentation and their subsequent response to treatment.

PROGNOSIS

Discussion of prognosis is difficult as it depends on the cause and patient-specific factors. Effective cerebral resuscitation with optimal oxygenation and minimization of intracerebral hypercarbia and acidosis will promote the best recovery potential while addressing the underlying disease process. Prognosis is naturally dependent on the degree of irreversible cellular damage and the ability to correct the primary insult while minimizing secondary brain injury.

CONTROVERSIES

❶ The utility of the 'coma cocktail' in the undifferentiated patient who presents with an altered conscious state.

❷ The timing of the lumbar puncture in an obtunded patient suspected of a central nervous system infection.

❸ The role of hyperventilation and mannitol in the management of acute elevation in intracranial pressure.

REFERENCES

1. Teasdale G, Jennett B 1974 Assessment of coma and impaired consciouness : a practical scale. Lancet 2(7872): 81–4
2. Teasdale G, Jennett B 1977 Aspects of coma after head injury. Lancet 1(8017): 878–81
3. Hoffman JR, Schriger DL, Votey SR, Luo JS 1992 The empiric use of hypertonic glucose in patients with altered mental status : a reappraisal. Annals of Emergency Medicine 21: 20–4
4. Hoffman JR, Schriger DL, Luo JS 1991 The empiric use of naloxone in patients with altered mental status: A reappraisal. Annals of Emergency Medicine 20: 246–52
5. Kelly AM, Koutsogiannis Z 2002 Intranasal naloxone for life threatening opioid toxicity. Emergency Medicine Journal 19: 375
6. Hoffman DS, Goldfrank LR 1995 The poisoned patient with altered consciousness: controversies in the use of a 'coma cocktail'. Journal of the American Medical Assocation 274: 562–9
7. Hasbun R, Abrahams J, Jekel J, Quagliarello VJ 2001 Computed tomography of the head before lumbar puncture in adults with suspected meningitis. New England Journal of Medicine 345(24): 1727–32

7.5 SEIZURES

GARRY J. WILKES

ESSENTIALS

1 Up to 10% of the population will have at least one seizure in their lifetime, but only 1–3% will develop epilepsy.

2 The management of an acute episode is directed at rapid control of seizures, identification of precipitating factors, and prevention/correction of complications.

3 Investigation of first seizures should be directed by historical and clinical findings. Routine laboratory and radiological investigations are not warranted for uncomplicated first seizures with full recovery.

4 Persistent confusion should not be assumed to be due to a postictal state until other causes are excluded.

5 Benzodiazepines and phenytoin are the principal anticonvulsant agents for acute seizures.

6 Status epilepticus and eclampsia are severe life threats. Management plans for these conditions should be developed in advance.

7 Pseudoseizures are important to distinguish from neurogenic seizures to prevent inadvertent harm to patients and allow appropriate psychotherapy treatment.

8 Management of drug (including alcohol)-related seizures includes measures to decrease drug absorption and enhance elimination. Specific therapy is available for only a few agents. Phenytoin is usually ineffective in the management of alcohol and drug-related seizures.

9 Severe head injuries are associated with an increased incidence of post-traumatic epilepsy, more than half of which will be manifest in the first year. Phenytoin is effective as prophylaxis for the first week only.

10 Patients with epilepsy should be encouraged to have ongoing care.

INTRODUCTION

The terms 'seizure', 'convulsion' and 'fit' are often used interchangeably and incorrectly. A *seizure* is an episode of abnormal neurological function caused by an abnormal electrical discharge of brain neurons. The seizure is also referred to as an *ictus* or the *ictal period*. A *convulsion* is an episode of excessive and abnormal motor activity. Seizures can occur without convulsions and convulsions can be caused by other conditions. The term 'fit' is best avoided in medical terminology, but is a useful term for non-medical personnel.

Seizures are common. It has been estimated that up to 10% of the population will have at least one seizure in their lifetime, and 1–3% of the population will develop epilepsy.[1] A single seizure may be a reaction to an underlying disorder, part of an established epileptic disorder, or an isolated event with no associated pathology. The challenge is rapidly to identify and treat life-threatening conditions as well as to identify benign conditions that require no further investigation or treatment.

The manifestations of epileptic disorders are extremely varied. Two international classifications have been developed: the International Classification of Epileptic Seizures, and the International Classification of Epilepsy and Epileptic Syndromes.[2,3] The International Classification of Epileptic Seizures divides epileptic seizures into two major categories: partial and generalized. Partial epileptic seizures are further classified according to the impairment or the preservation of consciousness into simple partial and complex partial seizures. Either condition may secondarily generalize into tonic-clonic seizures. Generalized seizures can be divided into convulsive and non-convulsive types.

Convulsive seizures are generalized tonic-clonic seizures or *grand mal* seizures. Non-convulsive generalized seizures include absence seizures (previously termed *petit mal* seizures), myoclonic, tonic and atonic seizures. Under the International Classification, epilepsy and epileptic syndromes are initially classified according to their corresponding types of seizures into localization-related and generalized disorders. Each disorder can be further classified according to its relationship to aetiological or predisposing factors into symptomatic, cryptogenic or idiopathic types.[3] Different seizure types are associated with differing aetiological and prognostic factors. The details of the classification systems are not as important in emergency medicine as the concept of recognizing the different seizure types and being aware of the accepted terminology when discussing and referring cases.

Given the high frequency of this condition in emergency departments it is important to have a management strategy formulated in advance. One such approach has been developed by the American College of Emergency Physicians.[4] The four main management concepts are as follows:

- Altered mental state should be thoroughly assessed and not assumed to be due to a postictal state.

tients with known epilepsy who have recovered completely from a typical seizure require little further investigation. If they remain obtunded or have atypical features they must be fully evaluated, e.g biochemical analysis, computerized tomography (CT) scan, etc.

- Patients with epilepsy should be encouraged to seek continuing care.
- Patients at risk of recurrent seizures should be advised about situations of increased personal risk, such as driving, operating power machinery or swimming alone.

FIRST SEIZURES

A generalized convulsion is a dramatic event. Patients and those accompanying them will often be frightened, anxious and concerned, not only for the acute event but for what it may signify. A diagnosis of epilepsy carries important implications. The patient's occupation, social activities, ability to drive a car and long-term health implications may all be profoundly influenced. It is, therefore, vital that the diagnosis is correct and explained fully to the patient and relatives.

The majority of patients will have completed the seizure before arrival in emergency department. Patients still seizing are treated immediately according to the guidelines below for status epilepticus.

The first and most important task is to determine whether a seizure has occurred. As the majority of patients will have returned to normal by the time they are reviewed in the emergency department, the diagnosis is primarily made on history. Patients will not remember seizures other than simple partial seizures, and the reports of witnesses may be unreliable or inconsistent. Generalized seizures are not accompanied by an aura, with the exception of partial seizures. Most seizures last less than 2 minutes, are associated with impaired consciousness, loss of memory for the event, purposeless movements, and a period of postictal confusion. Although witnesses may grossly over-

estimate the seizure duration, prolonged seizures, those occurring in association with a strong emotional event and those with full recall of events should be regarded with suspicion. Similarly, motor activity that is coordinated and not bilateral, such as side-to-side head movements, pelvic thrusting, directed violence and movement that changes in response to external cues, are less likely to be true seizures.

Conditions such as syncope may be accompanied by myoclonic activity and are important to distinguish from true seizures. Migraine, transient ischaemic attacks, hyperventilation episodes and vertigo are all important conditions to consider in the differential diagnosis. Pseudoseizures will be discussed below.

The history, examination and investigation process is aimed at identifying associated conditions and treatable causes of seizures. The aetiology of seizures can be classified into five groups on this basis:

- Acute symptomatic: occurring during an acute illness with a known CNS insult. Causes of this large, important group are listed in Table 7.5.1.

Table 7.5.1 Acute symptomatic causes of seizures
Hypoxia
Hypoglycaemia
Head trauma
Meningitis and encephalitis, including HIV disease
Metabolic, including hyponatraemia, hypocalcaemia, hyperthyroidism, uraemia and eclampsia
Drug overdose, including alcohol, tricyclics, theophylline, cocaine, amphetamine and isoniazid
Drug withdrawal, including alcohol, benzodiazepines, narcotics, cocaine and anticonvulsants
Cerebral tumour or stroke

(Reproduced with permission from Brown AF, Wilkes GJ 1994 Emergency department management of status epilepticus. Emergency Medicine 6: 49–61)

- Remote symptomatic: occurring without provocation in a patient with a prior CNS insult known to be associated with an increased risk of seizures, e.g. encephalopathy, meningitis, head trauma or stroke.
- Progressive encephalopathy: occurring in association with a progressive neurological disease, e.g. neurodegenerative diseases, neurocutaneous syndromes and malignancies not in remission.
- Febrile: patients whose sole provocation is fever. This is almost exclusively confined to children and as such is beyond the scope of this book;
- Idiopathic: patients who present de novo, or during the course of their illness, in the absence of an acute precipitating CNS insult. This is probably the most common group; however, this classification is by exclusion of the other causes.

A careful history is needed to decide whether this is part of an ongoing process or an isolated event. Patients may not recall previous events, may not recognize their significance, or may even avoid reporting previous episodes for fear of being labelled 'epileptic', with the associated consequences. Particular attention should be paid to any history of unexplained injuries, especially when occurring during blackouts or during sleep. Any history of childhood seizures, isolated myoclonic jerks and a positive family history increases the likelihood of epilepsy.

A complete physical and neurological examination is mandatory. Evidence of drug ingestion and head trauma is particularly important. A careful mental state examination in seemingly alert patients may reveal evidence of a resolving post-ictal state or of underlying encephalopathy. All patients not fully alert should not be assumed to simply be in a postictal state until other causes are excluded. Of particular importance is any evidence of underlying illness, such as fever, nuchal rigidity (meningitis) or cardiac murmurs (endocarditis). Needle tracks, evidence of chronic liver disease, dysmorphic features and marks such as *café-au-lait* spots (neurofibromatosis) are important aetiological clues. Complications such as tongue biting, broken teeth and peripheral injuries are common in generalized seizures. Stress fractures can occur, particularly in the elderly, and posterior dislocation of the shoulder is an uncommon, but significant and easily overlooked finding.

The investigations necessary following an uncomplicated seizure are minimal. Although it is common practice to order a variety of tests, such as electrolytes, blood sugar level and full blood counts, these are rarely of benefit in the fully recovered patient. Although abnormalities may cause seizures they are unlikely to be the cause if the patient has recovered. A serum prolactin level at 20 and 60 minutes post seizure may be helpful if the diagnosis is in doubt. Patients with abnormal physical or neurological examination should be managed according to clinical findings and the results of laboratory and radiological investigations. Findings suggestive of meningitis, encephalitis or subarachnoid haemorrhage are indications for cranial CT scan and lumbar puncture.

There are no clear guidelines to the routine need for or urgency of neuroimaging following a single uncomplicated seizure. Patients with focal neurological signs, those who do not recover to a normal examination, and those with a history of head trauma or intracranial pathology should all undergo cranial CT as soon as possible. The dilemma arises for patients with complete recovery and no focal signs. The incidence of abnormalities on CT in this group of patients is less than 1%.[5] The decision as to whether and when to scan patients in this group will be determined largely by local factors. Generally, a contrast CT (more sensitive for subtle lesions) is performed on an outpatient basis prior to review. MRI is more sensitive than CT for infarcts, tumours, inflammatory lesions and vascular lesions, but cost and availability limit its use as a primary investigative modality.

Electroencephalography (EEG) at the time of a seizure will make a definitive diagnosis. It is not usually performed in the acute setting except when nonconvulsive activity is suspected. Typically, an EEG is obtained electively on an outpatient basis, when it may still indicate an underlying focus of activity and may be able to detect specific conditions.

Once a diagnosis of first seizure is made and intercurrent conditions are excluded or treated, the patient may be discharged home. In most cases no treatment is needed. It must be stressed to the patient that a diagnosis of epilepsy has not been made but is being considered. When the suspicion is reasonable the patient should be given the same precautionary advice as epileptic patients with regard to driving and other activities that may place them or others at risk.

The planning of investigation and follow-up for patients suspected of having a first seizure is best done in conjunction with a neurology service. Planning and consultation will ensure that appropriate investigations are completed in a timely fashion. Generally, an interictal EEG and contrast CT are completed prior to review.

STATUS EPILEPTICUS

Status epilepticus (SE) may be defined as 'two or more seizures without full recovery of consciousness between seizures, or recurrent epileptic seizures for more than 30 minutes'.[6]

Status epilepticus accounts for 1–8% of all hospital admissions for epilepsy, 3.5% of admissions to neurological intensive care, and 0.13% of all visits to a university hospital emergency department. SE is more common at the extremes of age, with over 50% of all cases occurring in children and a disproportionately high incidence in those over 60 years of age. SE is also more frequent in the mentally handicapped and in those with structural cerebral pathology, especially of the frontal lobes. Four to 16% of adults and 10–25% of children with known epilepsy will have at least one episode of SE. However, SE occurs most commonly in patients with no previous history of epilepsy.[7]

Many compensatory physiological changes accompany seizures. As the duration is increased these mechanisms begin to fail, with an increased risk of permanent damage. There is mounting evidence that brain damage resulting from prolonged SE is in part caused by excitatory amino acid neurotransmitters such as glutamate and aspartate. These lead to an influx of calcium into neuronal cytoplasm and an osmotolysis with cell destruction. Continuing seizure activity itself contributes substantially to neuronal damage, which is further exacerbated by hypoxia, hypoglycaemia, lactic acidosis and hyperpyrexia. When seizures continue for over 60 minutes, the risk of neuronal injury increases despite optimal delivery of oxygen and glucose. The longer an episode of SE continues, the more refractory to treatment it becomes, and the more likely it is to result in permanent neuronal damage. Mortality increases from 2.7% with seizure duration under 1 hour, to 32% with seizure duration beyond this.[8] Generalized convulsive SE is, therefore, a medical emergency.

Treatment of SE is along the same lines as the resuscitation of all seriously ill patients. Management is in a resuscitation area with attention to four specific factors:

- Rapid stabilization of airway, breathing and circulation.
- Termination of seizure activity (clinical and electrical).
- Identification and treatment of precipitating and perpetuating factors.
- Identification and treatment of complications.

Each stage of resuscitation is made more difficult by the presence of active convulsions. No attempt should be made to prise clenched teeth apart to insert an oral airway: a soft nasal airway will suffice. Oxygen should be given by tight-fitting mask and the patient positioned in the left lateral position to minimize the risk of aspiration. IV access is important for drug treatment and fluid resuscitation, but may be difficult in actively seizing patients. Although SE cannot be diagnosed until seizures have persisted for 30 minutes, patients still seizing on arrival at emergency department should be treated with anticonvulsants immediately.

The principal pharmacological agents used are benzodiazepines and phenytoin. The particular benzodiazepine varies between countries, with little clinical evidence to support any particular one. In some Australasian centres midazolam is the preferred agent, in increments of 1–2 mg IV. If IV access cannot be rapidly secured, midazolam IM at a dose of 0.2 mg/kg will terminate most seizures.[8] Alternatives to midazolam are diazepam and clonazepam. Diazepam can be administered rectally if necessary, and this technique can be taught to parents with high-risk children. However, onset of action by this route in adults is slow and unpredictable. All benzodiazepines share the disadvantages of respiratory depression, hypotension and a short duration of clinical effect.

Phenytoin is usually used as a second-line agent (occasionally as a first-line agent) in a dose of 15–20 mg/kg at a rate of no more than 50 mg/min. Rapid administration is associated with brady-arrhythmias and hypotension. The common practice of administering 1 g is inadequate for most adults. Phenytoin does not commence its effect until 40% of the dose has been administered; for this reason it should be commenced at the same time that IV benzodiazepines are given. Most people on anticonvulsants who present in SE have negligible drug levels and the side effects from a full loading dose on top of a therapeutic level are minimal. The full loading dose should, therefore, be given even when the patient is known to be on therapy.[9]

The most common causes of failure to control seizures are:

- Inadequate antiepileptic drug therapy.
- Failure to initiate maintenance antiepileptic drug therapy.
- Hypoxia, hypotension, cardiorespiratory failure, metabolic disturbance, e.g. hypoglycaemia.
- Failure to identify an underlying cause.
- Failure to recognize medical complications, e.g. hyperpyrexia, hypoglycaemia.
- Misdiagnosis of pseudoseizures.

Causes of failure to regain consciousness following treatment of seizures include the medical consequences of SE (hypoxia, hypoglycaemia, cerebral oedema, hypotension, hyperpyrexia), sedation from antiepileptic medication, progression of the underlying disease process, non-convulsive SE and subtle generalized SE.

When benzodiazepines and phenytoin are ineffective, expert advice should be sought. Drugs that may be used in the control of SE are summarized in Table 7.5.2. Inhalational or barbiturate anaesthesia can also be used. Both require expert airway control and, in some cases, inotropic support. Management in an intensive care unit is advised.

For all patients with SE, early consultation with intensive care and neurology services is essential in planning definitive management and disposition.

NON-CONVULSIVE SEIZURES

Not all seizures are associated with convulsive activity. Convulsive seizures are generally easy to recognize, whereas non-convulsive seizures are more subtle and often require a high index of suspicion. These types of seizure are an important cause of alterations in behaviour and conscious level, and may precede or follow convulsive episodes. Seizures can involve any of the sensory modalities, vertiginous episodes, automatism, autonomic dysfunction or psychic disturbances, including *déjà vu* and *jamais vu* experiences. Non-convulsive seizures can easily be confused with migraine, cerebrovascular events or psychiatric conditions. The definitive diagnosis can only be made by EEG during the event.

Non-convulsive seizures may be partial (focal) or generalized. Complex partial seizures and focal seizures account for approximately one-third of all seizures, whereas primary generalized non-convulsive seizures (absence seizures) account for 6% of seizures.[10]

Non-convulsive status epilepticus (NCS) accounts for at least 25% of all cases of SE and is diagnosed more frequently when actively considered.[11] Absence seizures rarely result in complete unresponsiveness and patients may appear relatively normal to unfamiliar observers. NCS may precede or

Table 7.5.2 Doses of drugs used in refractory SE

Drug	Bolus (i.v. unless stated otherwise)	Maintenance Infusion
Midazolam	0.02–0.1mg/kg IV 0.15–0.3mg/kg IM	0.05–0.4mg/kg/hour
Phenytoin	15–20mg/kg at up to 50mg/minute, followed by further 5mg/kg	N/A
Phenobarbitone	10–20mg/kg at 60–100mg/minute	1–4mg/kg/day
Thiopentone	5mg/kg	1–3mg/kg/hour
Pentobarbitone (USA only)	5mg/kg at 25mg/minute	0.5–3mg/kg/hour
Propofol	2mg/kg	5–10mg/kg/hour
Lidocaine	2mg/kg	3–6mg/kg/hour
Chlormethiazole	0.8% solution, 40–100mL over 10 minute	0.8% solution 0.5–4mL/minute
Paraldehyde	0.15mL/kg im or 0.3–0.5mL/kg rectally diluted 1:1 with vegetable oil	

(Modified with permission from Brown AF, Wilkes GJ 1994 Emergency department management of status epilepticus. Emergency Medicine 6: 49–61)

follow convulsive seizures and may easily create the perception of a cerebral vascular or psychiatric event. The longest reported episode of absence status is 60 days, and that of complex partial status 28 days.[11]

Treatment of non-convulsive seizures in the acute setting is the same as for convulsive seizures. The event is terminated with benzodiazepines in most instances, and should be followed by a search for precipitating causes. An estimated 50% of patients with simple partial seizures have abnormal CT scans.[11] Long-term seizure control is with different agents from those used for convulsive seizures, highlighting the importance of involvement of a neurological service in planning follow-up.

PSEUDOSEIZURES

Pseudoseizures or psychogenic seizures are events simulating neurogenic seizures but without the accompanying abnormal neuronal activity. Differentiation from neurogenic seizures may be extremely difficult, even for experienced neurologists. Neurogenic and psychogenic seizures may coexist, making the diagnostic dilemma even more complex. Differentiation will often require video-EEG monitoring. In the emergency department this facility is not available and other methods must be used. It is important to recognize pseudoseizures so as to prevent the possible iatrogenic consequences of unnecessary treatment, while at the same time not withholding treatment from patients with neurogenic seizures.

Pseudoseizures are more common in women, less common after 35 years of age, and rare in patients aged over 50.[12] They may be associated with a conversion disorder, malingering, Munchausen syndrome or Munchausen syndrome by proxy. Patients with conversion disorder differ from malingerers by being unaware of the psychiatric cause of their actions.

Pseudoseizures typically last more than 5 minutes, compared to neurogenic seizures that usually terminate within 1 minute. Multiple patterns of seizures tend to occur in individual patients and postictal periods are either very brief or absent. Patients with recall of events during what appears to be a generalized convulsive seizure are likely to have had a psychogenic seizure. Extremity movement out of phase from one side to the other and head turning from side to side typify pseudoseizures. Forward pelvic thrusting occurs in 44% of patients with pseudoseizures and is highly suggestive of the diagnosis.[13]

Several manoeuvres are useful in identifying pseudoseizures. Eye opening and arm drop tests are accompanied by avoidance, eyes turning away from the moving examiner, and termination of the event when the mouth and nostrils are occluded are characteristic. Simple verbal suggestion and reassurance are also frequently successful.

The most definitive means of differentiating pseudoseizures is by ictal EEG or video-EEG monitoring. Unfortunately, this is of little value in the emergency department. Blood gas determinations demonstrate a degree of acidaemia in neurogenic tonic-clonic seizures, and not in patients with pseudoseizures. Pulse oximetry will detect a fall in SaO_2 during neurogenic but not pseudoseizures. Serum prolactin levels rise and peak 15–20 minutes after generalized tonic-clonic seizures, and then fall with a half life of 22 minutes. The levels do not consistently rise with partial seizures, and remain normal with pseudoseizures.[14]

Patients presenting with pseudoseizures are often treated with anticonvulsant medications both acutely and for maintenance. Such patients usually demonstrate resistance to anticonvulsant medication: many will, therefore, present with therapeutic or supratherapeutic levels. It is difficult to resist the temptation to immediately administer pharmacotherapy when confronted with a convulsing patient, but to do so will result in patients with pseudoseizures receiving unnecessary and potential harmful treatment.

Careful examination of eye movements, pupil reactions, asynchronous limb movements, rapid head turning from side to side, forward pelvic thrust movements, testing for avoidance manoeuvres and monitoring pulse oximetry may enable the diagnosis to be made and drug therapy avoided. In doubtful cases, blood gas determinations are helpful and serum prolactin levels can be collected for later analysis. Doubtful cases should be discussed with a neurology service and arrangements made for emergency EEG.

Once the diagnosis is confirmed it must be presented in an open and non-threatening manner. Patients often have underlying personal and/or family problems that will need to be addressed. Psychotherapy is effective, but seizures often relapse at times of stress.

ALCOHOL-RELATED SEIZURES

Seizures represent 0.7% of emergency department visits and alcohol contributes to 50% of these.[15] A study of 200 seizure visits to an urban community emergency department found that alcohol abuse was a significant factor in 41% of patients over the age of 18.[16] The majority of alcohol-related seizures occur as part of the alcohol withdrawal syndrome.

Although the precise pathophysiology of alcohol-related seizures has not been elucidated, it is clear that alcohol is a direct CNS toxin with direct epileptogenic effects. Acute toxicity and withdrawal are both associated with an increased incidence of seizures. Alcohol intoxication and chronic alcohol abuse are also associated with increased incidences of intercurrent disease, such as trauma, coagulopathy, falls, assaults and other drug intoxication, all of which further increase the likelihood of seizures. The management of seizures presumed to be alcohol related must include a search for associated disease and other causes.

Benzodiazepines are the principal anticonvulsant agent for acute seizures. These agents are also valuable in the treatment of withdrawal. Phenytoin is ineffective in the control of acute seizures or as a preventative.

DRUG-RELATED SEIZURES

Seizure activity in the setting of acute drug overdose is an ominous sign associated with greatly increased mortality and morbidity. The most commonly reported are in association with cyclic antidepressants (CA), antihistamines, theophylline, isoniazid, and drugs of addiction such as cocaine and amphetamines. The diagnosis and management of these toxic syndromes are discussed in the section on toxicology.

POST-TRAUMATIC SEIZURES

Post-traumatic epilepsy develops in 10–15% of serious head injury survivors.[17] More than half will have their first seizure within 1 year. Significant risk factors are central parietal injury, dural penetration, hemiplegia, missile wounds and intracerebral haematomas.[18] Early treatment with phenytoin for severe head injuries decreases the incidence of seizures in the first week only.[19]

Seizures developing after significant head trauma have a higher incidence of intracranial pathology. Contrast CT is the initial investigation of choice. MRI will demonstrate more abnormalities but has not been shown to affect outcome. Long-term treatment with anticonvulsants should be planned in conjunction with a neurosurgical service.

SEIZURES AND PREGNANCY

Seizures can occur during pregnancy as part of an established epileptic process, as new seizures, or induced by pregnancy. The most significant situations are eclampsia and generalized convulsive status epilepticus. At all times the management is directed at both mother and baby, with the realization that the best treatment for the baby will relate to optimized maternal care.

In previously diagnosed epileptics there is an increased risk of seizures during pregnancy of 17%.[20] Anticonvulsant levels are influenced by decreased protein binding, increased drug binding and decreased absorption of varying degrees. The final effect on free drug levels is unpredictable and is most variable around the time of delivery.[21] Careful clinical monitoring is essential, and monitoring of free drug levels rather than total serum levels may be necessary in selected patients. Anticonvulsants also interfere with the metabolism of vitamins D, K and folic acid. Supplementation is advisable.

Isolated simple seizures place both mother and fetus at increased danger of injury, but are otherwise generally well tolerated. Generalized seizures during labour cause transient fetal hypoxia and bradycardia of uncertain significance. Generalized convulsive SE is life-threatening to both mother and fetus at any stage of pregnancy.

All of the anticonvulsants cross the placenta and are potentially teratogenic. The risk of malformation in children of epileptic mothers is increased from 3.4% in the general population to 3.7%.[22] In general, the types of malformations associated are not drug specific, apart from the increased risk of neural tube defects associated with valproate and carbamazepine. Prenatal screening for such defects is advised in patients becoming pregnant while taking these agents. The risk from uncontrolled seizures greatly outweighs the risk from prophylactic medication in patients with good seizure control.[23]

The management of seizures in pregnant patients is along the same lines as for non-pregnant patients. After 20 weeks' gestation the patient should have a wedge placed under the right hip to prevent supine hypotension, and eclampsia must be considered (see below). Investigation will include an assessment of fetal well-being by heart rate, ultrasound and/ or tocography, as indicated. Management and disposition should be decided in consultation with neurology and obstetric services.

Eclampsia is the occurrence of seizures in patients with pregnancy-induced toxaemia occurring after the 20th week of pregnancy, consisting of a triad of hypertension, oedema and proteinuria. One in 300 women with pre-eclampsia progresses to eclampsia. Seizures are typically brief, self-terminating, usually preceded by headache and visual disturbances, and tend to occur without warning.[24] Treatment is directed at controlling the seizures and hypertension and expedient delivery of the baby. Magnesium sulphate is effective in seizure control and is associated with a better outcome for both mother and baby than standard anticonvulsant and antihypertensive therapy.[25–28] The mechanism of action is unclear.

Management of SE in pregnancy includes consideration of eclampsia, positioning in the left lateral position, and assessment and monitoring of fetal well-being. Urgent control of seizures is essential for both mother and baby. Phenobarbital may reduce the incidence of intraventricular haemorrhage in premature infants, and should be considered in place of phenytoin in this circumstance.[29] Early involvement of obstetric and neurology services is essential.

FUTURE DIRECTIONS

Non-invasive portable modalities allowing definitive precise diagnosis of seizures in the emergency department will decrease the need for subsequent investigations in the majority of patients who do not have true epilepsy, and permit early focused therapy. Advances in pharmacotherapy and neurosurgical techniques will also improve seizure control with minimal side-effects, allowing patients to more effectively resume normal activities.

CONTROVERSIES

❶ Investigation required for patients with first seizures.

❷ Place of lumbar puncture in the investigation of first seizures.

❸ Role of antipyretics in febrile seizures.

REFERENCES

1. Engel J Jr, Starkman S 1994 Overview of seizures. Emergency Medicine Clinics of North America 12(4): 895–923

2. Mosewich RK, So EL 1996 A clinical approach to the classification of seizures and epileptic syndromes [see Comments]. Mayo Clinic Proceedings 71(4): 405–14

3. So EL 1995 Classifications and epidemiologic considerations of epileptic seizures and epilepsy. Neuroimaging Clinics of North America 5(4): 513–26

4. American College of Emergency Physicians 1993 Clinical policy for the initial approach to patients presenting with a chief complaint of seizure, who are not in status epilepticus. Annals of Emergency Medicine 22(5): 875–83

5. Reinus WR, Wippold FJD, Erickson KK 1993 Seizure patient selection for emergency computed tomography. Annals of Emergency Medicine 22(8): 1298–303

6. Treiman DM 1995 Electroclinical features of status epilepticus. Journal of Clinical Neurophysiology 12(4): 343–62

7. Brown AF, Wilkes GJ 1994 Emergency department management of status epilepticus. Emergency Medicine 6: 49–61

8. McDonagh TJ, Jelinek GA, Galvin GM 1992 Intramuscular midazolam rapidly terminates seizures in children and adults. Emergency Medicine (4): 77–81

9. Lowenstein DH, Alldredge BK 1998 Status epilepticus. New England Journal of Medicine 338(14): 970–6

10. Hauser WA, Annegers JF, Kurland LT 1993 Incidence of epilepsy and unprovoked seizures in Rochester, Minnesota: 1935–1984. Epilepsia 34(3): 453–68

11. Jagoda A 1994 Nonconvulsive seizures. Emergency Medical Clinics of North America 12(4): 963–71

12. Riggio S 1994 Psychogenic seizures. Emergency Medicine Clinics of North America 12(4): 1001–12

13. Gates JR, Ramani V, Whalen S, Loewenson R 1985 Ictal characteristics of pseudoseizures. Archives of Neurology 42(12): 1183–7

14. Dana-Haeri J, Trimble MR 1984 Prolactin and gonadotrophin changes following partial seizures in epileptic patients with and without psychopathology. Biology Psychiatry 19(3): 329–36

15. Morris JC, Victor M 1987 Alcohol withdrawal seizures. Emergency Medicine Clinics of North America 5(4): 827–39

16. Krumholz A, Grufferman S, Orr ST, Stern BJ 1989 Seizures and seizure care in an emergency department. Epilepsia 30(2): 175–81

17. Dugan EM, Howell JM 1994 Posttraumatic seizures. Emergency Medicine Clinics of North America 12(4): 1081–7

18. Feeney DM, Walker AE 1979 The prediction of posttraumatic epilepsy. A mathematical approach. Archives of Neurology 36(1): 8–12

19. Temkin NR, Haglund MM, Winn HR 1995 Causes, prevention, and treatment of post-traumatic epilepsy. New Horizons 3(3): 518–22

20. Shuster EA 1994 Seizures in pregnancy. Emergency Medicine Clinics of North America 12(4): 1013–25

21. Yerby MS, Friel PN, McCormick K 1992 Antiepileptic drug disposition during pregnancy. Neurology 42(4 Suppl 5): 12–6

22. Stanley FJ, Priscott PK, Johnston R, Brooks B, Bower C 1985 Congenital malformations in infants of mothers with diabetes and epilepsy in Western Australia, 1980-1982. Medical Journal of Australia 143(10): 440–2

23. Yerby MS 1992 Risks of pregnancy in women with epilepsy. Epilepsia 33(Suppl 1): S23–26; discussion S26–27

24. Sibai BM 1991 Medical disorders in pregnancy, including hypertensive diseases. Current Opinion in Obstetrics and Gynaecology 3(1): 28–40

25. The Eclampsia Trial Collaborative Group 1995 Which anticonvulsant for women with eclampsia? Evidence from the Collaborative Eclampsia Trial [published erratum appears in Lancet 346(8969): 258]. Lancet 345(8963): 1455–63

26. Lucas MJ, Leveno KJ, Cunningham FG 1995 A comparison of magnesium sulfate with phenytoin for the prevention of eclampsia [see Comments]. New England Journal of Medicine 333(4): 201–5

27. Duggan K, Macdonald G 1997 Comparative study of different anticonvulsants in eclampsia. Journal of Obstetric and Gynaecological Research 23(3): 289–93

28. Jagoda A, Riggio S 1991 Emergency department approach to managing seizures in pregnancy. Annals of Emergency Medicine 20(1): 80–5

29. Morales WJ 1991 Antenatal therapy to minimize neonatal intraventricular hemorrhage. Clinical Obstetrics and Gynaecology 34(2): 328–35

SECTION

8

EDITED BY PETER CAMERON

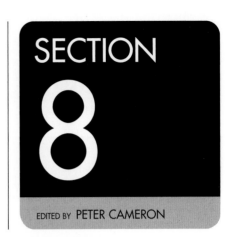

INFECTIOUS DISEASES

8.1 Approach to undifferentiated fever in adults 380

8.2 Meningitis 386

8.3 Septic arthritis 392

8.4 Osteomyelitis 394

8.5 Urinary-tract infection 396

8.6 Skin and soft-tissue infections 403

8.7 Hepatitis 410

8.8 HIV/AIDS 417

8.9 Antibiotics in the emergency department 424

8.10 Needlestick injuries 434

8.1 APPROACH TO UNDIFFERENTIATED FEVER IN ADULTS

ALLEN YUNG • JONATHAN KNOTT

ESSENTIALS

1 The first step in managing any febrile patient is to identify those patients in need of immediate resuscitation, urgent investigations and empirical therapy.

2 Over one-third of patients who have fever for more than a few days with no localizing symptoms and signs are likely to have a bacterial infection; half of these will be in the respiratory or urinary tracts.

3 An unexplained fever in a person over the age of 50 years should be regarded as due to a bacterial infection until proven otherwise.

4 An undifferentiated fever in an alcoholic patient, an intravenous drug user or an insulin-dependent diabetic patient is generally an indication for admission to hospital.

5 Any fever in a returned traveller from a malaria-endemic area should be regarded as due to malaria until proven otherwise.

6 Severe muscle pain, even in the absence of overt fever, may be an early symptom of meningococcaemia, staphylococcal or streptococcal bacteraemia.

7 An unexplained rash in a febrile patient should be regarded as meningococcaemia until proven otherwise.

8 The diagnosis of meningococcaemia should be considered in every patient with an undifferentiated fever.

9 Because there will always be some patients with unrecognized sepsis due to non-specific symptoms and a non-toxic appearance, all patients must be encouraged to seek review if they have any clinical deterioration.

INTRODUCTION

Fever is a common presenting symptom to the emergency department; about 5% of patients seen in an emergency department give fever as the reason for their visit. Most patients with fever have symptoms and signs that indicate the site or region of infection. A prospective study of patients aged 16 years or older who presented to an emergency department with fever greater than or equal to 37.9°C found that 85% of the patients had localizing symptoms and signs that suggested or identified a source of fever and only 15% had unexplained fever after the history and examination.[1]

Fever with no localizing symptoms or signs on presentation is often seen in the first day or two of the illness. Many patients with such a problem will ultimately prove to have self-limiting viral infections, but others will have non-viral infections requiring treatment. Among this latter group are illnesses that may be serious and even rapidly fatal.

Over one-third of patients who have fever for more than a few days with no localizing symptoms and signs are likely to have a bacterial infection.[1,2]

If no cause of fever is found in an adult with fever present for over 3 days there is a good chance the patient will have a bacterial infection that needs treatment.

Over half of these infections are likely to be in the respiratory or urinary tracts.[1]

The most important task in the emergency department for febrile patients without localizing features is not to miss early bacteraemia (especially meningococcal), bacterial meningitis or staphylococcal and streptococcal toxic-shock syndromes.

APPROACH

Management of febrile patients varies according to the severity, duration, rate of illness onset, patient characteristics and epidemiological settings. Although the steps in management of a febrile patient in the emergency department, listed below, may be set out in a sequential manner, in reality the mental processes involved occur simultaneously by the bedside.

- Step 1: Identify the very ill.
- Step 2: Find localizing symptoms and signs.
- Step 3: Look for 'at risk' patients.

Step 1: Identify the seriously ill who requires urgent intervention (Table 8.1.1)

The first step in managing any febrile patient is to identify those patients in need of immediate resuscitation, urgent

Table 8.1.1 Seriously ill patients requiring urgent intervention
Shock
Coma or stupor
Cyanosis
Profound dyspnoea
Continuous seizures
Severe dehydration.

investigations and empirical therapy. The presence of any of the following features justifies immediate intervention: shock, coma/stupor, cyanosis, profound dyspnoea, continuous seizures or severe dehydration.

Step 2: Identify those with localized infections or easily diagnosable diseases

Having excluded those who need urgent intervention, the doctor has more time to consider a diagnosis. The history and physical examination are usually sufficient to localize the source of community-acquired fever in most patients, especially if the illness has been present for several days.

HISTORY

A precise history remains the key to diagnosis of a febrile illness. An inability to give a history and to think clearly is a sign of potential sepsis.

Illness

An abrupt onset of fever, particularly when accompanied by chills or rigors and generalized aches, is highly suggestive of an infective illness.

Localizing symptoms, their evolution and relative severity helps to identify the site of infection; localized pain is particularly valuable in this way.

The severity and the course of the illness can be assessed by the patient's ability to work, to be up and about, to eat and sleep, and the amount of analgesics taken.

Previous state of health

Underlying diseases predispose patients to infections of certain sites or caused by certain specific organisms. Knowledge of any defects in the immune system is similarly helpful. For example, asplenic patients are more prone to overwhelming pneumococcal septicaemia and renal transplant patients to listeria meningitis.

Any past history of infectious diseases may be useful in excluding infections such as measles and hepatitis.

Predisposing events

Recent operations, accidents and injuries or medications may be the direct cause of the illness (e.g. drug fever or rash from co-trimoxazole, ampicillin) or may affect the resistance of the patient predisposing to certain infections. Concurrent menstruation raises the possibility of toxic-shock syndrome.

Epidemiology

Information on occupation, exposure to animals, hobbies, risk factors for blood borne viruses, and travel overseas or to rural areas may suggest certain specific infections, e.g. leptospirosis, acute HIV infection, hepatitis C and malaria.

Contact with similar diseases and known infectious diseases

This information is useful in the diagnosis of problems such as meningococcal infection, viral exanthema, respiratory infection, diarrhoea, and zoonosis.

EXAMINATION

Physical examination in the febrile patient serves two purposes: to assess the severity of the illness and to find a site of infection.

Bedside assessment of severity and 'toxicity' based on intuitive judgement is frequently wrong, and many patients with severe bacterial infections do not appear obviously ill or toxic.

Physical examination may yield a diagnosis in a febrile patient who has not complained of any localizing symptoms. A checklist of special areas to be examined is useful (Table 8.1.2):

- Marked muscle tenderness is a frequent sign of sepsis.
- Skin: rashes of any sort, especially petechial rash; cellulitis in the lower legs may present with fever and constitutional symptoms before pain in the leg develops. Evidence of intravenous drug use should be sought at the common injection sites.
- Lymph nodes: especially the posterior cervical glands. Tenderness

Table 8.1.2 Clinical pointers: non-specific clinical features ('alarm bells')
Severe pain in muscles, neck or back
Impairment of conscious state
Vomiting especially in association with headache or abdominal pain
Severe headache in the presence of a normal CSF
Unexplained rash
Jaundice
Severe sore throat or dysphagia with a normal looking throat
Repeated rigors

of the jugulo-digastric glands is a good sign of bacterial tonsillitis.
- Heart: murmurs and pericardial rubs
- Lungs: subtle crackles may be heard in pneumonic patients without respiratory symptoms.
- Abdominal organs: tenderness and enlargement without subjective pain may be the only clue to infections in those organs.
- Eyes: conjunctival haemorrhages are seen in staphylococcal endocarditis, and scleral jaundice may be present before cutaneous jaundice is obvious. Neck stiffness may be a clue to meningitis in a confused patient who cannot give a history.
- Sore throat may be absent in the first few hours of streptococcal tonsillitis. Examination of the throat may give the diagnosis. Oedema of the uvula is also a useful sign of bacterial infection in that region.
- Any area that is covered, e.g. under plasters or bandages for evidence of sepsis.

There are two caveats when assessing local symptoms and signs:

❶ Localizing features may not be present or obvious early in the course of a focal infection, e.g. the absence of cough in bacterial pneumonia, sore throat in tonsillitis or diarrhoea in gastrointestinal infections in the first 12–36 hours of the illness.

❷ Localizing features may occasionally be misleading. For example, diarrhoea, which suggests infection of the gastrointestinal tract, may be a manifestation of more generalized infection such as Gram-negative septicaemia and crepitations at the lung base may indicate a sub-diaphragmatic condition rather than a chest infection.

Step 3: Look for the 'at risk' patients

If no diagnosis is forthcoming after the first two steps, the next task is to identify the 'at risk' patient who may not appear overtly ill, but who, nonetheless, requires medical intervention. This applies particularly to those with treatable diseases that can progress rapidly such as bacterial meningitis, bacteraemia and toxic-shock syndromes.

Four sets of pointers are helpful in identifying these 'at risk' patients: the type of patients (host characteristics), exposure history, the nature of the non-specific symptoms and how rapidly the illness evolves.

Clinical pointers: type of patient

Clinical manifestations of infections are often subtle or non-specific in elderly and immunocompromised patients. The threshold for intervention in these patients should be lowered.

Elderly patients Elderly patients with infections often do not mount much of a febrile response and fever may be absent in 20–30% of elderly patients with a serious infection.[3]

Infectious diseases in the elderly often present with non-specific or atypical symptoms and signs that may rapidly progress.[4]

In patients with unexplained fever, up to one-third may have bacteraemia or focal bacterial infection. This proportion is even higher in those over the age of 50 years.[1] In the elderly, a fever higher than 38°C indicates a possible serious infection[5] and is associated with increasing risk of death.[6]

The urinary tract is the most frequent site of infection and source of bacteraemia; symptoms of urinary-tract infection are frequently absent in the elderly. The respiratory tract is the next most common site of infection; fever and malaise may be the only clues of pneumonia in the elderly. Urinalysis and chest X-ray will identify about half of the occult infections.[1]

An unexplained fever in a person over the age of 50 should be regarded as being caused by a bacterial infection until proved otherwise, and is generally an indication for admission to hospital.

Alcoholic patients Alcoholic patients present with multiple problems, many of which cause fever. Most are caused by infections, the commonest of which is pneumonia. Multiple infections may occur at the same time.[7]

Non-infectious causes of fever frequently co-exist with infections-conditions such as subarachnoid haemorrhage, alcoholic withdrawal and alcoholic hepatitis require admission.

The initial history and physical examination in the alcoholic may be unreliable and diagnosis may be difficult.

Alcoholic patients with fever for which no obvious cause is found should be admitted to the hospital for investigations and observation.

Injecting drug users The risk of acquiring serious or unusual infections in injecting drug users is high through repeated self injections with non-sterile, illicit substances; the use of contaminated needles and syringes; and poor attention to skin cleaning prior to injections.[8]

Most intravenous drug users presenting with fever have a serious infection. Some have obvious focal infections such as cellulitis and pneumonia. Others present simply with fever and the presence of bacteraemia and endocarditis must be suspected.

Clinical assessment cannot differentiate trivial from potentially serious conditions in these patients.[8] A history of chills, rigors and sweats strongly suggest the presence of a transient or ongoing bacteraemia. Back pain may be a subtle

symptom of endocarditis or vertebral osteomyelitis.

It is difficult to distinguish the patient with endocarditis from other drug users with fever due to another cause. Hospitalization of febrile injecting drug users is prudent if 24-hour follow-up is not possible. Intravenous drug use in the previous 5 days is a predictor of occult major infection, and is an indication for admission to hospital.[9]

Patients with diabetes mellitus Diabetic patients are more prone to developing certain bacterial infections.[1] A diabetic patient with an unexplained fever is more likely to have an occult bacterial infection than a non-diabetic patient. In general, an insulin-dependent diabetic patient, especially if over the age of 50 years, with fever and no obvious source of infection should be investigated and preferably admitted.

Febrile neutropenic patients Febrile neutropenic patients (absolute neutrophil count <500/mL, or <1000/mL and falling rapidly) must be hospitalized for intravenous antibiotics regardless of their clinical appearance. Infections may become fulminant within hours in these patients and the clinical manifestations of their infective illnesses are frequently modified by the underlying disease, therapy received and co-existing problems.

Splenectomized patients Splenectomized patients with fever must be very carefully assessed because of their increased risk of overwhelming bacterial infection. If the fever cannot be readily explained, admission for intravenous antibiotics is usually indicated.

Other immunocompromised patients Fever in transplant patients (renal, hepatic or cardiac) and those with HIV infection is not an absolute indication for admission but the threshold of interention should be considerably lowered in these patients and they are best assessed by their usual treating doctors.

Patients recently discharged from hospital may have hospital acquired infections or infections caused by multiresistant organisms. Recent operations or procedures may be a clue to the site of infections.

Clinical pointers: exposure history

Overseas travellers or visitors Returned travellers or overseas visitors may have diseases such as malaria and typhoid fever that need early diagnosis and treatment and rarely may have contagious diseases such as viral haemorrhagic fever. Any fever in a returned traveller from a malaria endemic area should be regarded as due to malaria until proven otherwise.

Contacts with animals A contact history with animals, either at work or at home, is frequently the clue to a zoonosis, particularly if the illness is a perplexing fever of several days' duration. The occurrence of multiple cases at work or at home should also make one suspect these infections early.

Contact with meningococcal and haemophilus meningitis Close contacts of patients with these infections have a high risk of acquiring the same infections. Early symptoms of these infections may be subtle and a high index of suspicion must be maintained.

Clinical pointers: non-specific clinical features (Table 8.1.2)

There are several non-specific clinical features whose presence should suggest the possibility of sepsis. These features warrant careful scrutiny even when the patient does not appear toxic. They are not specific indicators of serious problems and there will be many false positives. However, ignoring them is a cause of missed or delayed diagnosis of sepsis.

Severe pain in muscles, neck or back Severe muscle pain, even in the absence of overt fever, may be an early symptom of meningococcaemia, staphylococcal or streptococcal bacteraemia. It is also a feature of myositis and necrotizing fasciitis.

Impairment of conscious state A change in conscious state may be the sole

presenting manifestation of sepsis, especially in the elderly patients.

Vomiting Unexplained vomiting, especially in association with headache or abdominal pain should raise concern. Vomiting without diarrhoea should not be attributed to a gastrointestinal infection. It is a common symptom of CNS infections and occult sepsis.

Severe headache in the presence of a normal CSF This is especially important in a person who seldom gets headaches. Severe headache in a febrile patient with normal CSF should not be diagnosed as a viral infection; many focal infections, e.g. pneumonia and bacterial enteritis may also present in this manner. CSF may be normal in cerebral abscess and in the prodromal phase of bacterial meningitis.

Unexplained rash An unexplained rash in a febrile patient should be regarded as meningococcaemia until proved otherwise, even in the absence of headache or CSF pleocytosis.

Jaundice Jaundice in the febrile patients is associated with a greatly increased risk of death, admission to ICU and prolonged hospital stay.[6] In general, jaundice in a febrile patient is unlikely to be due to viral hepatitis—serious infections such as bacteraemia, cholangitis, pyogenic liver abscess and malaria must be ruled out.

Sore throat or dysphagia Severe sore throat or dysphagia with a normal-looking throat is frequently the presenting symptoms of *Haemophilus influenzae* epiglottitis in adults.

Repeated rigors Although repeated rigors may occur in some viral infections, they should generally be regarded as indicators of sepsis, in particular abscesses, bacteraemia, endocarditis, cholangitis, and pyelonephritis.

Clinical pointers: evolution of illness (Table 8.1.3)

How rapidly the illness evolves is often an indication of its severity. Previously

Table 8.1.3 Clinical pointers: evolution of illness
Those present early (<24 hours)
Those presenting with rapidly evolving symptoms
Patients presenting to emergency department on more than 1 occasion over a 24–48 hour period.

healthy individuals do not seek medical attention unless they are worried. Notice should be taken of any person seeking help within 24 hours of the onset illness or a person whose illness appears to have progressed rapidly within 24–48 hours.

Similarly, the patient who presents to the emergency department on more than one occasion over a 24–48 hour period warrants careful work-up.

Step 4: A final caveat - meningococcal infection

A major concern in the management of the undifferentiated fever in adult is missing the diagnosis of meningococcal bacteraemia when the patient does not appear ill on presentation.

There are a number of infections that must be treated rapidly to minimize morbidity and mortality (Table 8.1.4). With the exception of meningococcal bacteraemia, there are usually some clues in the history, physical examination or simple laboratory tests to suggest their presence.

Meningococcal infection is peculiar in its wide spectrum of severity and variable rate of progression in different individuals (Table 8.1.5). It may be fulminant and cause death within 12 hours or it may assume a chronic form that goes on for weeks.

The diagnosis meningococcal meningitis is simple when the patient presents with the typical clinical picture of bacterial meningitis.

When the patient presents with fever and a petechial rash meningococcaemia can be suspected easily if one remembers the golden rule that 'fever plus a petechial rash is meningococcaemia (or staphylococcal bacteraemia) until proved otherwise'. However, only about 50% of

Table 8.1.4 Infections requiring urgent treatment

Disease	Clues
Meningococcaemia	Myalgia, rash May be none
Falciparum malaria	Travel history, blood film
Bacterial meningitis	Headache, change in conscious state, CSF findings
Post-splenectomy sepsis	Past history, abdominal scar
Toxic shock syndromes	Presence of shock and usually a rash
Infections in the febrile neutropenic	Past history, blood film
Infective endocarditis	Past history, murmur, petechiae
Necrotising soft tissue infections	Pain, tenderness, erythema and swelling in skin/muscle, toxicity
Space occupying infection of head and neck	Localizing symptoms and signs
Focal intracranial infections	Headache, change in conscious state, neurological signs, CT findings.

Table 8.1.5 Presentations of meningococcal disease

Acute bacterial meningitis ± petechial rash
Fever + petechial rash
Fever + macular rash
Fever + alarm bells
Fever + contact history
Fever alone.

meningococcal disease present with a petechial rash.[10]

It is less well known that the early meningococcaemic rash may be macular, i.e. one that blanches with pressure. This is the basis of another golden rule in infectious disease: early meningococcal rash may resemble a non-specific viral rash.

The risk of missing the diagnosis increases markedly when the patient with meningococcal disease presents with fever and non-specific symptoms without a rash. Abrupt onset of fever and generalized aches may be due to influenza but it could be due to meningococcaemia.

It is prudent to single out meningococcal disease and ask oneself: could this patient have meningococcaemia? If in doubt, the safest course is to take cultures, give antibiotics and admit.

Investigations

Full blood examination is of limited use. White cell count ($>15 \times 10^9$/L), marked left shift, neutropenia or thrombocytopenia are pointers to a possible bacteraemia or occult bacterial infections, but they may also be seen in viral infections.[11] These tests may also be normal in the presence of systemic infection.

Urinalysis and urine culture should be done in febrile adults over the age of 50 years, unless pathology clearly lies elsewhere. However, if the history does not suggest urinary sepsis and the dip-stick urinalysis is normal, then urine cultures are usually negative.[12]

A chest X-ray is usually indicated unless a definite diagnosis has been made, e.g. chickenpox, tonsillitis.

Blood cultures should be undertaken in anyone suspected of having bacteraemia, endocarditis, or meningitis, in compromized patients with a fever, all febrile patients over the age of 50 and considered in anyone with an unexplained high fever. It should be noted that only 5% of blood cultures in this setting will be positive and less than 2% will alter clinical management.[13] In general, a patient considered 'sick enough' to warrant blood cultures should be admitted to hospital or followed up within 24 hours.

DISPOSITION

Patients who have any of the following features are in need of resuscitation, followed by work up and admission: shock, coma/stupor, cyanosis, profound dyspnoea, continuous seizures, and severe dehydration.

With few exceptions the following groups of febrile adults should be investigated and admitted:

- Those over 50 years of age.
- Patients with diabetes mellitus.
- Alcoholic patients.
- Injecting drug users.
- Immunologically compromised patients.
- Overseas travellers or visitors.
- Those with 'alarm bells'-see Table 8.1.2.

In general there should be close liaison with the admitting unit and the issue of empirical therapy for septic patients should be discussed. For the dangerously ill, e.g. those with septic shock or bacterial meningitis, antibiotics should be commenced immediately.

There is an increasing tendency to commence antibiotics in the emergency department as soon as possible to reduce hospital length of stay. Time to antibiotic therapy is often used as a key performance indicator for the emergency department, e.g. for febrile neutropenic patients. Antibiotic choice is influenced by the tissue infected, most likely organism, regional resistance patterns and patient co-morbidities.

Patients who do not require intervention after the basic work up in the emergency department are discharged home after a period of observation. Because of the time taken to interview the patient, perform investigations and wait for the results the patient usually would have been observed for 1–2 hours. The progression or lack of progression may be a help in deciding what to do. During observation one has to be aware that the apparent improvement of the patient may be the result of pain relief or fall in temperature due to antipyretics.

Arrangement must be made for the patient to be reviewed by the general practitioner or at the hospital. This is an essential component of the care of a febrile patient seen in the emergency department. The infectious process is a dynamic one and the doctor must maintain contact with the patient or family during the 24 to 72 hours following the initial visit. The establishment of emergency department short-stay units allows fast-track treatment and observation, usually for 24 to 48 hours, for carefully selected febrile patients that are not suitable for immediate discharge home. All febrile patients discharged from the emergency department should be encouraged to seek review if there is any adverse change to their condition.

CONTROVERSIES

❶ Whether empirical antibiotics should be given in order to minimize the risk of death from unrecognized sepsis or meningitis. No algorithms exist directing management of this problem.

❷ Determining which febrile patients should have blood cultures when most will be negative and few will change management.

❸ The role of emergency department short-stay units as an alternative to admission for selected patients. The safe and ideal course of action is to admit for observation all those patients who are ill enough to warrant a blood culture or a lumbar puncture. The limitation of hospital beds precludes this policy and there will be unnecessary admissions.

FUTURE RESEARCH DIRECTIONS

❶ The subject of undifferentiated fever of short duration in adults has not been well studied. There are little data on the spectrum of diseases producing this clinical problem.

REFERENCES

1. Mellors JW, et al 1987 A Simple Index to identify occult bacterial infection in adults with acute unexplained fever. Archives of Internal Medicine 147: 666–71
2. Gallagher EJ, Brooks F, Gennis P 1994 Identification of serious illness in febrile adults. American Journal of Emergency Medicine 12: 129–33
3. Norman DC, Yoshikawa TT 1996 Fever in the elderly. Infections Disease Clinics of North America 10: 93–9
4. Fontanarosa PB, Kaeberlein FJ, Gerson FW, et al 1992 Difficulty in Predicting Bacteraemia in Elderly Emergency Patients. Annals of Emergency Medicine 21: 842–8
5. Marco CA, et al 1995 Fever in Geriatric Emergency Patients: clinical features associated with serious illness. Annals of Emergency Medicine 26: 18–24
6. Tan SL, Knott JC, Street AC, et al 2002 Outcomes of febrile adults presenting to the emergency department. Emergency Medicine 14 (1): A22
7. Wrenn KD, Larson S 1991 The Febrile Alcoholic in the Emergency Department. American Journal of Emergency Medicine 9: 57–60
8. Marantz PR, Linzer M, Feines CJ, et al 1987 Inability to predict diagnosis in febrile intravenous drug abusers. Annals of Internal Medicine 106: 823–6
9. Samet JH, Shovitz A, Fowle J, et al 1990 Hospitalisation decisions in febrile intravenous drug users. American Journal of Medicine 89: 53–7
10. Tunkel AR, Scheld WM 1995 Acute bacterial meningitis. Lancet 346: 1675–80
11. Wasserman MR, Keller EL 1989 Fever, white blood cell count, and culture and sensitivity: their value in the evaluation of the emergency patient. Top Emergency Medicine 10: 81–8
12. Sultana RV, Zalotein S, Cameron PA, et al 2001 Dipstick urinalysis and the accuracy of the clinical diagnosis of urinary tract infection. Journal of Emergency Medicine 20(1): 13–9
13. Kelly A 1998 Clinical impact of blood cultures in the emergency department. Journal of Accident & Emergency Medicine 15: 254–6

FURTHER READING

Talan DA 1996 Infectious disease issues in the emergency department. Clinical Infectious Diseases 23: 1–14

INFECTIOUS DISEASES

8.2 MENINGITIS

ANDREW SINGER

ESSENTIALS

1 Bacterial meningitis can be a rapidly progressive and fatal illness. A high level of suspicion, as well as rapid diagnosis and treatment is necessary.

2 Eighty-five per cent of cases have headache, fever, meningism and mental obtundation, but these are often absent or diminished in very young or old patients, those partially treated with oral antibiotics or those with some form of immunocompromise.

3 Treatment should not be delayed if lumbar puncture cannot be performed within 20 minutes of arrival in the emergency department. Blood cultures should be taken prior to the first dose of antibiotics, if at all possible.

4 The combination of a third-generation cephalosporin and benzylpenicillin will treat most cases of suspected bacterial meningitis, and should be given as soon as the diagnosis is suspected (benzylpenicillin is sufficient in the pre-hospital setting).

5 Steroids appear to be of benefit to children with bacterial meningitis, and should be given either before or with the first dose of antibiotic.

INTRODUCTION

Definition

Meningitis is an inflammation of the leptomeninges, the membranes that line the central nervous system, as well as the cerebrospinal fluid (CSF) in the sub-arachnoid space. It is usually the result of an infection, but can be due to an inflammatory response to a localized or systemic insult.

Classification

Meningitis is usually classified according to the aetiology or location as bacterial, aseptic (viral, tuberculous, fungal, or chemical), or spinal (where the infection specifically affects the spinal meninges).

Aetiology

Bacterial

Bacterial meningitis is a serious cause of morbidity and mortality in all age groups. The bacterial causes vary according to age, as shown in Table 8.2.1. *N. meningitidis* serogroups A and C tend to cause endemic cases of meningitis, especially in Aboriginal populations, while serogroup B is more commonly associated with epidemics.[1] There has been an increase in the incidence of penicillin-resistant *S. pneumoniae*, especially in children.[2]

Aseptic

Aseptic meningitis may be either due to an immune response to a systemic infection (usually viral), or to a chemical insult.

Viral

Enteroviruses are the most common cause of meningitis, often in clusters of cases. Herpesviruses often cause meningitis as part of a more generalised infection of the brain (meningoencephalitis), or as part of an immune response to a systemic infection. A generalized viraemia may also cause aseptic meningitis, due to an immune reaction without direct infection.

Fungal

Fungal causes of meningitis, especially that due to *Cryptococcus neoformans* tends to occur in immunocompromised patients, such as those with HIV/AIDS, or those on immunosuppressant medication or cancer chemotherapy. It can occur in immunocompetent individuals as well, particularly the elderly.

Tuberculous

Tuberculous meningitis is rare in industrialized countries, but can occur in all age groups. It tends to follow an insidious course, with a lack of classical signs and symptoms. Diagnosis is often

Table 8.2.1 Causes of meningitis

Viral	Bacterial	Other
Echovirus 6, 9,11, 30 Coxsackie viruses A9, A16, B1, B5, B6 Enterovirus 71H Herpes simplex 1 & 2 Cytomegalovirus Varicella-zoster Epstein-Barr virus	**Neonates** (<3 months old): Group B streptococcus *Escherichia coli* *Listeria monocytogenes* Coagulase-negative *Staphylococcus aureus* *Pseudomonas aeruginosa* **Children** (<6 years old): *Haemophilus influenzae* type b *Neisseria meningitidis* *Streptococcus pneumoniae* **Adults** *Neisseria meningitidis* (especially in young adults) *Streptococcus pneumoniae* *Listeria monocytogenes* (especially in adults over 45) *Klebsiella pneumoniae* *Staphylococcus aureus* *Escherichia coli* (in the immunocompromised)	*Mycobacterium tuberculosis* *Cryptococcus neoformans* (especially in immunocompromised) Aseptic

difficult, due to the low yield from CSF staining, and the 4-week time frame required to culture the organism. Suspicion should be high in patients with immunocompromise or chronic illness. It tends to have a high mortality.

Spinal

Spinal meningitis is usually bacterial meningitis due to direct spread from a localized infection in the spine.

Epidemiology

The epidemiology of meningitis is different for groups according to age, as well as immunocompetence:

- Neonates: Table 8.2.1 shows the main causes of bacterial meningitis in neonates. There is an overall incidence of 0.17–0.32 cases per 1000 live births. There is 26% mortality, which is even higher in premature infants.[3]
- Children: Until the introduction of *Haemophilus influenzae* type b (Hib) immunization in the early 1990s, this organism was the major cause of bacterial meningitis in children under 5 years (up to 1990, the incidence of childhood Hib meningitis was 26.3 per 100 000 [152 per 100 000 in Aboriginal children]).[4] Between 1990 and 1996, there was a 94% reduction in the incidence of Hib disease. *N. meningitidis* and *S. pneumoniae* remain common causes, both of meningitis and generalized sepsis.[5]
- Adults: *N. meningitidis* and *S. pneumoniae* are a common cause in all age groups, with *N. meningitidis* predominating in adults under 24 years. *Listeria monocytogenes* is more common in adults over 45 years. The overall incidence in adults is 3.8 per 100 000 population.[6] More unusual organisms occur in patients following neurosurgery, or chronic illness, such as alcoholism, hepatic cirrhosis, chronic renal failure, and connective tissue disease [7](GNRs, coagulase-negative *S. aureus*, *M. tuberculosis*, *Klebsiella pneumoniae*).

- Patients with HIV/AIDS: *Cryptococcus neoformans* is relatively common with an incidence of 5 per million of population, or 10% of HIV-infected patients. Tuberculosis, *Listeria*, *Klebsiella* and syphilis are also causes of meningitis in this group, as well as viral causes of meningoencephalitis.[8]
- Tuberculous meningitis occurs in around 2% of patients with TB, and around 10% of HIV-infected patients with TB. It has a poor prognosis, with 20% mortality.

Pathogenesis

Initially, there is colonization of the infectious agent, commonly in the naso-pharynx in the case of the enteroviruses and bacteria such as meningococcus and Hib. Other infections may spread from already established foci such as otitis media, or sinusitis (e.g., pneumococcus). There is either haematogenous or local spread to the meninges and subarachnoid space, with inflammation of this area and the production of a purulent exudate, approximately 2 hours after invasion of the area. The inflammatory response is initiated by bacterial subcapsular components, such as lipoteichoic acid in *S. pneumoniae*, a lipo-oligosaccharide in *H. influenzae*, and other Gram-negative endotoxins. These substances stimulate the release of cytokines such as inter-leukin-1 and -6, tumour necrosis factor (TNF), arachidonic acid metabolites, as well as the complement cascade. There is a subsequent increase in neutrophil and platelet activity, with increased perme-ability of the blood-brain barrier. This response is often worse after the initial destruction of bacteria by antibiotics. If left untreated, fibrosis of the meninges may occur. In viral and aseptic menin-gitis, there is a more limited inflamma-tory response, with mild-to-moderate infiltration of lymphocytes. In the more chronic causes, such as fungi or tuber-culosis, the exudate is fibrinous, with the main cells being a mixture of lympho-cytes, monocytes/macrophages, and plasma cells. The base of the brain is most commonly affected.

PRESENTATION

History

There are some differences in the history with different causes of meningitis, which may allow an early differential diagnosis to be made. There are no pathognomonic single symptoms or signs for meningitis, so a high index of suspicion is necessary.

The combination of fever, headache, meningism and mental obtundation is found in approximately 85% of cases of bacterial meningitis.[9] It is also a common pattern in viral or aseptic meningitis, with obtundation being less of a feature. In fungal or tuberculous meningitis, these symptoms are much less common (less than 40% of cases of cryptococcal meningitis). Elderly patients or those who have had recent neurosurgery may present with subtle or mild symptoms, and lack a fever.[10]

The headache is usually severe and unrelenting. It may be either global, or located in a specific area. The main symptoms of meningism are nuchal rigidity (neck stiffness), and photo-phobia. The nuchal rigidity is something more than merely pain on movement of the neck. It is clinically important when the patient complains of a painful restriction of movement in the sagittal plane (i.e. forwards and backwards only). Up to 35% of cases have associated nausea and vomiting.

As a general rule, the height of the fever is a poor indication of the possible cause though, the fever may often only be mild in tuberculous or fungal meningitis, or in bacterial meningitis that has been partially treated by antibiotics. The spec-trum of mental obtundation can range from mild confusion, to bizarre behav-iour, delirium or coma. The severity of obtundation is a good indication of the severity of the illness.

Focal neurological signs occur in around 10–20% of cases of bacterial meningitis, but are also associated with cerebral mass lesions, such as toxoplas-mosis or brain abscess. They are also a feature of tuberculous meningitis. Seiz-ures are relatively uncommon (13–30%), but may occasionally be the only sign of meningitis if the patient has been partially treated with oral antibiotics.

There may also be associated systemic symptoms. Myalgias and arthralgias are often associated with viral causes, but may also be the sole presenting symptom in meningococcal meningitis. HIV/AIDS patients may show stigmata associated with that disease.

The course of the illness may also indicate the cause. Meningococcal or pneumoccal meningitis is often characterized by a rapid, fulminating course, often going from initial symptoms to death over an interval of hours. Viral causes tend to be a slower course over days. Fungal or tuberculous meningitis shows a more chronic course over days to weeks, with milder symptoms.

Risk factors for meningitis include the extremes of age, pre-existing sinusitis or otitis media, recent neurosurgery, CSF shunts, splenectomy, immunological compromise, and chronic diseases such as alcoholism, cancer, connective tissue disorders, chronic renal failure and hepatic cirrhosis.

Examination

The physical examination will often reflect symptoms elicited in the history, with fever, physical evidence of meningism, stigmata of AIDS, etc.

As stated above, neck stiffness is only clinically significant when it occurs in the sagittal plane. There will be a restriction of both passive and active movement. Other tests to elicit meningism include Kernig's sign and Brudzinski's sign, though these are only present in 50% of adult cases of bacterial meningitis. Kernig's sign is elicited by attempting extend the knee of a leg that has been flexed at the hip with the patient lying supine, and the other leg flat on the bed. The sign is positive if the knee cannot be fully extended due to spasm in the hamstrings. The test can be falsely positive in patients with shortening of the hamstrings, or other problems involving the legs or lumbar spine. In Brudzinski's sign, flexing the head causes the thighs and knees to also flex. It can also be tested in children by the inability to touch the nose with the flexed hips and knees in the sitting position. These are both late signs.

Focal neurological signs should be a cause for concern, as they can indicate a poor prognosis.

Papilloedema is rare and late, as is a bulging fontanelle in infants, and should alert one to alternative diagnoses.

A rash, often starting as a macular or petechial rash on the limbs, is seen in sepsis due to *N. meningitidis* and *S. pneumoniae*. A petechial rash is a particularly serious sign, and is an indication to start antibiotics immediately. A maculopapular rash is also a feature of viral causes.

INVESTIGATIONS

Lumbar puncture

A CSF sample via a lumbar puncture (LP) is an important source of information for making the diagnosis and determining the likely aetiology and treatment. As this procedure may be time consuming, treatment should not be delayed if there will be more than a 20-minute delay before the lumbar puncture and there is a reasonable clinical suspicion that a bacterial cause is present. Blood cultures should be taken prior to the administration of antibiotics.

Indications

- Symptoms suggestive of meningitis, especially the combination of fever, headache, neck stiffness and photophobia.
- Any patient with fever and an altered level of consciousness.
- Fever associated with seizures, especially in a neonate, older child or adult.
- Seizures in any patient who has been on oral antibiotics.

Precautions

- Deep coma: a patient with a Glasgow Coma Score (GCS) of 8 or less should have a computerized tomography (CT) scan first.
- Focal neurological signs: patient should have CT first, to exclude a space occupying lesion, which may increase the risk of cerebral herniation following the lumbar puncture.
- Surgery to the lumbar spine.
- Local skin infection around the lumbar spine.

The main features to note during the lumbar puncture are the opening pressure and the physical appearance of the CSF. The sample should be sent for Gram staining, culture, sensitivities, a cell count, and protein and glucose levels. If fungal meningitis is suspected, an India-ink stain and cryptococcal antigen screen should be requested. If tuberculous meningitis is suspected, multiple 5 mL samples of CSF will be required to increase the likelihood of a positive result. If there has been prior administration of antibiotics, a bacterial antigen screen should also be requested.

Turbid CSF is indicative of a significant number of pus cells, and is an indication for immediate administration of antibiotics. The patient should usually rest supine for a few hours following the procedure to prevent a worsening of the headache. This has been known to occur up to 24 hours following the procedure. The evidence for the benefits of enforced rest following lumbar puncture is equivocal.

The pattern of cell counts and glucose and protein levels is shown in Table 8.2.2. This can act as a guide only, and the clinician needs to be guided by the complete clinical picture.

A leukocyte count (WCC) of more than $1000/\mu L$ with a predominantly neutrophilic pleocytosis is considered positive for bacterial meningitis. Ten per cent of cases, especially if early in the course of the illness, may have a predominance of lymphocytes. As a general rule, bacterial meningitis is characterized by a raised CSF protein and a low CSF glucose level. The ratio of CSF:serum glucose levels is also lowered. The combination of CSF glucose <1.9 mmol/L, CSF to serum glucose ratio <0.23, CSF protein >2.2 g/L, and either a total WCC $>2000/\mu L$ or a neutrophil count of $>1180/\mu L$ has been shown to have a 99% certainty of diagnosing bacterial

Table 8.2.2 Expected CSF values in meningitis

Parameter	Normal range	Bacterial	Viral	Fungal or TB
Pressure (cm H$_2$O)	5–20	>30	Normal or mildly raised	
Protein (g/L)	0.18–0.45	>1.0–5.0	<1.0	0.1–0.5
Glucose (mmol/L)	2.5–3.5	<2.2	normal	1.6–2.5
Glucose ratio -CSF/serum	0.6 (0.8 in infants)	<0.4 (allow 2–4 h equilibration)	0.6	<0.4
White cell count/µL	<3, usually lymphocytes (if the tap is traumatic, allow 1 WBC for every 1000 RBC)	>500 (90% PMN)	<1000, predominantly monocytes (10% are >90% PMN, 30–40% >50% PMN)	100–500
Gram stain	No organisms	60–90% positive	No organisms	

meningitis.[11] Aseptic meningitis will often have cell counts near the normal range. This does not exclude infection with less common agents, such as herpesviruses, or *L. monocytogenes*.

CT scan

CT scanning of the brain is indicated as a prelude to lumbar puncture in the presence of focal neurological signs, mental obtundation, or abnormal posturing. It must be noted, though, that a normal CT does not exclude the risk of cerebral herniation in bacterial meningitis[12] and, therefore, those with the above signs should have lumbar puncture delayed until they are conscious and stable.

Microbiological diagnosis

Apart from microscopy and culture of CSF, there are a number of other methods that may allow identification of the causative organism to be made.

Skin lesion aspirate

In cases where a petechial rash is present, Gram staining or culture from some of the skin lesions may yield the causative organism. This has a reported sensitivity of 30–70%.

Throat swab

Throat swabs are useful in identifying a bacterial cause spread by nasopharyngeal carriage, and should be performed in a case of suspected bacterial meningitis.

Polymerase chain reaction

This is a relatively new technique that allows identification of the causative organism, and even the serotype for organisms like meningococcus. The test can be performed on CSF or EDTA blood samples, and may remain positive for up to 72 hours after the commencement of antibiotics. In CSF the reported sensitivity is 89% with a specificity of 100%, and in blood a sensitivity of 81% with a specificity of 97%.[13]

Serology

Tests to detect IgM to specific organisms are available for meningococcus and some viruses. For meningococcus, the test has a sensitivity and specificity of 97% and 95%, but is only reliable in adults and children over 4 years old, and takes 5–7 days after onset of the illness to reach diagnostic levels.

Antigenic studies

Latex agglutination, immunoelectrophoresis, or radioimmunoassay techniques can be used to screen for antigens from *S. pneumoniae*, Hib, group B streptococcus (*S. agalactiae*), *Escherichia coli* K1, *N. meningitidis*, and *C. neoformans*. The tests can be performed on serum, CSF or urine. Serum or urine samples tend to allow greater sensitivities (around 96–99%) than CSF (82–99%). The test is no more sensitive in untreated cases than either a positive Gram-stain or the presence of CSF pleocytosis.[14] The main purpose of antigenic studies is in

allowing rapid identification of the causative organism in cases confirmed by the CSF findings, or in cases where partial treatment with antibiotics renders the CSF sterile on culture. In many laboratories, these tests have been superseded by PCR methods.

General investigations

FBC, UEC, blood cultures, ESR and a throat swab can assist in building an overall picture.

Blood cultures should be taken prior to parenteral antibiotics, especially in patients where lumbar puncture has been delayed. One study found that blood cultures grew the causative organism in 86% of proven cases of bacterial meningitis, and that the combination of blood culture, CSF Gram's stain and antigen testing identified the cause in 92% of cases.[15]

DIFFERENTIAL

- Generalized viral infections, with meningism as a component.
- Encephalitis: this is a more generalized viral infection of the brain. Clinically, there may be no difference.
- Brain abscess: this tends to produce focal signs due to local pressure at the site of the abscess.
- Focal cerebral infections, such as those due to *Toxoplasma gondii* in HIV/AIDS patients.

- Subarachnoid haemorrhage: this will often produce identical symptoms of meningism, but generally without any other evidence of infection, such as fever.
- Migraine and other vascular headaches: again, meningism is a similar feature. The patient will often have a known history of the illness.
- Severe pharyngitis with cervical lymphadenopathy causing neck stiffness.

MANAGEMENT

Management depends on the likely causative agents, as well as the severity of the illness.

General

Patients should rest in bed, particularly following a lumbar puncture. A quiet, darkened room will be beneficial to those with headache or photophobia. Simple analgesics may be used for treatment of the headache, with or without codeine. Opiates may be required in severe headaches.

Sedation may be necessary if the patient is very agitated or delirious. Suitable drugs are diazepam 5–10 mg IV or midazolam 2–10 mg IV or IM, with or without the addition of a anti-psychotic such as haloperidol 5–20 mg IV or IM, or chlorpromazine 12.5–50 mg IV or IM.

Seizures should be treated appropriately, initially with a benzodiazepine, then maintenance with phenytoin or phenobarbitone. Meningitis can occasionally be associated with status epilepticus, which should be treated in the standard way.

Patients with raised intracranial pressure may need pressure monitoring, and measures to reduce the pressure, such as nursing the patient 30° head up, and the administration of hyperosmotic agents such as mannitol. Hyperventilation is controversial, as it may reduce intracerebral pressure at the expense of reduced cerebral perfusion. Obstructive hydrocephalus requires appropriate neurosurgical treatment with CSF shunting.

If septic shock has intervened, it should be treated in the usual way, with IV fluids and inotropes.

Antimicrobials

The choice of antimicrobial agent will be determined by the likely causative organism and, therefore, is primarily determined by age and immune status. It is important that antibiotic therapy is not delayed by investigations such as lumbar puncute or CT scan, and should be administered as soon as the diagnosis is made. Table 8.2.3 shows the recommended choice of antimicrobial for different situations and organisms. Table 8.2.4 shows the recommended dosage of each. As a general rule, the combination of a third-generation cephalosporin and benzylpenicillin will cover most organisms

in all age groups. It is important to note that there is emerging resistance in *S. pneumoniae* to penicillins (currently 7.6% of isolates in Australia). Moderately resistant strains (MIC 0.1–2.0 mg/L) may be treated with a third-generation cephalosporin. Highly resistant strains should be guided by specialist advice. A combination of vancomycin and rifampicin may be useful.

Steroids

Steroids have been shown to improve the prognosis of bacterial meningitis in children. The benefits are most marked in Hib infections (but note the marked reduction in Hib prevalence in Australia), but have also been shown, to a lesser extent, in meningococcus and pneumococcus infections. The main benefit is in reducing the longer-term complications, such as sensorineural deafness, and neurological deficits. There has been no demonstrable benefit in adults.

It is usually administered as dexamethasone 0.15 mg/kg IV q6h, commenced before or with the first dose of antibiotics, and continued for 2–4 days. The main adverse effect is gastrointestinal bleeding, which may be reduced by limiting treatment to 2 days.[16]

DISPOSITION

All cases of bacterial meningitis require admission for intravenous antibiotics, as

Table 8.2.3 Choice of antimicrobial in meningitis			
Organism	First-line drug	Second-line drug	Duration
Pre-hospital	Benzylpenicillin		
Organism unknown	Cefotaxime or ceftriaxone PLUS benzylpenicillin	Ampicillin instead of benzylpenicillin and gentamicin instead of a 3rd gen. cephalosporin in neonates	7–10 days
H. influenzae type b	Cefotaxime or ceftriaxone	Ampicillin or chloramphenicol	7–10 days
N. meningitidis	Benzylpenicillin or cefotaxime or ceftriaxone		5–7 days
S. pneumoniae	Benzylpenicillin	Cefotaxime or ceftriaxone or vancomycin	10 days
L. monocytogenes	Benzylpenicillin	Ampicillin	3–6 weeks
C. neoformans	Amphotericin PLUS flucytosine	Fluconazole	4–6 weeks
Herpes simplex	Aciclovir		14 days

Table 8.2.4 Antibiotic doses in treating meningitis[1]

Antibiotic	Daily dose mg/ kg/day	Max daily dose	Route	Divided doses
Cefotaxime	200	12 g	IV	50 mg/kg q6h
Ceftriaxone	100	4 g	IV	100 mg/kg once or twice daily
Benzylpenicillin	1080	12 g	IV	60 mg/kg q4h
Ampicillin	360	12 g	IV	50 mg/kg q4h
Chloramphenicol	80–100	4 g	IV	20–25 mg/kg q6h
Acyclovir	30	1500 mg/m²/day in children 2–12 years	IV	10 mg/kg q8h
Amphotericin B	0.5–0.7		IV	0.5–0.7 mg/kg daily
Flucytosine	100–150		po	100–150 mg/kg daily
Vancomycin	40	4 g	IV	10 mg/kg q6h

well as supportive therapy. They often require intensive therapy, especially if septic shock has supervened. Viral meningitis will usually require supportive therapy only, but this may require admission. Mild cases of viral or aseptic meningitis, with a clear diagnosis, can be safely sent home.

PROGNOSIS

Over the last 20 years, the mortality of bacterial meningitis has ranged from 6% to 20%. Mortality is higher in the very young or old. Meningitis in immuno-compromised individuals carries a high mortality of up to 50%. Bacterial meningitis in children can lead to a number of long-term sequelae, such as sensori-neural hearing loss, learning difficulties, motor problems, speech delay, hyper-activity, blindness, obstructive hydro-cephalus and recurrent seizures. These sequelae are less common in adults.

PREVENTION

Prophylaxis should be offered in cases of *Haemophilus influenzae* type b, or Meningococcus infection to:

- The index case.

- All household or child-care contacts who have either stayed overnight in the same house or have been in the same room as the index case for any period of 4 hours or more in the preceding 7 days (in Hib, if less than 24 months old, or less than 4 years and incompletely immunized against Hib).
- Passengers adjacent to the index case on a trip of 8 hours or longer duration
- Any person who has potentially shared saliva (such as eating utensils or drink bottles) with the index case.
- Health-care workers who have given mouth-to-mouth resuscitation to an index case.

Appropriate regimens are:

- For meningococcus:
  – Ciprofloxacin 500 mg orally as a single dose - preferred for females on oral contraceptives
  – Ceftriaxone 250 mg (125 mg in children <12 years) IM in 1% Lidocaine - preferred in pregnant females
  – Rifampicin 600 mg orally 12-hourly for 2 days (5 mg/kg in neonates <1 month, 10 mg/kg in children).
- For Hib:
  – Rifampicin 600 mg orally daily for

CONTROVERSIES

❶ Whether all patients should have a CT scan before lumbar puncture. In general it is safe without CT in those with a clear history consistent with meningitis and normal sensorium. Comatose patients should have lumbar puncture delayed until they are conscious.

❷ The use of steroids. Steroids have only been shown to improve outcome in *H. influenzae* infections.

4 days (10 mg/kg in neonates <1 month, 20 mg/kg in children)
– Ceftriaxone 1 g IM daily for 2 days (50 mg/kg in children).
– If the index case is <24 months old, Hib vaccination should be given as a full course as soon as possible after recovery. Unvaccinated contacts under 5 years of age should be immunized as soon as possible.

Casual, neighbourhood or hospital contacts are not required to receive prophylaxis.

Meningococcal vaccine should be considered in populations where cases are clustered. The vaccine is presently only available for Serogroup C.

REFERENCES

1. Munro R, Kociuba K, Jelfs J, Brown J, Crone S, Chant K 1996 Meningococcal disease in urban south western Sydney, 1990–1994. Australian and New Zealand Journal of Medicine 26: 526–32
2. Collignon PJ, Bell JM 1996 Drug-resistant Streptococcus pneumoniae: the beginning of the end for many antibiotics? Australian Group on Antimicrobial Resistance. Medical Journal of Australia 164: 64–67
3. Francis BM, Gilbert GL 1992 Survey of neonatal meningitis in Australia: 1987–1989. Medical Journal of Australia 156: 240–3
4. Bower C, Payne J, Condon R, Hendrie D, Harris A, Henderson R 1994 Sequelae of *Haemophilus influenzae* type b meningitis in aboriginal and non-aboriginal children under 5 years of age. Journal of Paediatric Child Health 30: 393–7
5. Herceg A 1997 The decline of Haemophilus influenzae type b disease in Australia. Communicable Diseases Intelligence 21: 173–6
6. Sigurdardottir B, Bjornsson OM, Jonsdottir KE, Erlendsdottir H, Gudmundsson S 1997 Acute bacterial meningitis in adults. A 20-year overview. Archives of Internal Medicine 157: 425–30
7. Segreti J, Harris AA 1996 Acute bacterial meningitis. Infectious of Disease Clinics of North America 10: 797–809
8. Jones PD, Beaman MH, Brew BJ 1996 Managing

HIV. Part 5: Treating secondary outcomes. 5.5 HIV and opportunistic neurological infections. Medical Journal of Australia 164: 418–21

9. Tunkel AR, Scheld WM 1995 Acute bacterial meningitis. Lancet 346: 1675–80

10. Miller LG, Choi C 1997 Meningitis in older patients: how to diagnose and treat a deadly infection. Geriatrics 52: 43–4

11. Spanos A, Harrell FE Jr, Durack DT 1989 Differential diagnosis of acute meningitis: an analysis of the predictive value of initial

observation. Journal of the American Medical Association 262: 2700–7

12. Rennick G, Shann F, de Campo J 1993 Cerebral herniation during bacterial meningitis in children. British Medical Journal 306: 953–5

13. Communicable Diseases Network Australia 2001 Guidelines for the early clinical and public health management of Meningococcal Disease in Australia

14. Feuerborn SA, Capps WI, Jones JC 1992 Use of latex agglutination testing in diagnosing pediatric meningitis. Journal of Family Practice 34: 176–9

15. Coant PN, Kornberg AE, Duffy LC, Dryja DM, Hassan SM 1992 Blood culture results as determinants in the organism identification of bacterial meningitis. Pediatric Emergency Care 8: 200–5

16. McIntyre PB, Berkey CS, King SM, Schaad UB, Kilpi T, Kanra GY, Perez CM 1997 Dexamethasone as adjunctive therapy in bacterial meningitis. A meta-analysis of randomized clinical trials since 1988. Journal of the American Medical Association 278: 925–31

8.3 SEPTIC ARTHRITIS

TREVOR JACKSON

ESSENTIALS

1 Delayed or inadequate treatment can lead to irreversible joint damage.

2 Diagnosis is usually straightforward, based on clinical features and synovial fluid examination; imaging techniques have a role in difficult cases.

3 *Staphylococcus aureus* and *Neisseria gonorrhoeae* are the most frequent pathogens.

4 Successful treatment hinges on rapid and complete joint drainage, and high-dose parenteral antibiotics guided by culture results.

5 Outcomes are good in paediatric and gonococcal subgroups, but the presence of chronic arthritis or polyarticular involvement is associated with up to 15% mortality and 50% chronic joint morbidity.

INTRODUCTION

Septic arthritis is defined as infection of the synovial lining and fluid of a joint. Bacteria are the usual pathogens by haematogenous seeding of the joint. Direct spread from adjacent infection or via trauma are less common routes of infection. Once established, phagocytic and neutrophil responses to the bacteria lead to proteolytic enzyme release and

cytokine production, resulting in synovial abscess formation and cartilage necrosis.[1]

Comorbidity or deficient host defences are risk factors for infection[2] and can be associated with more rapid and severe disease. (Table 8.3.1).

The majority of cases are community acquired and occur in children and young adults.[3] Prosthetic joint surgery and invasive management of chronic arthritis are factors in the increased prevalence observed in older age groups.

PRESENTATION

History

This will usually reveal the recent onset of a painful, hot and swollen joint, most commonly the hip or knee, although any joint may be affected. Systemic features of fever or rigors should be sought, and the presence of any risk factors.

Examination

Typical findings include a hot tender joint with marked limitation of passive or active movement due to pain. An effusion will be evident in most cases. A polyarticular presentation is more common in gonococcal infection or in the setting of chronic arthritis. In general, fever is low grade and few patients will appear 'toxic' and unwell. The elderly and immunosuppressed may present non-specifically with anorexia, vomiting, lethargy or fever.

INVESTIGATION

Synovial fluid examination and culture

Aspiration should be performed promptly with local anaesthetic and a large-bore needle to confirm the diagnosis and obtain a culture specimen. Typical findings in septic arthritis and its differential diagnoses are shown in Table 8.3.2.[4]

A Gram stain and culture should be performed immediately after aspiration to focus antibiotic therapy and maximize the yield of positive cultures. Most infections are acute and bacterial (Table 8.3.3),[4] although fungal and mycobacterial pathogens have been recognized in chronic infections.

Other laboratory investigations

Blood cultures should always be taken, and may be positive in up to 50%. Inflammatory markers are elevated (ESR and C-reactive protein), with typically a neutrophil-predominant leucocytosis. These are non-diagnostic, but aid in monitoring response to therapy.

Imaging studies

Plain radiographs should be performed in all cases: they may reveal effusions or local oedema, and help to exclude alternative conditions. Ultrasound is very sensitive in detecting effusions, and excellent for facilitating needle aspiration.

Fluoroscopy may also be used. Nuclear medical studies are very sensitive

Table 8.3.1 Risk factors for septic arthritis

Risk factors	Examples
Direct penetration	Trauma Medical (surgery, arthrocentesis) IV drug use
Joint disease	Chronic arthritis
Host immune deficit	Glucocorticoid, or immunosuppressive therapy HIV infection Chronic illness Cancer

Table 8.3.3 Bacterial causes of septic arthritis

Age group	Typical bacteria
Children	Staphylococcus aureus Group A streptococci (B in neonates) Haemophilus influenzae
Young adults	Neisseria gonorrhoeae Staphylococcus aureus
Older adults	Staphylococcus aureus Gram-negative species* Group A streptococci

*Pseudomonas sp. and Enterobacteriaceae

early, but not specific for sepsis. Computerized tomography (CT) and magnetic resonance imaging (MRI) have a small role in difficult joints (e.g. hip, sacroiliac).

DIFFERENTIAL DIAGNOSIS

Non-septic arthritis or synovitis may be differentiated on clinical features and joint fluid analysis. Fractures will generally be evident on joint radiographs whilst detection of osteomyelitis may require more advanced imaging techniques such as nuclear or CT scanning. Rheumatic fever and brucellosis are rare causes.

MANAGEMENT

Joint drainage and empiric parenteral antibiotic therapy must take place without delay. Surgical drainage is usually employed in children, with needle drainage more commonly first line in adult joints. Newer arthroscopic techniques are increasingly being used.[1,5,6] Repeated drainage procedures will often be necessary to ensure complete resolution of the infection.

Antibiotic therapy is initiated after culture specimens have been obtained, with clinical presentation and Gram stain guiding the choice of agents. All regimens must include an antistaphylococcal agent, with Gram-negative cover as indicated by the clinical setting.

Suggested regimen:

- Di(Flu)cloxacillin: 25–50 mg/kg up to 2 g intravenously, 6-hourly for 4 to 6 days, then 25 mg/kg up to 500 mg orally, 6-hourly for a total of at least 21 days.
- If Gram-negative cover indicated: Cefotaxime 25–50 mg/kg up to 1 g intravenously, 8-hourly OR Ceftriaxone 50–75 mg/kg up to 1 g intravenously, daily for 4 to 6 days.[7]

Suspicion of methicillin resistance should prompt the inclusion of vancomycin initially, with definitive therapy based on laboratory identification of the organism and its sensitivities.

The duration and route of therapy remain controversial, but in uncomplicated acute cases parenteral antibiotics will be required for at least 4 days, with a total treatment duration of 3–4 weeks.[7,9] Specific organisms such as Neisseria sp. will respond more rapidly, whereas chronic infections and co-morbidity will necessitate aggressive and more prolonged therapy.

General care, with joint rest, appropriate analgesia and physical therapy, is important.

DISPOSITION

All patients require admission until their joint sepsis is controlled. Thereafter, ongoing therapy may be monitored as an outpatient or via domiciliary hospital services.

PROGNOSIS

This depends upon the organism, patient comorbidity, and the adequacy and rapidity of treatment. Gonococcal and paediatric infections have a generally good response, with low rates of ensuing joint morbidity. Polyarticular sepsis in rheumatoid arthritis has been associated with mortality rates of up to 15%, and major morbidity in up to 50% of survivors.[1,4,8]

PREVENTION

Safe sexual practice can reduce gonorrhoeal infections. Strict aseptic technique, good patient selection and prophylactic antibiotics help prevent cases associated with invasive joint procedures. The overall incidence of infection after arthroplasty ranges from 0.5 to 2%.[1]

Table 8.3.2 Synovial fluid characteristics

Characteristic	Septic arthritis	Non-septic arthritis	Non-inflammatory effusion
Colour	Yellow/Green	Yellow	Colourless
Turbidity	Purulent, turbid	Turbid	Clear
Leucocytes/μl	10–100 000	5–10 000	<1000
Predominant cell	PMN*	PMN*	Monocyte

*PMN, Polymorphonuclear leucocyte

Infectious Diseases, 5th edn. JB Lippincott, Philadelphia, pp 1382–9
5. Stanitski CL, Harwell JC, Fu FH 1989 Arthroscopy in acute septic knees. Clinical Orthopaedics 241: 209
6. Broy SB, Schmid FR 1986 A comparison of medical drainage (needle aspiration) and surgical drainage (arthrotomy or arthroscopy) in the initial treatment of infected joints. Clinics in Rheumatological Disease 12: 501–22
7. Skin, muscle and bone infections 2000 In: Therapeutic Guidelines. Antibiotic, 11th edn. Therapeutic Guidelines Ltd
8. Youssef PP, York JR 1994 Septic arthritis: a second decade of experience. Australian and New Zealand Journal of Medicine 24: 307–11
9. Syrogiannopoulos GA, Nelson JD 1988 Duration of antimicrobial therapy for acute suppurative osteoarticular infections. Lancet 1(8575–6): 37–40

CONTROVERSIES

❶ Total duration of therapy has gradually been reduced but optimum duration is unclear, as is the balance between parenteral and oral routes.[9]

❷ Consensus has not been reached on the best method of joint drainage. Surgery is best for the hip and in children, but arthroscopic techniques are now being employed in many joints. Most centres still use repeated needle aspiration.

❸ Difficulties still exist with the differentiation of septic arthritis from new-onset non-septic arthritis, especially when polyarticular. Joint fluid analysis and medical imaging are utilized, but nuclear and CT scanning techniques may have difficulty in distinguishing infective from non-infective inflammation.

REFERENCES

1. Goldenberg DL 1993 Bacterial arthritis. In: Kelley WN, Harris ED, Ruddy S, Sledge CB (eds) Textbook of Rheumatology, 4th edn. WB Saunders, Philadelphia, pp 1449–66

2. Goldenberg DL, Reed JI 1985 Bacterial arthritis. New England Journal of Medicine 312: 764–71
3. Sonnen GM, Henry N 1996 Paediatric bone and joint infections. Paediatric Clinics of North America 4(4): 933–47
4. Brooks GF, Pons VG 1994 Septic arthritis. In: Hoeprich PD, Jordan MC, Ronald AR (eds)

8.4 OSTEOMYELITIS

TREVOR JACKSON

ESSENTIALS

1 *Staphylococcus aureus* is the most frequent pathogen in all age groups.

2 Surgery, trauma and diabetes predispose to chronic adult infections.

3 Diagnosis may be difficult, relying on the triad of clinical features, imaging studies and microbiological culture.

4 Successful treatment requires appropriate parenteral antibiotics and complete surgical clearance of necrotic bone.

INTRODUCTION

Infection of bone is an infrequent but important emergency department presentation. Most cases occur in children and the aged, with the former occurring via haematogenous spread and the latter associated with comorbidity such as trauma, surgery, vascular insufficiency and diabetes. Bacteria enter bone via the blood vessels, by direct spread from contiguous infection, or by direct inoculation during trauma or surgery. Initially metaphyseal, infection usually extends to the subperiosteal space, forming an abscess, stimulating new bone deposition known as an involucrum. Necrosis of cortical bone follows, whereby bone fragments or sequestra are formed that harbour bacteria.[1] Successful treatment requires eradication of the bacteria and complete removal of necrotic tissue.

PRESENTATION

History

New onset of localized bone pain and fever is typical. Inadequate vascular supply, diabetes, prior surgery such as arthroplasty or compound fracture, are all important risk factors. Chronic infections are commonly indolent, with few or no symptoms.

Examination

Most patients will not appear toxic or unwell. Typical findings include mild fever with warmth, tenderness and swelling at the site of pain. Joint movements may be restricted if osteomyelitis is periarticular or has involved the joint space. Chronic infections may present with overlying scars, ulcers or draining sinuses.

INVESTIGATIONS

General laboratory tests

Inflammatory markers (erythrocyte sedimentation rate and C-reactive protein) will be significantly elevated and are useful for monitoring the response to treatment. The white cell count is an unreliable guide to severity, typically showing low-grade neutrophil-predominant leucocytosis.

Imaging studies

Plain radiographs may reveal early soft tissue oedema and periosteal elevation, particularly in children. However, in adults, radiographs typically remain normal for at least 10–14 days; thereafter the findings reflect bony destruction. Cortical rarefaction, involucrum formation and sequestra may all be seen. In sub-acute infection, a bone abscess known as Brodie's abscess may appear as a lucent lesion at the metaphysis.

Nuclear medical scans with three-phase ^{99m}Tc MDP are sensitive early and well tolerated by children, but may lack specificity.[3] They are most useful when combined with clinical features and plain radiography. Computerized tomography (CT) and magnetic resonance imaging (MRI) studies are excellent for displaying the extent of established infection and soft tissue involvement, and for investigation of difficult sites (e.g. the spine).

Microbiology

Culture of infected bone obtained by needle aspiration or surgery[4] provides definitive evidence in up to 80% of cases. Blood cultures will be positive for a single bacterium in over 50% of infections, especially if established via haematogenous spread. Common bacterial pathogens are listed in Table 8.4.1. Polymicrobial infection will be encountered in the setting of chronic infection or compromised hosts (e.g. diabetic foot ulcers). Non-bacterial pathogens occur rarely.

Table 8.4.1 Bacterial causes of osteomyelitis

Age group	Typical bacteria
Children <2 years	Staphylococcus aureus Streptococcus spp.
Older children	Staphylococcus aureus
Adults	Staphylococcus aureus Streptococcus spp. Gram-negative species*

* Pseudomonas sp. and Enterobacteriaceae

DIFFERENTIAL DIAGNOSIS

Tumours such as Ewing's sarcoma or osteoid osteoma, traumatic injuries and septic arthritis are the most important. The latter may coexist with osteomyelitis in joints such as the hip and shoulder.

MANAGEMENT

After appropriate microbiological specimens have been obtained, treatment requires prolonged parenteral and oral antibiotics guided by the results of Gram stain and culture. All initial antibiotic regimens should include an anti-staphylococcal agent, with vancomycin if methicillin resistance is suspected. The duration and routes of therapy must be adjusted individually, but at least 3–4 weeks is necessary for acute uncomplicated cases.[5, 6]

Newer modalities of antibiotic delivery such as antibiotic impregnated beads are emerging, but are not yet in widespread use.

Suggested regimen:

- Di(Flu)cloxacillin: 25–50 mg/kg up to 2 g intravenously, 6-hourly for 4–6 days, then 25 mg/kg up to 500 mg orally, 6-hourly for a total of at least 21 days.[6]

In all cases, orthopaedic management will be essential to obtain culture specimens and ensure complete removal of necrotic bone at the site. The latter may be unnecessary in acute haematogenous cases in children, or complex in chronic postsurgical cases with prosthetic implants involving major revision.

DISPOSITION

Confirmed acute cases require admission. Unless the patient is toxic or immunosuppressed, antibiotic treatment should commence after a definitive diagnosis has been established. After in-patient investigation and stabilisation, patients may be able to complete antibiotic treatment at home.

PROGNOSIS

Acute osteomyelitis can be expected to resolve with few sequelae if prompt and adequate therapy is instituted. If epiphyses are involved, ongoing orthopaedic review will be necessary as bone growth may be impaired. Chronic osteomyelitis and sinus tracts will only be controlled with antibiotic therapy alone, surgery is necessary for eradication. Squamous cell carcinoma in the tract is a rare, long-term complication.

PREVENTION

Thorough debridement, careful wound management and antibiotic therapy are essential in the setting of open skeletal trauma. Careful patient selection, meticulous technique and antibiotic prophylaxis may all help to prevent infection following joint prosthetic surgery.

CONTROVERSIES

❶ The optimum duration for parenteral antibiotics, and the balance between parenteral and oral routes is still to be determined in complicated or atypical cases.[5]

REFERENCES

1. Brooks GF, Pons VG 1994 Septic arthritis. In: Hoeprich PD, Jordan MC, Ronald AR (eds) Infectious Diseases, 5th edn. JB Lippincott, Philadelphia, pp 1382–9
2. Sonnen GM, Henry NK 1996 Paediatric bone and joint infections. Paediatric Clinics of North America 43(4): 933–47
3. Boutin RD, Brossmann J, Sartoris DJ, Reilly D, Resnick D 1998 Update on imaging of orthopaedic infections. Orthopaedic Clinics of North America 29(1): 41–66
4. Weinstein SL, Buckwalter JA (eds) 1994 Turek's Orthopaedics, 5th edn. JB Lippincott, Philadelphia, pp 127–50
5. Syrogiannopoulos GA, Nelson JD 1998 Duration of antimicrobial therapy for acute suppurative osteoarticular infections. Lancet 1(8575–6): 37–40
6. Skin, muscle and bone infections 2000 In: Therapeutic Guidelines. Antibiotic, 11th edn. Therapeutic Guidelines Ltd

8.5 URINARY TRACT INFECTION

SALOMON ZALSTEIN

ESSENTIALS

1 Urinary tract infection (UTI) is the most common cause of Gram-negative sepsis.

2 Between 20% and 30% of women will have a UTI at some time in their lives.

3 Most UTIs are caused by *Escherichia coli*, but *Staphylococcus saprophyticus* is responsible for up to 15% of infections in young, sexually active women.

4 There is a genetic predisposition in some women to recurrent UTI.

5 There are specific bacterial virulence factors determining uropathogenic strains of bacteria.

6 The clinical differentiation of lower from upper urinary tract infection is inaccurate. Up to 50% of patients presenting with typical lower tract symptoms will have concurrent upper tract involvement.

7 Up to half of women presenting with dysuria and frequency will have fewer than 10^5 organisms/mL of urine, but about half of these do have bacterial UTI.

8 For the majority of outpatients with typical symptoms urine culture is not necessary.

9 In institutionalized elderly patients non-specific symptoms or decline in function correlate poorly with UTI despite the presence of pyuria and bacteriuria. Non-UTI causes must be sought.

INTRODUCTION

Urinary tract infections are the most common bacterial infections, and the major cause of Gram-negative sepsis in hospitalized patients.[1,2]

Definitions

The term 'urinary tract infection' (UTI) is commonly believed to represent a group of specific diagnoses with clear cut clinical syndromes, but this is not the case. The term is non-specific and may refer to a variety of clinical conditions, including asymptomatic bacteriuria, urethritis, cystitis, female urethral syndrome, and acute and chronic pyelonephritis. The most common clinical presentations are cystitis and acute pyelonephritis, although the clinical distinction between these diagnoses may not be as straightforward as the terms imply, with up to 50% of patients having unrecognized pyelonephritis.

Significant bacteriuria most commonly refers to more than 10^5 bacteria/mL of urine. This usually represents infection as opposed to contamination (see Quantitative culture). There are significant exceptions to this generalization (see Urethral syndrome). *Asymptomatic bacteriuria* refers to significant bacteriuria in the absence of symptoms.

UTI may be considered in two main groups: simple (or uncomplicated) and complicated. Simple UTIs occur in an otherwise healthy person with a normal urinary tract, most commonly a young non-pregnant female. A complicated UTI is one associated with anatomical abnormality, urinary obstruction or incomplete bladder emptying due to any cause: instrumentation or catheterization, pregnancy, or significant underlying disease such as immunosuppression or diabetes mellitus.

EPIDEMIOLOGY

In Australia, approximately 250 000 adults per year are diagnosed with urinary tract infection.[3] UTIs occur most commonly in women, in whom age, degree of sexual activity and the form of contraception used are all factors that affect the incidence and prevalence of infection.[4–6] At least 20% and up to 40–50% of women will have a UTI at some time in their life.[7,8] The overall rate of infection is, therefore, difficult to estimate, but in non-pregnant women aged 18–40 years has been stated to be between 0.5–0.7 per person per year.[6] Infection rates are much higher in pregnancy.

In males the prevalence of bacteriuria beyond infancy is 0.1% or less. Between the ages of 21 and 50, infection rates may be as low as 0.6–0.8/1000.[9] With increasing prostatic disease the frequency of bacteriuria may rise to 3.5% in healthy men and to more than 15% in hospitalized men by age 70.[10,11] Homosexual men are at increased risk of UTI.

In the presence of chronic disease and institutionalization in the elderly, the incidence of bacteriuria may be as high as 50%.[10, 12–14]

AETIOLOGY

More than 95% of all UTIs are caused by the Enterobacteriaceae and *E. faecalis*. Of these, *E. coli* accounts for about 90% of acute infections in outpatients and some 50% in inpatients. Which bacteria are isolated is influenced by factors such as whether the infection is initial or recurrent; the presence of obstruction, instrumentation or anatomical abnormalities; and whether the patient is an inpatient or outpatient. In simple acute cystitis, the most common presentation of UTI, a single organism is usually isolated. On the other hand, in the presence of structural abnormalities it is more common to isolate multiple organisms, and antibiotic resistance is frequently found. Perhaps surprisingly, the common skin commencal organism *Staphylococcus saprophyticus* causes infection in young, sexually active females and is responsible for 5–15% of acute cystitis.[7,15]

PATHOGENESIS

In healthy individuals the perineum, vagina, vaginal introitus and urethra and periurethral areas each have their respective flora and are normally colonized by bacteria different from those commonly associated with UTI. The periurethral area may become colonized by such UTI-causing (uropathogenic) bacteria, which then ascend via the urethra into the bladder, and thence may ascend further to the kidney, causing pyelonephritis. The reservoir for these bacteria is the gastrointestinal tract.[7] There are host and bacterial mechanisms involved in determining whether a UTI will occur.

Host mechanisms

Secretor/non-secretor status

The urethral and periurethral mucosae in women who do not secrete their blood group antigens (non-secretors) in their body fluids, have a higher affinity for bacterial adhesins (see below) than in other women. These women are more susceptible to recurrent infections.[7,16]

Contraceptive practices, use of diaphragm/spermicides

The use of a diaphragm with a spermicide (an inhibitor of normal vaginal flora) promotes vaginal colonization with uropathogenic bacteria.[5]

Anatomic considerations (men) and prostatic secretions

In males the length of the urethra, its separation from the anus and the presence of prostatic secretions all contribute to the prevention of colonization and subsequent UTI.

Entry of bacteria into the bladder

Instrumentation of the bladder (see below) is a well recognized mechanism by which bacteria are introduced into the bladder. Other factors have been considered but have not been conclusively demonstrated. These include sexual intercourse, frequency and timing of voiding, hormonal changes, and personal hygiene habits.[4,5,17]

Bladder defence mechanisms

The healthy bladder can normally clear itself of bacteria. There are three factors involved: voiding; urinary bacteriostatic substances such as organic acids, high urea concentrations and immunoglobulins; and active resistance by the bladder mucosa to bacterial adherence.

Obstruction

This may be extrarenal (congenital anomalies such as urethral valves, calculi, benign prostatic hypertrophy) or intrarenal (nephrocalcinosis, polycystic kidney disease, analgesic nephropathy). Complete obstruction of the urinary tract predisposes to infection by haematogenous spread. In the absence of such obstruction, haematogenous seeding of bacteria to the kidneys accounts for about 3% of infections. Partial obstruction does not have this effect.

Vesicoureteric reflux

Incompetence of the vesicoureteric valve is a congenital problem that is five times more common in boys than in girls, but tends not to be a significant factor in adults. It allows infected urine to ascend to the kidney and is the most common factor predisposing to chronic pyelonephritic scarring.

Instrumentation

Although any instrumentation of the urinary tract predisposes to infection, catheterization is the most common of these. A single catheterization will result in UTI in 1% of ambulatory patients, but in hospitalized patients 10% of women and 5% of men will develop a UTI after one catheterization. Once in place, catheters produce infection in up to 10% of patients per day, and nearly all catheterized patients will be bacteriuric by 1 month.[18] All chronically catheterized patients are bacteriuric.

Pregnancy

Changes to the urinary tract occur normally during pregnancy as a result of both anatomical alterations and hormonal effects: dilatation of the ureters and renal pelves, decreased peristalsis in the ureters and decreased bladder tone. These changes begin before the end of the second month. The prevalence of bacteriuria rises with age and parity. A large proportion of asymptomatic, bacteriuric women develop symptomatic pyelonephritis later in that pregnancy, with significant increases in toxaemia and prematurity.[19]

Diabetes mellitus

There is no epidemiological evidence to support the traditionally held belief that diabetics are more at risk of developing UTI. However, there is definite evidence that diabetics are at greater risk of developing complications of these infections, such as septicaemia, renal abscess and papillary necrosis.[20]

Bacterial factors

A number of studies[21–23] have shown that the strains of *E. coli* (and a number of other Gram-negative bacteria) that cause UTI are not just the most prevalent in the bowel of the patient at the time of the infection, but have specific characteristics, termed virulence factors, that give them certain capabilities: increased intestinal carriage, persistence in the vagina, and the ability to ascend and invade the normal urinary tract. Thus there are clearly uropathogenic strains of these bacteria. In cases of complicated UTI (e.g. those associated with reflux, obstruction or foreign body) these virulence factors are not significantly involved. The two most important virulence factors are resistance to phagocytosis – which is a function of O and K antigens on the bacterial surface – and adherence to uroepithelium – which is a function of adhesins, molecular components expressed on the tips of the pili of the bacteria, and receptors on the uroepithelium.

PRESENTATION

History

A careful history should be taken in any patient presenting with symptoms of apparent UTI, looking for risk factors for complicated or recurrent infection (such as previous UTIs and their treatment, the presence of known anatomical abnormalities and investigations or instrumentation, the possibility of pregnancy, and history of diabetes mellitus), as well as seeking to identify those patients with urethritis and vaginitis. In men, the most common cause of recurrent lower tract UTI is prostatitis, so evidence of prostatitis such as chills, dysuria and prostatic tenderness should be sought.

Lower tract infections typically present with irritative micturition symptoms such as dysuria and frequency, suprapubic discomfort, and sometimes macroscopic haematuria. There is usually no fever. The classic symptom complex of loin pain, fever and urinary symptoms is usually associated with pyelonephritis, but is not always present. It is important to note that the symptoms of pyelonephritis can be quite variable, and even absent. Studies have shown that, of patients presenting with typical lower tract symptoms and who have significant bacteriuria, 30–50% will have upper tract involvement in the infective process.[1,24,25] This has significant implications for treatment, particularly if short-course treatment is considered (see Treatment). Severe pain should raise the suspicion of a ureteric calculus that, combined with infection, poses a greater risk of sepsis and of permanent injury to the kidney.

Patients with chronic indwelling catheters usually have no lower tract symptoms at all, but may develop loin pain and fever.

In elderly patients, particularly in long-term care facilities, the long-held view that symptoms of increased confusion and reduced mobility in the absence of fever, are due to urinary tract infection have been put into doubt (see Treatment of specific groups: Elderly patients).[12,14,26]

Examination

The clinical signs of lower UTI are few and non-specific; however, patients should be examined to exclude other causes for their symptoms, particularly vaginitis in women and prostatitis in men. The presence of fever and renal angle tenderness both suggest pyelonephritis but, as previously indicated, their absence does not rule it out.

INVESTIGATIONS

The key step in the diagnosis of UTI is examination of the urine, most commonly a midstream specimen. Catheterization is appropriate in patients with altered mental state or who cannot void because of neurological or urological reasons. Suprapubic aspiration is commonly used in pediatric practice, but can be used in adults if other techniques have failed or are unable to be used.

The next step is to look for the presence of pyuria, and subsequently the specimen may be sent for quantitative culture. Testing for haematuria, proteinuria and nitrites may be of supportive value but is not diagnostic.

Pyuria

The 'gold standard' definition of pyuria is based on early work involving the measurement of the rate of excretion of polymorphs in the urine. This work showed that excretion of 400 000 polymorphs per hour was always associated with infection and was also found to be represented by 10 polymorphs per mm^3 in a single (unspun) mid-stream specimen of urine.[27] Using this definition, it has subsequently been shown that more than 96% of symptomatic patients who have significant bacteriuria have significant pyuria and less than 1% of asymptomatic people without bacteriuria have this degree of pyuria.[28] Other definitions of pyuria, such as >5 leucocytes/high power field are based on examination of either the urinary sediment or of centrifuged urine and are inherently inaccurate because they cannot be standardized, but are nevertheless often used.

Nitrites

This reagent strip-based test is dependent on the bacterial reduction of urinary nitrate to nitrite. The test has a low sensitivity (33–66%) and a high false-negative rate (about 45% in many studies). False-negative results are likely if the infecting organism is Gram positive or *Pseudomonas*, if the diet lacks nitrate, or if there is diuresis or extreme frequency, as a period of bladder incubation is necessary to form nitrites.[29] However, a positive result is highly specific (92–100%) for infection.[7,30]

Haematuria

Although a frequent accompaniment of UTI, this finding is non-specific as there are many other causes of haematuria.

Proteinuria

Most commonly with UTI protein excretion is less than 2 g/24 h. It is another common but non-specific finding.

Quantitative culture

In symptomatic patients a single specimen with a bacterial count >10^5/ mL has a 95% probability of representing infection, but in asymptomatic women one specimen with >10^5 bacteria/mL has only an 80% probability of indicating UTI, with the probability rising to 95% with two specimens showing the same organism in this concentration. However, about one-third of young females with symptoms will have bacterial counts less than 10^5/mL (see Urethral syndrome). In men, counts as low as 10^3/mL suggest infection.

Urethral syndrome or UTI with low numbers of bacteria

Up to half of women with typical lower tract symptoms will have fewer than 10^5 bacteria/mL. Of these, about one-half have bacterial UTI, with low numbers of bacteria. Of the rest, one group has urethritis due to *C. trachomatis* or *Neisseria gonorrhoeae*, and the other has negative cultures and may have *Ureaplasma urealyticum* urethritis. All except this last group have pyuria.[31,32]

Screening tests

In considering the use of reagent strips as screening tests for UTI it should be noted that variations in published sensitivity and specificity exist and are due to i) the use of different brands of reagent strips, ii) the use of different 'gold standards' against which comparison is made (e.g. counting chamber or cells/HPF counts), and most importantly, iii) the target population (e.g. symptomatic emergency department patients rather than an asymptomatic in-patient population). A reagent strip test for leucocyte esterase has gained popularity as a screening test for pyuria. This has a sensitivity of 75–96% and a specificity of 94–98% for detecting >10/mm³ of urine. This gives a positive predictive value (in symptomatic individuals) of 50% and a negative predictive value of 92% making it a valuable test for screening the emergency department population. More importantly, recent work by Sultana has shown that reagent strips significantly improve the clinician's accuracy in diagnosing UTI in symptomatic emergency-department patients.[33] The clinical probability of UTI must be considered when using such screening tests. In the patient with typical urinary tract symptoms it may provide an adequate screen. It should, however, be used with great caution in the presence of fever of unknown cause in the elderly, the patient with an indwelling catheter or the patient with an impaired mental state, as pyuria and the implied bacteriuria may not be the cause of the problem.

Blood cultures

Current evidence is that in pyelonephritis blood cultures add nothing to urine culture, which will identify the organism involved and its antibiotic sensitivities.[34] In cases of sepsis with unclear cause, blood cultures must still be taken.

IMAGING

Either ultrasound, non-contrast computerized tomography (CT) or IVP is required in case of clinical suspicion of a ureteric stone or obstruction with infection. Patients with pyelonephritis, in particular those who do not respond to treatment after 72 hours, or who suffer recurrent infection within 2 weeks, should have imaging of the urinary tract.[6,7,35]

MANAGEMENT

Ideally, treatment of UTI should rapidly relieve symptoms, prevent short-term complications such as progression from cystitis to pyelonephritis and subsequent sepsis, or long-term sequelae such as renal scarring, and prevent recurrences by eliminating uropathogenic bacteria from vaginal and perineal reservoirs. Treatment should be cost-effective and have few or no side-effects.

There is no evidence that non-specific treatments such as pushing fluids or attempting to alter urinary pH improve the outcome of normal antibiotic treatment.

Antibiotic treatment

Serum levels of antibiotics are largely irrelevant in the elimination of bacteriuria. Reduction in urinary bacterial numbers correlates with the sensitivity of the organism to the urinary concentration of the antibiotic. Inhibitory concentrations are usually achieved in the urine after oral doses of the commonly used antibiotics. On the other hand, blood levels are vitally important in the treatment of bacteraemic or septic patients, or those with renal parenchymal infections. The choice of antibiotic is based on the clinical presentation and the bacteria likely to be involved (Table 8.5.1).

Treatment of specific groups
(see Fig. 8.5.1)

Frequency dysuria syndrome: presumed simple UTI

A non-pregnant woman first presenting with typical lower urinary symptoms should have vulvovaginitis excluded and an MSU taken and examined (or tested by dipstick) for pyuria. If pyuria is confirmed, culture of the urine specimen is not necessary and treatment should be commenced empirically.

There is now good evidence that in this group of patients short course treatment is effective in both treating the infection and eradicating uropathogenic strains of bacteria from reservoirs. Three-day treatment is superior to a single dose in eradicating the reservoirs of uropathogenic organisms, thereby reducing the incidence of recurrence.[35] Longer courses have an increased incidence of side effects but not higher cure rates. The antibiotics of choice for 3-day treatment are trimethoprim or a fluoroquinolone, however, in order to postpone the emergence of bacterial resistance, the latter should only be used if an organism resistant to other agents is proven.[36,37] Amoxicillin/clavulanic acid, nitrofurantoin and cephalexin are suitable for 5-day therapy, but amoxicillin alone should not be used as there is a high incidence (25%–30%) of resistant *E. coli* in community-acquired UTI. If there is no clinical response, MSU should be sent for culture and, in sexually active women, treatment for *C. trachomatis* commenced (doxycycline 100 mg,bd). In non-sexually active women, further treatment is guided by the results of sensitivity testing. Short course treatment is inappropriate in women who are at risk of upper urinary tract infection (despite lower tract symptoms), which includes those with a history of previous infections due to resistant organisms or with symptoms for more than 1 week.

Males must have urine culture initially and should have at least 14 days of treatment with any of the agents used for treatment of young women with simple cystitis (Table 8.5.1). In men over 50 years there is a high probability of invasion of prostatic tissue and treatment may need to be continued for 4–6 weeks.

Recurrent UTI

A careful search for causes should be made together with urine culture and sensitivity testing. Treatment with an appropriate antibiotic (as for acute cystitis) for at least 10–14 days is required. The patient may benefit from maintenance prophylaxis with, e.g. nitrofurantoin or trimethoprim for several months (see host factors).

Acute pyelonephritis

Patients presenting with the typical symptoms of pyelonephritis are at risk of

Table 8.5.1 Choice of treatment depending on bacteria involved (see text)

Condition	Bacteria involved	Suggested treatment
Acute simple cystitis	E. coli, E. faecalis, S. saprophyticus, Proteus spp., Klebsiella spp., Pseudomonas spp., enterococci, staphylococci, Corynebacterium spp.	Trimethoprim for 3 days OR Amoxycillin/clavulanate 250 mg 8 hourly for 5 days OR cephalexin 500 mg 12 hourly for 5 days OR Nitrofurantoin 50mg 6 hourly for 5 days Males or patients with recurrent infection should be treated for up to 14 days Norfloxacin 400 mg 12 hourly for 3 days in resistant infection only
UTI with structural abnormalities (complicated) and inpatients	Increased frequency of Proteus spp. Pseudomonas spp., Klebsiella spp., enterococci, staphylococci, Corynebacterium spp.	Mild infection: trimethoprim or a fluoroquinolone Severe infection: aminoglycosides plus amoxycillin or imipenem/cilastatin Treatment may need to be continued (orally) for 4–6 weeks
Dysuria with low bacterial numbers (urethral syndrome)	Ureaplasma urealyticum*	Doxycycline in young women
Acute uncomplicated pyelonephritis	E. coli, Proteus spp., Klebsiella spp., S. saprophyticus	Mild infection: oral treatment with trimethoprim 300 mg/day, or amoxycillin/clavulanate 500 mg 8 hourly, or cephalexin 500 mg 6 hourly. Severe infection: parenteral treatment initially then oral, use aminoglycoside, plus amoxycillin or a 3rd generation cephalosporin. Consider piperacillin or fluoroquinolones. Treatment must be continued for 14 days in all patients
Malignancy causing obstruction/infection	Anaerobes	Add metronidazole or clindamycin
Pregnancy-associated cystitis	E. coli, E. faecalis, S. saprophyticus, Proteus spp., Klebsiella spp.	Nitrofurantoin 50 mg 6 hourly amoxycillin/clavulanate 250 mg 8 hourly or cephalexin 250 mg 6 hourly. Follow closely. Treat for 10–14 days
Catheter-associated	E. coli, Proteus spp., Klebsiella spp., Pseudomonas spp., enterococci, staphylococci	Treat only if symptomatic. Change catheter. Treat as for 'complicated UTI'

*May have chlamydial or gonococcal urethritis
Adapted from[35]

bacteraemia or sepsis syndrome and therefore must rapidly have adequate concentrations of appropriate antibiotics delivered to both the blood and the urine. In order to meet this requirement, particularly in patients who are vomiting, parenteral (intravenous) treatment is usually required initially, but seldom for longer than 24–48 hours, by which time the patient is usually afebrile and not vomiting.

The choice of antibiotics is of necessity empirical at this stage. In cases of mild-to-moderate infection, 14-day treatment with one of the antimicrobials used for simple cystitis is appropriate (with cipro-floxacin replacing norfloxacin for resistant organisms). For severe infections, parenteral amoxycillin together with gentamycin, both in high dose, are appropriate, with a third-generation cephalosporin as an alternative to genta-mycin when use of aminoglycosides is in-appropriate. Parenteral fluoroquinolone, and ureidopenicillins (e.g. piperacillin) may be appropriate for seriously ill patients with community-acquired infections. In patients with hospital-acquired infections and suspected Gram-negative sepsis, broader-spectrum agents such as cefta-zidime, ticarcillin/clavulanic acid and imipenem, perhaps in combination with aminoglycosides, may be required.

Parenteral treatment is followed by oral therapy for 2 weeks.[36, 37,38]

Economic imperatives have encouraged moves toward management strategies that avoid admission to in-patient beds. Emergency medicine has led this trend by establishment of observation (or short stay) units[39,40] and studies have demonstrated the safety and efficacy of treatment in such units with intravenous antibiotics and fluid administration, followed by oral therapy.[41] Many hospi-tals also have active 'hospital in the home' or 'out-patient antibiotic treatment (OPAT)' programmes, allowing close supervision of these patients by hospital-based staff and once- or twice-daily intravenous antibiotic administration at home.[42] This is a reasonable alternative to observation unit treatment suitable for milder cases, but requires careful patient selection to exclude those at risk of complicated infections. Appropriate follow-up is essential, with repeat urine cultures and imaging to exclude obstruction or anatomical abnormalities.

Pregnancy

UTI in pregnancy are associated with an increased incidence of premature delivery and low birthweight infants. This has also been demonstrated to occur with asymptomatic bacteriuria, although up to 40% of asymptomatic women develop acute pyelonephritis later in pregnancy. Therefore, screening for

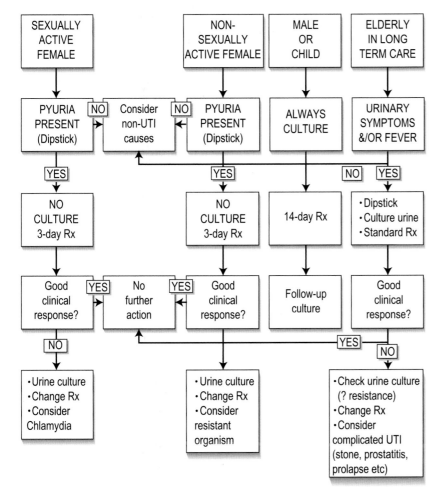

Fig. 8.5.1 Suggested management flow chart [S1]check.

Elderly patients

Asymptomatic bacteriuria is highly prevalent in residents of long-term care facilities with up to 30% of men and 50% of women showing bacteriuria, with a correlation between degree of functional impairment and likelihood of bacteriuria. There is good evidence that treatment of asymptomatic patients is of no benefit and may paradoxically be associated with increased morbidity. Conversely, symptomatic infection is a signficant cause of morbidity and mortality as this age group also has a higher incidence of bacteraemia associated with pyelonephritis, and septic shock commonly follows. Given the high rate of asymptomatic bacteriuria, the diagnosis of UTI in such individuals is difficult. The traditional view that non-specific symptoms such as increased confusion (without fever), falling or deteriorating mobility are due to UTI has been called into question and it is currently held that UTI should only be considered in patients with fever or specific genitourinary symptoms or both. In patients with non-specific symptoms, non-infective causes should be sought and in the case of fever alone, other potential sources of infection must be considered.[12,14,26]

Antibiotic treatment of symptomatic UTI in the elderly patient is no different initially to that of younger patients, however, it should be borne in mind that a greater variety of organisms may be cultured in this age group, and urine for culture should be obtained at the outset whenever possible.

DISPOSITION

Patients with simple UTI should have follow-up to confirm clinical cure. Failure of symptomatic improvement in 48 hours may indicate antibiotic resistance, which requires urine culture to elucidate. Recurrence of symptoms within 1–2 weeks may indicate occult renal infection, and necessitates urine culture and at least 7 days' treatment.

The follow-up of patients with pyelonephritis should include imaging to examine the collecting system and the

bacteriuria and treatment of pregnant women is essential, and urine must be sent for culture and antibiotic sensitivity testing. Three-day courses of treatment are not widely recommended, although it may be reasonable to use them with close follow-up in an effort to reduce antibiotic usage, however, 10–14-day treatment courses are the norm. Nitrofurantoin, amoxycillin/clavulanate or cephalexin are appropriate for use in pregnancy.

Complicated UTI

As there is a greater range of organisms causing infection in these circumstances, and a higher probability of antibiotic resistance, urine culture is essential and initial empiric treatment must cover the broader spectrum of organisms potentially involved. Trimethoprim or a quino-

lone is appropriate for mild infections. More serious infections may need combinations of agents, such as aminoglycosides with amoxycillin or imipenem/cilastatin.

Catheter-associated UTI

Urinary tract infections are the most common cause of nosocomial infections, most of which are due to the use of urinary catheters.[43] In patients with short-term catheters who develop infection, the catheter must be changed and treatment instituted as for complicated UTI. For those with chronic indwelling catheters (such as patients with spinal injuries), bacteriuria is universal and treatment is only indicated in the presence of symptoms such as fever, chills or loin pain. Antibiotic selection should again be based on culture.

CONTROVERSIES

❶ The role of screening, with dipstick methods, for leucocyte esterase vs urine microscopy.

❷ The role of blood cultures as part of the investigation of pyelonephritis. Although traditionally used, they add little or nothing to the diagnosis and management.

❸ The role of observation units and 'hospital in the home' or OPAT programmes.

renal parenchyma. Ultrasound is a good, rapid, non-invasive method that can be followed by IVP or contrast CT if indicated.

PROGNOSIS

In adults with normal urinary tracts UTI does not cause long-term sequelae. In the presence of urinary-tract abnormalities, infection may be a factor in producing renal damage or altering its rate of onset. Imaging of adults as part of their follow-up should detect this group of patients. In the elderly, bacteriuria may be a marker of functional deterioration. Opinion has been divided on whether or not asymptomatic bacteriuria leads to decreased survival in this age group. Treatment of asymptomatic bacteriuria in the elderly is not currently recommended, as there is no evidence of any benefit and some indication of increased morbidity due to antibiotic-related complications and emergence of resistant organisms.

REFERENCES

1. Bergeron M 1995 Treatment of pyelonephritis in adults. Medical Clinics of North America; 79: 619–49
2. Kreger B, Craven D, Carling P, McCabe W 1980 Gram - negative bacteremia iii. Reassessment of etiology, epidemiology & ecology in 612 patients. American Journal of Medicine 68: 332–43
3. Anonymous 2000 Urinary tract infections. Better Health Channel Website. Department of Human Services, State Government of Victoria; [cited May 13, 2002] Available from URL: http://www.betterhealth.vic.gov.au/bhcv2/bhcarticles.nsf/pages/Urinary_tract_infections
4. Kelsey M, Mead M, Gruneberg R, Oriel J 1979 Relationships between sexual intercourse and urinary tract infection in women attending a clinic for sexually transmitted diseases. Journal of Medical Microbiology 12: 511–2
5. Foxman B, Frerichs R 1985 Epidemiology of urinary tract infection: I. Diaphragm use and sexual intercourse. American Journal of Public Health 75: 1308–13
6. Hooton TM, Scholes D, Hughes JP, et al 1996 A prospective study of risk factors for symptomatic urinary tract infection in young women. New England Journal of Medicine 335: 468
7. Kunin C 1994 Urinary tract infections in females. Clinical Infectious Diseases 18: 1–12
8. Ronald A, Pattullo A 1991 The natural history of urinary infection in adults. Medical Clinics of North America 75: 299–312
9. Vorland L, Carlson K, Aalen O 1985 An epidemiological survey of urinary tract infections among outpatients in northern norway. Scandinavian Journal of Infectious Diseases 17: 277
10. Dontas A, Kasviki-Charvati P, Papanayiotou P, Marketos S 1981 Bacteriuria and survival in old age. New England Journal of Medicine 304: 939–43
11. Nicolle L, Bjornson J, Harding G, MacDonell J 1983 Bacteriuria in elderly institutionlaized men. New England Journal of Medicine 309: 1421–5
12. Nicolle L 2002 Urinary tract infection in geriatric and institutionalized patients. Current Opinion in Urology 12: 51–5
13. Nicolle L 1997 Asymptomatic bacteriuria in the elderly. Infectious Disease Clinics of North America 11(3): 647
14. Nicolle L 2000 Urinary tract infection in long-term-care facility residents. Clinical Infectious Diseases 31: 757–61
15. Jordan P, Iravani A, Richard G, Baer H 1980 Urinary tract infection caused by staphylococcus saprophyticus. Journal of Infectious Diseases 142: 510–5
16. Kinane D, Blackwell C, Brettle R et al 1982 Abo blood group, secretor state and susceptibility to recurrent urinary tract infection in women. British Medical Journal 285: 7–9
17. Bran J, Levinson M, Kaye D 1972 Entrance of bacteria into the female urinary bladder. New England Journal of Medicine 286: 626–9
18. Turck M, Goffe B, Petersdorf R 1962 The urethral catheter and urinary tract infection. Journal of Urology 88: 834–7
19. Kincaid-Smith P, Bullen M 1965 Bacteriuria in pregnancy. Lancet 1: 1312–4
20. O'Sullivan D, Fitzgerald M, Meyness M, Malins J 1961 Urinary tract infection, a comparative study in the diabetic and general population. British Jounal of Medicine 1: 786
21. Mabeck C, Orskov R, Orskov I 1971 Escherichia coli serotypes and renal involvement in urinary tract infection. Lancet 1: 1312–4
22. Hagberg L, Hull R, Hull S et al 1983 Contribution of adhesion to bacterial persistence in the mouse urinary tract. Infection and Immunity 40: 265–72
23. Svanborg-Eden C, Hausson S, Jodal Y, et al 1988 Host-parasite interactions in the urinary tract. Journal of Infectious Diseases 157: 421–6
24. Sandford J 1976 Urinary tract symptoms and infections. Annual Review of Medicine 26: 485–99
25. Rubin R, Cotran R, Tolkoff-Rubin N 1991 Urinary tract infection, pyelonephritis, and reflux nephropathy. In: Brenner B (ed.) The Kidney. WB Saunders, Philadelphia, pp 1597–1654
26. Bentley D, Bradley S, High K, Schoenbaum S, Taler G, Yoshikawa T 2000 Practice guidelines for evaluation of fever and infection in long-term care facilities. Clinical Infectious Diseases 31: 640–53
27. Brumfitt W 1965 Urinary cell counts and their value. Journal of Clinical Pathology 18: 550
28. Stamm W 1983 Measurement of pyuria and its relation to bacteriuria. American Journal of Medicine 75(1B): 53–8
29. Morgan M, McKenzie H 1993 Controversies in the laboratory diagnosis of community-acquired urinary tract infection. European Journal of Clinical Microbiology and Infectious Diseases 12: 491–504
30. Pappas P 1991 Laboratory in the diagnosis and management of urinary tract infections. Medical Clinics of North America 75: 313–25
31. Stamm W, Wagner K, Amsel R, et al 1980 Causes of the acute urethral syndrom in women. New England Journal of Medicine 303: 956–8
32. Stamm W, Running K, McKevitt M et al 1981 Treatment of the acute urethral syndrome. New England Journal of Medicine 303: 409–15
33. Sultana R, Zalstein S, Cameron P, Campbell D 2001 Dipstick urinalysis and the accuracy of the clinical diagnosis of urinary tract infection. Journal of Emergency Medicine 20: 13–9
34. McMurray B, Wrenn K, Wright S 1997 Usefulness of blood cultures in pyelonephritis. American Journal of Emergency Medicine 15: 137–40
35. Stamm W, Hooton T 1993 Management of urinary tract infections in adults. New England Journal of Medicine 329: 1328–34
36. Anonymous 2000 Urinary infections. In: Therapeutic Guidelines: Antibiotic. Version 11. North Melbourne: Therapeutic Guidelines Limited, pp 195–200
37. Warren J, Abrutyn E, Hebel J, Johnson J, Schaeffer A, Stamm W 1999 Guidelines for antimicrobial treatment of uncomplicated acute bacterial cystitis and acute pyelonephritis in women. Clinical Infectious Diseases 29: 745–58
38. Stamm W, McKevitt M, Counts G 1987 Acute renal infection in women: Treatment with trimethoprim-sulfamethoxazole or ampicillin for two or six weeks. Annals of Internal Medicine 106: 341–5
39. Williams A, Jelinek G, Rogers I, Wenban J, Jacobs IG 2000 The effect on hospital admission profiles of establishing an emergency department observation ward. Medical Journal of Australia 173: 411–4
40. Jelinek G, Galvin G 1989 Observation wards in australian hospitals. Medical Journal of Australia 151: 80–3
41. Ward G, Jorden R, Severance H 1991 Treatment of pyelonephritis in an observation unit. Annals of Emergency Medicine 20: 258–61
42. Montalto M, Dunt D 1997 Home and hospital intravenous therapy for two acute infections: An early study. Australian and New Zealand Journal of Medicne 27: 19–23
43. Haley R, Culver D, White J, Morgan W, Emori T 1985 The nationwide nosocomial infection rate. A new need for vital statistics. American Journal of Epidemiology 121: 159–67

FURTHER READING

Rubin RH, Cotran RS, Tolkoff-Rubin NE 1991 Urinary tract infection, pyelonephritis, and reflux nephropathy. In: Brenner BM (ed) The kidney, 5th edn. WB Saunders, Philadelphia, pp 1597–654
Sobel JD, Kaye D 1995 Urinary tract infections. In: Mandell GL, Bennett JE, Dolin R (eds) Principles and Practice of Infectious Diseases, 4th edn. Churchill Livingstone, New York, pp 662–90

8.6 SKIN AND SOFT-TISSUE INFECTIONS

JOHN VINEN

ESSENTIALS

1 The time-honoured principles of wound management, together with the judicious evidence-based use of antibiotics remain the basis for preventing and treating skin and soft-tissue infections.

2 All wounds, no matter how trivial, should be treated as tetanus prone wounds and treated accordingly.

3 Skin and soft-tissue infections are common and range from mild to life threatening, they occasionally require surgical intervention, and usually respond to narrow-spectrum antibiotics.

4 Deep soft-tissue infections have high morbidity and mortality and, unless treated aggressively, can rapidly result in loss of limb or death of the patient.

5 Infections due to unusual organisms, including organisms not usually considered to be pathogenic, frequently cause serious infections in the immunocompromised, diabetics and patients with hepatic disease.

INTRODUCTION

Infectious disease is one of the most common reasons for patients to present to the emergency department. Skin and soft-tissue infections make up an important subset of these. These are caused by a variety of agents, including bacteria, fungi, viruses and parasites. Cutaneous manifestations of infection can be the result of direct inoculation, release of a toxin, an immunologic process, or a combination of these. The management of skin and soft-tissue infections is reliant on accurate assessment of the problem,

an understanding of aetiology including the likely presence of bacterial pathogens, the type of bacteria likely to be involved and the appropriate use of antibiotic therapy. The wide range of antibiotics available, indications for specific antibiotics, the emergence and recognition of new infections and changing bacterial resistance patterns create a challenging scenario for the emergency physician.

WOUND MANAGEMENT/ PREVENT INFECTION

The goals of wound care are to avoid infection and to achieve a functional and cosmetically acceptable scar. Adequate wound management requires a thorough history with particular attention directed at factors adversely affecting wound healing. Factors such as the extremes of age, diabetes, chronic renal failure, malnutrition, alcoholism, obesity, and patients on immunosuppressive agents, cause an increased risk of infections and impaired wound healing.

Wounds located in highly vascular areas such as the scalp or face are less likely to become infected, compared to wounds in less vascular areas.

In order to reduce the incidence and severity of infections, wounds need to be thoroughly cleansed and irrigated. Devitalized tissue should be removed, injuries to associated structures need to be excluded and the wound closed appropriately. The method of wound closure is dependent on the location of the wound, the level of contamination of the wound and whether it is an 'old' wound (over 6 hours old). Wounds that should not be closed because of a high risk of infection, such as heavily contaminated wounds, should be treated by delayed primary closure 3–5 days after initial management. Where primary closure is possible the wound should be closed and a protective non-adherent

dressing applied for a minimum of 24 to 48 hours with the wound and dressing kept dry.[1]

The use of prophylactic antibiotics is not recommended except in situations where there is significant bacterial contamination, foreign materials present, the patient is immunosuppressed or the wound is the result of a bite (human or animal) or associated with an open fracture. Most wounds can be treated with first-generation cephalosporins or penicillinase-resistant penicillin. Broad-spectrum antibiotics should be limited to heavily contaminated and bite wounds, and immunosuppressed patients (Table 8.6.1).

INVESTIGATIONS

The Gram stain can be a useful test in identifying the organisms involved, though an adequate sample may be difficult to obtain where there is not a localized collection. Bacterial cultures are useful in differentiating anaerobic from aerobic organisms as well as assisting in the identification of the organisms present and their resistance patterns. Sensitivities to antibiotics can also be determined. It is important to test for diabetes mellitus in patients presenting with an abscess because of the strong association of the two. Patients with a chronic, recurrent or unusual infection should have their immune status checked, including serology for HIV.

INDICATIONS FOR ADMISSION

The need for hospital admission and parental therapy are relatively straightforward. Patients who have; systemic toxicity (febrile, tachycardia, rigors, confusion), involvement of vital structures (fingers, hand, face, genitourinary and anal regions) are unable to take oral

Table 8.6.1 Recommended empiric parenteral antibiotic therapy for serious wound infections[5]

Type of infection	Location	Immune status	Antibiotic	IV dose (adults)
Cellulitis/abscess	Extremities	Normal Immunocompromized diabetic, vascular insufficiency	Dicloxacillin metronidazole and cephalothin or cephazolin or Ampicillin	2 g 6-hourly 500 mg IV 12-hourly 1 g IV 4-hourly 1 g IV 8-hourly
	Perineal	All patients	Gentamicin Metronidazole Ticarcillin/potassium	2 g 6-hourly 5–7 mg/kg/day 500 mg IV 12-hourly
	All patients	Parenteral drug users	Drug users	3/0.1 g IV 6-hourly clavulanate
	Foot	All patients	Dicloxacillin	2 g 6-hourly
	Facial	All patients	Dicloxacillin	2 g 6-hourly
Bite wounds **Human**	All patients	All patients	Amoxycillin/ potassium clavulanate	1 g IV 6-hourly
Animal	All patients	All patients	For patients sensitive to penicillin, metronidazole and either doxycycline or co-trimoxazole or ceftriaxone or cefotaxime	400 mg orally 12-hourly 100 mg orally daily 160/180 mg orally hourly 1 g IV daily 1 g IV daily
Necrotizing fasciitis/ gas gangrene	All patients	All patients	Benzlypenicillin and gentamicin and metronidazole	2.4 g IV 4-hourly 5–7 mg/kg/day IV 500 mg IV 8-hourly
			For patients sensitive ot penicillin use clindamycin and gentamycin	600 mg IV 8-hourly slowly 5–7 mg/kg/day IV

medication, failed outpatient therapy or who are immunocompromised require admission (Table 8.6.1).

INDICATIONS FOR ANTIBIOTIC USE

Antibiotics are recommended for patients with: signs of systemic toxicity, high fever, tachycardia, flushed and who look unwell, who are immunocompromised, who have abscesses in high-risk areas (hands, perineal region or face) and where deep necrotizing infection is suspected.[2]

ANTIBIOTIC THERAPY

It is important for the emergency physician to recognize patients with serious skin and soft-tissue infections and to initiate appropriate care. Antibiotic therapy can be guided by Gram stain results, where possible, a Gram stain

should be done urgently as they may assist in the selection of appropriate antibiotics. Where this is not possible, the choice of antibiotic is empiric. Empiric therapy, to be effective must be guided by the patient's history, where they have been recently institutionalized and knowledge of the typical range of pathogens associated with each type of infection and their resistance patterns. The antibiotic of choice is the one that has proven efficacy against the range of expected pathogens, is associated with minimal toxicity and is cost effective. Where possible narrow spectrum antibiotics should be used in preference to broad spectrum antibiotics.[3]

TETANUS PROPHYLAXIS

All wounds should be considered to be tetanus prone wounds and treated accordingly. The patient's immunization status should be checked and where

appropriate tetanus toxoid + tetanus immunoglobulin should be administered. Deep and penetrating wounds and wounds that have significant tissue devitalization or where there is heavy contamination are best treated with prophylactic antibiotic cover, the antibiotic of choice is penicillin, patients who are allergic to penicillin should receive cephalexin (cephalothin if a parenteral drug is required). If there is a history of severe penicillin allergy, use erythromycin or vancomycin 1 g (40 mg/kg/day up to adult dose 1–2 divided doses IV slowly 12 hourly).

CUTANEOUS INFECTION

The outer keratin layer of skin serves as a mechanical barrier of bacterial invasion and provides protection from the development of skin infections and cutaneous abscesses. The continuous desquamation of the epidermis also contributes by shedding bacteria present on the skin.

Skin infections and abscesses can arise in skin that has been damaged. Patients who are immunosuppressed, diabetics and patients with chronic disease have a lower resistance to the development of skin infections and cutaneous abscesses.

The most common aerobic pathogen associated with a cutaneous infection (including abscesses associated with foreign bodies such as splinters) is *Staphylococcus aureus*. Other staphylococcus species, particularly *Staph. epidermidis* and *Staph. hominis* are also involved.[4] Streptococcus species, including *Streptococcus viridans* are commonly associated with staphylococcal skin infections and abscesses.

Abscesses involving the perianal, genital, buttocks, ungual and cervical areas are predominantly caused by anaerobic bacteria. Mixed flora, both aerobic and anaerobic, are usually found, with *Bacteroides fragilis* being the most common Gram-negative anaerobe. *Escherichia coli*, *Klebsiella* and *Proteus* are also common.

Organisms found in immunocompromised patients include *Cryptococccus neoformans*, *Coccidioides*, *Aspergillus*, *Mycobacterium kansasii*, *M. tuberculosis* and *Yersinia enterocolitica*.[5]

SUPERFICIAL SKIN INFECTIONS

Clinical presentation

Patients usually present with a complaint of localized pain, redness and swelling. The patient may have been self-treating or have had previous treatment with oral antibiotics without success. Frequently an abscess is fluctuant and indurated with surrounding erythema. The patient may also have associated lymphadenitis, regional lymphadenopathy and cellulitis. If the patient is febrile or there is systemic involvement, the patient's immune status needs to be examined.

The possibility of a foreign body associated with an abscess needs to be considered. A careful history needs to be taken to determine whether this is possible, radiography may be necessary.

The use of ultrasound can be useful in identifying the presence of a foreign body. The patient should also be questioned in relation to immunosuppressive agent use.

Folliculitis

A superficial infection characterized by reddened papules or pustules of the hair follicles.

Most cases are caused by *Staph.aureus*. *Pseudomonas aeroginosa* may be the cause following swimming pool or hot tub (spa) exposure. Treatment may only require the use of an antibacterial soap or solution. Removal of the hair in limited infections usually result in rapid resolution.

Erysipelas

Erysipelas is a rapidly progressive, erythmatous, indurated, painful, sharply demarcated superficial skin infection caused by *Strep. pyogenes* (other causes, non-group A streptococci, *H. Influenzae*, *Staph.aureus* and *Strep. pneumoniae*). It is common in young children and the elderly. Systemic symptoms (fever, chills, rigors and diaphresis) are common. 5% will have bacteriaemia.

Erysipelas may rapidly progress to cellulitis, abscess formation and occasionally fasciitis. Treatment consists of the use of antibacterial soap and oral penicillin.

Furuncle

A furuncle arises secondarily to an infected hair follicle. Furuncles most commonly occur on the back, axilla or lower extremities. *Staphylococcus* species are the most common organism associated with the condition.

Carbuncle

A carbuncle is a staphylococcal infection, most often occurring on the back of the neck. Carbuncles are larger than furuncles and often contain an interconnecting system of abscesses that can be quite extensive.

CELLULITIS

Cellulitis is the most common complication of wound infection. In patients with a normal immune system who are otherwise healthy, the infection is caused by bacteria that normally colonize skin, principally *Staph. aureus* and group A β-haemolytic streptococci. Clinically the two cannot be differentiated; commonly they occur simultaneously.[6] Treatment consists of elevation of the affected limb and administration of an anti-staphylococcal penicillin such as dicloxacillin or a first-generation cephalosporin. Patients suitable for outpatient treatment requiring parenteral therapy can be given ceftriaxone 1 g daily.[7]

Cellulitis may also be caused by Gram-negative organisms and anaerobes, particularly in diabetics. Anaerobes or Gram-negative organisms have been identified in 95% of affected diabetic foot ulcers with *Staph. aureus* found in approximately 33%. Broad-spectrum antibiotic treatment with metronidazole (400 mg orally 12-hourly) and cephalothin (1 g IV 4-hourly) or cephazolin (1 g IV 8-hourly) is recommended.

Infections that originate from wounds involving the feet may be due to *Pseudomonas aeruginosa*, this organism is also associated with osteomyelitis of the foot. Antibiotic treatment should consist of antipseudomonal β-lactam such as carbenacillin, or a third-generation cephlosporin such as ceftriaxone and an aminoglycoside.

Facial cellulitis, including periorbital and orbital cellulitis is a serious infection occurring in both adults and children.[8, 9] The causal organisms include *Staph. aureus*, *Haemophilus influenzae* type b and *Staph. pneumoniae*. This type of cellulitis may arise from an infected sinus. Broad-spectrum antibiotic therapy is required, the agent of choice being dicloxcillin 1 g IV 6-hourly. In children less than 5 years of age, because facial or parietal cellulitis can be due to *H. influenzae*, use cefotaxime 150 mg/kg/day up to a maximum of 2 g IV daily followed by amoxycillin/potassium clavulanate 75/18.75 mg/kg/day up to a maximum 1500/375 mg orally in three divided doses for 7 days.

In older children and adults where staphylococcal infection is more likely, flucloxacillin 500 mg (50 mg/kg/day up to adult dose, 6-hourly) orally,

6-hourly is recommended. If severe, use flucloxacilllin 2 g (150–200 mg/kg/day up to adult dose) IV 6-hourly.

Radiological evaluation including CT scanning may be necessary to identify underlying sinusitis.[10]

ABSCESSES

Pilonidal abscess

Pilonidal abscesses occur in the labial fold and arise from the disruption of the epithelium, leading to the formation of a pit lined with epithelial cells that may become plugged with hair and keratin, leading to an abscess. Treatment involves incision and drainage, usually in the operating theatre, although smaller abscesses can be drained in the emergency department under local anaesthetic. They are usually associated with mixed organisms, both aerobic and anaerobic.

Hidradenitis suppurativa

This is a chronic suppurative abscess of the upper apocrine sweat glands in the groin and axilla. It is much more common in females, also more common in obesity and in patients who have poor hygiene and who shave the region. Organisms include *Staph. aureus*, *Streptococcus viridans* and *Proteus*. The treatment required is incision and drainage, usually in the operating theatre. Definitive treatment may require removal of the apocrine sweat glands from the region.

Bartholin abscess

This occurs as a result of the obstruction of a Bartholin duct and usually is composed of mixed vaginal flora. *Neisseria gonorrhoeae* and *Chlamydia trachomatis* may also be involved. Treatment is incision, drainage and marsupialization of the cyst in the operating theatre.

Paronychia

This is a superficial abscess of the lateral aspect of the nail, commonly associated with patients whose hands are frequently wet. Common organisms involved are *Staph. aureus*, *Candida* and anaerobes. May require incision and drainage if fluctuant, with advice to keep the hands dry.

Perianal abscess

These are thought to originate in the anal crypts and extend into the ischiorectal space. Patients frequently complain of pain on defecation and sitting. Perianal abscesses may be associated with inflammatory bowel disease and fistula formation. Treatment should be incision and drainage in the operating theatre under general anaesthesia. When the abscess is superficial and 'pointing', drainage in the emergency department is possible.

Infected sebaceous cyst

Sebaceous cysts become infected when the duct is obstructed. They can occur anywhere on the body, but tend to favour the head and neck region. Treatment is incision and drainage, recurrence is not uncommon.

Treatment

Incision and drainage of cutaneous abscesses is the key to treatment. Some patients require oral antibiotic therapy (Table 8.6.2). Patients who are immunosuppressed or who have diabetes mellitus should be treated with appropriate antibiotic therapy based on the knowledge of the probable pathogen. Patients at risk of developing bacterial endocarditis also require antibiotics, including prophylactic antibiotics, prior to incision and drainage.

DEEP SOFT-TISSUE INFECTIONS

Necrotizing fasciitis

Necrotizing fasciitis is a life-threatening illness that has a sudden onset and that

Table 8.6.2 Oral therapy of soft tissue infections

Streptococcus - Group A
Phenoxymethyl Penicillin (V) 250 mg Q 6-hourly
Erythromycin 500 mg - 1 g Q 6-hourly

Staphylococcus aureus
Dicloxacillin 500 mg to 1 g Q 6-hourly
Erythromycin 500 mg to 1 g Q 6-hourly
Clindamycin 150 mg to 450 mg Q 6-hourly

may develop from simple wounds or sometimes without obvious injury.[11,12] Patients present with sudden onset of pain, swelling and fever with rapid development of extensive cellulitis. The skin frequently has a blue/brown discolouration, which progresses to necrosis.

Because of the involvement of cutaneous nerves numbness of the involved area is characteristic of advanced necrotizing fasciitis.[11] This is a result of infarction of the cutaneous nerve.

Patients appear extremely toxic with a high fever, tachycardia and malaise. Pathognomic features include; extensive undermining of the skin and subcutaneous tissues, with separation of the tissue planes. Crepitation may be evident, gas may be evident particularly on X-ray and is found in some 80% of patients radiologically. The gas is typically layered along fascial planes.

Bacteria involved in this infection is usually mixed; *Staph.aureus*, haemolytic streptococci, Gram-negative rods, and anaerobes. Sometimes only group A streptococci alone or in combination with *Staph. aureus*, are found. Aggressive therapy is essential, as mortality approaches 50%. Immediate surgical intervention to extensively open and debride the wound is required, myonecrosis may be present.[12] Appropriate antimicrobial therapy should be commenced immediately including high-dose penicillin G, antistaphylococcal penicillin, or first-generation cephalosporin, and an aminoglycoside. Hyperbaric oxygen therapy should be considered.

Gangrene

Gangrene is an acute life-and-limb threatening deep-tissue infection, also known as clostridial myonecrosis or gas gangrene. This infection is characterized by the rapid development (often within hours of injury) of intense pain in the region of a wound, followed by local swelling and a haemoserous exudate. A characteristic foul smell is also a good indication of the diagnosis. The area becomes tense and may become discoloured, developing a bluish and bronze or dusky discolouration. The presence of gas is typical though it may be a late finding. It is frequently found on X-ray, where it has a feathered pattern as a gas develops within the muscle itself. Aggressive treatment is required as the patient may present in an advanced stage of the infection with tachycardia, altered mental status, shock, and haemolytic anaemia.

Classically, the gas gangrene occurs in extensive and or deep wounds with predisposing factors including; vascular ischaemia, diabetes and presence of foreign bodies. Gram stain frequently reveals relatively few white blood cells and large numbers of club shaped Gram-positive rods.

Early surgical intervention is essential including wide debridement of necrotic muscle and other tissues, administration of high dose penicillin G, an aminoglycoside and hyperbaric oxygen therapy. Early hyperbaric oxygen therapy has been demonstrated to result in improved outcome.[2, 11–14]

Organisms commonly involved include Clostridium perfringens, C. novyi and C. septicum.

It is important to understand that whilst the presence of gas, may raise the suspicion of a deep-tissue infection including gas gangrene, it may also be present because of previous wound manipulation, self injection of air, localized gas abscess or other gas-producing organisms including: anaerobes, *E.coli*, *streptococci* and *staphylococci*.

TOXIC COMPLICATIONS OF WOUND INFECTIONS

A number of bacteria produce toxins that result in systemic symptoms.

Tetanus

Tetanus, whilst rare in developing countries, still occurs despite the fact that immunization is completely effective in preventing tetanus. All wounds should be treated as tetanus-prone wounds. Tetanus may occur with trivial wounds that may not even be apparent. The incubation period is variable, ranging from 3 days to several weeks after inocu-

lation, the disease is more severe at the extremes of age. Difficulty in swallowing and a fever with progression to stiffness and trismus is pathognomonic. It is also associated with autonomic nervous system dysfunction. Occasionally localized tetanus may occur with muscle spasm in the area adjacent to the wound. This is sometimes associated with cranial nerve dysfunction. Treatment is largely supportive, often requiring deep sedation, paralysis and ventilation for prolonged periods. Antibiotic therapy with high-dose penicillin should also be given in addition to tetanus immunization and tetanus immunoglobulin.

Botulism

Botulism is caused by *Clostridium botulinum* infection and subsequent toxin release. Wound botulism is rare. Most botulism is caused by ingested food, where toxin is ingested with symptoms appearing 2–18 hours later. Botulism is characterized by cranial nerve dysfunction, followed by progressive descending symmetrical paralysis with a mortality rate of approximately 16%.

Diphtheria

Diphtheria is rare though increasing in incidence. It is caused by toxicogenic strains of *Corynebacterium diphtheriae*. Pharyngeal diphtheria can result in airway obstruction with characteristic membrane formation. Complications include the development of myocarditis and peripheral neuritis. Treatment is with diphtheria anti-toxins and high-dose penicillin. Immunization is completely protective.

Toxic shock syndrome

Toxic shock syndrome (TSS) is due to toxogenic strains of *Staph. aureus*. TSS has been classically associated with the use of tampons, although of the 10% of non-menstrual related cases, cutaneous lesions such as lacerations, abscesses, burns and bites count for the majority of cases. It can also occur post operatively. Incubation period is generally 24–48 hours. The wound itself may look insignificant. There is a rapid onset of fever, hypotension and an initial diffuse

and later desquamating erythematous rash, and involvement of all organ systems. Occasionally *Staph. aureus* can be cultured locally, although blood cultures are rarely positive. Treatment is supportive, high-dose penicillin or a first-generation cephalosporin is required. Patients are frequently shocked requiring aggressive fluid resuscitation and inotropic support. Debridement of necrotic wounds, if present, should be done urgently. A similar syndrome can develop due to infection with group A β-haemolytic streptococci. This is known as 'wound' or 'surgical' scarlet fever. Treatment is the same as that for TSS.[13]

SPECIAL INFECTIONS

Water-related infections

Water-related infections may be caused by unusual organisms. *Vibrio vulnificus*, *V. alginolyticus* and other non-cholera vibrios are found in salt and brackish water. *Mycobacterium marinum*, *M. ulcerans*, *M. chelonei*, *M. gordanae*. and *M. fortuitum*, are found in fish tanks and can result in 'fish fancier's finger'.

Exposure to fresh or brackish water (rivers, mud and caving) can result in infection with *Aeromonas hydrophila*.[15]

Coral cuts are often infected with *Streptococcus pyogenes*; other marine pathogens may be involved (including *Vibrio* species). Treatment should consist of phenoxymethylpenicillin 500 mg 6-hourly.

Vibrio vulnificus and other *Vibrio* species may cause serious and life-threatening infections in patients with hepatic disease. Advanced infection may develop over 2–4 hours. It is associated with saltwater exposure or ingestion of raw shellfish. Infections can mimic gas gangrene, with rapid progression and tissue destruction; septicaemia may occur and can be fatal, particularly in immunocompromised patients and patients with hepatic disease.

Vibrio species are sensitive to tetracycline (500 mg orally, 6-hourly). If parenteral therapy is required, ceftriaxone 1–2 g IV daily, or cefotaxime 1 g IV 8-hourly.[16]

Aeromonas hydrophila infections can result in superficial skin infections, myositis and septicaemia. Treatment consists of administration of cefotaxime 1 g IV 8-hourly or ceftriaxone 1 g IV daily. If oral therapy is required ciprofloxacin 500 mg orally 12-hourly.[16]

Mastitis

Infections of the breast can occur in both sexes and in all ages; however, breast infections are most common in nursing mothers.

Treatment consists of regular emptying of the breast. Where breast-feeding needs to be stopped because of the severity of the infection or risk to the neonate, a pump should be employed (at least temporarily). Early antibiotic treatment is important to prevent abscess formation. Eleven per cent of patients who are not treated appropriately with antibiotics will develop an abscess. The antibiotic utilized should be an anti-staphylococcal agent such as dicloxacillin (250–500 mg orally 6-hourly) or a first-generation cephalorosporin such as cephalexin (250–500 mg orally 6-hourly). Erythromycin (250–500 mg orally 6-hourly) should be utilized in the patient who is allergic to penicillin. The duration of therapy required is 10 days. Severe infections may require parenteral or more prolonged therapy. Local care to the region is also important including warm compresses, breast support, analgesia and the application of a moisturizing cream to the nipple and areolar region. Patients who develop an abscess will require incision and drainage.[17]

Peritonsillar abscess (Quinsy)

Peritonsillar abscess is the most common deep head and neck infection. It occurs as a result of the spread of bacterial tonsillitis. It is most common in teenagers and young adults. It can also occur in immunosuppressed, immunodeficient and diabetic patients. Patients usually complain of dysphagia and appear toxic. Because of the difficulties associated with the examination CT scanning may be useful. Treatment consists of analgesia, hydration and 12–24 hours of high-dose parenteral antibiotics (clindamycin for those hypersensitive to penicillin) (e.g. penicillin 2 g IV 4 hourly). Patients with a significant abscess will benefit from either needle aspiration or surgical drainage.

Submandibular abscess (Ludwig's angina)

It is an infection of the submandibular space involving either the sublingual or submandibular compartment. Dental disease is the most common cause including recent extraction (lower second or third molars most commonly).

Most commonly occurs in ages 20–40 years with the patient appearing anxious and toxic. Rapid progression resulting in life-threatening upper airway obstruction can occur. CT imaging can be useful in indicating the extent and severity of the infection. Attention to the patient's airway is a priority (the patient may require airway intervention prior to the CT scanning).

Management of Ludwig's angina requires:

- airway protection
- parenteral antibiotics
- surgical drainage.

Once the airway is protected parenteral antibiotics alone may be adequate. Penicillin is recommended with some authorities recommending a third-generation cephalosporin together with anaerobic cover (metronidazole). Surgical drainage is usually reserved for refractory cases.

Retropharyngeal abscess

Most common in children with 95% in children <6 years and is usually followed by URTI. There may be a history of trauma to the mouth. The child appears toxic with limited neck mobility. They usually have dysphagia and trismus. Symptoms are often out of proportion to the findings on physical examination. A CT scan may be useful (essential where there is a history of trauma).

Management requires:

- airway control (paramount)
- parenteral antibiotics (third-generation cephalosporin and metronidazole)
- analgesia
- surgical drainage.

Epiglottitis (supraglottitis)

Epiglottitis is cellulitis of the supraglottic structures. In children the infection and oedema is usually confined to the epiglottis and closely surrounding structures. In adults the inflammation may also involve the prevertebral soft tissues, the valleculae, the base of the tongue and the soft palate. Epiglottitis should be considered, looked for and excluded in all patients with a sore throat who are toxic with dysphagia. Patients present with an abrupt onset of severe sore throat, fever, anxiety and drooling. The sore throat in children may manifest itself as refusal to eat.

The infection is rapidly progressive and may be fatal if untreated. There is a varying degree of respiratory distress, stridor (inspiratory), hoarseness, muffled voice and drooling. Patients want to sit in 'sniffing' position in order to protect their airway. Where the epiglottitis is suspected in children they should be taken to the operating theatre for gaseous induction by at least two practitioners experienced in airway management. The ability to do a surgical airway (crico-thyroidotomy or tracheostomy) should be available at all times.

Adults may not require airway intervention. They, however, need close monitoring. Once the airway has been managed patients require:

- rehydration
- parenteral antibiotics (third-generation cephalosporin or chloramphenicol for those who are penicillin hypersensitive).

Varicose/decubitus ulcers

Decubitus ulcers are cutaneous ulcerations caused by prolonged pressure that results in ischaemic necrosis of the skin and underlying soft tissue. They are most commonly found in patients who are bed bound, particularly elderly nursing home patients and patients with sensory deficits such as paraplegia and quadriplegia.

The combination of vascular insufficiency, neuropathy or immobility results in ulcer formation and unless treated aggressively, serious complications can follow.[18] Complications include cellulitis and deep soft tissue necrosis, osteomyelitis, septic thrombophlebitis, bacteraemia and sepsis. Culture of the ulcer invariably reveals a mixed bacterial flora of both aerobes and anaerobes, which do not distinguish between colonization and tissue infection. The most common organisms found are staphylococci, streptococci, coliforms and a variety of anaerobes.

Varicose ulcers are cutaneous ulcers caused by oedema and poor drainage of the tissues as a result of dysfunction of the venous system including varicose veins. These are more common in the elderly and obese. They may be chronic and very difficult to heal. They commonly have a range of organisms colonising the ulcer. Complications include cellulitis and occasionally bacteraemia. Culture of the ulcer variably reveals a mixed bacterial flora of both aerobes and anaerobes that cannot be distinguished between colonization and tissue infections. The most common organisms found are staphylococci, streptococci, coliforms and a variety of anaerobes.

Treatment consists of: debridement of necrotic tissue, pressure area and general nursing care as well as treatment of infection, if present. Antibiotic treatment is only indicated where there is systemic evidence of infection or where there is a complicating infection such as osteomyelitis or bacteraemia. Surgical debridement is frequently as important, if not more important than, antibiotic therapy particularly where the bacterial infection is localized.

Diabetic foot infections

Diabetic foot infections are a common complication of diabetes. Inadequately treated foot infections frequently results in amputation and instability of the patient's diabetes control. Once established, infections in diabetic patients are generally more severe and refractory to therapy. Patients who develop diabetic foot infections are frequently elderly, have a history of type 2 diabetes mellitus, are obese and have small and large vessel vascular disease.[19]

The peripheral neuropathy associated with the diabetes results in the loss of protective pain sensation and results in repetitive injuries, followed by the development of ulcers that become infected. Organisms involved are a mixed culture of anaerobes and aerobes with a mean of approximately five bacterial species per patient culture.[20] Aerobes include *Staph. aureus*, coagulase-negative staphylococci and streptococci. Enterobacteriaceae and *Corynebacterium* are not uncommon. Anaerobes which have been isolated from up to 48% of patients include *Bacteroides*, and *Clostridium* spp. The presence of anaerobes is associated with a high frequency of fever, foul-smelling lesions, and the presence of an ulcer.

Local signs and symptoms predominate, and include those secondary to infection, vasculopathy and neuropathy. Pain and tenderness is often minimal due to the neuropathy, pulses are frequently reduced or absent.

Underlying osteomyelitis must be looked for and excluded. This frequently requires radiography and/or a bone scan.

Treatment is multidisciplinary, involving surgeons and the patient's endocrinologist or physician.

Prolonged use of appropriate bactericidal antibiotics is essential for effective treatment. Where possible avoid nephrotoxic drugs. Therapy usually requires treatment with ampicillin, metronidazole and an aminoglycoside such as gentamicin. Glycaemic control is also important.

Zoonotic infections

Patients presenting with an infection should be asked for a detailed history, including the type of work they do and what they may have been in contact with. Saltwater fish handlers may develop infections due to *Erysipelothrix rhusiopathiae*; this causes erysipeloid, a type of cellulitis. It also causes infections in people handling fish, poultry, meat and hides. Patients with diabetes and hepatic disease are prone to serious infections due to *V. vulnificus*, a saltwater organism. The infection can be rapidly progressive and, unless recognized and treated

appropriately, can cause death from overwhelming sepsis.[15]

Intravenous drug users

Intravenous drug users frequently develop unusual infections because the needles and the drug paraphernalia used are contaminated. They also have alterations to their skin and flora and frequently have poor nutrition and immune function.[21] Many are hepatitis B, C and HIV positive. Rather than the Gram-positive organisms such as *Staph. aureus* found in non-IV drug users, IV drug users frequently have mixed organisms, particularly anaerobes, including: *Klebsiella, Entrobacter, Serratia,* and *Proteus*. They have mixed Gram-positive and Gram-negative infections. Some develop fungal infections, including candidaemia. Subacute bacterial endocarditis and endocarditis need to be considered in intravenous drug users. If endocarditis is not suspected, treatment should consist of flucloxacillin 2 g IV 6-hourly and gentamicin 5–7 mg/kg/day as a single daily dose.[21–23]

CONTROVERSIES

❶ The timing and method of wound closure of contaminated or 'old' (greater than 6 hours since injury) wounds.

❷ The prophylactic use of antibiotics in patients with 'clean' wounds.

❸ Which antibiotics to use in treating skin and soft tissue infections: narrow-spectrum, first generation cephalosporin or broad-spectrum third generation cephalosporin? Do you use antibiotics to cover both Gram-negative, Gram-positive organisms, anaerobes and aerobes?

❹ Do all patients with cellulitis and other soft tissue infections require inpatient therapy? Can more patients be treated wholly as outpatients utilizing parenteral therapy, or after early discharge once the acute toxic phase is over?

REFERENCES

1. Singer AJ, Hollander JE, Quinn JV 1997 Evaluation and management of traumatic lacerations. New England Journal of Medicine 337: 1142–8
2. Davidson J, Rotsein OD 1998 The diagnosis and management of common soft tissue infection. Canadian Journal of Surgery 31: 333–6
3. Victorian Postgraduate Medical Foundation Antibiotic Guidelines 2000
4. Trilla A, Miro JM 1995 Identifying high-risk patients for *Staphylococcus aureus* infections: skin and soft tissue infections. Journal of Chemotherapy 7 Supplement 3: 37–43
5. Heinz T, Perfect J, Schell W, Ritter E, Ruff G, Serafin D 1996 Soft-tissue fungal infections: surgical management of 12 immunocompromised patients. Plastic and Reconstrive Surgery 97(7): 1391–9
6. Aly AA, Roberts NM, Seipoks, MacLellan DG 1996 Case survey of management of cellulitis in a tertiary teaching hospital. Medical Journal of Australia 165: 555–6
7. Vinen J, Hudson B, Chan B, Fernandes C 1996 A randomised comparative study of once-daily ceftriaxone and 6-hourly flucloxacillin in the treatment of moderate to severe cellulitis. Clinical efficacy, safety and pharmacokenomic implications. Clinical Drug Investigation 12: 221–5
8. Ungkanont K, Yellon RF, Weissman JL, Casselbrant ML, Gonzalez-Valdepena H, Bluestone CD 1995 Head and neck space infections in infants and children. Otolaryngology–Head and Neck Surgery 112(3): 375–82
9. Leong WC, Lipman J, Hon H, Brouchaert NT 1997 Severe soft tissue infections: A diagnostic challenge. The need for early recognition and aggressive therapy. South Africa Medical Journal 87(5 Suppl): 648–52, 654
10. Becker M, Zbare P, Hermans R, Becker CD, Marchal F, Kurt AM, Marre S, Rufenacht DA, Terrier F 1997 Necrotizing fasciitis of the head and neck: role of CT in diagnosis and management. Radiology 202(2): 471–6
11. Talan DA 1989 Management of serious wound infections. Top Emergency Medicine 10(4): 33–41
12. Bosshardt TL, Henderson VJ, Organ Jr CH 1996 Necrotizing soft-tissue infections. Archives of Surgery 131(8): 845–52
13. Lille ST, Sato TT, Engrave LH, Foy H, Jurkovich GJ 1996 Necrotizing soft tissue infections:obstacles in diagnosis. Journal of the American College of Surgery 182(1): 7–11
14. Ben-Ahoaron U, Borenstein A, Eisenkraft S, Lifschitz O, Leviav A 1996 Extensive necrotizing soft tissue infection of the perineum. Israeli Journal of Medical Science 32(9): 745–9
15. Weber CA, Wertheimer SJ, Ognjan A 1995 Aeromonas hydrophila - its implications in freshwater injuries. Journal of Foot and Ankle Surgery 34(5): 442–6
16. Harlow KD, Harner RC, Fontenelle LJ 1996 Primary skin infections secondary to Vibrio vulnificus: the role of operative intervention. Journal of the American College of Surgery 183(4): 329–34
17. File TM Jr, Tan S 1995 Treatment of skin and soft tissue infections. American Journal of Surgery 169(5A Suppl): 26S–33S
18. Lertzman BH, Gaspari AA 1996 Drug treatment of skin and soft tissue infections in elderly long-term care residents. Drugs Aging 9(2): 109–21
19. Lavery LA, Harkless LB, Ashry HR, Felder Johnson K 1994 Infected puncture wounds in adults with diabetes:risk factors for osteomyelitis. Journal of Foot and Ankle Surgery 33(6): 561–6
20. Smith AJ, Daniels T, Bohnen JM 1996 Soft tissue infections and the diabetic foot. American Journal of Surgery 172(6A): 7S–12S
21. Henriksen BM., Albreksten SB., Simper LB., Gutschilk E 1994 Soft tissue infections from drug abuse. A clinical and microbiological review of 145 cases. Acta Orthopedica Scandinavia 65(6): 625–8
22. Bergstein JM, Baker EJ 4th, Aprahamian C, Schein M, Wittman DH 1995 Soft tissue abscesses associated with parenteral drug abuse: presentation, microbiology, and treatment. American Surgeon 61(12): 1105–8
23. Simmen HP, Givoanoli P, Battaglia H, Wust J, Meyer VE 1995 Soft tissue infections of the upper extremities with special consideration of abscesses in parenteral drug abusers. A prospective study. British Journal of Hand Surgery 20(6): 797–800

FURTHER READING

Falagas ME, Barefoot L, Griffith J, Ruthazar R, Syndman DR 1996 Risk factors leading to the clinical failure in the treatment of intra-abdominal or skin/soft tissue infections. European Journal of Clinical Microbiology and Infectious Diseases 15(12): 913–21

8.7 HEPATITIS

DEBORAH LEACH

ESSENTIALS

1 Most cases of acute hepatitis are caused by hepatitis A, B and C.

2 The diagnosis is made by a combination of the pattern of clinical illness, the elimination of other differential diagnoses, and serological evidence of infection.

3 Effective vaccination is available for hepatitis A and B.

4 Chronic viral hepatitis affects more than 1% of the population, most commonly due to hepatitis B and C.

5 Interferon therapy may be considered for selected cases of chronic hepatitis.

6 Rarer causes of hepatitis include toxins, drugs and autoimmune illnesses.

INTRODUCTION

Hepatitis is a spectrum of illnesses that exact an enormous toll worldwide in terms of morbidity and mortality.

Acute hepatitis produces inflammation of the liver with little or no fibrosis and little or no nodular regeneration. Minor distortion of the lobular architecture may occur. The aetiology includes:

- Infection
  - Viral, e.g. hepatitis A, B, C, D, E, G, GB
  - Other viruses as part of a systemic illness, e.g. EBV, CMV, yellow fever, herpes simplex, varicella zoster
  - Associated with septicaemia or leptospirosis
  - Associated with hepatic abcesses: either amoebic (seen in developing countries) or pyogenic (associated with extremes of age and biliary surgery)
  - Hepatitis A, B and C are the common agents (Table 8.7.1)
- Chemical or drug related, e.g. carbon tetrachloride, ethylene glycol, alcohol, halothane, isoniazid, rifampicin, methotrexate, MAO inhibitors, chlorpromazine and paracetamol[1,2] (Table 8.7.2)

Table 8.7.1 Characteristics of the hepatitis virus

Hepatitis	A	B	C	D	E	GB (A, B, C)	G
Virus	Picornavirus	Hepadnavirus	Flavivirus	RNA virus – classified with plant virus satellites	RNA virus	Flavi-like virus GBV – A & B closely related to HCV	Flavivirus distantly related to HCV
Transmission	Faecal–oral (person-person or epidemics)	Blood/body fluid Perinatal vertical transmission	Parenteral Possible other routes, e.g. sexual, perinatal	Parenteral (as for HBV) HDV requires HBV (enveloped with HbsAg)	Faecal–oral Central and South America, Asia and Africa	Blood, mainly coinfections with HBV & HCV	Blood and other parenteral routes High coinfection with HBV & HCV
Average incubation period	25 days	75 days	50 days	35 days	40 days	? Unknown	? Unknown
Hepatitis severity	Mild–moderate Increases with age	Moderate to severe 1% fulminant hepatic failure	Mild	Severe	Mild–moderate	? Unknown	Mild
Mortality	Overall <0.2% >40 years: 1%	0.2–2%	<1%	2–20%	0.2–1% in pregnancy up to 20%	? Unknown	? Unknown
Chronicity	No	2–7% in adults >90% in newborns	Up to 80%	1–3% of co-infections 70–80% of superinfection (with HBV)	No	Yes: GBV-C	Yes
Vaccination	Yes	Yes	No	Indirectly via HBV immunization	No	No	No

- Toxin related, e.g. *Amanita phalloides* mushrooms
- Miscellaneous, e.g. pregnancy, autoimmune, hyperthermia.

The spectrum of disease ranges from acute, subclinical, and self-limited to one with life-threatening complications such as fulminant hepatic failure or chronic hepatitis, with its associated risks of cirrhosis and hepatocellular carcinoma.

Chronic hepatitis causes even greater morbidity and mortality than acute hepatitis. It is diagnosed according to pathological criteria, but fairly clear clinical states occur.[3] Chronic hepatitis has been defined as the presence of raised ALT levels for longer than 6 months. In chronic persistent hepatitis the lobular architecture is preserved and overall there is an excellent prognosis. Chronic active hepatitis is characterized by periportal inflammation and piecemeal cellular necrosis with fibrosis. The natural history involves progression to cirrhosis. Hepatitis B and C cause more than 90% of cases of chronic hepatitis.

VIRAL HEPATITIS

During the last 50 years there has been an explosion in our knowledge of viral agents causing this disease. In the 1940s two viruses (hepatitis A and hepatitis B) were thought to account for all cases of the disease. In the 1970s, when diagnostic assays to detect these viruses were introduced, it became apparent that there were cases of parenterally transmitted hepatitis that were caused by one or more other viral agents. These were labelled under the umbrella term 'non-A, non-B' hepatitis. In the 1980s hepatitis D was described. Advances in molecular technology made possible the discovery in the late 1980s of hepatitis C, the major cause of parenterally transmitted non-A, non-B hepatitis, and

hepatitis E, the major cause of enterically transmitted non-A, non-B hepatitis. More recently, there has been the discovery of hepatitis G and the hepatitis GB group of viruses.[4] In 1994 it was claimed that an enteric non-A, non-E hepatitis had been discovered – hepatitis F. Further studies will elucidate the significance of this agent.[4]

The clinical pattern of disease is one of a systemic illness with an insidious or acute onset. The classic presentation is involves four phases:[1, 5–7]

- Phase I – Viral replication: while the patient is clinically asymptomatic, there is laboratory evidence of hepatitis
- Phase II – Prodromal phase: symptoms develop including anorexia, nausea, vomiting, arthralgisa, headache, coryza, fatigue and pruritis. Misdiagnosis as gastroenteritis or URTI may occur.
- Phase III – Icteric phase: occurs 1–2

Table 8.7.2 Drugs producing hepatitis

Drug	Pathology
Halothane (mild) Cloxacillin	Lobular hepatitis – resembles viral hepatitis
Isoniazid	
Paracetamol	Zonal hepatic necrosis with lesser inflammation
Halothane (severe)	
Non-steroidal	Acute fatty change
Agents	
Steroids	
Tetracycline	
Amiodarone	Resembles alcoholic hepatitis
Perhexaline	Clinically chronic liver disease
Phenytoin	Non-caseating granulomas with varying lobular hepatitis
Allopurinol	
Sulphonamides	
Chlorpromazine	
Erythromycin estolate	Cholestasis with hepatitis
Flucloxacillin	
α-methyldopa	Chronic active hepatitis
Nitrofurantoin	
Dantrolene	

weeks after the prodrome. There is development of jaundice, and right upper quadrant pain. There may be dark urine and pale stools.

- Phase IV – convalescent phase: symptoms resolve and lab enzymes normalize.

Cholestasis complicates 5–10% of cases of HAV and is characterized by persistent pruritus with or without jaundice for 2–6 weeks.

Warning signs of acute liver failure (incidence 0.1% in HAV and 0.5–1% in HBV) include persistent vomiting, worsening jaundice and prolonged prothrombin time.

The diagnosis of viral hepatitis depends on:[8]

- An appropriate clinical pattern of illness
- The elimination of other differential diagnoses
- Laboratory confirmation of acute infection with one of the hepatitis viruses.

Specialist referral should be made if the diagnosis is unclear or the course of the illness does not seem typical. Hospitalization should be considered for those with more severe illness or any warning signs of acute liver failure. The diagnostic process may become difficult in the presence of infection with more than one hepatic virus, or with a combination of autoimmune illness and viral infection.

Viral hepatitis is a notifiable disease with mandatory laboratory reporting in all Australian States and the UK.[5]

HEPATITIS A[1,5,9,10]

Virology

Hepatitis A (HAV), the predominant aetiologic agent in viral hepatitis, is caused by an RNA virus (family Picornaviridae, genus hepatovirus).

Epidemiology

Transmission is via the faecal-oral route, most commonly by person-to-person spread or by common-source epidemics caused by contamination of food or water. It is resistant to environmental factors such as temperature and certain chemicals. Viraemia occurs during the incubation period and the early acute phase of the illness, and there have been reports of transfusion-related transmission during this time.

The epidemiology of hepatitis A is highly influenced by personal and public hygiene, with a diminished incidence in developed countries. The secondary infection rate for household contacts of patients with acute HAV is 20%.

Clinical course

The incubation period is 15–45 days, followed by an acute onset of symptoms similar to those of gastroenteritis or a respiratory viral infection. Virus is shed in the stool 1–2 weeks prior to the onset of symptoms and for 1 week thereafter. Viral shedding ceases at about the time that the patient becomes icteric. The illness is mild to moderate in severity, with an overall mortality rate of less than 0.2%. Infection in younger age groups is usually not clinically apparent, and the disease is progressively more severe as age increases. Ten per cent of infected toddlers become symptomatic, whereas 50–70% of adults develop a clinical illness. In adults, 10–20% of cases develop a relapsing course over several months. Chronic hepatitis does not occur.

Laboratory tests[1]

IgM antibodies to the hepatitis A virus (IgM anti-HAV) in the presence of an acute hepatitis confirm the diagnosis. This test is positive from the onset of symptoms, and usually remains positive for 4 months. IgG anti-HAV becomes the predominant contributor to anti-HAV as the acute inflammatory response settles, and usually remains detectable for life, interpreted as evidence of a past infection and indicative of immunity.

Management[5]

Symptomatic management includes advice regarding fluid intake, avoidance of alcohol until resolution of symptoms, and eating a low-fat diet if nausea is present. Pruritus may be treated with local measures such as bathing and calamine lotion, or respond to antihistamines or cholestyramine. Steroids may be of use in cholestatic HAV. Transmission to close contacts is minimized by hygiene measures such as the use of personal eating utensils and strict handwashing procedures. Close contacts should be passively immunized with hepatitis A immunoglobulin and given the first dose of Hep A vaccine.

Immunization[5]

Effective, inactivated whole-virus vaccines have been developed. Vaccination should be considered for those at risk, including travellers, childcare staff, plumbers, those exposed during local epidemics, and patients with chronic liver disease. Food handlers who would represent a risk to the public should also be considered for vaccination.

Passive immunization is of temporary value and can be achieved with the use of pooled immunoglobulin.

HEPATITIS B[1,5,9,10]

Virology

Hepatitis B (HBV) is a highly infectious double-stranded DNA hepadnavirus, genus Orthohepadnavirus, with an antigenic inner core and outer coat.

Epidemiology

Transmission is primarily via exposure to blood or blood products; however, the virus is present in semen, saliva and other body fluids, leading to the risk of transmission by unprotected sex. Perinatal transmission at the time of birth from an infected mother to her child is a common mode of spread in Asia. The greatest risk occurs in babies born to HBeAg women. Antenatal screening for maternal hepatitis B enables vaccination of the newborn. Mandatory screening of blood donors has led to the virtual eradication of transfusion-related HBV. Unprotected sex and intravenous drug abuse are the most important current factors contributing to the spread of this virus. Percutaneous exposure via needle-stick injury in healthcare workers is another source of exposure.

Clinical course

The incubation period for HBV averages 75 days (range 70–160 days). The disease is usually not apparent and patients are anicteric. Acute hepatitis occurs in approximately 25%. This may be of moderate severity or severe, with a mortality rate of 0.2–2%. The illness is less likely to have a severe clinical course in the young, but more likely to become a chronic infection. Ninety per cent of those infected at birth develop chronic HBV versus the overall chronicity rate of 5–10%.

The onset of symptoms is usually insidious, and in 5–10% of cases is preceded by a serum-sickness type of illness with polyarthralgia, proteinuria and angio-oedema. The symptoms tend to be more severe and prolonged than those of hepatitis A. One per cent of patients develop fulminant hepatic failure.

Complete recovery from hepatitis B occurs in 90% of cases; 5–10% develop chronic hepatitis. Of these, 70–90% evolve into a clinically unaffected carrier state with the remainder developing progressive disease, with cirrhosis and the risk of hepatocellular carcinoma. Worldwide this virus is the major cause of hepatocellular carcinoma. Mild forms of chronic hepatitis may become more aggressive. Conversely, it is possible for a patient with chronic HBV to spontaneously clear the virus.

Laboratory tests[1,8]

Three different HBV antigens are used in the diagnosis of acute and chronic infection as well as the carrier state:

- Surface antigen: hepatitis B surface antigen (HBsAg) represents the outer coat of the virus. It appears in the serum prior to elevation in liver enzymes and persists until 1–2 months following the icteric phase (total duration about 6 months). The presence of HBsAg implies hepatitis or a carrier state.
- Antibodies to surface antigen: anti-HBs appear in the serum from 2 weeks to 6 months after HBsAg disappears. Their presence implies prior infection with HBV and current immunity. Chronic carriers of HBV do not clear HBsAg from the serum and do not develop anti-HBs. Anti-HBs remains detectable in the serum for decades after the initial infection.
- Core antigen (HBcAg):antibodies (anti-HBc) to the core of the HBV particle (HBcAg) appear in the serum 2 weeks after the appearance of HBsAg. High titres of IgM anti-HBc indicate high infectivity, whereas low levels persist in chronic disease. IgG anti-HBc may be detectable for decades after the initial infection.
- Hepatitis e antigen (HBeAg): the presence of HBeAg in the serum represents ongoing viral replication and high infectivity. It disappears on recovery, with the appearance of anti-HBe, but persists in chronic hepatitis.

HBV DNA

The presence of DNA in the serum is the most sensitive indicator of ongoing viral replication and hence a high risk of infectivity.

Hepatitis B serology

Diagnosis of acute hepatitis B

The standard for diagnosis is the detection of IgM anti-HBc in serum. Detecting HBsAg in a patient with acute hepatitis strongly suggests HBV as the causative agent, but this must be confirmed by the detection of anti-HBc, as a chronic HBV carrier (positive for HBsAg) may have an acute non-B hepatitis.

Ten to 20% of cases of acute hepatitis B have no detectable HBsAg. IgM anti-

HBc is useful in these cases. In rare cases the appearance of IgM anti-HBc is delayed or absent. These cases are difficult to evaluate.

Diagnosis of chronic hepatitis B

The carrier state is defined as the presence of HBsAg in the serum for longer than 6 months after initial detection. One to 2% of chronic carriers become HBsAg negative annually. When HBsAg persists without abnormal liver enzymes or obvious liver disease, the term 'healthy carrier' is used. Anti-HBs is absent in up to 80% of chronic carriers, with the remainder having detectable HBs in serum. HBeAg disappears in 50% of cases over time, and anti-HBe appears in the serum. This indicates that HBV replication has ceased and liver enzyme levels tends to normalize.

Reactivation of chronic hepatitis B

This may occur spontaneously or following treatment with immunosuppressive agents. HBsAg and IgM Anti-HBc may be detected and HBeAg may reappear. The diagnosis may be difficult, as it requires a knowledge of the previous HBsAg status of the patient.

Hepatitis B virus variants

Several variants of the virus have been identified, leading to different patterns of antigen and antibody response. One such variant involves an alteration in HBsAg that enables it to escape the effects of anti-HBs, thus rendering vaccination ineffective.

Immunity

The presence of anti-HBs.

Management[5,10]

Symptomatic management of acute HBV infection should be undertaken as for HAV. Sexual partners and household members should be vaccinated against HBV, and counselling regarding the avoidance of transmitting HBV should be undertaken. Liver function tests should be monitored each 1–2 weeks and HBV serology repeated monthly until the disappearance of HBsAg and the appearance of anti-HBs.

Some patients with chronic hepatitis B may benefit from drug treatment. Aims of treatment are a reduction in liver inflammation and fibrosis and prevetion of progression to cirrhosis. Many treatment regimes are being actively researched. α-interferon has been successfully used in these patients. Response to therapy is marked by an exacerbation of clinical symptoms. The side-effects of interferon include a severe flu-like illness, headache, weight loss, alopecia, bone marrow suppression and depression.[9] High liver ALT levels, recent acquisition of the virus and low HBV DNA levels are associated with a good response to therapy. Other drugs such as famcyclovir may be used. Liver transplantation may be considered in those with end-stage chronic hepatitis B. In those who are HBV DNA negative, a good response is possible. Conversely, in those who are HBV DNA positive, transplantation may be followed by severe recurrent disease and graft destruction.[1]

Immunization[5]

The first vaccines to be developed for the prevention of HBV were based on the purification of HBsAg from the blood of infected individuals. These were supplanted by HBsAg vaccines produced by recombinant DNA technology. Vaccination has proved to be highly effective in the prevention of hepatitis B in high-risk groups, including healthcare workers. Current Australian recommendations for vaccination include all infants and preadolescents, individuals with a high exposure risk and those with chronic liver disease.

Postexposure prophylaxis for HBV focuses on the immune status of the exposed patient, the relative risk of the source being HBsAg positive, and the mode of exposure (see Chapter 8.10).

HEPATITIS C[1,5,9,10,11]

Virology

Hepatitis C (HCV) is a single-stranded RNA virus, classified in the family flavivirus. There are several different subgroups of HCV. Infection with one virus does not protect the individual against becoming infected with another. In 1989 the virus was identified by cloning techniques.

Epidemiology

In 1975, when the newly developed diagnostic tests for HAV and HBV were used to examine serum from patients with transfusion-related hepatitis, it became apparent that most cases were 'non-A, non-B' hepatitis. Screening of blood donors has led to the virtual eradication of post-transfusion hepatitis related to this agent. Prior to screening, HCV had been responsible for 90% of cases of non-A, non-B hepatitis post transfusion. Intravenous drug use remains an important mode of transmission, and patients who abuse alcohol are at higher risk of HCV acquisition. Vertical transmission occurs in 5% of cases, and the risk of sexual transmission appears low. Needlestick injury among healthcare workers place them at significant risk. The incidence of infection approaches 10% in those with such an exposure to infected blood.

The chronic carrier rate in the Australian and UK population is 0.5–1%.

Clinical course

The incubation period of HCV averages 50 days. Acute hepatitis C is usually a subclinical or mild disease with <1% mortality rate; up to 80% of acute cases progress to chronicity. About 25% of these patients develop cirrhosis and the subsequent risk of hepatic failure and hepatocellular carcinoma. The measurement of liver enzymes is of limited value in the assessment of severity of the hepatitis, as significant liver injury can be present with variable or no alteration in ALT levels.

Laboratory tests[1,8]

Antibodies to HCV

IgM anti-HCV appear in the serum between 1 and 4 weeks after the onset of symptoms. In self-limiting disease it becomes undetectable by 6 months, but in contrast remains positive in those who develop chronicity. All patients' sera remain positive for IgG anti-HCV.

HCV RNA

This is detected by polymerase chain reaction and indicates the presence of the virus.

Management[5,10]

Management of the acute illness is symptomatic as for HAV and HBV. Counselling regarding the avoidance of transmission is important, particularly as there is no active or passive vaccination available.

Interferon therapy may be useful in certain patients with chronic HCV (see Side-effects: Hepatitis B treatment). Those with histologically less severe disease, shorter duration of disease and lower viral titres will have a better response. Antiviral agents such as amantadine may have a role in those who do not respond to interferon. Liver transplantation may be considered in end-stage HCV. Following transplantation, up to 90% of patients develop chronic HCV within 3 years.[1]

HEPATITIS D[9,10]

Virology

This virus is composed of the HDV antigen and a small piece of RNA enclosed by a coat of HBsAg. It is known as a 'defective' virus because it requires the presence of acute or chronic HBV infection to replicate.

Epidemiology

The mode of transmission of HDV is inextricably linked to HBV. HDV can occur as a coinfection with acute HBV, as a superinfection in chronic HBsAg carriers, or as a chronic infection with HBV and HDV.

Clinical course

HDV occurring as a coinfection with acute HBV is usually self-limiting, resolving as the HBV is cleared. Super-infection of HBsAg carriers is a more serious illness, with a higher mortality rate than acute HBV, and chronic HDV developing in 80%. These patients have a more rapid progression to cirrhosis.

Laboratory tests[1]

The diagnosis of HDV is made by detecting IgM anti-HDV in serum. This antibody appears in low titres in acute infections and is persistent in high titres in chronic infection. Newer assays can detect anti-HDV early in the course of the illness. IgG appears later and is the antibody found in convalescent serum.

The presence of the delta antigen indicates replication of HDV and can be detected in acute and chronic infections.

Immunization

Immunization against HBV affords protection against the development of HDV.

HEPATITIS E[1,9,10]

Virology

Hepatitis E is an enterically transmitted non-A, non-B RNA hepatitis virus. It appears to have a stable antigenic structure, allowing the possibility for an effective vaccine to be developed. In 1990 the genome of HEV was cloned. It resembles a calicivirus.

Epidemiology

This virus, first recognized as a unique entity in 1980, is seen mainly in developing countries, where it may occur as sporadic cases or as epidemics. Most cases found in Australia have been acquired during travel to endemic areas such as Asia and Africa. HEV is less readily transmitted than HAV, which explains why there may be recurring epidemics in adults living in areas where this virus is endemic.

Clinical course

The incubation period averages 40 days. Like HAV, the illness produced by HEV is self-limiting, with full recovery and no chronicity developing. Overall mortality rate is 0.2–1%, but the highest mortality rate, up to 20%, is in pregnant women. There are no reports of chronic infection.

Laboratory tests

The diagnosis is confirmed by the detection of IgM anti-HEV. IgG anti-HEV persists for at least 4 years following recovery from the illness.

NEW HEPATITIS VIRUSES

Several other proposed agents of viral hepatitis are referred to as non-ABCDE viral hepatitis.

Hepatitis GB, a flavi-like virus, was first described in 1968 in serum originating from a surgeon (GB) who had developed acute hepatitis.[12] Subsequently, attempts to identify the GB hepatitis agent revealed negative results for hepatitis A-E. More recently, sophisticated PCR techniques have revealed that the GB agent consists of three distinct viruses, GBV-A, GBV-B and GBV-C.[13]

Hepatitis G is an RNA flavivirus characterized in 1996 and distantly related to HCV. It is spread by blood and other parenteral routes.[1] There is a high co-infection rate with HBV and HCV. The severity of hepatitis is usually mild, but may progress to a chronic illness.

DRUG INDUCED HEPATITIS [14]

A variety of prescription agents cause hepatotoxicity either directly or via autoimmune mechanisms. Several drugs of abuse cause hepatic injury including cocaine, ecstasy, toluene and phencyclidine. Herbal medicines and toxic plants have also been implicated. The clinical syndrome has three phases:

- Phase I – GI phase: symptoms of nausea, vomiting, diarrhoea and abdominal pain.
- Phase II – Clinical resolution: 24–48 hours post exposure there is resolution of the GI symptoms.
- Phase III – Hepatic phase: 48–72 hours post exposure there is onset of hepatic failure.

ALCOHOLIC HEPATITIS[1]

Alcoholic hepatitis develops in about 10% of alcohol-dependent patients. The clinical picture varies from a mild illness to acute liver failure. Symptoms include anorexia, nausea, weight loss, weakness, abdominal pain, fever, dark urine and jaundice. Treatment involves supportive measures, correction of nutritional deficits as well as fluid and electrolyte abnormalities, and abstinence from alcohol. There may be a significant reversible component to the liver disease if alcohol use is ceased, but the overall mortality rate is 10–15%, related to liver failure, gastrointestinal haemorrhage and sepsis.

In patients with hepatitis C, ethanol abuse accelerates the viral-induced liver disease.

CHRONIC HEPATITIS

IDIOPATHIC AUTOIMMUNE CHRONIC ACTIVE HEPATITIS[1]

This rare condition affects mainly women between 10 and 40 years of age, and following an insidious onset characterized by fatigue, anorexia and jaundice, there is progression to cirrhosis and liver failure. Autoantibodies, antismooth muscle and antinuclear antibodies are usually present. Antiliver/kidney microsomal antibody may be found in an aggressive variant of this disease. Steroids and azathioprine are effective in reducing morbidity and mortality. Liver transplantation is considered in progressive disease. If the disease is untreated there is a mortality rate of 50% in 3–5 years.

FUTURE DIRECTIONS

❶ Improved public health measures to minimize the transmission of viral hepatitis.

❷ The development of more sensitive serological tests of viral hepatitis to allow earlier diagnosis.

❸ The development of a vaccine for hepatitis C.

❹ The development of more effective antiviral agents for the treatment of chronic hepatitis.

REFERENCES

1. Talley N, Martin C 1996 Clinical Gastroenterology: a Practical Problem-based Approach. MacLennan & Petty P/L, Sydney
2. Moseley R 1996 Evaluation of abnormal liver function tests. Medical Clinics of North America 80(5): 887–903
3. Farrell G 1998 Chronic viral hepatitis. Medical Journal of Australia 168(12): 619–26
4. Bowden DS, Moaven LD, Lucarnini SA 1996 New hepatitis viruses: are there enough letters in the alphabet? Medical Journal of Australia 164(2): 87–9
5. Farrell G 1998 Acute viral hepatitis. Medical Journal of Australia 168(11): 565–70
6. Martin P, Friedman L 1994 Viral hepatitis. Gastroenterology Clinics of North America 23: 429–614
7. Tintinalli J, Krome R, Ruiz E 1992 Acute jaundice and hepatitis. In: Emergency Medicine, a Comprehensive Study Guide, 3rd edn. McGraw-Hill, pp 356–62
8. Sjogren M 1996 Serologic diagnosis of viral hepatitis. Medical Clinics of North America 80(5): 929–56
9. Hirschmann S 1995 Current therapeutic approaches to viral hepatitis. Clinics in Infectious Diseases 20: 741–6
10. Purcell R 1994 Hepatitis viruses: changing patterns of human disease. Proceedings of the National Academy of Sciences USA 91: 2401–6
11. Danta M, et al 2002 factors associated with severity of hepatic fibrosis in people with chronic hepatitis C infection. MJA 177(5): 240–5
12. Rehermann B 1996 Immunopathogenesis of viral hepatitis. Baillière's Clinical Gastroenterology 10(3): 483–97
13. Schlauder G, Pilot-Matias TJ, Gabriel GS, et al 1995 Origin of GB-hepatitis viruses. Lancet 346: 447–8
14. Buggs A M 2002 e-Medicine - Hepatitis 3(7) 1–22

8.8 HIV/AIDS

ALAN C. STREET

ESSENTIALS

1 Globally, heterosexual transmission accounts for most HIV infections, but in Australia HIV infection remains predominantly a disease of homosexual and bisexual men.

2 Patients with previously undiagnosed HIV infection may present to the emergency department at any time during the course of HIV infection, from early (acute seroconversion illness) to late (opportunistic infection) stages.

3 Most serious HIV-related complications occur when the CD4 T-lymphocyte count is less than 0.2×10^9/L (bacterial pneumonia and tuberculosis are exceptions).

4 Measurement of the blood HIV RNA level provides important information about prognosis and response to antiviral therapy.

5 The emergency physician should be able to provide expert HIV pre- and post-test counselling in a sensitive and non-judgemental fashion.

6 Combination therapy with at least three antiretroviral drugs has dramatically reduced HIV mortality and morbidity, but at a cost in terms of drug toxicity, drug interactions and difficulty with adherence.

7 Close liaison between emergency department staff and the patient's hospital or local doctor is vital for optimal management of HIV-infected patients.

INTRODUCTION

HIV medicine is a complex and specialized field and emergency medicine physicians are not the usual primary care providers for people with HIV infection. However, the emergency department is often the first point of medical contact for patients presenting with acute HIV-related complications, whether or not the patient has been diagnosed with HIV infection previously.

Emergency medicine physicians do not need to be HIV experts, but they should:

- be familiar with the natural history and clinical manifestations of HIV infection
- understand the principles of HIV diagnosis, and be able to counsel patients before and after HIV testing
- know how to acutely manage

patients with common HIV-related disease syndromes
- have some knowledge of antiretroviral agents in current use.

The first cases of AIDS were recognized in the USA in 1981 and in Australia in 1982. The causative agent, human immunodeficiency virus (HIV), was discovered in 1984 and a diagnostic blood test developed soon thereafter. In 1986 the first effective antiviral drug (AZT, later renamed zidovudine) became available. More recently, use of combination antiretroviral therapy has led to dramatic reductions in HIV-associated morbidity and mortality in resource-rich countries. Unfortunately the global HIV situation is serious and rapidly worsening; in 2001, the World Health Organization (WHO) estimates were of 5 million new HIV infections, 3 million deaths, and 40

million people living with HIV infection, 28 million in sub-Saharan Africa and 7 million in Asia.[1] A major challenge in the coming years will be to develop an effective HIV vaccine.

EPIDEMIOLOGY

Globally, the great majority of HIV infections arise as a result of heterosexual transmission. In developed countries, injecting drug use and sex between men account for a greater proportion of HIV infections, although the contribution of specific behaviours to overall transmission varies greatly between countries and over time.

In Australia, almost 19 000 people have been diagnosed with HIV infection to December 2001. Of these, 8756 have progressed to AIDS, and 6152 have died. New South Wales has borne the brunt of the epidemic. Eighty-two per cent of people infected with HIV report male-to-male sex, 10% have become infected through heterosexual transmission, 5% of cases have occurred in injecting drug users, and 2% in recipients of contaminated blood or blood products. Women account for 6% of HIV-infected people and children for less than 1%.[2]

The number of annual Australian AIDS cases peaked at 955 in 1994 and fell to 143 in 2001.[2] At least 150–200 Australians become newly infected with HIV each year. In comparison to some other countries, the prevalence of HIV infection in injecting drug users has remained low, of the order of 2–3%.

PATHOGENESIS

Once HIV infection becomes established, one billion or more HIV virus particles are produced per day, chiefly in lymph nodes and other lymphoid tissue, accompanied by the daily turnover of up to 1 billion CD4 T-lymphocytes.[3]

417

Through direct infection of CD4 cells, and possibly other mechanisms, the number of CD4 cells falls, resulting in reduced helper function for cell-mediated and humoral immunity.

Viral replication occurs at a relatively constant rate, producing a stable level of HIV in the blood. This *viral load set point* can be measured with quantitative HIV RNA detection tests and is an important prognostic indicator because it determines the rate at which CD4 T-lymphocytes are lost. The HIV viral load is also measured to monitor antiretroviral therapy.

The peripheral blood CD4 T-lympho-cyte count is an accurate indicator of the degree of immunosuppression. The normal count is $0.5–1.5 \times 10^9/L$; susceptibility to opportunistic infection, and to most other serious HIV-related complications, is greatest when the CD4 cell count is less than $0.2 \times 10^9/L$.[4]

CLASSIFICATION AND NATURAL HISTORY

(Fig. 8.8.1)

HIV infection can be conveniently divided into four stages on the basis of time after infection, CD4 T-lymphocyte count and the presence of complications:[5]

❶ Acute infection: (discussed in more detail below) a febrile illness that occurs soon after infection
❷ Early infection: CD4 cell count $>0.5 \times 10^9/L$ - generally asymptomatic period
❸ Intermediate infection: CD4 cell count $0.2–0.5 \times 10^9/L$ - asymptomatic or less serious complications
❹ Late infection: CD4 cell count $<0.2 \times 10^9/L$ - susceptibility to opportunistic infections and malignancies.

Patients are categorized as having AIDS when they develop a defined opportunistic infection, an HIV-related malignancy, a wasting syndrome or AIDS dementia complex.

PRESENTATION

Emergency department doctors will deal with two fundamentally different groups of HIV patients.

First, some patients present with a manifestation of previously unrecognized HIV infection. To identify these patients, the physician must know who is potentially at risk of HIV infection (see Epidemiology above) and be aware of the many different ways in which previously undiagnosed HIV infection may present.[5] Prompt consideration of the possibility of HIV infection is important because the differential diagnosis will broaden to encompass a variety of other conditions, some of which may be life-threatening.

The second group of patients presenting to the emergency department are those who are already known to be HIV infected. They usually present with one of a limited number of syndromes, such as diarrhoea, fever or shortness of breath and cough. The initial diagnostic and treatment approach is based on a knowledge of the differential diagnosis for each of these syndromes.

Previously undiagnosed HIV infection

Primary infection (acute seroconversion illness) (see Table 8.8.1)

Up to 50% of patients will develop a glandular fever-like illness of varying severity 2–3 weeks after acquiring HIV. The most common features are fever, myalgia, headache, erythematous maculo-papular rash, diarrhoea, lymphadeno-pathy and mouth ulcers. Complications include aseptic meningitis, encephalitis and Guillain-Barré syndrome.[6] The diagnosis is often missed at this stage; patients may be considered to have infectious mononucleosis, or a 'viral illness' or the possibility of HIV infection is not considered in a patient with (for example) encephalitis.

Early infection (CD4 cell count $>0.5 \times 10^9/L$)

People are generally healthy during this phase. Thrombocytopenia may occur, and so HIV infection should be considered in appropriate patients with idiopathic thrombocytopenia.

Intermediate infection (CD4 cell count $0.2–0.5 \times 10^9/L$)

This is a phase when previously un-diagnosed HIV-infected patients often present, but the clues are often not recognized and diagnosis is missed. Manifestations include:

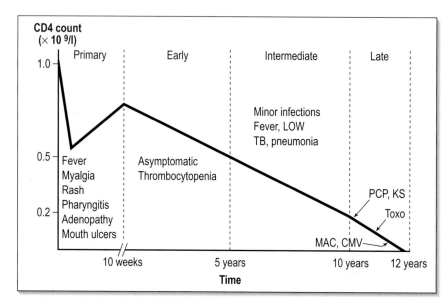

Fig. 8.8.1 Natural history of untreated HIV infection. 'Time' represents time after infection. (Modified with permission from Stewart G (ed.) 1997 Managing HIV. Australasian Medical Publishing Co Ltd, Sydney)

Table 8.8.1 Manifestations of primary HIV infection

Common (present in > 30% of patients)	Less common	Complications
Fever	Diarrhoea	Aseptic meningitis
Rash	Generalized lymphadenopathy	Guillain-Barré syndrome
Myalgia/arthralgia	Painful swallowing	Encephalitis
Headache	Abdominal pain	Interstitial pneumonitis
Pharyngitis	Cough	Rhabdomyolysis
Cervical lymphadenopathy	Photophobia	Haemophagocytic syndrome
Mouth ulcers	Tonsillitis	

Table 8.8.2 Respiratory complications in HIV-infected patients

Common	Uncommon
Pneumocystis carinii pneumonia (PCP)	Tuberculosis
Bacterial pneumonia:	Atypical mycobacteria
pneumococcus	Aspergillus pneumonia
Haemophilus influenzae	Other infections:
Bronchitis	Rhodococcus equi, CMV
	Non-infectious:
	Pulmonary Kaposi's sarcoma
	Lymphoma

- Minor infections: shingles, recurrent orolabial or genital herpes, oral thrush
- Skin conditions: extensive seborrhoeic dermatitis, worsening psoriasis
- Constitutional symptoms: fever, weight loss, diarrhoea
- Generalized lymphadenopathy
- More serious complications: bacterial pneumonia, tuberculosis and, rarely, Kaposi's sarcoma or non-Hodgkin's lymphoma.

Late-stage infection (CD4 cell count 0.2×10^9/L)

It is often not appreciated that patients may remain completely well during the early and intermediate stages of HIV infection, and only present when they develop a serious opportunistic infection. If the patient reveals that he or she is at risk of HIV infection, initial investigations can be directed at possible HIV-related diagnoses. However, if the patient does not volunteer this information, is not specifically asked about HIV risk factors, or does not belong to a conventional HIV risk group, diagnosis of the presenting illness and the underlying HIV infection is often delayed.

The following clinical situations should prompt consideration of the possibility of underlying HIV infection:

- Diffuse bilateral pulmonary infiltrates (as a manifestation of *Pneumocystis carinii* pneumonia, PCP) – often misdiagnosed as atypical pneumonia and treated with a macrolide agent or doxycycline.
- Ring-enhancing space-occupying cerebral lesion – misdiagnosed as brain abscess or tumour (if HIV infection considered, cerebral toxoplasmosis is the most likely diagnosis and brain biopsy can be avoided).
- Tuberculosis – although the overlap between those at risk for HIV and tuberculosis is not as great in Australia as in other countries, risk factors for HIV infection should be discussed with every tuberculosis patient and HIV testing encouraged after appropriate counselling.
- Kaposi's sarcoma – well-developed lesions (purple, oval and nodular) are easy to recognize, but early lesions are often non-descript (brown or pink and flat) and biopsy may be required for diagnosis.
- Other presentations – conditions such as cryptococcal meningitis, chronic cryptosporidial diarrhoea and AIDS dementia complex (manifesting as impaired cognition

and motor performance) are occasionally the first manifestation of HIV infection.

Disease syndromes in those with known HIV infection

Cough, shortness of breath, fever

Respiratory pathogens are listed in Table 8.8.2. The most important issue to decide is whether the patient has *Pneumocystis carinii* pneumonia (PCP) or not, because this complication is common and potentially serious. Tuberculosis must also be considered because of the need to place the patient in respiratory isolation.

- PCP (occurs in patients with $<0.2 \times 10^9$ CD4 cells/L): the presentation is subacute or chronic with a non-productive cough, dyspnoea, fever and chest tightness. Physical examination reveals fever, tachypnoea and reduced chest expansion, but chest auscultation is often normal. PCP is very unlikely in patients taking regular co-trimoxazole because this drug is virtually 100% effective as PCP prophylaxis.
- Bacterial pneumonia (may occur when the CD4 cell count is $>0.2 \times 10^9$/L): patients usually present with a short history, a productive cough and sometimes pleuritic chest pain. Physical examination varies from being normal to revealing signs of consolidation, with a pleural rub or effusion.
- Tuberculosis: the clinical features vary according to the degree of immunosuppression. If the CD4 cell count is $>0.2 \times 10^9$/L, patients present with typical symptoms and signs of tuberculosis (chronic cough, haemoptysis, fevers and weight loss), but in late-stage infection atypical manifestations such as disseminated disease are common and diagnosis is more difficult.

Focal neurological signs, convulsions or altered conscious state

These features generally indicate the presence of an intracerebral space occupying lesion, the most common causes of which are:

- Cerebral toxoplasmosis: this infection occurs when the CD4 cell count is $<0.2 \times 10^9/L$. The specific focal features depend on the site of the usually multiple lesions, and may include hemiparesis, visual field defects, personality change or cerebellar signs.
- Primary cerebral lymphoma: this complication occurs with advanced HIV infection (CD4 cell count usually $<0.05 \times 10^9/L$) and develops in 2–3% of AIDS patients. Clinical presentation is indistinguishable from that of cerebral toxoplasmosis.
- Progressive multifocal leucoencephalopathy: caused by a polyoma virus (JC virus); patients present with cognitive decline or focal signs. Seizures are relatively uncommon. Differentiation from cerebral toxoplasmosis and primary cerebral lymphoma requires computerized tomography (CT) or magnetic resonance imaging (MRI) scanning (see below).

Diarrhoea, with or without abdominal pain or fever

A wide range of gastrointestinal pathogens causes diarrhoea in HIV-infected patients (Table 8.8.3). Patients should be asked about recent travel or antibiotic use. Bloody diarrhoea is suggestive of a large bowel pathogen such as cytomegalovirus, *Entamoeba histolytica* or *Clostridium difficile*, whereas profuse watery diarrhoea suggests an infection of the small bowel, such as cryptosporidiosis. However, clinical features are often of limited diagnostic value and the specific diagnosis rests upon identification of the pathogen in a faecal or biopsy specimen.

Fever without localizing features

This is chiefly a problem in those with a CD4 cell count $<0.2 \times 10^9/L$. The differential diagnosis is extensive, the major causes being:

- Disseminated opportunistic infections: disseminated *Mycobacterium avium* complex

(MAC), disseminated tuberculosis, disseminated histoplasmosis (USA and South America), salmonella bacteraemia, CMV
- Focal opportunistic infections with non-focal presentation: PCP, cryptococcal meningitis, tuberculosis
- Bacterial infections: sinusitis, bacterial pneumonia, primary bacteraemia (especially in patients with an indwelling long-term intravenous device, or neutropenia)
- Non-HIV specific infections: right-sided endocarditis, secondary syphilis
- Non-infectious causes: non-Hodgkin's lymphoma, drug fever.

Difficult or painful swallowing

This is usually due to candida oesophagitis, in which case oral candidiasis is often present. Other causes include idiopathic aphthous ulceration, CMV oesophagitis and herpes simplex oesophagitis.

Headache, fever, neck stiffness

Cryptococcal meningitis is the most common cause of this syndrome, although headache may be mild and signs of meningism subtle or absent. Less common causes include tuberculous meningitis, syphilitic meningitis, HIV itself and lymphomatous meningitis.

Other presentations

- Abdominal pain: pancreatitis due to antiretroviral therapy, HIV cholangiopathy, intra-abdominal lymphadenopathy secondary to MAC or lymphoma
- Neuropsychiatric manifestations: depression, mania, cognitive decline
- Visual complaints: CMV retinitis (when CD4 cell count $<0.05 \times 10^9/L$), uveitis, rarely toxoplasma or cryptococcal chorioretinitis.

INVESTIGATION

Requesting an HIV antibody test

In Australia, doctors are legally obliged to counsel patients about the medical, psychological and social consequences of a positive or negative HIV antibody test. The counselling process involves the following:

- Asking the patient about risk factors for HIV infection
- Providing information about the test itself, including its limitations (e.g. 'window period') and the meaning of a positive or negative test
- Briely describing the natural history of HIV infection, including the improved outlook with modern antiretroviral therapy
- Addressing any concerns about confidentiality of results
- Reinforcing preventive messages, such as safer sexual practices.

Ideally, the patient should be counselled in a private and quiet environment. This is not always possible in an open-design, overcrowded and noisy emergency department!

The doctor who originally counsels the patient and requests the test is responsible for notifying the patient of the result, which should be done in person and not over the telephone or by post. This applies equally to positive and negative results.

Table 8.8.3 Gastrointestinal pathogens in HIV-infected patients

Bacterial	**Protozoal**
Salmonella, Campylobacter	Cryptosporidiosis
Clostridium difficile	Giardiasis
Mycobacterium avium complex (MAC)	*Entamoeba histolytica*
	Microsporidiosis
Viral	**Non-infectious**
CMV	Lactose intolerance
	Gastrointestinal
	Kaposi's sarcoma and lymphoma

Primary HIV infection

- Full blood examination, heterophile antibody test.
- HIV antibody: the antibody test may be negative initially, in which case it is vital to repeat the test in 2, 4 and 6 weeks.
- p24 antigen: this viral protein can be detected in blood during primary infection and has a diagnostic role in those with an initially negative antibody test. (At present, HIV RNA [viral load] tests are *not* recommended for diagnosis of primary HIV infection.)

Patients with previously unrecognized infection

The HIV antibody test will be positive in all patients, and other tests are not needed for diagnosis. As indicated in the previous section, appropriate pre- and post-test counselling is vital.

Specific investigations in patients known to be HIV infected

Cough, shortness of breath, fever

If the CD4 cell count is $>0.2 \times 10^9$/L, most patients can be managed as if they did not have HIV infection. Investigations required for patients with suspected bacterial pneumonia or tuberculosis include a chest X-ray, full blood examination, sputum examination and blood cultures.

If the CD4 cell count is $<0.2 \times 10^9$/L investigation is almost always indicated, the extent of which will be guided by the patient's condition and the likely diagnostic possibilities, and may include some or all of the following:

- Oxygen saturation
- Chest X-ray
- Blood cultures
- Sputum Gram stain, culture, and AFB smear and culture
- Induced sputum for detection (by microscopy) of PCP
- Bronchoscopy - rarely indicated nowadays.

A high index of suspicion for tuberculosis must be maintained. The diagnosis is generally suggested by one or more suggestive epidemiological, clinical or radiological features.

Focal neurological signs, convulsions or altered conscious state

CT scanning (with contrast) should be done in all patients, often as a matter of some urgency, and should always precede a lumbar puncture. A *Toxoplasma gondii* IgG test will have usually been performed in those with previously diagnosed HIV infection: if positive, this indicates a predisposition to the development of cerebral toxoplasmosis; if negative, toxoplasmosis is much less likely.

Diarrhoea, with or without abdominal pain and fever

Faecal examination (preferably three fresh specimens collected on different days) for:

- Microscopy for ova, cysts and parasites
- Cryptosporidium stain, microsporidium stain
- Culture for *Salmonella*, *Campylobacter* and *Shigella*
- *Clostridium difficile* culture and toxin if recent antibiotic therapy.

Selected patients with undiagnosed diarrhoea may require colonoscopy or upper GI endoscopy if conditions such as CMV, MAC or microsporidiosis are suspected.

Fever without localizing features

If the CD4 cell count is $>0.2 \times 10^9$/L serious HIV-related causes are uncommon, and so investigation will be guided by clinical features, severity of illness and so on.

If the CD4 cell count is $<0.2 \times 10^9$/L most patients will need investigation, beginning with the following basic work-up:

- Blood cultures, including mycobacterial blood cultures if CD4 cell count $<0.05 \times 10^9$/L
- Chest X-ray
- Serum cryptococcal antigen.

Additional tests for selected patients include faecal examination, sputum examination, abdominal ultrasonography or CT scanning, and occasionally bone marrow or liver biopsy.

Difficult or painful swallowing

Oesophagoscopy and biopsy are reserved for those who fail an empirical course of antifungal therapy (see below).

Headache, fever, neck stiffness

The serum cryptococcal antigen test is a useful screening test for cryptococcal meningitis because a negative result effectively excludes the diagnosis. A lumbar puncture should only be done after a brain CT scan, and if the CT does not show a space-occupying lesion or evidence of increased intracranial pressure. CSF should be routinely sent for the following:

- Protein and glucose
- Gram stain and culture (and AFB smear and culture if tuberculosis is suspected)
- India ink stain and cryptococcal antigen
- Cytology
- A CSF VDRL or RPR test should only be requested if the serum syphilis serology is positive.

MANAGEMENT

Primary HIV infection

- Symptomatic treatment
- Specific antiretroviral therapy – role not determined.

Specific HIV syndromes

Emergency department physicians should consult doctors experienced in treating HIV-infected patients for advice about the management of specific syndromes and opportunistic infections. The following guidelines focus on initial and empiric therapy and provide examples of treatment options, but detailed information about indications for specific agents, toxicity and so on is omitted. For more comprehensive treatment recommendations, a specialized text should be consulted.[7]

Cough, fever, shortness of breath
Any person with suspected pulmonary tuberculosis must be placed in respiratory isolation until the diagnosis is excluded. On the basis of the initial diagnostic evaluation, patients can be categorized and management proceed as follows:

- Significant infection unlikely: no treatment
- Possible PCP: empirical PCP therapy with co-trimoxazole, and steroids if P_aO_2 on room air <60 mmHg
- Possible bacterial pneumonia: oral amoxycillin (± clavulanic acid) or macrolide such as roxithromycin if mild, IV penicillin or ceftriaxone (plus or minus macrolide) if hospitalization required
- Possible tuberculosis: admission, respiratory isolation, empirical therapy (with isoniazid, rifampicin, pyrazinamide and ethambutol) considered.

Focal neurological signs, convulsions, altered conscious state
Treatment is guided by the results of the CT scan.

If a space-occupying lesion is found patients are treated empirically for cerebral toxoplasmosis with sulphadiazine and pyrimethamine. The CT scan is repeated after 2–3 weeks, and if no response is evident a biopsy might be considered in selected patients to diagnose cerebral lymphoma.

If the CT scan is normal, clinical circumstances will dictate whether no further action is taken or whether an MRI scan is indicated.

Diarrhoea, with or without abdominal pain and fever
Any infection identified on initial faecal examinations is treated on its merits. Symptomatic treatment with an antimotility agent such as loperamide can be given safely to most patients. Endoscopy is generally reserved for those in whom no specific cause is identified on initial evaluation, and whose diarrhoea persists despite antimotility therapy.

Fever without localizing features
Empirical antibacterial therapy (with an antipseudomonal agent such as ceftazidime, with or without an aminoglycoside or vancomycin) is indicated for patients with an absolute neutrophil count $<0.5 \times 10^9$/L. Otherwise the need for specific treatment is guided by the condition of the patient and the results of the diagnostic work-up. Treatment for disseminated MAC (with clarithromycin, ethambutol ± rifabutin) is generally given only after the organism has been isolated, although occasional patients with debilitating fevers, weight loss and no other diagnosis may be treated empirically.

Difficult or painful swallowing
Empirical antifungal therapy is started with an azole agent, usually oral fluconazole. Some patients with candida infections resistant to azoles need treatment with a short course of IV amphotericin B. Patients undergo endoscopy if they do not respond to antifungal treatment, and the results of histology and cultures determine subsequent treatment.

Headache, fever, neck stiffness
Patients with confirmed cryptococcal meningitis are treated with a combination of IV amphotericin B and oral 5-fluorocytosine for 1–2 weeks, then remain on suppressive therapy with oral fluconazole. If tuberculous meningitis is suspected empirical therapy should be started immediately pending the results of CSF cultures.

Specific treatment of other infections
- CMV infections: IV ganciclovir or IV foscarnet
- *Salmonella* infections: ciprofloxacin.

Antiretrovirals in the management of HIV infection
More potent antiretroviral drugs and the ability to measure HIV RNA levels have transformed the field of HIV therapeutics. However, antiretoviral therapy is not without its costs: difficulty in adhering to complicated drug regimens, short- and long-term toxicities of antiretroviral agents and the potential development of antiretroviral resistance.

The emergency medicine physician does not require a detailed knowledge of antiretroviral therapy, but should be aware of the agents that are used, their side effects, and the potential importance of drug–drug interactions.

Indications[8]
- Symptomatic HIV infection[9]
- Asymptomatic HIV infection – CD4 cell count less than 0.35×10^9/L, or viral load higher than 55 000 HIV RNA copies/mL
- Pregnant women with HIV infection[10]
- After significant HIV exposure sustained by healthcare worker.[11]

Classes of drugs
- Nucleoside reverse transcriptase inhibitors (NRTIs): zidovudine (ZDV or AZT), didanosine (ddI), zalcitabine (ddC), lamivudine (3TC), stavudine (d4T), abacavir
- Protease inhibitors (PIs): nelfinavir; indinavir, saquinavir, ritonavir, amprenavir, lopinavir/ritonavir[12]
- Non-nucleoside reverse transcriptase inhibitors (NNRTIs): nevirapine, efavirenz, delavirdine.

Regimens – at least three drugs
- Two NRTIs (ZDV+3TC *or* ZDV+ddI *or* d4T+3TC *plus* nevirapine or efavirenz
  OR
- Two NRTIs (as listed above) *plus* a PI (nelfinavir *or* indinavir *or* lopinavir/ritonavir).

Side-effects (see Table 8.8.4)

Drug–drug interactions
Many commonly used drugs metabolized by hepatic cytochrome P450 oxidases should not be used together with certain PIs or NNRTIs. The following list is not exhaustive, and physicians are urged to consult a pharmacist or HIV expert if there is any doubt about the potential for a drug interaction with an antiretroviral agent.

- Contraindicated with *all PIs*: astemizole, terfenadine, cisapride,

Table 8.8.4 Side effects of antiretroviral agents

Agent	Side effect
NRTI agents	
class effects	Hyperlactataemia, lactic acidosis
zidovudine	Nausea, headache, myalgia, anaemia, neutropenia
didanosine	Pancreatitis, diarrhoea, nausea, peripheral neuropathy
zalcitabine	Peripheral neuropathy, mouth ulcers, pancreatitis
lamivudine	Abnormal liver function, neutropenia, pancreatitis (all uncommon)
stavudine	Peripheral neuropathy, pancreatitis
abacavir	Hypersensitivity reaction (challenge contraindicated)
NNRTI agents	
nevirapine	Rash, hepatitis, fever
efavirenz	Neuropsychological (vivid dreams, insomnia, difficulty concentrating, light headedness), rash, abnormal liver function
delavirdine	Rash, abnormal liver function
Protease inhibitors	
class effects	Hyperglycaemia, hyperlipidaemia, redistribution of body fat, abnormal liver function
nelfinavir	Diarrhoea
indinavir	Renal calculi, back pain, nausea, hyperbilirubinaemia
ritonavir	Nausea, abdominal pain, diarrhoea, perioral paraesthesiae
saquinavir	Diarrhoea, nausea
lopinavir	Diarrhoea, nausea

rifampicin, midazolam, triazolam, simvastatin, ergotamine, dihydroergotamine
- Contraindicated with *saquinavir*: as for *all PIs*, plus rifabutin;
- Contraindicated with *ritonavir*: as for *all PIs*, plus pethidine, diazepam, amiodarone, quinidine, clozapine, pimozide;
- Contraindicated with efavirenz: as for *all PIs*, except rifampicin and simvastatin
- Contraindicated with delavirdine: as for *all PIs*, plus H2 receptor antagonists and proton pump inhibitors.

DISPOSITION

Patients with newly diagnosed HIV infection should be referred to a specialized HIV clinic, or to a doctor with expertise in HIV medicine.

HIV medicine is a complex and rapidly changing field. For this reason, the management of patients with known HIV infection presenting to the emergency department should always involve consultation with a hospital doctor knowledgeable about HIV infection, such as an infectious diseases physician or immunologist. In general, patients with a suspected or confirmed serious opportunistic infection will need to be admitted for investigation and management. Patients in the final stages of AIDS, or those with less serious complications, can often be managed in the community, in which case liaison with the local doctor, home-care nurses or community-care agencies is vital.

PROGNOSIS

Prior to the widespread use of opportunistic infection prophylaxis and better antiretroviral therapy, 50% of patients developed AIDS 10 years after becoming HIV infected, and 75% of patients after 13 years. Long-term non-progressors, who have a normal CD4 count and no HIV-related complications after 10 or more years of HIV infection, comprise less than 5% of patient cohorts.

The median survival after diagnosis of AIDS has improved from 10 months in the mid-1980s to over 2 years nowadays. With the emerging data on the clinical benefits of modern antiretroviral therapy, further improvements are expected.

Most AIDS-defining infections, such as PCP, have low mortality and high 1-year survival rates if treated appropriately, but survival rates following diagnosis of disseminated MAC and CMV end-organ disease are lower because these two opportunistic infections usually occur at a very advanced stage of HIV infection.

PREVENTION

Prevention of HIV transmission

- Educational efforts to encourage the adoption of safer sex practices
- HIV screening of blood and blood products
- Non-sharing and use of clean needles and syringes by injecting drug users
- Observance of standard precautions by workers in healthcare settings
- Use of antiretroviral prophylaxis to prevent transmission from mother to baby, and after significant exposures to HIV-infected blood.

Prevention of HIV-related complications[13]

Infection	Prevention
Pneumococcal pneumonia	Pneumococcal vaccination
Latent tuberculous infection	Isoniazid
PCP	Co-trimoxazole
Toxoplasmosis	Co-trimoxazole
MAC	Azithromycin or rifabutin

CONTROVERSIES

❶ Will HIV infection become more common among injecting drug users?

❷ Have the new antiretroviral agents converted HIV infection into a chronic medical condition (like hypertension), or will their beneficial effect wane with time because of the development of drug resistance?

❸ Can an effective HIV vaccine be developed?

REFERENCES

1. UNAIDS 2001 AIDS epidemic update 2001. Joint United Nations Programme on HIV/AIDS (UNAIDS) and World Health Organization (WHO), Geneva
2. National Centre in HIV Epidemiology and Clinical Research 2001 HIV/AIDS, viral hepatitis & sexually transmissible infections in Australia Annual Surveillance Report 2001. National Centre in HIV Epidemiology and Clinical Research, The University of New South Wales, Sydney
3. Havlir DV, Richman DD 1996 Viral dynamics of HIV: implications for drug development and therapeutic strategies. Annals of Internal Medicine 124: 984–94
4. Mellors JW, Rinaldo CR, Gupta P, et al 1996 Prognosis in HIV-1 infection predicted by the quantity of virus in the plasma. Science 272: 1167–70
5. Stewart G (ed.) 1994 Could it be HIV? Australasian Medical Publishing Company Ltd, Sydney
6. Carr A, Boyle MJ 1996 Primary HIV infection. In: Stewart G (ed.) Managing HIV. Australasian Medical Publishing Company Ltd, Sydney, pp 9–11
7. Crowe S, Hoy J, Mills J (eds) 2001 Medical Management of the HIV-infected Patient, 2nd edn. Martin Dunitz, Cambridge
8. Centers for Disease Control 2002 Guidelines for using antiretroviral agents among HIV-infected adults and adolescents: recommendations of the panel on clinical practices for treatment of HIV. Morbidity and Mortality Weekly Report 51(RR-7): 1–54
9. Hammer SM, Squires KE, Hughes MD, et al 1997 A controlled trial of 2 nucleoside analogues plus indinavir in persons with human immunodeficiency virus infection and CD4 cell counts of 200 per cubic millimeter or less. New England Journal of Medicine 337: 725–33
10. Watt DH 2002 Management of human immunodeficiency virus infection in pregnancy. New England Journal of Medicine 346: 1879–91
11. Centers for Disease Control 1995 Case-control study of HIV seroconversion in healthcare workers after percutaneous exposure to HIV-infected blood. Morbidity and Mortality Weekly Report 44: 929–33
12. Bartlett JG 1996 Protease inhibitors for HIV infection. Annals of Internal Medicine 124: 1086–8
13. Centers for Disease Control and Prevention 2002 Guidelines for preventing opportunistic infections among HIV-infected persons – 2002: recommendations of USPHS and IDSA. Morbidity and Mortality Weekly Report 51(No.RR-8): 1–27

8.9 ANTIBIOTICS IN THE EMERGENCY DEPARTMENT

DAVID MCD. TAYLOR • JOHN VINEN

ESSENTIALS

1 Patients with infectious disease are commonly seen in emergency departments.

2 There are changing patterns of infectious disease largely due to immunosuppression from chemotherapy and HIV disease.

3 Many bacteria are becoming increasingly resistant to available antimicrobials.

4 There are relatively few new antimicrobials to counter these changing patterns of resistance.

5 Antimicrobial prescribing should be evidence-based and in line with local guidelines.

6 Some patients with infection can be treated wholly as outpatients utililzing parenteral therapy, or after early discharge once the acute toxic phase is over.

PRINCIPLES OF ANTIMICROBIAL THERAPY

The first decision to be made regarding antimicrobial therapy is whether the administration of these agents is truly indicated. Their reflex prescription for patients with fever or presumed treatable infections is often irrational. This practice is potentially dangerous, as some agents can cause serious toxicity, diagnoses may be masked if appropriate cultures are not taken prior to therapy, and micro-organism resistance may emerge. The choice of an appropriate antimicrobial agent requires consideration of the following factors.

The micro-organism

The identity of the infecting organism must be known or suspected. In the emergency department setting most antimicrobial decisions will be made without the benefit of microbial culture, and the physician applies knowledge of the organisms most likely to cause infection in a given clinical setting.[1] However, certain 'rapid methods' of microbial identification may be employed. These include Gram-stain preparations (bacterial, some fungal and leucocyte identification) and immunological methods for antigen detection (enzyme-linked immunoabsorbent assay, latex agglutination, polymerase chain reactions).

Micro-organism susceptibility

The emergency physician is unlikely to have this information, and therapeutic decisions will generally be based upon a knowledge of likely susceptibilities.[1] For example, group A streptococci remain susceptible to the penicillins and cephalosporins, and virtually all anaerobes (except *Bacteroides* spp.) are susceptible to penicillin G. However, when the identity or susceptibility of the infecting organism is sufficiently in doubt, the patient's clinical condition is atypical, serious or potentially serious, or where antimicrobial resistance is suspected, it is good practice to obtain appropriate specimens for culture and susceptibility testing prior to empirical antimicrobial therapy (Table 8.9.1).

Host factors

An adequate history of previous drug allergies must be obtained in order to prevent the administration of an agent that may have serious or fatal consequences. The age of the patient may have clinically significant effects upon drug absorption (e.g. penicillin absorption is increased in the young and the elderly),[2] metabolism (e.g. reduced chloramphenicol metabolism in the neonate)[2] and excretion (e.g. declining renal function with age[3] may reduce the excretion of penicillins, cephalosporins and aminoglycosides). Furthermore, tetracyclines bind and discolour the developing bone and tooth structures in children aged 8 years or less.[2] Pregnant patients and nursing mothers may pose certain problems in the selection of appropriate antimicrobial agents, as all of these agents cross the placenta in varying degrees.[4] Other host factors that may require consideration include the patient's renal and hepatic function, their genetic (e.g. liver acetylation rate) or metabolic abnormalities (e.g. diabetes mellitus), and the site of the infection.[5]

Route of administration

In general, the oral route is chosen for infections that are mild and can be managed on an outpatient basis. In this situation, consideration needs to be given to compliance with treatment, the variability of absorption with food in the stomach, and interaction of the agent with concomitant medications.[5] The parenteral route is used for agents that are inefficiently absorbed from the gastrointestinal tract and for the treatment of patients with serious infections in whom high concentrations of antimicrobial agents are required.[5] Intramuscular administration will provide adequate serum concentrations for most infections, and may be appropriate where antimicrobial depots are desirable, e.g. procaine penicillin injections where patient compliance with oral medication is doubtful. Intravenous administration allows large doses of drugs to be given with a

minimal amount of discomfort to the patient, e.g. infection prophylaxis in compound fractures, life-threatening infections and shocked patients. With intravenous administration the use of large veins and saline flushing of the veins post-administration may help to minimize the incidence of venous irritation and phlebitis.

ANTIBIOTIC RESISTANCE

Bacteria can be resistant to an antimicrobial agent because the drug fails to reach the target or is inactivated, or because the target is altered.[6–8] Bacteria may produce enzymes that inactivate the drug, or have cell membranes impermeable to the drug. Having gained entry into the micro-organism, the drug must exert a deleterious effect. Natural variation or acquired changes at the target site that prevent drug binding or action can lead to resistance.

Resistance is most commonly acquired by horizontal transfer of resistance determinants from a donor cell, often of another bacterial species, by transformation, transduction or conjugation. Resistance may also be acquired by mutation, and passed vertically by selection to daughter cells. Antimicrobial agents can affect the emergence of resistance by exerting strong selective pressures upon bacterial populations favouring those organisms capable of resisting them.[9]

The recent emergence of antibiotic resistance is a very serious development that threatens the end of the antibiotic era. Penicillin-resistant strains of pneumococci account for 50% or more of isolates in some European countries. The worldwide emergence of *Haemophilus* and gonococci that produce β-lactamase is a major therapeutic problem.[10] Methicillin-resistant strains of *Staphylococcus aureus* are widely distributed among hospitals and are increasingly being isolated from community-acquired infections.[11] There are now strains of enterococci, pseudomonas and enterobacters that are resistant to all known

drugs.[12] Epidemics of multiply drug-resistant strains of *Mycobacterium tuberculosis* have been reported.[12]

A more responsible approach to the use of new and existing antimicrobial agents is essential to slow the development of multidrug-resistant organisms. Their use should be avoided in viral infections, and rational policies for their use in prophylaxis and in established bacterial infections must be developed and followed.[1] The use of narrow-spectrum antimicrobial agents to which the organism is susceptible is encouraged, and the use of combinations of agents may prevent the emergence of resistant mutants during therapy, in certain circumstances.

PROPHYLACTIC USE OF ANTIBIOTICS

Antimicrobial prophylaxis is the use of antimicrobial agents before infection takes place. It is indicated in many circumstances, including the prevention of recurrent rheumatic fever, endocarditis, meningitis, tuberculosis, and urinary-tract and surgical infections.[1] Antimicrobial prophylaxis in the emergency department is usually indicated to prevent trauma-related infection following contamination of soft tissue, crushing injuries, bites and clenched fist injuries, and compound fractures. Other risk factors for wound infection include shock, colon injury and massive haemorrhage.[13]

Antimicrobial prophylaxis should be considered where there is a significant risk of infection, but cannot be relied upon to overcome excessive soiling, damage to tissues, inadequate debridement or poor surgical technique. Proper wound care, with splinting and elevation of the affected area as indicated, will remain the most important factors in trauma-related infection prophylaxis.

Antimicrobial prophylaxis should be directed against the likely causative organism(s). However, an effective regimen need not necessarily include antimicrobials that are active against every potential pathogen. Regimens that only decrease the total number of

Table 8.9.1 Antimicrobial agents of choice in selected infections

Micro-organism	Diseases	First choice	Second choice
Gram-positive cocci			
Staphylococcus aureus*	Abscesses penicillinase-negative: Osteomyelitis	benzylpenicillin (penicillin G), phenoxymethylpenicillin (penicillin V)	cephalosporin (G1), clindamycin
	Bacteraemia penicillinase-positive: Endocarditis	nafcillin, oxacillin	cephalosporin (G1) vancomycin, clindamycin
	Pneumonia methicillin-resistant: Cellulitis	vancomycin ± rifampicin	co-trimoxazole + rifampicin ciprofloxacin + rifampicin
Streptococcus (A, B, C, G and bovis)	Pharyngitis, scarlet fever, otitis media, cellulitis, erysipelas, pneumonia, bacteraemia, endocarditis, meningitis	benzylpenicillin (penicillin G), phenoxymethylpenicillin (penicillin V), ampicillin	erythromycin, cephalosporin (G1) vancomycin
Streptococcus pneumoniae*	Pneumonia, arthritis, sinusitis, otitis media, meningitis, endocarditis	benzylpenicillin (penicillin G), phenoxymethylpenicillin (penicillin V), ampicillin, penicillin G	erythromycin, cephalosporin (G1–3) vancomycin + rifampicin, ceftriaxone
Streptococcus viridans*	Bacteraemia, endocarditis	benzylpenicillin (penicillin G) ± gentamicin	ceftriaxone, vancomycin ± gentamicin
Enterococcus	Bacteraemia, endocarditis, urinary tract infection	ampicillin + gentamicin, benzylpenicillin (penicillin G) + gentamicin	vancomycin + gentamicin, nitrofurantoin, fluoroquinolone, ampicillin + clavulanic acid
Gram-negative cocci			
Moraxella catarrhalis	Otitis, sinusitis, pneumonia	co-trimoxazole amoxycillin + clavulanic acid	cephalosporin (G2,3), erythromycin, tetracycline
Neisseria gonorrhoeae	Gonorrhoea, disseminated disease	ceftriaxone, ampicillin + probenecid	ciprofloxacin, doxycycline spectinomycin
Neisseria meningitidis	Meningitis, carrier state	benzylpenicillin (penicillin G) rifampicin	cephalosporin (G3), chloramphenicol
Gram-positive bacilli			
Clostridium perfringens*	Gas gangrene	benzylpenicillin (penicillin G)	clindamycin, metronidazole, cephalosporin
Clostridium tetani	Tetanus	benzylpenicillin (penicillin G), vancomycin	doxycycline, clindamycin
Clostridium difficile	Antimicrobial-associated colitis	metronidazole (oral)	vancomycin (oral)
Corynebacterium diphtheriae	Pharyngitis, tracheitis, pneumonia	erythromycin	benzylpenicillin (penicillin G), clindamycin
Listeria monocytogenes	Meningitis, bacteraemia	ampicillin ± gentamicin	co-trimoxazole, erythromycin
Gram-negative bacilli			
Brucella	Brucellosis	doxycycline + gentamicin	co-trimoxazole + gentamicin/rifampicin
Campylobacter jejuni*	Enteritis	fluoroquinolone	erythromycin, azithromycin
Escherichia coli*	Urinary tract infection, bacteraemia	ampicillin, co-trimoxazole cephalosporin (G1)	ampicillin + gentamicin, fluoroquinolone, nitrofurantoin
Enterobacter species	Urinary tract and other infections	fluoroquinolone imipenem	gentamicin + broad-spectrum penicillin, co-trimoxazole
Haemophilus influenzae*	Otitis, sinusitis, pneumonia	co-trimoxazole, ampicillin, amoxicillin	amoxicillin + clavulanic acid, azithromycin cefuroxime
	Epiglottitis, meningitis	cephalosporin (G3)	chloramphenicol
Klebsiella pneumoniae*	Urinary tract infection, pneumonia	cephalosporin ± gentamicin	co-trimoxazole, fluoroquinolone
Legionella pneumophila	Legionnaires' disease	erythromycin ± rifampicin	ciprofloxacin, azithromycin, co-trimoxazole
Pasteurella multocida	Animal bite infections, abscesses, bacteraemia, meningitis	benzylpenicillin (penicillin G), amoxicillin + clavulanic acid	doxycycline, cephalosporin
Proteus mirabilis*	Urinary tract and other infections	ampicillin, amoxycillin	cephalosporin, co-trimoxazole, gentamicin
Proteus (other species)*	Urinary tract and other infections	cephalosporin (G3), gentamicin	co-trimoxazole, fluoroquinolone
Pseudomonas aeruginosa*	Urinary tract infection, pneumonia, bacteraemia	broad-spectrum penicillin ± gentamicin	ceftazidime ± gentamicin fluoroquinolone ± gentamicin
Salmonella species*	Typhoid fever, paratyphoid fever, bacteraemia, gastroenteritis	fluoroquinolone, ceftriaxone	ampicillin, co-trimoxazole, chloramphenicol
Shigella*	Acute gastroenteritis	fluoroquinolone	ampicillin, co-trimoxazole
Vibrio cholerae	Cholera	doxycycline, fluoroquinolone	co-trimoxazole
Miscellaneous agents			
Chlamydia species	Pneumonia, trachoma, urethritis, cervicitis	doxycycline	azithromycin, erythromycin
Mycoplasma pneumoniae	Atypical pneumonia	erythromycin, doxycycline	azithromycin
Pneumocystis carinii	Pneumonia in impaired host	co-trimoxazole	trimethoprim + dapsone, pentamidine
Rickettsia	Typhus fever, Q fever, Rocky Mountain spotted fever	doxycycline	chloramphenicol
Treponema pallidum	Syphilis	benzylpenicillin (penicillin G)	ceftriaxone, doxycycline

* All strains should be examined in vitro for sensitivity to various antimicrobial agents.
G1, first-generation cephalosporin; G2, second-generation cephalosporin; G3, third-generation cephalosporin.

organisms may assist host defences and prevent infection.[1] The type, dose, duration and route of administration of antimicrobial therapy will vary according to the nature, site and aetiology of the injury, as well as host factors. In all cases of open traumatic injury, tetanus prophylaxis must be considered.

PENICILLINS

Chemistry and mechanism of action

The penicillins constitute one of the most important groups of antimicrobial agents and remain the drugs of choice for a large number of infectious diseases. The basic structure of the penicillins consists of a thiazolidine ring connected to a β-lactam ring, and a side chain. The penicillin nucleus is the chief structural requirement for biological activity, whereas the side chain determines many of the antibacterial and pharmacological characteristics of the particular type of penicillin.

Peptidoglycan is an essential component of the bacterial cell wall, and provides mechanical stability by virtue of its highly cross-linked latticework structure. Penicillin is thought to acetylate and inhibit a transpeptidase enzyme responsible for the final cross-linking of peptidoglycan layers. Penicillin also binds to penicillin-binding proteins (PBPs), causing further interference with cell wall synthesis and cell morphology. The lysis of bacteria is ultimately dependent upon the activity of cell wall autolytic enzymes - autolysins and murein hydrolases. Although the relationship between the inhibition of PBP activity and the activation of autolysins is unclear, the interference with peptidoglycan assembly in the face of ongoing autolysis activity might well lead to cell lysis and death.

Bacterial resistance to penicillins

Micro-organisms may be intrinsically resistant to the penicillins because of structural differences in PBPs. Resistance may be acquired by the development of high molecular weight PBPs that have

decreased affinity for the antibiotic.[8] Bacterial resistance can also be caused by the inability of the agent to penetrate to its site of action.[14] Unlike Gram-positive bacteria, Gram-negative bacteria have an outer membrane of lipopolysaccharide which functions as an impenetrable barrier to some antibiotics. However, some broader-spectrum penicillins, such as ampicillin and amoxicillin, can diffuse through aqueous channels (porins) of this outer membrane to reach their sites of action.

Bacteria can destroy penicillins enzymatically. Different bacteria elaborate a number of different β-lactamases and individual penicillins vary in their susceptibility to these enzymes. In general, Gram-positive bacteria produce a large amount of β-lactamase, which is secreted extracellularly. Most of these enzymes are penicillinases which disrupt the β-lactam ring and inactivate the drug. In Gram-negative bacteria, β-lactamases are found in relatively small amounts strategically located between the inner and outer bacterial membranes for maximal protection.

Classification of penicillins

Benzylpenicillin (penicillin G) and phenoxymethylpenicillin (penicillin V)

These drugs are the so-called 'natural penicillins'. The antimicrobial spectra of benzylpenicillin (penicillin G) and phenoxymethylpenicillin (penicillin V) are very similar for aerobic Gram-positive micro-organisms. Benzylpenicillin (penicillin G) is the drug of choice against many Gram-positive cocci (streptococci, penicillin-sensitive staphylococci), Gram-negative cocci (*Neisseria meningitidis* and *N. gonorrhoeae*), Gram-postive bacilli (*Bacillus anthracis*, *Cl. diphtheria*), anaerobes (peptostreptococcus, *Actinomyces israeli*, *Clostridium* and some *Bacteroides*), *Pasteurella multocida* and *Treponema pallidum*. Phenoxymethylpenicillin (Penicillin V) is an acceptable alternative for *Streptococcus pneumoniae*, *Strep. pyogenes* (A) and *Actinomyces israeli*.

The sole virtue of benzylpenicillin (penicillin V) compared to phenoxy-

methylpenicillin (penicillin G) is that it is more stable in an acid medium and, therefore, is much better absorbed from the gastrointestinal tract. Benzylpenicillin (penicillin G) is administered parenterally but has a half-life of only 30 minutes. Accordingly, repository preparations (penicillin G procaine, penicillin G benzathine) are often used and probenecid may be administered concurrently to block the renal tubular secretion of the drug. Once absorbed, both penicillins are distributed widely throughout the body. Significant amounts appear in the liver, bile, kidney, semen, joint fluid, lymph and intestine. Importantly, penicillin does not readily enter the CSF when the meninges are normal. However, when the meninges are acutely inflamed penicillin penetrates into the CSF more easily. Under normal circumstances, penicillin is eliminated unchanged by the kidney, mainly by tubular secretion.

The Penicillinase-resistant penicillins

These drugs remain the agents of choice for most staphylococcal disease. Methicillin is a penicillin resistant to staphylococcal β-lactamase, although the increasing incidence of isolates of methicillin-resistant micro-organisms is cause for concern. Methicillin-resistant *Staph. aureus* contain a high molecular weight PBP with a very low affinity for β-lactam antibiotics.[8] From 40 to 60% of strains of *Staph. epidermidis* are also resistant to penicillinase-resistant penicillins by the same mechanism. As bacterial sensitivities are usually not known in the emergency department, methicillin is rarely administered in this setting.

The isoxazolyl penicillins (oxacillin, cloxacillin, dicloxacillin and flucloxacillin) are congeneric semisynthetic penicillins which are pharmacologically similar. All are relatively stable in an acid medium and are adequately absorbed after oral administration. These penicillins undergo some metabolism but are excreted primarily by the kidney with some biliary excretion. All are remarkably resistant to cleavage by penicillinase, and inhibit both penicillin-sensitive and some penicillin-resistant staphylococci. Methicillin-resistant staphylococci are resistant to these penicillins. Isoxazolyl penicillins inhibit streptococci and pneumococci but are virtually inactive against Gram-negative bacilli.

The Aminopenicillins

Ampicillin is the prototypical agent in this group. It is stable in acid medium and, although well absorbed orally, is often administered parenterally. Amoxicillin is a close chemical and pharmacological relative of ampicillin. The drug is stable in acid and was designed for oral use. It is more rapidly and completely absorbed from the gastrointestinal tract than is ampicillin. The antimicrobial spectra of these agents are essentially identical, with the important exception that amoxicillin appears to be less effective for shigellosis. Ampicillin is the penicillin of choice for many Gram-negative bacilli (*H. influenzae*, *Escherichia coli*, *Proteus mirabilis*, *Salmonella typhi* and *Salmonella* spp.), some Gram-positive bacilli (*Listeria monocytogenes*) and some Gram-positive cocci (*Enterococcus faecalis*). It also has activity against *Pneumococcus* spp., *Neisseria* spp., *Peptostreptococcus*, *Fusobacterium*, *Clostridium* and *Erysipelothrix*.

Bacterial resistance to these drugs is becoming an increasing problem. Many pneumococcal isolates have varying levels of resistance to ampicillin. *H. influenzae* and the *viridans* group of streptococci are usually inhibited by very low concentrations of ampicillin. However, strains of *H. influenzae* (type b) that are highly resistant to ampicillin have been recovered from children with meningitis. It is estimated that 30% or more cases of *H. influenzae* meningitis are now caused by ampicillin-resistant strains. Similarly, ampicillin-resistant strains of *H. influenzae* have been increasingly isolated from cases of acute otitis media. An increasing percentage of *N. gonorrhoeae*, *E. coli*, *P. mirabilis*, *Salmonella* and *Shigella* are now resistant to ampicillin, and practically all species of *Enterobacter* are now insensitive.

β-lactamase inhibitors have been introduced to combat many penicillin-resistant micro-organisms. These molecules bind to β-lactamases and inactivate them, thereby preventing the destruction of β-lactamase antibiotics. Clavulanic acid binds to the β-lactamases produced by a wide range of Gram-positive and Gram-negative micro-organisms. It is well absorbed orally and can also be given parenterally. It has been combined with amoxicillin as an oral preparation (Augmentin®) and with ticarcillin as a parenteral preparation (Timentin®). Augmentin is effective for β-lactamase-producing strains of staphylococci, *H. influenzae*, gonococci and *E. coli*. Sulbactam is another β-lactamase inhibitor which also can be administered orally or parenterally. In combination with ampicillin (Unasyn®), good coverage is provided for Gram-positive cocci (including β-lactamase-producing strains of *Staph. aureus*), Gram-negative anaerobes (but not *Pseudomonas*) and anaerobes.

Adverse reactions to penicillin

Hypersensitivity reactions are the major adverse effects of penicillins. Penicillins are capable of acting as haptens to combine with proteins contaminating the solution, or with human protein after the penicillin has been administered. Penicilloyl and penicillanic derivatives are the major determinants of penicillin allergy. All acute hypersensitivity reactions to penicillin are mediated by the IgE antibody, and range in severity from rash to anaphylaxis. Anaphylatic reactions are uncommon, occurring in only 0.2% of 10 000 courses of treatment, with 0.001% out of 100 000 courses resulting in death.[15] Morbilliform eruptions that develop after penicillin therapy are likely to be mediated by IgM antibodies, and the uncommon serum sickness is likely to be mediated by IgG antibodies. All forms of penicillin are best avoided in patients with a history of penicillin allergy.

Otherwise, the penicillins are generally well tolerated. CNS toxicity, in the form of myoclonic seizures, can follow the administration of massive doses of benzylpenicillin (penicillin G), ampicillin or methicillin. Massive doses have also been associated with hypokalaemia. Haematological toxicity - usually neutropenia - and nephrotoxicity have also been reported. Gastrointestinal disturbances have followed the use of all oral penicillins, but have been most pronounced with ampicillin. Enterocolitis due to the overgrowth of *Cl. difficile* is well documented and abnormalities in liver function have been reported, especially with flucloxacillin.

CEPHALOSPORINS

The antimicrobial activity of cephalosporins, like that of other β-lactam antibiotics, results at least in part from their ability to interfere with the synthesis of the peptidoglycan component of the bacterial cell wall. However, the exact bactericidal and lytic effects of cephalosporins are not completely understood.

Classification and uses

The first-generation compounds (cephalothin, cefazolin, cefalexin) have a relatively narrow spectrum of activity focused primarily on the Gram-positive cocci, especially penicillin-sensitive streptococci and methicillin-sensitive *Staph. aureus*. These compounds have modest activity against Gram-negative organisms, including *E. coli* and *Klebsiella* spp. Cefaclor has extended Gram-negative activity and is active against *H. influenzae* and *M. catarrhalis*.

The second generation of cephalosporins (cefuroxime, cefamandole) are more stable against Gram-negative β-lactamases. They have variable activity against Gram-positive cocci but have increased activity against Gram-negative bacteria (*E. coli*, *Proteus*, *Klebsiella*). In spite of relatively increased potency against Gram-negative aerobic and anaerobic bacilli (*Bacteroides fragilis*), the cephamycins (cefoxitin, cefotetan) are included in this generation.

The third-generation cephalosporins (cefotaxime, ceftriaxone, ceftazidime, cefpirome) have very marked activity against Gram-negative bacteria. Most are useful against *Ps. aeruginosa*, *Serratia*, and *Neisseria* species and some Enterobacteriaceae. Some of these compounds have limited activity against Gram-positive cocci, particularly methicillin-sensitive *Staph. aureus*. This generation of cephalosporins is particularly effective in meningitis because of their better penetration into the CSF and higher intrinsic activity. However, as these third-generation drugs are expensive and have a wide antimicrobial spectrum, their use should be restricted.

Recently, several compounds have been considered as possibly meriting classification as a fourth generation. Cefepime has activity against Gram-positive cocci and a broad array of Gram-negative bacteria, including *Ps. aeruginosa* and many of the Enterobacteriaceae with inducible chromosomal β-lactamases.

Adverse reactions

Hypersensitivity reactions are the most common side-effects of the cephalosporins and all compounds have been implicated. The reactions appear to be identical to those caused by the penicillins. Immediate reactions such as anaphylaxis, bronchospasm and urticaria have been reported. More commonly a maculopapular rash develops, usually after several days of therapy. Because of the similarity in structure between the penicillins and the cephalosporins, patients allergic to one class of agents may manifest cross-reactivity when a member of the other class is administered. Studies indicate that about 1% of patients allergic to penicillin will demonstrate a clinically apparent reaction when a cephalosporin is administered.[16] Patients with a mild or temporarily distant reaction to penicillin appear to be at low risk of rash or other allergic reaction following the administration of a cephalosporin. However, subjects with a recent history of an immediate reaction to penicillin should not be given a cephalosporin. Other reactions to cephalosporins are uncommon and include diarrhoea, nephrotoxicity, intolerance of alcohol and bleeding disorders.

Bacterial resistance

The most prevalent mechanism for resistance to cephalosporins is their destruction by β-lactamase hydrolysis. The cephalosporins have variable susceptibility to β-lactamase, with the later-generation compounds being more resistant to the β-lactamases produced by Gram-negative bacteria. However, third-generation cephalosporins are susceptible to hydrolysis by inducible, chromosomally encoded (type 1) β-lactamases. The induction of type 1 β-lactamases by treatment of infections due to many aerobic Gram-negative bacilli with second- or third-generation cephalosporins may result in resistance to all third-generation cephalosporins.

MACROLIDES

Erythromycin was originally isolated from soil bacteria and contains a many-membered lactone ring to which are attached one or more deoxy sugars. Clarithromycin, azithromycin and roxithromycin are new semisynthetic derivatives of erythromycin. Clarithromycin differs only by methylation of a hydroxyl group and azithromycin contains a methyl-substituted nitrogen atom in the lactone ring. Roxithromycin is a good alternative to oral erythromycin, and has good oral bioavailability, but is more expensive. The macrolides are usually bacteriostatic and inhibit protein synthesis by binding reversibly to 50S ribosomal subunits of sensitive micro-organisms. They are thought to inhibit the translocation step wherein a newly synthesized peptidyl tRNA molecule moves from the acceptor site on the ribosome to the peptidyl (donor) site.

Clinical uses

Erythromycin is most effective against aerobic Gram-positive cocci and bacilli. It is active against *Strep. pyogenes*, *Strep. pneumoniae*, *Cl. perfringens*, *Cl. diphtheriae*, *L. monocytogenes* and some staphylococci. Useful activity has also been seen with *P. multocida*, *Borrelia* spp., *B. pertussis*, *Campylobacter jejuni*, *L. pneumophila*, *M. pneumoniae*, *C. trachomatis* and some atypical mycobacteria. It has modest activity in vitro against some Gram-negative organisms, including *H. influenzae* and *N. meningitidis*, and excellent activity against most strains of *N. gonorrhoeae*.

Clarithromycin is more potent against erythromycin-sensitive strains of streptococci and staphylococci, but has only modest activity against *H. influenzae* and *N. gonorrhoeae*. However, it has good activity against *M. catarrhalis*, *Chlamydia* spp., *L. pneumophila* and *M. pneumoniae*. Azithromycin is generally less active than erythromycin against the Gram-positive organisms and is more active than the other two macrolides against *H. influenzae* and *Campylobacter* spp. Azithromycin is very active against *M. catarrhalis*, *P. multocida*, *Chlamydia* spp., *M. pneumoniae*, *L. pneumophila* and *N. gonorrhoeae*.

Adverse reactions

Erythromycin is one of the safest antibiotics and causes serious adverse effects only rarely. Dose-related abdominal cramps, nausea, vomiting, diarrhoea and flatulence occur, but are common in children and young adults. Allergic reactions observed include fever, eosinophilia and skin eruptions. Cholestatic hepatitis, transient hearing loss, polymorphic ventricular tachycardia, superinfection of the gastrointestinal tract and pseudomembranous colitis have been reported. Intravenous use of erythromycin is often associated with thrombophlebitis, but the incidence of this complication can be decreased with appropriate dilution of the dose. Adverse reactions to the other macrolides, at the usual dose, are rare and usually confined to the gastrointestinal tract. For this reason roxithromycin is often prescribed instead of erythromycin.

Erythromycin and, to a lesser extent, the other macrolides, has been reported to cause clinically significant drug interactions.[17] Erythromycin has been reported to potentiate astemizole, terfenadine, carbamazepine, corticosteroids, digoxin, theophylline, valproate and warfarin, probably by interfering with cytochrome P450-mediated drug metabolism. Care should be used in the concurrent administration of the macrolides with these drugs.

Bacterial resistance

Resistance to erythromycin may be the result of decreased permeability through the cell envelope. This form of resistance is exhibited by the Enterobacteriaceae and *Pseudomonas* spp. Alteration of ribosomal proteins, especially the 50S protein, often affects binding of the drug and has led to the emergence of resistant strains of *B. subtilis*, *Strep. pyogenes* and *Strep. pneumoniae*, *Campylobacter* spp., *E. coli*, *Staph. aureus*, *Cl. perfringens*, *Listeria* spp. and *Legionella* spp. Finally, enzymatic degradation of the drug has conferred high-level resistance among strains of Enterobacteriaceae.

TETRACYCLINE

Tetracyclines are generally bacteriostatic and are thought to inhibit bacterial protein synthesis by binding to the 30S bacterial ribosome and preventing access of aminoacyl tRNA to its acceptor site.

Clinical uses

The antimicrobial spectra of all the tetracyclines are almost identical. They possess a wide range of antimicrobial activity against aerobic and anaerobic Gram-positive and Gram-negative bacteria. Clinically, the tetracyclines are useful against *Strep. pneumoniae*, *H. influenzae*, *Neisseria* spp., *E. coli*, *Brucella* spp., *H. ducreyi*, *Vibrio cholera*, *Campylobacter* spp., and some *Shigella* and *Mycobacterium* spp. Many pathogenic spirochaetes are susceptible, including *Borrelia burgdorferi*. They are also effective against some micro-organisms that are resistant to cell-wall active antimicrobial agents, such as *Rickettsia*, *Coxiella burnetti*, *Mycoplasma pneumonia*, *Chlamydia* spp., *Legionella* spp. and *Plasmodium* spp.

Adverse reactions

The tetracyclines all produce gastro-intestinal irritation in some individuals, although doxycycline is usually well tolerated. Epigastric discomfort, nausea, vomiting and diarrhoea are commonly reported. Renal and liver toxicity, and photosensitivity may occur. Tetracyclines are deposited in the skeleton and teeth during gestation and childhood, and can cause abnormalities of bone growth and discoloration of the teeth. It is, there-fore, prudent not to administer these agents to pregnant women or children under 8 years of age. Hypersensitivity reactions, including skin reactions, burning of the eyes, pruritus ani, vaginitis, angio-oedema and anaphylaxis, are rarely seen.

Bacterial resistance

Bacteria develop resistance to the tetra-cyclines predominantly by preventing the accumulation of the drug within the cell. This is accomplished by decreasing the influx or increasing the ability of the cell to export the antibiotic. Rarely, the tetracyclines are inactivated biologically or inhibited in their ribosomal attach-ment.[18] Resistance to one tetracycline usually means resistance to all. Clinically, most strains of enterococci are now resistant to tetracycline; group B strepto-cocci are 50% susceptible and only 65% of *Staph. aureus* remain susceptible. Resistant pneumococci are now found in many geographical areas, and many strains of *Neisseria* spp. are now resistant.

AMINOGLYCOSIDES

Each aminoglycoside demonstrates con-centration-dependent bactericidal activity against susceptible micro-organisms. Gentamicin is the most commonly administered aminoglycoside in the emergency department and is a mixture of three closely related constituents. It binds to a specific area on the interface between the smaller (30S) and the larger (50S) bacterial ribosomal subunits, causing an increase in misreading of messenger RNA and a measurable decrease in protein synthesis. However, these effects do not provide a complete explanation for the rapidly lethal effect of gentamicin on bacteria.

Clinical uses

The antibacterial activity of gentamicin is directed primarily against aerobic and facultative Gram-negative bacilli. It has little activity against anaerobic micro-organisms and facultative bacteria under anaerobic conditions, and its activity against most Gram-positive bacteria is very limited. Gentamicin is clinically effec-tive against *Pseudomonas aeruginosa*, *Proteus mirabilis*, *Klebsiella pneumoniae*, *E. coli*, *Enterobacter* spp. and *Serratia* spp. It is particularly effective when used in combination with cell-wall active antimicrobial agents, e.g. penicillin, cephalosporin. Interactions between these agents result in synergistic effects on bacterial death and may be useful against enterococci, *Strep. pyogenes*, some staphylococci, Enterobacteriaceae and *Pseudomonas aeruginosa*.

Adverse reactions

Gentamicin, like most other aminoglyco-sides, has the potential to cause injury to the renal proximal convoluted tubules, damage to the cochlear and/or vestibular apparatus, and neuromuscular blockade. As the drug is eliminated almost entirely by glomerular filtration, gentamicin dosing in renal failure must be undertaken with care and drug-level monitoring is recom-mended. Gentamicin has little allergenic potential. Anaphylaxis, rash and other hypersensitivity reactions are unusual.

Bacterial resistance

Bacteria defend themselves against the aminoglycosides by a combination of alteration of uptake, synthesis of modify-ing enzymes, and a change of ribosomal binding sites.

In several centres a significant per-centage of clinical isolates are highly resistant to all aminoglycosides.[19] At pre-sent, other widespread bacterial resist-ance to the aminoglycosides remains limited. However, there are reports of resistance emerging among some strains of *Ps. aeruginosa*, Enterobacteriaceae, *E. coli*, *Serratia* spp. and *Staph. aureus*.

METRONIDAZOLE

The toxicity of metronidazole is due to short-lived intermediate compounds or free radicals that produce damage by interaction with DNA and possibly other macromolecules.

Clinical uses

Metronidazole is active against a wide variety of anaerobic protozoal parasites.

It is directly trichomonacidal. Sensitive strains of *Trichomonas vaginalis* are killed by very low concentrations of the drug under anaerobic conditions. The drug also has potent amoebicidal activity against *E. histolytica*, even in mixed culture, and substantial activity against the trophozoites of *Giardia lamblia*. Metronidazole manifests antibacterial activity against all anaerobic cocci and both anaerobic Gram-negative bacilli and anaerobic spore-forming Gram-positive bacilli. *Bacteroides, Clostridium, Helicobacter, Fusobacterium, Peptococcus* and *Peptostreptococcus* spp. are all susceptible.

Adverse reactions

In general, metronidazole is well tolerated. The most common side effects are headache, nausea, dry mouth and a metallic taste. Vomiting, diarrhoea and abdominal distress are occasionally experienced.[20] Furry tongue, glossitis and stomatitis may occur during therapy, and are associated with a sudden intensification of moniliasis. Of clinical importance is metronidazole's well-documented disulfiram-like effect (Antabuse®). Some patients experience abdominal distress, vomiting, flushing or headache if they drink alcoholic beverages during therapy with this drug.

Bacterial resistance

Fortunately, very few strains of *Bacteroides* spp. have demonstrated resistance. Some resistant strains of *T. vaginalis* have been isolated from patients with refractory cases of trichomoniasis, but these patients have usually responded to higher doses of metronidazole and prolonged courses of therapy.[21]

CO-TRIMOXAZOLE

Co-trimoxazole is a combination of sulphamethoxazole, a sulphonamide antibiotic, and trimethoprim, a diaminopyrimidine. The antimicrobial activity of this combination results from actions on two steps of the enzymatic pathway for the synthesis of tetrahydrofolic acid. Sulfamethoxazole inhibits the incorporation of PABA into folic acid, and

trimethoprim prevents the reduction of dihydrofolate to tetrahydrofolate. The latter is the form of folate essential to bacteria for one-carbon transfer reactions. Mammalian cells utilize preformed folate from the diet and do not synthesize this compound. This combination has been associated with serious sulphonamide induced side effects. It has been recommended that the combination product be restricted to the few situations where combined use is the treatment of choice.[1]

Clinical uses

Trimethoprim alone is effective in the treatment of most urinary tract infections and should be used alone for this indication. However, co-trimoxazole is active against a wide range of Gram-positive and Gram-negative micro-organisms. *Cl. diphtheriae* and *N. meningitidis* are susceptible, as are most strains of *Strep. pneumoniae*. From 50% to 95% of strains of *H. influenzae*, *Staph. aureus* and *epidermidis*, *Strep. pyogenes* and *viridans*, *E. coli*, *Proteus mirabilis*, *Enterobacter* spp., *Salmonella*, *Shigella* and *Serratia* are inhibited. Also sensitive are *Klebsiella* spp., *Brucella abortis*, *Pasteurella haemolytica* and *Yersinia* spp. Co-trimoxazole has an important place in the treatment and prophylaxis of *P. carinii* infection, and the treatment of *L. monocytogenes* and *Norcardia* infection.

Adverse reactions

In routine use, the combination appears to produce little toxicity. About 75% of adverse reactions involve the skin. These reactions are typical of those produced by sulphonamides and include a wide variety of rashes, erythema nodosum, erythema multiforme of the Stevens-Johnson type, exfoliative dermatitis and photosensitivity. Severe reactions tend to be more common among the elderly and HIV-infected patients. Gastrointestinal reactions include nausea and vomiting, but rarely diarrhoea. Glossitis and stomatitis are relatively common. Central nervous system reactions (headache, depression and hallucinations) and haematological disorders (anaemias, coagulation disorders and granulocytopenia) have been reported.

Bacterial resistance

The frequency of development of bacterial resistance to co-trimoxazole is lower than it is to either of the constituent compounds alone. Resistance to sulfamethoxazole is presumed to originate by random mutation and selection, or by transfer of resistance by plasmids. Such resistance is usually persistent and irreversible. Resistance to all sulphonamides is now becoming widespread in both community and nosocomial strains of bacteria, including streptococci, staphylococci, Enterobacteriaceae, *Neisseria* spp. and *Pseudomonas* spp. Trimethoprim-resistant micro-organisms may arise by mutation, but resistance in Gram-negative bacteria is often associated with the acquisition of a plasmid that codes for an altered dihydrofolate reductase. Increasing incidences of resistance have been found in Enterobacteriaceae, *Ps. aeruginosa*, *Staph. aureus*, *E. coli*, *Salmonella* and *Shigella*.

QUINOLONES

The 4-quinolones, including naladixic acid, are a family of compounds that contain a carboxylic acid moiety attached to a basic ring structure. The newer fluoroquinolones also contain a fluorine substituent, e.g. ciprofloxacin, ofloxacin. Some may also contain a piperazine moiety. Bacterial DNA gyrase is an essential enzyme involved in DNA function. The quinolones inhibit the enzymatic activities of DNA gyrase and promote the cleavage of DNA within the enzyme-DNA complex.

Clinical uses

The early quinolones are most active against aerobic Gram-negative bacilli, particularly Enterobacteriaceae and *Haemophilus* spp., and against Gram-negative cocci such as *Neisseria* spp. and *M. catarrhalis*. The fluoroquinolones are significantly more potent and have a much broader spectrum of antimicrobial activity. Relative to naladixic acid, the fluoroquinolones also have additional activity against *Ps. aeruginosa* and some staphylococci. Ciprofloxacin remains the most potent fluoroquinolone against Gram-negative bacteria. Several intracellular bacteria are inhibited by the fluoroquinolones, including *Chlamydia, Mycoplasma, Legionella, Brucella* and some mycobacteria. Recently a new drug, moxifloxacin, has been released. It is useful for sinusitis, community-acquired pneumonia and acute bronchitis.

Adverse reactions

Generally, these drugs are well tolerated. Gastrointestinal symptoms of anorexia, nausea, vomiting, diarrhoea and abdominal discomfort are commonly seen, particularly with the older quinolones. Headache, dizziness, insomnia and alteration in mood are the next most commonly reported symptoms. Allergic and skin reactions, including phototoxicity, may occur. Rarely, arthralgias and joint swelling, leucopenia, eosinophilia, thrombocytopenia and haemolysis are reported.

Bacterial resistance

Resistance patterns over time indicated that resistance increased following the introduction of fluoroquinolones, and occurred most often with *Pseudomonas* spp. and staphylococci, and in soft-tissue infections and in infections associated with foreign bodies. Possibly reflecting the pressures of extensive use, increasing fluoroquinolone resistance has been reported among strains of *Cl. jejuni* and *E. coli*. Focused quinolone use should be considered to avoid compromising the utility of the fluoroquinolones.

NITROFURANTOIN

The mechanism of action is poorly understood, but activity in many cases appears to require enzymatic reduction within the bacterial cell.[22] The reduced derivatives are thought to bind to and damage intracellular proteins, including DNA, and inhibit bacterial respiration, pyruvate metabolism and the synthesis of inducible enzymes.

Clinical uses

Nitrofurantoin is active against over 90% of clinical strains of *E. coli, Citrobacter*

spp., *Staph. saprophyticus* and *E. faecalis*. However, most species of *Proteus, Pseudomonas, Serratia, Providencia, Morganella* and many *Enterobacter* and *Klebsiella* spp. are resistant. Given its spectrum of activity and concentration in the urine, nitrofurantoin is usually administered for the treatment of urinary-tract infections or for urinary antisepsis. However, it may have activity against bacteria not usually associated with urinary tract infections, including *Salmonella, Shigella, Staph. aureus, Strep. pneumoniae* and *pyogenes*, and *Bacteroides*. Fortunately, bacteria that are susceptible to nitrofurantoin rarely become resistant during therapy.

Adverse reactions

Gastrointestinal upsets, particularly nausea, vomiting and diarrhoea, are the commonest side-effects of nitrofurantoin. The frequency of these symptoms may be reduced if the macrocrystalline formulation is administered. Rashes, presumably allergic in nature, have been seen quite commonly. Cholestatic jaundice, acute and chronic hepatitis, pulmonary and haematological reactions, and peripheral neuropathies have all been reported.

ANTIVIRAL DRUGS

Several anitviral drugs are available although famciclovir, aciclovir and valaciclovir (prodrug of aciclovir that requires less dosage frequency) are the most frequently prescribed. Their mechanism of action is similar. Each drug targets virus-infected cells and inhibits viral DNA polymerase. Consequently, viral DNA synthesis and therefore viral replication are inhibited.

Clinical uses

These drugs are primarily used for the management of herpes zoster (within 72 hours of rash onset), treatment and suppression of genital herpes, and the management of patients with advanced symptomatic HIV disease. Famciclovir is well absorbed in the gut and has the advantage of three times daily dosage compared to five times daily for aciclovir.

Adverse reactions

These drugs are generally well tolerated. However, headache, gastrointestinal disturbance, dizziness and fatigue have been reported. Adverse efects are generally mild.

ANTIRETROVIRAL DRUGS

Emergency physicians are unlikely to initiate these drugs as they form the basis of HIV treatment. However, an appreciation of their uses and side effects is useful. Furthermore, the management of patients with HIV disease can be difficult and advice from an appropriate specialist source is recommended.

Clinical uses

The antiretroviral drugs are used in the treatment of established HIV infection. This includes patients with HIV-associated illnesses (e.g. CNS disease, malignancies, opportunistic diseases) and asymptomatic patients with low CD4 cell counts and/or high HIV viral loads. The drugs are also of use in the prevention of maternal-fetal transmission and as post-exposure prophylaxis for significant exposure from a known HIV-infected source.

Three major classes of antiretrovirals are available. For initial antiretroviral therapy, three drugs are generally used in combination. The recommended regimen is of use:

- Two nucleotiside reverse transcriptase inhibitors (NRTI) e.g. zidovudine, lamivudine, didanosine PLUS EITHER
- One protease inhibitor (PI) e.g. indinavir OR
- One non-nucleoside reverse transcriptase inhibitor (NNRTI) e.g. nevirapine.[1]

Adverse reactions

The toxicity associated with the different regimens stems from the component drugs. As classes, the NRTI drugs are associated with lactic acidosis and hepatic steatosis; the NNRTI drugs with rash, abnormal liver function tests and fever; the PI drugs with lipodystrophy, hyperglycaemia, hyperlipidaemia and abnormal liver function tests.

Importantly, the PI and NNRTI drugs are metabolized by the cytochrome P450 enzymes and interact with many other drugs. These drugs should not be prescribed with cisapride, dihydroergotamine, ergotamine, benzodiazepines and rifampicin. There are many other potential drug interactions with the antiretroviral agents and new prescriptions should be made with care.

OUTPATIENT PARENTERAL ANTIBIOTIC THERAPY

Outpatient parenteral antibiotic therapy (OPAT) has been widely used for the treatment of moderate to serious infections, either as an alternative to hospitalisation or following initial hospitalization and early discharge once the patient is over the toxic phase of the infection. A wide range of infections are suitable for OPAT therapy (Table 8.9.2).

Significant savings both in terms of direct and indirect costs are possible utilizing OPAT. Appropriate patient selection is essential for safe and effective outpatient parenteral therapy. (Table 8.9.3 and 8.9.4)

Table 8.9.3 Patient selection process

Condition suitable for outpatient therapy
Patient does not fulfil need to admit criteria (Table 8.9.5)
OR
Patient meets discharge criteria (Table 8.9.6)
Home environment suitable
Patient/family consent.

Table 8.9.4 Patient selection criteria

Able to give consent
Adequate social support at home
The antibiotic(s) chosen is appropriate for OPAT use
Patient's condition is stable
Concurrent illness does not require hospital care
Adequate venous access can be maintained
Patient is mobile
The infection is amenable to outpatient parenteral therapy
Adequate monitoring by the treating medical team is possible.

Table 8.9.5 Admission to hospital criteria

Confused
Persistent high fever
Systolic blood pressure <100 mmHg
Respiratory rate >30/min
Pulse rate >100/min
Requires specialized nursing care assistance with activities of daily living
Hypoxic on room air (PaO$_2$<60 mmHg)
Concurrent illness requiring inpatient care
Personal or social reasons
Consolidation in more than one lobe.

Table 8.9.6 Discharge criteria

Medical
Temperature settling
Clinical improvement
No specialized nursing care required
Stable
Bacterial pathogens identified
Response to inpatient therapy
Complications unlikely

Social
Parents interested and motivated
Parents capable
Home environment acceptable
Telephone and transport access.

Patients should be clinically stable, willing to participate and physically and mentally capable of being treated at home (Table 8.9.4).

Some patients require initial hospitalization (Table 8.9.5), following which they may be suitable for early discharge to continue treatment at home.

Once patients comply with predefined discharge criteria (Table 8.9.6) they may be able to be discharged into an outpatient parenteral therapy programme.

Close patient monitoring is essential with daily reviews by a nurse either by telephone or face to face whilst patients are in the programme. Patients should be reviewed at least weekly by a physician.

Table 8.9.2 Conditions that can be treated on an outpatient basis with parenteral antibiotic therapy

AIDS
Associated Infections

Cardiac
Endocarditis
Prosthetic-valve infections

Genitourinary
Pyelonephritis
Complicated urinary-tract infections
Prostatitis
Pelvic inflammatory disease

Respiratory
Pneumonia
Lung abscess

Soft-tissue infections
Cellulitis
Wound infections/abscesses

Bone and joint infections
Osteomyelitis
Septic arthritis
Prosthetic infections
Neurological infections
Meningitis

Other infections
Bacteraemia
Mastoiditis

The benefits of OPAT include a reduction in overall costs of patient care through avoidance or reduction in hospitalization, reduction of the costs associated with the hazards of hospitalization and increased patient satisfaction.

FUTURE DIRECTIONS

The most important challenge regarding infectious disease in the future will be the containment of antimicrobial resistance patterns. In part, these patterns have emerged as a result of poor prescribing habits. New antimicrobial drugs are being urgently sought, however, this process is difficult and slow. Until their development (in no way a certainty), physicians may be increasingly restricted in their prescribing patterns. This may take the form of widespread prescribing guidelines or more authoritative measures. In the meantime, it is incumbent upon all physicians to practice the most rational and responsible antimicrobial prescribing.

Detailed descriptions of the drugs described above are available on the Internet by accessing MIMS Online.[23]

REFERENCES

1. Therapeutic Guidelines Limited 2000 Therapeutic Guidelines: Antibiotic, Version 11, Therapeutic Guidelines Limited (pub), Melbourne
2. Weinstein L, Dalton AC 1968 Host determinants of response to antimicrobial agents. New England Journal of Medicine 279: 467
3. Moellering RC Jr 1978 Factors influencing the clinical use of antimicrobial agents in elderly patients. Geriatrics 33: 83
4. Philipson A 1983 The use of antibiotics in pregnancy. Journal of Antimicrobiological Chemotherapy 12: 101
5. Moellering RC Jr 1995 Principles of anti-infective therapy. In: Mandell GL, Bennett JE, Dolin R (eds) Principles and Practice of Infectious Diseases, 4th edn. Churchill Livingstone, New York, pp 199–212
6. Davies J 1994 Inactivation of antibiotics and the dissemination of resistance genes. Science 264: 375–82
7. Nikaido H 1994 Prevention of drug access to bacterial targets: permeability barriers and active efflux. Science 264: 382–8
8. Spratt BG 1994 Resistance to antibiotics mediated by target alterations. Science 264: 388–93
9. Kopecko D 1980 Specialized genetic recombination systems in bacteria: their involvement in gene expression and evolution. Proceedings in Molecular and Subcellular Biology 7: 135–243
10. Elwell LP, Roberts M, Mayer LW, Falkow S 1977 Plasmid-mediated beta-lactamase production in Neisseria gonorrhoeae. Antimicrobiological Agents and Chemotherapy 11: 528–33
11. Lyon BR, Skurray R 1987 Antimicrobial resistance of Staphylococcus aureus: genetic basis. Microbiology Review 5: 88–134
12. Chambers HF, Sande MA 1995 Antimicrobial agents. In: Goodman and Gilman's The Pharmacological Basis of Theraputics, 9th edn. McGraw-Hill, New York, pp. 1029–32
13. Stillwell M, Caplan ES 1989 The septic multiple-trauma patient. Infectious Diseases Clinics of North America 3: 155
14. Kobayashi Y, Takahashi T, Nakae T 1982 Diffusion of beta-lactam antibiotics through liposome membranes containing purified porins. Antimicrobiological Agents and Chemotherapy 2: 775–80
15. Idsoe O, Gothe T, Wilcox RR, et al 1968 Nature and extent of penicillin side reactions with particular reference to fatalities from anaphylactic shock. Bulletin of the WHO 38: 159
16. Saxon A, Hassner A, Swabb EA, Wheller B, Adkinson NF Jr 1984 Lack of cross-sensitivity between aztreonam, a monobactam antibiotic, and penicillin in penicillin-allergic subjects. Journal of Infectious Diseases 149: 16–22
17. Periti P, Mazzei T, Mini E, Novelli A 1992 Pharmacokinetic drug interactions of macrolides. Clinical Pharmacokinetics 23: 106–31
18. Speer BS, Shoemaker NB, Salyers AA 1992 Bacterial resistance to tetracycline: mechanisms, tranfer and clinical significance. Clinical Microbiology Review 5: 387–99
19. Spera RV Jr, Farber BF 1992 Multiply-resistant Enterococcus faecium. The nosocomial pathogen of the 1990s. Journal of the American Medical Association 268: 2563–4
20. Lau AH, Lam NP, Piscitelli SC, Wilkes L, Danzinger LH 1992 Clinical pharmacokinetics of metronidazole and other nitroimidazole anti-infectives. Clinical Pharmacokinetics 2: 328–64
21. Johnson PJ 1993 Metronidazole and drug resistance. Parasitology Today 9: 183–6
22. McCalla DR, Reuvers A, Kaiser C 1970 Mode of action of nitrofurazone. Journal of Bacteriology 104: 1126–34
23. MIMS Online. http://mims.hcn.net.au/ last accessed June 26, 2002

FURTHER READING

Vinen J, Hudson B, Chan B, Fernandes C A randomised comparative study of once-daily ceftriaxone and 6-hourly flucloxacillin in the treatment of moderate to severe cellulitis. Clinical efficacy, safety and parm

8.10 NEEDLESTICK INJURIES

FIONA NICHOLSON • ALAN C. STREET

ESSENTIALS

1 Avoiding blood and other body fluid exposure remains the primary means of preventing occupationally acquired blood-borne virus infections.

2 The risks of acquiring infection with a blood-borne virus from occupational exposure are: HIV 0.3%,[1] hepatitis B (HBV) 1–62%,[2] hepatitis C (HCV) 1.8%.[3,4]

3 HBV immunization is an integral part of workplace safety.

4 Effective post-exposure prophylaxis (PEP) is available for both HBV and HIV.

5 Significant emotional distress often complicates needlestick and related occupational injuries.

INTRODUCTION

Management of healthcare personnel (HCP) who sustain an occupational exposure to blood or other potentially infectious body fluids (e.g. semen, vaginal secretions, CSF and fluids containing visible blood,) has become a major concern. An estimated 800 000 such injuries each year in the USA.[5] HBV, HCV and HIV are the most important occupationally-acquired blood-borne pathogens, although many other organisms, including malaria, syphilis, cytomegalovirus, and possibly the agent of Creutzfeld–Jacob disease may also be transmissible via this route. Occupational exposure should be considered a medical emergency to ensure timely post-exposure management.

HEPATITIS B

The risk of acquiring HBV from occupational exposure is well recognized and is primarily related to the degree of contact with blood and the hepatitis B e antigen (HBeAg) status of the source. Following contact with a source positive for HBeAg, the risk of clinical hepatitis is 22–31% and serological evidence of HBV infection develops in 37–62% of exposed individuals. In contrast, after exposure to HBeAg negative blood, there is 1–6% risk of clinical hepatitis and a 23–37% risk of serological evidence of HBV infection.[2] Because of the high risk of HBV infection, routine vaccination against HBV has been recommended for HCP since the early 1980s[6] with a consequent marked decrease in the incidence of infection in this population.

Post-exposure management following an occupational blood/body fluid exposure to HBV requires evaluation of the source HBsAg status, and the HBV vaccination and vaccine response status of the exposed person.[7-8] HB Immune globulin (HBIG) is prepared from human plasma known to contain a high titre of antibody to HBsAg (antiHBs). It is screened for HBsAg and antibodies to HIV and HCV with the preparation process (since 1999) inactivating and eliminating HIV and HCV from the final product.[9] Table 8.10.1 provides more detailed information about specific indications for HBIG and hepatitis B vaccination following occupational exposures.

HEPATITIS C

HCV is not transmitted efficiently through occupational exposure to blood. Transmission to HCP has never been documented from skin contamination and rarely from mucous membrane exposure. Environmental contamination is not significant[10] in contrast to HBV.

Numerous studies and laboratory experiments have failed to demonstrate a role for either immune globulin[11] or antiviral agents (e.g. interferon and or ribavirin)[12] in post-exposure management. Recommendations for management of occupational exposures to HCV are aimed at achieving early identification of infection. A baseline serum is tested for anti-HCV and ALT with follow-up testing 3 and 6 months after the exposure.

HUMAN IMMUNODEFICIENCY VIRUS

The average risk of acquiring human immunodeficiency virus (HIV) infection from all types of reported percutaneous exposures to HIV-infected blood is 0.3%.[1] This is increased for exposures involving:

- A deep injury
- Visible blood on the device causing the injury
- A device previously placed in the source's artery or vein
- A source with terminal AIDS who is thereby presumed to have a high titre of HIV.[13]

These factors are also probably significant for mucous membrane and skin exposures to HIV-infected blood, where the average risk of HIV transmission is approximately 0.09% and <0.09% respectively.[14] Prolonged or extensive skin contact or visibly compromised skin integrity would also suggest a higher risk.

HCP potentially exposed to HIV need to be evaluated within hours. If the source is seronegative for HIV, baseline testing and further follow-up of the exposed person is normally not necessary. If the source HIV antibody test is positive or inconclusive, or the source is not available for testing, HIV antibody testing of the exposed person should be performed at 6 weeks, 12 weeks and 6 months post-exposure. Extended HIV follow-up testing (12 months) is recommended for HCP who become infected with HCV following exposure to a source co-infected with HIV/HCV.

Post-exposure prophylaxis (PEP) recommendations have been guided by a better understanding of the pathogenesis of primary HIV infection, which indicates

Table 8.10.1 HBV prophylaxis following occupational exposure		
Source	Healthcare worker	
	Unvaccinated	Vaccinated
HBs antigen positive	HBIG and commence vaccination series	1. If > 10 m IU/mL - reassure 2. If < 10 m IU/mL - HBIG and repeat vaccination 3. If result not available within 24 hours consider HBIG
HBs antigen negative	Course of vaccination	1. If > 10 m IU/mL – reassure 2. If < 10 m IU/mL - consider repeat vacc.
Unknown source	1. Consider HBIG 2. Commence vaccination	1. If > 10 m IU/mL - reassure 2. If < 10 m IU/mL - booster HBV vacc. +/– HBIG

HBIG if indicated should preferably be given within 24 hours;
HBV vaccine should also be administered as soon as possible (preferably within 24 hours);
Exposed HCP do not need to take any special precautions to prevent secondary transmission.[21]

that HIV infection does not become established immediately; this leaves a brief window of opportunity during which post-exposure antiretroviral intervention might modify or prevent viral replication. An early case/control study demonstrated that use of zidovudine decreased the risk of occupational HIV transmission by 81%,[15] and it is likely (but not proven) that combination antiretroviral therapy provides even greater protection. Failures of PEP are well documented with both single drug and combination drug regimens.[16]

PEP should be initiated promptly, preferably within 2 hours of the exposure, although it may still be effective for up to 48 hours. Recommendations for HIV PEP include a basic 4-week regimen of two drugs for most HIV exposures and an expanded regimen that includes the addition of a third drug for HIV exposures that pose an increased risk of transmission. When the source virus is known or suspected to be resistant to one or more of the drugs considered for the PEP regimen, the selection of drugs to which resistance is unlikely is recommended (Table 8.10.2).

Most occupational exposures do not result in transmission of HIV and the potential benefits of PEP need to be carefully weighed against the toxicity of the drugs involved. Nearly 50% of HCP taking PEP experience adverse symptoms (e.g. nausea, malaise, headache, diarrhoea and anorexia) and approximately 33% cease PEP because of side effects.[17,18] Whenever possible physicians with expertise in HIV transmission and anti-

retroviral therapy should be involved in implementation of PEP. The importance of completing the prescribed regimen needs to be stressed and measures taken to minimize side effects.

The emotional effect of an occupational HIV exposure is substantial[19,20] and is often underestimated. The exposed person may need time off work, short-term use of a night-time sedative or even referral for formal psychological or psychiatric counselling. Patients should be advised of measures to prevent secondary transmission (e.g. safer sexual practices) during the follow-up period, especially the first 6–12 weeks.

Maintaining confidentiality for the staff member sustaining exposure is a priority, as it may have lasting implications both personally and professionally.

Evaluation of the exposure source

Known source

- Inform of incident and discuss evidence of high-risk behaviours
- Obtain consent for testing (legal proceedings may follow if not consented)
- Test for HBsAg, anti-HCV and HIV antibody
- Refer for appropriate counselling and treatment
- Maintain confidentiality of source.

Unknown source or infection status not known (e.g. refuses testing)

- Evaluate individual likelihood of exposure to a source at high risk of

HIV infection, e.g. prevalence of intravenous drug use, history of risk behaviours, clinical symptoms
- Testing of needles is NOT recommended
- PEP rarely indicated and should be discussed with an infectious diseases physician

Although PEP is available and effective for both HBV and HIV it must be remembered that primary measures preventing blood exposure remain the most expedient in avoiding occupationally acquired infection.

Illustrative cases

Case 1

A 4-year-old child presents to the emergency department after stepping on a needle at the beach. The parents have the needle. The child has never been vaccinated against hepatitis B.

Management

❶ Reassurance: risk of transmission of HBV ~30%, HCV ~10%, HIV <0.3% **where source is known to be infected with these viruses.** With regard to HIV (usually the chief concern of parents), the needle is likely to have come from an injecting drug user and the prevalence of HIV in this population in Australia is currently 1–2%. So, the risk for transmission of HIV is 0.3% × 1% × unknown factor to allow for dried blood in the syringe = miniscule risk. Therefore, PEP is not indicated (but

Table 8.10.2 Recommended HIV post-exposure prophylaxis

Exposure type	HIV positive 1	HIV positive 11	HIV negative
Unknown source			
Less severe consider 2-drug PEP if HIV risk factors	2-drug PEP	3-drug PEP	reassure
More severe consider 2-drug PEP if HIV risk factors	3-drug PEP	3-drug PEP	reassure

HIV positive 1 = asymptomatic or low viral load; HIV positive 11 = symptomatic
Initiation of post-exposure prophylaxis (PEP) should not be delayed pending expert consultation.
Follow-up care and re-evaluation should occur within 72 hours post exposure.
If PEP is commenced and source is later determined to be HIV negative, then PEP should be discontinued.
Two-drug regimen: ZDV 300 mg bd+ 3TC 150 mg bd (available as Combivir® one tablet BD)
Alt :3TC 150 mg bd+ d4T 40 mg bd
d4T 40 mg bd + ddI 400 mg daily
3-drug regimen: Add indinavir 800 mg tds or nelfinavir 750 mg tds/1250 mg bd

note that PEP *may* be indicated in other countries if the risk of HIV in injecting drug users is higher).

❷ No benefit in testing needle.

❸ Obtain baseline serum specimen from child.

❹ Offer:
- Hep B Ig/Hep B vaccination
- Tetanus prophylaxis and vaccination if indicated.
- Advise parents of symptoms of hepatitis
- Serology for HIV at 6 weeks and 3 months, HCV at 3 months and 6 months, HBsAg at 6 months.

Case 2

A healthcare worker presents to the emergency department having had blood on her ungloved hands while caring for an HIV patient. She has no visible cuts or other skin defects on her hands. She received HBV vaccination some years previously and responded serologically. The source patient is known to be HBsAg and hepatitis C antibody negative.

Management

❶ Counselling regarding negligible risk of HIV transmission with intact skin exposures.

❷ Discuss with infectious disease physician (chiefly to reassure staff member) – very low risk exposure and PEP not indicated.

❸ Despite low risk, anticipate psychological distress.

❹ Reinforce practice of standard precautions (e.g. wearing gloves).

❺ Follow-up serology not necessary, unless specifically requested by exposed person.

REFERENCES

1. Bell DM 1997 Occupational risk of human immunodeficiency virus infection in health-care workers :an overview. American Journal of Medicine 102(suppl 5B): 9–15

2. Werner BG, Grady GF 1982 Accidental hepatitis-B-surface-antigen-positive innoculations: use of e antigen to estimate infectivity. Annals of Internal Medicine 97: 367–9

3. Lanphear BP, Linnemann CC Jr., Cannon CG, DeRonde MM, Pendy L, Kerley LM 1994 Hepatitis C virus infection in healthcare workers: risk of exposure and infection. Infection Control and Hospital Epidemiology 15: 745–570

4. Mitsiu T, Iwano K, Masuko K, et al 1992 Hepatitis C viral infection in medical personnel after needlestick accident. Hepatology 16: 1109–14

5. Jagger JI 1990 Preventing HIV transmission in health care workers with safer needle devices. 6th International Conference on AIDS, San Francisco, California, 22 June

6. CDC 1982 Recommendation of the Immunization Practices Advisory Commitee (ACIP) inactivated hepatitis B virus vaccine. MMWR 31: 317–28

7. Grady GF, Lee VA, Prince AM, et al 1978 Hepatitis B immune globulin for accidental exposures among medical personnel; final report of a multicenter controlled trial. Journal of Infectious Diseases 138: 625–38

8. Seeff LB, Zimmerman HJ, Wrught EC, et al 1977 A randomized, double blind controlled trial of the efficacy of immune serum globulin for the prevention of post-transfusion hepatitis: a Veterans Administation cooperative study. Gastroenterology 72: 111–21

9. CDC 1986 Safety of therapeutic immune globulin preparations with respect to transmission of human T-lymphotropic virus type III/lymphadenopathy-associated virus infection. MMWR 35: 231–3

10. Polish LB, Tong MJ, Co RL, Coleman PJ, Alter MJ 1993 Risk factors for hepatitis C virus infection among health care personnel in a community hospital. American Journal of Infection Control 21: 196–200

11. Alter MJ 1994 Occupational exposure to hepatitis C virus: a dilemma. Infection Control and Hospital Epidemiology 15: 742–4

12. Peters M, Davis GL, Dooley JS, Hoofnagle JH 1986 The interferon system in acute and chronic viral hepatitis. Progress in Liver Disease 8: 453–67

13. CDC 1995 Case-control study of HIV seroconversion in health care workers after percutaneous exposure to HIV-infected blood - France, United Kingdom and United States, Jan 1988-Aug 1994. MMWR 44: 929–33

14. Gerberding JL 1995 Management of occupational exposure to blood borne viruses. New England Journal of Medicine 332: 444–551

15. Cardo DM, Culver DH, Ciesielski CA, et al 1997 A case-control study of HIV seroconversion in health care workers after percutaneous exposure. New England Journal of Medicine 337: 1485–90

16. Jochimsen EM 1997 Failures of zidovudine postexposure prophylaxis. American Journal of Medicine 102(suppl 5B): 52–5

17. Wang SA, Panlilio AL, Doi PA, et al 2000 Experience of healthcare workers taking postexposure prophylaxis after occupational Hiv exposure: findings of the HIV postexposure prophylaxis registry. Infection Control and Hospital Epidemiology 21: 780–5

18. Parkin JM, Murphy M, Anderson J, El-Gadi S, Forster G, Pinching AJ 2000 Tolerability and side effects of post-exposure prophylaxis for HIV infection (Letter). Lancet 335: 722–3

19. Armstrong K, Gordon R, Santorella G 1995 Occupational exposures of health care workers (HCWs) to human immunodeficiency virus (HIV): stress reactions and counselling interventions. Soc Work Health Care 21: 61–80

20. Henry K, Campbell S, Jackson B, et al 1990 Long-term foolow-up of health care workers with work-site exposure to human immunodeficiency virus (Letter).Journal of the American Medical Association 236: 1765

21. CDC 1998 Recommendations for the prevention and control of hepatitis C virus (HCV) infection and HCV-related chronic disease. MMWR 47(No. RR-19)

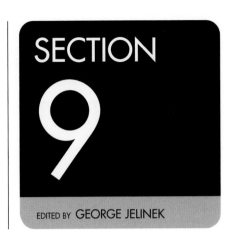

SECTION

9

EDITED BY GEORGE JELINEK

GENITOURINARY

9.1 Acute renal failure 440

9.2 The acute scrotum 453

9.3 Renal colic 457

9.1 ACUTE RENAL FAILURE

N. ADAMS • LINAS DZIUKAS

ESSENTIALS

1 The causes of acute renal failure (ARF) fall into three categories: pre-renal, renal and post-renal.

2 Pre-renal causes are mose common and mostly correctable.

3 Post-renal obstruction should always be excluded in patients with unexplained ARF.

4 Acute tubular necrosis is the most common renal cause of ARF, and the major mechanisms are renal ischaemia and renal toxins.

5 The absence of significant poteinuria, haematuria and red blood cell casts virtually excludes glomerulonephritis.

6 It is possible to lose up to 60% of renal function and have a normal serum creatinine.

7 The most important aspect of management of ARF is maintaining an adequate intravasuclar volume.

INTRODUCTION

Acute renal failure (ARF) is characterized by a sudden decline in the glomerular filtration rate (GFR), accumulation of nitrogenous wastes (resulting in rapid elevation of the plasma creatinine level [P_{CR}], the plasma urea concentration or the blood urea nitrogen [BUN]), impairment of normal regulation of electrolyte, acid-base and fluid balance, alterations in blood pressure and (frequently) oliguria. There is no consensus about the rate of increase in P_{CR} that constitutes ARF, with 35 separate definitions identified in a review.[1] A practical definition of ARF is a recent (days to weeks) increase in the P_{CR} of at least 0.05 mmol/L if the baseline P_{CR} is less than 0.3 mmol/L, and an increase of at least 0.1 mmol/L if the baseline P_{CR} is greater than 0.3 mmol/L.

INCIDENCE

The overall incidence of ARF in the general community is about 200 cases per million population per year.[2,3] About 1% of all hospital admissions have community acquired ARF, approximately 5% of hospital patients develop ARF, while 25–30% of patients admitted to a critical care unit develop ARF.[4–6]

CAUSES

More than 50 pathophysiologic processes are implicated in the aetiology of ARF.[7] These are divided into three categories: renal hypoperfusion/prerenal, renal, and postrenal. In community-acquired ARF, 50–70% of cases are due to pre-renal causes, 30–40% to intrinsic renal disorders, and 5–10% to urinary tract obstruction.[7] ARF developing in patients in a critical care unit often has multiple causes, with a nephrotoxic insult to an ischaemic kidney in the setting of pre-existing renal impairment, cardiac disease and sepsis.

HYPOPERFUSION (PRERENAL) CAUSES

The kidneys, which comprise 0.5% of the total body weight, receive 25% of the cardiac output. The high blood flow and the high filtration pressure produce a large-volume ultrafiltrate of plasma. Under normal circumstances renal plasma flow (RPF) and the GFR are relatively constant over a wide range of (systemic and renal) arterial pressures (autoregulation). Autoregulation is important in day-to-day, moment-to-moment control of renal haemodynamics in health, in hypertension, or in bilateral renal artery stenosis.

Adequate tissue perfusion ultimately depends on an adequate circulating volume, normal cardiac pump activity and the systemic vascular resistance. The total blood volume in a healthy 70 kg person is about 5650 mL, but it is the volume in the systemic arterial system (about 600–700 mL) that is most important in determining the adequacy of the circulation. This effective circulating volume is monitored by stretch receptors in the carotid sinus and the aortic arch, in the afferent arteriole of the glomerulus, and in the atria. Changes in the rate of discharge of these receptors alter systemic haemodynamics, intra-renal haemodynamics, glomerular haemodynamics, and renal sodium ion (Na^+) excretion.

The basic mechanism in prerenal ARF is impaired glomerular perfusion.[8,9] This can be preceded by renal hypoperfusion due to an absolute decrease in the effective circulating volume, or the volume is sensed as reduced because of a reduced cardiac output or reduced systemic resistance (Table 9.1.1). The decreased cardiac output can be due to chronic cardiac disease, but critically ill patients without pre-existing cardiac disease can develop reversible myocardial dysfunction.[10]

A reduction in the effective circulating blood volume produces systemic and renal vasoconstriction mediated by the sympathetic nervous system, antidiuretic hormone release, and the renin-angiotensin aldosterone axis. Renal blood flow decreases even if the systemic blood pressure is in the normal range. When the systemic arterial blood pressure falls below 75 mmHg, the renal autoregulatory system fails, and the GFR falls markedly.

Hypotension or a decrease in the effective circulating blood volume markedly increases the renal tubular reabsorption of water, sodium and urea. The urine output decreases, urine osmolality increases, and the sodium

Table 9.1.1 Conditions associated with an increased risk of prerenal azotaemia or prerenal ARF due to a decreased 'effective' circulating volume

Condition	ECF volume*	Cardiac output	SVR**	Other factors
Hypovolaemia	Reduced	Reduced	Increased	
Cardiac failure	Increased	Reduced	Increased	Afterload reduction with ACE inhibitors can improve cardiac output and reduce mortality, but may decrease the GFR and increase the risk of developing ARF if the intravascular volume is reduced
Sepsis	Normal or reduced Normal or reduced	Increased Decreased	Decreased Increased	Activation of leucocytes → release of tumor necrosis factor, interleukins Increased nitric oxide production Activation of coagulation cascade Activation of complement Intrarenal vasoconstriction due to endothelial cell production of endothelin, thromboxane A2, leukotrienes, and platelet activating factor Other organ damage or failure : pulmonary, hepatic, cardiac
Cirrhosis	Normal or increased	Increased	Reduced	Splanchnic vasodilation Low systemic mean arterial pressure Hypoalbuminemia Increased nitric oxide levels Increased intra-renal vasoconstrictors (endothelin, thromboxane A2, leukotrienes, platelet activating factor) Decreased intra-renal vasodilators
Nephrotic syndrome	Increased (overflow)	Normal	Normal	Renin-angiotensin suppressed Plasma ADH normal Plasma ANP elevated BP normal or ↑
	Decreased (underfill)	Decreased	Increased	Renin-angiotensin activated Plasma ADH ↑ Plasma ANP normal/low BP low normal or ↓

*The 'effective' circulating volume is sensed as decreased in all the conditions, even though the absolute volume of the extracellular fluid (ECF) can be normal, increased or reduced
** Systemic vascular resistance
The risk of developing prerenal ARF is increased in the above conditions if drugs are used that increase afferent arteriole vasoconstriction (e.g. noradrenaline (norepinephrine), nonsteroidal anti-inflammatory drugs, ciclosporin, tacrolimus) or impair efferent arteriole vasoconstriction (angiotensin-converting enzyme inhibitors, angiotensin AT1 receptor antagonists.

concentration of the urine falls. Because of increased tubular resorption of urea, the plasma urea concentration rises before the P_{CR}. Thus, the plasma urea/creatinine ratio is often greater than 100–150 in pre-renal failure.[7] The selective rise in the blood urea or the BUN concentration in the setting of reduced renal perfusion is referred to as prerenal azotemia.

Patients with prerenal azotemia have morphologically intact kidneys, and treatment of hypotension or the decreased effective circulating volume restores renal perfusion and the GFR to their previous levels. These compensatory mechanisms have their limits, and the patient with prerenal azotaemia may reach a point where ischaemic damage to the tubules results in acute tubular necrosis.

The prerenal causes of ARF are summarized in Table 9.1.2. Prerenal azotaemia is the most common form of acute renal impairment seen in the emergency department. Most of the underlying causes are potentially correctable. Timely and appropriate treatment can often restore normal renal perfusion and prevent the development of ischaemic acute tubular necrosis.

POSTRENAL CAUSES

Postrenal ARF occurs when there is obstruction of urinary outflow. Obstruction can be intrarenal, due to casts or crystals within the tubular lumen. Extrarenal obstruction can occur at the level of the urethra, bladder neck, bladder, ureter or pelvic-ureteric junction. In adults, obstruction is most commonly caused by either prostatic enlargement or retroperitoneal neoplasms (lymphoma, cancer of the cervix, uterus, bladder, ovary or colon, or metastatic cancer). A neurogenic bladder can produce functional obstruction. Other less common causes of postrenal ARF are bilateral renal calculi, papillary necrosis, and retroperitoneal fibrosis. Unilateral ureteric obstruction may cause ARF if there is a single functioning kidney

The immediate effect of renal obstruction is a rise in the intratubular pressure. There is an initial increase in renal blood flow, and a decrease in GFR. The renal hyperaemia lasts for several hours and is mediated by vasodilator prostaglandins. It is then followed by arterial vasoconstriction, which reduces renal blood flow below normal levels. The GFR continues to progressively

Table 9.1.2 Causes of pre-renal azotaemia and pre-renal acute renal failure

Intravascular volume depletion	Decreased cardiac output	Systemic vasodilation	Renal vasoconstriction
Haemorrhage : visible or concealed	Primary disease of: myocardium valves Conducting system Pericardium	Sepsis	Sepsis
Gastrointestinal losses	Extracardiac causes Sepsis Drug overdose	Liver disease	Hepatorenal failure
Renal losses	Pulmonary hypertension	Drugs Drug overdose Anaesthetics Afterload reduction	Drugs NSAIDS α-adrenergic agonists Radiocontrast agents Drug overdose
Skin losses Burns Third space losses Pancreatitis Burns	Positive pressure ventilation	Anaphylaxis	

decrease. The renal intratubular pressure increases transiently, and then falls. Tubular cells are injured, the interstitial tissue becomes oedematous, and there is an increase in the number of cells in the interstitium, followed by interstitial fibrosis.

The extent to which glomerular function recovers after the relief of obstruction depends on the duration of obstruction. Whole kidney function (measured as P_{CR}) may be unaffected by unilateral obstruction lasting up to 7 days, but during this time there is ongoing loss of nephrons. The ability of the tubules to conserve sodium, secrete potassium, or acidify the urine is impaired after the relief of longstanding obstruction.

Postrenal failure is an uncommon cause of ARF in the emergency department. However, the possibility must always be considered and excluded, because treatment by relief of the obstruction is usually fairly simple. The presence of severe oliguria, (<100 mL of urine per day), makes an obstructive cause for ARF more likely.[7]

RENAL CAUSES

The renal causes of ARF are categorized according to the primary anatomical site of the problem: acute tubular necrosis (ATN) (ischaemic or nephrotoxic or both), glomerular, vascular or interstitial (Table 9.1.3).

ACUTE TUBULAR NECROSIS

The most common renal cause of acute tubular necrosis (ARF) is ATN. Renal ischaemia or nephrotoxins or both, usually in the setting of sepsis, multi-organ failure (especially acute respiratory distress syndrome) or cardiac disease, cause most cases of ATN.

Ischaemic ATN

Experimental studies have increased understanding of the pathophysiology of ischaemic ATN.[11,12] The basic processes include: reduction in blood flow, hypoxia, ATP depletion, cytoplasmic and mitochondrial calcium ion (Ca^{2+}) overload following uncontrolled Ca^{2+} entry into cells, endothelial damage, tubular epithelial cell injury (leading to swelling, damage to cell membranes, loss of normal cell polarity, cytoskeleton injury, stimulation or induction of protein kinases), prolonged vasoconstriction, prolonged reduction in GFR, infiltration of polymorphs and lymphocytes, and the release of growth factors and cytokines. Vasoactive hormones and peptides that contribute to ATN include antidiuretic hormone (ADH), renin, aldosterone, atrial natriuretic peptide (ANP), endothelin, tumour necrosis factor (TNF), platelet aggregating factor (PAF), vasoactive intestinal peptide (VIP), nitric oxide, thromboxane and hepatocyte growth factor (HGF).

The proximal convoluted tubule and the medullary thick ascending limb of the loop of Henle are most susceptible to ischaemic and nephrotoxic injury. A spectrum of cell damage is seen, ranging from minimal to apoptosis to necrosis. The tubular damage causes obstruction, backflow of intraluminal fluid into the interstitium, and abnormal tubuloglomerular regulation. These effects of tubular injury reduce GFR.

Renal vasoconstriction and reduction in GFR is a major characteristic of ATN. This is a prolonged process, as ATN has an initiation phase (hours to days), a maintenance phase (a reduced GFR of about 5 to 10 mL/min persists for 1 to 2 weeks), and a recovery phase. An important cause of the vasoconstriction is sublethal endothelial cell injury, which increases the local formation of vasoconstrictors such as endothelin and adenosine, and reduces the local formation of nitric oxide, a major vasodilator.[12]

Recovery from ATN is accompanied by increased blood flow (reperfusion), resulting in the formation of potentially damaging reactive oxygen species by polymorphs and injured renal cells.

Table 9.1.3 Major renal causes of acute renal failure

Vascular causes
Large renal vessels*
Renal arteries : thrombosis, embolism, dissection, trauma
Renal veins: thrombosis, compression
Bilateral disease or a single functioning kidney

Renal microvasculature
Inflammatory : glomerulonephritis, vasculitis, radiation
Vasospastic : toxaemia of pregnancy, malignant hypertension, scleroderma
Thrombotic microangiopathies: haemolytic uraemic (HUS) syndromes:
1. Childhood HUS
2. Adult HUS
3. Pregnancy associated HUS
Thrombotic thrombocytopenic purpura
Disseminated intravascular coagulation
Hyperviscosity syndromes

Diseases of the glomeruli
Rapidly progressive glomerulonephritis (see Table 9.1.4)

Acute tubular necrosis (ATN)
Ischaemic ATN
Caused by renal hypoperfusion (see Table 9.1.1)
Nephrotoxic ATN
Endogenous toxins
Haemoglobin
Myoglobin
Uric acid
Myeloma light chains
Exogenous toxins
Antibiotics
Organic solvents : ethylene glycol
Poisons: snake venom, paraquat
Chemotherapeutic drugs : cisplatin
Anti-inflammatory drugs : NSAIDs
Immunosuppressive drugs : cyclosporin
Radiocontrast drugs

Tubulointerstitial disease
Acute tubulointerstitial nephritis (ATIN)

Drugs
Antibiotics: methicillin, rifampicin, cephalosporins, sulphonamides, NSAIDs
Other drugs: allopurinol, thiazide diuretics, furosemide
Infections: viral, bacterial, fungal
Infiltrations: lymphoma, leukaemia

Activation of polymorphs by dialyser membranes during haemodialysis may prolong ARF.[13] Reactive oxygen species may also be important agents of tissue injury in the ischaemic kidney if the function of endogenous free radical scavengers such as superoxide dismutase is impaired by hypoxia. These free radicals cause lipid peroxidation and breakdown of cell membranes, and play a major role in ARF caused by gentamicin or cyclosporine.[14]

Many clinical conditions are associated with renal ischaemia and multiple factors commonly contribute to the occurrence of ischaemic ATN (Table 9.1.3). Prerenal renal failure and ischaemic ATN form a continuum; ATN is distinguished by the failure of restoration of blood flow to improve the GFR, at least in the short term. The onset of ATN is also characterized by the development of tubular dysfunction. This usually manifests as an inappropriate increase in urinary sodium concentration and impairment in urinary concentrating capacity.

Toxic ATN[12,15]

Many medications and toxins are associated with ATN (Table 9.1.3). In most cases, several factors are needed to produce ATN, e.g. the combination of aminoglycoside use and hypovolemia. Idiosyncratic (allergic) drug reactions may be important in some individuals.

Radiocontrast agents account for 10% of cases of hospital-acquired ARF.[16,17] The newer non-ionic compounds are less toxic than the previously used ionic compounds, although they can also produce severe ATN. A group of patients are at high risk of developing ARF after radiocontrast administration. These include those with one or more of the following: pre-existing renal impairment, diabetes, hypertension, hypovolaemia, hyperuricaemia, proteinuria, and multiple myeloma. Large or repeated contrast loads also increase the risk of developing ATN. Renal damage due to radiocontrast agents includes vasoconstriction and direct damage to medullary tubules.

Haem pigment nephrotoxicity may complicate rhabdomyolysis (myoglobinuria), or intravascular haemolysis (haemoglobinuria). Rhabdomyolysis due to traumatic muscle damage may be seen in crush injuries, severe burns, electrocution, and after extreme exertion or prolonged seizures.[18–20] Non-traumatic rhabdomyolysis has been associated with drug overdose (usually pressure-induced), alcoholism, hyperthermia, hypothermia, hypokalaemia, and various envenomings. Ischaemic damage to muscles and subsequent rhabdomyolysis may complicate compartment syndrome, arterial occlusion, and some forms of vasculitis. Finally, rhabdomyolysis has been described in the setting of a number of viral and bacterial infections, and as an idiosyncratic reaction to various drugs (e.g. clofibrate). The incidence of ATN following rhabdomyolysis is about 10–15% but the severity of rhabdomyolysis does not readily correlate with the risk of developing ATN.[18,20] Intravascular haemolysis is rare but may occur in incompatible blood transfusion, envenoming, malaria, and exposure to certain drugs. The nephrotoxicity of haem pigments is enhanced by volume depletion, low urine flow rates and low urine pH.

Drugs that interfere with the normal intrarenal response to vasoconstriction (e.g. non-steroidal anti-inflammatory agents and angiotensin converting enzyme inhibitors) can cause ATN in susceptible persons.[21]

GLOMERULAR DISEASE[22,23]

Glomerulonephritis causes proteinuria or haematuria (with characteristic dysmorphic red cells or red cell casts) or both, often with hypertension. Glomerulonephritis has a limited number of clinical presentations: asymptomatic proteinuria or haematuria or both; macroscopic haematuria (recurrent, often associated with intercurrent infection); nephrotic syndrome; nephritic syndrome (abrupt onset, usually self limited, of oliguria, haematuria, proteinuria and hypertension), chronic glomerulonephritis (hypertension, renal insufficiency, proteinuria and/or haematuria), and rapidly progressive glomerulonephritis (RPG). Most forms of glomerulonephritis cause chronic renal failure, but RPG causes ARF (Table 9.1.4). The characteristic histological feature of RPG is the presence of large cellular crescents in Bowman's space, involving most of the glomeruli. RPG is a very uncommon condition that occurs in a number of

Table 9.1.4 Conditions associated with rapidly progressive glomerulonephritis (GN)

Condition	Serology and complement	Association
Antiglomerular basement membrane (anti-GBM) antibodies		
anti-GBM with lung involvement (Goodpasture disease) anti-GBM without lung involvement	anti-GBM antibody +ve C3 and C4 normal cytoplasmic ANCA +ve in 10-20 %	Goodpasture disease Present with haemoptysis and bilateral alveolar opacities on CXR Lung involvement may be mild or life threatening Other features are an iron deficiency anaemia, and increased CO uptake in pulmonary function tests
Vasculitis (ANCA +ve)		
Wegener granulomatosis	Cytoplasmic ANCA +ve C3 and C4 normal	Upper and lower respiratory involvement
Microscopic polyarteritis nodosa	Perinuclear ANCA +ve C3 and C4 normal	Multisystem involvement of skin and lung Fever, arthralgia, neuropathy No microaneurysms on angiography Rapidly progressive GN common
Renal limited cresentic GN	Perinuclear ANCA +ve C3 and C4 normal	Renal involvement only
Glomerular immune complex deposition, ↓ complement, ANCA -ve		
Systemic lupus erythematosis (SLE)	Anti-nuclear antibody Anti-double stranded DNA antibody ↓ C3, ↓ C4	Affects women of childbearing age Half of all SLE patients develop significant renal disease, usually in the first 5 years Skin involvement (malar rash, discoid rash, photosensitivity) Non-erosive arthritis Pleuropericarditis Fits or psychosis in the absence of precipitating causes Haemolytic anaemia, leukopenia/lymphopenia, thrombocytopenia
Post streptococcal GN	↓ C3, N C4, ↓ CH_{50} Positive ASOT Positive streptozyme test	Acute GN develops 2-3 weeks after pharyngitis or skin infection with certain Group A β-haemolytic streptococci
Subacute bacterial endocarditis (SBE)	↓ C3, ↓ C4, ↓CH_{50} Rheumatoid factor +ve Cryoglobulin +ve cytoplasmic-ANCA +ve (rarely)	
Membranoproliferative GN	Type I : C3 N or ↓, ↓C4, ↓CH_{50} Type II : ↓C3, N C4, ↓CH_{50}	
Absent anti-GBM antibody, ANCA -ve and normal complement		
Henoch-Schonlein purpura	Complement normal ↑ serum IgA levels in 50 % of cases Cryoglobulin +ve IgA rheumatoid factor +ve_	Non-thrombocytopenic vascular purpura Arthralgia Abdominal pain Skin biopsies contain capillary deposits of IgA, IgG and C3
Immunoglobulin A nephropathy	Complement normal ↑ serum IgA levels in 50 % of cases IgA rheumatoid factor +ve	Recurrent episodes of macroscopic haematuria May be familial Rarely may evolve into Henoch-Schonlein purpura
Classic polyarteritis nodosa	Complement normal ANCA rarely +ve	Non-specific symptoms (fever, weight loss, myalgias, raised ESR, anaemia, leucocytosis, thrombocytosis) Mononeuritis multiplex Microaneurysms on angiography Renal infarction is common Rapidly progressive GN is very rare

systemic diseases, or as a primary glomerulonephritis. Patients with RPG typically present as acute oliguric renal failure, which can progress to end-stage renal disease requiring dialysis within weeks. Early treatment may reduce or arrest the renal damage, so the diagnosis of this condition by serologic markers or renal biopsy is vitally important.

VASCULAR DISEASE

Both microvascular and macro vascular disease causes ARF. Macro vascular causes of ARF are acute thrombosis of the renal artery (usually after trauma), thromboembolism of the renal artery atheroembolic disease, renal artery dissection and renal vein thrombosis. Atheroembolic disease occurs when cholesterol emboli lodge in medium or small renal arteries, where they produce an inflammatory response and occlusion of the vessel.[24] Atheroembolic disease commonly complicates invasive intravascular procedures and may present after a delay of up to several weeks. Most patients are over 60 years of age and suffer from hypertension, peripheral vascular disease, ischaemic heart disease or diabetes. Evidence of atheroembolic damage to organs other than the kidney is often present. Skin involvement (presenting as livedo reticularis) is a characteristic feature.

Diseases that affect the renal microvasculature can produce ARF. These include inflammatory (e.g. glomerulonephritis or vasculitis) or non-inflammatory (e.g. malignant hypertension) disease of the vessel wall, hyperviscosity syndromes, and thrombotic microangiopathies. The possibility of thrombotic microangiopathy should be considered in ARF associated with vomiting or diarrhoea, neurologic signs, severe anaemia, thrombocytopenia and fragmented red blood cells in the peripheral blood film. Examples include haemolytic uremic syndrome (HUS), thrombotic thrombocytopenic purpura (TTP), or pregnancy-associated thrombotic microangiography.[25] The latter includes acute TTP, the HELLP syndrome (haemolysis, elevated liver enzymes, low platelets; this condition is severe pre-eclampsia [causing hypertension and renal impairment] associated with microangiopathic haemolysis and liver damage) and acute HUS.

INTERSTITIAL DISEASE[8,30]

Abnormalities of interstitial structure and function are important but secondary features of ARF due to ATN. However, ARF can be caused by a primary abnormality of the interstitial tissues: acute tubulointerstitial nephritis (ATIN). The morphological features of ATIN are interstitial oedema, mononuclear cell infiltration (predominately T-lymphocytes and macrophages) and tubular injury of variable severity. These changes are predominantly due to immunological mechanisms: anti-tubular basement membrane antibodies, immune complexes and cell-mediated immunity. The most important mechanism is cell-mediated immunity. ATIN is an uncommon cause of ARF, being found in only 2–3% of

renal biopsies.[26] Acute interstitial nephritis typically presents with fever, rash and eosinophilia. It is usually caused by an autoimmune reaction to certain drugs. Agents typically responsible are antibiotics (e.g. methicillin), diuretics, non-steroidal anti-inflammatory drugs, allopurinol, phenytoin and carbamazepine, but many other drugs have been implicated. It is important to identify the offending drug quickly, as withdrawal should lead to an improvement in renal function.

Infection may also cause ATIN, either by direct invasion of the kidney or indirectly through immunological mechanisms. ATIN can be caused by infection with hantavirus, a RNA virus that has a worldwide distribution and is the cause of so-called hemorrhagic fever with renal syndrome. Other infective causes of ATIN include leptospirosis, hepatitis A, infectious mononucleosis, cytomegalovirus, and human immunodeficiency virus (HIV) infection.

ARF in the renal transplant patient[23,31]

The assessment of ARF in the renal transplant recipient does not differ substantially from that of the general population. Obstruction may occur due to ureteric stenosis or compression by lymphocoele. Calcineurin inhibitors such as ciclosporin and tacrolimus may cause renal vasoconstriction, especially in the presence of hypovolaemia. Rejection of the transplant is a possible intrinsic renal cause of ARF, and transplant biopsy is often necessary to diagnose this.

RISK FACTORS FOR ACUTE RENAL FAILURE

The factors that are associated with an increased risk of developing ARF are listed in Table 9.1.5. The presence of multiple risk factors increases the number of non-renal complications in ARF, and in turn increases the mortality. Nearly half of hospital-acquired cases of ATN are seen in patients in the post-operative state. Acute hypotension due to haemorrhage will cause pre-renal

azotaemia, but the incidence of severe ARF is low in the absence of other risk factors. The incidence of ARF in major gastrointestinal bleeding is about 1.5%.[31] In severe trauma the incidence of ARF needing dialysis is about 0.1%.[37] Severe progressive ARF after cardiopulmonary resuscitation is rare, and pre-existing haemodynamics are more important than the actual hypoperfusion during resuscitation.[38]

CLINICAL PRESENTATION

ARF may have one or more of the following:

- Signs and symptoms of a decreased circulating blood volume or an increased circulating volume
- Signs and symptoms of renal tract obstruction
- Specific clinical situations
- Features due to the pathophysiologic effects of ARF itself.

HISTORY

A thorough review of the patient's history often reveals the likely cause of ARF. The history should include a detailed drug history, enquiry about recent invasive vascular or radiologic procedures, and any family history of renal disease. The past medical record should be thoroughly perused ('palpate the chart'). The drugs most commonly associated with ARF are angiotensin converting enzyme (ACE) inhibitors, and non-steroidal anti-inflammatory drugs (NSAIDs). NSAIDs can cause ATN in patients with a reduced effective circulating volume by decreasing the vasodilation effect of prostaglandins. This effect is most likely to occur in patients with severe cardiac failure, cirrhosis with ascites, nephrotic syndrome and sepsis. ARF caused by ACE inhibitors is most likely to develop in congestive cardiac failure, diabetic nephropathy, cirrhosis, polycystic kidney disease or bilateral renal artery stenosis. Diuretic-induced hypovolemia or chro-

Table 9.1.5 High-risk settings and risk factors for developing acute renal failure

Risk factors in the community	Risk factors in hospital-based patients[31]	Admission to intensive care unit[35,36]
Pre-existing renal impairment The GFR <80 mL/min/1.72 m² in 40% of non-diabetic adults, and <60 mL/min/1.72 m² in 13%[28]	Elective abdominal surgery Up to 25% of cases have an acute (usually mild and reversible) rise in P_{CR} Obstructive jaundice	25–30% of all admitted persons develop ARF
Age greater than 70 years ARF is more common in the elderly because of a higher incidence of systemic disease, polypharmacy and the effects of age on the kidney[29]	Cardiac disease Up to15% of patients have a >20% rise in P_{CR} after having cardiac surgery[32,33] 30% of patients with cardiogenic shock develop ARF in the first 24 hours[34]	Sepsis with multiorgan failure 20–50% develop ARF
Cirrhosis with ascites Over a 5 year period about 40% develop ARF[30]	Abdominal aorta surgery 5–30 % develop ARF	Risk factors for developing ARF are often present on admission to ICU and include: acute circulatory or respiratory failure, age >65 years, sepsis, past history of chronic heart failure, lymphoma or leukaemia and cirrhosis.

nic renal insufficiency are predisposing factors. ARF developing after recent invasive procedures suggests athero-embolic renal damage.

EXAMINATION

This is directed particularly toward the common and easily reversible causes of ARF – hypovolaemia and renal tract obstruction.

Decreased circulating blood volume

Changes in the effective circulating blood volume and the extravascular volume are not always the same. Under certain conditions (e.g. severe liver disease or nephrotic syndrome), an increased extravascular volume, manifested by peripheral oedema or ascites, is associated with a profound reduction in the circulating blood volume. It is thus important to evaluate the circulating blood volume separately from the extravascular fluid volume.

No single symptom or sign infallibly predicts a decreased circulating blood volume. A history of poor oral fluid intake and increased losses from vomiting, diarrhoea, diuresis or sweating is suggestive of fluid depletion but may not always be reliable. The presence of a dry axilla argues moderately for the presence of extravascular fluid depletion, whereas moist mucous membranes argue

moderately against extravascular fluid depletion. Reduced skin turgor, sunken eyes and capillary refill are not reliable signs of extravascular fluid depletion.[39] The most reliable signs of intravascular hypovolaemia are a postural (supine to standing) pulse increment of more than 30/minute or the inability to stand up long enough for vital signs to be taken due to light-headedness. Supine tachycardia, postural hypotension, supine hypotension and poorly filled neck veins are specific but not particularly sensitive signs of intravascular hypovolaemia.[39] When the signs of intravascular hypovolemia are difficult to interpret it may be useful to administer an intravenous fluid challenge of 250–500 mL of normal saline and then re-assess the patient.

Urinary tract obstruction

The symptoms and signs of urinary tract obstruction depend upon the site and cause, and the rapidity with which it develops. Pain is more common in acute obstruction and may be felt in the lower back, flank or suprapubic region, depending on the level of the obstruction. Chronic obstruction is usually painless. Symptoms of prostatic obstruction include frequency, nocturia, hesitancy, post-void dribbling, poor urinary stream and incontinence. Examination usually, but not always, reveals an enlarged bladder, whereas renal enlargement is not often felt. The presence or absence of prostatic enlargement on rectal

examination does not reliably predict ARF due to bladder neck obstruction.

Specific clinical situations

A patient with ARF who has hypertension, proteinuria and haematuria most likely has a nephritic syndrome due to glomerulonephritis. The presence of marked proteinuria (greater than 5 g/24 h), and peripheral oedema suggests nephrotic syndrome. ARF in a cancer patient is commonly due to prerenal fluid losses, nephrotoxicity of chemotherapeutic drugs or the products of tumour lysis. Other causes are sepsis due to immunosuppression, hypercalcaemia, tumour associated glomerulonephritis, and infiltration of the kidney or the urinary collecting system by tumour. Vasculitis due to infectious and non-infectious causes may involve large size, medium size or small renal vessels, and produce a variety of clinical features depending on organ involvement.[40]

Simultaneous involvement of the lungs and kidney (pulmonary renal-syndrome) can be caused by acute pulmonary oedema due to hypervolaemia in ARF of all types, infections (e.g. Legionnaire disease, mycoplasma infection), toxins (e.g. paraquat), in certain multisystem diseases (e.g. systemic lupus erythematosus, Wegener syndrome, microscopic polyarteritis), and classically in Goodpasture syndrome.

There is a high incidence of ARF in patients with HIV infection. Most occur during symptomatic HIV infection or as part of the acquired immune deficiency syndrome (AIDS). Predisposing factors are the nephrotoxicity of some antiviral drugs, and the wide range of antimicrobial agents used to treat opportunistic infections.

Acute liver damage may be accompanied by ARF during infections (hepatitis A, Epstein-Barr infection, cytomegalovirus infection, brucellosis, leptospirosis) or as a result of toxic damage (e.g. paracetamol poisoning). An allergic reaction to some drugs can simultaneously cause hepatitis and acute tubulointerstitial nephritis. Hepatorenal syndrome describes the development of progressive renal failure (with marked renal vasoconstriction, a benign urine sediment, concentrated urine and a low fractional excretion of sodium [FE_{Na}]) in patients with cirrhosis and a reduced effective circulating volume due to splanchnic pooling.

Clinical features of ARF

The clinical features of ARF itself are generally non-specific and may be non-existent. Symptoms include anorexia, fatigue, confusion, drowsiness, nausea and vomiting, and pruritus. Oliguria is a frequent but not invariable feature. Dyspnea, orthopnea, peripheral oedema and an elevated jugular venous pressure are present in intravascular and extravascular fluid overload.

Stress ulcers and gastritis are common in ARF, but life-threatening gastrointestinal bleeding is uncommon. Prolonged and severe ARF, or catabolic and anuric ARF, can lead to the development of the uremic syndrome. Clinical features include pericardial disease (pericarditis, pericardial effusion, tamponade, ileus, asterixis, psychosis, myoclonus and seizures. While septicaemia frequently causes ARF, the incidence of infection (especially involving the lungs and the urinary tract) is increased by ARF. Protein catabolism and malnutrition are very common and troublesome complications of ARF. Jaundice may develop in up to 40% of persons with ARF, and is due to multiple factors (e.g. sepsis, hepatic congestion, hypotension, blood transfusion).

On occasion it may be difficult to distinguish between chronic and acute renal impairment. The following features suggest the presence of chronic renal failure:

- Documented past history of renal impairment
- Family history of renal disease
- Polyuria or nocturia
- Uraemic pigmentation
- Normochromic, normocytic anaemia
- Radiologic evidence of renal osteodystrophy
- Bilateral small, scarred kidneys on ultrasound.

INVESTIGATIONS

Blood tests

The initial blood tests in a patient with ARF are a full blood examination, serum electrolyte concentration (sodium, potassium, bicarbonate, chloride, calcium, phosphate, magnesium), urea and creatinine concentrations, random blood glucose, liver function tests, coagulation tests and creatine kinase (CK) concentration.

Other tests that may be needed are:

- Serum troponin in suspected cardiac ischaemia
- Blood cultures in suspected sepsis
- ESR and CRP in vasculitis and endocarditis
- Serum cryoglobulin concentration in immunoproliferative disorders, SLE, polyarteritis nodosa, haemolytic anaemia, hepatitis B or hepatitis C infection
- Serum protein electrophoresis (suspected multiple myeloma)
- Complement C3, complement C4 and complement CH50 concentrations in suspected glomerulonephritis, vasculitis, endocarditis
- Anti-neutrophil cytoplasmic antibody (ANCA) in suspected endocarditis, vasculitis or glomerulonephritis
- Autoimmune disease serology: antinuclear antibody (ANA), anti-double-stranded DNA antibodies, rheumatoid factor
- Viral serology (hepatitis, HIV)

- Fibrin D-dimer levels, fibrinogen assay, thrombin time in suspected disseminated intravascular coagulopathy
- Anti-streptolysin O antibodies in glomerulonephritis
- Haptoglobin levels in microangiopathic anaemia, posttransfusion haemolysis, autoimmune haemolytic anaemia
- Arterial blood gases.

ARF typically causes an acute elevation in the plasma creatinine (P_{CR}) and blood urea concentrations, and is frequently accompanied by hyperkalaemia, hyponatraemia, hypocalcaemia, hypermagnesaemia, hyperphosphataemia and metabolic acidosis.

The P_{CR}, while widely used, is a suboptimal indicator of acute changes in renal function, starting to rise 24 to 48 hours after a reduction in the GFR. Creatinine levels are also influenced by muscle mass and the rate of muscle breakdown (e.g. rhabdomyolysis), and are susceptible to dilution effects in the presence of extracellular fluid overload. When the GFR is less than 20% of normal, P_{CR} can overestimate the GFR by a factor of two or more.

Urea levels are also usually elevated in ARF, but are more susceptible to influence by extra-renal factors. Urea production depends upon hepatic function and the hepatic protein load. Increased dietary protein, gastrointestinal haemorrhage, catabolic states (e.g. infection, trauma), and some medications (corticosteroids), increase urea production. Severe liver disease and protein malnutrition reduce urea production. The ratio of urea to creatinine may provide a clue to the aetiology of ARF. A ratio greater than 100:150 is associated with low urine flow states and suggests a pre-renal or post-renal cause.[41,42]

Hyponatraemia occurs in some cases of hypovolemia, where isotonic fluid losses are replaced by hypotonic fluid. This commonly occurs with diarrhoea, vomiting, or diuretic use. Hyponatraemia is also commonly seen in nephrotic syndrome, cirrhosis, and severe cardiac failure. Hypernatraemia may be seen in hypovolaemia, if water loss exceeds that of sodium

Hyperkalaemia is a common complication, with the serum K+ usually rising by 0.5 mmol/L/day in ARF. Mild hyperkalaemia (<6.0 mmol/L) is asymptomatic and does not need urgent treatment. Higher serum K+ levels can cause ECG abnormalities, life-threatening cardiac arrhythmias, paraesthesiae or weakness. Marked hyperkalaemia at the time of first presentation with ARF can occur in rhabdomyolysis, haemolysis, tumour lysis syndrome, and in patients on spironolactone. The serum Ca^{2+} concentration may be normal or reduced in ARF. Both hypocalcaemia and hypercalcaemia may occur at different stages of ARF in rhabdomyolysis

Rhabdomyolysis is characterised by a very high blood creatine kinase (CK) concentration. Abnormal liver function tests invariably accompany hepatorenal syndrome and hepatic cirrhosis. Hypoalbuminaemia will occur with prolonged or severe proteinuria in nephrotic syndrome.

Anaemia develops rapidly in ARF, but its presence or the degree of anaemia does not reliably distinguish between acute and chronic renal failure. Leukocytosis is usually seen if sepsis is the cause of ARF. Eosinophilia is often present in acute interstitial nephritis, polyarteritis nodosa and atheroembolic disease. Anaemia and rouleaux formation suggest a plasma cell dyscrasia. Thrombocytopenia and disseminated intravascular coagulation can complicate ARF due to rhabdomyolysis. A microangiopathic blood film associated with ARF suggests the presence of vasculitis.

Urine tests

Examination of the urinary sediment is a vital part of the investigation of a patient with ARF. Patients with prerenal ARF usually have no abnormal findings. Patients with ATN typically have large numbers of pigmented coarse granular casts, together with tubular epithelial cells and tubular casts. The presence of red cell casts and dysmorphic red cells is virtually diagnostic of glomerulonephritis (Table 9.1.6).

Measurement of urinary electrolyte concentrations and osmolality may give an indication of tubular function. A urinary sodium less than 10 mmol/L, urine osmolality greater than 500 mmol/kg water, and a serum urea/creatinine ratio greater than 100:1, all indicate appropriate tubular function and suggest a prerenal cause for ARF. With the development of ATN tubular function is impaired, resulting in urinary sodium greater than 10 mmol/L, urine osmolality less than 350 mmol/kg water, and a serum urea/creatinine ratio less than 100:1.

Patients with glomerulonephritis generally have normal tubular function and respond in a prerenal manner, whereas those with obstruction often have tubular dysfunction and behave like ATN.[43] Heavy proteinuria, glycosuria, radiocontrast media and some drugs may spuriously increase urine osmolality and specific gravity

The interpretation of urinary parameters is problematic in the presence of diuretics, cirrhosis or diabetes insipidus. Similarly, interpretation in patients with 'salt losing' states and concentrating defects (old age, hypokalaemia) may also be misleading.

Radiology

A chest X-ray is taken to assess the heart size and the presence of cardiac failure, infection, malignancy or other abnormalities. An abdominal X-ray focusing on the kidneys, ureter, and bladder (KUB) will reveal radiopaque calculi (calcium, cysteine or struvite stones), but not uric acid or xanthine calculi which are translucent. Ultrasound (US) examination is used to detect hydronephrosis.[44] The US investigation also provides information about bladder size. A normal US examination can occur in the very early stages of obstruction, or if the obstruction is due to retroperitoneal fibrosis or to infiltration of the ureters by tumour. Hydronephrosis not due to obstruction occurs in vesicoureteric reflux, in diabetes insipidus and in primary megaureter.

GENERAL MANAGEMENT

Prevention of acute renal failure

The principles are to prevent hypotension, maintain an effective circulating volume, avoid the use of drugs that interfere with the renal compensatory response to pre-renal azotaemia, minimize the use of exogenous nephrotoxins, reduce the toxicity of endogenous nephrotoxins (uric acid, haemoglobin, myoglobulin), minimize the develop-

Table 9.1.6 Urinary deposits in acute renal failure				
	Prerenal	*ATN*	*AIN*	*Acute nephritis*
Red blood cell	Occasional	+	Occasional	+++
White blood cell	Occasional	Occasional	+++ (± eosinophilis)	++
Casts				
Granular	Occasional	++	+	++
Epithelial	-	+++	-	++
Red blood cell	-	-	-	+++
Crystals				
Oxalate	Scanty	+++[1]	-	-
Urate	-	+++[2]	-	-

ATN: acute tubular necrosis; 1: ethylene glycol poisoning;
AIN: acute interstitial nephritis; 2: tumour lysis syndrome

ment of selective renal vasoconstriction, treat infection and correct obstruction.

Hypovolaemia is initially treated with crystalloid rather than colloid.[45] The rate and volume of crystalloid given depends on the initial blood pressure and heart rate, volume of fluid lost, cardiac function, and estimated ongoing fluid losses. The response to treatment is evaluated by simple bedside measurements (heart rate, blood pressure, urine output). Fluid replacement that is predominately determined by formulas (e.g. in burns) underestimates the fluid requirements.[46]

Preventative measures have been evaluated in certain high-risk situations. Diuretics do not protect against the development of radiocontrast ATN, and may even worsen the renal damage.[47] The administration of aminophylline, a non selective adenosine antagonist, does not protect against contrast induced ARF if the patient is adequately hydrated.[48] Prophylactic haemodialysis after radiocontrast use in high-risk patients is of no value.[49,50] Acetylcysteine can reduce the incidence of renal impairment after administration of radiocontrast.[51] Neither diuretics nor low dose dopamine are effective in reducing the incidence or severity of ARF in postoperative cardiac patients or in ICU patients.[52-54] Experimental studies and anecdotal experience in patients suggests that myoglobin nephrotoxicity is lessened by maintaining high urine flows through volume expansion and diuretic use (loop diuretics or mannitol). Alkalinization of the urine in this situation is also advocated, but has not been shown to be superior to saline diuresis. A preliminary study suggests that prostacycline reduces the incidence of ARF after cardiac surgery.[55]

Treatment of ATN[56-58]

Despite much experimental laboratory work and a number of large clinical trials in the last few decades, no therapeutic intervention has hastened the recovery of renal function in established ATN. Therapeutic trials of dopamine, atrial natriuretic peptide[59] and various growth factors have been uniformly disappoint-

ing. Administration of diuretics in hypervolaemia appears logical, as the aim is to increase salt and water excretion by increasing urine output in nonoliguric ARF or converting oliguric ARF to non-oliguric ARF. Other potential beneficial effects of diuretics are a reduction in intratubular cast formation, a reduction in the back leak of fluids, and a direct reduction in the degree of cellular damage. Both mannitol and frusemide cause renal vasodilation by a direct effect on arterioles or via increased prostaglandin production, and mannitol may reduce endothelial swelling. Administration of diuretics in the early stages of ATN (i.e. within the first 24–48 hours), produces a sustained increase in urine volume in about two-thirds of oliguric patients. However, administration of diuretics to critically ill patients with ARF is associated with an increased risk of death and non-recovery of renal function.[60] The conversion of oliguric ARF to non-oliguric ARF by dopamine or high-dose loop diuretics does not affect the duration of ATN, the need for dialysis or the outcome.[58] Therefore, treatment is supportive while awaiting the natural renal repair process. Early consultation with a nephrologist may improve the outcome in ARF.[61]

EMERGENCY DEPARTMENT MANAGEMENT

Hypovolemia and hypotension

Careful correction of hypovolemia is mandatory, using the appropriate fluid, crystalloid or blood. A prompt response to fluid challenge (with an increase in urine output and urinary sodium excretion, and a decrease in the serum creatinine and urea concentration) is strong evidence that prerenal ARF is present. Pulmonary oedema due to excessive fluid administration should be avoided. The role of invasive haemodynamic monitoring is controversial. Complications from central venous access may be higher in the patient with ARF, who is often at increased risk of

infection and bleeding. Close clinical observation and non-invasive monitoring is likely to be safer and just as effective in many patients.

Renal hypoperfusion may occur despite an adequate intravascular volume, especially in the presence of severe cardiac failure, sepsis or cirrhosis. Maintenance of cardiac output and renal perfusion may require inotropic support in these patients. The ideal inotropic agent for this is unclear, although dopamine has traditionally been used. It is difficult to justify the use of dopamine in ARF given the lack of evidence of benefit.[54] Of the other inotropic agents, vasopressin shows promise in sepsis, given its positive effect on systemic vascular resistance and its lack of α-adrenergic-mediated renal vasoconstrictor effect.[58]

Plasma electrolyte abnormalities

Potassium

Medications that increase the plasma potassium concentration (K^+) such as oral potassium tablets, ACE inhibitors and aldosterone antagonists should be stopped. ARF secondary to diarrhoea or diabetic ketoacidosis causes hypokalaemia and metabolic acidosis, while ARF due to vomiting or diuretic use can cause hypokalaemia with metabolic alkalosis. Marked hypokalaemia (K^+ <3.0 mmol/L) will need oral or intravenous potassium replacement. The K^+ in ARF is usually normal or elevated. The usual increase in K^+ in ARF is about 0.5 mmol/L/day, but a faster rate of increase (1–2 mmol/L/day) may occur is sepsis, rhabdomyolysis or extensive burns. All patients with hyperkalaemia should have a 12-lead electrocardiograph (ECG) looking for ECG changes of hyperkalaemia. Moderate hyperkalaemia (K^+ of 5.5–6.5 mmol/L) without clinical or ECG features of hyperkalaemia is treated with ion-exchange resins (oral or rectal resonium). Marked hyperkalaemia (K^+ >6.5 mmol/L) or the presence of ECG changes of hyperkalaemia in ARF are treated initially with intravenous drugs (calcium, insulin/glucose, salbutamol), followed by dialysis.

Sodium

Hyponatraemia in ARF is usually mild, and is treated by water restriction. Hypernatraemia is uncommon, but if marked is treated initially by oral administration of water or intravenous administration of hypotonic fluids or 5% dextrose.

Calcium, phosphate, uric acid and magnesium

Mild hypocalcaemia and hyperphosphataemia are common, but do not need treatment. Hyperuricaemia is common, is usually less than 600 mmol/L, and does not need treatment. Despite the hyperuricaemia, episodes of acute gout are very uncommon in ARF. Hypermagnesaemia is common, but is usually asymptomatic. Severe symptomatic hypermagnesaemia can occur if there is ongoing administration of magnesium during the course of ARF.[62]

Acid–base balance

A healthy person on a conventional diet produces about 50–100 mmol of non-volatile acid daily. The kidneys excrete this acid. ARF causes a mild-to-moderate metabolic acidosis with an increased anion gap. This acidosis does not usually require specific treatment. The development of very severe metabolic acidosis (pH<7.1 or serum bicarbonate <12 mmol/L) is uncommon unless an another disease process is present. Severe metabolic acidosis is an indication for dialysis.

Haematological changes

Anaemia is common in ARF, but does not need treatment. The role of erythropoietin in treating significant anaemia in ARF has not been established. Patients may have a prolongation of their bleeding time, but this is usually clinically insignificant. The bleeding abnormality can be corrected temporarily by desmopressin.

Hypervolaemia

Hypervolaemia is common in ARF, and can cause hypertension, raised jugular venous pressure, third heart sound, lung crackles, pleural effusion or ascites, peripheral oedema or acute pulmonary oedema. Fluid restriction minimizes the development of hypervolaemia: insensible losses are replaced by 400–600 mL of water per day, and measured losses (urine, nasogastric, diarrhoea) are replaced on a litre by litre basis with hypotonic saline.

The use of diuretics in hypervolaemic patients with ARF is problematic. Mannitol, which expands intravascular volume, worsens hypervolaemia and should be avoided. Furosemide has been given as an intravenous bolus at doses ranging from 1 to 5 mg/kg, or as a furosemide infusion. High doses of furosemide or a furosemide infusion increase the risk of deafness and of aminoglycoside induced renal toxicity. The use of loop diuretics worsens the outcome in ARF. The indications for furosemide are thus limited to patients with ARF complicated by acute pulmonary oedema. These patients are initially treated with continuous positive airway pressure (CPAP), intravenous glyceryl trinitrate if they are hypertensive, and a single dose of intravenous furosemide. These are interim treatment measures, and the definitive treatment is removal of fluid by ultrafiltration or dialysis or both.

Urinary-tract obstruction

Exclusion of urinary tract obstruction by ultrasound is essential. If present, obstruction must be promptly relieved by the appropriate means: bladder catheter, antegrade nephrostomy or urinary diversion.

Reduction of nephrotoxicity due to drugs

Agents such as NSAIDS, radiocontrast drugs, amphotericin, calcineurin inhibitors and aminoglycoside antibiotics should be avoided where possible. Adjustment of the dosage of drugs normally excreted by the kidney is likely to be necessary. If aminoglycosides need to be used they should be used at the low dosage range, and only given once per day.

Infection

Infection complicates 50–90% of cases of ARF. All patients with ARF should have urine and blood cultures, and other cultures as clinically indicated. Particular attention should be given to ensuring that invasive procedures are performed under the most sterile conditions possible. Prophylactic antibiotics are not indicated. Antibiotic use should be directed where possible by the results of cultures, and doses adjusted for the presence of renal failure.

Acute uraemic syndrome

This is due to retained nitrogenous wastes, and comprises one or more of the following: anorexia, nausea, hiccoughs, vomiting, ileus, confusion, myoclonus, asterixis, hyper-reflexia, seizures, pericarditis and pericardial effusion or pericardial tamponade. At a practical level the development of changes in mental state, seizures, asterixis or pericarditis are indications for urgent dialysis.

Nephrology consultation

Consultation with a nephrologist is mandatory in ARF thought to be due to glomerulonephritis (especially if there is a possibility of RPG), interstitial nephritis, vasculitis or thrombotic microangiopathy. The presence of one of the following suggests that dialysis (i.e. renal replacement treatment) will be required: oliguria or anuria, PCR >6–7 mmol/L, pulmonary oedema, encephalopathy, K^+ >6.5 mmol/L or severe metabolic acidosis. RRT is mandatory in patients with two or more of these features, or in patients with pericarditis.

INTENSIVE CARE UNIT MANAGEMENT

Patients with ARF in the setting of multiple organ dysfunction or severe sepsis or haemodynamic instability are treated in intensive care unit (ICU). One-third of these patients have pre-existing renal impairment, 80% need mechanical ventilation and 78% have continuous administration of vasoactive drugs.[63] In Australia critical care physicians control patient care and renal replacement therapy in 96% of cases.[63]

General measures

ARF is a complex process that involves simultaneous disturbances of renal blood flow, tubular integrity and leucocyte activation. The use of monotherapies that focused on vasodilatation, increased urine flow rate, protection of tubular cells from ongoing damage, accelerated regeneration of tubular cells or blocking leucocyte mediated injury has been unsuccessful, despite attractive theoretical rationales and promising experimental results. There has been increased interest in more general measures that reduce the length of stay and decrease the incidence of organ failure (including ARF) in ICU patients. Improved outcomes have been reported with insulin infusions,[64] early administration of antioxidants[65] and coupled plasma filtration and absorption of toxins by a hydrophobic resin.[66]

Renal replacement therapy[67]

Dialysis is required in about 85% of patients with oliguric ARF, and 30% of patients with non-oliguric ARF.

The principal types of dialysis or RRT are acute peritoneal dialysis (PD), acute intermittent haemodialysis (IHD) and various forms of continuous renal replacement treatment. Each modality has the capacity to achieve adequate clearance of uraemic toxins, to control uraemic complications and manage hypervolaemia. The choice of RRT is guided by the available resources, the expertise of the nephrologists and nephrologists, and the clinical condition of the patient.

PD is a relatively simple technique that does not need vascular access, avoids rapid changes in intravascular volume and does not need anticoagulation. The disadvantages of PD are the risk of bowel perforation, the development of peritonitis, and the loss of amino acids and proteins into the dialysate fluid.

IHD is typically performed for 3–4 hours daily or on alternate days. Direct percutaneous placement of double lumen, non-cuffed dialysis catheters into large vessels (typically the subclavian or internal jugular veins or the femoral vessels) is used to provide vascular access in ARF patients. Continuous renal replacement treatment is based on convective clearance of solute or diffusive clearance across a dialysis membrane or a combination of both techniques. Continuous venovenous haemofiltration (CVVH) and continuous arteriovenous haemofiltration (CAVH) are examples of the convective clearance, and continuous venovenous haemodialysis (CVVHD) is based on diffusive clearance. The two techniques are combined as continuous venovenous haemodiafiltration (CVVHDF) or continuous arteriovenous haemodiafiltration (CAVHDF). A new hybrid technique (sustained low-efficiency dialysis: SLED) has been used as an alternative to IHD and continuous RRT.[68] SLED involves the use of standard IHD equipment with reduced dialysate and blood flow rates for 12 hours a day. The most widely used techniques are CVVH and CVVHD.

At present IHD and continuous renal replacement treatment are regarded as equivalent methods for the treatment of ARF.[57] Continuous renal replacement treatment tends to be used for the very ill, and IHD for those less ill. The optimal technique of RRT in ARF is still being determined. PD is less effective than haemofiltration or haemodialysis in the treatment ARF.[69,70] Intensive (daily) IHD reduces mortality without increasing the incidence of haemodynamic complications.[71] Some studies have found that high levels of ultrafiltration in CVVH increase survival in critically ill patients with ARF compared to lower levels of ultrafiltration,[72] but this has not been confirmed by other studies.[73] Most studies have not found any clear-cut difference in outcome in ARF between IHD and continuous renal replacement.[74,75] Retrospective risk stratification studies have shown that continuous renal replacement is associated with a higher, unpredicted mortality rate at lower risk scores than is intermittent renal replacement treatment.[76]

PROGNOSIS

The prognosis of ARF is largely dependent on the underlying cause and the presence of co-morbidities. Mortality varies from about 40% in those with no co-morbidity to more than 80% in those who have three or more failed organ systems. Patients who die tend to have clinical courses complicated by sepsis, bleeding, delirium and respiratory failure. An independent association between ARF and mortality has been shown in certain patients. Following radiocontrast media the mortality of patients with ARF was increased fivefold and, following cardiac surgery, sixteen-fold as compared to patients with the same underlying disease without ARF.[77]

Patients with ATN have an average duration of ARF lasting 7–21 days. The renal failure phase is usually followed by a gradual improvement in renal function and a progressive increase in urine output. The GFR may increase before the renal tubules have recovered their full function, and the patient may lose excessive amounts of sodium and water during the recovery phase:

REFERENCES

1. Kellum JA, Levin N, Bouman C, Lameire N 2002 Developing a consensus classification system for acute renal failure Current Opinion in Critical Care 8: 509–14
2. Feest TG, Round A, Hamad S 1993 Incidence of severe acute renal failure in adults: results of a community based survey. British Medical Journal 306: 481–3
3. Liano F, Pascual J 1999 Epidemiology of acute renal failure : a prospective multicentre community-based study. Kidney International 50: 811–8
4. Kaufman J, Dhakal M, Patel B, Hamburger R 1991 Community-acquired acute renal failure. American Journal of Kidney Disease 17: 191–8
5. Brivet FG, Kleinknecht DJ, Loirat P, Landais PJM 1996 Acute renal failure in intensive care units: causes, outcome, and prognostic factors of hospital mortality. A prospective, multicentre study. Critical Care Medicine 24: 192–8
6. de Mendonca A, Vincent JL, Suter PM, et al 2000 Acute renal failure in the ICU: risk factors and outcome evaluated by the SOFA score. Intensive Care Medicine 26: 915–21
7. Agrawal M, Swartz R 2000 Acute renal failure. American Family Physician 61: 2077–88
8. Badr KE, Ichikawa I 1988 Prerenal failure: a deleterious shift from renal compensation to decompensation. New England Journal of Medicine 319: 623–9
9. Blantz RC 1998 Pathophysiology of pre-renal azotemia. Kidney International 53: 512–23
10. Bailen M R 2002 Reversible myocardial dysfunction in critically ill, noncardiac patients: A review. Critical Care Medicine 30: 1280–90
11. Ueda N, Kaush al GP, Shah SV 2000 Apoptotic mechanisms in acute renal failure. American Journal of Medicine 108: 403–15
12. Brady HR, Brenner BM, Clarkson MR, Lieberthal W 2000 Acute renal failure. Brenner & Rector's. The kidney 6th edn. WB Saunders Philadelphia, pp 1201–62
13. Rabb H, O'Meara YM, Maderna P, et al 1997 Leukocytes, cell adhesion molecules and ischemic

acute renal failure. Kidney International 51: 1463–8

14. Baliga R, Ueda X, Walker PD, Shah SV 1997 Oxidant mechanisms in toxic acute renal failure. American Journal of Kidney Diseases 29: 465–77

15. Wali R K, Henrich WL 2002 Recent developments in toxic nephropathy. Current Opinion in Nephrology & Hypertension 11: 155–63

16. Katzberg RW 1997 Urography into the 21st century: new contrast media, renal handling, imaging characteristics, and nephrotoxicity. Radiology 204: 297–312

17. Heyrnan SN, Reichrnan J, Brezis M 1999 Pathophysiology of radiocontrast nephropathy: a role for medullary hypoxia. Investigative Radiology 34: 685–91

18. Sinert R, Kohl L, Rainone T, Scalea T 1994 Exercise induced rhabdomyolysis. Annals of Emergency Medicine 23: 1301–6

19. Zager RA 1996 Rhabdomyolysis and myohemoglobinuric acute renal failure. Kidney International 49: 314–26

20. Pesik NT, Otten EJ 1996 Severe rhabdomyolysis following a viral illness: a case report and review of the literature. Journal of Emergency Medicine 14: 425–8

21. Schoolwerth AC, Sica DA, Ballermann BJ, Wilcox CS 2001 Renal considerations in angiotensin converting enzyme inhibitor therapy: a statement for healthcare professionals from the Council on the Kidney in Cardiovascular Disease and the Council for High Blood Pressure Research of the American Heart Association. Circulation 104: 1985–91

22. Miller S 1998 Acute oliguria. New England Journal of Medicine 338: 671–5

23. Albright R 2001 Acute renal failure: a practical update. Mayo Clinic Proceedings 76: 67–74

24. Modi K S, Rao, VK 2001 Atheroembolic renal disease. Journal of the American Society of Nephrology 12: 1781–7

25. Richards A, Goodship JA, Goodship THJ 2002 The genetics and pathogenesis of haemolytic uraemic syndrome and thrombotic thrombocytopenic purpura. Current Opinion in Nephrology & Hypertension 11: 431–5

26. Cameron JS 1988 Allergic interstitial nephritis: clinical features and pathogenesis. Quarterly Journal of Medicine 66: 97–115

27. de Fijter JW. Bruijn JA 1999 Acute nonoliguric renal failure after renal transplantation. American Journal of Kidney Diseases 33: 166–9

28. Chase CM, Garg AX, Kiberd BA 2002 Prevalence of low glomerular filtration rate in nondiabetic Americans: Third National Health and Nutrition Examination Survey (NHANES III). Journal of the American Society of Nephrology L3: 1338–49

29. Macias-Nunez JF, Lopez-Novoa JM, Martinez-Maldonado M 1996 Acute renal failure in the aged. Seminars in Nephrology 16: 330–8

30. Gines A, Escorsell A, Gines P, et al 1993 Incidence, predictive factors, and prognosis of the hepatorenal syndrome in cirrhosis with ascites. Gastroenterology 105: 229–36

31. Schrier RW, Gottschalk CW (eds) 1997 Acute renal failure. Diseases of the kidney, 6th edn. Little Brown and Company, Boston, pp 1069–1113

32. Zanarado G, Michielon P, Paccagnella A, et al 1994 Acute renal failure in patients undergoing cardiac operation: prevalence, mortality rate, and main risk factors. Journal of Thoracic Cardiovascular Surgery 107: 1489–95

33. Ryckwaert F, Boccara G, Frappier J, Colson PH 2002 Incidence, risk factors, and prognosis of a moderate increase in plasma creatinine early after cardiac surgery. Critical Care Medicine 30: 1495–8

34. Koreny M, Karth GD, Geppert A, et al 2002 Prognosis of patients who develop acute renal failure during the first 24 hours of cardiogenic shock after myocardial infarction. American Journal of Medicine 1l2: 115–9

35. Brivet FG, Kleinknecht DJ, Loirat P, Landais PJM I996 Acute renal failure in intensive care units: causes, outcome, and prognostic factors of hospital mortality. A prospective, multicentre study. Critical Care Medicine 24: 192–8

36. de Mendonca A, Vincent JL, Suter PM, et al 2000 Acute renal failure in the ICU: risk factors and outcome evaluated by the SOFA score. Intensive Care Medicine 26: 915–2l

37. Morris JA, Mucha P, Ross SE, et al 1991 Acute post traumatic renal failure : a multicentre perspective. Journal of Trauma 31: 1584–90

38. Domanovits H, Schillinger M, Mullner M, et al 2001 Acute renal failure after successful cardiopulmonary resuscitation. Intensive Care Medicine 27: 1194–9

39. McGee S, Abemethy W, Simel D 1999 Is this patient hypovolaemic? Journal of the American Medical Association 281: 1022–9

40. Jennette JC, Falk RJ 2000 Renal and systemic vasculitis. In: Johnson RJ, Feehally J (eds) Comprehensive clinical nephrology. Mosby, London, pp 1–28

41. Rose DR, Post TW 2001 Clinical physiology of acid-base and electrolyte disorders, 5th edn. McGraw-Hill, New York, pp 21–70, 258–84

42. Wolfson A, Paris P 1996 Diagnostic testing in emergency medicine. WB Saunders, Philadelphia

43. Miller T, Anderson R, Linas S, et al 1978 Urinary diagnostic indices in acute renal failure: a prospective study. Annals of Internal Medicine 89: 47–50

44. Platt JF 1996 Urinary obstruction. Radiological Clinics of North America 34: 1113–29

45. Schierhout G, Roberts I. 1998 Fluid resuscitation with colloid or crystalloid solutions in critically ill patients: a systematic review of randomised trials. British Medical Journal 316: 961–4

46. Cartotto RC, Innes MBA, Musgrave MA, et al 2002 How well does the Parkland formula estimate actual fluid resuscitation volumes? Journal of Burn Care & Rehabilitation 23: 258–65

47. Solomon R, Werner C, Mann D, et al 1994 Effects of saline, mannitol and furosemide on acute decreases in renal function induced by radiocontrast agents. New England Journal of Medicine 33: 1416–20

48. Venkataraman R, Kellum JA 2000 Novel approaches to the treatment of acute renal failure. Expert Opinion in Investigative Drugs 9: 2579–92

49. Vogt B, Ferrari P, Schonhoizer C, et al 2001 Prophylactic hemodialysis after radiocontrast media in patients with renal insufficiency is potentially harmful. American Journal of Medicine 111: 692–8

50. Huber W, Jeschke B, Kreymann B, et al 2002 Haemodialysis for the prevention of contrast-induced nephropathy: outcome of 31 patients with severely impaired renal function, comparison with patients at similar risk and review. Investigative Radiology 37: 471–81

51. Tepel M, vander Giet M, Schwarzfeld C, et al 2000 Prevention of radiographic-contrast-agent-induced reductions in renal failure by acetylcysteine New England Journal of Medicine 343: 180–4

52. Lassnigg A, Donner E, Grubhofer G, et al 2000 Lack of renoprotective effects of dopamine and furosemide during cardiac surgery. Journal of American Society of Nephrology 11: 97–104

53. Bellomo R, Chapman M, Finfer S, et al 2000 Low-dose dopamine in patients with early renal dysfunction: a placebo-controlled randomised trial Lancet 356: 2139–43

54. Kellum J A, Decker J 2001 Use of dopamine in acute renal failure : a meta-analysis. Critical Care Medicine 29: 1526–31

55. Morgera S, Woydt R, Kern H, et al 2002 Low-dose prostacyclin preserves renal function in high-risk patients after coronary bypass surgery. Critical Care Medicine 30: 107–12

56. Paller M 1998 Acute renal failure: controversies, clinical trials, and future directions. Seminars in Nephrology 18: 482–9

57. Star R. 1998 Treatment of acute renal failure. Kidney International 54: 1817–31

58. Esson M, Schrier R 2002 Diagnosis and treatment of acute tubular necrosis. Annals of Internal Medicine 137: 744–52

59. Lewis J, Salem MM, Chertow GM, et al 2000 Atrial natriuretic factor in oliguric acute renal failure. American Journal of Kidney Disease 36: 767–74

60. Mehta RL, Pascual MT, Soroko S, Chertow GM 2002 Diuretics, mortality, and nonrecovery of renal function in acute renal failure. Journal of American Medical Association 288: 2547–53

61. Mehta RL, McDonald B, Gabbai FB, et al 2002 Nephrology consultation in acute renal failure: does timing matter? American Journal of Medicine 113: 456–61

62. Schelling JR 2000 Fatal hypermagnesemia. Clinical Nephrology 53: 61–5

63. Silvester W, Bellomo R, Cole L 2001 Epidemiology, management , and outcome of severe acute renal failure of critical illness in Australia. Critical Care Medicine 29: 1910–5

64. Van den Berghe G, Wouters P, Weekers F, et al 2001 Intensive insulin therapy in critically ill patients. New England Journal of Medicine 345: 1359–67

65. Nathens AB, Neff MJ, Jurkovich GJ, et al 2002 Randomized, prospective trial of antioxidant supplementation in critically ill surgical patients. Annals of Surgery 236: 814–22

66. Ronco C, Brendolan A, Lonnemann G, et al 2002 A pilot study of coupled plasma filtration with absorption in septic shock. Critical Care Medicine 30: 1250–5

67. Pastan S, Bailey J 1998 Dialysis therapy. New England Journal of Medicine 338: 1428–37

68. Marshall MR, Golper TA, Shaver MJ, et al 2001 Sustained low-efficiency dialysis for critically ill patients requiring renal replacement therapy. Kidney International 60: 777–85

69. Phu NH, Hien TT, Mai N T H, et al 2002 Hemofiltration and peritoneal dialysis in infection-associated acute renal failure in Vietnam. New England Journal of Medicine 347: 895–902

70. Winkelmayer WC, Glynn RJ, Mittleman MA, et al 2002 Comparing mortality of elderly patients on hemodialysis versus peritoneal dialysis: a propensity score approach. Journal of the American Society of Nephrology 13: 2353–62

71. Schiffi H, Lang SM, Fischer R 2002 Daily hemodialysis and the outcome of acute renal failure. New England Journal of Medicine. 346: 305–10

72. Ronco C, Bellomo R, Homel P, et al 2000 Effects of different doses in continuous veno-venous haemofiltration on outcomes of acute renal failure: a prospective randomised trial Lancet 356: 26–30

73. Bouman CSC, Oudemans-van Straaten HM, Tijssen JGP, et al 2002 Effects of early high-volume continuous venovenous hemofiltration on survival and recovery of renal function in intensive care patients with acute renal failure: A prospective, randomized trial. Critical Care Medicine 30: 2205–11

74. Swartz RD, Messana JM, Orzol S, et al 1999 Comparing continuous hemofiltration with hemodialysis in patients with severe acute renal failure. American Journal of Kidney Disease 34: 424–32

75. Mehta RL, McDonald B, Gabbai FB, et al 2001 A randomozed clinical trial of continuous versus intermittent dialysis for acute renal failure. Kidney International 60: 1154–63

76. Martin C, Saran R, Leavey S, Swartz R 2002 Predicting the outcome of renal replacement therapy in severe acute renal failure. ASAIO Journal 48: 640–4

77. Kribben A, Edeistein CL, Schrier RW 1999 Pathophysiology of acute renal failure. Journal of Nephrology 12 Suppl 2: S142–51

9.2 THE ACUTE SCROTUM

GINO TONCICH

ESSENTIALS

1 Torsion is the most time-critical diagnosis in acute scrotal pain.

2 Early surgery is mandatory if the diagnosis is strongly suspected. No investigation should delay surgery.

3 Nuclear medicine and colour Doppler ultrasound are of limited use and are best used when testicular ischaemia needs to be excluded in an inflammatory mass.

4 Torsion of an appendage can be diagnosed by finding a small blue lump in the scotal sac and can be managed non-operatively.

5 Epididymo-orchitis is rare in adolescence and torsion should be suspected. Ancillary studies may be used to exclude torsion if suspicion remains.

6 Masses found on ultrasound should be followed up as traumatic injury can bring attention to an undiscovered tumour.

7 Ultrasound is unreliable in diagnosing testicular rupture.

8 Early surgery in scrotal trauma allows diagnosis and treatment of rupture, as well as early evacuation of other haematomas with shorter inpatient stays and less pain.

TORSION OF THE SPERMATIC CORD (TESTICLE)

Torsion is a twisting, not of the testicle (as is commonly described), but of the spermatic cord, which then interferes with the vascularity of the testicle, ultimately leading to infarction.

AETIOLOGY

Torsion is due to a powerful contraction of the cremaster muscles in an abnormally attached testis. A normal testis is anchored posterolaterally to the scrotal sac and is, therefore, fixed in place. The main abnormality found in patients with torsion is an enlarged tunica vaginalis, which surrounds the whole of the testes and epididymis, preventing the testis from creating any attachment to the scrotal wall. The testis, therefore, floats freely like a clapper inside a bell. The contraction of the cremaster causes the testes and adnexa to be rotated, thereby twisting the cord.[1]

PATHOLOGY

The twisting of the cord causes obstruction of the lymphatic and venous outflows, but allows arterial inflow, leading to venous engorgement. Eventually the pressure rises to occlude the arterial inflow.

The extent and rapidity of the damage depends on the degree of torsion, that is the number of turns. This can vary from one-quarter turn to three complete turns.

- Incomplete torsion (<360°) may not completely occlude arterial flow.
- One turn (360°) causes necrosis in 12–24 hours.
- Two or more (>720°) causes necrosis in less than 2 hours because arterial flow is completely obstructed.[1,2]

CLINICAL PRESENTATION

There is a sudden onset of severe scrotal or abdominal pain. There are no irritative voiding symptoms. Between 29 and 50% of patients have had previous episodes of acute scrotal pain.[3,4]

The patient looks pale and may vomit. The testis is tender and riding high in the scrotum. Other signs are loss of cremasteric reflex, scrotal oedema testicular swelling and retraction. One study in which all children had mandatory exploration found these clinical signs had sensitivities of 60–91% and specificities of 27–68%.[14]

Systemic signs such as fever are classically absent. Urinalysis is normal.

Intermittent torsion of the testis

This was first recognized in 1895, but not usually mentioned in reports on the acute scrotum. It is a syndrome of recurrent acute scrotal pain, usually lasting less than 2 hours, which resolves spontaneously. Creagh and McDermott[4] describe a series of 27 patients who underwent elective orchidopexy for these symptoms. Three patients developed acute torsion while on the waiting list; of those coming to operation, one had an atrophic testis and four had evidence of torsion of the appendages of the testis. One patient subsequently had torsion after surgery because absorbable sutures were used.[4]

DIFFERENTIAL DIAGNOSIS OF ACUTE TESTICULAR PAIN

Differential diagnoses to consider in acute testicular pain are listed in Table 9.2.1.

TRAPS IN THE CLINICAL DIAGNOSIS

There are many potential pitfalls in the clinical diagnosis of the acute scrotum:

- Age: The abnormality is present for life, so the torsion could potentially occur at any age. In those under 12 years of age an acutely painful scrotum should always be considered to be torsion.[3] Less than 4% of torsions occur in patients over 30 years. It is most common in

Table 9.2.1 Differential diagnosis of acute testicular pain

Epididymo-orchitis
Strangulated hernia
Haematocoele
Hydrocoele
Testicular tumour
Idiopathic scrotal oedema.

adolescence (12–18 years).[5] In teenagers there is an increasing amount of sexually transmitted disease, which may confuse the diagnosis. There is an old surgical aphorism: 'Question: When do you diagnose epididymo-orchitis in a teenager? Answer: After you have fixed the torsion'.

- Pain: In 25% there is no sudden onset of pain, nor is it necessarily severe. Some patients with epididymo-orchitis have severe pain.[1,3]
- Localization: Some patients may have no scrotal pain but may have all their pain referred to the lower abdomen or inguinal area. The scrotum must always be examined in males with lower abdominal pain.
- Abnormal position of testis: this is only seen if 360° or greater rotation occurs.[3]
- Previous repair: Torsion can occur in a testis that has previously been fixed, especially if absorbable sutures have been used.[4]
- Dysuria: Irritative voiding symptoms rarely occur with torsion and suggest infection.[3]
- Fever: Temperatures >102°F have been noted in up to 15% of torsion patients.[1]

INVESTIGATIONS

Surgical exploration of the scrotum

This is the investigation of choice where the diagnosis of torsion is likely, and maximizes the chance of saving the testis. Delaying the diagnosis is 'castration by neglect'.[3] Surgical exploration requires only a skin incision and has no major complications.[14]

Low rates of torsion diagnosed at operation have led to interest in other tests to predict torsion preoperatively.

Scintigraphic scanning

For the immediate distinction of testicular torsion from other aetiologies in the emergency situation scintigraphy has been more widely validated than ultrasound. Pertechnetate is injected intravenously. Perfusion of the testes by the isotope is in proportion to the blood flow to that testis. The whole procedure can be done in 15–20 minutes.[1] If there is no blood flow, a 'torted' testis should be 'cold' on the scan, while an inflammatory process should be 'hot' because of extra blood flow.

The findings depend on the stage of the torsion:

- Early on there is relatively increased activity in the testicular artery (normally invisible) up to the site of the twist, where the flow is abruptly cut off – 'the nubbin sign'. There is no activity in the region of the testis. Scrotal perfusion is still normal. At this stage there is 100% salvage if surgery is performed.
- Midphase or 'missed torsion' demonstrates increased blood flow in the scrotum and a deficient flow in the testis. The appearance is likened to a 'bull's eye' (a hot rim around a cold centre).
- Late-phase change is an increased scrotal halo in proportion to the testicular ischaemia.

The sensitivity of the scan is 93% meaning that 7% or 1 in 14 torsions will be missed. Specificity is in the order of 90%.

However, in incomplete torsion or spontaneous detorsion the scan may be normal or show reactive hyperaemia. This may remove the need for urgent exploration of the scrotum, but provides an indication for elective exploration.[1]

Colour Doppler imaging of the testis

This is the ultrasound examination of choice. It is useful in diagnosing torsion but also in elucidating other scrotal pathology. Comparison of blood flow to the asymptomatic side is crucial. If there is reduced flow to one side then some degree of torsion must be suspected. If the testis has untorted, hyperaemic flow may be noted. The sensitivity of colour Doppler imaging (CDI) for torsion can be as low as 82%, missing 1 in 5 cases, and is affected by:

- Lack of sensitivity in low flow states
- Inappropriate settings
- Inexperience of the operator
- Incomplete torsion
- Failure to compare low flow to the normal side
- Spontaneous untorting, giving an increased flow to the affected side, not reduced or absent flow.[2]

Role of investigations in suspected testicular torsion

When the diagnosis is probable then the only investigation is surgical exploration of the scrotum, and any investigations that delay theatre are unnecessary. If torsion is unlikely clinically, but needs to be excluded, then either CDI or scintigraphy can be used, provided they are available on an urgent basis. If this is not possible then surgical exploration may be necessary if the testis is to be saved.[1-3]

TREATMENT

Manual untwisting

The spermatic cord is infiltrated with local anaesthetic and the testis is untwisted. Untwisting is done by turning the left testis anticlockwise and the right one clockwise, like opening the pages of a book.[6] At best this is only a temporary measure, and surgical treatment should be planned. The manoeuvre is not universally recommended

Surgery

The scrotum is opened and the testis is delivered, untwisted and inspected for return of colour and bleeding. An obviously infarcted testis is removed at the initial surgery. A viable testis is sutured into place on the scrotal wall. The tunica should be inverted and also sutured to the scrotal wall. It is vital that the normal side is also explored and fixed to the scrotal wall, as the abnormality is bilateral in most cases. Retorsion following orchidopexy has occurred when absorbable sutures have been used.[1,3–5]

PROGNOSIS

Viability depends on the number of twists and the time taken to untwist the testis. There is 100% salvage if the testis is untwisted in less than 4 hours. Up to 24 hours the rate falls to 50%. Rare case reports of salvage after 30 hours have been reported.

Testicular salvage (return of circulation at surgery) does not mean no injury to the testicle. Long-term follow-up of salvaged testes shows that 75% have a reduction in volume. Abnormalities are also seen in sperm volume, motility and morphology. These abnormalities are not seen in patients who have had an infarcted testis removed at the initial operation. This suggests some anti-spermatogenesis effect caused by the damaged testicle.[1,3,4]

TORSION OF A TESTICULAR APPENDAGE

These are embryological remnants with no function. They are small (<5 mm) pedunculated structures that may twist on their pedicle. If the appendage can be isolated in the scrotum a small blue lump may be isolated: 'the blue dot sign'. These do not need surgery and can be treated with analgesia. Late presentations may have scrotal or testicular swelling, in which case they should be treated as torsion until proved otherwise.[1]

ACUTE EPIDIDYMO-ORCHITIS

INTRODUCTION

This is a clinical syndrome resulting from pain and swelling of the epididymis (and

Table 9.2.2 Causative agents in EDO
Bacterial: *Neisseria gonorrhoeae*, *Escherichia coli*, *Pseudomonas aeruginosa*, coliforms, *Klebsiella*, *Mycobacterium tuberculosis*
Chlamydial: *C. trachomatis*
Viral: mumps
Drugs: amiodarone epididymitis
Fungal: cryptococcal
Parasitic: filariasis (usually chronic).

the testis) of less than 6 weeks' duration. Chronic epididymitis is a long-standing condition of epididymal or testicular pain, usually without swelling.[2]

AETIOLOGY

A variety of organisms may be responsible for epididymo-orchitis (EDO) (Table 9.2.2).

The most likely cause depends on the patient's demographic group. For heterosexual males under 35 years of age, the agent is usually gonococcus or chlamydia. These organisms are also responsible for infection in homosexual males under 35 years (where anal sex is practised), but coliforms and even *Haemophilus* can cause infection. In males older than 35 years, EDO is usually due to obstructive urological disease, so coliforms predominate. EDO may also be part of a systemic disease, for example brucellosis or cryptococcus.

EDO is usually thought to be an ascending infection from the urethra or prostate, but it can be part of a generalized systemic disease. The infection spreads from epididymis to testicle, and eventually they may become one large inflammatory mass. Isolated orchitis is rare and usually due to viral causes, which are spread via the bloodstream.[7–9]

CLINICAL PRESENTATION

The exact features depend on the underlying cause and whether both the

epididymis and the testicle are involved. The pain may come on suddenly or slowly. There is scrotal swelling and tenderness that is relieved by elevating the testis. The spermatic cord is usually tender and swollen. Associated symptoms of urethritis are common. In younger males (under 35 years) a history of sexually transmitted disease may be elicited. In the older patient there is a history of instrumentation, intercurrent UTI or prostatism. Pyuria is common.

INVESTIGATIONS

Urethral swabs

Urethral discharge may not be seen if the patient has just voided, so a urethral swab and smear should be examined for white blood cells (WBC). If there are more than 5 WBC per high-powered field, then urethritis is likely. The presence of intracellular diplococci confirms the diagnosis of gonorrhoea; their absence suggests chlamydia.[7]

Midstream urine

Look for the presence of WBC or Gram-negative organisms.

DIFFERENTIAL DIAGNOSIS

In the acute non-traumatic setting the most important differential diagnosis is torsion of the testicle.[7] If the clinical features, urethral swabs or MSU do not differentiate, then ultrasound or isotope scans may help. In young men, if these are not available and there is no evidence of UTI or urethritis, then surgical exploration may be necessary. Ultrasound can help differentiate other causes of the acute scrotum.

TREATMENT

Symptomatic treatment consists of bed rest, analgesia and scrotal supports.

If the cause is secondary to a sexually transmitted disease, then appropriate antibiotics should be chosen after urethral swabs have been taken, for instance a single dose of ceftriaxone for gonorrhoea and a 10-day course of tetracycline for chlamydia. The patient's sexual partners should be investigated and treated. Tests for syphilis or HIV should be performed.

If the infection is secondary to urinary-tract infections then an appropriate antibioticlike amoxyl/clavulanic acid or trimethoprim should be used and treatment adjusted according to the urine culture results. Investigation for underlying urinary tract obstruction should be undertaken according to clinical features.

COMPLICATIONS

These include abscess formation, testicular infarction, chronic pain and infertility.

BLUNT TRAUMATIC INJURY TO THE TESTICLE

The mobility of the testicle, cremaster muscle contraction and the tough capsule usually protect the testicle from injury. However, a direct blow that drives the testicle against the symphysis pubis may result in contusion or rupture of the testicle. Typical mechanisms are a direct kick to the groin, or handlebar and straddle injuries.[10, 11]

The types of injury include scrotal-wall haematomas, tunica vaginalis haematoma (haematocoele) or intratesticular (subcapsular) haematoma.

The most serious is testicular rupture, where the tunica is split, allowing blood

CONTROVERSIES AND FUTURE DIRECTIONS

❶ There is still some controversy about the place of investigations in suspected torsion. The question remains whether all patients with suspected torsion should go straight to theatre or whether there is any role for investigations.

❷ There is debate about whether all patients with scotal and testicular trauma should have routine surgical exploration. Some recommend non-operative management.

❸ Attempts at testicular salvage may be abandoned in favour of orchidectomy of the affected side in order to preserve the spermatogenisis of the other side.

and seminiferous tubules to extrude into the tunica vaginalis. This occurs in up to 50% of blunt trauma. Complete disruption of the testis may occur.[10-12]

Ultrasound examination is not sensitive in detecting testicular rupture, so early surgical exploration is the investigation and treatment of choice.

It should be noted that 10–15% of testicular tumours present after an episode of trauma, and so any abnormalities on ultrasound examination should be followed to resolution if surgery is not performed.[13]

Early surgical exploration with evacuation of blood clots in the tunica vaginalis and repair of testicular rupture, if present, results in a shortened hospital stay, a greatly reduced period of disability and a faster return to normal activity compared to patients managed conservatively. Conservative management is complicated by secondary infection of the haematocoele, frank acute necrosis of the testis, and delayed atrophy due to pressure effects of haematoma. The orchidectomy rate for early exploration is only 9%, compared to 45% for those managed non-operatively.[11]

REFERENCES

1. Lutzker LG, Zuckier LS 1990 Testicular scanning and other applications of radionuclide imaging of the genital tract. Seminars in Nuclear Medicine XX: 159–88
2. Herbener TE 1996 Ultrasound in the assessment of the acute scrotum. Journal of Clinical Ultrasound 24: 405–21
3. Cass AS 1990 Torsion of the testis. Postgraduate Medicine 87: 69–74
4. Creagh TA, McDermott TE, et al 1988 Intermittent torsion of the testis. British Medical Journal 297: 525–6
5. Rajfer J 1997 Testicular torsion. In: Walsh PC, Retik AB, Darracott VE, Wein AJ (eds) Campbell's Urology, vol. 2, 7th edn. WB Saunders, London, pp. 2184–6
6. Schneider RE 1996 Testicular torsion. In: Tintinalli JE, Ruiz E, Krome RL (eds) Emergency medicine: a comprehensive study guide, 4th edn. McGraw-Hill, New York
7. Berger R 1997 Epididymitis. In: Walsh PC, Retik AB, Darracott VE, Wein AJ (eds) Campbell's Urology, vol. 1, 7th edn. WB Saunders, London pp 670–3
8. Tintinalli JE, Ruiz, E, Krome RL 1996 Epididymitis. In: Tintinalli JE, Krome RL (eds) Emergency Medicine: A Comprehensive Study Guide, 4th edn. McGraw-Hill, New York
9. Therapeutic Guidelines: Antibiotics, 10th edn. March 1998. Therapeutic Guidelines Limited, Melbourne
10. Bertini JE, Corriere JN 1990 The etiology and management of genital injuries. Journal of Trauma 28: 1278–81
11. Cass AS 1983 Testicular trauma. Journal of Urology 129: 299–300
12. Kukadia AN, Ercole CJ, et al 1996 Testicular trauma: potential impact on reproductive function. Journal of Urology 156: 1643–6
13. Cass AS, Luxenberg M 1991 Testicular injuries. Urology 38: 528–30
14. Van Glabeke E, Khairouni A, Larroquet M, Audry G, Gruner M 1999 Acute scrotal pain in children: results of 543 surgical explorations. Pediatric Surgery International 15: 353–7

9.3 RENAL COLIC

FIONA NICHOLSON

ESSENTIALS

1 Renal colic affects 2-5% of the population, with 50% of patients having a recurrence within 5 years.

2 Management includes adequate analgesia and hydration.

3 Intravenous pyelography or computerized tomography (CT) establish the diagnosis and evaluate the severity of obstruction.

4 Most stones (90%) are passed spontaneously within 1 month.

5 Obstruction, infection and intractable pain necessitate admission to hospital.

6 Urology follow-up is essential to minimize further episodes.

INTRODUCTION

Nephrolithiasis is a common disorder affecting 2–5% of the population at some point in their lives.[1] It occurs most frequently between the ages of 20 and 50 years, with a male:female ratio of approximately 3:1. About 50% of patients have a single episode but the remaining 50% have recurrent episodes within 5 years.[2]

Most calculi are believed to originate in the collecting system (renal calyces and pelvis) before passing into the ureter. Supersaturation with stone-forming substances (calcium, phosphate, oxalate, cystine or urate) combined with a decrease in urine volume and lack of chemicals that inhibit stone formation (such as magnesium, citrate and pyrophosphate) results in production of a calculus. In addition, infection with urea-splitting organisms that produce an alkaline urinary pH frequently contributes to the growth of 'struvite' or triple phosphate

(calcium, magnesium and ammonium phosphate) stones.

Less commonly, mixed stones occur via nucleation with sodium hydrogen, urate, uric acid and hydroxyapatite crystals providing a core to which calcium and oxalate ions adhere (heterogenous nucleation).

Approximately 75% of all stones are calcium based, consisting of calcium oxalate, calcium phosphate, or a mixture of the two. Another 10% are uric-acid based, 1% are cystine based and the remainder are primarily struvite.

Predisposing factors for stone formation include prolonged immobilization, hyperparathyroidism or peptic ulcer disease (hyperexcretion of calcium), small bowel disease, such as Crohn's disease or ulcerative colitis (hyperoxaluria), and gout (hyperuricaemia). Myeloproliferative disorders, malignancy, glycogen storage disorders and the use of certain medications (acetazolamide, vitamins C and D, antacids) may also be conducive to nephrolithiasis.[3]

PATHOPHYSIOLOGY OF PAIN

The mechanisms implicated in the production of the pain of renal colic are an increase in renal pelvic pressure, ureteric spasm and local inflammatory effects.

Acute obstruction of the upper urinary tract from a calculus results in increased pressure in the renal pelvis, which, in turn, induces the synthesis and secretion of renal prostaglandins, in particular PGE2. This promotes a diuresis by causing dilatation of the afferent arteriole that further elevates renal pelvic pressure.[4,5] The acute obstruction and renal capsular tension are believed to be the cause of the constant ache in the costovertebral angle.

In experiments with isolated ureteric smooth muscle, prostaglandins have also been shown to increase phasic and tonic

contractile activity[6] resulting in ureteric spasm and the severe, colicky pain.

PRESENTATION

The classic description of renal colic is severe, intermittent, flank pain of abrupt onset originating from the area of the costovertebral angle and radiating anteriorly to the lower abdominal and inguinal regions. Testicular or labial pain may be present and may suggest the location of the stone as a high ureteric position, with urinary frequency or urgency often developing as the stone nears the bladder. Nausea and vomiting frequently accompany the pain, and abdominal distension associated with ileus may also occur. One-third of patients complain of gross haematuria.[7]

Precipitating factors such as immobilization or a family history of renal disease should be sought, as well as complicating factors such as fever or single kidney.

Examination usually reveals an agitated, pacing patient unable to find a comfortable position. Pulse rate and blood pressure may be elevated secondary to the pain. Fever is unusual and suggests infection. The abdominal examination may only reveal signs of an early ileus with hypoactive bowel sounds, but is extremely useful in excluding intra-abdominal or retroperitoneal causes of the pain (such as pancreatitis, cholecystitis, appendicitis or leaking or rupture of the abdominal aorta).

Urinalysis may show red blood cells with an alkaline pH, nitrites, leukocytes or micro-organisms suggesting either the complication of infection or a diagnosis of acute pyelonephritis. Urine culture is indicated to rule out infection with urea-splitting organisms such as *Klebsiella* and *Proteus* spp. Electrolyte studies may demonstrate obstruction or suggest an underlying metabolic abnormality such as hypercalcaemia, hyperuricaemia or hypokalaemia. A slightly elevated white blood cell count may occur with renal colic, but a count greater than 15000/mm^3 suggests active infection.

RADIOLOGIC EXAMINATION

The intravenous pyelogram (IVP) remains the best radiological test to evaluate the upper urinary tract in patients with normal renal function and no history of hypersensitivity to contrast material. It establishes the diagnosis of calculus disease in 96% of cases and determines the severity of obstruction.[8] Classic findings of acute obstruction include a delay in the appearance of one kidney, a dilated ureter, and a dilated renal pelvis.[9] The IVP is useful in estimating the size of the stone, in identifying extravasation of dye, and in evaluating renal function.

A KUB (kidney, ureter and bladder) is the standard initial film performed before the injection of contrast media, and may provide presumptive evidence for a calculus. Most stones (90%) are radio-opaque and are seen as irregularly shaped densities on the KUB. Phlebitis in the pelvic veins and calcified mesenteric lymph nodes may add confusion, however, and small stones may be obscured by the bony density of the sacrum. Radio-opaque calculi are composed of calcium oxalate, cystine, calcium phosphate or magnesium-ammonium-phosphate. Uric acid stones, blood clots and sloughed papillae are lucent and seen as negative shadows on the IVP.

Ultrasonography is a useful alternative when renal function is impaired or contrast media contraindicated. It can identify the stone and its location, demonstrate proximal obstruction such as hydroureter or a dilated pelvis, and the size and configuration of each kidney. Computerized tomography (CT), with or without contrast, is the first-line test in many centres. with findings including demonstration of the stone, perinephric stranding, dilatation of the kidney (hydronephrosis) or ureter and low density of the kidney suggesting oedema. Cystoscopy with retrograde ureteropyelo-graphy is invasive and used as a last resort to delineate the renal tract.

MANAGEMENT

As 90% of stones are passed spontaneously, initial management is directed towards relief of pain and providing adequate hydration. Intravenous narcotics provide rapid analgesia and relieve anxiety in most cases. Parenteral non-steroidal anti-inflammatory agents appear to be equally effective. Intravenous crystalloid should be administered to ensure a urine volume of 100–200 mL/h in those unable to tolerate oral fluids.

Most patients with renal colic can be discharged with oral analgesia (codeine, paracetamol and nonsteroidals), hydration and a referral for outpatient urology. Rectal administration of indometacin is particularly effective if tolerated by the patient. Stones less than 5 mm in patients without associated infection or anatomic abnormality will pass within 1 month in 90% of cases, but only 5% of stones larger than 8 mm will pass, and hence will usually require elective surgical removal.[8]

Indications for admission to hospital are:

- Presence of infection
- Deteriorating renal function
- Persistent pain requiring parenteral narcotics
- Stone greater than 5 mm in diameter
- Extravasation of dye (uncommon).

Further intervention is required if obstruction with hydronephrosis is present, the stone is a large staghorn calculus or the patient continues to have pain and no stone is passed within 2–3 days. A percutaneous nephrostomy allows drainage of an obstructed kidney until the blockage can be removed, either by ureteroscopic procedures for low stones or by open surgery for large or infected stones. Extracorporeal shockwave lithotripsy (ESWL) is preferred for single or small (less than 2 cm) otherwise uncomplicated stones as it has minimal complications and morbidity.

Urology follow-up is essential for all patients, for elective removal of stones when complications have not ensued, and for the prevention of recurrence: 50% of all patients have a further episode within 5 years.

PRECAUTIONS

Renal colic, with its minimal findings on examination, is a commonly used presentation for those seeking narcotics or with Munchausen's syndrome and treating physicians must be aware of this. However, it is essential to give analgesia to those patients suffering from renal colic and it is probably preferable to give patients analgesia unnecessarily than cause unnecessary suffering. Features suggesting narcotic seeking include:

- Lack of cooperation
- Itinerant
- History of multiple narcotic 'allergies'
- History of contrast allergy
- Multiple prior stone events
- History of uric acid lithiasis (radiolucent)
- Factitious haematuria.

CONTROVERSIES AND FUTURE DIRECTIONS

❶ Controversies in the management of renal colic relate largely to analgesia. Traditionally, it has been taught that parenteral narcotics provide fast and effective pain relief, but with the advent of injectable non-steroidal anti-inflammatory drugs some argue that these should be first-line of care.

❷ Management of renal colic will be made much clearer with further research into appropriate analgesia and consideration of early and thorough investigation, whether intravenous pyelography or computerized tomography.

CONCLUSION

Renal colic is an acutely distressing medical condition that requires a careful evaluation of symptoms and signs to ensure timely analgesia, recognition of other causes of acute abdominal pain and avoidance of inappropriate narcotic usage.

REFERENCES

1. Lingeman J, et al 1991 Calculous disease of the kidney and bladder.In: Harwood-Nuss A (ed). The Clinical Practice of Emergency Medicine. JB Lippincott, Philadelphia
2. Trivedi BK. 1996 Nephrolithiasis. Postgraduate medicine 100(6): 3–78
3. Coe FL, Parks JH, Asplin JR 1992 The pathogenesis and treatment of kidney stones. New England Journal of Medicine 327(16): 1141–52
4. Holmlund D 1983 The pathophysiology of ureteric colic. Scandinavian Journal of Urology and Nephrology 75(Suppl): 25–27
5. Nishikawa K, Morrisin A, Needleman P 1977 Exaggerated prostaglandin biosynthesis and its influence on renal resistance in the isolated hydronephrotic rabbit kidney. Journal of Clinical Investigation 59: 1143–50
6. Cole RS, Fry CH, Shuttleworth KED 1988 The action of prostaglandins on isolated human ureteric smooth muscle. British Journal of Urology 61: 19–26
7. Smith DR 1978 General Urology, 9th edn. Lange Medical Publishers, Los Altos, California
8. Harrison JH, et al (eds) 1987 Campbell's Urology, vol 1, 4th edn. WB Saunders, Philadelphia
9. Samm BJ, Dmochowski RR 1996 Urologic emergencies. Postgraduate Medicine 100(4): 177–84

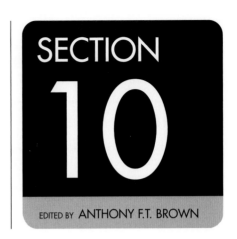

SECTION
10

EDITED BY ANTHONY F.T. BROWN

ENDOCRINE

10.1 **Diabetes mellitus** 462

10.2 **Thyroid and adrenal emergencies** 467

10.3 **Alcoholic ketoacidosis** 471

10.1 DIABETES MELLITUS

MICHAEL RAGG

ESSENTIALS

1 Diabetic ketoacidosis (DKA) is caused by a lack of insulin, either absolute or relative.

2 Infection is the precipitant in over 37% of cases of DKA.

3 Predictors of high mortality in DKA are sepsis or myocardial infarction as precipitants; increasing age, pre-existing cardiovascular or renal disease and coma on presentation.

4 An initial fluid rate of not more than 500 mL/h for 4 hours is recommended if shock is not present.

5 Not all patients with DKA require admission.[1]

6 Early diagnosis of hyperglycaemic, hyperosmolar non-ketotic syndrome (HHNS) requires a high index of suspicion. It is associated with a high mortality rate.

7 It is unclear why patients with HHNS do not develop ketoacidosis.

8 Altered conscious state and focal neurological signs are common on initial presentation of HHNS. Patients with HHNS are also at increased risk for arterial and venous thrombosis.

9 Hypoglycaemic coma requires immediate treatment with intravenous glucose. If liver glycogen stores are adequate, intramuscular glucagon can be used, and may be given prehospital.

INTRODUCTION

General concepts of diabetes mellitus

In 1996 the classification system and diagnostic criteria for diabetes were re-examined by the American Diabetes Association and the World Health Organization.[2] The classification of type I and type II diabetes mellitus has been retained; however, the recommended criterion for a diagnosis of diabetes is now a fasting plasma glucose of 7 mmol/L or greater. The oral glucose tolerance test is no longer recommended.

Secondary diabetes mellitus can occur in the following conditions: pancreatitis and pancreatectomy, haemochromatosis, Cushing's syndrome, acromegaly, phaeochromocytoma and glucagonoma.

The exact aetiology of diabetes is unclear. Evidence regarding type I diabetes suggests genetic and environmental factors, associated with certain HLA types (90% of patients are HLA-DR3 or DR4 or both) and abnormal immune responses. Increasing evidence now also implicates certain genes as possible contributors, particularly sites on chromosomes 6, 7, 11, 14 and 18. With type II diabetes genetic factors are implied by familial aggregation of cases. Environmental factors in the context of genetic susceptibility as well as obesity are also implicated.

In Australia, diabetes is more common in the Aboriginal community. Other groups with high prevalence include Native Americans and Pacific Islanders. Type I diabetes occurs most frequently among caucasians throughout the world. Diabetic ketoacidosis (DKA) and hyperglycaemic hyperosmolar non ketotic syndrome (HHNS) are both life-threatening acute complications of diabetes mellitus. Though some important differences do exist, the pathophysiology and treatment have many similarities.[3] DKA is usually seen in type 1 diabetes and HHNS in patients with type 2, however, both complications can occur in type 1 and 2 diabetes.[3]

DIABETIC KETOACIDOSIS

The clinical presentation of diabetic ketoacidosis (DKA) was first described almost 2000 years ago: 'The patients never stop making water and the flow is incessant ... life is short, unpleasant and painful, thirst unquenchable, drinking excessive ... if for a while they abstain from drinking, their mouths become parched and their bodies dry; the viscera seem scorched up; the patients are affected by nausea, restlessness and a burning thirst, and within a short time, they expire'.[4]

DKA has been described as starvation in the midst of plenty. Cells are unable to utilize glucose owing to a lack of insulin, either absolute or relative. Glucose transporters (GLUT) in the cell membrane require insulin to create glucose channels. GLUT 2 and 4 appear to be important in DKA. Physiological mechanisms are activated to provide greater quantities of glucose, which leads to hyperglycaemia and excessive production of alternative fuels (ketoacids and fatty acids). Glucagon is a major stimulus to these processes. The hyperglycaemia leads to an osmotic diuresis, and severe dehydration with hypokalaemia results.

Precipitants of DKA in one study were as follows:[5]

- Infection 37%
- Treatment error 21%
- Unknown in 14%

- Endocrine and miscellaneous 8%
- Pancreatitis and other abdominal disorders 5%
- AMI 5%.

Suggested diagnostic criteria for DKA:[6]

- Glucose >13.8 mmol/L
- pH <7.35
- Low HCO_3
- High anion gap
- Positive serum ketones.

HYPERGLYCAEMIC, HYPEROSMOLAR NON-KETOTIC SYNDROME

In patients with HHNS, ketosis is less marked or absent, glucose levels are higher, and insulin deficiency is relative rather than absolute. Table 10.1.1 outlines the major differences between the two conditions.

Infections and other acute illnesses, particularly cardiovascular, are the usual precipitant for HHNS. Certain drugs may also precipitate HHNS (e.g. β-blockers, calcium channel-blockers, diuretics, glucocorticoids, phenytoin).

The exact reason why patients with HHNS do not develop ketoacidosis is not fully understood. Relative insulin deficiency, in combination with markedly elevated glucagon levels, causes hyperglycaemia. One theory suggests that there remains sufficient insulin peripherally to prevent lipolysis but not enough to cause glucose uptake into cells. Another theory is that the hyperosmolar state, coupled with dehydration, inhibits lipolysis and ketogenesis.

DIABETIC HYPOGLYCAEMIA

Hypoglycaemia most commonly occurs in the type I diabetic. The critical plasma level at which hypoglycaemia occurs varies between different individuals. Common precipitants include exercise, late meals, inadequate carbohydrate intake, ethanol ingestion and errors of insulin dosage.

PRESENTATION

The classic presentation of diabetes includes the characteristic symptoms of thirst, polyuria and weight loss. Other indicators, such as impairment of visual acuity, repeated skin sepsis, pain and paraesthesia in the limbs and genital pruritus, may occur. In approximately 10% of cases of type I diabetes, diabetic ketoacidosis is the initial presentation. In type II patients symptoms of diabetes are now known to occur late in the natural history of the disease. In the USA it has been estimated that type II diabetes is present for an average of 10–12 years before the diagnosis is made. Although uncommon, hyperglycaemic, hyperosmolar non-ketotic syndrome can be the initial presentation in type II diabetics.

The clinical presentation of DKA typically consists of nausea, vomiting, abdominal pain (thought to be due to the ketosis), polyuria, thirst, polydipsia, tiredness and malaise. Patients may notice the smell and taste of ketones. With increasing severity, drowsiness progressing to coma (directly related to serum osmolality), severe dehydration, hypotension, tachycardia and marked Kussmaul respiration develop.

In HHNS, the history is usually that of a prolonged illness over days or even weeks. Increasing lethargy, polyuria and polydipsia are often not appreciated by the patient, and the initial presentation is of increasing stupor, drowsiness or coma. Examination reveals severe dehydration, hypotension, neurological deficits such as hemiplegia or hemisensory loss, seizures and obtundation. The latter is related directly to the serum osmolality. Patients with HHNS may be labelled as having had a stroke. A high index of suspicion is necessary to make the diagnosis in the early stages of this illness.

Hypoglycaemia produces neurological and mental dysfunction. Less commonly, it can present as hypothermia, depression and psychosis. In some instances hypoglycaemia is entirely asymptomatic.

INVESTIGATIONS

Essential investigations in patients with DKA include: full blood examination; urea and electrolytes; glucose level; calcium, magnesium and phosphorus; arterial blood gases; CXR and ECG; urinalysis and blood cultures.

The nitroprusside test for measuring serum or urinary ketones detects aceto-

Table 10.1.1 Comparison of diabetic ketoacidosis (DKA) and hyperglycaemic, hyperosmolar non-ketotic syndrome (HHNS)

Characteristic	DKA	HHNS
Presentation	90% occur in known diabetics	Often initial
Frequency	Common	Uncommon
Usual type	Type I	Type II
Precipitant	>1/3 due to infection	More severe illness (e.g. AMI, sepsis)
Blood glucose	Often >16 mmol/L	Often >40 mmol/L
Serum osmolality	Usually <350 mmol/L	Usually >350 mmol/L
Fluid deficit	5–8 L	8–12 L
Ketoacidosis	Present	Absent
Prodrome	Short time frame	Long time frame
Mortality rate	5–10%	40–60%
Age range	Peak range 20–29 years	Peak range 57–70 years

acetate and acetone. It does not accurately detect b-hydroxybutyrate. The latter may be the predominant ketoacid in sepsis, hypotension or shock. Accordngly, if one of these conditions coexists with DKA, a negative nitroprusside test may obscure the diagnosis.

Investigations in the patient with HHNS are similar to those required for DKA. Calculated serum osmolality in HHNS is greater than 350 mmol/L in most patients.

DIFFERENTIAL DIAGNOSIS

Diabetes mellitus

Polyuria and polydipsia are cardinal presenting symptoms of diabetes mellitus. Other causes include:

- Diabetes insipidus
- Psychogenic polydipsia
- Electrolyte abnormalities: hypercalcaemia, hypokalaemia
- Thyrotoxicosis
- Drugs: TCAs, lithium, diuretics.

Diabetic ketoacidosis

- Hyperglycaemic, hyperosmolar non-ketotic syndrome
- Lactic acidosis (e.g. metformin)
- Alcoholic ketoacidosis
- Hypoglycaemic coma
- Other causes of anion-gap metabolic acidosis, e.g. anaemia, drugs (aspirin).

Hyperglycaemic, hyperosmolar non-ketotic syndrome

- DKA
- Cerebrovascular accident
- Sepsis
- Other metabolic causes of coma (e.g. hypothyroidism)
- Overdose.

MANAGEMENT

General management of diabetes mellitus

The Diabetes Control and Complications Trial (DCCT) Research Group published a landmark article in 1993[7] showing that intensive therapy in insulin-dependant diabetes mellitus (IDDM) patients effectively delays the onset and slows the progression of diabetic retinopathy, nephropathy and neuropathy. The findings from the DCCT have been incorporated with other education programmes to provide the following current recommendations for standards of care in patients with diabetes:

- Preprandial blood glucose between 4.4 and 6.6 mmol/L
- HbA$_1$C <7% (normal range 4–6%)
- Lipids: total cholesterol <200 mg/dL
- Fasting triglycerides <200 mg/dL
- Systolic BP <140 mmHg and diastolic BP <90 mmHg
- Urine albumin <30 mg/24 h.

Other important recent advances include the results of the Scandinavian Simvastatin Survival Study,[8] which showed that the use of simvastatin in diabetic patients with previous coronary heart disease significantly reduced the risk of future coronary heart disease, thus highlighting the importance of strict treatment of dyslipidaemia in diabetic patients. Also, the use of ACE inhibitors, even in normotensive patients with diabetes, delays the onset of diabetic nephropathy.

The sulphonylurea group of drugs and the biguanide metformin remain an important part of the management of type II diabetes. They are both oral hypoglycaemic agents that act by stimulating the pancreatic secretion of insulin in the case of the sulphonylurea group, and by suppressing hepatic glucose production and enhancing the peripheral use of glucose in the case of metformin.

Two new types of oral agents are now available for the treatment of diabetes. The alpha-glucosidase inhibitor acarbose and the thiazolidinediones pioglitazone and rosiglitazone, which now have a defined role in management and are available in Australia. Acarbose acts on the gastrointestinal tract to interfere with carbohydrate digestion. The thiazolidinediones act primarily by reducing insulin resistance thereby enhancing the effect of circulating insulin.[9]

Insulin was first administered to humans in 1922. Animal insulins (bovine, porcine) have been used for many years; however, in the 1980s human insulins were first made commercially available. Today, with the widespread availability of human insulins, animal insulins are of historical interest only. Table 10.1.2 illustrates the different types of insulins and the important parameters of each type.

Mixtures of short- and intermediate-acting insulins are also available: 70/30 (70% NPH/30% regular) and 50/50 (50% NPH/50% regular).

Insulin delivery is an area of much interest. Jet injectors reduce the pain of injection and medical waste, but the problems associated with subcutaneous injection remain. Intranasal administration has the problem of variability of absorption. In addition, unmodified

Table 10.1.2 Pharmacokinetic characteristics of currently available human insulins			
Insulin	Onset of action	Peak of action	Duration of action
Lispro*	5–15 minutes	1–2 hours	4–5 hours
Regular	30–60 minutes	2–4 hours	6–8 hours
NPH	1–2 hours	5–7 hours	13–18 hours
Lente	1–3 hours	4–8 hours	13–20 hours
Ultralente	2–4 hours	8–10 hours	18–30 hours

*Lispro insulin (Humalog®) is the first rapidly acting insulin analogue. It produces a peak blood insulin level 2–3 times higher than regular insulin.

insulin is poorly absorbed across mucous membranes, and, therefore, requires the addition of penetrating-enhancing vehicles (e.g. sodium glycocholate), the safety of which is yet to be established. Intrapulmonary administration is currently being studied in several large-scale trials. Finally, oral insulin (encapsulated in a liposomal envelope) has been incorporated into the Diabetes Prevention Trial.[7] It may have a role in diabetes prevention, possibly via an immune tolerance mechanism.

The first pancreas transplant for type I diabetes occurred in 1966. Over the 20-year period, 1977–1996, there have been approximately 8000 such transplants worldwide. Today, patients undergoing simultaneous pancreas and renal transplants have a 74% chance of pancreas graft survival and a 92% chance of renal graft survival at 1 year.

Current indications for pancreas transplantation are:

- Type I diabetes plus ESRF requiring renal transplant
- Type I diabetes, where insulin therapy is unreasonable or consistently fails to prevent metabolic complications.

Management of diabetic ketoacidosis

Initial resuscitation
- ABC approach
- Rapid colloid or crystalloid infusion for hypotension, shock.

Fluids
If hypotension is not present, give 0.9% saline at 500 mL/h for first 4 hours followed by 0.9% or 0.45% saline at 250 mL/h for next 4 hours. The decision to switch to a hypotonic solution (i.e. 0.45% saline) will depend on the serum sodium level and the rate of decrease of the serum osmolality.

Continue until serum glucose reaches 14 mmol/L, then change to 5% or 10% glucose.

In certain subgroups (e.g. haemodynamically unstable, CVS disease, elderly), CVP and PAWP monitoring may be required.

Insulin
A loading dose of 0.1–0.2 U/kg of regular insulin IV is followed by an infusion of regular insulin at a rate of 0.1 U/kg/hour. During the first 4–8 hours of treatment, blood glucose should be monitored hourly.

Reduce the infusion rate when the blood glucose reaches 14 mmol/L. However, the insulin must not be halted when euglycaemia is reached as in most cases, euglycaemia occurs before the ketosis is cleared.

If >100 U/h is required, administration of steroids is recommended.

Potassium
The whole body deficit is typically 3–5 mEq/kg. Despite this, patients frequently have elevated plasma potassium levels initially. The aim is to anticipate potassium shifts and maintain normal serum levels during treatment.

Other electrolytes
Although deficits of magnesium, calcium and phosphate exist, current literature does not support their routine replacement.

Management of hyperglycaemic, hyperosmolar non-ketotic syndrome
The principles of management of HHNS are similar to that of DKA. The following points, however, are unique to HHNS:

- The degree of dehydration is usually greater (the average fluid deficit is approximately 9 L of fluid). Losses of water exceed those of sodium, resulting in hypertonic dehydration. Significant fluid replacement is required early in the management of HHNS. How rapidly fluid is given depends on the response to therapy, blood pressure and urine output.
- Hypotensive patients should receive 0.9% saline initially unless they are severely hyperosmolar (>330 mOsm/L), in which case they should be given 0.45% saline.

- Once the patient is stable, 0.45% saline is used to replace the total deficit over 24 hours.
- As these patients are often older, with coexisting disease, early use of invasive monitoring is important.
- Insulin should be given as an infusion at 0.1 U/kg/h (i.e. similar to DKA). Concerns about insulin sensitivity and, therefore, the need for lower insulin doses has been questioned.
- Patients with HHNS are at particular risk of arterial and venous thrombosis and heparin prophylaxis should be given.

Management of hypoglycaemic coma
- The ABC approach is important in the patient with coma.
- 50 mL of 50% glucose should be given IV initially; further glucose administration is often necessary.
- 0.5–2 mg of glucagon can be given IV or IM in the patient with adequate liver glycogen stores. It would thus be unhelpful in the alcoholic patient.

DISPOSITION

Patients with DKA have historically required hospital admission, however, the role of outpatient management for a certain small subset of less sick patients has been defined. Suggested parameters permitting initial treatment in the emergency department, followed by early discharge home, include the following:[4]

- On presentation: pH >7.20, HCO$_3$ >10 mEq/L
- At 4 hours: pH >7.35, HCO$_3$ >20mEq/L, ability to take oral fluids, normal physical findings, ability to dipstick urine frequently for ketones and monitor fingerprick glucoses.

All patients diagnosed with HHNS should be admitted to hospital. Intensive care management is indicated for the initial phase of this illness.

CONTROVERSIES

❶ Fluid management: unless shock is present, the initial fluid rate should be slower than previously recommended for DKA management – 500 mL/h of 0.9% saline for the first 4 hours.

❷ Phosphate replacement: the routine replacement of phosphate in DKA is not recommended.

❸ Not all patients with DKA need admission: a subset of patients with DKA can be managed in the emergency department.

❹ Previously HHNS and DKA insulin infusion rates were different: the insulin infusion rate in HHNS should initially be the same as that for DKA.

PROGNOSIS

In DKA, infection and myocardial infarction are the two precipitants associated with a high mortality. Other factors associated with a worse outcome include increasing age, coma, and underlying cardiovascular and renal disease. One study showed that of deaths due to DKA, patient neglect contributed in 40% of cases, delay by the family doctor in 36%, and of those who died in hospital, poor management occurred in 46% of cases.[11]

Mortality remains high for HHNS: rates from 40 to 60% are quoted.

REFERENCES

1. Bonando WA, Gutzeit MF, Losek JD, et al 1988 Outpatient management of diabetic ketoacidosis. American Journal of Disease 142: 488–50
2. Alberti KGMM, DeFronzo RA, Keen H, Zimmet P 1992 International Textbook of Diabetes Mellitus. John Wiley & Sons Ltd, Chichester
3. Delaney MF, et al 2000 Diabetic ketoacidosis and hyperglycaemic hyperosmolar non-ketotic syndrome. Endocrinology and Metabolism Clinics of North America 29(4): 683–705
4. Fleckman AM 1993 Diabetic ketoacidosis. Endocrinology and Metabolism Clinics of North America 22(2): 181–207
5. Snorgard O 1989 diabetic ketoacidosis in Denmark. Journal of Intensive Medicine 226: 223–8
6. Fleckman AM 1991 Diabetic ketoacidosis. Practical Diabetology 10: 3
7. The Diabetes Control and Complications Trial Research Group 1993 The effect of intensive treatment of diabetes on the development and progression of long-term complications in insulin-dependent diabetes mellitus. New England Journal of Medicine 329: 977–88
8. Pyroala K, Pedersen TR, Kjekshus J, et al 1997 Cholesterol lowering with simvastatin improves prognosis of diabetic patients with coronary heart disease. A subgroup analysis of the Scandinavian Simvastatin Survival Study. Diabetes Care 20: 814–20
9. Lebovitz HE 1997 Alpha-glucosidase inhibitor in endocrine and metabolism. Clinics of North America 28(3): 547
10. Marshall SM, et al 1997 Diabetic ketoacidosis and hypoglycaemia in non ketotic comas. In: Alberti KGMM, DeFronzo RA, Zimmet P (eds) International Textbook of Diabetes Mellitus. John Wiley & Sons, pp. 1159–60
11. Deaths due to diabetic ketoacidosis 1981 Quarterly Journal of Medicine 50: 502–3

10.2 THYROID AND ADRENAL EMERGENCIES

ANDREW MACLEAN • PAMELA ROSENGARTEN

ESSENTIALS

1 The thyroid and adrenal emergencies posing an acute threat to life are thyroid storm, myxoedema coma and acute adrenal insufficiency. Diagnosis of these conditions requires a high index of suspicion and treatment frequently must be initiated upon clinical rather than laboratory diagnosis.

2 The usual features of thyroid storm are fever, alteration in mental state, cardiovascular complications such as tachyarrhythmias and cardiac failure, and signs of hyperthyroidism. Treatment is with β-blockers, drugs that block thyroid hormone synthesis and release, and corticosteroids.

3 The usual clinical features of myxoedema coma are an alteration in conscious state, hypothermia and features of hypothyroidism. Treatment is with intravenous tri-iodothyronine (T3) and corticosteroids.

4 The most important clinical feature of acute adrenal insufficiency is hypotension unresponsive to fluid therapy. Although hyponatraemia and hyperkalaemia are usual in acute adrenal insufficiency, electrolytes may be normal. Treatment is with intravenous corticosteroid replacement on suspicion of the diagnosis.

5 In all of these conditions general supportive measures and treatment of precipitating events must parallel the specific treatment regimes.

Table 10.2.1 Causes of thyrotoxicosis

Primary hyperthyroidism Graves disease Toxic multinodular goitre
Thyroiditis de Quervains Postpartum Radiation
Central hyperthyroidism Pituitary adenoma
Ectopic thyroid tissue
Metastatic thyroid tissue
Drug induced Lithium Iodine (including radiographic contrast) Amiodarone

INTRODUCTION

Three conditions are covered in this chapter – thyrotoxicosis, hypothyroidism and adrenal insufficiency. They present relatively infrequently to emergency departments but all are potentially fatal if they go unrecognized and untreated.

THYROTOXICOSIS

AETIOLOGY

There are a number of pathological causes for thyrotoxicosis (see Table 10.2.1).

CLINICAL FEATURES

The signs and symptoms of hyperthyroidism are secondary to the effects of excess thyroid hormone in the circula-tion. The severity of signs and symptoms may be related to the duration of the illness, the magnitude of the hormone excess, as well the age of the patient. The symptoms and signs summarized in Table 10.2.2 illustrate the spectrum of possible clinical features associated with the various causes of hyperthyroidism.

DIAGNOSIS

A comprehensive history and physical examination should be performed with particular attention to weight, blood pressure, pulse rate and rhythm, palpa-tion and auscultation of the thyroid to determine thyroid size, nodularity, and vascularity, neuromuscular examination, eye examination for evidence of exoph-thalmos or ophthalmopathy, and cardi-ascular examination looking specifically for cardiac failure.

Laboratory evaluation

The thyroid stimulating hormone (TSH) level is the single best screening test for hyperthyroidism. The recent development of sensitive TSH assays has greatly facilitated the diagnosis of hyperthyroid-ism. Hyperthyroidism of any cause (except excess TSH production) results in a lower than normal TSH.

Other laboratory and isotope tests may include:

- Free T4(thyroxine) or free T3(triiodothyronine) assay when the TSH is high or high normal and there is strong clinical suspicion of hyperthyroidism.
- Thyroid autoantibodies including TSH receptor antibody. These are not routinely necessary but may be helpful in selected cases.
- Radioactive iodine uptake and/or thyroid scan. These tests may be helpful in establishing the cause of hyperthyroidism but are not part of the emergency department assessment.

Table 10.2.2 Clinical features of thyrotoxicosis
Nervousness, irritability
Palpitations and tachycardia, in particular atrial fibrillation
Heat intolerance and increased sweating
Tremor
Weight loss and alterations in appetite
Frequent bowel movements
Fatigue and muscle weakness
Thyroid enlargement (depending on cause)
Pretibial myxoedema (with Graves disease)
Exertional intolerance and dyspnoea
Menstrual disturbance and impaired fertility
Mental disturbances
Sleep disturbances
Changes in vision, photophobia, eye irritation, diplopia or exophthalmos
Dependent lower extremity oedema
Sudden paralysis.

(Reproduced with permission from AACE Guidelines for the evaluation and Treatment of Hyperthyroidism and Hypothyroidism 1999. American Association of Clinical Endocrinologists)

TREATMENT

Mild hyperthyroidism does not require any treatment in the emergency department and may simply be referred to an appropriate outpatient setting. Any features of thyroid storm (see below) mandate admission, as does any significant intercurrent illness. Atrial arrhythmias should be controlled by the use of β-blockers. The aim is to achieve a rate of less than 100 beats per minute.

If thyroid blocking drugs are to be commenced in the emergency department ensure that all bloods have been collected first. High doses are often required initially to gain a response. The dose can then be tapered. Carbimazole 5–15 mg tds or propylthiouracil 50–150 mg qid is a reasonable starting dose with the larger doses being used for the more severe cases. It is preferable to discuss initiation of these agents with the physician who will be managing the patient after their discharge from emergency.

THYROID STORM

Thyroid storm occurs in about 1% of patients with hyperthyroidism. In most cases it occurs as an acute deterioration in a patient with poorly controlled or undiagnosed hyperthyroidism precipitated by factors such as surgery, trauma, infection, radioiodine, iodinated contrast, thyroxine ingestion or any other significant stressor.

The mortality rate in untreated patients is 90% and with treatment 10 to 15%.

The diagnosis is entirely clinical, as there is no test to differentiate it from thyrotoxicosis.

Clinical presentation
- Abrupt onset.
- Fever -> 37.6°C up to 41°C
- Cardiovascular complications -
  - tachycardia with pulse rates up to 200 to 300/min
  - atrial fibrillation
  - wide pulse pressure
  - high output cardiac failure

- Alteration in mental state is always present, varying from agitation and restlessness to delirium, coma and seizures.
- Abdominal pain with vomiting and diarrhoea is frequent.
- Features of thyrotoxicosis are present and are significantly exaggerated.
- Death is usually due to cardiovascular collapse.

Treatment
Treatment of thyroid storm is directed to blocking the peripheral effects of thyroid hormones, blocking thyroid hormone synthesis and release and corticosteroids.

β-blockers β blockade is the most important factor in decreasing morbidity and mortality. Many of the peripheral manifestations of hyperthyroidism, in particular the cardiovascular effects, can be reduced by the use of propranolol. As well as antagonizing the effects of thyroid hormones and the hypersensitivity to catecholamines, propranolol inhibits the peripheral conversion of T_4 to T_3. Intravenous increments of 0.5 mg should be given initially up to 10 mg in total. Continuous cardiovascular monitoring is essential. Subsequent doses of 40–120 mg 6 hourly can be given orally. β-blockers should effectively treat the cardiac failure secondary to the tachyarrhythmia or high cardiac output, but may cause complications in patients with pre-existing heart disease or asthma. In this situation esmolol may be used, as any adverse effects will be of brief duration due to its short half-life. A 250–500 µg/kg bolus is followed by an infusion starting at 50–100 µg/kg/min that can then be titrated to effect. Another option is to carefully use a combination of a β-blocker and digoxin.

Thyroid blocking drugs Propylthiouracil (900–1200 mg loading dose) is given orally or via a nasogastric tube if necessary. The loading dose is followed by 200–300 mg, 4–6 hourly. Propylthiouracil acts by preventing hormone synthesis by blocking the iodination of tyrosine and also inhibits the peripheral conversion of T_4 to T_3. Iodine in large doses inhibits the synthesis and release of thyroid hormones. It can be given either orally as Lugol's iodine, 30–60 drops daily in divided doses, or intravenously as sodium iodide, 1 g IV 12 hourly. Lithium carbonate can be used in patients are allergic to iodine.

General supportive measures Dehydration and electrolyte disturbances need correction. Aggressive treatment of hyperthermia with paracetamol and cooling measures is necessary but induction of shivering should be avoided. Salicylates are contraindicated as they displace T_4 from binding proteins.

Corticosteroids are given, as a relative deficiency may be present and also to inhibit the peripheral conversion of T_4 to T_3. Hydrocortisone 100 mg IV 6 hourly or dexamethasone 2 mg IV 6 hourly are used.

Treatment of the precipitating cause A meticulous search for a cause is vital, as correct treatment will improve the prognosis.

APATHETIC HYPERTHYROIDISM

Patients with this condition are generally older, although it has been recorded in all age groups. The clinical picture is of depressed mental state and cardiac complications, in particular cardiac failure. Weight loss is usually significant and eye signs are rare. Most of the usual hyperkinetic manifestations of hyperthyroidism are absent. Treatment is as for standard hyperthyroidism.

HYPOTHYROIDISM

Hypothyroidism results from undersecretion of thyroid hormone from the thyroid gland. Causes of primary hypothyroidism include chronic autoimmune thyroiditis (Hashimoto's thyroiditis), surgical removal of the thyroid gland, radioactive iodine, thyroid gland ablation

and external irradiation. A significant number of cases are idiopathic. Secondary causes of hypothyroidism include pituitary and hypothalamic disease.

CLINICAL FEATURES

The symptoms are generally related to the duration and severity of hypothyroidism, the rapidity with which hypothyroidism occurs and the psychological characteristics of the patient. These are summarized in Table 10.2.3.

When a patient has a goitre, a complete evaluation including a comprehensive history and physical examination and appropriate laboratory evaluation should be performed. Patients with chronic thyroiditis have a higher incidence of other associated autoimmune diseases such as vitiligo, rheumatoid arthritis, Addison's disease, diabetes mellitus, and pernicious anaemia.

DIAGNOSIS

Laboratory evaluation

A TSH assay should always be used as the primary test to establish the diagnosis of hypothyroidism.

Additional tests may include free thyroxine assay, thyroid autoantibodies, thyroid scan and/or ultrasound if structural thyroid abnormalities are suspected.

Thyroid autoantibodies are positive in 95% of patients with autoimmune thyroiditis (Hashimoto's thyroiditis) and high titres are of great value in making this specific diagnosis. Thyroid nodules are not uncommon with chronic thyroiditis and carry a small risk of thyroid cancer.

TREATMENT

Rapid commencement of full thyroid hormone replacement can result in myocardial ischaemia because of an increase of myocardial oxygen consumption without a corresponding increase in cardiac output. In adults the initial daily

Table 10.2.3 Clinical features of hypothyroidism
Fatigue
Constipation
Weight gain/obesity
Memory and mental impairment, decreased concentration
Depression, personality changes
Dry skin and cold intolerance
Yellow skin
Coarse facial features
Enlarged tongue
Coarse brittle hair or loss of hair, loss outer 1/3 eyebrows
Irregular or heavy menses and infertility
Hoarseness
Myalgias
Goitre
Hyperlipidaemia
Delayed relaxation phase of tendon reflexes, ataxia
Bradycardia and hypothermia.

(Reproduced with permission from AACE Guidelines for the evaluation and Treatment of Hyperthyroidism and Hypothyroidism 1999. American Association of Clinical Endocrinologists)

replacement dose is therefore 25 μg of T_4, which should remain unchanged for 3–4 weeks to allow a steady state to be reached. It is appropriate to start this in the emergency department if a firm diagnosis has been made and appropriate follow-up arranged. The dose is then increased at 25–50 μg increments until the optimum dose is reached as determined by clinical response and TSH level. Admission should be considered for any patient with coexistent unstable angina to monitor cardiac function. Any features of myxoedema coma (see below) mandate admission.

MYXOEDEMA COMA

The clinical syndrome of altered mental state, features of hypothyroidism and hypothermia is referred to as myxoedema coma. There is usually a precipitating event such as infection, stroke, trauma, myocardial infarction or administration of drugs particularly phenothiazines, phenytoin, amiodarone, propranolol or lithium that initiates this terminal decompensation phase of hypothyroidism.

The mortality for myxoedema coma remains up to 50% despite aggressive treatment.

CLINICAL PRESENTATION

- Altered mental state, usually coma due to cerebral oedema, hypoxia and hypercarbia.
- Seizures may precede coma in 25% patients.
- Hypothermia with temperature usually less that 32.2°C. Notably patients do not shiver.
- Hypoventilation resulting in hypoxia and hypercarbia.
- Cardiovascular complications including hypotension and bradycardia, with heart rate inappropriate to the hypotension. Pericardial effusion, rarely tamponade.
- Hypoglycaemia is common.
- Hyponatraemia.
- Paralytic ileus, megacolon, urinary retention.
- Clinical features of hypothyroidism.

Treatment should commence on clinical suspicion:

- Administration of thyroid hormones - there is no consensus as to whether T_3 or T_4 replacement is preferable.[6,13] Intravenous T_3 being the active form of the hormone may give a faster clinical response in myxoedema coma. It is given as an initial bolus of 25–50 μg followed by 10–20 μg 8 hourly. Some clinicians prefer a continuous infusion with a lower total dose of 20 μg per day, as large initial doses may not be necessary for recovery and may in fact be harmful. Oral or nasogastric replacement of T_3 is not recommended in the initial phase of management because of unreliable gastrointestinal absorption.

The use of T_4 is supported on the grounds that the gradual delivery of T_3 through the peripheral conversion of T_4 is better tolerated and that the onset of action is more predictable. A 400–500 μg bolus (300 g/m²) followed by 50 μg IV daily until oral therapy is tolerated is recommended. Combined approaches are now also described.

- Corticosteroids are given as there is impaired response to stress and potential co-existent adrenal insufficiency. Hydrocortisone 100 mg 6 hourly is recommended.
- General supportive measures including correction of ventilatory, circulatory, temperature and metabolic abnormalities. Use of warm humidified oxygen is beneficial.
- Treat the precipitating cause.
- Any sedating drugs should be avoided and great care needs to be taken not to water overload the patient.

ADRENOCORTICAL INSUFFICIENCY

AETIOLOGY

The majority of presentations of acute adrenal insufficiency occur as an exacerbation of a chronic disease process. Acute precipitating factors include sepsis, major injury, surgery and acute myocardial infarction. These do not normally lead to an acute crisis but will do so where there is a malfunctioning adrenal system.

CAUSES

The causes of primary adrenocortical insufficiency include autoimmune (Addison's disease – 80%), primary or secondary malignancy, infection such as tuberculosis, Freidrich-Waterhouse syndrome from meningococcaemia or severe sepsis, haemorrhage into the adrenal glands and drugs. Secondary causes include pituitary failure and the most common cause of adrenocortical insufficiency, which is suppression of adrenopituitary axis by long-term steroid therapy.

CLINICAL PRESENTATION

- Hypotension: suspect adrenocortical failure in the hypotensive patient without an apparent cause who is unresponsive to fluid therapy. Orthostatic hypotension is almost always present.
- Abdominal pain which may be severe, with vomiting.
- Other features including weakness, postural syncope, anorexia, mucocutaneous pigmentation/ vitiligo (if primary adrenal disease) and mental state alteration.

This diagnosis should be suspected in any patient with refractory hypotension.

LABORATORY INVESTIGATIONS

The classical laboratory findings are hyponatraemia (due to sodium depletion and the intracellular movement of sodium), hypochloraemia and hyperkalaemia (due to acidosis and aldosterone deficiency). Mild hypercalcaemia (in 10–20% of cases) and a non-anion gap metabolic acidosis may be present. Hypoglycaemia if present is usually mild. However, all basic laboratory investigations may be normal in the presence of an Addisonian crisis.

DIAGNOSIS

Baseline cortisol and ACTH levels should be taken prior to treatment. ACTH may be high in primary adrenal disease or low in pituitary disease. The Synacthen® stimulation test is the definitive test and may be required subsequently if the initial test results are not diagnostic. Anti-adrenal antibodies are positive in 70% of patients with autoimmune adrenalitis.

TREATMENT

If the acute adrenal insufficiency is suspected treatment should not be delayed awaiting confirmatory results:

- Corticosteroid replacement with either intravenous hydrocortisone or dexamethasone is essential. Dexamethasone is given as 10 mg stat followed by 4 mg 8 hourly, whereas hydrocortisone is given in a dose of 250 mg stat followed by 100 mg 6 hourly. Dexamethasone is recommended where the diagnosis has not been confirmed by laboratory investigations as it does not interfere with cortisol assay.[12]
- Fluid replacement therapy: normal saline infusion 1 L stat, then titrated to response (volume deficit rarely greater than 10%). Intravenous 5%

dextrose should be given at the same time either separately or as 5% dextrose in normal saline.

- General supportive measures including treatment of hypoglycaemia and any symptomatic electrolyte abnormalities. Most of these will be corrected with saline rehydration alone.
- Mineralocorticoid replacement is usually not necessary in the acute crisis if salt and water replacement is adequate.
- Once the crisis has been successfully treated it is important to investigate and manage the cause and develop a maintenance regime.

FURTHER READING

AACE Guidelines for the Evaluation and Treatment of Hyperthyroidism and Hypothyroidism 1999 American Association of Clinical Endocrinologists

Edwards CRW, Baird JD, Toft AD 1991 Endocrine and metabolic diseases. In: Davidson's Principles and Practice of Medicine. Churchill Livingstone, Edinburgh

Frederick R 1991 Addisonian Crisis: Emergency presentation of primary adrenal insufficiency. Annals Emergency Medicine 20: 802–6

Franklin JA 1994 The management of hyperthyroidism. New England Journal Medicine 330: 1731–8

Hurlburt K, Iserson K 1990 Adrenal emergencies In: Wolfson AB (ed.) Endocrine and Metabolic Emergencies. Churchill Livingstone, New York

Jordan RM 1995 Myxedema coma. Medical Clinics of North America 79: 185–94

The Royal College of Pathologists of Australia 1997 Manual of the Use and Interpretation of Pathology Tests, 2nd edn. The Royal College of Pathologists of Australia, Sydney

Mitchell JM, Almquist T 1990 Thyroid disease in the emergency department. In: Wolfson AB (ed.) Endocrine and Metabolic Emergencies. Churchill Livingstone, New York

Rao RH 1995 Bilateral massive adrenal haemorrhage. Med Clin North Am,79: 107–29

Stockigt JR 1993 Thyroid disease. Medical Journal of Australia 158: 770–4

Tietgens ST, Leinung MC 1995 Thyroid storm. Medical Clinics of North America 79: 169–84

Vedig AE 1997 Adrenocortical insufficiency. In: Oh TE (ed.) Intensive Care Manual, 4th edn. Butterworths, London

Vedig AE 1997 Thyroid emergencies. In: Oh TE (ed.) Intensive Care Manual, 4th edn. Butterworths, London

Wartofsky L 1998 Diseases of the thyroid. In: Wilson JD, Braunwald E, et al (eds) Harrisons Principles of Internal Medicine, 14th edn. McGraw-Hill, New York

Williams GH, Dluhy RG 1998 Diseases of the adrenal cortex. In: Wilson JD, Braunwald E, et al (eds) Harrisons Principles of Internal Medicine, 14th edn. McGraw-Hill, New York

10.3 ALCOHOLIC KETOACIDOSIS

MICHAEL RAGG

ESSENTIALS

1 Alcoholic ketoacidosis (AKA) usually occurs in the chronic alcohol abuser who has experienced vomiting and reduced food intake prior to presentation.

2 AKA causes an anion-gap metabolic acidosis, but the exact pathophysiological basis for this condition is not completely understood.

3 β-Hydroxybutyrate is the predominant ketoacid found in AKA. The nitroprusside test does not detect this, and so early in this condition urinalysis may be negative for ketones. In reality this is uncommon.

4 The principles of management are replacement of fluid and electrolyte deficits, provision of thiamine, and treatment of the intercurrent illness.

5 A subset of patients with AKA can be managed in the emergency department.

INTRODUCTION

Alcoholic ketoacidosis (AKA) was first described by Dillon et al in 1940.[1] The disorder usually (but not invariably) occurs in poorly nourished chronic alcohol abusers who have experienced vomiting and decreased food intake prior to presentation. Precipitants, such as 'binge drinking' and intercurrent illness are often involved. In one study of 74 patients with AKA, the most common intercurrent illnesses were pancreatitis (36%), myopathy/rhabdomyolysis (18%), gastritis/upper GI bleeding (16%), seizures (15%), hepatitis/cirrhosis (12%), alcohol withdrawal (11%), hypoglycaemia (8%) and infection (8%).

It is important to note, however, that AKA can occur in first-time drinkers who are starved, although this is rare.

The pathophysiological basis for AKA is complex and not completely understood. Although the physiological factors that exist with AKA are known, the exact reason why it begins and why not all people are affected is unknown. In all people who are starved, the liver will produce ketones from fatty acids to supply the brain, kidney and other organs with metabolic fuel. Here ketones replace glucose as a substrate for oxidative phosphorylation. In AKA the production is not balanced by removal, and thus accumulation occurs.

The chronic consumption of alcohol leads to an elevation of the ratio of dihydronicotinamide (NADH) to nicotinamide adenine dinucleotide (NAD). This occurs through a reduction reaction in the metabolism of ethanol in the hepatic cell. It is this increased ratio that is thought to limit gluconeogenesis via the inhibition of the enzyme pyruvate carboxylase. This, added to the patient's starved state, leads to the rapid depletion of glycogen stores. An increase in lipolysis occurs in response, leading to high levels of circulating free fatty acids and hence ketogenesis. The principal ketocid produced is β-hydroxybutyrate.

Other factors are also important in the pathogenesis of AKA. The underlying illness causes vomiting and eventually dehydration. Once this state is reached, an increase in circulating catecholamine and cortisol levels occurs that will also stimulate lipolysis and hence ketogenesis. In addition, an extracellular fluid deficit causes a decrease in renal perfusion and thus impairs the body's ability to excrete ketoacids. It is, therefore, this combination of factors that leads to ketoacidosis in these patients.

The metabolic acidosis found in the patient with AKA is usually not entirely due to ketoacids. Lactic acidosis is often present to some degree. Thiamin deficiency, severe dehydration leading to shock, and intercurrent illnesses such as rhabdomyolysis may all directly cause increased levels of lactic acid.

PRESENTATION

AKA is generally seen in the chronic alcohol abuser, who has recently abruptly ceased or decreased their intake of alcohol. The common presenting symptoms are nausea, vomiting, anorexia, abdominal pains and poor caloric intake. Other symptoms include shortness of breath, tremulousness, dizziness, fever, haematemesis and muscle pains. Of these, the most common are nausea, vomiting and abdominal pain.

Examination usually reveals no alteration or a slight impairment in conscious state, in contrast to hyperosmolar non-ketotic coma in diabetics. Patients may rarely present comatose, in which case alcohol-induced hypoglycaemia and other causes of altered conscious state such as head injury need to be excluded. Vital signs vary according to the degree of dehydration and the nature of the precipitating illness.

Other findings on physical examination include abdominal tenderness secondary to such conditions as gastritis, pancreatitis, peptic ulcer disease and alcoholic hepatitis. Abdominal findings other than tenderness are uncommon, although signs of an acute abdomen may reflect a coexisting surgical intraperitoneal process. Signs of chronic liver disease or alcohol withdrawal syndrome may also be present.

INVESTIGATIONS

The laboratory findings in AKA reflect acidosis secondary to ketoacids and electrolyte changes as a consequence of vomiting and dehydration. The two major ketoacids in this condition are β-hydroxybutyrate (BOHB) and aceto-acetate (AcAc). The ratio of BOHB to acetoacetate is typically elevated, as the elevated $NADH/NAD^+$ ratio favours the formation of BOHB rather than AcAc. Acetone levels are not increased. The importance of this is that when urine or blood ketones are qualitatively measured, a nitroprusside test is commonly used. This is most sensitive to acetoacetate, less sensitive to acetone, and not at all to BOHB. Therefore, the initial testing of a patient with AKA may be negative or weakly positive, although the results of the largest study to date suggest that this is in fact uncommon.[3]

Although a raised anion-gap metabolic acidosis is the most common abnormality found in AKA, other mixed pictures may also occur:

- Primary metabolic acidosis plus primary respiratory alkalosis, the latter as a result of abdominal pain or alcohol withdrawal syndrome
- Primary metabolic acidosis plus primary metabolic alkalosis, the latter due to severe vomiting
- Triple acid-base disorder, i.e. primary metabolic acidosis, primary metabolic alkalosis and primary respiratory alkalosis.

The raised anion gap in AKA is largely due to BOHB and acetoacetate. However, in the volume-depleted alcohol patient, electrolyte abnormalities may contribute to the anion gap.

Biochemical parameters will often reveal an initial serum potassium level within normal limits, despite these patients having a total body potassium depletion. Indeed, if gastrointestinal losses are large, this deficit may be severe. Both serum chloride and bicarbonate levels are usually low. Hypophosphataemia was found in 25% of patients in one study.[2]

Serum glucose levels are variable, ranging from hypoglycaemia to mild hyperglycaemia. Marked hyperglycaemia usually indicates diabetic ketoacidosis; however, if it is observed during an episode of AKA, an erroneous diagnosis of diabetic ketoacidosis may be made.

Liver function tests will often reveal some abnormalities, although marked changes are uncommon. Similarly, serum lactate levels in patients with AKA are usually only mildly elevated. Serum ethanol levels are often low or undetectable. Haematological indices are nonspecific.

DIFFERENTIAL DIAGNOSIS

The differential diagnosis of AKA is that of a raised anion-gap metabolic acidosis, where there is a history of chronic alcohol consumption, and includes:

- Diabetic ketoacidosis
- Lactic acidosis
- Ingestion of alcohols other than ethanol such as ethylene glycol, methanol or isopropyl alcohol
- Salicylate intoxication
- Uraemia
- Other rarer causes, including inhaled industrial acetylene, cyanide, toluene, formaldehyde, nalidixic acid, hippuric acid and oxalic acid.

A mild degree of lactic acidosis often accompanies AKA, as previously mentioned. Other alternative diagnoses such as severe pancreatitis, serious acute illness associated with circulatory collapse, a postictal state, or even thiamine deficiency should be excluded if a severe lactic acidosis is detected.

TREATMENT

The treatment of AKA includes:

- Correction of immediately life-threatening problems
- Restoration of extracellular fluid deficit
- Treatment of the electrolyte and metabolic derangement
- Provision of thiamine to prevent Wernicke's encephalopathy
- Treatment of any intercurrent illness.

The immediate treatment of imminent or actual circulatory collapse is rapid intravenous fluid administration. If frank hypotension is present, the use of a colloid is appropriate. Otherwise, 0.9% saline not only replaces the volume deficit, but may also promote renal excretion of ketone bodies. Following the administration of 0.9% saline, the next type of intravenous fluid to continue management is a mixture of sodium chloride and glucose. One study has compared the effect of treatment with saline alone with that of glucose administration (5% dextrose).[3] In this study it was noted that the group treated with glucose alone had a more rapid correction of their acidosis and a faster decline in levels of β-hydroxybutyrate and acetoacetate. Glucose is believed to be essential in terminating ketogenesis and repleting glycogen stores.

The patient with AKA is usually potassium and phosphorus depleted. Potassium replacement should be given if the serum potassium level is low, or if a normal serum potassium level exists in the presence of acidaemia. Routine replacement of phosphorus is not recommended. Magnesium helps restore calcium and potassium homoeostasis, and may also help prevent the alcohol-withdrawal syndrome.[4-6] In addition, these patients are often magnesium depleted as a result of chronic alcohol consumption. Therefore, magnesium should also be replaced in patients with AKA.

Finally, thiamine must be given to all patients with AKA. It is necessary to prevent Wernicke's encephalopathy and is also an essential cofactor for the decarboxylation of pyruvate in the metabolism of glucose. Other essential vitamins, in the form of multivitamin preparations, may be given in addition.

DISPOSITION

Any intercurrent or precipitating illness must be treated. As the acidosis of AKA usually clears in 12–24 hours it may be possible to manage some of these patients in the emergency department. However, if the underlying condition is serious (e.g. acute pancreatitis) the patient must be admitted.

Patients with AKA that are appropriate for discharge include those that are able to tolerate oral fluids, are haemodynamically stable with no orthostatic hypotension, and in whom both the metabolic abnormalities and the underlying illness have resolved.

PROGNOSIS

The prognosis of AKA is related to the underlying intercurrent illness. AKA itself is associated with a good prognosis.

REFERENCES

1. Dilon ES, Dyer WW, Smelo LS 1940 Ketone acidosis in non-diabetic adults. Medical Clinics of North America 24: 1813
2. Wrenn K, Slovis C, Minion G, et al 1991 The syndrome of alcoholic ketoacidosis. American Journal of Medicine 91: 119–28
3. Fullop M 1993 Alcoholic ketoacidosis. Endocrinology and Metabolism Clinics of North America 22: 209–19
4. Tso EL, Barish RA 1992 Magnesium: Clinical considerations. Emergency Medicine in Review 10: 735–45
5. Lim P, Jacob E 1972 Magnesium status of alcoholic patients. Metabolism 21: 1045–8
6. Berkelhammer C, Bear RA 1985 A clinical approach to common electrolyte problems: Hypomagnesemia. Canadian Medical Association Journal 132: 360–8

FURTHER READING

Fulop M 1993 Alcoholic ketoacidosis. Endocrinology and Metabolism Clinics of North America 22(2): 209–12
Ragg MA, Eddey D 1995 Does alcoholic ketoacidosis go undetected? Emergency Medicine 7(4): 31–5

SECTION

11

EDITED BY LINDSAY MURRAY

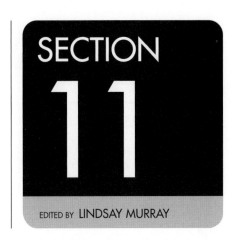

METABOLIC

11.1 **Acid-base disorders** 476

11.2 **Electrolyte disturbances** 481

11.1 ACID-BASE DISORDERS

ROBERT DUNN

ESSENTIALS

1 Acid-base disorders are classified according to the major abnormality (acidosis or alkalosis) and its origin (metabolic or respiratory). Mixed disorders are common.

2 Calculation of the 'anion gap' may be useful in determining the origin of a metabolic acidosis.

3 Lactic acidosis is the most common cause of metabolic acidosis.

4 Treatment of acidosis is directed toward correction of the underlying cause; administration of $NaHCO_3$ is indicated in a small number of conditions.

5 Metabolic alkalosis in the emergency department is usually secondary to prolonged vomiting, and its management is directed towards rehydration with normal saline and correction of the underlying cause.

6 The alveolar gas equation allows comparison of arterial and alveolar partial pressures of oxygen; a higher than expected value is indicative of a ventilation-perfusion defect.

INTRODUCTION

Acid-base disorders are commonly encountered in the emergency department, and their recognition is important for the diagnosis, assessment of severity and monitoring of many disease processes. Although these disorders are usually classified according to the major metabolic abnormality present (acidosis or alkalosis) and its origin (metabolic or respiratory), it is important to realize that acid-base disorders of a mixed type commonly occur and that the recognition and assessment of these is more complex.

NORMAL VALUES

To interpret acid-base disorders one must be familiar with the concept of pH and aware of the normal ranges for pH, P_aCO_2, and HCO_3^-. The pH is the log $[H^+]$ and may be derived from a number of formulae, such as:

$$pH = 6.1 + \log[HCO_3^-]/(0.03 \times P_{CO_2})$$

or

$$pH = pK + \log[A^-]/[HA]$$

(the Henderson Hasselbalch equation).[1]

The serum pH is normally maintained between 7.35 and 7.45, which represents an $[H^+]$ of approximately 40 nmol/L. The normal range of arterial P_{CO_2} is between 35 and 45 mmHg and the arterial $[HCO_3^-]$ is between 22 and 26 mmol/L. Venous HCO_3^- has a normal range of 24–28 mmol/L and is higher than that of arterial blood due to the exchange of HCO_3^- for Cl^- (the 'chloride shift') that occurs as a result of CO_2 transport by haemoglobin from the tissues. Oxygen saturation is calculated by many blood gas analyzers and assumes that the oxygen-haemoglobin dissociation curve is in a 'normal' position. This calculation may be inaccurate in the presence of chronic hypoxia where increased levels of 2-3DPG will alter the position of the curve. Measurement of haemoglobin saturation by co-oximetry is the 'gold standard', however, this is uncommonly used.

DEFINITIONS AND CONVENTIONS

The P_{O_2} and P_{CO_2} are the partial pressures of oxygen and carbon dioxide, and the site to which this refers to is denoted by various prefixes. The symbol 'i' indicates inspired gas, 'a' indicates arterial blood and 'A' indicates alveolar gas. Where no prefix is used, it is usually

assumed that the value relates to arterial blood. The base excess is defined as the number of mmol of acid needed to be added to 1 L of whole blood (at STP) to return it to a pH of 7.4. The standard base excess is the number of mmol of acid needed to be added to 1 L of whole blood with a P_{CO_2} of 40 mmHg (at STP) to return it to a pH of 7.4.

VENOUS GAS CORRELATION

In many situations, arterial blood sampling is not needed to provide the information required regarding the patient's acid base status. If an arterial blood sample is difficult to obtain or the determination of P_{O_2} or P_{CO_2} are not important, the measurement of either venous or capillary pH and HCO_3^- are acceptable alternatives.[2,3] In the absence of shock, the venous pH is approximately 0.05 less than the arterial pH. Venous blood for pH determination should be obtained as close as possible to the central venous system.[3]

ARTERIAL BLOOD GAS SPECIMEN COLLECTION

When attempting arterial blood gas specimen collection, the non-dominant limb should be used whenever possible. The radial artery at the wrist is the most commonly used site for specimen collection in adults, as it is easily accessible with the patient sitting upright. This is particularly useful when the patient is in respiratory distress.

Before attempting radial arterial puncture, an Allen's test should be performed to confirm the patency of the ulnar artery. To perform this test, the patient is asked to elevate the selected arm and make a tight fist while both the radial and ulnar arteries are occluded with firm pressure from the thumbs of the examiner. After a few minutes the arm is lowered to waist level and the patient opens the hand. The pressure over the ulnar artery is then released while that over the radial artery is maintained. In a negative test, normal skin colour returns to the palm within 2 seconds. In a positive test the hand remains white for longer than 2 seconds. A positive test indicates that the flow in the ulnar artery may be insufficient to maintain the viability of the hand should the radial artery become thrombosed following arterial puncture. In the presence of a positive test another site for arterial puncture should be used.

Following skin preparation with antiseptic, a needle attached to a heparinized syringe is inserted along the line of the artery at an angle of 45° to the skin and with the bevel pointing upwards in order to maximize the area of the needle inlet exposed to arterial blood flow. Although flow may be less, a 25G needle is the preferred size in the well-perfused patient as it causes significantly less pain and vascular trauma than larger needle sizes. In the presence of hypotension, a 23G needle should be used to enable filling of the syringe. Once in the artery, arterial blood should fill the syringe against gravity. Slow filling in the well-perfused patient suggests incorrect needle position and sampling of accompanying veins. Some syringes may also require the barrel to be withdrawn to the desired amount to be collected. Once at least 0.25 mL, and preferably 0.5 mL, of blood has been collected the needle is removed quickly and direct pressure applied over the puncture site for at least 5 minutes. All air bubbles should be expelled from the sample prior to capping the syringe with an airtight stopper and the specimen immediately transported to the point of analysis. The temperature of the patient should be noted for entry into the analyzer. If a delay in analysis of more than 15 minutes is likely, or an arterial lactate measurement is required, the specimen should be packed in ice.[4]

If the radial artery is unsuitable, the brachial artery at the cubital fossa may be used. This approach requires the elbow to remain extended throughout the procedure. The femoral artery is an acceptable alternative, however, in infants, the close proximity of the femoral head to the femoral artery makes this a less desirable site. To perform femoral arterial puncture, the patient must be supine and the needle should be at least 23G in size.

The contraindications for arterial puncture are a positive Allen's test (for the radial artery approach), an absent pulse or cellulitis at the insertion site, or severe coagulopathy (relative contraindication only). Complications are rare following a single small-bore needle arterial puncture, but include local or generalized sepsis, arterial thrombosis and distal tissue ischaemia.

An arterial catheter should be inserted if repeated arterial or venous punctures are required, invasive blood pressure monitoring indicated, or access for arteriovenous haemofiltration is required. The approaches used for arterial catheter insertion are the same as those for arterial puncture, and Seldinger or non-Seldinger techniques can be used. Whenever possible, femoral artery catheterization should be avoided due to the high incidence of infective and thromboembolic complications. Local anaesthesia should be used prior to arterial catheter insertion; the catheter should be sutured in place after insertion and connected to a line pressurized to 250–300 mmHg. The appropriate catheter sizes for insertion are 18–20G for the radial artery, 16G for the femoral artery and 12G for arteriovenous haemofiltration.

ACIDOSIS

Systemic acidosis is defined as the presence of an increased concentration of H+ ions in the blood. The physiological effects of acidosis are a decrease in the affinity of haemoglobin for oxygen and an increase in serum K+ of approximately 0.4–0.6 mmol/L for each decrease in pH of 0.1. It is commonly believed that acidosis decreases myocardial contractility, but this is usually of little clinical significance at a pH of more than 7.1. Although the presence of acidosis is often associated with a poor prognosis, the presence of acidosis per se usually has little clinically significant effects, and it is the nature and severity of the underlying illness that determines outcome. In certain situations, such as in pregnant women and in the neonate, increased acid production may result in a greater change in serum pH (and possibly greater adverse physiological effects) than expected, owing to the decreased buffering capacity of the plasma. A decrease in measured serum HCO_3^- of up to 5 mmol/L has also been reported as a result of underfilling of vacuum-type specimen tubes.[5]

METABOLIC ACIDOSIS

Metabolic acidosis is defined as an increase in the [H+] of the blood as a result of increased acid production or decreased acid elimination by routes other than the lungs. The cause is often multifactorial and can be further classified into 'anion-gap' and 'non-anion gap' metabolic acidosis.

Anion gap

As electroneutrality must exist in all solutions, the 'anion gap' represents the concentration of anions that are not commonly measured. The most commonly used formula for the calculation of the 'anion gap' is:

$$\text{Anion gap} = ([Na] + [K]) - ([Cl] + [HCO_3])$$

The normal value for the anion gap depends on the analyser used and whilst the upper limit of normal has been commonly quoted as being 18, the mean range with some modern analyzers is only 5–12.[6-7] In the normal resting state this is mostly accounted for the concentration of ionic proteins in the serum, with a lesser contribution from other 'unmeasured' anions such as PO_4^- and SO_4^-. In pathological conditions where there is an increase in the concentration of 'unmeasured' anions, an 'anion-gap' metabolic acidosis results. The anions responsible for the increase in the 'anion gap' depend on the aetiology of the acidosis. Lactic acid is the predominant anion in hypoxia and shock, PO_4^- and SO_4^- in renal failure, ketoacids in diabetic and alcoholic ketoacidosis, oxalic acid in ethylene glycol poisoning, and formic acid in methanol poisoning.[8]

Of the causes of an anion-gap metabolic acidosis, lactic acidosis is the most commonly encountered in the emergency department and is defined as a serum lactate of greater than 2.5 mmol/L. The causes of lactic acidosis can be broadly grouped into conditions of increased lactate production or decreased metabolism. In the seriously ill patient it is common for both of these to be present simultaneously. Tissue hypoxia of any cause decreases oxidative phosphorylation and results in the increased conversion of pyruvate to lactate. This is commonly seen in major haemorrhage and in the presence of severe cardiorespiratory disease. An alternative cause for increased lactate production may be the uncoupling of oxidative phosphorylation following exposure to toxins, such as cyanide, salicylates, metformin and iron.[8] Severe thiamine deficiency may result in a marked increase in lactate production known as warm beri-beri. Metabolism of lactic acid occurs in the liver and kidney and is reduced when these organs are diseased or in the presence of alkalosis, hypothermia and diabetes mellitus.

It is important to realize that, in many conditions, a variety of factors may produce the acidosis, and that multiple anions may be involved in the production of an 'anion-gap' acidosis. For example, in a patient with severe diabetic ketoacidosis, poor tissue perfusion, renal failure, increased lactic and ketoacid production, decreased SO_4^- and PO_4^- elimination and decreased lactic acid metabolism may all be present. Lactic acidosis is generally considered to be severe if serum lactate is >4 mmol/L. Serum lactate should be measured by immediate assay of arterial blood, as levels decrease rapidly following sampling.

Non-anion gap

Non-anion gap metabolic acidosis is a result of loss of HCO_3^- from the body, rather than increased acid production. To maintain electroneutrality, chloride is usually retained as HCO_3^- is lost, and the hallmark of non-anion gap acidosis is an elevation of the serum chloride. The causes of non-anion gap metabolic acidosis are further classified according to the site of HCO_3^- loss. Gastrointestinal losses can occur with lower GIT fluid losses that are rich in HCO_3^-, or with cholestyramine ingestion due to binding of HCO_3^- in the gut. Renal losses can occur with renal tubular acidosis, carbonic anhydrase inhibitor therapy or adrenocortical insufficiency. Acid is rarely ingested in sufficient quantity so as to cause systemic acidosis.

RENAL TUBULAR ACIDOSIS (RTA)

This is a group of conditions where there is an impaired ability to secrete H^+ in the distal convoluted tubule or absorb HCO_3^- in the proximal convoluted tubule. This may result in a chronic metabolic acidosis, with hypokalaemia, nephrocalcinosis, rickets or osteomalacia. There are many subtypes of RTA and many different aetiologies. Those most commonly encountered in the emergency department are due to inherited renal tubular transportation disorders, chronic renal diseases, toluene toxicity, heavy metal toxicity, or therapy with various drugs, including lithium. Chronic treatment of type I RTA with citrated HCO_3^- decreases the systemic acidosis and may prevent renal calculi formation, and progression of renal and secondary bone disease.

MANAGEMENT OF ACIDOSIS

The treatment of acidosis should usually be directed primarily towards correction of the underlying cause. Intravenous HCO_3^- is of use in the presence of acidosis and severe hyperkalaemia; severe tricyclic antidepressant, salicylate, methanol or ethylene glycol toxicity; and cardiac arrest in young children or pregnant women. The use of HCO_3^- in patients with diabetic ketoacidosis and lactic acidosis associated with sepsis or severe cardiorespiratory disease does not appear to improve outcome.[9,10] The potential hazards of HCO_3^- therapy include a high solute load, hyperosmolarity, hypokalaemia, decreased ionized serum calcium, worsening of CSF acidosis (which may precipitate hepatic encephalopathy in susceptible patients), and decreased metabolic degradation of citrate, lactate and ketone bodies in the liver.[11]

RESPIRATORY ACIDOSIS

Respiratory acidosis is defined as an elevation of the arterial P_{CO_2} and can only be due to alveolar hypoventilation. The effects of mild-to-moderate hypercarbia are usually confined to its effect on decreasing the alveolar partial pressure of oxygen (see alveolar gas equation). With more significant elevations, sweating, tachycardia, confusion and mydriasis occur. When the P_{CO_2} is greater than 80 mmHg, the level of consciousness is usually depressed. There are many possible causes of alveolar hypoventilation. CNS causes include severe hypotension, drugs with respiratory depressant effects (especially opioids and sedatives), cerebrovascular events, tumours, infections, neurotrauma and metabolic derangements. Lesions of the spinal cord, such as tumours, infections, trauma or demyelination, may also result in alveolar hypoventilation if the lesion is above C4. Lower in the afferent limb of respiratory muscle innervation, lesions of peripheral nerves such as Guillain–Barré syndrome or trauma to both phrenic nerves may also be causative. Neuromuscular junction dysfunction following postsynaptic destruction of acetylcholine receptors in myasthenia gravis, inactivation of cholinesterase in organophosphate poisoning, or the effects of spider or snake venoms and muscle relaxant drugs may also cause ventilatory failure. Muscular dystrophy, myopathies and severe electrolyte disorders may cause muscular weakness, and lesions of the chest wall, such as flail chest, severe kyphoscoliosis or arthritis, may also impair effective ventilation.

Pleural abnormalities, such as tension pneumothorax, massive haemothorax/pleural effusion, pulmonary conditions, such as severe fibrosis, pulmonary oedema or pneumonia, and severe airway obstruction due to severe croup, asthma or the inhalation of a foreign body are additional causes. In the intubated patient, causes such as the improper connection of the anaesthetic circuit, mechanical ventilator failure and the use of inappropriate equipment in small children should be considered.[1]

The treatment of respiratory acidosis is directed towards reversal of the causative factors. Ventilatory assistance is usually indicated in the presence of severe hypoxia, depressed level of consciousness or an acute elevation of $P\text{CO}_2$ levels greater than 80 mmHg.

ALKALOSIS

Alkalosis is defined as a decrease in $[\text{H}^+]$ in the blood. The physiological effects of this are the same as the effects of the administration of HCO_3 as described previously. In very severe cases altered mental state, seizures and respiratory depression may also occur. The most common symptoms of metabolic alkalosis are related to a decrease in the concentration of ionized calcium, and are more commonly present in respiratory alkalosis due to anxiety, than in other aetiologies. Reduced levels of ionized calcium may cause neurological symptoms such as lightheadedness, dizziness, chest tightness and difficulty swallowing. On examination, the respiratory rate is elevated, muscular tremor is often present and, if severe, carpopedal spasm may also be observed. Chovstek's and Trousseau's signs may also be present.

METABOLIC ALKALOSIS

This is caused by loss of acid from the gastrointestinal tract or kidney, or the addition of exogenous alkali. Upper GIT acid losses as the result of severe and prolonged vomiting are the most common cause encountered in the emergency department. Other causes, such as hyperaldosteronism, Bartter's and Gitelman's syndromes, and severe hypokalaemia, result in the loss of H^+ in the urine due to increased H^+–K^+ exchange in the distal convoluted tubule. Diuretics may also induce alkalosis by the same mechanism, but the pH is rarely raised to more than 7.5.

Alkali may be added to the body in the form of citrate in red cell transfusions, intravenous NaHCO_3 administration, or as urinary alkalinizers. The milk alkali syndrome may occur as a result of the chronic ingestion of more than 2 g of calcium salts each day (commonly in conjunction with vitamin D).[12] The metabolic derangement known as post-hypercapnoeic alkalosis is caused by the decrease of a chronically elevated $P\text{CO}_2$ to normal levels, as occurs in relative hyperventilation. In such patients the HCO_3^- is usually elevated as a result of chronic hypercarbia, and when the $P\text{CO}_2$ is acutely lowered to normal levels, the appearance on blood gas analysis is that of a metabolic alkalosis, rather than that of a relative respiratory alkalosis. The ingestion of strong alkali is almost never a cause of systemic alkalosis.

The causes of metabolic alkalosis can be further classified according to their response to intravenous saline (which also correlates with the urinary chloride concentration). If the urinary Cl is <10 mmol/L, this is considered to be saline responsive and is usually caused by GIT losses, diuretics or the acute correction of chronic hypercapnoea. If the urinary Cl is >10 mmol/L, the metabolic alkalosis is considered to be saline resistant and is usually caused by mineralocorticoid excess, oedema states or renal failure.

The treatment of metabolic alkalosis should be directed primarily towards correction of the underlying cause. In the presence of upper gastrointestinal fluid losses, intravenous fluids with a high chloride content (such as 0.9% saline) should be used initially for rehydration, and correction of hypokalaemia may also be required.

RESPIRATORY ALKALOSIS

This is the only acid-base disturbance in which compensation may be complete. In a fully compensated chronic respiratory alkalosis the pH will return to 7.4 in approximately 4 days, and the reduction in serum HCO_3^- that occurs results in an increase in the anion gap.

Common causes of respiratory alkalosis in the general population include exercise, altitude-related hypoxia, and stimulation of the medullary respiratory centre by progesterones during pregnancy. In the emergency department setting, causes such as anxiety, hypoxia, early sepsis, cerebral oedema, hepatic cirrhosis, mechanical ventilation, and salicylate, theophylline and carbon monoxide toxicity should be considered.[8] Treatment is directed towards correction of the underlying cause and the treatment of hypokalaemia or hypocalcaemia as required. Hydrochloric acid can be administered to correct the metabolic abnormality, but is rarely required. A dose of 1–3 mmol/kg of hydrochloric acid can be given through a central venous line at a rate of no faster than 1 mEq/min.[13]

ARTERIAL BLOOD GAS INTERPRETATION

Alveolar gas equation

One of the most commonly used physiological equations in emergency medicine practice is the alveolar gas equation. This is represented as follows:

$$P_{\text{alveolar}}\text{O}_2 = P_i\text{O}_2 - (P_A\text{CO}_2/R)$$

where R = respiratory quotient (usually 0.8), $P_A\text{CO}_2$ is approximated by $P_a\text{CO}_2$ and $P_i\text{O}_2$ = (atmospheric pressure − partial pressure of water vapour) × Fio_2.

At sea level the partial pressure of water vapour is 47 mmHg, and if breathing room air (at a Fio_2 of 0.21) then $P_i\text{O}_2$ = 150 mmHg.

The alveolar gas equation is used as it allows comparison of the actual $P_a\text{O}_2$ with the calculated alveolar value to derive the alveolar-arterial gradient, elevation of which indicates an abnormal ventilation-perfusion relationship in the lungs. The normal range of the alveolar-arterial gradient in the erect patient is age (in years)/4.[13] The usefulness of the equation for the detection of pulmonary disease is decreased if the patient is supine or the FiO_2 is high. In addition, the respiratory quotient varies with the composition of the patient's diet, approaching 0.95 in a high-carbohydrate diet and as low as 0.6 if the diet is high in fat or ethanol. As the exact composition of the patient's diet is rarely known in the emergency setting, the results of the alveolar gas equation should be interpreted with caution. In addition, adjustment should also be made for the changes in inspired P_iO_2 due to changes in barometric pressure that can occur due to altitudes above and below sea level, meteorological effects and diurnal variation.

RULES FOR COMPLEX ACID-BASE DISORDERS

Comparison of actual and calculated values of pH, PCO_2 and HCO_3^- may be of some use in determining the presence of more than one type of acid-base abnormality. These calculations are based on the assumption that 'normal' pH is 7.4, PCO_2 = 40 mmHg and HCO_3^- (arterial) = 24 mmol/L. They are more of theoretical interest than of significant practical value. In the presence of a simple metabolic acidosis of >24 hours' duration, the expected PCO_2 should equal $1.5 \times HCO_3^- + 8$ (± 2), with the lower limit of compensation being 10 mmHg.[14] In addition, the PCO_2 should equal the last two digits of the pH in a pH range between 7.4 and 7.1. In the presence of a simple metabolic alkalosis the PCO_2 should equal $0.9 \times HCO_3^- + 9$, and the PCO_2 should equal the last two digits of the pH in a pH range between 7.4 and 7.6.[14] As a compensatory mechanism, the PCO_2 will not increase to more than 60 mmHg. In the presence of a simple respiratory acidosis it is expected that for every 10 mmHg increase in PCO_2 the HCO_3^- should increase by 1 mmol/L within 10 minutes, and, if sustained, by up to 4 mmol/L by 4 days. In the presence of a simple respiratory alkalosis it is expected that each 10 mmHg decrease in PCO_2 should decrease HCO_3^- by 1 mmol/L within 10 minutes and, if sustained, by up to 2 mmol/L by 4 days. In addition, the PCO_2 will only compensate to partial pressures between 10 and 60 mmHg, and the HCO_3^- will only compensate for a chronic respiratory acidosis to concentrations between 18 and 45 mmol/L.

REFERENCES

1. Ganong WF 1997 Medical Physiology, 7th edn. Appleton & Lange, New Jersey
2. Dar K, Williams T, Aitken R, Woods KL, Fletcher S 1995 Arterial versus capillary sampling for analysing blood gas pressures. British Medical Journal 309: 6971
3. Kelly A-M, McAlpine R, Kyle E 2001 Venous pH can safely replace arterial pH in the initial evaluation of patients in the emergency department. Emergency Medicine Journal 18: 340–2
4. Liss HP, Payne CP Jr 1993 Stability of blood gases in ice and at room temperature. Chest 103(4): 1120
5. Herr RD, Swanson T 1992 Pseudometabolic acidosis caused by underfill of vacutainer tubes. Annals of Emergency Medicine 21(2): 177
6. Lolekha PH, Vanavanan S, Lolekha S 2001 Update on value of the anion gap in clinical diagnosis and laboratory evaluation. Clinica Chimica Acta 307(1–2): 33–6
7. Paulson WD, Roberts WL, Lurie AA, Koch DD, Butch AW, Aguanno JJ 1998 Wide variation in serum anion gap measurements by chemistry analyzers. American Journal Clinical Pathology 110(6): 735–42
8. Dunn R, Dilley S, Brookes J, et al (eds) 2000 The Emergency Medicine Manual, 2nd edn. Venom Publishing Adelaide
9. Cooper DJ, Walley KR, Wiggs BR, Russell JA 1990 Bicarbonate does not improve hemodynamics in critically ill patients who have lactic acidosis: a prospective controlled clinical study. Annals of Internal Medicine 112: 492–8
10. Mathieu D, Neviere R, Billard V, Fleyfel M, Wattel F 1991 Effects of bicarbonate therapy on hemodynamics and tissue oxygenation in patients with lactic acidosis: a prospective, controlled clinical study. Critical Care Medicine 19(11): 1352
11. Okuda Y, Adrogue HJ, Field JB, Nohara H, Yamashita K 1996 Counterproductive effects of sodium bicarbonate in diabetic ketoacidosis. Journal of Clinical Endocrinological Metabolism 81(1): 314
12. Whiting SJ, Kim K, Wood R 1997 Calcium supplementation. Journal of the American Academy of Nursing Practice 9(4): 187–92
13. Rippe J 1993 Manual of intensive care medicine. Little, Brown and Company, Boston
14. Walmsley R, White G (eds) 1988 A Guide to Diagnostic Clinical Chemistry, 2nd edn. Blackwell, Oxford

11.2 ELECTROLYTE DISTURBANCES

JOHN PASCO

ESSENTIALS

1 The brain is most at risk from hyponatraemia because the osmotically expanded intracellular volume may induce increased intracranial pressure (hyponatraemic encephalopathy).

2 Treatment of hyponatraemia is controversial and needs to be carefully individualized because of the risk of central pontine myelinolysis (CPM).

3 Hypernatraemia has a high in-hospital mortality rate, which often reflects severe associated medical conditions.

4 Although usually benign, hypokalaemia may cause cardiac arrhythmias and rhabdomyolysis. Oral replacement is usually sufficient, except where there is severe myopathy or cardiac arrhythmias.

5 ECG changes in the presence of hyperkalaemia require urgent potassium-lowering measures and myocardial protection with calcium.

6 Management of severe hypercalcaemia includes enhancement of renal excretion of calcium, inhibition of osteoclast activity and treatment of the underlying condition.

7 Acute symptomatic hypocalcaemia should be treated with IV calcium.

8 Hypomagnesaemia is difficult to diagnose because its symptoms are non-specific and the serum level often does not reflect the true magnesium status of the patient. It usually exists as a 'deficiency triad' with hypokalaemia and hypocalcaemia.

9 Hypermagnesaemia is often iatrogenic particularly in elderly patients or patients with renal impairment and/or chronic bowel conditions receiving magnesium therapy.

HYPONATRAEMIA

INTRODUCTION

Hyponatraemia, defined as serum sodium concentration of less than 130 mmol/L, is a common condition.

PATHOPHYSIOLOGY

Hyponatraemia is almost always associated with extracellular hypotonicity, with an excess of total body water relative to sodium. The exceptions are:

- Normotonic hyponatraemia (pseudohyponatraemia): an artefactually low sodium measurement seen in hyperlipidaemia and hyperproteinaemia. It is rarely seen now because of the routine use of direct ion-selective electrodes to measure sodium.
- Hypertonic hyponatraemia: a dilutional lowering of the measured serum sodium concentration in the presence of osmotically active substances, most commonly glucose, but also mannitol, glycerol and sorbitol. In the presence of hyperglycaemia the true serum sodium can be estimated by

adjusting the measured serum sodium upwards by 1 mmol/L for each 3 mmol/L rise in glucose.

Hyponatraemia causes cellular swelling as water moves down an osmotic gradient into the intracellular fluid. Most of the symptomatology of hyponatraemia is produced in the CNS by the swelling of brain cells within the rigid calvarium, causing raised intracranial pressure (hyponatraemic encephalopathy). As intracranial pressure rises, adaptive responses come into play. Initially there is a reduction of the cerebral blood and CSF pools. Later, neuronal intracellular osmolality is reduced by extrusion of potassium, followed within hours to days by organic solutes such as amino acids, phosphocreatine and myoinositol. These processes return brain volume towards normal and restore cellular function.

Patients become symptomatic when hyponatraemia develops rapidly and the adaptive responses have not had time to develop, or when the adaptive responses fail.

AETIOLOGY AND CLASSIFICATION

Hypotonic hyponatraemia may be classified according to the volume status of the patient (hypovolaemic, euvolaemic or hypervolaemic).

Hypovolaemic hyponatraemia

These patients have deficits in both total body sodium and total body water, but the sodium deficit exceeds the water deficit. Causes include renal and extra-renal fluid losses, and are listed in Table 11.2.1.[1] Determination of the urinary sodium concentration can differentiate these two groups. Extrarenal losses are associated with low urinary sodium concentrations (<20 mmol/L) and hyperosmolar urine. The exception is with

Table 11.2.1 Causes of hypovolaemic hyponatraemia
Renal losses (urinary [Na] >20 mmol/L) Diuretics – thiazides Mineralocorticoid deficiency – Addison's disease Salt-losing nephropathy Ketonuria Osmotic diuresis – glucose, mannitol, urea Bicarbonaturia with metabolic alkalosis
Extrarenal losses (urinary [Na] <20 mmol/L) Vomiting – self-induced, gastroenteritis, pyloric obstruction Diarrhoea Third-space fluid loss – burns, pancreatitis, trauma

Table 11.2.2 Causes of euvolaemic hyponatraemia
Psychogenic polydipsia
Iatrogenic water intoxication Absorption of hypotonic irrigation fluids during TURP Inappropriate intravenous fluid administration
Postoperative hyponatraemia (elevated ADH levels)
Non-osmotic ADH secretion Glucocorticoid deficiency Severe hypothyroidism Thiazide diuretics
Drugs (ADH analogues, potentiation of ADH release, unknown mechanisms) Psychoactive agents: fluoxetine, sertraline, thiothixene, haloperidol, amitriptyline, 'Ecstasy', MAOI, tricyclic antidepressants Oxytocin Anticancer agents: cyclophosphamide, vincristine, vinblastine NSAIDs Carbamazepine Chlorpropamide
SIADH

Table 11.2.3 Clinical manifestations of hyponatraemia
Anorexia
Nausea
Vomiting
Lethargy
Muscle cramps
Muscle weakness
Headache
Confusion/agitation
Altered conscious state
Seizures
Coma

Table 11.2.4 Patient groups at risk of hyponatraemia
Postoperative
Menstruating females
Elderly women on thiazide diuretics
Prepubescent children
Psychiatric polydipsic patients
Hypoxaemic patients
AIDS patients
Patients taking 'Ecstasy' (MDMA)

severe vomiting and metabolic alkalosis, where bicarbonaturia obligates renal sodium loss and urinary sodium is high (>20 mmol/L), despite volume depletion. However, urinary chloride, a better indicator of ECF fluid volume, is low.

Euvolaemic hyponatraemia

Total body water is increased with only minimal change in total body sodium. Volume expansion is mild and usually not clinically detectable. Causes are listed in Table 11.2.2.

Hypervolaemic hyponatraemia

Total body water is increased in excess of total body sodium. Causes include congestive cardiac failure, hepatic cirrhosis with ascites, nephrotic syndrome and chronic renal failure.

CLINICAL PRESENTATION

In addition to the features of the underlying medical condition and alteration in extracellular volume, clinical manifestations of hyponatraemia per se usually develop when serum sodium is less than 130 mmol/L. The severity of symptoms depends partly on the absolute serum sodium concentration and partly on its rate of fall. At sodium concentrations from 125 to 130 mmol/L the symptoms are principally gastrointestinal, whereas at concentrations below

125 mmol/L the symptoms are predominantly neuropsychiatric. The principal signs and symptoms of hyponatraemia are listed in Table 11.2.3.

Hyponatraemic encephalopathy carries a high mortality (50%) if left untreated.[1] Population groups prone to hyponatraemic encephalopathy have been identified (Table 11.2.4).[1–5]

Premenstrual patients appear at risk of developing hyponatraemic encephalopathy because oestrogen and progesterone are thought to inhibit the brain Na-K ATPase and increase circulating levels of ADH.[3]

Psychogenic polydipsia occurs primarily in patients with schizophrenia or bipolar disorder. These patients develop hyponatraemia with a far lower fluid intake than is usually necessary (over 20 L of water/day in a 60 kg man, in the absence of elevated levels of ADH)[2,3] and it may arise through a combination of factors: antipsychotics, increased thirst perception, enhanced renal response to ADH and a mild defect in osmoregulation.

Hyponatraemia in AIDS is common and associated with a high mortality. It may be secondary to SIADH, adrenal

insufficiency or volume deficiency with hypotonic fluid replacement.[2]

The use of 'Ecstasy' at 'rave' parties has been associated with acute hyponatraemia.[4,5] This may be due to a combination of drug effect and drinking large quantities of water in an attempt to prevent dehydration.

SYNDROME OF INAPPROPRIATE ADH SECRETION

This is a diagnosis of exclusion and is characterized by inappropriately concentrated urine in the setting of hypotonicity. It accounts for approximately 50% of all cases of hyponatraemia. These patients have elevated serum ADH levels without an obvious volume or osmotic stimulus. The diagnostic criteria for syndrome of inappropriate ADH secretion are shown in Table 11.2.5 and conditions associated with the syndrome are listed in Table 11.2.6.

Table 11.2.5 Diagnostic criteria for SIADH

Hypotonic hyponatraemia

Urine osmolality >100 mmol/kg (i.e. inappropriately concentrated)

Urine sodium >20 mmol/mL while on a normal salt and water intake

Absence of extracellular volume depletion

Normal thyroid and adrenal function

Normal cardiac, hepatic and renal function

No diuretic use

Table 11.2.6 Conditions associated with SIADH

Neoplasms (ectopic ADH production)
  Bronchogenic carcinoma
  Pancreatic carcinoma
  Prostate carcinoma
  Lymphoma
  Mesothelioma
  Thymoma
  Carcinoma of the bladder

Pulmonary disease
  Pneumonia
  Tuberculosis
  Aspergillosis
  Cystic fibrosis
  COAD
  Positive-pressure ventilation

CNS disease
  Encephalitis
  Acute psychosis
  Head trauma
  Brain abscess
  Meningitis
  Hydrocephalus
  Brain tumour
  Delirium tremens
  Guillain–Barré syndrome
  Stroke
  Subdural or subarachnoid bleed

HIV infection

Pneumocystis carinii pneumonia

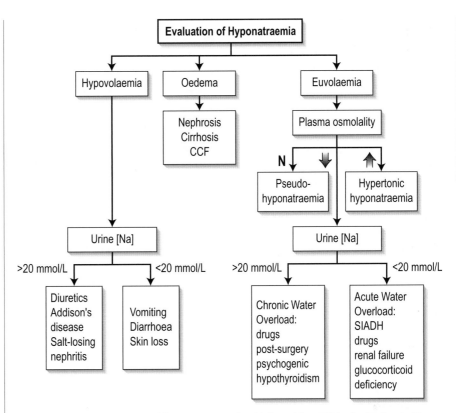

Fig. 11.2.1 Assessment of hyponatraemia. (Adapted from Walmsley R, Guerin M 1984 Disorders of fluid and electrolyte balance. John Wright & Sons, Bristol)

ASSESSMENT

This should include an assessment of the patient's volume status and serum and urine sodium concentrations and osmolalities (Fig. 11.2.1).

MANAGEMENT

There is ongoing controversy over the treatment of hyponatraemia because of the risk of central pontine myelinolysis (CPM), which is discussed below.

Treatment should be carefully individualized and depends on the presence of symptoms, the duration of the hyponatraemia and the absolute value of sodium. Treatment of the underlying cause is obviously essential and may correct the hyponatraemia. For hypovolaemic hyponatraemia, adequate volume replacement is essential.

Acute symptomatic hyponatraemia

Symptomatic hyponatraemia developing within 48 hours should be treated promptly and aggressively because the risk of developing osmotic demyelination is clearly outweighed by the encephalopathy.[2] Hypertonic saline (3% NaCl) should be infused at a rate of 1–2 mL/kg/h to raise the serum sodium by 1–2 mmol/L/h. Where neurological symptoms are severe, hypertonic saline can be infused at 4–6 mL/kg/h. Other measures to reduce intracranial pressure, such as intubation and IPPV, may also be required.

Chronic symptomatic hyponatraemia

Hyponatraemia present for more than 48 hours, or where the duration is unknown, presents the greatest dilemma. Care must be taken with correction of sodium as these patients are at the greatest risk of developing CPM, yet the presence of encephalopathy mandates urgent treatment.[2,3,6] Hypertonic saline can be infused so that a correction rate of no more than 1–1.5 mmol/L/h is maintained. Therapy with hypertonic saline should be discontinued when (a) the patient becomes asymptomatic; (b) the serum sodium has risen by 20 mmol/L; or (c) the serum sodium reaches 120–125 mmol/L. Thereafter, slower correction with water restriction should follow. The serum sodium should never be acutely elevated to hypernatraemic or normonatraemic levels, and should not be elevated by more than 25 mmol/L during the first 48 hours of therapy.

Chronic asymptomatic hyponatraemia

In this situation saline infusion is usually not required, and patients can be managed by treating the underlying disorder, discontinuing diuretic therapy or restricting fluids. Fluid restriction is inexpensive and effective but is often limited by patient non-compliance. Other treatment options include pharmacological inhibition of ADH with demeclocycline, which is limited by its neuro- and nephrotoxic side-effects, or increasing solute with the use of frusemide or urea.[2,7]

Central pontine myelinolyis

This is an iatrogenic disorder which develops progressively over 3–5 days following the correction of hyponatraemia. It is characterized initially by dysarthria, mutism, lethargy and affective changes, which may be mistaken for psychiatric illness. Classically, pseudobulbar palsy and spastic quadriparesis are observed. Demyelination in the central pons and extrapontine sites is demonstrated on magnetic resonance imaging (MRI) scan and at autopsy.[8]

It appears that the risk of developing central pontine myelinolyis (CPM) is highest when hyponatraemia has been present for more than 48 hours. In these patients the adaptive response has been effective but the brain is not well protected from the osmotic stresses of sodium correction. Alcoholics, malnourished patients, hypokalaemic patients, burn victims and elderly patients on thiazides seem to be most at risk of developing osmotic demyelination.[1,2]

Both the rate and the magnitude of sodium correction appear important in the development of CPM. Although there is as yet no agreed rate of correction that is regarded as completely safe, most authorities suggest that the serum sodium concentration should not rise by more than 10–14 mmol/L during any 24-hour period.[2,3,6]

HYPERNATRAEMIA

INTRODUCTION

Hypernatraemia is less common than hyponatraemia and may be defined as a serum sodium concentration greater than 150 mmol/L.

It is important to recognize hypernatraemia because it is usually associated with severe underlying medical illness. It is a condition of hospitalized patients, elderly and dependent people. The incidence of hypernatraemia in hospitalized patients ranges from 0.3 to 1%, with from 60 to 80% of these developing hypernatraemia after admission.[7] In-hospital mortality is high (40–55%) and may be due to a combination of hypernatraemia and the severity of the underlying disease.[7,9]

PATHOPHYSIOLOGY

Hypernatraemia is a relative deficiency of total body water compared to total body sodium, thus rendering the body fluids hypertonic. The normal compensatory response includes stimulated thirst – the most important response – and renal water conservation through ADH secretion. In the absence of ADH water intake can match urinary losses because of increased thirst, but where the thirst mechanism is absent or defective, patients become hypernatraemic even in the presence of maximal ADH stimulation. Therefore, hypernatraemia is usually seen where water intake is inadequate – i.e. in patients too young, too old, too sick to drink, with no access to water, or with a defective thirst mechanism.

Extracellular hypertonicity causes a shift of water from the intracellular space until there is osmotic equilibrium. The resultant cellular contraction may explain some of the clinical features of hypernatraemia. The brain is especially at risk from shrinkage because of its vascular attachments to the calvarium. Haemorrhage may occur if these vascular attachments tear.

As with hyponatraemia, the rate and magnitude of the rise in sodium determine the severity of symptoms, which is a reflection of the brain's capacity to adapt to the deranged osmotic conditions.[7]

AETIOLOGY AND CLASSIFICATION

The clinical causes of hypernatraemia are listed in Table 11.2.7. Population groups at particular risk of developing hypernatraemia are listed in Table 11.2.8.[2,7]

Hypernatraemia is classified into three categories based on extracellular volume status: hypovolaemic, hypervolaemic and euvolaemic.[2,7,10]

Hypovolaemic hypernatraemia

This occurs where there is loss of both total body water and sodium, but with a greater loss of water. Renal causes include osmotic diuresis and diuretic excess.

Table 11.2.7 Causes of hypernatraemia

Altered perception of thirst
  Osmoreceptor damage/destruction
  exogenous: trauma, hydrocephalus
  endogenous: vasculitis, carcinoma,
  granuloma
  Idiopathic: psychogenic, head injury
  Drugs

Normal perception of thirst
  Poor intake
    Confusion
    Coma
    Depression
    Dysphagia
    Odynophagia

Increased water loss and decreased intake
  Diuresis
  Renal loss
  Diabetes insipidus
  Chronic renal failure

Diuretic excess
GIT loss: fistulae, diarrhoea
Exogenous increase in salt intake

Table 11.2.8 Groups at particular risk for hypernatraemia

Elderly or disabled, unable to obtain oral fluids independently
Infants

Inpatients receiving
  Hypertonic infusions
  Tube feedings
  Osmotic diuretics
  Lactulose
  Mechanical ventilation

Altered mental status
Uncontrolled diabetes mellitus
Underlying polyuric disorders

Urinary sodium is usually greater than 20 mmol/L. Extrarenal causes include profuse diarrhoea, sweating, burns and fistulae. Urinary sodium is usually less than 20 mmol/L.

Euvolaemic hypernatraemia

This is the most common form of hypernatraemia. Patients have pure water losses, with intracellular dehydration as water shifts according to the osmotic gradient. Hypernatraemia in these patients occurs only when there is no accompanying water intake, i.e. restricted access to water or a defect in thirst sensation.

Extrarenal losses are usually seen in skin losses in burns patients and via the respiratory system in respiratory infections and at high altitude. Renal water loss is usually due to diabetes insipidus – a failure of ADH production or secretion (central diabetes insipidus), or a failure of the collecting duct of the kidney to respond to ADH (nephrogenic diabetes insipidus).

Hypervolaemic hypernatraemia

This is not very common. These patients are typically extracellular volume expanded but intracellular volume depleted. It is seen following resuscitation with sodium bicarbonate, with the use of hypertonic saline solutions, with excess salt intake, in primary hyperaldosteronism and in Cushing syndrome.

CLINICAL PRESENTATION

In addition to the features of the underlying medical condition and alteration in extracellular volume, the clinical features of hypernatraemia *per se* are primarily CNS. Early symptoms are anorexia, nausea and vomiting; lethargy, hyperreflexia, confusion, seizures and coma occur later.

MANAGEMENT

The speed at which hypernatraemia is corrected should take into account the rate of development and severity of symptoms. Too rapid correction, especially in chronic hypernatraemia, can cause cerebral oedema or isotonic water intoxication. The rate of correction of chronic hypernatraemia should not exceed 0.5–0.7 mmol/L/h.

Treatment is based on clinical assessment of the patient's volume status.

Hypovolaemic hypernatraemia

These patients require restoration of the volume deficit with isotonic saline, colloid or blood in the first instance, to prevent peripheral vascular collapse, and treatment of the underlying cause. Following this, the water deficit is corrected with 0.45% saline, 5% dextrose or oral water.[2,7]

The water deficit is calculated as follows:

$$\text{Water deficit} = \text{total body water} \times (1 - Na2/Na1)$$

where Na2 = desired sodium, Na1 = actual sodium. Total body water is usually 60% of the body weight.

The calculated normal daily maintenance fluids should be added to the above volumes.

Euvolaemic hypernatraemia

Calculate the water deficit as above and replace the deficit and ongoing losses with 5% dextrose, 0.45% saline or oral water.[2,7] To avoid cerebral oedema, particularly in chronic hypernatraemia,

50% of the water deficit should be replaced over the first 6–12 hours and the rest given slowly over 1–2 days. Serum sodium estimations should be repeated at regular intervals.

Hypervolaemic hypernatraemia

Removal of sodium is required with the use of diuretics such as furosemide and discontinuation of causative agents. Furosemide causes excretion of more water than sodium, so a hypotonic fluid such as 5% dextrose may need to be infused. In severe cases, or in renal failure, dialysis may be required.

HYPOKALAEMIA

INTRODUCTION

Hypokalaemia may be defined as a serum potassium concentration of less than 3.5 mmol/L. It is usually considered to be severe when this is less than 2.4 mmol/L.

PATHOPHYSIOLOGY

Hypokalaemia may develop as a consequence of potassium depletion or shift of potassium into cells. In either case there is an increase in the ratio of intracellular to extracellular potassium concentrations. This in turn produces hyperpolarization across excitable membranes, and is responsible for the effects of hypokalaemia on striated muscle and the cardiac conducting system.

AETIOLOGY

The causes of hypokalaemia are listed in Table 11.2.9.

CLINICAL PRESENTATION

Hypokalaemia commonly produces no symptoms in otherwise healthy subjects.

Table 11.2.9 Causes of hypokalaemia

Inadequate dietary intake

Abnormal losses
  GI
    Vomiting, nasogastric aspiration
    Diarrhoea, fistula loss
    Villous adenoma of the colon
    Laxative abuse

Renal

Mineralocorticoid excess
  Conn syndrome
  Bartter syndrome
  Ectopic ACTH syndrome
  Small cell carcinoma of the lung
  Pancreatic carcinoma
  Carcinoma of the thymus
  Renal tubular acidosis
  Magnesium deficiency

Drugs
  Diuretics
  Corticosteroids
  Gentamicin, amphotericin B
  Cisplatin

Compartmental shift
  Alkalosis
  Insulin
  Na K-ATPase stimulation
  Sympathomimetic agents with β_2 effect
  Methylxanthines
  Barium poisoning
  Hypothermia
  Toluene intoxication
  Hypokalaemic periodic paralysis

Clinical features may include weakness, constipation, ileus and ventilatory failure. Myopathy may develop, with weakness of the extremities which characteristically worsens with exercise. If the hypokalaemia is severe and untreated, rhabdomyolysis may occur. Polyuria and polydipsia may result from the effect of hypokalaemia on the distal renal tubule (nephrogenic diabetes insipidus of hypokalaemia). Cardiac effects include ventricular tachycardias and atrial tachycardias, with or without block. Characteristic ECG changes include PR prolongation, T-wave flattening and inversion, and prominent U waves.[11]

MANAGEMENT

Oral replacement is safe for asymptomatic patients and 40–60 mmol of potassium every 1–4 hours is usually well tolerated.

Intravenous administration of potassium is recommended when hypokalaemia is associated with cardiac arrhythmias, familial periodic paralysis or severe myopathy. Usual infusion rates are 10–20 mmol/h. Rates greater than 40 mmol/h are not recommended. Potassium is a sclerosant and should, therefore, be given via a large peripheral or central vein. Lidocaine, heparin and hydrocortisone can be used to ameliorate symptoms. Serum potassium estimations every 1–4 hours and continuous cardiac monitoring are mandatory.

HYPERKALAEMIA

INTRODUCTION

Hyperkalaemia, defined as a serum potassium concentration greater than 5.5 mmol/L, is less common than hypokalaemia. Moderate (6.1–6.9 mmol/L) and severe (>7 mmol/L) hyperkalaemia can have grave consequences, particularly if acute.

PATHOPHYSIOLOGY

Two homoeostatic mechanisms are responsible for maintaining potassium balance. The renal system maintains external potassium balance by excreting 90–95% of the average daily potassium load (100 mmol/day); the gut excretes the remainder. This is a relatively slow process: only half an administered load of potassium will have been excreted in the urine after 3–6 hours.[12,13] The extrarenal system involves hormonal and acid-base mechanisms that rapidly translocate potassium intracellularly. This system is critical in the management of acute hyperkalaemia.

AETIOLOGY

The causes of hyperkalaemia are listed in Table 11.2.10.

Table 11.2.10 Causes of hyperkalaemia

Pseudohyperkalaemia
  Delay in separating red cells
  Specimen haemolysis during or after venesection
  Severe leucocytosis/thrombocytosis

Excessive intake
  Exogenous: IV or oral KCl, massive blood transfusion
  Endogenous: tissue damage
    Burns
    Trauma
    Rhabdomyolysis
    Tumour lysis

Decrease in renal excretion
  Drugs
    Spironolactone, triamterene, amiloride
    Indometacin
    Captopril, enalapril
  Renal failure
  Addison's disease
  Hyporeninaemic hypoaldosteronism

Compartmental shift
  Acidosis
  Insulin deficiency
  Digoxin overdose
  Succinylcholine
  Fluoride poisoning
  Hyperkalaemic periodic paralysis

CLINICAL PRESENTATION

The clinical features of hyperkalaemia are often non-specific. Diagnosis depends on clinical suspicion, measurement of potassium concentration in the plasma, and the characteristic changes on the ECG.

Generalized muscle weakness, flaccid paralysis and paraesthesiae of the hands and feet are common, but there is poor correlation between the degree of muscle weakness and serum potassium concentration.

The ECG changes (Table 11.2.11) are characteristic, but are an insensitive method of evaluating hyperkalaemia.

Serum biochemistry in almost all patients with hyperkalaemia shows some degree of renal impairment and metabolic acidosis. In dialysis patients hyperkalaemia may develop without concomitant metabolic acidosis.

Table 11.2.11 ECG changes of hyperkalaemia

Plasma potassium (mmol/L)	ECG characteristics
6–7	Tall peaked T waves (>5 mm)
7–8	QRS widening, small-amplitude P waves
8–9	Fusion of QRS complex with T wave producing sinewave
>9	AV dissociation, ventricular tachycardia, ventricular fibrillation

MANAGEMENT

Pseudohyperkalaemia is common and, if hyperkalaemia is an unexpected finding, the serum potassium should be remeasured.

Hyperkalaemia with ECG changes requires urgent management. The priorities are as follows:[11,14]

❶ Antagonize potassium cardiac toxicity:
 • IV calcium chloride 10%, 5–10 mL or
 • IV calcium gluconate 10%, 5–10 mL. The effects of calcium should be evident within minutes and last for 30–60 minutes. A calcium infusion may be required. Calcium antagonizes the myocardial membrane excitability induced by hyperkalaemia. It does not lower serum potassium levels.

❷ Shift potassium into cells:
 • IV soluble insulin, 20U with dextrose 50g or
 • salbutamol nebulized (10–20 mg) or IV (0.5 mg diluted in 100 mL over 10–15 minutes)[11,15] or
 • IV sodium bicarbonate, 50–200 mmol.

❸ Enhance potassium excretion.
 • Oral and/or rectal resonium A 50 g. This is a cation exchange resin; as the resin passes through the gastrointestinal tract Na and K are exchanged and the cationically modified resin is then excreted in the faeces.
 • Furosemide diuresis.
 • Haemodialysis. This is usually reserved for cases of acute renal failure or end-stage renal disease.

It is the most effective treatment for acutely lowering serum potassium, but there is usually a time delay in instituting dialysis and the temporizing measures outlined above must be employed in the interim.

The usefulness of bicarbonate for the acute therapy of hyperkalaemia has recently been questioned. A number of studies have shown that bicarbonate fails to lower potassium levels sufficiently in the acute, life-threatening situation to justify its use as first-line treatment.[12,13] It is still recommended, however, when hyperkalaemia is associated with severe metabolic acidosis (pH <7.20).

The use of insulin and glucose is well supported in the literature.[12,13] A response is usually seen within 20–30 minutes, with lowering of plasma potassium by up to 1 mmol/L and reversal of ECG changes. Transient hypoglycaemia may be observed within 15 minutes of insulin administration. In some patients, particularly those with end-stage renal failure, late hypoglycaemia may develop. For this reason, a 10% dextrose infusion at 50 mL/h is recommended and the blood glucose should be monitored closely. The exact mechanism by which insulin translocates potassium is not known: it is thought to be stimulation of Na-K-ATPase independent of cAMP.

β_2-Agonists significantly lower plasma potassium when given intravenously or via a nebulizer.[12,13] Potassium levels are reduced by up to 1.00 mmol/L within 30 minutes following 10–20 mg of nebulized salbutamol. The effect is sustained for up to 2 hours. Adverse effects of salbutamol administration include tachyarrhythmias and precipitation of angina

in patients with coronary artery disease. Patients on non-selective β-blockers may not respond. Some patients with end-stage renal disease are also resistant to this therapy. The reason for this is unknown. Greater decreases in potassium have been observed when salbutamol treatment is combined with insulin and glucose. The additive effect is thought to be due to stimulation of Na-K-ATPase via different pathways. Transient hyperglycaemia may occur with combined therapy, but delayed hypoglycaemia does not occur.

HYPOCALCAEMIA

INTRODUCTION

A reduction in serum calcium concentration manifests principally as abnormal neuromuscular function.

PATHOPHYSIOLOGY

Calcium is involved in smooth and skeletal muscle contraction and relaxation, platelet aggregation, neurotransmission, hepatic and adipose glycogenolysis, thermogenesis and neutrophil function. In addition, most endocrine and exocrine gland function is calcium dependent. Hypocalcaemia occurs when calcium is lost from the extracellular fluid at a rate greater than can be replaced by the intestine or bone.

AETIOLOGY

The major cause of severe hypocalcaemia is hypoparathyroidism, as a result of surgery for thyroid disease, autoimmune destruction, or from developmental abnormalities of the parathyroid glands. Other causes are listed in Table 11.2.12.

CLINICAL PRESENTATION

Patients with acute hypocalcaemia are more likely to be symptomatic than those with chronic hypocalcaemia. Symp-

Table 11.2.12 Causes of hypocalcaemia

Factitious EDTA contamination

Hypoalbuminaemia

Decreased PTH activity
  Hypoparathyroidism
  Pseudohypoparathyroidism
  Hypomagnesaemia

Decreased vitamin D activity

Acute pancreatitis

Hyperphosphataemia
  Renal failure
  Phosphate supplements

'Hungry bone' syndrome

Drugs
  Mithramycin
  Diuretics: furosemide, ethacrynic acid

tomatic hypocalcaemia is characterized by abnormal neuromuscular excitability and neurologic sensations.[15] Early signs are perioral numbness and paraesthesia of distal extremities. Hyperreflexia, muscle cramps, and carpopedal spasm follow. Chvostek's sign – ipsilateral contraction of the facial muscles elicited by tapping the facial nerve just anterior to the ear – and Trousseau's sign – carpopedal spasm with inflation of a blood pressure cuff for 3–5 minutes – are signs of neuromuscular irritability. If muscle contractions become uncontrollable tetany results, and this can prove fatal if laryngospasm occurs. Seizures may occur when there is CNS instability. Cardiovascular manifestations include hypotension, bradycardia, impaired cardiac contractility and arrhythmias. ECG evidence of hypocalcaemia includes prolonged QT interval, and possibly ST prolongation and T-wave abnormalities.

MANAGEMENT

Acute symptomatic hypocalcaemia

In the emergency situation where seizures, tetany, life-threatening hypotension or arrhythmias are present, IV calcium is the treatment of choice. Infusion of 15 mg/kg of elemental cal-

cium over 4–6 hours increases the total serum calcium by 0.5–0.75 mmol/L.[15]

Administration of 10–20 mL of 10% calcium gluconate (89 mg elemental calcium per 10 mL) IV over 5–10 minutes is recommended. This should be followed by a continuous infusion, because the effects of a single IV dose last only about 2 hours. The infusion rate should be adjusted according to serial calcium measurements obtained every 2–4 hours. Over-rapid infusion may cause facial flushing, headache and arrhythmias.

Calcium chloride 10% may also be used. This contains more calcium per ampoule (272 mg in 10 mL), resulting in a more rapid rise in serum calcium, but is more irritant to veins and can cause thrombophlebitis with extravasation.

Where hypocalcaemia and metabolic acidosis are present (usually in sepsis or renal failure) correction of the acidosis with bicarbonate may result in a rapid fall in ionized calcium as the number of calcium-binding sites is increased. Therefore, hypocalcaemia must be corrected before the acidosis. Bicarbonate or phosphate should not be infused with calcium because of possible precipitation of calcium salts.

Cardiac monitoring is recommended during rapid calcium administration, especially if the patient is taking digoxin, when calcium administration may precipitate digitalis toxicity.

If coexisting magnesium deficiency is suspected, or when symptoms do not improve after calcium administration, MgSO$_4$ 1–5 mmol IV over 15 minutes may be given.

Chronic asymptomatic hypocalcaemia

These patients are usually managed with oral calcium supplements taken between meals. Calcitriol, the active hormonal form of vitamin D, 0.5–1.5 mg daily, can also be given.

HYPERCALCAEMIA

INTRODUCTION

The normal total serum calcium concentration is from 2.15 to 2.55 mmol/L.

Hypercalcaemia is a relatively common condition with a frequency estimated at 1:1000–1:10 000.[16] Although there are many causes, the most frequent are malignancy and hyperparathyroidism, with the former the most likely to cause hypercalcaemia requiring urgent attention.[16]

PATHOPHYSIOLOGY

Total serum calcium is made up of protein-bound calcium (40%, mostly albumin and not filterable by the kidneys), ion-bound complexes (13%, bound to anions such as bicarbonate, lactate, citrate and phosphate), and the unbound, ionized fraction (47%). The ionized fraction is the biologically active component of calcium and is closely regulated by parathyroid hormone (PTH). Total serum calcium is affected by albumin and does not necessarily reflect the level of plasma ionized calcium. Normal ionized calcium levels are from 1.14 to 1.30 mmol/L. Protein binding in turn is influenced by extracellular fluid pH and alterations in serum albumin. Acidaemia decreases protein binding and increases the level of ionized calcium.

To correct for pH:

Ionized calcium rises 0.05mmol/L for each 0.1 decrease in pH.

To correct for serum albumin:

Corrected $[Ca^+]$ = measured $[Ca^+]$ + (40 – albumin g/L) × 0.02 mmol/L.

Corrected calcium is used for all treatment decisions except where direct measurement of ionized calcium using an ion-specific electrode is available.

Three pathophysiological mechanisms may produce hypercalcaemia:[16]

- Accelerated osteoclastic bone resorption. This is the most common cause of severe hypercalcaemia. Osteoclasts are activated by PTH and various humoral tumour products, the most common being parathyroid hormone-related protein (PTHRP).

- Increased gastrointestinal absorption (rarely important).
- Decreased renal excretion of calcium. PTH and PTHRP stimulate renal tubular reabsorption of calcium. Hypercalcaemia per se causes polyuria by interfering with renal mechanisms for reabsorption of water and sodium. If there is inadequate fluid intake to compensate, extracellular volume depletion occurs, reducing glomerular filtration and exacerbating the hypercalcaemia.

AETIOLOGY

The majority of cases of hypercalcaemia requiring urgent treatment are due to malignancy or, less commonly, primary hyperparathyroidism (parathyroid crisis). Malignant hypercalcaemia is most commonly seen with the solid tumours: lung and breast cancer, squamous cell carcinoma of the head and neck and cholangiocarcinoma, and the haematological malignancies multiple myeloma and lymphoma.[15] Other causes of hypercalcaemia are uncommon (Table 11.2.13).

Table 11.2.13 Causes of hypercalcaemia
Factitious Haemoconcentration Postprandial
Malignancy
Primary hyperparathyroidism Drugs Thiazides Vitamin D Lithium Vitamin A
Hormonal Thyrotoxicosis Acromegaly Hypoadrenalism Phaeochromocytoma
Granulomas Tuberculosis Sarcoidosis
Renal failure
Milk alkali syndrome
Immobilization

CLINICAL FEATURES

Hypercalcaemia causes disturbances of the gastrointestinal, cardiovascular, renal and central nervous systems.[15,17]

Gastrointestinal manifestations include anorexia, nausea, vomiting and constipation. Cardiovascular manifestations include hypertension and a shortened QT interval on the ECG. Renal manifestations include polyuria, polydipsia and nephrocalcinosis (rare). CNS symptoms include psychotic behaviour, seizures, apathy, cognitive difficulties, obtundation and coma. Renal elimination of digoxin is also impaired.

Moderately elevated total serum calcium (3.00–3.50 mmol/L) is usually associated with symptoms. Markedly elevated total serum calcium (>3.5 mmol/L) mandates urgent treatment regardless of symptoms.

MANAGEMENT

Irrespective of the cause, the management of hypercalcaemic crisis is the same. There are four primary treatment goals:[17–20]

1. Hydration of the patient
2. Enhancement of renal excretion of calcium
3. Inhibition of accelerated bone resorption
4. Treatment of the underlying problem.

Hydration and diuresis

Hydration expands intravascular volume, dilutes calcium and increases calcium clearance. Infusion rates of 200–300 mL/h of 0.9% saline, depending on the degree of hypovolaemia and the ability of the patient to tolerate fluid, may be required.

Furosemide 20–40 mg IV every 1–4 hours, or by infusion, is usually added once the patient is adequately hydrated. This inhibits the function of the ascending loop of Henle and increases the excretion of calcium and sodium. This treatment, although effective, results in a relatively modest reduction in serum calcium, and patients with severe hypercalcaemia usually require additional treatment.

Inhibition of bone resorption

Pharmacological inhibition of osteoclastic bone resorption is the most effective treatment for hypercalcaemia, particularly hypercalcaemia of malignancy. Bisphosphonates, analogues of pyrophosphate, are the principal agents used. They inhibit osteoclast function and hydroxyapatite crystal dissolution. Unfortunately, normalization of calcium levels may take from 3 to 6 days, which is too slow in critically ill patients.

Etidronate given as a dose of 7.5 mg/kg daily over 4 hours for 3–7 days produces normocalcaemia in most patients after a 7-day course. Adverse reactions include a transient elevation in serum creatinine, a metallic taste and transient hyperphosphataemia.

Disodium pamidronate is more potent and lowers serum calcium more rapidly and predictably than etidronate. It is currently the bisphosphonate of choice. The dose is 60 mg IV (in 500 mL 0.9% saline over 4 hours) if serum calcium is less than 3.5 mmol/L, and 90 mg IV if serum calcium is more than 3.5 mmol/L. Calcium levels normalize in up to 80% of patients within 7 days, and this effect can persist for up to a month. Common adverse reactions include a mild transient elevation in temperature, local infusion site reactions, mild GI symptoms and mild hypophosphataemia, hypokalaemia and hypomagnesaemia.

An alternative treatment to pamidronate is sodium clodronate 1500 mg in 500 mL 0.9% saline IV (4–6 mg/kg daily) over 4 hours.

Glucocorticoids are the treatment of choice in selected patient populations where the production of 1,25-dihydroxyvitamin D is the known mechanism for causing hypercalcaemia. Such conditions include vitamin D toxicity, sarcoidosis, other granulomatous diseases, and haematological malignancies such as multiple myeloma and lymphoma. The usual dose is 200–300 mg hydrocortisone IV for 3–5 days. However, the maximal calcium-lowering effect does not occur for several days, and glucocorticoids should only be regarded as adjunctive therapy in hypercalcaemic crises.

The use of other agents, such as calcitonin, mithramycin and gallium nitrate, is now largely obsolete.

Treat the underlying disorder

The definitive treatment for hypercalcaemia is to treat the underlying disease: surgery for hyperparathyroidism, and tumour-specific therapy for hypercalcaemia of malignancy.

HYPOMAGNESAEMIA

INTRODUCTION

The diagnosis of magnesium deficiency is difficult and often overlooked largely because the symptoms are non-specific and do not usually appear until the patient is severely deficient.

Serum magnesium concentration (normal range: 0.76–0.96 mmol/L) is not a sensitive indicator of magnesium deficiency as is may not truly reflect total body stores. However, it is commonly used in the absence of other reliable methods to estimate the 'true' magnesium status. A low serum magnesium concentration is usually present in symptomatic magnesium deficiency, but it is important to remember that it may be normal in the presence of significant intracellular depletion.

PATHOPHYSIOLOGY

Magnesium plays a critical role in metabolism; as an enzyme cofactor, in the maintenance of cell membranes and in electrolyte balance. It is the fourth most common cation in the body and is predominantly an intracellular ion with the majority found in bone (>50%) and soft tissue. Only 0.3% of total body magnesium is located extracellularly, of which 33% is protein bound, 12% is complexed to anions such as citrate, bicarbonate and phosphate, and 55% is found in the free ionized form.

Hypokalaemia is present in 40-60% of cases of magnesium deficiency, due to renal wasting of potassium. The hypokalaemia is resistant to potassium replacement alone, as a result of a combination of factors including impaired cellular cation pump activity, decreased Na/K pump activity and increased cellular permeability to potassium.

Hypocalcaemia is usually present at serum magnesium concentrations below 0.49 mmol/L. This may be due to impaired PTH synthesis or secretion, or to PTH resistance as a result of magnesium deficiency.

AETIOLOGY

From an emergency medicine perspective, hypomagnesaemia is most frequently encountered in the context of acute and chronic diarrhoea, acute pancreatitis, diuretic use, in alcoholics and in diabetic ketoacidosis, secondary to glycosuria and osmotic diuresis. Table 11.2.14 details causes of magnesium deficiency.

Hypomagnesaemia has been found in 30% of alcoholics admitted to hospital and results from a combination of the direct effect of alcohol on the renal tubule, which increases magnesium excretion, and associated malnutrition, diarrhoea and metabolic acidosis.[21]

CLINICAL PRESENTATION

The clinical manifestations of severe magnesium deficiency include metabolic, neurological and cardiac effects (Table 11.2.15).

The presenting symptoms are non-specific and can be attributed to associated metabolic abnormalities such as hypocalcaemia, hypokalaemia and metabolic alkalosis. In particular, patients may present with symptoms of hypocalcaemia - neuromuscular hyperexcitability, carpopedal spasm and positive Chvostek's and Trousseau's signs.

Early ECG changes of magnesium deficiency include prolongation of the PR and QT intervals, with progressive

Table 11.2.14 Causes of magnesium deficiency[22]

Gastrointestinal losses
Acute and chronic diarrhoea
Acute pancreatitis
Severe malnutrition
Intestinal fistulae
Extensive bowel resection
Prolonged nasogastric suction

Renal losses
Osmotic diuresis – diabetes, urea, mannitol
Hypercalcaemia and hypercalcuiria
Volume expanded states
Chronic parenteral fluid therapy

Drugs
ACE inhibitors
Alcohol
Aminoglycosides
Amphotericin B
Cisplatin
Ciclosporin

Diuretics – thiazide or loop

Other
Phosphate depletion

QRS widening and U wave appearance as severity progresses. Changes in cardiac automaticity and conduction, atrial and ventricular arrhythmias including torsades de points can occur. Administration of a magnesium bolus can abolish torsades de pointes, even in the presence of normal serum magnesium levels.[22] Magnesium is a cofactor in the Na/K ATPase system and so magnesium deficiency enhances myocardial sensitivity to digitalis and may precipitate digitalis toxicity. Digitalis-toxic arrhythmias, in turn, can be terminated with intravenous magnesium.

MANAGEMENT

Oral replacement is the preferred option in asymptomatic patients, although this route takes longer.

Symptomatic moderate-to-severe magnesium deficiency should be treated with parenteral magnesium salts. The patient should be closely monitored and therapy discontinued if deep tendon reflexes disappear or serum magnesium exceeds 2.5 mmol/L.[22] Suggested dosing regimes are outlined in Table 11.2.16.

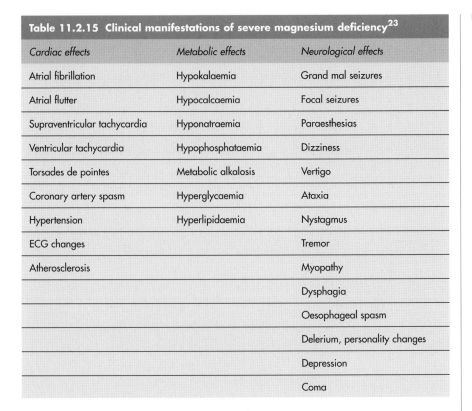

Table 11.2.15 Clinical manifestations of severe magnesium deficiency[23]

Cardiac effects	Metabolic effects	Neurological effects
Atrial fibrillation	Hypokalaemia	Grand mal seizures
Atrial flutter	Hypocalcaemia	Focal seizures
Supraventricular tachycardia	Hyponatraemia	Paraesthesias
Ventricular tachycardia	Hypophosphataemia	Dizziness
Torsades de pointes	Metabolic alkalosis	Vertigo
Coronary artery spasm	Hyperglycaemia	Ataxia
Hypertension	Hyperlipidaemia	Nystagmus
ECG changes		Tremor
Atherosclerosis		Myopathy
		Dysphagia
		Oesophageal spasm
		Delerium, personality changes
		Depression
		Coma

Table 11.2.16 Magnesium doses (in mmol magnesium)

Emergency – IV route
8–16 mmol statim
40 mmol over next 5 hours

Severely ill – IM route
48 mmol on day 1
17–25 mmol on days 2–5

Asymptomatic – oral route
15 mmol/day

HYPERMAGNESAEMIA

Hypermagnesaemia (serum magnesium above 0.95 mmol/L) is rare and usually iatrogenic.

The elderly and patients with renal impairment or chronic bowel disorders are particularly at risk, especially when IV magnesium or magnesium-containing cathartics or antacids are used.

Clinical manifestations include mental obtundation progressing to coma, cardiac arrhythmias, loss of deep tendon reflexes, refractory hypotension and respiratory arrest, nausea and vomiting, muscle paralysis, and flushing.

Magnesium administration should be immediately discontinued. Further management is largely supportive. Maintain urine output at greater than 60 mL/h with fluid administration to enhance renal excretion. Frusemide (40–80 mg IV) may also given once the patient is adequately hydrated. Haemodialysis may be of benefit in severe cases, particularly if there is impaired renal function.

REFERENCES

1. Berl T 1990 Treating hyponatremia: what is all the controversy about? Annals of Internal Medicine 113: 417–9
2. Kumar S, Berl T 1998 Sodium-electrolyte quintet. Lancet 352: 220–8
3. Fraser C, Arieff A 1997 Epidemiology, pathophysiology, and management of hyponatremic encephalopathy. American Journal of Medicine 102: 67–77
4. Maxwell D, Polkey M, Henry J 1993 Hyponatraemia and catatonic stupor after taking 'ecstasy'. British Medical Journal 307: 1399
5. Box SA, Prescott LF, Freestone S 1997 Hyponatraemia at a rave. Postgraduate Medical Journal 73(855): 53–4
6. Cluitmans F, Meinders A 1990 Management of severe hyponatremia: rapid or slow correction? American Journal of Medicine 88: 161–6
7. Fried L, Palevsky P 1997 Hyponatremia and hypernatremia. Medical Clinics of North America 3: 585–609
8. Laureno R, Illowsky B 1997 Myelinolysis after correction of hyponatremia. Annals of Internal Medicine 126(1): 57–62
9. Long C, Marin P, Byer A, Shetty H, Pathy M 1991 Hypernatraemia in an adult in-patient population. Postgraduate Medical Journal 67: 643–5
10. DeVita M, Michelis M 1993 Perturbations in sodium balance. Clinics in Laboratory Medicine 13(1): 135–48
11. Mandel A 1997 Hypokalemia and hyperkalemia. Medical Clinics of North America 81(3): 611–39
12. Allon M 1993 Treatment and prevention of hyperkalemia in end-stage renal disease. Kidney International 43: 1197–209
13. Salem MM, Rosa RM, Batlle DC 1991 Extrarenal potassium tolerance in chronic renal failure: implications for the treatment of acute hyperkalemia. American Journal of Kidney Disease 18: 421–40
14. Halperin M, Kamel K 1998 Potassium-electrolyte quintet. Lancet 352: 135–40
15. Bourke E, Delaney V 1993 Assessment of hypocalcemia and hypercalcemia. Clinics in Laboratory Medicine 13(1): 157–77
16. Deftos L 1996 Hypercalcemia. Postgraduate Medicine 100(6): 119–26
17. Bushinskey D, Monk R 1998 Calcium-electrolyte quintet. Lancet 352: 306–11
18. Chisholm M, Mulloy A, Taylor T 1996 Acute management of cancer-related hypercalcemia. Annals of Pharmacotherapy 30: 507–13
19. Bilezikian J 1992 Management of acute hypercalcemia. New England Journal of Medicine 326(18): 1196–203
20. Falk S, Fallon M 1997 Emergencies - ABC of palliative care. British Medical Journal 315: 1525–8
21. Weisinger JR, Bellorin-Font E 1998 Magnesium and Phosphorus - electrolyte quintet. The Lancet 352: 391–6
22. Fawcett WJ, Haxby EJ, Male DA 1999 Magnesium: physiology and pharmacology. British Journal of Anaesthesia 83(2): 302–20
23. Fox C, Ramsoomair D, Carter C 2001 Magnesium: its proven and potential clinical significance. Southern Medical Journal 94(12): 1195–201

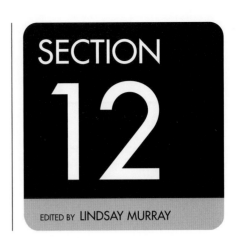

EDITED BY LINDSAY MURRAY

HAEMATOLOGY

12.1 **Blood transfusion** 494

12.2 **Neutropenia** 499

12.3 **Haemophillia** 501

12.4 **Anaemia** 503

12.5 **Thrombocytopenia** 511

12.1 BLOOD TRANSFUSION

HAMISH MACLAREN

ESSENTIALS

1 In prescribing blood products the emergency physician should always be sure that the potential benefits outweigh the potential risks.

2 The risk of viral transmission via blood transfusion cannot be completely eliminated.

3 The decision to transfuse packed red cells should ultimately be based on the knowledge that the patient's own oxygen-carrying capacity has dropped to an unacceptably low level.

4 Meticulous documentation and vigilant monitoring are keys to the avoidance of serious adverse reactions.

INTRODUCTION

Probably the earliest successful blood transfusions were carried out by the Incas, who had the advantage of being virtually all group O Rh-positive. Attempts at transfusion in the early 17th century by the Italian physician Giovanni Colle were thwarted by adverse reactions, and the procedure was banned across much of Europe. It was Karl Landsteiner's work at the beginning of the 20th century that demonstrated the ABO blood group system and explained many of the observed severe incompatibility reactions (Table 12.1.1). He won the Nobel Prize for medicine or physiology in 1930, and went on to discover the Rhesus factor in 1940.

Transfusion of blood and blood products is now routine and vital to the practice of emergency medicine. As with any prescription drug, these therapeutic products are associated with potential hazards as well as advantages. The hazards are more likely to be encountered when blood products are used during emergencies.

With the exception of exchange transfusions in the neonate, whole blood is rarely transfused in current practice, as the product is expensive, difficult to store, and offers no advantage over a product containing the particular components the patient requires. It also exposes the patient to an unnecessarily high number of foreign antigens.

PACKED RED BLOOD CELLS

Red cell concentrates are centrifuged from whole blood donations and preserved in an additive solution of sodium chloride, adenine, glucose and mannitol, with a packed cell volume of between 50 and 70%. If stored at 4°C, this preparation has a shelf-life exceeding 4–5 weeks. Transfusion of one unit in an adult can be expected to raise the haemoglobin by approximately 1 g/dL and the haematocrit by about 3%.

Packed red cells are the product most commonly prescribed in the emergency department, the usual indication being acute haemorrhage. Transfusion of packed red cells is indicated where the patient's oxygen-carrying capacity is so impaired that control of bleeding alone, if, indeed, that can readily be achieved, is regarded as insufficient to take the patient out of danger. Occasionally it may be necessary to transfuse a patient with a primary haematological condition, a failure of erythropoiesis or a haemolytic process. The indication for transfusion is the same as for haemorrhage: a severe reduction in oxygen-carrying capacity. Complex multisystem failure, such as DIC or septic shock, may result in simultaneous blood loss, circulatory collapse, haemolysis and a coagulopathy. Transfusion therapy may be life-saving in this context (Table 12.1.2).

In deciding which patients require transfusion of packed red cells, important considerations include:

- The extent of the blood loss
- The rapidity of onset: as a very rough rule of thumb, patients will collapse when they lose 40% of blood volume acutely
- Evidence of impaired tissue oxygenation: poor capillary refill, pallor, restlessness and apprehension, obtundation and confusion, poor urine output, air hunger, metabolic acidosis
- Evidence of impending circulatory collapse: tachycardia and hypotension.

Table 12.1.2 Potential indications for red cell transfusion

Haemorrhage
Dilutional anaemia following severe burns
Iron-deficiency anaemia
Megaloblastic anaemia
Anaemia of chronic disorders
Chronic renal failure
Failure of erythropoiesis
Sickle cell disease
Septic shock
DIC

Table 12.1.1 The ABO blood group system

ABO blood group	O	A	B	AB
Antigens on red cells	None	A	B	A, B
Antibody in serum	Anti-A, Anti-B	Anti-B	Anti-A	None

Transfusion should not be undertaken when alternative haematinic therapy is deemed safe and appropriate. A moderately anaemic patient who is asymptomatic and not bleeding, with some reserve oxygen-carrying capacity, does not require blood transfusion. A haemoglobin of 7 g/dL is sometimes taken as the failsafe point in the decision whether to transfuse, though of course the patient's unique circumstances need to be taken into account: treat the patient, not the numbers. The National Health and Medical Research Council together with the Australasian Society of Blood Transfusion recently published transfusion guidelines for red blood cells and other products (Table 12.1.3).

Single unit transfusion has traditionally been regarded as unnecessary. A recently observed trend towards giving patients one unit of red cells particularly in the operating theatre may reflect a growing confidence in the safety of blood products but is unlikely to be justified in the emergency department setting.

Except in the extreme emergency setting, prior to transfusion, the patient's informed consent should be sought, obtained, and documented. Patients may be encountered who refuse transfusion, either on religious grounds or for fear of adverse reactions, particularly with respect to the transfer of viral agents. This can pose problems if the patient appears incompetent to give or withhold informed consent. The situation of an exsanguinating minor whose parents refuse permission to transfuse is particularly difficult. Court orders can be obtained to treat minors without parental consent, and in such an extreme situation many doctors would feel justified in applying to obtain one, even retrospectively.

PRECAUTIONS WHEN CROSS-MATCHING AND TRANSFUSING BLOOD

Although most patients do not require transfusion in the emergency department, it is often appropriate to 'group and hold' or cross-match the patient while in the department. Many hospitals have written protocols stating the anticipated requirements for a given surgical procedure. Documentation should be meticulous. It is preferable that the person drawing the blood for cross-matching should also fill in and sign the laboratory request form. Most severe incompatibility reactions to blood trans-

Table 12.1.3 Guidelines for transfusion of blood components

Indications	Considerations
Red blood cells	
Hb	
<70 g/L	Lower thresholds may be acceptable in patients without symptoms and/or where specific therapy is available.
70–100 g/L	Likely to be appropriate during surgery associated with major blood loss or if there are signs or symptoms of impaired oxygen transport.
>80 g/L	May be appropriate to control anaemia-related symptoms in a patient on a chronic transfusion regimen or during marrow suppressive therapy.
>100 g/L	Not likely to be appropriate unless there are specific indications.
Platelets	
Bone marrow failure	At a platelet count of $<10 \times 10^9$ in the absence of risk factors and $<20 \times 10^9$ in the presence of risk factors (e.g. fever, antibiotics, evidence of systemic haemostatic failure).
Surgery/invasive procedure	To maintain platelet count at $>50 \times 10^9$. For surgical procedures with high risk of bleeding (e.g. ocular or neurosurgery) it may be appropriate to maintain at 100.
Platelet function disorders	May be appropriate in inherited or acquired disorders, depending on clinical features and setting. In this situation, platelet count is not a reliable indicator.
Bleeding	May be appropriate in any patient in whom thrombocytopenia is considered a major contributory factor.
Massive haemorrhage/transfusion	Use should be confined to patients with thrombocytopenia and/or functional abnormalities who have significant bleeding from this cause. May be appropriate when the platelet count is $<50 \times 10^9$ ($<100 \times 10^9$ in the presence of diffuse microvascular bleeding).
Fresh frozen plasma	
Single factor deficiencies	Use specific factors if available.
Warfarin effect	In the presence of life-threatening bleeding. Use in addition to vitamin-K-dependent concentrates.
Acute DIC	Indicated where there is bleeding and abnormal coagulation. Not indicated for chronic DIC.
TTP	Accepted treatment.
Coagulation inhibitor deficiencies	May be appropriate in patients undergoing high-risk procedures. Use specific factors if available.
Following massive transfusion or cardiac bypass	May be appropriate in the presence of bleeding and abnormal coagulation.
Liver disease	May be appropriate in the presence of bleeding and abnormal coagulation.
Cryoprecipitate	
Fibrinogen deficiency	May be appropriate where there is clinical bleeding, an invasive procedure, trauma or DIC.

(Adapted from the National Health and Medical Research Council and Australasian Society Clinical Practice Guidelines on appropriate use of blood components http://www.health.gov.au/nhmrc/publications/pdf/cp82.pdf)

fusion result not from exposure to unusual antigens but from an administrative error. Any systematic change in documentation protocols, for example the adoption of an electronic record, needs to be accompanied by an obsessive risk management strategy.

The checking of the compatibility details of blood to be transfused must be meticulous. Blood products should not be left lying around workbenches. Universal precautions must be observed by staff setting up transfusions. Rapid or large transfusions should be via a blood warmer. Blood is transfused intravenously through sterile giving sets containing 170 µm filters. Alternative routes, arterial, intraperitoneal, or intraosseous, are only used in exceptional circumstances. Lines for transfusion should be dedicated lines; drugs and other additives should be administered at separate sites. Normal saline is compatible with all blood components.

Pulse, blood pressure and temperature are measured at regular intervals, and particular attention is paid to the patient during the first 15 minutes of the transfusion. The transfusion is started slowly. The rate at which it continues depends upon the clinical urgency. The usual regime is 500 mL over 1–2 hours. As a general rule, the faster the anaemia has developed the more rapidly it needs to be corrected. Rapid infusion techniques may be indicated in patients who appear to be exsanguinating, but over-rapid infusion can precipitate cardiac failure in the elderly. Hypothermia may be a problem if a blood warmer is not used.

ADVERSE REACTIONS

Immediate

Left ventricular failure

This may be precipitated, especially in elderly patients, by excessive volume expansion with colloid and/or crystalloid prior to transfusion of packed red cells. Elderly patients with acute GI haemorrhage should be transfused early in order to avoid this complication.

Non-haemolytic reaction

This usually consists of mild fever and/or urticaria, beginning shortly after commencement of the transfusion. It may represent a reaction between antibodies in the patient's plasma and donor white cell antigens. In the absence of circulatory collapse it is usually possible to continue the transfusion. Aspirin or antihistamines can attenuate the clinical response, and it may also be useful to slow the transfusion. If significant symptoms such as wheeze or anaphylaxis persist, it may be necessary to transfuse leucocyte-depleted red cells. Rarely, incompatibility to leukocyte antigens can cause pulmonary hypersensitivity and non-cardiogenic pulmonary oedema. Therapy is supportive.

Haemolytic reaction

This is a severe incompatibility reaction commencing within minutes of the start of the transfusion. There may be headache, chest, loin and abdominal pain, shortness of breath, fever, tachycardia and circulatory collapse, progressing to acute renal failure and disseminated intravascular coagulation (DIC).

The transfusion should be ceased immediately. The laboratory must be informed of the incompatibility reaction, and both the donor blood and further blood samples from the patient sent for rescreening. Further action depends on the patient's condition. Intensive-care admission may be required to manage complications. The need for transfusion should be reassessed. Specific therapies that have proved useful include heparin in the context of DIC, and mannitol and loop diuretics in the maintenance of adequate renal output.

Hyperkalaemia

Although potassium leaks out of stored red cells, hyperkalaemia is not usually a problem unless the transfusion is massive. In such cases serum potassium levels should be monitored.

Delayed

Delayed transfusion reaction

In these reactions a previously undetected antibody is boosted in response

Table 12.1.4 Pathogens transmissible by blood transfusion
Bacteria
Pseudomonas
Salmonella
Treponema pallidum
Brucella
Parasites
Plasmodium
Trypanosoma
Toxoplasma
Babesia
Viruses
Hepatitis B and delta agent
Hepatitis A (rare)
Hepatitis C
Other hepatitis 'non-A, non-B'
Parvovirus
HIV-1 and HIV-2
CMV
EEB
HTLV-I
HTLV-II

to a red cell antigen. The features are those of an intravascular haemolytic anaemia, and include fever, jaundice and a falling haemoglobin. These reactions may develop within a week of the transfusion, are usually self-limiting, and rarely severe.

Infection

Table 12.1.4 lists some of the pathogens known to be transmissible through transfusion of blood products. Blood transfusion services combat these potential hazards by using rigorous selection and screening procedures of donors and donor blood. Blood banks have rigorous protocols with respect to storage. In the emergency department it is essential that packs be inspected for tears or pinholes prior to transfusion. The pack content should be inspected for evidence of haemolysis or clotting. The establishment of ever more rigorous screening methods is making the risk of transmission of some viral agents vanishingly small, but it cannot be completely eliminated (Table 12.1.5). The decision to transfuse is never trivial, and transfusion should only proceed when it is considered that the risk of not transfusing is greater than that of doing so.

The potential for prions, thought to be the infective molecules in the new

Table 12.1.5 Transfusion risks (UK figures)	
Risk	Incidence
Transmission of HIV	1 in 10^7
Transmission of Hep B	1 in 10^5
Transmission of Hep C	1 in 10^5
Fatal haemolytic transfusion error	1 in 600 000
Severe non-haemolytic reaction	1 in 1000
Bacterial contamination	1 in 10^6

variant form of Creutzfeldt–Jakob disease (CJD), to be transmitted by blood transfusion has become a subject of intense scrutiny for transfusion medicine.

MASSIVE TRANSFUSION

In the emergency department massive transfusion takes place in the context of uncontrolled bleeding, often as a result of major trauma. Between the patient's arrival in the department and departure to the operating theatre, a combination of colloid, crystalloid and blood products well in excess of the patient's blood volume may have been given. In the operating theatre, and subsequently in intensive care, the blood volume might be replaced more than 20 times.

All such patients develop a coagulopathy and are specifically at risk of disseminated intravascular coagulation and adult respiratory distress syndrome (ARDS). The development of these and other life-threatening complications is specifically related to inadequate resuscitation, as well as to delays in definitive surgical treatment. Victims of blunt and penetrating trauma show different characteristics in this respect, but in both groups untreated hypovolaemic shock and widespread cellular anoxia predict a poor outcome. Occasionally under these circumstances it may be necessary to transfuse 'universal donor' O-negative blood, or red cells that are grouped but not cross-matched. This is done when it is the view of the resuscitation team leader that the risk of delay outweighs the risk of transfusing incompatible

blood products. Blood bank technicians are reluctant to issue uncross-matched blood. Unless there is prior communication between clinicians and blood bank, unexpected calls for urgently needed blood can go badly wrong, with unnecessary delays in transfusion. Some of these problems can be overcome by installing a dedicated blood fridge in the emergency department, regularly maintained, supplied and serviced by the blood bank. Another approach is to organize regular 'blood drills', where team players rehearse the steps necessary for the timely delivery of uncross-matched blood.

It is in the context of massive transfusion that blood products other than packed red cells are most often used in the emergency department. There are practically no platelets left in stored blood after 48 hours. Once a patient is well into the replacement of his second blood volume it is common to observe ooze from raw surfaces, mucous membranes and cannula sites. It can be anticipated that these patients will require platelet supplements, but best practice is to monitor replacement needs using full blood count (FBC), platelet and coagulation studies, as well as observing the patient's clinical response. In the context of massive transfusion a platelet count below 50×10^9/L warrants replacement therapy. Give one unit of concentrate per 10 kg body weight.

Haemostatic concentrations of plasma coagulation factors tend to be maintained better than effective platelet concentrations during massive transfusion, and again, fresh frozen plasma (or cryoprecipitate) should be given according to

need rather than prophylactically, and monitored according to the results of coagulation studies.

Hyperkalaemia may complicate massive transfusion and is discussed above. Other metabolic abnormalities, such as hypocalcaemia and citrate toxicity, are encountered rarely.

PLATELETS

Platelets are obtained from whole blood donations or by plateletpheresis from a single donor. The indications for platelet transfusion include:

- Bone marrow failure
- Platelet dysfunction
- Dilutional thrombocytopenia (see Massive transfusion)
- Cardiopulmonary bypass
- Life-threatening autoimmune thrombocytopenia.

Patients whose platelets fall below 50×10^9/L are at risk of bleeding, and below 10×10^9/L they definitely require platelet transfusion. In autoimmune thrombocytopenia the benefit is likely to be short-lived because of continued autoimmune platelet destruction. Ideally, patients should be given ABO and Rh-specific platelets. Patients who receive multiple platelet transfusions can become refractory to treatment because they mount an immune response to HLA.

GRANULOCYTES

These are rarely given in the emergency department. Indications include severe persistent neutropenia and infection, and abnormal leucocyte function and infection. Adverse effects include alloimmunization, CMV (cytomegalovirus) infection in the immunocompromised, pulmonary infiltrations, and graft-versus-host disease.

FRESH FROZEN PLASMA

This entity is collected from whole blood or through plasmapheresis. It is not used as a plasma expander but as replacement therapy for coagulation factors. Indications for its use include disseminated intravascular coagulation (DIC), liver disease, massive transfusion coagulopathy, reversal of oral anticoagulation, rare factor replacement, thrombotic thrombocytopenic purpura (TTP), and occasionally post thrombolysis. Each millilitre of fresh frozen plasma (FFP) contains one unit of a given coagulation factor. Dosage can be calculated by estimating the patient's plasma volume and incremental factor activity requirements.

CRYOPRECIPITATE

This is prepared through slow thawing of FFP and separation of the precipitate. It contains Factor VIIIC, vWF, fibrinogen, Factor XIII, and fibronectin. Indications for use include low plasma fibrinogen levels. Its use in von Willebrand's disease and the haemophilias has been largely superseded by specific treatments.

PROTHROMBINEX HT

Prothrombinex HT is a Commonwealth Serum Laboratories blood product that contains factors II, IX, and X (approximately 600U of each). It is lyophilized and has been heat-treated to inactivate viruses. The main indication for its use is reversal of over-anticoagulation with warfarin in a bleeding patient.

FURTHER READING

Adebamowo CA, Shokunbi W, Lawal B 1996 Predeposit autologous blood transfusion in a tropical surgical practice. British Journal of Surgery 83(8): 1158–9

FUTURE DIRECTIONS

❶ The practice of patients donating their own blood ahead of their own elective surgery is not really applicable in emergency medicine. However, other techniques of autologous transfusion involving salvage and reinfusion of shed blood (e.g. the Haemonetics cell saver salvage system and the Solcotrans autologous whole blood transfusion system) could well play a role under certain conditions in resuscitation medicine. Of course utilization of such techniques introduces new and characteristic hazards.

❷ Meanwhile, the search for a viable red cell substitute goes on. It needs to pick up oxygen easily from the lungs, deliver oxygen easily to the tissues, and be stable, antigenically inert and relatively cheap. Possible contenders include modified haemoglobin, encapsulated haemoglobin and perfluorochemicals. The ready availability of a safely transfusable oxygen carrier will revolutionize emergency medicine.

Allen JG, 1972 The case for the single transfusion. New England Journal of Medicine 287: 984

Baumann MA, Menitove JE, Aster RH, Anderson T 1986 Urgent treatment of idiopathic thrombocytopenic purpura with single-dose gammaglobulin infusion followed by platelet transfusion. Annals of Internal Medicine 104(6): 808–9

Buchman TG, Bulkley GB 1987 Current management of patients with lower gastrointestinal bleeding. Surgical Clinics of North America 67(3): 651–64

Bull BS, Bull MH, 1994 Hypothesis: disseminated intravascular inflammation as the inflammatory counterpart to disseminated intravascular coagulation. Proceedings of the National Academy of Science USA 91: 8190

Du Hadway H 1995 Transfusion reaction. Home Health Nurse 13(6): 73–4

Fontanarosa PB, Giorgio GT 1989 The role of the emergency physician in the management of Jehovah's Witnesses. Annals of Emergency Medicine 18(10): 1089–95

Greenburg AG 1997 New transfusion strategies. American Journal of Surgery 173(1): 49–52

Gregory SA, McKenna R, Sassetti RJ, Knospe WH 1986 Hematologic emergencies. Medical Clinics of North America 70(5): 1129–49

Grupp-Phelan J, Tanz RR 1996 How rational is the crossmatching of blood in a pediatric emergency department? Archives of Pediatric and Adolescent Medicine 150(11): 1140–4

Hamilton SM 1993 The use of blood in resuscitation of the trauma patient. Canadian Journal of Surgery 36(1): 21–7

Hooker EA, Miller FB, Hollander JL, Burkowski EM 1994 Do all trauma patients need early crossmatching for blood? Journal of Emergency Medicine 112(4): 447–51

Iserson KV, Knauf MA, Anhalt D 1990 Rapid admixture blood warming: technical advances. Critical Care Medicine 18(10): 1138–41

Kelen GD, Green GB, Purcell RH, et al 1992 Hepatitis B and hepatitis C in emergency department patients. New England Journal of Medicine 326(21): 1399–404

Kruskall MS, Mintz PD, Bergin JJ, et al 1988 Transfusion therapy in emergency medicine. Annals of Emergency Medicine 17(4): 327–35

Loo S, Low TC 1997 Perioperative transfusion strategies: a national survey among anaesthetists. Annals of the Academy of Medicine 26(2): 193–9

Moore FA, Moore EE, Sauaia A 1997 Blood transfusion. An independent risk factor for postinjury multiple organ failure. Archives of Surgery 132(6): 620–4

Phillips GR III, Kauder DR, Schwab CW 1994 Massive blood loss in trauma patients. The benefits and dangers of transfusion therapy. Postgraduate Medicine 95(4): 61–72

Prusiner SB, 1991 Molecular biology of prion diseases. Science 252: 1515

Roberts WE 1995 Emergent obstetric management of postpartumhemorrhage. Obstetrics and Gynecology Clinics of North America 22(2): 283–302

Schmidt PJ, Leparc GF, Samia CT 1988 Use of Rh positive blood in emergency situations. Surgery, Gynecology and Obstetrics 167(3): 229–33

Schwab CW, Shayne JP, Turner J 1986 Immediate trauma resuscitation with type O uncrossmatched blood: a two year prospective experience. Journal of Trauma 26(10): 897–902

Simon TL, Smith KJ 1989 The issues in autologous transfusion. Human Pathology 20(1): 3–6

Spence RK, Cernaianu AC, Carson J, Del Rossi AJ 1993 Transfusion and surgery. Current Problems in Surgery 30(12): 1101–80

Woodcock BE, Walker S, Adams K 1993 Haemolytic transfusion reaction – successful attenuation with methylprednisolone and high dose immunoglobulin. Clinical Laboratory Haematology 15(1): 59–61

12.2 NEUTROPENIA

HAMISH MACLAREN

ESSENTIALS

1 The risk of infection increases significantly as the absolute neutrophil count drops below $1.0 \times 10^9/L$.

2 Life-threatening neutropenia is likely to be due to impaired haematopoiesis.

3 A detailed medications history is vital to the 'work-up' of neutropenia.

4 Significant neutropenia in the presence of fever mandates admission to hospital.

INTRODUCTION

'A 21-year-old male presents to the emergency department with a history of fever, chills and rigors. He has a temperature of 39.9°C. His full blood count reveals an absolute neutrophil count of $0.2 \times 10^9/L$'.

Such an encounter presents the emergency physician with two challenges, to determine the aetiology of the neutropenia, and simultaneously to prevent the patient succumbing to overwhelming bacterial or fungal infection.

Neutropenia is a decrease in the number of circulating neutrophils. The neutrophil count varies with age, sex and racial grouping. In practice, the increased risk of infection only becomes significant as the neutrophil count drops below 1.0 $\times 10^9/L$. This risk can be stratified as follows:

- 500–1000/microl: significant risk
- 200–500/microl: highly significant risk
- <200/microl: dangerous.

In addition, neutropenic patients are at greater risk of overwhelming infection if the onset of the neutropenia is acute rather than chronic, and – in the case of patients receiving cancer chemotherapy –

if the absolute neutrophil count is in the process of falling rather than rising.

PATHOPHYSIOLOGY AND AETIOLOGY

Polymorphonuclear neutrophils are formed in marrow from the myelogenous cell series. Pluripotent haematopoietic stem cells are committed to a particular cell lineage through the formation of colony-forming units, which further differentiate to form given white cell precursors. The mature neutrophil has a multilobed nucleus and granules in the cytoplasm. The cells are termed 'neutrophilic' because of the lilac colour of the granules caused by the uptake of both acidic and basic dyes.

The neutrophils leave the marrow and enter the circulation, where they have a lifespan of only 6–10 hours before entering the tissues. Here, they migrate by chemotaxis to sites of infection and injury, and then phagocytose and destroy foreign material. In health, about half of the available mature neutrophils are in the circulation. 'Marginal' cells are adherent to vascular endothelium or in the tissues and are not measured by the full blood count. Some individuals have fixed increased marginal neutrophil pools and decreased circulating pools; they are said to have benign idiopathic neutropenia.

For a previously normal individual to become neutropenic there must be decreased production of neutrophils in the marrow, decreased survival of mature neutrophils, or a redistribution of neutrophils from the circulating pool. The important causes are shown in Table 12.2.1.

It is a defect in neutrophil production that is most likely to prove life threatening. Consumption of neutrophils in the periphery is likely to be rapidly compensated for by a functioning marrow. Fortunately, most of the primary diseases of haematopoiesis are rare, and in prac-

tice many of the acquired neutropenias are drug induced. Processes interfering with haematopoiesis, often involving autoimmune mechanisms, may affect neutrophils both in the marrow and in the periphery. Some drugs cause neutropenia universally, but many more reactions are idiosyncratic, be they dose-related or independent of dose. Some commonly implicated drugs are listed in Table 12.2.2. Cancer chemotherapy drugs are now recognized as the commonest cause of neutropenia.

CLINICAL PRESENTATION

Patients with marked neutropenia are liable to present febrile and constitutionally unwell, with manifestations of infection. They may have a sore throat, and ulcerating lesions of the mouth and gingiva. Evidence of pallor and bleeding is suggestive of pancytopenia.

The history of the mode of onset and duration of the illness is important. Systems enquiry may reveal cough, headache and photophobia, a diarrhoeal

Table 12.1.1 Important causes of neutropenia

Decreased production
Aplastic anaemia
Leukaemias
Lymphomas
Metastatic cancer
Drug-induced agranulocytosis
Megaloblastic anaemias
    Vitamin B_{12} deficiency
    Folate deficiency
CD8 + large granular lymphocytosis
Myelodysplastic syndromes

Decreased survival
Idiopathic immune mediated
SLE
Felty syndrome
Drugs

Redistribution
Sequestration in the spleen (hypersplenism)
Increased utilization: overwhelming sepsis
Viraemia

Table 12.2.2 Drugs commonly associated with neutropenia
Antibiotics: chloramphenicol, sulphonamides, isoniazid, rifampicin, β-lactams, carbenicillin
Antidysrhythmic agents: quinidine, procainamide
Antiepileptics: phenytoin, carbamazepine
Antihypertensives: thiazides, ethacrynic acid, captopril, methyldopa, hydralazine
Antithyroid agents
Chemotherapeutic agents: especially methotrexate, cytosine arabinoside, 5-azacytidine, azothiaprine, doxorubicine, daunorubicine, hydroxyurea, alkylating agents
Connective tissue disorder agents: phenylbutazone, penicillamine, gold
H_2-receptor antagonists
Phenothiazines, especially chlorpromazine
Miscellaneous: imipramine, allopurinol, clozapine, ticlopidine, tolbutamide

illness, or urinary symptoms. The past history may reveal a known haematological abnormality or previous evidence of immunosuppression. A detailed drug history is vital. Most neutropenic drug reactions occur within the first 3 months of taking a drug. In the emergency department vital signs include pulse, blood pressure, temperature, respiratory rate and pulse oximetry reading. Some febrile illnesses show characteristic periodicity in temperature changes, and these should be recorded.

Physical examination may reveal necrotizing mucosal lesions, pallor, petechial rashes, lymphadenopathy, bone tenderness, abnormal tonsillar or respiratory findings, spleno- or other organomegaly. Careful examination of the skin of the back, the lower limbs and the perineum for evidence of infection is important.

INVESTIGATIONS

The work-up in the emergency department proceeds as for any unspecified febrile illness. Investigations include a full blood count, platelets and blood film, and a coagulation profile. Anaemic patients may require a group-and-hold or a cross-match. Blood cultures are taken prior to the instigation of antibiotic therapy. Other investigations which may be appropriate include a chest X-ray, throat swab, swabs of skin lesions, MSU for urinalysis and culture, and biochemistry, including electrolytes and creatinine, glucose and liver function tests. Patients with apparent CNS infections might require a lumbar puncture at some stage, but this should be postponed or even cancelled in the presence of an uncorrected coagulopathy. Antibiotics, if clinically indicated, should be commenced prior to lumbar puncture.

MANAGEMENT AND DISPOSITION

Evidence of circulatory collapse warrants immediate aggressive resuscitation. The presence of neutropenia with fever mandates admission to hospital. Both the haematological abnormality and the likely presence of infection require investigation. Sometimes the aetiology of the neutropenia will be evident; on other occasions marrow aspiration and biopsy will be required. On admission, all drug therapies should be stopped wherever possible. With high fevers, low cell counts and constitutional symptoms, broad-spectrum antibiotic therapy should be started in the emergency department after drawing blood for culture. The choice of antibiotics is empirical, depending on the clinical and laboratory findings at the time and the likely pathogen. Regimens change with time and differ between regions. One possible approach might be to obtain good Gram-negative cover with a quinolone such as ciprofloxacin, and Gram-positive cover with either teicoplanin or vancomycin. The possibility of fungal infection might prompt the use of amphotericin B. Emergency resuscitation is continued and unstable patients are admitted to intensive care. The use of granulocyte infusions is rarely adopted, although growth factor infusions such as G-CSF have been shown to shorten the period of neutropenia.

FURTHER READING

Bochud PY, Calandra T, Francioli P 1994 Bacteremia due to viridans streptococci in neutropenic patients: a review. American Journal of Medicine 97(3): 256–64

Brandt B 1990 Nursing protocol for the patient with neutropenia. Oncologist Nursing Forum 17(1 Suppl): 9–15

Chanock SJ, Pizzo PA 1996 Fever in the neutropenic host. Infectious Disease Clinics of North America 10(4): 777–96

Gulick PG 1990 Update on infections in neutropenic hosts. Journal of the American Osteopathic Association 90(10): 920–5

Kemp SF, Lockey RF 1995 Amphotericin B: emergency challenge in a neutropenic, asthmatic patient with fungal sepsis. Journal of Allergy and Clinical Immunology 96(3): 425–7

Lauter CB 1989 Antibiotic therapy of life-threatening infectious diseases in the emergency department. Annals of Emergency Medicine 18(12): 1339–43

Lazarus HM, Creger RJ, Gerson SL 1989 Infectious emergencies in oncology patients. Seminars in Oncology 16(6): 543–60

12.3 HAEMOPHILIA

HAMISH MACLAREN

ESSENTIALS

The emergency physician needs to be aware of the following complications of haemophilia:

1 Haemarthroses

2 Compartment syndrome

3 Bleeding into the neck

4 Intracranial bleeding

5 Retroperitoneal bleeding.

INTRODUCTION

Haemophilia is a disorder of coagulation. Haemophilia A is due to a deficiency of Factor VIII, haemophilia B (Christmas disease) to a deficiency of Factor IX. The general term 'haemophilia' usually refers to Factor VIII deficiency as an inherited disorder, although an acquired form is also recognized.

PATHOPHYSIOLOGY

The defective gene is at the tip of the long arm of the X chromosome. A wide variety of genetic mutations lead to underproduction of Factor VIII: 50% of haemophiliac families have an inversion of the factor VIII gene. However, up to 30% of new cases may be due to sporadic genetic mutations. Transmission is X-linked recessive; female carriers have at least 50% factor VIII activity and usually do not express the disease. Haemophilia B is also transmitted by an X-linked recessive gene. Haemophilia A is the commoner disease, with an incidence of 1 in 8000–10 000 live male births, compared to an incidence of 1 in 25 000–30 000 for haemophilia B.

The severity of the bleeding disorder depends on how much Factor VIII activity is present:

- 6–60%: mild
- 1–5%: moderate
- <1%: severe.

The traditional model of the coagulation cascade considers clotting as the result of the activation of one of two series of reactions, termed the intrinsic and the extrinsic pathways, culminating in the final common pathway. However, more recent work suggests that the interrelationship of the two pathways in the activation of Factors IX and X is far more complex in vivo. Activated Factor X releases an inhibitor of activated Factor VII, and for coagulation to continue there has to be stimulation via the IX/VIII pathway, which can continue without VIIa stimulus, perhaps stimulated by thrombin and Factor XI. This explains why Factors VIII and IX are so critical to clot formation.

The traditional model of the coagulation cascade is still useful in describing routine laboratory tests of coagulation. The prothrombin time(PT) measures primarily Factors II, VII, V and X. The partial thromboplastin time (PPT) measures primarily Factors XII, XI, IX, VIII, X and V. Factor VIII has an intimate association with von Willebrand factor, an adhesive glycoprotein secreted by endothelium and megakaryocytes, and required for the normal instigation of platelet plug formation. In addition, von Willebrand factor is required for the stabilization and transport of Factor VIII within the circulation. Thus von Willebrand disease is associated with low Factor VIII activity.

CLINICAL PRESENTATION

Children with haemophilia manifest the disease when they begin to crawl, and patients who are severely affected may present with bleeding episodes on a weekly basis. However, first-time presentations in adulthood are not unknown and the bleeding may even then be severe.

Bleeding tends to be spontaneous or following minor trauma. It may be a 'gush' rather than an 'ooze', implying a clotting rather than a platelet plug problem. Bleeding is from vessels rather than capillary beds, and haemarthroses and haematomata are formed. The following bleeding patterns each constitute an emergency:

- Haemarthroses. If not treated properly, these lead to arthropathies and joint destruction.
- Bleeding into tissue planes. Tense flexor haematomas in limbs can cause compartment syndromes.
- Bleeding into the neck. May cause airway compromise.
- CNS bleeding. Haemophiliac patients with even apparently minor head trauma need hospital assessment and computerized tomgraphy (CT) head scanning. Beware subtle signs of a developing subdural haematoma. If an intracranial bleed is suspected, replacement therapy should be initiated prior to radiological investigation.
- Retroperitoneal bleeding. If there is evidence of acute blood loss and the source cannot be found, consider the retroperitoneal space.

Patients may also present with a complication of therapy. Most haemophiliac patients treated before 1985 have been exposed to pathogenic viruses, of which the most important are hepatitis C, hepatitis B and the superimposed delta agent, and HIV. Of those who received plasma prior to the mid-1980s, 90% are Hep B positive, 85–100% are Hep C positive, and 60–90% are HIV positive. In some studies HIV is now the leading cause of death in the haemophiliac population.

Recently it has been postulated that the new variant form of Creutzfeldt–

Jakob disease (CJD) might be transmissable by transfusion of blood and blood products. The infective agent or prion is a protein devoid of nucleic acid genome, which is resistant to all currently available techniques of eradication. The implications for all forms of transfusion medicine are daunting.

INVESTIGATIONS

These will be tailored to individual presentations and may include plain radiography of affected joints and CT scanning of the head and trunk looking for fluid collections. A full blood count, blood film and coagulation profiles are useful in the evaluation of first presentations.

Patients with both haemophilia A and B have a normal prothrombin time, a normal thrombin clot time, and a prolonged activated partial thromboplastin time (although it can be normal if factor activity exceeds 30%). Specific factor assays are required to distinguish between haemophilias A and B.

MANAGEMENT

Treatment of acute bleeding episodes involves replacement therapy, adjunctive therapies such as pain relief, rest and mobilization, and treatment of the complications of the bleed. In the context of pain relief aspirin (or other platelet-modifying drugs) should be avoided, and NSAIDs used with caution. In major bleeds there may be a requirement for red cell transfusion. Developing limb compartment syndromes may require surgical decompression. Intracranial bleeds may require neurosurgical intervention. In all of these cases factor replacement must commence as quickly as possible. Management of complex presentations requires a multidisciplinary approach.

Replacement therapy

Some patients with Factor VIII levels higher than 10% may be successfully treated with 1-amino-8-d-arginine vaso-pressin (DDAVP), which can be given intravenously, subcutaneously, or even inhaled. The exact mechanism of action is unclear, but it appears to mobilize available Factor VIII stores and may raise the Factor VIII activity by a factor of 3. The parenteral dose is 0.3 mg/kg 12-hourly, and a response should be evident within the first hour. Side-effects, including facial flushing and headache, are usually well tolerated. Tachyphylaxis tends to develop after three or four doses.

Antifibrinolytic agents such as tranexamic acid and epsilon-aminocaproic acid have been used as adjunctive therapy in minor episodes of bleeding, say, following dental extraction. Fibrin tissue adhesives containing fibrinogen, thrombin, and Factor XIII have also been successfully placed in tooth sockets and similar surgical sites.

Patients with moderate and severe deficiencies require Factor VIII concentrate. Many patients can administer this at home, 'on demand'. Indeed, the availability of Factor VIII and the ease of administration has revolutionized the care of haemophiliac patients in the community. However, the following are indications for hospital admission:

- A big bleed
- Ongoing bleed
- Possible bleeding into the head or neck
- Need for ongoing pain relief
- Need for ongoing therapy, especially infusions
- Possibility of compartment syndrome
- Inadequate social circumstances.

If Factor VIII concentrate is unavailable cryoprecipitate or fresh frozen plasma can be given, but these products continue to pose a small risk of viral transmission. A bag of cryoprecipitate holds 100 units of Factor VIII, whereas FFP contains 1 unit of Factor VIII/mL.

Determining the dose of Factor VIII concentrate

One unit of Factor VIII concentrate is the amount of Factor VIII activity in 1 mL of normal plasma. Given that a 70 kg adult has a plasma volume of 3500 mL, we can expect that an infusion of 3500 units of Factor VIII will produce 100% Factor VIII activity in a haemophiliac with negligible activity prior to treatment. The half-life of Factor VIII is approximately 12 hours. Accordingly, a further dose of 1750 units in 12 hours' time will again restore 100% activity.

It is not always necessary to provide 100% Factor VIII activity in order to ensure haemostasis: levels of 30–50% may be sufficient in the context of haemarthrosis, or dental extraction. Larger infusions should be reserved for life-threatening situations.

Inhibitors

Some patients develop antibodies to Factor VIII, known as 'inhibitors'. Treatment has to be modified according to the titre of inhibitor present (measured by the Bethesda Inhibitor Assay or BIA concentrate). Patients are classified as 'high responders' if their baseline inhibitor titre exceeds 10 Bethesda Units (BU) or if the titre rises above 10 BU on exposure to Factor VIII. Different management strategies are employed according to the severity of the bleed. Either the dose of Factor VIII can be increased (although this may result in a further rise in inhibitor titre) or alternative therapies or 'bypassing agents' such as prothrombin complex, activated prothrombin complex, porcine Factor VIII or recombinant Factor VIIa can be used. Factor VIIa is administered in doses of 90–120 microg/kg 2–3 hourly.

Most patients who develop inhibitors do so early in life and are known to have severe hereditary haemophilia, but inhibitors can also arise in previously normal individuals to produce an acquired haemophilia. The incidence of this phenomenon is from 0.2 to 1/1 000 000/year. Patients tend to be elderly and some have autoimmune disease, but there is also an association with pregnancy as well as with some drugs, notably penicillin. Patients haemorrhage into muscle and soft tissues, and may present with haematemesis, or with unusual postoperative bleeding. In the laboratory the patient's blood shows a prolonged APPT that is not corrected by 'mixing', that is, by the addition of normal plasma. Factor VIII levels are low. Management is directed towards control of the bleeding episode, replacement therapy, and the prevention of further reactions using a variety of immunosuppressive remedies.

HAEMOPHILIA B

Treatment strategies for haemophilia B are similar to those for haemophilia A except that the principal replacement therapy involves Factor IX. One unit/kg of Factor IX raises the level of factor activity by 1% and, as with haemophilia A, life-threatening conditions require higher doses, sustained over a longer period.

FURTHER READING

Bell BA, Birch K, Glazer S 1993 Experience with recombinant factor VIIA in an infant with hemophilia with inhibitors to FVIII:C undergoing emergency central line placement. A case report. American Journal of Pediatrics, Hematology and Oncology 15(1): 77–9

Bush MT, Roy N 1995 Hemophilia emergencies. Journal of Emergency Nursing 21(6): 531–8

De Behnke DJ, Angelos MG 1990 Intracranial hemorrhage and hemophilia: case report and management guidelines. Journal of Emergency Medicine 8(4): 423–7

Gregory SA, McKenna R, Sassetti RJ, Knospe WH 1986 Hematologic emergencies. Medical Clinics of North America 70(5): 1129–49

Pfaff JA, Geninatti M 1993 Hemophilia. Emergency Medicine Clinics of North America 11(2): 337–63

Warrier I, Ewenstein BM, Koerper MA, et al 1997 Factor IX inhibitors and anaphylaxis in hemophilia B. Journal of Pediatrics, Hematology and Oncology 19(1): 23–7

12.4 ANAEMIA

HAMISH MACLAREN

ESSENTIALS

1 Anaemia is a condition in which the absolute number of red cells in the circulation is abnormally low.

2 Anaemia is not a diagnosis: it is a finding, which should prompt the search for an underlying cause.

3 The anaemic patient is doing at least one of three things: not producing enough red cells, destroying them too quickly, or bleeding.

4 Bleeding is the most common cause of severe anaemia encountered in the emergency department.

INTRODUCTION

Anaemia is a condition in which the absolute number of red cells in the circulation is abnormally low. The diagnosis is usually made on the basis of the full blood count (FBC). This, together with the blood film, offers qualitative as well as quantitative data on the blood components, and a set of normal values is shown in Table 12.4.1.

The average lifespan of a normal red blood cell in the circulation is from 100 to 120 days. Aged red cells are removed by the reticuloendothelial system, but under normal conditions are replaced by the marrow such that a dynamic equilibrium is maintained. Anaemia develops when red cell loss exceeds red cell production. It follows that the anaemic patient is doing at least one of three things: not producing enough red cells, destroying them too quickly, or bleeding.

The overriding functional importance of the red cell resides in its ability to transport oxygen, bound to the haemoglobin molecule, from the lungs to the tissues. Functionally, anaemia may be regarded as an impairment in the supply of oxygen to the tissues and the adverse effects of anaemia, from whatever cause, are a consequence of the resultant tissue hypoxia. Anaemia is not a diagnosis: rather, it is a clinical or a laboratory finding that should prompt the search for an underlying cause (Table 12.4.2).

HAEMORRHAGE

AETIOLOGY

By far the most common cause of severe anaemia encountered in the emergency department is haemorrhage. Therefore, the assessment of the anaemic patient is

Table 12.4.1 Full blood count (FBC): normal parameters

Haemoglobin (Hb)	
Males	13.5–18 g/dL
Females	11.5–16.5 g/dL
RBC count	
Males	4500–6500×10^9/L
Females	3900–5600×10^9/L
Haematocrit	
Males	42–54%
Females	37–47%
MCH	27–32 pg
MCHC	32–36 g/dl
MCV	76–98 fl
Reticulocytes	0.2–2%
WBC	4–11×10^9/L
Neutrophils	1.8–8×10^9/L
Eosinophils	0–0.6×10^9/L
Basophils	0–0.2×10^9/L
Lymphocytes	1–5×10^9/L
Monocytes	0–0.8×10^9/L
Platelets	150–400×10^9/L
MCV = HCT divided by RBC	
MCH = Hb divided by RBC	
MCHC = Hb divided by Hct	

Most automated counting machines now give the red cell distribution width (RDW), a measure of degree of variation of cell size

often chiefly concerned with the search for a site of blood loss. The most common causes of haemorrhage are outlined in Table 12.4.3. However, the emergency physician must always be alert to the possibility that the patient is not bleeding but is manifesting a rarer pathologic condition.

Table 12.4.2 Causes of anaemia

Haemorrhage
Traumatic
Non-traumatic
  acute or chronic

Production defect
Megaloblastic anaemia
  Vitamin B_{12} deficiency
  Folate deficiency
Aplastic anaemia
Pure red cell aplasia
Myelodysplastic syndromes
Invasive marrow diseases
Chronic renal failure

Decreased RBC survival (haemolytic anaemia)
Congenital
  Spherocytosis
  Elliptocytosis
  Glucose-6-phosphate-dehydrogenase deficiency
  Pyruvate kinase deficiency
  Haemoglobinopathies: sickle cell disease
  Thalassaemias
Acquired
  Autoimmune haemolytic anaemia
    Warm
  Cold
  Microangiopathic haemolytic anaemias
  RBC mechanical trauma
  Infections
  Paroxysmal nocturnal haemoglobinuria

Table 12.4.3 Common causes of haemorrhage in the emergency department

Trauma
Blunt trauma to mediastinum
Pulmonary contusions/haemopneumothorax
Intraperitoneal injury
Retroperitoneal injury
Pelvic disruption
Long bone injury
Open wounds: inadequate first aid

Non-trauma
GI haemorrhage
  Oesophageal varices
  Peptic ulcer
  Gastritis/Mallory-Weiss
  Colonic/rectal bleeding
Obstetric/gynaecological bleeding
  Ruptured ectopic pregnancy
  Menorrhagia
  Threatened miscarriage
  Antepartum haemorrhage
  Postpartum haemorrhage
Other
  Epistaxis
  Postoperative
  Secondary to bleeding diathesis

CLINICAL PRESENTATION

While it may be obvious on history and examination that a patient is bleeding, occasionally the source of blood loss is occult and the extent of loss underestimated.

In the context of trauma the history often gives clear pointers to both sites and extent of blood loss. Consideration of the mechanism of injury may allow anticipation of occult pelvic, intraperitoneal or retroperitoneal bleeding. Intracranial bleeding is never an explanation for hypovolaemic shock in an adult. In the context of non-trauma it is essential to obtain an obstetric and gynaecological history in women of childbearing age. The remainder of the formal history may supply information essential in determining the aetiology of anaemia. The past medical history may point to a known haematological abnormality or to a chronic disease process. A drug and allergy history is always relevant. Many drugs cause marrow suppression, haemolytic anaemia and bleeding. The family history points to hereditary disease; the social history may alert the clinician to an unusual occupational exposure in the patient's past or, more likely, to recreational activities liable to exacerbate an ongoing disease process. The systems review is particularly relevant to the consultation with middle-aged or elderly male patients, who must be asked about symptoms of altered bowel habit and weight loss.

The symptomatology of anaemia proceeds from vague complaints of tiredness, lethargy and impaired performance through to more sharply defined entities such as shortness of breath on exertion, giddiness, restlessness, apprehension, confusion and collapse. Comorbid conditions may be exacerbated (the dyspnoea of chronic obstructive airway disease) and occult pathologies unmasked (exertional angina in ischaemic heart disease). Anaemia of insidious onset is generally better tolerated than that of rapid onset, because of cardiovascular and other compensatory mechanisms. Acute loss of 40% of the blood volume may result in collapse, whereas in certain developing countries it is not rare for patients with haemoglobin concentrations 10% of normal to be ambulant. Trauma superimposed on an already established anaemia can lead to rapid decompensation.

The cardinal sign of anaemia is pallor. This can be seen in the skin, the lips, the mucous membranes and the conjunctival reflections. Yet not all anaemic patients are pallid, and not all patients with a pale complexion are anaemic. Patients who have suffered an acute haemorrhage may show evidence of hypovolaemia: tachycardia, hypotension, cold peripheries, sluggish capillary refill. The detection of postural hypotension is an important pointer towards occult blood loss. Conversely, patients with anaemia of insidious onset are not hypovolaemic and may manifest high-output cardiac failure as a physiological response to hypoxia.

Other features of the physical examination may provide clues to the aetiology of anaemia. The glossitis, angular stomatitis, koilonychia and oesophageal web of iron-deficiency anaemia are uncommon findings. Bone tenderness, lymphadenopathy, hepatomegaly and splenomegaly may point to an underlying haematological abnormality. The rectal and gynaecological examinations can sometimes be diagnostic.

INVESTIGATIONS

The full blood count often reveals an anaemia that has not been clinically suspected and that must be interpreted in the light of the history and examination. If the anaemia is mild it may be a chance finding with little relevance to the patient's presenting complaint, but such a finding should never be ignored. At the very least a follow-up blood count should be arranged.

Anaemic patients have a low red cell count, a low haematocrit and a low haemoglobin, but some caveats need to be borne in mind:

- Patients who are bleeding acutely may initially have a normal FBC.
- Normal or high haematocrits may reflect haemoconcentration.

- Mixed pictures can be difficult to interpret, e.g. that of a polycythaemic patient who is bleeding.

Red cell morphology, particularly the MCV (mean corpuscular volume), can help elucidate the cause of an anaemia. The finding of a pancytopenia suggests a problem in haematopoiesis, rather than haemolysis or blood loss. In women of childbearing age, assay of blood or urine β-HCG is important.

MANAGEMENT

The principles of management of haemorrhage are as follows:

- Maintain the circulation.
- Identify the site of bleeding.
- Control the bleeding.
- Identify the underlying pathological process.
- Arrange for definitive treatment.
- Restore the blood volume.

The indications for red cell transfusion are discussed in Chapter 12.1. The faster the onset of the anaemia, the greater the need for urgent replacement. Patients who are tolerating their anaemia may require no more than an appropriate diet with or without the addition of haematinics. Elderly patients with severe bleeding often need red cells urgently. Excessive administration of colloid and/or crystalloid precipitates left ventricular failure, and it can then be difficult to administer red cells.

Chronic haemorrhage

The finding of a hypochromic microcytic anaemia on blood film is usually indicative of iron deficiency and, in the absence of an overt history of bleeding, should prompt the search for occult blood loss. Iron-deficiency anaemia may be due to malnutrition, but inadequate dietary intake of iron is not usually the sole cause of anaemia in developed countries: much more commonly it is the result of chronic blood loss from the GI tract, the uterus or the renal tract. More unusual causes are haemoptysis and recurrent epistaxes.

Patients present with insidious and rather vague symptoms. They may be unaware that they are bleeding and will probably show none of the trophic skin, nail and mucosal changes of iron deficiency. The automated cell count, in addition to showing a hypochromic, microcytic picture, may also show a raised RDW (red cell distribution width), which reflects anisocytosis on the blood film.

Iron studies may confirm the diagnosis of iron deficiency without pointing to the underlying cause. Serum iron and ferritin are low and total iron-binding capacity is high.

DISPOSITION

If the source of blood loss is obvious, for example heavy menstrual bleeding, then appropriate referral may be all that is indicated. If the source is not obvious, particularly in older patients, then sequential investigation of the GI tract and the renal tract may be indicated. Decisions to admit or discharge these patients depend on the red cell reserves, the patient's cardiorespiratory status, home circumstances, and the likelihood of compliance with follow-up.

The anaemia itself can be corrected with oral iron supplements: 200 mg of ferrous sulphate three times daily is an appropriate regimen, although single daily doses are often more acceptable to the patient and have fewer gastrointestinal side effects.

ANAEMIA OWING TO DECREASED RED CELL PRODUCTION

MEGALOBLASTIC ANAEMIA

The finding of a raised mass cell volume (MCV) is common in the presence or absence of anaemia. Alcohol abuse is a frequent underlying cause, and other causes are listed in Table 12.4.4. MCVs greater than 115 fL are usually due to megaloblastic anaemia, which in turn is usually due to either vitamin B_{12} or folate deficiency. Vitamin B_{12} and folate are essential to DNA synthesis in all cells. Deficiencies manifest principally in red cell production because of the sheer number of red cells that are produced. B_{12} deficiency is usually the result of a malabsorption syndrome, whereas folate deficiency is of dietary origin. Tetrahydrofolate is a cofactor in DNA synthesis and, in turn, the formation of tetrahydrofolate from its methylated precursor is B_{12}-dependent. Unabated cytoplasmic production of RNA in the context of impaired DNA synthesis appears to produce the enlarged nucleus and abundant cytoplasm of the megaloblast. These cells, when released to the periphery, have poor function and poor survival.

B_{12} deficiency is an autoimmune disorder in which autoantibodies to gastric parietal cells and the B_{12} transport factor (intrinsic factor) interfere with B_{12} absorption in the terminal ileum. Patients have achlorhydria, mucosal atrophy (a painful smooth tongue), and sometimes evidence of other autoimmune disorders, such as vitiligo, thyroid disease and Addison's disease. This is so-called 'pernicious anaemia'.

A rare, but important, manifestation of this disease is 'subacute combined degeneration of the spinal cord'. Demyelination of the posterior and lateral columns of the spinal cord manifests as a peripheral neuropathy and an abnormal gait. The CNS abnormalities worsen and

Table 12.4.4 Some causes of a raised MCV
Reticulocytosis
Liver disease
Alcohol
Myelodysplasia
Drugs
Megaloblastic anaemias (B_{12} and folate deficiency)
Pregnancy
Hypothyroidism

become irreversible in the absence of B_{12} supplementation. Treatment of B_{12} deficient patients with folate alone may accelerate the onset of this condition.

Undiagnosed untreated pernicious anaemia is not a common finding in the emergency department, but the laboratory finding of anaemia and megaloblastosis should prompt haematological consultation. The investigative work-up, which includes B_{12} and red cell folate levels, autoantibodies to parietal cells and intrinsic factor, a marrow aspirate, and Schilling's test of B_{12} absorption, may well necessitate hospital admission.

The work-up for folate deficiency is similar to that for B_{12}. Occasionally patients require investigation for a malabsorption syndrome (tropical sprue, coeliac disease), which includes jejunal biopsy. Folate deficiency is common in pregnancy because of the large folate requirements of the growing foetus. It can be difficult to diagnose because of the maternal physiological expansion of plasma volume and also of red cell mass, but diagnosis and treatment with oral folate supplements are important because of the risk of associated neural tube defects.

Both B_{12} and folate deficiency are usually manifestations of chronic disease processes. Rarely, an acute megaloblastic anaemia and pancytopaenia can develop over the course of days and nitrous oxide therapy has been identified as a principal cause of this condition.

ANAEMIA OF CHRONIC DISORDERS

Patients with chronic infective, malignant or connective tissue disorders can develop a mild-to-moderate normochromic normocytic anaemia. Evidence of bleeding or haemolysis is absent, and there is no response to haematinic therapy. The pathophysiology of this anaemia is complex and probably involves both decreased red cell production and survival. Possible underlying mechanisms include reticuloendothelial overactivity in chronic inflammation, and defects in iron metabolism mediated by a variety of acute-phase reactants and cytokines such as interleukin-1, tumour necrosis factor, and interferon γ, which impair renal erythropoietin production and function.

Anaemia of chronic disorders (ACD) is generally not so severe as to warrant emergency therapy. The importance of ACD in the emergency department lies in its recognition as a pointer towards an underlying chronic process. Difficulties can arise in distinguishing ACD from iron deficiency, and the two conditions may coexist – in rheumatoid arthritis, for example. Iron studies generally elucidate the nature of the anaemia. In iron deficiency, iron and ferritin are low and total iron binding is high, whereas in ACD iron and total iron binding are low and ferritin is normal or high.

There has been a recent explosion of interest in improving the well-being of cancer patients by treating an associated anaemia with recombinant erythropoietin.

OTHER CAUSES OF DECREASED RED CELL PRODUCTION

Bone marrow failure is rarely encountered in emergency medicine practice. The physician must be alert to the unusual, insidious or sinister presentation and particularly attuned to the triad of decreased tissue oxygenation, immunocompromise, and a bleeding diathesis that may herald a pancytopenia. An FBC may dictate the need for haematological consultation, hospital admission and further investigation.

Among the entities to be considered are the aplastic anaemias, characterized by a pancytopenia secondary to failure of pluripotent myeloid stem cells. Half of cases are idiopathic, but important aetiologies are infections (e.g. non-A, non-B hepatitis), inherited diseases (e.g. Fanconi's anaemia), irradiation, therapeutic or otherwise, and – most important in the emergency setting – drugs. Drugs that have been implicated in the development of aplastic anaemia include, in addition to antimetabolites and alkylating agents, chloramphenicol, chlorpromazine and streptomycin.

Characteristic of patients with a primary marrow failure is the absence of splenomegaly and the absence of a reticulocyte response. There is a correlation between prognosis and the severity of the pancytopenia. Platelet counts less than $20 \times 10^9/L$ and neutrophil counts less than $500/mL$ equate to severe disease. Depending on the severity of the accompanying anaemia, patients may require red cell and sometimes platelet transfusion in the emergency department, as well as broad-spectrum antibiotic cover. It is imperative to stop all medications that might be causing the marrow failure. Other forms of marrow failure include pure red cell aplasia (PRCA), where marrow red cell precursors are absent or diminished. This can be a complication of haemolytic states in which a viral insult leads to an aplastic crisis (see Haemolytic anaemias).

The myelodysplastic syndromes are a group of disorders primarily affecting the elderly. In these states there is no reduction in marrow cellularity but the mature red cells, granulocytes and platelets generated from an abnormal clone of stem cells are disordered and dysfunctional. There is peripheral pancytopenia. These disorders are classified according to observed cellular morphology (Table 12.4.5). These conditions were once termed 'preleukaemia', and one-third of patients progress to acute myeloid leukaemia.

Two more causes of failure of erythropoiesis might be mentioned. One is due to invasion of the marrow and disruption of its architecture by extraneous tissue, the commonest cause being metastatic cancer. Finally, and by no means uncommon, is the anaemia of chronic renal

Table 12.4.5 Classification of the myelodysplastic syndromes
Refractory anaemia (RA)
Refractory anaemia with ringed sideroblasts (RARS)
Refractory anaemia with excess of blasts (RAEB)
Chronic myelomonocytic leukaemia (CMML)

failure, where deficient erythropoiesis is attributed to decreased production of erythropoietin. Most patients with chronic renal failure on dialysis treatment tolerate a moderate degree of anaemia, but occasionally require either transfusion or treatment with erythropoietin. Emergency physicians should recognize anaemia as a predictable entity in patients with chronic renal failure, usually not requiring any action.

DECREASED RED CELL SURVIVAL: THE HAEMOLYTIC ANAEMIAS

Patients whose main problem is haemolysis are encountered rarely in the emergency department. The most fulminant haemolytic emergency one could envisage is that following transfusion of ABO-incompatible blood (discussed in Chapter 12.1), a vanishingly rare event where proper procedures are followed. Haemolysis and haemolytic anaemia are occasionally encountered in decompensating patients with multisystem problems. Rarely, first presentations of unusual haematological conditions occur.

Some of the haemolytic anaemias are hereditary conditions in which the inherited disorder is an abnormality intrinsic to the red cell, its membrane, its metabolic pathways, or the structure of the haemoglobin contained in the cells. Such red cells are liable to be dysfunctional, and to have increased fragility and a shortened lifespan. Lysis in the circulation may lead to clinical jaundice as bilirubin is formed from the breakdown of haemoglobin. Lysis in the reticuloendothelial system generally does not cause jaundice but may produce splenomegaly. The anaemia tends to be normochromic normocytic; sometimes a mildly raised MCV is due to an appropriate reticulocyte response from a normally functioning marrow. Serum bilirubin may be raised even in the absence of jaundice. Urinary urobilinogen and faecal stercobilinogen are detectable and serum haptoglobin is depleted. The anti-globulin (Coombs') test is important in the elucidation of some haemolytic anaemias. In this test, red cells coated in vivo (direct test) or in vitro (indirect test) with IgG antibodies are washed to remove unbound antibodies, then incubated with an antihuman globulin reagent. The resultant agglutination is a positive test.

Any chronic haemolytic process may be complicated by an 'aplastic crisis'. This is a usually transient marrow suppression brought on by a viral infection which can result in a severe and life-threatening anaemia. Red cell transfusion in these circumstances may be life-saving.

HEREDITARY SPHEROCYTOSIS

A deficiency of the red cell wall protein, spectrin, leads to loss of deformability and increased red cell fragility. These cells are destroyed prematurely in the spleen. The condition may present at any age, with anaemia, intermittent jaundice and cholelithiasis. Patients are Coombs' negative and show normal red cell osmotic fragility. Splenectomy radically improves general health. Hereditary elliptocytosis is a similar disease, with usually a milder course.

GLUCOSE-6-PHOSPHATE DEHYDROGENASE DEFICIENCY

Glucose-6-phosphate dehydrogenase (G6PD) generates reduced glutathione, which protects the red cell from oxidant stress. G6PD deficiency is an X-linked disorder present in heterozygous males and homozygous females. The disorder is commonly seen in West Africa, southern Europe, the Middle East and South East Asia. Oxidant stress leads to severe haemolytic anaemia. Precipitants include fava beans, antimalarial and analgesic drugs, and infections. The enzyme deficiency can be demonstrated by direct assay, and treatment is supportive.

SICKLE CELL ANAEMIA

Whereas in the thalassaemias there is a deficiency in a given globin chain within the haemoglobin molecule, in the haemoglobinopathies a given globin chain is present but structurally abnormal. HbS differs from normal HbA by one amino acid residue: valine replaces glutamic acid at the sixth amino acid from the N-terminus of the β-globin chain. Red cells containing HbS tend to 'sickle' at states of low oxygen tension. The deformed sickle-shaped red cell has increased rigidity, which causes it to lodge in the microcirculation and sequester in the reticuloendothelial system – the cause of a haemolytic anaemia.

Sickle cell disease is encountered in Afro-Caribbean people. The higher incidence in tropical areas is attributed to the survival value of the β-S gene against falciparum malaria. Heterozygous individuals have 'sickle trait' and are usually asymptomatic. Homozygous (HbSS) individuals manifest the disease in varying degrees. The haemolytic anaemia is usually in the range 60–100 g/L and can be well tolerated because HbS offloads oxygen to the tissues more efficiently than HbA.

A patient with sickle cell disease may occasionally develop a rapidly worsening anaemia. This may be due to:

- A production defect. Reduced marrow erythropoiesis may be secondary to folate deficiency or to a parvovirus infection. This is an aplastic crisis.
- A survival defect. Increased haemolysis is usually secondary to infection.
- Splenic sequestration.

In any of these circumstances transfusion may be life-saving. However, these events are unusual and more commonly encountered is the vaso-occlusive crisis. A stressor – for example infection, dehydration or cold – causes sickle cells to lodge in the microcirculation. Bone marrow infarction is one well recognized complication of the phenomenon, but virtually any body system can be affected.

Common presenting complaints include acute spinal pain, abdominal pain (the mesenteric occlusion of 'girdle sequestration'), chest pain (pulmonary vascular occlusion), joint pain, fever (secondary to tissue necrosis), neurological involvement (TIAs, strokes, seizures, obtundation, coma), respiratory embarrassment and hypoxia, priapism, 'hand-foot syndrome' (dactylitis of infancy), haematuria (nephrotic syndrome, papillary necrosis), skin ulcers of the lower limbs, retinopathies, glaucoma and gallstones.

Most patients presenting with a vaso-occlusive crisis know they have the disease but otherwise the differential diagnosis is difficult. Sickle cells may be seen on the blood film, and can also be induced by deoxygenating the sample. Hb electrophoresis can establish the type of Hb present. Other investigations are dictated by the presentation, and may include blood cultures, urinalysis and culture, chest X-ray, arterial blood gases and ECG.

Pain relief should commence early. A morphine infusion may be required for patients with severe ongoing pain. Other supportive measures are dictated by the presentation. Intravenous fluids are particularly important for patients with renal involvement. Aim to establish a urine output in excess of 100 mL/h in adults. Antibiotic cover may be required in the case of febrile patients with lung involvement. It may be impossible to differentiate between pulmonary vaso-occlusion and pneumonia. Many patients with sickle cell disease are effectively splenectomized owing to chronic splenic sequestration with infarction, and are prone to infection from encapsulated bacteria. The choice of antibiotic depends on the clinical presentation. Indications for exchange transfusion are shown in Table 12.4.6. The efficacy of exchange transfusion in painful crises remains unproven.

Haemoglobin S-C disease
Sickle trait or Hb S-C disease occurs in up to 10% in the black population. The clinical presentation resembles that of sickle cell disease but is usually less severe.

Table 12.4.6 Indications for exchange transfusion in sickle cell crisis
Neurological presentations: TIAs, stroke, seizures
Lung involvement ($PaO_2 < 65$ mmHg with FiO_2 60%)
Sequestration syndromes
Priapism

Haemoglobin C disease
In HbC, lysine replaces glutamic acid in the sixth position from the N terminus of the β-chain. Red cells containing HbC tend to be abnormally rigid, but the cells do not sickle. Homozygotes manifest a normocytic anaemia but there is no specific treatment and transfusion is seldom required.

THALASSAEMIAS

There is a high incidence of β-thalassaemia trait among people of Mediterranean origin, although in fact the region of high frequency extends in a broad band east to South East Asia.

Thalassaemias are disorders of haemoglobin synthesis. In the haemoglobin molecule, four haem molecules are attached to four long polypeptide globin chains. Four globin chain types (each with their own minor variations in amino acid order) are designated α, β, γ and δ. Haemoglobin A comprises two α and two β chains; 97% of adult haemoglobin is HbA. In thalassaemia there is diminished or absent production of either the α chain (α-thalassaemia) or the β chain (β-thalassaemia). Most patients are heterozygous and have a mild asymptomatic anaemia, although the red cells are small. In fact, the finding of a marked microcytosis in conjunction with a mild anaemia suggests the diagnosis.

There are four genes on paired chromosome 16 coding for α-globin and two genes on paired chromosomes 11 coding for β-globin. α-Thalassaemias are associated with patterns of gene deletion as follows: (—/—) = Hb-Barts hydrops syndrome, incompatible with life. (-α/—) is HbH disease.

Patients who are heterozygous for β-thalassaemia have β-thalassaemia minor or thalassaemia trait. They are usually symptomless. Homozygous patients have β-thalassaemia major.

Diagnosis of the major clinical syndromes is usually possible through consideration of the presenting features in conjunction with an FBC, blood film and Hb electrophoresis.

HbH disease patients present with moderate haemolytic anaemia and splenomegaly. The HbH molecule is detectable on electrophoresis and comprises unstable β tetramers. α Trait occurs with deletion of one or two genes. Hb, MCV and MCH are low, but the patient is often asymptomatic.

β-Thalassaemia major becomes apparent in the first 6 months of life with the decline of fetal Hb. There is a severe haemolytic anaemia, ineffective erythropoiesis, hepatosplenomegaly and failure to thrive. With improved care many of these patients are surviving to adulthood, and may possibly present to the emergency department, where transfusion could be life-saving. Patients with β-thalassaemia trait may be encountered in the emergency department relatively frequently. They are generally asymptomatic, with a mild hypochromic microcytic anaemia. It is important not to work these patients up continually for iron deficiency, and not to subject them to inappropriate haematinic therapy.

ACQUIRED HAEMOLYTIC ANAEMIAS

Many of the acquired haemolytic anaemias are autoimmune in nature, a manifestation of a type II (cytotoxic) hypersensitivity reaction. Here, normal red cells are attacked by aberrant autoantibodies targeting antigens on the red cell membrane. These reactions may occur more readily at 37°C (warm autoimmune haemolytic anaemia, or AIHA), or at 4°C (cold AIHA). Warm AIHA is more common. Red cells are coated with IgG, complement, or both. The cells are destroyed in the reticuloendothelial system. Fifty per cent of cases are idiopathic, but other recognized causes include lymphoproliferative disorders, neoplasms, connective tissue disorders, infections and drugs (notably methyldopa and penicillin). Patients have haemolytic anaemia, splenomegaly and a positive Coombs' test. In the emergency department setting, it is important to stop any potentially offending drugs and search for the underlying disease. The idiopathic group may respond to steroids, other immunosuppressive or cytotoxic drugs, or splenectomy.

In cold AIHA, IgM attaches to the I red cell antigen in the cooler peripheries. Primary cold antibody AIHA is known as cold haemagglutinin disease. Other causes include lymphoproliferative disorders, infections such as mycoplasma, and paroxysmal cold haemoglobinuria. Patients sometimes manifest Reynaud's disease and other manifestations of circulatory obstruction. Symptoms worsen in winter. Red cell lysis leads to haemoglobinuria.

MICROANGIOPATHIC HAEMOLYTIC ANAEMIA

In this important group of conditions intravascular haemolysis occurs in conjunction with a disorder of microcirculation. Important causes are shown in Table 12.4.7.

Table 12.4.7 Causes of microangiopathic haemolytic anaemia
Thrombotic thrombocytopenic purpura (TTP)
Haemolytic uraemic syndrome (HUS)
HELLP
DIC
Malignancy
Vasculitis
Malignant hypertension

HAEMOLYTIC URAEMIC SYNDROME AND THROMBOTIC THROMBOCYTOPENIC PURPURA

These are probably manifestations of the same pathological entity, with haemolytic uraemic syndrome (HUS) occurring in children and thrombotic thrombocytopenic purpura (TTP) most commonly in the fourth decade, especially in women. The primary lesion is likely to be in the vascular endothelium. Fibrin and platelet microthrombi are laid down in arterioles and capillaries, possibly as an autoimmune reaction. The clotting system is not activated. Haemolytic anaemia, thrombocytopenia and acute renal failure are sometimes accompanied by fever and neurological deficits.

In adults, the presentation is usually one of a neurological disturbance (headache, confusion, obtundation, seizures or focal signs). The blood film reveals anaemia, thrombocytopenia, reticulocytosis and schistocytes. Coombs' test is negative.

Patients require hospital admission. Adults with this condition may require aggressive therapy with prednisone, antiplatelet therapy, further immunosuppressive therapy, and plasma exchange transfusions.

HELLP SYNDROME

HELLP stands for haemolysis, elevated liver enzymes and a low platelet count, and is seen in pregnant women in the context of pre-eclampsia. Treatment is as for pre-eclampsia, early delivery of the baby being of paramount importance.

DISSEMINATED INTRAVASCULAR COAGULATION

The introduction of procoagulants into the circulation resulting in the overwhelming of anticoagulant control systems may occur as a consequence of a substantial number of pathophysiological insults - obstetric, infective, malignant, and traumatic. Disseminated intravascular coagulation (DIC) has an intimate association with shock, from any cause. The widespread production of thrombin leads to deposition of microthrombi, bleeding secondary to thrombocytopaenia and a consumption coagulopathy, and red cell damage within abnormal vasculature leading to a haemolytic anaemia.

Recognition of this condition prompts intensive care admission and aggressive therapy. Principles of treatment include definitive management of the underlying cause and, from the haematological point of view, replacement therapy that may involve transfusion of red cells, platelets, FFP, and cryoprecipitate. There may be a role for heparin and other anticoagulant treatments if specific tissue and organ survival is threatened by thrombus.

PAROXYSMAL NOCTURAL HAEMOGLOBINURIA

This entity is unusual in that an intrinsic red cell defect is seen in the context of an acquired haemolytic anaemia. A somatic stem cell mutation results in a clonal disorder. A family of membrane proteins (CD55, CD59 and C8 binding protein) are deficient and render cells prone to complement-mediated lysis. Because the same proteins are deficient in white cells and platelets, in addition to being anaemic patients are prone to infections and haemostatic abnormalities. They may go on to develop aplastic anaemia or leukaemia. Treatment is supportive. Marrow transplant can be curative.

OTHER CAUSES OF HAEMOLYSIS

Haemolysis may be due to mechanical trauma, as in 'March haemoglobinuria'. Artificial heart valves can potentially traumatize red cells. Historically, ball-and-cage type valves have been most prone to cause haemolysis, whereas disc

Table 12.4.8 Infections associated with haemolysis
Malaria, especially *Plasmodium falciparum* (blackwater fever)
Babesiosis
Bartonella
Haemophilus
Clostridia
Mycoplasma
EBV
Measles
CMV
Varicella
Herpes simplex
Coxsackie virus
HIV

Table 12.4.9 Drugs and toxins associated with haemolysis
Arsine (arsenic hydride)
Lead (plumbism)
Bites: bees, wasps, spiders, snakes
Copper toxicity
Local anaesthetics: lidocaine, benzocaine
Nitrates, nitrites
Sulphonamides
Antimalarials
Dapsone

valves are more thrombogenic. Improvements in design have made cardiac haemolytic anaemia very rare. Haemolysis is sometimes seen in association with a number of infectious diseases, notably malaria. Other infections that have been implicated are listed in Table 12.4.8. Certain drugs and toxins are associated with haemolytic anaemia (Table 12.4.9). The haemolytic anaemia that is commonly seen in patients with severe burns is attributed to direct damage to the red cells by heat.

FURTHER READING

Bayless PA 1993 Selected red cell disorders. Emergency Medicine Clinics of North America 11(2): 481–93

Bojanowski C 1989 Use of protocols for ED patients with sickle cell anaemia. Journal of Emergency Nursing 15: 83–7

Brookoff D, Polomano R 1992 Treating sickle cell pain like cancer pain. Annals of Internal Medicine 116(5): 364–8

Carbrow MB, Wilkins JC 1993 Haematologic emergencies. Management of transfusion reactions and crises in sickle cell disease. Postgraduate Medicine 93(5): 183–90

Egbert D, Hendricksen DK 1988 Congestive heart failure and respiratory arrest secondary to methyldopa-induced hemolytic anaemia. Annals of Emergency Medicine 17(5): 526–68

Erslev AJ, 1991 Erythropoietin. New England Journal of Mediicine 316: 101

Evans TC, Jehle D 1991 The red blood cell distribution width. Journal of Emergency Medicine 9 (Suppl 1): 71–4

Friedman EW, Webber AB, Osborn HH, Schwartz S 1986 Oral analgesia for treatment of painful crisis in sickle cell anaemia. Annals of Emergency Medicine 15: 787–91

Gaillard HM, Hamilton GC 1986 Hemoglobin/hematocrit and other erythrocyte parameters. Emergency Medicine Clinics of North America 4(1): 15–40

Gregory SA, McKenna R, Sassetti RJ, Knospe WH 1986 Hematologic emergencies. Medical Clinics of North America 70(5): 1129–49

Hedberg K, Shaffer N, Davachi F, et al 1993 Plasmodium falciparum-associated anaemia in children at a large urban hospital in Zaire. American Journal of Tropical Medicine and Hygiene 48(3): 365–71

Losek JD, Hellmich TR, Hoffman GM 1992 Diagnostic value of anemia, red blood cell morphology, and reticulocyte count for sickle cell disease. Annals of Emergency Medicine 21(8): 915–8

Naidorf JS, Kennedy JM, Becher JW Jr 1990 Methyldopa-induced anaemia in a 15 year old presenting as near-syncope. Pediatric Emergency Care 6(1): 29–32

O'Sullivan H, Jennings F, Ward K, et al 1981 Human bone marrow biochemical function and megaloblastic haematopoiesis after nitrous oxide anaesthesia. Anaesthesiology 55: 645

Pollack CV Jr 1993 Emergencies in sickle cell disease. Emergency Medicine Clinics of North America 11(2): 365–78

Powers RD 1986 Management protocol for sickle-cell disease patients with acute pain: impact of emergency department and narcotic use. American Journal of Emergency Medicine 4(3): 267–8

12.5 THROMBOCYTOPENIA

SIMON WOOD

ESSENTIALS

1 A low platelet count detected on automated blood count should always be confirmed by examination of the blood film prior to further investigation or treatment.

2 The cause of isolated thrombocytopenia can often be determined by a careful history and physical examination in addition to assessment of the full blood count and blood film.

3 Platelet transfusion is unnecessary in the management of the thrombocytopenic patient unless the platelet count is extremely low or there is ongoing bleeding.

4 In the absence of other clotting disorders or abnormal platelet function, bleeding in the thrombocytopenic patient is often amenable to local measures of haemostasis.

INTRODUCTION

Thrombocytopenia is defined as a reduction in the number of circulating platelets, the normal circulating platelet count being $150–400 \times 10^9/L$. It is the most common cause of abnormal bleeding.[1] Like anaemia, thrombocytopenia itself is not a diagnosis, but rather a manifestation of another underlying disease process.

In the emergency department setting, thrombocytopenia may present as an incidental finding on a routine blood count or may be diagnosed in the context of abnormal bleeding. In most cases, the underlying aetiology can be determined by a careful history and physical examination combined with interpretation of the blood count.

AETIOLOGY

The clinically important causes of thrombocytopaenia are outlined in Table 12.5.1. Diagnoses are classified by pathological process. It should be noted that more than one pathological process may be present.

ARTIFACTUAL THROMBOCYTOPENIA

Artifactual thrombocytopenia results from an underestimation of the platelet count as measured by an automated particle counter. The most common mechanism is platelet clumping. Clumping is most often due to the anticoagulant EDTA, but may also result from autoantibodies such as cold agglutinins. The presence of giant platelets and platelet satellitism may also yield falsely low automated platelet counts.[2]

Artifactual thrombocytopenia should be suspected when the automated platelet count is low in the absence of symptoms or signs of abnormal bleeding or disorders associated with thrombocytopenia. It is best excluded by examination

Table 12.5.1 Causes of thrombocytopenia

Pseudothrombocytopenia
Platelet clumping
Collection into anticoagulant (EDTA)
Platelet agglutinins
Giant platelets

Increased platelet destruction
Immune
  Primary
    Idiopathic thrombocytopenic purpura (ITP)
  Secondary
    Autoimmune thrombocytopenia associated with other disorders
    Grave's disease, Hashimoto's thyroiditis, systemic lupus erythematosus
    HIV-related thrombocytopenia
    Drug-induced thrombocytopenia
    Heparin, gold salts, quinine / quinidine, sulphonamides, rifampicin, H2 –blockers, indomethacin, carbamazepine, valproic acid
    Post-transfusion purpura
Non-immune
  Thrombotic thrombocytopenic purpura – haemolytic uraemic syndrome
  Pregnancy
  Gestational benign thrombocytopenia
  Preeclampsia/HELLP
  Disseminated intravascular coagulation

Decreased platelet production
Congenital
  TAR (thrombocytopenia with absent radius), Wiskott-Aldrich syndrome, Fanconi anaemia
Acquired
  Viral infection
  Epstein-Barr virus, rubella, dengue fever
  Marrow aplasia
  Malignant bone marrow infiltrates
  Chemotherapeutic agents
  Radiation therapy

Abnormal distribution and dilution
Splenic sequestration (hypersplenism)
Splenic enlargement
Hypothermia
Massive blood transfusion

of the blood film by an experienced observer. Any case of thrombocytopenia found on an automated blood count should be confirmed by examination of the peripheral smear prior to further investigation or treatment.

IMMUNE-RELATED THROMBOCYTOPENIA

Idiopathic thrombocytopenic purpura

Idiopathic thrombocytopenic purpura (ITP) is defined as an isolated thrombocytopenia (low platelet count with an otherwise normal complete blood count and peripheral blood smear) in a patient with no clinically apparent associated conditions that can cause thrombocytopenia.[3] It is a common cause of low platelet count and abnormal bleeding in both children and adults. ITP is thought to be caused by the development of autoantibodies to platelet membrane antigens.

Treatment is aimed at modulating the immune response and reducing the rate of platelet destruction and is indicated in all patients who have counts less than 20 $\times 10^9$/L, and those with counts less than 50 $\times 10^9$/L accompanied by significant mucous membrane bleeding. First phase treatment includes parenteral glucocorticoids and intravenous IgG. Splenectomy is usually reserved for patients who do not respond to medical therapy and have ongoing bleeding symptoms.[3] Platelet transfusions may cause temporary increases in platelet count and may be used in cases of life-threatening haemorrhage but are otherwise not usually indicated.[4]

In addition to the primary idiopathic form, immune thrombocytopenic purpura may also accompany autoimmune disorders such as Grave's disease and systemic lupus erythematosus. It is the main mechanism of the thrombocytopenia related to HIV infection.

Drug-related thrombocytopenia

A large number of drugs have been reported to cause immune-related thrombocytopenia. By far the most commonly implicated are quinine, quinidine, and heparin. Heparin is associated with a syndrome of thrombosis due to diffuse platelet activation accompanied by a consumptive thrombocytopenia.

In most cases of drug-related thrombocytopenia, recovery occurs rapidly after withdrawal of the offending agent. The exception is patients with gold sensitivity who may remain thrombocytopenic for months due to the slow clearance of this drug.[5]

Post-transfusion purpura

Post-transfusion purpura is clinically distinct from thrombocytopenia due to dilution of platelets following massive transfusion. It is an acute, severe thrombocytopenia occurring about one week after blood transfusion and is associated with a high-titre of platelet-specific alloantibodies. It is most commonly reported in multiparous women following their first blood transfusion. The mechanism for alloantibody formation is unclear. Spontaneous recovery occurs within weeks, although fatalities from severe haemorrhage have been reported.[5]

NON-IMMUNE PLATELET DESTRUCTION

Thrombotic thrombocytopenic purpura

Thrombotic thrombocytopenic purpura (TTP) is considered to be the adult form of the haemolytic uraemic syndrome (HUS). Essentially, a thrombotic microangiopathy the classic pentad of clinical findings is: 1) fever, 2) thrombocytopenia, 3) microangiopathic haemolytic anaemia, 4) neurologic abnormalities, and 5) renal involvement.

TTP can occur sporadically as an idiopathic disorder or may be associated with pregnancy, epidemics of verotoxin-producing *Escherichia coli* and *Shigella dysenteriae*, malignancy, chemotherapy, marrow transplantation, and drug-dependant antibodies. Treatment with plasma exchange has dramatically influenced the outcome of TTP. Mortality has fallen from more than 90% prior to introduction of plasma exchange to less than 20% with this treatment.[6]

Thrombocytopenia in pregnancy

Gestational thrombocytopenia develops during an otherwise normal pregnancy and is clinically distinct from autoimmune thrombocytopenias such as ITP. It is thought to be due to decreased platelet survival consequent to activation of the coagulation system. Thrombocytopenia is usually mild and there is no corresponding thrombocytopenia in the infant. The platelet count returns to normal after delivery, although thrombocytopenia may recur in subsequent pregnancies.[7]

Autoimmune thrombocytopenias, on the other hand, are often associated with more severe reductions in the platelet count. Antiplatelet antibodies are capable of crossing the placenta and may result in significant thrombocytopenia in the foetus and newborn. This can lead to complications, such as intracranial haemorrhage, during the delivery. Treatment of the mother with autoimmune thrombocytopenia is similar in principle to the treatment of non-pregnant cases.[7]

In the context of pregnancy, thrombocytopenia may also be seen as part of the HELLP (haemolysis, elevated liver enzymes, low platelets) and pre-eclampsia syndromes. The two syndromes are thought to be related. Common to both is a process of microvascular endothelial damage and intravascular platelet activation. This leads to release of thromboxane A and serotonin, which provoke vasospasm, platelet aggregation and further endothelial damage.[8] In both syndromes, the process is terminated by delivery.

Disseminated intravascular coagulation (see Chapter 12.4)

Thrombocytopaenia is one manifestation of the syndrome of disseminated intravascular coagulation (DIC). DIC is an acquired syndrome of diffuse intravascular coagulation up to the level of fibrin formation, accompanied by secondary fibrinolysis or inhibited fibrinolysis.[9] It occurs in the course of severe systemic diseases or may be provoked by toxins such as snake venoms.

THROMBOCYTOPENIA DUE TO IMPAIRED PLATELET PRODUCTION

Congenital disorders of impaired platelet production usually present in childhood and will not be discussed.

Of the acquired disorders of impaired platelet production, the most commonly seen in the emergency setting is the incidental finding of reduced platelet count in patients suffering viral illness. Causative viruses include Epstein-Barr virus, rubella, and dengue fever. Thrombocytopenia in these cases is reversible and requires no specific therapy other than monitoring of the platelet count to ensure normalization.

Disorders of bone marrow dysfunction, such as malignant infiltration and bone marrow suppression, cause thrombocytopenia accompanied by reductions in numbers of other blood components. Examination of the full blood count (FBC) and blood film usually distinguishes these from other causes of isolated thrombocytopenia. Further investigation is best referred to a haematologist.

MASSIVE BLOOD TRANSFUSION AND THROMBOCYTOPENIA

Massive blood transfusion is defined as the transfusion of a volume equivalent to the patient's normal blood volume within a 24-hour period. Thrombocytopenia results from dilution of the patient's remaining platelets and, where whole blood is used, decreased survival of platelets in stored blood. It is possibly the most important factor contributing to the haemostatic abnormality seen in massively transfused patients. Platelet transfusion should be reserved for cases where the platelet count falls below $50 \times 10^9/L$.[4]

HYPERSPLENISM

Hypersplenism refers to the thrombocytopenia due to pooling in patients with splenic enlargement. It is the primary cause of thrombocytopenia in hepatic cirrhosis, portal venous hypertension, and congestive splenomegaly. In these cases, thrombocytopenia is rarely severe and not usually of clinical importance.[2]

Transient thrombocytopenia has been described in patients suffering severe hypothermia and is due to splenic sequestration. Platelet counts usually return to normal within days of rewarming.[2]

CLINICAL PRESENTATION

Thrombocytopenia may be an incidental finding on the FBC or may be diagnosed in the context of abnormal bleeding. There are distinct differences in the patterns of abnormal bleeding associated with disorders of platelet deficiency and disorders of impaired coagulation.

Spontaneous bleeding related to thrombocytopenia typically manifests as cutaneous petechiae and/or purpura, most commonly in dependent areas such as the legs and buttocks.[1,3] Other spontaneous manifestations include multiple small retinal haemorrhages, epistaxis, gingival and gastrointestinal bleeding. Bleeding following trauma or surgery in thrombocytopenic patients is often immediate and may respond to local methods of haemostasis. In contradistinction to this the bleeding associated with coagulation disorders is most commonly in the form of large haematomata or haemarthroses that occur spontaneously or develop hours to days following trauma.[1]

In addition to the haemorrhagic manifestations of platelet insufficiency, patients with thrombocytopenia may present with the clinical features of the underlying causative disorder. Splenic enlargement may be present in cases where thrombocytopenia is due to

hypersplenism but is not a feature of immune-related thrombocytopenia.

The level of platelets associated with clinically significant abnormal bleeding is not precisely defined. It will vary depending on the platelets' functional integrity, and with the presence or absence of other risk factors, such as coagulation disorder, trauma, and surgery. There is evidence that platelet counts above $5 \times 10^9/L$ are sufficient to prevent bleeding when the platelets are functionally normal and there are no other risk factors. Severe haemorrhage is uncommon at platelet counts above $20 \times 10^9/L$ and in the setting of surgery the risk of abnormal haemorrhage is reduced at counts above $50 \times 10^9/L$.[4]

INVESTIGATIONS

The FBC and examination of the blood film is diagnostic of thrombocytopenia. The pattern of deficiency should be considered. Isolated thrombocytopenia refers to a low platelet count in the presence of an otherwise normal FBC and blood film. In these cases, FBC combined with a careful clinical history and examination is often sufficient to lead to a final diagnosis.[3] Coexistent anaemia and/or leukopenia suggest bone marrow dysfunction as the primary aetiological process.

Other useful investigations may include coagulation studies and d-dimer (DIC, preeclampsia), electrolytes, urea and creatinine (TTP), liver function tests (HELLP, liver disease), and thyroid function tests (autoimmune thyroid disorders). Platelet antibody titres are indicated in the workup of pregnancy related thrombocytopenia, and bone marrow aspirate may be indicated in investigation of thrombocytopenia due to bone marrow dysfunction, but neither of these tests is useful in the emergency department setting.

TREATMENT

Treatment for specific causes of thrombocytopenia has already been discussed.

Bleeding in the face of low platelet count may be responsive to local methods of haemostasis if the remaining platelets are functionally normal and there is no other disorder of coagulation present. Platelet transfusion may be helpful in cases of severe haemorrhage and is sometimes used prophylactically to prevent bleeding in patients with very low platelet counts.

Platelet transfusion is primarily indicated in patients in whom thrombocytopenia is due to impaired platelet production and who are bleeding or have very low counts. The threshold for prophylactic transfusion in these patients is controversial. It is indicated when the platelet count is below $5 \times 10^9/L$, but is probably not indicated above this level unless other risk factors for bleeding are present.[4]

Platelet transfusion is rarely indicated in immune-related thrombocytopenias as the transfused platelets are rapidly destroyed. Transfusion of platelets may aggravate TTP.[4] In DIC, platelet transfusion has not been proven to be effective but may be indicated in bleeding patients. There is little evidence to support the suggestion that blood component therapy aggravates DIC.[10] In cases of massive blood transfusion, platelets are not routinely indicated unless there is ongoing bleeding and the platelet count is below $50 \times 10^9/L$.[4]

Raising the platelet count to $20–50 \times 10^9/L$ is sufficient to prevent serious bleeding. In patients undergoing surgery or other invasive procedures counts up to $60–100 \times 10^9/L$ may be required. A useful rule of thumb is that in a 70 kg adult, transfusion of one unit of platelets

CONTROVERSIES AND FUTURE DIRECTIONS

❶ The platelet count at which prophylactic platelet transfusion is indicated.

❷ The development and clinical testing of alternative methods of platelet preparation and platelet substitutes.

will increase the platelet count by $11 \times 10^9/L$.[4]

At present, platelet preparations for transfusion are stored in liquid at 22°C. Problems include the continued risk of febrile non-haemolytic reactions, transmission of infectious agents, and graft-versus-host disease. Alternatives to conventional liquid storage include frozen storage, cold liquid storage, photochemical treatment and lyophilized platelets. None of these methods is currently widely available. Several platelet substitutes have been developed but remain untested in the clinical setting. Some examples are red cells with surface-bound fibrinogen, fibrinogen-coated albumin microcapsules (FAMs), and liposome-based haemostatic agents.[11]

DISPOSITION

Disposition will depend on the presence and extent of abnormal bleeding, the degree of thrombocytopenia, and the underlying aetiology. In general, patients who present with abnormal bleeding and

a low platelet count should be admitted for further evaluation and treatment. In the absence of bleeding, patients who have isolated thrombocytopenia with counts above $20 \times 10^9/L$ may be investigated on an outpatient basis.[3]

REFERENCES

1. Rodgers GM, Bithell TC 1999 The diagnostic approach to the bleeding disorders. In: Lee GR, Wintrobe MM, Lee GR et al (eds) Wintrobe's Clinical Hematology, 10th edn. Lippincott Williams & Wilkins, Maryland, pp 1557–78
2. George JN 1995 Thrombocytopenia: pseudothrombocytopenia, hypersplenism, and thrombocytopenia associated with massive transfusion. In: Beutler E, et al Beutler E, Williams WJ (eds) Williams Hematology, 5th edn. McGraw-Hill, New York, pp 1355–60
3. American Society of Hematolgy ITP Practice Guideline Panel 1996 Diagnosis and treatment of idiopathic thrombocytopenic purpura. Am Fam Physician 54(8): 2437–47, 2451–2
4. Mollison PL, Engelfriet CP, Contreras M 1997 Blood transfusions. In: Clinical medicine, 10th edn. Blackwell Science, Oxford
5. George JN, El-Harake M, Aster RH 1995 Thrombocytopenia due to enhanced platelet destruction by immunological mechanisms. In: Beutler E, et al (eds) Williams Hematology, 5th edn. McGraw-Hill, New York, pp 1315–54
6. George JN, El-Harake M 1995 Thrombocytopenia due to enhanced platelet destruction by nonimmunological mechanisms. In: Beutler E, et al (eds) Williams Hematology, 5th edn. McGraw-Hill, New York, pp 1290–314
7. Schwartz KA 2000 Gestational thrombocytopenia and immune thrombocytopenias in pregnancy. Hematology and Oncology Clinics of North America 14(5):1101–16
8. Padden MO 1999 HELLP syndrome: recognition and perinatal management. American Family Physician 60(3): 829–36
9. Ten Cate H 2000 Pathophysiology of disseminated intravascular coagulation in sepsis. Critical Care Medicine 28(9 Suppl): S9–S11
10. Levi M, de Jonge E, van der Poll T, ten Cate H 2000 Novel approaches to the management of disseminated intravascular coagulation. Critical Care Medicine 28(9 Suppl): S20–S24
11. Lee DH, Blajchman MA 2001 Novel treatment modalities: new platelet preparations and substitutes. British Journal of Haematology 114: 496–505

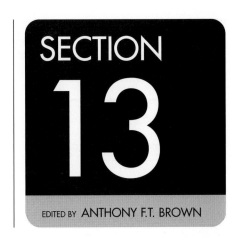

SECTION

13

EDITED BY ANTHONY F.T. BROWN

RHEUMATOLOGY

13.1 **Rheumatological emergencies** 516

13.1 RHEUMATOLOGICAL EMERGENCIES

SHAMEEM SAFIH

ESSENTIALS

1 Discriminating between articular, periarticular and non-articular syndromes is critical to the management of rheumatological emergencies.

2 The most useful tests are FBC, ESR, X-ray and analysis of joint fluid.

3 Treatment of rheumatological emergencies involves relief of inflammation and pain control by rest, analgesia, NSAIDs and steroids.

4 Acute low back pain should be managed with early mobilization.

INTRODUCTION

Rheumatological illnesses are common in the general population. Although life-threatening emergencies are rare, patients often present to the emergency department with related conditions. These may include a clinical manifestation of arthritis, a complication of the primary disorder, or a complication associated with therapy. In most cases the primary goal of treatment is relief of pain and inflammation. Long-term therapy is also aimed at maintaining or increasing joint function and rehabilitating the patient. Multidisciplinary input is usually required.

The most common acute presentation is an episode of acute inflammation of one or more joints. It is essential to determine whether or not sepsis is present. Most rheumatological diseases are multisystem and, although uncommon, the patient may present with an extra-articular complication such as temporal arteritis, alveolar haemorrhage, pericarditis, or instability of the cervical spine. Complications of therapy include bone marrow depression, immune suppression and opportunistic infection. Investiga-

tions essential to the diagnosis include a full blood count (FBC), erythrocyte sedimentation rate (ESR), radiographs and analysis of joint fluid.

Resolution of inflammation and pain control are achieved mainly through rest, analgesia, non-steroidal anti-inflammatory drugs (NSAIDs) and steroids.

Rheumatological disorders primarily involve the joints and can be characterized as mono- or polyarticular, although there may be considerable overlap between conditions. Rheumatological soft tissue disorders such as bursitis and tendinitis, or nerve entrapments such as carpal tunnel syndrome form a spectrum of related disorders.

ACUTE MONOARTICULAR ARTHRITIS

Pain is the most common presentation. The causes of inflammation in a single joint are:

- Septic arthritis (see Chapter 8.3)
- Gout
- Crystal deposition diseases such as pseudogout
- Haemarthrosis from clotting disorders such as haemophilia, warfarin therapy, trauma
- Mechanical internal derangement or an exacerbation of osteoarthritis
- Immune-mediated arthritis, which may occasionally present with single joint involvement such as rheumatoid arthritis, systemic lupus erythematosus (SLE), Reiter's disease, serum sickness, and psoriatic disease.

An appropriate history is taken inquiring into the mode of onset of pain, the presence and duration of constitutional symptoms, any history of trauma to the joint, known arthritic disorder, recent gastroenteritis, genitourinary symptoms,

known haematological disease, a family history and a history of drug therapy.

When examining a painful joint the main objective is to identify the exact anatomical site of pathology to determine whether the joint is involved or the extra-articular structures (extracapsular) (Table 13.1.1).

GOUT

Gout is a complication of hyperuricaemia and is classified as primary or secondary. Primary gout is characterized by a genetic tendency to overproduction (10%) or renal tubular underexcretion (90%) of uric acid. The acquired hyperuricaemia of secondary gout has multiple causes, such as conditions associated with an increased production of uric acid including excessive dietary purine intake, myeloproliferative and lymphoproliferative disorders, haemolytic disease, psoriasis, severe muscle exertion and alcohol abuse. Decreased excretion of uric acid is seen with impaired renal function, dehydration, diuretics and acidosis. Secondary gout is also associated with hyperparathyroidism, hypertension, lead nephropathy and the use of ciclosporin, pyrazinamide, ethambutol and low-dose salicylate.

Tissue deposition of monosodium urate crystals results in gouty arthritis, tophi or nephropathy. Urinary calculi also result from hyperuricaemia. Gout is the most common inflammatory arthritis in adult males (peak incidence in the fifth decade), with an incidence of 0.2% in the general population. There is a family history of gout in 50% of cases. Beyond 60 years of age the incidence is similar in males and females. In America the black races are more frequently affected. In New Zealand gout is commoner in male Maoris (incidence 10%) than in male caucasians (incidence 3%). Obesity is a predisposing factor. The risk of coronary artery disease is increased.

Table 13.1.1 Regional periarticular syndromes

Region	Periarticular syndrome	Non-articular syndrome
Jaw	Temporomandibular joint (TMJ) dysfunction 'myofascial pain syndrome'	Temporal arteritis Dental molar problems Parotid swellings Preauricular lymphadenitis
Shoulder	Subacromial bursitis Long-head bicipital tendinitis Rotator cuff tear	Brachial plexopathy Cervical nerve root injury Pancoast tumour
Elbow	Olecranon bursitis Epicondylitis	Ulnar nerve entrapment
Wrist	Extensor tendinitis, including de Quervain's synovitis	Carpal tunnel syndrome
Hip	Greater trochanteric bursitis Adductor syndrome Ischial bursitis Fascia lata syndrome	Meralgia paraesthetica Deep infection Paget's disease Neoplasm
Knee	Anserine bursitis Prepatellar bursitis Meniscal or ligamentous injury Baker's cyst	Neoplasm Osteomyelitis
Ankle	Peroneal tendinitis Achilles tendinitis Retrocalcaneal bursitis Calcaneal fasciitis Sprain Erythema nodosum	Hypertrophic pulmonary osteoarthropathy Tarsal tunnel syndrome
Foot	Plantar fasciitis Pes planus Cellulitis	Morton's neuroma Vascular insufficiency

CLINICAL FEATURES

The metatarsophalangeal joint of the big toe is the joint most commonly involved in the initial attack (70%), followed by the ankle, the tarsus and the knee. The hand or the fingers may be affected in subsequent attacks. Mild trauma, a dietary excess of purines, an alcohol binge or some form of stress, illness or surgery may precipitate the attack. In 5% of patients the onset will be polyarticular. The joint is inflamed, swollen, painful and tender, with barely any motion. The skin over the affected joint becomes shiny, red or purple. Fever up to 38°C may be present.

INVESTIGATIONS

The white cell count (WCC) and the ESR are non-specific markers that may be raised. Serum uric acid is normal in up to 40% of cases. Asymptomatic hyperuricaemia is not uncommon in the general population. Synovial fluid analysis is the definitive diagnostic test (Table 13.1.2). It also excludes concomitant or primary sepsis. In most cases the clinical history and examination are sufficient to make the diagnosis. However, where there is doubt, joint aspiration is essential. Negatively birefringent crystals of sodium urate are seen under polarized light microscopy.

MANAGEMENT

Rest, immobilization, NSAIDs and analgesia are the mainstay of therapy.

NSAIDs
An NSAID regimen such as naproxen 750 mg stat, followed by 500 mg in 8 hours, followed by 250 mg 8-hourly should be instituted. Contraindications to NSAIDs such as active peptic ulceration, and relative contraindications such as history of peptic ulcer disease, asthma, congestive heart failure, hypertension, renal impairment and concomitant anticoagulant therapy should be considered. Aspirin is avoided in low doses as it increases serum uric acid levels.

Colchicine
Colchicine administered orally has an 85–90% response rate. However, toxicity is high, with early gastrointestinal side effects. The drug is best reserved for patients in whom NSAIDs are contraindicated and who have normal liver and kidney function. The usual dosage regimen is 500 µg, one to two taken orally every hour, to a maximum of 8 mg in 24 hours, or until gastrointestinal side effects such as diarrhoea or evidence of clinical improvement occurs.

Corticosteroids
Oral corticosteroids are used as alternative second-line therapy having excluded sepsis first. Prednisone is given at 30–50 mg daily, tapered off over 2 weeks. An alternative is to inject hydrocortisone into the joint following aspiration. This is particularly useful if NSAIDs are contraindicated.

Allopurinol
Preventative therapy should not be started during an acute attack, but is left until 1–2 weeks after resolution of symptoms. However, if a patient is already on allopurinol it should be continued at the same dose.

Other measures
Rest, simple analgesia and patient education on diet, weight loss and the avoidance of alcohol.

ACUTE PSEUDOGOUT

This is one of the spectrum of calcium pyrophosphate dihydrate (CPPD) deposition diseases. The aetiology is classified into:

Table 13.1.2 Synovial fluid findings

Diagnosis	Appearance	WBC/mm³	Polymorphonuclear leucocytes (%)	Crystals under polarized light	Gram stain
Normal	Clear	<200	<25	None	Neg
Osteoarthritis	Clear	<4000	<25	None	Neg
Trauma	Blood, fat droplets from articular fractures	<4000	<25	None	Neg
Acute gout	Turbid	2000–50 000	>75	Needle-like crystals with negative birefringence*	Neg
Pseudogout	Turbid	2000–40 000	>75	Positive birefringence* Rhomboid crystals	Neg
Septic arthritis Rheumatoid arthritis/	Purulent / turbid	5000–150 000	>75	None	Positive in up to 75%
Seronegative arthritis	Turbid	2000–50 000	50–75	None	Neg

- Hereditary
- Idiopathic, which increases with age
- Associated with metabolic disease such as hyperparathyroidism, familial hypercalciuric hypercalcaemia, gout, haemochromatosis, haemosiderosis, hypothyroidism, hypomagnesaemia, hypophosphatasia and amyloidosis
- Associated with joint trauma and surgery.

Pseudogout is more common in the middle-aged and the elderly, especially those over 65 years, and is slightly more common in males.

CLINICAL FEATURES

The onset is abrupt, severe, and may last several days. The knee is the most commonly affected joint being involved in 50% of cases, followed by the wrist. The onset is polyarticular in 5% of cases. Tophi are absent. The clinical presentation includes:

- Progressive osteoarthritis
- Pseudorheumatoid arthritis
- Pseudoneuropathic joints.

The serum uric acid is normal. X-rays show linear calcification within joints and there may be X-ray evidence of periarticular calcification. Synovial fluid shows rhomboid birefringent crystals of calcium pyrophosphate. The CPPD disease spectrum includes asymptomatic chondrocalcinosis characterized by X-ray calcification of the acromioclavicular joint, the verterbral discs, pubic symphysis, knee, hip and wrist joints.

In 5% of patients the ESR is raised, and in 10% the IgM rheumatoid factor is positive.

TREATMENT

NSAIDs are useful, but response to colchicine is uncommon. In some patients aspiration will provide relief (and make the diagnosis). Intra-articular steroids are also used. The disease is self-limiting.

ACUTE HAEMARTHROSIS

Acute haemarthrosis in a joint may be traumatic or due to a bleeding disorder. Traumatic haemarthrosis is caused by intra-articular fractures or ligamentous tears such as the anterior cruciate in the knee. A severely osteoarthritic joint may develop an acute haemarthrosis following minimal trauma. An X-ray of the joint should be taken. Non-traumatic haemarthrosis may occur secondary to a clotting factor deficiency. A relevant family history and haematologic and drug histories are important. The patient is usually a male with a history of haemophilia. The knee, elbow or ankle are most commonly involved. A platelet count, bleeding time and APTT should be performed.

TREATMENT

In non-traumatic haemarthrosis the underlying cause is addressed. Appropriate factor replacement with fresh frozen plasma or factor concentrate, or antidotes such as vitamin K for warfarin toxicity are given, in consultation with the patient's haematologist where relevant. Analgesia, rest and immobilization are indicated. Aspiration is usually unnecessary. Selective aspiration of a tense and painful haemarthrosis less than 24 hours old may be performed followed with pressure bandaging with crepe bandage After this period the blood has usually clotted. Aspiration may be performed during or after infusion of the deficient factor.

In all cases of trauma an X-ray is necessary. The history and a careful examination of the joint may suggest the nature of the injury. If there is no obvious bony injury and no apparent significant soft tissue injury, the joint is immobilised, analgesia prescribed, and for a lower extremity injury, crutches are given. Referral is made to an orthopaedic clinic. If there is a significant fracture or soft tissue injury then acute orthopaedic consultation is required. Aspiration is not routine because of the risk of infection, but as for the non-traumatic haemarthosis, a particularly tense and painful traumatic haemarthosis with no underlying fracture on X-ray may be aspirated and pressure bandaged.

ACUTE POLYARTHRITIS

Polyarthritis syndromes are often gradual in onset and difficult to diagnose. The important issues remain to consider are infection, underlying inflammation and whether the structures involved are intra-articular or extra-articular.

Important aspects of the history include:

- The mode of onset
- Acute (less than 6 weeks): gonococcal, viral, Lyme disease, Reiter's syndrome, rheumatic fever
- Chronic: rheumatoid arthritis, SLE, sclerodema, psoriatic arthritis, dermatomyositis, other autoimmune disease
- Course: progressive, intermittent or migratory
- Joints involved: symmetric or asymmetric
- Constitutional symptoms: fever, night sweats, generalized stiffness, fatigue and weight loss that may accompany the insidious onset of the rheumatoid-like conditions
- Rheumatological disease systems review: rash, alopecia, Raynaud's phenomenon, sicca syndrome, uveitis, scleritis, oral and genital ulcers, urethritis, cervicitis, chronic bowel symptoms and pleuropericardial symptoms
- History of recent sore throat, febrile illness, venereal disease, sexual contact, diarrhoea, rash or uveitis
- Past history of rheumatic fever and juvenile polyarthritis
- Family history of psoriasis, inflammatory bowel disease, uveitis

or chronic back pain (ankylosing spondylitis).

Physical examination must include the vital signs and a search for stigmata of underlying diseases such as psoriatic nails or skin lesions, oral and genital ulcers, and cardiovascular features such as murmurs, rubs, bruits and evidence of vasculitis.

INVESTIGATIONS

Blood is taken for full blood count (FBC) and ESR and renal function tests. Aspiration of joint and analysis of synovial fluid may be indicated. Other investigations include rheumatoid factor, C-reactive protein and a serum auto-antibody profile.

RHEUMATOID ARTHRITIS

Rheumatoid arthritis occurs in 2% of the general population and is two to three times more common in females. It is a chronic systemic inflammatory disorder of unknown aetiology characterized by symmetric synovitis, destructive polyarthritis and widespread extra-articular manifestations. A much less common form is juvenile rheumatoid arthritis. The initial clinical presentation is usually with an insidious onset of symptoms, often lacking the characteristic symmetry of joint involvement, although it may present as a palindromic arthritis or, uncommonly, as an acute monoarthritis.

CLINICAL FEATURES

The diagnosis in adults requires four of the American Rheumatism Association criteria:

- Morning stiffness lasting at least 1 hour
- Arthritis of three or more joints
- Swelling of proximal interphalangeal or metacarpophalangeal or wrist joints

- Symmetrical involvement
- Rheumatoid nodules
- Abnormal level of serum rheumatoid factor
- Radiological erosion or periarticular osteoporosis in hand or wrist joints.

Other features are malaise, fatigue and raised ESR. Progressive joint destruction may contribute to the pain of synovitis, although pain occurs without synovitis.

Specific articular manifestations

Cervical spine
Instability, decreased motion and myelopathy result from longstanding joint involvement. Degeneration of the transverse ligament of the C1 vertebra produces C1–C2 instability.

Upper limb
The shoulders have restricted motion leading to a frozen shoulder with characteristic nocturnal exacerbations of pain. The limbs may have a flexion deformity, and compression ulnar neuropathy may result. The wrist, metacarpophalangeal and proximal interphalangeal joints are typically affected, with the distal interphalangeal joints spared. There is ulnar drift at the metacarpophalangeal joints. swan-neck and boutonnière deformity are common. Tenosynovitis may lead to tendon rupture, particularly of the extensor pollicis longus. Rupture by attrition of the long extensors of the middle, ring and the little fingers may occur.

Lower limb
The hip and knee are frequently involved. Rheumatoid arthritis is one of the causes of a Baker's cyst, due to a posterior herniation of the joint capsule of the knee joint. In the foot and ankle the metatarsophalangeal joint, talonavicular joint and ankle joint are involved, in decreasing order of frequency. Metatarsophalangeal joint subluxation may occur. There is talonavicular joint inflammation resulting in pronation and eversion deformity secondary to muscle spasm. A posterior tibial nerve neuropathy may occur, causing burning paraesthesiae on the sole of the foot.

Extra-articular manifestations

Rheumatoid arthritis causes a large number of extra-articular manifestations involving all organ systems. These may be due to joint inflammation causing secondary functional or neurological defects, resulting from vasculitis or inflammation distant from the joint, or caused by the treatment. A thorough examination of the entire patient is essential.

TREATMENT

The goals of long term therapy are pain relief, reduction of joint inflammation, maintenance or restoration of joint function, and prevention of bone and cartilage destruction.

Education, rest and exercise, NSAIDs, occupational and rehabilitative therapy are the main modes of therapy. Medication is either for symptomatic relief (aspirin, NSAIDs) or aimed at disease process modification.

NSAIDs

Any NSAID may be used with particular attention to contraindications and side effects. Some suggested regimens are:

Aspirin 600–1200 mg every 4–6 hours
or
Indometacin 75–200 mg daily in
    divided doses
or
Naproxen 750–1500 mg per day
or
Ibuprofen 1600–2400 mg per day.

Disease-modifying anti-rheumatic drugs

These are not considered emergency drugs and are best prescribed by the rheumatologist or local doctor with long-term care. There is a higher risk of side effects to the bone marrow, liver and kidneys that should be regularly monitored.

- Antimalarials: hydroxychloroquine which necessitates a 6-monthly eye check to exclude the development of retinopathy

- Sulphasalazine: common side effects of nausea and gastric intolerance
- Cytotoxics: methotrexate, which has good efficacy and a relatively low toxicity profile, or D-penicillamine, which has a similar efficacy to gold
- Gold salts
- Corticosteroids, which may be injected intra-articularly and are effective in reducing inflammation in a single large joint. Oral corticosteroids are used in the management of vasculitis, pericarditis and pleuritis
- Immunosuppressives such as cyclophosphamide and azathioprine, which are third-line drugs carrying a high risk of bone marrow suppression, infection, mutagenesis and carcinogenesis.

Other interventions:
- Orthopaedic and orthotic interventions are often required. Surgery involving joint fusion, synovectomy, total joint arthroplasty and reconstruction may be required.

Emergency therapy

Early consultation with a rheumatologist is essential especially in a pateint with an acute first presentation. For mild or moderate presentations, it is important to exclude infection, control symptoms with simple analgesics including NSAIDs, and discharge for local doctor or specialist follow-up. The patient should be admitted if there is a severe exacerbation, and any acute complications should be recognized and treated (Table 13.1.3).

Table 13.1.3 Rheumatological emergencies associated with the risk of death or significant morbidity

Pulmonary haemorrhage	SLE, Wegener disease, Goodpasture syndrome, other vasculitis
Respiratory failure, pulmonary fibrosis	Acute spondylitis, scleroderma, rheumatoid arthritis
Cervical spine instability	Rheumatoid arthritis
Cricoarytenoid obstruction	Rheumatoid arthritis
Tracheobronchial collapse	Relapsing polychondritis
Cardiac tamponade	SLE
Aortic dissection	Ankylosing spondylitis, relapsing polychrondritis
Cardiac arrhythmia, myocarditis (arrhythmias)	Polymyositis, dermatomyositis, scleroderma
Angina	Vasculitides
Myocardial infarction	SLE
Pericarditis	SLE, Rh A
Pancarditis	Acute rheumatic fever, SLE
Adrenal insufficiency	Cessation of long-term glucocorticoid therapy
Transverse myelitis	SLE
Sudden blindness	Temporal arteritis
Renal failure (nephritis)	SLE, diffuse cutaneous scleroderma, rhabdomyolysis occurring in dermatomyositis and polymyositis
Malignant hypertension	Scleroderma
Septic shock	Bacterial endocarditis with damaged cardiac valves
Cerebrovascular event	SLE
GI bleed, aplastic marrow crisis	Side effect of drug therapy

COURSE AND PROGNOSIS

The spontaneous remission rate is a less than 10%. High titres of rheumatoid factor (which are positive in 75% of cases), the presence of nodules, and HLA- DR4 haplotype are markers of severity. The patient's life expectancy is shortened by 10–15 years by infection, pulmonary and renal disease, and gastrointestinal bleeding.

SYSTEMIC LUPUS ERYTHEMATOSUS

This is a chronic inflammatory auto-immune multisystem disease character-ized by spontaneous remission and relapses. Its severity ranges from mild episodes to a rapidly fatal illness. Lupus-like syndromes may be caused by drugs such as chlorpromazine, hydralazine, isoniazid, methyldopa, procainamide and quinine.

Systemic lupus erythematosus (SLE) is a disease of young women with 85% of patients being female. Blacks are affected more often (1 in 250 black females) than whites (1 in 1000 white females). There is a familial tendency, with specific genes being involved. Autoimmune serologic markers are positive.

CLINICAL FEATURES

Systemic constitutional symptoms of ma-laise, weight loss and fever of unknown origin are common. A non-specific photo-sensitive rash, alopecia, urticaria, Raynaud's phenomenon and mucocutaneous ulcers occur. The typical malar or butterfly rash occurs in less than 50% of patients. Joint symptoms occur in over 90% of patients, with arthritis, arthralgia or myalgia.

The lungs may be involved with pleuritis, pleural effusion, pneumonitis or bronchopneumonia. Cardiac compli-cations include pericarditis, myocarditis, valvulitis, aseptic (Libman-Sacks) endo-carditis and cardiac failure. There is often a vasculitis. Neurological involvement includes encephalopathy, psychosis, organic brain syndrome, seizure, neuro-pathy, transverse myelitis and stroke. Eye complications such as conjunctivitis, transient blindness and cottonwool retinal bodies are seen. Finally there may be renal involvement and haematological effects such as purpura, splenomegaly, anaemia, leucopenia, thrombocytopenia and pancytopenia.

INVESTIGATIONS

FBC and ESR , liver and renal function tests should be performed. Antinuclear antibodies are positive in 95% of cases. Antidouble-stranded DNA antibodies and anti-Smith antibodies are specific for SLE. Serum C3 and C4 complement levels are low during an exacerbation. C-reactive protein is usually low. There may be a false positive VDRL test. Urinalysis may reveal protein, red cells or casts indicating glomerular disease.

MANAGEMENT

Life-threatening complications such as infection and cardiac complications should be identified and treated urgently. Fatigue and stress exacerbate the con-dition and should be avoided. Sunlight exposure should be minimized and a sunscreen used.

Pharmacological agents include NSAIDs, antimalarials, corticosteroids and immunosuppressants, often needed in high doses. Symptomatic treatment may be required with antiepileptics, anti-hypertensives, antipsychotics and antide-pressants. In acute exacerbations infection must be actively sought out, particularly SBE. Early consultation with a rheuma-tologist, and counselling and support services are essential.

PROGNOSIS

The prognosis has improved dramatically with a 10- and 15-year survival of 90% and 80% respectively.

GONOCOCCAL ARTHRITIS

One per cent of gonococcal infections become complicated by septic arthritis. Typically the hands, wrists, elbows, knees and ankles are involved. Sexually active females are four times more commonly affected. The presentation is with fever, rigors, fleeting migratory polyarthralgia, tenosynovitis, and skin lesions such as embolic haemorrhagic necrotic pustules, followed by a septic mono- or oligoarth-ritis. Blood cultures are positive in only 10–50% of cases. Throat, cervical and urethral swabs should be taken, as these have a higher positive yield (75–86%).

Synovial fluid culture for the gono-coccus is positive in fewer than half of the cases. although there is a higher posi-tive yield with a gram stain of the fluid. The white cell count in the fluid is between 30 000 and 100 000/mL. Management consists of intravenous ceftriaxone or cefotaxime, plus azithromycin or doxy-cycline with daily joint aspiration, in consultation with an infectious disease specialist and orthopaedic service.

PSORIATIC ARTHRITIS

Psoriatic arthritis occurs in 5–10% of patients with psoriasis with 95% of the joint involvement peripheral, most often in the upper limb. The pattern may be pauciarticular, but in the majority more than five joints are involved.

There are five clinical subtypes recognized:

- Asymmetric oligoarthritis
- Predominant distal interphalangeal joint involvement
- Psoriatic spondyloarthropathy
- Symmetrical small joint polyarthritis
- Arthritis mutilans.

Rheumatoid factor seropositivity is usually absent, and nodules and vasculitis do not occur. The arthritis is destructive in a small percentage of patients and can lead to severe joint deformity 'arthritis mutilans'. Psoriatic skin disease is a diagnostic feature that should be sought in the scalp, behind the elbows or around the umbilicus and natal cleft when not obvious. Nail changes include pitting and onycholysis.

Sausage digits are produced by arthritis, periostitis and tenosynovitis in the fingers. Epicondylitis and plantar fasciitis may occur. Thirty per cent of patients have mild inflammation at the eye, most commonly conjunctivitis.

DIAGNOSIS

This is essentially clinical, requiring the demonstration of coexisting synovitis and psoriasis. ESR and CRP are raised. Patients are rheumatoid factor and autoantibody negative.

TREATMENT

NSAIDs, sulphasalazine, methotrexate and intra-articular corticosteroids are used in consultation with a rheumatologist. Oral corticosteroids are avoided, as their cessation often exacerbates the psoriasis.

REITER SYNDROME

This consists of arthritis, urethritis, conjunctivitis, and skin and mucosal lesions. In 80% of cases there is an association with HLA-B27 antigens. Males are affected 15 times more often than females and there is an association with HIV disease. The syndrome follows infection by *Chlamydia* in the genitourinary tract, or *Salmonella*, *Shigella*, *Yersinia* or *Campylobacter* in the gastrointestinal tract. Fever, weight loss and malaise are present to varying degrees. Arthritis occurs within 1–3 weeks of urethritis or diarrhoea. Joint involvement is asymmetrical. The knees, ankles, feet and wrists are commonly involved. Joint stiffness, myalgia and low back pain occur with inflammation located at the insertion of tendons. Chronic heel pain of Achilles tendinitis or plantar fasciitis may be present. Urethritis, cervicitis, cystitis and

prostatitis are usually transient. In the eye there is uni- or bilateral non-infectious conjunctivitis, keratitis, iritis and rarely optic neuritis. Diarrhoea precedes the syndrome by 1–3 weeks, and is often mild or transient.

Laboratory investigations include urethral swabs, urinalysis, stool cultures, a full blood count and ESR, and joint fluid analysis. X-rays show sacroiliitis in 70% of patients. Symptoms may last from 6 weeks to 6 months, and 15–50% of patients have recurring bouts. Heel pain is associated with a worse prognosis. Two per cent develop chronic arthritis and 3% develop an ankylosing spondylitis syndrome. Treatment is with reassurance and NSAIDs. Bed rest is sometimes useful. Refractory cases are treated with sulphasalazine and even methotrexate.

RHEUMATIC FEVER

Although this is now rare in developed countries, acute rheumatic fever is still seen in Maori and Polynesian New Zealanders at a rate of 65–70 per 100 000 children per year between the ages of 5 and 14, and is also more prevalent in aboriginal communities. Migratory polyarthritis affecting the large joints such as the knees, elbows, ankles and shoulder is present in 85–95% of cases at initial presentation. Other features are carditis, chorea, erythema marginatum, subcutaneous nodules, fever, arthralgia, a prior history of rheumatic fever, prolonged PR interval on ECG, and a raised ESR. The aetiology is thought to be autoimmune following group A β-haemolytic streptococcus throat infection. The affected age group is between 5 and 20 years. Treatment consists of monitoring for complications, aspirin, NSAIDs, and penicillin or erythromycin to eradicate the causative bacteria.

SCLERODERMA

This term encompasses a spectrum of disorders with two main subsets:

- Limited cutaneous scleroderma, previously called the CREST syndrome, with calcinosis, Raynaud's disease, oesophageal dysmotility, sclerodactyly and telangiectasia. In this variation Raynaud's phenomenon usually precedes the skin changes by several years, and the skin is affected only at the extremities or not at all.

- Diffuse cutaneous scleroderma, with skin changes beginning within 1 year of the onset of Raynaud's phenomenon, affecting the skin of the extremities and the trunk, with early visceral involvement such as interstitial lung disease, oliguric renal failure, diffuse gastrointestinal tract disease and myocardial disease. The aetiology is thought to be autoimmune microvessel disease causing widespread and unregulated fibrosis.

VIRAL ARTHRITIS

PARVOVIRUS B$_{19}$

Twelve per cent of patients with recent-onset polyarthralgia/arthritis will have this aetiology. In adults a 'flu-like illness occurs, with arthralgia being more common than arthritis. Joint involvement is similar to that in rheumatoid arthritis. There is morning stiffness, and in half the patients they will have the diagnostic criteria for rheumatoid arthritis. Specific antibodies to the parvovirus are detectable for the first 2 months after infection. The disease is self-limiting, but may last up to 5 years.

HEPATITIS B VIRUS

This may cause severe arthritis of the hand, knee or a large joint. Onset is usually pre-icteric, but the duration is variable.

ALPHAVIRUS

These are mosquito-borne viruses of the Togaviridiae family that cause a febrile polyarthritis. The Ross River virus causes involvement of the wrist, MCP joint, IP joint and knees associated with a macular or maculopapular rash.

Most of the other viruses such as mumps, adenovirus, Coxsackie virus, Epstein-Barr virus, herpes simplex, CMV and rubella cause an arthritis/arthralgia syndrome. Arthritis is also be associated with vaccines and with HIV disease.

OTHER INFECTIONS

Other infective causes of arthritis include syphilis, TB, leprosy, brucella and *Mycoplasma pneumoniae.*

BACK PAIN

Back pain is one of the most common presentations encountered in the emergency department. It is often complex to sort out as:

- An exact anatomical diagnosis is elusive.
- The pain is often chronic.
- Pain control is difficult.
- Patient mobilization, and hence discharge from the emergency department, is difficult.
- Patients' expectations of immediate resolution of symptoms are unrealistic.
- It may be a manifestation of depression or other psychological disorder.
- Compensation-related matters influence the presentation.

However, serious pathological causes of back pain that may be life-threatening or, for instance, affect spinal cord function may be present and must be actively excluded.

PATHOLOGY

There are many aetiological and pathological processes that cause back pain. The pain may arise primarily in the back, or it may be referred from abdominal visceral conditions such as an abdominal aortic aneurysm and pyelonephritis. Locally, the pain arises in the soft tissues, intervertebral discs, facet joints and bone. It may be due to trauma, inflammation secondary to arthritic disease of any origin, degenerative disease, primary or secondary malignancy, infection, metabolic bone disease such as Paget's disease and osteoporosis, and congenital or developmental abnormality.

Disc disease ranges from a bulge to protrusion, extrusion and sequestration. A significant central disc bulge causes low back pain, whereas a posterolaterally prolapsed disc may cause sciatica. Spinal stenosis, which can be degenerative, developmental or discogenic in aetiology, causes radicular symptoms. Spinal claudication may be associated with spinal stenosis.

Spondylolysis is a congenital defect in the pars articularis, which can lead to spondylolisthesis or forward slip of a vertebra on the one below. There are four stages of slipping: less than 25%, less than 50%, less than 75% and more than 75%. The most common spondylolisthesis is of the L5 on the S1 vertebra. Half the patients develop symptoms at some stage.

Alternatively, tumours either primary, such as multiple myeloma, or more commonly secondary from the prostate, breast, lung, kidney or thyroid may affect the back. Infective causes include discitis, osteomyelitis and epidural abscess. Finally, back pain is common in pregnancy and is multifactorial in origin. Psychosomatic back pain should only be considered when all other reasonable causes have been excluded.

HISTORY

An accurate history determines the likely cause in the majority of cases. Serious underlying pathology must be excluded and may be related to the age of the patient. When enquiring about the pain the onset, site, radiation, character and aggravating and relieving factors should be sought. Sciatica is indicated by radiation of the pain below the knees. Pain temporally related to physical activity such as lifting implies a mechanical cause. Coughing, sneezing or straining increase pressure in the spinal canal, and will aggravate pain if there is compromise of the canal space.

Boring pain, worse at night and unrelieved by simple analgesics in an older individual suggests malignancy, as does a pain that is of long standing, associated with weight loss, altered bowel habit, indigestion, prostatic or gynaecological symptoms. Pain that makes the patient restless occurs with aortic aneurysm, pancreatitis or renal colic.

Bowel and bladder function and uni- or bilateral loss of power or sensation in the legs must always be assessed for. Fever may indicate infection, malignancy or a connective tissue disorder. If fever is present, a search must be made for a possible primary source of sepsis, including the use of intravenous drugs.

PHYSICAL EXAMINATION

Vital signs must be taken carefully. An accurate temperature reading is important. A systematic examination is essential to avoid missing a potentially serious condition. This includes examining spinal-cord function, eliminating the presence of a malignancy and infection, and ruling out secondary causes such as an abdominal aortic aneurysm and acute pancreatitis.

Local examination of the back includes observation for deformity and scoliosis. Palpation may reveal tenderness. Distally, evidence of nerve root irritation may be found in the straight leg-raising test, bowstring sign and Lasegue's sign.

The cross-over sign or a positive crossed leg-raise test is considered diagnostic of discogenic sciatica. Sensation should be carefully tested, especially in the perineal region including anal tone. Saddle anaesthesia and loss of anal and urethral sphincter control occur in cauda equina compression and constitute a surgical emergency. Deep tendon and plantar reflexes, power and gait should be examined.

INVESTIGATIONS

Investigations are performed according to the findings on history and examination. FBC and ESR are sent if an infection is suspected. Radiographs are of limited value and should only be taken if there has been trauma with a mechanism to suggest a fracture, or if the history is suggestive of malignancy. Computerized tomography (CT) bone scans and magnetic resonance imaging (MRI) may be indicated. For acute back pain of probable musculo-ligamentous cause no investigation is indicated.

MANAGEMENT

The most important role of the emergency physician is to rule out an immediate threat to life or spinal cord function. Back pain in the elderly should immediately raise the suspicion of a vascular problem such as a leaking aortic aneurysm or a dissection of the aorta, regardless of how benign the history or findings on examination.

For acute non-specific back pain without any serious underlying aetiology it is important to educate the patient and create an expectation of a return to normal function. Analgesia such as panadol or codeine, warm compresses, and NSAIDs such as naproxen or diclofenac are useful. There is some evidence that benzodiazepines are useful in the acute stage for soft tissue back injury, although intravenous narcotics should be avoided, except as an occasional one-off to give the patient the confidence to mobilize. Early mobilization within −2 days and early graduated exercises promote a faster recovery and earlier return to work. The management of chronic back pain is outside the scope of the emergency department, and involves modalities such as ultrasound, manipulation, physiotherapy, TENS and steroid injections.

REGIONAL SOFT-TISSUE RHEUMATIC CONDITIONS

Periarticular pain may be caused by inflammation in bursal sacs, tendon sheaths or tendons. Contributory or aetiologic factors include excessive use of the joint causing soft-tissue trauma due to friction; acute trauma; arthritic disease, as in rheumatoid arthritis or gout (crystal deposits), chronic degenerative processes and infection.

SHOULDER PAIN

Rotator cuff tendinitis

The rotator cuff is made up of supraspinatus, infraspinatus, teres minor and subscapularis muscles. Any of these may be involved.

Clinical features

There is usually a history of excessive use. The onset of pain in the shoulder may be acute or chronic. Tenderness is elicited by palpation of the inflamed tendons. With supraspinatus tendinitis abduction produces a painful arc from 60° to 120°. The impingement sign is positive with impingement pain disappearing on local anaesthetic injection into the subacromial bursa.

Investigations

X-rays may reveal the presence of calcification in calcific tendinitis, which may be asymptomatic or may cause severe subacromial bursitis.

Management

Rest, hot or cold packs, analgesia and NSAIDs are prescribed. Depot corticosteroid injections, ultrasound therapy and specific exercise are useful.

Rotator cuff tear

Acute tears are caused by minor trauma in the over-40 year old with degenerative changes. In the fit under-40 age group, more significant trauma is involved. The mechanism of injury is forced abduction against resistance, as may happen when breaking a fall with the outstretched hand. However, 50% of patients recall no trauma, implying a gradual attrition of the tendon culminating in a sudden and complete tear.

Rotator cuff tears may be partial or complete. Clinically, there is pain, weak-ness or loss of abduction, and failure to externally rotate or be able to maintain the arm in extreme external rotation. The drop arm test may be positive. Injection of the tender area with local anaesthetic relieves the pain and allows more accurate examination of the shoulder. The patient should be referred to an orthopaedic surgeon after a diagnostic ultrasound, MRI or arthrogram. Acute tears in young people require early surgical repair with conservative treatment preferred in the elderly.

Bicipital tendinitis and rupture

The long head of the biceps is intracapsular and extrasynovial. The diagnosis of bicipital tendinitis is based on localization of tenderness. Rupture of the long head is readily diagnosed by the 'Popeye' sign, that is, bulging of the muscle belly distally. Acute rupture in young individuals is best treated surgically. In the older patient conservative management is more appropriate.

ELBOW

Lateral (tennis elbow) or medial (golfers elbow) epicondylitis and olecranon bursitis are common. Degenerative disease, trauma and gout are implicated in the latter. Olecranon bursitis may also be secondary to infection, when diagnostic and therapeutic aspiration and antibiotics are indicated. Surgical drainage may be required if infection is found.

WRIST

De Quervain's tenosynovitis is inflammation of the abductor and extensor pollicis longus tendons on the radial aspect of the wrist, causing tenderness, swelling and motion crepitus over the tendons. Finkelstein's test is usually positive, with an increase in pain on passive ulnar deviation of wrist with the thumb folded across the palm and the fingers flexed over it. Treatment is conservative with NSAIDS, splint or local steroid injection. Occasionally, if conservative management fails, surgical treatment is indicated with release of the tendon sheaths.

Any of the other long tendons around the wrist may become inflamed following minor trauma or repetitive injury. Infection of the flexor digitorum superficialis (FDS) or flexor digitorum profundus (FDP) tendon sheaths in the palm requires aggressive treatment with immediate surgical drainage and antibiotics.

CARPAL TUNNEL SYNDROME

Median nerve compression in the carpal tunnel may be idiopathic or secondary to rheumatoid arthritis, a scaphoid or Colles' fracture, other trauma and fluid retention in pregnancy or with the use of the contraceptive pill. Myxoedema, acromegaly and amyloidosis are rarer causes. Typically there is nocturnal pain or discomfort, with relief by hanging the arm over the bed. Sensory disturbance occurs in the middle and index fingers and thumb, although pain may radiate up the forearm. The thenar muscles are wasted if the entrapment is long standing. Tinel's sign may be positive with tapping over the median nerve at the wrist reproducing paraesthesiae in its distal distribution, as may be Phalen's sign with the same symptoms on full active flexion of the elevated wrist. Management includes NSAIDS, splinting, steroid injection and surgical decompression of the tunnel.

PERIARTICULAR HIP CONDITIONS

Trochanteric bursitis is common. Others conditions recognized are iliopsoas bursitis, ischial bursitis and meralgia paraesthetica causing paraesthesiae or numbness over the sensory distribution of the lateral cutaneous nerve of the thigh.

KNEE

BAKER'S CYST

This is a popliteal cyst or cystic swelling of the semimembranous gastrocnemius bursa, which communicates with the knee joint in 40% of the population. Increasing size of the bursa is associated with increasing discomfort. Rheumatoid arthritis, osteoarthritis, internal knee derangements, gout and Reiter's syndrome predispose to formation of the cyst. The patient may present acutely with rupture of the cyst, with a warm, tender, painful, swollen calf simulating a deep vein thrombosis. Ultrasound is indicated for differentiation. The management of a symptomatic cyst is conservative.

ANSERINE BURSITIS

The typical patient is an older, overweight female with osteoarthritis of the knees. Pain and tenderness occur on the medial aspect of the knee, approximately 5 cm below the joint line, at the insertion of the tendons. Relief occurs with rest, muscle stretching, analgesia and steroid injection of the bursa.

PREPATELLAR BURSITIS

The cause is inflammatory usually secondary to kneeling. If there is an overlying abrasion and there is concern about sepsis, or there is fever with inflammation, immediate aspiration, drainage and antibiotics are indicated.

RUPTURE OF QUADRICEPS AND PATELLAR TENDONS

Quadriceps tendon rupture is caused by sudden violent contraction of the quadriceps with the knee flexed. Spontaneous rupture occurs in patients with chronic renal failure, rheumatoid arthritis, hyperparathyroidism, gout, and in SLE patients on steroids. It is usually seen in the elderly. Infrapatellar tendon rupture is usually traumatic in origin occurring in the young sports person, but may occur for the same reasons as rupture of the quadriceps tendon. Clinically there is failure of extension of the knee, a palpable gap, and on X-ray a high-riding patella. Surgery is indicated.

FURTHER READING

Butler RC, Jayson IV 1996 Collected reports on the rheumatic diseases. The Arthritis and Rheumatism Council for Research, Chesterfield, Derbyshire, UK

Kelley WN, Harris E, Ruddy S, Sledge CB 1997 Textbook of Rheumatology, 5th edn. WB Saunders, London

Snaith ML 1996 ABC of Rheumatology. BMJ Publishing Group, London

Tintinalli JE, Ruiz E, Krome RL 1996 Emergency Medicine: A Comprehensive Study Guide, 4th edn. McGraw-Hill, New York

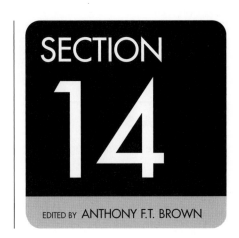

DERMATOLOGY

14.1 **Emergency dermatology** 528

14.1 EMERGENCY DERMATOLOGY

GEORGE VARIGOS • VANESSA MORGAN

ESSENTIALS

1 Emergency dermatology presentations may be divided into three major groups: acute on chronic, new localized and new generalized.

2 Acute on chronic complications can be due to compliance failure or a complication of the specific skin disease. A careful history will usually differentiate.

3 The new acute rash may have a pattern that is localized, sharply defined or grouped. Look for the following forms of lesions: papules, purpura, nodules, pustules, vesicles and blisters.

4 A generalized new acute rash should be differentiated according to duration, targetoid lesions, associated pustules, purpura, scaling, weeping or blisters.

INTRODUCTION

The pattern and form of acute dermatological conditions that present to the emergency department are confusing in that the presenting clinical features, such as vasodilatation, exfoliation, blistering or necrosis are the common end-point of inflammatory processes in the skin. The pathological response involves cytokines or chemokines, and their effects give the visible responses. The important clinical differences seen in these acute reactions should be recognized by the trained observer (see Table 14.1.1 and 14.1.2).

This chapter aims to provide a clinical pathway from taking the appropriate history and having a knowledge of the distinguishing clinical features of the likely differential diagnoses. The conditions discussed are limited to specific dermatological states that may present to the emergency department as a true urgency. The presentation of skin infections and anaphylaxis are covered elsewhere. It is important to use other resources as well as this book, such as an atlas and dermatology texts, to provide details of the conditions mentioned.

CLINICAL PRESENTATION

Emergency presentations may be divided into three major groups:

- Acute on chronic
- New localized
- New generalized.

Acute on chronic rash with a past skin condition

The presentation to emergency is usually the patient with progressive lack of control, worsening status or treatment failure. Consider the following reasons:

- Compliance failure, elicited by a careful, detailed history

- Complications of the specific skin disease in question. Examples below are discussed for the following conditions: atopic eczema, psoriasis, and the autoimmune blistering diseases
- A new skin condition.

The clinical presentations and management of atopic eczema (Table 14.1.3 and Fig. 14.1.1), psoriasis and autoimmune blistering diseases are presented below.

Table 14.1.2 Definition of patterns in skin disorders

Annular	Ring like or part of a circle
Linear	Line like
Arcuate	Arch like
Grouped	Local collection of similar lesions
Unilateral	One side
Symmetrical	Both sides

Table 14.1.1 Definition of macroscopic skin pathological lesions

Papule	Circumscribed firm raised elevation, less than 0.5 cm in diameter.
Nodule	A solid or firm mass more than 0.5 cm in the skin which can be observed as an elevation or can be palpated.
Purpura	Discolouration of skin or mucous membranes due to extravasation of red blood cells.
Pustule	A visible accumulation of fluid, usually yellow, in the form of a vesicle or papule containing the fluid. It may be centred around a pore such as a hair follicle or sweat glands and sometimes appear in normal skin, not uncommonly palmar/plantar.
Vesicle	A visible accumulation of fluid in a papule of <5 mm. The fluid is clear, serous-like and is located within or beneath the epidermis.
Blister or bullae	Large fluid containing lesions of more than 5 mm.
Plaque	An area or sheet of skin elevated and with a distinct edge, of any shape and usually wider than 1 cm.

(Diagnosis of Skin Disease, Rook AJ, Burton JL, Champion RH, Ebling FJG 1992 Textbook of Dermatology. Blackwell Scientific, Oxford)

Table 14.1.3 Atopic eczema: acute attacks and complications

	Infective eczema *Eczema herpeticum*	Erythroderma *Impetiginized eczema*	*Unstable eczema*	Acute eczema *Psychological*	*Contact*
Cause	Infection with herpes simplex, Varicella, which can rapidly disseminate over the skin	Staphylococcal	Due to many factors Systemic or external	Stressors	Allergen?
Examination	Grouped locally or generally Pinhead-sized papules or vesicles Clear or closed pustules Excoriated sharply defined circular erosions	Discharge and weeping Yellow and crusted blisters or erosions	Total body redness Scale or weeping pruritus Hypothermia Fever, sepsis	Severe Red Pruritus Disturbed sleep	Sharp edges Localized
Management	Antivirals if severe, early, and eyes at risk	Oral antibiotics Antiseptic (triclosan) soaks and wet dressings	Admission Oral steroids Ciclosporin	Admission topicals Oral steroids Paraffin etc.	Oral steroids Admission

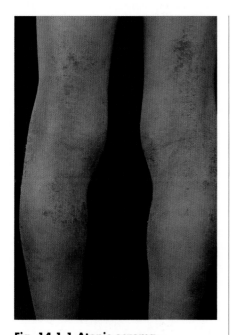

Fig. 14.1.1 Atopic eczema.

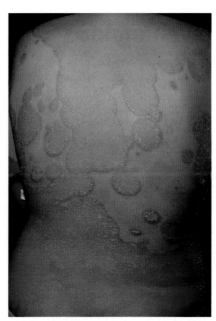

Fig. 14.1.2 Psoriasis.

- Immune activated psoriasis flares: these are caused by bacterial or viral infective foci in respiratory, bowel, gallbladder or bladder sites, and rarely with malignancy. Typically there are new guttate lesions or flares in old plaques. Often there have been similar triggered attacks in the past.

INVESTIGATIONS

Skin biopsy is usually performed in the ward or clinic to confirm the diagnosis. Further investigations for systemic monitoring of complications such as infection, metabolic and fluid balance changes, blood film changes, renal and liver function are indicated, as well as monitoring for the side effects of therapy.

PSORIASIS: ACUTE ATTACKS AND COMPLICATIONS

Psoriasis (Fig. 14.1.2) may present acutely in the following patterns:

- Erythroderma: this is an unstable state that may be caused by systemic or external factors, including treatment. Clinically it is indistinguishable, as there is total body redness with no typical features

of psoriasis. At presentation, hypothermia and sepsis must be considered.

- Pustular psoriasis : this is triggered by systemic or external factors, including topical treatments, medication and oral steroids. Examination reveals yellow sterile pustules on plaques, diffuse generalized or localized red areas, beginning around the paronychium of the digits or pulp. Arthritis may be present. If it is generalized consider Reiter's syndrome or hypocalcaemia.

MANAGEMENT

Admission is required if the patient has extensive areas involved, is systemically unwell or unable to cope. Treatments include antibiotics, ultraviolet therapy, methotrexate, ciclosporin or etretinate that require a dermatology consultation and careful review of past treatment. There is now clinical evidence of the benefit of rotating therapies in psoriasis and that a past failed treatment should not subsequently be considered ineffective.

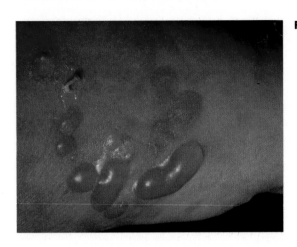

Fig. 14.1.3 Pemphigoid.

AUTOIMMUNE BLISTERING DISEASES

Acute new blistering lesions may be a result of:

- The immune-suppressive drugs being reduced or withdrawn inappropriately;
- Triggers such as infections, i.e. herpes or a general illness, or stressors.

Clinical presentations of the specific blistering diseases include:

- Pemphigus: flaccid crusted lesions and impetiginized erosions, mucosal ulceration
- Bullous pemphigoid (Fig. 14.1.3): tense blisters, some on plaques of redness; also urticarial lesions with pruritus
- Cicatricial pemphigoid: results in scarring, areas often involve mucosa and affect swallowing, rarely causing stridor. Erosive areas in mucosa and skin
- Epidermolysis bullosa acquisita: fragility of skin with erosions and blisters on minor trauma, commonly on the limbs
- Linear IgA bullous disease: onset often in childhood, but seen in adults as fragility of skin and mucosa with characteristic new blisters surrounding the edges of older, recently healed areas.

INVESTIGATIONS

- Systemic monitoring of complications such as local infection, sepsis, metabolic and fluid balance, blood film changes, renal and liver function
- Monitoring the side effects of therapy, such as X-ray for crush fractures.

MANAGEMENT

These are serious and life-threatening conditions requiring admission or urgent consultation with the dermatology unit. The specific immunosuppressive treatments used are oral steroids, in combination with azathioprine and, less often, ciclosporin or cyclophosphamide. General management includes monitoring for the side effects of these drugs, including systemic infection, sepsis, blood film changes, renal or liver toxicity.

Paraneoplastic pemphigus and pemphigoid require follow-up and investigation for occult malignancies.

NEW AND LOCALIZED

Consider the new acute rash, which may be localized, sharply defined or grouped. The following conditions must be carefully looked for by their distinguishing morphologies such as papules, purpura, vesicles, bullae, nodules or pustules (see Table 14.1.1 for definitions).

New papular rash

Bites These are typically single or grouped, and may be seen as linear lesions or new groups in different areas. Each bite has a central pinpoint vesicle on a red papule. Sometimes the single lesions have central darkening, and even necrosis with blackening. Old bite areas can flare with new episodes of bites, called papular urticaria, and is often seen in children. Management is to find the likely vector and remove or treat. Suspect pets, bird mites and sandpits.

Purpuric and papular rashes

Vasculitis (Fig. 14.1.4) This is clinically diagnosable when palpable and on the lower limbs. A biopsy is required if not palpable but vasculitis is suspected.

Fig. 14.1.4 Vasculitis.

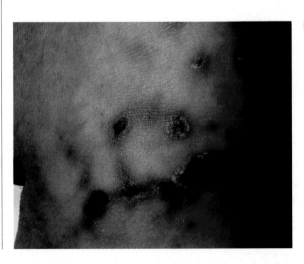

This is usually after admission or referral to clinic.

Management

This includes investigations for triggers such as an infective focus (viral and bacterial), autoimmune diseases, vasculitis such as Wegener's granulomatosis, polyarteritis nodosa and inflammatory bowel diseases. Rarely internal tumours and leukaemia may present with vasculitis. Sharp edges with stellate or irregular shapes depict full thickness ischaemia and are seen in septic embolic lesions or meningococcal infections, and in thrombotic occlusion states such as calciphilaxis.

New vesicular or blistering rashes

Viruses Often grouped vesicles in a region or dermatome are seen, with a history of recurrences as in herpes simplex or varicella zoster. New contacts are important in molluscum virus; also commonly associated with contact in swimming pools, baths at home, etc.

Management

Direct immunofluorescence testing for herpes is helpful. Appropriate oral antivirals such as acyclovir are given if within 72 hours of onset. However, there is no strict time limit if the patient is immunosuppressed or systemically unwell, and tests for herpes are positive. Molluscum virus is treated with a variety of locally inducing irritants, including cryotherapy; if disseminated, consider immune suppression.

Contact allergic dermatitis

This is clinically acutely eczematous, with oedema, redness, blisters and weeping areas from small vesicles or bullous lesions with a linear or sharply defined edge. It is considered because of the sharp-edged pattern and history of external precipitants, i.e. photosensitive distribution, airborne, plant or other contacts including medications. It is important to remember the differential diagnoses of contact dermatitis such as cellulitis, erysipelas, varicose dermatitis

and self-inflicted states (artefacta) or abuse causes. The latter present with sharply defined and often bizarre shapes.

Management

Management of allergic contact dermatitis is to suspect and remove any cause. If none is elucidated, arrange a review for patch testing by a dermatologist. The preferred emergency medication is a short course of oral steroids, reducing from 25–50 mg for 3–6 days, topical wet dressings for the usually weeping and blistering state, and topical steroid creams.

Nodules

Single or multiple nodular lesions include the following important conditions:

- Lymphoma or secondary tumours as single or multiple, deeply plum-coloured nodules and purpuric lesions.
- Erythema nodosum has multiple and especially tender dermal lesions over the legs and thighs, but not restricted to these sites, with associated joint aches. Consider the common causes, including hormonal medications, infections and sarcoid.
- Fixed drug eruptions classically lead to recurring nodules in the same sites, usually purple oval lesions, sometimes with blisters and erosions. Remember to consider the additives in foods, herbal substances, chemist products, laxatives, etc., and non-proprietary medications as well as prescription drugs as causal.
- Infections cause linear and erythematous nodules. Consider atypical *Mycobacterium marinum* and deep fungal infection. Single nodules may occur with infections such as milker's nodules, or leishmaniasis. Dermatophyte, tinea infection has a slow onset and may present as a deep nodular grouped appearance especially after topical steroid use (tinea incognito).

The history and medical status of the patient are important, as immune suppressed patients present with skin infections. Take a careful history of

contacts and activities, such as hobbies, fishtanks and animals. Multiple lesions may be a feature of sepsis such as meningococcal, prior to the more purpuric feature of vasculitis. Livedo with nodules is a reticulate eruption classically seen in polyarteritis nodosa occuring on the lower legs with nodules in a purple net-like (livedo reticular) pattern. Consider also the autoimmune states, lupus anticoagulant and immune complex diseases.

Management

Each specific state requires work-up and the cause elicited.

Pustular

Multiple pustular lesions

- Sweet's syndrome causes pustules on plaques, with fever and a neutrophilia, and is often confused with sepsis (see below).
- Pyoderma gangrenosum (Fig. 14.1.5) often begins as single or grouped and later symmetrical pustular lesions which rapidly ulcerate, usually but not exclusively involving the lower legs. The clinical characteristic is a pustule evolving into a deep ulcer with an undermined dark purple edge. Rapid progress is also a feature, and an underlying cause, such as

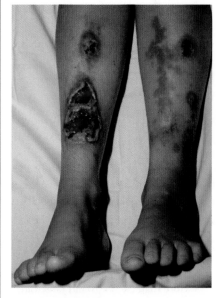

Fig. 14.1.5 Pyoderma.

inflammatory bowel disease, rheumatoid arthritis or tumours must be considered.

Management

Admission if severe or the cause requires investigation. Cultures to exclude unusual infections, if appropriate, and biopsy is helpful but not diagnostic. Systemic steroids are usually the preferred treatment, with prednisolone 50–60 mg daily. Other medications include minocycline, dapsone and immunosuppressants.

Grouped pustules

Impetigo is caused by *Staphylococcus aureus* and *Streptococcus pyogenes* in grouped patterns around the nose and flexures, with the typical yellow, often acneform, crusts. A contact history is relevant.

Management

Antibiotics, see Chapter 8.10.

Candida

This can manifest as disseminated pustules in an emergency patient presenting generally unwell with sepsis.

Management

Usually admission for rapid assessment and systemic treatment.

Less acute conditions, such as acne, acne rosacea and fungal infection are often pustular but generally present as a chronic state.

NEW AND GENERALIZED

Consider the new acute rash with a pattern consisting of 90–100% skin involvement.

It is vital to ask what the form of the lesion is in the generalized or diffuse rash, and the duration, onset and offset:

- Redness
  - less than 24 hours
  - more than 24 hours and several colours
  - more than 24 hours and targetoid, with four rings of colour

- with pustules
- with purpura
- with scale and/or weeping
- with blisters less than or more than 30% cover.

Reactions may be broadly grouped as either autoimmune, infection, malignancy, inflammatory bowel, or drug/allergy-induced.

The differential diagnosis includes the following:

- Urticaria (Fig. 14.1.6)
- Toxic erythema, usually infective or drug induced
- Erythema multiforme (Fig. 14.1.7)
- Toxic epidermal necrolysis (TEN) (Fig. 14.1.8)
- Acute febrile neutrophilic dermatoses (Sweet syndrome) (Fig. 14.1.9)
- Vasculitis
- Erythroderma or exfoliative dermatitis
- Erythrosquamous disorder such as eczematous, from drug allergy or infestations, i.e. scabies, psoriasis, and rare disorders of cornification such as pityriasis rubra pilaris
- Autoimmune blistering disorders: pemphigus, pemphigoid, epidermolysis bullosa acquisita, linear IgA bullous disease.

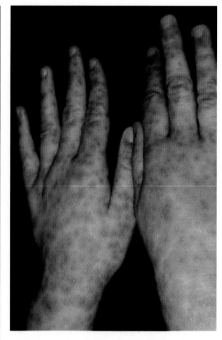

Fig. 14.1.7 Erythema multiforme.

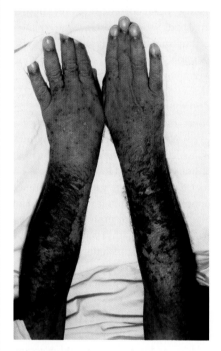

Fig. 14.1.8 Toxic epidermal necrolysis.

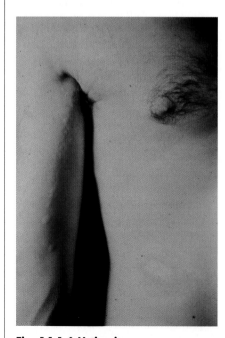

Fig. 14.1.6 Urticaria.

Areas of redness only

- Consider urticaria if each 'lesion' on history clears within 24 hours, and look in particular for raised red areas with a halo of vasoconstriction, various shapes, and a tendency to stay in the same areas or region, i.e.

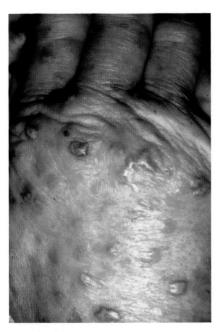

Fig. 14.1.9 Sweet syndrome

non-mucosal or involving the mucosa. Sometimes redness may vary in areas, even look paler in the centre and be mistaken as targetoid.

- Consider toxic erythema if the 'lesions' on history stay for more than 24 hours often due to a viral or drug cause, and also consider urticarial vasculitis if they fade from urticarial areas to leave pigmentation.
- Consider angio-oedema if the skin is pink to normal colour and there is swelling of the deeper skin. Sometimes urticaria will be visible. Rarely α_1-antitrypsin deficiency may begin in this form.

Management

Urticaria is usually caused by foods or medications, and may be due to more than one substance at a time that degranulates mast cells. Stop all likely foods and avoid aspirin. Treat with oral antihistamines and consider combined H_1 and H_2 receptor blockers, or doxepin may be trialled as a strong anti-H_1 and H_2 inhibitor. Investigations are usually unhelpful and clinic referral is needed if the cause is not easily determined.

Urticarial vasculitis may present with a low complement level, and lupus must then be considered. Consider other causes of vasculitis and treat with antimalarials, colchicine, steroids or dapsone.

Redness with added colour changes within lesions, lasting several days

'Targetoid' is defined as three or four concentric rings of colour changes and is typical of erythema multiforme (EM). It is often seen with a darker centre or sometimes blistering and with erosions, especially in the mucosal sites. Usually only 30% of the skin surface is seen as blistering in EM. Otherwise, if more than 30% of the surface is blistered then by definition the diagnosis is labelled as toxic epidermal necrolysis (TEN, see below).

Vasculitis may present with less typical target lesions, with no rings but blurring or shades of red with central darkening.

Management

Admission and biopsy are often required in ill patients and those with extensive disease. Specific treatment of the cause is essential. TEN is usually due to a drug such as sulphonamides or anticonvulsants. General treatment is supportive care with fluids and antibiotics if exposed surfaces are present. The skin requires dressings as for burns. Systemic steroid use is likely to only be helpful in the early stages of EM, but is contraindicated in TEN, although this is still controversial.[1–5]

Redness with blistering or pustular changes seen within lesions lasting several days

- **Sweet syndrome**.[6] This is blisters or pustules, sometimes with a purpuric ring or redness, on a base of red raised areas (acute febrile neutrophilic dermatoses). Usually it presents with fever, peripheral neutrophilia and non-infective sterile pustules on plaques or nodules over upper limbs, head and trunk. Acute generalized exanthematous pustulosis (AGEP) without purpura is a differential diagnosis, with a drug as a likely cause.

Management

These cases may mistakenly be admitted to intensive care as clinical signs suggest sepsis. When the patient does not improve on antibiotics, skin biopsy is required. Causes include carcinoma and leukaemia, as well as infections and autoimmune diseases. Oral steroids and dapsone are usually effective. Recurrent attacks each lasting several (5–6) weeks have been described, and malignancies are seen more in the blistering forms.

Redness with purpura and palpable lesions

Clinically these features represent a vasculitis and are immune-complex mediated. They are seen particularly on the lower limbs. If black and irregular stellate shapes of purpuric lesions appear, this indicates many vessel sizes are involved and no collateral circulation with ischaemia Therefore, suspect septicaemia such as meningococcal or generalized increased thrombotic states. Deeper lesions may be due to a panniculitis affecting the subcuticular fatty layer.

Management

Determine the likely cause and systemic involvement for example renal, bowel or brain. Generalized vasculitis requires medical assessment and admission. Panniculitis may be infective or systemic due to vasculitis in the septa or lobular areas.

Diffuse redness and scaly rashes

This may also include weeping areas with itching. This is an erythroderma or exfoliative dermatitis.

Management

Investigate the cause including drug hypersensitivity syndrome, and look for lymphadenopathy, hepatic enlargement and peripheral eosinophilia. Obtain a history of likely drugs such as phenytoin, carbamazepine and other antiepileptics. Malignancies include leukaemia and Sézary syndrome, and solid cell carcinoma. Nutritional deficiency states and infective causes or complications should also be excluded.

Treat both the causes and complications, including assessment of hydration, sepsis, temperature control and general medical and cardiac state in the elderly. Topical therapy includes emollients and measures to treat or prevent infection. Systemic steroids may be needed and infection should be controlled.

Emergency management and treatment of erythroderma

The causes include eczema (40%), psoriasis (22%), drugs (15%), lymphoma (Sezary syndrome) (10%), and idiopathic (8%). Complications include:

- High output cardiac failure
- Dehydration – renal failure may result
- Protein loss – oedema often occurs and contributes to renal failure with fluid loss
- Hypothermia/temperature dysregulation
- Thrombophlebitis/DVT
- Infection – cutaneous and respiratory (pneumonia major cause of death)
- Side effects of treatment.

Admit the patient, obtain any history of previous skin disease, recent medications, recent changes to skin management and assess hydration and cardiac status, check for oedema, respiratory infection, DVT. Send investigations for FBC with film and differential, ELFTs, blood cultures if temp >38 or if unwell and having rigors even if the temperature is normal, skin swabs and a chest X-ray.

CONTROVERSIES

❶ The use of steroids. TEN may become worse with steroids and have a poorer prognosis. If given early in erythema multiforme steroids are helpful but equivocal.

❷ Pooled human intravenous immnoglobulin for toxic epidermal necrolysis treatment is now regarded first choice with a short course of ciclosporin.[7]

Treatment is general with attention to temperature control avoiding hypothermia, fluid balance chart if necessary with IV fluid replacement, referral to dietician for high protein diet in the first 24 hours, chest physiotherapy and DVT prophylaxis. Specific treatment includes bath oil daily in bath or shower, 50% soft and liquid paraffin all over strictly qid, and antibiotics only if there is proven infection. Dermatology referral and supervision is essential.

Diffuse and severe blistering rashes

There is extensive skin involvement over large areas, with flaccid blisters and loss of roof, leaving raw areas >30%. Consider toxic epidermal necrolysis (TEN) if it is likely caused by drugs such as sulphonamides, anticonvulsants including sodium valproate and lamotrigine and non-steroidal anti-inflammatory drugs (NSAIDs).

Other blistering conditions to be considered include pemphigus, pemphigoid, epidermolysis bullosa acquisita and linear IgA bullous disease.

Management

The most likley drug cause must be ceased. Skin biopsy is required. General nursing requires burns dressing and care in the severe acute stages.

REFERENCES

1. Kakourou T, Klontza D, Soteropoulou F, Kattamis C 1997 Corticosteroid treatment of erythema multiforme major (Stevens-Johnson syndrome) in children. European Journal of Paediatrics 156(2): 90–3
2. Eastham JH, Segal JL, Gomez MF, Cole GW 1996 Reversal of erythema multiforme major with cyclophosphamide and prednisone. Annals of Pharmacotherapy 30(6): 606–7
3. Criton S, Devi K, Srideva PK, Asokan PU 1997 Toxic epidermal necrolysis - a retrospective study. International Journal of Dermatology 36(12): 923–5
4. Engelhardt SL, Schurr MJ, Helgerson RB 1997 Toxic epidermal necrolysis: an analysis of referral patterns and steroid usage. Journal of Burn Care and Rehabilitation 18(6): 520–4
5. Fine JD 1995 Management of acquired bullous skin diseases. New England Journal of Medicine 333(22): 1475–84
6. Von den Driesch P 1994 Sweet's syndrome (acute febrile neutrophilic dermatosis). Journal of the American Academy of Dermatology 31(4): 53
7. Viard I, Werlhrl P, Bullani R, et al 1998 Inhibition of TEN by blockage of CD95 with human intravenous immmunoglobulin. Science 282: 490–3

FURTHER READING

Du Vivier A 1993 Atlas of Clinical Dermatology. Gower Medical Publishers, Aldershot
Rook AJ, Burton JL, Champion RH, Ebling FJG 1992 Textbook of Dermatology. Blackwell Scientific, Oxford

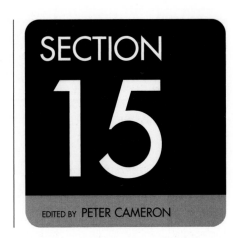

EYES

15.1   Ocular emergencies   536

15.1 OCULAR EMERGENCIES

DAVID V. KAUFMAN • JAMES K. GALBRAITH • MARK J. WALLAND

ESSENTIALS

Injuries

1 Always assess and record vision.

2 Gentle examination with magnification is essential.

3 X-ray/computerized tomography where bony or penetration injury is suspected.

4 For caustic burns free irrigation with water is the principal first aid measure with subsequent removal of any particulate matter.

Painful loss of vision

1 Bacterial keratitis requires intensive, specific, topical antibiotic therapy.

2 Acute angle closure glaucoma produces a rock-hard inflamed eye with a fixed mid-dilated pupil.

Painless loss of vision

1 The relative afferent pupillary defect ('Marcus-Gunn pupil') is an objective sign of neuroretinal dysfunction and must be actively sought.

2 Central retinal artery occlusion requires attempts to lower intraocular pressure acutely and immediate referral is, therefore, required.

3 Elderly patients with acute visual failure have giant cell arteritis until proven otherwise, and need oral steroid cover until the diagnosis is excluded.

4 Recent onset of distorted vision requires ophthalmic review within 1–2 days to exclude exudative age-related macular degeneration.

5 New onset of floaters, particularly in association with flashes, requires early ophthalmic review to exclude retinal detachment.

INTRODUCTION

Ocular emergencies are common. A relatively trivial traumatic presentation may mask a more serious underlying injury. Similarly, a relatively transient episode of visual loss with no abnomality found on examination may indicate potentially life-threatening cerebrovascular disease. Therefore, all eye presentations in an emergency department should be carefully evaluated with the necessary equipment.

Basic sight testing equipment should include a Snellen 6-metre chart and a black occlusive paddle with multiple pin-hole perforations. A slit-lamp bio-microscope is needed for examination of the anterior segment and the removal of foreign bodies.

Emergency eye trolley setup

Examining equipment

- Torch
- Magnifying loupe
- Desmarres lid retractors/lid speculum
- Sterile dressing packs
- Normal saline for irrigation
- Fluorescein strips (sterile)
- Topical anaesthetic (e.g. amethocaine 1%).

Treating

- Mydriatics (dilating): tropicamide 1%, homatropine 2%
- Miotic (constricting): pilocarpine 2%
- Pressure control: acetazolamide 250 mg tablets; ampoules 500 mg (Diamox®)
- Eye pads, plastic shields, tape
- Cotton-tipped applicators (sterile)
- 25G, 23G disposable hypodermic needles (foreign body removal).

A portable slit lamp for examining reclining patients is valuable. A pressure-measuring device, such as a Tono-pen®, which is portable, accurate and easily used, is desirable.

OCULAR TRAUMA

HISTORY

Ocular injuries, however, trivial, are a frightening experience for the patient, who may have a deep-rooted fear of blindness. The incidence of injuries varies with the environment and protective measures taken. The major injuries result from blunt trauma or penetrating injuries to the globe, with or without the retention of a foreign body. Mechanical interference with eye movement may result from orbital injury, either haematoma or interference with muscle function. Similarly, neuro-trauma may disturb the visual pathways or ocular motor nerves.

It is necessary to elicit a history of the patient's prior visual status, including the wearing of glasses or contact lenses and ocular medication.

EXAMINATION

Visual acuity

After an eye toilet to remove any debris from the eyelids, vision is tested by a distance Snellen chart, if necessary using a pinhole device as a rough focusing aid. Vision less than 6/60 Snellen may be graded by the patient's ability to count fingers at a measured distance, discern hand movements or to project the direction of a light from various angles. The eye not being tested must be completely shielded by an opaque occluder.

It is essential to assess early whether the patient has sustained a relatively minor superficial injury or a severe injury which may be either blunt or penetrating. Reassurance and extreme gentleness in examining the eye, using topical anaesthetic, will allow a more definite assessment to be made in the emergency department. With penetrating trauma any external pressure on the eye may result in ocular structures being squeezed out of the wound, drastically worsening the prognosis.

To open lids that are adherent due to blood or discharge, gently bathe with sterile saline. Wipe the eyelid skin dry and apply gentle distractive pressure to skin below the brow and below the lower lid; i.e. over bony orbital rim to open the lids. Note that no pressure should be applied to the globe.

INVESTIGATION

All patients in whom a penetrating injury is suspected require X-ray or computerized tomography (CT) scanning to exclude a radio-opaque intraocular foreign body (IOFB). If there is any possibility of metallic IOFB, magnetic resonance imaging (MRI) scans are contra-indicated. When an adequate examination cannot be made, or where occult perforation is suspected, examination under anaesthesia is mandatory.

MANAGEMENT OF SPECIFIC INJURIES

Superficial injury

Corneal abrasion
The corneal epithelium is easily dislodged by a glancing blow from fingers, twigs, stones or a paper edge. The trauma produces an acute sensation of a

foreign body, with light sensitivity and excessive tearing.

After fluorescein staining, the size of the epithelial defect is recorded. Antibiotic ointment (chloramphenicol) is instilled and an eye pad applied if local anaesthetic is used. The condition heals spontaneously within 24–48hours. Large abrasions produce reflex ciliary spasm, which may require short-acting mydratics such as homatropine 2% in addition to oral analgesia to relieve the pain.

Corneal foreign body
Small ferrous particles rapidly oxidize when adherent to the corneal epithelium, producing a surrounding rust ring within hours. The rusted particle requires removal under adequate topical anaesthesia using a slit–lamp microscope. An adherent rust ring may be loosened by the application of antibiotic ointment and padding for 24 hours, after which it is easily shelled out with the edge of a fine hypodermic needle. Mechanical dental burrs may cause large areas of epithelial removal and delay return to work. Wooden splinters are particularly dangerous as they may easily penetrate the eye and cause violent suppuration. In all suspected foreign body injury, the upper and lower lids should be everted and examined with suitable lighting and magnification. The conjunctival fornices may be swept gently with a moist cotton bud under topical anaesthesia.

Penetrating injury
A careful history is important in assessing penetrating injury, including prior visual status and the use of contact lenses or spectacles. Occupational trauma may be due to high speed penetrating metal fragments. Agricultural trauma often involves heavily contaminated implements.

Examination of the eye involves the instillation of sterile topical anaesthetic drops, followed by a gentle eye toilet removing debris, clot and glass from the face and lids. The lids should be opened without pressure (Fig. 15.1.1). The penetration may be evidenced by an obvious laceration or presence of prolapsed tissue with collapse of the globe. Conjunctival oedema (chemosis) and low intraocular

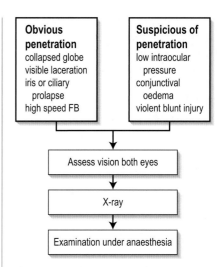

Fig. 15.1.1 Emergency department diagnosis of penetrating injury.

pressure may indicate an occult perforation or bursting injury.

When a penetrating injury is either suspected or established, the patient must be transferred without delay to a centre where appropriate surgical facilities are available. During transport, the eye should be covered with a sterile pad and a plastic cone. Vomiting should be prevented with antiemetics, and the fasted patient given intravenous fluids as necessary.

Penetrating trauma involving the cornea has the best prognosis. Lens involvement requires removal of the tramatised lens and usually a staged implantation of an intraocular lens. Posterior segment trauma involving tears or perforation of the choroid and retina requires staged vitreo-retinal surgery and has a guarded prognosis. Uncommonly, penetrating trauma excites an autoimmune reaction resulting in a destructive inflammation involving the uninjured fellow eye – sympathetic ophthalmitis. Long-term follow-up of all ocular trauma is mandatory.

Blunt trauma
Concussion of the globe may cause tearing of the iris root, resulting in blood in the anterior chamber. A hyphema greater than one-third of the anterior chamber usually indicates some damage to the drainage angle, and may also be associated with concussive lens damage. Uninterrupted absorption of the hyphema

is essential, and is aided by sedation and admission to hospital. The affected eye is padded and the patient nursed semi-recumbent to encourage sedimentation of the blood in the anterior chamber to clear as much of the angle as possible. A hyphema may cause considerable pain due to raised intraocular pressure. To lower the pressure, oral or intravenous acetazolamide 500 mg initially is required.

Pain is relieved by paracetamol or narcotics, with antiemetics if necessary. Aspirin in any form should be avoided as it increases the risk of secondary haemorrhage. The patient should remain in bed until the blood has completely cleared from the anterior chamber. Bleeding recurs in up to 10% of patients, usually due to early mobilization in those with extensive iris damage. Total hyphema has a poor prognosis because of secondary glaucoma, field loss and corneal opacification. When angle damage occurs, long-term follow-up after hyphema is required to determine whether the intraocular pressure is raised. The fundus requires careful examination after the hyphema has cleared completely, to exclude a traumatic retinal tear, which may be heralded by sudden onset of flashes and floaters.

Chemical burns

Chemical trauma requires priority assesment on arrival at an emergency centre.

Alcohol and solvent burns occur from splashes while painting and cleaning. Although the epithelium is frequently burnt, it regenerates rapidly. The condition is very painful initially, but heals with topical antibiotic and patching for 48 hours.

Alkali and acid burns are potentially more serious because of the ability of the burning agent to alter the pH in the anterior chamber of the eye and inflict chemical damage on the iris and lens. Caustic soda, lime and plaster, commonly used in industry, may inflict painful, deep and destructive ocular burns. Splashes of acids, such as sulphuric and hydrochloric, if concentrated, will cause equally destructive injury.

The first principle of management at the injury site is copious irrigation of the eyes for at least 10 minutes with running water. Assessment of the ocular burn should be done using topical anaesthetic drops and fluorescein staining to determine the area of surface injury. The eyelids should be everted and the fornices carefully examined and swept gently with a cotton bud to ensure there is no particulate caustic agent remaining.

Chemical burns where the epithelium is intact or minimally disturbed can usually wait 24 hours before review by an ophthalmologist. Burns involving more than one-third of the epithelium and the corneal edge, with any clouding of the cornea, are potentially more serious as subsequent melting of the cornea by collagenase action may ensue. These burns should all be further irrigated in the emergency department with a buffered sterile solution such as lactated Ringer's (Hartmann's). The irrigation should continue until the tears are neutral to litmus testing.

More serious caustic injuries have shown a significant improvement in outcome with the introduction of 10% citrate and ascorbate drops, commencing 2-hourly for 48 hours and reducing over the week, in combination with 1 g oral ascorbic acid daily. This regimen has an inhibitory effect on corneal melting. Topical antibiotic (chloramphenicol) and soluble steroids such as prednisolone phosphate 0.5% decrease inflammation.

Initial treatment of caustic injury

- Immediate flooding of the eye with fresh water for 10 minutes
- Transfer to medical centre
- Assess visual acuity in both eyes
- Ascertain chemical agent and time of injury
- Sterile topical anaesthetic, e.g. teracaine (amethocaine)
- Stain with fluorescein
- Examine the cornea and conjunctiva
- Evert lids and sweep tarsal plate with cotton bud
- Reirrigate.

A minor injury is defined as less than one-third epithelial loss and a clear cornea. A major injury is a large epithelial defect, a conjunctival burn and hazy media.

For major injury commence ascorbic acid 1 g daily and 10% topical ascorbate hourly.

Prevention

Children are constantly exposed to domestic hazards, particularly household utensils with sharp points and caustic substances in spray cans, which need to be kept out of reach. The well-known workshop injuries caused by iron fragments created while hammering or chipping, exploding car batteries and carbonated drinks bottles cause significant trauma. Protective glasses – preferably polycarbonate – may provide protection in racquet sports. Contact lenses do not protect.

Australian seatbelt legislation has markedly reduced the incidence of penetrating eye injuries in road trauma, but eye problems still occur from violent head and facial trauma in addition to the neurological complications of head injury.[1,2]

INFLAMMATORY EYE CONDITIONS

ACUTE ANGLE-CLOSURE GLAUCOMA

Acute angle-closure glaucoma (AACG) is characterized by an acute impairment of the outflow of aqueous from the anterior chamber in an anatomically predisposed eye. This results in a rapid and severe elevation in intraocular pressure (IOP). Normal IOP lies between 10 and 20 mmHg, but in cases of AACG can rise to greater than 60 mmHg. This is manifested as severe pain, blurring of vision and redness. The pain may be severe enough to cause nausea and vomiting, and may be poorly localized to the eye. Visual disturbance can be preceded by halos around lights, and in established cases is due to corneal oedema. Relative hypoxia of the pupillary sphincter due to elevated pressure results in a pupil unresponsive to light stimulation and classically fixed and mid-dilated. The associated inflammation induces congestion of conjunctival and episcleral vessels.

Treatment of AACG is aimed at lowering the intraocular pressure and allowing the flow of aqueous from the posterior to the anterior chamber. Acetazolamide 500 mg IV may be effective in acutely lowering the pressure and thereby reducing pain. Constriction of the pupil with 2% pilocarpine, a parasympathomimetic, 'breaks' the pupil block and re-establishes the flow. The forward bowing of the iris is relieved and the angle opens to allow aqueous to leave the eye. One drop is initially instilled every 5 minutes for 30 minutes, and then half-hourly. However, if the pressure is very high the anoxia induced will render the pupillary sphincter unresponsive to the pilocarpine. In these cases it is necessary to further lower the intraocular pressure to allow perfusion and function of the sphincter.

After pressure reduction a peripheral iridotomy is performed using the YAG laser to allow aqueous permanently to bypass the pupil and remove the risk of further episodes of AACG. The anatomical predisposition to AACG is usually bilateral, and a peripheral iridotomy is also performed in the other eye as an elective procedure. Until this is done miotics are instilled (G. pilocarpine 2% qid) in the unaffected eye to avoid the risk of AACG.

An alternative treatment is to perform a YAG laser peripheral iridotomy in the affected eye in the acute phase to immediately bypass the pupil block and allow aqueous access to the angle, but this is often hampered by corneal oedema.

ACUTE IRITIS

Acute iritis is an inflammatory response in the ciliary body and the iris. As part of this response there is an increase in vascular dilation and permeability, with release of inflammatory mediators and cells that can damage intraocular structures.

Acute iritis is usually an idiopathic condition with no cause or systemic association. Less commonly associated conditions may include HLA B27-related disease, sarcoidosis, inflammatory bowel disease, including ulcerative colitis and Crohn's disease, connective tissue disorders such as ankylosing spondylitis, and ocular infection including herpetic disease or toxoplasmosis. A complete history will often give clues to these associations.

Acute anterior iritis is generally unilateral, although bilateral involvement is seen. It is characterized by pain, redness and visual disturbance. The pain is constant and exacerbated by light owing to movement of the inflamed iris. Dilation of the conjunctival and episcleral vessels is apparent, particularly in the vessels adjacent to the corneal limbus, often referred to as limbal flush. Visual acuity can be reduced by varying degrees depending on the severity of inflammation. The pupil is constricted due to irritation.

Examination of the anterior segment with the slit lamp will reveal evidence of increased vascular permeability, seen as fibrin clumps, flare and inflammatory cells in the aqueous released from the vessels. In some cases small collections of neutrophils can be seen aggregating on the posterior surface of the cornea as keratic precipitates. In cases of severe inflammation cells can accumulate in the inferior anterior chamber and a sediment level can be seen as a hypopyon. The intraocular pressure may be raised.

Treatment of acute iritis is directed towards resolution of the inflammatory response and limiting the ocular effects of this response. The mainstay of treatment is intensive topical steroid eye drops (prednisolone acetate 1%, up to hourly in severe cases). In severe cases orbital steroid injections or oral steroids may be necessary. Mydriatic eye drops (G. homatropine 2% qid) are used to break any lens-iris adhesions and to limit the extent of permanent adhesions.

In 'splinting' the iris these drops also provide pain relief by limiting pupil movement. As the degree of inflammation decreases as seen with slit-lamp examination the topical treatment is decreased in frequency. The long-term use of topical steroid drops is not without risk, and can be associated with the development of glaucoma, cataract and concurrent ocular surface infection, such as herpes simplex keratitis.

ACUTE INFECTIOUS KERATITIS

The surface of the eye is protected by several mechanisms from penetration by infectious agents, both bacterial and viral. The flow of tears over the surface washes debris away and contains antibodies and lysozymes. The smooth surface of the corneal epithelium hinders the adherence of infectious agents, and the rapid repair of any defect in the epithelium limits the likelihood of penetration by such agents. If these defences are impaired in any way there is the possibility of penetration into the corneal stroma, and active infection may occur.

Bacterial keratitis is characterized by a focus of infection with an associated inflammatory response. Patients complain of pain, redness, watering, and a decrease in visual acuity. Fluorescein staining shows an area of ulceration over the infection, which appears as an opacity or area of whiteness within the cornea. Marked conjunctival and episcleral injection results in a unilateral red eye. Evidence of intraocular inflammation is usually present, with cells and flare being seen in the anterior chamber on slit-lamp examination. In severe cases a collection of inflammatory cells can be seen in the inferior part of the anterior chamber as sediment, called a hypopyon.

The most important aspect of management is to identify the infectious agent and to commence appropriate antibiotic treatment. A specimen is taken as a scraping for microbiological assessment, including Gram staining and culture. Under topical anaesthetic, using a preservative-free single-use dispenser of benoxinate or tetracaine (amethocaine), a sterile 23G needle is used to gather a small specimen. This is transferred directly to glass slides and also plated on to HB and chocolate agar plates for culture. Antibiotic therapy is not delayed until the results are available, but is commenced on a broad-spectrum basis such as the intensive use of a single fluoro-quinolone (G. ciprofloxacin) on an hourly basis. Daily monitoring with slit-lamp examination is mandatory and severe infections require hospital admission. This regimen can be modified when culture and sensitivity results are available. It is sometimes necessary to add a topical steroid when the active infection is under control, to limit the amount of inflammation and hence the damage to the cornea.

Herpes simplex infection of the cornea usually presents initially as an infection of the epithelial cell layer, although with recurrent episodes stromal involvement may be seen. It is most often a unilateral infection. As with other herpetic infections it is not possible to eradicate the virus, but limitation of inflammatory-mediated damage is important. Patients complain of foreign body sensation, redness, watering, and a variable decrease in visual acuity. On examination the areas of infected epithelium can be seen as a branching irregularity or dendrite on the surface of the eye. Multiple dendrites may be scattered over the surface, particularly in immunocompromised patients. These are best seen when the cornea is stained with fluorescein or Rose Bengal stains and viewed under the slit lamp.

Treatment is directed to clearing the virus from the cornea to promote epithelial healing and limit stromal involvement and damaging corneal inflammation. An antiviral ointment, acyclovir, is instilled five times daily until there is resolution of the epithelial lesions, and then ceased as long-term usage may be toxic to the unaffected corneal epithelium.

ACUTE VISUAL FAILURE

INTRODUCTION

Acute visual failure is an acute change in visual acuity or visual field. Effective emergency management depends upon rapid recognition of those conditions for which acute therapy is available (Table

Table 15.1.1 Acute visual failure for which acute therapy is available

Condition	Therapy
Central (or branch) retinal artery occlusion	Acetazolamide Pulsed ocular compression Anterior chamber paracentesis
Anterior ischaemic optic neuropathy (arteritic)	Steroids
Retinal detachment	Surgery
Exudative age-related macular degeneration	Retinal laser

Table 15.1.2 Symptoms significant for cause in acute visual failure

Symptom	Condition
Floaters (if recent onset)	Vitreous haemorrhage Retinal detachment
Flashes (especially temporal)	Retinal detachment Migraine aura
Shadow (billowing curtain/cloud)	Retinal detachment
Distortion	Exudative macular degeneration
Amaurosis fugax	Retinal artery occlusion Anterior ischaemic optic neuropathy
Hemifield loss of vision Horizontal hemifield (if previous amaurosis fugax) (if flashes/floaters) Vertical hemifield (usually bilateral)	 Anterior ischaemic optic neuropathy Branch retinal vein occlusion Branch retinal artery occlusion Retinal detachment Retrochiasmal CVA/compression
Whole-field loss of vision Sudden loss of vision (if previous amaurosis fugax) Rapid loss of vision (systemic symptoms in GCA) Gradual (sub-total) loss of vision Pain on eye movement	 Vitreous haemorrhage Central retinal artery occlusion Anterior ischaemic optic neuropathy Optic neuritis Central retinal vein occlusion Optic neuritis

15.1.1); some conditions have no effective therapy, or are more appropriately managed on an outpatient basis.

CLINICAL ASSESSMENT

History

Particular attention should be paid to the rapidity of onset, degree of visual loss, previous episodes and associated symptoms. An absence of pain in the presentation of acute visual failure is no indication that the problem is insignificant (Table 15.1.2).

One should distinguish on history between acute onset or acute discovery of visual loss, as a patient may discover decreased vision from, for example, cataract, or retinal venous occlusion, by inadvertently covering one eye for the first time.

Examination

Testing of the visual acuity and visual field will clarify uni- or binocular involvement.

Examination of the pupils is mandatory before pharmacologic dilation. Test for a relative afferent pupillary defect

(RAPD), one of the few objective signs. When required, pupils will dilate in 10–15 minutes with tropicamide 1.0% drops, which last 2–4 hours.

Bilateral visual field loss usually implicates a retrochiasmal – and, therefore, non-ocular – cause. This visual field defect, however, respects a vertical midline. In contrast, the retinal nerve fibre layer and retinal vascular elements within the eye are distributed around a horizontal midline, and may thus involve a superior or inferior hemifield. Localized ocular pathology does not cause a visual field defect respecting a vertical midline.

Bilateral acute complete visual failure is uncommon. Bilateral occipital infarction may present with bilateral blindness, but pupil responses would be expected to be intact. Rapidly progressive bilateral sequential visual loss from temporal arteritis is occasionally encountered. Other prechiasmal causes of bilateral simultaneous ocular involvement include toxic causes, such as poisoning with either quinine or methanol, where the patient presents with bilateral blindness and fixed, widely dilated pupils. Visual recovery in these cases is variable, and the efficacy of a range of therapeutic interventions is uncertain and controversial.[3-5]

CENTRAL RETINAL ARTERY OCCLUSION

The history is typically of sudden, painless loss of vision in the affected eye over seconds. This may have been preceded by episodes of transient loss of vision (amaurosis fugax) in the previous days or weeks. Mean age of presentation is in the 60s. Men are more frequently affected, and the history may include evidence of previous cardiac or cerebrovascular disease. Systemic arterial hypertension and diabetes mellitus are frequent associations. Carotid disease is frequently implicated, with emboli often being the cause of the obstruction, but their absence does not preclude the diagnosis, as the obstruction may lie behind the lamina cribrosa.

The visual acuity is drastically reduced, often to the level of light perception, with a relative afferent pupillary defect (RAPD) present on the affected side. Fundus examination shows creamy-white retinal oedema (cloudy swelling) with a central red fovea – the 'cherry-red spot' – caused by the absence of oedema in the thinner retina at the fovea. The arterioles may be attenuated. An embolus may be seen at any point along the retinal arterioles, from the disc to the periphery.

Acute treatment proceeds on the assumption that the cause is embolic. The principles of therapy are, therefore, to vasodilate the retinal arterial circulation in order to promote dislodgement of the embolus from a proximal position and its movement downstream to a less strategic site. All the measures currently used are directed to lowering the intraocular pressure (IOP), thereby relieving the compressive effect on the intraocular vasculature. Intravenous or oral acetazolamide 500 mg will lower IOP within 15–30 minutes; pulsed ocular compression ('ocular massage') involves cyclical sustained compression of the globe for 10–15 seconds before sudden release of this compression, continuing for 5–10 minutes. The release of pressure may result in a momentary marked increase in the perfusion pressure gradient and dislodge an embolus. Definitive reduction of IOP is achieved with anterior chamber paracentesis by the removal of aqueous from the eye (see Anterior chamber paracentesis). Visual outcomes are generally poor in CRAO, but occasional successes justify aggressive intervention if the patient presents within 12 hours.

Intra-arterial fibrinolytic therapy is a promising technique that is not widely available at present and requires the services of an experienced interventional neuroradiology team.[6-9] The place of hyperbaric therapy is uncertain at this time.[10] The use of carbogen gas (95% oxygen/5% carbon dioxide) is now largely historical.

Long-term management must include attempts to define the embolic source. Investigations may include Doppler and cardiac ultrasound, and perhaps angiography (including aortic arch studies), as well as assessment of cardiac and cerebro-

vascular risk factors. An ESR should exclude temporal arteritis – which causes 5% of cases of CRAO – as a non-embolic cause.

Anterior chamber paracentesis

The eye is anaesthetized with topical, unpreserved drops from single-use dispensers - amethocaine 1%. The fornices and globe are prepared with a drop of 10% povidone-iodine. An assistant is useful to steady the patient's head at the slit lamp. With toothed forceps to provide counterpressure opposite the site of entry into the anterior chamber, a 27 G needle on an insulin syringe with the plunger removed, is inserted parallel to the iris plane: if the eye is phakic (i.e. natural lens present), then the needle course must be only over the iris, below the margin of the pupil, to avoid contact with the lens. Aqueous will drain along the barrel of the syringe and should be allowed to continue until the cornea starts to wrinkle. The needle is then withdrawn, taking great care not to allow the needle point to tip backwards against the lens in the softened eye. The entry wound is self-sealing. Antibiotic drops such as chloramphenicol should be commenced and used four times a day for 4 days. Vision will be worse immediately after the procedure.

ANTERIOR ISCHAEMIC OPTIC NEUROPATHY

Arteritic anterior ischaemic optic neuropathy (AION) is the feared visual loss of giant cell (temporal) arteritis (GCA). The patient is usually mid-60s or older, and more commonly female. Presentation is with profound vision loss in one eye. This may have been preceded by premonitory visual obscurations or double vision, to which the patient may not have ascribed significance. Systematic questioning may reveal specific features such as jaw claudication, headache, scalp tenderness, anorexia, malaise, weight loss or night sweats, and there may be a history of polymyalgia rheumatica in up to 50% of cases. GCA is a systemic illness with the potential for devastating visual loss, as well as long-term life-threatening non-ophthalmic complications.

Vision may be reduced at presentation to the level of perception of light only. An RAPD will be present. Total field loss in the affected eye is usual. Fundus examination will almost invariably show disc oedema, but the fundus may be otherwise normal. Evidence of decreased acuity, colour vision deficits and disc oedema should also be sought in the other eye. Palpation of the temporal arteries will often be abnormal, with the pulses perhaps absent or the arteries thickened and tender.

Treatment should be started on an urgent basis on clinical suspicion in conjunction with the ESR (>60 mm/h), and must not be delayed or deferred until temporal artery biopsy: the biopsy will remain positive for at least several days, despite steroids. Elevation of both ESR and C-reactive protein (CRP) is highly specific for a diagnosis of GCA, but does not avoid the need for biopsy.[11] Urgent referral to an ophthalmologist is required.

Prednisolone 1 mg/kg daily is an accepted dose, although recent experience has suggested that 'pulse' methylprednisolone 500 mg intravenously daily or twice daily over 1–2 hours is safe and more efficacious in suppressing the inflammation, and this has become standard therapy in a number of centres. This is generally used for 3 days, and oral prednisolone is then substituted.[12–14] Treatment will be prolonged (at least 6 months) and should be undertaken in co-operation with a physician. Attention should also be directed to the avoidance – in this aged patient group – of the legion steroid complications.

Non-arteritic AION is classically seen in males in the late 50s and 60s, who have a history of cardiac or vascular disease, hypertension, diabetes or smoking. The presentation may be similar to that seen with GCA – although the visual acuity and field loss may not be as profound and the specific systemic symptoms are absent – so that management must be as for arteritic AION until GCA is excluded.

RETINAL DETACHMENT

Retinal detachment is usually a result of retinal hole formation, with seepage of fluid into the subretinal space and lifting of the retina. This may occur as a result of trauma, but is more often seen in an older age group as a result of vitreous traction in spontaneous posterior vitreous detachment, and is predisposed to by high myopia (short-sightedness).

Posterior vitreous detachment

Shrinkage and detachment of the vitreous is common in the older population, and produces a new onset of floaters – wispy spots, threads or 'spider webs' in the vision. As part of this process, vitreous traction on the retina may produce flashes of light (photopsia) – which can usually be distinguished from the visual aura of migraine – seen particularly in the temporal periphery of vision in that eye. While posterior vitreous detachment (PVD) is usually not serious in its own right, early elective ophthalmic review is required as it is not possible to exclude related changes predisposing to retinal detachment without dilated examination of the retinal periphery.

Retinal detachment

With a history of flashes and floaters, the presence of pigmented cells in the anterior vitreous should alert one to the possibility of a retinal hole and subsequent retinal detachment. A detached retina shows a visual field defect, which will be described as a shadow or curtain, corresponding to the area of detachment, e.g. inferior field defect equals superior retinal detachment. The visual acuity may be normal. There may be an RAPD, depending on the amount of retina involved. Vision loss is painless. These features require urgent ophthalmic consultation with a view to surgery.

VITREOUS HAEMORRHAGE

The most common causes are proliferative diabetic retinopathy, chronic branch retinal vein occlusion, posterior vitreous detachment or trauma. Patients with an acute vitreous haemorrhage may have symptoms varying from a few floaters causing blurred vision to a total loss of vision to a level of light perception, depending on the density of the haemorrhage. Any loss of vision is painless. The red reflex may be poor and the view of the retina may be similarly variably impaired. There should be no RAPD, unless the underlying retina is damaged or detached.

The patient should be referred for early ophthalmic assessment - urgent if an RAPD is present – which may include B scan ultrasonography to exclude retinal detachment if the retinal view is inadequate. Aspirin should be avoided.

AGE-RELATED MACULAR DEGENERATION

In 20% of cases of age-related macular degeneration an exudative-type disease is seen, and in its most sinister form this will involve subretinal neovascularization (SRNV). These patients may present with painless distortion of vision, particularly metamorphopsia – a complaint that objects which they know to be straight appear curved. Visual acuity is reduced, depending on the stage of the disease; an RAPD is rarely seen owing to the relatively small area of retina involved, which manifests as a central scotoma on field testing. Macular drusen (yellow spots) and haemorrhage may be seen, with at least drusen usually also seen in the fellow eye.

Acute symptoms must not be dismissed. With appropriate laser photocoagulation central vision may be preserved in a proportion of these patients, but treatment must be undertaken, following fundus fluorescein angiography, within about 3 days. Urgent ophthalmic review is therefore appropriate.

CENTRAL (BRANCH) RETINAL VEIN OCCLUSION

Central or branch retinal vein occlusion may present as a painless blurring of vision that is not sudden. Patients are usually in the older age group, often with systemic hypertension, diabetes mellitus and glaucoma. Visual acuity varies with severity, as does the presence of an RAPD. The characteristic fundus appearance is of extensive intraretinal haemorrhage with a variable number of cottonwool spots. There may be disc oedema, with venous tortuosity and a generally congested appearance.

There is no emergency management specific to the vein occlusion that will positively influence the visual outcome, and the patient should, therefore, be referred to the next ophthalmic out-patient clinic. Systemic hypertension and raised intraocular pressure rarely require acute control.

OPTIC NEURITIS

Optic neuritis classically presents in young females, and may be the first presentation of a demyelinating illness. Visual symptoms are not usually sudden, and presentation is thus seldom acute. The vision declines gradually over days, perhaps to the level of 6/36–6/60, with loss of colour vision being prominent. The common visual field defect is a central scotoma and an RAPD should always be present. If disc oedema is not seen the diagnosis may be retrobulbar neuritis. There may be pain on eye movement.

CONTROVERSIES

❶ What are the roles of hyperbaric oxygen and intra-arterial fibrinolytic therapy in central retinal artery occlusion?

❷ What is the appropriate therapy for acute optic neuritis: oral steroid, intravenous steroid, or no treatment?

Good spontaneous recovery has made the value of treating optic neuritis controversial: the results of the Optic Neuritis Treatment Trial[15] would suggest that there is no place for oral predniso-lone alone in management. The benefit of 'pulse' intravenous methylprednisolone seems restricted to shortening the acute episode, without influencing the possi-bility of progression to multiple sclerosis or the final visual outcome.[16] However, there is usually no role for acute inter-vention, and referral within a day or two to a neurologist or an ophthalmologist is satisfactory.

REFERENCES

1. McCarty CA, Fu CLH, Taylor HR 1999 Epidemiology of ocular trauma in Australia. Opthamology 106: 1847–52
2. Colby K 1999 Management of open globe injuries. Int Opthalmol Clin 39: 59–69
3. Canning CR, Hague S 1988 Ocular quinine toxicity. British Journal of Ophthalmology 72: 23–6
4. Bacon P, Spalton DJ, Smith SE 1988 Blindness from quinine toxicity. British Journal of Ophthalmology 72: 219–24
5. Stelmach MZ, O'Day J 1992 Partly reversible visual failure with methanol toxicity. Australia and New Zealand Journal of Ophthalmology 20: 57–64
6. Watson PG 1969 The treatment of acute retinal arterial occlusion. In: Cant JS (ed.) The Ocular Circulation in Health and Disease. Mosby Year Book, St Louis, pp 243–5
7. Schmidt D, Schumacher M, Wakhloo AK 1992 Microcatheter urokinase infusion in central retinal artery occlusion. American Journal of Ophthalmology 113: 429–34
8. Weber J, Remonda L, Mattle HP, et al 1998 Selective intra-arterial fibrinolysis of acute central retinal artery occlusion. Stroke 29: 2076–9
9. Beatty S, Au Eong KG 2000 Local intra-arterial fibrinolysis for acute occlusion of the central retinal artery: a meta-analysis of the published data. British Journal of Ophthalmology 84: 914–6
10. Beirna I, Reissman P, Scharf J, et al 1993 Hyperbaric oxygenation combined with nifedipine treatment for recent-onset retinal occlusion. European Journal of Ophthalmology 3: 89–4
11. Hayreh SS, Podhajsky PA, Raman R, Zimmerman B 1997 Giant cell arteritis: validity and reliability of various diagnostic criteria. American Journal of Ophthalmology 123: 285–96
12. Hayreh SS 1990 Anterior ischaemic optic neuropathy. Differentiation of arteritic from non-arteritic type and its management. Eye 4: 25–41
13. Liu GT, Glaser JS, Schatz NJ, Smith JL 1994 Visual morbidity in giant cell arteritis. Clinical characteristics and prognosis for vision. Ophthalmology 101: 1779–85
14. Cornblath WT, Eggenberger ER 1997 Progressive visual loss from giant cell arteritis despite high-dose intravenous methylprednisolone. Ophthalmology 104: 854–8
15. Beck RW, Cleary PA, Anderson MA, et al 1992 A randomized controlled trial of corticosteroids in the treatment of acute optic neuritis. New England Journal of Medicine 326: 581–8
16. Kapoor R, Miller DH, Jones SJ, et al 1998 Effects of intravenous methylprednisolone on outcome in MRI-based prognostic subgroups in acute optic neuritis. Neurology 50: 230–7

FURTHER READING

Phillips C 1994 Ophthalmology. Baillière Tindall, London

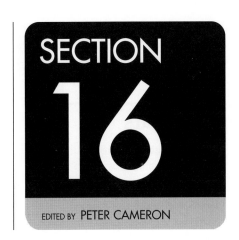

DENTAL

16.1 Dental emergencies 546

16.1 DENTAL EMERGENCIES

SASHI KUMAR

ESSENTIALS

1 An avulsed tooth reimplanted within 30 minutes has a 90% survival rate.

2 Dental caries are the most common cause of dental emergency attendance.

3 Dental caries require analgesia in the emergency department and referral to a dentist for definitive care. Antibiotics are not required unless complicated by abscess.

ANATOMY

The tooth consists of the crown, which is exposed, and the root, which lies within the socket covered by the gum and serves to anchor the tooth. The gingival pulp carries the neurovascular structures via the root canal and is covered by dentine, which in turn is covered by enamel; the hardest substance in the body (Fig. 16.1.1).

The deciduous teeth are 20 in number and erupt between the ages of 6 months and 2 years. The permanent dentition begins to erupt at around age 6 and in the adult consists of 32 teeth.

DENTAL CARIES

The commonest cause of toothache or odontalgia is caries. Dental caries-related emergencies account for up to 52% of first contact with a dentist for children below the age of 3 years.[1] Dental caries is the cause of emergency visits to a dentist in 73% of paediatric patients.[2] Pain associated with dental caries is of a dull, throbbing nature, localized to a specific area and aggravated by changes in temperature in the oral cavity.

Examination reveals tenderness of the offending tooth when tapped with a tongue depressor or a mirror. Management includes symptomatic pain relief using analgesics such as paracetamol with or without codeine, and urgent referral to the dentist.

PERIODONTAL EMERGENCIES

Pain is the most common cause of self-referral to the emergency department for dental problems. The common conditions causing dental pain are acute apical periodontitis and reversible and irreversible pulpitis resulting from dental caries.[3] Symptoms include painful swollen gums with or without halitosis. On occasions frank pus or bleeding from the gums may be the presenting symptom. At all stages varying degrees of pain associated with inflammation are invariably present.[4]

Management includes diagnosis of the periodontal disease and the offending tooth. Symptomatic pain relief can be achieved with analgesics, non-steroidal inflammatory agents and warm saline rinses. Routine antibiotic therapy is not required unless there is evidence of gross infection locally, regional lymphadenopathy, or fever. In all cases urgent review by the dentist is mandatory.

ALVEOLAR OSTEITIS

This condition, commonly referred to as 'dry socket', occurs between 3 and 5 days following dental extraction. The dull throbbing pain is due to the collection of necrotic clot and debris in the socket. The condition is diagnosed on the history and examination, which confirms the acutely tender extraction site.

Treatment consists of irrigation of the extraction site to remove the necrotic material and packing the socket with sterile gauze soaked in local anaesthetic, followed by urgent dental review.[5]

TRAUMATIC DENTAL EMERGENCIES

Tooth avulsion is probably the most serious tooth injury. An avulsed tooth, if reimplanted in the socket within 30 minutes, has a 90% survival rate.[6] The mechanism of injury in such cases is usually either accidental sports-related facial injuries or assault.

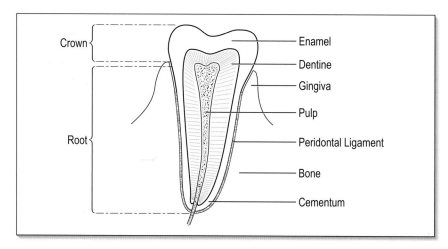

Fig. 16.1.1 The anatomy of the tooth. (From an original drawing by Ian Miller RN)

Crown — Enamel — Dentine — Gingiva — Pulp — Peridontal Ligament — Bone — Cementum — Root

Management

If the patient makes telephone contact with the emergency department he is advised to locate the tooth because, even if the crown is broken, the root may be intact. The tooth should not be handled by the root to avoid damage to the periodontal ligament fibres; it is washed in running cold water and replaced in the socket. If this is not possible, place the tooth in the cheek or under the tongue and proceed immediately to the dentist. Do not scrub the tooth.[7,8]

The best transportation medium for an avulsed tooth is saliva. Cold milk or iced salt water are suitable alternatives.

If the patient arrives in the emergency department with the tooth, clean it by holding it by the crown in cold running water; any foreign debris should be removed with forceps. The tooth should not be allowed to dry. Following irrigation the tooth should be placed in the socket as near the original position as possible, and the patient referred to a dentist for stabilization with an archbar or orthodontic bands.

Deciduous teeth are treated in the same manner, but if the reimplanted tooth remains mobile after 2 weeks it should be extracted. The complications of reimplantation are ankylosis and loss of viability.

DENTAL FRACTURES

The incidence of fractured teeth is reported to be 5 and 4.4 per 100 adults per year for all teeth and posterior teeth respectively.[9] Based on the above statistics, it can be deduced that the likelihood of experiencing a fractured frontal/ anterior tooth is about 1 in 20 in a given year in adults, and in 1 in 23 for posterior teeth.

Traumatic injuries to the teeth have been classified as follows:[10]

Class I: Simple fracture of the enamel of the crown
Class II: Extensive fracture of the crown involving dentine;
Class III: Extensive fracture of the crown involving dentine and dental pulp;

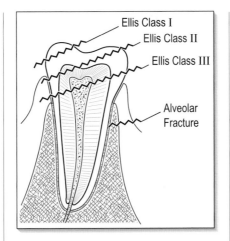

Fig. 16.1.2 Ellis classification. (From an original drawing by Ian Miller RN)

Class IV: Extensive involvement and exposure of the entire pulp;
Class V: Totally avulsed or luxated teeth;
Class VI: Fracture of the root with or without loss of crown structure;
Class VII: Displacement of tooth without fracture of crown or root;
Class VIII: Fracture of the crown in its entirety (Fig. 16.1.2).

Management

Emergency management includes reassurance, adequate analgesia, replacement of an avulsed tooth in the socket, and immediate referral to a dentist for further evaluation and appropriate management.

Specific treatment depends on the type of fracture:[11]

- Class I Treated by smoothing the enamel margins and applying topical fluoride to the fracture site.
- Class II A calcium hydroxide dressing is applied as a bandage to provide a stable form of temporary restoration, which will be replaced by a more aesthetic restoration as soon as the vitality of the pulp is assured.
- Class III If seen within 6 hours of the accident, calcium hydroxide direct pulp capping. If more than 6 hours but less than 24 hours,

pulpotomy. If more than 24 hours since the accident, total pulpectomy.
- Class IV Conventional filling for permanent teeth and total pulpectomy for a primary tooth.
- Class V Managed as for an avulsed tooth.
- Class VI If the pulp is necrotic, pulpectomy and root canal therapy.
- Class VII If the tooth is intruded it should be extracted. If driven through the labial plate of bone, extraction; if not, it should be left alone to re-erupt. If the tooth is extruded, slowly move it back to its original position using finger pressure. Primary teeth, if mobile after 2 weeks after the injury, should be extracted. Parents should be warned about possible damage to the developing permanent tooth.
- Class VIII In a permanent tooth, pulpotomy or pulpectomy. Primary teeth with this amount of destruction should be extracted.
- When a tooth is missing following facial trauma a thorough intraoral examination is followed by appropriate radiographs to avoid missing an intruded tooth. When full intrusion of a tooth is suspected a facial computerized tomography (CT) scan may aid definite diagnosis.[12]

TEMPOROMANDIBULAR DISLOCATION

Temporomandibular dislocation can result from congenital weakness of ligaments, iatrogenic causes (traumatic extractions, prolonged dental procedures and direct laryngoscopy), trauma, drugs, epilepsy, and even simple yawning. The dislocation may be unilateral, but is more commonly bilateral. The condyle is most frequently dislocated anterior to the articular eminence.

The patient presents with an open bite and malocclusion. If unilateral, the mandible deviates to the unaffected side. The patient complains of severe pain in the ear and is unable to fully open or close the mouth. Management includes diagnosis and reduction. The patient is seated, with posterior head support, and the muscle spasm is overcome by using intravenous benzodiazepines, such as midazolam, and narcotic analgesia such as fentanyl.

The mandible is held by the clinician by both hands with the gloved thumbs intraorally just lateral to the lower molars. The mandibular condyle is then manipulated in a downward and backward direction below the articular eminence. In bilateral dislocation it may be easier to reduce one side at a time using a lateral rocking motion.

Following the procedure a postreduction radiograph is taken to confirm enlocation. The patient is discharged with a supportive bandage to the mandible and a soft diet advised for the next few days. Follow-up by the maxillofacial surgeon is essential, as temporomandi-

---

CONTROVERSIES

❶ Dental services are generally not part of acute health service funding. Therefore, low-income patients may have to wait for medical complications of poor dental hygiene before being able to access appropriate care.

---

bular dysfunction due to damage to the fibrous cartilage can lead to ongoing symptoms or recurrent dislocations.

REFERENCES

1. Sheller B, Williams BJ, Lombardi SSM 1997 Diagnosis and treatment of dental caries related emergencies in a children's hospital. American Academy of Pediatric Dentistry 19(8): 470–5
2. Wilson S, Smith GA, Preisch J, Casamassimo PS 1997 Non traumatic dental emergencies in a pediatric emergency department. Clinical Pediatrics 36(6): 333–7
3. Matthews RW, Peak JD, Skully C 1994 The efficacy of management of acute dental pain. British Dental Journal 176: 413–6
4. Ahl DR, Hidgeman JL, Snyder JD 1986 Periodontal emergencies. Dental Clinics of North America 30: 459–72
5. Laskin DM, Steinberg B 1984 Diagnosis and treatment of common dental emergencies. Medicine of Dentistry 84. A.O., 77: 41–52
6. Gaedeve Norris MK 1992 Emergency treatment for tooth avulsion. Action stat! Nursing 92, March: 33
7. Scheer B 1990 Emergency treatment of avulsed incisor teeth. British Medical Journal 301: 4
8. Rice RT, Bulford OG Jr 1988 Clinical notebook. Emergency treatment of injured teeth. Journal of Emergency Nursing 14(1): 32–3
9. Bader JD, Martin JA, Shugars DA 1995 Preliminary estimates of the incidence and consequences of tooth fracture. Journal of the American Dental Association 126: 1650–4
10. Ellis RG, Davey KW 1970 The Classification and Treatment of Injuries to the Teeth of Children, 5th edn. Yearbook Medical Publishers, Chicago
11. Braham RL, Roberts MW, Morris ME 1977 Management of dental trauma in children and adolescents. Journal of Trauma 17(11): 857–65
12. Tung-Chain Tung, Yu-Ray Chen, Chien-Tzung Chen, Chia-Jung Lin 1977 Full intrusion of a tooth after facial trauma. Journal of Trauma 2: 357–9

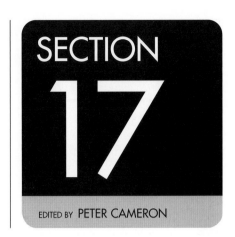

SECTION
17

EDITED BY PETER CAMERON

ENT

17.1 Ears, nose and throat   550

17.1 EARS, NOSE AND THROAT

SASHI KUMAR

ESSENTIALS

1 Removal of foreign bodies from the ear requires good lighting, a cooperative or fully restrained patient, and a patient/gentle approach by the clinician.

2 Ot haematoma requires urgent release by aseptic incision and immediate application of a firm mastoid bandage.

3 It is important to exclude septal haematoma in patients with a fractured nose. In general X-rays are not warranted.

4 Patients presenting with odynophagia but no dysphagia following ingestion of a fish bone, and negative physical examination and radiology, can be safely discharged for review within 48 hours.

THE EAR

INTRODUCTION

Emergency presentations for ear, nose and throat (ENT) problems are common and all emergency physicians need to be familiar with the basic skills required for assessment and management of these problems.

FOREIGN BODY

Foreign bodies in the ear are most common in children under the age of 5 and in adults with learning difficulties. Animate objects such as insects in the ear can affect all ages, especially adults who enjoy the outdoors, particularly at dusk.

Accidental foreign bodies, such as the end of a cotton bud or a matchstick, occur in people obsessed with cleaning their ears with such objects.

Management

Two simple rules in managing foreign bodies in the ear are:

- Do not attempt to remove a foreign body that is not there! (Identify the foreign body prior to attempts at removal.)
- Unless the object is alive, there is no emergency to remove it if it can be done safely at a later time under better conditions.

Removal of a live foreign body

This is a true ENT emergency. The insect should be killed as a matter of urgency, as considerable damage is being done to the sensitive skin of the bony meatus and the tympanic membrane by the flapping wings and appendages of the desperate insect trying to escape.

The movement of the insect also causes intense pain and tinnitus, thereby creating further anxiety and distress.

Any liquid used to kill the insect should be carefully chosen so as to avoid damage to the sensitive skin and tympanic membrane: strong corrosive agents, knockdown spray or alcohol should be avoided. The common agents of choice are lidocaine 2%, olive oil, water for injection or normal saline.

One of the preferred methods is to instill some water for injection from a 10 ml plastic ampoule and leave an examination light on the pinna. The insect swims up to surface towards the light and can be helped to safety by holding the tip of the ampoule.

Removal of a foreign body in a child or a mentally handicapped adult may be done in one of two ways. The patient is either cooperative and unrestrained or fully restrained. It is vital not to attempt any procedure with partial restraint, as any movement of the patient during the attempt could cause trauma to the ear canal and the tympanic membrane.

The techniques used are the dry method using an alligator forceps or a Jobson Horne probe, or the wet method, which is to syringe the ear canal with tepid water. The water should be close to body temperature to avoid caloric effect, which produces nystagmus and dizziness.

The key to success is good lighting, preferably through a head lamp, a co-operative or fully restrained patient, and a patient, gentle approach by the clinician, who knows when to stop if unsuccessful.

TRAUMA

Penetrating trauma can cause perforation of the eardrum and occasionally disruption of the ossicular chain. Dislocation of the footplate of the stapes following such an injury can cause permanent sensori-neural hearing loss. Referral to an ENT specialist is essential in all cases of traumatic perforation.

Blunt trauma

Boxing and other contact sports can lead to blunt trauma to the pinna. Accumulation of blood under the perichondrium produces a 'cauliflower ear' or 'ot haematoma'. A slap on the ear can also produce a ruptured tympanic membrane with or without ossicular chain disruption.

Assessment

Assessment of the injury includes a clinical assessment of the hearing loss. A ruptured eardrum without ossicular chain disruption does not usually cause a significant hearing loss. Any evidence of nystagmus or tinnitus suggests damage to the inner ear.

Management

A simple traumatic perforation of the eardrum is managed by simple analgesics and keeping the ear dry. On no account should any drops or water be allowed into the ear, as this may precipitate otitis media.

If occular chain disruption or inner ear trauma is suspected, an urgent ENT opinion is required to assess the need for urgent tympanotomy and repair.

Ot haematoma requires urgent release of the accumulated blood by aseptic incision and drainage and the immediate application of a firm mastoid bandage to prevent reaccumulation. The patient should be placed on broad-spectrum antibiotics to prevent infection.

INFECTION

Otitis externa

Infection of the external ear is common and affects between 3 and 10% of the patient population.[1] It can be localized (furuncle) or diffuse. The symptoms are pain, itching and tenderness to palpation, followed by aural fullness, hearing loss and discharge. The common pathogens responsible are *Pseudomonas aeruginosa*, *Proteus* spp. and *Staphylococcus aureus*.[2]

The diagnosis is usually self-evident, but the diagnostic sign of otitis externa is tenderness on pulling the pinna or pressing on the tragus.

Management

The most important step in the treatment is thorough and atraumatic cleansing of the ear canal.[3] Tolerance and cooperation between the patient and the clinician is vital. Pope Otowick (Xomed)® is very useful in the management of this condition. This is a semirigid tube that, when inserted into the ear canal, swells, absorbing moisture to increase the size of the ear canal. Topical otic drops, such as Sofradex® (Roussel), are used three to four times a day and the patient is reviewed on a daily basis to change the wick and continue the ear toilet. Occasionally oral antibiotics such as ciprofloxacin or flucloxacillin may be required,[4] particularly if there is evidence of cellulitis. The patient is advised to keep the ear clear of any water.

Fungal infection of the external auditory meatus is treated with ear toilet as described, and topical antifungal otic medication.

Otitis media

Acute otitis media is a common infection and is due to eustachian catarrh blocking of the eustachian tube, and negative pressure in the middle ear cavity. Although viral in origin, secondary bacterial infection often supervenes. The most frequently isolated pathogens are *Streptococcus pneumoniae*, *Haemophilus influenzae* and *Moraxella catarrhalis*.[5] The symptoms are earache, fullness, hearing loss and fever, with ear discharge if the drum has perforated.

The clinical findings vary from a retracted dull eardrum to a congested bulging drum, and a perforated tympanic membrane with discharge in the ear canal.

Management

Treatment is almost always empiric and amoxycillin is a good first-line therapy. Cephalosporins and trimethoprim/sulpha are also used with considerable success. The newer macrolides, such as azithromycin and clarithromycin, are rational alternatives.[5]

In otitis media with a perforated eardrum the mainstay of treatment should be toilet by dry mopping followed by antibiotic drops such as Sofradex®. The ear should be kept dry and regular follow-up arranged until the perforation has healed.

Labyrinthitis

Acute labyrinthitis usually has cochlear symptoms such as hearing loss and tinnitus. If the symptoms are limited to vertigo and nystagmus, it is more likely to be due to acute vestibular neuronitis.

Management

The management of labyrinthitis includes bed rest, antiemetics, e.g. stemetil, benzodiazepine, e.g. valium, and admission if severely debilitating.

Otitis media with effusion (glue ear)

This is most common in children in developed countries. The symptoms are fullness and hearing loss, and occasionally pain. Management includes the diagnosis based on history and examination, which reveals a dull, retracted drum or fluid behind the drum without redness. Repeated attacks of glue ear are an indication for the insertion of tympanostomy tubes.

Mastoiditis

Acute mastoiditis is a complication of acute or chronic otitis media. Extension of infection can cause meningitis or cerebral abscess, with life-threatening complications if untreated.

Examination reveals infection in the middle ear cavity by way of an injected drum or a perforated drum with discharge. The cardinal sign of acute mastoiditis is tenderness at the base of the mastoid on digital pressure. The diagnosis is confirmed by CT scan.

Management

Admission, intravenous antibiotics and surgical intervention to drain the abscess.

THE NOSE

FOREIGN BODY

A foreign body in the nose is common in preschool children and adults with learning difficulties. The most common types of foreign body are beads, buttons and pieces of paper.

The diagnostic sign of a neglected nasal foreign body is a unilateral foul-smelling nasal discharge. The patient or the parent usually provides the history as to the type of foreign body and for how long present.

Management

The removal of the foreign body follows the same rules as for a foreign body in the ear. An additional method is to blow forcefully through the patient's mouth while occluding the unaffected nostril. This could be done by the parent with instruction.

The suggested method of removal is to pass the ring end of a Jobson Horne probe above and behind the foreign body and to roll it along the floor of the nose. This patient should be cooperative and unrestrained, or fully restrained. At the first sign of trauma or bleeding removal should be organized under general anaesthesia as soon as possible.

TRAUMA

Fractured nose

This is a common presentation in the emergency department. The history is often quite clear and the findings include pain and tenderness over the nasal bones with or without crepitus, and swelling at the bridge of the nose with or without epistaxis.

Careful examination will usually rule out CSF rhinorrhoea due to cribriform plate fracture and any external deformity. Active bleeding from the nostril should be controlled by direct pressure by pinching the nostril; if it does not settle it may require nasal packing.

Radiographs are not indicated for nasal bone fracture as this is a clinical diagnosis and it is often difficult to visualize the fracture line on the X-rays; radiographs do not help in management. If associated facial fractures are suspected, facial views should be taken.

Management

Acute intervention is required in the following circumstances:

- Continuing epistaxis should be managed along the lines described later.
- Obvious external deformity of the nose needs cosmetic correction, either by immediate reduction under local anaesthetic or by referral to an otolaryngologist for review and reduction in 7–10 days' time. A formal rhinoplasty may be required in severe cases. The acute management of a fractured nose is reassurance, analgesia and ice packs, followed by a review by the general practitioner or otolaryngologist in 7–10 days. The patient is advised to avoid any form of contact sport for a week.

- CSF rhinorrhoea requires a CT scan and neurosurgical referral.
- A septal haematoma can become infected, causing a septal abscess that could result in the collapse of the external nose. The diagnosis is made by visualizing the boggy swelling on one or both sides of the septum, and management requires admission, drainage under local or general anaesthesia, followed by nasal packing.

SINUSITIS

Approximately 90% of upper respiratory infections have associated sinus cavity disease.[6] Viral rhinosinusitis is the most common cause and is associated with the common cold. Approximately 0.5–2% of these cases progress to bacterial sinusitis.

Clinical features

Symptoms of viral sinusitis are rhinorrhoea, nasal obstruction and sneezing, and facial pressure with or without headache. With bacterial superinfection a purulent or coloured nasal discharge and fever of 38°C or higher develop. Significant facial pain and maxillary toothache with no obvious dental cause also occurs. The common organisms involved are *Streptococcus pneumoniae* and *H. influenzae*. Patients with allergic sinusitis typically have sneezing and itching, with watery eyes, as a leading symptom.

Radiographs of the sinus are not very helpful unless they demonstrate a distinct air-fluid level, as this increases with the likelihood of bacterial sinusitis. CT can indicate the presence of sinus abnormalities and evidence of infection. A raised white cell count is neither sensitive nor specific in the diagnosis of bacterial sinusitis.

Management of viral rhinosinusitis is symptomatic and it is generally self-limiting. Bacterial sinusitis must be treated with antibiotics: amoxicillin, augmentin or keflex could be used as first-line drugs. Although of unproven value, an oral decongestant or antihistamine is commonly used. Complications of sinus disease include meningitis, orbital extension and brain abscess.

Diagnosis is by CT scan and treatment is intravenous antibiotics with surgical intervention by an otolaryngologist.

EPISTAXIS

Nose bleeding is the most common ENT emergency: a Scottish study reported an incidence of 30/100 000 people[7] in which the cause could only be found in 15%.[8] The common identified causes are trauma, blood dyscrasias, anticoagulation therapy, and occasionally hereditary haemorrhagic telangiectasia.[9] Although hypertension has been traditionally labelled as a cause of epistaxis, studies have shown that blood pressure in these patients is no higher than in the control population.[10,11]

Management

The control of epistaxis due to a general cause such as uncontrolled warfarin therapy or a bleeding disorder is to reverse the cause. Local measures can still be used to stem the flow.

Idiopathic epistaxis, or that due to a local cause such as trauma, can be dealt with using local measures. The most common cause of anterior epistaxis is bleeding from Kiesselbach's plexus of the septum[12] (Fig. 17.1.1), which can easily be controlled by simple measures in the emergency department. Careful examination of a seated patient applying direct pressure to the bleeding vessel by pinching the anterior nares with the thumb and forefinger for up to 10 minutes will usually slow or cease the bleeding. Following this, the application of cotton pledgets soaked in 5% cocaine or lidocaine with adrenaline will provide analgesia and vasoconstriction to the septum and the anterior part of the lateral wall.

Examination may reveal the bleeding vessel on the septum, which can be cauterized under direct vision using silver nitrate sticks. Following this the patient is observed for a short time and can be discharged from the emergency department.

If the bleeding cannot be controlled by the above measures, or the bleeding

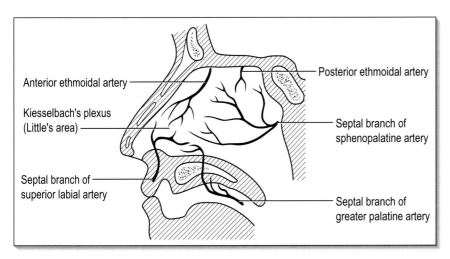

Fig. 17.1.1 Arterial supply to the nasal septum. (From an original drawing by Ian Miller RN)

Anterior ethmoidal artery

Kiesselbach's plexus (Little's area)

Septal branch of superior labial artery

Posterior ethmoidal artery

Septal branch of sphenopalatine artery

Septal branch of greater palatine artery

point is posteriorly placed, the nasal cavity should be packed. There are several ways to pack the nose, the most traditional being to use ribbon gauze to fill the entire nasal cavity in layers (Fig. 17.1.2). Brighton's epistaxis catheter, which has a double balloon for anterior and posterior tamponade, or a Merocel® nasal pack (Xomed), which can be used as a nasal tampon, are both quite useful. Almost all patients with nasal packing need admission and observation. When the above measures are unsuccessful, further invasive procedures such as postnasal packing, examination under anaesthesia and septal surgery or arterial ligation may be required under general anaesthesia.

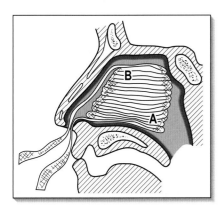

Fig 17.1.2 Insertion of anterior nasal pack (begin at A and finish at B). (From an original drawing by Ian Miller RN)

SUMMARY

Patients with anterior nasal bleeds can usually be managed by chemical cautery with silver nitrate and then be discharged. Posterior bleeding or failure to control by simple measures may require nasal packing and admission for further invasive procedures.

THE THROAT

FOREIGN BODY

Coins are a common oesophageal foreign body in children. In adults the foreign body is usually a fish, chicken or meat bone, and occasionally objects such as partial dentures, safety pins, etc.

The common lodgement sites include the cricopharynx, the oesophagus at the level of the aortic arch, and the gastro-oesophageal junction. Fish bones can lodge in the tonsil, the posterior third of the tongue or the vallecula prior to entering the oesophagus.

Management

Careful examination of the oropharynx initially, especially if the patient localizes the foreign body above the level of the hyoid and to one side. If the foreign body is found it should be removed under direct vision.

A foreign body at or below the cricopharynx requires general anaesthesia and endoscopy.

Lateral X-ray of the neck is useful in identifying and localizing radio-opaque foreign bodies, such as coins and bones, including large fish bones.

Patients presenting with odynophagia but no dysphagia following the ingestion of a fish bone, and a negative physical examination, can be discharged safely for review in 48 hours. Symptoms of increasing odynophagia, fever, haematemesis or dysphagia warrant admission for endoscopy. Patients with a confirmed foreign body should be admitted for endoscopy and removal.

INFECTION

Tonsillitis

Patients with acute tonsillitis present to the general practitioner and occasionally to the emergency department. The emergency department patient usually has severe symptoms or is not responding to oral antibiotics. They are often dehydrated, toxic, with a high temperature and unable to take adequate oral fluids. Treatment includes intravenous penicillin in high doses (e.g. 2MU 4-hourly), intravenous fluids and adequate analgesia.

Quinsy

Peritonsillar abscess or quinsy is a condition in which the infection in the tonsil has breached the capsule and caused cellulitis in the adjacent soft palate (peritonsillitis), and eventually a collection of pus (quinsy).

Examination reveals a congested tonsil being pushed medially and downwards by a diffuse swelling of the soft palate. The opposite tonsil may look injected. There are often unilateral or bilateral enlarged and tender jugulodigastric lymph nodes in the neck.

Management includes admission to hospital for intravenous fluids, penicillin or cephalosporin, and adequate analgesia. Incision and drainage of the quinsy can be done in the emergency department under local anaesthesia in a conscious patient sitting up, to avoid aspiration of pus. Sometimes this needs general anaesthesia. Intubation of such patients should be performed by a skilled anaesthetist and every effort must be made to avoid rupturing the abscess to avoid aspiration of pus.

Retropharyngeal abscess

This is predominantly a disease of young children, as the retropharyngeal lymph nodes atrophy after the age of 5. In older patients it could be secondary to trauma or lodgement of a foreign body, such as a fish bone. Diagnosis is made on symptoms of fever, swelling of the neck due to cervical lymphadenopathy and, especially in young children, stridor. Clinical suspicion leads to imaging procedures such as CT, which is diagnostic.

Management includes admission to hospital, intravenous antibiotics (e.g. ceftriaxone 2 g) and urgent ENT consultation. Treatment is incision and drainage of the abscess under general anaesthesia.

Post-tonsillectomy bleed

Haemorrhage from the tonsillar fossa that occurs 24 hours after tonsillectomy is termed secondary haemorrhage. This

---

CONTROVERSIES

❶ Timing of nasal fracture reduction. This may be performed either immediately or after 7–10 days.

❷ The method used for control of epistaxis. There is no clear advantage in using one method over another.

---

differs from primary, which happens during surgery and reactionary haemorrhage, which occurs within 24 hours after surgery whilst the patient is still in the hospital. The cause of secondary haemorrhage is usually infection and this occurs classically 10 days postoperatively. This incidence is about 1% and is usually not very severe. The management is intravenous antibiotics, usually penicillin. The patient should be admitted and bloods taken for estimation of haemoglobin and a group and held. Application of a swab soaked in 1 in 1000 adrenaline (epinephrine) to the tonsillar fossa after removal of the clot and may help to stop the bleeding. Rarely the patient may need to have a general anaesthetic to cauterize/ligate the bleeder.[13]

REFERENCES

1. Bojrab DI, Bruderly T, Razzak YA 1996 Otitis externa. Otolaryngology Clinics of North America 29(5): 761–82
2. Briggs RJ 1995 Otitis externa: presentation and management. Australian Family Physician 24(10): 1859–64
3. Ali Raza S, Denholm SW, Wong JCH 1995 An audit of the management of acute otitis externa in an ENT casualty clinic. Journal of Laryngology and Otology 109: 130–3
4. Mirza N 1996 Otitis externa - management in the primary care office. Postgraduate Medicine 99(5): 153–8
5. Block SL 1997 Causative pathogens, antibiotic resistance and therapeutic considerations in acute otitis media. Paediatric Infectious Diseases Journal 16(4): 449–56
6. Bukata R 1997 Sinusitis, a ubiquitous, yet enigmatic disease. Emergency Medicine and Acute Care Essays 21(3): 1–4
7. Kotecha B, Fowler S, Harkness P, Walmsley J, Brown P, Topham J 1996 Management of epistaxis: a national survey. Annals of the Royal College of Surgeons of England 78: 444–6
8. Small M, Maran AGD 1984 Epistaxis and arterial ligation. Journal of Laryngology and Otology 98: 281–4
9. Juselius H 1974 Epistaxis. Journal of Laryngology and Otology 88: 317
10. Shaheen OH 1970 Studies of nasal vasculature and problems of arterial ligation for epistaxis. Annals of the Royal College of Surgeons of England 47: 30
11. Weiss NS 1972 The relation of high blood pressure to headache and epistaxis and selected other symptoms. New England Journal of Medicine 287: 631
12. Darry KW, Barlow F, Deleyiannis WB, Pinczower EF 1997 Effectiveness of surgical management of epistaxis at a tertiary care center. Laryngoscope 107: 21–4
13. Evans JNG (ed.) 1987 Scott Brown's Otolaryngology, 5th edn. Butterworth, London, p. 96

SECTION

18

EDITED BY ANTHONY F.T. BROWN

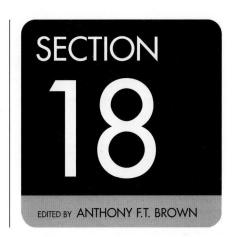

OBSTETRICS AND GYNAECOLOGY

18.1 Emergency delivery 556

18.2 Ectopic pregnancy and bleeding in early pregnancy 561

18.3 Bleeding after the first trimester of pregnancy 564

18.4 Abnormal vaginal bleeding in the non-pregnant patient 567

18.5 Pelvic inflammatory disease 570

18.6 Pelvic pain 572

18.1 EMERGENCY DELIVERY

STEPHEN PRIESTLEY

ESSENTIALS

1 A rapid assessment of pregnant patients in labour arriving at the emergency department must be performed in order to decide on the most appropriate site for management.

2 Equipment, drugs and protocols must be in place within emergency departments so that unexpected deliveries can be managed safely.

3 Lines of communication with regional obstetric services should be established and maintained so that decisions regarding management of labour and transfer of mothers and babies are optimum.

INTRODUCTION

Occasionally doctors working in emergency departments are faced with managing a patient in labour and are required to manage a spontaneous vaginal delivery. This situation is generally accompanied by much anxiety on the part of the emergency department medical and nursing staff but it is important that a calm, systematic approach to this situation is taken to minimize the risk of adverse foetal or maternal outcome. This chapter describes the management of normal delivery in an emergency department.

THE SETTING

There are a number of settings where the conduct of childbirth may need to occur in an emergency department. Pregnant patients at different gestational ages may present in varying stages of labour to the emergency department. Management will depend on the availability of obstetric services, the gestational age, and on both the stage of labour and its anticipated speed of progression. Safe transfer to a delivery suite when there is adequate time is always preferable to delivery in the emergency department. If there is no delivery suite available and there is no time for transfer to an appropriate facility, or the patient arrives with full cervical dilatation and the foetal presenting part on the perineal verge then rapid arrangements need to be made to perform the delivery in the emergency department. Patients who have precipitate labour – an extremely rapid labour lasting less than 4 hours that is more common in the multiparous – may have to attend the emergency department even when en route to the delivery suite or another hospital because of the rapidity of the labour.

The diagnosis of a concealed or unrecognized pregnancy may also be made in the emergency department. Concealed pregnancies occur most commonly in teenage girls who do not tell anyone that they are pregnant and receive no antenatal care, whilst unrecognized pregnancies occur most commonly in obese females who may present to the emergency department complaining of abdominal pains or a vaginal discharge and are found to be pregnant and/or in labour. Women with intellectual impairment or mental illness are another group that may present with an unrecognized pregnancy.

The term precipitous birth or 'born before arrival' (BBA) is commonly associated with precipitate labour and refers to women who deliver their baby prior to arrival at a hospital, usually without the assistance of a trained person. Both the mother and the baby require assessment and may need resuscitation and completion of the third stage of labour on arrival in the emergency department.

The incidence of BBA is low and in Weir's series was found to be 1 in 695 births (0.14%), whilst the incidence of precipitate labour is 17 % in the total hospital population.[1]

HISTORY

Assessment of the patient in labour in the emergency department includes obtaining information regarding gestational age, antenatal care, progression of the pregnancy, past obstetric and a medical history. This is accompanied by a physical and obstetric examination to confirm the progression of labour, the number of babies and the presence or absence of any complications related to the pregnancy and labour.

In hospitals where there is a delivery suite a member of that unit should attend the emergency department to assist with the assessment and conduct of the labour. Delivery in hospitals where there is no delivery suite should include immediate contact by telephone with the nearest or most appropriate obstetric unit in order to obtain advice and organize the transfer of the mother and newborn.

Gestational age may be determined from the last normal menstrual period (LNMP) if this is known. The due date (estimated date of confinement – EDC) can be calculated by adding 9 months and seven days to the date of the LNMP. Ultrasound performed antenatally is also useful in estimating the EDC where dates are uncertain, remembering that those performed later in the pregnancy are less accurate in dating the gestational age of the baby than those performed early in the pregnancy. Additionally, an estimation of the gestational age of the baby can be made by abdominal examination – between 20 and 35 weeks there is a rough correlation between gestational age and the height of the uterine fundus measured in centimetres from the pubic symphysis.

Past obstetric history including duration and description of previous labours, the types of deliveries and the sizes of previous babies should be obtained in addition to a history of caesarian section, use of forceps, neonatal death and history of postpartum haemorrhage, abnormal presentations, shoulder dystocia or prolonged delivery of the placenta. Maternal conditions such as cardiac and respiratory disease, diabetes, bleeding diatheses, hepatitis B and herpes simplex should be documented. All drugs whether prescribed, over-the-counter or illicit that the patient is taking should be noted. The presence of any bleeding or other complications during the pregnancy should also be noted. Results of investigations performed antenatally should be obtained including blood count, blood group and hepatitis B status.

A careful history regarding the onset and timing of contractions and the presence and nature of foetal movements must be sought in addition to a history of vaginal bleeding or discharge which may represent the rupture of membranes.

EXAMINATION

A general examination is carried out with particular emphasis on vital signs, and abdominal and pelvic examination. The breast, nipples, heart and chest should be examined and a urinalysis performed looking for evidence of infection, glucose or proteinuria which may be associated with pre eclampsia.

Abdominal examination is performed to ascertain the height of the fundus, the lie and presentation of the baby and to make an assessment of the engagement of the presenting part. The presence of scars and extrauterine masses should be noted.

The frequency, regularity, duration and intensity of uterine contractions should be assessed. The foetal heart should be counted for one minute using an ordinary stethoscope, Pinard or a doppler stethoscope and should be between 120 and 160 beats per minute. The foetal heart should be counted for at least a 30 second period following a contraction and if bradycardia is detected the mother should be given oxygen and positioned in the left lateral position to ensure that uterine blood flow and foetal oxygenation is optimized. If post contraction bradycardias persist despite these measures then an intravenous fluid bolus should be given and specialist obstetric advice sought. Vaginal bleeding or discharge should be noted and the amount recorded remembering haemorrhage may also be concealed. The colour and character of any amniotic fluid should be assessed looking for evidence of meconium staining.

An aseptic vaginal examination with the patient in the dorsal lithotomy position should be performed to assess the effacement, consistency and dilatation of the cervix, the nature and position of the presenting part (i.e. vertex or breech) and to exclude a cord prolapse. If unsure of the nature of the presenting part a portable ultrasound can aid in diagnosis. The exception to the performance of a vaginal examination is the gravid patient with active vaginal bleeding who should be evaluated with an ultrasound to exclude placenta praevia before *any* pelvic examination is performed. If the membranes are intact, there is no indication to rupture them if the labour is progressing satisfactorily because of the risk of cord prolapse if the presenting part is not well engaged in the pelvis. An assessment can also be made of the size of the pelvis and an attempt to gauge the general 'degree of fit' between the presenting part and the pelvis.

After the vaginal examination a sterile perineal pad is applied and the patient is able to assume whichever position gives her the most comfort.

After this assessment the decision whether to transfer the patient to a delivery suite either within the hospital or at a distant hospital must be made. Cervical dilatation greater than 6 cm in a multiparous patient and 7–8 cm in the primiparous makes transfer to a distant hospital an increasingly hazardous procedure because of the risk of rapid progression to full cervical dilatation and delivery of the baby. The availability and type of transport and personnel and distance to be travelled must be carefully considered and consultation with an obstetric unit regarding the safety of transfer and arrangements for reception of the patient must occur.

MANAGEMENT

Preparation for delivery

Ongoing assessment of maternal temperature, blood pressure, heart rate and contractions should be performed and recorded. Foetal heart rate should be counted every 15 minutes up to full cervical dilatation and every 5 minutes thereafter.

Unless there is a clear indication for an intravenous line such as history of postpartum haemorrhage or antepartum haemorrhage, bleeding tendency, evidence of preeclampsia or history of a previous caesarian section then placement for the normal delivery is unnecessary. Venepuncture should be performed for haemoglobin and blood group and some set aside for crossmatching.

A delivery pack, sterile surgical instruments and oxytocics should be obtained and placed close by (see Table 18.1.1). Resuscitation equipment and drugs should be available.

Assembling personnel with clear task delegation is essential. It is important to remember that reassurance and emotional support for the mother is crucial during the entire labour and the mother's partner. A specific member of staff may be delegated to provide this.

If a midwife or doctor experienced in delivery is available then they should assume control of the procedure and continue the assessment of the progression of labour and conduct the delivery of both the baby and the placenta. A doctor or nurse with some experience in neonatal or paediatric resuscitation should perform a rapid assessment of the need for intervention immediately after the delivery of the baby.

Conduct of labour

Labour is divided into three stages: The first stage is from the onset of regular contractions to full dilatation (10 cm) of the cervix. The second stage is from full

Table 18.1.1 Equipment and drugs required for emergency delivery

Equipment	Drugs	
Three clamps - straight or curved (e.g Pean)	Adrenaline (epinephrine)	1:1000
Episiotomy scissors	Syntocinon	10 units
Scissors	Ergometrine	250 µg
Suture repair set	Vitamin K	1 mg
Absorbable suture material (e.g Vicryl Rapide®)	Lidocaine	1%
Neonatal resuscitation equipment		
Blanket		
Warmer		
Sterile drapes		
Huck towels		
Sterile gloves		
Soap solution		
Sterile bowls		

dilatation of the cervix to delivery of the baby and the third stage is from the birth of the baby until delivery of the placenta.

A full description of the detailed management of the three stages is beyond the scope of this chapter – rather a brief summary of the management of a normal vertex delivery is described.

First stage

The patient should be examined abdominally and vaginally as necessary to follow the progress of the labour. As mentioned earlier measurement and recording of maternal vital signs and foetal heart rate are performed.

The perineum should be gently washed with a nonirritating soap solution such as 0.1% chlorhexidine. Neither shaving, urinary catheterization nor enema administration are required.

Analgesics are helpful for the patient with significant discomfort and are not injurious to the foetus. The timing and dose of analgesia must be decided with due regard to the stage and rate of progression of labour. Intramuscular pethidine (1–1.5 mg/kg) is commonly used and generally provides good analgaesia. The provision of other forms of analgaesia such as epidural anaesthesia is beyond the scope of this chapter.

Sedatives and analgesics drugs should not be given immediately before anticipated delivery because of possible depressive effects on the baby.

The average duration of the first stage of labour in primiparous patients is 8–12 hours; in subsequent pregnancies, 6–8 hours.

Second stage

Spontaneous delivery of the foetus presenting by vertex is divided into three phases: delivery of the head, delivery of the shoulders and delivery of the body and legs. The second stage of labour begins when the cervix is fully dilated and delivery will occur when the presenting part reaches the pelvic floor. The normal duration of this stage ranges from 20 to 60 minutes in the primiparous to 10 to 30 minutes in the multiparous patient. Preparations for delivery including cleansing must be made as described earlier. The patient should be draped in such a manner that there is a clear view of the perineum. Either a dorsal lithotomy or lateral Sims' position may be used for the actual delivery. The dorsal lithotomy position is recommended for inexperienced operators as it is easier to visualize and manually control the delivery process and perform episiotomy. In the dorsal lithotomy position the mother should be tilted slightly over to the left side using a pillow or soft wedge to avoid compression of the inferior vena cava by the gravid uterus and possible maternal hypotension and foetal hypoxia.

When the presenting part distends the perineum delivery is imminent and anaesthesia may be administered. Lidocaine 1% 5–10 mL may be injected in the posterior area of the perineum at this time to facilitate episiotomy. Episiotomy is carried out when delivery is imminent to minimize the risk of the perineum tearing with delivery of the head. A mediolateral perineal incision is made beginning at the frenulum of the labia minora and extending towards the ischiorectal fossa. A midline episiotomy is no longer recommended due to an increased risk of tears extending through to the rectum. The patient should be encouraged to bear down during contractions and rest in between.

Delivery of the head must be controlled by the accoucheur so that it extends slowly after delivery and does not pop out of the vagina. Placing the palm of one hand over the head to control its extension most easily effects this. At this point the patient should cease actively pushing and may need to be instructed to pant or breathe through her nose in order to overcome her desire to push. The accoucheur's second hand (covered with a sterile gauze pad or towel) may be used to gently lift the baby's chin, which can be felt in the space between the anus and the coccyx.

As the occiput descends under the symphysis pubis, extension occurs and progressively the forehead, nose, mouth and finally chin emerge. If there is evidence of meconium staining of the liquor, the baby's nose and mouth should be gently suctioned.

In 25–30% of patients the umbilical cord is looped around the neck, which should be checked for. Generally it is only loosely looped and can be drawn over the head. If there is tension, two clamps should be placed on the cord 2–3 cm apart and the cord cut in between them. Release of additional loops is now straightforward by unwinding the clamped ends around the neck. The baby's head, having been delivered face down (the most common occipito-anterior position) is allowed to 'restitute' to one or the other lateral positions.

Once the head has restituted, the shoulders will lie in an anteroposterior plane within the pelvis, and delivery of the shoulders is now effected taking great care not to allow the perineum to tear. Usually the anterior shoulder slips under the symphysis pubis with the next contraction by exerting downward and backward traction on the head to facilitate this. Excessive force must not be used as this may result in a brachial plexus injury. Additional pressure may be exerted just above the symphysis pubis by an assistant to push the shoulder downward to come from under the symphysis.

On delivery of the anterior shoulder, lifting the baby up will result in delivery of the posterior shoulder followed by the body and lower limbs. Grasp the baby firmly with one hand securing the infant behind the neck and the other encircling both ankles and place on the mother's abdomen. The baby is slippery as a result of being covered with vernix and should never be held with one hand alone. Record the time of birth. Dry the baby and wrap in a warm, dry blanket to minimize heat loss.

If the baby is breathing spontaneously and is close to term, there is no need to immediately cut the cord. An assessment of the baby with Apgar scoring should be done to determine the need for resuscitation. If the baby is preterm or requires resuscitation the cord should be quickly clamped following delivery and the baby transferred to a resuscitation trolley that has a radiant heat source for further assessment and resuscitation.

To cut the umbilical cord an umbilical clamp is applied 1–2 cm from the baby's abdomen and the cord is trimmed approximately 0.5 cm above the plastic clamp.

Following the birth of the baby, the woman's abdomen is palpated to exclude the possibility of a second foetus and an oxytocic agent is administered. The commonest is oxytocin at a dose of 10 units given intramuscularly or intravenously as a slow bolus. An alternative is ergometrine in a dose of 250 μg intramuscularly or slowly intravenously over 2 minutes. If there is evidence of pre-eclampsia, eclampsia or hypertension then ergometrine should not be used.

Third stage

After administration of the oxytocic agent signs of separation of the placenta from the uterine wall should be looked for. These include a gush of blood from the vagina, lengthening of the cord and rising of the contracted and globular uterine fundus as the placenta passes down the birth canal. Following separation, traction on the cord in a backward and downward direction should be applied with one hand whilst the other is placed on the woman's lower abdomen to support the uterus. Traction must cease if the cord feels as though it is tearing. As the placenta appears at the introitus traction is then applied in an upward direction and the placenta is grasped and gently rotated to ensure that the membranes are delivered without tearing. The placenta should be inspected to look for any missing segments or cotyledons that may prevent the uterus from contracting properly if they remain within the uterus.

PROCEDURE POST DELIVERY

The uterus should be rubbed to facilitate contraction and expulsion of clots. The usual causes of post partum haemorrhage include incomplete uterine contraction as a result of clots or tissue remaining within the cavity, which must be expelled by massaging the fundus or by manual removal. Further oxytocics may be necessary. Bleeding may also occur from other sites and a careful examination of the cervix, vagina, episiotomy wound and perineum should always be performed following delivery. The episiotomy wound and any other lacerations may be repaired with an absorbable suture material such as Vicryl Rapide.

The baby should be kept warm and dry and both mother, and baby should have vital signs measured and recorded. Regular observations of the maternal fundal height, uterine tone and vaginal loss should also be made.

If vitamin K is available it should be administered to the baby as a deep intramuscular injection of 1 mg.

DISPOSITION

Disposition of mother and baby to an obstetric unit either within the hospital or at a distant hospital should then be made when both are stable. The important information that must be provided includes the time of birth, drugs given to either mother or baby and the Apgar scores of the baby. Results of any blood tests and a copy of the observations should also be communicated.

If either mother or baby is unstable then early consultation with the appropriate referral service is mandatory regarding the optimum timing and nature of the transfer.

COMPLICATIONS OF DELIVERY

Breech delivery

Breech presentation occurs in 3–4% of all deliveries, reducing in incidence with advancing gestation. Most breech presentations are delivered by caesarean section. There is evidence that neonatal morbidity and mortality are worse in a breech group than in those foetuses delivering by cephalic presentation.[2] The object is safe delivery of the foetus.

In delivery, minimal interference is best. Allow the foetus to deliver spontaneously to the umbilicus. Deliver the foetus until the scapulae are visible with gentle traction applied to the hips. Then rotate the trunk until the anterior shoulder delivers, with subsequent rotation of the trunk in the opposite direction results in delivery of the posterior shoulder. Once the shoulders are delivered the accoucheur delivers the head either with the application of forceps or by placing the index finger in the baby's mouth and flexing the head resulting in delivery.

Shoulder dystocia

Shoulder dystocia can be one of the most frightening complications of vaginal delivery and is frequently unexpected. The important steps in management are: recognizing the at-risk patient, getting assistance early and understanding the manoeuvres to deliver the foetus. The at-risk patient may have a large baby or have had a previous shoulder dystocia or gestational diabetes (or have no predisposing factor).

The problem encountered in shoulder dystocia is following delivery of the foetal head; the anterior shoulder does not deliver spontaneously, or with gentle traction by the accoucheur. The anterior shoulder is caught immediately above the symphysis. The rate is approx 1:300 deliveries.

Foetal morbidity and mortality rates are significant. The effects of prolonged asphyxia include neuropsychiatric dysfunction. Brachial plexus injuries result from lateral traction on the foetal head during delivery. Erbs palsy arises from damage to the C5 and C6 nerve roots, with paralysis of the deltoid and short muscles of the shoulder, and of brachialis and biceps, which flex and supinate the elbow. The arm hangs limply by the side with the forearm pronated and the palm facing backwards. Ninety per cent of these lesions recover fully or almost fully.

The first sign of shoulder dystocia is retraction of the foetal chin into the perineum, following the delivery of the head. Delivery in under 5 minutes is essential to prevent asphyxia.

Measures for treatment of shoulder dystocia:

- McRoberts manoeuvre: exaggerated flexion of maternal legs resulting in widening of the pelvic diameter.
- Suprapubic pressure (these two usually result in delivery of the foetus).
- Woods corkscrew manoeuvre: the shoulders are rotated to a transverse position freeing the obstruction.

- Delivery of the posterior shoulder (may result in clavicular or humeral fracture).
- Zavanelli's procedure: replacing the head in the uterus and performing a caesarean section.

Post-partum haemorrhage

A post-partum haemorrhage (PPH) is defined as loss of 500 mL or greater after delivery of the foetus. Based on recent statistics, haemorrhage was a major factor in 1/3 of maternal deaths in Australia.

Causes of PPH

- Retained placenta or products of conception
- Uterine atony
- Soft-tissue laceration
- Coagulopathy
- Uterine rupture

Risk factors

- Retained placenta
- Grand multiparity (reduced muscular tissue in uterus)
- Antepartum haemorrhage
- Over distension of the uterus from polyhydramnios or multiple pregnancy
- Large placental site associated with multiple pregnancy, molar pregnancy
- Past history of PPH or haemorrhagic disorders
- Fibroid uterus
- Precipitate labour
- Prolonged labour
- Chorioamnionitis
- Tocolytic agents, inhalational anaesthetics
- Twenty per cent occur in the absence of any risk factors.

Management of PPH

- Prevention is the mainstay of treatment by identifying the at-risk patient and the aggressive use of oxytocin, with active management of third stage. These measures reduce the incidence of PPH by 40%. Resuscitate the patient with IV fluids and cross-match blood.
- If a coagulation or platelet defect is present then correct with either FFP or platelets.

- Medical treatment of uterine atony.
- Give intravenous oxytocin 10 units or ergometrine 250 mg, as well as ergometrine 250 mg IM followed by an infusion of either 40IU of oxytocin or 1 mg of ergometrine.
- Remember to rub up the fundus and deliver the placenta if undelivered. Examine the lower genital tract for tears. Suspect uterine rupture in patients with severe abdominal pain.
- If uterine atony persists further measures may be required. Exploration of the uterine cavity may be required.
- Further medical treatment includes PG F2a 2.5 mg in aliquots. It is successful in 60–85% cases of refractory uterine atony. Side effects include nausea, vomiting, diarrhoea, pyrexia, hypertension and bronchoconstriction. Its use is contra-indicated in women with asthma and hypertension.
- Surgical management of continuing postpartum haemorrhage.
- Uterine artery ligation has minimal complications and reduces the pulse pressure by 60–70% to allow endogenous haemostatic mechanisms to control bleeding. Failing this, internal iliac artery ligation may be performed usually bilaterally. Hysterectomy is the operation of last resort. It may be necessary in uterine atony or rupture as well as in placenta praevia, and be the operation of choice in women of higher parity.

ACKNOWLEDGEMENT

The author would like to acknowledge the assistance of Dr Ian Barabash, Senior Obsteric Registrar at Sunshine Hospital, in completion of this chapter.

REFERENCES

1. Weir PE, Beischer NA 1980 Birth before arrival in hospital. Medical Journal of Australia 2: 31
2. Brenner WE, et al 1974 The characteristics and perils of breech presentation. American Journal of Obstetrics and Gynecology 118: 700

OBSTETRICS AND GYNAECOLOGY

FURTHER READING

Beischer NA, Mackay EV, Colditz P (eds) 1997 Obstetrics and the Newborn: an Illustrated Textbook, 3rd edn. W.B.Saunders, Pennsylvania

Decherny AH, Perroll MH (eds) 1994 Current Obstetrics and Gynaecologic Diagnosis and Treatment, 8th edn. Appleton and Lange, New Jersey

Gianopoulos JG 1994 Emergency complications of labour and delivery. Emergency Medical Clinics of North America 12(1): 201–17

Jensen MD, Bobak IM (eds) 1984 Essentials of Maternity Nursing. The CV Mosby Company, St Louis

Llewellyn-Jones D (ed.) 1994 Fundamentals of Obstetrics and Gynaecology, 6th edn. Mosby, St Louis

Tintinalli JE, Krome RL, Ruiz E 1993 Emergency Medicine. A Comprehensive Study Guide, 3rd edn. McGraw-Hill Inc, New York

18.2 ECTOPIC PREGNANCY AND BLEEDING IN EARLY PREGNANCY

SHEILA BRYAN

ESSENTIALS

1 Approximately 25% of all clinically diagnosed pregnancies are associated with bleeding in the first 12 weeks.

2 Ectopic pregnancy occurs at a rate of about 11 per 1000 diagnosed pregnancies.

3 Ultrasound is the single most useful investigation in the assessment of early pregnancy bleeding.

4 Rh(D) immunoglobulin should be considered for all patients with Rhesus negative blood group.

INTRODUCTION

Bleeding in early pregnancy is a common problem affecting approximately 25% of clinically diagnosed pregnancies, and of these women approximately 50% will have bleeding due to a failed pregnancy.[1] Causes of bleeding include incidental, which has no bearing on the outcome of the pregnancy, failed pregnancy and ectopic pregnancy. With few exceptions, history and examination are usually unhelpful in reaching a diagnosis or in guiding management of these patients. Ultrasound is the single most useful tool in the assessment of bleeding in early pregnancy and has significantly changed the emergency approach to these patients.

HISTORY

History should include the date of the last normal period, the outcomes of previous pregnancies and the use of assisted reproductive techniques.

When estimating the amount of vaginal bleeding it is useful to quantify the blood loss compared to the woman's normal menstrual loss. Bleeding heavier than a normal period is a poor prognostic sign.

The history of passage of fetal products should not be used as a basis for a diagnosis. Blood clots or a decidual cast may be misinterpreted as fetal products. In addition, the correct identification of a fetus does not exclude the possibility of a live second twin or of a coexistent ectopic pregnancy.

History and examination are not reliable in the diagnosis of an ectopic pregnancy.[2] However, a high index of suspicion is required in patients with known risk factors, such as a past history of tubal damage secondary to ectopic pregnancy, infection or surgery; assisted reproductive techniques; increased age; smoking and progesterone-only contraception. Intrauterine contraceptive devices not only decrease the chance of intrauterine pregnancies, but increase the likelihood of an ectopic.[3]

EXAMINATION

Determination of the patient's hemodynamic status and the rate of ongoing bleeding are essential. Hypotension, tachycardia and signs of peritoneal irritation on abdominal examination suggest a ruptured ectopic pregnancy or bleeding from a corpus luteal cyst. These two conditions are often not associated with heavy vaginal blood loss.

Hypotension, relative bradycardia and heavy vaginal bleeding is usually caused by the products of conception dilating the cervix and causing cervical shock with a vagal response.

The vast majority of patients presenting with bleeding in early pregnancy will have bleeding lighter than their normal period and many will present with just spotting. In patients with a first presentation of light bleeding and with no history to suggest trauma or infection, and in whom the PAP smear is up to date, the value of vaginal examination is limited. Vaginal examination is, however, recommended for heavy bleeding and for recurrent presentations.

Two important factors guide the management of a hemodynamically stable patient with vaginal bleeding; they are the anatomical location of the pregnancy (intrauterine or ectopic) and the viability of the pregnancy (presence of a fetal heart beat). Neither of these factors is reliably ascertained on clinical examination.

Before the widespread availability of ultrasound, examination was performed to assess the cervical os and to look for the products of conception. An open internal cervical os was thought to be diagnostic of an inevitable miscarriage, and the identification of products of conception was suggestive of a complete miscarriage. However, both of these clinical signs are difficult to determine and, alone, are no longer used to guide the management of patients.

The management options for ectopic pregnancy, failed pregnancy and incomplete miscarriage may be either surgical, medical or conservative. The treatment method is based on the ultrasound findings and the preference of the patient and the treating doctor.[3,4]

A complete physical examination should be performed including an assessment of the patient's mental state, as pregnancy loss has a profound psychological impact on some women.

INVESTIGATIONS

Biochemistry

Urine pregnancy tests are sensitive to a level of 25–60 IU/L. False negatives may occur in the setting of early pregnancy or dilute urine.

The beta subunit of human chorionic gonadotrophin (β-hCG) is produced by the outer layer of cells of the gestational sac (syncytiotrophoblast) and may be detected as early as 9 days after fertilization.[5] The β-hCG level increases by approximately 1.66 times every 48 hours, then plateaus before falling to a lower level at around 12 weeks. The half life of β-hCG is approximately 36 hours, so the level will remain elevated for a number of weeks following a miscarriage or termination. A positive pregnancy test or a single β-hCG level is, therefore, unreliable to confirm ongoing pregnancy, and cannot be used to identify the retained products of conception.[6] High levels of β-hCG can be associated with multiple and molar pregnancies.

Haematology

A full blood count and cross match should be arranged for haemodynamically unstable patients. Blood group and Rhesus factor should be determined on all patients.

Ultrasound

Routine early pregnancy ultrasound should be performed on *every* patient in order to locate the pregnancy anatomically and to assess its viability. The introduction of emergency department ultrasound provides a cost-effective method for the assessment of patients presenting with bleeding in early pregnancy.[6]

A developing pregnancy may be expected to be reliably identified by transvaginal ultrasound at a β-hCG level of greater than 1000 IU/L.[7] However in certain clinical settings ultrasound is still valuable when the hormone level is less then 1000 IU/L.[8]

A gestational sac can be identified as early as 31 days gestation. Embryonic cardiac activity can be identified at approximately 39 days (5.5 weeks) gestation, at which stage the crown rump length of the embryo is approximately 5 mm and the β-hCG is approximately 12 050 IU/L (range 5280–22950 IU/L).[7]

MANAGEMENT

Haemodynamically unstable patients

Haemodynamically unstable patients with suspected ectopic pregnancy should be resuscitated and transferred to theatre for surgical intervention as soon as possible. Ultrasound can assist in the diagnosis of a ruptured ectopic if free fluid is identified in the pouch of Douglas and no pregnancy is identified in the uterus. The identification of an interuterine pregnancy does not exclude an ectopic pregnancy. Ectopic pregnancy may coexist with an intrauterine pregnancy (heterotopic pregnancy). The incidence of heterotopic pregnancy in the general population is up to 1:3889 but occurs in up to 1:100–1:500 in patients who have undergone assisted reproduction.[9] A ruptured corpus leuteal cyst may also cause haemodynamic compromise and is often diagnosed laparoscopically.

Patients with heavy bleeding, hypotension and bradycardia should be examined with a speculum, and if tissue is lodged in the cervical os it should gently be removed.

Haemodynamically stable patients

The management of haemodynamically stable patients is dependent upon the findings at ultrasound. In a patient with early pregnancy bleeding and an ultrasound confirming a live intrauterine gestation, there is a 85–90% chance of the pregnancy progressing to term. Poor prognostic indicators include the ultrasound findings of an enlarged yolk sac, gestational sac greater than 20 mm mean diameter and fetal bradycardia after 7 weeks gestation.[10] In the absence of the above indicators, patients may be reassured and discharged for review by their treating obstetrician.

All other ultrasound diagnoses will require consultation with the obstetric and gynaecology service to develop a management plan. The range of ultrasound results and management options are outlined in Table 18.2.1.

Rh (D) immunoglobulin

All patients should have their blood group and Rhesus (Rh) factor determined. As little as 0.1 mL of Rh(D) positive fetal blood will cause maternal Rh immunization. In early pregnancy bleeding, a dose of 250 IU of Rh(D) immunoglobulin should be given to Rh-negative women as soon as possible and within 72 hours of onset of the bleeding. This dose will prevent immunization by a feto-maternal hemorrhage of up to 2.5 mL of fetal cells. In the case of repeat or prolonged bleeding further doses may be required.[11] In multiple pregnancies or a gestation greater than 13 weeks a dose of 625 IU is recommended. The

Table 18.2.1 Management options for haemodynamically stable patients with light vaginal bleeding in early pregnancy

Ultrasound findings	Differential diagnosis / comments	Management options in discussion with obstetric team
Live intrauterine pregnancy	95% chance of pregnancy progressing to term	Refer to obstetrician for ongoing care Review if increased bleeding or pain
Ectopic pregnancy	Ectopic pregnancy	Conservative (observation) Medical (methotrexate) Surgical (salpingectomy/salpingostomy)
Intrauterine gestational sac with no fetal pole	Early pregnancy Failed pregnancy (anembryonic or blighted ovum)	Repeat scan in 1 week Review if increased pain or bleeding
Fetus with no fetal heart beat or retained products of conception	Failed pregnancy Incomplete miscarriage	Conservative (observation) Medical (vaginal ± oral misoprostol) Surgical (dilation and curettage)
Empty uterus	Early pregnancy Complete miscarriage Ectopic pregnancy	Serial β-hCG levels Repeat scan when level >1000 IU/L or if levels stabilize If β-hCG falling then monitor to level <5 IU/L
Molar pregnancy	Partial mole Complete mole	Surgery (dilation and curettage) ± methotrexate Monitor for up to 12 months

Kleihauer test is used in later pregnancy to quantify the amount of fetal cells in the maternal circulation, but is unreliable in early pregnancy.

PROGNOSIS

Approximately 50% of patients with bleeding in early pregnancy will proceed to term. Only 60% of women with an ectopic pregnancy will conceive naturally again with an ectopic rate of 25–30% in subsequent pregnancies.

DISPOSITION

Patients with a live intrauterine gestation may be discharged home with advice to avoid sexual intercourse and not to use tampons until after the bleeding has settled. All other patients should be referred to the obstetric and gynecology service.

A referral for counseling or psychological support may be indicated in some women.

CONTROVERSIES

❶ The role of emergency department ultrasound.

❷ The management of patients with no intrauterine pregnancy identified on ultrasound.

❸ The indications for anti D immunoglobulin.

❹ The best method of emptying the uterus following a failed pregnancy.

❺ The best method of managing an ectopic pregnancy.

Due to the high frequency of first trimester miscarriage, investigation for an underlying cause is generally not indicated until after the third consecutive miscarriage.

REFERENCES

1. Beischer NA, MacKay EV, Colditz PB 1997 Obstetrics and the Newborn, 3rd edn. WB Saunders, Pennsylvania, p. 176

2. Dart R, Kaplan B, Varakis K 1999 Predictive value of history and physical examination in patients with suspected ectopic pregnancy. Annals of Emergency Medicine 33(3): 283–90

3. Tay JI, Moore J, Walker JJ, 2000 Ectopic pregnancy. British Medical Journal 320: 916–9

4. Ankum WM, Waard MW, Bindels PJE 2001 Management of spontaneous miscarriage in the first trimester: an example of putting informed shared decision making into practice. British Medical Journal 322: 1343–6

5. Guyton AC, Hall JE 1996 Textbook of Medical Physiology, 9th edn. WB Saunders, Pennsylvania, pp 1037–9

6. Durston W, Carl M, Guerra W, et al 2000 Ultrasound availability in the evaluation of ectopic pregnancy in the ED: comparison of quality and cost effectiveness with different approaches. American Journal of Emergency Medicine 18(4): 408–17

7. Cacciatore B, Titinen A, Stenman U-H, et al 1990 Normal early pregnancy: Serum hCG levels and vaginal ultrasonography findings. British Journal of Obstetrics and Gynecology 97: 899–903

8. Dart RG, Kaplan B, Cox C 1997 Transvaginal ultrasound in patients with low beta-human chorionic gonadotropin values: how often is the study diagnostic. Annals of Emergency Medicine 30(2): 135–40

9. In vitro fertilization-embryo transfer (IVF-ET) in the Unites States 1990 results from the IVF-ET registry of the Medical Research International and Society for Assisted Reproductive Technology (SART)/The American Fertility Society Fertility and Sterility 1992, 57: 15–24

10. Filly RA 1994 Ultrasound evaluation during the first trimester. In: Callen PW (ed.) Ultrasonography in Obstetrics and Gynecology, 3rd edn. WB Saunders, Pennsylvania

11. Guidelines on the prophylactic use of Rh D immunoglobulin (Anti-D) in obstetrics NHMRC, 1999

18.3 BLEEDING AFTER THE FIRST TRIMESTER OF PREGNANCY

JENNY DOWD • SHEILA BRYAN

ESSENTIALS

1 Up to 4% of pregnant women will have significant bleeding after 20 weeks gestation.

2 Resuscitation of the mother followed by ultrasound localization of the placenta are the priorities of management for patients with heavy vaginal bleeding.

3 Secondary post-partum haemorrhage is commonly caused by endometritis or retained products of conception.

INTRODUCTION

Vaginal bleeding after the first trimester may be due to a number of causes. The most common are classified as incidental, whereby the bleeding is not directly related to pregnancy. Obstetric causes of bleeding include placenta praevia, accidental haemorrhage or abruption and vasa praevia. Bleeding that occurs after 20 weeks' gestation is classified as an ante-partum haemorrhage (APH).

Primary post-partum haemorrhage (PPH) is defined as heavy (greater than 600 mL) vaginal bleeding within 24 hours of delivery and is discussed in the chapter on emergency delivery. Secondary PPH is most commonly due to infection and/or retained tissue, and may cause significant bleeding up to 6 weeks post partum.

ANTEPARTUM HEMORRHAGE

DIFFERENTIAL DIAGNOSIS

Incidental causes

These include bleeding from the lower genital tract most commonly from physiological cervical erosion or eversion, which may be either spontaneous or post-traumatic such as post coital. Other causes that need to be excluded include bleeding from cervical polyps, cervical malignancy and cervical or vaginal infections.

Bleeding from haemorrhoids or vulval varices may also mistakenly be reported as vaginal bleeding.

Placenta praevia

Placenta praevia occurs when the placenta is situated in the lower part of the uterus and thus in front of the presenting part of the fetus. It occurs in 0.5% of pregnancies.[1] Bleeding in this situation is usually painless unless associated with labour contractions and often presents with several small, warning bleeds.

Accidental haemorrhage

This is bleeding from a normally situated placenta. This may be from the edge of the placenta known as a marginal bleed or from behind the placenta associated with placental separation or abruption. Vaginal bleeding may not always be present with a placental abruption; it is, however, usually associated with pain. An abruption that causes significant detachment of the placenta may cause fetal compromise and fetal death in up to 30% cases.[2] The retroplacental clot is comprised of maternal blood and up to 2–4 litres may be concealed behind the placenta without vaginal loss. An abruption may follow relatively minor blunt trauma such as a fall onto the abdomen or a shearing force such as that applied in motor vehicle deceleration accidents. It may also occur spontaneously in women with hypertension, inherited disorders of coagulation or in association with cocaine use.[3]

Vasa praevia

This is the presence of fetal vessels running in the amniotic membranes distant from the placental mass and across the cervical os. These vessels occasionally rupture, often in association with rupture of the amniotic membranes. When this happens the bleeding is from the fetus, which may quickly lead to fetal compromise. The first indication of this may be fetal bradycardia or other abnormalities of the fetal heart rate seen on cardiotocographic (CTG) tracing.

Physiological

Vaginal blood mixed with mucus is called a 'show' and is due to the mucus plug (operculum) within the endocervical canal dislodging as the cervix begins to dilate. This usually occurs at the time of, or within a few days of the onset of labour, and is not significant unless the pregnancy is pre-term or associated with rupture of the membranes. As a general guide if the woman needs to wear a pad to soak up blood she should be assessed as having an APH.

HISTORY

The history should specifically include details of recent abdominal trauma or drug use suggesting a diagnosis of placental abruption. A history of recent coitus is commonly identified in bleeding from a cervical erosion.

Constant pain over the uterus or sometimes the back from separation of a posteriorly situated placenta is suggestive of abruption. Intermittent pains in the lower abdomen or back may represent uterine contractions. Women may describe this as period pains or tighenings and may notice a general hardening over the whole uterus associated with the pain. Painless bleeding is suggestive of either an incidental cause or of placenta praevia.

The history should also include details regarding the presence and quality of fetal movements.

An increase in pelvic pressure associated with vaginal fluid loss associated with spotting or mild bleeding suggests cervical incompetence. This usually presents between 14–22 weeks gestation. Prior cervical damage secondary to either a cone biopsy or a cervical tear is a risk factor for cervical incompetence.

EXAMINATION

Assessment of the mother is the priority. A relatively low blood pressure with a systolic of 90 mmHg and a resting tachycardia of up to 100 bpm may be normal in pregnancy.

Examination after 30 weeks' gestation should be performed with the right hip elevated by a pillow to give a 15° degree tilt of the pelvis to the left. This avoids the problem of vena caval compression.

Speculum or digital vaginal examination should *not* be performed until the site of the placenta is determined (by ultrasound) to avoid disrupting a low-lying placenta.

A sterile speculum examination should be performed when there is a possibility of rupture of the membranes, or the cervix needs to be visualized to exclude a local cause of bleeding and to look for cervical dilatation. The safest way to visualize the cervix is with the woman in the left lateral position using a Simm's speculum. Digital vaginal examination should be performed if the possibility of cervical change due to labour needs to be assessed.

Ideally, an external cardiotocograph (CTG) should be applied to assess the status of the fetus. If this is not available, auscultating the fetal heart for several minutes should be attempted, noting any major variations in rate, particularly decelerations after uterine tightenings.

The normal range of the fetal heart rate is 120–160 bpm, but a healthy term or post-term fetus may have a heart rate of between 100 and 120 bpm.

INVESTIGATIONS

Blood should be taken for a baseline haemoglobin, coagulation screen, Kleihauer test, blood group, Rhesus factor, rhesus antibodies and a cross match.

If the patient is hypertensive a pre-eclampsia screen should be ordered. This includes liver function test, uric acid and platelet count.

Ultrasound is used to assess fetal gestation, presentation, liquor volume and placental position. Many 'low-lying' placentas at 18 weeks are no longer classified as placenta praevia by 30–32 weeks, owing to the differential growth of the lower uterine segment as pregnancy progresses. As only 50% of placental abruptions will be seen on ultrasound, it is not a reliable test for excluding this problem and the diagnosis is usually made on clinical grounds alone.

MANAGEMENT

Incidental causes of bleeding usually require no specific therapy appart from explanation and reassurance. Cervical polyps are rarely removed during pregnancy due to the risk of heavy bleeding.

Minor amounts of bleeding due to placenta praevia distant from term are managed by close observation either as an inpatient or an outpatient.

Small abruptions may also be managed conservatively, with serial ultrasounds to check fetal growth and regular CTG assessments until around 37 weeks, when delivery is usually advised (to pre-empt a massive abruption). Sometimes a small retroplacental clot will cause weakening of the amniotic membranes and subsequent rupture of the amniotic sac 1–2 weeks after the initial bleed.

Massive antepartum haemorrhage, often with fetal demise when associated with placental separation, requires urgent delivery, possibly by caesarean section.

Hypovolemia and coagulopathies should be treated as per usual guidelines.

PROGNOSIS

In a hospital where there are no obstetric or neonatal facilities a decision will need to be made about when to transfer the patient to an obstetric hospital. If the fetus is between 23 and 34 weeks, and delivery can be delayed for 24 hours, then corticosteroids should be administered to the mother. Two intramuscular doses of betamethasone or dexamethasone given over 24 hours decreases the baby's risk of respiratory distress syndrome, necrotizing enterocolitis and intraventricular haemorrhages.[4] The current survival rate of a 23-week fetus born in good conditions in a tertiary centre is 35%.[4]

DISPOSITION

Admission and observation is recommended if immediate delivery is not indicated for fetal or maternal reasons.

SECONDARY PPH

INTRODUCTION

Secondary PPH is defined as excessive or prolonged bleeding from 24 hours to 6 weeks post partum. Normal lochia is moderately heavy and red for some days but settles to lightish bleeding or spotting after 2–4 weeks. Some women have a persistent brownish discharge for up to 8 weeks.

DIFFERENTIAL DIAGNOSIS

Common causes of secondary PPH include retained products of conception and endometritis. The bleeding is usually prolonged moderate blood loss or a recurrence of blood loss after an initial decline. Less common causes include trophoblastic disease, uterine arterio-venous malformations (AVMs) and any of the incidental causes outlined in the previous section. Annoying spotting may occur for weeks in women using progestogen-only contraception in the setting of an oestrogen-deficient endo-metrium.

HISTORY

Distinguishing endometritis from retained products may be difficult clin-ically and the two conditions often coexist. Endometritis can follow any type of delivery, but is more commonly seen in women with a history of prolonged rupture of the membranes and multiple vaginal examinations during labour.

EXAMINATION

Abdominal examination may show sub-involution of the uterus with retained tissue while offensive lochia, uterine tenderness and systemic signs of infection support the diagnosis of endometritis.

AVMs present with heavy vaginal bleeding and, occasionally, haemodynamic compromise.

CONTROVERSIES

❶ The timing of delivery in patients with mild antepartum haemorrhage due to placental abruption.

❷ Suppression of labour in patients with APH.

❸ The timing and interpretation of ultrasound investigation in patients with secondary PPH.

INVESTIGATIONS

Cervical swabs for microscopy and cul-ture and *Chlamydia trachomatis* detec-tion will help guide the management of endometritis. Full blood examination and blood cultures are indicated if the woman is clinically septic. Ultrasound is used to diagnose AVMs and can quantify the amount of retained products of conception.

TREATMENT

If endometritis is suspected and the woman is systemically well, empirical outpatient treatment with amoxicillin/ clavulanic acid 875 mg/125 mg bd for 5–7 days is appropriate. Erythromycin can be substituted in penicillin sensitive patients. If clinically septic, admission and intravenous antibiotics are required.

If bleeding persists ultrasound exami-nation should be performed to look for retained products of conception. Patients with small amounts of retained products of conception may be treated conser-vatively. Uterine curettage in the post-partum period is associated with the risks of uterine perforation or Asherman syndrome, from traumatic removal of all endometrium leading to intra-uterine adhesions, and, therefore, should only be performed by experienced operators.

REFERENCES

1. Cotton D, Ead J, Paul R, Quilligan E 1980 The conservative aggressive management of placenta praevia. American Journal of Obstetrics and Gynecology 17: 687–9
2. Saftlas A, Olsen D, Atras H, et al 1991 National trends in the incidence of abruptio placenta. Obstetrics and Gynecology 78: 1081–6
3. Paterson M 1986 The aetiology and outcome of abruptio placentae in Sweden. Obstetrics and Gynaecology 67: 523–8
4. Hack M, Fanaroff AA 1999 Outcomes of children of extremely low birthweight and gestational age in the 1990s. Early Human Development 53(3): 193–218
5. Bonnar J 2000 Massive obstetric haemorrhage. Best Practice & Research in Clinical Obstetrics and Gynaecology 14(1): 1–18

18.4 ABNORMAL VAGINAL BLEEDING IN THE NON-PREGNANT PATIENT

MEL E. HERBERT • MARY L. LANCTOT

ESSENTIALS

1 The most important part of the assessment of a patient with vaginal bleeding is the exclusion of pregnancy.

2 Treatment is based on the degree of haemodynamic stability and the most likely diagnosis.

3 Lesions that are bleeding excessively are best treated by local measures, such as suturing and packing.

4 Empiric hormonal manipulation is appropriate in patients with a clinical diagnosis of dysfunctional uterine bleeding (DUB) after a reasonable search for an alternative diagnosis. The use of oral contraceptives remains a simple and effective therapy for most patients with DUB.

5 In patients over 35 years of age endometrial biopsy should precede oestrogen therapy.

6 NSAIDs are also effective for many forms of uterine bleeding.

INTRODUCTION

Vaginal bleeding can be divided into two major categories: that which occurs in pregnancy and that which occurs in the non-pregnant patient. Therefore, the first step in diagnosing a patient who presents with vaginal bleeding is to determine whether or not she is pregnant. Non-pregnancy-related vaginal bleeding is caused by multiple aetiologies with significantly different prognoses and therapies than pregnancy-related bleeding. This chapter deals exclusively with bleeding in non-pregnant women.

DEFINITIONS

- *Menorrhagia:* menstrual cycles that are either excessive or prolonged.
- *Metromenorrhagia:* prolonged or excessive bleeding that occurs at irregular intervals.
- *Oligomenorrhoea:* interval between uterine bleeding from 35 days to 6 months.
- *Polymenorrhoea:* regular bleeding that occurs at intervals shorter than 21 days.
- *Amenorrhoea:* the absence of bleeding for more than 6 months.
- *Intermenstrual bleeding:* bleeding that occurs between otherwise regular menstrual periods.

CAUSES OF ABNORMAL VAGINAL BLEEDING

Dysfunctional uterine bleeding (DUB) is the term used for bleeding in patients who are not taking exogenous hormones and have no causative structural lesions. DUB is usually the result of anovulatory cycles causing oestrogen overstimulation and proliferation of the uterine lining. Anovulatory DUB is responsive to hormonal manipulation. However, in 10–15% of cases of DUB the cycles are

ovulatory and the hormonal therapy is less effective.[1] The differentiation of ovulatory from anovulatory bleeding can usually be made on the history alone. Anovulatory bleeding is irregular in timing and amount, whereas ovulatory bleeding follows the usual cyclic periodicity, but is heavy in nature. Other causes of vaginal bleeding can be divided by anatomical location, as in Table 18.4.1.

It is helpful to consider the causes of bleeding by age group. In adolescence, anovulatory DUB is extremely common.[2] In perimenopausal patients anovulatory DUB is also common, as is uterine and cervical malignancy. In the postmenopausal patient always consider uterine and cervical malignancy. In patients of all ages consider exogenous hormone use and coagulopathies.

HISTORY

A menstrual history is important in determining the cause of vaginal bleeding. This should focus on cycle length, regularity, the presence of inter-menstrual bleeding and the presence of clots. Patient estimates of the amount of vaginal bleeding are inaccurate and, therefore, have limited use in diagnosis, but the presence of clots is abnormal

Table 18.4.1 Causes of vaginal bleeding by anatomical site			
Vulva	*Vagina*	*Cervix*	*Uterine*
Neoplasm	Neoplasm	Neoplasm	Endometrial cancer
Trauma	Trauma	Cervical polyps	Uterine polyps
Infectious lesions	Vaginitis	Cervicitis	Fibroids
	Foreign body	Ectropion	Endometritis Intra-uterine device (IUD) Dysfunctional uterine bleeding (DUB)

and suggests heavy bleeding.[3] Other historical information should include evidence of a cancer, familial bleeding disorders, a bleeding diathesis, sexually transmitted diseases, trauma and exogenous steroid use. Classically, the diagnosis of anovulatory bleeding is made from the history of irregular menses with periods of amenorrhoea followed by heavy bleeding. Some clinicians suggest that these historical features alone may confirm this diagnosis.

PHYSICAL EXAMINATION

Determination of the haemodynamic stability of the patient is essential. Search for evidence of anaemia, bleeding disorders and endocrinopathies. Many local causes of bleeding, such as trauma or malignancy, can be excluded by careful pelvic examination. This examination should focus on the presence and amount of bleeding, cervical lesions, evidence of STD or trauma, and the size of the uterus.

INVESTIGATIONS

- Pregnancy test: this should be performed immediately on all women of childbearing age, even in the face of assurances from the patient that pregnancy could not be a possibility. These tests are highly sensitive: a negative test excludes pregnancy with 99% accuracy.[4]
- Haematocrit: there should be a low threshold for performing this test, as an abnormal result may alter management and the clinical estimation of anaemia is unreliable.[5]
- Tests for bleeding disorders: these tests are directed by the presence and type of bleeding disorder elicited on history and physical examination.
- Ultrasound: when the diagnosis is unclear or the uterus is enlarged, ultrasound is essential in diagnosing anatomical causes of bleeding such as fibroids.

MANAGEMENT

General measures

Determination of the patient's haemodynamic stability is the first step in the management of vaginal bleeding. Resuscitation should proceed in the usual manner. The initial specific therapy instituted is determined by the degree of patient stability.

Specific treatments

Therapy for DUB

Conjugated oestrogens In unstable patients with DUB, bleeding can be controlled with either a D and C or intravenous conjugated oestrogen at a dose of 25 µg q6h until bleeding stops, commonly between 24 and 48 hours. This appears effective in both ovulatory and anovulatory bleeding.[6]

Oral contraceptives In patients under 35 years of age with no evidence of uterine malignancy or other pathology a presumptive diagnosis of DUB may be followed by the institution of hormonal manipulation. A simple and effective regimen is to prescribe oral contraceptives (OCPs), which decrease menstrual bleeding by 50%, reduce dysmenorrhoea and may be effective in some patients with fibroids.[8] In patients over 35 years of age no hormonal therapy should be instituted until a biopsy of the endometrial tissue has been taken to exclude uterine cancer. Standard dosing involves three to four progestogen-dominant monophasic OCPs each day for 5 to 7 days. The patient is then asked to take a single tablet per day for 3 weeks, when the medication is withdrawn and bleeding ensues.

NSAIDs Cyclo-oxygenase prostaglandin inhibitors are also effective in the therapy of menorrhagia associated with DUB. NSAIDs block prostaglandin PGE$_2$, a vasodilator in the endometrium that may be found in excess in patients with menorrhagia. NSAIDs have been associated with a 30–50% reduction in bleeding in patients with menorrhagia.[8]

This class of drugs has the added benefit of providing analgesia, as many of these patients also experience concurrent dysmenorrhoea. An inexpensive and effective regimen is ibuprofen 600 mg q6h. The agent most studied is mefenamic acid, but it is unclear if any particular NSAID is superior to another.

Progesterone agents Progesterone antagonizes the effects of oestrogen on the uterus. Progesterones can be used to reduce bleeding in the acute setting, and then on a regular basis to prevent uterine endometrial overgrowth. A number of regimens are frequently used. It is important to remember that progesterone alone is not an effective contraceptive in many patients.

Some progesterone regimens are as follows:

- *Medroxyprogesterone acetate*: 30–40 mg/day for 1 week, then decrease the dose by 10 mg/day each week until 10 mg/day is reached. Bleeding usually stops in the first few days. After 3–4 weeks the progesterone can be removed. The patient should be advised that a withdrawal bleed will occur.
- *Progesterone* may be given in a dose of 10 mg/day, with daily dose increases until bleeding stops. Maintain the dose for 3–4 weeks, then withdraw the medication, again informing the patient that a withdrawal bleed will occur. Patients with ongoing anovulatory cycles may have progesterone for 10 days per month to ensure cyclic shedding and prevent overgrowth of the endometrium.

Other agents Tranexamic acid has been shown to reduce menstrual blood flow when compared to placebo. This plasminogen acitvator inhibitor acts by promoting local haemostasis. Clinically significant reductions (40–60%) in menstrual blood loss have been consistently reported. Dosing regimes vary. One regime is 1 g q6h for 4 days. Nausea and leg cramps have been described in up to one-third of patients taking this medication making its side-effect profile less desirable.

Danazol has been shown to reduce menstrual blood loss, but again 40% of women taking this agent report an unacceptable adverse effects, such as weight gain, oily skin, acne, and deepening of the voice. As this drug adds little benefit over and above the therapies previously discussed, the role in the emergency department setting is limited.

Iron therapy   The anaemic patient will require treatment with iron therapy. Doses in the range of 60–180 mg of elemental iron are sufficent and in some cases the only therapy required.[9]

Therapy of structural lesions

- Traumatic cervical bleeding that requires immediate therapy is best controlled by a simple stitch with a nylon suture. This is also appropriate for bleeding polyps or other well-defined anatomical lesions. Cautery or adrenaline (epinephrine) injection may be useful in patients with less brisk bleeding.
- Cervical bleeding from malignancy is harder to control because the lesions tend to be friable and sutures frequently pull through. Most cases do not require therapy in the emergency department but, if needed, cautery with silver nitrate or electricity may be sufficient. Brisk bleeding that cannot be controlled is best treated with vaginal packing with 1:200 000 adrenaline (epinephrine)-soaked gauze and immediate gynaecology consultation.
- Uterine bleeding that is thought to be from trauma or malignancy is diffcult to control. In extreme cases temporary uterine packing may be indicated. Gynaecology consultation should be sought immediately.

CONTROVERSIES

❶ The absolute degree of anaemia, in an otherwise stable patient, which requires transfusion.

❷ In DUB, the selection of hormonal therapy varies greatly between institutions and physicians.

- Fibroid bleeding is best controlled with NSAIDs and hormonal therapy. In rare cases where the bleeding is brisk, a gynaecology consultation in the emergency department should be obtained.
- Infections are treated on their own merits.
- Exogenous steroids are a frequent cause of abnormal bleeding that is rarely ever life-threatening. These patients are best treated by referral to their gynaecologist.

All invasive interventions are preceded by appropriate analgesia and, if necessary, sedation. The statement that the 'cervix does not feel pain' is a myth.

DISPOSITION

Patients with haemodynamic instability or profound anaemia need to be admitted for blood transfusion and other therapies directed at the cause of the bleeding. Consultation and further investigation may be delayed in patients who are stable, who have a small amount of bleeding or bleeding that is controlled in the emergency department, and have no significant anaemia. The majority of cases of DUB are controlled with hormonal therapy.

CONCLUSION

A systematic approach to vaginal bleeding must include the exclusion of pregnancy and the search for anatomical lesions. In patients with DUB, hormonal therapy and NSAIDs are usually effective.

REFERENCES

1. Altchek A 1977 Dysfunctional uterine bleeding in adolescence. Clinical Obstetrics and Gynecology 20: 633–50
2. Brennan DF 1995 Ectopic pregnancy - Part I: Clinical and laboratory diagnosis. Academy of Emergency Medicine 2(12): 1081–9
3. Cartwright PS 1995 Diagnosis of early pregnancy and early complications. Medical Clinics of North America 79(6): 1319–33
4. Rayburn WF, Carey JC 1996 Normal and abnormal menses. In: Obstetrics and gynecology. Williams & Wilkins, Baltimore, p. 337
5. Sheth TN, et al 1997 The relation of conjunctival pallor to the presence of anemia. Journal of General Internal Medicine 12(2): 102
6. De Vore GR, Owens O, Kase N 1982 Use of intravenous Premarin in the treatment of dysfunctional uterine bleeding: a double-blind randomized control study. Obstetrics and Gynecology 59: 285–91
7. van Eijkeren MA, Christiaens GCML, Scholten PC, et al 1992 Menorrhagia: current drug treatment concepts. Drugs 43: 201–9
8. Walthen PI, Henderson MC, Witz CA 1995 Abnormal uterine bleeding. Medical Clinics of North America 79: 329–42
9. Munro MG 2000 Medical management of abnormal uterine bleeding. Obstetric and Gynecology Clinics of North America 27(2): 287–304

FURTHER READING

Jennings JC 1995 Abnormal uterine bleeding. Medical Clinics of North America 79: 1357–76
MacKay HT 1996 Non-pregnancy related vaginal bleeding. In: Harwood-Nuss, Linden CH, Luten R (eds) The Clinical Practice of Emergency Medicine, 2nd edn. Lippincott-Raven, Philadelphia
Seamens C, Slovis CM 1996 Abnormal vaginal bleeding in the nonpregnant patient. Emergency Medicine Reports 17(22): 219–28

18.5 PELVIC INFLAMMATORY DISEASE

SHEILA BRYAN

ESSENTIALS

1 Pelvic inflammatory disease (PID) is an inflammation of the upper genital tract. The clinical presentation ranges from mild or atypical disease through to peritonitis.

2 Sequelae of PID include infertility, chronic pelvic pain and ectopic pregnancy. The severity of the initial infection does not relate to the risk of late complications.

3 Chlamydia trachomatis is the most common pathogen identified in PID. Other pathogens include Neisseria gonorrhoeae and mixed anaerobes. Screening high-risk patients for sexually transmitted infections reduces the incidence of PID.

4 Owing to the high incidence of significant long-term sequelae and the difficulty of clinical diagnosis, empirical treatment should be initiated on the basis of minimal diagnostic criteria.

5 Management includes antibiotics to cover N. gonorrhoeae, C. trachomatis and anaerobes.

INTRODUCTION

Pelvic inflammatory disease (PID) refers to a clinical syndrome resulting from infection or inflammation involving the endometrium, fallopian tubes, ovaries, broad ligaments and/or contiguous structures.

Most cases of PID are caused by the ascent of microorganisms from the endocervix and occasionally the vagina into the upper genital tract.[1] Sexually transmitted N. gonorrhoeae and C. trachomatis are the most common organisms involved with C. trachomatis being the most prevalent in Australia.[2] Many cases are polymicrobial with both aerobic and anaerobic bacteria being involved, although the role of anaerobes in the pathogenesis is unsure.

Although it is clear that the pathogenesis of many cases of PID involves the ascent of infection, the precise mechanism determining the spread of microorganisms from the lower to the upper genital tract remains unknown. The mechanism of tubular damage is direct cellular toxicity by N. gonorrhoeae and in the case of C. trachomatis the damage is secondary to a host immune response.[3,4]

The clinical diagnosis of acute PID is hampered by the wide range of associated clinical symptoms ranging from non-specific pelvic pain through to acute peritonitis.

EPIDEMIOLOGY

The exact incidence of PID is unknown due to the difficulty in clinical diagnosis. In 1999 an estimated 268 018 cases of PID were diagnosed in American emergency departments.[5]

Risk factors for PID include sexually transmitted infections and procedures that involve instrumentation of the cervix, for example dilation and curettage or termination of pregnancy. The presence of intrauterine contraceptive device (IUCD) does not increase the risk of PID except in the 20 days following their insertion.[6] The use of combined oral contraceptives is associated with an increased risk of colonization of the cervix with C. trachomatis and N. gonorrhoeae, but current data are unclear regarding the increased risk of PID.[7,8] There is also an increased risk of PID during or shortly after the menses.[9]

PRESENTATION

In an attempt to improve the sensitivity and specificity of the clinical diagnosis of PID, a number of combinations of clinical and laboratory features have been used as minimum criteria on which to diagnose PID and initiate treatment.[10] However, the minimum diagnostic criteria appear to lack sensitivity in identifying mild or atypical disease. Current recommendations are to initiate treatment for PID in any woman with either uterine or adnexal tenderness, or cervical motion tenderness if no other cause for the signs can be found.[11,12]

History

Abdominal pain is the most sensitive symptom of PID but as an isolated symptom it lacks specificity. Other symptoms may include abnormal vaginal bleeding, dyspareunia or vaginal discharge. The history should also assess for the recognized risk factors for PID such as younger age, young age at first sexual intercourse, multiple sexual partners and high frequency of sexual intercourse and instrumentation of the cervix.

Examination

The finding of adnexal tenderness has a sensitivity of 95% for the diagnosis of PID. An elevated oral temperature and the presence of vaginal discharge are also supportive of the diagnosis of PID.

A thorough examination should be performed to look for alternative causes for the symptoms. The presence of right upper quadrant pain in a patient with PID should raise the possibility of the Fitz-Hugh-Curtis syndrome (FHCS), which is an extra pelvic manifestation of PID involving both an acute and chronic phase. In the acute phase there is perihepatitis and focal peritonitis resulting from the transport of inflammatory peritoneal fluid to the subphrenic and subdiagphragmatic spaces. FHCS is usually an incidental finding in patients with PID but occasionally acute right upper quadrant pain may be the presenting complaint mimicking biliary disease.[13]

INVESTIGATIONS

Biochemical tests

A pregnancy test should be performed on all women of childbearing age. PID in pregnancy is rare but has significant implications for the fetus. Pelvic pain secondary to a complication of pregnancy is an important differential diagnosis.

Haematological tests

White cell count (WCC), erythrocyte sedimentation rate (ESR) and C-reactive protein (CRP) are all non-specific markers of inflammation that lack sensitivity and specificity in the diagnosis.[14]

Microbiology

Cervical cultures for *N. gonorrhoeae* and *C. trachomatis* should be taken. The delay required to identify pathogens limits the value of these tests in the initial diagnosis, although they have a role in retrospectively supporting the diagnosis of PID, defining antibiotic sensitivities and identifying the need to treat sexual partners.

The presence of either mucopus or white blood cells in the vaginal discharge is a sensitive marker for PID. If the cervical discharge appears normal and there are no white blood cells in the wet prep the diagnosis of PID is unlikely.[15]

Ultrasound

Ultrasound has an important role in assessing patients with pelvic pain. While vaginal ultrasound lacks sensitivity in the diagnosis of mild-to-moderate PID, it is valuable in the assessment of patients with tubo ovarian abscesses and in excluding other forms of pelvic pathology. Power Doppler transvaginal ultrasound has recently been shown to have a positive predictive value of 91% and a negative predictive value of 100% for mild PID. However, the technique has yet to be trialed further and may be of limited value due to the need for experienced operators.[16]

Other imaging techniques

Computerized tomography (CT), magnetic resonance imaging (MRI) and radiolabelled leucocyte scans have all been used to investigate pelvic pain. While they all appear to have good sensitivity and specificity in identification of PID they are not currently performed routinely.

Laparoscopy

Laparoscopy was previously considered to be the gold standard for diagnosing PID. Over the last few years the limitations of laparoscopy in the identification of mild disease have been highlighted and the new gold standard for diagnosis of PID is now a combination of laparoscopy and endometrial biopsy. However, the cost and the risk of even laparoscopy cannot always be justified, and so it is generally reserved for patients with either severe or chronic pelvic pain in whom a definitive diagnosis is sought.

DIFFERENTIAL DIAGNOSIS

Important differential diagnoses include appendicitis, diverticulitis, ectopic pregnancy, endometriosis, complications of ovarian cysts and ovarian tumours.

MANAGEMENT

Many patients with the clinical diagnosis of PID may be treated as outpatients. The main indications for hospital admission are:

- Clinically severe PID with temp >38°C.
- Oral antibiotics not appropriate either due to vomiting or unpredictable compliance.
- Failure to respond to 24–48 hours of outpatient therapy.
- Surgical emergencies such as appendicitis or ectopic pregnancy cannot be excluded.
- Coexistent medical problems such as pregnancy or diabetes mellitus.
- Adolescent age due to problems with compliance and the potential for severe consequences.

Antibiotic therapy[17]

Mild to moderate infection (non-sexually acquired):

- Amoxicillin plus clavulanate 875/125 mg orally 12 hourly for 7–10 days plus doxycycline 100 mg orally 12 hourly for 7–10 days. In pregnant or breast-feeding women doxycycline is contraindicated, and roxithromycin 300 mg orally for 14 days (category B1) is substituted.

Mild-to-moderate (sexually acquired) PID:

- Doxycycline 100 mg orally 12 hourly for 14 days plus metronidazole 400 mg orally 12 hourly for 14 days. Ceftriaxone 250 mg IM or IV plus 1 g azithromycin orally.

Severe infection (sexually acquired):

- Cefotaxime 1 g intravenously 8 hourly or ceftriaxone 1 g intravenously daily plus metronidazole 500 mg intravenously 12 hourly and doxycycline 100 mg orally 12 hourly.

Parenteral therapy should be continued until there is substantial improvement when an oral regimen can be commenced to complete 14 days of treatment.

In all proven cases of *N. gonorrhoeae* and *C. trachomatis* sexual partners should be treated.

DISPOSITION

All patients discharged on oral medication should be reviewed in 24–48 hours to assess the response to therapy.

CONTROVERSIES

❶ The indications for laparoscopy.

❷ Clinical criteria on which to initiate treatment.

❸ Oral vs parenteral therapy.

❹ The duration of therapy.

PROGNOSIS

Women with PID are at increased risk of chronic pelvic pain, ectopic pregnancy and infertility.[18]

REFERENCES

1. Cunningham FG, Hauth JC, Gilstrap LC 1978 The bacterial pathogenesis of acute pelvic inflammatory disease. Obstetrics and Gynecology 52(2): 161–4
2. Wang IR, Fraser IS 1997 Diagnosing and treating pelvic infections. Current Therapeutics 38(7): 37–45
3. Melly MA, Gregg CR, McGee ZA 1981 Studies on the toxicity of Neisseria gonorrhoeae for human fallopian tube mucosa. Journal of Infectious Diseases 143: 432–431
4. Paton DL Kuo CC Wang SP, Halbert SA 1987 Distal obstruction induced by repeated chlamydia trachomatis salpingeal infection in pig-tailed macaques. Journal of Infectious Diseases 155: 1292–9
5. Centers for Disease Control STD Surveillance 2000 Special focus profiles, STD's in women and infants.
6. Farley TM, Rosenberg MJ, Rowe PJ, Chen JH, Meink O 1992 Intrauterine devices and pelvic inflammatory disease: an international perspective. Lancet 339: 785–8
7. Barten JM, Nyange, PM, Richardson BA, et al 2001 Hormonal contraception and risk of sexually transmitted disease acquisition: results from a prospective study. American Journal of Obstetrics and Gynecology 185(20): 380–5
8. Ness RB, Soper DE, Holley RL, et al 2001 Hormonal and barrier contraception and risk of upper genital tract disease in the PID Evaluation and Clinical Health (PEACH) study. American Journal of Obstetrics and Gynecology 185(1): 121–7
9. Nowicki S, Tassell AH, Nowiki B 2000 Susceptibility to gonococcal infection during the menstrual cycle. Journal of the American Medical Association 283(10): 1291–2
10. Centers for Disease Control and Prevention 1998 Guidelines for treatment of sexually transmitted diseases. MMWR 47(No. RR-1): 79–85
11. Peipert JF, Ness RB, Blume J, et al 2001 Clinical predictors of endometritis in women with symptoms and signs of pelvic inflammatory disease.
American Journal of Obstetrics and Gynecology 184(5): 856–63
12. Centers for Disease Control and Prevention 2002 Sexually transmitted diseases treatment guidelines 2002. MMWR 51(NoRR-6): 32–6
13. Lopez-Zeno JA, Keith LG, Berger 1985 The Fitz-Hugh-Curtis syndrome revisited. Changing perspectives after half a century. Journal of Reproductive Medicine 30: 567–82
14. Peipert JF, Boardman J, Hogan JW, Sung J, Mayer KH 1996 Laboratory evaluation of acute upper genital tract infection. Obstetrics and Gynecology 87(5): 730–6
15. Peipert JF, Ness RB, Soper DE, Bass D 2000 Association of lower genital tract inflammation with objective evidence of endometritis. Infectious Diseases Obstetrics and Gynecology 8: 83–7
16. Molander P, Sjoberg J, Paavonen J, et al 2001 Transvaginal power doppler findings in laparoscopically proven acute pelvic inflammatory disease. Ultrasound Obstetrics and Gynecology 17: 233–8
17. Therapeutic Guidelines: Antibiotic Version 12, 2003. Therapeutic Guidelines Limited, Australia 69–71
18. Westrom L, Joesoef R, Reynolds G, et al 1991 Pelvic inflammatory disease and fertility. Sexually Transmitted Diseases 19(4): 185–92

18.6 PELVIC PAIN

MICHAEL CADOGAN • ANUSCH YAZDANI • JAMES TAYLOR

ESSENTIALS

1 The possibility of pregnancy must be considered in all patients of reproductive age with abdominal or pelvic pain.

2 Effective analgesia mandates the regular administration of non-steroidal anti-inflammatory (NSAID) drugs.

3 A negative pelvic examination even in the absence of other findings should not preclude a gynaecological referral.

4 Psychogenic pain is a diagnosis of exclusion.

INTRODUCTION

Pelvic and lower abdominal pain in female patients is a complex and challenging complaint. It is the second most common gynaecological symptom after vaginal bleeding. The large differential diagnosis for female pelvic pain makes a conclusive diagnosis in the emergency department difficult and, therefore, a systematic evaluation is essential. Within the emergency department, the emergency physician aims to identify and stabilize the critically ill patient, identify those conditions that require early surgical intervention and to expedite the investigation and further management of the female patient with pelvic pain, following adequate analgesia.

Conditions causing pelvic pain may be acute or chronic; gynaecological, non-gynaecological or non-organic and cyclical or acyclic. They may be life threatening and are often complex requiring ongoing care and management by other specialties. This chapter outlines the initial investigation and management of those gynaecological conditions most commonly associated with acute and chronic pelvic pain.

HISTORY

It is essential to take a thorough history to help determine the potential cause(s) of the patient's pain. Parietal pelvic pain may be well localized and occurs secondary to peritoneal irritation such as in appendicitis and Mittelschmerz. Generalized and diffuse abdominal pain is associated with significant amounts of intraperitoneal blood or pus resulting from the rupture of an ectopic pregnancy or tubo-ovarian abscess.

Pain of sudden onset is often associated with ovarian cyst rupture or adnexal torsion. Gradually worsening pain is more suggestive of a long-term process, such as endometriosis or chronic pelvic inflammatory disease. Pain with sexual intercourse (dyspareunia) may be associated with adnexal pathology and endometriosis.

An evaluation of the patient's sexual and menstrual history determines the potential for pregnancy-related problems or sexually-transmitted diseases (STD) and defines chronic pain as cyclic or acyclic. Particular details should include possible physical and sexual abuse; menarche; menopause; contraception; LMP; previous STD; gravida, parity, tubal surgery and previous ectopic pregnancy.

Careful consideration of the pain's radiation may provide clues as to the underlying origin of the pelvic pain. The uterine fundus, adnexae and bladder dome may be associated with pain referred to the lower abdomen via the hypogastric nerve plexus.

The S2–4 sacral nerve roots transmit pain from the lower uterine segment, cervix, bladder trigone and rectum to the lower back, buttocks, perineum and legs. It is also important to ask about associated urological, gastrointestinal and musculoskeletal symptoms.

Finally, psychosocial factors are particularly relevant in the evaluation of chronic pelvic pain (CPP). The symptoms of fatigue, loss of energy and depressed mood are commonly associated with chronic pelvic pain, and a screen for anxiety, depressive and somatoform disorders is essential. Enquiries about marital distress, the spouse's response to pain and the familial response to handling pain are all important.

EXAMINATION

The emergency physician must record the vital signs, consider early analgesia and establish rapport with the patient who may be reticent, frightened or embarrassed. The pulse, blood pressure and temperature are important in evaluating the potential for life-threatening haemorrhage such as an ectopic pregnancy or overwhelming sepsis associated with tubo-ovarian abscess.

Abdominal examination commences with inspection for distension associated with obstruction, ascites or abdominal masses. Palpation and percussion may delineate areas of generalized or localized tenderness and aim to replicate the patient's pain. At the same time, it is important to check for hernias, inguinal nodes and other non-gynaecological causes for the patient's symptoms (see Table 18.6.1).

A pelvic examination is essential in the sexually active patient. This should be performed in the presence of a chaperone after providing adequate explanation of the procedure and gaining verbal consent. The examination includes:

- **Visual examination** of the vulva and urethral meatus to identify varicosities, infection or abnormal lesions.
- **Speculum examination** aiming to directly visualize the cervix, cervical os and the vaginal vault. This allows the physician to note vaginal discharge, take endocervical and vaginal swabs and perform a PAP smear.
- **Bimanual (vagino-abdominal)** examination that examines the cervix, uterus and adnexae.

The normal uterus is mobile, but conditions such as endometriosis or adhesions may cause fixation. An enlarged uterus may be associated with pregnancy, fibroids and adenomyosis. The uterine axis is dependent on a number of other local pelvic factors, such as the relative content of the bladder or bowel. A retroverted uterus is usually normal, but a fixed retroverted uterus is classically associated with pouch of Douglas pathology such as endometriosis.

Uterine tenderness may occur with any pelvic peritonism, adenomyosis or fibroid degeneration. An open cervix may be associated with the passage of intrauterine pathology such as a failed pregnancy or clots. Cervical excitation is a non-specific sign associated with conditions that produce pelvic peritonism such as blood or other irritants in the peritoneal cavity. Palpable adnexal masses are associated with gross pathology, such as ovarian cysts and endometriomas, often associated with adnexal tenderness.

A rectovaginal examination allows palpation of the posterior cul-de-sac for ovarian masses, the posterior wall of the uterus and the uterosacral ligaments for nodularity and tenderness associated with endometriosis. It is best performed only once, preferably by the doctor with ongoing clinical care. The rectal examination completes the pelvic examination taking note of stool consistency, faecal occult blood and the presence of mass lesions.

A normal pelvic examination does not exclude pelvic pathology. It may still provide valuable information and helps in the selection of further definitive investigations, such as ultrasound scan (USS) and laparoscopy.

LABORATORY INVESTIGATIONS

Laboratory studies depend on the history and physical examination and are

Table 18.6.1 Causes of acute pelvic pain

Gynaecological	Intestinal	Non-gynaecological Urological	Other
Complication of pregnancy: ectopic, miscarriage	Appendicitis	Cystitis	Hernia
Complication of ovarian and adnexal cysts and masses	Diverticulitis	Acute urinary retention	Porphyria
Pelvic inflammatory disease	Inflammatory bowel disease	Urolithiasis	Pelvic vein thrombophlebitis
Adnexal torsion	Gastroenteritis	Pyelonephritis	
Leiomyoma complication	Bowel obstruction Constipation		

tailored to the individual patient. They include the following:

Urinalysis

Urinary β hCG is fast, cheap and reasonably accurate. It should be peformed in all sexually active patients. The presence of leucocytes in the urine may indicate infection, but can also be associated with inflammation of adjacent pelvic organs. The urine should still be sent for microscopy, culture and sensitivity if urinary-tract pathology is suspected, as dipstick sensitivities are only 70–75%. The urine may also be sent for chlamydial PCR, and the presence of red cells and casts noted in the consideration of urolithiasis.

Swabs

During the speculum examination, endocervical swabs for chlamydia, gonorrhoea and ureaplasma and a swab of the introitus for agents associated with vulvar vestibulitis, a cause of dyspareunia, should be taken.

A PAP smear test is of little benefit in the patient with acute pelvic pain, and the inability to guarantee adequate follow-up of the result excludes its performance.

Blood tests

Serum β hCG is usually positive 14 days post conception. Screening for pregnancy is an essential investigation with patients of reproductive age and a serum (or urine) pregnancy test should be performed. False-positive and -negative serum and urine tests do occur, but are rare.

A full blood count may be helpful in identifying the presence and likely type of anaemia, but does not determine the cause. A leucocytosis may indicate underlying infection or inflammation. An elevated ESR or CRP may indicate inflammation and acute pathology, and are included in the clinical diagnosis of PID in some centres. They must not be sent 'routinely'.

Tumour markers have a limited role in the evaluation of pelvic pain within the emergency department. Markers such as the CA 125 have a role in the evaluation of pelvic pain when an adnexal masses or endometriosis is suspected, and serial

levels improve the sensitivity and specificity of such markers, usually carried out on an outpatient basis.

IMAGING

Ultrasound assessment

This should now be regarded as a non-invasive extension of the physical examination. It is the single most useful test in diagnosing acute gynaecological presentations within the emergency department.

Ultrasound (USS) can determine the uterine size, presence of fibroids, and the thickness and characteristics of the endometrium and myometrium. It may delineate adnexal pathology such as ovarian cysts, endometriomata, hydro/pyosalpinx, tubo-ovarian abscess and tumours.

USS is a more accurate predictor of abnormal pelvic pathology, as confirmed by laparoscopy than pelvic examination alone. However, studies using laparoscopy as the gold standard still found that half of the patients with either a normal pelvic examination or ultrasound scan had abnormal laparoscopic findings.

Computerized tomography

Computerized tomography (CT) is helpful to delineate further pelvic masses such as malignancy or abscess formation. It may also be helpful in identifying urinary calculi, Spigelian hernias, abdominal tuberculosis and appendicitis.

Magnetic resonance imaging

Magnetic resonance imaging (MRI) may define adenomyosis and obstructive uterine anomalies associated with endometriosis. The high cost, limited availability and the requirement of specific rectal and vaginal coils currently limit its use.

DIFFERENTIAL DIAGNOSIS

Patients attending the emergency department may present with:

- Acute pelvic pain
- An acute presentation of chronic pelvic pain (acute-on-chronic)
- Chronic pelvic pain.

Acute pelvic pain

Table 18.6.1 summarizes the conditions that present to the emergency department with acute pelvic pain. The causes may be broken down into the following:

Pregnancy related

Pregnancy must be excluded in all women of reproductive age and, if diagnosed, ectopic pregnancy must then be excluded. See Chapter 18.2.

Pelvic inflammatory disease

See Chapter 18.5 on the evaluation of pelvic inflammatory disease.

Adnexal pathology

Ovarian

- Functional ovarian cysts are either follicular ovarian cysts that develop during the first 14 days of the menstrual cycle prior to ovulation, or corpus luteum cysts that develop during the last 14 days after ovulation. Functional cysts are usually asymptomatic unless complications occur. As these cysts are related to normal ovarian activity, ovarian cysts in the postmenopausal woman are never considered 'functional'.
- Neoplastic masses may be either benign or malignant. Features that increase the risk of malignancy include being postmenopausal, the presence of ascites and increasing size or complexity.
- Infective masses usually arise as part of a tubo-ovarian mass in association with PID.
- Endometriomata are deposits of endometriosis in association with the ovary, forming a collection of altered blood and cellular debris, hence the term 'chocolate cyst'.

Non-ovarian adnexal masses

- Para-ovarian and paratubal cysts are related to either the ovary or, more commonly, the Fallopian tube.

- Hydrosalpinx arises in the blocked fallopian tube.

Any of these structures may present acutely due to rupture, haemorrhage or torsion.

Rupture of ovarian cyst Follicular cyst rupture at ovulation may be accompanied by ovarian bleeding and peritoneal irritation during the mid-cycle known as Mittelschmerz. The rupture of a corpus luteum cyst usually occurs between days 20 and 26 of the menstrual cycle and is associated with intraperitoneal bleeding. This bleeding may be catastrophic depending on the size of the torn ovarian blood vessel. USS helps differentiate a ruptured ectopic pregnancy from a corpus luteum cyst, although they can coexist.

Intraovarian haemorrhage Haemorrhage may occur into a cyst or a tumour. The symptoms of sudden onset, sharp unilateral pain with increasing intensity result from ovarian capsule distension. There may be localized or generalized peritonism dependent on the degree of peritoneal irritation and haemorrhage extravasation. Pelvic examination may reveal a focal expanding adnexal mass, which is confirmed by USS.

Haemorrhagic ovarian cysts may be managed conservatively. Indications for intervention include failure to obtain adequate analgesia; failure of rapid symptom resolution and haemodynamic instability.

Torsion of adnexae The adnexae include the ovary and fallopian tube. Torsion occurs when these structures twist on their supportive appendages causing compromise of their vascular supply. It most commonly occurs in the third decade of life and accounts for 3–5% of emergency gynaecological surgery.

Over 90% of cases of adnexal torsion are associated with cystic tumours or simple cysts of the ovary. Torsion of the fallopian tube is less common and is associated with hydrosalpinx, tubal ligation and pelvic adhesions. Both of these conditions are often associated with an enlarging adnexal mass secondary to venous obstruction and secondary oedema.

Pain associated with adnexal torsion is commonly sudden in onset, sharp, unilateral and increasingly severe on a background of a dull pelvic ache. It is associated with nausea, vomiting, low-grade pyrexia and with urinary symptoms secondary to bladder irritation. Late presentations may be associated with ovarian necrosis, frank peritonitis and shock.

Pelvic examination reveals cervical motion tenderness, adnexal tenderness and a discrete adnexal mass in the majority of patients. USS usually confirms the underlying pathology and defines the adnexal mass.

Definitive diagnosis and treatment can be laparoscopically or via laparotomy.

Ovarian infection This may occur rarely as a primary event with mumps or tuberculosis, but usually occurs in the setting of PID with the formation of a tubo-ovarian abscess. See Chapter 18.5.

Chronic pelvic pain

Chronic pelvic pain is defined as pain lasting greater than 6 months, localized to the anatomic pelvis causing functional disability requiring medical or surgical treatment. It affects up to 15 million women worldwide and accounts for 10% of gynaecology outpatient attendances.

Patients usually present to the emergency department with an acute exacerbation of their chronic condition; an acute unrelated cause of pelvic pain or an inability to cope with their debilitating condition. The commonest diagnoses associated with chronic pelvic pain are endometriosis and pelvic adhesions, however, up to 60% of patients have no visible pathology at laparoscopy and 25% of patients remain without a definitive diagnosis.

Cyclic pelvic pain

Cyclic pelvic pain (see Table 18.6.2) occurs in 30–50% of reproductive age women and interferes with normal daily activities in up to 12% of cases. It is usually related to ovulation or menstruation. Many conditions that cause cyclic pain may ultimately cause acyclic pain, such as endometriosis.

Mittelschmerz Mittelschmerz is defined as a transient mid-cycle pain occurring at or after ovulation. Increasing ovarian capsular pressure is associated with poorly localized pain, which becomes localized following follicular rupture and the release of fluid and/or blood that causes peritoneal irritation.

Table 18.6.2 Causes of chronic pelvic pain	
Cyclic	*Acyclic*
Mittelschmerz	Chronic PID
Endometriosis *	Pelvic adhesions
Adenomyosis	Uterine prolapse
Cervical stenosis *	Chronic urethritis
Intra-uterine device	Diverticulitis
Leiomyoma (fibroids)	Irritable bowel syndrome
Primary and secondary dysmenorrhoea	Levator syndrome of the perirectal area
Pelvic congestion *	Detrusor instability
	Interstitial cystitis
	Abdominal hernias
	Abdominal wall myofascial pain
	Abuse syndromes: physical and sexual
	Depression
* May become acyclic	

There are usually minimal findings on physical examination, but a thorough evaluation is essential to rule out other pelvic pathology. A slightly enlarged ovary may be palpated on the affected side.

Mittelschmerz is a clinical diagnosis, but USS may reveal the presence of a recently ruptured follicle. Regular non-steroidal anti-inflammatory (NSAID) tablets and reassurance are the mainstay of treatment. Although the pain on presentation may be severe, it usually resolves spontaneously.

Endometriosis Endometriosis occurs when ectopic endometrial glands and stroma are present outside the uterine cavity. Initially the pain is cyclic and associated with menses, but as pelvic adhesions develop the pain often becomes continuous and acyclic.

Endometriosis affects women aged 20–45 and is the second most common cause of cyclic pain in reproductive age females. Over 70% of sufferers are nulliparous and up to 60% of patients investigated for infertility are found to have endometriosis.

Typically, the pain commences a few days prior to menses and extends variably into or beyond the period. Persistent, unilateral mid-cycle pain is suggestive of an endometrioma. Patients may also commonly present with dysmenorrhoea (75%), dyspareunia (20%), tenesmus or following the finding of an adnexal mass (endometrioma).

In the vast majority of women with endometriosis, the physical examination is completely normal. Findings suggestive of endometriosis include adnexal tenderness during menses and a fixed retroverted uterus with posterior tenderness. In addition, uterosacral ligament and posterior uterus nodularity with tenderness on rectovaginal examination is characteristic, but may not always be present.

USS may reveal endometriomas but not focal endometriotic lesions. The diagnosis may only be made definitively on histology. Laparoscopic excision is both diagnostic and therapeutic.

Adenomyosis Adenomyosis is a benign condition characterized by the ingrowth of the endometrial glands and stroma into the myometrium. The majority (>80%) of cases involve multiparous women in the fourth and fifth decade of life. Patients usually present with menorrhagia and dysmenorrhoea.

Pelvic examination reveals a symmetrically enlarged, slightly tender uterus with a diffusely boggy consistency. Rarely, a large mass (adenomyoma) may be palpated.

USS may reveal generalized uterine enlargement with indistinct myo-endometrial margins. However, MRI will clearly demonstrate the pathology.

Hysteroscopy and endometrial biopsy may demonstrate adenomyosis, but definitive diagnosis is usually made at hysterectomy.

Leiomyomata (fibroids) Leiomyomas or fibroids are benign tumours of myometrial origin. They are the commonest pelvic tumour and occur in 25% of Caucasian women and 50% of black women. Their aetiology is unknown but they are seen to recede in the climacteric and enlarge in pregnancy.

Symptoms are usually associated with chronic cyclic pelvic pain with or without bleeding. Acute pain occurs with torsion or degeneration. Torsion usually involves pedunculated subserosal lesions. Degeneration is usually associated with pregnancy and results from the rapidly expanding lesion restricting its own blood supply.

Fibroids may be palpated on bimanual pelvic examination. The lesions are usually painless unless associated with acute degeneration when uterine tenderness, pyrexia and leucocytosis may be seen.

Treatment of chronic leiomyomata is usually conservative unless associated with marked anaemia. The patient with acute torsion or degeneration of a fibroid requires opiate analgesia and urgent gynaecological review for definitive management.

Dysmenorrhoea

Primary dysmenorrhoea This is painful menstruation in the absence of pelvic pathology and is a diagnosis of exclusion. Primary dysmenorrhoea is associated with the release of prostaglandins, principally PGF2α, from the endometrium during menstruation. This causes abnormal uterine contractions, arteriolar vasoconstriction and uterine ischaemia with the most intense pain occurring as the menstrual flow is subsiding. It usually coincides with the onset of ovulatory cycles 4–12 months after menarche and affects up to 10% of young nulliparous women.

Primary dysmenorrhoea is associated with spasmodic, crampy lower abdominal pain radiating to the lower back and upper thighs, and usually lasts 24–48 hours. Associated symptoms include headache, nausea and vomiting.

The symptoms of primary dysmenorrhoea may be alleviated by regular administration of non-steroidal anti-inflammatory (NSAID) drugs or by suppressing ovulation with the oral contraceptive pill.

Secondary dysmenorrhoea This is painful menstruation associated with pelvic pathology including cervical stenosis, adenomyosis, leiomyomata, pelvic congestion syndrome and the intra-uterine contraceptive device. It usually affects women later in life and symptoms often start earlier in the menstrual cycle and can precede menstruation.

Acyclic pelvic pain

Pelvic adhesions Adhesions occur when anatomic structures are abnormally bound to one another by bands of fibrous tissue. They are believed to account for the pain suffered by up to 33% of patients with chronic pelvic pain, although their exact role is uncertain. They are associated with PID, endometriosis, abdominal surgery, perforated appendix and inflammatory bowel disease.

Adhesions contain their own nerve fibres and the pain perceived by patients is thought to originate within the fibrous tissue when it is under tension. The pain is often consistent in location and aggravated by sudden movements, intercourse or physical activity. Laparoscopy is the gold standard for diagnosis and treatment.

Pelvic congestion syndrome Pelvic congestion syndrome is characterized by dilation, congestion and venous stasis of the pelvic veins. This syndrome is associated with multiparity, polycystic ovarian syndrome, tubal ligation and lower limb varicosities.

Patients commonly present with a chronic, dull ache localized to the pelvis and lower back with exacerbations of sharp stabbing pain. Other symptoms include dyspareunia (75%), dysfunctional uterine bleeding (54%) and mucoid vaginal discharge (47%).

Deep abdominal palpation, particularly over the adnexae, usually reproduces the patients' pain. Superficial vulval varices are often seen on external examination and speculum examination may reveal a bluish tinge to the engorged cervix.

Pelvic venography can establish the size of varicosities and the site of incompetence. Ultrasound may demonstrate uterine enlargement and venous incompetence.

CONTROVERSIES

❶ Focused ultrasound scan training of emergency physicians to evaluate pelvic pain

---

Psychological There is an association between chronic pelvic pain and somatization disorders. In addition, many women with chronic pelvic pain have suffered physical, sexual and emotional abuse, and psychiatric disease is often missed.

CONCLUSION

Pelvic pain in the female patient presents a complex and challenging problem to the emergency physician. Systematic evaluation may be rewarded with a diagnosis in acute pelvic pain, but chronic conditions require review and follow-up with a specialist unit.

The exclusion of pregnancy-related problems, provision of adequate analgesia, resuscitation of the acutely unwell patient, prompt initiation of appropriate investigations and specialist referral for ongoing evaluation are paramount to the management of gynaecological pelvic pain.

FURTHER READING

Berchuk A, Boente MP, Bast RB 1992 The use of tumour markers in the management of patients with gynaecological carcinomas. Clinical Obstetrics and Gynaecology 35(1): 45–54

Carter JE 1993 A systematic history for the patient with pelvic pain. JSLS 3: 245–52

Howard FM 1993 The role of laparoscopy in chronic pelvic pain: promise and pitfalls. Obstetrics and Gynaecology Surv 48: 357–87

Howard FM, Perry CP, Carter JE, El-Minawi AM 2000 Pelvic Pain: Diagnosis and Management. Lippincott, New York

Muse KN 1990 Cyclic pelvic pain. Obstetrics and Gynaecology Clinics of North America 17: 427

Scialli AR, Barbieri RL, Glasser MH, Olive DL, Winkel CA 2000 Chronic pelvic pain: An integrated approach. Medical Education Collaborative, Association of Professors of Gynaecology and Obstetrics: 3–9

OBSTETRICS AND GYNAECOLOGY

18

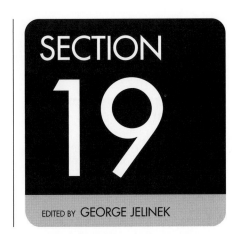

EDITED BY GEORGE JELINEK

PSYCHIATRIC EMERGENCIES

19.1 Mental state assessment *580*

19.2 Distinguishing medical from psychiatric causes of mental disorder presentations *584*

19.3 The violent patient *590*

19.4 Deliberate self harm/suicide *597*

19.1 MENTAL STATE ASSESSMENT

SYLVIA ANDREW-STARKEY

ESSENTIALS

1 The mental state examination should form part of the examination of any patient who has neurological impairment, altered level of consciousness or behavioural disturbance, for whatever reason.

2 Safety for all concerned is paramount.

3 The use of a standard format ensures consistency and understanding between healthcare professionals.

4 The mental state examination should be followed by a physical examination, and investigations if necessary, to exclude organic illness.

INTRODUCTION

About 1–2% of emergency department patients require a formal mental state assessment.[1] These are usually patients being assessed after a toxic ingestion, other act of self-harm, or unusual or aggressive behaviour. Generally these assessments are performed after hours, are difficult to organize, and utilize considerable resources. Staff in the emergency department, surrounded by the physically ill or injured, may not be enthusiastic about seeing patients requiring a mental-state assessment. Patients are often reluctant to disclose intimate feelings to a medical team, and can be uncooperative or abusive, particularly when intoxicated. It is not surprising that some emergency department personnel find the assessment of behaviourally disturbed patients unrewarding.

MENTAL STATE EXAMINATION

The psychiatric mental state examination (MSE) is an orderly method of recording a psychiatric interview. Useful information can be gathered and MSE can be performed on any uncooperative patient, even if totally mute. Careful observation, active listening to what the patient says, gathering information from relatives and friends, and an organized and systematic approach to documentation are paramount to the success of the psychiatric assessment. As other people are usually involved in the person's crisis, it is important to listen to relatives, friends or caregivers, and to police or ambulance officers. MSE is a fluid process: a patient's response may change with time.[2] Some of the major components of the MSE are listed in Table 19.1.1.[2–4]

The two key elements to an MSE are the actual interview itself and observations made during the interview. Following an MSE, the interviewer should be able to answer a number of questions (Table 19.1.2). The answers will determine the patient's appropriate disposition.

It is vital to ensure that an opinion regarding treatment and management is not based on factors such as religious beliefs, political opinion, sexual preference or promiscuity, intellectual or physical disability, or acute intoxication due to the influence of drugs or alcohol (Table 19.1.3). The interviewer should also be aware of personal feelings towards behaviourally disturbed patients. These may stem from experience, both professional and personal, and may influence management and treatment. They may also influence the way in which a patient interacts with the interviewer, and can be the difference between a successful and an unsuccessful MSE.

After performing a complete MSE the emergency physician can make a reasonable assessment of the likely problem, the likelihood of cooperation with treatment, and the appropriate disposition.

Table 19.1.1 Overview of a mental state examination

General description
    Appearance
    Behaviour
    Attitudes

Mood and affect
    Mood
    Affect
    Appropriateness

Speech

Perception

Thought processes
    Content
    Form

Cognition
    Consciousness
    Orientation
    Memory
    Intelligence

Insight and judgement

Impulse control

Table 19.1.2 Criteria determining management and disposition

Does the patient have an illness?

Is there a question of safety for the patient or for the protection of others?

Does the patient have insight into the illness?

Will the patient comply with suggested treatment?

Can the patient be managed in the community or is hospitalization required?

Table 19.1.3 Factors that should not influence a psychiatric opinion

Religious beliefs

Political opinion

Philosophical beliefs

Sexual preference or orientation

Promiscuity or immorality

Intellectual disability

Intoxication with drugs or alcohol

SECURITY AND SAFETY

Before entering the interview area it is important to determine its safety. Risk factors for violence should be considered (see Chapter 19.3). If any risk factors are present, the interviewer must have security guards or police present or close at hand to ensure the safety of all concerned.

Before commencing an interview, the interviewer should inform nursing or medical staff of the location and approximate length of time for the interview. The interviewer may choose to wear a personal alarm. Important aspects to note upon entering the room are the nearest exit, and items of furniture that could be used as weapons. The interviewer should sit between the patient and the door, and should never be boxed into a corner. If the interviewer begins to feel uncomfortable at any stage, the option of leaving and returning at a later stage should be open. All threats, attempts and gestures should be treated seriously.[5,6]

BEGINNING THE MSE

The MSE should begin with an introduction and with the interviewer establishing rapport. Behaviourally disturbed patients are unable to tolerate noise, and so should be in a private and safe environment. The patient should feel secure.[1,7] The patient may have a short concentration span, and so interruptions should be avoided as they disrupt the flow of the interview. Body language is important, and so the interviewer should try to impart an air of empathy regardless of personal feelings. The interviewer should sit on the same level as the patient and explain the process that is going to occur. The voice should be quiet and calm. A warm, caring attitude should be conveyed, with genuine concern for the person and their problems. Open-ended questions should be used. Deception should be avoided and promises should not be made unless they can be kept.

THE FORMAL PSYCHIATRIC INTERVIEW

Basic demographic information

The interviewer can begin by asking a series of non-threatening questions to create a profile of the lifestyle and thought processes of the patient. Very basic information about the patient and the home situation is collected, including data about significant persons in the circle of family and friends and the quality of relationships with these persons. Ask also about family history of disease (both medical and psychiatric).

Questions should be asked about previous history (medical as well as psychiatric) and drug or alcohol use (prescription or illicit). Previous medical history and regular medications should be noted, as a number of organic disorders and the drugs used to treat them have side effects that include behaviour and mood changes. A summary of these is given in Table 19.1.4.

Table 19.1.4 Demographic information
Age
Address
Other persons (and relationship to the patient) at home address
Social resources: family, friends, and their location and relationship with them
Occupation and occupational history
Past medical history
Previous hospital admissions

Previous psychiatric hospital admissions
    Length of stay in hospital
    Type of treatment (medication or ECT)
    Medications on discharge
    Follow-up arrangements
    Family history of illness

Alcohol
Drug use
Tobacco use
Hobbies

Presenting complaint

The patient should provide a recollection of the day's events. The interviewer should establish why the patient has presented at just this moment, and what precipitated events. A crisis that is part of a long-standing life struggle is not likely to benefit from intervention, whereas a fundamental change which has occurred in a patient's life may.[7]

Method of transportation to the emergency department is important in determining compliance with treatment and management. A patient voluntarily attending the emergency department may have some insight and is likely to request treatment; a patient restrained and handcuffed by police is unlikely to comply with community management.

Mood and affect

The interviewer should ask questions regarding the patient's mood (internal feelings) and whether it is in keeping with affect (external expression). The mood may be incongruent with affect, swing wildly between extremes (labile), or be completely inappropriate.

Usually, mood is assessed by asking about the patient's ability to cope with activities of daily living, such as eating, weight loss or gain, sleep disturbance (early morning wakening or trouble getting to sleep) and general hygiene. The patient's ability to concentrate may also diminish with increasing mood disturbance, reflected by the ability to perform normal work duties.

This may lead to direct questioning regarding mood and thoughts of suicide. Be direct in asking the patient about suicide and a formulated plan. A well-thought-out plan with a clear means of carrying out threats is of great concern.

Delusions and hallucinations

Delusions and hallucinations are often very personal, and the patient may not wish to disclose intimate thoughts and beliefs to the interviewer. Hallucinations can be auditory, visual, tactile, olfactory, somatic or gustatory. The context in which they occur should be explored. Hypnagogic (occurring just before sleep) and hypnopompic (occurring on awakening) hallucinations are more benign than others. Common themes for all types of hallucinations include suicide, persecution, control, reference, religion, grandeur or somatization.

Impulsivity

The interviewer should ask if the patient has been in trouble with police before, or if there is a criminal record. Patients with poor impulse control tend to have multiple dealings with law enforcement agencies. They often are incapable of controlling aggressive, hostile, guilty, affectionate or sexual impulses appropriately. The method of expression of these impulses (verbal or behavioural) is also important in determining the ultimate disposition for the patient.[2] A patient who is impulsive and has poor judgement is likely to need a great deal of supervision, and may be more appropriately managed in a psychiatric hospital, whereas someone who gives careful thought before acting may suitably remain at the usual place of residence with minimal supervision.

Insight and judgement

Insight is the degree of understanding of what is happening and why.[3] This may vary as follows:

- Complete denial of illness
- Slight awareness of being sick and needing help, but denying it at the same time
- Awareness of being sick but blaming it on others or external factors
- Awareness that illness is due to something unknown within the patient
- Intellectual insight: admission that the patient is ill and that symptoms are due to their own irrational feelings, but without being able to apply this to the future
- True insight: being aware of motives and feelings and being aware of what can lead to changes in behaviour.

It is important to determine the patient's level of insight, if any: it is a determinant of appropriate management and treatment, the level of supervision required, and the likelihood of compliance with treatment.

OBSERVATIONS DURING THE INTERVIEW

The next part of the MSE consists of documenting observations made during the interview. The interviewer should be aware of what the patient is saying, how it is said, and what the patient is doing. The interviewer should be a participant observer, participating with and actively observing the actions of the patient.[1]

Appearance, attitude and behaviour[8]

The interviewer should determine the overall physical and emotional impression conveyed by the patient. This is an important indication of the patient's ability to self-care. Table 19.1.5 lists features requiring particular attention. Attitude to the interviewer is important, and may indicate whether the patient will be compliant with management and treatment.

Abnormal posturing or repetitive behaviours should be noted. These may indicate increasing thought disturbance. With increasing aggression and agitation there may be motor restlessness, pacing and hand-wringing. Tension in this situation may escalate rapidly, and steps should be taken early to defuse the situation.

The interviewer should note the rate, volume and rhythmicity of speech. This can range from completely mute, through monosyllabic answers to rapid, loud speech indicative of pressure of speech. The tone, inflection, content and structure of speech should also be noted. The interviewer should determine if the speech is fluent, if the thoughts behind it are logical, and whether it flows appropriately for the situation.

Thought disorder

Behaviourally disturbed patients show many patterns of thought disorder. A brief list and explanation is given in Table 19.1.6. Speech in behaviourally disturbed patients often does not reach its goal, is not fluent, and is interrupted

Table 19.1.5 General appearance and behaviour

General
  Clothes
  Application
  Appropriate for climate

Cleanliness
  General grooming (hair, nails)
  Tattoos, track marks in arms

Eye contact
  Avoids direct gaze
  Decreases with increasing anxiety

Facial expression   Variation in facial expression, voice, use of hands and body movements
Reaction to the interviewer   Aggressive, submissive, cooperative, guarded, evasive, passive or hostile

Motor
  Restless
  Repetitive behaviour, e.g. rocking, hand-wringing
  Tremor
  Posturing
  Tics
  Tardive dyskinesia

Speech
  Rate, volume and rhythm
  Mute
  Poverty of speech (slow, monosyllabic responses)
  Pressure of speech (extremely rapid, loud speech)
  Normal inflection or flat and monotonous

Table 19.1.6 Thought disorder

Circumstantiality	Delays in reaching goals by long-winded explanations, but eventually gets there
Distractible speech	Changes topic according to what is happening around the patient
Loosening of associations	Thought pattern where logical progression
'Cottonwool thinking'	Does not occur and ideas shift from one subject to another with little or no association between them
Flight of ideas	Fragmented, rapid thoughts that the patient cannot express fully as they are occurring at such a rapid rate
Tangentiality	Responses that superficially appear appropriate, but which are completely irrelevant or oblique
Clanging	Speech where words are chosen because they rhyme and do not make sense
Neologisms	Creation of new words with no meaning except to the patient
Thought blocking	Interruption to thought process where thoughts are absent for a few seconds and are unable to be retrieved

with many pauses and changes in direction.

Thought content[8]

Often there are recurrent themes in the patient's speech, indicative of ruminations and preoccupations. These may revolve around suicide, persecution, control, reference, religion or somaticism (the extremes of which are nihilistic delusions – the belief that part of the self does not exist, or is dead or decaying), or they may be grandiose in nature.

Perception

Despite denial of hallucinations, the patient's eyes may suddenly switch direction for no apparent reason during a psychiatric interview, or they may appear to be listening to a voice. These observations may indicate active hallucinations. Patients may even hold conversations with their auditory hallucinations. These are important observations, and are often quite subtle and missed if no effort is made to be an active observer.

Orientation, sensorium and cognition

A formal examination of cognitive function should be part of the full psychiatric assessment. The interviewer should ensure that the patient does not have an acute confusional state that may account for a behavioural problem. An assessment of a patient's cognitive functioning and intelligence may assist in deciding the best way to deal with their problems.

A number of tools may be used to assess cognitive functioning. These should include assessments of orientation, concentration, memory, language, abstraction and judgement.

PHYSICAL EXAMINATION

The MSE is only the first part of a patient's assessment. Each patient should have a thorough physical examination, and possibly a neurological examination, upon arrival in the emergency department. This is particularly important on first psychiatric presentation.

Approximately 20% of psychiatric patients have a concurrent medical disorder requiring treatment, and possibly contributing to the acute behaviour problem. Investigations depend on physical findings, but may include CK, CT, EEG, urine drug screen and lumbar puncture. Only after this can the emergency department doctor make an informed assessment of the patient and plan the most appropriate management.

REFERENCES

1. Rosen P, et al 1992 Emergency Medicine. Concepts and Clinical Practice. Mosby Year Book, St Louis
2. Mackinnon RA, Yudofsky SC 1991 Principles of Psychiatric Evaluation. JB Lippincott, Philadelphia
3. Kaplan HI, Sadock BJ 1993 Pocket Handbook of Emergency Psychiatric Medicine. Williams & Wilkins, Baltimore
4. Reeves RR, Bulleen JA 1995 A standardised form for the DSM-IV review of symptoms and mental status examination for students and residents. Journal of the American Osteopathic Association 95: 381–7
5. Hyman SE 1991 A Manual of Psychiatric Emergencies, 2nd edn. Little, Brown & Company, Boston
6. Phelan M, Strathdee G, Thornicroft G 1995 Emergency Mental Health Services in the Community. Cambridge University Press, Cambridge
7. Vaccaro JV, Clark GH 1996 Practising Psychiatry in the Community - a Manual. American Psychiatric Press, Washington, DC
8. Waldinger RJ 1990 Psychiatry for Medical Students, 2nd edn. American Psychiatric Press, Washington, DC

FURTHER READING

Cummings JL 1993 The mental status examination. Hospital Practice 28: 56–68
Dingemans PMAJ, et al 1995 Component structure of the brief psychiatric rating scale (BPRS-E). Psychopharmacology 122: 263–7
Holecz S 1993 The emergency department's system for tracking mental status changes in psychiatric patients, with guidelines for the care of violent patients. Emergency Nursing 19: 412–6
Kaufman DM, Zun L 1995 A quantifiable, brief mental status examination for emergency patients. Journal of Emergency Medicine 12: 449–56
Maclean A, Andrew-Starkey S 1993 The impact on the emergency department of integrating psychiatric services into a general hospital. Emergency Medicine 5: 276–81
Stuart GW, Sundeen SJ 1991 Principles and Practice of Psychiatric Nursing, 4th edn. Mosby Year Book, St Louis

19.2 DISTINGUISHING MEDICAL FROM PSYCHIATRIC CAUSES OF MENTAL DISORDER PRESENTATIONS

DAVID SPAIN

ESSENTIALS

1　Morbidity and health costs are reduced by correctly distinguishing between medical and psychiatric causes of mental disorder in patients presenting to emergency departments.

2　The triage nurse or medical officer should ask the patient whether any medical conditions exist in addition to the psychiatric complaints. This will identify most medical causes of mental disturbance.

3　Missed medical diagnosis is most commonly associated with failure to undertake an adequate medical history, mental-state examination and physical examination.

4　Substance-related disorders are most easily identified on direct or collateral history.

5　The presence of delirium or other significant cognitive defects makes an organic or substance-related illness almost certain.

INTRODUCTION

Emergency physicians are facing a significantly increased volume and complexity of mental-disorder presentations. Increased numbers of previously institutionalized chronically mentally ill patients are now in the community. Further, in the last several years an alarming increase of presentations has occurred from substance-abuse disorders. Intoxicated patients, with and without mental disorder, are increasingly being presented to emergency departments for assessment due to concerns about patient or community safety. ED resources are increasingly being tested as we attempt to care for these patients who frequently display impulsive, suicidal or violent behaviour. A thorough understanding of the assessment and appropriate disposition of mental-disorder presentations is essential knowledge for all emergency physicians.

The concept of differentiating an organic from a psychiatric basis for a mental disorder is becoming increasingly blurred as research shows the biological and genetic basis of many traditional psychiatric illnesses. The accepted terminology for classification of mental disorder is also rapidly changing. One accepted Western standard is the *Diagnostic and Statistical Manual of Mental Disorders, 4th Edition* (DSM-IV).[1] To emphasize the biological basis of many traditional psychiatric illnesses, DSM-IV no longer uses the term 'organic mental disorder'. Despite this change, current clinical management and disposition still revolve around the traditional distinction of organic (medical) from psychiatric problems.

In practice emergency physicians need a simple classification defining the principle diagnosis of the presenting mental disorder consistent with current DSM-IV terminology. This should assist diagnostic, management and disposition accuracy. Table 19.2.1 is such a suggested classification. A more simplistic grouping into psychiatric, medical, substance-related or anti-social behaviour may even suffice. Correct assignment by the emergency physician to the appropriate classification, and hence appropriate disposition reduces medical costs and morbidity.[2]

GENERAL APPROACH

Patients with abnormal behaviour labelled as psychiatric after routine medical and psychiatric assessment frequently have a final diagnosis of a medical cause or precipitant for the mental disorder. The incidence of missed

Table 19.2.1 A simple classification of principal diagnosis of mental disorder for emergency physicians

DSM-IV terminology	Broad traditional clinical grouping	Likely principal management and disposition
Axis 1		
Clinical disorder due to a general medical disorder	Organic	Medical
Delirium, dementia and amnestic and other cognitive disorders	Organic	Medical
Substance-related disorder – intoxication or withdrawal disorder.	Organic	Medical
Substance-related disorder – substance induced persistent disorder.	Organic	Psychiatric
Clinical disorder (not identified to above or axis II principal diagnosis).	Psychiatric	Psychiatric

medical diagnosis ranges between 8 and 46%.[2–4] A prospective study of emergency department patients in the USA showed a medical diagnosis in 63% of patients with first psychiatric presentations.[5] Deciding whether a particular presentation of mental disorder is medical or psychiatric is often difficult, as there are very few absolutes that distinguish medical from psychiatric illness. Careful collection and weighing of appropriate information commonly leads to an accurate differential diagnosis.

Some diagnoses and dispositions can be determined quickly after a medical and psychiatric history, with the addition of a mental state and full physical examination. This may sometimes take place without expensive diagnostic procedures.[6] Other presentations are difficult and require extensive and intensive evaluation, repeat evaluation, observation in hospital and significant investigations before the diagnosis is clear.

Many initial assessments in emergency departments are difficult and inaccurate owing to the presence of intoxicating substances or difficult patient factors. The latter may include poor communication ability, poor hygiene making examination unpleasant, antisocial behaviour, intentional obscuring of information, or denial of problems. Intoxicated patients may have other complex and distracting issues, such as threats of violence or self-harm, possible head injury, possible unknown substance overdose, and poor cooperation with necessary history, examination and investigations. A nonjudgemental approach with prudent intervention based on known or likely risks, close monitoring in a safe environment, and repeated reassessment of physical and mental state over time are necessary to obtain an accurate diagnosis and optimal outcome.

Studies on medical clearance by emergency department staff, primary-care physicians and psychiatrists have repeatedly shown a poor ability to discover medical conditions. This failure is commonly due to one or more of the following factors: inadequate history; failure to seek alternative information from relatives, carers and old records;

poor attention to physical examination, including vital signs; absence of a reasonable mental state examination; uncritical acceptance of medical clearance by receiving psychiatric staff; and failure to re-evaluate over time.[7] A recent study noted that medical conditions were most easily identified in the emergency department by the triage nurse or medical officer asking whether any medical conditions existed in addition to the patient's psychiatric complaints.[8]

Conversely, studies have shown that many patients admitted with a medical diagnosis frequently have a physical presentation of a classic psychiatric disorder. In addition, patients who frequently present to emergency departments with physical problems commonly have abnormal illness behaviour. Inability to recognize this leads to inappropriate diagnosis and management, with subsequent treatment failure.

Psychiatric patients also have a higher incidence of physical illness than the general population. The co-morbid illness may not have been diagnosed previously in this socially disadvantaged population.

Evaluation requires a thorough approach and a commitment of time and effort. Special skills are required for medical clearance and psychiatric interview. A coordinated and focused medical and psychiatric assessment has the highest yield of correct diagnoses.[2] Proformas may improve compliance and documentation of important details.

TRIAGE

Triage is vital, as many patients presenting with apparent psychiatric problems have medical conditions. The patient previously labelled psychiatric must be carefully triaged to avoid any new medical problems being overlooked. Psychiatric patients have been found to express their physical illnesses in different ways from those without mental illness. They may be suffering from severe or life-threatening illness, but fail to communicate this to their medical carers. Correct identification at the point of entry by nursing staff facilitates correct

Table 19.2.2 Triage safety questions[10]
Is the patient a danger to him or herself?
Is the patient at risk of leaving before assessment?
Is the patient a danger to others?
Is the area safe?

Table 19.2.3 High-yield indicators of organic illness
First presentation of mental disorder

Delirium
  Abrupt onset change in mental state
    Hours to days
    Fluctuates
  Change in cognition
    Disorientation
    Memory deficit
    Language disturbance.
  Disturbance of consciousness
    Fluctuating or decreased
    Poor attention
  Perceptual disturbance
    Hallucinations (especially visual)
    Illusions
    Misinterpretations

Drug use
  Recreational/illicit
  Overdose
  Prescribed or over-the-counter

Recent or new medical problems
Neurological signs or symptoms
Abnormal vital signs

management and reduces morbidity and mortality.[9] Many patients with psychiatric illness are also a significant risk to themselves or others, and require urgent intervention. Questions regarding safety should always be raised[10] (Table 19.2.2).

Nursing staff should use a triage checklist to identify likely organic presentations (Table 19.2.3). These are indications for urgent medical assessment. If these are absent and a psychiatric diagnosis is likely, then an appropriate urgency rating by Australasian Triage Scale for psychiatric presentations should be applied. This triage categorization for psychiatric presentations has been developed and verified, and allows reasonable waiting time standards for urgency to be applied (Table 19.2.4).[11]

Table 19.2.4 Guidelines for Australasian Triage Scale coding for psychiatric presentations[11]

Emergency: Category 2
Patient is violent, aggressive or suicidal, or is a danger to self or others, or requires police escort.

Urgent: Category 3
Very distressed or acutely psychotic, likely to become aggressive, may be a danger to self or others. Experiencing a situation crisis.

Semiurgent: Category 4
Long-standing or semi-urgent mental health disorder and/or has a supporting agency/escort present (e.g. community psychiatric nurse*)

Non-urgent: Category 5
Long-standing or non-acute mental disorder or problem, but the patient has no supportive agency or escort. Many require a referral to an appropriate community resource.

* It is considered advantageous to 'up triage' mental health patients with carers present because carers' assistance facilitates more rapid assessment.

Triage should consider patient privacy issues if the history obtained is to be accurate. Collateral information from the carers with the patient should always be diligently obtained, carefully considered and documented. Integration of all this information should allow the patient to be placed in an appropriate and safe environment where continuing visual and nursing observations can occur while medical assessment is awaited.

THE INTERVIEW ENVIRONMENT

A climate of trust is very important, as many details of the psychiatric interview are quite intimate. The psychiatric interview should take place in as quiet and private an environment as possible. The choice of the interview site may be limited in emergencies to ensure safety for both patient and staff.

HISTORY

A careful traditional medical history is the most common identifier of medical illness as a cause of a mental disorder presentation. Substance-related disorders are also most easily identified on history. A careful drug history, including prescribed, recreational and over-the-counter medications, should always be included. A slow onset and a previous psychiatric history are more commonly associated with psychiatric illness. Conversely, rapid onset, no premorbid decline and no past psychiatric history favours a medical cause. Poor recall of recent events may indicate delirium.

Family history is often a key indicator of psychiatric or medical cause. For example, a depressed 30-year-old man with a family history of Huntington's disease or porphyria is more likely to have a physical cause. Conversely, an 18-year-old man with a hypomanic presentation and a strong family history of bipolar disorder more likely has a psychiatric cause. Suicidal and homicidal risk should be assessed routinely to ensure safety. Escalating immediate risk can often be recognized by combining patient perceived lethality and inquiry about any transition from thoughts, to actual plans and finally to actions.

For patients with previous psychiatric illness the system review is a useful screen for organic illness.

HIV is an increasingly important area as HIV-related illness becomes the new great mimic of modern psychiatry and medicine. Practices likely to have put the patient at risk should be explored. These may have been in the distant past. Known HIV status always warrants assessment for an organic cause of any new behavioural disturbance. Clinically, these problems often initially present with symptoms of mild anxiety or depression.

Many treatable medical causes are only evident after significant investigations.[12]

Delirium, a highly specific but not absolute indicator of medical or substance-induced disorders, should always be sought. By definition this requires a history of recent onset and of fluctuation over the course of the day. Patients may not be able to attend sufficiently to give this history if delirious. The psychiatric history, including life profile, may give evidence of the presence or absence of premorbid decline. An abrupt onset of abnormal behaviour with no premorbid decline is more suggestive of an organic cause.

COLLATERAL HISTORY

Collateral history is important as the patient is not always capable of or willing to give full information. This history often crystallizes a diagnosis that would otherwise be uncertain or completely missed. Previous discharge summaries may provide relevant information regarding alcohol and drug use, previous behaviour and diagnosis. The family should be asked to bring in all medications, including over-the-counter items. Family, friends and caregivers may give more rapid access to collateral history than waiting for past admission details. Family and friends may be the only source for obtaining a history of a patient's fluctuating mental status, even when the patients appears quite lucid in the emergency department. This should raise strong suspicion of an organic illness.

EXAMINATION

Lack of attention to important details of the examination is a frequently identified cause of missed medical illness. Areas that commonly yield positive findings, but which are frequently omitted are the neurological examination, a search for general or specific appearances of endocrine disease, the toxidromes, examination for signs of malignancy, drugs or alcohol abuse, and vital sign examination.

Vital signs

Abnormal vital signs are frequently the only abnormality found on examination of patients with serious underlying medical disease. They must always be acknowledged and explained. Pulse oximetry should be included to rapidly exclude hypoxia. A bedside blood sugar level should be routine for patients with abnormal behaviour.

Mental state examination

This is an account of objective findings of mental state signs made at the time of interview. It is the psychiatric equivalent of the medical examination, and specifically details the current status.[13] Observations made by other staff in the department, such as hallucinations, may be very significant and can be included with the source identified. Careful consideration of the mental status frequently clearly distinguishes medical from psychiatric illness, and guides further investigation and management. For example, the presence of delirium or other significant cognitive defects make an organic illness almost certain. Delirium can be very subtle. Sometimes, owing to the fluctuating nature, the patient may appear normal on a single interview. Other less obvious features, such as lability of mood, variability of motor activity or lapses in patient concentration making the interview more difficult, can be the only clues and can be easily overlooked. The importance of formulation using collateral history and repeated mental-state examination is stressed. Documentation is important so that mental status changes with time can be appreciated.

Examination tools

Cognitive defects may be rapidly and reliably identified in emergency department during mental-status examination by the use of Folstein's Mini Mental State Examination[14] (Table 19.2.5). A score of less than 20 suggests an organic aetiology. Elderly patients with delirium or cognitive defects are frequently not recognized by emergency physicians.[15] These patients are at high risk of morbidity and mortality.[16] Simple assessment

Table 19.2.5 Mini-mental state examination[15]

Date of assessment Cognition			Points
Orientation			
1. What is the date?			1
What is the day?			1
What is the month?			1
What is the year?			1
What is the season?			1
2. What is the name of this building?			1
What floor of the building are we on?			1
What city are we in?			1
What state are we in?			1
What country are we in?			1
Registration			
3. I am going to name three objects. After I have said them I want you to repeat them. Remember what they are because I am going to ask you to name them in a few minutes. APPLE TABLE PENNY		APPLE	1
		TABLE	1
		PENNY	1
Code first attempt and then repeat the answers until the patient learns all three			
Attention and calculation			
4. Can you subtract 7 from 100, and then subtract 7 from the answer you get and keep subtracting until I tell you to stop?		93	1
		86	1
		79	1
		72	1
		65	1
	OR		
5. I am going to spell a word forwards and I want you to spell it backwards. The word is 'WORLD'. Now you spell it backwards. Repeat if necessary.		D	1
		L	1
		R	1
		O	1
		W	1
Recall			
6. Now what are the three objects I asked you to remember?		APPLE	1
		TABLE	1
		PENNY	1
Language			
7. Interviewer: Show wristwatch What is it called? Interviewer: Show pencil What is it called?			2
8. I'd like you to repeat a phrase after me. 'NO IFS ANDS OR BUTS'			1
9. Read the words on the bottom of this Table and do what is says.			1
10. Interviewer: Read the full statement below before handing the respondent a piece of paper. 'Do not repeat or coach.' I am going to give you a piece of paper. What I want you to do is take the paper in your right hand, fold it in half and put the paper on your lap.		Takes with R hand	1
		Folds in half	1
		Puts on lap	1

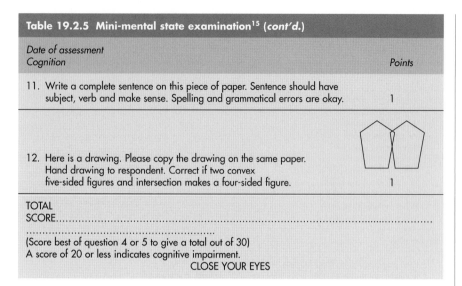

Table 19.2.5 Mini-mental state examination[15] (cont'd.)

Date of assessment Cognition	Points
11. Write a complete sentence on this piece of paper. Sentence should have subject, verb and make sense. Spelling and grammatical errors are okay.	1
12. Here is a drawing. Please copy the drawing on the same paper. Hand drawing to respondent. Correct if two convex five-sided figures and intersection makes a four-sided figure.	1
TOTAL SCORE..	

(Score best of question 4 or 5 to give a total out of 30)
A score of 20 or less indicates cognitive impairment.
CLOSE YOUR EYES

methods such as the Confusion Assessment Method (CAM) are rapid reliable methods of identifying delerium in older patients suitable for emergency department use.[17] Use of such simple methods should be encouraged to reduce inappropriate disposition. The screening tests above are suitable screening tools for emergency departments but are not intended to replace formal neuropsychological assessment. Proformas of medical history, mental-state examination and physical examination may improve thoroughness of assessment and documentation.

INVESTIGATIONS

Investigations should always be guided by clinical findings and must be tailored to each individual presentation. First presentations and suspicion of a medical cause that needs to be confirmed or excluded are the major indications. Baseline blood tests, such as FBP, BSL, electrolytes, LFTs, calcium and TFTs, may at times detect clinically unsuspected problems. Examination and culture of urine and CSF should be undertaken if occult infection is considered a possible cause. A urine drug screen may on occasions be the only way to confirm clinical suspicions of drug-related illness. Time delays for results, low specificity from cross-reactivity, and uncertainty caused by drugs with long half-lives limit

their usefulness. Newer drug screening stat tests at the bedside may improve their usefulness in the emergency department. Mandatory brain CT is not indicated,[18–20] but the threshold for imaging in first presentations of altered mental state without obvious cause should be low. HIV and syphilis testing should be done on all patients with significant risk profile. Newer modalities such as MRI, MR spectroscopy, positron emission tomography (PET) and single-photon emission CT (SPECT) may have a role in the future. EEG examination is rarely a current emergency department test for psychiatric patients.

DIAGNOSTIC FORMULATION

Emergency physicians should suspect organic disease until proved otherwise. In particular, reversible medical causes of abnormal mental state should be sought. Proformas improve documentation and summation.[21] Consideration of the factors in Table 19.2.6 may help determine doubtful cases. There are few absolutes that distinguish organic from psychiatric patients. Use of the five-axis DSM-IV system improves the ability to look at the patient's presentation in the context of total functioning.[1] It also allows emergency physicians to communicate with psychiatric peers in the recognized language.

Some patients require periods of observation, re-examination and further investigations before a definitive answer is obtained. Intoxicated patients frequently are not assessable till sober. Interim care and disposition varies depending on presentation, prior history and facilities available.

A common expectation of emergency physicians for patients referred to psychiatrists is to document that the patient is 'medically cleared'. The assessment is known to be imprecise and difficult.[2–5,7–9,21] Better documentation is

CONTROVERSIES AND FUTURE DIRECTIONS

❶ Significant controversy currently revolves around where assessment should take place. Should this be in the traditional hospital-based general emergency department, or is an alternative psychiatric assessment centre an option? The traditional model has a better safety-net function for those with organic illness.

❷ Should all patients receive initial assessment by a doctor, or can nurse practitioners provide this role with medical supervision? There are no significant outcome studies to date. Many believe that an adult assessment unit with psychiatrically trained nurses has produced significant benefits to patients, with shorter waiting times and better psychiatric assessments when compared to junior medical staff. However, there may be weaknesses in the recognition and comprehension of medical problems, occasionally leading to initial misclassification of medical patients as psychiatric.

❸ Providing adequate resources and a safe physical environment for assessment, management and disposition of the rapidly escalating number of patients with substance-related disorder is the greatest current challenge.

Table 19.2.6 Factors influencing the likelihood of medical or psychiatric illness as the principal diagnosis

Organic	Psychiatric
Abnormal vital signs	Family history of psychiatry disorder
Age > 40 with first psychosis	Past psychiatric illness
Delirium	Fully orientated
Conscious level fluctuates	Clear sensorium
Inability to attend	
Memory impaired	
Impaired cognitive abilities	Intact cognition
Neurological signs, e.g. dysarthria	
Abnormal physical signs	
Abrupt onset	Slow onset
Dramatic change in general status (hours to days)	Premorbid slow deterioration in employment/family/socially
Recent medical problem	Recent significant life event
Medication, drugs/alcohol/withdrawal	Non-compliance psychiatric medication
Marked new personality changes.	
Visual, tactile or olfactory hallucinations more common. Agitation/irritability HIV/AIDS Failed psychiatric treatment	Auditory hallucinations more common especially: Voices arguing Voices commentary Two voices discussing Audible thoughts
Disorganized delusions	Structured delusions.
Movement disorders	Somatic passivity experiences.
Perseveration	
Confabulation	
Illusions or misinterpretations	
Circumstantiality	
Concretism	Thought withdrawal, insertion or broadcasting
FH degenerative brain disease	
FH heritable metabolic	

to state that the emergency department assessment has revealed no evidence of an emergent medical problem.

CONCLUSION

A thorough medical history, psychiatric history, collateral history, physical examination, mental state examination and judicious specific investigation will identify most patients likely to have an underlying physical cause for a mental disorder presentation. Omission of any of these steps inevitably leads to missed medical diagnosis and incorrect disposition.

REFERENCES

1. American Psychiatric Association Task Force on DSM-IV 1994 Diagnostic and Statistical Manual of Mental Disorders, 4th edn.
2. Hoffman RS 1982 Diagnostic errors in the evaluation of behavioural disorders. Journal of the American Medical Association 248: 964–7
3. Koranyi EK 1979 Morbidity and rate of undiagnosed physical illness in a psychiatric clinic population. Archives of General Psychiatry 36: 414–9
3. Paul RC, Popkin MK, Devaul RA, et al 1978 Physical Illness presenting as psychiatric disease. Archives of General Psychiatry 35: 1315–20
4. Hennemann P, Mendoza R, Lewis RS 1994 Prospective evaluation of emergency department medical clearance. Annals of Emergency Medicine 24: 672–7
5. Allen MH, Faumann MA, Morin FX 1995 Emergency Psychiatric Evaluation of 'organic' mental disorders. New Directions for Mental Health Services 67: 45–55
6. Tintinalli JE, Peacock FW, Wright MA 1994 Emergency medical evaluation of psychiatric patients. Annals of Emergency Medicine 23: 859–62
7. Olshaker JS, Browne B, et al 1997 Medical Clearance and screening of psychiatric patients in the emergency department. Academic Emergency Medicine 4: 124–8
8. Ferrerra PC, Chan L 1997 Initial Management of the patient with altered mental status. American Family Physician 55: 1773–80
9. Pollard C 1994 Psychiatry Reference Book - nursing staff. Department of Emergency Medicine Royal Hobart Hospital
10. Smart D, Pollard C, Walpole B 1999 Mental health triage in emergency medicine. Australian and New Zealand Journal of Psychiatry 33: 57–66
11. Sternberg DE 1986 Testing for physical illness in psychiatric patients. Journal of Clinical Psychiatry 447(Supp 1): 3–9
12. Dakis J, Singh B 1994 Making sense of the psychiatric patient. Foundations of clinical psychiatry, Melbourne University Press, p. 79
13. Folstein MF, Folstein SE, McHugh PR 1975 'Mini Mental State': A practical method for grading the cognitive state of patients for the clinician. Journal of Psychiatric Research 12: 189–98
14. Hustey FM, Meldon SW 2002 The prevalence and documentation of impaired mental status in elderly emergency department patients. Annals of Emergency Medicine 39:3 248–52
15. Inouye SK, van Dyck CH, et al 1990 Clarifying confusion. The confusion assessment method. A new method for detection of delirium. Annals of Emergency Medicine 24: 672–7
16. Trzepacz P, McIntyre, Charles SC, et al 1999 Practice Guideline for the Treatment of Patients with Delirium. American Journal of Psychiatry 156:5 (Supplement) 1–20
17. Weinberger DR 1984 Brain disease and psychiatric illness: When should a psychiatrist order a CAT scan? American Journal of Psychiatry 41: 1521–7
18. Sata LS 1970 Diagnosing organic psychosis. Maryland State Medical Journal 19(2) 61–4
19. Ananth J, Gamal R, et al 1993 Is routine CT head scan justified for psychiatric patients? A prospective study. Journal of Psychiatry and Neuroscience 18: 69–73
20. Riba M, Mahlon H 1990 Medical clearance: fact or fiction in the hospital emergency room. Psychosomatics 31: 400–4

19.3 THE VIOLENT PATIENT

JENNIFER G BROOKES

ESSENTIALS

1 Knowledge of the dynamics of violence, differential diagnosis, management, ethical and legal considerations is required for the comprehensive care of violent patients in the emergency department.

2 A major concern in the assessment of violent patients in the emergency department is the need to determine the presence of organic disease.

3 The interventions used should be those that are most effective in achieving control but the least restrictive to the patient.

INTRODUCTION

Emergency department violence is a significant problem.[1-3] Violent incidents place a heavy demand on hospital and departmental resources, as well as placing patients, staff and visitors at risk. Patient violence in the general hospital setting, including the emergency department, may be associated with a wide range of pathology, including organic disorders, psychiatric illness and substance abuse. The emergency department is susceptible to violence because of a number of factors including 24-hour accessibility, easy access, a wide range of patients, patients with undifferentiated problems, patients in crisis situations, long waiting times, overcrowding and inadequate security.[1,4] The stress experienced by staff working in such an environment is considerable.[5] The effective management of violent patients requires education and training of staff in the prevention and management of violent incidents, an effective response to such incidents (such as an aggression control team), adequate staffing and resources to ensure a safe working environment, and specific emergency department design features. In addition, there must be adequate documentation and monitoring of violent incidents. The underreporting of violent incidents remains a problem, and until there is comprehensive reporting of all types of violence then research into the cause, effects and management of violent behaviour in the emergency department will be hampered. A knowledge of the dynamics of violence, differential diagnosis, management, and ethical and legal considerations is required for the comprehensive care of violent patients in the emergency department.

PREDICTION OF VIOLENCE

There is a consistent association between violence and young males or a past history of violence, but these factors alone are insufficient predictors to allow the early recognition of most potentially violent patients.[3] A past history of violence is cited as the most consistent risk factor for violent behavior,[6,7] and for this reason a medical record alert system for documenting and alerting staff to patients with prior emergency department violence is advocated. Most violent behaviour occurs in the setting of recognizable and escalating features of patient behaviour, which should alert staff to the possibility of impending violence. The early recognition of the potential for violence should allow effective interventions, which may minimize or avert the risk. The prodromal syndrome of impending violence is characterized by increasing anxiety and tension, verbal abuse and profanity, and increasing hyperactivity.[8] In particular, increasing hyperactivity (e.g. pacing, inability to keep still) should be recognized as a predictor of imminent violence and the patient should be evaluated immediately.[8] Nevertheless, some episodes of violence may be sudden and unexpected, and there should be the capacity for staff and/or an aggression-control team to respond immediately, akin to a cardiac arrest team. If the patient states that violence is probable, this should never be ignored.

DIAGNOSIS

Psychiatric disorders, situational crises, antisocial behaviour and organic states, including disease or drug-related disorders (including alcohol use), are the main underlying problems associated with violence. Psychiatric conditions commonly associated with violence are schizophrenia, personality disorder and mania.[9] A major concern in the assessment of violent patients in the emergency department is the need to determine whether there is organic disease, and this may be particularly difficult in a patient with pre-existing psychiatric illness. The following general conditions should be considered in the evaluation of any violent patient:

- Hypoxia
- Hypoglycaemia
- Trauma
- Sepsis
- Metabolic disorders
- CNS conditions (infection, trauma, seizure disorder, cerebrovascular accident)
- Endocrine disorders
- Acute intoxication or withdrawal
- Medications (side effects, toxicity).

Failure to diagnose organic illness may result in failure to deliver specific treatment, inappropriate disposition of the patient and a high risk of morbidity and mortality. One Australian study found that organic disorders were the most frequent cause of violent behaviour requiring the violence management team in a general hospital setting, with hypoxia, head injury and dementia being the most frequently identified organic mental disorders.[2] A recent study of restraint practices in Australasian emergency departments found that violence or threatened violence was the most common indication for restraint.[10] This highlights the need for comprehensive medical evaluation of violent patients, and an awareness of the potential deleterious effects of physical and chemical restraint.

ASSESSMENT

The goals of assessment in the emergency department are to stabilize the patient, exclude life-threatening disorders, identify and treat organic disorders, and to determine whether the behavioural disorder is functional (such as schizophrenia or mania). It is usually not possible to arrive at a specific psychiatric diagnosis in the emergency setting.

Assessment of the violent patient is frequently hampered by the inability to undertake a comprehensive history and examination. Information should be obtained from as many sources as possible, such as past medical records, family, friends, local medical officer, mental health workers, social workers, police, ambulance officers and treating specialists. Details of the violent events, the time course of physical or mental deterioration, previous level of function, psychiatric history and medical history, including drug and alcohol use, are important. Information gained from the history will also contribute to the prediction of risk and danger. Physical examination should be performed with particular emphasis on vital signs, oxygen saturation, cardiovascular and neurological systems, and mental status examination. Organic illness should be suspected when the patient is aged over 40 years, or there is disorientation, altered conscious state and abnormal vital signs.[11] Additional features suggesting organic disorder are sudden onset (hours to days), visual hallucinations, delusions, no past psychiatric history, or a history of substance abuse or toxins.[11,12] When physical examination is not possible, direct observation of the patient may provide considerable information. Features to note include general appearance, gait, posture, speech, motor function, affect, odour, pupil size, respiration, lacrimation, skin colour, skin condition and diaphoresis.

Investigations in the violent patient include glucose, full blood count, electrolytes, renal function, urinalysis and therapeutic drug levels. Additional investigations may be indicated in selected patients. These include arterial blood gas, ethanol level, other blood and urine drug screens, thyroid function, septic screen including lumbar puncture, ECG, chest X-ray and CT scan.

MANAGEMENT

General management

As a general rule the intervention used should be effective in achieving control but least restrictive to the patient. Where the potential for violence exists, staff must act in a defensive and anticipatory fashion, at all times ready for the level of violence to escalate. Staff should heed intuitive feelings of escalating danger and act accordingly. Nevertheless, staff should not assume that intuition alone will reliably detect danger. Every threat must be taken seriously and every fearful feeling acknowledged, if assault and injury are to be prevented.[9]

Efforts must be made to ensure that the environment and management of the patient do not contribute to the escalation of violence. The patient should be placed in a quiet and secure area, removed from other patients and members of the public, but not isolated from supervision. The patient should be constantly observed, to protect against self-harm, harm to others or self-discharge. Observation also allows early detection of signs of impending violence. Security staff should be forewarned and nearby. Staff should not interview the patient alone, or out of earshot or sight of support staff. Junior staff should not be involved in the assessment and management of patients with the potential for violence, unless the supervising clinician deems it appropriate and safe. Staff should use a manner that is courteous, helpful and non-judgemental, but firm in the provision of explanation and guidelines for the patient's behaviour. The patient's demands, if unable to be fulfilled, should be acknowledged and an explanation provided. Similarly, unnecessary delay in assessment should be avoided.

Different patient disorders may respond variably to different intervention techniques. In organic mental disorder verbal intervention is rarely effective and restraint is usually required to allow evaluation and investigation to proceed.[13] Treatment of underlying organic pathology is necessary and the administration of chemical or physical restraint must be tempered by the likelihood of adverse effects. Similarly, patients with functional psychoses, such as schizophrenia or mania, may be difficult to influence verbally and chemical restraint is often required, sometimes combined with physical methods.[13] Verbal intervention is often effective for patients with non-psychotic, non-organic disorders, such as personality disorder,[2,13] and the patient may accept offers of medication.

The general indications for the use of chemical or physical restraint are:[8,14]

- To prevent imminent harm to the patient or to others, if other means are not effective or appropriate
- To allow evaluation, investigation and treatment of the patient
- At the patient's request
- To prevent significant harm to the environment of the emergency department.

If staff believe that there is a risk of imminent violence then immediate action is indicated. It is arguable whether chemical or physical restraint is more restrictive and intrusive to the patient,[15,16] and either may be contraindicated depending on the patient's clinical condition.

Verbal intervention

All patients should receive some form of verbal intervention, and the development of staff-patient rapport is an important component of effective management.

Empathetic verbal intervention is the most effective way to calm an agitated, fearful, panicky patient.[8] Treating the patient with courtesy and respect, encouraging them to express feelings, acknowledging their affect and demonstrating patient advocacy may encourage rapport and effective communication. Limits of acceptable behaviour should be set and explained to the patient. Violence is a defence against passivity and helplessness,[17] and offering the patient acceptable alternatives for behaviour or treatment may allow them to retain a sense of control.

Physical restraint

Physical restraint should only be used when absolutely necessary and may be indicated in the following situations:

- To allow adequate assessment and treatment of the patient
- To prevent the patient from self-harm or harm to others
- After failure of verbal or chemical means of restraint
- In order to allow the administration of chemical restraint.

Physical restraints should never be used as a punitive action or solely for the convenience of staff. The use of physical restraint is maximally restrictive of the patient's freedom and may place the patient and staff at risk of injury. Although physical restraint may prevent injury and reduce agitation, it can have substantial deleterious physical and psychological effects on both patients and staff.[14,18] Restraints should not be used in unstable patients with organic illness.

Physical restraint is always combined with verbal interventions, and often with chemical restraint. A pre-emptive 'show of force' may result in the patient achieving control of behaviour. Attempts to gain physical control of a violent and combative patient should not be undertaken unless adequate numbers of staff are available. Staff should have received specific training in this aspect of aggression control, and, ideally, a hospital aggression control team should be used. A minimum of five persons is required for the safe physical restraint of a patient. The handling and immobilization of the patient's head and neck, trunk and limbs must be undertaken in a controlled and safe manner at all times. As for the team management of trauma or cardiac arrest, an experienced team leader should be present and team members allocated specific tasks. The treating physician may best preserve the therapeutic relationship with the patient by avoiding physical participation in the restraint process. The patient should be addressed throughout, with calm explanation of the procedure. Where mechanical restraints are used, non-locking restraints are preferred, as the need for keys may be dangerous in the event of fire or a deteriorating medical condition.[16] Close monitoring of the patient is essential following the application of physical restraints. The patient should be supervised at all times, either directly or via closed-circuit television. A physical check of the patient, including vital signs, should be undertaken every 15 minutes. Examination of restraint sites for pressure areas or other soft-tissue injuries, and turning of the patient should be undertaken regularly. Aspiration is a risk when the patient is restrained in the supine position, but this may more readily permit medical treatment.[16] Nursing care should emphasize feeding, hydration, toileting, periodic restraint release and continued interaction with the patient.[14] Temporary relief of one of the four-point restraints every 15 minutes minimizes the risk of neurovascular compromise. Documentation of authorization for restraint, the type of restraint used, the timing, rationale, patient's condition, patient's reaction to restraint, observations and release of restraint should be made for each episode of restraint.[14,19]

There is no place for the use of 'seclusion' in the emergency department if this involves placing the patient in a locked, secluded and unobserved environment.

Chemical restraint

Chemical restraint may be requested by the patient, or be indicated to allow evaluation, treatment or control of the violent patient. Chemical restraint may allow for more rapid control of a violent situation, with a safer and shorter duration of physical restraint.

Choice of agent (Table 19.3.1)

Drugs most often used in the management of the acutely disturbed patient are benzodiazepines and antipsychotic agents. In organic brain syndrome any sedating agent may result in increased patient agitation or confusion. Antipsychotic agents or benzodiazepines, alone or in combination, may be used for functional psychoses. The administration of chemical restraint is aimed at controlling violent, extremely agitated or hyperactive behaviour. It is not intended to treat core psychiatric symptoms, such as hallucinations and delusions, which usually require 2–6 weeks of adequate drug treatment for remission to occur.[17] The end-point for rapid tranquillization is not sedation, but the alleviation of

Table 19.3.1 Commonly used agents for chemical restraint of the violent patient

Drug	Initial adult dose* (mg)	Route of administration	Half-life (hours)[28,29]
Midazolam	2.5–10	IM, IV	2 ± 0.6
Diazepam	2.5–10	Oral, IV	43 ± 13
Haloperidol	2.5–10	Oral, IM, IV	18 ± 5
Droperidol	2.5–10	IM, IV	2 ± 0.2
Chlorpromazine	25–100	Oral, IM, IV	30 ± 7

*In the elderly and patients with organic disorders smaller doses should be used and titrated to effect

anxiety, tension and motor excitement.[17] The physician's experience and familiarity with an agent may outweigh other considerations in the choice of drug.

Route of administration

If circumstances permit, oral medication should be offered to the patient, allowing them a choice in their treatment. The intramuscular route is the simplest and most expeditious route in the uncooperative patient.[15] Although the intravenous route has the advantage of rapid onset of action and ease of titration, the placement of an intravenous cannula in the combative patient is problematic. The risk to staff and patient during placement, and the difficulties in retention of the cannula, may render attempted cannulation hazardous or impossible. However, placement and retention of intravenous access may be important for the treatment of coexisting medical problems or to allow the treatment of side effects of chemical restraint, such as hypotension. Dosing intervals are usually 30–60 minutes, and dose and time intervals should be manipulated so that the lowest effective dose is given.[20] Most patients respond after one to three doses at 30–60-minute intervals,[20] but shorter intervals may be required when using the intravenous route. For patients with an underlying organic disorder smaller doses should be used and titrated to effect. Likewise, elderly patients require judicious administration of doses one-half or less than those required in the young adult.

Benzodiazepines: diazepam, midazolam

These agents have fewer serious side effects and interactions than the antipsychotic agents. The cardiovascular effects of the benzodiazepines are mild, allowing their use in patients with underlying medical illness. Hypotension, respiratory depression and apnoea may occur. Diazepam is poorly and inconsistently absorbed following intramuscular injection, and should be administered by the oral or intravenous routes. Its long half-life is a disadvantage, particularly in the elderly. Midazolam is readily and rapidly absorbed by the intramuscular route. Uncommonly, benzodiazepines may cause disinhibition or may be insufficient to control combative behaviour. Disinhibition, increasing agitation and confusion or oversedation are a risk in the elderly demented patient, and so low-dose short-acting drugs are preferred.[21] An advantage of the benzodiazepines is their wide safety margin, and the availability of flumazenil as an antagonist. The possibility of alcohol or sedative drug withdrawal would favour the use of benzodiazepines. Benzodiazepines may be combined with antipsychotic agents both safely and effectively.

Antipsychotic agents: haloperidol, droperidol, chlorpromazine

These agents are the treatment of choice in aggression due to psychosis, although their use is limited by adverse reactions. Side effects include dystonic reactions, anticholinergic symptoms, hypotension and neuroleptic malignant syndrome. These agents should not be used in seizure-prone patients, such as those with untreated epilepsy or withdrawing from central depressants such as alcohol or benzodiazepines. This precaution is based on the theoretical consideration of the lowering of the seizure threshold by antipsychotic agents, although this may not be borne out in clinical practice.[10] They should also be avoided in patients suffering from drug intoxications with anticholinergic side effects. Chlorpromazine is a low-potency highly sedating agent. It has significant α-adrenergic antagonist activity and some direct negative inotropic action, whereas haloperidol has less antiadrenergic activity. As a result, orthostatic hypotension is more common with chlorpromazine than with haloperidol, and is the most troublesome cardiovascular side effect, particularly in the hypovolaemic patient. Higher potency agents such as haloperidol have less propensity to cause sedation, anticholinergic and cardiovascular side effects,[15] and so are preferable if sedation is not desired, e.g. in the elderly or in patients at risk of significant hypotension. Droperidol has no antipsychotic properties, is very sedating and causes orthostatic hypotension. The neurological side effects of antipsychotic agents particularly relevant to their use in the emergency department include acute dystonia, akathisia, and neuroleptic malignant syndrome. Akathisia may be associated with increased aggression. Extrapyramidal side effects are most likely with haloperidol, and are readily treated with benzatropine 1–2 mg by the intramuscular or intravenous routes, followed by oral medication as required. Neuroleptic malignant syndrome is a rare occurrence, associated with a high mortality and requiring immediate treatment. Small doses of more potent agents such as haloperidol are preferable in the elderly and in organic brain syndrome, provided seizures are not a threat. The potent antipsychotic agents are less likely than sedating agents to increase confusion in delirious or demented patients.

WEAPONS

There is no place for heroics in the management of violent patients in the emergency department. For patients threatening violence with a weapon of any nature, immediate security staff and police involvement is indicated. Consideration may be given to attempting to isolate the patient or allowing them to leave the department pending police or security attendance, provided this can be achieved without posing an additional threat to other patients, staff and visitors.

STAFF PREPARATION

All staff who may be involved in the management of violent or potentially violent patients should have received specific training in this area, including recognition of the non-verbal indicators of escalating aggression, self-defence, and techniques of verbal, chemical and physical intervention. Prior to approaching a potentially violent patient staff should remove all jewellery, pens, stethoscopes, neck ties, name badges and other items of equipment that may be used to harm them or the patient, inadvertently or otherwise. Universal precautions (gloves, gown, goggles, mask) are appropriate to protect staff from body fluid contact. The area in which the patient is to be restrained should be of an adequate size to allow the entry of a unified aggression control team at a safe distance from the patient. Equipment such as oxygen cylinders, light stands, chairs, trolleys and any other item that may be used for self-harm or harm to others must be removed. Standard emergency department cubicles are usually inadequate for the safe undertaking of team restraint of the violent patient. Staff should remain at a safe distance from the patient and should not place themselves in a situation with the patient where they are alone and unobserved, or with no ready access to exit from the interview room.

DISPOSITION

The choice of disposition depends on the primary diagnosis, associated medical or psychiatric conditions, and the requirement for continuing restraint or involuntary detention of the patient. The prime consideration is the placement of any organically impaired patient in an environment providing safe medical and nursing care. Similarly, patients who remain significantly under the influence of drugs administered for chemical restraint should not be transferred to an area unable to provide appropriate supervision. Patients detained involuntarily need a high level of supervision in order to meet the requirements of the detention order. In the transfer of any violent or potentially violent patient, staff have an obligation to pass relevant information to the receiving area to ensure the potential risk to receiving staff has been conveyed.

POST-INCIDENT MANAGEMENT

Issues to be considered following a violent event include formal incident reporting, identification of staff members and others who may be adversely affected by the incident, and the provision of medical care to injured staff. Immediate staff support, staff respite, formal debriefing, counselling and return to work support may be required.[22] Clinical review of specific incidents and violence management strategies should be part of quality improvement, risk management or occupational health and safety undertakings. The existence of a standardized reporting procedure is critical to allow formal review of the incident, to maintain a comprehensive record of incidents to determine the extent of the problem of violence, and to contribute to the development of preventative measures.[4]

LEGAL CONSIDERATIONS: CONSENT AND COMPETENCE

The management of the violent patient may involve legal and ethical dilemmas. Consideration of the principle of respect for patient autonomy must be balanced with the principles of beneficence and non-maleficence. In particular, the physician has a responsibility to protect the welfare of both the patient and the community. The primary legal considerations in caring for the violent patient are the rights of the patient, the duties of the healthcare providers, and concern for third parties.[9] The need to obtain informed consent or respect for the patient's refusal of treatment necessitates assessment of the patient's capacity (competence) to make such decisions. Competent patients have the right to refuse medical treatment and the use of restraints cannot be justified as a means of forcing treatment on a competent patient who is refusing treatment.[18] If detainment, restraint and treatment are carried out inappropriately, staff may be liable for charges of assault and unlawful imprisonment. Conversely, injury to the patient, staff or members of the public by a patient may result in charges of negligence against staff.

In practice, many violent patients refuse initial requests to participate in the assessment and management process. Thus, the initial management of many violent patients in the emergency department may include the decision to initiate measures to control patient behaviour and institute patient care prior to any assessment. This is necessary in order to undertake assessment and treatment, including the assessment of competence. Unfortunately, it may only be with hindsight, when outcome is determined, that the physician knows whether the patient was, indeed, competent or incompetent to refuse care. It is suggested that, on balance, if the patient is significantly impaired and a serious danger to self or others, he or she should be detained.[23] In general, the more life-threatening or limb-threatening the emergency, the more preferable it is for the physician to err in favour of detention and treatment of the patient.

When time is of the essence and formal assessment of competence impossible (e.g. patient refuses to communicate), the physician should consider the following parameters:[24]

- The risk involved in refusal of care by the patient
- The risk involved in restraint, investigation and treatment
- The presence of any information that would guide the doctor as to this patient's usual autonomous wishes (e.g. advance directives, opinions of relatives)
- The presence, or suspicion of presence, of pathological processes that might impinge on the patient's competence.

In an emergency situation, treatment of the organically impaired patient should be limited to measures designed to preserve life or prevent serious medical consequences, and additional treatment deferred until actual consent is obtained.[23] Restraint should be used only for the shortest time possible and with the least restriction possible.[18]

Every department that uses chemical or physical restraint should have written guidelines approved by the emergency department executive, and by the hospital administration and legal services.

Documentation should be comprehensive; clinical reasoning must be clearly recorded, and collaboration from other health professionals or sources in other disciplines is highly desirable.[25] Clinicians should be familiar with the local legal requirements and institutional policies with regard to consent, involuntary detainment, and mental health and other relevant legislation (such as that relating to refusal of treatment and occupational health and safety). The reporting to police of assaults and damage to property should be encouraged, ideally supported by hospital guidelines.

PREVENTION OF VIOLENCE

A preventative approach to occupational aggression and violence should address several key areas: physical environment, organizational environment, clinical issues, policies, and procedures and training.[22] All hospitals should consider the need for precautions tailored to their particular circumstances. A number of security measures may be considered in an effort to deter violence in emergency depart-

ments. The presence of a well-trained hospital security force on a 24-hour basis may be invaluable. Controlling access to the department, metal detectors, closed circuit or video surveillance, emergency alarm systems, personal duress alarms and secure examination rooms are some measures that can be used.[4] In addition, a regularly reviewed alert system to identify patients who have a previous history of violence should be considered. There is some evidence that the training of staff in violence management may result in a reduction in the incidence of assault on staff.[26] In addition to reducing staff and patient injuries, staff training may be effective in reducing rates of physical restraint and reducing inappropriate restraint.[14] Common problems in the management of the violent patient are detailed in Table 19.3.2.

THE IMPACT OF VIOLENCE ON STAFF

In order to successfully manage violent patients, staff must have confidence in their own safety and that of team members. In addition, staff need to have some understanding of their own

responses to violence. They may experience feelings of fear, anxiety, helplessness, vulnerability or anger. Denial is the ubiquitous defence against anxiety generated by a violent patient,[27] but may result in a serious underestimation of the risk. In its most common form denial manifests as the clinician's failure to gather anxiety-provoking data, such as inquiring about patients' ownership of weapons.[27] On the other hand, staff may have prejudicial attitudes which contribute to an overestimation of the patient's risk for violence. Staff may feel fear or anger at the patient, which may result in a distortion of their perceived danger.[27] Reactions of staff to violence may range from short-term psychological trauma to post-traumatic stress disorder, and there may be adverse effects on job performance and staff–patient relationships.[5] Violence may affect staff members by both an acute and a cumulative effect.[5] The impact of all types of violence on staff, even in the absence of physical injury, should not be underestimated. A not uncommon, but rarely cited, source of stress for staff is exposure to body fluids during violent incidents, which has the potential to result in considerable psychological or physical morbidity.

CONCLUSION

Management of the violent patient presents one of the most difficult problems in emergency medicine. Difficulties in evaluation and treatment, threats to the safety of the patient, self and others, and medicolegal considerations, make for a complex clinical challenge. A successful outcome depends on the individual skills of treating staff, effective team management, and the judicious use of interventions.

Table 19.3.2 Deficiencies in the management of violent patients	
Unnecessary delay in assessment	Undertaking restraint in an unsafe environment
Ignoring past history of violence	Failure to consider weapon possession on the patient or in patient belongings
Ignoring signs of impending violence	Failure to exclude organic disorders
Denial reactions in staff	Inadequate documentation of restraint
Confrontational attitude	Inadequate monitoring following physical or chemical restraint
Issuing threats	Premature transfer of violent patients to psychiatric unit without medical evaluation
Interacting with the patient in an unnecessarily isolated environment	Delay in transfer to secure unit resulting in prolonged emergency department restraint
Lack of understanding of the relevant ethical and legal issues	Failure to inform other emergency department staff of risk of violence
Using inadequate staff numbers for restraint	Failure to inform receiving ward staff of risk of patient violence
	Underreporting of violent incidents

REFERENCES

1. Lavoie FW, Carter GL, Danzyl DF, Berg RL 1988 Emergency department violence in US teaching hospitals. Annals of Emergency Medicine 17: 1227–33
2. Brayley J, Lange R, Baggoley C, Bond M, Harvey P 1994 The violence management team. An approach to aggressive behaviour in a general

CONTROVERSIES AND FUTURE DIRECTIONS

❶ Emergency department design and staffing should specifically address the need for 24-hour protection against violence.

❷ There is a need for prospective controlled studies of the use of physical and chemical restraint in the emergency department.

❸ Research into emergency department violence should explore the use of standardized methods of reporting of all types of emergency department violence, the short- and long-term impact of violence on staff, and the effectiveness of measures aimed at the prevention of violence.

hospital. Medical Journal of Australia 161: 254–8

3. Brookes JG, Dunn RJ 1997 The incidence, severity and nature of violent incidents in the emergency department. Emergency Medicine 9: 5–9

4. American Medical Association Young Physicians Section 1995 Violence in the medical workplace: prevention strategies. American Medical Association, Chicago

5. Brookes JG 1997 The impact of violence on emergency department staff. Emergency Medicine 9: 117–21

6. Atakan Z, Davies T 1997 ABC of mental health: Mental health Emergencies. British Medical Journal 314: 1740

7. Hill S, Petit J 2000 Psychiatric emergencies. The violent patient. Emergency Medicine Clinics of North America 18(2): 301–15

8. Dubin WR 1992 Overcoming danger with violent patients: guidelines for safe and effective management. Emergency Medicine Reports 13: 105–12

9. Rice MM, Moore GP 1991 Management of the violent patient: therapeutic and legal considerations. Psychiatric Aspects of emergency medicine. Emergency Medicine Clinics of North America 9(1): 13–30

10. Cannon ME, Sprivulis P, McCarthy J 2001 Restraint practices in Australasian emergency departments. Australian and New Zealand Journal of Psychiatry 35(4): 464

11. Dubin WR, Weiss KJ, Zeccardi JA 1983 Organic brain syndrome. The psychiatric impostor. Journal of the American Medical Association 249: 60–2

12. Williams ER, Shepherd SM 2000. Psychiatric emergencies. Medical clearance of psychiatric patients. Emergency Medicine Clinics of North America 18(2): 185–98

13 Tardiff K 1988 Management of the violent patient in an emergency situation. The violent patient. Psychiatric Clinics of North America 11(4): 539–49

14. Fisher WA 1994 Restraint and seclusion: a review of the literature. American Journal of Psychiatry 151: 1584–91

15. Clinton JE, Sterner S, Stelmachers Z, Ruiz E 1987 Haloperidol for sedation of disruptive emergency patients. Annals of Emergency Medicine 16: 319–22

16. Lavoie FW 1992 Consent, involuntary treatment and the use of force in an urban emergency department. Annals of Emergency Medicine 21: 25–32

17. Dubin WR, Feld JA 1989 Rapid tranquillisation of the violent patient. American Journal of Emergency Medicine 7(3): 313–20

18. AnnasG 1999 The last resort – the use of physical restraints in medical emergencies. The New England Journal of Medicine 341(18): 1408–12

19. Splawn G 1991 Restraining potentially violent patients. Journal of Emergency Nursing 17: 316–7

20. Dubin WR 1988 Rapid tranquillisation: antipsychotics or benzodiazepines? Journal of Clinical Psychiatry 49(Suppl 12): 5–11

21. Salzman C 1988 Treatment of the agitated demented elderly patient. Hospital and Community Psychiatry 39: 1143–4

22. Victorian Health Industry Occupational Health and Safety and Workcover Advisory Committee 1995 Guidelines for the prevention and management of occupational aggression and violence in the Victorian health industry. Health and Community Services Promotion Unit

23. Griglak MJ, Bucci RL 1985 Medicolegal management of the organically impaired patient in the emergency department. Annals of Emergency Medicine 14: 685–9

24. Ben-Meir M 2000 Competency assessments and the justifications for the use of restraint in the emergency department. Minor research thesis. Masters of heatlh ethics. University of Melbourne

25. Citrome L, Green L 1990 The dangerous agitated patient. Postgraduate Medicine 87: 231–6

26. Infantino JA, Musingo S 1985 Assaults and injuries among staff with and without training in aggression control techniques. Hospital and Community Psychiatry 36: 1312–4

27. Lion JR, Pasternak SA 1973 Countertransference reactions to violent patients. American Journal of Psychiatry 130: 207–10

28. Hardman JG, Limbird LE, Molinoff PB, Ruddon RW, Gilman AG (eds) 1995 The Pharmacological Basis of Therapeutics, 9th edn. McGraw-Hill, New York

29. Thomas J (ed) 1998 Australian Prescription Products Guide, 1998, 27th edn. Australian Pharmaceutical Publishing Company Ltd

19.4 DELIBERATE SELF HARM/SUICIDE

ANTONIO CELENZA

ESSENTIALS

1 Patients present frequently to emergency departments following acts of deliberate self harm. These patients form a heterogeneous group, most of whom do not have ongoing suicidal behaviour and have an excellent prognosis.

2 Management requires many resources including emergency staff, observation wards, medical teams, social workers and psychiatrists. There needs to be a planned strategy to deal with these patients addressing triage, restraint and observation, assessment, treatment and disposition.

3 Assessment of suicide risk following deliberate self harm is difficult. It involves assessment of background demographic, psychiatric, medical and social factors as well as assessing the suicidal behaviour itself and the current situation. Patients can then be stratified into risk groups and managed accordingly.

4 The most consistent factors predicting suicide following deliberate self harm are psychiatric illness, personality disorder, substance abuse, multiple previous attempts, and current suicidality and hopelessness.

5 Discharge following crisis intervention or brief problem-solving treatments can be helpful to many low-risk patients, however, short-stay or overnight admission and psychiatric assessment should be encouraged for all patients.

INTRODUCTION

Suicide is a deliberate act of intentional self-inflicted death. Emergency departments play a key role in management of deliberate self-harm (DSH) and suicide. Ten per cent of people who commit suicide are seen in an emergency department in the month prior to death, thus providing an opportunity for intervention.[1] The major impact, however, is in the assessment of large numbers of suicidal patients who will not come to harm, and the accurate risk stratification of these patients to maximize resource utilization and help prevent suicide or repetition of self-harm.

A person who expresses suicidal ideation or commits an act of DSH is sending a distress signal that emergency physicians must recognize. Suicidality should also be assessed in patients with symptoms or signs of depression, unusual behavioural changes, those with substance abuse or other psychiatric disorders, and

those who present with injuries of questionable or inconsistent mechanism, such as self inflicted lacerations and gunshot wounds or motor vehicle accidents involving one victim.

INCIDENCE

In Australia there are over 2500 deaths a year from suicide (approximately 1 in 7500 of the Australian population with a similar rate in the UK, New Zealand and the USA) and it is now the leading cause of death in people under 30 years of age.[2] The rate of suicide in developed countries varies: Scandinavian and Eastern European countries have rates as high as 1 in 2500, whereas Greece, Spain, Italy and Ireland have rates less than 1 in 10 000.[3] Suicide attempts occur in approximately 1 in 400, suicidal threats occur in 1 in 100, and suicidal thoughts can occur as frequently as one in four.[4]

The most frequent methods of suicide in Australia are hanging, firearms, carbon-monoxide poisoning and drug ingestions. Proportions due to each method vary according to region, residence, age and sex.[1,5] Most cases of DSH are due to self-poisoning with 90% associated with alcohol intoxication. The most common drugs are non-prescription analgesics and psychotropic drugs. Self-injury usually involves cutting of the wrist or forearm. Cutting is usually done in private with a knife, broken glass or razor blade. More violent forms of self-injury are less common and suggest serious suicidal intent.

AETIOLOGY

Suicide occurs across diagnostic groups. No specific psychological or personality structure is associated with suicide, and patients who commit suicide or DSH do so for many unrelated reasons. The precipitant may be a personal crisis or life change that may be amplified by poor social support, substance abuse or psychiatric disorder. Intoxication may decrease inhibitions enough to allow an act to proceed.

One-third of patients with DSH express a wish to die, however, this intent may not be serious. Most seek attention or want to communicate the extent of their distress and express a need to be helped to live. Other reasons include release of tension, escape from a stressful situation, blotting out distressing thoughts, eliciting guilt or manipulating others, expressing anger or grief, or escaping from custody. Many patients threaten suicide or exaggerate suicidality to increase the likelihood of admission to hospital. These patients are more likely to be substance dependent, antisocial, homeless, unmarried and in legal difficulty. However, these instances of secondary gain should not be assumed to be the cause of the suicide attempt and the suicidal behaviour should be taken seriously.

Some acts are not associated with any suicidality. Many overdoses are related to recreational drug use and not associated with an attempt to die. Bizarre self-mutilation may occur in psychotic patients and may not necessarily involve an attempt at suicide.

PATIENT CHARACTERISTICS

Demographic factors

Age

Suicide and DSH are rare in children under 12 years of age. Historically, suicide rates increased with age reaching a peak after age 45 in males and 55 in females. However, recent data suggest similar rates of suicide from the age of 15 onwards, with a peak at 25–34 years in males and 35–44 in females.[2,6] Suicide in males aged 15–24 years is thought to be associated with substance abuse and psychiatric disorders such as schizophrenia. The incidence of DSH increases throughout puberty reaching a peak at 15–24 years of age and decreasing thereafter.

Gender

The overall rate for male suicide is 21 per 100 000 population and 5.5 per 100 000 for females. The rate for male DSH has been increasing recently with the male to female ratio now 1:1.3.

Marital status

Marriage reinforced by children decreases the risk of suicidal behaviour. Being single, separated, divorced or widowed increases the risk of suicide two- to threefold.

Employment

Unemployment increases the risk of DSH by 10–15 times, with the risk increasing with duration of unemployment. This may not be a cause or effect, but may be due to some underlying factor such as a psychiatric condition, personality disorder or substance abuse.

Social factors

Suicide rates are higher in those who live alone or are in a lower social group, especially in urban areas characterized by social deprivation and overcrowding. Recent data in Australian Aboriginal people suggest substantially higher suicide rates that commence at a lower age than the non-Aboriginal population.[6] This is likely to be similar in indigenous groups of other developed countries. Some higher social status groups such as doctors, dentists, musicians, lawyers and law-enforcement officers are more prone to suicide.[7] Most adults (75%) with DSH have relationship problems with their partners and teenagers with their parents. A major argument or separation often precedes the act on a background of ongoing social difficulties.

Medical factors

There is an increased rate of medical illness in patients who commit suicide, especially epilepsy, chronic ill health, terminal illness or chronic pain. The majority of such patients will have sought medical advice in the 6 months before suicide. Most patients with DSH have good health.

Psychiatric factors

There is a pre-existing psychiatric disorder in 90–100% of cases of suicide,[8,9] of which depression accounts for 66–80%, however, this rate may be based on retrospective psychological analysis. Psychiatric disorders are present in 5–10% of patients who commit DSH, but may be secondary to social difficulties. The rate of suicide among psychiatric inpatients is 3–12 times higher than the general population and involves more violent methods such as jumping from buildings, hanging or jumping in front of vehicles. One-third of these episodes occurs after self-discharge from hospital, with another third occuring during approved leave. The high-risk time is the first week of admission and during the first 3 months after discharge.[10]

Affective disorders

The psychiatric diagnosis that carries the greatest risk of suicide is mood disorder, particularly major depression if associated with borderline personality disorder, anxiety or agitation.[11] Fifteen per cent of these high-risk patients commit suicide over a lifetime. Depression correlates well with the occurrence of suicidal desire and ideation, but may not be as strong a predictor of planning and preparation (intense thoughts, plans, courage and capability),[9] and, therefore, suicide completion. Hopelessness is the most important factor associated with suicide completion and may be of greater importance than suicidal ideation or depression itself.[9] A high degree of hopelessness during an episode of depression increases the current risk of suicide, but also of future feelings of hopelessness and, therefore, of future risk of suicide. Depressed patients should, therefore, have their attitudes towards the future carefully assessed.

Substance abuse

Fifteen per cent of alcohol dependent persons eventually commit suicide. The majority of these are also depressed. The risk is higher if associated with social isolation, poor physical health, unemployment and previous suicidal behaviour. There is an increased risk of suicide in patients who use recreational drugs. Young male heroin addicts may have 20 times the risk of the general population. Alcohol dependence is uncommon in DSH, but alcohol intoxication is involved in 50–90% of suicide attempts.

Schizophrenia

Up to 10% of schizophrenics die by suicide. Young adult males are at high risk especially if there is associated depression, previous suicidal behaviour or unemployment, or if they live alone or were recently discharged from hospital. Most suicides occur during a relatively chronic or non-psychotic phase of the illness associated with some degree of insight into possible mental deterioration or with feelings of hopelessness.

Personality disorders

Patients with antisocial and borderline personality disorders are at high risk of DSH and suicide, especially if associated with labile mood, impulsivity, alienation from peers and associated substance abuse. This may be due to precipitation of undesirable life events, predisposition to psychiatric and substance-abuse disrders, and social isolation. Adjustment disorders are common in adolescents (associated with 25% of adolescent suicide).[8]

Neuroses

Multiple attenders to emergency departments are also at high risk. This group has seven times the risk of the general population and rates of suicide similar to clinical psychiatric populations. This risk is particularly pronounced in patients who present with panic attacks, especially if associated with depressive symptoms.

ASSESSMENT

This requires a systematic, multidisciplinary approach involving prior staff education; appropriate triage, observation and restraint procedures; and a planned strategy for assessment followed by appropriate treatment and disposition. The overall priorities are to define the physical sequelae of the act, risk of further suicidal behaviour, and any psychiatric diagnoses. These three aspects are those that can then be targeted for short-term interventions.

Triage

In a patient who has attempted DSH, initial management involves resuscitation, treatment of immediate life threats and preventing complications. The patient should be triaged according to both the physical problem as well as current suicidality, aggressiveness and mental state. The mental health triage scale can be used for this purpose.[12] A triage score of 2 or 3 should be applied if the patient is violent to themselves or others, actively suicidal, is psychotic or distressed or at risk of leaving before full assessment. Constant observation is required at this point and nursing staff, orderlies, security or police may be needed.

Medical assessment

The patient should be prevented from doing further harm by limiting availability of drugs, removing sharp implements, removing car keys, ropes, belts or sheets and securing nearby windows. Other concurrent and concealed methods of self-harm should be sought. Assessment of the patient may be difficult either due to an organic cause, they may still be unsettled from the precipitant of the act, or from genuinely not wanting to be in hospital or allow medical intervention. This may necessitate the physical or chemical restraint of the patient if they are at a high risk or cannot be fully assessed and want to self-discharge. Emotional support of patient, friends and relatives is required during this phase.

Suicide risk assessment

Initially, this needs to be done in the emergency department so as to determine patient disposition, however, full psychiatric assessment may need to wait until drug effects wear off. Other sources of information need to be accessed since patient history can be unreliable or incomplete. Friends, family, local doctor, ambulance officers, helping agencies already involved and previous presentations documented in the medical record can all add useful information in order to complete an assessment. A therapeutic relationship should be formed and the clinician should be non-judgmental, non-threatening and clearly willing to help. A negative attitude is common among emergency personnel, especially with repeat attenders. This may intensify the patient's already low self esteem, increasing future suicide potential and making a therapeutic relationship difficult to establish.[13] When managing a patient who may be suicidal, the suicidal ideation should be discussed openly. This does not increase the likelihood of attempted suicide and may make the patient realize there are other options.

Assessment of suicide risk involves assessing background demographic, psychiatric, medical and social factors, as well as the current circumstances and suicidal behaviour itself as outlined in

Table 19.4.1. There are epidemiological differences between people who attempt suicide and those who complete suicide. Although the groups are different, there is an important overlap. The more an individual's characteristics resemble the profile of a suicide completer, the higher the risk of future suicide or suicide attempts. Despite this, in long-term follow-up studies, very few of these factors have been shown to be good predictors of suicide following DSH. The most consistent factors are psychiatric illness, personality disorder, substance abuse, multiple previous attempts, and current suicidality and hopelessness. Guidelines are available to assist in suicide-risk stratification and describe characteristics associated with suicide-risk levels and the appropriate further assessment and disposition for each group.[14]

Use of scales

Many screens have been devised to identify high-risk groups within those presenting with DSH. PATHOS,[15] Suicidal Intent Scale,[16] Sad Persons Scale[17] and other scoring systems have been devised to complement medical assessment of suicide risk. The modified Sad Persons Scale (Table 19.4.2) incorporates some high-risk characteristics to predict suicide risk in patients with suicidal ideation or behaviour. However, many of these scales use outdated risk factors and patient populations unrepresentative of what we see in emergency departments. Scales need to be sensitive, however, this misclassifies a large number of individuals as potentially suicidal. These deficiencies need to be considered when applying suicide risk scales in the emergency department and these scales should not be used as an absolute assessment of suicide risk or of the need for psychiatric assessment. The problems associated with suicide-risk assessment are summarized in Table 19.4.3.

DEFINITIVE TREATMENT AND DISPOSITION

Following necessary medical treatment and suicide-risk stratification, disposition

Table 19.4.1 Factors associated with suicide[13]

Variable	High risk	Low risk
Background factors		
Gender	Male	Female
Marital Status	Single, separated, divorced, widowed	Married
Employment	Unemployed or retired	Employed
Medical factors	Chronic illness, chronic pain, epilepsy	Good health
Psychiatric factors	Depression, schizophrenia, previous psychiatric inpatient, substance abuse, personality disorder	No psychiatric history, mild depression, normally robust personality
Social background	Unresponsive family, socially isolated, indigenous background	Supportive family, socially stable and integrated
Current factors		
Ideation	Frequent, prolonged, pervasive	Infrequent, transient
Attempts	Multiple	First attempt
Lethality	Violent, lethal and available method, aware of medical dangerousness	Low lethality, poor availability
Planning	Planned, active preparation, extensive premeditation, telling others prior to act	Impulsive
Rescue	Act performed in isolation, event timed to avoid intervention, precautions taken to avoid discovery	Rescue inevitable, obtained help afterwards
Final acts	Wills, insurance, giving away property, suicide notes	
Coping skills	Unwilling to seek help, feels unable to cope with present difficulties	Can easily turn to others for help, can plan to overcome present difficulties, willing to become involved in aftercare
Current ideation	Admitting act was intended to cause death, no remorse or guilt, continued suicidal ideation, hopelessness	Primary wish to change, pleased to recover, suicidal ideation resolved by act, optimism
Precipitant	Similar circumstances can recur, acute precipitant not resolved	Stressful but transient life event, acute precipitant addressed

Table 19.4.2 Modified Sad Persons Scale[17]

Variable	Score
Gender: male	1
Age: <19 or >45 years	1
Depression: hopelessness, despair especially if associated with physiological shift symptoms	2
Psychiatric care: previous DSH, psychiatric care or severe personality disorder	1
Excessive drug use	1
Rational thinking loss: severe depression with psychotic features, organic brain syndrome, delusions	2
Single, separated, divorced, widowed	1
Organized attempt: planned, premeditated, lethal and available method	2
No life supports: social isolation, homeless, unemployed	1
States future intent: continued suicidal ideation	2

may involve involuntary or voluntary admission to a psychiatric or medical ward, short-term or overnight observation with psychiatric or social worker review, or discharge with appropriate follow-up. Restraint and involuntary admission may be necessary for the high-risk patient who wishes to self-discharge.

Overnight observation is required for many patients to allow drug intoxication to resolve so that proper psychiatric assessment can take place. An overnight stay in hospital can also help resolution of many areas of conflict. Important elements of management involve neutralizing the precipitating problem, treatment of psychiatric illness and environmental interventions such as family counselling, encouraging a support network, and developing coping and problem-solving skills.[19] Open discussion about suicide should be undertaken and a firm stance should be maintained that suicide is an ineffective solution. Alternative, non-suicide solutions should be reinforced. Other factors that should be addressed whilst patients are in hospital include problems with relationships, employment, finances, housing, legal problems, social isolation, alcohol and drug abuse, and bereavement. In this regard, medical social workers are invaluable. For repeat attenders or manipulative patients who are often socially isolated, hospitalization should not be a substitute for social services, substance-abuse treatment and legal assistance,[20] although admission may be necessary while appropriate supports are put in place.

Discharge is appropriate for the low-risk patient who is cooperative, no longer suicidal, not intoxicated, has no underlying psychiatric or substance abuse disorder, and has strong social support with the precipitating problem having resolved due to the act or subsequent assessment and intervention in hospital. Discharged patients should make a

Table 19.4.3 Problems in assessing suicide risk

Suicide is rare, even in high-risk groups, so it cannot be predicted without a high rate of false-negative or false-positive errors

Suicidality presents in heterogeneous ways that may not be recognized

Suicidality is transient and affected by intoxication, stress and being in hospital

The patient may be reluctant, oppositional or manipulative

The patient may present in an atypical fashion, especially the elderly with physical complaints[18]

Suicide risk factors identify high-risk subgroups but not individuals

The demographic factors associated with suicide have changed recently thus changing the make-up of risk groups

Risk factors are based on studies of long-term follow-up and, therefore, long-term risk

Subtle changes in mental status and behaviour may be missed if not assessed by the usual doctor

Unexplained improvement in psychological status may be the result of increased motivation to die

Patients may deny their true intentions due to embarrassment, fear of being stopped in carrying out their own wishes, fear of being institutionalized, or fear of the confidentiality of the interview

Patients may say life is not worth living or that they feel they would be better off dead, but not necessarily have an increased risk of suicide, unless they have made suicidal plans or attempts or if they have pervasive hopelessness

Correlation between medical danger and suicidal intent is low unless the patient can accurately assess the probable outcome of their attempts if treatment had not been received

---

commitment to seek help if they reach a crisis point, and the physician should be available to help. This can be part of a commitment to a non-suicidal behavioural plan between the patient and clinician. This contract should be with the clinician who will arrange definitive care. Contracts may delay the patient's suicidal impulses so that other treatment strategies can be implemented. If discharged, there should be liaison with the patient's general practitioner and therapist, and follow-up should be confirmed where possible within 1–2 days.

Pharmacotherapy involves the treatment of the underlying psychiatric disorder. Antidepressants decrease the risk of attempting suicide, although the lethality of suicide attempts is increased if tricyclic antidepressants are taken in overdose. Selective serotonin reuptake inhibitors may have a more selective effect in decreasing suicidal behaviour and are less toxic in overdose. These factors make this class of drugs an attractive choice for depressed patients who are suicidal,[21] however, any long-term therapeutic drug should, ideally, be prescribed by the doctor who will provide definitive follow-up.

CONSEQUENCES

Risk of suicide

Approximately 1% of patients commit suicide during the year following an attempt and in approximately 40% of suicides there is a history of a previous attempt. In a prospective 18-year follow-up study, the rate of suicide after an episode of DSH was 4.0% at 5 years and 6.7% at 18 years.[22]

DSH usually invokes help from friends, family and the medical profession so that the patient's social situation and psychological well-being tends to improve. However, the risk of repetition is 12–15% in the following year with 10% of these occurring in the first week.[19] This is more likely in females who are unemployed, have a personality disorder or substance-abuse problems. Hospitalization and aftercare decrease short-term risk of suicide, but have little impact on long-term risk of suicide. Howeve, this may be due to under-treatment of psychiatric illness.[8,23,24] There is limited evidence that special aftercare reduces repetition of DSH, but these services can have a positive effect on psychological and social functioning, especially for female patients.

Exposure to suicide in adolescents tends not to cause an increased risk of suicide among friends but may cause an increased incidence of depression, anxiety, and post-traumatic stress disorder.[25]

Repeated episodes of DSH

These may be due to loneliness, attention-seeking behaviour, poor coping mechanisms or manipulation of family, friends or health carers. Some patients may use repeated DSH or continued suicidal ideation as a means of fighting off a sense of hopelessness or boredom. Chronic repeaters may suffer from personality disorders, recreational drug use, and violent behaviour. These patients place a heavy burden on hospital resources, are difficult to treat and have a high rate of eventual suicide.

PREVENTION

Comprehensive strategies for prevention of suicide have been or are being developed in Finland, Norway, Sweden, Australia and New Zealand.[3] Suicide prevention focuses on psychiatric, social and medical aspects, and usually involve public education, media restrictions on reporting of suicide, school-based programmes with teacher education, training of doctors in detection and treatment of depression and other psychiatric disorders, alcohol and drug-abuse information, enhanced access to the mental-health system and supportive counselling after episodes of DSH. Decreasing the availability of lethal methods may involve legislative changes such as more stringent gun control, restricting access to well known jumping sites or changes to availability or packaging of tablets.[26,27] Overall, studies into the effectiveness of suicide-prevention strategies have shown uncertain estimated reductions in suicide rates following interventions.[28]

Proper recognition and treatment of mental illness, improved social services, and drug- and alcohol-support services may be of greater benefit than specific suicide-prevention strategies.

CONCLUSION

Assessment of suicide risk is an important skill in emergency medicine since many patients present to emergency departments with suicidal behaviour. Athough the risk of suicide for an individual patient cannot be forecast, emergency physicians can provide a system for assessment and identifying of risk groups. We can attempt acute interventions to prevent short-term completion of suicide or repetition of DSH, since emergency physicians are predominantly involved in the care of these patients, often using short-stay wards. A team approach involving psychiatry and social work is necessary in most cases with many minor problems resolved by a short-term hospital admission, brief crisis intervention and intense short-term follow-up.

CONTROVERSIES AND FUTURE DIRECTIONS

❶ Although in most cultures suicide has been considered morally wrong since ancient times, there are arguments that it may be rational, especially if active voluntary euthanasia is considered a suicidal act.

❷ The legal position is clear in not assisting suicide, and we have a duty of care for people who are suicidal. However, the question of how long doctors should have the power to keep suicidal people alive against their will remains controversial.[29]

❸ Emergency departments have an important role in the epidemiological monitoring and further research of patient risk factors.

❹ Clinical trials of emergency-department assessment and brief intervention strategies, including short-stay admissions need to occur since more patients are managed entirely in emergency departments.

❺ Currently available guidelines need to be validated and refined, and current, local scales produced.

REFERENCES

1. Salter A, Pielage P 2000 Emergency departments have a role in the prevention of suicide. Emergency Medicine 12: 198–203
2. Australian Bureau of Statistics 2000 Suicides Australia 1921–1998. Canberra: ABS, 2000.
3. Taylor SJ, Kingdom D, Jenkins R 1997 How are nations trying to prevent suicide? An analysis of national suicide prevention strategies. Acta Psychiatrica Scandinavia 95: 457–63
4. McKelvey RS, Pfaff JJ, Acres JG 2001 The relationship between chief complaints, psychological distress, and suicidal ideation in 15–24 year-old patients presenting to general practitioners. Medical Journal of Australia 175: 550–2
5. Dudley MJ, Kelk NJ, Florio TM, Howard JP, Waters BGH 1998 Suicide among young Australians, 1964–1993: an interstate comparison of metropolitan and rural trends. Medical Journal of Australia 169: 77–80
6. Baume P 1996 Suicide in Australia: do we really have a problem? Australian Journal of Education & Developmental Psychology 13: 3–39
7. Kaplan HI, Sadock BJ, Grebb JA 1994 Kaplan and Sadock's Synopsis of Psychiatry, 7th edn. Williams & Wilkins, Baltimore pp 803–9
8. Lonnqvist JK, et al 1995 Mental disorders and suicide prevention. Psychiatry and Clinical Neurosciences 49: S111–S116
9. Hawton K 1987 Assessment of suicide risk. British Journal of Psychiatry 150: 145–53
10. Shah AK, Ganesvaran T 1997 Inpatient suicides in an Australian mental hospital. Australia and New Zealand Journal of Psychiatry 31(2): 291–8
11. Gilbody S, House A, Owens D 1997 The early repetition of deliberate self harm. Journal of the Royal College of Physicians London 31(2): 171–2
12. Smart D, Pollard C, Walpole B 1999 Mental health triage in emergency medicine. Australian and New Zealand Journal of Psychiatry 33: 57–66
13. Hutzler JC, Rund DA 1996 Behavioral disorders: emergency assessment and stabilization. In: Tintinalli JE, Krome RL, Ruiz E (eds) Emergency Medicine: A Comprehensive Study Guide, 4th edn. American College of Emergency Physicians, New York pp 1337–40
14. Australasian College for Emergency Medicine and the Royal Australian and New Zealand College of Psychiatrists 2000 Guidelines for the management of deliberate self harm in young people. ACEM and RANZCP, Victoria
15. Kingsbury S 1996 PATHOS: a screening instrument for adolescent overdose: a research note. Journal of Child Psychology and Psychiatry and Allied Disciplines 37(5): 609–11
16. Beck AT, Schuyler D, Herman J 1974 Development of suicidal intent scales. In: Beck AT, Resruk HLP, Lettieri DJ (eds) The Prediction of Suicide. Charles Press, Maryland
17. Hockberger RS, Rothstein RJ 1988 Assessment of suicide potential by nonpsychiatrists using the SAD PERSONS score. Journal of Emergency Medicine 6(2): 99–107
18. Johnston M, Walker M 1996 Suicide in the elderly. Recognizing the signs. General Hospital Psychiatry 18(4): 257–60
19. Brent DA 1997 The aftercare of adolescents with deliberate self harm. Journal of Child Psychology and Psychiatry and Allied Disciplines 38(3): 277–86
20. Lambert MT, Bonner J 1996 Characteristics and six-month outcome of patients who use suicide threats to seek hospital admission. Psychiatric Services 47(8): 871–3
21. Kasper S, Schindler S, Neumeister A 1996 Risk of suicide in depression and its implication for psychopharmacological treatment. International Journal of Psychopharmacology 11(2): 71–9
22. De Moore GM, Robertson AR 1996 Suicide in the 18 years after deliberate self harm. British Journal of Psychiatry 169: 489–94
23. Kurz A, Moller HJ 1995 Attempted suicide: efficacy of treatment programs. Psychiatry and Clinical Neurosciences 49: S99–S103
24. McNeil DE, Binder RL 1997 The impact of hospitalization on clinical assessments of suicide risk. Psychiatric Services 48(2): 204–8
25. Brent DA, Moritz G, Bridge J, Perper J, Canobbio R 1996 Long-term impact of exposure to suicide: a three-year controlled follow-up. Journal of the American Academy of Child and Adolescent Psychiatry 35(5): 646–53
26. Cantor CH, Baume PJM 1998 Access to methods of suicide: what impact? Australian and New Zealand Journal of Psychiatry 32: 8–14
27. Hawton K, Mistry H, et al 1996 Paracetamol self-poisoning. Characteristics, prevention and harm reduction. British Journal of Psychiatry 168: 43–8
28. Gunnell D, Frankel S 1994 Prevention of suicide: aspirations and evidence. British Medical Journal 308: 1227–33
29. Wilkinson G 1994 Can suicide be prevented? British Medical Journal 309: 860–1

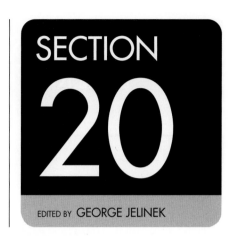

CRISIS INTERVENTION

20.1 Crisis intervention in the emergency department 604

20.2 Death and dying 608

20.3 Sexual assault 612

20.4 Domestic violence 619

20.1 CRISIS INTERVENTION IN THE EMERGENCY DEPARTMENT

JENNIFER G. BROOKES • DEBORAH S. LEACH

ESSENTIALS

1 A crisis occurs when an individual faces a problem not readily manageable using usual coping mechanisms.

2 Crisis intervention focuses on managing the immediate problem and aims to resolve the crisis and restore psychological equilibrium.

3 Timely management of a crisis may prevent the later emergence of chronic psychiatric or psychological problems.

4 The steps of crisis management include assessment, planning, intervention and follow-up.

INTRODUCTION

A crisis occurs when an individual faces a problem not readily manageable using usual coping mechanisms. It is characterized initially by increased tension and anxiety, with a state of disequilibrium, great emotional upset and a feeling of helplessness. This phase is followed by the development of problem-solving mechanisms that may or may not be successful in resolving the crisis. These mechanisms may alleviate the acute discomfort, restore emotional equilibrium and enable the person to learn adaptive reactions for use in future situations. If the mechanisms are maladaptive, the crisis worsens and functioning deteriorates. A crisis can also be seen as a turning point. The Chinese define crisis in terms of two characters: the first is WEI, which equates to danger; the second is CHI, or opportunity. The danger is self-destructive behaviour and the opportunity is to learn new and improved problem-solving techniques.[1]

Crisis intervention focuses on managing the immediate problem and aims to resolve the crisis and restore psychological equilibrium, ideally, converting failure into coping as soon as possible. Timely management of a crisis may prevent the later emergence of chronic psychiatric or psychological problems. Although many hospitals provide crisis intervention services, such as social work and pastoral counselling, some emergency departments lack specific services in crisis intervention, particularly after hours. In either case, caregivers in the emergency department need to be at least familiar with the process of crisis intervention, if not practitioners in the process itself.

THE CRISIS PROCESS

It is useful to consider the crisis process as neither pathological nor an illness, although patients with underlying psychopathology may be more vulnerable to such situations. It is not necessarily the events themselves, but rather how one experiences those events, and how one responds to the experience, that constitutes a crisis. Personality variables and prior life experience determine the perception and interpretation of the critical event, and this, in turn, determines its stressfulness. Factors involved in the event itself may compromise one's ability to cope. These include an unfamiliar situation or a sudden, unanticipated event, such as job loss, illness or relationship breakdown. The level of social support available is important in mediating the ability to cope. A person encountering crisis tends to react in a characteristic way. The initial event may result in feelings of loss, deprivation or threat to personal integrity.[2] The response results in a high degree of anxiety, tension, and a sense of loss and emptiness. A variety of feelings may occur, such as fear, shock, anger or guilt. There may be associated physical symptoms, such as sweating, tachycardia, frequency of urination, gastrointestinal disturbance or chest pain. The usual coping and problem-solving mechanisms may fail, and if the precipitating stressors continue this results in further anxiety. Unfortunately, the state of anguish and confusion experienced in crisis impairs the ability to make decisions and solve problems, the very skills needed during the crisis. When an effective solution is found using previously or newly developed coping skills, the person may return to the pre-crisis level of functioning, ideally, with improved coping skills for the future. Failure to resolve the problem leads to progressive deterioration. A state of active crisis results when internal strength and social supports are lacking, the problem remains unresolved, and tension and anxiety rise to an unbearable degree.[3] Thus, the characteristics of the individual, the nature of the precipitating stressful event and the adequacy of supports may determine the individual's success or failure in dealing with stressful events.[4]

There are a number of circumstances in which crisis intervention may be required in the emergency department, for either patients, family, friends or staff:[4]

- Crises associated with loss: bereavement, sudden infant death syndrome, separation or divorce, loss of body function, acute illness, miscarriage, loss of self-esteem, job or financial resources
- Crises associated with change: transitional or maturational crises (midlife crisis, adolescence to adulthood crises), role changes (changes in work, marital status and parenthood)

- Crises associated with interpersonal problems: assault, domestic violence, elder abuse or a child at risk
- Crises associated with marked internal conflict: when a patient may be faced with a seemingly impossible decision between two or more alternatives.

Caregivers should be alert to the need for crisis intervention in patients, families or witnesses to traumatic events and be familiar with referral agencies appropriate to their needs.

CRISIS INTERVENTION

Current crisis intervention theory and practice owe a large debt to Lindemann for his classic paper on the acute grief process in survivors following the Coconut Grove Nightclub fire in Boston in 1942, in which more than 400 people died and many more suffered burns.[5] Lindemann described the responses of survivors to this shocking loss, and is considered a paradigm for grief reactions to situational loss. His work led to the development of crisis intervention techniques. Gerald Caplan, a pioneer in preventative psychiatry, laid the foundations for crisis theory, practice and intervention.[6]

Crisis intervention is a short-term helping process that focuses on resolution of the immediate problem through the use of personal, social and environmental resources. The minimum therapeutic goal of crisis intervention is psychological resolution of the individual's immediate crisis and restoration to their previous level of functioning.[7] The maximum goal is improvement in the individual's functioning over the pre-crisis level.[7] Classic crisis intervention refers to specific intervention, usually over a 4–6-week period, although treatment may range from one to six sessions. For patients whose reactions persist beyond 6 weeks more specific therapy may be required. The physician must be aware that the goal of crisis intervention is short-term and task-oriented management to restore the individual to a level

of emotional functioning adequate for their immediate needs. Underlying psychopathology or other chronic problems may require later specific therapy.[8]

The following are goals for caregivers in crisis intervention:

- Assist people to return to their pre-crisis level of functioning.
- Improve coping skills for use in the future.
- Prevent negative outcomes resulting from the crisis.

The steps of crisis management include:[3]

- Assessment
- Planning
- Intervention
- Follow-up.

Assessment

After medical aspects of the patient's presentation have been addressed, a psychosocial assessment of the crisis situation should be undertaken. The precipitating event should be determined: this event has usually occurred within the previous 10–14 days, and frequently in the previous 24 hours.[7] The individual's perception of the event should be sought. An assessment should be made of the person's coping skills and the adequacy of supports. The presence of adequate social supports significantly influences the outcome of the crisis. Signals suggesting that a person is coping ineffectively and needs intervention to forestall a negative outcome include suicidal or homicidal ideation, difficulty in managing feelings, alcohol or drug abuse, trouble with the law, or an inability to effectively use available help. A mandatory component of assessment of individuals in crisis is determination of the risk of suicide, assault or homicide. Information from other sources should be sought, preferably with the permission of the patient. Information gathered from family, friends, police, ambulance officers or treating doctors may prove valuable. Crisis assessment is incomplete without evaluating the person's social resources and cultural milieu. Additional information that should be gathered includes the

extent to which the crisis has disrupted normal life patterns, the ability to continue normal daily activities, and the impact of the crisis on others, including support persons.

Effective interview techniques require a straightforward approach, including direct and specific questions, particularly when assessing suicidal or homicidal intent.[7] Intervention strategies include listening actively and with concern; encouraging the open expression of feelings; helping the person gain an understanding of the crisis; help with the gradual acceptance of reality and exploration of new ways of coping with problems; linking the person to a social network; and reinforcing newly learned coping strategies.[3] The provision of reassurance, explanation and information may assist in alleviating patients' misconceptions and anxieties. Similarly, the provision of clear limits for disruptive or threatening behaviour may be necessary.

Strategic steps in this phase of management include:

- Developing an empathic alliance with the patient, identifying as closely as possible with their feeling state and reflecting this back to them, e.g. 'You look terribly upset'
- Prevention of rapid and ineffective movement from one advice giver to another
- Discovering the issues
- Discovering and affirming resources: personal, family, friends, professionals.

Planning

Following assessment, a plan should be developed for the person or family in crisis, based on the information gathered. The plan should be developed in active collaboration with the person in crisis and significant others. It should be appropriate to their functional level and dependency needs, be consistent with culture and lifestyle, inclusive of significant others and the social network, be realistic, time limited and concrete, yet dynamic and renegotiable, and inclusive of follow-up.[3] If there is a significant threat to the safety of the person in crisis or others, then hospitalization is necessary. Social support is one of the most important variables influencing crisis outcome; it is the quality rather than the quantity of support that is important.[9] The person in crisis should be helped to help themselves, with the assistance of others. The plan should focus on immediate problems that directly contribute to the crisis. The mode of assessment and planning should inspire confidence, and restore a sense of order and independence to the individual in crisis, helping them, with support, to find their own solution.

Implementation

Intervention is initiated with the expectation that it is a planned action with an expected result. The problem is defined and specific direction may be given regarding alternative solutions, including mechanisms for alternatives if there are difficulties adhering to the original plan. The patient is encouraged to take responsibility for initiating positive action in developing coping skills to deal with the crisis.[3]

Follow-up

The last step includes the arrangement of appropriate follow-up and evaluation of the crisis management process, through to the resolution of the crisis. Follow-up is more likely to be successful and less likely to be viewed as an unwanted intrusion if it is incorporated into the total management plan, and assumes the individual's retention of self-determination, even in a crisis situation.[3] Although at times little more than guidance, advice or education may be required to assist the individual in the successful resolution of crisis,[2] referral for ongoing intervention may frequently be required from the emergency department. To reduce challenge and stress for the patient, the physician should take responsibility for arranging follow-up appointments.[1] Resources in the emergency department should be available to allow the caregiver to arrange appropriate referral.

It is important to remember that the crisis assessment process itself is a component of resolution. Orderly history taking and a structured interview process allow the person in crisis to identify with, and incorporate the ordered approach shown by the physician, and to regain a sense of self-control with improved understanding of the events.[1] Working through the crisis with the patient and other participants fosters confidence in the ability of those concerned to bring about a successful resolution.

CRISIS INTERVENTION FOR THOSE AROUND THE PATIENT

The care of family and friends of the person in crisis may be relatively neglected in the intervention process unless specific evaluation of those at risk is sought. It is not uncommon to find that it is not just the individual who is in crisis, but the whole family. In crisis intervention a broad base must be used to identify the need for intervention in those associated with the patient, such as family, witnesses, survivors and perpetrators of interpersonal violence.[10] Intervention with survivors of patients who have died in the emergency department, or relatives of seriously injured or ill patients, may alleviate some of the adverse effects experienced as a result of the crisis.[11-14] Specific staff employed as family advocates can form a key point in the communication loop that comprises patient, family, doctor and nurse.[14] The provision of care to those providing support to the patient further enhances the ability of supporters to assist the patient through his or her own crisis. The importance of effective communication cannot be over-emphasized. Factors such as uninterrupted time in an appropriate setting, communication style, timing, patience and content should all be considered.[15]

THE IMPACT ON STAFF

Events in the emergency department and patients' own crises may adversely affect staff. There is the risk that through direct or indirect exposure to stressful events, such as violence or victims of violence, staff may themselves become secondary victims.[16] Emergency department staff must be vigilant in detecting any adverse effect, which may occur as an inevitable part of emergency medicine practice on self, colleagues and other team members. The impact on staff of dealing with patients in crisis situations may manifest in two detrimental ways. First, it may interfere with the ability to deal with the patient appropriately in the immediate setting, and second, it may continue to adversely affect the staff member in the future. The emotional reaction of a physician to a patient is termed countertransference, and may engender feelings in the physician such as anger, anxiety, sexual arousal, sympathy or warmth.[2] Being aware of one's reactions to patients better enables an objective approach to management. Staff should hold realistic expectations in their dealings with patients. There will be many circumstances in which the shortcomings of the patient, the staff or the system result in the provision of a less than ideal service. It is not possible to provide perfect solutions all of the time.

SUPPORT FOR STAFF

Support should be provided for staff dealing with critical incidents in the emergency department or providing support for patients in crisis. Formal support may include the provision of crisis intervention, support groups, psychological debriefing, or specific counselling such as stress management. Hospitals should be vigilant in providing systems to support potentially vulnerable groups such as medical students and junior doctors. Independence of support persons from both medical power structures and direct involvement in staff evaluation strengthens their role.[17] It remains debatable as to which is the best form of intervention for particular groups and incidents. There is some controversy regarding the effectiveness of psychological debriefing for people exposed to unpleasant psychological

CONTROVERSIES AND FUTURE DIRECTIONS

❶ The provision of 24-hour crisis intervention should become standard in emergency departments.

❷ The care of patients in crisis and their families should be an area of special strength and knowledge for emergency department staff.

❸ Further research is needed to evaluate the effectiveness of interventions provided for staff following traumatic events.

experience, and further research is needed to evaluate the effectiveness of professional interventions such as psychological debriefing and more individualized counselling.[18–20]

CONCLUSION

Staff in the emergency department are frequently called upon to assist patients experiencing a crisis situation in which a problem has emerged that cannot be managed by the usual coping mechanisms. Staff must be aware of patients at risk and be able to respond in an appropriate manner to their needs. This includes identification of the patient at risk of immediate self-harm or violence, identification of available supports, initiation of crisis management, and appropriate disposition and referral. There needs to be an awareness of the impact on staff of caring for patients in crisis, and appropriate supports should be available.

REFERENCES

1. Rabin PL, Hussain G 1983 Crisis intervention in an emergency setting. Annals of Emergency Medicine 12: 300–2
2. Kercher EE 1991 Crisis intervention in the emergency department. Emergency Medicine Clinics of North America 9: 219–32
3. Hoff LA 1995 People In Crisis - Understanding and Helping, 4th edn. Jossey-Bass, San Francisco
4. Ingamells D 1988 The crisis practitioner (Editorial). Australian Family Physician 17(6): 417
5. Lindemann E 1944 Symptomatology and management of acute grief. American Journal of Psychiatry 101: 141–8
6. Caplan G 1964 Principles of Preventive Psychiatry. Basis, New York
7. Aguilera DC 1994 Crisis Intervention, 7th edn. Theory and Methodology. Mosby, St Louis
8. Kaplan H, Saddock B 1989 Comprehensive Textbook of Psychiatry, 5th edn. Williams & Wilkins, Baltimore, pp 1563–7
9. Stelmachers ZT 1996 Crisis intervention. In: Tintinelli JE, Ruiz ER, Krome RL (eds) Emergency Medicine - A Comprehensive Study Guide, 4th edn. McGraw-Hill, New York, pp 1352–6
10. Bell CC, Jenkins EJ, Kpo W, Rhodes H 1994 Response of emergency rooms to victims of interpersonal violence. Hospital and Community Psychiatry 45: 142–6
11. Adamowski K, Dickinson G, Weitzman B, Roessler C, Carter-Snell C 1993 Sudden unexpected death in the emergency department: caring for the survivors. Canadian Medical Association Journal 149: 1445–51
12. Bunn TA, Clarke AM 1979 Crisis intervention: an experimental study of the effects of a brief period of counselling on the anxiety of relatives of seriously injured or ill hospital patients. British Journal of Medical Psychology 52: 191–5
13. Yates D, Ellison G, McGuiness 1990 Care of the suddenly bereaved. British Medical Journal 301: 29–31
14. Washington G 2001 Family advocates: caring for families in crisis. Dimensions of Critical Care Nursing 20(1): 36–40
15. Reever M, Lyon D 2002 Communication in crisis. In: Lifford K et al Emedicine http:/www.emedicine.com
16. Brookes JG 1997 The impact of violence on emergency department staff. Emergency Medicine 9: 117–21
17. Grace K 2002 The junior doctor in distress: the role of the medical education officer at the individual level. Medical Journal of Australia 177(1 Suppl): S22–S24
18. Bisson JI, Deahl MP 1994 Psychological debriefing and prevention of post-traumatic stress. British Journal of Psychiatry 165: 717–20
19. Del Mar CB 2002 Should we debrief and counsel people who have had psychological shock? Medical Journal of Australia 177: 258–9
20. Raphael B, Meldrum L, McFarlane AC 1995 Does debriefing after psychological trauma work? British Medical Journal 310: 1479–80

20.2 DEATH AND DYING

BRYAN WALPOLE

ESSENTIALS

1 Death and dying are an inevitable part of emergency medicine practice.

2 Emergency physicians have a responsibility to initiate grief management.

3 The interview with the family of the recently deceased, can be a positive start to successful grieving and recovery.

4 Information about a death should not be given over the telephone.

5 In talking to relatives of the newly deceased, the word 'dead' should be used, as the grieving process can start when there is an acknowledgment of death.

6 Reactions to death include disbelief, numbness, expressive reactions, guilt and displacement activity. There should be no timelines set on recovery.

7 Relatives and their invited friends should be encouraged to view the body.

8 Organ donation services should be offered unless there are clinical contraindications.

9 Caring for the carers is often overlooked.

10 Emergency physicians should regularly self assess for emotional fatigue.

INTRODUCTION

As a truly universal human custom, dying is one of those rare things. We all do it sooner or later, however, inexpertly. All societies mark it, some heavily, some lightly. Whole religions have been invented to militate against its all too evident, shocking finality. It happens more secretly in Western societies than most, but although it happens in every community we do not talk about it as we talk about politics, sex, religion and the economy. Many cultures, not all of them ancient, are on cosier terms with death than us.

Death and dying patients are an inevitable part of emergency medicine practice. Facing a surviving family, or counselling a dying patient, may for some symbolize failure in the battle against disease. In emergency medicine practice, one does not have the benefit of a long-standing doctor–patient relationship. The support and mutual understanding that are the cornerstones of family practice are missing, and so rapport has to be forged in the heat of the moment. Families need space and time to come to grips with death, but time, and space are a precious commodity in the emergency department. Access block, and overcrowding should not preclude sensitive, empathetic grief management.

The cold, clean and sterile surroundings of a hospital morgue, or the shambles of a recently deserted resuscitation room, stand in stark contrast to the comfort, soft furnishings, and music of the funeral parlour. To follow the heat and adrenaline rush of a difficult resuscitation with the grace and emotional energy required to care for a family who have now become patients, requires considerable effort. The survivors, however, deserve our care and compassion as much as did the recently deceased.

Similarly, management of the patient brought to the emergency department in extremis, even when death is anticipated, can be a complex and challenging task, as families, baling out either through exhaustion, fear or ignorance, call an ambulance in the few hours prior to death, often in the middle of the night.

As a multicultural society we have no single distinct death ritual, nor a standard way of expressing loss and grief, as in monocultures. This, combined with the fact that most emergency department deaths are unexpected, places a significant responsibility on emergency physicians to initiate grief management and refer for continuing care.

Quality management of grief states can prevent significant morbidity, as unresolved grief can lead to later problems with physical and mental health.

THE DEATH PROCESS

Death does not occur at a finite moment. Cardiac death, cerebral death, brain-stem death and cellular death form a continuum over minutes or hours. The legal definition of death varies between regions. The diagnosis of brain death can be made accurately and positively by appropriately qualified and experienced people using relatively simple bedside tests.[1] It is imperative, however, that any reversible condition producing depression of the brain must first be excluded. The time of death is the time when brain death is established, not the time when life support is ceased. Persons considered dead may continue to breathe for a considerable length of time, and faint cardiac action that cannot be detected in major vessels, or by auscultation, can continue to provide sufficient oxygen for vital organs to survive for some hours. So it is important that relatives are not informed of death until all breathing and cardiac activity have ceased. A second opinion and cardiac monitor can help verify this.

Illustrative case

A 90-year-old man collapsed in the community and was attended by an emergency physician. Despite 15 minutes of advanced cardiac life support (including high-dose adrenaline (epinephrine)) the patient remained in persistent asystole, with no respiratory effort. Ambulance staff withdrew, the coroner was notified, but during family bereavement counselling, the emergency physician noticed the endotracheal tube moving rhythmically against the shroud. Closer inspection revealed good colour, a pulse and breathing. After 4 days in hospital the patient recovered completely, to live another 2 years, and to receive a national award for services to the country. The important principle of waiting 5–10 minutes before announcing death, and confirming the persistent cessation of vital signs, was not taken into consideration, much to the embarrassment of the doctor concerned.

This period may be used to clean the site, cut off unsightly tubes inside their orifice, and tape together or use adhesive on unsightly wounds, prior to family viewing the body. Such activities must be negotiated with forensic services beforehand, so that all requirements of the local Evidence Act can be met.

DYING PERSONS

The dying and their families face numerous psychological issues as death draws nigh. Sometimes it can be difficult to counteract the tendency to focus on the physical and tactical needs of care, rather than the emotional, spiritual and cultural dimensions of human experience. A large family may need significant space, which can interfere with the routine work of the emergency department so a private room should be available. Dying persons can have a deep-seated fear of abandonment, accepting further treatment for the sake of the family or doctor, knowing it will be of little personal benefit. Open communication and congruent goals for care should be forged early, and links with family doctor, caring specialist teams or hospice care should be established so that everyone feels safe and secure, with the proposed regimen, pending ward admission. Then all can pay special attention to physical comfort, symptom management, privacy and the confidentiality of the patient and family. Extensive references are immediately available on the Internet, for staff and family.[2]

BREAKING BAD NEWS

Most emergency department deaths are unanticipated, and informing families can be a harrowing experience. If the opportunity presents, it is essential that the family be well briefed during resuscitation and, where practicable, involved in the process. A member of the family can be invited into the resuscitation room, where the senior emergency physician present should discuss the procedures under way and provide encouragement to touch, speak to and kiss the patient. This is not only reassuring, but the presence of numerous competent staff with an array of sophisticated equipment reassures family members that the healthcare team has not let them down, and this can prevent many doubts and questions later. If the outcome is hopeless this can be discussed with the family, perhaps asking their permission before abandoning resuscitation. Even if they do not wish to accept such responsibility they will remember these moments for the rest of their lives. Having participated in the resuscitation, and in the decision to stop can be helpful, even when the request has been declined.

The interview with the family of the recently deceased can be more difficult than the resuscitation. Handled with sensitivity, however, it can be a positive start to successful grieving and recovery.

Illustrative case

A 5-year-old child was crushed by a falling goalpost during a primary school soccer game. He was brought to hospital with severe (unsurvivable) head injuries and rapidly intubated. His mother arrived shortly afterwards, and despite the gross facial deformation with brain visible, she came to the resuscitation room and had some time with her son before resuscitation was ceased. On the anniversary of his death she came to the emergency department with flowers and a request to speak to the staff who had been there on the day. She expressed her gratitude for the sensitivity and tact shown in allowing her to be part of his final moments, and stated how much this had supported her, as she knew he had never suffered and

that the final words he received prior to death were hers.

The room in which such information is given should be private, comfortable, and contain a telephone. Tea, coffee, iced water and simple food should be readily available. If refreshments arrive soon after the news has been broken, this can help diffuse tension. The offering of food is a time-honoured expression of warmth and comfort, facilitates communication and the grieving process.

Only in very exceptional cases should any information about death be given over the telephone by hospital staff. Cases abound of misidentification, and of people becoming involved in road trauma while rushing to hospital. A polite request to attend hospital as a relative is ill, should bring them in a more orderly, safe fashion. A taxi (paid for on arrival, for indigent persons) should be available.

Illustrative case

A 22-year-old man was killed when bricks being carried in a station wagon crushed his upper torso after a head-on car crash. He was identified from a driver's licence photograph, as his face was grossly distorted. The family was grieving and about to attend the bedside when a brother claimed the deceased must be someone else carrying the licence of his brother, as he had seen his brother in the past hour. It transpired that the deceased was currently suspended for drink-driving, and had borrowed a licence.

The emergency physician should greet the family by name, confirm the relationship of each with the patient, and shake hands or touch them gently. All parties should be seated, and a helpful way to start is to ask the family what they know. They may have been present at the scene, where CPR was under way, or have come to hospital independently with no preconceived ideas. Then a short résumé of the resuscitation should be given, such as:

He collapsed at work and his
workmates started resuscitation,
which was continued in the
ambulance. On arrival at hospital
he was gravely ill, we were

breathing for him, and pumping his heart for almost an hour; however, he has failed to respond to resuscitation. We ceased a short while ago, and I am afraid he is dead.

or

She was involved in a car crash on the outskirts of town. She sustained very serious head injuries and on arrival at hospital was completely unresponsive, with severe brain and neck injuries. Shortly after arrival her heart stopped and we were unable to resuscitate her further. She died a few moments ago.

It is important to use the word 'dead' or 'died'; euphemisms such as 'passed away', 'she's gone', 'departed this life', are unclear messages that can mislead. The grieving process cannot start until there is acknowledgement of death. A truthful explanation can be comforting.

Reactions

There are a range of responses to the information that a close relative has died. The mode of death can be a guide. Homicide can lead to great distress, along with suicide and unintended injury. Some common reactions are:

- Disbelief: some will immediately deny the event, claiming it must be somebody else, or that they are dreaming. Reinforcement is required.
- Numbness: some sit mute, appearing not to take in the information. They need time to absorb it.
- Expressive: a sudden flood of tears or loud cries (a Latin cultural response) with upsetting or disturbing noises should be allowed to run its course. Such acknowledgement can be a positive response.
- Guilt: particularly with homicide and suicide, such news is often followed by 'if only', or 'why couldn't I have'. Here, gentle repeated reassurance and discussion can be important. These people are at risk for pathological grief reactions, and can be helped by seeing the body and talking to it.
- Displacement activity: an immediate

call to inform relatives, organize the funeral and discuss family matters is a poor prognostic sign. These people are often seen as mature, rational, and born organizers, but they are at serious risk for pathological grief reactions months later. They will need careful follow-up to see that they grieve eventually.

Grief is not like an illness, to be fought and cured as so often is the case in Western medicine. Generalizations can be made about human behavioural tendencies, and time lines can be drawn for predicted recovery, but each person's grieving process is unique.

Some people never get better and nobody survives grief unchanged.

All relatives need time to receive the clear message of death, which they may need to be given again and again. Some need to make meaning of the event, and the clinical art of managing perceptions is paramount.

VIEWING THE BODY

Relatives and their invited friends should be encouraged to view the body. By seeing the body, by feeling and touching, the grieving process, separation and rebuilding can start. People should be encouraged to speak to, touch, kiss, stroke, caress, even to argue, negotiate and cajole in private for as long as they wish. Without this time, weeks or months later, delusions can persist that the person might not have died, and conspiracy theories can emerge. The presence of a bereavement or viewing room can make this process much easier as, particularly with children, visiting can go on for several hours. A hospital morgue may be used, some have a purpose-built facility and appropriate staff support. Relatives should be informed of the necessity for police presence if the matter has been referred to the coroner.

LEGAL ISSUES

By law, in all Australian States a body belongs to the Crown until a death

certificate is issued. This is issued by the Registrar General after satisfactory details are supplied by a medical practitioner on the medical certificate as to the reasons for death. This is a legal document, and is the source of information for the preparation of national mortality statistics. The quality of these statistics, and subsequent public-health interventions, depend largely on the ability of doctors to present accurate information.

DEATH CERTIFICATES

Cases where a death must be referred to the coroner are usually detailed on the inside of the death certificate book. Any death suspected to be not entirely from natural causes, requires reporting. The coroners office will assist.

Unless the emergency physician is thoroughly familiar with the patient and the medical history, and saw the patient prior to death, the opinion as to whether a death certificate should be issued should be left to the family practitioner, specialist or hospital unit normally caring for the patient. Where the cause of death is unclear, or no doctor has sufficient information to fill out a death certificate, an autopsy is required. Although this may cause distress to some families (and particular ethnic groups), any bona fide cultural concern can be referred to the coroner, where such matters are usually dealt with sensitively. Under the requirements of the Evidence Act, a body must be under the jurisdiction of the police from as soon as practicable after death until the coroner states that it is no longer required for legal purposes. Thus, any interference with the body is illegal, unless it is with the assent of the police officer in charge. The coroner's office should be notified as soon as practicable after death, so a police officer, if required, can attend.

ORGAN DONATION

Although parenchymal organs are generally taken from beating-heart donors, the recently dead can be corneal or occasionally renal donors. Organ donation should be mentioned unless there are clinical contraindications, such as hepatitis B, HIV or malignancy. Relatives can ask later why donation was not suggested, and some really appreciate the opportunity to contribute to the welfare of others. A routine check of the driver's licence, or at the donor registry can help clarify the issue. All Australian States have access to professional transplant coordinators to facilitate the process once permission has been obtained.

BEREAVEMENT COUNSELLING

Most hospitals have qualified practitioners to support the recently bereaved. Referral should be arranged prior to departure if counsellors have not already made contact. Ministers of religion are trained in grief counselling, and are usually available after hours. People can feel unprepared to ask for them, and it is not necessary for the deceased to have had any religious affiliation to make use of such counsellors. The family doctor is also a useful resource, and should always be informed promptly, of the death of a practice patient. Social workers are expert in grief counselling, and many funeral companies now provide counselling services.

SUBSEQUENT ISSUES

Permission to leave

Recently bereaved people are sometimes confused, frightened, stunned, and at a loss as to what to do next. When forensic issues (identification, statements) and viewing have been completed, they can be given the dead person's possessions and politely given permission to leave the hospital. 'There is nothing more you can do', or 'Can I phone someone or get a taxi to take you home' may be usefully offered.

Information about contacting a funeral office to arrange for collection of the death certificate and the body, and to

discuss burial rites, should be in an explanatory leaflet, readily available.

Tranquillizers

Requests for tranquillizers can come from survivors or a third party, who may ask that the bereaved be given sedation. Most experts involved in loss and grief counselling agree that early sedation is contraindicated. It may be part of the management of morbid grief weeks or months later, but has no place in early management. Anxiety, sadness and insomnia can be a natural part of early grief.

Follow-up

For most people the normal expectations are that they will live the allotted 3 score years and 10, according to the biblical principle, that parents will predecease their children, and that the dying person will be able to deal with any unfinished business and die surrounded by loved ones, as seen on TV, video and film. There is an expectation that death will be natural, peaceful and, for the majority, pain free. In marked contrast to such expectations is the unexpected death of a loved one at an emergency department, where rape, murder, or innocent victims of armed hold-ups, terrorists or love-struck psychopaths are regular realities. The mode of death has major implications for the resolution of grief. Iserson describes four modes of death often referred to as the NASH categories (natural, abuse, suicide, and homicide), of which the latter three particularly require careful follow-up for abnormal bereavement reactions. Shame, guilt, morbid hatred, outrage and resignation often follow deaths where there has been violence, violation or other wilful intent. Following receipt of the autopsy report, a follow-up interview can be arranged with the family, when matters surrounding death can be discussed.

Where deaths have been witnessed, post-traumatic stress disorder may occur. This is defined in DSM-III-R as the development of characteristic symptoms following a psychologically distressing event outside the range of usual human

experience. Early treatment is controversial, and may produce a better outcome, but it is almost always welcome. The concept of trauma debriefing is now well established, not only in the literature but in clinical practice throughout the world. It is a legal requirement in some occupational health and safety legislation. Some organizations offer telephone counselling and meetings.

It is also important to educate significant others in a person's life as to the symptoms of pathological grief, so that appropriate support can be offered.

PROFESSIONAL ISSUES

One of the important aspects of looking after survivors is caring for the carers, who are often overlooked. Those involved in caring for others who have experienced trauma need support and the opportunity to vent thoughts and feelings. Many authorities, including the National Association for Loss and Grief (NALAG), consider it imperative that formal diffusing and debriefing should be provided to any worker involved either at the scene of trauma or with surviving victims, or with family members of victims. The mental health of professionals is an important consideration, and due recognition should be given to this aspect so as to offset possible burnout. Emergency department managers need to give attention to thresholds for adding debriefing to standing orders, as mandated in some hospitals. Junior and rotating staff may be less resistant than professional practitioners of emergency medicine. There is, however, a distinct propensity for those who spend their lives among misery to become cynical and full of black humour. The cultural norms of emergency medicine can become so integrated into personal values that the physician does not even recognize their presence. We should regularly assess our own emotional fatigue, and if there is a significant divergence between our personal values and career activities, we may be motivated to seek support from a trusted source.

CONTROVERSIES AND FUTURE

❶ The challenge for emergency physicians is to further develop departmental policies and procedures relating to death and dying in the emergency department, and to ensure that staff are well versed in these procedures. Departments need to work on improving communication with community health practitioners.

❷ There is a growing debate about whether the witholding of information about the death of a loved one over the telephone constitutes medical paternalism, and takes away people's autonomy. Currently, however, it is still accepted that such information should be witheld.

❸ Increasingly attention will be paid to ensuring the well-being of staff who are constantly exposed to death and dying in the course of their duties.

FURTHER READING

Carey G, Sorensen R (eds) 1997 The Penguin Book of Death. Penguin Books, Melbourne University Press, Melbourne

Iserson KV 1999 Grave Words; Notifying Survivors About Sudden Unexpected Deaths. Galen Press Ltd., Tucson, AZ
Plueckhahn VD, Breen K J, Cordner S M 1994 Law and Ethics in Medicine for Doctors in Victoria. Melbourne University Press, Melbourne

Selby H 1992 (ed.) The Aftermath of Death. Federation Press, Ananndale, Australia
Tintinalli J, Ruiz E, Krome RL (eds) 1996 Emergency Medicine: a Comprehensive Study Guide, 4th edn. McGraw-Hill, New York

WEBSITES

http://www.findingourway.net/ An American site, extensive links for bereavement information.
http://www.compassionatefriends.org/ An international organisation, offering support for parents that have children die. "Unconditional love with no timeline."
http://www.compassionate friendsvictoria.org.au/ The Victorian site for the above. Qld, WA and NSW are linked from the site.
http://www.nalagvic.org.au/ The Victorian site of a national organisation, set up after the Granville train crash. Has a number of good specific links, mostly Australian.
http://www.grief.org.au/ Site for assistance, support, education, claiming to prevent poor outcomes. Partly government funded.

20.3 SEXUAL ASSAULT

IAN KNOX • ROSLYN CRAMPTON

ESSENTIALS

1 Rape is an assault in which a sexual act is used as a means of humiliating or controlling the victim. The perceived stigma to the victim caused by cultural myths results in underreporting of this criminal offence.

2 The complex medical, legal and psychological sequelae mandate a team-based approach involving doctors, police and counsellors in a collaborative effort. Allowing the victim to control the pace and extent of the caregiver's response is an important aspect of the victim's recovery.

3 The medical evaluation is specifically directed at the issues of injury assessment and management, infection risk and emergency contraception. The forensic aspects of the examination have specific objectives.

INTRODUCTION

Rape, and all its variations and sub-entities, is an act of violence in which a sexual act is part of the assault. Sexual pleasure, in the way the general community would perceive this pleasure, is not the objective of the rapist. The intention is to subjugate, humiliate or control the victim, and the sexual act is the means by which this is achieved.[1]

The failure to understand this fundamental distinction has allowed a host of misconceptions and myths to arise that not only tend to exonerate the perpetrator but transfer blame to the victim. Over 90% of the victims of adult sexual assault are women and 98% of the offenders are men. Therefore, for the purposes of this review, the victim is referred to as if female and the offender as if male.

DEFINITIONS

As the word *rape* is surrounded by legal and emotional issues, the term *sexual assault* is preferable to change the focus to the assaultive nature of the act.

Sexual assault is a crime, with a legal definition, which may vary between states and territories. Section 347 of the Queensland Criminal Code is a typical example. Rape is defined as:

Sexual intercourse (carnal knowledge) without consent of the woman or with consent if consent was obtained by force, threat, fear of bodily harm or by fraudulent misrepresentation.

Each part of this definition has accumulated further legal interpretation and case law. However, it is phrased, sexual assault has a number of elements. It is an act of a sexual nature, which is carried out against the will of the victim. The victim either does not give consent, is intimidated to consent, or is legally incapable of giving consent because of youth or incapacity. It includes attempts to force the victim into sexual activity and also includes rape, attempted rape, aggravated sexual assault (assault with a weapon or infliction of injury), indecent assault (oral or anal intercourse), penetration by objects and forced sexual activity that did not result in penetration. These incidents represent offences in every Australian state and territory.

Penetration is not an essential element to sexual assault. Indeed, in many sexual assaults, the assailant is unable to initiate or complete sexual intercourse.[2]

The absence of physical resistance by the victim is not regarded as consent. Consent by intimidation or coercive conduct without physical threat is also a criminal act.

Sexual assault by a carer upon a child is termed sexual abuse. This is sexual activity in which consent is not an issue and involves the child in sexual activity that is either beyond the child's understanding or is contrary to accepted community standards. There are legal definitions regarding age, generally in the order of 15–17 years depending on the state or territory. Sexual violence involving a disabled person may also be either abuse or assault depending on the nature of the act or the circumstances of the victim.

EPIDEMIOLOGY

In the year 2000, 15 630 victims of sexual assault were reported to Australian police.[3] This represented a 10% increase on the preceding year; and represents a rate of 82 victims/100 000 persons. The reported incidence of sexual assault reflects only a fraction of the actual frequency of the crime. Victims hesitate reporting because of humiliation, fear of retribution and lack of understanding with the criminal justice system. Once an incident of sexual assault has been reported to the police, 22% of cases result in the perpetrator being charged.[4]

In order to assess the nature and extent of violence against women, the Australian Bureau of Statistics in 1996 undertook a survey of 6300 women, a sample representative of the almost seven million Australian women over the age of 18 years.[5]

The investigators reported that almost 100 000 Australian women over the age of 18 years were victims of a sexual assault in the preceding 12 months. This represents 1.4% of the adult female population. Overall, 18% had experienced sexual violence during their lifetime and for almost half of these, this had occurred on more than one occasion. This is consistent with American statistics that one in five women in the USA will suffer a sexual assault and that one in 17 will suffer forced sexual intercourse in their lifetime.[6]

Overwhelmingly, the offender is known to the victim. In the ABS study, only 22.7% of the sexual assaults were committed by strangers. Her assailant was most likely to be her boyfriend or date (34%), a friend (27%) or a previous partner (21%). The violation of trust that this represents also has a significant effect on the victim. Spousal rape is often more violent and repetitive than other rape, and is less commonly reported, in part because of economic dependency.[7]

The victim's response to the assault is also important. The ABS study confirmed the belief that only a small minority of women ever report to the police. Overall, this was 10%, with 8.5% reporting to a doctor and another 13% seeking the help of professional counselling. Most women look for the support of family, friends, neighbours and workmates. For whatever reason, 22% of women who suffered a sexual assault had spoken to no one, sought no help and had taken no action as a result of the assault.

RAPE MYTHS AND BARRIERS TO CARE

Any review of the literature on sexual assault will uncover discussions regarding social attitudes and preconceptions, often called rape myths.

In general, these myths reflect positions, values, or feelings that are not based on fact. Many of the rape myths arise and are perpetuated by socialization processes that specify sex-role behaviours and attitudes towards women. Date rape

is thought to be exceedingly under-reported because the victim believes she contributed to the act because she participated in foreplay. Acceptance of these rape myths can convey that victims are responsible for the assault. This results in ignoring the multifaceted nature of the problem, blaming the rape victim, and reinforcing her guilt and shame. Indeed, the ABS study found that 12.5% of women did not report the assault to the police because of shame and embarrassment.

When considering how to approach the sexual assault victim, emergency physicians and nurses need to be aware of these attitudes that the victim and they themselves may have. A non-judgmental, accepting stance by care providers is essential. The victim will have enough self-doubt without carers adding to that. It is not the health professional's role to make a judgement as to whether the rape occurred; the courts will decide this. False allegations of rape are made but given the perceived penalties associated with reporting a rape, such a person is likely to be disturbed and in need of help anyway.

MEDICAL CARE FOR THE VICTIM

The objective for the attending doctor is firstly to provide for the medical needs of the victim and also, if required, to collect forensic evidence to assist in any police investigation. The history taken from the victim must be very specific and questions should be restricted to obtaining information for these purposes only. Questions should not lead into other aspects of the assault which are not relevant to the examining doctor's involvement. It is important not to prolong the examination for the victim. Furthermore, undirected questioning risks bringing inconsistencies into the description of the assault that may hinder subsequent criminal proceedings.

In general terms, there are three matters which need attention when assessing the medical needs of the sexual assault victim. These are the risk of:

1. Physical injury
2. Acquiring an infection
3. Pregnancy.

The literature typically describes about half the victims having some sort of physical injury,[8–12] although less than 5% of victims require admission to hospital for treatment. A recent analysis of over 1000 cases[13] revealed that physical examination shows evidence of general body trauma in 64% of victims. Genital trauma was noted in 52% of victims, while 20.4% of patients had no injuries documented. These findings indicate that many sexual assault victims may not have either general or genital trauma on examination, and this absence does not mean that an assault did not occur.

Studies of the genital injuries of victims using colposcopy[14] have revealed that up to 87% of patients have some type of injury. More conventional examination of the pre-menopausal victim will reveal that only around a third have genital injuries documented, usually cervical erosions, abrasions, bruising and swelling. Generally, such injuries do not require specific treatment with up to one-third being asymptomatic. Nonetheless, they should be assessed and documented. Toluidine blue staining may also increase the detection rate of perineal lacerations in adult victims.

If injuries are photographed, this is best done by a police photographer qualified in forensic photography. The victim may not give an accurate indication of her injuries such may be the emotional impact of the assault. Some victims are unable to recall even if penetration occurred.

Most non-genital injuries are found on the head, neck and face. One-third are on the extremities and 15% on the trunk. Again, the large majority of these injuries require either symptomatic or outpatient care (abrasions, lacerations and minor fractures). Less than 1% are serious enough to warrant admission. Very occasionally, rape may turn into murder. A study from Florida found that one in 1500 sexual assaults resulted in the death of the victim, with asphyxiation as the most common cause of death.[15] While there has been no comparable Australian study, the Australian Institute of Criminology reports that there were 351 homicides committed in Australia in 1990–91 and a sexual assault was the precipitating factor in 11 (3.1%).[16]

Providing accurate advice to a woman on the risk of acquiring a sexually transmitted disease is made difficult by a number of factors. First, published data are only a guide in the settings in which the studies were done. Second, all studies acknowledge the difficulty of distinguishing between pre-existing infection and infection acquired as a result of the assault. One study found that 43% of victims had evidence of pre-existing infection.[17] Third, only a very small percentage of women actually report being sexually assaulted and are, therefore, available to study relative risks. Finally, poor follow-up rates are the norm, making assessment of risk of those diseases with long incubation periods, typically the viral sexually transmitted diseases (STDs), difficult.

It is the rapist, of course, who is the source of such infections but there is little, if any, literature regarding the incidence of STD infection in rapists. While the documented sexual activities of rapists tend to be high risk in respect of acquiring STD,[18] there is a high rate of sexual dysfunction in rapists in their ability to maintain an erection and ejaculate.[2]

While the risk of acquiring an infection is difficult to define, women will generally accept an offer of antibiotics. Intramuscular ceftriaxone is the antibiotic of choice,[19] in combination with either oral doxycycline or erythromycin depending on whether the victim is pregnant. Ceftriaxone can be mixed with lidocaine to reduce the pain of the injection.[20] Oral antibiotic alternatives include ciprofloxacin and amoxicillin (plus probenecid) depending on local resistance patterns.

Given the low prevalence of syphilis in the general community,[20] it may be reasonable not to give benzathine penicillin routinely, but to have syphilis serology performed at 3 months depending on the circumstances and whether follow-up can be assured.

Hepatitis B virus can be transmitted by sexual intercourse,[21–23] but the risk of transmission is undefined. By comparison, the risk of infection following a percutaneous needlestick from a HBAg-positive individual to a HBAb-negative recipient is 5–43%.[24] There is very little mention of HBV testing in the literature relating to rape management programs but it has been advocated for victims of both sexes.[25,26]

HBV vaccination and immunoglobulin should be available where the assailant is either known to be HBV+ve or the woman is considered to be particularly at risk of infection. Hepatitis B vaccination without HBIG is highly effective in preventing HBV infection in sexual contacts of persons who have chronic HBV infection. Persons exposed to an assailant with acute HB V infection additionally require HBIG which prevents 75% of such infections.[27]

It is likely that the victim will be concerned about HIV or will become concerned at a later date. The offer of HIV testing should be made accompanied by the usual, full explanation and written consent needs to be obtained if the test is done. A prospective study from the Royal London Hospital of 124 victims found one case of HIV seroconversion that could have been a result of a sexual assault.[28] Risk assessment includes the probability the source is infected, the likelihood of transmission at that exposure, the interval before therapy, the efficacy of the drugs, and adherence to therapy. The risk of transmission of HIV following percutaneous needlestick exposure from a known HIV-positive source is considered to be 0.4%. The risk for HIV transmission per episode of receptive penile anal exposure is 0.1–3%. The risk per episode of receptive vaginal exposure is 0.1–0.2%.[29] The risk following exposure to other body fluids is not known but should be lower. Prophylaxis against HIV using retroviral or other agents has not been shown to be effective in protecting sexual assault victims and is not generally recommended.[17] Studies on health care workers are not applicable as they had rapid access to HIV status of the contaminant and access to antiviral agents often within 1–2 hours. Note as many as 35% of health care workers do not finish the course due to side effects. However, the circumstances of the victim or the assault may necessitate the consideration of HIV prophylaxis, for example a male rape in a prison setting. Of the agents available, zidovudine is the best studied and most effective[30] despite uncertainties about teratogenicity and mutagenicity. The dose and administration follows the recommendations for occupational exposure.[31]

Tetanus prophylaxis must be considered as part of the management of any injuries in the normal way.

The risk of pregnancy following a single unprotected coitus has proven difficult to define. However, a large prospective study from North America rated the risk of pregnancy from rape as 5%.[32]

There are a variety of emergency contraception options and, until recently, the most widely used was the so-called Yuzpe regimen. This consists of two doses of a combination of ethinyl oestradiol 100 g and levonorgestrel 0.5 mg, the first dose taken within 72 hours of intercourse and the second 12 hours later. This regimen is not provided as a distinct formulation but is conveniently obtained by using appropriately dosed oral contraceptive pills. The failure rate is variously estimated at between 2%[33] and 25%.[34] Many women experience nausea and vomiting after taking this combination and while there is no evidence that this reduces its efficacy, a concurrent anti-emetic is usually prescribed. Pregnancy is the only absolute contraindication with a history of thrombo-embolic disease being a relative contraindication. The 1998 WHO taskforce[35] compared the Yutzpe with the use of the progestagen, levonorgestrel, used alone in two separate doses each of 0.75 mg given 12 hours apart. If given within 72 hours the proportion of pregnancies prevented was 85% compared with 57% with Yutzpe regimen, and nausea and vomiting were significantly less frequent. With either regimen, the earlier it is given, the more effective it is. The formulation of 0.75 mg levonorgestrel is now available in Australasia.

Insertion of an intrauterine contraceptive device is a highly effective, if less convenient alternative. Its failure rate is less than 1%, but is associated with pelvic infection and medico-legal uncertainties.

Treatment/prophylaxis options for victims are summarized in Table 20.3.1.

The literature demonstrates that there is poor compliance with follow-up instructions. Arrangements for follow-up testing for pregnancy, STDs, HIV and hepatitis B vaccination should be supplied as written instructions as victims may subsequently remember little of their interview.

THE FORENSIC EXAMINATION

The forensic examination is carried out at the request of the police for the purpose of obtaining evidence of the rape or assault that could be used in a prosecution. Police services produce kits that give a comprehensive guide to the examinations required for the various aspects of the prosecution. These kits also contain a comprehensive range of swabs, slides and specimen containers for the collection of this evidence. It is important for the examining doctor to

Table 20.3.1 Treatment options for the sexual assault victim
Antibiotic prophylaxis Ceftriaxone 250 mg i.m. plus doxycycline 100 mg b.d. for 7 days or erythromycin 500 mg q.i.d. for 7 days, or Ciprofloxacin 250 mg p.o. as an alternative to ceftriaxone
Antiviral prophylaxis Protection against Hepatitis B or HIV transmission should follow institutional treatment guidelines for occupational exposure to these agents.
Emergency contraception Levonorgestrel 0.75 mg in two separate doses 12 hours apart **or** Two oral contraceptive pills (containing ethinyl oestradiol 50 μgm) and repeated 12 hours later. May be preceded by an anti-emetic (e.g. metoclopramide 10 mg) taken 30 minutes beforehand

be very familiar with the contents of these kits and have an organized approach to collection of all specimens. This familiarization must occur beforehand and should not be left until the time of the examination to sort what needs to be done. Careful documentation of all general and genital injuries is valuable, and may be aided by use of a body map. Grey-Euram et al[36] found that evidence of genital and non-genital trauma was significantly associated with successful prosecution.

It is important to recognize that the victim may not be able to make an immediate decision as to whether to proceed to making a formal statement to the police. However, there are time constraints on the collection of forensic evidence. A solution may be to collect the evidence and have the police store it. The victim can then make an unhurried decision over the next few days as to whether she wishes to proceed. The forensic examination should also be guided by the history. For example, if anal intercourse has not occurred, there is no point in putting the victim through a rectal examination.

It is always the victim's prerogative as to whether the examination is to occur and whether all parts of the examination are to be performed. The legal concept of 'the chain of evidence' must be followed in the handling of forensic specimens. The chain of evidence does not require a police officer to be present during the examination, but the specimens should be handed to the police after the examination is concluded.

The objectives of the forensic examination are quite specific. They are to collect evidence regarding:

- Proof of sexual contact
- Consent or the use of force
- The identity of the assailant.

Proof of sexual contact

Proof of sexual contact is established by the detection of spermatozoa or semen either on or within the victim or on her clothes. In general only 50% of sexual assault cases have seminal evidence recovered, and this rate decreases after

24 hours. The likelihood of detecting spermatozoa or semen from the vagina is generally very low by 72 hours.[37] However, under some circumstances, spermatozoa may persist for days longer and can be obtained from cervical mucous. The detection of sperm or semen from the rectum or mouth is possible but very dependent on the actions of the victim after the assault. A dry swab as well as a fresh slide is taken to calculate the number of complete sperm at the time of examination as their concentration may be useful as a guide to the time the assault occurred.

Certain chemicals are detectable in seminal fluid and can be used as proof of sexual contact even when sperm cannot be identified, or after vasectomy. Prostatic acid phosphatase can be detected in significant levels for up to 14 hours and sometimes longer in the vagina following sexual intercourse.[38] Acid phosphatase is normally found in vaginal fluid but at levels only 5–10% of seminal fluid. Prostate specific antigen (PSA) is a male specific glycoprotein found in semen and may be detected in the vagina for up to 48 hours after intercourse and may be detected when acid phosphatase cannot be found.[39]

It is not necessary to prove sexual contact to prove rape. Legally, penetration is said to have occurred once the tip of the penis has entered the labia majora and ejaculation does not have to occur. In a review of 372 female rape victims in Detroit, Tintinalli and Hoelzer found no correlation between the finding of sperm or acid phosphatase activity and the recording of a conviction.[40]

Consent

Evidence of the lack of consent may be found by indications of the use of force. This may be deduced from the state of the victim's clothes or by the presence of injuries. Again, most studies of rape victims record that only about half the victims show any signs of physical injury.

Identification of the assailant

The most accurate laboratory method currently available to identify the assailant is DNA testing.[41,42] The chance of incorrectly identifying an alleged assailant as the source of DNA material is infinitely small, literally one in several trillion. Any sample collected from the victim that contains cellular material from her assailant can be used for DNA testing. This includes spermatozoa, semen if it contains cells, or blood or tissue from under fingernails.

Stray hair follicles, for example combed from the pubic region of the victim may yield DNA to identify an assailant if the sheath cells are still present. Such hair that also includes the shaft and the follicle can also be used for a direct visual comparison under a microscope with hair from a suspect. As an investigation, however, this has a low return and requires the collection of plucked hair from the head and pubic region of the victim. Plucking the hair from the victim can be done at any time if it becomes important rather than in the aftermath of the assault.

Care must be taken when the victim undresses for the examination. Hair or clothes fibres from the offender or other tracers from the crime scene may have adhered to the body or clothes of the victim. She should undress standing over a drop sheet, which should then be included in a bag into which her clothes are placed. This becomes part of the physical evidence. The victim should then be able to shower with simple toiletries provided for her. She will need a change of clothes, fresh underwear and loose-fitting comfortable outerwear such a track suit and slippers. Such simple provisions are inexpensive but begin to give the victim the sense of re-establishing control.

PSYCHOLOGICAL IMPACT OF A SEXUAL ASSAULT

The predominant psychological reaction of the sexual assault victim is a devastating and profound sense of loss.[43] There are two major causes of this. First, throughout the assault the victim may well be in grave fear for her own survival. It is common knowledge that rapists sometimes murder their victims and the use of actual or threatened violence possibly supported by a weapon is an almost universal feature of rape. Second, the victim suffers a gross invasion of bodily boundaries in a manner that removes her control over that which she holds most personal to her.

As a result, sexual assault survivors show the features of post-traumatic stress disorder that has been termed the rape trauma syndrome.[42]

Following a sexual assault, the victim can show a wide range of emotional responses but these can generally be characterized in one of two broad types, expressed or controlled. In the expressed style, the victim's fear and anxiety may be shown by crying and obvious distress. In the controlled style, the victim will be outwardly calm, even appearing detached or nonchalant. It is important for care givers to recognize these emotional styles exist and not to make value judgements about victim's credibility on the basis of their emotional presentation.

After this comes a reorganization phase in which the victim attempts to assimilate the event and recover her lifestyle. Continuing counselling can assist the victim during this phase by providing an opportunity for ventilation of feelings, providing reassurance and support of adaptive behaviour and education.

Up to 95% of victims may meet the criteria of post-traumatic stress disorder following the rape[44] and as a many as 16.5% of victims still show stress-related symptoms 17 years after the attack.[45] Survivors report a variety of emotional changes in the longer term following the assault including fear, anxiety and depression. Many report sexual dysfunction and disruption of relationships,[43] a finding that has also been noted in male victims.[46] On the other hand, appropriate interventions and support can lead to better outcomes including changes that could be viewed as positive. One cohort of survivors saw themselves as stronger, more careful, more self-reliant, independent or thoughtful.[47]

Even though the emergency physician plays a brief role in the care of the victim, they can also have an important impact on her psychological recovery. It has been found that the greater the support the doctor provides to the victim, the better the outcome,[48] and that the victims consider the manner in which the medical examination is performed as more important than other factors such as the gender of the doctor. However, the same study found doctors to be the least supportive in comparison to other health professionals, families, friends and social service agencies.

SEXUAL ASSAULT IN SPECIAL CIRCUMSTANCES

Pregnancy

A study from Texas found no difference in the frequency of sexual assault for women who were less than 15 weeks pregnant.[49] Beyond then, she was less likely to be raped leading the authors to theorize that being obviously pregnant might be protective against rape or if she was raped, she was less likely to be seriously physically injured. There were no premature deliveries in the 4 weeks following the rape and no adverse foetal effects were detected.

Postmenopausal women

It is one of the myths associated with rape that victims are young and physically attractive or dress or behave in a way which provokes the attacks.[50] The reality is that the victim may be any age including elderly. This is consistent with the view that rape is an act of subjugation and asserting control rather than of sexual passion. In terms of physical injury, the injury patterns are similar except that postmenopausal women are significantly more likely to need surgical management and repair of genital injuries than are younger women.[51]

Children

The circumstances regarding children who are the victims of sexual assault differ from those relating to adults. First, the child is likely to have been the victim of chronic abuse rather than an attack by a stranger. Second, almost always the offender will be a man known to the child, often in a position of authority and trust.[52] This introduces the issue of protecting the child from further molestation. The injury pattern is highly variable. Chronic sexual abuse tends to develop as a pattern of behaviour between the victim and the offender beginning with touching and possibly leading to penetrative intercourse. This escalation of activity may evolve over a lengthy period and physical trauma may not be a feature. If the child has been the victim of a stranger assault, the risk of physical injury is greater than for an adult victim.[53]

Child sexual assault is ideally managed by a team with specific paediatric expertise.

Men

Male rape outside institutional settings is largely unrecognized and under reported, but males may comprise up to 10% of rape victims.[55–56] Males may be more likely to suffer significant physical injury during an assault even though their ability to resist may be no different to that of a female victim.[55] Male victims may carry additional burdens of guilt arising from concerns about their sexual orientation, which result from the attack and from the reaction of the police if they report. This concern will be heightened if they find themselves physically sexually stimulated during the assault as can also occur with female victims.[47]

In general, the short-term and long-term psychological consequences of sexual assault are no different between male and female victims. Apart from the obvious physiological and anatomical differences, there is no difference in the medical consequences of sexual assault for male and female victims.

CONCLUSION

While a sexual assault is an act of violence, the consequences for the survivor are primarily emotional and psychological rather than physical. Nonetheless, the emergency physician may well be expected to provide an initial medical assessment and may be asked to assist the police in the collection of forensic evidence. Therefore, this doctor will be amongst the first to attend to the victim in the aftermath of the assault. It is obvious that the doctor must have a clear understanding of the technical aspects of his or her role. It is just as important for the doctor to have an accepting, non-prejudicial attitude that places the well-being of the victim ahead of any other considerations, including apprehension about becoming involved in subsequent legal processes. In this way, survivors may be given the best opportunity to recover from an event which will change their lives.

CONTROVERSIES AND FUTURE DIRECTIONS

❶ The continuing challenge to the medical profession and the community in general in regard to sexual assault is overcoming deeply imbedded myths and misconceptions. Some distance has been covered in this regard such that services for most sexual assault victims have improved in the past few years. However, those barriers persist in a number of areas in which the incidence of sexual assault is only starting to become recognized and which will test our ability to respond. These areas include institutional and educational settings, which also includes the special problem of sexual assault of the disabled, inmates, military and police academies and the general issue of male rape victims.

❷ Domestic violence remains an issue for major public concern.

❸ Finally, one of the most challenging areas to confront us is the endemic problem of violence including sexual violence inflicted on indigenous women. Some groups of aboriginal girls and women report that half of them had been the victim of incest or sexual assault.[57]

REFERENCES

1. Groth AN, Burgess AW, Holmstrom LL 1977 Rape: power, anger and sexuality. American Journal of Psychiatry 134(11): 1239–43
2. Groth AN, Burgess AW 1977 Sexual dysfunction during rape. New England Journal of Medicine 297: 764–7
3. Australian Bureau of Statistics. Recorded Crime, Australia. ABS catalogue no. 4510.0 Commonwealth of Australia 2000
4. Australian Bureau of Statistics 1997 Australian Social Trends. Crime and Justice-Violent Crime: Violence against Women. Commonwealth of Australia
5. Australian Bureau of Statistics 1996 Women's Safety Australia. ABS catalogue no. 41280.0. Commonwealth of Australia
6. Moscarello R 1990 Psychological management of victims of sexual assault. Canadian Journal of Psychiatry. 35(1): 25–30
7. Hampton HL 1995 Care of the woman who has been raped. New England Journal of Medicine 332: 234–7
8. Rambow B, Adkinson C, Frost TH, et al 1992 Female sexual assault: Medical and legal implications. Annals of Emergency Medicine 21: 727–31
9. McCauley J, Guzinski G, Welch R, et al 1987 Toluidine blue in the corroboration of rape in the adult victim. American Journal of Emergency Medicine 5(2): 105–8
10. Beebe D 1991 Emergency management of the adult female rape victim. American Family Physician 43(6): 2041–6
11. Tucker S, Ledray LE, Werner JS 1990 Sexual assault evidence collection. Wisconsin Medical Journal 89(7): 407–11
12. Geist RF 1988 Sexually related trauma. In: Stewart G (ed.) Emergency Medicine Clinics of North America 6(3): 439–66
13. Riggs N, Houry D, Long G et al 2000 Analysis of 1076 Cases of Sexual Assault. Annals of Emergency Medicine 35: 358–62
14. Slaughter L, Brown CR 1992 Colposcopy to establish physical findings in rape victims. American Journal of Obstetrics and Gynecology 166: 83–86
15. Deming JE, Mittleman RE, Wetli CV 1983 Forensic science aspects of fatal sexual assaults on women. Journal of Forensic Sciences 28(3): 572–6
16. Strang H 1992 Characteristics of homicide in Australia 1990–91. In: Strang H, Gerull S-A (eds) Conference proceedings No 17-Homicide: patterns, prevention and control. Canberra: Australian Institute of Criminology 5–20
17. Jenny C, Hooten TM, Bowers A, et al 1990 Sexually transmitted diseases in victims of rape. New England Journal of Medicine 322: 713–6
18. Abel GG, Becker JV, Mittleman M, et al 1987 Self reported sex crimes in non-incarcerated paraphiliacs. Journal of Interpersonal Violence 2: 3–25
19.
20. Patel IH, Weinfeld RE, Konikoff J, et al 1982 Pharmacokinetics and tolerance of ceftriaxone in humans after single dose administration in water and lidocaine diluents. Antimicrobial Agents Chemother 21: 957–62
21. Szmuness W, Much MI, Prince AM, et al 1975 On the role of sexual behaviour in the spread of hepatitis B infection. Annals of Internal Medicine 83: 489–95
22. Schreeder MT, Thompson SE Hadler SC, et al 1982 Hepatitis B in homosexual men: prevalence of infection and factors related to transmission. Journal of Infectious Diseases 146: 7–15
23. Alter MJ, Ahtone J, Weisfuse I, et al 1986 Hepatitis B transmission between heterosexuals. Journal of the American Medical Association 256: 1307–10
24. Gerberding JL, Henderson DK 1992 Management of occupational exposures to bloodborne pathogens: Hepatitis B virus, hepatitis C virus, and human immunodeficiency virus. Clinical Infectious Diseases 14: 1179–85
25. Glaser JB, Hammerschlag MR, McCormack WM 1986 Sexually transmitted diseases in victims of sexual assault. New England Journal of Medicine 315: 625–7
26. Osterholm MT, MacDonald KL, Danila RN 1987 Sexually transmitted diseases in victims of sexual assault. New England Journal of Medicine 316: 1024
27. Centre for Disease Control 1997 Postexposure prophylaxis Hepatitis B.Recommendations and Reports. MMWR 47: 101–4
28. Estrich S, Forster GE, Robinson A 1990 Sexually transmitted diseases in rape victims. Genitourinary Medicine 66: 433–8
29. Centre for Disease Control 1998 Management of possible sexual or injecting drug use or other non occupational exposure to HIV. MMWR 47: 1–14
30. Cardo DM, Culver DH, Ciesielka CA, et al 1997 A case-control study of HIV seroconversion in healthcare workers after percutaneous exposure. New England Journal of Medicine 337: 1485–90
31. Jeffries DJ 1991 Zidovudine after occupational exposure to HIV. British Medical Journal 302: 1349–51
32. Holmes MM, Resnick HS, Kilpatrick DG, et al 1996 Rape-related pregnancy: Estimates and descriptive characteristics from a national sample of women. American Journal of Obstetrics and Gynecology 175: 320–5
33. Reader FC 1991 Emergency contraception. British Medical Journal 302: 801
34. Glasier A 1997 Emergency postcoital contraception. New England Journal of Medicine 337: 1058–64
35. Task Force on Postovulatory Methods of Fertility Regulation 1998 Randomized controlled trial of levonorgestrel versus the Yutzpe regimen of combined oral contraceptives for emergency contraception. Lancet 352: 428–33
36. Grey-Eurom K, Seaberg D 2002 The Prosecution of Sexual Assault Cases; Correlation with Forensic Evidence. Annals of Emergency Medicine 39: 39–63
37. Greydanus DE, Shaw RD, Kennedy EL 1987 Examination of sexually abused adolescents. Seminars in Adolescent Medicine 3: 59–65
38. Ricci LR 1982 Prostatic acid phosphatase and sperm in the post-coital vagina. Annals Emergency Medicine 11: 530–4
39. Graves HCB, Sensabaugh GF, Blake ET 1985 Post-coital detection of a male-specific semen protein: application to the investigation of rape. New England Journal of Medicine 312: 338–43
40. Tintinalli JE, Hoelzer M 1985 Clinical findings and legal resolution in sexual assault. Annals of Emergency Medicine 14: 447–53
41. Gill P, Jeffreys AJ, Werrett DJ 1985 Forensic application of DNA fingerprints. Nature 318: 577–9
42. Marx JL 1988 DNA fingerprinting takes the witness stand. Science 240: 1616–8
43. Rose DS 1986 Worse than death: Psychodynamics of rape victims and the need for psychotherapy. American Journal of Psychiatry 143: 817–24
44. Foa EB, Rothbaum BO, Riggs DS, et al 1991 Treatment of post-traumatic stress disorder in rape victims: A comparison between cognitive behavioural procedures and counselling. Journal of Consulting and Clinical Psychology 59: 715–23
45. Kilpatrick DG, Saunders BE, Veronen LJ, et al 1987 Criminal victimisation: Lifetime prevalence, reporting to police, and psychological impact. Crime and Delinquency 33: 479–89
46. Mezey G, King M 1989 The effects of sexual assault on men: A survey of 22 victims. Psychological Medicine 19: 205–9
47. Nadelson CC, Notman M, Zackson H, et al 1982 A follow-up study of rape victims. American Journal of Psychiatry 139: 1266–70
48. Popiel DA, Susskind EC 1985 The impact of the rape: Social support as the moderator of stress. American Journal of Community Psychology 13: 645–76
49. Satin AJ, Hemsell DL, Stone IC, et al 1991 Sexual assault in pregnancy. Obstetrics and Gynecology 77: 710–4
50. Mazelam PM 1980 Stereotypes and perceptions in the victims of rape. Victimology 5: 121–231
51. Ramin SM, Satin AJ, Stone IC, et al 1992 Sexual assault in postmenopausal women. Obstetrics and Gynecology 80: 860–4
52. Ricci LR 1985 Child sexual abuse: The emergency cdepartment response. Annals of Emergency Medicine 15: 711–6
53. Cartwright PS, and the Sexual Assault Study Group 1987 Factors that correlate with injury sustained by survivors of sexual assault. Obstetrics and Gynecology 70: 44–6
54. Kaufman A, DiVasto P, Jackson R, et al 1980 Male rape victims: Non-institutionalised assault. American Journal of Psychiatry 137: 221–3
55. King MB 1990 Male rape. British Medical Journal 301: 1345–6
56. Lipscomb GH, Muram D, Speck PM, et al 1992 Male victims of sexual assault. Journal of the American Medical Association 267: 3064–6
57. Atkinson J 1990 Aboriginal and Islander Health Worker 14: 4–27

20.4 DOMESTIC VIOLENCE

SANDRA NEATE

ESSENTIALS

1 Domestic violence encompasses physical, psychological and sexual violence.

2 All forms of domestic violence are inter-related in a complex way. Victims of violence may suffer many forms of abuse over their lives.

3 Between 30 and 50% of women and approximately 15% of men experience domestic violence over their lifetime.

4 Domestic violence occurs across all socio-economic, religious and cultural groups.

5 Predisposing factors for being a perpetrator or victim of violence may begin as early as childhood.

6 Disclosure of violence is rare and detection is difficult.

7 Treatment requires a coordinated approach from health practitioners, social services, the police and judicial system.

DEFINITION

Domestic violence in its broadest sense includes all types of violence within intimate or family relationships. Domestic violence can be physical, emotional or sexual and can occur during childhood, adulthood or both. Physical violence is when physical force such as pushing, hitting, biting, punching or assault with a weapon is used to control a person. Non-personal physical violence such as damage to property, punching holes in walls, throwing objects or brandishing weapons, can be equally intimidating. Sexual violence or abuse involves coercing a partner into engaging in sexual activity against his or her will by

using intimidation, threats or physical harm.[1] Psychological abuse consists of verbal harassment, ridicule, threats of physical harm and behaviours designed to intimidate, humiliate, control and isolate. Isolation can involve prevention of family contact, attendance at work, or contact with medical practitioners and others whom the perpetrator fears may uncover the violence. Psychological abuse nearly always precedes physical abuse.[2]

Violence is traditionally assumed to be perpetrated by men against women but may be by women against men or by partners in same-sex relationships. The partnership may be current or past. Other family members related by blood or law may be perpetrators of domestic violence. Domestic violence also includes abuse of the elderly by either spouse or other family member and may involve physical and psychological abuse, neglect and exploitation. Child abuse falls within the spectrum of domestic violence but is usually considered a separate issue.

Most studies of domestic violence concentrate on violence between partners in a committed relationship. In the USA the alternative term of intimate partner violence is frequently used. The common factor in violent intimate relationships is an imbalance of power with one person exerting coercive control over the other by some means of violence whether physical, psychological or sexual, either actual or threatened. The subjective experience and definition of domestic violence is strongly influenced by cultural beliefs and previous life experiences and the individual's perceptions of their experience may vary greatly from standard clinical definitions.[3]

INCIDENCE

The prevalence of domestic violence varies according to definition (whether emotional and sexual abuse are in-

cluded), timing of the abuse (immediate, during adult life or cumulative life time prevalence) and whether the violence is actual or threatened. Prevalence surveys within Australian emergency departments, where domestic violence was defined as an adult being afraid of or actually being physically hurt by a partner, indicate that approximately 30% of women and 15% of men report a lifetime history of domestic violence, with 19–24% of women and 8% of men disclosing a history of domestic violence during their adult life.[4–6] US studies report a higher cumulative lifetime prevalence of approximately 50% but include actual and threatened personal and non-personal violence.[7]

Overall, women have four times the risk of experiencing domestic violence than men and those who have been victims of child abuse have six times the risk of experiencing adult domestic violence. Men and women report similar incidences of approximately 7% of childhood abuse alone.[4] Pregnancy represents a high-risk time for being the victim of domestic violence. Six per cent of pregnant women are battered during their pregnancy.[8] The incidence of abuse towards women with mental or physical disabilities is between 33 and 83% depending on the severity of disability and the definition of abuse.[8] In the USA approximately one million elderly people per year are physically assaulted, neglected or exploited.[9]

Approximately 2% of women presenting to emergency departments have experienced physical violence within the 24 hours preceding the presentation.[4,6] The incidence is approximately 10% if psychological abuse is included.[7]

PREDICTORS OF DOMESTIC VIOLENCE

Several demographic factors may be associated with an increased risk of being a perpetrator or victim of domestic violence. Characteristics associated with an increased risk of a male inflicting injury on a female partner are alcohol abuse, drug use, low education standards (not finishing secondary school), unemployment, and being a former rather than current partner. Alcohol abuse is the most identifiable risk factor and has a clear dose–response relationship.[10,11] One half of victims report that their male partners were intoxicated at the time of assault.[11] However, the relationship between alcohol and abuse is not necessarily cause and effect. An asymmetric power balance between the perpetrator and victim remains the main determinant of conflict in violent intimate relationships. The association between alcohol and domestic violence may be that alcohol abuse makes physical assault more likely within the context of these relationships.[10]

The greatest risk for being a female victim of domestic violence is having a former partner, with an even higher risk if the woman is currently living with this former partner. Separated or divorced women are four times more likely to be abused than women who have never married or are married or widowed.[12] Other demographic factors for women do not show statistically significant predictive value.[10] Male victims of violence in the USA tend to be younger, single and African American,[13] and the perpetrators are more likely to be de-facto partners and family members other than spouses.[4] Men who are abused are commonly assaulted by the women whom they abuse.[14]

Despite these trends in demographics, domestic violence occurs across all socio-economic groups, races and religions and demographic characteristics are not sensitive or predictive indicators of domestic violence.[10,15] Clinical presentations such as injury pattern, specific obstetric and gynaecological symptoms, psychiatric symptoms and substance abuse have all been examined for sensitivity as predictors of domestic violence. None of these presentations has been found to have a significant sensitivity or positive predictive value for detecting domestic violence.[16]

OUTCOMES

Domestic violence affects the victim's health in a multitude of physical and psychological ways. Despite the emphasis on physical injury, most presentations to health professionals by domestic violence victims are a complex mix of indirectly related physical and psychological problems and are not trauma related.[7]

Physical injury and illness

Physical injuries resulting from domestic violence follow some patterns. Injuries inflicted on females are likely to be contusions, abrasions, lacerations, fractures and dislocations. Women are more likely to be choked, beaten or sexually abused.[4,10] Men have a greater risk of having objects thrown at them or weapons used against them. Features suggestive of intentional injury include history inconsistent with the injury, injuries in varying temporal stages, or unreasonable delay in presentation. Non-accidental injuries are often in central compared with peripheral regions of the body. Injuries to defensive areas of the body or to the back, legs, buttocks, back of the head and soles of the feet suggest an attempt at self protection. Although domestic-violence-related injuries follow certain patterns, injury pattern is of low positive predictive value when attempting to identify domestic violence.[17]

Abuse before, during and after pregnancy represents a threat to mother and foetus. Approximately 40% of women who are physically abused are forced into non-consensual sex at some stage, highlighting the link between physical and sexual violence. This results in high rates of sexually transmitted disease, unintended and adolescent pregnancy, and elective termination of pregnancy.[18] There is also an established complex link between domestic violence and preterm labour, low-birth-weight babies and postnatal depression.[3,19] Prevention of antenatal care, due to the perpetrator's fear of disclosure of violence, is common.

Children who live in violent households are at risk of both emotional and physical injury. The majority of physical injuries are inadvertent as children are held during the violent episode or as they attempt to intervene to save a parent from harm.[20]

Death is the ultimate physical injury. Approximately 25% of USA female homicides are domestic-violence related.[21] One USA study examining female homicides over a 5-year period found that 44% of homicide victims had presented to an emergency deparment in the 2 years preceding their death. Despite 28 injury-related visits and 48 total visits, domestic violence was documented in only two cases and intervention occurred in none.[21]

Psychological impact

Domestic violence is a strong independent risk factor for the development of mental illness. Women experiencing domestic violence have an approximately 11-fold increase of dissociation (often a defence mechanism to rise above the pain of physical and emotional injury), are at six times the risk of developing somatization symptoms, are five times as likely to suffer anxiety and are three times as likely to suffer depression, phobias and drug dependence. Abused women have twice the rates of hazardous alcohol consumption and dependence as non-abused women.[12] 'Double abuse' occurring in childhood and adulthood causes yet another significant increase in these psychiatric diagnoses.[22] Women experiencing psychological abuse may suffer greater psychological distress and illness than those who experience physical violence. Ridicule and humiliation are particularly responsible for causing low self esteem in the victim.[2]

The emotional impact of witnessing family violence is a significant independent factor for lifetime psychiatric diagnoses in women.[22] Children living in a home where violence is perpetrated against a parent are themselves 15 times more likely to be a victim of abuse or neglect, as domestic violence and child abuse are each predictors of the other.[3] Domestic violence is a risk factor for becoming a perpetrator of homicide in the pre-teenage group.[23] The outcome of the experience of violence is directly proportional to the duration and frequency of violent episodes.[3] Overall, approximately one-third of the population risk for all psychiatric diagnoses is attributable to domestic violence.[22]

Seeking treatment for mental-health problems can further add to the abused woman's burden, as a psychiatric history may be used against her by the perpetrator in dealings with police or in custody disputes.[14]

Social

Control by the abuser who fears disclosure by the victim leads to social isolation such as loss of contact with friends and family, and prevention from paid employment. Financial dependence on the abuser together with the responsibility of children add to isolation, loss of choices and difficulties of separation from the abuser. Poverty is prevalent and multifactorial. Separation from or incarceration of the abuser may lead to further loss of income. In the case of the elderly, finances may be improperly used by the legal guardian

Homelessness may be relative, where there is no sense of safety or security in the home, or absolute where there is need for interim accommodation, emergency shelters or, in extreme cases, families may be living on the streets. Children or elderly people living in violent circumstances may find themselves institutionalized by authorities or carers.

Outcomes for male victims of domestic violence differ from outcomes for female victims in several significant ways. Men are more likely to suffer serious physical injury than women. However, male victims express fewer feelings of fear and terror, and less frequently feel trapped and controlled. Men are also generally less constrained by financial dependence. As fear, control, dependence and isolation contribute greatly to the psychological outcomes of domestic violence, women still suffer approximately 95% of the serious physical and psychological consequences of domestic violence.[14]

BARRIERS TO DETECTION

Detection rates of domestic violence are low. Only 10% of people presenting with acute domestic-violence-related injuries or issues will be directly asked by the attending nurse or physician or volunteer information regarding the violence issue. Documentation of violence in the medical record is rare.[7] After an education programme to promote detection of domestic violence, only 50% of those who reported domestic violence on screening questionnaire had violence documented in their medical records.[24]

Barriers to detection include system and patient factors. System factors include the physical environment such as inadequate privacy and inadequate staffing resulting in time constraints. Health-practitioner-related factors such as lack of time and education, inappropriate attitudes or frustration at the patient's inability to effect change, and cultural, social and gender issues contribute further barriers. Patient factors include feelings of shame and humiliation, cultural taboos, confidentiality concerns, fear of reprisals from the perpetrator and safety issues, both personal and relating to children. Reluctance to involve the police, children's services and the judicial system may result from fear of removal of children and other legal ramifications.[8]

Indigenous women report violence rarely. Historical interactions with police such as forcible removal of children and high rates of aboriginal death in custody result in indigenous women fearing for the safety of themselves and their families when police or social services are involved.[3] The elderly may be prevented from reporting by fear of further abuse, neglect or the threat of institutionalization.[3]

SCREENING

Between 30 and 50% of women presenting to emergency departments have been the victim of domestic violence in their lifetime, 2–10% within the preceding 24 hours. The high prevalence of domestic violence, low positive predictive values of demographic factors and clinical presentations, low detection rates and high incidence of subsequent physical and psychological illness have supported the argument for universal screening. Opportunistic screening may increase detection rates of domestic violence.[25] Detection rates without screening are in the order of 0.4% increasing to approximately 14% with the use of simple direct questioning.[25] Screening may indicate to the victim that channels of communication are open and that help will be available when she is ready to disclose information. It educates women about violence, its nature and prevalence. Screening may also be important in detection of perpetrators. Approximately 40% of domestic violence perpetrators have sought medical attention in the preceding 6 months with half having attended an emergency department.[26]

Many methods of screening are described. The use of a single screening question may be as effective as asking several questions. Screening questions should be simple and direct such as 'Have you been hit, kicked, punched or otherwise hurt by someone in the last year?', 'Do you feel safe at home?' or 'Are you afraid of your partner?'[27][28] Explanation that these questions are routine may improve patient comfort.

Most women find screening an acceptable practice. Up to two-thirds of medical practitioners and 50% of nurses are not in favour of screening because of demands on time and feelings of burnout associated with constantly discussing the issue. In the USA the legal implications of mandatory reporting add to reluctance to screen.

Screening may improve detection rates. Increased detection rates have been shown to increase referral rates to external agencies. Confounding the whole issue is the fact that despite much research into the ideal screening tool and how to implement screening in emergency departments, currently no evidence exists that screening leads to improved health outcomes for victims.[29,30]

MANAGEMENT

The management of domestic violence is complex. Common misconceptions include that the woman is best leaving her situation immediately, reporting to police and involving legal services. Simply leaving a violent relationship is no guarantee of safety. Involvement of police or the judicial system is no guarantee of a positive outcome for the individual. Conversely, leaving and reporting may lead to adverse outcomes such as increased levels of violence. It can be difficult for health practitioners, especially those accustomed to 'fixing' life-threatening conditions, to let go of the concept of fixing or curing the problem or even knowing for certain that the problem exists. The goal should not be to persuade the woman to leave the violent relationship. Leaving a violent relationship is a process and not an event, and requires support through all phases. Help may best be offered by expressing concern, listening, providing support and offering a bridge to services.

Understanding

Interviews with survivors of domestic violence have provided a framework for understanding the stages through which a victim must work before being ready to leave a violent relationship.[31] These phases are first a precontemplative phase where the woman is not consciously aware of or is in denial about the abuse. She then moves through a contemplation phase where the abuse is acknowledged, but she is unable to decide to leave. A preparation stage follows where the woman takes small steps in preparation to leave and prepares for significant action. This is a period of increased danger for the woman and safety is paramount. This may well be the period where the victim faces the greatest obstacles to leaving. She may have been isolated from friends and family, and be financially dependent and concerned for her ability to survive and protect her children. The action stage when she finally leaves can be prolonged and is typically characterized by relapses where she returns to the relationship. After a period of 6 months without return to the relationship she is then said to be in a maintenance phase.

Listening and understanding where the woman is in terms of progress through these phases will assist in assessing readiness for change and guide intervention.[8] The aim is to validate the patient's experience, emphasize that she does not deserve the abuse nor is it her fault and empower her to improve her own safety and well-being. Her own decision-making should be supported, with the emphasis that she is in control of her choices. The doctor or nurse is not there to advise the patient what is best.

Referral

There are multiple agencies to assist victims of domestic violence. Community services include hotlines for emergency advice through to counseling services, emergency shelters, police and legal services. Up to 50% of domestic-violence-related emergency department presentations occur between the hours of 8 pm and 8 am.[23] Emergency department staff need to be aware of how to access these community services 24 hours a day.

Safety

Immediate action may be required in the form of not returning home, or staying with friends or relatives or in emergency accommodation. If the victim judges it safe to return home, a safety plan can be organized including readily accessible emergency contact numbers and an emergency bag with identification, money, credit cards, legal documents and medication relating to both the woman and her children. Safety is an on-going issue as a woman leaving an abusive relationship is at greatest risk of injury as she is leaving the relationship. Seventy per cent of domestic violence murders occur as the woman is leaving or has left the home.[32] On-going contact due to custody arrangements make the risk of abuse a continuing one.

Reporting

Seven states in the USA mandate reporting of injuries resulting from domestic violence specifically. In total, 45 states have laws that require reporting of injuries caused by weapons, major crimes or domestic violence.[33] Reporting of domestic violence is not mandatory in Australasia. Mandatory reporting remains controversial. Arguments in favour of reporting are based on the assumption that reporting will stop the violence. Arguments against reporting are that victims will be deterred from disclosure and that health practitioners will avoid asking about violence due to concerns about their legal responsibility to report even if uncertain.

Documentation

Documentation in the medical record may provide vital legal evidence and should be objective and accurate. Direct quotes should be used rather than paraphrasing, and descriptions of behaviours and appearances rather than interpretation add objectivity. Body maps assist documentation of physical injury. Photographs may be of assistance. When sexual assault is suspected, the involvement of specific sexual-assault-centre staff will ensure legally admissible evidence is obtained.

The perpetrator

Many perpetrators suffer from depression, alcohol and substance dependency, and post-traumatic stress disorder.[26] Some of these conditions may be amenable to treatment. Batterers with antisocial personality disorder are less amenable to treatment. The management of perpetrators of physical and sexual assault still remains largely the domain of the police and criminal justice system.

The management of domestic violence requires a co-ordinated response from all practitioners and service providers involved from the moment the victim first discloses the violence. This includes the health system, social services, and the police and judicial system if the victim chooses to pursue this course of action. At all times, the victim's wishes must be paramount and the service providers should do their utmost to support these wishes.

CONCLUSION

Domestic violence is a complex issue with risk factors for being a perpetrator or a victim beginning in childhood and continuing through adult life. Factors such as the childhood environment, whether there is violence experienced personally or witnessed, the gaining of self-esteem, education level, drug and alcohol abuse, and mental health and personality issues all impact. Domestic violence is extremely common and frequently remains undetected, but interventions aimed at increased detection and referral may not improve outcomes for the individual. Expressing concern and willingness to listen, being non-judgemental, supporting and stage-appropriate referral are the mainstays of management.

CONTROVERSIES AND FUTURE DIRECTIONS

❶ While there has been considerable research on the ideal screening tool for domestic violence in emergency departments, until it can be shown that screening is useful and, more particularly, not harmful, emergency departments should not routinely screen for domestic violence. More research is urgently needed on the outcomes after screening interventions.

❷ Mandatory reporting of violence of all types remains controversial. Breach of confidentiality remains a concern.

❸ Management strategies should not be aimed at encouraging the woman to leave the violent relationship. Support and stage-appropriate referral are the mainstays of management.

REFERENCES

1. Burke LK, Follingstad DR 1999 Violence in lesbian and gay relationships: theory, prevalence, and correlational factors. Clinical Psychology Review 19: 487–512
2. O'Leary KD 1999 Psychological abuse: a variable deserving critical attention in domestic violence. Violence and Victims 14: 3–23
3. Astbury J, Atkinson J, Duke JE, et al 2000 The impact of domestic violence on individuals. Medical Journal of Australia 173: 427–31
4. Roberts GL, O'Toole BI, Raphael B, Lawrence JM, Ashby R 1996 Prevalence study of domestic violence victims in an emergency department. Annals of Emergency Medicine 27: 741–53
5. de Vries Robbe M, March L, Vinen J, Horner D, Roberts G 1996 Prevalence of domestic violence among patients attending a hospital emergency department. Australian and New Zealand Journal of Public Health 20: 364–8
6. Bates L, Redman S, Brown W, Hancock L 1995 Domestic violence experienced by women attending an accident and emergency department. Australian Journal of Public Health 19: 293–9
7. Abbott J, Johnson R, Koziol-McLain J, Lowenstein SR 1995 Domestic violence against women. Incidence and prevalence in an emergency department population. Journal of the American Medical Association 273: 1763–7
8. Kramer A 2002 Domestic violence: how to ask and how to listen. Nursing Clinics of North America 37: 189–210, ix

9. Jones J, Dougherty J, Schelble D, Cunningham W 1988 Emergency department protocol for the diagnosis and evaluation of geriatric abuse. Annals of Emergency Medicine 17: 1006–15
10. Kyriacou DN, Anglin D, Taliaferro E, et al 1999 Risk factors for injury to women from domestic violence against women. New England Journal of Medicine 341: 1892–8
11. Kyriacou DN, McCabe F, Anglin D, Lapesarde K, Winer MR 1998 Emergency department-based study of risk factors for acute injury from domestic violence against women. Annals of Emergency Medicine 31: 502–6
12. Roberts GL, Williams GM, Lawrence JM, Raphael B 1998 How does domestic violence affect women's mental health? Women Health 28: 117–29
13. Mechem CC, Shofer FS, Reinhard SS, Hornig S, Datner E 1999 History of domestic violence among male patients presenting to an urban emergency department. Academic Emergency Medicine 6: 786–91
14. Frank JB, Rodowski MF 1999 Review of psychological issues in victims of domestic violence seen in emergency settings. Emergency Medical Clinics of North America 17: 657–77, vii
15. Fanslow JL, Norton RN, Robinson EM 1999 One

year follow-up of an emergency department protocol for abused women. Australian and New Zealand Journal of Public Health 23: 418–20
16. Zachary MJ, Mulvihill MN, Burton WB, Goldfrank LR 2001 Domestic abuse in the emergency department: can a risk profile be defined? Academy of Emergency Medicine 8: 796–803
17. Muelleman RL, Lenaghan PA, Pakieser RA 1996 Battered women: injury locations and types. Annals of Emergency Medicine 28: 486–92
18. Campbell JC, Coben JH, McLoughlin E, et al 2001 An evaluation of a system-change training model to improve emergency department response to battered women. Academy of Emergency Medicine 8: 131–8
19. Gazmararian JA, Petersen R, Spitz AM, Goodwin MM, Saltzman LE, Marks JS 2000 Violence and reproductive health: current knowledge and future research directions. Maternal and Child Health Journal 4: 79–84
20. Christian CW, Scribano P, Seidl T, Pinto-Martin JA 1997 Pediatric injury resulting from family violence. Pediatrics 99: E8
21. Wadman MC, Muelleman RL 1999 Domestic violence homicides: ED use before victimization. American Journal of Emergency Medicine 17: 689–91
22. Roberts GL, Lawrence JM, Williams GM, Raphael B 1998 The impact of domestic violence on women's mental health. Australian and New Zealand Journal of Public Health 22: 796–801
23. Shumaker DM, Prinz RJ 2000 Children who murder: a review. Clinical Child Family Psychological Review 3: 97–115
24. Roberts GL, Lawrence JM, O'Toole BI, Raphael B 1997 Domestic violence in the Emergency Department: 2. Detection by doctors and nurses. Annals of General Hospital Psychiatry 19: 12–5
25. Morrison LJ, Allan R, Grunfeld A 2000 Improving the emergency department detection rate of domestic violence using direct questioning. Journal of Emergency Medicine 19: 117–24
26. Coben JH, Friedman DI 2002 Health care use by perpetrators of domestic violence. Journal of Emergency Medicine 22: 313–7
27. Gerard M 2000 Domestic violence. How to screen & intervene. RN 2000; 63: 52–6; quiz 58.
28. Chescheir N 1996 Violence against women: response from clinicians. Annals of Emergency Medicine 27: 766–8
29. Ramsay J, Richardson J, Carter YH, Davidson LL, Feder G 2002 Should health professionals screen women for domestic violence? Systematic review. British Medical Journal 325: 314
30. Cole TB 2000 Is domestic violence screening helpful? Journal of the American Medical Association 284: 551–3
31. Gerbert B, Caspers N, Bronstone A, Moe J, Abercrombie P 1999 A qualitative analysis of how physicians with expertise in domestic violence approach the identification of victims. Annals of Internal Medicine 131: 578–84
32. Haywood YC, Haile-Mariam T 1999 Violence against women. Emergency Medical Clinics of North America 17: 603–15, vi
33. Houry D, Sachs CJ, Feldhaus KM, Linden J 2002 Violence-inflicted injuries: reporting laws in the fifty states. Annals of Emergency Medicine 39: 56–60

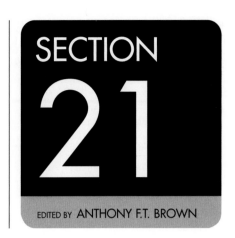

PAIN RELIEF

21.1 Pain relief in emergency medicine 626

21.1 PAIN RELIEF IN EMERGENCY MEDICINE

DANIEL M. FATOVICH • ANTHONY F. T. BROWN

ESSENTIALS

1 Acute pain is the most common complaint presenting to an emergency department.

2 Pain is a complex, multidimensional, subjective phenomenon.

3 Patient self-reporting is the most reliable indicator of the existence and intensity of pain.

4 Patients in pain should receive timely, effective and appropriate analgesia, titrated according to response.

5 There is a wide range of pharmacological and non-pharmacological techniques available for the treatment of acute pain. Effective pain relief should always be achievable.

6 Local anaesthetic nerve blocks should be considered as an analgesic supplement or as an alternative method of achieving analgesia, particularly where pain is localized.

7 Toxicity may occur with inadvertent rapid intravenous injection, or exceeding the recommended safe maximum dose. Neurological and cardiovascular effects predominate and may be lethal. Resuscitation equipment should always be available when using local anaesthetic agents.

8 Intravenous regional anaesthesia with prilocaine for Bier's block is a simple, safe technique commonly used for reduction of forearm fractures.

INTRODUCTION

Pain is defined by the International Association for the Study of Pain as 'an unpleasant sensory and emotional experience associated with actual or potential tissue damage or described in terms of such damage'.[1] However, once a patient presents for medical care, severe acute pain has ceased to serve a useful purpose. Whereas in some conditions the nature and progression of the pain may be helpful in making the diagnosis of the underlying pathology, too great a reliance has been placed upon this feature, thereby allowing the patient to suffer needlessly for long periods.[2,3]

When severe pain is inadequately relieved it produces pathophysiological and abnormal psychological reactions that often lead to complications. This is important because acute pain is the most common presenting complaint to an emergency department[4] and forms part of the daily practice of emergency medicine. It should be considered poor patient care not to treat pain while attempting to arrive at a diagnosis. There can be no greater gift to one's neighbour than to practise, teach and discover more effective methods to relieve pain and suffering.[2,3] Unfortunately, the management of acute pain is not a specific component of medical training.

PHYSIOLOGY

Pain is one of the most complex aspects of an already intricate nervous system. A number of theories have been developed to explain the physiology of pain, but none is proven or complete.

In 1965, the Melzack-Wall Gate Control Theory emphasized mechanisms in the central nervous system that control the perception of a noxious stimulus, and thus integrated afferent, upstream processes with downstream modulation from the brain.[5] However, this theory did not incorporate long-term changes in the central nervous system to the noxious input and to other external factors that impinge upon the individual.[5] It is now widely recognized that nociceptor function is altered by the 'inflammatory soup' that characterizes a region of tissue injury.[5]

The final pain experience is subject to a complex series of facilitatory and inhibitory events that precede pain awareness, such as past experience, anxiety or expectation.[6]

Most pain originates when specific nerve endings (nociceptors) are stimulated, producing nerve impulses that are transmitted to the brain. Nociception is the detection of tissue damage by specialized transducers.[5] There are two types of nociceptor:[7]

1. Mechanoreceptors that are present mainly in the skin and respond rapidly to pinprick or heat via Aδ, myelinated afferent neurons
2. Polymodal, which are the nerve endings of unmyelinated C-type afferent neurons and are widely distributed throughout most tissues; they respond to tissue damage caused by mechanical, thermal or chemical insults, and are responsible for the slow onset, prolonged, poorly localized, aching pain following an injury.

A number of chemicals are involved in the transmission of pain to the ascending pathways in the spinothalamic tract. The principal neurotransmitter is thought to be the peptide substance P, but many others have been identified.[8,9] Opioid receptors are present in the dorsal horn, and it is thought that encephalins (endogenous opioid peptides) are neurotransmitters in the inhibitory interneurons.[7]

Phospholipids released from damaged cell membranes trigger a cascade of reactions, culminating in the production of prostaglandins that sensitize nociceptors to other inflammatory mediators, such as histamine, serotonin and bradykinin.[7]

The threshold for the perception of a painful stimulus is similar in everyone, and may be lowered by certain chemicals such as the mediators of inflammation. The discrete cognitive processes and pathways involved in the interpretation of painful stimuli remain a mystery. The cognitive and emotional reactions to a given painful stimulus are variable among individuals, and may be affected by culture, personality, past experiences and underlying emotional state.[3,5,10] Pain is a complex, multidimensional, subjective phenomenon.[10]

ASSESSMENT OF PAIN AND PAIN SCALES

There is no objective measure of pain. Doctors use a variety of methods for determining how much pain a patient feels. These include the nature of the illness or injury, the patient's appearance and behaviour, and physiological concomitants. None of these is reliable.

Because there are no accurate physiologic or clinical signs to objectively measure pain, pain scales have been developed. Three scales have become popular tools to quantify pain intensity:[11,12] These are the visual analogue scale (VAS), the numeric rating scale and the verbal rating scale.

The VAS usually consists of a 100 mm line with one end indicating no pain and the other end indicating the worst pain imaginable. The patient simply indicates a point on the line that best indicates the amount of pain experienced.

In the numeric rating scale the patient is asked to choose a number from a range (usually 0–10) that best describes the amount of pain experienced, with zero being no pain and 10 being the worst pain imaginable. This has been used for ischaemic chest pain and is more useful in illiterate patients. The verbal rating scale simply asks a patient to choose a phrase that best describes the pain, usually mild, moderate or severe.

The use of pain scales has been restricted predominantly to research, where experimental pain is not associated with the strong emotional component of acute pain. In the clinical setting, anxiety, sleep disruption and illness burden are present.[9] It is difficult to use a unidimensional pain scale to measure a multidimensional process. Using intensity only will often fail to capture the many qualities of pain and the pain experience. The best illustration of this problem is that the same pain stimulus can be applied to two different people with dramatically different pain scores and analgesic requirements.[13] At best, the use of pain scales is an indirect reflection of 'real' pain, with patient self-reporting being the most reliable indicator of the existence and intensity of pain.[14]

Nevertheless, pain scales are simple and easy to use and are becoming routine in emergency departments, with some recommendations that they should be a standard part of triage.[4]

GENERAL PRINCIPLES

Patients in pain should receive timely, effective and appropriate analgesia, titrated according to response.[3] There is, therefore, almost no role for intramuscular analgesia. The following points should be stressed:

- The correct dose is enough.
- A patient's analgesic requirements should be reviewed frequently.
- Emergency departments should have specific policies relating to pain and analgesia.
- Senior clinicians should lead by example.

SPECIFIC AGENTS

Opioids
The term opioid refers to all naturally occurring and synthetic drugs producing morphine-like effects. Morphine is the standard opioid agonist against which others are judged.[15] These drugs are the most powerful agents available in the treatment of acute pain. Unfortunately, many doctors use them inappropriately and there are particular concerns regarding respiratory depression and iatrogenic addiction.

Less than 1% of patients who receive opioids for pain develop respiratory depression.[16] Tolerance to this side-effect develops simultaneously with tolerance to the analgesic effect. If the opioid dose is increased so that at least half the pain is relieved, the chance of respiratory depression is small. Further, naloxone will reverse the effects of opioids. In relation to fears of addiction, large studies have shown that iatrogenic opioid abuse is exceedingly rare.[17]

A number of specific opioid receptors have been identified. They are responsible for a variety of effects, including analgesia, euphoria, respiratory depression (μ receptor); cough suppression, sedation (κ); dysphoria, hallucinations (σ); nausea and vomiting, and pruritus (δ).[7]

Opioids act on injured tissue to reduce inflammation, in the dorsal horn to impede transmission of nociception, and supraspinally to activate inhibitory pathways that descend to the spinal segment.[9]

Patients who require opioid analgesia often require admission to hospital. This is because:

- If the patient's condition is so painful that it requires intravenous opioid, then there will be ongoing opioid requirements that can only be administered in hospital.
- There have been occasions where patients have received opioid analgesia that has relieved their pain, and they have then been discharged without a final diagnosis. This is a dangerous practice. A patient may present with abdominal pain with vomiting for instance, and a provisional diagnosis of gastroenteritis is made. After opioid analgesia is given the patient may feel better and be discharged. A diagnosis such as appendicitis or bowel obstruction has not been excluded. For patients where the

final diagnosis is certain, such as in anterior shoulder dislocation, discharge is appropriate after a suitable period of observation until the patient is deemed clinically fit for discharge. This is a different scenario from that described previously, as it is a single system problem in which there is no doubt about the diagnosis.

Side effects

All potent opioid analgesics have the potential to depress the level of consciousness, protective reflexes and vital functions. It is mandatory that these are closely monitored during and after administration.[7] Specific side effects include:

- Respiratory depression
- Nausea and vomiting: nausea occurs in approximately 40% and vomiting in 15%[7]
- Hypotension: opioids may provoke histamine release
- Constipation
- Spasm of the sphincter of Oddi. Therefore, patients with biliary colic may initially experience more pain. There is no good evidence to suggest that pethidine has any clinically significant advantage at equi-analgaesic doses over other opioids for biliary or renal colic[15]
- Meiosis.

Route of administration

Opioids may be administered by many routes, including oral, SC, IM, IV, epidural, nebulized, intrapleural, intranasal and transdermal. All may have a role in a specific clinical situation.[4] Doses and duration of effect are given in Table 21.1.1. There is a good rationale for the use of the IV route in moderate-to-severe pain.[4] Rapid pain relief and titration to effect are obvious advantages. Intramuscular administration results in unreliable and variable absorption, and older practices of routinely prescribing '75 mg pethidine IM' are deplorable and take no account of an individual's requirements.[7]

Special considerations

Allergic reactions are extremely rare with opioids.

Pethidine should be used with caution in patients with renal failure, as there is increased risk of CNS toxicity due to the toxic metabolite, norpethidine. Norpethidine causes tremor, twitching, agitation and convulsions.[15] Also pethidine is contraindicated in patients receiving MAO inhibitors, as they interfere with pethidine metabolism, increasing the likelihood of toxicity.[18] Finally, pethidine may trigger the serotonin syndrome if used concomitantly with SSRIs. Its general use is declining.

Fentanyl does not release histamine making it ideal for treating patients with reactive airways disease. There are advantages in using this drug for brief procedures in the emergency department because of its short half-life. High doses of fentanyl may produce muscular rigidity, which may be so severe as to make ventilation difficult, but which responds to naloxone or muscle relaxants.

Codeine is the most commonly utilised oral opioid. Prescribed alone in doses as high as 120 mg, codeine has been demonstrated to be no more effective than placebo in both the adult and geriatric populations, while causing important gastrointestinal side effects such as nausea, vomiting and constipation.[4] However, in combination with paracetamol or aspirin, it has been shown to be superior to either agent alone, with analgesia equivalent to that provided by NSAIDs.

Tramadol is a new opioid, with novel non-opioid properties.[19] Its efficacy lies between codeine and morphine. It has a relative lack of serious side effects such as respiratory depression, and the potential for abuse and psychological dependence is low.[19] Other side effects include, nausea, vomiting, dizziness and somnolence.[19] It should be avoided or used with caution in patients who are taking tricyclic antidepressants, and other drugs such as SSRIs that reduce the seizure threshold. Also the concomitant administration of tramadol with monoamine oxidase inhibitors, or within 2 weeks of their withdrawal, is contraindicated.[19]

Non-opioid analgesics

Non-steroidal anti-inflammatory drugs

Non-steroidal anti-inflammatory drugs (NSAIDs) are either non-selective cyclo-oxygenase (COX) inhibitors or selective inhibitors of COX-2 (COX-2 inhibitors). NSAIDs have been demonstrated in numerous trials to be effective analgesic agents for moderate pain, specifically when there is associated inflammation.[4] As with opioids there are multiple routes of administration available. Unfortunately, their use in acute severe pain is limited by the length of time to onset of 20–30 minutes. There is no clear superiority of one agent over another.

Caution should be used in the elderly and in patients with renal disease, hypertension and heart failure. In patients with asthma, 2–20% are aspirin sensitive and there is a 50–100% cross-sensitivity with NSAIDs. There is up to a 30% incidence of upper gastrointestinal bleeding when NSAIDs are used for over 1–2 weeks. The risk of bleeding in the elderly for short (3–5 days) acute therapy appears to be minimal.[4] NSAID use in pregnancy (especially late), is not recommended. Ibuprofen is considered the NSAID of choice in lactation.

Ketorolac is a parenteral NSAID that is equianalgesic to opioids with clinical research showing that ketorolac and morphine are equivalent in reducing pain. There is a distinct benefit favouring ketorolac in terms of side effects, when

Table 21.1.1 Doses and duration of effect of opioid analgesics

Drug	Dose	Duration (h)
Pethidine	1–1.5 mg/kg or more	3–5
Morphine	0.1–0.2 mg/kg or more	2–3
Fentanyl	1–2 μg/kg or more	0.5–1

ketorolac is titrated intravenously for isolated limb injuries.[20,21]

Simple analgesics

Agents such as paracetamol and aspirin are effective for mild pain and have useful antipyretic activity. Paracetamol has no gastrointestinal side effects of note and may be prescribed safely in patients with peptic ulcer disease or gastritis.[4] Aspirin has the risk of gastrointestinal side effects, such as ulceration and bleeding. It also has an antiplatelet effect, which lasts for the life of the platelet.

Other agents

Nitrous oxide

Nitrous oxide is an inhalational analgesic and sedative which, in a 50% mixture with oxygen (Entonox®) has equivalent potency to 10 mg morphine in an adult.[7] The delivery system uses a preferential inhalational demand arrangement for self-administration, which requires an airtight fit between the mask and face. As the patient holds the mask their grip will relax if drowsiness occurs, the airtight seal will be lost and the gas flow stops.

This system requires a degree of patient involvement and cooperation, and is useful for patients who have difficult IV access or are needlephobic. Patients who are elderly, young, confused or uncooperative will not find the technique effective. Nitrous oxide increases the volume of a pneumothorax or any other gas-filled cavity.

Sumatriptan

Sumatriptan is a $5HT_1$ receptor agonist that is effective for the treatment of acute migraine in a high proportion of patients. The dose is 50 mg orally, or 6 mg subcutaneously if the patient is vomiting. Ideally, it should be taken at the onset of headache, but is still effective when the headache is established. In about one-third to one-half of patients the headache returns within 24 hours, but is almost always responsive to a second tablet.[22]

Sumatriptan is not an analgesic and should not be used for non-vascular headache, for migraine aura with early evolving headache, or as a diagnostic test for migraine. Contraindications include pregnancy, ischaemic heart disease or chest pain with previous use, uncontrolled hypertension, ergotamine in the previous 24 hours, and current or recent (within 2 weeks) therapy with MAOIs.

Conscious sedation

Conscious sedation is defined as a medically controlled state of depressed consciousness that permits appropriate response by the patient to verbal command. Stable vital signs are maintained, along with an independent airway and adequate spontaneous respirations.[23]

The properties of the ideal analgesic and sedative agent for conscious sedation include minimal serious side effects, uniform efficacy, easy and painless administration, controllable duration of action, amnestic effects, short onset and duration of action, small dose range for effectiveness, economical cost, and few contraindications.[24]

Several agents have been used either singly or in combination in an attempt to meet these goals. These include nitrous oxide, ketamine, and combinations of a benzodiazepine with an opioid, such as midazolam/fentanyl. Equipment and personnel for monitoring and resuscitation must always be at hand for patients undergoing conscious sedation.

Conscious sedation is an effective technique for performing painful procedures in the emergency department, such as reduction of a joint dislocation. Patients are fit for discharge when the conscious state has returned to normal and transport has been arranged with appropriate follow-up arrangements, including a warning not to drive or consume alcohol.

Ketamine

Ketamine, an NMDA [N-methyl-D-aspartate] antagonist, is a unique anaesthetic that induces a state of dissociation between the cortical and limbic systems to produce a state of dissociative anaesthesia. It induces analgesia, amnesia, mild sedation and immobilization. It does not impair protective reflexes, but random or purposeful movements are frequently observed in patients after administration. Side effects include hypersalivation, vomiting, emergence reactions, nightmares, laryngospasm, hypertension, tachycardia and increased intracranial pressure.[24]

Unfortunately, there are, therefore, many contraindications to ketamine including upper or lower respiratory infection, procedures involving the posterior pharynx, cystic fibrosis, age younger than 3 months, head injury, increased intracranial pressure, acute glaucoma or globe penetration, uncontrolled hypertension, congestive cardiac failure, arterial aneurysm, acute intermittent porphyria and thyrotoxicosis. Despite this, ketamine is used increasingly in emergency departments.

PAIN RELIEF IN PREGNANCY

Many analgesics are safe in pregnancy. A *Medicines in Pregnancy* booklet has been produced by the Commonwealth Department of Health and Family Services (Australian Drug Evaluation Committee) and should be referred to as necessary.[25]

Paracetamol, opioids and local anaesthetics are safe and allow for a flexible approach to most painful conditions in pregnancy. NSAIDs should not be given in the latter part of pregnancy.

NON-PHARMACOLOGIC THERAPIES

Although pain perception involves neuroanatomical processes, the other interrelated component, pain reaction, is psychophysiological. Therefore, the use of non-pharmacologic techniques is vitally important. These include empathy, a compassionate approach, a calm manner and reassurance. Immobilization of fractures with splinting is effective, as is the application of ice to a wound. Other techniques, such as hypnosis, transcutaneous nerve stimulation and manipulation have not been widely studied in the emergency department setting.

SPECIAL PAIN SITUATIONS AND NON-ANALGESIC AGENTS

Whilst this chapter has focused on analgesic agents, there are many non-analgesics that are effective in providing analgesia. Examples of this include:

- Glyceryl trinitrate and beta blockers for acute myocardial infarction
- Redback spider antivenom for latrodectism
- Antiviral agents for herpes zoster
- Antidepressants or anticonvulsants for neuropathic pain
- Oxygen therapy for cluster headache
- Calcium gluconate for hydrofluoric acid burns
- Hot water (43°C) for venomous marine stings.

In addition, adjuvant therapy with anxiolytics such as midazolam contributes to pain relief.

Acute migraine headache requires a stepwise approach to the use of pharmacologic agents. Moderate-to-severe migraine may warrant the use of specific antimigraine medications such as ergotamine or sumatriptan, unless contraindicated.[3] The combination of aspirin (900 mg) and metoclopramide is as effective as sumatriptan in the treatment of migraine, is better tolerated and also cheaper.[3] Intravenous prochlorperazine is more effective than metoclopramide or rectal prochlorperazine.[3] The use of opioids is not recommended.[3]

Obtaining a definitive diagnosis allows directed therapy that contributes to pain relief. If specific treatments appear to be ineffective, then the diagnosis should be reconsidered.

PAIN RELIEF IN CHILDREN

Children commonly suffer pain that is even more difficult to evaluate and there

is evidence that children are routinely undertreated for painful conditions.[24] There are many situational, behavioural and emotional factors affecting a child's pain. Anxiety is perhaps the most important, and it is difficult to separate 'true pain' from simple anxiety. There are many pain scales available for use in children, but none has been validated in the emergency setting.[10] The best method is one that is appropriate for the age and cognitive level of the child.

In children, all doses must be calculated on a mg/kg basis. Otherwise, the general principles are similar to those for adults, except for the following:

- Non-pharmacologic manoeuvres are particularly important such as hiding needles and distraction.
- Intravenous access is not always easily obtained and there is hesitancy to induce pain, as children are particularly fearful of needles. Unfortunately, insertion of an IV line in a struggling toddler may be more distressing than a single IM injection.
- There is an expectation that children will cry during evaluation and treatment. Further, in the past, there was a myth that neonates and children did not perceive pain!

It is difficult to compare paediatric with adult pain. There is inadequate information about how children perceive, remember and react to pain. Children may have qualitatively and quantitatively different responses. There is virtually no study of analgesic practices or effects in children treated in emergency departments.[26] Children may experience more pain for the same pain stimulus, such as local anaesthetic infiltration, than do adults.[13]

LOCAL ANAESTHESIA

Local anaesthetic agents should always be considered for patients presenting to the emergency department with pain, either to supplement other analgesia or for definitive pain relief. This is particularly appropriate where the pain is quite

localized, as in certain fractures and wounds.

Pharmacology

Local anaesthetic agents inactivate sodium channels, temporarily blocking membrane depolarization and preventing nerve impulse transmission. Those containing ester bonds include cocaine, procaine and tetracaine (amethocaine), which undergo hydrolysis by plasma pseudocholinesterase, whereas amide-type agents include lidocaine, prilocaine and bupivacaine and undergo hepatic metabolism.

Local anaesthetics are available in single or multidose vials, with or without dilute adrenaline at 1:200 000 (containing 5 µg adrenaline (epinephrine) per mL) to prolong the duration of action. Antioxidants such as sodium bisulphite or metabisulphite are added to adrenaline (epinephrine)-containing solutions and preservative such as methylparaben to multidose vials, and are implicated in some allergic reactions to the anaesthetics. True allergy to local anaesthetics is extremely rare when verified by progressive challenge testing.[27]

The duration of action of local anaesthetics is related to the degree of protein binding, vasoactivity, concentration and possibly pH, although the addition of adrenaline (epinephrine) is the most practical way to prolong their effect. Table 21.1.2 gives typical maximum safe doses and duration of action of commonly used agents. Solutions containing adrenaline (epinephrine) should never be injected near end arteries, such as in the fingers, toes, nose or penis.

ADVERSE EFFECTS

Systemic toxicity (Table 21.1.3)

Systemic toxicity occurs after inadvertently rapid intravenous injection or exceeding the recommended safe maximum dose. Symptoms and signs of toxicity are related to plasma drug levels, and progress from circumoral tingling, dizziness, tinnitus and visual disturbance to muscular twitching, confusion, convulsions, coma and apnoea. Cardio-

Table 21.1.2 Maximum safe dose and duration of action of common local anaesthetics

Drug	Dose (mg/kg)*	Duration (h)
Lidocaine	3	0.5–1
Lidocaine with adrenaline (epinephrine)	7	2–5
Bupivacaine	2	2–4
Prilocaine	6	0.5–1.5

*1% solution contains 10 mg/mL

Table 21.1.3 Features of systemic local anaesthetic toxicity (in order of increasing plasma levels)

Circumoral tingling

Dizziness

Tinnitus

Visual disturbance

Muscular twitching

Confusion

Convulsions

Coma

Apnoea

Cardiovascular collapse (highest plasma levels)

Table 21.1.4 Adverse reactions to local anaesthetics (other than systemic toxicity)

Allergy: Esters > amides
Additives - methylparaben, sodium metabisulphite

Catecholamine effects from added adrenaline (epinephrine)

Vasovagal

Delayed wound healing

Malignant hyperthermia

Methaemoglobinaemia – prilocaine, benzocaine

vascular effects are also seen with high plasma levels, including bradycardia, hypotension and cardiovascular collapse, which are all exacerbated by associated hypoxia.

The management of systemic toxicity includes immediate cessation of the drug, airway maintenance, supplemental oxygen and incremental doses of an intravenous benzodiazepine such as midazolam 0.05–0.1 mg/kg for seizures. Major reactions may require endotracheal intubation, fluids, vasopressors and inotropic support. As reactions occur immediately or within minutes after local anaesthetic use, medical expertise, resuscitation equipment and monitoring facilities must always be available.

Other reactions (Table 21.1.4)

Other adverse reactions to local anaesthetics include allergy, catecholamine effects from added adrenaline (epinephrine), vasovagal reactions when the patient is upright, such as during a dental procedure, cytotoxic delayed wound healing, malignant hyperthermia from amide use, and methaemoglobinaemia due to excessive prilocaine or benzocaine.

SPECIFIC NERVE BLOCKS

The following nerve blocks are contraindicated in uncooperative patients and in patients with local anaesthetic allergy. Care must be taken not to exceed the recommended maximum local anaesthetic doses (Table 21.1.2), and monitoring facilities, resuscitation equipment and medical expertise must be available at all times.

Digital nerve block (ring block)

Indications

Wound debridement, suturing, drainage of infection, fracture or dislocation reduction around the nail, fingertip and distal finger or toe.

Contraindications

Local sepsis, Raynaud's phenomenon and peripheral vascular disease.

Technique

Use 2% plain lidocaine. Inject 1–1.5 mL using a 25 gauge needle into the palmar aspect of the base of the finger or toe, approaching from the dorsum. Withdraw the needle until subcutaneous and rotate until pointing to the extensor surface of the digit, and inject a further 0.5 mL. Perform the same procedure on the other side of the digit. Allow at least 5 minutes for the block to work.

Complications

Avoid intravascular injection by aspirating prior to injection. Do not use a tourniquet or more than 4 mL total volume, to avoid impairing the circulation due to high local tissue pressures.

Ulnar nerve wrist block (lateral approach)

Indications

Procedures on the medial border of the hand and medial 1.5 digits, or combined with median and radial nerve blocks for hand anaesthesia.

Contraindications

Local sepsis, neuritis.

Technique

Identify the flexor carpi ulnaris tendon at the proximal palmar crease. Introduce a 25 gauge needle on the ulnar aspect of the tendon, directed horizontally and laterally for 1 cm under the tendon. Inject 4 mL of 1% lidocaine. Withdraw the needle until subcutaneous then inject 5 mL of 1% lidocaine fanwise to the dorsal midline, to block superficial cutaneous branches.

Median nerve wrist block

Indications

Procedures on the lateral border of the hand in the territory supplied by the median nerve, excluding the medial

1.5 digits, or combined with ulnar and radial nerve blocks for hand anaesthesia.

Contraindications

Local sepsis, carpal tunnel syndrome or neuritis.

Technique

Identify the tendons of the flexor carpi radialis and palmaris longus at the proximal wrist crease. Introduce a 25 gauge needle vertically 0.5–1 cm lateral to the palmaris longus (or 0.5 cm medial to the flexor carpi radialis in the 10% of individuals lacking a palmaris longus). Inject 5 mL of 1% lidocaine when the needle gives as it penetrates the flexor retinaculum or paraesthesiae are elicited, at a depth of approximately 1 cm to the skin. Avoid injecting into the nerve itself, as it may lie more superficial than this.

Radial nerve wrist block

Indications

Procedures on the dorsal radial aspect of the hand, or combined with ulnar and median nerve blocks for hand anaesthesia.

Contraindications

Local sepsis, neuritis.

Technique

Identify the tendon of the extensor carpi radialis, and infiltrate 5–10 mL of 1% lidocaine subcutaneously in a ring around the radial border of the wrist to the area overlying the radial pulse, at the level of the proximal palmar crease.

Femoral nerve block

Indications

Analgesia for fractured shaft of femur, especially for applying splintage.

Contraindications

Local sepsis, bleeding tendency.

Technique

Palpate the femoral artery below the midpoint of the inguinal ligament, which extends from the pubic tubercle to the anterior superior iliac spine. Insert a 21 gauge needle 1 cm lateral to this point, perpendicular to the skin. Advance until

paraesthesiae are elicited down the leg and withdraw slightly, aspirate to exclude intravascular placement, and inject 10 mL of 0.5% bupivacaine. Alternatively, feel for a give as the needle punctures the fascia lata, aspirate, then inject 10 mL of 0.5% bupivacaine fanwise laterally away from the artery.

Complications

Puncture of femoral artery.

Foot blocks at the ankle

Indications

Where local anaesthetic infiltration of the foot is awkward or difficult because of thick sole skin or pain, or when excessive amounts of anaesthetic would otherwise be required.

Contraindications

Local sepsis, peripheral vascular disease.

Technique

Three superficial nerves, the sural, superficial peroneal and saphenous, are blocked by subcutaneous infiltration in a band around 75% of the ankle circumference. Two deeper nerves – the posterior tibial by the posterior tibial artery and the deep peroneal (anterior tibial) nerve by the dorsalis pedis artery – are blocked, usually in combinations with the superficial ones, according to the area of anaesthesia required:

- The sural nerve is blocked by injecting 3–5 mL of 1% lidocaine subcutaneously between the Achilles tendon and the lateral malleolus, 1 cm above the malleolus.
- Superficial peroneal nerves are blocked by injecting 4–6 mL of 1% lidocaine subcutaneously in a band between the extensor hallucis longus tendon and the lateral malleolus, on the anterior aspect of the ankle.
- The saphenous nerve is blocked by injecting 3–5 mL of 1% lidocaine subcutaneously above the medial malleolus, laterally until over the tibialis anterior tendon.
- The posterior tibial nerve is blocked by infiltrating 3–5 mL of 1% lidocaine immediately lateral to the

posterior tibial artery as it passes behind the medial malleolus, at a depth of 0.5–1 cm to the skin.
- The deep peroneal (anterior tibial) nerve is blocked by infiltrating 1–2 mL of 1% lidocaine just above the base of the medial malleolus, lateral and behind the extensor hallucis longus by the dorsalis pedis pulse at a depth of 0.5 cm.

Complications

Exceeding a total volume of 20 mL of 1% lidocaine local anaesthetic, with the risks of systemic toxicity or poor peripheral perfusion due to raised tissue pressures.

Intravenous regional anaesthesia or Bier's block

Indications

Operative procedures such as debridement, tendon repair and foreign body removal in the forearm and hand. Reduction of fractures and dislocations, typically Colles' fracture of the wrist.

Contraindications

Local anaesthetic sensitivity; peripheral vascular disease, including Raynaud's; sickle-cell disease; local infection such as cellulitis; uncooperative patients, including children; hypertension with systolic blood pressure over 200 mmHg; severe liver disease; and unstable epilepsy.

Technique

Two doctors are required, allowing one to perform the manipulation and the other, with training in the procedure and resuscitation skills, to perform the block. Explain the procedure to the patient and obtain informed consent. Assemble and check all equipment, and apply standard monitoring, including ECG, non-invasive blood pressure and pulse oximetry.

Use a specifically designed and maintained single 15 cm adult cuff, placed over cottonwool padding to the upper arm. Double-cuff tourniquets require higher inflation pressures as they are narrower. The upper cuff is inflated first, followed by the lower cuff 15 minutes later, after injection of the prilocaine, thereby causing less discomfort to the patient. The upper cuff is then released. The use of a double cuff does not always reduce the ischaemia pain, and predisposes to accidental cuff release.

Insert a small intravenous cannula into the dorsum of the hand of the injured limb and a second cannula in the other hand or wrist as emergency access to the venous circulation. Exsanguinate the injured limb by simple elevation and direct brachial artery compression for 2–3 minutes, carefully supporting the limb at the site of any fracture. An Esmarch bandage may be used instead, in the absence of a painful wrist fracture.

Keep the arm elevated and inflate the cuff to 100 mmHg above systolic blood pressure. The radial artery pulse should be absent and the veins remain empty. If this is not the case, do not inject anaesthetic but repeat the exsanguination procedure and cuff inflation. Lower the arm and inject 2.5 mg/kg (0.5 mL/kg) of 0.5% prilocaine slowly over 90 seconds and record the time.

Continuously monitor the cuff pressure and wait at least 5–10 minutes to confirm the adequacy of analgesia before removing the cannula on the injured limb. Perform the surgical procedure. Keep the tourniquet inflated for a minimum of 20 minutes and a maximum of 60 minutes.

Monitor the patient carefully for any signs of anaesthetic toxicity (see Table 21.1.3) over the next 15 minutes following cuff release, while organizing discharge from the monitored area.

Complications

No severe cardiac complications, deaths or methaemoglobinaemia have been reported using 0.5% prilocaine at the maximum dose of 2.5 mg/kg.[28] Discomfort from the cuff is possible, but rarely significant. The IVRA technique is preferred to haematoma block for

CONTROVERSIES AND FUTURE DIRECTIONS

❶ A uniform approach to pain research needs to be developed in order to make meaningful comparisons between studies.

❷ Further study should be undertaken of the role and utility of pain scores in the emergency department.

❸ The application of new analgesic drugs in the emergency department should be studied, along with alternative administration techniques, including needleless systems.

❹ An objective measure of pain should be developed.

Colles' fracture, which provides poorer analgesia that may compromise the reduction.[29]

REFERENCES

1. International Association for the Study of Pain 1979 Pain terms: a list with definitions and notes on usage. Pain 6: 249–52
2. Bonica JJ 1987 Foreword. In: Paris PM, Stewart RD (eds) Pain Management in Emergency Medicine. Appleton & Lange, Norwalk, pp xi–xii
3. National Health and Medical Research Council. Acute pain management: scientific evidence. Endorsed November 1998. Published Feb 1999. Available at: http://www.nhmrc.health.gov.au/ publicat/pdf/cp57.pdf Accessed June 2002
4. Ducharme J 1994 Emergency pain management: a Canadian Association of Emergency Physicians (CAEP) consensus document. Journal of Emergency Medicine 12: 855–66
5. Loeser JD, Melzack R 1999 Pain: an overview. Lancet 353: 1607–9
6. Paris PM, Uram M, Ginsburg MJ 1987 Physiological mechanisms of pain. In: Paris PM, Stewart RD (eds) Pain Management in Emergency Medicine. Appleton & Lange, Norwalk
7. Nolan JP, Baskett PJF 1997 Analgesia and anaesthesia. In: Skinner D, Swain A, Peyton R, Robertson C (eds) The Cambridge Textbook of Accident and Emergency Medicine. Cambridge University Press, Cambridge
8. Besson JM 1999 The neurobiology of pain. Lancet 353: 1610–5
9. Carr DB, Goudas LC 1999 Acute pain. Lancet 353: 2051–8

10. Turk DC, Melzack R 1992 The measurement of pain and the assessment of people experiencing pain. In: Turk DC, Melzack R (eds) Handbook of Pain Assessment. Guildford Press, New York, pp 3–12
11. Ho K, Spence J, Murphy MF 1996 Review of pain-measurement tools. Annals of Emergency Medicine 27: 427–32
12. Turk DC, Okifuji A 1999 Assessment of patients' reporting of pain: an integrated perspective. Lancet 353: 1784–8
13. Fatovich DM 1998 The validity of pain scales in the emergency setting (abstract). Journal of Emergency Medicine 16: 347
14. Acute Pain Management Guideline Panel 1992 Acute pain management: operative or medical procedures and trauma: clinical practice guideline. US Department of Health and Human Services, Washington, DC
15. McQuay H 1999 Opioids in pain management. Lancet 353: 2229–32
16. Miller RR 1976 Analgesics. In: Miller RR, Greenblatt DH (eds) Drug Effects in Hospitalized Patients. Wiley, New York
17. Porter J, Jick H 1980 Addiction rate in patients treated with narcotics. New England Journal of Medicine 302: 1238
18. Meyer D, Halfin V 1981 Toxicity secondary to meperidine in patients on monoamine oxidase inhibitors: a case report and review. Journal of Clinical Psychopharmacology 1: 319–21
19. Bamigbade TA, Langford RM 1998 The clinical use of tramadol hydrochloride. Pain Reviews 5: 155–82
20. Rainer TH, Jacobs P, Ng YC, et al 2000 Cost effectiveness analysis of intravenous ketorolac and morphine for treating pain after limb injury: double blind randomised controlled trial. British Medical Journal 321: 1247–51
21. Jelinek GA 2000 Ketorolac versus morphine for severe pain. [editorial] British Medical Journal 321: 1236–7
22. Goadsby PJ 1992 Sumatriptan and migraine: breakthrough therapy. Current Therapeutics 33: 11–8
23. Fatovich DM, Jacobs IG 1995 A randomized, controlled trial of oral midazolam and buffered lidocaine for suturing lacerations in children (the SLIC Trial). Annals of Emergency Medicine 25: 209–14
24. Terndrup TE 1992 Pain control, analgesia, and sedation. In: Barkin RM (ed.) Pediatric Emergency Medicine: Concepts and Clinical Practice. Mosby Year Book, St Louis
25. Commonwealth Department of Health and Family Services (Australian Drug Evaluation Committee) 1996 Medicines in Pregnancy, 3rd edn. Australian Government Publishing Service
26. Thomson AE, Frader JE 1987 Pain management in children. In: Paris PM, Stewart RD (eds) Pain Management in Emergency Medicine. Appleton & Lange, Norwalk
27. Fisher MM, Bowey CJ 1997 Alleged allergy to local anaesthetics. Anaesthesia and Intensive Care 25: 611–8
28. Lowen R, Taylor J 1994 Bier's block - the experience of Australian emergency departments. Medical Journal of Australia 160: 108–11
29. Handoll HHG, Madhok R, Dodds C 2002 Anaesthesia for treating distal radial fractures in adults (Cochrane Review). The Cochrane Library Issue 3, Oxford: Update Software

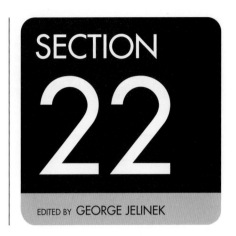

ULTRASOUND

22.1 Emergency department ultrasound 636

22.1 EMERGENCY DEPARTMENT ULTRASOUND

TONY JOSEPH

ESSENTIALS

The Australasian College for Emergency Medicine (ACEM) supports the following principles:

1 Ultrasound examination, interpretation and clinical correlation should be available in a timely manner 24 hours a day for emergency department patients.

2 Emergency physicians providing emergency ultrasound services should possess appropriate training and hands-on experience to perform and interpret limited bedside ultrasound imaging.

3 ACEM specifically supports the use of ultrasound imaging by emergency physicians for at least the following clinical indications: traumatic hemoperitoneum, abdominal aortic aneurysm, pericardial fluid, ectopic pregnancy and evaluation of renal and biliary tract disease.

4 ACEM encourages continued research in the area of ultrasound imaging and any other or evolving bedside imaging techniques and modalities.

5 ACEM encourages emergency medicine training programmes to provide instruction and experience in bedside ultrasound imaging for their trainees.

BACKGROUND

Diagnostic medical ultrasound developed initially from the use of sonar in the 1950s. It was discovered that sound waves (or echoes) could be reflected from distant objects and, provided the speed that sound travelled in a particular medium was known, the distance of the object from the source of the sound waves could be calculated.

Modern transducers can transmit sound waves (pulse-echoes) generated from electric signals by a piezo-electric crystal through body tissues and interfaces, and these waves are reflected by the tissues back to the same transducer. The sound waves or echoes are then converted back to electrical signals by the piezo-electric crystal. The echo signals are then amplified, processed and displayed on the ultrasound screen.

The usual type of ultrasound is B-mode (brightness modulation), which means that the amplitude of the echoes reflected back to the transducer determines the brightness of the display on the screen.

The technology originally was used only by radiology departments, but was quickly embraced by obstetricians in the 1970s when they found the technology allowed them to easily assess their patients in their offices. Since the 1980s, ultrasonography has been used by European and Japanese surgeons to assess trauma patients and by USA emergency and surgical specialties. Emergency-department ultrasound (EDUS) was first introduced in Australasia in the late 1990s.

The 1999 position statement on ultrasound of the Australasian College for Emergency Medicine[1] is as follows:

Ultrasound imaging has been shown to enhance the clinician's ability to assess and manage patients with a variety of acute illnesses and injuries. As ultrasound examinations can be performed at the bedside, this diagnostic modality is of great use for unstable patients who may not be candidates for other imaging procedures. Focused bedside ultrasound examinations performed by trained emergency physicians in order to answer specific clinical questions have been shown to improve patient outcomes.

The emergency department is ideal for clinical ultrasound use with rapid patient turnover and the requirement to differentiate many aspects of disease presentation at the bedside. This may include the trauma patient with potential intra-abdominal haemorrhage, the woman with a threatened miscarriage or the elderly patient with a potential abdominal aortic aneurysm (AAA). These patients require a single answer to a single question: is there haemoperitoneum, is there a viable intrauterine pregnancy or is there an AAA?

The equipment has changed markedly over the last decade from large and relatively immobile machines to smaller and more robust ones with excellent image reproduction.

The American College of Physicians published a position statement on emergency ultrasound in 1990 that stated that emergency ultrasound should be performed by appropriately trained and credentialled physicians.[2] This was followed by the development of a 'model curriculum' by the Society for Academic Emergency Medicine in 1994.[3] The clinical indications and training guidelines were further refined by an ACEP endorsed 'scope of practice' working party in 2001.[4]

The current core indications for the EDUS are seen in Table 22.1.1.

INTRODUCTORY PHYSICS OF ULTRASOUND

Sound is produced by mechanical energy that causes molecules to vibrate. It

Table 22.1.1 Current core indications for emergency ultrasound
Trauma (haemoperitoneum and haemopericardium)
Pregnancy
Biliary tract
Renal tract
Abdominal aortic aneurysm
Echocardiography
Procedural

requires a medium to travel through such as air, liquid or solid material and cannot travel in a vacuum. Humans are able to detect sound in the frequency range of 20–20 000 Hz. The definition of ultrasound is sound with a frequency greater than 20 000 Hz. Medical ultrasound is usually in the frequency range of 2.5 to 10 MHz (2.5–10.0×10^6 Hz).

Medical sonography uses a pulse-echo technique for imaging sections of the human body. A transducer sends the sound waves through the body and listens to or receives the echoes, which are transmitted back to the source. The main component of the transducer that allows this characteristic is a piezo-electric crystal, which has the peculiar property that allows for electro-mechanical conversion of energy. In other words, this allows the transducer to convert electrical energy into sound (mechanical energy) and sound waves (echoes) back to electrical energy. The transducer spends most of the time (99%) 'listening' for returning sound echoes and only 1% of the time in sound transmission. The pulse waves of sound are transmitted to the patient and are either transmitted through the tissue or reflected back to the transducer depending on the acoustic impedance that differs for each tissue. Interfaces between tissues can be strongly echogenic depending on the magnitude of the acoustic impedance mismatch between tissues. This is a particular advantage for viewing Morison's pouch, which is the interface between the liver and the right

kidney where blood commonly accumulates in blunt abdominal trauma.

The main physical sound wave properties of interest to the medical sonographer are the frequency and wavelength. The higher the frequency, the better the resolution of the object being imaged, but this is at a price of decreased depth of penetration.

Each tissue has its own acoustic impedence that is reflected in the image quality after the echoes are transformed back to electrical energy, amplified and then processed electronically to a display that uses a range of shades of grey. The stronger reflected wave is represented by brighter shades of grey approaching white.

Medical ultrasound images are classified as either B-mode (brightness modulation), where the amplitude of the incoming echoes is used to modulate the brightness of the display and a 2-dimensional image is produced, or M-mode. The latter mode is a continuously updated B-mode display of echoes from a single line of sight from the same position in the patient that results in a 1-dimensional image progressing across the display screen.

Tissue that does not generate echoes (anechoic) appears black on the screen,

for instance fluid such as blood or urine. Hence, fluid in Morison's pouch appears as black on the screen and contrasts with the increased reflectivity of the images from the tissue interface. Tissue such a bone that reflects all ultrasound waves appears as extremely white on the display monitor. Doppler refers to the behaviour of high-frequency sound waves as they are reflected off moving fluid. The colour of the wave as in colour doppler depends on whether the fluid is moving towards or away from the transducer.

It is necessary to have an understanding of some of the properties of ultrasound in order to manipulate the images to obtain the best quality.

Refraction refers to the bending of the sound waves at the interface of two mediums when the sound waves cross at an oblique angle. Attenuation is the decrease in signal energy as it passes through a medium. Scatter is the reflection of sound waves off objects that are irregular or smaller than the ultrasound beam, for instance bowel gas, and this makes ultrasound difficult to interpret. Resolution of the image refers to the minimal properties of the sound waves required to produce separate reflections of two images. This may be axial and relates to the ability of the ultrasound to

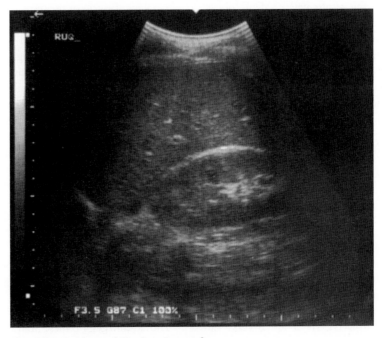

Fig. 22.1.1 Normal Morison's pouch.

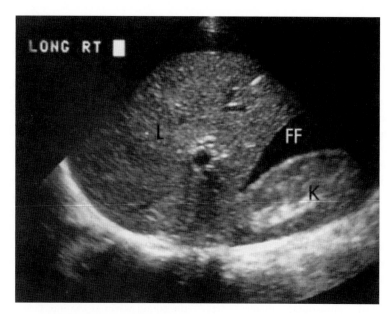

Fig. 22.1.2 Fluid in Morison's pouch.

produce separate images of two objects along the path of the sound wave. This is dependent on the frequency and wavelength. Lateral resolution depends on the beam width and is the minimum distance two objects are separated perpendicular to the beam path. The beam width is determined by the focal zone of the transducer.

There are also artifacts associated with ultrasound scanning. The commonest are shadowing and enhancement. Shadowing results when a dense object such as bone blocks signal transmission. Enhancement refers to the fact that signals that pass through a cystic fluid-filled structure such as the bladder, are subject to attenuation as they pass around the structure compared to the signals which pass through the fluid-filled structure. When the signal has passed through the fluid and reaches the opposite wall, it reaches a denser structure compared to the sound waves, which have been attenuated by travelling around the side. Hence the reflection from the tissue behind the structure appears brighter and denser than the surrounding tissue. This property is utilized when visualizing the uterus and its contents through a full bladder in early pregnancy. There are a number of other artifacts, which are beyond the scope of this introductory chapter.

TRANSDUCERS

There are linear, curved, phased array and special transducers.[5] Linear array transducers are made up of small rectangular crystals arranged side by side in a straight line. They are usually relatively small and high frequency (7.0–10.0 MH) and produce high-resolution images of superficial tissues. Hence they are useful for imaging small parts such as the internal jugular vein or the testis. Phased array transducers have sequential firing of the elements from one end to the other and this results in steering of the beam. The small footprint and diverging field of view make these transducers suitable for limited access areas such as between the ribs or through fontanelles. Curved array transducers have the crystals arranged in a convex arc. These have large fields of view with good detail but are limited in some areas due to difficult skin contact. They are the commonest types of transducer (3.5–5.0 MHz probes) and are used for abdominal scanning.

There are other specialized types of transducers that include endovaginal, transrectal, transoesophageal and intravascular.

The advantages of these transducers include:

- Close proximity to the organ of interest allowing the use of higher frequency crystals with better resolution
- Smaller fields of view and less beam distortion
- Less impediments
- Independence from other organs such as the urinary bladder, which does not need to be full with endovaginal transducer use.

THE SCOPE OF EMERGENCY DEPARTMENT ULTRASOUND

Focused assessment by sonography for trauma exam

Ultrasound was first used for the assessment of blunt abdominal trauma (BAT) by Kristensen et al[6] in Germany in 1971, and in 1988 it was compulsory for German surgical trainees to demonstrate proficiency in the use of ultrasound. In the USA, Tso et al first reported on the evaluation of BAT by ultrasound in 1992.[7] After minimal training they found that trauma fellows could diagnose haemoperitoneum with a sensitivity of 91% and a specificity of 99%. It is important to understand that the ability to diagnose parenchymal injury by ultrasound is very limited.

Computerized tomography (CT) of the abdomen is still required to make the diagnosis of solid intra-abdominal organ injury in the era of conservative management of stable, blunt abdominal trauma.

The focused assessment by sonography for trauma (FAST) study essentially looks at four intra-abdominal areas (Table 22.1.2) and this examination can

Table 22.1.2 FAST Study
Morison's pouch (Hepato-renal space)
Spleno-renal space
Subxiphiod pericardium
Suprapubic

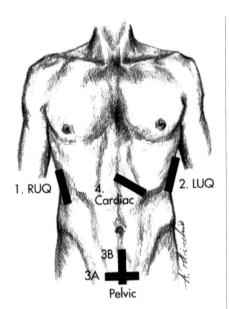

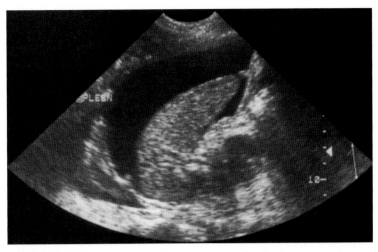

Fig. 22.1.4 Fluid in splenorenal area. (Note free fluid superior to the spleen)

Fig. 22.1.3 Transducer placement for fast and accurate assessment of the four areas.

be completed in 2–5 minutes. The aim of FAST is to detect haemoperitoneum, haemopericardium or haemothorax.

Conditions in BAT that require further ultrasonographic evaluation include: where abdominal examination is reliable but equivocal for injury, e.g. tenderness without peritonism; examination is unreliable on the basis of head or spinal injury; intoxication; language difficulties; or when clinical examination is negative but the patient requires prolonged anaesthesia such as for orthopaedic procedures.

Unfortunately, more than 60% of trauma patients fall into one of the above categories and require a diagnostic investigation to exclude significant intra-abdominal injury.[8]

Diagnostic peritoneal lavage (DPL) has been largely replaced in those centres that use FAST for assessment of blunt abdominal trauma. While DPL is very sensitive with a low specificity, it may result in a high negative laparotomy rate. It requires experience, is invasive and takes a minimum of 15 minutes to perform in the most experienced hands.

Abdominal CT scan is also very sensitive and specific for intra-abdominal bleeding as well as very accurate for retroperitoneal and bony pelvic injuries.

The disadvantages of CT include its unsuitability for haemodynamically unstable patients, lack of accuracy in hollow viscus injury and provision of large amounts of ionizing radiation. However, in those centres that use FAST to assess BAT, there is a definite role for abdominal CT in those patients with a negative FAST examination who may have a solid organ laceration without significant haemoperitoneum. It is important to accurately diagnose these patients as they will require a period of observation in hospital in case of potentially catastrophic secondary haemorrhage.

The FAST examination can be generally completed in less than 3–5 minutes for the detection of significant intra-abdominal bleeding and in less than 1 minute if Morison's pouch alone is imaged.[9] It can be performed at the same time as the initial resuscitation, requires no special patient preparation and is easily repeatable. There are no contraindications but interpretation is difficult in the obese patient, those with large amounts of subcutaneous air or bowel gas and, occasionally, in those with large retroperitoneal haematomas, which may spread anteriorly.

The accuracy of FAST for the detection of haemoperitoneum and visceral injuries as performed by surgeons is well documented by Rozycki et al, with a collected series of 4941 patients demonstrating a sensitivity of 93.4%, a

specificity of 98.7% and an accuracy of 97.5%.[10] This compared favourably to a series of 997 patients on whom FAST was performed by radiologists with a sensitivity of 90.8%, specificity of 99.2% and accuracy of 97.8%.

One of the first studies reporting on the use of ultrasound for the assessment of blunt abdominal trauma was by Tso et al in 1992.[7] They reported on 163 patients who had FAST scans performed by trauma fellows who had 1 hour of didactic and 1 hour of practical training. The overall sensitivity for the detection of parenchymal injury was 69% with a specificity of 99%. All false-negative exams occurred in patients with organ injury who had minimal or no haemoperitoneum detected by DPL or CT. They concluded that a negative FAST did not rule out parenchymal injury.

There have been many studies validating the accuracy of the FAST by non-radiologists for the detection of haemoperitoneum in BAT. The sensitivity varies from 80 to 100% and the specificity from 88 to 100%.[11,12,13]

FAST has also been validated for use in paediatric trauma patients with sensitivity from 89 to 100% and specificity of 96–98%.[14] Children are a very easy group to scan due to a generally low body fat content. Also FAST has been shown to be useful in pregnant trauma patients[15] as it can give valuable information about both mother and baby.

Further, Boulanger et al[16] have validated the use of trauma ultrasonography as part of a diagnostic algorithm with selective use of DPL and abdominal CT. They found that this use of ultrasound was a rapid and accurate test for intraperitoneal fluid and the need for laparotomy in patients with a negative scan was very rare.

Some authors have also proposed the use of a scoring system for quantification of intraperitoneal fluid volume, which can be a predictor of the need for surgery. McKenny et al[17] measured the depth of the largest collection of fluid from anterior to posterior in centimeters and noted each additional site of fluid seen on US. The total score was equal to the depth of the largest volume in cm plus 1 point for each additional positive site. They found that 9 out of 10 patients with a score of 2 or less did not require a laparotomy and 35/46 patients with a score greater than 2 required a laparotomy.

It would seem that the place of the FAST examination in the evaluation of the trauma patient is in the rapid assessment of the haemodynamically unstable patient, thus replacing the diagnostic peritoneal lavage. There is also a role in the patient with a low clinical risk for intraperitoneal bleeding who may spend a long period of time in the operating theatre, for instance patients with orthopaedic or head injuries.

The sonographer should be aware of the limitations of FAST, which include a low sensitivity for isolated solid organ and hollow viscus injury as well as the technical difficulties in obese patients and those with large amounts of intraperitoneal or subcutaneous air.

USE OF ULTRASOUND IN EARLY PREGNANCY

Ultrasound in the first trimester is useful in the investigation of abdominal pain and vaginal bleeding. In the context of a positive pregnancy test, ultrasound can distinguish between intrauterine and ectopic pregnancy. If an intrauterine pregnancy can be identified, then ectopic pregnancy can be safely excluded as the risk of heterotopic pregnancy is 1/30 000 in the general population and 1/5000 in patients on fertility treatment.

Transabdominal ultrasonography (TAS) is performed with a full bladder to enable better visualization of the intrauterine structures. If the uterine contents are not identifiable, then a transvaginal ultrasound (TVS) should be performed as this does not require a full bladder.

TVS allows the visualization of intrauterine structures and diagnosis of intrauterine pregnancy 1–2 weeks earlier than TAS. TVS should be able to diagnose intrauterine pregnancy by 5 weeks gestation with a quantitative βHCG level of 1500–2000 mIU/mL.

The transvaginal probe (5.0–7.5 MHz) is covered by a sterile condom and placed inside the vagina. The orientation of the probe is different to that of the transabdominal probe in that, while longitudinal and transverse images are obtained, the sonographer must orientate to the proximity of the organs being imaged.

Features of normal pregnancy visible on transvaginal ultrasound[19] (see Table 22.1.3)

The earliest ultrasound sign of intrauterine pregnancy is the presence of a yolk sac within the gestational sac or a double decidual (ring) sign. The sonographer must be wary of incorrectly labelling the pseudogestational sac of an ectopic pregnancy as a gestational sac. The most reliable sign of an intrauterine pregnancy is the identification of a fetus with a detectable heart beat. The risk of miscarriage at 7–12 weeks' gestation with an intrauterine foetus plus heartbeat is approximately 2%.[19]

Table 22.1.3 Timing of transvaginal findings in normal pregnancy
Gestational sac: 4.5–5 weeks
Yolk sac: 5 weeks
Foetal pole: 5–6 weeks
Cardiac activity: 6 weeks
Foetal parts: 8 weeks

The diagnosis of ectopic pregnancy in the emergency department is suspected by the ultrasound findings of an empty uterus in a pregnant patient. This will require a formal radiology department ultrasound that may visualize the ectopic pregnancy or a complex mass in the fallopian tube.

The level of the β-HCG can also be used as a risk stratification measure in the evaluation of the pregnant patient with abdominal pain or vaginal bleeding. In the first trimester, β-HCG doubles every 24–36 hours in a normal pregnancy to a maximum of 10 000 to 100 000 mIU/mL. The patient with an ectopic pregnancy has a low, normal β-HCG level that either plateaus, increases slowly, or declines and doesn't follow the normal doubling time frame. If the patient has a β-HCG level above the discriminatory level of 1500–2000 mIU/mL, an intrauterine pregnancy should be visualized on TVS. If the level is below the discriminatory level and no intrauterine pregnancy is seen in an otherwise normal uterus, the patient may be safely discharged to return in 24–48 hours for repeat β-HCG and ultrasound. They should be instructed to return to the emergency department if there is an increase in abdominal pain or vaginal bleeding.

If the level is above the discriminatory range (>1500 mIU/mL) and no intrauterine or ectopic pregnancy is seen, the patient is assumed to have an ectopic pregnancy and should have an obstetric/gynaecology consultation. If a mass is seen in the adnexae or there is fluid in the cul-de-sac, an urgent obstetric/gynaecology consultation is required as the positive predictive value for ectopic pregnancy is 94%.[19] Care must also be taken to ensure that a foetal pole with a heartbeat is located within the uterine cavity, as a late ectopic pregnancy can survive in the fallopian tube or myometrium.

An interstitial pregnancy (2–3% of all ectopic pregnancies) is located in the fallopian tube as it traverses the uterine wall with the main part of the gestational sac located outside the uterine cavity. The mortality rate is more than twice that of other tubal pregnancies (2%) as

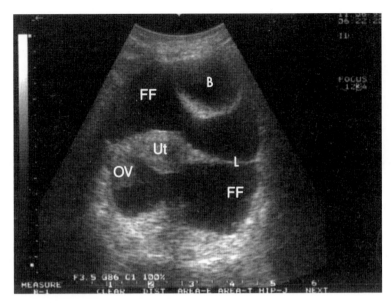

Fig. 22.1.5 Fluid in pouch of Douglas.

Shock
Syncope
Hypotension
Abdominal pain
Abdominal mass
Flank pain
Back pain (especially in the older population)

they tend to rupture later (at 8–16 weeks duration). These pregnancies may be difficult for the most experienced sonographer to diagnose and often require laparoscopy in order to make the diagnosis. Clues which may help in the diagnosis of this abnormality include blood in the peritoneal cavity (in an apparent intrauterine pregnancy), a thin asymmetric myometrium and an eccentrically located gestational sac.[20] If there is any doubt as to the presence or not of intrauterine pregnancy, Obstetrics should be consulted and a formal radiology ultrasound organized.

Durham et al[21] were able to demonstrate an acceptable accuracy for emergency physicians (EPs) in the detection of ectopic pregnancy in the first trimester. They found a 96% agreement between the EPs and radiology department findings in the evaluation of first trimester bleeding. They concluded that those patients, in whom they were unable to make a diagnosis, could be identified and appropriate diagnostic follow-up arranged.

There have also been a number of studies which show that EP pelvic ultrasound results in a significantly decreased length of stay when compared to those scans done by radiologists especially in those patients with a normal intrauterine pregnancy.[22,23]

There are significant training issues associated with the development of the skills necessary to perform accurate pelvic ultrasound in the first trimester especially with regard to transvaginal ultrasound. With assistance from other EPs who have acquired the necessary experience, as well as radiology and obstetric sonographers, it is possible to acquire the skills necessary to perform accurate and safe first trimester ultrasonography.

Emergency ultrasonography in the second and third trimesters is done by the transabdominal route. This focuses on the detection of foetal movement, detection of foetal heartbeat, state of the placenta and evaluation of the pregnant trauma patient. Obvious foetal abnormalities may be detected but this is best left to radiology and obstetric/gynaecology sonographers as a definitive examination is beyond the scope of emergency department ultrasonography.

ULTRASOUND OF THE ABDOMINAL AORTA

EDUS of abdominal aortic aneurysm (AAA) can be one of the easiest and most beneficial examinations for the patient. The accuracy of US for AAA is 97%.[24] Indications are listed in Table 22.1.4.

Saccular dilatation of the aorta greater than 3 cm is abnormal and occurs in approximately 2% of the population. Rupture is more likely in aneurysms greater than 5.0–6.0 cm and these patients are candidates for surgery as the mortality of elective repair is 3.5% compared to 50% for a ruptured AAA.[24]

The aorta enters the abdominal cavity at the level of the diaphragm and travels to the left of the inferior vena cava (IVC) anterior to the vertebral column. It bifurcates at the level of L4 and 1–2 cm below the umbilicus into left and right common iliac arteries. It should be visualized in both transverse and longitudinal planes along its entire length using a 2.5–3.5 mHz probe. It should be easily distinguishable from the IVC as the latter is easily compressible and the aorta is pulsatile and non-compressible.

Detection of an AAA in a haemodynamically unstable patient, who is hypotensive with severe back pain, should result in immediate transfer to the operating suite for laparotomy and resection or grafting. The sensitivity for EDUS diagnosis of AAA is 97–100% with very high specificity[25]. Large amounts of bowel gas and obesity can hinder the detection and diagnosis of AAA. Other limitations of EDUS include the difficulty in detection of retroperitoneal rupture and aortic dissection.

Those patients who are symptomatic but haemodynamically stable (with AAA seen on US) still require abdominal CT for accurate detection of the upper and lower limits of the AAA, which assists

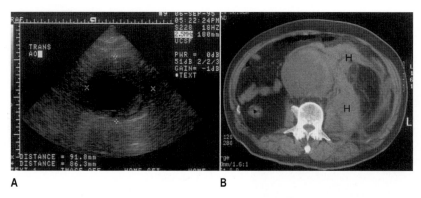

A   B

Fig. 22.1.6 A shows a 9 x 8 cm abdominal aortic aneurysm with some clot in the cavity. B shows a CT of the same patient with extensive retroperitoneal haemorrhage not seen on the ultrasound.

surgical planning and assesses for a retroperitoneal, contained rupture.

US is also very useful for ruling out AAA as a cause of abdominal pain (especially renal colic) in an otherwise well elderly patient. US is not only accurate in diagnosing those who need to go to the operating theatre urgently for repair but also in triaging those who do need immediate operative intervention. Scanning for AAA is a very easy skill to learn and the novice user commences on a very steep learning curve with very few false negatives and false positives.[26]

Kuhn et al[27] found in a study of novice emergency physician ultrasonographers who scanned patients with potential AAA, an accuracy of 100% in scan interpretation. They included 68 patients with potential AAA and found 26 positive, 40 negative and two indeterminate. They concluded that EDUS would have improved the care in 46 patients without adverse sequelae.

GALLBLADDER ULTRASOUND

Epigastric and right upper quadrant pain are common presenting symptoms to the emergency department. The normal gallbladder, a pear-shaped cystic structure, is 7–10 cm long and 2–3 cm in transverse diameter. It is best imaged by a 3.5 or 5.0 MHz transducer in the right subcostal area in the mid-clavicular line. While most patients are supine, good views may also be obtained in the left lateral decubitus or upright positions.

Acute cholecystitis is often associated with gallstones, which are echogenic with a well seen shadow. Gallstones are the most common finding in acute cholecystitis, but alone are not sufficient to make the diagnosis (see Table 22.1.5).

Gallstones associated with wall thickening have a 95.2% positive predictive value for acute cholecystitis.[28] Mean gallbladder thickness is 9 mm for acute cholecystitis and 5 mm for chronic cholecystitis.[28] Common bile duct dilatation greater than 7 mm (or >10 mm in those with prior biliary surgery) occurs in biliary obstruction. This is relevant because stones in the common bile duct, cystic duct and gallbladder neck may be difficult to see. Approximately 5–10 % of gallbladders are not seen due to postprandial contraction and 5–10% of acute cholecystitis cases are acalculous.[29]

RENAL ULTRASOUND

While CT is the optimal method to evaluate the renal tract in the patient

Table 22.1.5 Sonographic features of acute cholecystitis
Gallstones
Sludge
Wall thickening
Pericholestatic fluid
Sonographic Murphy's sign

with renal colic, it takes time to organize and may not be readily available out of normal hours. Ultrasound is a rapid and non-invasive way to assess the renal tract for obstruction in the patient with loin pain suggestive of renal colic.

The normal kidney is 9–12 cm long, 2.5–3.0 cm thick and 4–5 cm wide. It is bean-shaped along its long axis that is tilted posteriorly with the superior pole heading posteriorly.

The kidney is scanned in the long and transverse axes using a 3.5 or 5.0 MHz probe. The patient should be well hydrated to allow for optimal views of the renal pelvis and vesicoureteric junction. The renal capsule is highly echogenic, the parenchyma homogeneous and the renal sinus (collecting system) highly echogenic. The purpose of emergency department renal sonography is to look for calculi, hydronephrosis and peri-renal fluid.

Hydronephrosis is caused by any obstruction to the renal outflow tract through the ureters or urethra. The usual cause is a stone in the ureter, but it may also be due to prostate enlargement or bladder outlet obstruction. Hydronephrosis is defined as separation of the highly echogenic renal sinuses by interconnected fluid-filled areas. As the obstruction progesses, the renal cortex becomes compressed. Obstruction is classified from Grade 1 (minimal calyceal separation) to Grade 3 (severe dilatation of the calyces with loss of renal parenchyma). Calculi may be visualized within the kidney, bladder and vesicoureteric junction but they are more difficult to see than gallstones and can be obscured by bowel gas.

Incidental findings on renal sonography may include renal masses that can be classified as cystic or solid. These will usually require further evaluation by CT.

OTHER USES FOR EMERGENCY DEPARTMENT ULTRASOUND

Central line placement

Central venous access may be required in critically ill patients who present to the emergency department. These patients require timely venous access often for the administration of fluids, blood and ionotropes. Traditional central access routes use a Seldinger (percutaneous) approach via the internal jugular, subclavian and femoral veins. The success often depends on operator experience and patient body habitus.

It has been shown that the use of an ultrasound-guided technique can significantly improve the success rate along with decreased time to completion of the procedure and a lesser complication rate. The easiest method for internal jugular cannulation utilizing a two-person technique is with one person holding the sterile-covered probe while the proceduralist cannulates the internal jugular vein under direct vision. The probe should be a high frequency 7.5 or 10-MHz linear probe with a sterile cover.

Denys et al[30] demonstrated in a study of 1226 patients with internal jugular access, using ultrasound as a guide, an overall success rate of 100% compares to 81% in those with no ultrasound. Their first pass success was double that of the conventional technique and the time to access was 9.8 seconds compared to 44.5 seconds. They also showed a significant decrease in complication rates. Others[31] have used ultrasound guidance for subclavian vein cannulation (92% vs 44%), despite the interference from ribs and clavicle.

Hilty et al[32] have used ultrasound-guidance for femoral vein cannulation. Their overall success rate was 90% versus 65%, there were less needle passes and no instances of femoral arterial catheterization.

Ultrasound guidance for central access should become a standard of care and be included in the training curriculum for emergency medicine.

Testicular imaging

Acute testicular and scrotal pain is a relatively common presenting symptom to the emergency department. Acute scrotal pain may be due to testicular torsion or epididymo-orchitis. Scrotal swelling or mass may be due to hydrocele, hernia or testicular mass. Scrotal trauma may be associated with testicular rupture.

Ultrasound of the testicle has become a standard of care for the evaluation of testicular pain. It gives excellent visualization of the anatomy, is non-invasive and is reproducible at the bedside.

Torsion of the testis (or more correctly the spermatic cord) is detected by bedside US.

It is important to make this diagnosis in the emergency department as the testicular salvage rate by surgical correction is 80–100% if surgery occurs within 6 hours, 70% if within 6–12 hours and 20% after 12 hours. Hence early diagnosis is important.

Blood flow can be detected by colour doppler that shows direction of flow. Power doppler, while not able to show direction of flow, is up to five times more sensitive that colour doppler. Decreased or absent blood flow compared to the asymptomatic testicle is the principal diagnostic feature.

A hydrocele is an abnormal collection of fluid between the two layers of the tunica vaginalis. It may be congenital or may be associated with trauma, tumours, torsion or epididymo-orchitis. It appears as an anechoic collection on ultrasound.

Epididymo-orchitis appears in older men (40–50 years) and is infective in origin. Ultrasound findings include a thickened epididymis with decreased echogenicity, but an increased blood flow in the epididymis and testicle when compared to the other side.

Deep vein thrombosis

Physical examination for the presence of deep vein thrombosis (DVT) in the legs is notoriously unreliable and only 30–37% of patients referred to vascular labs for suspected DVT have the diagnosis confirmed.[33]

Compression ultrasound is the investigation of choice for proximal DVT and it is superior to both plethysmography and doppler ultrasound with a sensitivity of 93–100% and specificity of 97–100%.

The technique involves using a 3 to 7 MHz transducer. With the patient supine, the common femoral artery and vein are identified just below the inguinal ligament. The vein is followed to the superficial femoral and down to the trifurcation of the popliteal vein. Gentle pressure is exerted on the vein, which should be easily compressible compared to the artery. Non-compressibility of the vein indicates the presence of a clot below the transducer. If compressibility can be demonstrated at both the common femoral and popliteal veins, this reliably excludes proximal DVT.

Lensing et al[34] demonstrated a sensitivity of 100% for compression ultrasound in detecting proximal DVT when compared to venography where they used compressibility of the common femoral or popliteal veins as the sole criteria for a positive test.

Blaivas et al[35] confirmed these findings in a study that examined emergency physicians who had undergone a standardized course in order to identify thrombus in the common femoral or popliteal veins. They performed colour duplex doppler examinations on patients with leg pain and swelling; and found a very high agreement with formal vascular studies with a κ 0.8 and 98% agreement with the diagnosis.

Much of the literature on ultrasound of the leg has referred to duplex scanning that involves B-Mode and pulsed doppler. Colour doppler identifies artery and vein and thus facilitates correct identification of the vessel in question.

Echocardiography

While a formal evaluation of cardiac muscle and valve function is beyond the scope of the focussed exam required by the emergency physician, important information can be derived from a brief, goal orientated cardiac study.

Echocardiography makes use of two types of image production: motion or M-mode and the usual 2-D echocardiography. M-Mode uses a very thin band of echo signal that is imaged against time. This produces accurate measurement of cardiac wall thickness, and good resolution of small, high-velocity structures such as cardiac valves. 2-D echocardiography produces the usual echo images allowing detection of cardiac wall abnormalities, ejection fraction and abnormal fluid accumulation. M-mode and 2-D can be combined to view a particular structure (such as a valve) and colour Doppler can be used to calculate stroke volume and pressure gradients across valves.

Cardiac transducers vary from 2.5 to 5 MHz and usually have a smaller footprint than used for the usual FAST exam so that they may fit between the ribs. However, conventional transducers are usually adequate. The views most easily obtained are subcostal or apical 4-chamber and long-axis parasternal views.

Pericardial effusions especially those causing cardiac tamponade are easily seen on these views. Small and medium size effusions (<300 mL) may be only visible in the posterior pericardium, while larger effusions (>300 mL) are visible in both anterior and posterior pericardial sacs. This study provides valuable information in the assessment of the patient with penetrating chest trauma and enables the clinicians to make rapid decisions regarding the need for urgent thoracotomy. With transmural tears of the right ventricle, pericardial haemorrhage may not accumulate immediately and a repeat examination is worthwhile. The ultrasound demonstration of pericardial effusions may also guide the insertion of pericardial drains in the non-trauma patient.

Another useful emergency application of echocardiography is in the assessment of the cardiac-arrest patient with pulseless electrical activity. Visible cardiac contractions, if present, may encourage the continuation of the resuscitation looking for a reversible cause such as hypovolaemia or pulmonary embolism, and if absent, allow cessation of further resuscitation due to a poor prognosis.

In the patient with massive pulmonary embolism, cardiac ultrasound may also demonstrate a dilated, hypokinetic right ventricle which, in the clinical setting of pulmonary embolism, may guide the decision for thrombolysis.

The assessment of valve, wall motion and detailed cardiac function are beyond the scope of this chapter.

Appendicitis

Ultrasound of the right lower quadrant is difficult at the best of times and in the hands of the most experienced sonographers. The normal appendix can be difficult to view sonographically as it is a small tubular structure about 6 mm in diameter surrounded by bowel gas. It has been shown that a high level of clinical suspicion and the use of a scoring system such as the Mantrels criteria [36] has a sensitivity of 91.6% and a specificity of 84.7%. When ultrasound has been compared to CT for accuracy in the diagnosis of appendicitis, the average sensitivity and specificity has been 92% and 85% respectively[37] compared to CT, which showed a sensitivity of 90–100% and specificity of 95–97%.

The appendix is best visualized by the linear probe 3.5 to 7.5 MHz. In the right iliac fossa the normal appendix will be easily compressible whereas the inflamed appendix will not compress. On transverse scan the classic bulls-eye or target appearance has a diagnostic accuracy rate of 95%.[38] This consists of a hypoechoic, fluid-filled lumen, surrounded by a hyperechoic inner ring and a hypoechoic outer ring and the diameter is >6 mm.

Miscellaneous applications

Ultrasound can offer invaluable assistance in both diagnostic and therapeutic procedures in the emergency department.

Suprapubic bladder aspiration or catheter placement

The probe is placed transversely over the suprapubic region and angled caudally to bring into view the bladder. The operator is then in a position to apply a sterile cover to the proble and, using a sterile technique, enter the bladder with a needle and either aspirate the bladder or pass a wire to introduce a catheter via the Seldinger technique.

Abscesses

A linear tranducer (7.5–10 MHz) may be useful in localizing superficial abscesses that require drainage. The abscess should be imaged in two planes and the depth under the skin noted and marked. Fluid in the abscess will appear hypoechoic within an abscess wall, although there may be necrotic debris floating in the purulent fluid. The ultrasound may also guide surgical drainage of the lesion. Blaivas[39] describes a case where ultrasound-guided drainage of a breast abscess in the emergency department was successful after blind attempts at surgical drainage. This form of imaging may obviate the need surgical exploration and drainage.

Foreign bodies

Glass, plastic, wood and metal can all be seen on ultrasound using a high frequency linear probe 5–10 MHz. Glass and metal are particularly echogenic and may generate an acoustic shadow. Wood splinters may generate a slightly hyperechoic signal when compared to surrounding tissue.[40]

TRAINING AND CREDENTIALING

In 1999, the Australasian College for Emergency Medicine (ACEM) proposed a policy document supporting the use of emergency department ultrasound (EDUS) for trauma, abdominal aortic aneurysm (AAA), early pregnancy, renal and biliary disease.[1] The College supported a policy document regarding the credentialing process for training in evaluation of the FAST exam and detecting an abdominal aortic aneurysm.[1] The policy detailed attendance at a workshop that would cover basic information to equip the physician's performance and interpretation of both FAST and AAA. The College also mandated that, during the training process, the novice sonographer should perform a minimum of 25 trauma exams with five positives and 15 AAA exams with five positives. All of the training exams should be confirmed by another study and a record kept.

In 2001, ACEM approved the Ultrasound Special Interest Group recommendations for Minimum standards for an Ultrasound Workshop. The College also stressed that the credentialing guidelines were recommendations only and it was the responsibility of each individual hospital to have credentialing arrangements in place for the local practitioners.

It is unclear how much training

emergency physicians (and other non-radiologists) require in order to become proficient in all the indications for EDUS. The model curriculum as proposed by Mateer et al[3] suggested an introductory course of 40 hours duration and 150 examinations during the residency (including 50 abdominal, 50 echocardiographic and 50 obstetric/gynaecological scans).

The object was to obtain competency in identification of:

- Haemoperitoneum in abdominal trauma
- Intrauterine pregnancy in 1st trimester bleeding
- Abdominal aortic aneurysm
- Pericardial effusion/pulseless electrical activity
- Hydronephrosis or hydroureter
- Gallstones, biliary sludge, gallbladder wall thickening and pericholecystic fluid.

The ACEP Emergency Ultrasound Guidelines – 2001[4] reviewed the previous criteria for achievement of ultrasound proficiency. The taskforce recommended that a 16-hour introductory course was reasonable as long as it covered all aspects of machine technology and ultrasound scanning techniques for the six primary modalities. They suggested that emergency physicians should obtain a minimum of 25 ultrasound exams for each primary modality (see above) with a range of 25–50 in total. They also suggested that there should be some positives, but that number was not specified. The ACEM ultrasound sub-committee agreed, but still felt that a certain number of positives (a minimum of three for each modality) was reasonable as it was essential that each novice be able to demonstrate an ability to recognize abnormal findings.

It seems reasonable that a 16 hour introductory course is sufficient as an introduction to the use of EDUS as demonstrated in a study by Mandevia et al[41] They presented a 16-hour emergency ultrasound curriculum (lectures and hands-on) to a mixed group of ultrasound novices (mainly residents). They also gave a pre- and post-ultrasound interpretation test to all the participants. The mean pre-test score was 65% and post-test 84%. They followed up the residents over 10 months to check the accuracy of their scans, which showed a mean sensitivity of 92.4% and specificity of 96.1%. They concluded that a 16-hour course is a sufficient introductory basis and that focussed sonography can be taught with accuracy and success.

The focus for Australasian EDUS will be to train and credential both residents and consultants in the use of sonography in order to answer a specific question. It cannot, and was never intended to, be a definitive examination. This will remain the realm of the radiology department. Instead, it is an extension of the clinical examination and should be used with that aim in mind.

The credentialing process will involve attendance at a workshop that covers in sufficient detail all aspects of the modality being studied followed by a proctored performance of at least 25 scans for each indication, which are reviewed and compared to a gold standard study. There will be a requirement for a minimum of at least three positive results before the individual is said to be credentialed for that particular indication. The individual will also be required to keep a log book and show evidence of on-going skills maintenance and professional development in that discipline.

EDUS is a rapidly changing field with new developments occurring in machine and probe technology, doppler capability, image quality and resolution.

CONTROVERSIES AND FUTURE DIRECTIONS

❶ Training and maintaining skills in the other primary indications for EDUS besides trauma and AAA may be difficult for emergency physicians.

❷ Maintaining skills once credentialing is achieved in certain EDUS modalities may also be problematic.

❸ It is important that emergency physicians retain awareness of the limitations of EDUS especially in the obese and those with excess bowel gas or subcutaneous air.

❹ Newer ultrasound technologies, such as colour and power doppler, 3-dimensional ultrasound, tissue harmonic imaging and telemedicine will rapidly change this area of emergency medicine.

REFERENCES

1. ACEM Policy Document : www.acem.org.au
2. American College of Emergency Physicians 1990 Council Resolution on Ultrasound. ACEP News November
3. Mateer J, Plummer D, Heller M, et al 1994 Model curriculum for physician training in emergency ultrasonography. Annals of Emergency Medicine 23: 95–102
4. ACEP 2001 Emergency ultrasound guidelines – 2001. Annals of Emergency Medicine 38(4): 470–81
5. Gent R 1997 Applied Physics and Technology of Diagnostic Ultrasound. Openbook Publishers
6. Kristensen JK, Buemann B, Kuehl E. 1971 Ultrasonic scanning in the diagnosis of splenic haematomas. Atcta Chirurgie Scandinavia 137: 653–6
7. Tso P, Rodriguez A, Cooper C, et al 1992 Sonography in blunt abdominal trauma: A preliminary progress report. Journal of Trauma 33: 39–43
8. Boulanger BR, McLellan BA 1996 Blunt abdominal trauma. Emergency Clinics of North America 14 (1): 151–71
9. Jones R 2000 Clinical use of ultrasound in thoracoabdominal trauma. Trauma Reports. Special Supplement, Volume 1, No 2.
10. Rozycki GS, Shackford SR 1996 Ultrasound, what every Trauma Surgeon should know. Journal of Trauma 40(1): 1–4
11. Boulanger B, McLellan B, Brenneman F, et al 1996 Emergent abdominal sonography as a screening test in a new diagnostic algorithm for blunt trauma. Journal of Trauma 40: 867
12. Rozycki GS, Ochsner MG, Schmidt JA, et al 1995 A prospective study of surgeon-performed ultrasound as the primary adjuvant modality for injured patient assessment. Journal of Trauma 39: 492–8
13. McKenney MG, Martin L, Lentz K, et al 1996 1000 consecutive ultrasounds for blunt abdominal trauma. Journal of Trauma 40: 607
14. Luks FL, Lemire A, St-Vil D, et al 1993 Blunt abdominal trauma in children: the practical value of ultrasonography. Journal of Trauma 34: 607
15. Ma OJ, Mateer JR, DeBehnke DJ 1996 Use of ultrasonography for the evaluation of pregnant trauma patients. Journal of Trauma 40: 665
16. Boulanger BR, McLellan BA, Brenneman FD, et al 1996 Emergent abdominal sonography as a screening test in a new diagnostic algorithm for blunt trauma. Journal of Trauma 40: 867–73
17. McKenny KL, McKenny MG, Nunez DB, et al 1996 Interpreting the trauma ultrasound: Observations in 62 positive cases. Emerg Rad 3: 113–6
18. Simon BC, Snoey ER. 1997 Ultrasound in Emergency and Ambulatory Medicine. Mosby – Year Book Inc, St Louis
19. Cattanach S 1994 Ectopic pregnancy: we can still miss the diagnosis. Australian Family Physician 23(2): 190–2, 196

20. DeWitt C, Abbott J 2002 Interstitial Pregnancy; a potential for misdiagnosis on ectopic pregnancy with emergency department ultrasonography. Annals of Emergency Medicine 40 (1): 106–9

21. Durham B, Lane B, et al 1997 Pelvic ultrasound performed by emergency physicians for the detection of ectopic pregnancy in complicated first – trimester pregnancies. Annals of Emergency Medicine 29(3): 338–47

22. Burgher S, Tandy TK, et al 1998 Transvaginal ultrasonography by emergency physicians decreases patient time in the emergency department. Acad Emerg Med 5(8): 802–7

23. Shih C 1996 Effect of emergency physician-performed sonography on length of stay in the Emergency Department 29 (3): 348–52

24. Beede SD, Ballard DJ, James EM, et al 1990 Positive predictive value of clinical suspicion of abdominal aortic aneurysm: Implications for efficient use of abdominal ultrasonography. Archives of Internal Medicine 150: 549

25. Hollier LH, Taylor LM, Oshsner J 1992 Recommended indications for treatment of abdominal aortic aneurysms. Journal of Vascular Surgery 15(6): 1046–56

26. Shuman WP, Hastrup W, Kohler TR, et al 1998 Suspected leaking abdominal aortic aneurysm: use of sonography in the emergency room. Radiology 168 (1): 117–9

27. Kuhn M, Bonin RL, Davey MJ, et al 2000 Emergency Department ultrasound scanning for abdominal aortic aneurysm: accessible, accurate and advantageous. Annals of Emergency Medicine 36(3): 219–23

28. Mittelstaedt CA 1992 Biliary system. In: Mittelstaedt CA (ed.) General Ultrasound. Churchill Livingstone, New York, pp 249–335

29. Abrams BJ 1996 Bedside ultrasonography: the utility in emergency medicine. Emergency Medicine 17(15): 151–60

30. Denys BG, Uretsky BF, Reddy PS 1993 Ultrasound- assisted cannulation of the internal jugular vein. A prospective comparison to the external landmark-guided technique. Circulation 87(5): 1557–62

31. Gualtieri E, et al 1995 Subclavian venous catheterisation: greater success rate for less experienced operators using ultrasound guidance. Critical Care Medicine 23 (4): 692

32. Hilty WM, Hudson PA, Levitt MA, et al 1997 Real-time ultrasound-guided femoral vein catheterisation during cardiopulmonary resuscitation. Annals of Emergency Medicine 29(3): 331–7

33. Hirsch J, Hull RD, Rascob GE 1986 Clinical features and diagnosis of venous thrombosis. Journal of the American College of Cardiology 8: 114B–127B

34. Lensing AWA, Prandone P, Brandjes D, et al 1989 Detection of deep -vein thrombosis by real-time B-mode ultrsonography. New England Journal of Medicine 320: 324–5

35. Blaivas M, Lambert MJ, Howard RA, et al 2000 Lower extremity doppler for deep vein thrombosis – can emergency physicians be accurate and fast? Academic Emergency Medicine 7(2): 120–6

36. Alvarado A 1986 A practical score for the early diagnosis of acute appendicitis. Annals of Emergency Medicine 15: 557–64

37. Gwynn LK 2002 The diagnosis of acute appendicitis: clinical assessment versus computed tomography evaluation. Journal of Emergency Medicine 21: 119–23

38. Jeffrey RB, Laing FC, Townsend RR, et al 1988 Acute appendicitis: sonographic criteria based on 250 cases. Radiology 167: 327–9

39. Blaivas M 2001 Ultrasound – guided breast abscess aspiration in a difficult case. Academic Emergency Medicine 8: 398–401

40. Orlinsky M, Knittel P, Feit T, et al 2000 The comparative accuracy of radiolucent foreign body detection using ultrasonography. American Journal of Emergency Medicine 18: 401–3

41. Mandevia DP, Aragona J, Chan L, et al 2000 Ultrasound Training for Emergency Physicians – a prospective study. Academic Emergency Medicine 7(9): 1008–14

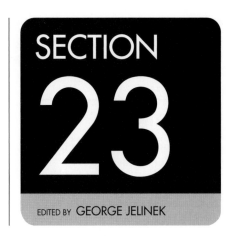

RESEARCH METHODOLOGY

23.1 Research methodology   648

23.1 RESEARCH METHODOLOGY

DAVID MCD. TAYLOR

ESSENTIALS

1 Research projects should be designed and undertaken in a structured, predetermined fashion.

2 The study protocol should be written well in advance of data collection and adhered to throughout the project.

3 Most research mistakes relate to inadequate sample size calculations and selection bias in subject recruitment.

4 During the study design phase, assistance from a statistician is highly recommended.

5 Ethical issues related to research are becoming more important, especially since the introduction of new Privacy Legislation.

INTRODUCTION

The basic strategy of clinical research is to compare groups of people. These might be different groups or the same group pre- and post-intervention. The methods used are mainly non-experimental, that is observational. They are based on what we can observe and compare of groups of people within populations. By comparing the characteristics (such as behaviours and exposures) and the health experiences of these groups of people, it is possible to identify associations that might be responsible for the cause of a disease.

INITIATING THE RESEARCH PROJECT

The research question

The research question forms the basis of every research study and the reason that it is undertaken. It is the scientific, clinical, practical or hypothetical question that, when answered, will allow the researcher to apply newly found knowledge for some useful purpose. The researcher should always aim to undertake studies that will impact upon clinical practice.

The research question may be generated from many sources including questions raised by clinical observations, the published medical literature, scientific conferences, seminars and discussions, or the effectiveness of currently used or new treatment.

Example: Is drug A better than drug B?

The study hypothesis

A hypothesis is a bold statement of what we think the answer to the research question is. Essentially, it is our best guess of what the underlying reality is. As such, it has a pivotal role in any study. The purpose of a research study is to weigh the evidence for and against the study hypothesis. Accordingly, the hypothesis is directly related to the research question.

Example: Directional hypothesis:
Drug A is *better* than drug B
Null hypothesis: Drug A is *as good as* drug B

In expressing a hypothesis, the researcher needs to be very specific about who or what is to be observed and under what conditions. A failure to define clearly the study groups and the study endpoints often leads to sloppy research.

The study aims

The aims of a study are a description of what the researcher hopes to do in order to weigh up the evidence regarding the study hypothesis.

Example: To determine which is the better drug, drug A or drug B.

Just as the research question begs the hypothesis, the hypothesis begs the study aims. The examples above demonstrate clearly the natural progression from research question through to the study aims. This is a simple, yet important process, and time spent defining these components will greatly assist in clarifying the study's objectives. These concepts are discussed more fully elsewhere.[1,2]

ASSEMBLING THE RESEARCH TEAM

All but the smallest of research projects are undertaken as a collaborative effort with the co-investigators each contributing in their area of expertise. Co-investigators should meet the criteria for co-authorship of the publication reporting the studies findings.[3]

Usually, the person who has developed the research question takes the role of principal investigator (team leader) for the project. Among the first tasks is to assemble the research team. Ideally, the principal investigator determines the areas of expertise required for successful completion of the project (e.g. biostatistics) and invites appropriately skilled personnel to join the team.[1] It is advisable to keep the numbers within the team to a minimum. In most cases, three or four persons are adequate to provide a range of expertise without the team becoming cumbersome. It is recommended that nursing staff be invited to join the team, if this is appropriate. This may foster research interest among these staff, improve departmental morale and may greatly assist data collection and patient enrolment.

All co-investigators are expected to contribute time and effort to the project, although the extent of this contribution will vary. The temptation to include very senior staff or department heads simply to bolster the profile of the project should be avoided if possible. It is recommended that personality and track record for 'pulling one's weight' be considered when assembling the team. There is little more frustrating than having poor contributors impede the progress of a study. Assigning specific responsibilities, in writing, to each member of the team is a useful tactic in dealing with this potential problem. However, care should be taken to ensure that the timelines for assignment completion are reasonable.

The importance of good communication within the research team cannot be overemphasized. This is usually the responsibility of the principal investigator and may involve regular meetings or reports. At the risk of flooding each co-investigator with excessive or trivial communications (e.g. e-mail), selected important communications should be forwarded as they appear, for instance, notification of ethics committee approval and updates on enrolment.

DEVELOPMENT OF THE STUDY PROTOCOL

The protocol is the blue print or recipe of a research study. It is a document drawn up prior to commencement of data collection that is a complete description of study to be undertaken.[4] Every member of the study team should be in possession of an up-to-date copy. Furthermore, an outside researcher should be able to pick up the protocol and successfully undertake the study without additional instruction.

Purpose of the study protocol

Research protocols are required:

- For the ethics committee application
- For applications for research funding
- To facilitate the smooth and efficient running of the study through the provision of well-researched and documented information
- For the basis of the Introduction and Methods sections of the final research report.

Protocol structure

The protocol should be structured largely in the style of a journal article's Introduction and Methods sections.[4] Hence, the general structure is as follows:

Introduction

- Background, including a brief summary of the literature
- Research question
- Hypothesis
- Aims
- Need for the proposed research, that is the purpose of the study.

Methods

- Study design – a simple description of the design of the proposed study, e.g. randomized clinical trial, cohort study, cross-sectional survey.
- Study setting – a description of where and when the study will take place.
- Study subjects – inclusion and exclusion criteria and a description of how participants are to be recruited.
- Procedures and interventions – the nature of any interventions to be used, including information on safety, necessary precautions and rationale for the choice of dose(s).
- Study endpoints – data-collection instruments, e.g. questionnaires, proformas, equipment.
- Data-collection procedures – including quality-control procedures to ensure integrity of data.
- Data management – including a description of how data will be handled, how privacy concerns will be addressed and how storage and back up of data will be undertaken.
- Bias and confounding control – sources of bias and variability, and measures to be taken to address them.
- Ethical issues – subject confidentiality, safety, security and access to data.
- Statistical analysis – (a) sample size: a description of calculations used to determine sample size and assumptions included in the process should be included. This should

include power calculations where appropriate to ensure that it is clear that the study can recruit a sufficient number of patients to achieve a significant result. (b) data analysis: this should include a description of the primary variables to be analysed, a specification of any *a priori* subgroup analyses and the statistical methods to be used. Few researchers are adequately trained in research statistical methods to undertake their own data analysis. It is highly recommended that a statistician be consulted during protocol development and data analysis.

This general plan should be followed in the preparation of any study protocol. However, the final protocol will vary from study to study.

STUDY DESIGN

Study design, in its broadest sense, is the method used to obtain data to prove or disprove the study hypothesis. Many factors influence the decision to use a particular study design and each design has important advantages and disadvantages. For a more extensive discussion on study design the reader is referred elsewhere.[1,5]

Observational studies

In general, research studies examine the relationship between an exposure or risk factor (e.g. smoking, obesity, vaccination) and an outcome of interest (e.g. lung cancer, cardiac disease, protection from infection).

In observational (non-experimental) studies, the principal challenge is to find a *naturally occurring* experiment, i.e. a comparison of two or more populations that enables the investigator to address an hypothesis about the outcome of interest.

Cross-sectional studies

Cross-sectional studies examine the present association between two variables. For example, within a population you could take a single random sample of all persons, measure some current characteristic (e.g. lung function) and then correlate that characteristic with the presence or absence of lung cancer. Data are often collected in surveys and the information on exposure and outcome of interest is collected from each subject at one point in time. The main outcome measure obtained from a cross-sectional study is prevalence.

Ecological studies

Ecological studies relate the rate of an outcome of interest to an average level of exposure that is presumed to apply to all persons in the population or group under investigation. So, for example, we could determine the association between the average amount smoked per capita in different countries and the incidence of lung cancer in each country.

Cohort studies

In a cohort study, a group of individuals, in whom the personal exposures to a risk factor have been documented, are followed over time. The rate of disease that subsequently occurs is examined in relation to the individuals' exposure levels. For example, within a population you could take a sample (cohort) of healthy individuals, document their personal past and ongoing smoking history, and relate that to the subsequent occurrence of lung cancer in that same sample. Although not as powerful a study design as clinical trials (see below), cohort studies are able to provide valuable data relating to the causation of disease.

Case-control studies

Case-control studies involve a comparison between a representative sample of people with an outcome of interest (cases) and another sample of people without the outcome (controls). If an antecedent feature (exposure) is found to be more common in the cases than the controls, this suggests an association between that exposure and the development of the outcome. The frequencies of past exposures to risk factors of interest are compared in each group. Case-control studies provide only medium level evidence of an association between exposure and outcome of interest.

Case reports and case series

This study design is often employed in emergency medicine research. The clinical details (history, management, outcome) of interesting or similar patients are described. This study design provides weak evidence for an association between exposure and outcome of interest and is best employed for hypothesis generation. For example, a series of patients who all developed skin necrosis after being bitten by a certain spider would reasonably lead to the hypothesis that the venom of the spider of interest contained a particular tissue necrosis factor. However, this hypothesis would need to be proven by the isolation of the factor and experimental demonstration of its effects.

Data for case reports/series are often extracted from medical record reviews or existing databases. This is one reason for the weakness of this study design insofar as the data were most likely collected for purposes other than the research study. Accordingly, such data are often of low quality and may suffer from inaccuracies, incompleteness and measurement bias.

Experimental studies

In an experimental study, the researcher is more than a mere observer, and actively manipulates the exposure of study subjects to an exposure of interest (risk) and measures the effects (outcomes) of this manipulation.

The preferred form of experimental study is currently the randomized, controlled trial, in which the intervention is randomly assigned at the level of the individual study subject. Although the most scientifically rigorous design, other study designs must often be used for a number of reasons including:

- The state of knowledge about a disease process
- Real-world opportunities
- Logistics and costs
- Ethical considerations.

For ethical reasons, we cannot easily use experimental studies to study factors that are thought to increase the risk of disease in humans. For example, you could not do a study where you ask half of the group to smoke for 10 years and half of the group to remain non-smokers.

Types of clinical trials

- Parallel group trials – these are the most common type of clinical trial and involve two or more groups of patients treated separately, but concurrently.
- Two-period crossover trial – patients are treated for two periods using a different treatment in each period. Patients are randomly allocated to the two possible orders of treatment so that half the patients receive the treatments in the sequence of AB and the other half in the sequence BA.
- Other types – factorial trials, N-of-one trials and sequential trials are used much less frequently.

Key features of clinical trials

- Randomization – this is a process by which patients are allocated to one of two or more study groups, purely by chance. The overwhelming advantage of randomization is that it prevents any manipulation by the investigators or treating doctors in the creation of the treatment groups. This prevents a situation whereby a doctor can, for example, allocate the sicker (or not so sick) patients to a new treatment. Randomization also has the benefit of producing study groups comparable to one another with respect to known, as well as unknown risk factors, and guarantees that statistical tests will have valid significance levels. The most convenient methods of randomizing patients are random number tables in statistical textbooks or computerized random-number-generating programs.

    A fundamental aspect of randomization is that it must only take place after the commitment to participate has been made (enrolment taken place). Another important principle is that randomized patients are irrevocably committed to follow-up and must not be excluded from, or lost to follow-up, regardless of their subsequent compliance or progress ('intention to treat analysis').

- Blinding – blinding is the most effective method of minimizing systematic error (bias) in clinical trials. In single-blinded studies, patients participating in the trial are unaware which treatment they are receiving but the investigators do know. In double-blind studies, neither the subjects nor the investigators know which patient is receiving which treatment. This type of study is usually only feasible with drug studies where it is possible to provide identically appearing medication. This is often achieved using the double dummy approach in which patients receive two medications, one active and the other placebo. The alternative treatment involves a swap-over of the active and placebo medications. Even in apparently blinded studies, there may be various indicators that allow the patient or investigator to determine which treatment they are receiving. In this circumstance, additional methods of bias control may be needed.

CONCEPTS OF METHODOLOGY

Validity and repeatability of the study methods

It is essential that the study uses valid and repeatable methods, that is, measurements that measure what they purport to measure. Ideally, the validity of each of the measurements used in any study should be tested, during the design stage of the study, against another method of measuring the same thing that is known to be valid.

Two types of validity are described:

❶ Internal validity means that, within the confines of the study, the results appear to be accurate, the methods and analysis used bear up to scrutiny, and the interpretation of the investigators appears supported.

❷ External validity is the extent to which the results of a study can be generalized to other samples or situations.

Again, for all types of study, it is important that repeatable methods are used, e.g. measurements that are closely similar when repeated under the same circumstances. Thus, if someone is asked the same question twice about a characteristic that has not changed in the meantime (such as their height), it would be said to be repeatable if they always (or almost always) answered in the same way. Repeatability of the question should be tested during the design phase, though it is also useful to monitor it during the main study. A good example would be a haemoglobino-meter that consistently measured the haemoglobin level 2 g/dL too low. Although the haemoglobin measurements would be repeatable, they would be wrong (invalid).

Response rate

Non-response is a problem for many types of observational study. Almost invariably, people who respond to, or participate in, a study (responders) have different characteristics from those who do not (non-responders). This can introduce substantial selection bias into the prevalence estimates of a cross-sectional study. In order to minimize this bias, as large a sample as possible is required. To this end, investigators undertaking cross-sectional surveys aim for at least 70% of invited participants to actually respond. Unfortunately, a target response rate of 70% is often not met and low response rates are likely to impact significantly upon bias and validity of the study.

Study variables

A variable is a property or parameter that may vary from patient to patient. The framework for the study hypothesis is the independent variable. This variable is often the factor that is thought to affect the measurable endpoints, or dependent variables, in the study. For example, cigarette smoking causes lung cancer. In this example, cigarette smoking is the independent variable and lung cancer is the dependent variable, as its incidence and nature depends upon cigarette smoking.

Study endpoints

Study endpoints are variables that are impacted upon by the factors under investigation. It is the extent to which the endpoints are affected, as measured statistically, that will allow us to accept or reject the hypothesis. For example, a researcher wishes to examine the effects of a new anti-hypertensive drug. It is known that this drug has minor side effects of impotence and nightmares. A study of this new drug would have a primary endpoint of blood pressure drop and secondary endpoints of the incidence of the known side effects.

A good hypothesis predicts what we would find if we were to measure certain endpoints. The testing of the hypothesis involves seeing whether or not the endpoint measurements confirm these predictions. Accordingly, the careful selection of appropriate endpoints is of vital importance, as is the accurate measurements of those endpoints.

Essentially, all forms of investigation involve counting or measuring to quantify the study endpoints. In doing so, there is always the opportunity for error, either in the measurement itself or in the observer who makes the measurement. Such errors (measurement bias) can invalidate the study findings and render the conclusions worthless.

SAMPLING STUDY SUBJECTS

There are several important principles in sampling study subjects:

- The sample must be representative of the study population. If the study population comprises all people living in a certain area, the study sample should include a representative sample of all members of the population. Certain groups are frequently left out (for instance the homeless, squatters, people in institutions, or people with no telephone). Such groups must be thought of in advance, and steps taken to ensure their inclusion.

- The sample must be derived from the population randomly. The way in which the sample is drawn from the study population is critical to how well the sample represents that population. This determines how 'generalizable' the results will be. Although there are many alternative ways to maximize sample representativeness, as a general rule, a random sample is preferred. A random sample is one in which each member of the population has an equal likelihood or probability of being selected.
- Loss to follow-up. The researcher must avoid loss of members from the sample once it has been taken, for two reasons. First, loss of subjects will effectively decrease the study sample size and may impact adversely on the power of the study to generate statistically significant results. Second, if subjects lost to follow-up differ in important ways from subjects who remain in the study, then the study results may be affected by selection bias.

Sampling frame

This is a list of all members (for instance, persons, households, businesses) of the target population that can be used as a basis for selecting a sample. For example, a sampling frame might be the electoral role, the membership list of a club, or a register of schools. It is important to ensure that the sampling frame is complete, that all known deficiencies are identified and that flaws have been considered (omissions, duplications, incorrect entries).

Sampling methodology

Probability sampling

When every member of the population has some known probability of inclusion in the sample, we have probability sampling. There are several varieties:

❶ Simple random sampling – in this type of sampling, every element has

an equal chance of being selected and every possible sample has an equal chance of being selected. This technique is simple and easy to apply when small numbers are involved, but requires a complete list of members of the target population and it is very cumbersome to use with large populations.

❷ Systematic sampling – this employs a fixed interval to select members from a sampling frame. For example, every twentieth member can be chosen from the sampling frame. It is often used as an alternative to simple random sampling as it is easier to apply and less likely to make mistakes. Furthermore, the cost is less, its process can be easily checked and it can increase the accuracy and decrease the standard errors of the estimate.

❸ Stratified sampling – a stratified sample is obtained by separating population elements into non-overlapping groups (strata) and by selecting a single random (or systematic) sample from each stratum. This may be done to:
   a. gain precision – this is possible by dividing a heterogeneous population into strata in such a way that each stratum is internally homogeneous
   b. accommodate administrative convenience – field work is organized by strata, which usually results in cost savings
   c. obtain separate estimates for each stratum
   d. accommodate different sampling plans in different strata, e.g. over sampling.
   However, the strata should be designed so that they collectively include all members of the target population, each member must appear in only one stratum and the definitions or boundaries of the strata should be precise and unambiguous.

Non-probability sampling

Convenience sampling is an example of non-probability sampling. This tech-

nique is used when patients are sampled during periods convenient for the investigators. For example, patients presenting to an emergency department after midnight are much less likely to be sampled if research staff are not present. This technique is less preferred than probability sampling, as there is less confidence that a non-probability sample will be representative of the population of interest or can be generalized to it. However, it does have its uses, such as in in-depth interviews for groups difficult to find, and for pilot studies.

DATA-COLLECTION INSTRUMENTS

Surveys

Surveys are one of the most commonly used means of obtaining research data. While seemingly simple in concept, the execution of a well-designed, questionnaire-based survey can be difficult.

Designing a survey

From a practical point of view, the following points are suggested:

Before a survey
- Define the research question(s) to be answered
- Determine the sampling strategy
- Design, test and revise the questionnaire (validation)
- Train the data collectors
- Determine the technique for cross-validation
- Define the methods of data analysis.

During the survey
- Verify and cross-validate the questionnaire
- Check timetables and budget.

After the survey
- Cross-check all the data again
- Perform the main data analysis
- Perform any other exploratory data analysis
- Write the report.

If possible, incorporate commonly asked questions into your questionnaire. One good source of such questions is standard surveys (such as Australian Bureau of Statistics). There are many other sources of pre-validated questions (for instance measures on quality of life, functional ability, disease specific symptoms). The scientific literature, accessible through MEDLINE and other databases is a good start. This is particularly important if you want to compare the sample with other surveys or, in general, if you want to be able to compare the sample's responses to previously completed work.

Also, previously used questionnaires for similar topics are very helpful and often can be used directly. The advantage to doing this is that these questionnaires' reliability and validity are established.

The wording of a question can affect its interpretation. Attitude questions with slightly different wordings can elicit differing responses. So several questions on the same topic may be helpful to be certain that the 'true attitude' of the respondent is obtained. This technique can enhance internal validity and consistency.

Pre-testing of a questionnaire is most important. Consider the following points:

- Assess face validity of all questions
- Is the wording clear?
- Do different people have similar interpretations of questions?
- Do closed questions have appropriate possible answers?
- Does the questionnaire give a positive impression?
- Is there any bias in the questions?

It is always worth checking with your colleagues to determine whether the questionnaire will answer the study question. Also, trial a cross-section of potential respondents of differing reading levels and background. There can be a few surprises, and several revisions may be required before the final questionnaire is determined.

Data-collection proformas

These documents are generally used to record individual case data that are latter transferred to electronic databases. These data may be obtained from the patient directly (e.g. vital sign measurements) or extracted from the medical records or similar source.

While simple in concept, careful design of a data-collection proforma should be undertaken. First, a list of the data required should be drafted and translated into data fields on the proforma. These fields should be clearly laid out and well separated. Prior to data collection, the proforma should be trialed on a small selection of subjects. In such an exercise, it is commonly found that the data fields are not adequate for the collection of the required data. Hence, revision of proforma is often required.

Consideration should be given to the ease of data entry and extraction from the proforma. Data entry should progress logically from the top to the bottom of the document without interruption. This is particularly important for data extraction from medical records. Data extracted from the front of the record should be entered at the top of the proforma and so on. Consideration should also be given to later translation of the data to an electronic database. This should follow the same principles as described above. If possible, design a proforma that will allow data to be scanned directly into an electronic database.

BIAS AND CONFOUNDING

Study design errors

In any study design, errors may occur. This is particularly so for observational studies. When interpreting findings from an observational study, it is essential to consider how much of the association between the exposure (risk factor) and the outcome may have resulted from errors in the design, conduct or analysis of the study.[5] The following questions should be addressed when considering the association between an exposure and outcome:

- Could the observed association be due to bias (systematic errors) in the way subjects were selected for the study or in the way information was obtained from them?
- Can the result be explained by confounding factors?
- Could the result be due to chance?

Systematic error (bias)

Bias in the way a study is designed or carried out can result in an incorrect conclusion about the relationship between an exposure (risk factor) and an outcome (such as a disease) of interest.[5] Small degrees of systematic error may result in high degrees of inaccuracy. It is important to note that systematic error is not a function of sample size. Many types of bias can be identified:

- Selection bias occurs when there is a difference between the people selected for a study (study sample) and those who are not; for instance, employed versus unemployed. Only proportional representation of all groups can, in a way, indicate the absence of selection bias.
- Non-response bias is a function of two components: the non-response rate and the extent to which non-respondents systematically differ from respondents. We may need to ask why the question was not answered. Is it not clear? Is it too personal? Is there a negative interaction with the interviewer? Is the subject afraid of answering 'yes'? Non-response bias may be a type of selection bias.
- Measurement bias may result from faulty methods to measure study endpoints. These may include poorly calibrated machines or stretched measuring tapes, for example. Strictly speaking, the following examples of bias are all types of measurement bias.
- Prevarication bias relates to subjects purposely giving incorrect answers and may result from threatening or insensitive questions.
- Interviewer bias results from the incorrect interpretations by the interviewer of the responses made by the interviewee. This is often an unconscious process, but may result if the interviewer expects, or would like, certain responses.

- Interpretation bias may result from questions that are not clear enough or that the subject does not understand. Some subjects may 'interpret' the question differently from others; for instance, does 'teeth' include 'dentures'?
- Recall bias may result when asking about events that happened a long time ago. For example, Were you ever vaccinated against tetanus? Every effort to avoid historical questions should be made.

Confounding

This is not the same as bias. A confounding factor can be described as one that is associated with the exposure under study and independently affects the risk of developing the outcome.[5] Thus, it may offer an alternative explanation for an association that is found and, as such, must be taken into account when collecting and analyzing the study results.

Confounding may be a very important problem in all study designs. Confounding factors themselves affect the risk of disease and if they are unequally distributed between the groups of people being compared, a wrong conclusion about an association between a risk factor and a disease may be made. A lot of the effort put into designing non-experimental studies is in addressing potential bias and confounding. For example, in an often-cited case-control study on the relationship between coffee drinking and pancreatic cancer, the association between exposure and disease was found to be confounded by smoking. Smoking is a risk factor for pancreatic cancer; it is also known that coffee drinkers are more likely to smoke than non-coffee drinkers. These two points create a situation in which the proportion of smokers will be higher in those who drink coffee than in those who do not. The uneven distribution of smokers then creates the impression that coffee drinking is associated with an increased rate of pancreatic cancer when it is smoking (related to those who drink coffee and to pancreatic cancer) that underlies the apparent association.

Common confounders

Common confounders that need to be considered in almost every study include age, gender, ethnicity and socioeconomic status. Age is associated with increased rates of many diseases. If the age distribution in the exposure groups differs (such as where the exposed group is older than the non-exposed group) then the exposed group will appear to be at increased risk for the disease. However, this relationship would be confounded by age. Age would be the factor that underlies the apparent, observed, association between the exposure and disease. Although age is a common confounder, it is the biologic and perhaps social changes that occur with age that may be the true causes that increase the rate of disease.

There are several ways to 'control for' the effect of confounding. To control for confounding during the design of the study, there are several possible alternatives:

- Randomization – random assignment into treatment groups, the cornerstone of a randomized, controlled trial, randomly distributes potential confounding factors between the control and intervention groups.
- Restriction – restricting the participants to one level of a potentially confounding variable is another method used in the design of a study to control for confounding, for instance only enrolling patients aged 60 years or more.
- Matching – matching subjects on potential confounding variables ensures that these variables are evenly distributed between cases and controls, especially in case-control studies.

In the analysis phase of a study, one can use:

- Stratification – during the analysis phase of a study, the effect of potential confounders can be assessed within separate strata of the confounding variable.
- Statistical modelling – regression models offer the benefit of controlling for multiple confounders simultaneously.

PRINCIPLES OF CLINICAL RESEARCH STATISTICS

Sample size

The sample must be sufficiently large to give adequate precision in the prevalence estimates obtained by the study for the purposes required. On the other hand, any increase in the sample size increases the study's cost, so an excessive sample size, though a much rarer event, should also be avoided.

The most common mistake made by inexperienced researchers is to underestimate the sample sizes required for their study. As a result, the sample sizes used may be too small and not representative of the population that the sample is meant to represent. This usually leads to outcome measures that have very wide 95% confidence intervals and, hence, statistically significant differences between study groups may not be found.

To ensure that a study has adequate sample sizes to show statistically significant differences, if they are there, sample sizes should be calculated prior to the study commencement. In reality, sample size is often determined by logistic and financial considerations, that is a trade off between sample size and costs.

Study power

The power of a study is the chance of correctly identifying, as statistically significant, an effect that truly exists. If we increase the sample size, we increase the power. As a general rule, the closer the power of a study is to 1.0, the better. This means that the 'type II error' will be small and there will be only a small chance of not finding a statistical difference when there really is one. Usually, a power of 0.8 or more is sufficient.

Statistical versus clinical significance

To determine 'statistical significance', we can obtain a P-value, relative risk or some other statistical parameter that is indicative of a difference between study groups. However, a statistical difference (e.g. *P*<0.05) between groups may be found if the study is highly powered (many subjects), even though the absolute difference between the groups is very small and not a clinically significant or meaningful difference.

This difference is important for two reasons. First, it forms the basis of sample size calculations. These calculations include consideration of what is thought to be a clinically significant difference between study groups. The resulting sample sizes adequately power the study to demonstrate a statistically and clinically significant difference between the study groups, if one exists. Second, when reviewing a research report, the absolute differences between the study groups should be compared. Whether or not these differences are statistically significant is of little importance if the difference is not clinically relevant. For example, a study might find an absolute difference in blood pressure between two groups of 3 mmHg. This difference may be statistically significant, but too small to be clinically relevant.

DATABASES AND PRINCIPLES OF DATA MANAGEMENT

The fundamental objective of any research project is to collect information (data) to analyze statistically and, eventually, produce a result or report. Data can come in many forms (lab results, personal details) and is the raw material from which information is generated. Therefore, how data are managed is an essential part of any research project.[4]

Defining data to be collected

Many a study has foundered because the wrong data were collected or important data were not collected. Generally, data fall into the following groups with examples:

- Identification data: personal information needed to link to the appropriate patient

- Research data: provides the information that is analyzed to answer the study question
- Administrative data: initials of the data collector, the study centre if multi-centred trial.

Collect only the research data that are essential to answer the study objective. It is important to avoid collecting data that will not be of use. This is time-consuming, expensive and may detract from the quality of the remaining data. However, there will usually be a minimum of data that must be collected. If these data are not collected, then the remaining data may not be analyzed adequately. This relates particularly to data on confounding factors.

Database design

A database is a specific collection of data that is organized in a structured fashion. In other words, database software provides us with a way of organizing the data we collect from a research project in a systematic way.

Good database design will:

- Reduce repetitiveness, for instance entering in an address or age for a patient many times
- Include validation
- Have data in a convenient form for analysis
- Be pilot tested.

Data entry

This refers to the entry of data into the electronic database, e.g. Access®, Excel®. Even if the study design and the data collection have been well done, the final data set may contain inaccurate data if the data-entry process is inadequate. This relates particularly to manually entered data where mistakes are bound to happen.

Data entry can be achieved in many ways:

- Manual data entry – this may be single entry undertaken by one person. Alternatively, double entry involves two independent people entering the same data. Any differences between the two are reconciled. This is a form of

double-checking but is clearly more time-consuming and, therefore, expensive.
- Direct data entry – this can be achieved by having database forms (proformas) on a computer screen. Direct entry of data via an Internet web page is one form of direct data entry. Alternatively, scannable forms can be fed into a scanner, avoiding the need for manual transcription.

Data validation

Effectively, this is a quality assurance process that confirms the accuracy of the data during its various phases of the study. Data validation can be done in the following ways:

- Visual review: matching data on questionnaires with medical records (source data)
- Value range checks: cholesterol levels should be >0 and <20 mmol/L (that is, do the numbers in the database make sense?)
- Field type checks: text should not be entered into numerical field
- Logical checks (if, then): if classed as a non-smoker, then cigarettes/day should be 0.

RESEARCH ETHICS

Participation in a clinical trial involves a sacrifice, by the participant, of some of the privileges of normal medical care for the benefit of other individuals with the same illness. The privileges foregone might include:

- The right to have treatment decided entirely on the basis of the treating doctor's judgement rather than by random allocation
- The right to have concomitant therapy according to requirements, rather than be standardized for all trial participants.

Participation also requires the discomfort and inconvenience associated with additional investigations and the potential incursion on privacy. Without the willingness of some individuals to make the sacrifices associated with participation in clinical trials, progress in clinical medicine would be greatly impaired. Most individuals who now expect to receive safe and effective medical care are benefiting by the sacrifices previously made by other individuals.

Some have argued in contrast, that enrolment into clinical trials ensures the absolute best care currently available, with greater involvement and scrutiny by attending healthcare teams.

If one accepts that clinical trials are morally appropriate, then the ethical challenge is to ensure a proper balance between the degree of individual sacrifice and the extent of the community benefit. However, it is a widely accepted community standard that no individual should be asked to undergo any significant degree of risk regardless of the community benefit involved; that is, the balance of risks and benefits must be firmly biased towards an individual participant. According to the Physician's Oath of the World Medical Association 'concern for the interests of the subject must always prevail over the interests of science and society.'

Because of the trade-offs required and because of the spectrum of views about the degree of personal sacrifice that might be justified by a given community benefit, it is accepted that all clinical trials should be reviewed by an ethics committee that should have as a minimum:

- Sufficient technical expertise to quantify the risks and benefits involved
- Adequate community representation so that any decisions are in keeping with community standards.

Scientific value

It is unethical to request individuals to undergo the risks, inconvenience and expense of a study that is unlikely to provide a scientifically worthwhile answer. It is also unethical to request sacrifices from volunteers that are out of keeping with the value of the research being undertaken. In keeping with this principle, studies that suffer from substantial

design errors or are susceptible to serious bias in event recording or measurement, should not be approved until these deficiencies are remedied.

It is unethical to allow scientifically invalid studies to proceed. Sample-size calculations should be scrutinized because of the ethical undesirability of including too few subjects to provide an answer or many more than is needed to provide a convincing answer. Another safeguard to ensure that the research will be valuable, is that the investigator should be qualified, experienced and competent, with a good knowledge of the area of study, and have adequate resources to ensure its completion.

Benefits foregone

It is unethical to require any patient to forego proven effective treatment during the course of a trial. It follows that clinical trials should only be undertaken when each of the treatments being compared is equally likely to have the more favourable outcome.

Very commonly, however, there is an expectation that one or other treatment is the more beneficial before a trial is commenced. This may be based on results of uncontrolled studies or even on biochemical or physiological expectations. The large number of times such expectations have been proven wrong can still provide strong justification for a trial.

If such an expectation of benefits is held strongly by an individual, it is probably not ethical for that individual to participate in a study. Furthermore, it is the responsibility of an ethics committee to assess the strength of the presumptive evidence facing one or other treatment, and consider whether any substantial imbalance in likely outcome exists. This must be considered in relation to the importance of the question being addressed.

Informed consent

Participants in clinical trials have a fundamental right to be fully informed about the nature of a clinical trial and to be free to choose whether or not to take part. Ethical principles also dictate that prospective participants be:

- Told they are taking place in a clinical trial and have an unambiguous right to decline to participate or to withdraw at any time
- Provided with a full explanation about the discomforts and inconvenience associated with the

CONTROVERSIES AND FUTURE DIRECTIONS

❶ The momentum of change in clinical research is accelerating. Complicated and ambitious study designs have brought to light ethical issues previously not considered. In particular, is the issue of consent of patients requiring resuscitation. In this circumstance, the patient is clearly unable to give consent and some argue that this automatically precludes their enrollment in studies investigating resuscitation techniques. Others disagree and note that such a position would terminate much research in this difficult area.

❷ Other ethical issues related to clinical research are also being addressed. Strict new confidentiality requirements have recently been legislated at both Federal and State level in Australia. Furthermore, good clinical research practice guidelines and research-risk-management strategies are being developed at various levels. Furthermore, the issue of research authorship integrity is being revisited and there is the development of Ethics Committee streamlining and standardization of application forms at State level.

❸ Meanwhile, emergency medicine research faces many difficulties, not least of which is resource limitation. Substantial clinical research requires skilled personnel, time, funding and a supportive infrastructure. Emergency medicine in Australasia has established a respected clinical practice. However, among its present challenges is the establishment of a culture of research with the resource to support and promote it.

study, and a description of all risks that may reasonably be considered likely to influence the decision whether or not to participate.[4]

It is usual practice to provide prospective participants with a Plain Language Statement that provides a simple, easy to understand account of the purposes, risks and benefits associated with participation in the study. Ethics committees are required to review these statements and confirm that they provide a reasonable account.

In practice the procedures involved in obtaining informed consent are often problematic. Considering the dependence of sick patients on the health system, their anxiety and their desire to cooperate with their physicians, it is doubtful whether informed consent is every 'freely given'. When ethics committees identify situations where this scenario is likely to be a particular problem, the involvement of an independent uninvolved person to explain the study may be useful.

REFERENCES

1. Taylor D McD 1999 Practical issues in the design and execution of an emergency medicine research study. Emergency Medicine 11: 167–74
2. Hall GM (ed.) 1999 How to Write a Paper, 2nd edn. BMJ Publishing Group, London
3. Uniform requirements for manuscripts submitted to biomedical journals. Available at: http://www.jama. ama-assn.org/info/auinst_req.html (last accessed March 8, 2002)
4. Good Research Practice Committee (eds) 2001 A Guide to Good Research Practice. Department of Epidemiology and Preventive Medicine, Monash University, Melbourne
5. Jekel JF, Katz DL, Elmore JG (eds) 2001 Epidemiology, Biostatistics, and Preventive Medicine, 2nd edn. WB Saunders Company, Philadelphia

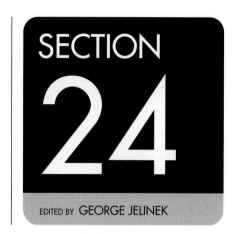

EDITED BY GEORGE JELINEK

EMERGENCY MEDICINE AND THE LAW

24.1 Mental health and the law: the Australasian and UK perspectives 660

24.2 The coroner: the Australasian and UK perspectives 667

24.3 Consent and competence: the Australasian and UK perspectives 674

24.1 MENTAL HEALTH AND THE LAW: THE AUSTRALASIAN AND UK PERSPECTIVES

DAVID EDDEY • SUZANNE MASON

ESSENTIALS

1 The emergency department is frequently the point of access to the mental health system.

2 Emergency physicians need to be able to distinguish between patients with physical and those with psychiatric illness.

3 Patients should only be committed involuntarily to an approved hospital if they have a mental illness requiring immediate treatment for their own health or safety or the protection of others, and if adequate treatment cannot be obtained in a less restrictive manner

4 Emergency physicians need to have a sound working knowledge of mental health legislation as it relates to their practice and to the jurisdiction in which they work.

INTRODUCTION

The emergency department is frequently the interface between the community and the mental-health system. In recent years changes in health policy have resulted in 'mainstreaming' of mental health services, so that stand alone psychiatric services are less common and services are more likely to be provided in a general hospital setting. Linked to this has been a move away from managing long-term psychiatric patients in institutional settings, so that many of these former patients are now living in the community with or without support from mental health services.

Traditionally, by virtue of their accessibility, emergency departments have been a point of access to mental health services for persons with acute psychiatric illness, whether this be self or family referral or by referral from ambulance, police or outside medical practitioners. An important function of an emergency department is to differentiate between those who require psychiatric care for a psychiatric illness, and those who present with a psychiatric manifestation of a physical illness and who require medical care. Admission of a patient with a psychiatric manifestation of a physical illness to a psychiatric unit may result in further harm to or death of the patient.

In the UK and Australasia, doctors in general are empowered by legislation to detain a mentally ill person who is in need of treatment. Mental illness is a common emergency department presentation (in the UK, making up around 1–2% of new patient attendances), and emergency physicians require, not only the clinical skills to distinguish between those who require psychiatric or medical intervention, but also a sound working knowledge of the mental health legislation and services relevant to the state where they practice. This ensures that patients with psychiatric illness are managed in the most appropriate way, with optimal utilization of mental health resources and with the best interests and rights of the patient and the community taken into consideration.

VARIATIONS IN PRACTICE

MENTAL HEALTH ACT: ENGLAND AND WALES

Definition of mentally ill or mental illness

According to the 1983 Mental Health Act, mental illness is undefined. However, in practice it includes conditions such as schizophrenia, manic depressive psychosis and organic brain syndromes. Mental impairment is defined as 'a state of arrested or incomplete development of mind which includes significant impairment of intelligence and social functioning and is associated with abnormally aggressive or seriously irresponsible conduct on the part of the person concerned'. A psychopathic disorder is defined as 'a persistent disorder or disability of mind which results in abnormally aggressive or seriously irresponsible conduct on the part of the person concerned'. The Act does not cover promiscuity or other immoral conduct, sexual deviancy, or dependence on drugs or alcohol.

Detention of patients with mental illness

The Mental Health Act 1983 provides legislation with regard to the management of patients with a mental illness unwilling to be admitted or detained in hospital voluntarily, where this would be in the best interests of the health and safety of patients and others. Patients in the emergency department are not considered in-patients until they are admitted onto a ward. In order for legislation to be imposed it is necessary for two conditions to be satisfied:

❶ The patient must be suffering from a mental illness

❷ Emergency hospital admission is required because the patient is considered to be a danger to themselves or others.

Detention under the Mental Health Act does not permit treatment for psychiatric or physical illness. Treatment can be given under common law where the patient is considered to pose a serious threat to themselves or others. Otherwise all treatment must be with the patients' consent.

Section 2 of the Mental Health Act facilitates compulsory admission to hospital for assessment and treatment for up to 28 days. The application is usually made by an approved social worker or the patients' nearest relative and requires two medical recommendations, usually from the patient's general practitioner and the duty senior psychiatrist (who is approved under Section 12 of the Mental Health Act). In the emergency department, the responsibility for co-ordinating the procedure often lies with the emergency physician.

Section 3 of the Mental Health Act covers compulsory admission for treatment. Once again, recommendations must be made by two doctors, one of whom is usually the general practitioner and the other a psychiatrist approved under Section 12 of the Act. The application is usually made by an approved social worker or the patients' nearest relative. Detention is for up to 6 months, but can be renewed.

Section 4 of the Mental Health Act covers emergency admission for assessment, and attempts to avoid delay in emergency situations when obtaining a second recommendation could be dangerous. It requires the recommendation of only one doctor, who may be any registered medical practitioner who must have seen the patient within the previous 24 hours. The order lasts for 72 hours. Application can be made by the patients' nearest relative or an approved social worker. In practice, the application of Section 4 of the Mental Health Act rarely happens. Usually Sections 2 or 3 are the preferred options.

Section 136 of the Act authorizes the police to remove patients who are believed to be mentally disordered and causing a public disturbance to a place of safety. The place of safety referred to in the Act is defined in Section 135 as 'residential accommodation provided by a local authority under Part III of the National Assistance Act 1948, or under Paragraph 2, Schedule 8 of the National Health Service Act 1977, a hospital as

defined by this Act, a police station, a mental nursing home or residential home for mentally disordered persons or any other suitable place, the occupier of which is willing temporarily to receive the patient'. In practice, the police often transport these patients to local emergency departments. The patient must be assessed by an approved social worker and a registered doctor. The order lasts for 72 hours.

Section 5 (2) of the Act allows the detention of patients who are already admitted to hospital. Unfortunately, presence in the emergency department is not considered to constitute admission to hospital, and this section is, therefore, not applicable to the emergency department.

The National Service Framework for Mental Health

The National Service Framework for Mental Health produced by the Department of Health in the UK (1999) is aimed at improving quality and addresses the mental health needs of working age adults up to 65 years. It states as one of its standards that:

> Any individual with a common mental health problem should be able to make contact round the clock with the local services necessary to meet their needs and receive adequate care.

Although emergency departments do not provide the ideal environment for a mental-health assessment, they are likely to continue to provide an entry point for people with mental health problems. Easy access to the emergency department can lead to individuals with acute mental-health problems seeking help directly, making up to perhaps 5% of emergency department attenders.

Use of sedation or physical restraint

From time to time doctors in the emergency department may need to sedate or even restrain a patient. It must be remembered that causes for acute

agitation or violent behaviour must be assumed to be surgical or medical until proven otherwise. Wherever possible, non-drug measures should be used to calm situations such as using 'talk down' methods. However, there are occasions where physical or pharmacological restraint is needed. Sedation or restraint must be the minimum necessary to prevent the patient from self-harm or harming others. Generally, a patient committed involuntarily is subject to treatment necessary for their care and control, and this may reasonably include the administration of sedative or anti-psychotic medication as emergency treatment.

Patients who are physically or pharmacologically restrained must be closely supervised and not left alone, or in the care of persons not trained or equipped to deal with the potential complications of these procedures. Transporting these patients to a mental-health service should be done by suitably trained medical or ambulance staff, and not delegated to police officers or other persons acting alone.

Emergency treatment

In England and Wales treatment of any condition cannot be given without the consent of the patient. The majority of patients detained under the Mental Health Act consent to treatment. However, under common law, emergency life-saving treatment can be given where patients do not have the capactiy to consent. Deciding on whether patients have such capacity may be difficult. It is advisable to involve other doctors, espcially a psychiatrist, when making this decision. In addition, the next of kin should be informed of any decisions made in relation to the patient. If lacking the mental capacity to consent, then treatment can be provided in the best interests of the patient.

Powers of the police

The police have powers in relation to mentally ill persons who may or may not have been assessed by a doctor. They can operate under the following sections of the Mental Health Act:

Section 135: removing patients to hospital. The police may enter premises to remove a patient believed to be suffering from a mental disorder to a place of safety for up to 72 hours.

Section 136: persons in public places (see above).

MENTAL HEALTH LEGISLATION IN AUSTRALASIA

In Australia mental health legislation is a State jurisdiction, and among the various States there is considerable variation in the scope of mental health acts, and between definitions and applications of the various sections. Specific issues should, therefore, be referred to the Mental Health Act relevant to the emergency physician's practice location.

The Australian mental health acts referred to in this chapter are:

ACT – Mental Health (Treatment and Care) Act 1994

New South Wales – Mental Health Act 1990

New Zealand – Mental Health Act 1992

Northern Territory – Mental Health Act 1992

Queensland – Mental Health Act 1974 and amendments 1993

South Australia – Mental Health Act 1990

Tasmania – Mental Health Act 1963 and amendments 1996

Victoria – Mental Health Act 1986 and amendments 1997

Western Australia – Mental Health Act 1996.

Sections of the various mental health acts relevant to emergency medicine include those dealing with:

- The definition of mentally ill
- The effects of drugs or alcohol
- Criteria for detention and admission as an involuntary patient
- Involuntary admission
- Persons unable to recommend a patient for involuntary admission
- Physical restraint and sedation
- Emergency treatment
- Powers of police
- Amendment of documents
- Offences in relation to documents
- Deaths.

Definition of mentally ill or mental illness

For the purposes of their respective Mental Health Acts all the States, except for the Northern Territory and Queensland, define mental illness or disorder as follows:

ACT

The ACT defines a psychiatric illness as a condition that seriously impairs (either temporarily or permanently) the mental functioning of a person and is characterized by the presence in the person of any of the following symptoms: delusions, hallucinations, serious disorder of thought form, a severe disturbance of mood or sustained or repeated irrational behaviour indicating the presence of these symptoms.

The ACT Mental Health Act also defines 'mental dysfunction' as a 'disturbance or defect, to a substantially disabling degree, of perceptual interpretation, comprehension, reasoning, learning, judgement, memory, motivation or emotion'.

New South Wales

The New South Wales Act defines mental illness in the same way as the ACT, but in addition distinguishes between a mentally ill person and a mentally disordered person.

A person is a mentally ill if suffering from mental illness and, owing to that illness, requires care, treatment or control in order to protect the patient or others from serious physical harm. A person is also considered to be mentally ill if suffering from a mental illness that is characterized by a severe disturbance of mood or sustained or repeated irrational behaviour, and requires care, treatment or control to protect the person from serious financial harm or damage to the person's reputation.

A person (whether or not the person is suffering from mental illness) is mentally disordered if the person's behaviour for the time being is so irrational as to justify conclusion on reasonable grounds that temporary care, treatment or control of the person is necessary for the person's own protection from serious physical harm, or for the protection of others from serious physical harm.

New Zealand

In New Zealand the Mental Health Act defines a mentally disordered person as possessing an abnormal state of mind, whether continuous or intermittent, characterized by delusions or by disorders of mood, perception, volition or cognition to such a degree that it poses a danger to the health or safety of the person or others, or seriously diminishes the capacity of the person to take care of themselves.

South Australia

In the South Australian Act mental illness means any illness or disorder of the mind.

Tasmania

Mental disorder means mental illness, arrested or incomplete development of mind, psychopathic disorder and any other disorder or disability of the mind.

Victoria

A person is mentally ill if they have a mental illness, being a medical condition characterized by a significant disturbance of thought, mood, perception or memory.

Western Australia

A person has a mental illness if they suffer from a disturbance of thought, mood, volition, perception, orientation or memory that impairs judgement or behaviour to a significant extent.

Safeguards against prejudice

New Zealand and all Australian States, except South Australia, include a number of criteria which, alone, cannot be used to determine that a person has a mental illness and requires involuntary admission. These generally include the expression of or refusal to express particular religious, political and philosophical beliefs; cultural or racial origin; sexual promiscuity or preference; intellectual disability; drug or alcohol taking; economic or social status; immoral or indecent conduct; illegal conduct; and antisocial behaviour. Tasmania only refers to promiscuity or immoral conduct.

Effects of drugs or alcohol

In most Australian States and New Zealand the taking of drugs or alcohol cannot, of itself, be taken as an indication of mental illness. However, the mental health acts of New South Wales, Northern Territory and Victoria specify that this does not prevent the serious temporary or permanent physiological, biochemical or psychological effects of alcohol or drug taking from being regarded as an indication that a person is mentally ill.

The remaining States do not specifically exclude the temporary or permanent effects of drugs or alcohol, but use definitions of mental or psychiatric illness that are broad enough to cover this.

Criteria for admission and detention as an involuntary patient

All States require that an involuntary patient has a mental illness that requires treatment while detained in an in-patient setting for the health (mental or physical) and safety of that patient or for the protection of others. Victoria, Western Australia and the ACT also require that the patient has refused or is unable to consent to voluntary admission.

Both New South Wales and Western Australia include the protection of the patient from self-inflicted harm to the patient's reputation, relationships or finances as grounds for involuntary admission.

In New Zealand the doctor must have reasonable grounds for believing that the person may be mentally disordered, and that it is desirable that in the interests of that person, or of any other person or of the public, that an assessment, examination and treatment of the person is conducted as a matter of urgency.

Involuntary admission

The process of involuntary admission varies quite markedly across the States. It is variously known as recommendation, certification or committal.

ACT

In the ACT a medical or police officer is able to apprehend a mentally ill person who requires involuntary admission, and is able to use reasonable force and enter premises in order to do so. The officer is required, as soon as possible, to provide a written statement to the person in charge of the mental health facility giving patient details and the reasons for taking the action.

A doctor employed by the mental health facility must examine the patient within 4 hours of arrival, and may authorize detention for up to 3 days. The doctor must inform the Community Advocate and Mental Health Tribunal of the patient's admission within 12 hours, and the patient must receive a physical and psychiatric examination within 24 hours of detention.

New South Wales

The Mental Health Act in New South Wales allows for a patient requiring involuntary admission to be detained in hospital on the certificate of a doctor who has personally examined the patient immediately or shortly before completing the certificate.

For a mentally ill patient the certificate is valid for 5 days from the time of writing, whereas for a mentally disordered patient the certificate is valid for 1 day from the time of writing. Mentally disordered patients cannot be detained on the grounds of being mentally disordered on more than three occasions in any 1 month.

Part of the certificate, if completed, directs the police to apprehend and bring the patient to hospital, and also enables them to enter premises without a warrant.

An involuntary patient must be examined by the 'medical superintendent' as soon as practicable, but within 12 hours of admission. The patient cannot be detained unless further certified that they are mentally ill or disordered. This doctor cannot be the same doctor who requested admission or certified the patient. If the 'medical superintendent' does not feel that the patient is mentally ill or disordered then they must arrange for examination by a psychiatrist as soon as practicable.

A patient who has been certified as mentally disordered, but not subsequently found to be mentally ill, cannot be detained for more than 3 days and must be examined by the 'medical superintendent' at least once every 24 hours, and discharged if they are no longer mentally ill or disordered, or if appropriate and less restrictive care is available.

New Zealand

In New Zealand a doctor who believes that a person requires compulsory assessment and treatment must have examined the 'proposed patient' within the preceding 3 days and must give a certificate stating the reasons for the opinion and that the patient is not a relative. Once this is done, the area mental health service must arrange an assessment examination by a psychiatrist or other suitable person forthwith. If the assessing doctor considers that the patient requires compulsory treatment, the patient may be detained for up to 5 days. Subsequent assessment may result in detention for up to 14 more days, after which a 'compulsory treatment order' must be issued by a family court judge.

Northern Territory

In the Northern Territory a police officer or medical practitioner who believes that a person requires involuntary admission is able to take that person into custody in a mental health facility. The chief medical officer must make an application to a magistrate to keep the patient in custody within 24 hours, and again within 3 days if the person requires further detention.

Queensland

In Queensland the recommendation to admit an involuntary patient must be made by a doctor who has personally examined the patient, and is valid for 14 days from the day the patient was last examined by the doctor making the recommendation, and for 7 days from the time the recommendation was made.

The recommendation needs to be accompanied by an 'application' for admission made by a person over the age of 18 who has seen the patient within 7 days. The person making the application cannot be the doctor making the recommendation. The recommendation can be endorsed by the recommending doctor to direct a police officer to convey the patient to hospital.

The patient may be detained for up to 3 days, after which time a second recommendation needs to be made by a doctor who has examined the patient subsequent to admission.

South Australia

In South Australia a doctor who considers that a patient requires involuntary admission is required to fill in the appropriate order for admission and detention in an approved treatment centre. This is valid for 3 days, unless revoked, and requires that the person is examined by a psychiatrist as soon as practicable but within 24 hours. The psychiatrist may revoke the order or may order further detention of up to 21 days.

The South Australian Mental Health Act enables police to enter premises, apprehend and convey a mentally ill person to a medical practitioner for examination. It also enables ambulance officers to convey, using reasonable force if necessary, a mentally ill person to a place for assessment or care.

Tasmania

In Tasmania, involuntary admission usually requires an 'application' and the 'recommendation' of two doctors; however, in urgent cases an emergency application that is valid for 72 hours can be made by one doctor. This is valid for 3 days from the time of admission. A second recommendation made within this time means that the patient can be held for up to 28 days, provided that the original grounds for recommendation are sufficient to support an application for admission.

An 'application' for admission can be made by the nearest relative or an 'authorized officer', who must have personally seen the patient, and general applications for admission are valid for 14 days from when the patient was last examined by a recommending medical practitioner. In situations other than an emergency, the medical 'recommendation' is made by two medical practitioners who have personally examined the patient, either together or independently, within the previous 7 days. One of the recommending doctors is required to have had previous acquaintance with the patient, and only one can be on the staff of the public hospital to which the patient is being referred.

The Tasmanian Act allows for admission for observation or for treatment. An application for admission for observation is made on the grounds that the patient is suffering from a mental disorder that warrants detention under observation for at least a limited period of time, in the interests of the health and safety of the patient or others. The patient can be detained for up to 28 days.

An application for admission for treatment is made on the grounds that a patient is suffering from 'mental illness or subnormality or psychopathic disorder' that warrants detention in hospital for treatment, in the interests of the health and safety of the patient or others.

Victoria

A person may be admitted to and detained in an approved mental health service once the 'request' and the 'recommendation' have been completed. The request can be completed by any person over 18 years of age, including relatives of the patient, but cannot be completed by the recommending doctor. The recommendation is valid for 3 days after completion, and the recommending doctor must have personally examined or observed the patient.

The request and recommendation are sufficient authority for the medical practitioner, a police or ambulance officer to take the person to a mental health service, or to enter premises without a warrant and to use reasonable force or restraint in order to take the person to a mental health service. Prescribed medical practitioners (psychiatrists, forensic physicians, doctors employed by a mental health service, the head of an emergency department of a general hospital or the regular treating doctor in a remote area) are also enabled to use sedation or restraint to enable a person to be taken safely to a mental health service.

Once admitted, the patient must be seen by a medical practitioner employed by the mental health service as soon as possible, but must be seen by a registered psychiatrist within 24 hours of admission, or as soon as practicable within 24 hours if the admitting doctor considers that the patient does not meet the criteria for involuntary admission. The psychiatrist can then either authorize further detention, place the patient on a community treatment order, or discharge them.

Western Australia

In Western Australia a patient who requires involuntary admission is referred, in writing, for examination by a psychiatrist. The referring doctor must have personally examined the patient within the previous 48 hours. The referral allows the patient to be admitted as an involuntary patient for 7 days after the referral was made. The patient must be examined by a psychiatrist within 24 hours of admission, and cannot be detained further if not examined. The patient can be detained for a further 3 days on the order of the psychiatrist, after which time another order needs to be made. If no suitable alternatives are available and the condition of the patient requires their involvement, the referring doctor may direct police to apprehend the patient, by writing a 'transport order'. This enables police to apprehend, enter premises, and search the patient or premises. It is valid for 7 days after the referral was made.

Persons unable to recommend a patient for involuntary admission

New Zealand and most States, except for the Northern Territory and the ACT, specify that certain relationships prevent a doctor from requesting or recommending a patient for involuntary admission.

The recommending doctor cannot be a relative or guardian of the patient and, in addition, in Queensland, Tasmania and Western Australia, the doctor cannot be a business partner or assistant of the patient. In Queensland and Tasmania, the recommending doctor cannot be in receipt of payments for the maintenance of the patient.

In New South Wales, the doctor must declare, on the schedule, any direct or indirect pecuniary interest, or those of their relatives, partners or assistants, in an 'authorized hospital'. In Tasmania, the doctor cannot be on the staff of a private hospital to which the patient will be admitted, and in Western Australia, the doctor cannot hold a licence from or have a family or financial relationship with the licence holder of a private hospital in which the patient will be treated, nor can the doctor be a board member of a public hospital treating the patient.

Use of sedation or physical restraint

From time to time the emergency department may need to sedate or even restrain a patient. The various mental health acts vary considerably in dealing with this issue.

Generally, a patient committed involuntarily is subject to treatment necessary for their care and control, and this may reasonably include the administration of sedative or antipsychotic medication as emergency treatment. In general, sedation or restraint must be the minimum necessary to prevent the patient from self-harm or harming others.

Patients who are physically or pharmacologically restrained must be closely supervised and not left alone or in the care of persons not trained or equipped to deal with the potential complications of these procedures. Transporting these patients to a mental health service should be done by suitably trained medical or ambulance staff, and not delegated to police officers or other persons acting alone.

The ACT specifies that sedation may be used to prevent harm, whereas Western Australia specifies that sedation can be used for emergency treatment without consent, and that the details must be recorded in a report to the Mental Health Review Board.

Victoria specifically permits the administration of sedative medication by a 'prescribed medical practitioner' to allow for the safe transport of a patient to a mental health service. There is a schedule to complete if this is undertaken.

The legislation is more specific with regard to the use of physical restraint. In the ACT this can be done to prevent harm to the patient or others, or to keep the patient in custody.

Queensland requires that restraint used for the protection of others can only be done on an 'order', but is permissible for the purposes of treatment. Tasmania permits its use, on the approval of the responsible medical officer, for the protection of the patient, other persons or property. Victoria permits the restraint of involuntary patients for the purposes of medical treatment and the prevention of injury or persistent property destruction. Victoria also allows the use of restraint by ambulance officers, police or doctors in order to safely transport the patient to a mental health service, but this must be documented in the recommendation schedule.

Western Australia permits the use of restraint for the purposes of medical treatment and for the protection of the patient, other persons or property. This authorization must be in writing and must be notified to the senior psychiatrist as soon as possible.

The New Zealand Mental Health Act makes no specific reference to restraint or sedation, but enables any urgent treatment to protect the patient or others.

Emergency treatment and surgery

On occasions, involuntary patients may require emergency medical or surgical treatment. Most States and New Zealand, except for Queensland and Tasmania, make provision for this in their legislation, in that patients can undergo emergency treatment without consent. In New Zealand treatment that is immediately necessary to save life, prevent serious damage to health or to prevent injury to the person or others, can be undertaken without consent.

Victoria has the most specific reference to this treatment by making special allowance for a patient requiring treatment that is life sustaining or preventing serious physical deterioration to be admitted as an involuntary patient to a general hospital or emergency department for the purposes of receiving treatment. The patient is deemed to be on leave from the mental health service, and all the other provisions of the Act apply.

Apprehension of absent involuntary patients

Involuntary patients who escape from custody or who fail to return from 'leave' are considered in most State mental health acts to be 'absent without leave' (AWOL) or 'unlawfully at large', although the ACT and the Northern Territories make no reference to this in their acts. In the remaining States authorized persons, including staff of the mental health service and police, have the same powers of entry and apprehension as for other persons to whom a recommendation or certificate relates. In Queensland and Tasmania these powers exist for 28 days from the time of going AWOL, whereas in Victoria they apply for 12 months, after which time the patient is automatically discharged unless the chief psychiatrist considers it appropriate for the patient to remain, theoretically at least, in custody. New South Wales, South Australia and Western Australia do not specify a time limit for the return of AWOL patients.

In New Zealand any compulsory patient who becomes AWOL may be 'retaken' by any person within 3 months of becoming absent. If not returned after 3 months the patient is deemed to be released from compulsory status.

Powers of the police

The police in all States and New Zealand have powers in relation to mentally ill persons who may or may not have been assessed by a doctor. For someone who is not already an involuntary patient and who is reasonably believed to be mentally ill and requiring care, police are able to enter premises and apprehend, without a warrant, and to use reasonable force if necessary, in order to remove the person to a 'place of safety'. Generally, this means taking the person to a medical practitioner or a mental health service for examination without undue delay.

The same powers apply to involuntary patients who abscond or are absent without leave, although some States have specific schedules or orders to complete for this to be done. In general, once police become aware of the patient they are obliged to make attempts to find and return them to what can be viewed as lawful custody.

Amendment of documents

Four States (New South Wales, Tasmania, Victoria and Western Australia) specify that the amendment or correction of documents in relation to the admission of an involuntary patient is permissible, without the patient being discharged, returned to the recommending doctor, or their status being changed. Western Australia does not specify a time limit for this to be done, but in Tasmania it must be done within 14 days, in Victoria within 21 days, and in New South Wales within 28 days. The New Zealand Act makes no reference to the amendment of documents.

Offences in relation to certificates

Most States and New Zealand specify in their respective mental health acts that it is an offence to wilfully make a false or misleading statement in regard to the certification of an involuntary patient.

Some States (New South Wales, South Australia and Victoria), except in certain circumstances, also regard failure to personally examine or observe the patient as an offence.

Protection from suit or liability

New Zealand and all Australian States, except the Northern Territory, specify in their mental health acts that legal proceedings cannot be brought against

doctors acting in good faith and with reasonable care within the provisions of the Mental Health Act relevant to their practice.

Deaths

Involuntary patients should be considered to be held in lawful custody, whether in an emergency department, as an in-patient in a general hospital or psychiatric hospital, or AWOL. As such, the death of such a patient must be referred for a coroner's investigation.

CONTROVERSIES AND FUTURE DIRECTIONS IN THE UK

❶ In the UK the most commonly used places of safety for individuals deemed to be a danger to themselves or the public are the emergency department, police stations and psychiatric units. Concern exists about the suitability of emergency departments for acting as places of safety. The Royal College of Psychiatrists jointly with the British Association for Accident and Emergency Medicine stated in 1996 that emergency departments were inappropriately staffed and equipped to supervise such individuals. However, the National Service Framework on Mental Health states that hospitals should be used in preference to police stations. To date, there has been no national consensus on the future use of the emergency department as a place of safety. Currently, individual departments are entering into local policy agreements with other agencies on their use.

❷ As the specialty of emergency medicine expands, health professionals such as emergency nurse practitioners and paramedics are increasingly making clinical decisions about patients. This presents a challenge to the specialty in ensuring that all are appropriately trained and informed of the law relating to patients with mental health problems. A recent study has found that knowledge of Section 136 (Mental Health Act for England and Wales) among health professionals is lacking. In addition, few health-care professionals surveyed had received formal training on the subject. It is vital that training and education continues to be central to delivering an appropriate service in often difficult circumstances.

❸ In the UK, a new draft Mental Health Bill was published in 2002. It introduced a new legal framework for the compulsory treatment of people with mental disorders in hospitals and the community. The new procedure involves a single pathway in three stages: a preliminary examination, a period of formal assessment lasting up to 28 days and treatment under a Mental Health Act order. In order for the compulsory process to be used, four conditions must be satisfied: the patient must have a mental disorder, the disorder must warrant medical treatment, treatment must be necessary for the health and safety of the patient or others, and an appropriate treatment for the disorder must be available. The draft bill makes provision for treatment without consent as it is justified under the European Convention on Human Rights Article 8 (2) in the interests of public safety or to protect health or moral standards. Exactly how the bill when published in its final format will affect practice in the emergency department is unclear. However, it is essential that specialists are informed of changes to the law that they may come across when dealing with other agencies in trying to provide the most appropriate care for patients.

FURTHER READING

Barker A 1997 Mental health and the law. British Medical Journal 315: 590–1

Birmingham L 2002 Detaining dangerous people with mental disorders: New legal framework is open for consultation. British Medical Journal 325: 2–3

Department of Health 1983 The Mental Health Act (England and Wales). HMSO, London

Department of Health 1999 Mental Health – national service framework. Modern standards and service models. HMSO, London

Drug and Therpeutics Bulletin 1997 Managing self-harm: The Legal Issues. Vol 35(6): 41–3

Hughes J 1987 An Outline of Modern Psychiatry, 2nd edn. Wiley and Sons, Brisbane

Lynch RM, Simpson M, Higson M, Grout P 2002 Section 136, The Mental Health Act 1983; Levels

of knowledge among accident and emergency doctors, senior nurses and police constables. Emergency Medicine Journal 19: 295–300
Royal College of Psychiatrists 1996 Psychiatric services

to accident and emergency departments. Council Report CR43
Royal College of Psychiatrists 1996 Report of a joint working party of the Royal College of Psychiatrists

and British Association for Accident and Emergency Medicine. (Council Report CR43). RCP, London

24.2 THE CORONER: THE AUSTRALASIAN AND UK PERSPECTIVES

SIMON YOUNG • HELEN L PARKER

AUSTRALASIA

ESSENTIALS

1 The function of the coroner is to investigate and report on a person's death. Where possible, the coroner must determine the identity of the deceased, the circumstances surrounding the death, the medical cause of death, and the identity of any person who contributed to that death. The coroner may also comment on matters of public health and safety.

2 Each jurisdiction has a number of defined circumstances in which a death must be reported to the coroner. Commonly these are when the death appears to have been caused by violent, unnatural or accidental means, or has occurred in suspicious circumstances, or when the cause is unknown.

3 Preparation for a coronial investigation starts as soon as someone dies in reportable circumstances. The body, medical notes, and details of all investigations and procedures may be required by the coroner. Accurate and complete medical notes are an essential part of this process.

4 A coronial inquest is a public inquiry into a death to which a medical practitioner may be subpoenaed. The doctor may be required to give evidence of fact regarding what happened or expert opinion.

5 The findings of a coronial inquest in which the performance of an emergency physician or department has been examined should be carefully scrutinized. They may contain important statements regarding the practice of the emergency physician, the functioning of the emergency department, and the emergency medical system as a whole.

6 Coronial findings may be used constructively to effect positive change within a department, institution or system.

INTRODUCTION

The function of the coroner is to investigate and report the circumstances surrounding a person's death. A coronial inquest is a public inquiry into one or more deaths conducted by a coroner within a court of law. Legislation in each Australian State and Territory defines the powers of this office and the obligations of medical practitioners and the public towards it. The process effectively puts details concerning a death on the public record, and is being increasingly used to provide information and recommendations for future injury prevention.

As many people die each year either in an emergency department or having attended an emergency department during their last illness, it is almost inevitable that emergency physicians will become involved in the coronial process at some stage during their career. Such involvement may be brief, such as the discharge of a legal obligation by reporting a death, or may extend further to providing statements to the coroner regarding deaths of which they have some direct knowledge. Later, the coroner may require them to appear at an inquest to give evidence regarding the facts of the case, and possibly their opinion. Occasionally, the coroner requires a suitably experienced emergency physician to provide an expert opinion regarding aspects of a patient's emergency care.

Although the inquisitorial nature of the coronial process is sometimes threatening to medical practitioners, their involvement is a valuable community service. In addition, they may obtain important information regarding aspects of a patient's clinical diagnoses and emergency care.

LEGISLATION

The office of the coroner, and its functions, procedures and powers, is created by State and Territory legislation. The legislation also creates obligations on medical practitioners to notify the coroner of reportable deaths, and to cooperate with the coroner by providing certain information in the course of an inquiry. The normal constraints of obtaining consent for the provision of clinical information to a third party do not apply in these circumstances.

The coroner is vested with wide-ranging powers to assist in obtaining information. In practice, the police are most commonly used to conduct the investigation. Under the various Coroners Acts they have the power to enter and inspect buildings or places, take possession of and copy documents or other articles, take statements, and require people to appear in court. The coroner has control of a body whose death has been reported, and may direct that an autopsy be performed.

As each Australian State and Territory legislation is different, emergency physicians must be familiar with the details in their particular jurisdiction. The current legislation in each State and Territory is the following:

Australian Capital Territory – *Coroners Act 1997*
New South Wales – *Coroners Act 1980*
New Zealand – *Coroners Act 1988*
Northern Territory – *Coroners Act 1993*
Queensland – *Coroners Act 1958–1977*
South Australia – *Coroners Act 1975*
Tasmania – *Coroners Act 1995*
Western Australia – *Coroners Act 1996*
Victoria – *Coroners Act 1985*.

REPORTABLE DEATHS

Most deaths that occur in the community are not reported to a coroner and, consequently, are not investigated. The coroner has no power to initiate an investigation unless a death is reported. If a medical practitioner is able to issue a medical certificate of the cause of death, the Registrars-General of that State or Territory may issue a death certificate and the body of the deceased may be lawfully disposed of without coronial involvement.

In general, to issue a certificate of the cause of death, a doctor must have attended the deceased during the last illness, and the death must not be encompassed by that jurisdiction's definition of a reportable death. It is essential that every medical practitioner has a precise knowledge of what constitutes a reportable death within the jurisdiction.

It is uncommon for a doctor who is working in an emergency department to have had prior contact with a patient during the last illness. Therefore, even if sure of the reason why the patient died, the doctor is often unable to complete a medical certificate of the cause of death. It is quite permissible, and even desirable, under these circumstances, to contact the patient's treating doctor to inquire as to whether that doctor is able to complete the certificate. This process reduces the number of deaths that must be reported and assists families who may be distressed about coronial involvement.

All Australian Coroners Acts contain a definition of the deaths that must be reported. Although the precise terminology varies, there are many similarities between them. In general, each Act has provisions for inquiring into deaths that are of unknown cause or that appear to have been caused by violent, unnatural or accidental means. Many Acts also refer to deaths that occur in suspicious circumstances, and some specifically mention killing, drowning, dependence on non-therapeutic drugs, and deaths occurring while under anaesthesia. The Tasmanian Act goes further, to specify deaths that occur under sedation.

As an example, the *Victorian Coroners Act* 1985 defines a reportable death as one: a) where the body is in Victoria, b) that occurred in Victoria, c) the cause of which occurred in Victoria, d) of a person who ordinarily resided in Victoria at the time of death, e) that appears to have been unexpected, unnatural or violent, or to have resulted, directly or indirectly, from accident or injury, f) that occurs during an anaesthetic, g) that occurs as a result of an anaesthetic and is not due to natural causes, h) that occurs in prescribed circumstances, i) of a person who immediately before death was a person held in care, j) of a person whose identity is unknown, k) that occurs in Victoria where a notice under Section 19(1)(b) of the *Registration of Births Deaths and Marriages Act 1959* has not been signed, or l) that occurs at a place outside Victoria where the cause of death is not certified by a person who, under the law in force in that place, is authorized to certify that death.

Despite the seemingly straightforward definitions given in the various Acts, there are many instances where it may not be clear whether a death is reportable or not. Emergency physicians are often faced with situations where there is a paucity of information regarding the circumstances of an event, and where the cause of death may be difficult to deduce. Correlation between the clinical diagnoses recorded on death certificates and subsequent autopsies has been consistently shown to be poor. What exactly constitutes unexpected, unnatural or unknown is open to debate, and may require some judgement. In all cases the coroner expects the doctor to act with common sense and integrity. If at all in doubt it is wise to discuss the circumstances with the coroner or assistant, and to seek advice. This conversation and the advice given must be recorded in the medical notes.

The process of reporting a death is generally a matter of speaking to the coroner's assistants (often referred to as coroner's clerks), who will record pertinent details and, if necessary, investigate. The report should be made as soon as practicable after the death. A medical practitioner who does not report a reportable death is liable to a penalty.

Even though coroners' offices and the police work closely together, reporting a death to the coroner is not necessarily equivalent to reporting an event to the police. If it is possible that a person has died or been seriously injured in suspicious circumstances, then it is prudent to ensure the police are also notified.

A CORONIAL INVESTIGATION

After a death has been reported, the coroner or designated assistant may initiate an investigation. This is most commonly conducted by the police assisting the coroner, with an autopsy conducted by a forensic pathologist.

The body, once certified dead, becomes part of that investigation and should be left as far as possible in the condition at death. If the body is to be viewed by relatives immediately it is often necessary to make it presentable. This must be done carefully, so as to not remove or change anything that may be of importance to the coroner. If a resuscitation was attempted all cannulae, endotracheal tubes and catheters should be left in situ. All clothing and objects that were on (or in) the deceased should be collected, bagged and labelled. All medical and nursing notes, radiographs, electrocardiographs and blood tests should accompany the body if it is to be transported to a place as directed by the coroner.

Medical notes taken during or soon after the activity of a busy resuscitation are often incomplete. It is not easy to accurately recall procedures, times and events when the main task is to prevent someone from dying. Similarly, after death there are many urgent tasks, such as talking to relatives, notifying treating or referring doctors, and debriefing staff. It is essential, however, that the documentation is completed as accurately and thoroughly as possible. The notes must contain a date and time, and clearly specify the identity of the author. If points are recalled after completing the notes these may be added at the end of the previous notes, again with a time and a date added. Do not under any circumstances change or add to the body of the previous notes.

In addition to completing the medical notes, a medical practitioner may be requested to provide a statement to the coroner regarding the doctor's involvement with the deceased, and an opinion on certain matters. Such a statement should be carefully prepared from the original notes and written in a structured fashion, using non-medical terminology where possible. The statement often gives the opportunity for the medical practitioner to give further information to the coroner regarding medical qualifications and experience, the position fulfilled in the department at the time of the death, and a more detailed interpretation of the events. If a statement

is requested from junior emergency department staff, it is strongly advisable for these to be read by someone both clinically and medicolegally experienced.

Providing honest, accurate and expeditious information to relatives when a death occurs assists in preventing misunderstandings and serious issues arising in the course of a coronial investigation. Relatives vary enormously in the quantity and depth of medical information they request or can assimilate after an unexpected death. It is wise not only to talk to the relatives present at the death, but also offer to meet later with selected family members. Clarification with the family of what actually occurred, what diagnoses were entertained, and what investigations and procedures were performed is not only good medical practice, but can allay concerns regarding management.

If a significant diagnosis was missed, inappropriate or inadequate treatment given, or a serious complication of an investigation or procedure occurred, assistance and advice from the hospital insurers and medical defence organizations should be sought before talking to the family. However difficult it may be, it is far better that the family is aware of any adverse occurrences before the inquest than for them to harbour suspicions or to get a feeling something is being covered up. The coroner is far more likely to be sympathetic to a genuine mistake or omission when it has been discussed with the family and the hospital has taken steps to prevent a recurrence.

EXPERT OPINION

Having gathered all the available information regarding a death the coroner may decide that expert opinion is necessary on one or more points. Commonly, this involves the standard of care afforded to the deceased. It may, however, also include issues such as the seniority of doctors involved, the use of appropriate investigations, the interpretation of investigations, and the occurrence of complications of a procedure. The coroner relies heavily on such

opinions for the findings, and the selection of an appropriate expert is essential.

The person selected by the coroner to give this opinion should possess postgraduate specialist medical qualifications and be broadly experienced in the relevant medical specialty. For events occurring in the emergency department a senior emergency physician with over 5 years' experience is usually most appropriate. The specialist medical colleges may be requested to nominate such a person.

The emergency physician requested to give expert opinion must have access to a be able to review all of the available relevant information. Such a person must also consider him or herself adequately qualified and experienced to provide an opinion, and to answer any specific questions the coroner may have requested to be addressed. The doctor must have the time and ability to provide a comprehensive statement and to appear as a witness at the inquest if requested, and to act impartially. The doctor should decline involvement if an interest in the outcome of the case could be implied.

A CORONIAL INQUEST

A coronial inquest is a public inquiry into one or more deaths. Deaths may be grouped together if they occurred in the same instance, or in apparently similar circumstances. The purpose of the inquest is to put findings on the public record. These may include the identity of the deceased, the circumstances surrounding the death, the medical cause of death, and the identity of any person who contributed to the death. The coroner may also make comments and recommendations concerning matters of health and safety. In some jurisdictions these are termed 'riders'. In addition, as His Honour B.R. Thorley pointed out, the inquest serves to:

> ... include the satisfaction of legitimate concerns of relatives, the concern of the public in the proper administration of institutions and matters of public and private interest ...

The inquest does not serve to commit people for trial, nor to provide information for a subsequent criminal investigation.

With broad terms of reference, and the ability to admit testimony that may not be allowed in criminal courts, inquests interest many people, not only those who may have been directly involved. They are often highly publicized media events and may provoke political comment, especially where government bodies are involved. A medical practitioner served a subpoena to attend should prepare carefully, both individually and in conjunction with the hospital.

Preparation for an inquest begins at the time of the death. Complete and accurate medical notes, together with a carefully considered statement, provide a solid foundation for giving evidence and handling any subsequent issues. Statements containing complex medical terminology, ambiguities or omissions only serve to create confusion. Discuss the case with colleagues who are not directly involved, the hospital medical administration, and a medical defence organization. Legal advice and representation are essential to any doctor appearing in an inquest, even though the case may appear straightforward. It is wise for any areas of damaging evidence or potential conflict to be identified and managed accordingly.

Appearing at an inquest can be a stressful event, especially if on a review of the circumstances a doctor's actions or judgement may be called into question. Professional peer support, as well as legal advice, should be offered to all medical staff. Simple actions, such as a briefing on court procedures and some advice on how to deal with cross-examination, can be of immense value.

A coroner's court is conducted with a mix of 'inquisitorial' and 'adversarial' legal styles. It is inquisitorial in that the coroner may take part in and direct proceedings, and can question witnesses and appoint court advisers. It is adversarial in that parties with a legitimate interest can be represented in proceedings, and can challenge and test witnesses' evidence, especially where it differs from what they would like presented. The 'rules of evidence' are more relaxed in the coroner's court than in a criminal court. Hearsay evidence – that is, evidence of what someone else said to a witness – is generally admissible. Despite these differences, it is important to remember it is no less a court than a criminal court, and demands the same degree of respect and professional conduct one would accord to the latter.

CORONIAL FINDINGS

At the conclusion of an inquest the coroner makes a number of findings directed at satisfying the aims of that inquest. These findings are made public, and are often of interest to those who are directly involved, as well as to a wider audience.

The findings of an inquest in which the conduct of a particular emergency physician, emergency department or hospital have been scrutinized will be of particular interest. Although it is always pleasing to have either positive or a lack of negative comment delivered in the finding, criticism of some aspect of the conduct of an individual, department, hospital or the medical system in general is not uncommon. Unfortunately, it is often this criticism that attracts the most public attention and, somewhat unfairly, the public perception of our acute healthcare system is shaped by the media's attention to coronial findings.

In the recent past, coroners have commented on inadequate training, experience and supervision of junior doctors, inadequate systems of organization within departments, and poor communication between doctors and family members.

Although adverse or critical findings have no legal weight or penalties attached to them, they are in many respects a considered community response to a situation in which the wider population has a vested interest. Used constructively they can be extremely useful in convincing hospital management that a problem exists and beginning a process for effecting positive change within a department or institution.

UK

ESSENTIALS

1 The coroner, or procurator fiscal in Scotland, is responsible for the investigation of circumstances surrounding death in particular situations.

2 Emergency physicians should be familiar with the types of death which require referral to the coroner/procurator fiscal. These include deaths due to any trauma, poisoning or other unnatural causes, deaths related to medical procedures and deaths whose cause is unknown. Deaths that occur whilst detained under the mental health act or in custody of police should also be reported. Several other specific circumstances exist and in doubtful cases, discussion with the district coroner's office should occur.

3 The body remains under the control of the coroner once death has been reported. Medical devices should be left in-situ and the body should receive minimal handling, particularly in suspicious or violent deaths, in order to preserve forensic trace evidence.

4 Concise documentation of the clinical circumstances surrounding the death may direct the pathologist towards a detailed examination of the relevant organ or system, and acts as a solid basis for the emergency physician for the preparation of a subsequent statement and examination at an inquest.

5 Emergency physicians should seek assistance from senior colleagues and legal advice when asked to prepare a statement for the coroner, or attend an inquest.

INTRODUCTION

The investigation into circumstances surrounding deaths is an important part of civilized society. Accurate recording of cause of death serves many purposes including accurate disease surveillance, the detection of secret homicide, and the detection of potentially avoidable factors that have contributed to a death. Various death investigation systems exist around the world. The UK uses the coronial system, Scotland the procurator fiscal. By virtue of the patient population encountered by emergency physicians, and the types of deaths that are subject to investigation, emergency physicians may expect to find themselves in contact with either the coroner or procurator fiscal system during their working lives, thus necessitating an understanding of the workings of these systems.

HISTORY OF THE CORONER

The history of the coroner's office is an interesting reflection of events that shaped our civilization and is in constant evolution. The Shipman Inquiry is the most recent event that will shape the coroner's role. The office of the coroner was established in 1194 and its primary function then was that of protection of the crown's pecuniary interests in criminal proceedings. The coroner was involved when a death was sudden or unexpected, or a body was found in the open; however, aside from the duty to ensure the arrest of anyone involved in homicide, the coroner held a significant role in the collection of the deceased's chattels and collection of various fines.[1]

Introduction of *The Births and Deaths Registration Act* in 1836, mandated registration of all deaths before burial could legally occur. This may have arisen out of concern regarding the accurate statistical information concerning deaths, but also concern about hidden homicide. Another Act introduced the same year enabled coroners to order a medical practitioner to attend an inquest and perform an autopsy in equivocal cases.

The Coroners Act of 1887 saw a shift of emphasis from protection of financial interests to the emphasis that remains today – the medical cause of death and its surrounding circumstances with eventual community benefit in mind.

The Broderick committee was appointed in 1965 to review death certification in response to adverse publicity about inquests and pressures to improve death certification. Their report published in 1971 contained 114 recommendations, many of which were enacted. Table 24.2.1 lists the reasons the Broderick Committee considered the purpose of an inquest.[2]

The current *Coroners Act* (1988) states that a coroner shall hold an inquest into a death when there is '... reasonable cause to suspect that the deceased has died a violent or unnatural death, has died a sudden death of which the cause is unknown, or has died in prison or in a such place or circumstances as to require an inquest under any Act'.[3]

STRUCTURE OF THE CORONER SYSTEM IN THE UK

Coroners are independent judicial officers who mostly have a legal background (some also have a medical background) and must possess at least 5 years' post-qualification experience. They are responsible only to the Crown, this being an important safeguard for society; however, their administration is largely the responsibility of the Home Office. They must work within the laws

Table 24.2.1 Reasons for an inquest (according to the Broderick Committee)

- To determine the medical cause of death
- To allay rumours or suspicion
- To draw attention to the existence of circumstances which if unremedied might lead to further deaths
- To advance medical knowledge
- To preserve the legal interests of the deceased person's family, heirs or other interested parties[2]

and regulations that apply to them: *The Coroners Act 1988, Coroners Rules 1984* and the *Model Coroners Charter*. There are approximately 148 coroner's districts throughout England and Wales, and each district has a coroner, a deputy and possibly several assistant deputy coroners. Coroners are assisted in their duties by coroner's officers, who are frequently police officers or ex-police officers, whose work is dedicated solely to coronial matters. This follows long-established practice and has probably arisen because of the significant proportion of cases in which police are the notifying agent. The nature of a coronial investigation also frequently requires a person to possess knowledge about legal matters and skill in information gathering. From a practical viewpoint, the coroner's assistants may be responsible for performing such duties as attending the scene of a death, arranging transport of the body to the mortuary, notification of the next of kin and obtaining statements from relevant parties. Clearly, variation in the structure of the service between regions is inevitable and reflects the size, composition and workload within the district.[4]

OVERVIEW OF THE CORONIAL PROCESS

Upon notification of a death, the coroner makes initial inquiries and may direct a pathologist to perform a post-mortem. Sometimes it becomes clear at this early point that the death is a natural one and does not fall within the *Coroners Act*, thus no inquest is required and a death certificate is issued. In other circumstances, further investigations occur and relevant information is gathered. If the coroner is subsequently satisfied that the death is natural, again no inquest is required. In other cases, or in certain prescribed circumstances, an inquest is held. At the conclusion of an inquest, a finding or verdict is delivered. This verdict must not be framed in a way that implies civil or criminal liability.

Table 24.2.2 Circumstances in which a death should be reported to the Coroner

- The cause of death is unknown
- The deceased was not seen by the certifying doctor either after death or within the 14 days before the death
- The death was violent or unnatural or suspicious
- The death may be due to an accident (whenever it occurred)
- The death may be due to self-neglect or neglect by others
- The death may be due to an industrial disease or related to the deceased's employment
- The death may be due to an abortion
- The death occurred during an operation or before recovery of the effects of an anaesthetic
- The death may be a suicide
- The death occurred during or shortly after detention in police or prison custody

Table 24.2.3 Specific guidelines regarding deaths related to medical management in Scotland

- Deaths which occur unexpectedly having regard to the clinical condition of the deceased prior to his receiving medical care
- Deaths which are clinically unexplained
- Deaths seemingly attributable to a therapeutic or diagnostic hazard
- Deaths which are apparently associated with lack of medical care
- Deaths which occur during the actual administration of general or local anaesthetic

REPORTABLE DEATHS

There is no statutory obligation in the UK for a doctor or any member of the public to report certain deaths to the coroner. However, an ethical responsibility exists and it is recognized practice to do so in particular circumstances. A 1996 letter from the Deputy Chief Medical Satistician to all doctors outlined these circumstances (Table 24.2.2).[5]

Each booklet of medical death certificates also contains a reminder of the deaths that a coroner needs to consider. The list is not exhaustive. Other circumstances include where the deceased was detained under the Mental Health Act, the death may be related to a medical procedure or treatment, or there is an allegation of medical mismanagement.

SCOTLAND

In Scotland, the role of death investigation is undertaken by the procurator fiscal's office, which is also responsible for the investigation and prosecution of crime. The spectrum of deaths investigated is essentially the same as in England and Wales, however, more specific guidelines regarding deaths possibly related to medical mismanagement are provided (Table 24.2.3).

How to report to a death

Having determined that a death is reportable, the emergency physician should contact the district coroner's office and notify the details of the deceased. Where doubt exists about the necessity, or otherwise, to report a death, a doctor should contact that office to discuss the matter further. This may avoid undue distress to relatives should the death be subsequently referred by the registrar of births and deaths. The discussion, and subsequent decision should be recorded in the patient's clinical notes. A death certificate should not be written.

HANDLING THE BODY

There appear to be no official guidelines in place regarding handling of the body once death has been reported to the coroner, however, this aspect may be an important component of the subsequent investigation. Any therapeutic and monitoring devices such as endotracheal tubes, intercostal catheters and intravascular catheters should be left in-situ, as determination of their correct placement or otherwise may be relevant to the death investigation. In a similar line, it may be important to isolate any equipment (e.g. intravenous infusion pump devices) suspected of being faulty and contributing to the death. In circumstances of suspicious, or violent deaths in particular, the body should be not be handled unnecessarily nor should the body be washed. Important trace evidence that may be crucial for subsequent criminal proceedings could conceivably be lost. For example, in deaths involving firearms, it may be useful for a forensic scientist to swab the deceased's hands for gunshot residue to help confirm or refute the notion of a self-inflicted injury.

Clothing removed from the deceased during resuscitation efforts should be set aside and preferably placed into individual paper bags. Any remaining clothing on the deceased should be left in-situ.[6] Blood taken during resuscitation attempts, regardless of whether it was processed or not, should not be discarded, but kept refrigerated and its existence indicated to the coroner. The examination of ante-mortem blood samples can provide valuable information, particularly with respect to electrolyte and glucose concentrations, drug concentrations, and in deaths possibly attributable to anaphylaxis, tryptase assay.[7]

DOCUMENTATION

The clinical record of the deceased will usually accompany the body to the mortuary and is frequently perused by the pathologist. Clinical information is crucial in consideration of the cause of death and may help direct the pathologist towards an appropriately detailed examination of the relevant system or organ. The guidelines for appropriate documentation in reportable cases are really the same that apply in medical record-keeping in general. They should be made contemporaneously, or as close to as is possible in a resuscitation environment. Each entry should be dated and the time recorded. They must be legible, objective and the sources of information identified. Any errors made should be crossed out, dated and signed. Likewise, if information comes to hand or is recalled at a later date, that entry should be dated and timed. Never add an entry or alter notes without identifying that it is, indeed, so. Finally, the author's name and designation should be clear, and all entries signed.

INFORMATION FOR FAMILIES

The next-of-kin of the deceased must be informed that the death has been reported to the coroner and the requirement or reasons for doing so. It is important to inform them that police may be involved in the investigation of the death on behalf of the coroner, but that this does not imply a criminal wrong doing. An information leaflet explaining the coroner's work and rights of the next-of-kin is available from the Home Office[8] and should be available in every emergency department to pass on to bereaved families. Another useful publication written for bereaved families provides information regarding postmortems and is available from the Royal College of Pathologists.[9]

POSTMORTEMS

The coroner may decide upon the initial report of a death that a postmortem is necessary in order to determine the cause of death, or resolve an issue relevant to a coronial inquiry. In the year 2000, postmortem examinations were conducted in 62% of cases reported to the coroner, continuing a steady downward trend in the proportion of postmortems conducted out of reported cases.[10] Having decided upon the necessity for a postmortem, the coroner directs a pathologist to conduct a postmortem. The Coroners Act states that, in fact, the coroner may 'direct any legally qualified medical practitioner' to conduct the postmortem; however, the Coroners Rules 1984 direct that they should be performed 'whenever practicable by a pathologist with suitable qualifications and experience', and, in practice, most are conducted by Home-Office-accredited forensic pathologists. Clearly, if the standard of medical care provided by the hospital in which the death occurred is in question, it is inappropriate for a pathologist employed by that hospital to conduct the postmortem.

Consent from relatives to conduct the postmortem is not required in coroner's cases. In the event that relatives object to the postmortem examination, the coroner may delay it to allow them time to obtain legal advice. However, if the death does fall within the coroner's jurisdiction, and is deemed to be necessary, their objection would be overridden. Relatives may request a second postmortem; however, this seldom occurs in practice.

The coroner must, in theory, notify certain persons, including the usual medical attendant of the deceased or the hospital in which the death occurred, of the time and date of the postmortem (Rule 7, The Coroners Rules 1984). In practice, this tends to occur when a desire to be represented at the examination has been expressed to the coroner, and in that instance a nominated, medically qualified representative (not a doctor whose practice may be in question) may be present to observe the postmortem.

The issue of tissue retention at autopsy has received recent worldwide attention. Rule 9 of The Coroner's Rules 1984 is quite broad allowing the pathologist to retain 'material which in his opinion bears upon the cause of death, for such a period as the Coroner sees fit'. Guidelines issued by The Royal College of Pathologists[11] recommend that in coroner's cases, clear protocols between the coroner and the pathologist should exist, and retention of tissues outside of the above-mentioned context should occur with the agreement of both the relatives of the deceased and the coroner.

PREPARING A STATEMENT FOR THE CORONER

The coroner may request a statement from a doctor involved in the care of the deceased and, while there is no obligation to comply with this request, it is generally in the doctor's interest to do so. The coroner, otherwise, has no option but to compel the doctor to attend court and answer questions. A statement, therefore, that has been carefully prepared with due thought to any issues identified may, indeed, avert the need for an inquest, or at least will act as a solid base upon which the examination in court will occur. It is important that the doctor writing the statement understands the circumstances of the death; thus, access to the postmortem report is often vital and is allowable under Rule 57 of the Coroner's Rules. It is generally advisable, except perhaps in circumstances where it is clear that simple, factual background information only is required, to seek legal advice early when requested to provide a statement or attend an inquest.

The statement should be typewritten and contain the author's qualifications, work experience and current employment post. The sources from which the report is prepared (e.g. clinical notes, pathology reports) should be acknowledged, and it should be set out in a logical manner in chronological order. Technical terms should be qualified with an explanation readily understood by a lay person. It is advisable to have a senior colleague review the statement before submission to the legal representative for final review. The final statement should be dated and signed, and a copy kept for future reference.

INQUEST

An inquest is a public hearing at which the identity of the deceased and how, when and where the deceased came by his/her death are to be determined. In the year 2000 only 12% of reported deaths proceeded to inquest, the remainder being examined 'in chambers'. Inquests (or Fatal Accident Inquiries in Scotland) are mandatory in certain prescribed circumstances, including deaths in prison or police custody, and deaths resulting from workplace incidents. In certain circumstances inquests are held with a jury who are responsible for the final verdict.

The inquest is inquisitorial in nature,

where the truth surrounding the circumstances of the death is sought, rather than adversarial, where two or more parties have a particular claim to prove. As with the preparation of a statement for the coroner, it is wise for a medical witness to seek legal advice and possibly representation prior to attendance at an inquest. The legal arena in which they are held is unfamiliar territory to most doctors and they frequently attract intense media scrutiny; thus, involvement in an inquest may be a daunting and stressful experience requiring support from colleagues and friends.

CONTROVERSIES AND FUTURE DIRECTIONS

❶ The current Coronial system in the UK is under fundamental review.

REFERENCES

1. Knapman P, Powers M 1985 The Law and Practice on Coroners. Barry Rose, Chichester
2. Cordner S, Loff B 1994 800 years of coroners: have they a future? The Lancet 344: 799–801
3. Coroners Act 1988 (c.13) www.hmso.gov.uk
4. Tarling R 1998 Coroner Service Survey: A research and Statistics Directorate Report. Home Office, London
5. Dorries C 1999 Coroner's Courts – a Guide to Law and Practice. Wiley, Chichester
6. Dimond B 1995 Death in accident and emergency. Accident and Emergency Nursing 3: 38–41
7. Burton J, Rutty G 2001 The Hospital Autopsy, 2nd edn. Arnold, London
8. Home Office 2002 When sudden death occurs- Coroners and Inquests. Home Office, London
9. The Royal College of Pathologists 2000 Examination of the body after death – information about post-mortem examination for relatives. The Royal College of Pathologists, London www.rcpath.org
10. Allen R 2000 Deaths reported to coroners England and Wales 2000. Home Office Research Development and Statistics Directorate, London
11. The Royal College of Pathologists 2000 Guidelines for the retention of tissues and organs at post-mortem examination. The Royal College of Pathologists, London www.rcpath.org

24.3 CONSENT AND COMPETENCE: THE AUSTRALASIAN AND UK PERSPECTIVES

EDWARD BRENTNALL • G. MICHAEL GALVIN • HELEN L. PARKER

AUSTRALASIA

ESSENTIALS

1 Patient consent is essential for medical treatment.

2 Consent may be implied, verbal or written.

3 Consent must be informed, specific, freely given, and cover that which is actually done.

4 The patient must be capable of giving the consent.

5 Occasionally, treatment may be given without consent, if the patient is not competent to give that consent.

6 Emergency physicians must know when these exceptions apply, and what to do in those circumstances.

INTRODUCTION

Consent lies at the heart of the medical contract between the doctor and the patient. Medical investigation and treatment are essentially voluntary acts, which the patient consents to the doctor performing. Great attention has been placed on the issue of consent since the *Rogers v Whittaker* case in which consent given by the patient was held to be invalid. The issue revolved around whether or not disclosure by the surgeon was sufficiently detailed to allow the consent to be informed.

FIVE ESSENTIALS OF VALID CONSENT

There are five elements of valid consent. These are:

- The patient must be legally capable of giving consent.
- Consent must be informed.
- Consent must be specific.
- Consent must be freely given.
- Consent must cover that which is actually done.

HOW IS CONSENT GIVEN?

Consent may be given in one of three ways.

Implied consent

This is the simplest form of consent and is the form used, for example, when a patient allows blood to be taken or an intravenous line inserted. As it is an assault to touch another person without their consent, the practice of medicine requires a great deal of implied consent. The experienced practitioner develops a technique to facilitate obtaining this consent. There is a simple explanation of what is proposed and why it is necessary. This may be as simple as 'I need to insert this line into a vein to give you some extra fluids'. Implied consent is sufficient for many purposes, but not for more major procedures, for which formal consent should be obtained.

Verbal consent

Verbal consent is just as valid as written consent, but it may be more difficult to establish the basic elements. Documentation should indicate that the patient did consent. The doctor obtaining the consent, together with any witness, should sign the medical record. Additional strength is given to such consent if the doctor appends a note that the patient appears to fully understand what has been consented. The documentation must be completed at the time.

Written consent

In some ways written consent is the most difficult to establish. It is impossible to cover every outcome. The difficulties lie with being specific and with the patient being informed. For simpler procedures it may be better to have implied or verbal consent, rather than written consent.

PATIENTS WHO ARE NOT LEGALLY ABLE TO GIVE CONSENT

Children and adolescents

The legal age of consent in Australasia has changed in the last quarter century from 21 to 18 years, and in some circumstances to 16 years or less. This has occurred against a background of differing ages at which persons may vote, buy tobacco or alcohol, drive cars or engage in sexual activity.

The most important factor to be considered by the emergency physician is the competence of the patient to understand what is wrong and what the treatment entails. This has more to do with intellectual and emotional maturity than chronological age. It would be reasonable for a 14-year-old girl to consent to appendicectomy, but quite unreasonable to expect the same person to understand the consequences of a hysterectomy.

In a genuine emergency the care of the patient is the most important factor and the absence of a parent or guardian is not a bar to an emergency procedure. Should treatment of a minor be required and valid consent not obtainable, the emergency physician must document the steps taken to obtain consent and the reason why the treatment must be carried out. If at all possible the opinion of a second doctor should also be attached, provided that the second doctor approximates the first in seniority. Many hospitals require that in such circumstance the director of clinical services or delegate give 'approval'. This is simply a means of ensuring that the

hospital is aware of the situation and accepts responsibility.

A special situation occurs for children whose parents hold religious beliefs that proscribe blood transfusion or the administration of blood products. This creates a situation where the child is incompetent and the parents do not consent. There is now almost standard legislation that allows the attending doctors to certify that blood transfusion is required to sustain life, and to then administer the treatment in the face of active opposition from the parents. The relevant legislation protects the doctor, who acts out of a duty of care to the patient.

INTELLECTUALLY DISABLED

For consent to be valid, the patient must be able to understand the nature of the condition, the options available and the treatment being recommended. In addition there must be an understanding of the material risks and the possible outcome of any potential treatments. The mildly disabled may be able to satisfy these criteria, but the more severely disabled will not be in a position to give valid consent. In the latter situation the guardian or Guardianship Board would have to be involved in all but the most urgent cases.

MENTALLY ILL

A diagnosis of mental illness does not automatically preclude a patient from giving consent. The attending doctor must decide on the competence of the patient to consent. The attending psychiatrist may be in a position to assist. If the patient is not competent then the relevant mental health legislation must be considered. In an emergency where life or quality of life is seriously threatened and time is of the essence, the facts should be recorded and treatment commenced. A sound knowledge of the mental health and guardianship legislation relevant to the region is essential.

PATIENT DISABLED BY DRUGS OR ALCOHOL

When a patient is temporarily disabled by drugs or alcohol the situation is less clear. In some Australian States persons who have committed serious assault may escape conviction because the law considers them incapable of forming the intention to commit the act. Legal and medical opinions do not always agree, especially in respect of 'capacity' and blood alcohol readings. The absolute legal position is unclear as to whether an intoxicated person can give consent, but there is no doubt that any doctor who acts in the best interest of the patient will always be on solid ground in the event of an action. Restraint may be justified in order to prevent a patient taking his or her own discharge when that might have adverse medical results. There are no simple rules, but it is worth considering whether it is better to be sued for assault and wrongful imprisonment, or to be sued for the damage that followed to the patient who was allowed to leave. It may be possible to ask the Guardianship Board for help, but there will be occasions in which immediate decisions must be taken, and the best rule is to do whatever will be the best for the patient in the longer term. Again, documentation

CONTROVERSIES

❶ Arguments abound over what constitutes lack of competence. Is alcohol intoxication sufficient reason for overriding the patient's failure to consent to necessary treatment?

❷ The age at which minors are entitled to give consent for treatment is contentious, and varies with the treatment proposed, its consequences, and the maturity of the child.

❸ The question of seeking consent for ceasing treatment, particularly apparently futile treatment such as CPR in certain circumstances, is difficult to answer.

at the time, and the signatures of witnesses, will help if the court is involved.

EMERGENCY PATIENT

There has been little written about the patient who requires emergency care but is temporarily incapable of providing consent. The overriding principle, however, is one of the duty of care owed by the doctor to the patient. The duty is to provide an appropriate standard of care commensurate with the skill and experience of the doctor. There is an obligation to explain to the patient what has been done as early as is reasonable in the recovery phase.

GUARDIANSHIP BOARDS

In every State and Territory of Australia there is legislation that covers the protection and administration of incompetent patients. All of these bodies are available to give timely help and, if necessary, hold a formal hearing. Whenever possible, this avenue of assistance should be used. The Boards have the authority to conduct hearings, receive evidence and make decisions on behalf of incompetent persons. These decisions have the authority of law and provide protection for the patient and the doctor. Emergency physicians should ensure that they are aware of how to contact their local Board, both in and out of working hours.

SUMMARY

- The emergency physician must know the five essentials of consent.
- The emergency physician must understand:
  – Implied consent
  – Verbal consent
  – Written consent.
- There must be adequate and contemporaneous documentation of decisions.
- A sound working knowledge of mental health and guardianship legislation is required.

- Doctors' primary responsibility to their patients is their duty of care. A doctor acting in the best interests of the patient is unlikely to be successfully sued.

UK

ESSENTIALS

1 Accepted ethical principles mandate that consent or agreement should be sought from patients prior to initiating medical interventions. In emergencies, when a patient's consent cannot be sought, however, medical practitioners may provide care that is necessary to preserve life or prevent deterioration.

2 Consent can only be provided or denied by persons deemed competent to do so. The legal principles used to judge the competence of a person incorporate the elements of comprehension, appreciation, reasoning and choice. Emergency physicians should be conversant with the steps necessary to assess a patient's competence within this framework.

3 Where a patient is deemed incompetent to refuse medical treatment, the treatment provided must satisfy the 'best interests' principle and take into consideration all relevant factors.

4 The provision of clear, accurate and relevant information to patients is vital if they are to make an informed decision. Recent legal judgements have underscored the importance of considering what may be 'material' or 'significant' to that particular individual when disclosing information.

5 Consent may be implied, verbal or written. Documentation pertaining to the discussion and process surrounding the consent process is more important and useful than a solitary signature on a consent to treatment form.

INTRODUCTION AND ETHICAL CONSIDERATIONS

Central to consideration of the subject of consent and competence is an appreciation of the principles of medical and clinical ethics. These codes of behaviour act as guidelines for the medical profession with respect to what is considered proper conduct.

The four basic ethical principles relevant to the practice of medicine are often cited as:[1]

- Autonomy – the rights of individuals to make decisions on their own behalf.
- Beneficence – the duty to do the best for the patient.
- Non-maleficence – the duty to do no harm to the patient.
- Justice – the fair distribution of resources incorporating the notion of responsibility to the wider community.

It is also useful to consider The World Medical Association's International Code of Medical Ethics, which cites a fundamental principle: 'A Physician shall respect the rights of patients ...'.[2] These rights are enumerated in the World Medical Association's Declaration of Lisbon and include the:

Right to self-determination
a. The patient has the right to self-determination, to make free decisions regarding himself/ herself. The physician will inform the patient of the consequences of his/her decisions.
b. A mentally competent adult patient has the right to give or withhold consent to any diagnostic procedure or therapy. The patient has the right to the information necessary to make his/her decisions. The patient should understand clearly what is the purpose of any test or treatment, what the results would imply, and what

would be the implications of withholding consent.

c. The patient has the right to refuse to participate in research or the teaching of medicine.[3]

In consideration of these rights of patients, it clearly behoves the physician from an ethical viewpoint, to obtain consent or agreement from patients prior to initiating diagnostic and therapeutic procedures and pathways. There are also legal obligations that should be borne in mind.

The emergency physician, however, works in an environment where time-critical interventions may be required to save life or prevent deterioration in health, and patients requiring these may not be in a position to provide consent. In these situations it is not only common sense that dictates that such interventions should be provided without having obtained consent, but it is a legal duty to do so and one that also satisfies ethical considerations. The General Medical Council's guidance to doctors stipulates that: 'In an emergency, where consent cannot be obtained, you may provide medical treatment to anyone who needs it, provided the treatment is limited to what is immediately necessary to save life or avoid significant deterioration in the patient's health. However, you must still respect the terms of any valid advance refusal which you know about, or is drawn to your attention. You should tell the patient what has been done and why, as soon as the patient is sufficiently recovered to understand.'[4]

In other situations where an intervention is proposed, agreement of the patient should be sought. The term 'informed decision making' is preferred by some to 'informed consent' as it reflects consideration of patient autonomy.[5] It is also important to consider consent as a two-way process, with an exchange of knowledge between a patient and a doctor.[6] The concepts of competence, provision of adequate information and the voluntariness with which consent is given, are crucial in the consideration of obtaining valid consent or seeking an informed decision.

COMPETENCE

Ethical codes dictate that for consent to be valid it must be given by a person who has the capacity to make that decision. In the UK all persons aged 16 years and over are presumed to possess that capacity unless proven otherwise.[7] The assessment of the competence, or capacity of an adult to make decisions on their own behalf, is a functional one that requires more than cognitive testing with a tool such as the 'mini-mental status examination',[8] although this should be performed and documented as part of the assessment process.[9] Assessment of competence should be sought and conducted by the doctor proposing the treatment or investigation.

Several concepts of decision-making capacity should be considered. A 'sliding-scale' concept with three progressive levels was suggested by Drane, essentially proposing that the clinician would expect a more stringent standard of capacity in situations where the proposed treatment carried greater risk.[10] This concept formally describes a process that clinicians probably already incorporate subconsciously into their daily practice. It has, however, also been described in legal judgements: 'What matters is that the doctors should consider whether at the time he had a capacity which was commensurate with the gravity of the decision which he purported to make. The more serious the decision, the greater the capacity required.'[11]

Applebaum and Grisso described a method of assessment reflecting the legal standards for determination of competence.[12] The elements of their approach correlate with those described in the Re C judgement, a UK case that examined the competence of a long-term schizophrenic patient to refuse medical treatment. The essential elements required to demonstrate competence are described as:

- The ability to maintain and communicate a choice
- The ability to understand the relevant information
- An ability to appreciate the situation and its consequences
- The ability to manipulate the information in a rational fashion.[10]

These elements are expounded in various guides written for the medical profession.

From a practical viewpoint, the questions listed in Table 24.3.1 suggested by Biegler and Stewart are useful in determining a patient's competence.

A truncated version involving similar questions was proposed by Annas and Densburger[13] (Table 24.3.2).

Recording the questions asked and answers received provides comprehensive

---

Table 24.3.1 Questions for determining competence

Comprehension
Ask patient to recall and paraphrase information related to proposed treatment, including risks and benefits of treatment, alternative treatment and consequences of no treatment at all. Retest later to check for stability.

Belief
Tell me what you really believe is wrong with your health now.
Do you believe that you need some kind of treatment?
What is the treatment likely to do for you?
Why do you think it will have that effect?
What do you believe will happen if you are not treated?
Why do you think the doctor has recommended this treatment for you?

Weighing
Tell me how you reached the decision to accept (reject) treatment.
What things were important to you in reaching the decision?
How do you balance those things?

Choice
Have you decided whether to go along with your doctor's suggestion for treatment?
Can you tell me what your treatment decision is?

Table 24.3.2 Simplified questions for assessing competence
What is your present physical condition?
What is the treatment being recommended for you?
What do you and the doctor think might happen to you if you decide to accept the treatment?
What do you and your doctor think might happen if you decide not to accept the recommended treatment?
What are the alternatives available (including no treatment) and what are the possible consequences of accepting each?

Table 24.3.3 People considered to have parental responsibility
The child's parents if married to each other at the time of conception or birth.
The child's mother, but not the father if they were not so married, unless the father has acquired parental responsibility via a court order or a parental responsibility agreement or the couple subsequently marry.
The child's legally appointed guardian.
A person in whose favour the court has made a residence order concerning the child.
A local authority designated in a care order in respect of the child.
A local authority or other authorized person who holds an emergency protection order in respect of the child.

documentation of the process by which the assessment outcome was reached.

Whilst a third party, such as a relative, is unable to legally provide consent for an incompetent adult, it is long established practice and frequently a useful exercise, to involve relatives in the process of determining what the patient would have wanted in a particular circumstance. They may also provide valuable information during the process of competence assessment regarding a person's set of values and beliefs, and usual behaviour, particularly if the patient appears to have elected a path at odds with a previously expressed wish or one that might appear imprudent or irrational.

PATIENTS WHO MIGHT NOT BE ABLE TO CONSENT

Children and young adults

At the age of 16 years, under the Family Law Reform Act 1969, there is a pre-sumption that the patient is competent to give consent on their own behalf. However, up to the age of 18 years, if the person is found to lack competence, a parent or person with parental capacity can give consent on behalf of that patient. Those persons considered to have parental responsibility are detailed in the Children act 1989 and are listed in Table 24.3.3.

With respect to children under the age of 16 years, the influence of the case of Gillick must be considered. The courts hold that children who possess sufficient understanding and intelligence to enable them to fully understand what a proposed intervention entails, should be considered competent to consent to that intervention.

Patients detained under the Mental Health Act

Patients detained under the Mental Health Act 1983 may receive treatment without consent for their mental disorder, however, this does not automatically extend to interventions pertaining to physical disorders unrelated to the mental disorder. Neither the presence of a mental disorder nor detention under the act should be taken in themselves to indicate incompetence and a patient in this situation should be assessed in relation to the intervention proposed in the usual manner.

Intellectually impaired persons

An adult may be deemed to lack competence by virtue of a permanent intellectual impairment. In this instance it is lawful for a doctor to provide treatment that is in the patient's 'best interests'. The views of people close to the patient should be taken into consideration, whilst mindful of the fact that these third parties lack legal status to actually make decisions on that patient's behalf. In Scotland, a proxy decision maker may be appointed under the Adults with Incapacity (Scotland) Act. Enduring power of attorney empowers legal status with respect to financial and legal affairs but not medical treatment decisions.

Patients who are temporarily impaired

Adults may temporarily lack competence by virtue of a number of factors and conditions including drug and alcohol intoxication, and head injury. In these circumstances it is lawful to provide treatment 'necessary and no more than is reasonably required in the patient's best interests pending the recovery of capacity.'[14]

Advance directives or statements

Patients may make an advance statement or living will detailing their wishes for medical treatment should they become incapacitated at a later date. These may take the form of a written document or witnessed oral statement. They are legally binding provided the patient is an adult, was competent at the time made, and the statement clearly applies to the current circumstances.[14] If doubt exists about its validity, a court ruling should be sought.

Table 24.3.4 Information to provide patients so that consent is informed

Details of the diagnosis including any uncertainties and thus differentials.
Likely prognosis of the condition both treated and untreated.
Intervention options including option of no treatment or investigation, and the likely benefits and probabilities of success of each of these interventions.
Risks of each intervention, including serious or frequently occurring risks and their likely impact upon that patient.
Whether or not the intervention is experimental.
How the patient's condition will be monitored and re-assessed.
The identity of the responsible doctor(s) and other members of the health care team.
Whether trainee doctors will be involved and the extent of their involvement.
Where applicable, details of costs or charges that will apply.

INFORMATION REQUIRED TO MAKE AN INFORMED DECISION

Information is a cornerstone on which we base our decisions, and patients must be equipped with clear, accurate and relevant information if they are to make informed decisions about their medical care. In considering what information is relevant to provide to a patient, it is useful to consider legal judgements arising from medical negligence cases. The Sidaway case in 1985 considered that the standard used should be the same as that used when judging whether a doctor was negligent in their care of a patient. That standard was referred to as the 'Bolam' test and essentially held that a doctor's actions should be judged against 'that of a responsible body of medical opinion held by practitioners skilled in the field in question'.[14] This test, however, has been criticized in subsequent judgements and The Department of Health Reference Guide to Consent for Examination and Treatment states: 'It is therefore advisable to inform the patient of any "material" or "significant" risks in the proposed treatment'; it also points out that the General Medical Council states that doctors should 'find out about patient's individual needs and priorities when providing information about treatment options'.

Patients should receive information as listed in Table 24.3.4 (adapted from 'Seeking patients' consent: the ethical considerations'[4]).

Clearly, this information should be conveyed in unambiguous terms and in a manner that is likely to be understood by a patient. Language and other communication needs must be met and there must be an opportunity for patients to ask questions and reflect upon the information given to them. The information should be given by the doctor responsible for providing the intervention, or a delegate who is suitably qualified and has sufficient knowledge of the proposed intervention.

VOLUNTARINESS OF CONSENT

Aside from satisfying the criteria that a person who is making an informed decision must be competent and that the decision is based upon the provision of adequate information, a valid decision must be made freely, without undue pressure or influence from outside sources. When considering this, it may appear proper to refrain from recommending a particular course of treatment to a patient for fear of unduly influencing their decision. This thinking is, however, flawed. A physician's recommendation is frequently expected and desired by patients, and unless information has been presented in a manipulative fashion to specifically elicit a particular choice, this recommendation cannot be considered coercive.[15] Physicians should be aware of those aspects that might unduly influence a decision and should be reminded that these considerations are particularly relevant to persons in police custody.[16]

FORMS OF CONSENT AND DOCUMENTATION

The form in which consent is expressed by a patient is variable and may be implied, verbal or written. Implied consent describes everyday practices in which the body language or similar of a patient indicates their agreement to the procedure, for instance, putting out their arm for blood pressure measurement. Verbal and written forms of consent are self-explanatory, and much emphasis has traditionally been placed upon obtaining the latter. Excepting some requirements of the Human Fertilisation and Embryology Act and the Mental Health Act, a signature or mark of a patient on a consent form is not a legal requirement. Nor does the signature influence the validity of that consent, it simply serves as evidence that consent was sought. It is good practice to document the content of the discussion with the patient, the conclusion reached, details of the assessment of capacity and the names of other persons present who were witness to the discussion.

COURSE OF ACTION WHEN A PATIENT IS DEEMED INCOMPETENT

The law is clear about the provision of treatment in emergencies and this has been addressed already. What of the situation that is not immediately life threatening but where the patient is not competent to make a decision and there is no advance directive? As alluded to already, the physician may resort to

Table 24.3.5 Factors to be considered when acting in the patient's best interests without consent

The patient's own wishes and values (where these can be ascertained) including any advance statement.
Clinical judgement about the effectiveness of the proposed treatment, particularly in relation to other options.
Where there is more than one option, which option is least restrictive of the patient's future choices.
The likelihood and extent of any degree of improvement in the patient's condition if treatment is provided.
The views of the parents if the patient is a child.
The views of people close to the patient, especially close relatives, partners, carers or proxy decision-makers about what the patient is likely to see as beneficial and;
Any knowledge of the patient's religious, cultural and other non-medical views that might have an impact upon the patient's wishes.

acting in the patient's best interests, or may obtain authority from a court. The latter is particularly desirable in circumstances where a declaration or order from a court will protect the physician from adverse criticism and claims with respect to possible unlawful action, but courts can also safeguard a patient's welfare.[17] Guidelines for applications to the court can be accessed in the Department of Health guidelines.

When acting in a patients 'best interests' it is important to acknowledge:

- Intervention options
- Evidence of the patient's previously expressed preferences, including information from third parties
- Knowledge of the patient's background.[4]

Given that this is a situation likely to be frequently encountered by the emergency physician Table 24.3.5 lists the factors that should be considered as set down by the British Medical Association Consent Tool Kit.[18]

UNIQUE CONSIDERATIONS FOR THE EMERGENCY DEPARTMENT

Emergency physicians work in an environment where multiple simultaneous demands are placed upon them. Particularly with respect to critically ill and injured patients, detailed information regarding their presentation, past history and usual level of functioning is often lacking, incomplete and may, in fact, be wrong. A physician may suspect that a patient might be impaired, but have little time to make a detailed assessment before a treatment decision is required. Similarly, the information available to the physician at a point in time might suggest that a particular diagnosis and course of action is warranted, and this might change markedly upon receipt of further information. In short, the emergency physician must frequently make complex decisions at short notice with little background information. In situations where decisions have been made on behalf a patient who is felt to be incompetent, it is important to document carefully the information available to the physician, and the possible diagnoses and their sequelae entertained at that time, and the reasons for the course taken. It is good practice also to seek the assistance and advice of a colleague where the competence of a patient is in doubt and significant interventions are deemed necessary.

CONTROVERSIES AND FUTURE DIRECTIONS

❶ English medical law is likely to be influenced in the future by the recent introduction of The Human Rights Act 1998, with courts having to take into consideration case law of the European Court of Human Rights.

❷ Case law on the issue of what is considered appropriate information to give to patients regarding treatment options is evolving.

❸ One philosopher proposed that patients in emergency departments already have their freedom of choice restricted because they have not chosen their site of treatment, and treatment choices are restricted to institutional policies.

REFERENCES

1. Breen K, Plueckhahn V, Cordner S 1997 Ethics Law and Medical Practice. Allen and Unwin, St Leonards
2. World Medical Association International Code of Medical Ethics www.wma.net/e/policy/17-a e.html
3. World Medical Association Declaration on the Rights of the Patient www.net/e/policy/17-h e.html
4. General Medical Council 1998 Seeking Patient's Consent: the ethical considerations. www.gmc-uk.org/standards/consent.htm
5. Skene L, Nisselle P 2001 High Court warns of the 'retrospectoscope' in informed consent cases: Rosenberg v. Percival. Medicine Today 2001 October, pp 79–82
6. Alderson P, Goodey C 1998 Theories of consent. British Medical Journal 317: 1313–5
7. British Medical Association Consent Tool Kit Card 5 Assessment of Competence
8. Savulescu J, Kerridge I 2001 Competence and consent. Medical Journal of Australia 175: 313–5
9. Biegler P, Stewart C 2001 Assessing competence to refuse medical treatment. Medical Journal of Australia 174: 522–5
10. Miller S, Marin D 2000 Assessing capacity. Emergency Medicine Clinics of North America 18 (2): 233–42
11. BMA 1995 Assessment of mental capacity. BMA and the Law Society. Chapter 10 on www.bma.org.uk
12. Appelbaum P, Grisso T 1988 Assessing patients' capacities to consent to treatment. New England Journal of Medicine 319(25): 1635–8
13. Annas GJ, Densberger JE 1984 Competence to refuse medical treatment: autonomy vs. paternalism. Toledo Law Review 15: 561–92. Quoted in: Miller S, Marin D 2000 Assessing capacity. Emergency Medicine Clinics of North America 18(2): 233–42
14. British Medical Association Consent Tool Kit Card 9 Advance Statements
15. Moskop J 1999 Informed consent in the emergency department. Emergency Medicine Clinics of North America 17(2): 327–39
16. Pownall M. 1999 Doctors should obtain informed consent for intimate body searches. British Medical Journal 318: 1310
17. Oats L 2000 The courts' role in decisions about medical treatment. British Medical Journal 321: 1282–4
18. British Medical Association Consent Tool Kit Card 8 Determining 'Best Interests'

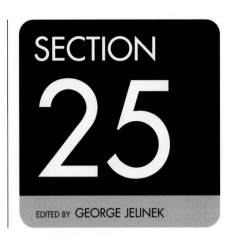

EMERGENCY MEDICINE SYSTEMS

25.1 Prehospital emergency medicine 682

25.2 Retrieval 686

25.3 Medical issues in disasters 694

25.4 Triage 702

25.5 Refugee health 706

25.6 Emergency department observation wards 710

STEPHEN BERNARD

ESSENTIALS

1 Ambulance officers are trained to administer a range of life-saving emergency medical interventions.

2 Ambulance dispatch is increasingly computerized and this allows for medical determination of response type and quality assurance.

3 Ambulance care of the trauma patient is similar to initial evaluation by the emergency physician, with emphasis on basic life-support measures.

4 Current survival rates from pre-hospital cardiac arrest are low and first responder programmes would appear to be a cost-effective solution.

5 Ambulance paramedics may treat many complications of acute coronary syndromes, including pain, cardiac arrhythmias and pulmonary oedema.

6 Ambulance paramedics effectively treat pre-hospital medical emergencies including seizures, hypoglycaemia and anaphylaxis.

INTRODUCTION

Ambulance services have the primary role of providing rapid transport of patients to an emergency department (ED). In addition, ambulance officers are trained to administer emergency medical care to patients with life-threatening illnesses.

DISPATCH

Many countries now have a single telephone number for immediate access to the ambulance service in cases of emergency, such as 911 in North

America, 999 in the UK and 000 in Australasia.

However, the dispatch of the correct ambulance resource in the optimal time-frame is a complex exercise. It is inappropriate to dispatch all ambulances on a 'code 1' (lights and sirens) response, since this entails some level of risk to the crew and other road users. On the other hand, it may be difficult to accurately identify life-threatening illnesses or injuries using information gained from telephone communication alone. It is also inappropriate to dispatch highly trained advanced life-support paramedics to routine cases where these skills are not required.

In order to have consistent, accurate dispatch of the appropriate resource in the optimal time-frame, many ambulance services are now using computer-aided dispatch programs. These computer programs have structured questions for use by call-takers with minimal medical training to rapidly identify a chief complaint, followed by subsequent yes/no questions to determine the acuity and severity of the illness. The answers to these questions allow the call taker or dispatcher to recommend the optimal skill level and speed of response. This computer algorithm is medically determined according to local protocols and practices, provides consistency of dispatch, and allows audit of protocol compliance for quality-assurance purposes.

Most ambulance services generally have at least four dispatch codes. A code 1 (or local equivalent terminology) is used for conditions that are considered immediately life threatening. For these, emergency warning devices (lights and sirens) are routinely used. The possibility of life-saving therapy arriving as soon as possible is judged as outweighing the potential hazard of a rapid response. In a code 2 (or equivalent) response, the condition is regarded as being urgent and emergency warning devices are used

only when traffic is heavy. In a code 3 response, an attendance by ambulance within an hour is deemed medically appropriate. Finally, non-emergency or booked calls are arranged at a designated time agreed by the caller and the ambulance service dispatcher.

CLINICAL SKILLS

Ambulance service protocols vary considerably around the world. In Australia, protocols are determined on a state-by-state basis by medical advisory committees. Since there are few randomized, controlled trials to provide evidence-based guidance for pre-hospital care, there is still much controversy and considerable variation in the ambulance skill set in different ambulance services, both in Australia and internationally.

Many ambulance services divide the medical response into a number of levels, dispatching ambulance officers trained in basic life support (including defibrillation) only to non-emergency or urgent cases and more highly trained ambulance officers (designated as advanced life-support paramedics or intensive-care paramedics) only to patients who are considered to have a life-threatening condition for which advanced life-support skills may be appropriate. In addition, ambulances services may co-respond with other emergency services (such as fire fighters) to provide rapid-response defibrillation.

The rationale for some of the pre-hospital interventions is outlined in the following sections.

TRAUMA CARE

Pre-hospital trauma care may be considered as either basic trauma life support (which includes clearing of the airway, administration of supplemental oxygen, control of external haemorrhage, spinal immobilization, splinting of fractures and the administration of inhaled analgesics) or advanced life support (ALS), which includes intubation of the airway, intravenous cannulation and fluid therapy, and the administration of intravenous analgesia.

Basic trauma life support

On arrival at the scene of the patient with suspected major trauma, ambulance officers are trained to perform an initial evaluation, which is similar to the approach that has been developed for physicians, namely consideration of dangers, response, airway, breathing, circulation, disability and exposure.

The initial assessment of the airway and breathing includes the application of cervical immobilization in patients who have a mechanism of injury that suggests a risk of spinal column instability. However, spinal immobilization of many patients with minimal risk of spinal cord injury is uncomfortable and possibly leads to unnecessary radiographic studies. Although decision instruments have been developed to identify patients in the emergency department who require radiographic imaging,[1] the extension of these guidelines to the pre-hospital setting is controversial. Therefore, ambulance officers are generally instructed to immobilize the neck in all cases of suspected spinal-column injury without reference to a clinical algorithm.

Advanced trauma life support

The role of advanced trauma life support, particularly intubation of the trachea and intravenous cannulation and fluid therapy by ambulance paramedics, is controversial.[2] Although these interventions may seem to be intuitively beneficial in the severely injured patient, there have been no studies that indicate that these improve patient outcome. Researchers for the Cochrane Library have examined the literature relating to trials of ALS in trauma and concluded that there is no evidence of benefit of pre-hospital ALS.[3] In fact, one meta-analysis of the available literature has indicated that the provision of advanced life support in trauma patients is associated with a significant increase in mortality rate.[4] The authors proposed that the performance of pre-hospital ALS skills leads to an increase in scene time and, thus, a delay in definite surgical care of the patient. On the other hand, none of the studies conducted has been sufficiently rigorous to allow definitive conclusions. Therefore, many ambulance services continue to authorize advanced airway management and intravenous fluid resuscitation in blunt trauma patients.

Airway management in severe head injury

Following severe head injury, many unconscious patients have decreased oxygenation and ventilation during pre-hospital care.[5] This may cause a secondary brain injury, leading to a worse neurological outcome. In addition, a depressed gag or cough reflex may lead to aspiration of vomit and this may cause a severe pneumonitis, which may be fatal or result in a prolonged stay in an intensive care unit. To prevent these complications of severe head injury, endotracheal intubation (ETI) may be performed. This facilitates the control of pO2 and pCO2, provides protection for the airway and is regarded as the standard of care for patients with Glasgow Coma Score <9 following severe head trauma after admission to hospital.[6]

Whilst it is intuitively beneficial that patients with severe head injury should undergo ETI as soon as possible following injury, the technique and timing of this procedure is controversial and the usefulness of ETI in the pre-hospital setting is uncertain. For example, in a retrospective study of 671 patients with severe head injury, ETI in the field was associated with a decrease in mortality rate from 56% to 36%.[7] On the other hand, another study showed that pre-hospital ETI was associated with worse outcome in trauma patients.[8] However, both of these studies were retrospective analyses of databases. Also, the use of drugs to facilitate ETI was not allowed. Therefore, it would be presumed that only the most severely head injured patients were able to be intubated. Another study of 456 patients with severe head injury who underwent pre-hospital ETI without any use of drugs showed that there were almost no survivors with good outcome.[9]

Most patients with severe head injury maintain a gag or cough reflex, and ETI requires the use of drugs to facilitate laryngoscopy and placement of the endotracheal tube. The usual approach involves the administration of both a sedative drug and a rapidly acting muscle-relaxant such as suxamethonium. In the USA, many ambulance services allow the use of suxamethonium.[10] However, this drug has not been introduced in most ambulance services in Australia or the UK. The perceived difficulty with the introduction of pre-hospital muscle-relaxants is the cost of the provision of initial training and skills maintenance to enable ambulance paramedics to undertake this complex procedure safely. There are also concerns that failed intubation in the pharmacologically paralyzed patient or unrecognized oesophageal intubation could worsen outcome or prove fatal.

It is unclear from the literature as to whether ETI using suxamethonium should be performed pre-hospital by ambulance paramedics or, alternatively, be performed in an emergency department by appropriately trained physicians. The studies currently available are case series. For example, a review of 1657 pre-hospital intubations using suxamethonium in a North American ambulance service showed that this was successful in 95.5%.[11] The patients with unsuccessful ETI (4.5%) were successfully managed with other means, such as bag/mask ventilation or cricothyroidotomy. Unrecognized oesophageal intubation occurred in 0.3%, prior to the introduction of capnography. The use of suxamethonium by ambulance paramedics on a helicopter emergency medical service in Victoria, Australia has also been reported.[12] This study found that 107/110 (97%) intubations using RSI were successful, and that failed intubations were satisfactorily managed using an alternative airway technique.

Although this evidence supports the relative safety of RSI in selected ambulance services, further studies are needed to demonstrate that this approach improves outcome, compared with RSI in the emergency department by physicians.

Intravenous fluid resuscitation for hypotension following trauma

Whereas intravenous (IV) fluid resuscitation has been shown to worsen outcome in penetrating trauma,[13] most major trauma in Australasia and the UK is blunt rather than penetrating and few patients require urgent surgical control of haemorrhage. Nevertheless, pre-hospital IV fluid resuscitation for patients with bleeding following blunt trauma remains controversial.[14]

Supporters of pre-hospital IV fluid therapy suggest that this treatment is intuitively beneficial and that any delay of this therapy increases the adverse effects of prolonged hypotension, which may result in end-organ ischaemia, leading to multi-organ system failure and increased morbidity and mortality. In particular, hypotension after severe head injury is associated with an adverse outcome.[5]

Opponents of pre-hospital IV fluid therapy suggest that IV fluid therapy prior to surgical control in patients with uncontrolled bleeding increases blood loss because of increased blood pressure, dilution coagulopathy and hypothermia from large volumes of unwarmed fluid. Any additional blood loss would increase transfusion requirements and could be associated with increased morbidity and mortality. Since it may be difficult for paramedics to determine whether bleeding following blunt trauma is controlled or uncontrolled in the pre-hospital setting, and the additional scene time for IV insertion may delay definitive surgical care, it has been proposed that IV fluid therapy should be delayed until arrival at the emergency department and surgical assessment.[14] In addition, ambulance paramedic training and skills maintenance in pre-hospital fluid therapy is very costly and may not be justified without some evidence of patient benefit.

Evidence for benefit of the administration of IV fluid to bleeding patients in the pre-hospital setting is lacking. Researchers for the Cochrane Library have reviewed the literature and found no evidence from any studies to support early or large volume IV fluid administration in trauma patients with suspected bleeding.[15] In addition, a meta-analysis of the available literature on pre-hospital IV fluid found an increase in mortality rates if pre-hospital IV fluid was given.[4]

On the other hand, animal models of uncontrolled bleeding suggest that minimum volume resuscitation (where fluid therapy is limited to a mean arterial blood pressure of 40 mmHg) is associated with improved outcome compared with either no IV fluid or standard resuscitation.[16] Therefore, it has been proposed that limited IV fluid be administered by paramedics to patients with hypotension following trauma.[17] This approach has been studied in the UK in 1309 patients where paramedics were randomly allocated to two groups, one administering 1000 mL of IV fluid to patients with suspected bleeding following trauma, to be repeated if necessary, and the other group to administering a 250 mL bolus of IV fluid only if the radial pulse was absent.[18] There was no difference overall in outcome between the groups.

Trauma analgesia

The administration of effective analgesia in the pre-hospital setting for traumatic pain remains a difficult issue for ambulance services. Many ambulance officers are not trained to administer IV therapy, and treatment options are, therefore, limited to inhaled or topical therapy.

Inhaled analgesic treatments include methoxyflurane and oxygen/nitrous oxide. However, while these are reasonably effective, there are concerns with the administration of these drugs in enclosed spaces such as ambulances because of the unquantified risk of repeated exposures of these analgesics to the ambulance officers.

Alternatively, the training of ambulance officers in the insertion of an IV cannula and administration of small increments of IV morphine is increasingly regarded as a feasible alternative to inhalation analgesia. Alternative routes of narcotic administration such as intranasal administration of fentanyl are the subject of current studies.[19]

Triage to a trauma service

Following initial assessment and treatment, the patient must be transported to an appropriate emergency department. In many cities, the patient is triaged to an emergency department that is staffed and equipped to provide definitive care. However, the accurate triage of patients for bypass of closer emergency departments requires the use of accurate scoring systems to avoid inappropriate transfer of minimally injured patients to trauma centres, or patients with occult serious injuries to centres which are unable to deliver definitive care.[20]

CARDIAC CARE

Cardiac arrest

In 1967, external defibrillation was introduced into pre-hospital care[21] and this led to the development of mobile coronary care units in many countries for the delivery of advanced cardiac care for the patient with suspected myocardial ischaemia. Protocols for the management of pre-hospital cardiac arrest are based on the concept of the 'chain of survival', which includes an immediate call to the emergency medical service, the performance of bystander CPR, early defibrillation and advanced cardiac life support (intubation and drug therapy).[22]

The patient in cardiac arrest represents the most time-critical patient attended by ambulance services. For the patient with ventricular fibrillation, each minute increase from time of collapse to defibrillation is associated with an increase in mortality of approximately 10%, with few survivors if the ambulance response is longer than 12 minutes.[23]

However, most ambulance services in Australia and the UK have response times that average 8–9 minutes. Since there may be 2 minutes between collapse and dispatch, and 2 minutes from arrival at the scene to delivery of the first defibrillation, overall times from collapse to defibrillation are approximately 12 minutes. Therefore, current survival rates for witnessed cardiac arrest due to defibrillation in most countries are low.[24] On the other hand, decreases in ambulance response times require very significant increases in ambulance resources and this is an expensive strategy in terms of cost per life saved.

Alternatively, response times to cardiac arrest patients may be reduced with the use of co-response by first responders equipped with defibrillators. Such first responder programmes have been introduced in Australia[25] and Canada[26] with promising results.

Acute coronary syndromes

Most ambulance services have protocols for the management of the patient with chest pain where the cause is suspected as an acute coronary syndrome. These protocols usually include supplemental oxygen, administration of glyceryl trinitrates and aspirin, followed by rapid transfer to an emergency department for definitive diagnosis and management. In addition, pain relief using morphine may be given by advanced life-support paramedics.

In order to decrease the time between symptom onset and administration of thrombolysis, the role of pre-hospital thrombolysis is currently being examined. While this may have a role in more rural and remote services, the current trend is the rapid transfer of appropriate patients to centres for interventional therapies.[27]

Cardiac arrhythmias arrhythmias

Some patients with an acute coronary syndrome develop a cardiac arrhythmia during ambulance care. Pulseless ventricular tachycardia is treated with immediate defibrillation, and lidocaine is commonly authorized for ventricular tachycardia where a pulse is palpable. However, the drug treatment of supraventricular tachycardia is more contro-

versial. Whilst the use of verapamil or adenosine appears to be equivalent in efficacy,[28] many ambulance services require the patient to be transported for 12-lead electrocardiography and management of the arrhythmia in an emergency department. Patients with bradycardia are safely treated with atropine.[29]

Pulmonary oedema

During myocardial ischaemia, the patient may develop pulmonary oedema and in these patients the use of oxygen, diuretics and glyceryl trinitrates is regarded as useful.

OTHER MEDICAL EMERGENCIES

Ambulance officers attend a wide range of other medical emergencies where pre-hospital treatment is considered life saving.

Hypoglycaemia

The patient with hypoglycaemia due to relative excess of exogenous insulin may be satisfactorily treated with dextrose, administered orally or intravenously. For ambulance officers who are not authorized to insert IV lines, or where IV access is not possible, the administration of intramuscular glucagon is also effective, although this is associated with an increase in the time to full consciousness.[30]

Narcotic overdose

Patients who illegally inject narcotic drugs may suffer coma and respiratory depression and this is readily reversed by naloxone. However, the administration of IV naloxone by paramedics is somewhat problematic, since IV access may be difficult and the half-life of IV naloxone may be shorter than the injected narcotic. If the patient awakens and leaves, there may also be a recurrence of sedation. Therefore, many ambulance services administer naloxone via the intramuscular or subcutaneous route. Whilst the absorption via this route may be slower, overall the time to return of normal respirations is equivalent.[31]

CONTROVERSIES AND FUTURE DIRECTIONS

❶ Advanced life support including intubation and intravenous fluid therapy by ambulance paramedics for the severe trauma patient is unproven and expensive.

❷ Advanced life support including intubation and anti-arrhythmic drug therapy by ambulance paramedics for the cardiac arrest patient is also unproven.

❸ The current provision of pre-hospital analgesia using inhaled analgesic drugs is not ideal, however, the use of alternatives such as intravenous or intranasal narcotics requires considerable training.

Anaphylaxis

Many patients with known severe anaphylaxis are prescribed adrenaline (epinephrine) by their physician for self-administration. The use of intramuscular adrenaline (epinephrine) by ambulance paramedics is also supported by studies that show that this is a safe and effective pre-hospital therapy.[32]

Seizures

Out-of-hospital status epilepticus is also regarded as a time critical medical emergency. The first-line treatment of status epilepticus is usually a benzodiazepine and the pre-hospital treatment using an IV benzodiazepine has been shown to be safe and effective.[33] There are also supportive data on the use of intramuscular midazolam[34] and there is now considerable experience of intramuscular midazolam in Australia suggesting that this is a safe and effective approach for seizures in adults.

REFERENCES

1. Hoffman JR, Mower WR, Wolfson AB, et al 2000 Validity of a set of clinical criteria to rule out injury to the cervical spine in patients with blunt trauma. National Emergency X-Radiography Utilization study (NEXUS) Group. New England Journal of Medicine 343: 94–9
2. Pepe PE 2000 Controversies in the pre-hospital

management of major trauma. Emergency Medicine 12: 180–9

3. Sethi D, Kwan I, Kelly AM, et al 2002 Advanced trauma life support training for ambulance crews (Cochrane Review). In: The Cochrane Library, Issue 2

4. Liberman M, Mulder D, Sampalis J, et al 2000 Advanced or basic life support for trauma: Meta-analysis and critical review of the literature. Journal of Trauma 49: 584–7

5. Chesnut RM 1997 Avoidance of hypotension: Conditio sine qua non of successful severe head-injury management. Journal of Trauma 42: S4–S9

6. The Brain Trauma Foundation 2000 The American Association of Neurological Surgeons. The Joint Section on Neurotrauma and Critical Care. Resuscitation of blood pressure and oxygenation. Journal of Neurotrauma 17: 471–8

7. Winchell RJ, Hoyt DB 1997 Endotracheal intubation in the field improves survival in patients with severe head injury. Archives of Surgery 132: 592–7

8. Murray JA, Demetriades D, Berne TV, et al 2000 Prehospital intubation in patients with severe head injury. Journal of Trauma 49: 1065–70

9. Lockey DJ, Davies G, Coats T 2001 Survival of trauma patients who have prehospital tracheal intubation without anaesthesia or muscle relaxants: observational study. British Medical Journal 323: 141

10. McDonald CC, Bailey B 1998 Out-of-hospital use of neuromuscular-blocking agents in the United States. Prehospital Emergency Care 2: 29–32

11. Wayne MA, Friedland E 1999 Prehospital use of succinylcholine: a 20 year review. Prehospital Emergency Care 3: 107–9

12. Bernard SA, Smith K, Foster S, Hogan P, Patrick I 2002 The use of rapid sequence intubation by ambulance paramedics for patients with severe head injury. Emergency Medicine 14: 406–11

13. Bickell W, Pepe P, Mattox K, et al 1994 Immediate versus delayed fluid resuscitation for hypotensive patients with penetrating torso injuries. New England Journal of Medicine 331: 1105

14. Roberts I, Evans P, Bunn F, Kwan I, Crowhurst E 2001 is the normalization of blood pressure in bleeding trauma patients harmful? Lancet 357: 385–7

15. Kwan I, Bunn F, Roberts I, et al 2002 Timing and volume of fluid administration for patients with bleeding following trauma (Cochrane Review). In: The Cochrane Library, Issue 2

16. Capone A 1995 Treatment of uncontrolled hemorrhagic shock: Improved outcome with fluid restriction. Journal of American College of Surgeons 180: 49

17. Greaves I, Porter KM, Revell MP 2002 Fluid resuscitation in pre-hospital trauma care: A consensus view. Journal of the Royal College of Surgeons, Edinburgh 47: 451–7

18. Turner J, Nicholl J, Webber L, et al 2000 A randomized, controlled trial of prehospital intravenous fluid replacement therapy in serious trauma. Health Technology Assessment 4: 1–57

19. DeVellis P, Thomas SH, Wedel SK 1998 Prehospital and emergency department analgesia for air-transported patients with fractures. Prehospital Emergency Care 2: 293–6

20. Tamim H, Joseph L, Mulder D, Battista RN, Lavoie A, Sampalis JS 2002 field triage of trauma patients: improving on the Prehospital Index. American Journal of Emergency Medicine 20: 170–6

21. Baskett TF, Baskett PJ 2001 Frank Pantridge and mobile coronary care. Resuscitation 48: 99–104

22. Cummins RO, Ornato JP, Thies WH, Pepe PE 1991 Improving survival from sudden cardiac arrest: The "chain of survival" concept. A statement for health professionals from the advanced cardiac life-support subcommittee and the emergency cardiac care committee, American Heart Association. Circulation 83: 1832–47

23. Larsen MP, Kizenberg MS, Cummins RO, Hallestrom AP, et al 1993 Predicting survival from out-of-hospital cardiac arrest: A graphic model. Annals of Emergency Medicine 22: 1652–8

24. Bernard SA 1998 Outcome from prehospital cardiac arrest in Melbourne, Australia. Emergency Medicine 10: 25–9

25. Smith KL, McNeill JJ and the Emergency Medical Response Steering Committee, et al 2002 Cardiac arrests treated by ambulance paramedics and fire fighters. Medical Journal of Australia 177: 305–9

26. Stiells IG, Wells GA, Field BJ, et al 1999 Improved out-of-hospital cardiac arrest survival through the inexpensive optimization of an existing defibrillation program. Journal of the American Medical Association 281: 1175–81

27. Stone GW 2002 Primary angioplasty versus "earlier" thrombolysis-time for a wake-up call. Lancet 360: 814–5

28. Madsen CD, Pointer JE, Lynch TG 1995 A comparison of adenosine and verapamil for the treatment of supraventricular tachycardia in the prehospital setting. Annals of Emergency Medicine 25: 649–55

29. Swart G, Brady WJ Jr, DeBehnke DJ, Ma OJ, Aufderheide TP 1999 Acute myocardial infarction complicated by hemodynamically unstable bradyarrhythmia: prehospital and ED treatment with atropine. American Journal of Emergency Medicine 17: 647–52

30. Howell MA, Guly HR 1997 A comparison of glucagon and glucose in prehospital hypoglycaemia. Journal of Accident and Emergency Medicine 14: 30–2

31. Wanger K, Brough L, Macmillan I, Goulding J, MacPhail I, Christenson JM 1998 Intravenous vs subcutaneous naloxone for out-of-hospital management of presumed opioid overdose. Academic Emergency Medicine 5: 293–9

32. Barton ED, Ramos J, Colwell C, Benson J, Baily J, Dunn W 2002 Intranasal administration of naloxone by paramedics. Prehospital Emergency Care 6: 54–8

33. Safdar B, Cone DC, Pham KT 2001 Subcutaneous epinephrine in the prehospital setting. Prehospital Emergency Care 5: 200–7

34. Alldredge BK., Gelb AM., Isaacs SM, et al 2001 A Comparison of lorazepam, diazepam, and placebo for the treatment of out-of-hospital status epilepticus. New England Journal of Medicine 345: 631–7

35. Vilke GM, Sharieff GQ, Marino A, Gerhart AE, Chan TC 2002 Midazolam for the treatment of out-of-hospital pediatric seizures. Prehospital Emergency Care 6: 215–7

25.2 RETRIEVAL

SALOMON ZALSTEIN

ESSENTIALS

1 Transport of critically ill or injured patients is associated with significant adverse events and physiological derangements.

2 Such events are minimized if the patient is transferred after careful assessment and preparation by a specifically trained medical team.

3 The decision to transfer should be made as early as possible.

4 Good communication between all those involved in the retrieval process is the key to efficient transfer.

5 All procedures likely to be needed during transport should be performed prior to moving the patient.

6 Retrieval teams are intended to augment the capabilities of ambulance personnel and to integrate with ambulance services.

DEFINITION

The verb retrieve has several meanings: to find and bring in; to recover or rescue; to repair or set right; or to restore to a flourishing state.[1] In the context of medical care, retrieval may be seen to be consistent with the spirit of all these definitions. Generally, the term is used to indicate the use of an expert team to assess, stabilize, transport and escort patients with severe injury or critical illness. An essential part of the retrieval process is early provision of specialized advice to the health-care providers at the patient's side.

Retrieval may at times be continuous with rescue and is occasionally qualified by the description 'primary' and 'secondary' to indicate those patients who are still at 'scene' on the one hand, and those who have received initial attention at a health-care facility of some sort, on the other. While such differentiation is generally of value in assessing the need for and urgency of transfer, and potentially the composition of the retrieval team, rigid adherence to such a classification can have a negative impact. It may be incorrectly considered that secondary retrieval missions are always less urgent than primary missions, whereas experience has shown that secondary retrievals may, on occasion, be that in name only due to the poor level of care available at the referring facility.

INDICATIONS FOR RETRIEVAL

Transfer of patients is common and occurs for a variety of reasons. These usually are based on the need for care not commonly available in remote and rural areas (such as major trauma services, burns, neurosurgery, cardiac surgery, renal medicine, transplantation, interventional cardiology or high level intensive care) due to centralization of advanced services. Non-clinical reasons for retrieval include considerations such as equity of access to specialized health services, support of local health service providers and avoidance of depletion of local resources in the process of transferring the patient.

Implicit in all cases is that the patient is being transferred to a higher level of care, or for specialized or definitive care. Selection of patients for retrieval and determining its priority or urgency is an area open to discussion. There are few if any clear-cut rules. The decision to use a retrieval team must be based on a sound knowledge of the clinical capabilities and training of local ambulance personnel, the clinical condition of the patient in the context of local medical resources, indicating both the urgency and complexity of the retrieval, and the time

required, distance to be travelled and mode of transport available. The use of physiologically based sickness scoring systems, common in intensive care units, has been studied but not widely adopted as a triaging tool for patients requiring transport.[2–5] Such scoring systems may be of use in quality-assurance processes.[6,7] The use of simpler classification systems has been described, but these have been used for retrospective analysis rather than triage.[8,9]

Thus retrieval should be considered for patients with severe injury or illness who require highly specialized management not available at the point of referral and whose condition is of such complexity as to require a level of care during the transport phase that cannot be provided by ambulance personnel within their normal scope of practice (see below).

LEVEL OF CARE AND TEAM COMPOSITION

Patients are transferred between hospitals so they may be provided with a higher level of care than is available at the source.

Patients with serious illness exhibit pathophysiological responses to movement, either within hospital or between them. Several studies over many years have shown that transporting critically ill or injured patients may be associated with adverse events during transport and with adverse outcomes. Such negative events are more likely when patients are transported in the care of junior staff and are avoided by the use of a specialist transport (retrieval) team, which has training and experience in advanced critical care management in addition to the specific problems of the transport environment.[2,6,10–16] Others have commented that inter-hospital transport is dangerous because the patient's illness may be incompletely defined and the degree of physiological stability not established. Added to this is the difficulty of managing a critically ill patient in the transport environment.[5] Conversely, it has been shown that potentially unstable

patients with severe illness can be safely transferred by highly skilled medical staff employing adequate preparation and an appropriate vehicle and equipment.[9,17,18] At times this may require very complex equipment and logistics, such as an extracorporeal membrane oxygenator (ECMO), a perfusionist team member and multi-vehicle support.[19,20]

The level of training and scope of practice of paramedics varies among ambulance services from different regions within Australasia, and more so among countries internationally. This makes applicability of studies difficult; however, in general, pre-hospital provider education is not directed at the care of the patient with complex multi-system physiological derangements.

There is wide acceptance of the principle that the patient with critical illness or injury undergoing interhospital transport to a higher level of care should receive a standard of care during that transport that exceeds that available at the referring hospital and approaches that of the receiving facility, in other words, the care provided by medical staffed retrieval teams specifically trained and equipped for this purpose. This principle is accepted internationally and published in the guidelines of various overseas organizations,[22–24] and within Australasia in the joint document of the Joint Faculty of Intensive Care Medicine, the Australian and New Zealand College of Anaesthetists and the Australasian College for Emergency Medicine (JFICM/ANZCA/ACEM).[25] Thus, while retrieval teams are not intended to replace ambulance and paramedic services, a medically staffed retrieval team has a wider range of management options available to them and is able to perform major procedures in rural hospitals.[21] It is, therefore, intended to augment and integrate with paramedic capabilities. Medical retrieval should be considered the appropriate level of care during transport of the critically ill.

What is far less clear is ideal team composition in cases of primary retrieval, particularly in trauma. Examination of the literature shows that the debate is not concluded.[26-29] Different systems in different States and countries make valid comparisons problematic and hence definite conclusions are difficult to draw.

TRANSPORT PLATFORMS

There are three platforms commonly used in retrieval: road vehicle, fixed wing aircraft and rotary wing aircraft.

Each transport platform has specific advantages and disadvantages (Table 25.2.1).[30] Consideration of these should be an integral part of both the establishment of a retrieval service or system and the planning of individual retrieval missions. A mature retrieval service will have predetermined mission criteria for the use of each of these platforms and these will vary with local conditions.

The most important factors in developing these predetermined criteria are distance and time, such that there are three concentric zones:

1. Road – within 50 km, or 60 minutes
2. Helicopter – usually between 50 to 400 km
3. Fixed wing – generally greater than 400 km.

Local factors such as road system, time of day and anticipated traffic conditions, relative availability of different transport assets, proximity to airports, and availability of hospital helipads mean that each system must develop its own vehicle selection criteria.

Superimposed on these general and predetermined criteria are specific issues such as weather conditions, and individual patient or mission requirements. For instance, very obese patients may be too large for some helicopters.

Ideally, charges to the users of the system (that is the referring and receiving hospitals) should be the same for all transport platforms. In this way, decisions can be made on clinical and operational factors, not primarily on cost.

Regardless of the platform type, the retrieval service should have access to vehicles or aircraft specifically configured for transport of critically ill patients. Decisions about platform are not simply medical but must be made with full knowledge and understanding of operational constraints and availability.

Table 25.2.1 Transport platforms advantages and disadvantages		
Platform	Advantages	Disadvantages
Road vehicle - may be a standard ambulance vehicle or a vehicle specifically built or modified for retrieval missions	Able to provide 'door-to-door' service Commonly available including occasional need for multiple vehicles Requires minimal training/orientation of retrieval team Relatively inexpensive to acquire, modify equipment and operate No limitations or exclusions regarding illness or injury type Able to function in virtually all weather conditions Able to travel at very slow speed if required Able to stop if necessary for patient care Can easily divert to another facility Can be fitted out to accommodate specific requirements or equipment	Prolonged transport/out of hospital time, dependent on traffic and road conditions, with implications for equipment battery life and alterations in patient status Noise and vibration make some assessments impossible Repetitive acceleration/deceleration with implications on alterations to patient physiology or pain Limitation of AC power supply, particularly for long transfers
Rotary wing aircraft	Relatively high speed (2–3 times ground vehicle) No runway/airport requirement Rapid initiation (short time to launch) Able to access remote or difficulty locations Can be 'door-to-door' if helipad access available	High acquisition, fit out and operating cost Requires helipad or unobstructed landing area Space and weight limitations Limited access to patient Major weather and altitude limitations Unable to be pressurized Noise and vibration can interfere with patient physiology, assessment and monitoring equipment Limitations of electrical supply All crew members must be appropriately trained
Fixed wing aircraft	High speed/long range Generally smooth transport (if pressurized) May be able to be pressurized Less noise and vibration than rotary wing	Longer time to initiation of flight due to airport location, flight plan requirements Requires runway, loading/unloading and additional road transport to/from aircraft Some weather limitations Potential impact of altitude and hypoxia on some illnesses/injuries, and retrieval team Significant acquisition, fit out and operating cost All crew members must be appropriately trained Aircraft not dedicated to the task may have electrical supply limitations Space more limited than in road vehicle

EMERGENCY MEDICINE SYSTEMS

Road vehicle

One of the main advantages of this platform is the ready availability of the standard ambulance, however, a vehicle specifically equipped and configured for retrieval is preferable (see Equipment and vehicle fit out). The major disadvantage is dependence on traffic and road conditions, often resulting in long response times (the time taken for the retrieval team to arrive at the point of referral) and prolonged periods during which the patient is outside hospital. Consequently, road transport becomes less desirable where the transport time for each of the outbound and inbound legs of the retrieval exceed 60 minutes. However, in poor weather, road transport may be the only option.

Helicopter (rotary wing aircraft)

This is the most expensive mode of transport. The operating range (the radius or outward leg only) is dependent on type and model, flight and weather conditions, load carried and re-fuelling availability, but is usually considered to be 50 to 400 km at speeds of 120 to 150 knots (approx. 200 to 280 km/h). Although its flight speed is less than that of fixed wing aircraft, by eliminating the need for additional road transfer, this platform can provide the fastest 'door-to-door' transport even at the limit of its operating range. It is, thus, ideally suited for transfer of the sickest patients provided helicopter access exists at both referring and receiving hospital. Conversely, it is generally operationally and economically unwarranted to use this mode of transport for distances of less than 50 km or flight times of less than 30 minutes. This is particularly true in the absence of a hospital helicopter landing area as the additional transfers by road may negate the speed advantage over road transport. However, local geography, road and traffic conditions may mean that flights of only 10 or 15 minutes are necessary for expeditious transfer. The decision to use helicopter or fixed wing aircraft in any given circumstance must be based on a thorough understanding of the operational capabilities of the particular aircraft to be used and on a detailed knowledge of local facilities.

Fixed wing aircraft

This mode provides the fastest transport over the longest distances. Turboprop aircraft commonly used in Australasia cruise at speeds of 250 knots, while small jets are capable of speeds in excess of 400 knots. The major disadvantages are the need for additional road transport to and from the aircraft and the long initiation time. Over longer distances this factor is offset by the faster speed. Careful consideration must be given to the patient's clinical condition as some may be negatively affected by altitude (Table 25.2.2). Many aircraft are now capable of having the cabin pressurized to sea level pressure, circumventing these problems.

EQUIPMENT AND VEHICLE FIT OUT

In order to provide the level of care required, a retrieval service (and the platforms used) must be appropriately equipped. The joint policy statement of JFICM/ANZCA/ACEM[25] includes an equipment list which is quite comprehensive. Others have published standards on vehicle fit out as well as equipment.[23,24,31]

Oxygen

Adequate oxygen must be available. If the patient is mechanically ventilated at the referral source then simple calculation of the minute volume and the expected duration of the transfer permits an estimate of the volume of oxygen required. A safety margin of at least 100% should be factored in to the calculation, keeping in mind that transport times are often greatly underestimated by those not regularly involved in transport

Ventilator

Several transport ventilators are commercially available. Ideally, these should be lightweight, simple to operate, robust and reliable. They should permit different ventilation modes, varying FiO_2, addition of PEEP and have disconnect, low supply pressure, high airway pressure alarms as a minimum.

Monitor/defibrillator

Monitoring of vital parameters as recommended by JFICM/ANZCA/ACEM[25] is essential: ECG, SaO_2, and $ETCO_2$ for ventilated patients, invasive BP, CVP and temperature. The ability to record is highly desirable. Defibrillation in aircraft can be dangerous because of interference with avionics. The pilot must be informed if the patient requires defibrillation. In any transport vehicle it is safest to use adhesive defibrillator pads

Table 25.2.2 Conditions which may be adversely affected by altitude

Condition	Effect of altitude
Dysbarism	Reduced pressure increases nitrogen coming out of solution
Dependence on high oxygen concentration	Falling pO_2 with altitude increases need for supplemental oxygen or endotracheal intubation
Penetrating eye injury	Extrusion of eye contents*
Bowel obstruction	Worsening dilatation/distension
Air in body cavity (without drainage): Pneumothorax Pneumocranium Pneumoperitoneum	Increase size and pressure in the cavity concerned
Use of cylindrical splints (casts)	May cause compartment syndrome

* May also occur with vomiting because of motion sickness in flight, pain, or analgaesic medication

and 'hands-free' defibrillation, allowing the person performing the defibrillation to remain at a distance from the patient.

Electrical power

Adequate electrical power to allow continuous operation of all equipment for the full duration of the retrieval should be available. This may be from a generator or AC inverter.

Infusion pumps

Syringe pumps are smaller and lighter but less accurate than large infusion pumps, and spring operated syringe drivers are suitable only for non-critical infusions of medications the rate of which is to be constant throughout the transfer.

Suction

Suction must be constantly available. Some systems lose power when motors are switched off. Ideally, a second system, which is not reliant on electrical or motor power of the transport platform, should be available in case the primary system fails.

Seating

There must be adequate seating for all members. This must allow the occupants to provide care to the patient while remaining seat-belted.[31]

Lighting

This must be adequate for providing care and completing documentation but should also be able to be dimmed or turned off for patient comfort and must be able to be screened from the driver or pilot for safe night operations.

Alarms

In helicopters with high levels of ambient noise, consideration should be given to wiring audio alarms of monitors through the intercom system. It has been repeatedly demonstrated that audio alarms are perceived far sooner than visual alarms.

Mounting for equipment

Equipment restraint is covered by existing ambulance standards.[32] The mounting mechanism must be stable enough to withstand sudden direction changes or collision while remaining accessible to retrieval team members during transport. A device, which enables equipment to be moved together with the patient at loading and unloading, reduces the risk of equipment disconnection and enhances efficient operation, but total weight and weight distribution must be considered in design and use of such devices.[33–35]

Equipment in aircraft

All equipment to be used or carried in aircraft must be certified as meeting the standards set by aviation authorities relating to adequate fixation and absence of electrical interference with avionics.

ORGANIZATION, STAFFING AND FUNDING

Several different models exist within Australasia and internationally. Each model has its unique attractions and disadvantages. Staffing based on an individual hospital unit or department (such as intensive care or emergency department) allows communication and co-ordination and the concentration of equipment, training, expertise and research in one area. The disadvantage for the department is the necessity of ensuring that there is sufficient staffing for retrieval supernumerary to the normal requirements of that department, which may pose an organizational and financial burden. In order to economize, extra staff may not be employed and staff may be expected to undertake other duties between retrievals. While this mode of staffing is less expensive, it can lead to considerable disruption to the parent unit if retrievals are frequent. This model is, therefore, most suitable for small volume systems. Similar arguments apply to trans-departmental services within single institutions. In some States, the retrieval service is centrally co-ordinated and tasked by a State supported authority with retrieval staff being employed by that authority or by individual organizations that are not institution based. Funding in these circumstances is entirely by State government in some cases or supported by corporate sponsorship to varying degrees in others. The advantage of a non-institutional organization is that retrieval staff are not caught in the dilemma of divided responsibility and are able to dedicate their attention entirely to retrieval when on duty. This mode of staffing will result in shorter response times, but is more expensive. It is, therefore, more appropriate for larger retrieval systems, where there are economies of scale. This mode of staffing is also more appropriate if the system undertakes primary missions which are usually time critical in nature. As with any other emergency service, there is a compromise between immediate availability and efficiency, and it is accepted that there is not full utilization of the staff.

An important part of a retrieval system is the education of practitioners in the service area of the system to seek consultation early and thus allow the earliest possible mobilization of the retrieval team. The referring practitioners, conversely, must be secure in the knowledge that the system will provide a timely and efficient service when called upon.

STAFF TRAINING

Retrieval services generally draw their physician team members from amongst specialty groups that commonly manage critically ill patients. Emergency physicians, intensive-care physicians and anaesthetists are particularly suited to such work on the basis of their specialist training, knowledge and skills. The retrieval setting, however, is significantly different from the normal occupational environment of these specialists and poses specific challenges. The retrieval team member must be capable of working in an unusual environment, with unfamiliar staff and often in the cramped surroundings of a transport vehicle or aircraft.[21] Furthermore, the equipment used in retrieval may be unique to that environment and unfamiliarity reduces the effectiveness and efficiency of the team and increases risks to the patient and the crew. Thus, regardless of the medical specialty, specific training in retrieval is essential. The aircraft environment poses challenges and risks of its own (see Risks of Retrieval) and all crew members involved in aeromedical work must be physically capable and appropriately trained to work in this environment without posing an increased risk to their patient, other crew members or themselves.

THE RETRIEVAL PROCESS

Co-ordnation

This may be central or institutionally based. Central co-ordination reduces inter-institutional rivalries and allows for the most efficient use of all available hospital and transport resources and eliminates confusion at the point of referral regarding which organization to contact. Regardless of the model, an ideal system must be well co-ordinated and have a single, well publicized telephone number for access to the service. This number must be operational on a 24 hour, 7-day basis and calling the number should allow rapid access to the three major components of a modern retrieval service:

- Specialist advice (which may avoid the need for retrieval)
- Bed finding of an appropriate bed and specialist service
- Initiation of retrieval when necessary.

It should be stressed that these three processes often occur concurrently. Since the transport phase itself cannot be significantly shortened, it is imperative that this be commenced as soon as possible, and not wait until allocation of a hospital or a bed.

Communication

High-quality communication throughout all phases is essential for the smooth conduct of a retrieval mission. Automatic recording of all communications is ideal for audit and review purposes. Effective co-ordination of a retrieval mission requires good communication between all those involved in the mission: the mission co-ordinator, the referral source, the retrieval organization and team members, ambulance service(s) that may be required for some or all phases of the transfer, and the receiving institution and physician. This may best be achieved by a conference call system, allowing the referring doctor to make a single call rather than a frustrating and time-consuming series of calls, while often simultaneously trying to care for the patient.

It is essential that the retrieval team be in direct and constant communication with the referring practitioner. Prior to their arrival, direct discussion of the case between the referring practitioner and the retrieval team may lead to changes in treatment and preparations which expedite the transfer. It is also vital that during all phases of the mission there is the capability for direct and efficient communication between the retrieval doctor, the referring hospital and the receiving unit. This is particularly important where the patient may need urgent treatment or intervention upon arrival at the receiving hospital.

Handover

A careful and thorough handover of the patient should occur upon arrival of the retrieval team. The team should thoroughly understand all the case history, pre-existing medical conditions of relevance and all interventions and management thus far. Investigation results available and imaging should be examined. A similar process will occur at the receiving hospital.

Patient preparation

The retrieval doctor must make a thorough assessment of the patient. A useful format is the standard 'airway, breathing, circulation' approach as for resuscitation. At each step assessment of the adequacy or stability of the particular area, whether intervention is necessary or whether the intervention already provided is sufficiently stable for transport. While undertaking this process, the retrieval doctor must keep in mind the principles of safe transport of critically ill patients that have been articulated by others:[36,37]

- Treatment is not possible in a moving vehicle.
  The simplest tasks, such as measuring blood pressure by auscultation or listening to breath sounds, become extremely difficult or impossible in a moving vehicle due to noise, movement and vibration. Insertion of intravenous cannulae or an endotracheal tube is even more testing.
- Any procedures that may be needed should be completed before moving the patient.
  This is the corollary of the first principle. Other procedures which may be termed 'safety measures' should also be performed. These include extra intravenous access lines for emergencies, and definitive airway management (see below).
- Careful and unhurried assessment, stabilization and preparation are necessary before transfer. The aim is to move the patient at normal road speeds (for road transfers) rather than using 'lights and sirens'. However, prolonged time at the scene may also be counterproductive. The time spent assessing and stabilizing the patient should be balanced against the priority of minimizing the time until the patient arrives at the receiving hospital, keeping in mind the expected duration of the journey and the ability to stop for management procedures or divert to an alternate destination.
- Full monitoring is essential. Monitoring as recommended by JFICM/ANZCA /ACEM guidelines should be commenced as early as possible during the preparation phase and continued throughout the transfer.

Assessment and stabilization

Airway and breathing

The patient must have a clear and adequately protected airway. Patients who may not need endotracheal intubation while being closely observed in the emergency department or intensive care unit often need intubation during transport, in line with the first principle above. Similarly, patients who may be appropriately managed with the use of devices to provide high inspired oxygen or by non-invasive ventilation often need mechanical ventilation during transport. This is particularly so during air transport. While pressurized aircraft are capable of cabin pressurization to sea level pressure, this is at the cost of increased fuel consumption. Thus, the cabin is usually kept at a pressure equivalent to an altitude of 6000 or 7000 feet (while flying at altitudes in excess of 20 000 feet), producing a PaO_2 of about 60 mmHg in the normal subject. Any special requirements regarding pressurisation should be anticipated and communicated to the pilot as soon as possible.

Oxygen supplies must be adequate (see Equipment and vehicle fit out) and, with mechanically ventilated patients, an alternative means of ventilation such as a bag-valve device must be always to hand.

In making respiratory system assessment, the potential need for an intercostal catheter should be considered in patients such as those with chest trauma who are mechanically ventilated. At the cabin pressures mentioned, a pneumothorax will increase in size by about one-third. In patients with intercostal catheters in place, there is often insufficient height between the stretcher and the floor of the vehicle to permit safe use of an under water seal drain. A Heimlich valve is usually required.

Circulation

Patients must have adequate venous access to permit fluid and drug administration. At least two peripheral cannulae should be available and checked for patency, ensuring that at least one will be usable should one fail in an emergency. Whenever possible, central access should be used to make accurate assessment of volume status as such an assessment, including the possible need for blood, is crucial to safe transport. Critically ill patients tolerate movement poorly and are prone to episodes of hypotension unless hypervolaemic.[38] Concurrently with fluid resuscitation is the need to ensure that all haemorrhage is adequately controlled. In cases where the patient must be transported over long distances, a surgical procedure may be required to achieve such control before transport. The need for pharmacological support of blood pressure must be carefully considered before departing. Blood pressure cannot be accurately measured without an arterial line for direct measurement, so this must also be established.

Disability

The patient's baseline neurological status should be documented. Patients who are adequately sedated experience less blood pressure and possibly ICP fluctuation, so attention must be given to ensuring that this is done. Protection of the spine in trauma patients is essential as it is assumed that proper clearance of the spine is not possible without adequate imaging and clinical assessment of the conscious, co-operative patient.

Extremities

All injured limbs must be splinted or bandaged while permitting observation of vascular status. During air transport, cylindrical splints (such as plaster casts) may predispose to compartment syndrome due to swelling of the limb beneath the cast.

Exposure

Transport increases the likelihood of hyper- or hypothermia in the patient. This is particularly true for sedated or pharmacologically paralyzed patients who are functionally poikilothermic, and even more so for those transported by air. Patients must be appropriately 'packaged' in sheets and blankets while still permitting rapid access to venous access points or to injuries for observation.

Tubes

Intubated patients must have gastric and bladder catheters. A careful check should be made of all lines and tubes to ensure that they are patent and properly secured. Any line not required should be either removed or capped.

Infusions

There must be an adequate supply of all fluids and infusions, clearly labelled.

Documentation

Prior to departing the point of referral, a check should be made that all documentation and X-rays have been packaged with the patient. An accurate record of all interventions and observations en route is essential.

LIMITATIONS

There is good evidence that, given adequate time and sufficient resources, retrieval services can transfer even the most critically ill patients requiring the highest level of technological support in transit.[19,20] Retrieval is, therefore, limited only by the flexibility of the organization and the availability of adequate support.

RISKS OF RETRIEVAL

All forms of patient transport are associated with risks. Patient transfer itself poses a risk of physiological deterioration. This is minimized by appropriate preparation, stabilization and en-route monitoring by a highly trained and experienced retrieval team.

There are risks specific to the mode of transport and the way that such transport is used. Ambulances, like all vehicles, are at risk of collision whenever on the road. However, operation of ambulances in emergency mode (with use of lights and sirens and without strict adherence to road laws) is associated with increased collision risk, particularly at intersections. Furthermore, those in the rear compartment of the ambulance, often not adequately restrained, have a 2.8 times greater risk of death or injury than those seated in the front of the vehicle.[39]

There are physical and emotional pressures that are peculiar to the aviation environment know as the 'stresses of

Table 25.2.3 The stresses of flight[43]
1 Hypoxia
2 Temperature
3 Vibration
4 Noise
5 Acceleration/deceleration forces
6 Third spacing
7 Barotrauma
8 Dehydration/humidity
9 Fatigue

flight' (Table 25.2.3). These affect both the patient and the personnel conducting the transfer. Transfer by air is particularly hazardous to patients with conditions that may be aggravated by changes in altitude, in particular those in which gas entrapment in body cavities or organs is a feature (Table 25.2.2). The use of pressurized fixed-wing aircraft or flight at low altitude may avoid altitude-related complications.

Among air transports, helicopters have long been viewed as the most dangerous. In the USA, where helicopters are widely used in emergency medical services (or ambulance) work, several studies have shown that the risk is significant. The accident rate for emergency medical sevice helicopters is 2 to 3 times the rate for commercial (air taxi) operations.[40,41] It has also been shown that over 60% of these are due to pilot-associated (rather than mechanical) factors, that organizations that fly often are less likely to have accidents, and that, of those crashes occurring on missions classified as inter-hospital transfers, over 80% were during the phase of travelling to the patient or returning to the receiving hospital with the patient on board. Only 16% occurred during the 'return to base' leg of the mission. The implication that the sense of urgency involved played a part in these crashes is quite apparent.[40,42] It is imperative that neither the medical team nor the organization's management place pressure on the pilot to undertake a mission in marginal weather conditions.

CONTROVERSIES AND FUTURE DIRECTIONS

❶ The optimal retrieval team composition for primary transport of trauma patients is controversial. The debate rages as some argue that trauma patients are more dependent on time to definitive treatment and others contend that medical personnel can provide better care at the scene than paramedics.

❷ The use of scarce intensive care resources for the 'hopeless' patient is debated. The questions being asked are 'should these patients be admitted to an intensive care unit?', which leads to the question of whether such patients should be retrieved. An appropriate triaging tool would assist in making such difficult decisions.

❸ The optimal staffing models of retrieval services remain to be determined. Should these be centrally based or hospital based? Both models operate successfully in Australasia.

The decision when to fly (and when not to fly) must remain solely with the pilot. Clinical urgency does not make unsafe conditions safe.

REFERENCES

1. Hughes J, Michell P, Ramson W (eds) 1992 The Australian Concise Oxford Dictionary. Oxford University Press, Melbourne
2. Bion J, Edlin S, Ramsay G, McCabe S, Ledingham I M 1985 Validation of a prognostic score in critically ill patients undergoing transport. British Medical Journal 291: 432–4
3. Pollack M, Ruttimann U, Getson P 1988 Pediatric risk of mortality (PRISM) score. Critical Care Medicine 16: 1110–6
4. Orr R, Venkataraman S, Cinoman M, Hogue B, Singleton C, McCloskey K 1994 Pretransport pediatric risk of mortality (PRISM) score underestimates the requirement for intensive care or major interventions during interhospital transport. Critical Care Medicine 22: 101–7
5. Kanter R, Tompkins J 1989 Adverse events during interhospital transport: Physiological deterioration associated with pretransport severity of illness. Paediatrics 84: 43–48
6. Bion J, Wilson I, Taylor P 1988 Transporting critically ill patients by ambulance: Audit by sickness scoring. British Medical Journal 296: 170
7. Reeve W, Runcie C, Reidy J, Wallace P 1990 Current practice in transferring critically ill patients among hospitals in the West of Scotland. British Medical Journal 300: 85–7
8. Smith D, Hackel A 1983 Selection criteria for pediatric critical care transport teams. Critical Care Medicine 11(1): 10–2
9. Ehrenwerth J, Sorbo S, Hackel A 1986 Transport of critically ill adults. Critical Care Medicine 14(6): 543–7
10. Gentleman D, Jennett B 1981 Hazards of inter-hospital transfer of comatose head-injured patients. The Lancet 2: 853–5
11. Waddell G, Scott P, Lees N, Ledingham I M 1975 Effects of ambulance transport in critically ill patients. British Medical Journal 1: 386–9
12. Ridley S, Carter R 1989 The effects of secondary transfer on critically ill patients. Anaesthesia 44: 822–7
13. Smith I, Fleming S, Cernaianu A 1990 Mishaps during transport from the intensive care unit. Critical Care Medicine 18: 278–81
14. Deane S, Gaudry P, Woods W, Read C, McNeil R 1990 Interhospital transfer in the management of acute trauma. Australia and New Zealand Journal of Surgery 60: 441–6
15. Andrews P, Piper I, Dearden N, Miller J 1990 Secondary insults during intrahospital transport of head-injured patients. The Lancet 335: 327–30
16. Lambert S, Willett K1 1993 Transfer of multiply-injured patients for neurosurgical opinion: A study of the adequacy of assessment and resuscitation. Injury 24: 333–6
17. Gebremichael M, Borg U, Habashi N, et al 2000 Interhospital transport of the extremely ill patient: The mobile intensive care unit. Critical Care Medicine 28: 79–85
18. Valenzuela R, Criss E A, Copass M K, Luna G, Rice C 1990 Critical care air transportation of the severely injured: Does long distance transport adversely affect survival? Annals of Emergency Medicine 19: 169–72
19. Rosengarten A, Rosalion A, Epstein J, Kelly A 2000 Management of a patient with complete rupture of a main bronchus in a community hospital. Medical Journal of Australia 172: 430–3
20. Rosengarten A, Elmore P, Epstein J 2002 Long distance road transport of a patient with Wegener's granulomatosis and respiratory failure using extracorporeal membrane oxygenation. Emergency Medicine 14: 181–7
21. Gilligan J, Griggs W, Jelly M, et al 1999 Mobile intensive care services in rural South Australia. Medical Journal of Australia 171: 617–20
22. Jastremski M, Hitchens M, Thompson M et al. 1993 Guidelines Committee of the American College of Critical Care Medicine; Society of Critical Care Medicine and American Association of Critical-care Nurses Transfer Guidelines Taskforce. Guidelines for transfer of critically ill patients. Critical Care Medicine 21: 931–7
23. Bristow A, Baskett P, Dalton M, Ediss P 1991 Medical helicopter systems-recommended minimum standards for patient management. Journal of the Royal Society of Medicine 84f: 242–4
24. Bristow A, Baskett P, Byrne N, Craig K 1992 A report-recommended standards for UK fixed wing medical transport systems and for patient management during transfer by fixed wing aircraft. Journal of the Royal Society of Medicine 85: 767–71
25. Joint Faculty of Intensive Care Medicine and Australian and New Zealand College of Anaesthetists and Australasian College for Emergency Medicine. Draft recommendations on standards for transport of critically ill patients. [Cited 29 June 2002] Available from URL http://www.acem.org.au/facem/ic-10_draftpolicy.pdf
26. Baxt W, Moody P 1987 The impact of a physician as part of the aeromedical prehospital team in patients with blunt trauma. Journal of the American Medical Association 257(23): 3246–50

27. Bartolacci R, Munford B, Lee A, McDougall P 1998 Air medical scene response to blunt trauma: Effect on early survival. Medical Journal of Australia 169: 612–6

28. Cameron P, Zalstein S 1998 Transport of the critically ill. Is there a doctor in the helicopter? Medical Journal of Australia 169: 610–1

29. Cameron P, Flett K, Kaan E, Atkin C, Dziukas L 1993 Helicopter retrieval of primary trauma patients by a paramedic helicopter service. Australia and New Zealand Journal of Surgery 63: 790–7

30. Shneider C, Gomez M, Lee R 1992 Evaluation of ground ambulance, rotor-wing and fixed-wing aircraft services. Critical Care Clinics 8(3): 533–64

31. Commission on Accreditation of Medical Transport Systems (CAMTS) 1999 Accreditation Standards, 4 edn. CAMTS, Anderson, South Carolina

32. Australian/New Zealand Standard. Ambulance restraint systems AS/NZ 4535:1999. Homebush, NSW: Standards Australia/Standards New Zealand

33. Nagappan R, Riddell T, Barker J, Maiden N, Lindsay S 2000 Patient care bridge – mobile ICU for transit care of the critically ill. Anaesthesia and Intensive Care 28: 684–6

34. Wishaw K, Munford B 1990 The CareFlight stretcher bridge: A compact mobile intensive care unit. Anaesthesia and Intensive Care 18: 234–8

35. Evans J, Hotte A 1994 A novel equipment bridge for helicopter transport of critically ill patients. Anaesthesia and Intensive Care 22: 284–7

36. Runcie C 1997 Principles of safe transport. In: Morton N, Pollack M, Wallace P (eds). Stabilization and Transport of the Critically Ill. Churchill Livingstone, New York, pp 31–47

37. Wallace P, Ridley S 1999 ABC of intensive care: Transport of the critically ill patient. British Medical Journal 319: 368–71

38. Runcie C 1997 Resuscitation, stabilization and preparation for transport. In: Morton N, Pollack M, Wallace P (eds) Stabilization and Transport of the Critically Ill. Churchill Livingstone, New York, pp 49–64

39. Kahn C, Pirrallo R, Kuhn E 2001 Characteristics of fatal ambulance crashes in the United States: an 11-year retrospective analysis. Prehospital Emergency Care 5: 261–9

40. Low R, Dunne M, Blumen I, Tagney G 1991 Factors associated with the safety of EMS helicopters. American Journal of Emergency Medicine 9: 103–6

41. Rhee K, Baxt W, Mackenzie J, et al 1990 Differences in air ambulance patient mix demonstrated by physiologic scoring. Annals of Emergency Medicine 19: 552–6

42. Frazer R 1999 Air medical accidents. A 20-year search for information. Air Medicine 5 :34–39

43. Blumen I 1994 Altitude and flight physiology: A reference for air medical physicians. In: Blumen I, Rodenberg H (eds) Air Medical Physician Handbook. Salt Lake City: Air Medical Physician Association, pp V.1. 1–V.1.23

FURTHER READING

Morton N, Pollack M, Wallace P 1997 Stabilization and Transport of the Critically Ill. Churchill Livingstone, London

25.3 MEDICAL ISSUES IN DISASTERS

RICHARD J. BRENNAN • DAVID A. BRADT • JONATHAN ABRAHAMS

ESSENTIALS

1 Effective disaster planning requires knowledge of a community's major risks, disaster types, and their associated patterns of morbidity and mortality.

2 Emergency physicians and other health professionals have a vital role in disaster management arrangements. They contribute most significantly to disaster preparedness and response activities.

3 Emergency physicians are most likely to respond to disasters associated with multiple casualties. Effective management of mass casualty incidents requires knowledge of the regional disaster plan, scene assessment issues, site management, communications, casualty flow plans, field triage, and the clinical management of unique clinical entities, including crush injury and blast injury.

4 New and emerging threats, including those due to acts of terrorism and climate change, must be addressed in updated disaster plans.

5 Public health interventions become high priorities following disasters that disrupt the social and public health infrastructure (e.g. cyclone, flooding), disasters that result in significant population displacement and disasters that involve chemical, biological or radiological agents.

INTRODUCTION

Disaster preparedness and response involve a complex, multidisciplinary process of which emergency medicine comprises one component. Government agencies, fire fighters, law enforcement, ambulance services, civil defence, the Red Cross and other aid organizations may all have a role to play. The health and medical management of disasters can also cut across professional disciplines, and require contributions from emergency medicine, public health, primary care, surgery, anaesthetics, and intensive care.

From the perspective of health, different types of disasters are frequently associated with different patterns of morbidity and mortality. The clinical and public health needs of an affected community will, therefore, also vary according to the type and extent of disaster. Emergency physicians should understand the health and medical consequences of the various types of disasters in order to determine their own roles in preparedness and response. In practice, emergency physicians will be most actively involved in the response to an acute-onset disaster that involves multiple casualties, such as a transportation incident. Several other types of disasters, including floods and cyclones, are generally associated with few, if any, casualties. The health and medical needs in these settings usually involve augmenting public health and primary care services.

The aims of this chapter are to familiarize emergency physicians with disaster management arrangements, and to provide an overview of the medical response to a disaster involving multiple casualties. While the chapter focuses on health and medical issues, it should be remembered that the effects of disasters are often widespread and long term. Disasters cause significant social, economic and environmental losses that can have a devastating effect on the general well-being of the affected community.

DEFINITIONS AND CLASSIFICATION

There is no international standardization of disaster definitions or classifications. Common to most definitions is the concept that following a disaster the capacity of the impacted community to respond is exceeded, and there is, therefore, a need for external assistance. The World Health Organization characterizes a disaster as a phenomenon that produces large-scale disruption of the normal health-care system, presents an immediate threat to public health, and requires external assistance for response. The Australian Emergency Manual defines *disaster* as an event that overwhelms normal community and organizational arrangements, and requires extraordinary responses to be instituted.

Disaster management is the range of activities designed to maintain control over disaster and emergency situations, and to provide a framework for helping at-risk populations avoid or recover from the impact of a disaster. It addresses a much broader array of issues than health alone, including hazard identification, vulnerability analysis and risk assessment. Disaster medicine can be defined as the study and application of various health disciplines to the prevention, preparedness, response and recovery from the health problems arising from disasters. This must be achieved in cooperation with other agencies and disciplines involved in comprehensive disaster management. In practice, emergency medicine and public health are the two specialties most intimately involved in disaster medicine.

The term emergency is frequently used when referring to disasters, as in the Australian Federal Government agency Emergency Management Australia. The Australasian College for Emergency

Medicine, however, defines an emergency as an acute illness or injury in an individual patient that requires medical care within 1 hour. A mass casualty incident is an event causing illness or injury in multiple patients simultaneously through a similar mechanism, such as a major vehicular crash, structural collapse, explosion or exposure to a hazardous material.

Disasters may be classified in several ways. Most commonly disasters are divided into two broad categories: natural and human-generated (Table 25.3.1). Disasters may also be classified according to other characteristics, including acute versus gradual onset, short versus long duration, unifocal versus multifocal distribution, common versus rare, and primary versus secondary. Currently there is no standard classification of disaster impact severity.

EPIDEMIOLOGY

Globally, the types of disasters associated with the greatest numbers of deaths are complex humanitarian emergencies (CHEs). These are humanitarian crises characterized by political instability, armed conflict, large population displacements, food shortages and collapse of public health infrastructure. Because of insecurity and poor access to the affected population, aggregate epidemiological data for CHEs are somewhat limited. However, between 1998 and 2002 more than 3.3 million people in the eastern region of the Democratic Republic of Congo lost their lives due to the consequences of the major humanitarian crisis afflicting that country. Incredibly, this was more than three times the total number of deaths globally due to natural and technological disasters during the decade of the 1990s. United Nations data demonstrate that over 100 million people are directly impacted by CHEs and more than 310 million people live in countries that are currently experiencing CHEs.

According to information compiled by the International Federation of the Red Cross, there has been a significant increase in the total number of natural and technological disasters worldwide during the past 30 years. From 1992 to 2001, an average of approximately 499 such disasters were documented annually, with 712 recorded in 2001. While the total number of people killed by natural and technological disasters has stabilized at approximately 80 000 per year, the total number affected has almost trebled over the past 3 decades. It is estimated that approximately 200 million people are directly affected on an annual basis.

The commonest types of disasters across the globe are: transportation incidents, floods, windstorms, industrial incidents, droughts/famines, and earthquakes (see Table 25.3.2). Asia is the region of the world most prone to disasters, followed by the Americas, Africa, Europe and Oceania (Table

Table 25.3.1 Classification of disasters

Natural disasters	Human-generated disasters
Acute onset	
Floods	Transportation/vehicular crashes
Cyclones/hurricanes	Structural fires
Heatwaves	Structural collapses
Bushfires	Mining accidents
Earthquakes	Hazardous material releases
Landslides	Radiation accidents
Tornadoes	Terrorism
Volcanic eruptions	War/complex humanitarian emergencies
Epidemics	
Gradual/chronic onset	
Drought	
Desertification	
Pest infestations (e.g. locusts)	

Table 25.3.2 Total numbers of documented disasters, by continent and phenomenon, 1992–2001 (Adapted from: International Federation of the Red Cross and Red Crescent Societies. World Disasters Report 2001. Geneva, IFRC, 2002)

	Asia	Americas	Africa	Europe	Oceania	Total
Transport incidents	668	233	437	186	11	1535
Floods	362	216	207	153	25	963
Windstorms	322	283	49	71	58	783
Industrial incidents	225	55	37	67	2	386
Miscellaneous accidents	178	45	57	53	5	338
Droughts/famines	77	39	113	13	11	253
Earthquakes	112	48	10	37	8	215
Avalanches/landslides	101	40	12	25	5	183
Forest/bush fire	18	55	11	39	9	132
Extreme temperatures	35	30	6	51	4	126
Volcanic eruptions	16	23	3	2	6	50
Other national disasters	14	4	4	1	2	25
Total	2128	1071	946	698	146	4989

Table 25.3.3 Disaster incidence and sequelae, Australasia and Oceania, 1992–2001 (Adapted from: International Federation of the Red Cross and Red Crescent Societies. World Disasters Report 2001. Geneva, IFRC, 2001)

Natural disasters	(n)	Human-generated disasters	(n)
High winds	58	Transportation	11
Floods	25	Industrial accidents	2
Droughts	11	Other	5
Earthquakes	8		
Forest fires	9		
Landslides	5		
Volcanoes	6		
Other	6		
Total events	128	Total events	18
Killed	2718	Killed	601
Affected	17 990 000	Affected	12 000

25.3.2). Compared with other regions of the world, Australasia and Oceania have a relatively low incidence of disasters (Table 25.3.2). Over the past 10 years the commonest causes of natural disasters in Australia have been floods, severe storms, and cyclones. Nationally, an average of 40 lives is lost per year due to disasters in Australia (Table 25.3.3). In addition, over 1 565 000 people are affected annually, through injury, displacement, financial loss, damage or loss of homes and businesses. Historically, the leading causes of death from natural disasters have been heatwaves, followed by cyclones, floods and bushfires. Human-generated disasters resulting in multiple casualties have occurred more frequently in Australia in recent years. The commonest causes of mass casualty incidents have been bus crashes, structural fires, mining incidents, aviation incidents and train crashes.

The impact of disasters has been less in New Zealand, where only four lives were lost among 2026 persons annually affected over the last decade. The pattern of natural disasters also differs, with the commonest major events being floods, earthquakes and landslides. The North Island of New Zealand has six active volcanoes, with the last attributed loss of life occurring in 1953.

Disaster epidemiology globally, including the Australasian region, is expected to be affected by climate change and the El Nino effect. El Nino is an alteration in the temperature and flow of Pacific Ocean currents, leading to a redistribution of water in the global water cycle. Global warming is likely to be associated with an increase in the frequency and unpredictability of cyclones. Rising temperatures have already been implicated in the spread of infectious disease vectors, including malaria-carrying mosquitoes. Droughts and bushfires are also expected to become more frequent in some regions. Rising sea levels and other disasters associated with global warming are particularly likely to threaten the lives and livelihoods of coastal communities and those living in low-lying islands.

SOCIO-ECONOMIC IMPACT

Disasters have the potential for major socio-economic impact, costing the international community billions of dollars annually. In developing countries, years of development work and investment can be devastated by a single disaster. During the 10 years to 2001, disasters caused an average of approximately

$US 69.4 billion damage per year. The types of disasters associated with the greatest economic impact are earthquakes, floods and windstorms. Terrorist attacks on major financial centres, such as the World Trade Center in New York and to major tourist destinations, such as Bali, have the potential for enormous and increasing social, economic and political impact.

In Australia, disasters cost an average of $A 1.14 billion annually. Over the past 30 years, floods, storms, then cyclones have caused the greatest disaster-related economic losses in Australia. The most economically costly disasters were Cyclone Tracy (1974), the Newcastle earthquake (1989), and the Sydney hailstorm (1999).

Economic estimates, of course, are unable to reflect the true scale of human suffering associated with disasters. While we can often document the mortality, morbidity, and financial losses associated with disasters, it is impossible to quantify the associated personal, psychological, social, cultural, and political losses. In response to the global suffering and losses from disasters, the United Nations General Assembly declared the 1990s as the International Decade for Natural Disaster Reduction.

DISASTER MANAGEMENT/ EMERGENCY MANAGEMENT

As emergency physicians play a vital role in the medical aspects of disaster management, they should be familiar with the four underlying concepts on which these arrangements are based.

All agencies (integrated) approach
The basis for the Australian system for managing disasters is a partnership between the Commonwealth, State/ Territory and local governments, and the community. Under legislation, State and Territory governments have the primary responsibility for coordinating disaster-management activities. The major role of

the Australian Federal Government is to assist State and Territory governments in developing their capacity to deal with disasters, for example by providing training courses and developing manuals of best practice. The Commonwealth also provides physical assistance to a State or Territory in the event that a disaster exceeds that State or Territory's response capability. Federal assistance in the area of health would most likely be medical resources provided by the Australian Defense Force (ADF). The ADF also has special expertise in the management of incidents involving chemical and biological agents.

Comprehensive approach
The comprehensive approach to disaster management encompasses prevention, preparedness, response and recovery. Health and medical professionals contribute most significantly to disaster preparedness and response. Prevention activities include regulatory and physical measures that prevent or mitigate the effects of disasters. Preparedness involves arrangements to ensure that resources and services which may be needed can be rapidly mobilized and deployed. Response activities are those actions taken during and immediately after impact to ensure that the disaster's effects are minimized. Recovery involves strategies and services that support affected communities in reconstructing their physical infrastructure and restoration of their social, economic, physical and emotional well-being.

All hazards approach
Different types of disasters can cause similar problems. Therefore, disaster management plans are based on a core set of arrangements and measures that can be applied to all hazards. Many risks, however, including acts of terrorism, will also require specific prevention, preparedness, response and recovery measures.

The prepared community
The prepared community is the focus of Australia's disaster management arrangements. Local governments, voluntary

organizations and individuals all play a critical role in this area. Experience has demonstrated that individual and community self-help can often provide the most immediate, decisive and effective relief following a disaster, as it cannot be assumed that assistance from external sources will always arrive promptly, particularly in remote area communities.

DISASTER PLANNING

Disaster planning is the process by which a community develops a comprehensive strategy to effectively manage and respond to disasters. It is a collaborative effort that requires cooperation between government agencies, community services and private organizations. The ultimate goals of the planning process include clarification of the capabilities, roles and responsibilities of responding agencies, and the strengthening of emergency networks. Other operational issues, such as emergency communications and public warning systems, will also be addressed.

A critical concept in disaster planning is the graduated response. The initial response to an event begins at the local level. More resources can subsequently be requested from regional, state or national levels, as required, to supplement those of the local providers. Compatibility between plans at the different levels is therefore necessary. A hierarchy of disaster management plans exists in which plans at lower levels dovetail with those of the next highest level. Command and control arrangements, as well as the roles and responsibilities described in a particular plan, must be compatible with the other plans to which it relates. Emergency physicians must be aware of these requirements if they are to constructively contribute to the development of state, regional and hospital disaster plans.

The Sydney 2000 Olympic Games in Australia and several high-profile terrorist events, particularly the World Trade Center attack in New York City and the bombings in Bali, have accelerated disaster management planning for terrorist events. In the USA, the use of commercial jet liners and anthrax-laced mail as weapons of mass terror have revealed a number of hazards and vulnerabilities that were previously not well recognized. Their exploitation by terrorists has resulted in a major re-evaluation of the disaster risk assessment process by intelligence, security, disaster management, and public health agencies across the USA. A similar review of terrorist threats and domestic vulner-abilities is now an essential component of disaster planning in Australia and New Zealand. Although terrorists are most likely to use conventional weapons, they clearly now have access to weapons of mass destruction (i.e. chemical, biolo-gical and radiological agents). Incidents involving these agents must therefore be addressed during the disaster planning process.

Disaster exercises must be conducted regularly to test the response and recov-ery aspects of the plan. Exercises range from desktop simulations to realistic scenarios with moulaged patients in the field. If conducted appropriately, they should effectively test whether the objectives of the plan have been met, and provide the opportunity for disaster response training. Disaster planning is a continuous process, and plans need to be regularly reviewed and updated. Disaster exercises may provide insights into areas in which the plan needs to be improved.

DISASTER RESPONSE ACTIVITIES

Incident management

Scene assessment and stabilization

The initial scene assessment will be conducted by first responders, such as police or ambulance personnel. It is im-portant for the first medical responder, generally an ambulance officer, to rapidly report findings to the Ambulance Communications Centre. An accurate, timely assessment is critical to initiating an appropriate and effective response. Key information that should be related from the scene includes the nature and magnitude of the disaster, the presence of ongoing hazards, the estimated number of deaths and injuries, the need for further assistance, and the most appropriate routes of access to the scene. In large-scale disasters that affect entire populations, such as cyclone or earth-quake, a broader epidemiological assess-ment will be required including an evaluation of the impact on the health infrastructure, public utilities and shelter.

Site security and safety procedures must be observed to ensure that rescuers and bystanders do not become victims. This is particularly relevant when a terrorist incident is suspected, because of the threats posed by a secondary attack on responders or the potential use of weapons of mass destruction. The police should establish a perimeter around the scene of a multiple casualty incident and allow access only to authorized personnel. If a hazardous material is involved, rescuers may be required to wear specialized personal protective equipment (PPE) to protect their airways, eyes and skin. Electrical hazards, fires, explosions, leaking gases and unstable structures may all pose signifi-cant threats to rescue personnel. These hazards must be eliminated or controlled prior to initiating rescue operations.

Hazard-specific issues

While the all-hazards approach remains fundamental to disaster management, a unifying approach for undifferentiated hazards has been developed for the management of incidents involving chemical, biological or radiological agents. Basic principles of awareness include: recognition of potential terrorist events, avoidance of the affected area, isolation of the affected area, and notification of proper authorities. Basic principles for first responders include the four don'ts: don't become a victim, don't rush in, don't TEST (taste, eat, smell, touch) anything, and don't assume anything. Only properly trained and equipped hazardous material per-sonnel should be in contaminated areas.

Site arrangements

Regardless of the nature of the incident, a Forward Command Post should be set up at or near the disaster site at the beginning of the emergency operation. The Command Post will have represen-tatives from the major responding services, and report back to the regional or State Emergency Operations Centre. The function of the Command Post is to coordinate the activities of the various services during the rescue operations. It also provides a central point for the submission of requests for assistance by each of the responding services. Medical and ambulance commanders will be located at the Command Post to direct and coordinate medical care to victims at the scene, patient transportation, hospital communications, provision of medical supplies, and medical air operations.

Communications

Good communications are vital to ensure appropriate command, control and coordination during a disaster. Communication problems are often cited as a major cause of suboptimal disaster response. There are many factors that may contribute to poor communica-tions at the scene. Damaged equipment and overloaded telephone systems indicate the need for back-up systems, including cellular phones. The use of different radio frequencies by different agencies may lead to poor coordination, and an inability to communicate vital information. Compatible frequencies need to be identified and utilized. Megaphones may be required to overcome noise at the scene due to heavy extrication equipment, helicopters and general rescue activities. Information overload may also hamper the rescue effort. Radio and telephone reports should be kept brief, relevant and suc-cinct. Professional jargon is frequently misunderstood or misinterpreted by other agencies, and is best avoided.

Hospitals must also have reliable communications systems. Designated phone lines, cellular phones and back-up radio networks may augment the existing system during a disaster. It is essential for hospitals to remain in regular contact with the incident medical director, to provide information regarding medical capabilities, bed capacity and bed availability.

Medical management

Personnel

The role of doctors and nurses at a disaster scene is somewhat controversial. Emergency responders generally respond best when their disaster roles are similar to their daily professional practice. Medical and nursing personnel are best suited to staffing emergency rooms and hospitals, where they have the advantage of working in a familiar, more stable environment. Ambulance personnel have more experience in pre-hospital settings and are usually responsible for conducting the initial medical assessment and triage. In situations where there are multiple casualties, it may be appropriate to send a hospital team to the scene of a disaster, where their main functions will be to perform primary and secondary triage, and to provide medical care at the Patient Treatment Post. Only doctors and nurses specifically trained to work in the field environment should be deployed to the disaster scene, as inexperienced personnel may well hinder the medical response.

Casualty-flow plan

A casualty-flow plan needs to be defined to optimize patient care and transportation. A Casualty Collection Area should be established at a site that is close enough to the disaster scene to allow easy access, but far enough away to ensure protection from potential hazards. Patients are assembled and triaged here prior to transfer to a nearby Patient Treatment Post, where they are once again triaged, and basic medical care provided. An Ambulance Loading Point and Ambulance Holding Point also need to be clearly marked so that patient transportation is conducted efficiently, and to ensure that scene convergence and congestion is minimized. Landing zones for helicopters are established away from the incident site for safety reasons, to limit noise, and to reduce down-wash from rotor blades. A temporary morgue may need to be established in a nearby area when many fatalities have occurred.

Triage

The aim of triage is to allocate medical resources, including personnel, supplies and facilities, in a manner that provides the greatest good to the greatest number. The emphasis is not on providing optimal care to each individual patient, but rather on directing limited medical resources to those who are most likely to benefit. Triage is the single most important medical activity at the disaster site. It is a dynamic, ongoing process that occurs at every stage of patient management, from the disaster site, to the Casualty Collection Area, Patient Treatment Post and again at the hospital. Patients are rapidly assessed and categorized according to priority of treatment and transport. The condition of patients frequently changes, and repeated examinations are required so that patients may be moved up or down in the order of priority. Triage is a learned skill and should be conducted by the most experienced medical or ambulance officer at the scene.

The number of triage categories used during a disaster varies from two to five. In general, most systems recognize that there are categories of patients who require immediate care, delayed care, minimal care, and those that are expectant or unsalvageable. Patients requiring immediate care are individuals who are in critical condition, but to whom simple life-saving procedures may be successfully applied, such as the manual clearing of the airway. Patients classified as requiring delayed care may have significant injuries, but are likely to survive if treatment is postponed for several hours. Minimal care patients are generally ambulatory and their treatment may be delayed until other patients have been appropriately treated. Expectant or unsalvageable patients are those that have acutely life-threatening injuries requiring advanced resuscitation, or those that have non-survivable injuries, such as massive head trauma. Advanced life support measures, such as cardiopulmonary resuscitation, are rarely indicated at a scene with multiple casualties. Instead, these patients generally receive palliative care, but only after patients in the immediate category have received appropriate treatment.

Stabilization

Following triage of the affected patients, rapid stabilization of airway, breathing and circulation is provided to those with the greatest potential for survival. Definitive care is not generally provided at the scene. On-scene medical care concentrates on securing the airway, administration of oxygen, external pressure to control haemorrhage, and insertion of intravenous catheters for volume expansion prior to hospital transportation. Medical care should generally be provided at the Patient Treatment Post, but during prolonged rescues resuscitative procedures may be required prior to extrication. Appropriate use of analgesia, including parenteral narcotics and regional nerve blocks, may assist with the extrication of trapped individuals. Special on-scene procedures are sometimes required for those with crush injury, blast injury, burns or hypothermia. Amputation of a mangled limb, although rarely indicated, may be a life-saving procedure for an entrapped patient.

Decontamination

Industrial accidents and terrorist events may result in exposure to hazardous chemical agents. Evacuation of victims from the contaminated area and removal of contaminated clothes should be conducted as a matter of urgency. Rapid decontamination of the skin is especially necessary following exposure to the liquid or aerosolized form of an agent. It is most useful when conducted within 1 minute of exposure, but in practice this is rarely possible. When indicated, decontamination should be conducted close to the scene (i.e. in the 'warm zone'), and, ideally, prior to transportation. Commonly used agents for decontamination include soap and water, and hypochlorite (household bleach) in concentrations of 0.5–2.0%. Steps must be taken to ensure that emergency responders, health personnel and other patients are not at risk of secondary exposure to the chemical agent. Decontamination after exposure to a biological agent is less important, as most biological agents are not dermally active. But decontamination may be an effective way to limit the spread of the agent from potential secondary aerosolization.

Transportation

Efficient and rational transportation of patients to appropriate health facilities is dependent on good communications between hospitals and the incident Transport Officer. Capabilities of the affected community's hospitals should be identified and documented in the regional disaster plan. Hospitals will be required to regularly update the Incident Commander and Transport Officer of their bed availability status. The closest hospitals are often flooded by 'walking wounded' who have made their own way from the scene, and by victims transported by well-meaning civilians. This has the potential of overwhelming local emergency departments, and the Transport Officer must take this into consideration when determining the appropriate distribution of patients. It is essential that the disaster not be relocated to the nearest hospitals.

A number of factors need to be considered when determining the most appropriate hospital for a particular patient, including the patient's triage category, the hospital's capabilities (e.g. trauma, burns), transportation times, distance from the scene, and the available transportation modalities. Medical helicopters may be able to transport patients to more distant hospitals, to relieve pressure on nearby facilities.

Hospitals

Emergency physicians are expected to be familiar with their own hospital disaster plan, and have contributed significantly to its development. It is the responsibility of hospital administration to establish a control centre with adequate communication resources. The emergency department needs to be cleared of non-critical patients, and steps taken to expedite appropriate discharge of stable ward patients, so that bed capacity may be optimized. The emergency department

should be well stocked with supplies. A recall system for additional medical and nursing staff mobilized in a disaster needs to be incorporated into the plan. Extra security staff should be on standby to assist with the control of patients, families, friends and the media.

Patients require re-triage by a senior medical officer as they arrive at the emergency department. Those with acutely life-threatening injuries are immediately resuscitated. Less severely injured patients need to be regularly reviewed while awaiting definitive care, to monitor for a potential deterioration in their condition. Expectant, unsalvageable patients are provided appropriate palliative care, and their condition clearly explained to their families. Documentation is kept succinct, and should generally be limited to the essential points about each patient's condition and treatment.

URBAN SEARCH AND RESCUE

Urban search and rescue (USAR) is the science of locating, reaching, treating and safely extricating survivors who remain trapped following a structural collapse. Search and rescue response capabilities have increased significantly in recent years, due to advances in rescue technology and in emergency services. USAR is one of the most visible aspects of the disaster response operation and attracts a significant degree of media and public attention. This point was illustrated by the extrication of a lone survivor following a major landslide in Thredbo, New South Wales in 1997, and the public euphoria that was associated with his successful rescue.

In the period immediately following a structural collapse, many survivors are rescued by uninjured bystanders. Those who remain trapped generally need the assistance of specially trained and equipped units from fire, ambulance or police services in order to be safely extricated. Medical members of search and rescue teams are tasked to provide medical care to the victims and medical support to the rescuers. They are not

involved in the actual extrication process. Potential hazards to victims and rescuers are numerous, and scene safety is of critical importance. The identification and extrication of victims following a major structural collapse is one of the most physically and emotionally challenging tasks of any rescue operation. The shock of dealing with scenes of carnage and mutilation may render some rescue personnel ineffective. These teams must therefore be trained and prepared to deal with the emotional strains of working in such a demanding environment.

MENTAL HEALTH

It is easy to overlook the mental health needs of affected individuals during the emergency response, when rescue and life-saving interventions receive top priority. Emergency physicians should be aware of the significant psychological impact of disasters on victims, families and rescue personnel. Mental health consequences, such as depression, anxiety states, and post-traumatic stress syndrome, are well described following disasters and need to be considered when developing the disaster plan. Crisis counseling may play an important role in the overall medical care provided to patients following a disaster. Rescue personnel should be provided with the opportunity to attend critical incident stress debriefing, which aims to provide them with the opportunity to discuss and examine their own reactions to the disaster.

MASS GATHERINGS

Social and cultural events can result in the gathering of many people in one place at a particular time, sometimes over several days. Common examples include rock concerts, sporting events, fairs and parades. The organization of medical services for mass gatherings is generally designed to address minor medical needs, but must also take into consideration medical emergencies, such as cardiac arrests, and disaster planning, for incidents such as fire, structural collapse or terrorism. Medical services developed for the mass gathering must be linked to local emergency medical systems. Public health services, such as food safety and environmental health measures, must be consistent with local regulations.

PUBLIC HEALTH ISSUES IN DISASTERS

Public health professionals are involved in all phases of the disaster cycle, and it is important for emergency physicians to understand the role of public health in disaster medicine and disaster management. Epidemiological studies that have identified risk factors for illness and injury following disasters have contributed greatly to disaster planning, mitigation, response and recovery. These investigations have been central to the development of the science of disaster medicine. They have led to key strategies that have been effective in reducing disaster-related morbidity and mortality.

Public health interventions become high priorities following disasters that disrupt the social infrastructure (for instance cyclone, flooding, earthquake), and disasters that result in significant population displacement (such as complex humanitarian emergencies). Priorities for the affected population include the provision of adequate water quantity and quality, sanitation, food, shelter, infectious disease control, and disease surveillance. The role of public health following a mass casualty incident includes injury control, occupational health and safety measures for responders, and injury surveillance.

The interface between emergency medicine and public health becomes increasingly important following technological disasters or terrorist events involving biological, chemical or nuclear agents. The terrorist attacks with anthrax in the USA during 2001 and their aftermath demonstrated the vital importance of key public health tools such as disease surveillance and outbreak investigation and control. Following incidents with chemical or radiological agents, public health officials may be required to provide guidance on issues such as evacuation of the public, mass decontamination and the mass distribution of iodine. Emergency physicians should become more familiar with the skills, roles, and responsibilities of their public health colleagues, especially as they relate to disaster management and infectious disease control.

CONCLUSION

Emergency physicians contribute most significantly to the preparedness and response aspects of disaster management. The increased threats posed by terrorists, including the use of weapons of mass destruction, requires a revision of disaster risk-assessment processes and disaster planning. Disasters associated with multiple casualties provide unique challenges to the health and medical communities. Curative medical skills and public health principles are both critical to the comprehensive management of a community affected by a disaster.

CONTROVERSIES AND FUTURE DIRECTIONS

❶ Well-conceived disaster planning is the most effective means of mitigating the adverse effects of disasters. As the spectrum of potential hazards has now expanded to include threats of terrorism utilizing weapons of mass destruction, emergency physicians will have an increased role in helping communities make informed choices about the risks that they face and the appropriate levels of preparedness in which they must invest.

❷ Recent experience with terrorist attacks and other disasters has demonstrated that the capacity of many emergency medical and public health personnel to respond effectively to the large variety of potential events remains limited. It is clear that greater investment is still required in the training of relevant personnel, the development of specialized response teams, the reinforcement of public health surveillance, and the review and refinement of disaster response plans.

❸ Internationally, minimum standards in disaster response have recently been developed by the Sphere Project. The goals of Sphere are to increase the quality of assistance provided to populations affected by disasters and to ensure the accountability of responding agencies. Minimum standards have been established for the five main sectors of disaster response, health services, nutrition, food aid, water and sanitation, and shelter and site planning. These standards will be revised by 2003, following an extensive review of current advances in the fields of disaster management and disaster medicine. Thereafter, it is expected that they will be more widely accepted, promoted and applied by disaster response agencies.

REFERENCES

1. Abrahams J 2001 Disaster management in Australia: The national emergency management system. Emergency Medicine (Fremantle) 13: 165–73
2. Barbera JA, Macintyre A 1996 Urban search and rescue. Emergency Medical Clinics of North America 14: 399–412
3. Bissell RA, Becker BM, Burkle FM 1996 Health care personnel in disaster response: reversible roles or territorial imperatives? Emergency Medical Clinics of North America 14: 267–88
4. Brennan RJ, Nandy R 2001 Complex humanitarian emergencies : a major global health challenge. Emergency Medicine (Fremantle) 13: 147–56
5. Brennan RJ, Waeckerle JF, Sharp TW, et al 1999 Chemical warfare agents: emergency medical and emergency public health issues. Annals of Emergency Medicine 34: 191–204
6. Coates L 1996 An overview of fatalities from some natural hazards in Australia. In: Proceedings of the conference on Natural Disaster Reduction 1996. Institution of Engineers, Barton, ACT, Australia
7. Emergency Management Australia 1994 Australian emergency manual - disaster medicine. Commonwealth of Australia, Canberra
8. Emergency Management Australia 1994 Australian Counter-Disaster Handbook Vol 2. Australian Emergency Management Arrangements. Commonwealth of Australia, Canberra
9. Emergency Management Australia 1997 Hazards, disasters and survival. Commonwealth of Australia, Canberra
10. Henderson AK, Lillibridge SR, Salinas C, et al 1994 Disaster Medical Assistance Teams: Providing health care to a community struck by hurricane Iniki. Annals of Emergency Medicine 23: 726–30
11. Hirshberg A, Holcomb JB, Mattox KL 2001 Hospital trauma care in multiple casualty incidents:

a critical view. Annals of Emergency Medicine 37: 647–52

12. International Federation of the Red Cross and Red Crescent Societies 2001 World Disasters Report 2001. IFRC, Geneva

13. Keim M, Kaufmann AF 1999 Principles for emergency response to bioterrorism. Annals of Emergency Medicine 34: 177–82

14. Leonard RB 1996 Medical support for mass gatherings. Emergency Medicals Clinics of North America 14: 383–98

15. Lillibridge SR, Noji EK, Burkle FM 1993 The emergency assessment of a population affected by a disaster. Annals of Emergency Medicine 22: 1715–20

16. Noji EK (ed.) 1997 The Public Health Consequences of Disasters. Oxford University Press, New York

17. Society for Academic Emergency Medicine 1995 Disaster medicine: current assessment and blueprint for the future. Academic Emergency Medicine 2: 1068–76

18. Stein M, Hirshberg A 1999 Medical consequences of terrorism. The conventional weapon threat. Surgery Clinics of North America 79: 1537–52

25.4 TRIAGE

DREW RICHARDSON

ESSENTIALS

1 Triage is the ongoing process of sorting patients on the basis of the urgency of their need for medical care.

2 Urgency is distinct from both severity and complexity.

3 Triage categorization has been found to strongly relate to both resource use and patient outcome.

4 The five-level Australasian Triage Scale (ATS) forms the basis of emergency department triage in Australasia.

5 The ATS is also used in casemix funding models and important performance measures.

6 Similar triage scales have been developed and adopted in other jurisdictions.

INTRODUCTION

Provision of high-availability quality medical care is expensive and has been traditionally limited to the very wealthy or to situations of great demand, such as the military in battle. Even today, well-organized emergency medical systems are concentrated in societies sufficiently affluent to spend 5% or more of GDP on health. Some form of rationing is required whenever an expensive resource is coupled with fluctuating demand. Price, queuing and denial are all used in different areas of medicine. Simple application of any of these methods in emergency medicine would not be efficient nor equitable, so the majority of emergency medical systems use a triage process to sort patients into a number of queues.

Triage, the sorting of patients on the basis of urgency, is an ongoing process that, nevertheless, requires formal structures at different points within the continuum of care. In the emergency-department setting there is considerable evidence that urgency can be assigned reliably and distinctly on a five level scale, and that this categorization is applicable and useful beyond the concept of 'urgency' into other aspects of hospital care.

ORIGINS OF TRIAGE

The word 'triage', arising from the French 'trier' meaning 'to sort' has its origins in Latin. It has entered English at least three times: from the 18th century wood industry, the 19th century coffee industry, and from 20th century emergency medicine. The process understood today as triage was first described by Baron Dominique Jean-Larrey (1766–1842)[1], the surgeon to Napoleon, who also developed the ambulance volante, the first field ambulance. This delivered large numbers of injured but salvageable cases to medical units, mandating a more efficient system than treatment in order of military rank. Jean-Larrey's 'order of dressing and arrangement' by urgency was also in keeping with the egalitarian spirit of the French revolution, although there is no evidence that he actually used the word triage. His concept was embraced and refined by military surgeons over the next 150 years, usually with the primary intent of returning soldiers to battle in the most efficient manner.

CIVILIAN TRIAGE DEVELOPMENT

There was certainly some sorting of patients from the moment 'casual wards' opened in 19th century hospitals, but the first systematic description in civilian medicine was by E Richard Weinerman in Baltimore in 1966.[2] Since that time, there has been a huge growth in emergency medicine as a specialty and a number of workers have undertaken formal investigation of triage, particularly in Australasia. The Australasian experience formed the basis of emergency department triage development in Canada and the UK, whilst some other jurisdictions have developed systems independently.

PROCESS OF TRIAGE

The underlying principles of triage are those of equity (or justice) and efficiency. Emergency departments experience potentially overwhelming demand from patients with an enormous range of conditions. Equity demands that the distribution of resources for treatment is fair in the broadest sense. The concept of urgency is well understood by the population who generally accept that it is fair to treat those in the greatest need ahead of those who arrived before them. Efficiency demands that best use is made of available resources. In the setting of emergency medicine cost and resource pressures prevent all demand being satisfied simultaneously. The overall philosophy of 'doing the greatest good for the greatest number' requires resource allocation on the basis of need, which in turn requires a process to identify and prioritize the needs of the presenting population.

In the emergency department, urgency is distinct from severity and prognosis, although a correlation exists. Some urgent problems (for example, upper airway obstruction) have a poor outcome without rapid intervention but are not severe in the sense of requiring long-term care, other severe problems (for example life-threatening malignancy) may not require any treatment in the emergency department time frame.

Triage is an ongoing process that may change in response to alterations in patient status and resource availability, but it is efficient to undertake a formal process once, early in the patient's encounter, and then review only as necessary. Emergency department triage is normally undertaken by trained nursing staff at the time of arrival, and the assigned urgency is then used to guide treatment order. The overall efficiency and effectiveness of such a system depends not only on the allocated priority but also on the treatment strategy, that is, the way in which the next patient is chosen from the different queues. A more urgent case should wait less time than a less urgent case, but when resources become available to treat the next patient, choice may still be required between a new arrival and a slightly less urgent patient who has already been waiting for some time.

AUSTRALASIAN TRIAGE DEVELOPMENT

The first Australasian description was of the Box Hill Triage Scale by Pink and Brentnall in 1977.[3] They used verbal descriptions without time consideration, and classified patients into five categories: immediate, urgent, prompt, non-urgent and routine. Fitzgerald modified this scale in 1989,[4] to produce the Ipswich Triage Scale. This used five colours to categorize patients according to the statement: 'This patient should under optimal circumstances be seen within ...'. The five categories were seconds, minutes, an hour, hours and days. Fitzgerald found his triage scale to have good inter-observer reliability on formal testing, and to be a practical predictor of emergency department outcome and length of intensive care unit stay, but a relatively poor predictor of outcome at hospital discharge.

Jelinek[5] investigated the relationship between the Ipswich Triage Scale and resource use in a stratified sample of 2900 presentations. He observed a strong correlation between triage categorisation and overall use of resources in the emergency department, and validated possible funding models. He proposed two possible casemix classifications: urgency and disposition groups (UDGs – 12 groups), and urgency-related groups (URGs – 73 groups) based on urgency, disposition and diagnosis. After trimming for outliers, these were found to account for 47% and 58% of the cost variance in large hospitals.

In 1994, the Australasian College for Emergency Medicine formalized the National Triage Scale,[6] derived from the Ipswich Triage Scale. This used colours, names or numerical categories to represent five groups, based on the answer to the statement: 'This patient should wait for medical care no longer than ...'. The categories were: immediate, 10 minutes, 30 minutes, 1 hour and 2 hours. The definition document also proposed Jelinek's concept[5] of performance indicators based on the proportion of patients whose care fell within the desired time threshold, and audit by means of admission rates and sentinel diagnoses. It influenced treatment strategies by indicating the need to achieve performance indicators in a high proportion of patients in every category (higher in the more urgent) and it clearly established the need for emergency departments to employ systematic, accountable and audited triage processes.

Over the next few years the National Triage Scale was widely accepted, and recognized by all Australian State Governments as an appropriate measure of access to emergency care. It was also adopted in the performance indicators promulgated by the Australian Council on Healthcare Standards.[7] Research repeated the findings of Fitzgerald and Jelinek with reference to the new five-point scale and investigated many more of the subtleties of triage scale use.

AUSTRALASIAN TRIAGE SCALE

The Australasian Triage Scale (ATS)[8] is the current refinement of the National Triage Scale. It has been jointly developed by the Australasian College for Emergency Medicine, emergency nursing organizations, and other interested parties. For practical purposes the scale concept itself is unchanged, but the ATS uses numeric classification only, better defines waiting time, and includes associated implementation guidelines and educational material.

The ATS categorizes patients presenting to emergency departments in response to the statement: 'This patient should wait for medical assessment and treatment no longer than ...'.

ATS category:
Treatment acuity (maximum waiting time)
ATS 1 Immediate
ATS 2 10 minutes
ATS 3 30 minutes
ATS 4 60 minutes
ATS 5 120 minutes

OTHER TRIAGE SCALES

The concept of desirable waiting time must include some subjective component, but has nevertheless been found to be reliable and reproducible. Achievement of ATS waiting times has proven to be a useful performance indicator, but remains a measure of process rather than emergency-department outcome. Concerns have been expressed in some jurisdictions about the medicolegal implications of a time-based threshold which will not always be met, and other systems have taken different approaches in development of their own emergency-department triage systems. Nevertheless, most have developed five-level triage systems along the Australasian model. Major validated triage scales include:

- The Canadian Emergency Department Triage and Acuity Scale (CTAS): derived from the ATS but using a 15 minute threshold in category 2.[9]
- The Manchester Triage Scale: uses an algorithmic approach to the United Kingdom Triage scale, similar to the ATS but with longer thresholds in the lower acuity categories.[10]
- The ESI Triage algorithm: developed in the USA without any time thresholds, but using a simple approach to classifying urgency.[11]

USES OF THE TRIAGE SCALE BEYOND WAITING TIME

Triage is based on a brief assessment, and an individual triage categorization can reflect only the probability of certain outcomes. Large populations of triaged patients, however, exhibit predictable patterns. There is a very strong, almost linear relationship between triage category and total rate of admission, transfer, or death, ranging from 80–100% in ATS 1 to 0–20% in ATS 5. This pattern is repeated across hospitals of different size and different patient mix.[12] Admission rates by triage category follow the pattern of overall admission rates in relation to age, giving a flattened 'U shaped' distribution. The inter-rater reliability studies performed using the Ipswich Triage Scale have been repeated using the NTS/ATS, and it has been found to be slightly better.[13] Further, admission rates by triage category have been shown to be constant over time in individual institutions.[14]

The NTS/ATS has been extensively studied as a casemix tool. Emergency department outcome (admission/transfer/death versus discharge) accounts for the largest variance in cost, but triage categorization comes a close second, with age third. The mean cost of care for a category 1 patient is approximately ten times that of a category 5 patient. UDGs, described by Jelinek using the Ipswich Triage Scale, have been validated using the National Triage Scale by Erwich on 17 819 attendances.[15] Age has been included to derive urgency, disposition, and age groups (UDAGs – 32 groups), which account for 51% of the cost variance, and are not susceptible to different diagnostic approaches.[13]

Triage categorization is a very strong predictor of emergency department outcome, and a good predictor of utilization of critical care resources. However, it is a relatively poor predictor of outcome at hospital discharge.[17] Many patients with chronic or sub-acute conditions that frequently cause death are triaged to less urgent categories because there is no benefit from earlier treatment within the time scales available in the emergency department.

Lastly, attainment of performance indicators for patients seen within triage thresholds has been shown to be a measure of resource allocation within the emergency department. A longitudinal comparative study has demonstrated a significant improvement with an increase in emergency department staff and funding.[18]

STRUCTURE AND FUNCTION OF A TRIAGE SYSTEM

The exact requirements for triage vary with the role, location, and size of the hospital, but effective systems share a number of important features, mostly derived from experience:

- A single point in the emergency department near the entrance where triage is undertaken so that all patients will be exposed to the nurse undertaking triage

- Appropriate facilities for undertaking brief assessment and limited treatment (first aid) including relevant equipment and washing facilities for staff and patients
- A balance between competing concerns of accessibility, confidentiality, and security
- A means of recording assessment and triage categorization that will 'follow' the patient through their time in the emergency department and be available for review afterwards. In most large departments this is now a computerized information system
- Contemporary data on the state of the emergency department and the expected patients, such as the information system and ambulance and police radio systems.

PRE-HOSPITAL TRIAGE

The principle of making best use of available resources to maximize patient outcome remains the basis of triage in any setting. Relatively less therapeutic options are available to pre-hospital providers and patient disposition is generally limited to transport and sometimes choice of hospitals. The initial pre-hospital phase, the travel to the patient, must be undertaken on the basis of minimal information. Allocation of resources through a structured triage system remains important, but data may not be sufficient for a five level scale, although this is currently being studied in Western Australia. Most pre-hospital systems are strongly protocol driven, and tend towards three or four level assessment: rapid response (lights and sirens), immediate response, routine response, or no transport.

MILITARY AND DISASTER TRIAGE

In situations of overwhelming imbalance between resources and demand, triage remains critical in ensuring that available resources are used to achieve the greatest good. The principles of rapid assessment, documentation, and multiple queues for care remain the same, but competing demands on resources may mean triaging cases to receive minimal or no care, or treating first those who can return to work or duty. The need for both human and physical resources for more important tasks may profoundly limit individual patient care.

Military and disaster triage require seniority and experience (which by definition is rarely available), the ability to make and defend rapid decisions, and a successful liaison with other players outside the medical or nursing hierarchy. Senior personnel with significant experience and preferably with additional training should be chosen for this role if possible. Formal triage and documentation must be brief and will use different scales from those appropriate in the emergency department.

CONTROVERSIES AND FUTURE DIRECTIONS

❶ The research base undertaken on the National Triage Scale showed it to be relatively reliable and reproducible, but identified some areas for improvement. The Australasian Triage Scale and its associated guidelines and educational materials were designed to address some of the recognised problems with the NTS, but revision and improvement of the Scale will continue. Further study is required to assess the impact of the ATS on issues including:
– Variation in implementation between sites, particularly hospitals of different role delineation[12]
– Variation associated with activity – there is evidence of consistency in some hospitals[14], but changes in others[19]
– Variation in approach to paediatric triage, especially between mixed and paediatric emergency departments[20]
– Marked differences in education practice for triage nurses.[21]

❷ The role of the ATS is still under assessment in prehospital and disaster triage, and the process of triage in emergency departments continues to evolve. The importance of triage as a management tool and the demand for greater reliability and consistency will continue to increase in line with the pressure of emergency department workload.

REFERENCES

1. Larrey DJ 1832 Surgical Memoirs of the Campaigns in Russia, Germany, and France. Translated Mercer JC. Carey and Lea, Philadelphia. Cited in Winslow G Triage and Justice. University of California Press, CA
2. Weinerman ER, Rateen RS, Robbins A 1966 Yale studies in Ambulatory care V. Determinants of use of hospital emergency services. American Journal of Public Health Nations Health 56(7): 1037–56
3. Pink N 1977 Triage in the accident and emergency department. Australian Nurses' Journal 6(9): 35–6
4. Fitzgerald GJ 1989 Emergency department triage. Doctor of Medicine Thesis. University of Queensland, Australia
5. Jelinek GA 1995 Casemix classification of patients attending hospital emergency departments in Perth, Western Australia. Doctor of Medicine Thesis, University of Western Australia
6. Australasian College for Emergency Medicine 1994 National Triage Scale. Emergency Medicine (Freemantle) 6(2): 145–6
7. Australian Council on Healthcare Standards 1996 Clinical Indicators – a User's Manual. ACHS, Zetland NSW
8. Australasian College for Emergency Medicine 2002 Australasian Triage Scale. Emergency Medicine (Freemantle)14: 335–6
9. Beveridge R, Ducharme J, James L, Beaulieu S, Walter S 1999 Reliability of the Canadian Emergency Department Triage and acuity scale: interrater agreement. Annals of Emergency Medicine 34(2): 155–9
10. Manchester Triage Group 1997 Emergency triage. Publishing Group, London
11. Wuerz RC, Milne LW, Eitel DR, Travers D, Gilboy N. Reliability and validity of a new five-level triage instrument. Academic Emergency Medicine 2000 Mar; 7(3): 236–42
12. Whitby S, Ieraci S, Johnson D, Mohsin M 1997 Analysis of the process of triage: the use and outcome of the National Triage Scale. Liverpool Health Service, Liverpool NSW
13. Jelinek GA, Little M 1996 Inter-rater reliability of the National Triage Scale over 11 500 simulated occasions of triage. Emergency Medicine (Freemantle) 8: 226–30
14. Richardson DB 1998 No relationship between emergency department activity and triage categorization. Academic Emergency Medicine 5: 141–5
15. Erwich MA, Bond MJ, Phillips DG, Baggoley CJ 1997 The identification of costs associated with Emergency Department attendances. Emergency Medicine (Freemantle) 9: 181–7
16. Erwich MA, Bond MJ, Baggoley CJ 1996 Costings in the emergency department. Report to the Commonwealth Department of Health and Human Services (Australia)
17. Dent A, Rofe G, Sansom G 1999 Which Triage category patients die in hospital after being admitted through emergency departments? A study in one teaching hospital. Emergency Medicine (Freemantle) 11: 68–71
18. Rogers IR, Evans L, Jelinek GA, Jacobs I, Inkpen C, Mountain D 1999 Using clinical indicators in emergency medicine: documenting performance improvements to justify increased resource allocation. Journal of Accident and Emergency Medicine 16: 319–21
19. Richardson DB, Kelly AM, Baggoley CJ, Fulde GWO, Rogers IJ, Ieraci S 1999 Variation in Triage Categorisation: Does daily activity make a difference? [abstract] Academic Emergency Medicine 6: 397–8
20. Durojaive L, O'Meara M 2002 A study of triage in paediatric patients in Australia. Emergency Medicine (Freemantle) 14: 67–76
21. Kelly AM, Richardson D 2001 Training for the role of Triage in Australasia. Emergency Medicine (Freemantle) 13: 230–2

25.5 REFUGEE HEALTH

ALED WILLIAMS • MARK LITTLE

ESSENTIALS

1 The worldwide refugee problem is massive and likely to increase.

2 Overall reponsibility for refugees lies with the United Nations High Commision for Refugees (UNHCR) though numerous other organizations also assist.

3 The most familiar scenario is the movements of large populations across a border into a 'refugee camp'.

4 The response to a refugee crisis consists of an emergency phase where acute needs are met and a post emergency phase when mortality levels in the camp approach those of the local area.

5 The basics of nutrition, shelter, clean water and sanitation are always the most important.

6 There are well-documented standards in all areas of refugee care.

7 For individual refugees the outcomes are either resettlement in their country of origin, integration into the new host country or resettlement into a third country.

8 Ultimately, solutions to refugee movements are political.

INTRODUCTION

Caring for refugees is not a new problem. Since World War II up to 100 000 000 civilians have been forced to flee their homes due to unrest. The major factors that cause people to flee their country, conflict, political repression and persecution are as old as humanity. The term 'refugee' was first coined in 1573 and used to describe Calvinists fleeing political repression in the Spanish-controlled Netherlands. Refugee numbers are now higher than ever and seem to be relentlessly increasing. The United Nations High Commission for Refugees is currently responsible for the welfare of some 12 million refugees worldwide and there are an estimated further 7 million 'persons of concern'. These consist mostly of internally displaced persons (refugees inside their country of origin), asylum seekers and recently returned refugees. This equates to about 1:300 persons on the planet. The problem is massive.

The solution to any refugee problem is, ultimately, political and non-medical. Even in the acute phases of refugee movement the most important things are simple, such as food, shelter and clean water. Physicians, however, can play a considerable role especially if they are adaptable and able to use simple cheap and effective solutions to problems.

This chapter provides an understanding of the issues and possible solutions to the refugee health problem, a bibliography for further reading, an outline of the essential attributes of refugee doctors, and links to appropriate organizations for the interested reader.

RESPONSIBILITY FOR REFUGEE CARE

Until the end of the World War I, the response to refugees was from philanthropic sections of the community. The formation of the League of Nations began the process of the international community assuming responsibility for refugees. In 1921 a High Commission for Refugees was established with a mandate to look after refugees fleeing the Russian and Armenian wars. Its first Commissioner was Fridtjof Nansen who established a special identity document, the 'Nansen Passport', as refugees frequently had no means of identification.

In the wake of World War II, the United Nations established the International Refugee Organization to assist the millions of displaced persons in Europe. Between 1947 and 1951 it helped 1.6 million people mainly Germans and Austrians.

The modern response to refugees started in 1951 with the establishment of the United Nations High Commission for Refugees (UNHCR) and the Convention Relating to the Status of Refugees which has the force of law and has been ratified by 120 countries. With some fine-tuning over the years this remains the cornerstone of International Refugee Law. It defines a refugee as:

> ... any person who, owing to a well founded fear of being persecuted for reasons of race, religion, nationality, member of a particular social group or political opinion, is outside the country of his nationality and is unable or, owing to such a fear, unwilling to avail himself of the protection of that country.

The UNHCR also encourages countries to receive refugees and to provide them with assistance and protection. One of the major points of the Convention is the principle of 'non-refoulement', which means that refugees cannot be forcibly returned to their countries of origin.

REFUGEE CAMPS

Persons fleeing war or persecution escape in many different ways and may live in host countries in several different arrangements, for instance integration with local community or staying with relatives. The typical image of refugees is of mass movements of populations across borders into temporary accommodations or 'refugee camps'. It is under these circumstances refuges are most at risk. Importantly, the populations in refugee camps do not exist in isolation. There are always interactions with the local population, and these may not always be beneficial. Also important are political and ethnic factors within the refugee population. These can lead to tensions or even violence in the camps, as was demonstrated tragically in the post Rwandan holocaust camps in 1994. Camps themselves can even sustain conflict in some areas, for instance in the West Bank or in the camps on the Thai Cambodian border, which were used by the Khmer Rouge as refugees from which to carry on a war.

EMERGENCY PHASE

As a result of a crisis, either due to war, or acts of nature, large populations can be displaced from their normal environment. This often results in large numbers of people, with minimal or none of the basic life needs, descending on a region. Where the people congregate is usually where refugee camps evolve. Most population movements into refugee camps occur in third world countries, which have limited resources to deal with them. Pre-planning by aid agencies and governments is, therefore, essential so that humanitarian responses can be quick and coordinated. Considerable expertise in responding to refugee emergencies has been gained and the main priorities are now well recognized. These are outlined below, as per Medecins Sans Frontieres (MSF) guidelines.

Initial assessment

A rapid assessment of the population structure, their medical and other needs is essential in the very early stages to enable planning and appropriate delivery of resources.

Measles immunization

Conditions in refugee camps can facilitate large-scale measles epidemics, which in an at-risk population can have devastating consequences. In Tuareg refugee camp in Mauritania in 1992, in a 5-month period, 40% of the paediatric deaths was due to measles. Mass vaccina-tion of all children from 6 months to 15 years is essential and is usually combined with administration of vitamin A, which reduces the under 5 years mortality rate and the measles case fatality rate.

Water and sanitation

Poor water supply and sanitation plays a major role in the spread of diarrhoeal diseases. Well-defined standards that can be checked with simple kits now exist for acceptable water quality. Standards for quantity are 5 litres/person/day initially rising to 15 litres/person/day when possible. Similarly set standards apply to the location, type and number of latrines and washing facilities.

Food and nutrition

Malnutrition is common in refugee populations especially in the at risk young and elderly groups. The initial food ration recommended is 2100 kilo-calories/person/day. It is also important to undertake surveys for specific nutritional deficiencies such as scurvy or pellagra and treat accordingly.

Assessment of nutrition in the popu-lation is an ongoing process and special feeding programmes may need to be set up for at-risk groups. Generally, there are specific agencies such as the United Nations World Food Program, which specialize in this area.

Shelter and site planning

Proper shelter and adequate clothing are essential early priorities. Overcrowding can lead to or worsen disease outbreaks as well as affecting the mental health of refugees. Protection from the elements is also essential for well-being especially in extreme climates. Again well-defined standards for living space and shelter construction exist. Planning the location of the camp is also essential. A good site needs to be large enough, secure, and have adequate infrastructure like good road or air access. It should also have access to a water supply and be relatively protected from the elements.

General health care

Organizing a system to deal with common infections and diseases is essential. There may be numerous organizations involved in the refugee camp and so there is a need for coordination. Medical needs of the population are rapidly assessed and locally occurring diseases taken into account. Experience has led to the creation of medical kits intended to cover the needs of 1000 refugees for a 3-month period. There are also manuals and guidelines available.

Control of infectious disease

The four most frequent infectious diseases in the emergency phase are measles, diarrhoea, respiratory infections and malaria. Providing good basic living conditions will help ward off these and other illnesses but once an outbreak has occurred there is potential for high mortality rates so aggressive treatment and decisive public health measures are essential. As diarrhoea is a major cause of death, early establishment of oral rehydration centres is essential.

Public health surveillance

Collecting epidemiological data on a daily basis provides essential information to those in charge of a camp so that interventions can be planned and disease outbreaks rapidly recognized. The most useful health indicator is the daily crude mortality rate (CMR), which is normally expressed as deaths/10 000 population/ day. A CMR of over 1 is an indicator of an emergency situation. Disease specific mortality rates may also be useful.

Human resources and training

Administering a refugee camp is very complex and requires a variety of skilled personnel including doctors, water/ sanitation experts, nutritionist, logisticians and others. First, the need for different types of personnel needs to be assessed then their activities need to be co-ordinated and managed. Local staff and some of the refugees need to be trained to help in essential tasks.

Coordination

Any refugee action may have a large number of agencies assisting. There may be UN agencies, military forces, international non-government organizations (NGOs), such as MSF, Oxfam and local agencies like the National Red Cross societies. The host country's government and local authority also have an important role to play. Coordinating many diverse agencies, some of whom have conflicting agendas, is a huge challenge and means that one agency needs to take on a leadership role, good communication needs to be established early and overall goals must be established.

POST-EMERGENCY PHASE

This phase begins when the basic needs of the population are met (food, shelter, water and so on) and the CMR is less then 1 per day, which is roughly similar to that of the local population. The situation in the post-emergency phase is complex and fluid. Some of the refugees may become quite settled and start to work locally or farm some land. The health and nutritional status of refugees may even surpass those of local population because of large amounts of overseas aid. This may lead to resentment. Complex political issues may arise. Descent back into the emergency phase may occur with an epidemic outbreak or fresh influx of refugees.

In general, though, the post emergency phase is concerned with consolidation of what has been achieved, preparation for possible new emergencies, and sustainability.

There needs to be continuing monitoring of water quality, public health and nutritional status. Health-care issues in the post emergency phase are complex. Some of the issues that may need to be addressed include:

- Standardization of training, supervision and delivery of health services
- Curative health-care services
- Reproductive health care, including, antenatal and delivery, post natal family planning, STD and HIV/ AIDS
- Child health activities such as EPI programmes

- Specific HIV/AIDS/STD programmes
- TB programmes
- Psychosocial and mental health.

PERMANENT SOLUTIONS

There are three possible solutions to any refugee situation, repatriation, integration, or resettlement in another country.

Repatriation is the preferred option but is often quite complex. First, there needs to be a solution to the problem that caused the refugees to leave initially. This may take years. Persons returning need a lot of extra support in order to rebuild their lives. Some refugees remain in the host countries and integrate into local communities. This was commonplace in African nations, but is increasingly difficult, especially when African governments look at the reluctance of affluent Western countries to accept refugees.

The minority of refugees who cannot return are resettled in third (mostly Western) countries. Many countries have quotas, and will only admit once a person is assessed by the UNHCR as having a valid claim. In 2001 the number resettled was 100 000. Of these, the USA took 68 500, Canada took 12 200 and Australia received 6500.

PAST PROBLEMS

In the past there have been important problems with the response to a refugee crisis. Often these have their root in poor coordination between the agencies that respond to a particular crisis, which may lead to inappropriate interventions and even frank competition. Often in a dramatic disaster such as an earthquake, which has considerable media coverage there is a frenzy of intervention as agencies attempt to get their image across to international viewers to assist in fundraising. In the 2001 earthquake in Gujarat province, India, it was estimated that there were as many as 200 different government and non-government agencies in the field. There is no doubt that

this has resulted in unnecessary death, most notably in the great lakes region of Africa following the Rwandan genocide.

INNOVATIONS IN REFUGEE CARE

Overcoming the problems of lack of planning and coordination have been the major thrust of more recent developments. Importantly, in 1997 it was decided to establish a set of minimum standards and rights to which refugees were entitled. The collaborative project called Sphere involved numerous organizations involved in humanitarian care including Red Cross, MSF, and Oxfam. It produced a manual that is available at no cost from the website www.sphere.org. Individual organizations, such as MSF, have several excellent manuals describing in detail the approach to humanitarian emergencies.

The UN in conjunction with other agencies has been refining its disaster response capabilities. Through the office for the coordination of humanitarian affairs (OCHA) there is now a system of stockpiling supplies, cash reserves and ability for rapid assessment and deployment. The UN works in partnership with several NGOs and the Federation of Red Cross and Red Crescent Societies who have also been developing rapid response field assessment and coordination teams (FACTs). There is now a system of coordination through the field Coordina-

Table 25.5.1 At-risk groups within a refugee population
Females (especially pregnant)
Head of household
Young (<5 years)
Elderly
Chronically sick
Disabled
Ethnic, religious or political minority groups
Urban refugees in a rural environment

tion Support Section (FCSS) of OCHA and the ability to appoint 'lead agency' status to a particular organization.

The Internet and electronic media are also being increasingly used in innovative ways by humanitarian agencies. It is now possible to follow evolving disasters on several websites (e.g. United Nations affiliated sites, Red Cross sites and MSF sites) and explore what that particular organization is doing. OCHA is also exploring the use of a Virtual Operations Coordination Center which is an online resource that can be accessed by registered users from various agencies to coordinate their approach to a particular disaster.

ATTRIBUTES OF A REFUGEE DOCTOR

Working under the special conditions imposed by a refugee camp demands special qualities. It is certainly not a glamorous job and often much of what has been learned from training and practice in the West is either not relevant or needs much modification to suit local conditions and resources. In general the main requirements are:

- Flexibility, versatility and ability to improvize
- Ability to work independently
- Ability to work under extreme circumstances

CONTROVERSIES AND FUTURE DIRECTIONS

❶ There is often a lack of coordination between agencies involved in refugee care leading to adverse outcomes. The challenge is to coordinate the response and maximize efficiencies and outcomes.

❷ There is often a reluctance by Western countries to accept refugees from the developing world.

❸ Improving standards and training in refugee care is a high priority.

❹ Arguably, the response would be considerably improved with the formation of rapid assessment and deployment teams.

❺ There is a need for better coordination between the UN and other agencies.

❻ Much could be gained from increased preparedness of the international community in holding cash reserves and humanitarian stockpiles.

- Cultural sensitivity
- Getting on with all types of people
- Ability to follow leadership and direction
- Acceptance of security and health risks
- A family willing to accept risks.

FURTHER READING

Medecins Sans Frontieres 1997 Refugee health, an approach to emergency situations. McMillan Education Ltd. This and many other invaluable MSF texts on treatment protocols, basic kits are all available free on the MSF website: www.msf.org
Humanitarian Charter and Minimum Standards in Disaster Response 2000 The Sphere Project. Oxfam Publishing. Available free on website www.shpere.org

Emergency relief items, vol 1 & 2 2000 United Nations Development Program
Hospitals for war wounded 1998 International Committee of the Red Cross
www.refiefweb.int. This is the entry point into the UN agencies such as OCHA and its various branches. Also publishes situation reports of evolving disasters
www.unhcr.org. refugee facts, figures and histories
www.ifrc.org. International federation of Red Cross and Red Crescent societies
www.icrc.org. International committee of the Red Cross site. This is more concerned with war zones
www.msf.org. the MSF website which is a very useful resource with several free publications on refugee health care
www.oxfam.org
www.sphere.org. From which you can download the sphere manual
www.redcross.org.au. The Australian Red Cross Site for information on where Australians are currently posted overseas. www.msf.org.au has similar data for MSF

ALED WILLIAMS

ESSENTIALS

1 Observation wards are an integral part of modern emergency departments.

2 They are run by emergency-department staff according to strict policies and protocols.

3 The spectrum of conditions considered suitable for observation ward care is increasing.

4 Intensive treatment, frequent reassessment and rapid turnover leads to great efficiency in patient care.

5 Overall effects are to reduce admission length of stay for conditions suitable for observation ward treatment.

6 Inappropriate discharges from the emergency department are reduced.

7 The overall standing of the emergency department is enhanced.

INTRODUCTION

An observation ward (OW) is an essential part of a modern emergency department. OWs are a valuable tool in the safe and efficient management of patients and are rapidly being embraced by emergency departments worldwide. In a 1989 survey it was found that of 44 emergency departments in major Australian hospital emergency departments 50% had beds designated as an OW. A further 25% expressed an intention to establish one.[1] Though there is much local variability, they are defined by the following general characteristics:

- They are run and staffed by emergency-department personnel

- They are separate from main patient assessment and treatment areas but remain either attached or in close proximity to the main body of the emergency department
- Specific policies exist as to the type of patients who can and cannot be admitted
- Admitting rights lie with emergency department staff only
- Admissions are time limited after which patients are either discharged or transferred to the care of another specialist team
- Frequent ward rounds by senior medical staff are conducted
- OW patients have preferential access to acute diagnostic, referral and paramedical services.

The primary role of OWs is to provide rapid turnover intensive observation and treatment to patients with suitable medical conditions. This increases efficiency of both the emergency departments and the hospital overall. OWs have additional benefits, which may include improving patient flow through a busy emergency department by providing a temporary 'holding area' for admissions, temporary accommodation for patients for whom discharge at an antisocial hour would be inappropriate (such as the elderly) or acute situational crises at antisocial hours. They may also function as a 'safety net' for patients seen at night by junior medical staff who are uncertain of the diagnosis for review by senior staff in the morning thus possibly reducing inappropriate discharges.

OW POLICIES AND PROTOCOLS

OWs function well under the umbrella of firm policies and protocols. These of course vary according to the institution, the number of beds in the OW, medical

and nursing staff levels and the main perceived functions of the OW in a particular emergency department. In general, though, the following issues need to be addressed:

Admission process

To avoid confusion requests for admission to the OW should go through a specific doctor nominated on each shift to have overall responsibility for OW patients. All patients need to have a clear treatment plan with defined objectives for the admission. Any treatment to be given during the admission such as IV fluids or medications needs to be clearly documented. If the patient is admitted for observation then what is required should also be clearly documented as well as action to be taken if there is any deterioration.

Admission criteria

Only some types of patients are suitable for OW management. The list below is not comprehensive and varies from institution to institution. The general principle is that the admitting doctor expects that the patient will be admitted for a definite and limited time (usually 24 hours):

Time-limited intensive treatment
- Analgesia for renal colic
- Mild-to-moderate asthma
- Rehydration after gastroenteritis
- Migraine headache
- Some cases of envenoming, e.g. red back spider, brown snake envenoming with coagulopathy only
- Analgesia and mobilization after soft-tissue injuries
- Commencement of therapies that are to be continued out of hospital by either the patient's GP or home care nurses (e.g. IV antibiotics for cellulitis or fractionated heparin for deep vein thrombosis).

Patients requiring a period of observation before a decision about final disposition is made

- Post minor head injury with GCS of 14–15
- Possible snakebite victims with no evidence of envenoming who are awaiting repeated blood tests
- Post procedure, e.g. lumbar puncture or Bier's block
- Many toxicology patients if ventilation or specific intensive care procedures are not required
- Alcohol intoxication
- Abdominal pain without specific signs in otherwise well patients.

Patients for whom discharge is inappropriate for social or other reasons

- Elderly isolated or vulnerable patients at antisocial hours
- Acute situational crises out of hours that could benefit from social work or psychiatric input in the morning.

'Safety net' for junior staff working out of hours

- There are some patients in whom junior staff may be unclear as to a diagnosis but there is no definite indication to admit, inpatient teams refuse admission or the junior doctor 'is just not sure'. Such patients can be admitted and observed overnight for review by senior staff in the morning. As well as being a useful teaching exercise, the potential for 'missing' a diagnosis is reduced, but a clear management plan needs to be in place and the patient regularly reviewed so that deterioration is not missed.

'Bed management' issues

- 'Holding bay' for patients admitted to other wards where there is a delay in availability of the bed. This can ease congestion in the emergency department
- Patients awaiting an investigation, e.g. CT or ultrasound where there is an expected delay.

Special 'institution specific' cases

- Some institutions may develop more complex uses for OWs in order to capitalise on their efficiencies. Some examples are:
  – Chest pain assessment units
  – Toxicology units for treatment of more complex overdoses eg paracetamol toxicity requiring NAC, prolonged anticholinergic delirium, etc.

Exclusion criteria

In order for the OW to work efficiently it is also necessary to have exclusion criteria for some types of patient. Again these vary from institution to institution but in general terms should include the following:

Patients who will clearly need >24 hours admission

- These are patients who should be admitted to inpatient wards, e.g. those with complex medical problems
- Greater than one problem, especially in the elderly
- Patients who cannot be given a clear treatment plan.

Patients who require intensive nursing care

- Because of the nature of OWs nursing time is at a premium. Patients who are a heavy nursing load are therefore not suitable. For similar reasons, as well as safety issues, OWs are generally not suitable for psychotic, violent or disruptive patients.

Admission means that proper assessments are not done

- 'Can't you just put them in the obs ward and I'll see them in the morning' is a frequently heard plea from tired inpatient registrars. Although, at times, some flexibility is needed, this practice can be dangerous if appropriate intervention is delayed. The decision to admit to the OW should always lie with emergency department staff only.

EFFICIENCY OF PATIENT CARE

Efficiency is essential if an observation ward is to maintain rapid patient turn-over and treat patients within defined time criteria. This is achieved by a combination of factors:

- Frequent reassessments are complimented by regular ward rounds with senior staff such as experienced registrars or consultants. This results in rapid decision-making and referral if necessary. Frequency and seniority of ward rounds is not affected by weekends or public holidays as is often the case in other inpatient wards. Typically ward rounds are conducted at shift change times when the responsibility for the patients in the ward is passed form one senior doctor to another (e.g. at commencement of morning, afternoon and night shifts).
- There is preferential access to diagnostic services such as radiology to expedite diagnosis and treatment.
- Typically, a large number of observation ward patients require the services of a social worker, alcohol and drug councillor or other paramedical service. Streamlining the referral process to these services greatly increases the efficiency of the OW. Ideally, this is done by their attendance on morning ward rounds.
- Depending on criteria for admission and discharge about 10–20% of patients admitted to the OW need to be referred to another specialist team for admission and others may need a specialist opinion before discharge. Again preferential access is important to ensure smooth and efficient patient flow. Because in general a large proportion of OW patients require psychiatric input (e.g. post minor overdose, situational crisis) it is especially important to have an arrangement with the psychiatry department.

STAFFING

OWs are staffed by emergency-department personnel. As mentioned, a senior doctor is nominated to have responsibility for the ward during each shift. It is preferable to allocate nursing staff from each shift to the OW from the general emergency deparment pool of nurses rather than employ nurses only for the OW. This leads to increased flexibility with staffing and demonstrates that the OW is an integral part of the emergency department. The nursing establishment of an emergency department needs to take into account commitment to the OW and will need to be increased when it is initially set up. Some units, however, find that a stable, OW-experienced nursing workforce responsible for the ward facilitates greater efficiency. This is a matter for individual units.

AUDIT AND FEEDBACK

As with any other medical activity auditing admissions to the OW and monitoring adverse events is important. Results can then be fed back through emergency department doctors as a quality improvement exercise. firm key performance indicators for OWs have not been established yet but data worth collecting and analyzing might include numbers of OW admissions subsequently admitted under an inpatient team (internationally 10–20% is considered acceptable[2]), patients discharged who re-present within 48 hours, and adverse events and outcomes.

OVERALL IMPACT OF OBSERVATION WARDS

OWs are generally well accepted by emergency department staff who easily see the benefits to efficient functioning of the department. The improved efficiency, however, goes beyond the emergency department and can affect the hospital as a whole. In a recent study performed in a major Australian emergency department[3] it was found that the introduction of an OW had significant effects on the

hospital as a whole. Using DRG codes for the most frequently admitted OW patient types a comparison on numbers admitted to OW and inpatient wards was done. Total inpatient days for these groups were also analyzed. It was found that the introduction of an OW resulted in a decrease of these patients admitted to the inpatient wards associated with an increase in admissions to the OW. Overall the total numbers of patients increased, but, despite this increase, the total number of bed days decreased. Effectively, more patients were treated using fewer days in hospital, a clear indication of increased efficiency throughout the hospital.

The safety net function in reducing inappropriate discharges and picking up missed diagnoses has an effect on patient well being as well as potentially reducing litigation and adverse publicity against the hospital. Less tangible results are an increase in staff satisfaction, an increase in patient satisfaction because of fewer days in hospital and an improvement in the 'public image' of the emergency department within the hospital.

SHORT-STAY MEDICINE

Much of the difference between emergency physicians and their colleagues lies in their approach to a patient or a problem. To some extent, emergency medicine is a method of practice rather than a set of skills and clinical knowledge. A similar comparison can be drawn between standard inpatient wards and an observation ward. The main difference is in the high efficiency; rapid turnover, problem-based approach. The 'technique' of observation medicine can be applied to situations other than emergency departments. The examples of chest pain assessment units and toxicology units as an extension of observation wards have already been mentioned.

CONTROVERSIES AND FUTURE DIRECTIONS

❶ There is potential for expansion of the observation ward concept to increase hospital efficiency, and many hospitals now have short-stay medical wards (acute assessment units, emergency medicine units) modelled on these wards.

❷ This provides new roles for emergency physicians in chest-pain units, toxicology units and other short-stay areas.

❸ There is a gradual blurring of the boundaries between the emergency department and inpatient units as a result.

In the increasing drive for efficiency and cost effectiveness it is likely that more variations on the technique of 'OW' medicine will appear. Medical acute assessment units and short stay wards have already made an appearance in some Australasian hospitals and it is likely that their numbers will increase. What role there will be for emergency physicians in this treatment model remains to be seem but there is a large potential for at least some expansion of emergency medicine beyond its traditional boundaries with positive effects on both job satisfaction and professional longevity.

REFERENCES

1. Jelinek GA, Galvin GM 1989 Observation wards in Australian hospitals. Medical Journal of Australia 151: 509–11
2. Brillman J, Mathers-Dunbar L, Graff L, et al 1995 Management of observation units. American College of Emergency Physicians. Annals of Emergency Medicine 25: 823–30
3. Williams A, Jelinek GA, Rogers IR, Wenban JA, Jacobs IG 2000 The effect of establishment of an observation ward on hospital admission profiles. Medical Journal of Australia 173: 411–4

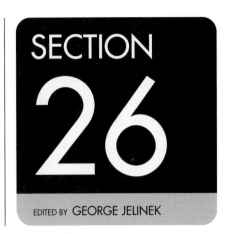

SECTION

26

EDITED BY GEORGE JELINEK

ADMINISTRATION

26.1 Emergency department staffing 714

26.2 Emergency department layout 716

26.3 Quality assurance/quality improvement 720

26.4 Business planning 723

26.5 Accreditation, specialist training and recognition in Australasia 726

26.6 Specialist recognition and training in emergency medicine: the UK view 731

26.7 Complaints 733

26.8 Clinical risk management in the emergency department 739

26.1 EMERGENCY DEPARTMENT STAFFING

SUE IERACI

ESSENTIALS

1 Emergency departments should be staffed so as to provide high-quality clinical care and sustainable working conditions, and to achieve performance benchmarks.

2 Senior medical staff should have protected non-clinical time for administrative, educational and research roles.

3 Clinical work for senior medical staff includes not only direct patient care, but also supervision and teaching of junior staff, coordination of patient flow and liaison with other clinicians.

4 In calculating staff numbers required, it is essential to consider not only the extent of senior cover required, but also the volume of the clinical and non-clinical workload.

5 Precise numbers and types of staff required depend on individual and institutional work practices and hospital roles.

GENERAL PRINCIPLES

The random presentation of undifferentiated patients to emergency departments necessitates a clinical and ancillary staff mix with the structure, organization and training necessary to recognize, triage, evaluate and provide initial management for the full spectrum of acute illness and injury.

Patients requiring emergency care have the right to timely care by skilled staff. The aim of staffing an emergency department is ultimately to provide care in an acceptable time according to the patient's clinical urgency (triage category). Staff working in the department also have the right to safe and manageable working conditions and reasonable job satisfaction.

As the activity of an emergency department fluctuates in both volume and acuity, a threshold level of staffing and resources is required in order to be prepared for likely influxes of patients. In addition, the staffing number and mix needs to take account of the important teaching role of emergency departments.

The precise numbers and designation of medical and other staff employed will be determined by the local workpractices (what tasks are carried out and by whom). This chapter discusses staffing requirements under the current Australasian model of emergency department workpractices. This includes a major supervisory and teaching role for consultants, and a significant proportion of specialist trainees and junior medical staff in the medical workforce, with a range of tasks, including venepuncture, test requisitioning and written documentation.

In the UK, there is a move away from the traditional model of staffing based on enthusiastic and committed, but relatively inexperienced senior house officers, towards more care being delivered by senior medical staff: consultants, registrars, staff grades and associate specialists. There is significant expansion under way in the numbers of registrar training posts and consultants in emergency departments.

This expansion will ensure that more care is delivered by experienced medical staff in conjunction with nursing colleagues, particularly in the enhanced nurse practitioner role. The concept is of an experienced team of clinicians delivering care.

CALCULATING CLINICAL WORKLOAD

Emergency department casemix and costing studies have sought to measure the medical time commitment for

Table 26.1.1 Australasian Triage Scale Categories	
NTS category	Medical time
Category 1	160 min
Category 2	80 min
Category 3	60 min
Category 4	40 min
Category 5	20 min

various clinical conditions. Table 26.1.1 describes the approximate average medical time commitment for each of the Australasian Triage Scale categories:[1]

- The direct clinical workload can then be calculated from census data (number of presentations by triage category).
- The workforce should be resourced and organized so that patients are treated within the benchmark times for their clinical acuity (triage category). The Australasian College for Emergency Medicine has defined the following benchmarks for waiting time by triage category (see Table 26.1.2).[2]
- Staffing should be adequate to achieve benchmark clinical performance, as well as providing for the various clinical and non-clinical medical roles that supplement direct patient care.

MEDICAL STAFF

The medical workforce of Australasian emergency departments currently includes the following categories:

- Consultants (specialist emergency physicians), including a medical director
- Registrars (specialist trainees)
- Senior non-specialist staff: experienced hospital medical officers

26

ADMINISTRATION

Table 26.1.2 Benchmarks for waiting time by triage category					
	Category 1	Category 2	Category 3	Category 4	Category 5
Treatment acuity	Immediate	Within 10 min	Within 30 min	Within 60 min	Within 120 min
Benchmark performance	98%	95%	90%	90%	85%

- Junior medical staff: interns and resident medical officers who have not yet started specialty training.

The specialist practice of emergency medicine includes non-clinical roles (including departmental management and administration, planning, education, research and medicopolitical activities) as well as clinical roles. The non-clinical workload of an individual department varies with its size and role, the structure of its staffing and the other management systems within the institution. For senior staff, clinical work generally includes co-ordination of patient flow, bed management and supervision, and bedside teaching of junior staff, in addition to direct patient care. Some emergency physicians may have other particular roles, such as retrieval and hyperbaric medicine or toxicology services. The increasing number of academic staff may have major research and teaching commitments.

To cover these roles, the ACEM recommends a minimum of 30% non-clinical time for staff specialists (more for directors of departments) and 15% non-clinical time for registrars.

In its 1997 report on the emergency medicine specialist workforce, the Australian Medical Workforce Advisory Committee (AMWAC Report 1997, 1 February 1997) recommended 24-hour 7-day consultant cover for major referral hospitals, and 16-hour 7-day consultant cover for urban district and major rural/regional centres. The projections based on these figures are currently being revised. The calculation of medical staff numbers required for a particular department must include not only the extent of consultant cover required, but also the clinical workload and performance, local workpractices, and the nature of clinical and non-clinical roles. Because of variations in roles and work-practices between sites, it is not possible to devise a staffing profile that is universally appropriate.

ANCILLARY STAFF

Clerical, paramedical and other ancillary staff are essential to the efficient provision of emergency medical services. They should be specifically trained and experienced for emergency department work. Clerical staff have a crucial role, encompassing reception, registration, data entry and communications within and outside the department, as well as maintenance of medical records. Dedicated paramedical staff, including therapists and social workers, are important in providing thorough assessment and management of patients, including participating in disposition decisions and discharge support. Other staff such as porters and ward assistants play an important role in releasing clinical staff from non-clinical roles.

OPTIMIZING WORK PRACTICES

Traditional hospital work practices involve systems and tasks that are inefficient for the smooth running of modern, busy emergency departments. In a work environment with a rapid patient throughput and large numbers of staff, efficient work practices are crucial in optimizing clinical performance as well as job satisfaction. A review of staff numbers and seniority cannot provide maximum benefit without consideration of the way the work is done, what tasks are done, and by whom.

A review of emergency department work practices can encompass the following principles:

- Re-allocation or deletion of inefficient tasks
- Optimal use of ancillary and technical staff
- An extended clinical nursing role
- Use of communication technology and data systems.

As the emergency department workforce develops greater seniority and specialization, and the demands of patient care increase, it is no longer possible to justify outdated work practices. Local research has shown that it is possible to improve clinical service provision by re-organising roles and tasks in a sustainable way.[3] The opportunity exists to create a work environment that both delivers good clinical service and is rewarding and satisfying for staff.

REFERENCES

1. Bond MJ, Erwich-Nijout MA, Phillips D, Baggoley C 1998 Urgency, disposition and age groups: a casemix model for emergency medicine. Emergency Medicine 10: 103–10
2. Australasian College for Emergency Medicine 2000
3. Morris J, Ieraci S, Bauman A, Mohsin M 2001 Emergency department workpractice review project: introduction of workpractice model and development of clinical documentation system specifications. Project report

26.2 EMERGENCY DEPARTMENT LAYOUT

MATTHEW W. G. CHU • ROBERT DUNN

ESSENTIALS

1 The layout of the emergency department should maximize access to every space with the minimum of cross-traffic.

2 The triage location should enable staff to directly observe and gain access to both the ambulance entry and the patient waiting areas.

3 The acute area should be open, with all spaces directly observable from the staff station.

4 Supporting areas, such as the clean and dirty utilities, the medication room and equipment stores, should be centrally located.

5 Areas often poorly planned include office and clinical spaces and tutorial rooms. Computer and telephone entry points and storage space are often underestimated.

6 Planning should consider the implications on night staffing when minimal staff are on duty.

7 The security of both staff and patients is paramount in planning an emergency department.

INTRODUCTION

The major role of an emergency department is the effective provision of acute care. It has a key role within a hospital, as it may be the source of between 15 and 75% of the hospital's total number of admissions. It has a vital role in a hospital's trauma services, and in disaster and fire planning. As a consequence, the department should be purpose-built to facilitate the provision of effective emergency care and ensure the safety of patients, staff and their property. The physical environment includes an effective communication system, appro-priate signposting, adequate ambulance access and clear observation of relevant areas from the triage area. There should be easy access to the resuscitation area, and quiet and private areas should cater for patients and relatives. Adequate staffroom and tutorial areas should be available. Clean and dirty utilities and storage areas are also required.

DESIGN CONSIDERATIONS

The design of the department should promote rapid access to every area with the minimum of cross-traffic. There must be proximity between the resuscitation and the acute treatment areas for non-ambulant patients. Supporting areas, such as clean and dirty utilities, the pharmacy room and equipment stores, should be centrally located to prevent staff traversing long distances. The main aggregation of clinical staff will be at the staff station in the acute treatment area. This is the focus around which the other clinical areas are grouped.

Lighting should conform to Australian standards and clinical care areas should have exposure to daylight whenever possible to minimize patient disorienta-tion. Climate control is essential for the comfort of both patients and staff. Each clinical area needs to be serviced with medical gases, suction, scavenging units and power outlets. The minimum suggested configuration for each type of clinical area is outlined in Table 26.2.1.

Medical gases should be internally piped to all patient care areas, and adequate cabling should ensure the availability of power outlets to all clerical and non-clerical areas. Although patient and emergency call facilities are often considered, there is often inadequate provision for telephone and data-entry ports. Emergency power must be available to all lights and power outlets in the resuscitation and acute treatment areas. All computer terminals in the department should have access to emer-gency power, and emergency lighting should be available in all other areas. The electricity supply should be surge protected to protect electronic and computer equipment, with physiological monitoring areas being cardiac pro-tected, and other patient care areas being body protected.

A factor involving a 35–45% increase to the room requirements is necessary to account for circulation space. Such examples include the provision of corri-dors (though this should be minimized) wide enough to allow the easy passage of two hospital beds with attached intra-venous fluids. The floor covering in all patient care areas should be durable and non slip, easy to clean, impermeable to

Table 26.2.1 Configurations for clinical areas				
	Resuscitation	Acute treatment	Specialty	Consultation room (plaster/procedure)
Oxygen outlets	3	2	2	1
Medical air outlets	2	1	1	–
Suction outlets		2	2	1
Nitrous oxide	1	1	1	–
Scavenging unit	1	1	1	–
Power outlets	14	8	8	4

water and body fluids, and with properties that reduce sound transmission and absorb shocks. Administrative, interview and distressed relatives areas should be carpeted.

SIZE AND COMPOSITION OF THE EMERGENCY DEPARTMENT

The appropriate size of the emergency department depends on a number of factors: the number and acuity of patient attendances, the admission rate, the degree of 'access block' experienced and the speed of patient throughput all contribute to the determination of optimum department size. Departments of inadequate size often function inefficiently, are uncomfortable for patients, and significantly impair patient care. For the average Australasian emergency department with an admission rate of approximately 25–30%, its total internal area (excluding departmental radiology facilities and observation/holding ward) should be approximately 50 m^2/1000 yearly attendances. The total number of patient treatment areas (excluding interview, plaster and procedure rooms) should be at least 1/1300 yearly attendances, and the number of resuscitation areas should be at least one for every 15 000 yearly attendances. It is recommended that, for departments with average patient acuity, at least half the total number of treatment areas should have physiological monitoring available.

CLINICAL AREAS

Individual treatment areas

The design of individual treatment areas should be determined by their specific functions. Adequate space should be allowed around the bed for patient transfer, assessment, performance of procedures and storage of commonly used items. The use of modular storage bins or other materials employing a similar design concept should be considered.

To prevent transmission of confidential information, each area should be separated by solid partitions that extend from floor to ceiling. The entrance to each area should be able to be closed by a movable partition or curtain.

Each acute treatment bed should have access to a physiological monitor. Central monitoring is recommended and monitors should ideally be of the modular type, with print and monitoring modules. The minimum physiological parameters monitored should be ECG, NIBP, temperature and SaO$_2$. Monitors may be mounted adjacent to the bed on an appropriate pivoting bracket, or be movable.

All patient care areas, including toilets and bathrooms, require individual patient call facilities and emergency call facilities, so that staff can summon urgent assistance. In addition, an examination light, a sphygmomanometer (preferably wall mounted), ophthalmoscope, otoscope, waste bins and footstool should all be immediately available. Basins for hand washing should be readily available.

Resuscitation area

This area is used for the resuscitation and treatment of critically ill or injured patients. It must be large enough to fit a standard resuscitation bed, allow access to all parts of the patient, and allow movement of staff and equipment around the work area. As space must also be provided for equipment, monitors, storage, wash-up and disposal facilities, the minimum suitable size for such a room is usually 40 m^2 (including bedside storage), or 25 m^2 (if not including bedside storage) for each bed space in a multibedded room. The area should also have visual and auditory privacy for both the occupants of the room and other patients and their relatives. The resuscitation area should be easily accessible from the ambulance entrance and the staff station, and be separate from patient circulation areas. In addition to standard physiological monitoring, invasive pressure and capnography monitoring should be available. Other desirable features include a ceiling-mounted operating theatre light, a radiolucent resuscitation

trolley with cassette trays, overhead X-ray and lead lining of walls and partitions between beds.

Acute treatment area

This area is used for the assessment, treatment and observation of patients with acute medical or surgical illnesses. Each bed space must be large enough to fit a standard mobile bed, with adequate storage and circulation space. The recommended minimum space between beds is 2.5 m and each treatment area should be at least 10 m^2. All of these beds should be positioned to enable direct observation from the staff station and easy access to the clean and dirty utility rooms, procedure room, pharmacy room, and patient shower and toilet.

Single rooms

These rooms should be used for the management of patients who require isolation, privacy, or who are a source of visual, olfactory or auditory distress to others. Deceased patients may also be placed there for the convenience of grieving relatives. These rooms must be completely enclosed by floor-to-ceiling partitions and have a solid door. Each department should have at least two such rooms. Isolation rooms should be used to treat patients with conditions that require separation from other patients. Each room should have negative-pressure ventilation and an en-suite toilet so that isolation procedures may be maintained for infective patients. A decontamination room should be available for patients contaminated with toxic substances. In addition to the requirements of an isolation room, this room must have a floor drain and contaminated water trap. Single rooms should otherwise have the same requirements as acute treatment area bed spaces.

Seclusion room

This is a type of single room designed specifically for the assessment and containment of patients with actual or potential behavioural disturbances. It should have two doors large enough to allow a patient to be carried through, and must be lockable only from the outside. One of the doors may be of the 'barn door' type, enabling the lower section to be closed while the upper section remains open. This allows direct observation of, and communication with, the patient without requiring staff to enter the room. The room should be shielded from external noise and must be designed in such a way that direct observation of the patient by staff outside the room is possible at all times. Services such as electricity or medical gases should not be accessible to the patient and no materials should be present that could be used as weapons or for actions of self-harm. It is preferable that furniture should be made of foam rubber and the design ensure that patients have no access to air vents or hanging points. A smoke detector should be fitted, and closed-circuit television may be used in addition to direct visual monitoring.

Consultation area

Consultation rooms are provided for the examination and treatment of ambulant patients who are not suffering a major or serious illness. These rooms have similar space requirements to acute treatment area bed spaces. Consultation rooms may be adapted and equipped to serve specific functions, such as ENT or ophthalmology treatment.

Plaster room

The plaster room allows for the application of plaster of Paris and for the closed reduction of displaced fractures or dislocations, and should be at least 15 m^2 in size. Physiological monitoring during procedures involving regional anaesthesia or sedation is required. Specific features of such a room include a storage area for plaster and bandages; X-ray viewing panels; provision of oxygen and suction; a nitrous oxide delivery system; plaster trolley with plaster instruments; and a sink and drainer with a plaster trap. Ideally, a splint and crutch store should be directly accessible from the plaster room.

Procedure room

Procedure room(s) may be required for the performance of procedures such as lumbar puncture, tube thoracostomy, thoracocentesis, diagnostic peritoneal lavage, bladder catheterization or suturing. It requires noise insulation and should be at least 15 m^2 in size.

Staff station

A single central staff area is recommended for staff servicing the different treatment areas, as this enables better communication between, and coordination of, staff members. The staff station in the acute treatment area should be the major staff area within the department. The staff area should be of an 'arena' or 'semiarena' design, whereby the main areas of clinical activity are directly observable. The station may be raised in order to give uninterrupted vision of patients, and should be centrally located. It should be constructed to ensure that confidential information can be conveyed without breach of privacy. The use of sliding windows and adjustable blinds may be used to modulate external stimuli, and a separate write-up area may be considered. Other features should include an adequate number of telephones, computer terminals and X-ray viewing boxes; dangerous drug/medication cupboards; emergency and patient call displays; under-desk duress alarm; valuables storage; police blood alcohol sample safe; stationery store; and writing and workbenches. Direct telephone lines, bypassing the hospital switchboard, should be available to allow staff to receive admitting requests from outside medical practitioners or to participate in internal or external emergencies when the need arises. A dedicated line to the ambulance and police service is essential, as is the provision of a facsimile line. A pneumatic tube system for sending specimens to pathology and transferring medical records and imaging requests may also be located in this area.

CLINICAL SUPPORT AREAS

The clean utility area requires sufficient space for the storage of clean and sterile supplies and procedural equipment, and benchtops to prepare procedure trays.

The dirty utility should have sufficient space to house a stainless steel benchtop with sink and drainer, pan and bottle rack, bowl and basin rack, utensil washer, pan/bowl washer/sanitizer, and slop hopper and storage space for testing equipment (such as for urinalysis). A separate store room may be used for the storage of equipment and disposable medical supplies. It is a common design error to underestimate the amount of storage space required for a modern department. A pharmacy/medication room may be used for the storage of medications used by the department, and should be accessible to all clinical areas. Entry should be secure with a self-closing door, and the area should have sufficient space to house a refrigerator for the storage of heat-sensitive drugs. Other design features should include spaces for a linen trolley, mobile radiology equipment, patient trolleys and wheelchairs. Beverage-making facilities for patients and relatives, a blanket-warming cupboard, disaster equipment store, a cleaners' room and shower and toilet facilities also need to be accommodated. An interview room may be designated for the interviewing or counselling of relatives in private. It should be acoustically treated and removed from the main clinical area of the department. A distressed relatives' room should be designated for the relatives of seriously ill or deceased patients. Consideration for two such rooms should be given in larger departments to allow the separation of relatives of patients who have been protagonists in violent incidents or clashes. They should be acoustically insulated and have access to beverage-making facilities, a toilet and telephones. A single-room treatment area should be in close proximity to these rooms to enable relatives to be with dying patients, and should be of a size appropriate to local cultural practices.

NON-CLINICAL AREAS

Waiting area

The waiting area should provide sufficient space for waiting patients as well as relatives or escorts, and should be open and easily observed from the triage and reception areas. Seating should be comfortable and adequate space should be allowed for wheelchairs, prams, walking aids and patients being assisted. There should be an area where children may play, and support facilities such as television should be available. Easy access from the waiting room to the triage and reception area, toilets and baby change rooms, and light refreshment should be possible. Public telephones should be accessible and dedicated telephones with direct lines to taxi firms should be encouraged. The area should be monitored to safeguard security and patient well-being, and it is desirable to have a separate waiting area for children. The waiting area should be at least 4.4 m^2/1000 yearly attendances, and should contain at least one seat per 1000 yearly attendances.

Reception/triage area

The department should be accessed by two separate entrances: one for ambulance patients and the other for ambulant patients. It is recommended that each contain a separate foyer that can be sealed by the remote activation of security doors. Access to treatment areas should also be restricted by the use of security doors. Both entrances should direct the patient flow towards the reception/triage area, which should have clear vision to the waiting room and the ambulance entrance. The triage area should have access to a pulse oximeter, a computer terminal, a hand basin, examination light, telephones, chairs and desk, and patient weighing scales, and should have adequate storage space for bandages, medical equipment and stationery.

Reception/clerical office

Staff at the reception counter receive patients arriving for treatment and direct them to the triage area. After assessment there, patients or relatives will generally be directed back to the reception/clerical area, where clerical staff will conduct registration interviews, collate the medical record and print identification labels. When a decision to admit has been made, clerks also interview patients or relatives at the bedside or at the reception counter to finalize admission details. The counter should provide seating and be partitioned for privacy at the interview. There should be direct communication with the reception/triage area, the staff station in the acute treatment area, and the design should take due consideration of the safety of staff. This area should have access to an adequate number of telephones, computer terminals, printers, facsimile machines and photocopier. It should also have sufficient storage space for stationery and medical records.

Tutorial room

This room provides facilities for formal undergraduate and postgraduate education and meetings. It should be in a quiet, non-clinical area near the staff room and offices. Provision should be made for a VCR, television, slide projector, overhead projector, whiteboard, power outlets, projection screen, tube X-ray viewer, telephone and examination couch.

Telemedicine area

Departments using telemedicine facilities should have a dedicated, fully enclosed room with appropriate power and communications cabling. This room should be of suitable size to allow simultaneous viewing by members of multiple service teams, and should, ideally, be close to the staff station.

Offices

Offices provide space for the administrative, managerial, quality assurance, teaching and research roles of the emergency department. The number of offices required will be determined by the number and type of staff. In a large department offices may be needed for the director, deputy director, nursing manager, nurse educator, academic staff, staff specialists, registrars, secretary, social worker/mental health crisis worker, information support officer, research and projects officers and clerical supervisor. Larger departments may consider the incorporation of a meeting room into the office area.

Staff facilities

A room should be provided within the department to enable staff to relax during rest periods. Food and drink should be able to be prepared and appropriate table and seating arrangements should be provided. It should be located away from patient care areas and have access to natural lighting and appropriate floor and wall coverings. A staff changing area with lockers, toilets and shower facilities should also be provided.

THE FUTURE

Over the last 20 years emergency departments have been providing care of an ever-increasing complexity. Changes in technology have enabled the management of greater numbers of patients in the community who would previously have required hospitalization. As financial pressures on hospitals have also increased, the importance of the emergency department has grown considerably, and modern departments have significantly expanded facilities. Future design considerations are likely to centre on advances in the areas of information technology, telecommunications and new non-invasive diagnostic modalities. In addition to these technologically driven changes, it is likely that a greater emphasis will be placed on developing emergency department design configurations that maximize efficient work practices. Computerized patient tracking systems using electronic tags and built-in sensors will provide additional information that may further improve operational efficiency. The electronic medical record will make detailed medical information immediately available and will greatly facilitate quality improvement and research activities. Digital radiography, personal communication devices, voice recognition systems and expanded telemedicine facilities will make the emergency department of the future as reliant on electricity and cabling as it is on oxygen and suction. In the UK, new guidance has recently been issued by the Department of Health.

26.3 QUALITY ASSURANCE/QUALITY IMPROVEMENT

DIANE KING

ESSENTIALS

1 Quality management plays a pivotal role in the running of an emergency department.

2 All staff must be engaged in the process of quality improvement.

3 Performance measures are an integral part of the quality cycle.

INTRODUCTION

A primary role of the emergency department is to deliver the best possible care to presenting patients. In order to deliver optimal care a system of quality management must be part of the culture for all staff and must be applied to all functions of the department. Quality management requires effective leadership, organizational vision, strategic development, commitment to improving processes and systems, accountability, communication, support for staff development and commitment to analysis, change and review. This is a continuous cycle, with measurement and monitoring

required to establish that change has indeed been an improvement. Consumer involvement is a fundamental part of quality management. In the emergency setting consumers include patients, staff, and the other clinical and hospital staff who interface with the emergency department.

HISTORY

The traditional approach of quality assurance involves a number of retrospective attempts to police various activities of the emergency department. The types of tools used in this approach are pathology result checking, missed fractures, medical record reviews, death audits and patient complaints. Although these checks are essential, it must be recognized that the traditional quality-assurance (QA) philosophy involves crisis management and implies 'fault', and the apportioning of blame. The trend currently involves movement from the QA model to the philosophy of total quality improvement and total quality management.[1] This management system has been adopted from industrial

models, and applied to hospitals.[2] The basic philosophies are being adopted both by national bodies and individual departments. Much of the change has been triggered by the climate of accountability and clinical governance.

DEFINITIONS

- Quality – 'doing those things necessary to meet the needs and reasonable expectations of those we service, and doing those things right every time.'[2]
- Quality assurance (QA) – 'a system used to establish standards for patient care, to monitor how well standards of care are met, and to correct unwarranted deviations from the standards.'[3] This implies intervention to correct deficiencies, and is often externally driven.
- Quality improvement (QI) – raising quality performance to ever increasing levels.
- Continuous quality improvement (CQI) – a management approach that focuses on providing a service that meets the 'customer's' needs in

such a fashion that the process itself leads to continuous improvement. This uses data collection, statistical tools, and team dynamics to develop quality processes.

- Total quality management (TQM) – uses the management approach of continuous quality improvement, and implies the commitment of the whole organization to the implementation of a quality plan. This involves the crossing of boundaries, and traditional spheres of activity.

- Clinical indicators – measures of the clinical outcomes of care. They are population-based screens that help point to potential problems. They also allow comparative data to be collected nationally and benchmarking to occur.

- Clinical guidelines – are reference tools which help guide clinical practice. They provide a focus, or reference point for peer review, but should not be seen as immutable, and their appropriate use requires considerable clinical expertise.

- Benchmarking – the use of the best practices in a field to act as a marker and goal for improvement.[4]

CONTINUOUS QUALITY IMPROVEMENT

The Deming cycle (described by WE Deming) is a fundamental tool for the approach to quality in any system. The PDCA (plan, do, check, act) cycle should incorporate the important principles of planning, staff engagement, measurement, implementation, remeasurement, and reevaluation.

A QI system covers a number of dimensions. These are

- Access – e.g. waiting times and access to inpatient beds
- Safety – e.g. body fluid exposures, work-related injury, stress
- Acceptability – e.g. complaint rates, staff and patient satisfaction surveys
- Effectiveness – e.g. time to thrombolysis, admission rates and unplanned representations

- Continuity – e.g. discharge letters to GPs, wound, plaster and head-injury advice.

Joseph Juran has identified three universal processes of quality management:[5]

❶ Quality planning
Involves the identification of customers, both internal and external, determining the customers' needs, developing services that are responsive to those needs, developing processes that produce those services, and then putting the plans into action.

❷ Quality control
Involves choosing the areas to be measured, establishing the methods of measurement, establishing the standards of performance (benchmarking), measuring actual performance, and then taking action on the difference between the actual and the standard.

❸ QI
Involves establishing the infrastructure for improvement, identifying specific needs for improvement (such as waiting times), establish a project team with clear responsibilities, and provide the necessary resources, motivation and training. The teams use the performance measures to evaluate processes and develop ways to improve performance. These are then instituted, and the process re-evaluated to assess improvement.

There are a number of vital characteristics of a CQI programme that are necessary for its successful operation.[1] A CQI programme:

- Requires leadership (management) commitment
- Is 'customer' focused. Customers include patients primarily, but also include relatives, staff, other departments within the hospital, students, ambulance personnel, and anyone who is involved with the functioning of the emergency department.
- Is performance based. This requires accurate and relevant performance measures.

- Is internally driven, not externally mandated.
- Focuses on systems first, and individuals second. This acknowledges the fact that a perfect world does not exist, but that quality can always be improved within a system (improving the norm), and takes the emphasis away from apportioning blame.
- Is a hospital-wide set of activities.

A more detailed outline of TQM is beyond the scope of this book, however, the recent literature abounds with discussion on the various tools used, pitfalls in introduction, and so on.[6–14]

NATIONAL BODIES

The push to TQM has been facilitated by various bodies, in particular The Australian Council on Healthcare Standards (ACHS) that, in 1997, introduced its Evaluation and Quality Improvement Program (EQuIP) as a framework for hospitals to establish quality processes.[15] This is a requirement for accreditation with the ACHS. In the USA the Joint Commission on Accreditation of Healthcare Organizations (JCAHO) has also led the way, in the move from QA to QI.[16]

The Australasian College for Emergency Medicine, the American College of Emergency Physicians and the British Association for Accident and Emergency Medicine are facilitating the process of QI by their training role, introduction of clinical indicators, policy development and standards for emergency departments.[17] In Australasia the introduction of the Australasian Triage Scale, which has been widely adopted in emergency departments, has been a critical step forward in the process of benchmarking, and the development of standards.[18]

QUALITY IN THE EMERGENCY DEPARTMENT

The emergency department is a complex environment, which involves close interaction with the rest of the hospital and the community. The inputs are uncontrollable and unregulated, and the 'customers' are under a high level of stress because of the nature of their problems, the unfamiliarity of the environment, and the lack of control they perceive at a time when they are feeling personally vulnerable.

The emergency department is dealing simultaneously with life-threatening illness and minor complaints. It is an area under a high level of scrutiny from all quarters, the patients, the families and friends, the other departments in the hospital, and the wider community – both medical and non-medical. This in itself is stressful, and is compounded by the fact that many of the staff working in the emergency department are rotating through the department for relatively short periods of time, are often relatively junior and are undergoing training themselves. This training role is of critical importance in most emergency departments, and must not be forgotten in any process dealing with quality issues. All these aspects of an emergency department make the maintenance of quality difficult and all the more imperative. In order to establish a system where quality care can be delivered with any degree of reliability, it is important that all staff are committed to the process, and that management provide appropriate leadership and resources. The delivery of quality involves a continuing process of data collection (performance measures), analysis, feedback and introduction of strategies to improve the system, followed by re-analysis of the performance measures(the quality cycle).

COMMON MEASURES OF CLINICAL PERFORMANCE OR OUTCOME

The following are commonly used measures:

- Time to thrombolysis
- Waiting time by triage category
- Death audits
- Admission rates by triage category
- Access block measures
- Chart audits
- Total emergency department treatment time
- Trauma audits – missed cervical fractures, delay in craniotomy, waiting times versus triage category, and death audits are the ACHS trauma clinical indicators
- Patient satisfaction surveys
- Staff satisfaction surveys
- X-ray and pathology report follow-up
- Patient complaints audits
- Equipment functioning and supply
- Safety of the working environment
- Staff retention.

The first three of these are the current ACHS/ACEM Clinical Indicators for Emergency Medicine.[17]

It is clear from the list, that the measures are potentially innumerable, and that local factors must dictate those areas of special interest, and that this will vary from hospital to hospital. In deciding on which areas should be measured it is important to focus on areas that have been targeted as requiring improvement.

It is also evident that all emergency departments have common areas where there is high potential for problems to develop, and that these areas should be routinely monitored. The mechanism for doing this will vary from institution to institution.

Another aspect of the measuring of performance is that the process is one in evolution. Not only should the quality of the service improve as the measures are improved and re-assessed, but the areas for attention can change and develop with the whole system. Again, this process must be internally driven to be effective. There is little point in collecting an enormous amount of data, unless the process is useful to the improved functioning of the whole system. Those best able to make those improvements should be an integral part of the system.

REFERENCES

1. O'Leary DS, O'Leary MR 1992 From quality assurance to quality improvement. The Joint Commission on Accreditation of Healthcare Organizations and Emergency Care. Emergency Medicine Clinics of North America 10(3): 447–91
2. Mayer TA 1992 Industrial models of continuous quality improvement. Implications for emergency medicine. Emergency Medicine Clinics of North America 10(3): 523–47
3. American College of Emergency Physicians 1986 Quality assurance manual for emergency medicine. ACEP, Dallas
4. American College of Emergency Physicians 1997 Benchmarking in emergency medicine: an information paper. ACEP, Dallas
5. Juran JM 1986 The quality trilogy: a universal approach to managing for quality. Quality Progress, August, 19–24
6. Allison EJ 1992 Continuous Quality Improvement in Emergency Medicine. ACEP News, pp 4–5
7. Carlin E, et al 1996 Using continuous quality improvement tools to improve pediatric immunization rates. Journal on Quality Improvement 22: 277–87
8. Fernades C, Christenson J 1995 Use of CQI to facilitate patient flow throughout the triage and fast-track areas of an ED. Journal of Emergency Medicine. 13(6): 847–55
9. Howland R, Decker M 1992 Continuous quality improvement and hospital epidemiology: common themes: quality management in health care 1: 9–12
10. Kaissier JP 1993 The quality of care and the quality of measuring it. New England Journal of Medicine 329: 1263–4
11. Brown MG, Hitchcock DE, Willard ML 1994 Why TQM Fails. Irwin Pulishing, Toronto
12. Berwick DM 1996 Quality comes home. Annals of Internal Medicine 125: 839–43
13. Berwick DM 1989 Continuous improvement as an ideal in health care. New England Journal of Medicine 320: 53–56
14. Kennedy MP, Cleaton PGA, Harrington AP, et al 1997 Quality Assurance to Continuous Quality Improvement: Development of an Emergency department system. Emergency Medicine 9: 247–53
15. Australian Council on Healthcare Standards 1996 The EQuIP Guide: Standards and Guidelines for the ACHS Evaluation and Quality Improvement Program. Australian Council on Healthcare Standards, Melbourne
16. Joint Commission on Accreditation of Health Care Organizations 1991 Accreditation manual for hospitals. Joint Commission on Accreditation for Health Care Organizations
17. The Australian Council on Healthcare Standards 1998 Clinical indicators, a users' manual. Emergency medicine indicators, version 2. The Australian Council on Healthcare Standards, Melbourne
18. Standards Committee Australasian College for Emergency Medicine 1994 National Triage Scale. Emergency Medicine 6: 145–6

26.4 BUSINESS PLANNING

RICHARD H. ASHBY

ADMINISTRATION

ESSENTIALS

1 The business plan is an important multipurpose document developed annually by the emergency department management group, to inform the organization about the agreed performance dimensions of expenditure, activity, efficiency and quality of services proposed for the next financial year.

2 The basic content of the business plan should include a projection and analysis of the current year's performance, together with proposed budget, activity, efficiency and quality targets for the next financial year.

3 Once approved by the hospital executive, the emergency-department management group should regularly monitor actual outcomes against the targets and take remedial action where necessary.

INTRODUCTION

Emergency departments in public sector health services in Australasia are typically mid-sized clinical units within the organizational structures of hospitals. Staff numbers may range from 20 to over 200 and expenditure budgets from $1 m to over $15 m per annum. Emergency department efficiency directly affects the global efficiency of the healthcare process in the hospital, and purchasers are therefore increasingly interested in the value and performance of emergency medicine services. Emergency department managers are being required to report on the dimensions of cost, output, quality and efficiency through a business planning process and other reporting mechanisms in order to justify their level of resourcing.

TYPES OF PLANS

Emergency department plans are relatively low in a hierarchy of planning instruments that begin with national and state health policy, health departments' strategic and corporate plans, regional and hospital strategic and business plans, and, finally, the business and project plans of individual clinical units and departments. Strategic plans describe how organizations propose to respond to changing technology, altered demographics, shifting paradigms of care and industrial and regulatory reform, as well as issues associated with the cost, quality and accessibility of health care. These plans typically look 5–10 years into the future, and the emergency department should reasonably expect to have input at a variety of levels into the strategic planning process.

Project plans, on the other hand, are highly focused on a particular objective outcome to be achieved within a given timeframe, and with a specified level of resources. Project plans may need to be created by an emergency department for the implementation of a new and significant piece of technology, major refurbishment or redevelopment, or some types of work practice reform. However, the most important planning instrument for an emergency department is its annual business plan.

THE BUSINESS PLAN

The business plan is an important multipurpose document that needs to be developed by the emergency department management group, in consultation with hospital management, on an annual basis. At one level the business plan represents a management contract between the executive of the hospital and the emergency department. At another level the business plan provides information to the staff of the department about the agreed targets for expenditure, activity, efficiency and quality of services to be provided in the next financial year.

PLANNING PROCESS

The plan should be developed by the medical director, business manager and nurse manager of the emergency department. It is often useful to include a representative from the hospital's financial services department early in the process, so that there is a clear understanding of the financial framework for the plan. It is vitally important that the process be informed with as much useful data as possible, including accurate and up-to-date financial and activity statistics, and quality and efficiency indicators. The premises, or context, of the business plan need to be established. Unless there are specific reasons for change it can usually be assumed that purchasers will require that the business plan be based on management of the same level of activity at a similar quality to the previous year. Other premises, relating to estimated wages growth, non-labour cost escalations, leave requirements and so on, should be stated.

The timing of business plan development depends on the government budget cycle for public sector emergency departments and the timing of the financial year for private sector emergency departments. In most jurisdictions this process needs to commence in early January, with the draft business plan available for the hospital executive by the end of February. The process may need to begin much earlier if significant additional or special funding is being sought. Such requests are best handled as separate submissions, which will then need to pass through the various evaluation and approval steps to be finally included in the government's forward estimates and budget. It is uncommon for special projects requiring substantial funds to be

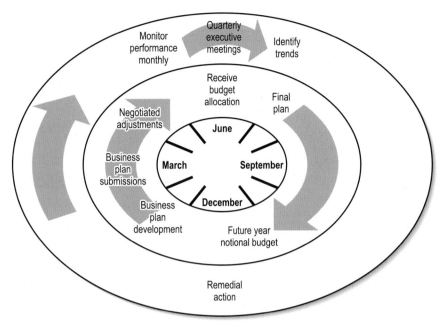

Fig. 26.4.1 Business plan cycle.

Table 26.4.1 Typical business plan index
Smithfield Hospital Emergency Department
Business Plan 2003/2004
Table of Contents
1.0 Introduction Mission, role, objectives
2.0 Executive summary
3.0 Projected outcomes 2002/2003
3.1 Budget
3.2 Budget variance analysis
3.3 Staffing profile
3.4 Activity
3.5 Quality Efficiency indicators Clinical indicators Consumer indicators
4.0 Budget estimates 2003/2004
5.0 Special issues 2003/2004 Equipment <$5000 >$5000 Maintenance Projects Information system Short-stay unit Head injury research

approved and funded within one budget cycle.

A typical business planning cycle is illustrated in Figure 26.4.1.

Business plan content

The emergency department business plan must address, as a minimum, each of the dimensions of performance, that is, expenditure, activity, quality and efficiency. A typical index is illustrated in Table 26.4.1. Some hospitals may require that their own format be used.

The introduction to the business plan should be brief. It is often useful to restate the role and objectives of the emergency department, and of any of its subunits. The executive summary should present an overview of the business plan, including a general perspective on the integrity of the budget and activity targets for the current year, and outlining any premises used in the creation of the current plan. Special issues may be highlighted.

Budget

The projected financial outcomes for the current financial year should have been carefully estimated. This projected end-of-year position should be shown in a tabular format against the agreed targets from the previous year's business plan, as well as the actual outcomes of the previous year. In government organizations adherence to budget is the highest priority and, therefore, the budget details should be presented first. The management group should have a detailed understanding of every variance from the budget that has occurred in the current year, and a note of explanation of variance on every line item should be provided. Because the high fixed costs associated with operating an emergency department are related to the labour intensity of the service, it is useful to include a section tracking paid full-time equivalent staff, by month, for the current year compared to the previous financial year. This is especially important if there has been an overrun in the labour budget, as the hospital executive will wish to be reassured that this is not due to the employment of excess staff.

Activity

The activity of the emergency department may be shown as total attendances and attendances by category of the Australasian Triage Scale. The admission rate by triage category should also be shown, and all values should be tabulated against the previous year's activity levels.

Where an emergency department operates a short-stay ward or observation unit, the top 20 diagnosis-related groups (DRGs) by volume should be shown, together with the number of total separations, weighted separations and the case-mix index. This information should be available from the financial services department. Again, the data should be benchmarked to the previous year. Additional relevant activity data, such as interhospital transfers, retrievals and so on, should be included.

Quality

Waiting time by triage category is the key quality and efficiency indicator for an emergency department. The average waiting time per patient in each triage category should be shown, together with the percentage of patients in each triage category who are seen within the timeframe specified by the Australasian Triage Scale. This data should be benchmarked against the previous year's performance and, ideally, also against published data from similar hospitals elsewhere. Performance against clinical indicators recommended by the Australian Council on Healthcare Standards should also be reported. Additional access indicators include the frequency of ambulance bypass (occasions per month), and admission access block (percentage of total admitted patients spending longer than 8 hours in the emergency department) should be provided. Some units use additional quality indicators, such as the percentage of correct diagnoses made on admitted patients by the emergency department, and the mortality rate of sentinel diagnoses (for instance poisoning and overdose, major trauma), among others.

The written complaint rate (per 10 000 attendances) about emergency department services should be known and reported.

It is appropriate in the section on 'quality' that research and educational achievements should be succinctly reported, together with any innovative projects.

Projections

Having summarized the current year's performance, the remainder of the business plan should be used to present the emergency department's projections and estimates for the next financial year. Again, the projected budget should be presented first. This is best done in a tabular format and compared to the previous year's budget and projected actual expenditure. Any premises, assumptions or caveats related to the projected budget should be included as footnotes to the table. The most common premise relates to the volume and quality of services to be provided, and the usual approach is iso-volume/iso-quality; this should not be varied in the business plan unless previously agreed by the hospital executive. Periodically circumstances will dictate that a hospital vary the desired quality of

services, perhaps as part of a strategic initiative to develop the emergency department, or the volume of services in response to changing demographic projections. Apart from anticipated wages growth, it is important for the management group to make reasonable enquiries about predictable leave (such as sabbaticals or long-service leave), and these should be appropriately costed. In the non-labour budget possible variations in the cost of overseas-sourced clinical supplies or pharmaceuticals due to re-valuation of the currency should be considered, although in some jurisdictions non-labour increments are specified, for budget purposes, across the whole of government.

Realistically, most hospital executives will reject a budget proposal that exceeds the previous year's expenditure, escalated by projected wages growth, unless there are special mitigating factors, or a source of funds for the predicted additional expenditure has been identified. For this reason, it is often useful to have three additional sections in the business plan addressing equipment needs, facility maintenance needs, and a projects summary.

Equipment

The emergency department management group should canvass widely among the staff about perceived equipment needs. It is important that the totality of clinical and non-clinical equipment needs is understood and equitably prioritized in order to optimize the efficiency of the whole department. Most hospitals require that equipment requests be stratified according to cost, with items less than $5000 typically being met from a global allocation to the department. Apart from tabulating the need for this lower-priced equipment, a few lines of narrative about each item often assists the executive in ensuring the reasonableness of the request. The table should indicate whether the equipment is new or replacement. High-cost equipment (e.g. ultrasound machines, CT scanners or arterial blood gas machines) will almost always require the presentation of a full business case and economic analysis

in line with whole of government procurement instructions.

Facility maintenance

All but the newest departments will require some expenditure on maintenance each year. Again, it is useful for the emergency department management group to undertake a focused tour of all areas of the department to establish an inventory of maintenance needs. Reasonably accurate costings can be obtained from hospital engineering services or external contractors.

Projects

This final section can be used to describe and cost small or large projects to enhance the emergency department facilities, infrastructure or services. For example, there may be a proposal to establish a 10-bed short-stay unit adjacent to the emergency department, involving facility redevelopment, the acquisition of clinical and non-clinical equipment (including information systems), staff resourcing and business process reform. This is best presented in a project format, including a clear description of the business need (supported by all available, relevant data), a business case outlining all the costs and benefits and, if possible, additional material such as architects' sketches and a project implementation plan, including a project timetable.

PRIVATE EMERGENCY DEPARTMENTS

The overview of business planning presented above is equally relevant to emergency departments in private hospitals. However, private emergency departments also need to develop a revenue budget and marketing plan appropriate to their circumstances. The marketing plan will usually be a part of the hospital's overall arrangements, but the emergency department should be in a position to report on any changes in referral pattern or on any opportunities to expand the business.

BUSINESS PLAN IMPLEMENTATION AND MONITORING

Soon after the hospital receives its global budget and activity targets from government, a short process of negotiation between the hospital executive and the emergency department management group should take place. This will fine-tune the business plan and, ultimately, permit authorization of the plan and the appropriate delegation for its implementation.

The emergency department management group should meet at least monthly to review actual performance against the outcomes predicted by the plan. Any variance from the budget in particular should be studied and understood. Remedial action should be taken wherever possible to maintain budget integrity. In many places the emergency department management group would meet with the hospital executive at least quarterly to review department performance and to deal with any variation that may have occurred.

26.5 ACCREDITATION, SPECIALIST TRAINING AND RECOGNITION IN AUSTRALASIA

ALLEN YUEN • ANDREW SINGER

ESSENTIALS

1 Specialist training in emergency medicine in Australia and New Zealand is the responsibility of the Australasian College for Emergency Medicine (ACEM).

2 Overseas-trained doctors also require recognition from either the Australian Medical Council (AMC) or the Medical Council of New Zealand (MCNZ).

3 Specialist training in emergency medicine under ACEM occurs in three phases: basic, provisional and advanced training.

4 Provisional trainees must complete the ACEM Primary Examination and Advanced Trainees the Fellowship Examination.

5 Advanced trainees must complete a minimum paediatric requirement, as well as a research paper.

6 Overseas-trained specialists must undergo an assessment by ACEM in order to be recognized as specialist emergency physicians in either country

7 Accreditation is awarded to hospitals if they satisfy predetermined criteria.

8 Emergency department criteria here are set by the Australasian College for Emergency Medicine (ACEM), and concentrate on standards of care for patients, and the supervision and training of registrars.

9 Hospitals are inspected at regular intervals to determine whether standards are being maintained to allow continuation of accreditation.

10 Recommendations are made to correct identified deficiencies.

11 The accreditation process is an important component in improving performance.

SPECIALIST RECOGNITION AND REGISTRATION

Specialist recognition in New Zealand and Australia is handled by the respective medical councils in each country – the Medical Council of New Zealand (MCNZ) and the Australian Medical Council (AMC). In New Zealand, MCNZ handles both specialist recognition (termed vocational registration) and general medical registration. In Australia, AMC has responsibility of specialist recognition of overseas-trained doctors and the accreditation of specialist medical colleges. Medical registration (both general and specialist where applicable) is the responsibility of the eight state and territory medical boards. All medical practitioners must be both recognized by AMC if their primary medical degree has been obtained outside of Australia or New Zealand, and registered with the medical board of the state or territory in which they are practising. Medical registration is also required for specialist training. State and territory medical boards also have provision for temporary registration for training purposes under an occupational training visa, which allows up to 4 years of training in Australia. These require sponsorship by an Australian employing hospital, as well as ACEM.

SPECIALIST TRAINING IN EMERGENCY MEDICINE

Specialist medical training is the responsibility of the various specialist medical colleges. Most of these organizations are trans-national, covering both Australia and New Zealand. They are accredited by AMC. Specialist training in emergency medicine is covered by the Australasian College for Emergency Medicine (ACEM). The college provides the framework, standards and supervision for specialist training in emergency medicine, and successful trainees are granted fellowship of ACEM (FACEM). This is the recognized specialist qualification in emergency medicine in Australia and New Zealand.

Training occurs in hospitals and rotations accredited by ACEM for training. Each accredited emergency department appoints a director of emergency medical training (DEMT). This is a Fellow of ACEM with the responsibility of running the training programme in that department, as well as coordinating and controlling both emergency department and non-emergency department rotations. The description below of the training programme reflects the situation at January 2003. The training programme undergoes regular review and revision.

Specialist training in emergency medicine is divided into three phases:

❶ Basic training
❷ Provisional training
❸ Advanced training.

Basic training

This usually consists of the pre-registration year of practice (internship) and the second year of practice following a doctor's primary medical degree. It must occur in a variety of clinical rota-

tions, and be signed off by the administration of the employing institution.

Provisional training

This usually occurs in the third postgraduate year. There are three requirements of provisional training:

❶ Completion of 12 months of training in approved rotations. At least 6 months of this must be in emergency medicine. Each rotation is assessed and signed-off by the DEMT or local supervisor (for non-emergency department rotations) at its completion.
❷ Successful completion of the ACEM primary examination. The ACEM primary examination is a basic science examination covering four subjects: anatomy, pathology, physiology and pharmacology. Each subject consists of a 90-minute multiple-choice examination and a 10-minute viva voce examination. The examination is conducted twice a year in a number of locations across Australia and New Zealand. Each subject may be attempted multiple times, but each subject must be passed to successfully complete the examination.
❸ Provision of three structured references and completion of the trainee selection process. Each trainee must obtain three structured references (as supplied by ACEM). These assess the trainee's potential for a career in emergency medicine, and are reviewed by the Trainee Selection Committee.

Advanced training

Advanced training occurs once the trainee has completed all the requirements of provisional training. ACEM has a detailed curriculum outlining the knowledge and skills required by the completion of advanced training. The main elements are emergency department training, non-emergency-department advanced training, the minimum paediatric requirement, a research paper and completion of the fellowship examination.

Emergency department training

Trainees must complete 30 months of training in accredited emergency departments. Each accredited emergency department is allowed to provide training for a specific trainee up to a specified maximum amount of time (either 6, 12 or 24 months). Training must be in a minimum of 3-month rotations, and is assessed and signed off by the DEMT at the end of each rotation or every 6 months.

Hospitals are also assigned a role delineation (major referral, urban district, rural/regional) when they are inspected for training accreditation. Trainees must complete at least 6 months in a major referral hospital and either an urban district or rural/regional hospital.

Non-emergency-department training

Trainees must complete 18 months of training in approved non-emergency department rotations. These are usually in hospitals accredited for training by the respective college for that specialty. It is highly recommended that at least 6 months be spent in critical-care rotations (anaesthesia and intensive care).

Up to 6 months of non-emergency department training can be gained in designated special skills rotations, such as retrieval, toxicology, rural critical care, research and general practice.

Minimum paediatric requirement

This is gained concurrently during emergency department and non-emergency department advanced training. Trainees must log at least 400 substantive encounters with paediatric (aged 15 years and under) patients, as well as complete a number of procedures on paediatric patients under supervision. Emergency departments are given specific accreditation for this minimum paediatric requirement.

Research paper

Each trainee must publish or present a research paper, to the satisfaction of ACEM.

Fellowship examination

Trainees may attempt the fellowship examination when they are within 1 year of completion of their training. The examination consists of three written sections (multiple choice, short-answer questions and visual aid questions) and three clinical sections (long case, short cases and structured clinical examination). It is run twice a year in various locations across Australia and New Zealand.

Variations to training

Up to 2 years of advanced training (up to 1 year of which can be in emergency medicine) can be gained overseas, with the prior approval of ACEM.

Training can also be completed on a part-time basis (at least 20 hours per week), and trainees can suspend training for up to 2 years.

RECOGNITION OF SPECIALIST TRAINING OBTAINED OUTSIDE OF ACEM

This can essentially be divided into two groups: 1) training in emergency medicine obtained outside of Australia and New Zealand and 2) training obtained outside of emergency medicine.

Overseas-trained specialists (OTSs) in emergency medicine must apply for specialist recognition from either AMC or MCNZ. In both cases, once the documentation and English language status has been confirmed, the OTS is referred to ACEM for assessment. ACEM reviews the applicant's training, qualifications and experience and conducts a structured interview. ACEM then makes a recommendation to AMC or MCNZ for either specialist recognition or further training and assessment.

Those applicants with training within Australia or New Zealand, but outside of ACEM must apply to ACEM for recognition. ACEM reviews the applicant's training qualifications and experience and may conduct an interview. The college then makes a ruling on required further training and assessment, if any.

Doctors who have only partially completed a training programme outside of ACEM either in Australia and New Zealand or overseas are only eligible for a partial credit for training, and usually will need to start at least part way through provisional training.

There are currently discussions with the UK Faculty of Accident and Emergency Medicine (FAEM) to streamline the recognition and training process, so that movement of trainees and specialists between Australia or New Zealand and the UK will be easier. There are also moves to create an international core curriculum that will lead to a number of common aims and elements of training across the world.

ACEM has a comprehensive web site (www.acem.org.au) that provides up-to-date information on all aspects of training and other college matters.

AMC (www.amc.org.au) and MCNZ (www.mcnz.org.nz) also have web sites with useful information for overseas-trained doctors wishing to work in either country.

ACCREDITATION

Hospitals seeking accreditation for defined purposes such as service provision or training must comply with set standards determined by external institutions which oversee the criteria applicable to such hospitals.

In the case of hospitals overall, The Australian Council on Healthcare Standards (ACHS)[1,2] determines the service standards of patient care provided by a hospital and its individual departments. The process focuses on improving performance, continuum of care, leadership and management, human resource management, information management, safe practice and environment, utilizing audits and key performance indicators in their assessments (see Chapter 25.3 on Quality Assurance/ Quality Improvement).

The learned Colleges, including the Australasian College for Emergency Medicine, separately accredit hospitals for their ability to provide postgraduate training, taking the above criteria into account, but placing greater emphasis on the quality of experience, education and supervision for trainees.

The accreditation process plays an important role in the identification of problems and guiding subsequent actions taken to correct these deficiencies.[2]

College Procedure

The ACEM[3,4] conducts regular (at least 5 yearly) inspections of emergency departments (EDs), to ensure that standards are maintained and that the various criteria for accreditation are met.

The completed hospital information questionnaire and accompanying documents, supplied to the team before the inspection, are carefully studied, and interviews with administration, department heads, specialists, trainees, nurse managers and educators contribute significantly to the decisions made.

Levels of accreditation

There are three levels of accreditation awarded: 6 months, 12 months or 2 years. These periods refer to the amount of accredited time recognized as a part of a trainee's compulsory emergency medicine training in that particular ED. The trainee may spend more time in the that department, but the extra time will not count towards training requirements. The trainee may spend more time within the same hospital accruing non-ED time in accredited rotations in other specialties relevant to emergency medicine.

The greater the value for trainees, the more likely a hospital will attain full accreditation of 2 years. These are hospitals, usually tertiary university teaching hospitals, with wide range of specialties, services and education resources. District and rural base hospitals can also achieve full accreditation if they meet the requirements. Other hospitals may be given 12 or 6 months accreditation, because of their size, specialized nature or casemix or caseload limitations.

Since the period of advanced training is 4 years after success in the primary examination, the above periods of accreditation ensure that trainees rotate through at least two hospitals, benefiting from the particular strengths of each. It is desirable, although not compulsory, for trainees to gain experience in a large teaching hospital and a small, preferably rural, hospital.

Requirements

To be accredited for training,[3,4] a hospital's ED must demonstrate adequate senior supervision, an adequate range and number of patients, medical, nursing and clerical staffing with appropriate rosters, a department design and equipment which allow good work practices, diagnostic and inpatient support services and particularly a commitment to education and training with resources such as a library, manuals, computer access to updated medical and drug information, data collection and retrieval, audits and research.

There needs to be a supportive hospital administration, which gives access to inpatient beds and operating theatres for emergency admissions by having appropriately defined policies. It must provide resources to maintain clinical standards in the ED.

Adequate senior staffing with emergency physicians is essential, as it is mandatory for trainees to be well-supervised, particularly after-hours during busy evening and weekend periods. Trainees need to be given increasing levels of responsibility,[5] including administrative, as they advanced in their training, as some may be appointed to director positions at smaller hospitals soon after attaining their specialist qualification.[6]

The College takes note of departmental teamwork, the quality and

Table 26.5.1 Criteria for accreditation
Trainee supervision
Patient casemix and caseload
Department staffing
Workflow patterns
Administrative support
Diagnostic and inpatient support services
Education and training
Audits and research

currency of equipment and the functional design which result in good workflow patterns and efficient patient care.

Structured education programs with interactive tutorials and teaching sessions directed at the primary and fellowship examinations for trainees, as well as programs for junior doctors, must be in place. These programs may be shared between a network of hospitals, and trainees must be rostered dedicated teaching time to allow them to attend education sessions.

The participation of the ED in undergraduate education is important, and it is expected that the registrars, as advanced trainees, will be involved in student teaching. The senior consultant staff must show a commitment to undergraduate education, and this should be recognized by university academic appointments.

The increasing rationalization of hospital services may result in specialties such as paediatrics, obstetrics, neurosurgery, thoracics and orthopaedics being located in only one hospital in each region. Trainees would be expected to rotate between these hospitals to gain the desired breadth of experience, and the accreditation inspection may encompass a network of hospitals over a number of days.

The ability of a hospital to provide rotations for emergency medicine trainees to training positions at registrar level in such terms as medicine, surgery, cardiology, anaesthesia, intensive care, paediatrics, retrieval medicine, psychiatry and toxicology enhances a hospital's chances of attaining full accreditation. Special accreditation has been given to terms such as transfusion, simulation, rural critical care and forensic medicine.

ACEM regulations are relatively flexible, and allow trainees to design significant parts of their programs. They may work part (at least half) time, which suits trainees with family commitments. They are encouraged to work in a variety of hospitals, both in Australia and New Zealand as well as overseas,[7] preferably in centres with prior College specialist training accreditation. So far, these have been in the UK and US.[8]

Research and quality assurance projects[9] provide a framework for improving performance, and the College examines the department's commitment to research particularly, and also to key clinical indicators such as waiting times by triage category, time to thrombolysis or angioplasty for patients with acute myocardial infarction and death audits.

Recommendations

Following an accreditation inspection, a detailed report is forwarded to the College's Board of Censors and Council for discussion.

Recommendations are then made regarding level of accreditation, suitability for paediatric training, accreditable rotations, and the number of advanced training positions the particular ED can sustain.

Identified problems are listed, and it is expected the hospital will rectify these. Over 90% of the recommendations made by ACHS surveyors prior to 1990 were implemented.[2] It is probable that the compliance would be even better now with both ACHS and ACEM accreditation reports having a greater impact on hospitals.

Failure to meet the standards may mean a loss of accreditation or accreditation at a lower levels.

Implications

The accreditation process is comprehensive, fair and important; it can also be intimidating.[10] Hospitals will retain their accreditation as long as they maintain the desired standards. Inspections by either the ACHS or College can highlight a department's or hospital's shortcomings to administrators, so that attention can be paid to correcting the deficiencies.[2,4]

While there has been criticism that a single visit may not be sufficient to adequately assess an emergency hospital and its back-up resources, there has been, in fact, little disagreement with the recommendations made, and where there has been dispute, changes have been implemented within the hospital or department to allow early reinspection to determine whether the desired accreditation level can be restored. The College does not base its recommendations on the inspection alone, although it behoves a hospital to prepare well for the inspection and ensure key personnel, documentation and supporting data are available for the inspection team.

Loss of accreditation can occur at any time, even between the regular inspections, if, for instance, reports are received from trainees of unsatisfactory training or supervision, staff specialist resignations or substantiated evidence of poor patient care. Losing accreditation can have adverse long-term consequences in terms of loss of reputation and lack of good applicants for positions in these departments.

In order to protect the trainees at an institution that loses accreditation, the College's recommendations allow trainees credentialed training time pending corrective measures within that hospital or suitable alternatives elsewhere.

Success with accreditation ensures a continuation or upgrading of an ED's reputation, and makes that hospital more attractive for prospective trainees and staff specialists. Quality departments attract quality staff, with continuing improving performance. Hospitals therefore have strong incentives to maintain high standards in their EDs.

CONTROVERSIES

❶ Logbooks will probably become an integral part of ACEM training.

❷ Partial training in another specialty or another country only allows limited credentialing of past training and experience.

❸ In the future there may be joint training programmes with related specialties such as paediatrics and intensive care.

❹ There are discussions in progress to create a more international training programme, with easier movement of trainees and specialists between countries.

❺ There is considerable debate over whether a fair accreditation assessment be made on the basis of a single inspection. Many argue that a single snapshot of an ED in time cannot adequately represent the complex pattern of functions and activities going on within that department, and that longer inspections over a period of time may be necessary. This needs to be balanced against the drain on College resources this would entail.

❻ The question of what happens to trainees if a department loses its accreditation status needs to be asked. The ACEM is very mindful of the interests of its trainees, and puts in place conditions around the accreditation recommendations which safeguard the training requirements of trainees.

REFERENCES

1. Australian Council on Healthcare Standards. The EquIP Guide 1998 Standards and guidelines for the ACHS evaluation and quality improvement program
2. Holt PE, Darby DN 1992 ACHS surveyor recommendations: recent trends in the accident and emergency service. Australian Clinical Reviews 12(1): 29–3
3. Australasian College for Emergency Medicine 2002 Training and Examination Handbook Melbourne, The College
4. Yuen A 1996 A review of ACEM accreditation: 1986–1995. Emergency medicine 8(3): 152–62.
5. Gaudry PL 1992 Did you pass accreditation? Emergency Medicine 4(1): 29
6. Baggoley C 1999 Emergency medicine. Where to from here? The College. Emergency Medicine 11: 234–237
7. Taylor DMcD, Jelinek GA 1999. A comparison of Australasian and United Sates emergency medicine training programmes. Emergency Medicine 11(1): 49–56
8. Hamilton G 1999 Emergency medicine: where to from here? Overseas viewpoint. Emergency Medicine 11: 229–33
9. O'Leary DS, O'Leary MR 1992. From quality assurance to quality improvement. The Joint Commission on Accreditation of Healthcare Organizations and Emergency Care. Emergency Medicine Clinics North America 10(3): 477–92
10. Vinen J 1992 Accreditation – was it worth it? Emergency medicine 4(1): 30

26.6 SPECIALIST RECOGNITION AND TRAINING IN EMERGENCY MEDICINE: THE UK VIEW

ALASTAIR MCGOWAN

ESSENTIALS

1 Specialist training in emergency medicine in the UK is the responsibility of the Faculty of Accident and Emergency Medicine.

2 Regulations concerning specialist training in the UK are being fundamentally reviewed. A new supervising Board is being developed.

3 The processes and duration of specialist training are likely to change. The duration is likely to come more in to line with Europe, North America and Australasia.

4 Basic specialty training is followed by higher specialist training.

5 Overseas candidates must have completed 3 years in a programme acceptable to the Faculty of Accident and Emergency Medicine.

INTRODUCTION

Regulation of postgraduate training from October 2003 will be under the control of a newly formed Postgraduate Medical Education and Training Board. This will be the competent authority to accredit training. It will also be the authority that will ultimately consider equivalence of overseas training, taking advice from the Faculty of Accident and Emergency (A&E) Medicine.

The relationship between the Royal Colleges and their Faculties, and this new board, and between this new board and the General Medical Council (GMC), are still being clarified.

GENERAL MEDICAL COUNCIL REGISTRATION

Doctors who wish to practice medicine in the UK need to be registered with the General Medical Council. There are four different types of registration with the GMC: provisional, limited, full and specialist.

Provisional registration allows doctors who have qualified in the UK and European Economic Area (EEA; who are also EEA nationals) and those qualified in Australia, Hong Kong, New Zealand, Singapore, South Africa and the West Indies to work in pre-registration house officers posts which are approved for the purpose of pre-registration service.

Limited registration allows overseas qualified doctors who hold an acceptable qualification (included in the World Health Organization's list of medical schools) to practice in supervised National Health Service (NHS) training posts which are educationally approved. It is also granted for locum posts at these grades.

Full registration allows doctors to practice in unsupervised medical practice in any post in the NHS and in private practice. This type of registration is needed to work as a General Practitioner.

Specialist registration allows doctors to take up a substantive or honorary consultant post in the NHS. No doctor can take up these appointments unless they are on the specialist register.

The GMC will only grant registration to an overseas doctor provided that he or she has passed or been exempted from the Professional and Linguistic Assessments Board (PLAB) test. Doctors are exempt from the PLAB test if they qualified as follows:

- In Australia, New Zealand or the West Indies
- At the Universities of Cape Ton, Natal or the Witwatersrand in South Africa
- At certain Universities in Hong Kong or Singapore where the language of instruction is English
- At the University of Malaya, on or before 31 December 1987.

Rules on immigration define an overseas doctor as:

One who regardless of where he/she may have obtained his/her primary qualification, does not have the right of indefinite residence or is not settled in the United Kingdom, or who does not benefit from European community rights.

BASIC SPECIALTY TRAINING (previously called General Professional Training)

After qualification from medical school, and completing the pre-registration year, a UK graduate will be fully registered with the GMC. An overseas graduate, having successfully completed the PLAB test or been exempted from it, may have obtained full or limited registration.

Before entering higher specialist training all trainees must undertake a minimum of 2 years of basic specialty training. During this time they should obtain a wide range of experience at Senior House Officer (SHO) level in a variety of specialties, of which a minimum of 6 months must be spent in emergency medicine. At least half of the 2-year period should include responsibility for the management of patients admitted to hospitals as emergencies.

All doctors entering Higher Specialist Training (HST) in emergency medicine must hold an appropriate higher qualification. During this period of basic specialty training therefore, trainees are expected to successfully complete Membership of the Royal College of Physicians (MRCP, UK or Ireland), Membership of the Royal College of Surgeons (MRCS Edinburgh, Glasgow, England or Ireland), or Part II of Fellowship of the Royal College of Anaesthetists (FRCA). A new qualification, Membership of the Faculty of A&E Medicine, will be available from April 2003. This period of basic specialty training is currently under review.

SHO training in the future will be more structured, will be programme based, and progression through the programmes, which may be either 2 or 3 years, will be subject to satisfactory annual assessments.

Candidates from overseas wishing to enter higher specialist training in emergency medicine and holding overseas qualifications they consider equivalent to those listed above, must apply to the Joint Committee of Higher Training in A&E Medicine for recognition of these qualifications.

Formal reciprocity agreements with overseas centres are being explored but are some way from being finalized. It may be that the new Postgraduate Medical Education and Training Board will require each case to be considered individually.

HIGHER SPECIALIST TRAINING

Higher specialist training in emergency medicine is normally of 5 years duration, although some retrospective recognition may be made of time spent in a relevant specialty for doctors who have completed more than 2 years in training posts at Basic Specialist Training level.

Training of UK graduates in overseas hospitals may be recognized as Higher Specialist Training provided the training hospital is itself recognized by the competent local authority and the period

of experience overseas has been previously agreed by the supervising Postgraduate Dean in the UK.

The 5 years of higher specialist training must include a minimum of 36-months in emergency medicine and must include experience of at least 3-months duration in:

- General paediatrics
- General medicine (including cardiology)
- Anaesthesia and intensive care
- Trauma and orthopaedic surgery
- General surgery (and/or plastic surgery, neurosurgery, cardiothoracic surgery including experience in the care of surgical emergencies)

where these attachments have not been covered during basic specialist training.

A relevant period of research may contribute up to a maximum of 12 months towards the total duration of higher specialist training in emergency medicine.

Progression through each of these 5 years of higher specialist training is dependent on a satisfactory assessment. A Record of In-Service Training Assessment (RITA) is completed for each trainee by the regional training committee at the end of each year.

A satisfactory 4th year RITA must be registered with the Faculty of A&E Medicine before a trainee is eligible to sit the specialty examination in emergency medicine.

The specialty examination in emergency medicine is taken by UK graduates during the 5th year of their Higher Specialist Training period.

Overseas candidates who wish to sit the examination must have completed 3 years in a programme of specialty training acceptable to the examination committee of the Faculty of A&E Medicine. At least 1 year of this training must have been spent in an approved higher specialist training post in Great Britain or Ireland.

The specialty examination measures competence in four domains of practice. Clinical competence is measured by a data interpretation section and OSCE section. These two sections account for

50% of the overall mark. Competence in literature appraisal is assessed by each candidate preparing one clinical topic review of 3000 words. Managerial competence is assessed by an in-tray exercise in which several problems or scenarios are presented for prioritization and management.

All four sections of the examination must be passed. After successful completion of the specialty examination, and the programme of training, a trainee's name will be forwarded to the Postgraduate Medical Education and Training Board for award of a certificate of completion of training.

Details of the curriculum for Higher Specialist Training in the UK can be obtained from: www.faem.org.uk

ENTRY ON TO THE SPECIALIST REGISTER FOR APPLICANTS FROM OVERSEAS

Doctors who have completed specialist training in emergency medicine outside the European Community may apply for entry to the UK specialist Register. To be recommended for entry as a Specialist in Accident & Emergency Medicine such doctors should satisfy all the following requirements.

It is the responsibility of applicants to provide validated evidence that they:

- hold Full or Limited Registration with the GMC or confirmation of eligibility for such registration.
- be registered as a Medical Practitioner with the competent body in the country, or countries, where they have previously practised and undergone training.
- have completed general professional training in supervised training posts (or equivalent). This should be of at least 2 years duration. It must lead to the acquisition of one of the diplomas allowing entry to Higher Specialist Training in the UK, or an acceptable overseas equivalent. Time in non-training posts where the applicant has independence of action (e.g. Consultant or Locum

Consultant posts) cannot be taken in to consideration.

- have completed Specialist Training in Emergency Medicine of at least 5 years duration. It is recognized that the balance of general and specialist training may vary between countries. The overall duration of training from Medical Registration to completion of Specialist Training must be at least 7 years.
- be able to provide names and addresses of three professional referees.

MAINTENANCE OF SPECIALIST REGISTRATION

The GMC is developing a procedure of revalidation. This will comprise a 5-year cycle of annual appraisal by peers and/or managers. Details are still being elaborated. Annual appraisal is compulsory for all Consultants in the NHS as of 2002. Such appraisal will include verification that the Consultant is participating in a programme of Continuing Professional Development (CPD). Each College currently runs its own programme of CPD which generally involves participating in 50 hours of educational activity per year.

Further details on revalidation will be available from: www.revalidationuk.info

CONTROVERSIES AND FUTURE DIRECTIONS

❶ Reforms of the NHS are underway. The Government's NHS Plan represents the most radical re-thinking of the provision of medical care in the UK since the inception of the NHS in 1948.

❷ The structure and duration of basic specialist training as a Senior House Officer, and the structure and duration of higher specialist training as a Registrar are under review.

❸ The role of the Royal Colleges and their Faculties in the setting of the assessment of trainees against these standards is set to be brought under the quality assurance and overall supervision of the new Postgraduate Medical Education and Training Board.

❹ It is likely that the future pattern of training and assessment in the UK will be of a competency based programme likely of shorter duration than at present and leading to certification as a specialist rather than as a consultant.

❺ Such changes would bring the UK's training programme more in to line with programmes of training currently pursued in Australasia and in the USA.

❻ Against this background discussions concerning reciprocity of training are ongoing.

26.7 COMPLAINTS

ALLEN YUEN

ESSENTIALS

1 Complaints occur in every emergency department.

2 They indicate dissatisfaction with some aspect of a patient's attendance.

3 The majority of complaints are justified.

4 They warrant acceptance, apology and investigation.

5 A timely report of findings and recommendations must follow.

6 The complaint should be resolved satisfactorily.

7 Lessons learnt should be audited and used in quality improvement.

INTRODUCTION

Complaints are inevitable in the setting of busy emergency departments and high patient expectations. Emergency-department staff are well aware of what constitutes optimal care. However, emergency departments are areas where there is little control over the cases which present and the timing and volume of new arrivals, where unexpected scenarios can develop at any time, where caseload and casemix are to an extent unpredictable, and where there is a mixture of staff with different levels of experience. Improvements in clinical care resulting from advances in emergency medicine and nursing have set new standards, which the public has become familiar with, through the media.

Patients and their relatives have much higher expectations of emergency departments than previously. They are better informed, and more litigious, encouraged by legal firms advertising to patients that they have a right to complain and to take legal advice if they have any cause for dissatisfaction. Nevertheless, many patients, who may have legitimate cause for complaint, do not. The level of complaints is not an accurate gauge of patient satisfaction.

Patients have a right to complain if they feel dissatisfied about any aspect of their attendance, and it is appropriate to acknowledge this, note the complaint, apologize for their disappointment and take any corrective measure that will help at the time. If there is no immediate remedial action available, then the complainant should be given an undertaking that the problem will be investigated with those involved, and any appropriate actions taken. Once it is decided what measures are needed, the complainant is contacted to resolve the matter satisfactorily. If this cannot be achieved for whatever reason, wider consultation may be required, and this will often involve the hospital's legal advisers and the doctor's medical defence organization.

INCIDENCE

Complaint rates vary from 0.26 to 3.8 complaints/1000 patients.[1,2] Some hospitals only record written complaints, while others include verbal in their data. Often the complaints contain more than one issue. More complaints relate to paediatric patients, and more may be made by the literate.

In a recent Victorian study of 2419 emergency department-related complaints from 36 hospitals over 5 years, 37% were made by the patient while 48% were from relatives. Friends accounted for 3%, and the rest included GPs, specialists, government representatives and lawyers. Emergency department complaints were 14.3% of the total 16901 hospital complaints.[1]

It is likely that all reports of rate of complaints are underestimates.

REASONS FOR COMPLAINTS

One Australasian study identified four main reasons for complaint: problems relating to care – inadequate treatment, diagnosis or follow-up (33.5%); poor communication skills – rudeness and discourtesy (31.5%); delays (26%); and administrative deficiencies – incorrect documentation, inability to obtain previous records, lack of privacy or confidentiality and loss of property (7%).[1] In private hospitals, fees are an increasing source of complaint (for a more detailed list see Table 26.7.1).

Complaints may be classified into two main groups. The first involves problems

Table 26.7.1 Contributing factors and reasons for complaints
Unpredictability of casemix and caseload
Variation in attendance rates
Long waiting times
Insufficient staffing for unexpected peaks
Junior staff with variable experience and supervision
Deficiencies in treatment (real or perceived)
Inadequate assessment and missed diagnosis (real or perceived)
Poor attitudes, lack of professionalism
Poor communication, lack of information or consent
Interruptions , multiple concurrent tasks
Delays in investigations, consultations
Access block to inpatient beds
No appropriate follow-up
Inappropriate or premature discharge
Unmet expectations
Invasion of privacy
Fees in private hospital emergency departments
Litigation for compensation

in clinical care, including alleged medical negligence, in which compensation may be sought and litigation threatened. Second are those in which the patient or relative has a grievance for a variety of reasons, and seek assurance that corrective measures will be made to ensure that no one else has a similar unpleasant experience.[3]

Problems in clinical care

About 50% of complaints claiming inadequate medical assessment and treatment are substantiated.[2]

Inadequate physical examination followed by a missed diagnosis found on a later visit may be a source of complaint and can only be refuted if relevant positives and negatives, found at the initial visit, are documented accurately.

Medicine is not an exact science, and the early clinical features may be atypical or overlap with other causes that seem unlikely at initial presentation. To try to explain this to an anxious patient who simply wants a quick diagnosis and symptom-relief can pose difficulties to a busy doctor. Still, efforts need to be made to help the patient to understand.

'Missed' fractures are the most frequent 'misdiagnosis'. Some 'misdiagnoses' as perceived by patients result from poor communication, with lack of explanation by the treating doctor of possible causes, and what to do if there is no improvement, such as to attend their local doctor, or to have an outpatient appointment arranged.[2]

Lack of treatment includes insufficient or no analgesia, lack of X-rays, blood tests, urine culture or antibiotics (where an initial presentation, particularly in a child, may have suggested a viral illness with eventual progression to a bacterial infection), or lack of a splint for a 'soft-tissue injury' that is subsequently diagnosed as a fracture.

Rough, unskilled or incompetent treatment still occurs despite advances in training of both doctors and nurses. A heavy workload is not an acceptable excuse for this. With the reduction in allowable weekly labour hours for hospital-employed doctors, emergency departments rely, to some extent on junior staff and locums, under variable levels of senior supervision on some rosters.

Unprofessional conduct and refusal to refer to a specialist or to a previous treating doctor are unacceptable causes of complaint.

Cases of sexual misconduct are very rare in emergency departments, and would be referred to a medical board.

Communication problems

Failures of communication feature prominently in all complaints.[4]

Failure of doctors to introduce themselves and to explain the reasons for examination, investigations, treatment, admission or discharge, referrals or delays are all easily avoidable causes of complaints.[2]

Abruptness, rudeness, discourtesy, insensitivity, absence of caring and other aspects of poor attitude used to be the main reason for complaints, but no longer, perhaps because the public is now more accustomed to this, as standards in general society have decreased. In emergency departments, when people are rightfully anxious about their medical condition, such attitudes should not be tolerated.

Failure to obtain consent in the case of minors, to gain informed consent for procedures and to warn about risks, occurs commonly in emergency departments, where it is assumed that their attendance gives implied consent, but this can be challenged if the patient is brought to hospital by ambulance or other means.

Incorrect documentation is a significant cause for complaint, particularly when it results in the wrong treatment. Doctors may miss significant clues, if they ignore aspects of a patient's history that do not fit in with a presumed working diagnosis. This may also occur if the history is rushed and overly brief.

Reliance on referring letters or ambulance sheets, without checking with the patient, often results in transcribing incorrect past history, medication charts and allergies. It cannot be assumed that referral details or old case histories are correct.

Conflicting, wrong and misleading information may be related to differences in the information supplied by various sources, but is more reason for being meticulous in ensuring their accuracy. Sometimes this is impossible to do, because the reliable sources cannot be contacted. At times, it is due to 'doctor-shopping', a trend that sees patients attend the most convenient bulk-billing family medicine clinic, where their past history is unknown, hoping for a quick cure for acute problems, while reserving attendances at their usual general practitioner for their more complicated ongoing illnesses.

Clinical staff in emergency departments are commonly faced with excessive communication loads. The combination of interruptions and multiple concurrent tasks resulted in 36 communication events an hour in one study, and this may produce clinical errors by disrupting memory processes.[5]

Problems with delays

Difficulty with access to health care is a worldwide problem, even in developed countries where economic rationalism and changing government policies have resulted in closure of hospital beds, mental-health institutions and community resources. Lifestyle and industrial issues have decreased the numbers of medical and nursing staff in hospitals, particularly after hours.

Diminished outpatient services means that patients need to be referred to private consultants' rooms where appointments may not be readily available. Fewer general practices open in the evenings or weekends. Some patients want a one-stop service for their medical consultation, their laboratory tests and their radiology. These social reasons make unnecessary use of scarce resources, and despite strategies such as telephone triage services and hospital-run after hours GP clinics. All the above have contributed to increased emergency department attendances, in combination with the effects of an ageing population with more complex medical problems.

Delays in triage, time seen by doctor, treatment, investigations, consultations, admission or discharge therefore occur. Measures to decrease these are only partially successful, because there is generally no excess of staff or resources to call upon when there are unexpected peaks in workload.

Particularly in the case of children, long delays cannot be easily tolerated, and a significant number 'walk out' without being seen. The majority of these do not generate a complaint, but some lead on to increased morbidity.[8]

The elderly are less likely to complain, but suffer in silence, such that any pain they have may be unrecognized and untreated until late in the management.[9]

Administrative problems

Incorrect documentation by clerical, nursing or medical staff, lack of privacy or confidentiality, loss of valuables, poor cleaning or other environmental issues and queries regarding billing in private hospitals comprise the majority of administrative complaints.[1,2]

Errors are made by doctors in giving advice regarding a patient's right to claim compensation, since the full circumstances cannot easily be ascertained at the time of consultation. Doctors should not advise patients regarding entitlements to worker's or traffic crash compensation, but should complete the necessary documentation objectively. Care should be taken with accuracy in completing medical certificates.

Poor department design, lack of an accessible staff room or little adherence to departmental policy may cause complaints about staff socializing, eating or drinking.

Their laughter is seen by some patients as inappropriate, and by others as a sign of good staff morale.

Lack of formality, addressing older patients by their given name and casual dress standards without identification have become the accepted norm in many Australasian hospitals, but still upset some of our senior citizens and immigrants.

The Federal Privacy Act 1988 was

recently amended, and became effective in December 2001.[6,7] It has resulted in removal of prominent whiteboards detailing patient information in view of other patients and visitors. Computers are now used in most departments, but even these may be visible to passersby.

The Federal Privacy Act gives patients a general right of access to information held about them. However, the doctor still has ownership of his clinical notes and specialists have legal rights over their reports. While patients have right of access, they must obtain consent from the doctors for further reproduction of the material. Ethics are involved, in that relevant material must be made available to another doctor. Refusal of access must be based on reasonable grounds, such as access posing a serious threat to the life or health of any person.[7] In contrast, information on a patient must not be divulged to third parties without patient consent, unless compelled by law, such as with mandatory reporting of child abuse. Disputes may need to be settled in court.

Unmet expectations

Patient satisfaction surveys have ranked waiting times, symptom relief, a caring and concerned attitude and correct diagnosis as their priorities when attending an emergency department. However, there is a mismatch when compared with staff, who agree with the same priorities, but rank waiting time fourth.[10]

Patients expect emergency department doctors to identify serious or dangerous conditions and to treat these appropriately. Explanation and reassurance is needed. They expect investigations and admission as indicated.[3]

PRESSURE FOR LITIGATION AND COMPENSATION

Legal firms now advertise in the lay press that patients dissatisfied with any aspect of their health care should seek legal advice as they may be entitled to compensation, and some recent large awards may encourage more patients to take this course. While progression to litigation is relatively rare, this has resulted in increasing rates of medical indemnity insurance and has contributed to the practice of 'defensive medicine'.[4]

PROCEDURE

All verbal complaints need to be responded to immediately by the person to whom the complaint is made, and subsequently by a senior person, the department director, nurse unit manager, or, in the case of financial disputes, the business manager. An appropriate immediate response is preferable, as this helps to defuse any anger (Table 26.7.2). The complainant should be interviewed in a private office or cubicle away from distractions.

The basis of the patient's grievance must be fully understood, and addressed. It may be that one has to deal with a patient's misperception of what has happened. Empathy is more likely to lead to a successful outcome than an aggressive denial.[13] How to do this without further alienating the patient requires good rapport and skill.

Understanding and patience is required in handling complaints. Verbal complaints must be listened to attentively,

Table 26.7.2 Procedure
Accept the complaint
Apologize for the complainant's dissatisfaction
Defuse any anger
Record the details
Undertake to investigate
Arrange follow-up
Investigate
Discuss with staff
Inform administration
Consider legal implications
Follow-up with complainant
Resolve complaint
Lessons to be learnt

and a record made of the complainant's name and contact details, the nature of the complaint, the patient's name and other relevant information. If the complaint is abusive, there is no point in reacting likewise, as this will only escalate the hostility. State that you would like to help, but can only do so if you are permitted to record the details, without undue pressure.

For written complaints, a written acknowledgement of the complaint together with an apology for their dissatisfaction should be sent within 3 days with an undertaking to have the matter investigated and measures taken to address the problem.

Some experienced directors thank patients for their complaints, on the basis that these provide an opportunity for improving the service. An initial apology that they have been dissatisfied acknowledges the complaint; it does not admit error. Nor does it admit that the complaint is correct; it recognizes that the complainant is aggrieved, and that the complaint will be investigated and appropriate action taken to address the grievance.

If the complaint is of an obviously serious nature, such as a fatal outcome, an apology, such as 'I'm terribly sorry that you have lost your wife/father', is appropriate. It does not admit liability, but empathizes with the relative and allows the hospital to undertake to investigate the circumstances, and then to discuss the matter further after obtaining additional information, so as to understand the cause of death or establish whether management was appropriate. It is important to respect the grief and the need to know as much as possible about the circumstances. It may be that the grief reaction includes a need to blame. Counselling support may be offered (pastoral care, social work, stress psychologists, etc.).[10] Arrangements for a follow-up appointment, telephone call or letter should be made.

If there is a ready explanation, then this can be given, and may often be sufficient. Complaints about waiting times may be easily dealt with in most instances by a courteous explanation of the triage process, the current caseload, the priorities within the department, the staffing, cubicle and bed availability and reassurance that they will be seen as soon as possible. If they are not satisfied, then alternatives such as attending another emergency department or medical centre can be offered.

Complaints relating to 'misdiagnosis', may be due rather to natural progression of a disease. For instance, meningococcal septicaemia may present in its early stages as a non-specific viral-like illness, only to deteriorate rapidly and sometimes fatally over the next few hours. Likewise subarachnoid haemorrhage does not always present with classical sudden onset of headache with neck stiffness and photophobia. Even more frequently, pulmonary embolism can be present without the usual classical features. The patients themselves, previously relatively young and healthy, tend to deny their symptomatology, and may not give a full history, making it extremely difficult for the doctor to make an accurate diagnosis in such situations.

Failure to spot a borderline fracture or pneumonia on a film may not be classed as negligent, but failure to follow-up on a positive radiological report could well be.[11]

While some complaints may appear trivial, the underlying reasons for the complaints must be investigated, and causes identified, so that corrective measures can be taken to prevent recurrences. Patients must feel that their complaints are taken seriously, and appropriate action taken. Making flimsy excuses without looking properly into the matter will not help. The responses must not be seen as arrogant, defensive or dismissive, and any of these could merely exacerbate the problem. The concept of establishing an adult-adult relationship with the complainant is a good basis for continuing useful discussion.

If a complaint has medicolegal implications, then the medical director, chief executive or hospital legal liaison officer need to be informed and the matter discussed with a view to appropriate responses.

If the complaint has come indirectly from the Health Complaints Commissioner (or equivalent), a legal firm, a parliamentarian or the medical board, these usually go to the medical director or the chief executive, seeking information for their client, so that they can decide whether the matter can be resolved by mediation or conciliation, rather than proceeding to litigation. [4]

Any doctor involved should decide whether medical defence/indemnity insurance organization needs to be informed, and where doubt exists, it should.

Check with the involved staff, record notes and charts. Establish facts regarding assessment, treatment and follow-up.

If it is established that there is justification for the complaint, then involved staff may need debriefing and counselling.[12] This is often overlooked, as doctors and nurses have left clinical medicine or nursing following a complaint, even though they may not have been directly responsible for the outcome.

When the complaint is a result of human error, the doctor or nurse must accept that no one can always function at optimal capacity in such an unpredictable area as an emergency department, nor can they be responsible for unexpected changes or serious deterioration in a patient's illness. There are many mitigating circumstances in patient care that can affect outcome, such as distractions, simultaneous care of patients, other priorities, inability to contact the patient's usual doctor to obtain important information and so on.

Once the facts have been established and a report formulated, contact the complainant for further discussion. This must be a factual interview with a frank discussion of the situation, and the actions that are recommended.

RESOLUTION

In one Victorian study, about 75% of complaints were resolved,[1] usually by explanation or apology. As a result, changes in procedure or policy occurred (2%). Remedial action took place in 5%

of cases. Only a small percentage (less than 1%) proceeded to the courts. Compensation was rare (0.2%).

The complaint was not upheld, was unsubstantiated, was frivolous or vexatious, or lapsed in up to 15% of cases. In 1% there was not enough detail to investigate.

Fees were refunded, waived or reduced in less than 1% of cases, but this could well rise with changes in societal expectations.

The majority of complainants who go to state Health Complaints Commissioners (or equivalent) are not seeking revenge or compensation. Most of their cases are resolved by enquiry, assessment and investigation of the complaint, and then conciliation with the affected parties.[4]

PREVENTION

A well-equipped emergency department that has adequate numbers of senior staff supervising junior staff with strict lines of responsibility will have fewer adverse events and complaints.

Verbal and printed explanations of triage, department assessment procedure and investigation turn-around times must be provided to patients, particularly when waiting times are excessive. Children and psychiatric patients tolerate long waits least well, and need to be seen earlier. If the situation changes, triage staff should give updated waiting times to patients who have still not been seen.[2]

If the doctor makes a point of describing to the patient, the findings during the examination, and records this in the notes, this may overcome complaints that certain areas were not examined. Patients may be unaware of, or not remember, which areas have been examined. Patient notes should be contemporaneous, but if additions or alterations are appropriate in order to clarify a matter, they may be added and dated as such.

Guidelines and protocols of recommended management should be available in all emergency departments to ensure maintenance of standards.[11]

When an adverse event occurs,

medical defence organizations now advise that staff should disclose it fully, apologize early and sincerely, with a statement of genuine and empathic regret, and acknowledgement of the patient or relative's distress,[13] and then discuss the circumstances with them giving an undertaking to take corrective measures. They should not be seen as avoiding the patient, otherwise anger and suspicion will arise.[4] An apology is much more likely to defuse rather than inflame the situation. It is a pity that this principle appears not to be well understood by hospital administrators. Early crisis counselling and psychological support may be offered to patient, relatives and affected staff.[12]

Staff should be encouraged to report any incident or adverse outcome that might generate a complaint, so that the appropriate manager can investigate with staff, prepare a report and convey lessons to be learnt to prevent a recurrence. If the expected complaint then eventuates, a ready response may well reassure the complainant that the hospital takes its work seriously, and the patient may find the actions already taken are adequate to address the issues.

Addressing senior citizens by their prefixed surname may avert complaints of lack of respect or overfamiliarity. These patients and many of those from overseas still prefer doctors to wear white coats, but professional attire and an identification badge will suffice.[14]

Better communication by either or both medical and nursing staff of reasons for delays, examination, investigations, treatment, consultations, admission or discharge, referrals and choice of specialist will prevent a large proportion of the complaints relating to actual patient care.

Good documentation may provide the only means to resolve a dispute, as stressed patients are not good listeners, the use of medical jargon tends to con-fuse patients and the drama and trauma of the emergency can distort perceptions of what actually occurred.[4]

Systems must be in place to check and take appropriate action on abnormal pathology and imaging results, which often return after the treating doctor has finished a rostered shift. Misdiagnoses need to be audited and used as educational tools.

Care with department design is a necessity, so that the waiting and resuscitation areas are visible, patient privacy is maintained, temperature is comfortable, rest rooms are accessible and staff have tea and tutorial rooms adjacent to the main clinical area.[15]

The lessons to be learnt after investigation of a complaint should be discussed with all those concerned, and then presented to all staff to reinforce the issues and solutions. In doing so, anonymity of patient and staff involved should be preserved.

Specific training on how to relate to patients in the pressures of the emergency department environment should be incorporated into orientation and graduate programmes for both doctors and nurses.[1]

Complaints are opportunities for learning, as few lessons are better learnt than those which threaten one's self-esteem. Debriefing and counselling should be offered to affected staff. Objective and supportive feedback will facilitate improved staff performance.[2]

All complaints should be audited, and the results summarized for presentation at a department meeting for discussion. These should form part of a quality improvement programme.

CONTROVERSIES

❶ While there is still some controversy about whether an apology should be made, particularly amongst lawyers and hospital administrators, the evidence strongly suggests that apology, without admission of liability, actually reduces the risk of litigation. It also more often results in patient satisfaction.

❷ The question of how to approach an abusive complainant is difficult. Self-protection and empathy are important aspects of any approach.

REFERENCES

1. Taylor DMcD, Wolfe R, Cameron PA 2002 Complaints from emergency department patients largely result from treatment and communication problems. Emergency Medicine 14: 43–9
2. Brookes J 2000 Complaints. In: Dunn R (ed.) The Emergency Medicine Manual, 2nd edn. Venom Publishing, Adelaide, pp 27–9
3. Bartley B, Cameron PA 2000 QUEST: Questionnaire relating to patients' understanding and expectations of their symptoms and treatment. Emergency Medicine 12: 123–7
4. Wilson B 1998 Using complaints constructively. Australasian Journal of Emergency Care 5(4): 26–9
5. Coiera A, Jayasuriya R, Hardy J, Bannan A, Thorpe M 2002 Communication loads on clinical staff in the emergency department. Medical Journal of Australia 176: 415–8
6. Burton P 2002 Privacy an ongoing concern. Aust Med 18 Mar: 10
7. Federal Privacy Commissioner 2001 Guidelines on privacy in the private health sector. 8 November 2001
8. Hanson R, Clifton-Smith B, Fasher B 1994 Patient dissatisfaction in a paediatric accident and emergency department. Journal of Quality Clinical Practice 14: 137–43
9. Nerney M, Chin M, Lei Jin et al Factors associated with older patients' satisfaction with care in an inner-city emergency department. Annals of Emergency Medicine 38: 140–5
10. Holden D, Smart D 1999 Adding value to the patient experience in emergency medicine: What features of the emergency department visit are most important to patients? Emergency Medicine 11(1): 3–8
11. Bryce G 1998 Complaints – how to deal with them. Journal of Accident and Emergency Medicine 15: 63–4
12. Valent P 1998 Treating helper stresses and illnesses. In: Valent P (ed.) Trauma and Fulfillment Therapy Brunner/Mazel, Philadelphia pp 153–6
13. Nisselle P 2002 Crisis management: honest and open disclosure. Australian Medical Journal April: 9
14. Hertzberg S 2000 Attitudes to dress standards of medical officers (Abstract) Emergency Medicine Mar 12: A10.
15. Chu M, Dunn R 2003 Emergency department layout. Textbook of Adult Emergency Medicine. Churchill Livingstone, Edinburgh, p 20

26.8 CLINICAL RISK MANAGEMENT IN THE EMERGENCY DEPARTMENT

JOHN VINEN

ESSENTIALS

1 Awareness by all emergency department (ED) staff of the concept of patient safety and factors affecting the delivery of safe care is an essential component of the ED's clinical risk management (CRM) strategy.

2 The delivery of safe and effective patient care is reliant on a culture of safety within the ED.

3 To be effective and not intrusive CRM strategies must be incorporated into every aspect of ED operations.

4 The use of common definitions and data sets is essential if factors compromising patient safety in the ED are to be understood.

5 In order to study, monitor and analyse incidents occurring in the ED a good understanding of the process of patient care is essential.

6 Quality indicators facilitate the monitoring of patient safety in the ED and assist in the establishment of benchmarks.

INTRODUCTION

The emergency department (ED) environment is complex, time-pressured and dynamic. The random presentation of a broad spectrum of undifferentiated conditions of varying acuity from trivial to immediately life-threatening is unique to the practice of emergency medicine (EM). Nowhere else in medical practice are staff required to make (often critical) decisions with high levels of uncertainty, minimal information and significant time pressure. Attending to multiple patients simultaneously in a noisy ever-changing environment with constant interruptions and the frequent need to interrupt what one is doing in order to attend to a new arrival or the sudden deterioration of an existing patient leads to the creation of an environment of error.

The ED is a recognized high-risk environment 'perfectly designed' for errors to occur.[1,2] Clinical risk management (CRM) of necessity needs to be part of the day-to-day activities within the ED. CRM needs to be incorporated into all aspects of the delivery of emergency care if it is to be effective and not intrusive. CRM is a comprehensive yet focused strategy aimed at the three components of the delivery of care in the ED; the system, the process and the individual. CRM is aimed at ensuring the delivery of safe error-free patient care[3].

To be effective CRM also requires a culture of safety rather than a culture of blame. CRM encompasses the entire 'episode of care' involving all phases of emergency care (Fig. 26.8.1).[2]

THE EXTENT OF THE PROBLEM

In order to understand both the need and the focus of a CRM program it is necessary to understand the extent and nature of problems related to patient safety in the ED. In the USA medical error in the ED compromises an estimated 21.9% of medical liability based on location of the incident. Failure to diagnose myocardial infarction is the fifth most costly based on average cost with the majority of cases involving serious injury or death. Risk increases after hours with the majority of cases involving patients discharged from the ED, of whom 50% fulfilled the criteria for admission.[4–7]

Studies utilizing differing methodologies (retrospective criteria-based chart review, study of closed claims, longitudinal surveys and prospective anonymous privileged incident reporting) identified that the majority of incidents occurring in the ED are preventable with a high risk of an adverse outcome (AO) and with a significant chance of legal action being taken.[1,8–13] The Critical Incident Monitoring Study (CIMS) study in Australia found that the majority of incidents involved junior inexperienced staff when the ED was busy, after-hours when senior experienced staff were not available to supervise.[5]

Recognition of problem areas in the ED from the literature facilitates the recognition and implementation of corrective strategies (Table 26.8.1).

CIMS evaluated data from six Australian EDs, and found that 78% of reported incidents were due to 'systems' factors, ranging from 54% for medication errors to 96.2% for 'failure to admit.' Nearly all (96.6%) of the incidents in the CIMS study were considered to be preventable. The Quality in Australian Health Care Study (QAHS) found that 70% of adverse events were due to systems factors and demonstrated high preventability, with preventability higher than average for family practice, internal medicine, and EM.

CIMS determined that four system factors are associated with the incidents: junior or very junior medical and nursing staff, on night duty or on duty on the weekend with no senior cover (i.e. staff with wider clinical experience on whom they could call) and a busier than usual ED and where there was a comparative shortage of senior and experienced ED staff[5].

INCIDENTS, ERRORS, ADVERSE EVENTS AND ADVERSE OUTCOMES

In order to ensure consistency and to allow for accurate data collection,

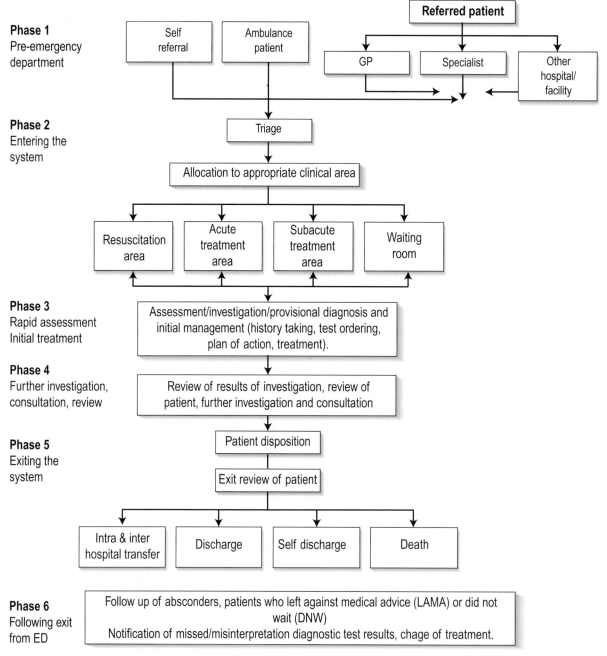

Figure 26.8.1 Six-phase model of emergency patient care.

analysis and interpretation, standard definitions and data sets must be used (Table 26.8.2).

To identify, monitor and correct problem areas it is essential that all EDs incorporate into their CRM program an incident reporting and analysis process. An incident reporting system is essential because:

- It draws attention to the problems that are occurring.
- Data are essential for an effective CRM system.
- It highlights to staff that patient safety is important, that it is a focus of the department and that action is being taken to address the problems.[2,5]

CAUSE AND EFFECT

It needs to be clearly understood that rarely is there only one cause of an incident. Most of the incidents have multiple causes, the majority of which include system failures (Fig. 26.8.2).

Also, the vast majority of incidents do not result in actual harm, that is an

Table 26.8.1 Examples of incidences/errors

PROBLEM	CORRECTIVE STRATEGY
Phase 1: • Failure to accept/transfer care Direct line to ED Admitting Officer • Delayed transfer/acceptance • Incorrect medical advice – EMS – other hospitals/facilities – family practitioners – phone advice to patient/relatives • Incidents involving external medical teams – Medical emergency on campus (e.g. cardiac arrest team) – Disaster teams	Pre-Emergency Department (Duty Consultant) and pre-determined transfer agreement
Phase 2: • Failure to triage • Delayed triage • Incorrect triage [under triage] • Incorrect allocation to Clinical Area • Vital signs not done	**Entering the System** Backup staff for busy periods Experienced trained triage nurse at all times
Phase 3: • Delayed assessment • Failure to adequately manage airway • Inadequate fluid administration	**Rapid Assessment / Initial Treatment** Trauma Team/activation criteria Priority assessment process for patients presenting with chest pain/ACS
Phase 4: • Failure to order required investigation • Failure to consult • Delayed consultation	**Further Investigation, Consultation and Review** Senior experienced staff on duty Senior experienced staff on duty Senior experienced staff on duty
Phase 5: • Failure to admit / inappropriate discharge • No discharge instructions • Failure to refer	**Exiting the System** EGAIRT Nurse Appointment made prior to discharge followed by reminder contact
Phase 6: Failure to follow-up – LAMA – DNW Failure to ensure follow-up – Timely – At all Failure to notify missed abnormality – X-ray – Pathology – ECG Failure to contact re: – Change of treatment - resistant organisms – Delayed return of abnormal result	**Following exit from the ED** Patient contact ASAP after leaving Patient contact ASAP after leaving Recalled for treatment Patient contacted to arrange change in therapy
All Phases • Medication error • Incorrect / failure to accurately interpret diagnostic test / X-ray • Failure to act on abnormal result • Inadequate documentation In order to improve patient safety and the quality of care it is first essential to understand the issues by studying the problems utilising standard definitions and a defined minimum data set followed by analysis of the findings looking at causation with the aim of introducing corrective strategies.	

adverse event (AE) or AO. Because of the potential for an AE or AO from each and every incident no incident can be considered to be trivial (Figure 26.8.3).

Incidents are indicators of a failure in patient safety and should be treated as such. Incidents are also frequent, and most go unnoticed or are accepted as part of doing business in the ED. Unless documented and analyzed problem areas cannot be readily identified. Trends are important.

PRACTICAL APPLICATION OF CRM STRATEGIES

CRM strategies can be practically applied based on the system, process, and indivi-

Table 26.8.2 Standard definitions and data sets

DEFINITIONS

Incidents:
... are 'any unintended event which is inconsistent with routine hospital practice or of the quality of patient care which has had or could have had a demonstrable adverse outcome for a patient. Incidents may or may not result in an adverse event.'[2]

Adverse Event:
... is 'where an incident has resulted in a demonstrable impact on the quality of patient care. An adverse event in turn may or may not result in an adverse outcome.'[2]

Adverse Outcome:
... is 'where an incident has occurred and resulted in and undesirable event (adverse event) leading to harm to the patient.'[2]

Medical Errors:
... are 'failure of a planned action to be completed as intended (error of execution) or use of a wrong plan to achieve an aim (error of planning)'.[14]
It may be a simple mistake or due to lack of expertise, negligence or other cause.

Malpractice/Negligence:
'Negligence' is the failure to use reasonable care under the circumstances as determined by the courts. It is doing, or not doing, something that a reasonably prudent doctor would do (or not do) under the same circumstances. It is a deviation, or departure, from accepted practice. 'Malpractice' is professional negligence, with medical malpractice the negligence of a doctor.[16]
The term 'medical negligence' or 'malpractice' should not be used to describe an incident, adverse event, or adverse outcome unless judgement on a particular case has been handed down.

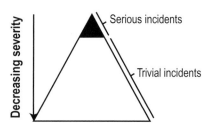

Fig. 26.8.3 Incidents.

dual, and the phase of care (Fig. 26.8.1). System strategies for applying CRM are detailed in Table 26.8.3. Process strategies are listed in Table 26.8.4. Individual strategies are noted in Table 26.8.5. Strategies for applying CRM based on phase of care can be found in Table 26.8.6.

Role of the 'reverse triage' nurse

An important part of the CRM process is the role of the 'EGAIRT' or reverse triage nurse (Table 26.8.7). This pre-exit review ensures all patients leave the ED with minimal potential for adverse events and outcomes.

CRM and major incidents/disaster response

In order for the ED to respond to major incidents (internal and external) a number of requirements need to be met (Table 26.8.8).

Clinical guidelines/reference databases

The use of assessment and management charts utilizing clinical guidelines has been demonstrated to improve clinical decision-making and documentation.

On-line reference databases (with a down time manual backup system) facilitate clinical decision-making and drug administration. The availability of comprehensive up-to-date information on the range of conditions presenting to the ED is now a reality. Not only should this information and the technology to support it be available, staff should be required to use it (e.g. MIMS on-line, New South Wales DOH Clinical Information Access Program (CIAP) website,[17] etc.).

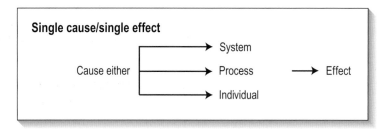

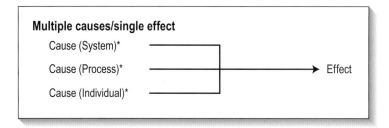

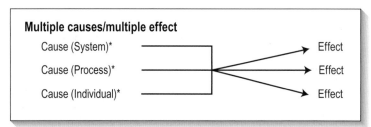

* Any combination possible

Fig. 26.8.2 Cause and effect of incidents.

Table 26.8.3 System strategies

- ➤ Adequate resourcing
- ➤ Adequate facilities
- ➤ Equipment – checklist/maintenance and replacement program
- ➤ Staffing (numbers and seniority)
  – extended hours cover by consultants
- ➤ Fully integrated IT system
- ➤ Reference databases/decision support systems
  – protocols/guidelines/algorithms
- ➤ Communication process/system
  – communication clerk
- ➤ Effective and efficient patient processing system
- ➤ Environmental – temperature, light and noise
- ➤ Emergency Department Information System (EDIS)
  – system
  – alerting
  – overview of department activity
  – patient tracking
  – full interface with PMI, pathology, radiology, pharmacy systems
- ➤ Support systems (diagnostic radiology, pathology, supplies department, bed management, etc.)
  – need to be responsive/responsible
- ➤ Crisis response process – access block, major incidents/disasters
- ➤ Standardization – equipment, processes
- ➤ Teamwork – shift times/formal handover/transfer of care
- ➤ Essential power supply
- ➤ Needleless system/sharps disposal system

Table 26.8.4 Process strategies

- Direct line to ED Admitting Officer (AO), cordless phone
- 'Patient expects' database (patients referred/transferred to the ED)
- Triage process:
  – Utilisation of the Australasian Triage Scale (ATS)[16]
  – Back up for busy periods
  – Allocation to appropriate clinical area
- Patient senior staff review process
- Structured handover process for each and every patient
- Pre-exit review of all patients – the 'EGAIRT '(Reverse Triage) Nurse (Table 26.7.8)
- Senior staff real time review of ECGs, X-rays, abnormal pathology results
- Timely review of post discharge and transfer radiology/pathology results
- Timely review of DNWs, LAMAs
- Proforma – assessment/admission, ODs, chest pain, traumas.

Table 26.8.5 Individiual strategies

- Recruitment/selection/appointment
- Orientation
- Credentialing and accreditation
- Training – 'error training' – increased awareness of problems/high risk conditions/situations, recurrent incidents and corrective strategies ('share the lesson').
- Supervision
- CME/MOPS
- Performance appraisal

Facilities

The ED should be purpose-designed and built and large enough to meet peak period demand and comply with the Australasian College for Emergency Medicine Emergency Department Design Guidelines.[18] Environmental and other services need to comply with Australian Standards. A communication system separate from the PABX should also be available. Security and OHSS requirements should be in place.

QA/Audit/CRM review

In order to ensure that all aspects of ED operations are monitored as part of a comprehensive CRM program, a range of structured activities is essential.

The activities that are required to be monitored on a continuous basis range from overall ED efficiency in managing patients to ensuring individual patients receive the care that they require. The focus of these strategies is patients' safety and the delivery of timely appropriate care.

INDICATORS/ BENCHMARKS

The utilization of performance and quality indicators (QIs) to monitor performance and measure quality allows for benchmarking and the identification of problem areas and trends.

All indicators are inter-related as a result of the complexity of care in the ED with a number of indicators func-

Table 26.8.6 Phase of care strategies

Phase 1

- Referral/transfer agreements
- Medical advice policies and protocol
- Medical emergency team(s):
  – policies and protocols
  – training

Phase 2
- 24/7 trained triage nurse available
- Back up triage staff for busy periods
- Link triage category with clinical area role
- Measurement and documentation of vital signs
- Availability of medical records
- Immediate availability of MRN/labels

Phase 3
- Immediate bed availability for all triage category 1 & 2 patients
- Triage category 1/trauma/cardiac arrest team

Phase 4
- Timely senior staff review of all patients post-assessment by junior staff
- Regular review of status of all patients in the ED by senior staff on duty

Phase 5
- Pre-exit review all patients by senior (EGAIRT) nurse and MO
- Appropriate referral of discharged patients
- Written discharge instructions, all discharged patients

Phase 6
- Timely review of all discharged patients – radiology, ECG and pathology results
- Review of LAMAs, and DNWs

All Phases
- Documentation
- Incident/error reports
- Complaints
- Documentation of interpretation of ECG/X-ray findings
- Date and signing each and every diagnostic report form indicating that it has been reviewed in a timely manner

Table 26.8.7 Role of the 'EGAIRT' (reverse triage) nurse

E	ducation of patient
G	uarantee that treatment is complete
A	dmission not indicated
I	nformation (documentation) complete
R	eview (follow-up) arranged
T	ransport arranged

tioning as both performance (PIs) and quality indicators (QIs) (Table 26.7.9).

INDICATORS AND AUDIT

A number of the data elements utilized in studying incidents, AEs, error and ED

Table 26.8.8 Essentials for CRM in disasters

- Entire ED on essential power supply/ backup via generator

- Key support services (pathology, diagnostic imaging, operating theatres, lift (at least one), etc. also need to be on essential power supply service

- Bottled oxygen cylinders to be available for supply failure

- Back-up suction equipment essential

- Non-PABX communication system

- Back-up manual patient registration and tracking system

performance/operations can be used as quality indicators.[19]

QIs are a subset of safety indicators and measure and monitor the quality of

Table 26.8.9 Performance and quality indicators

PERFORMANCE INDICATORS
- Triage waiting times
- Treatment time
- Access block (a hospital bed management PI)

QUALITY INDICATORS
- Time to 1st ECG for patient with chest pain
- Measurement and documentation of vital signs
- Pregnancy test for female patient of child bearing age with abdominal pain
- Time to thrombolysis or angioplasty/stenting for patients with AMI
- Weight (in Kg) measured for all children

Failure to:
- Investigate
- Interpret X-rays correctly
- Act on abnormal results

Delay in:
- Administering
  – thrombolysis
  – antibiotics for
    • meningitis
    • sespis
    • compound fractures

care in the ED. QIs must meet the requirement of an indicator, reflect the environment, be directly relevant to clinical practice and reflect the quality of care in the ED no matter what the circumstances (resource constraint, overcrowding, etc.).

QIs assist in improving quality through a number of mechanisms (Table 26.8.10). Few QIs are pure. All ED QIs are impacted by external (to the ED) factors.

Some QIs can be considered to be relatively pure (Table 26.8.11).

There is also an overlap of many indicators. Triage waiting times are both PIs and QIs. When used as PIs triage waiting times measure the system's ability to attend to the medical assessment of new arrivals based on the urgency for medical care (based on the ATS). When used as QIs triage waiting times measure the quality of care of a range of medical conditions where there is good evidence that outcome (morbidity and mortality) is directly influenced by time to medical treatment (Table 26.8.12).

Table 26.8.10 Mechanisms by which QIs improve quality

➤ Providing a better understanding of the process of care

➤ Increasing understanding of the variation that exists in a process and measuring the variation

➤ Monitoring a process over time

➤ Providing a common reference point and allowing comparisons/benchmarking

➤ Allowing the documentation and analysis of failures in the quality of care and facilitating the development of preventative strategies aimed at reducing the frequency of quality of care failure

➤ Seeing the effect of change in a process

➤ Establishing a more accurate basis for further research

Table 26.8.11 Pure ED QI's

Arrival time to:
➤ Medical assessment/resuscitation for triage category 1

➤ Initial ECG in chest pain/suspected AMI

➤ Administration of aspirin and thrombolysis/angioplasty for AMI

➤ Administration of antibiotics in:
 – suspected bacterial meningitis
 – compound fractures[20]

➤ Defibrillation for VF

➤ Ventilation for respiratory arrest

➤ Airway management for GCS ≤8

Table 26.8.12 Triage waiting times QIs

Time to thrombolysis/angiogram for AMI

➤ Time to intervention for compromised airway

➤ Time to DC shock for VF

Table 26.8.13 System, process and individual aspects of care indicators

System
➤ Triage waiting times
➤ Senior staff review of all patients

Process
➤ Triage process/accuracy
➤ Patient tracking during treatment
➤ Measurement of vital signs

Individual
➤ Errors
➤ Failure to consult
➤ Failure to refer
➤ Failure to admit

Table 26.8.14 Phase of care indicators

Phase 1
➤ Failure to accept urgent transfer
➤ Delayed transfer
➤ Failure to give treatment advice (administer penicillin for suspected meningitis)
➤ Increased transport time/patient taken to inappropriate facility because ED on bypass status

Phase 2
➤ Failure to triage
➤ Delayed triage
➤ Incorrect triage (under triage)
➤ Incorrect allocation of treatment area

Phase 3
➤ Delayed assessment/treatment
 – excessive waiting time
➤ Failure to protect/establish airway
➤ Inadequate resuscitation fluids

Phase 4
➤ Required investigation not done
➤ Failure to consult
➤ Incorrect diagnosis
➤ Missed diagnosis
➤ Missed injuries

Phase 5
➤ Failure to admit
➤ LAMA
➤ DNW

Phase 6
➤ Death after discharge
➤ Recalls
➤ No or delayed follow-up
➤ Failure to refer
➤ Inappropriate escort during transfer
➤ Incorrect mode of transport during transfer
➤ Failure to notify re missed abnormality
➤ Failure to contact re required change of treatment

All Phases
➤ Died in the ED
➤ Misinterpretation or failure to act on abnormal diagnostic investigation findings
➤ Incident reports
➤ Medication errors
➤ Failure to document
➤ Complications of procedures

26.8.15). Because of the complexity of the ED, studying QIs by phase of care allows for identification of causal factors in a manageable way.

Access block is a hospital PI and not an ED PI but has a very significant impact on ED PIs and QIs.

The audit process whilst time consuming is an essential component of the ED's CRM program. Some of the important operations that need to be audited function as QIs (Table 26.8.16).

QIs can be categorized in several ways. They can be indicators of system, process or individual aspects of care (Table 26.8.13), indicators of phase of care (Table 26.8.14), or indicators of the problem (disease specific) (Table

Table 26.8.15 Problem (disease specific) indicators

Problem/Disease Specific

➤ Failure to use spirometric based management of acute asthma
➤ Pre-eclampsia – failure to:
  – Measure BP
  – Examine for oedema
  – Examine for proteinuria
➤ Time to thrombolysis/angioplasty
➤ Time to antibiotic administration
  – Meningitis
  – Compound fractures
➤ Pregnancy test
  – Females with abdominal pain

Table 26.8.16 Potential targets for audit

➤ Accuracy of triage category allocation

➤ Accuracy of allocation to clinical areas

➤ Chart audits:
  – adequacy of documentation
  – documentation of :
    • vital signs
    • weight in Kg (children)

➤ Review of results of diagnostic investigations

➤ Representations within 7 days

➤ LAMAs

➤ DNWs

➤ Deaths (DIED)

➤ Recalls for:
  – treatment
  – admission

CONTROVERSIES

❶ There is still not a consensus on patient safety terminology. The commonly used term 'error' is judgemental and a process of attribution based on outcome. Its use compromises staff commitment to incident reporting activities.

❷ Hindsight bias remains a problem even with those that are supposedly well informed.

❸ It remains to be proved whether incident reporting and the implementation of many CRM strategies actually reduce the frequency of incidents and increase patient safety.

❹ It is unclear whether lessons learned from other high risk industries can be used to improve the safety of patient care.

❺ Research into patient safety in the ED is in its infancy. What is required is a concerted effort to study the relationship between the unique environment in the ED and factors compromising patient safety.

REFERENCES

1. Brennan TA, Leape LL, Laird NM, et al 1991 Incidence of adverse events and negligence in hospitalized patients: results of the Harvard Medical Practice Study I. New England Journal of Medicine 324: 370–6

2. Vinen JD 2000 Incident monitoring in emergency departments: an Australian model. AEM. 2000; 7: 1290–7
3. Australasian College for Emergency Medicine Policy on Quality 2002 Improvement in Emergency Medicine www.acem.org.au/open/documents/quality.pdf
4. Annual Report to Policy Holders: Physicians and Surgeons 1991, St Paul, MN St Paul Fire and Marine Insurance Company
5. Vinen JD, Gaudry PL, Ashby R, Epstein J, Blizard PJ 1994 Critical incident monitoring study in emergency medicine (CIMS) interim report. Australasian College for Emergency Medicine and Commonwealth Department of Human Services and Health, Sydney
6. Rusnak RA, Stair TO, Hansen K, Fastow JS 1989 Litigation against the emergency physician: common features in cases of missed myocardial infarction. Annals in Emergency Medicine 1029–34
7. Trautlein JJ, Lambert RL, Miller J Malpractice in the emergency department – review of 200 cases 1984 Annals of Emergency Medicine 13: 709–11
8. Leape LL, Breanan, TA, Laird NM, et al 1991 The nature of adverse events in hospitalized patients: results of the Harvard Medical Practice Study II. New England Journal of Medicine 324: 377–84
9. Thomas EJ, Studdert DM, Burstin HR, et al Incidence and types of adverse events and negligent care in Utah and Colorado in 1992 2000. Medicine Care 38: 261–71
10. California Medical Association Medical Feasability Study 1977. In: Mills DH, Boxden JS, Rubsamen, PS (eds). Sutter, San Francisco

11. Wilson R McL, Runciman WB, Gibberd RW, Harison BT, Newby L, Hamiton JD 1995 The quality in Australian Health Care Study. Medical Journal of Australia 163: 458–71
12. Thomas EJ, Studdert DM, Runciman WB, et al 2000 A comparison of iatrogenic injury studies in Australia and the USA, I: context, methods, casemix, population, patients and hospital characteristics 2000 International Journal of Quality Health Care. 12: 371–8
13. Runciman WB, Webb RK, Helps SC, et al 2000 A comparison of iatrogneic injury studies in Australia and the USA II. Reviewer behaviour and quality of care. International Journal of Quality Health Care 12: 379–8
14. Kohn LT, Corrigan JM, Donaldson MS (eds) 1999 To err is human: building a safer health system. Institute of Medicine Report. National Academy Press, Washington, DC
15. Mackauf SH 1999 Neurologic malpractice. Neurological Clinics 17: 345–53
16. Australasian College for Emergency Medicine National Triage Scale 1994. Emergency Medicine 6: 145–6
17. www.ciap.health.nsw.gov.au/index.html
18. www.acem.org.au/open/documents/ed-design_htm
19. Vinen JD 2002 Time to initiation of thrombolysis after myocardial infarction: quality indicators. Emergency Medicine 32: 125–6
20. McCaskill ME, Little DG 1993 Time to definitive management of open fractures of long bones. Emergency Medicine 5: 272–5

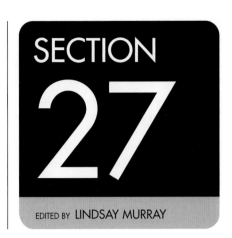

EDITED BY LINDSAY MURRAY

ENVIRONMENTAL

27.1 Heat-related illness 748

27.2 Hypothermia 752

27.3 Dysbarism 756

27.4 Radiation accidents 763

27.5 Near-drowning 769

27.6 Electric shock and lightning injury 774

27.7 Anaphylaxis 779

27.8 Altitude illness 784

27.1 HEAT-RELATED ILLNESS

IAN ROGERS • ALED WILLIAMS

ESSENTIALS

1 Heat exhaustion is largely a manifestation of intravascular volume depletion and usually responds simply to rest and intravenous fluids.

2 Heatstroke is a true medical emergency, where rapid cooling using tepid spraying, fanning and ice packs is essential to minimize morbidity and mortality.

3 Patients with drug-related hyperthermias die from the complications of the high temperatures, not from direct drug toxicity. Early and aggressive treatment of hyperthermia before complications occur is vital.

4 With more widespread use of potent serotoninergic agents we can expect the numbers of patients presenting to emergency departments with serotonin syndrome to increase. A high index of suspicion needs to be maintained.

INTRODUCTION

Heat-related disorders have a broad range of potential aetiologies and manifestations. In some the primary disorder is a failure of thermal homoeostasis, whereas in others the hyperthermia is secondary to other processes. The major heat-related illnesses to consider are heat exhaustion, heatstroke, neuroleptic malignant syndrome, serotonin syndrome and malignant hyperthermia. Although of different aetiologies they share much common ground, particularly with regard to complications and treatment.

EPIDEMIOLOGY AND PATHOPHYSIOLOGY

Heat exhaustion is the most common heat-related illness presenting to emergency departments. It occurs where substantial losses of fluid and electrolytes as sweat are inadequately replaced, and is most commonly observed in athletes and manual workers. The primary pathophysiologic mechanisms are dehydration and intravascular volume depletion, but may include electrolyte loss and exercise-induced respiratory alkalosis.[1]

The other, more serious, heat-related disorders are all associated with hyperthermia, which if not treated promptly results in similar pathophysiology at a cellular and organ system level. A core body temperature greater than 41°C results in progressive denaturing of a number of vital cellular proteins, failure of vital energy-producing processes, and loss of cell membrane function. At a cellular level the exact mechanisms leading to loss of cell membrane function and cell death in heat illness remain uncertain. Proposed theories include increased ion fluxes, particularly of Na^+ and K^+, futile cycling of the Ca^{2+} ATPase, enhanced glycolysis, Na^+ and K^+ depletion, and altered neurotransmitter release.[1-4] At an organ system level these changes may manifest as rhabdomyolysis, acute pulmonary oedema, disseminated intravascular coagulation, cardiovascular dysfunction, electrolyte disturbance, renal failure, liver failure and permanent neurologic damage.[5] Any or all of these complications must be expected in severe heat illness.

Heatstroke shares some pathophysiologic similarities with heat exhaustion, and in practice it may be difficult to distinguish between the two entities. The hallmark of heatstroke is failure of the hypothalamic thermostat, leading to hyperthermia and the associated additional pathophysiologic features described above. Clinically, heatstroke can be

Table 27.1.1 Heatstroke risk factors

Behavioural
Exertion
Athletes
Manual workers
Army recruits
Pilgrims
Inappropriate clothing
   Elderly
Inappropriate exposure
   Babies left in cars

Drugs
Anticholinergics
Stimulants/hallucinogens
Salicylates
Phenothiazines
Diuretics

Illness
Seizures
Delirium tremens
Infections
Dystonias

divided into 'exertional heatstroke' due to exercise in a thermally stressful environment, and 'classic heatstroke', which occurs in patients with impaired thermostatic mechanisms. Common risk factors for heatstroke are listed in Table 27.1.1.

Certain drugs produce hyperthermia by mechanisms in addition to interference with thermostatic function. In the related serotonin and neuroleptic malignant syndromes, increased motor activity and central resetting of the hypothalamic thermostat combine to produce hyperthermia. In the case of serotonin syndrome these effects are a consequence of a relative excess of central nervous system serotonin, whereas in neuroleptic malignant syndrome dopamine depletion or dopamine receptor blockade is responsible.

The elevation of central nervous system serotonin in serotonin syndrome is usually associated with combinations of serotoninergically active drugs, taken either therapeutically or in overdose. The incidence of serotonin syndrome when such combinations are taken is not known, but is low, and there is much individual variation in susceptibility.[6,7] The syndrome is rarely precipitated by a single serotoninergic agent.[8] Drugs associated with the serotonin syndrome are listed in Table 27.1.2. The most commonly implicated combinations are MAOI with SSRI, MAOI with tricyclics, and MAOI with pethidine.[6]

Neuroleptic malignant syndrome (NMS) is a rare idiosyncratic reaction to neuroleptic agents with an incidence of between 0.02% and 3.0%, depending on the diagnostic criteria used. It occurs in response to a single agent, usually at therapeutic dosage. In individuals the occurrence may be dose-related. Certain at-risk groups have been identified and are listed in Table 27.1.3.[9]

Table 27.1.2 Drugs causing serotonin syndrome

Antidepressants
Selective serotonin reuptake inhibitors (SSRI)
Selective serotonin and noradrenaline (norepinephrine) reuptake inhibitors (SSNRI)
Tricyclics
Monoamine oxidase inhibitors (MAOI)
Trazodone
Lithium
Buspirone

Analgesics
Pethidine
Pentazocine

Antiparkinsonian agents
L-Dopa
Bromocriptine

OTC preparations
Dextromethorphan

Recreational drugs
'Ecstasy'

Table 27.1.3 Risk factors for neuroleptic malignant syndrome

Patient factors
Male sex (male:female = 2:1)
Dehydration
Agitation
Organic brain disease

Drug dosing factors
High initial neuroleptic dose
High-potency neuroleptic (e.g. haloperidol)
Rapid dosage increase
Depot neuroleptics

NB: Duration of drug exposure and toxic overdose are not related to risk of developing NMS.

Malignant hyperthermia is a genetically inherited disorder in which triggering agents cause a release of sarcoplasmic Ca^{2+} stores. The resulting elevation of myoplasmic Ca^{2+} stimulates many intercellular processes, including glycolysis, muscle contraction and an uncoupling of oxidative phosphorylation. This leads to hyperthermia which, in contrast to neuroleptic malignant and serotonin syndromes, is purely peripheral in origin.

CLINICAL SYNDROMES

Heat exhaustion

The clinical presentation of heat exhaustion will be familiar to all emergency practitioners as it mirrors that of dehydration from any other cause. Patients complain of headache, nausea, vomiting, malaise and dizziness. There may be a history of collapse, and there is likely to be a tachycardia and (orthostatic) hypotension. The orthostatic hypotension may manifest at the end of physical exertion (such as running) by collapse with brief loss of consciousness. The collapse is due to a sudden drop in cardiac output from loss of muscle pumping that has been maintaining venous return in a hypovolaemic subject. This syndrome has been labelled as 'exercise-associated collapse'. In distinction to heatstroke, the core temperature will be less than 40°C and neurological function will rapidly return to normal once the patient is lying down.

Heatstroke

The classic clinical features of heatstroke are neurological dysfunction, core temperature above 41°C and hot, dry skin. However, relying on this classic triad to make the diagnosis will result in a number of cases being missed. Loss of consciousness is a constant feature of heatstroke,[5] but by the time of emergency-department presentation conscious state may be improving, although some neurological abnormality will persist. Temperature readings may be misleadingly low, due either to effective pre-hospital care or to measurements at inappropriate sites, such as the oral cavity or axilla. Profuse sweating is, in fact, a

Table 27.1.4 Features of the serotonin syndrome

Central nervous system
Agitation
Confusion
Decreased level of consciousness
Seizures

Motor
Hyperreflexia
Myoclonus
Incoordination
Tremor

Autonomic
Diaphoresis
Diarrhoea
Fever
Hypertension

common feature.[5] Other clinical features may include tachycardia, hyperventilation, seizures, vomiting and hypotension.

Serotonin syndrome

Serotonin syndrome is characterized by a triad of CNS, autonomic and motor dysfunction (Table 27.1.4). It develops after a latent period, which is normally a few hours but may be as long as several days.[10] The spectrum of illness produced is broad. Most patients are only mildly affected and may escape clinical detection. Only the most serious develop hyperthermia severe enough to produce the complications of rhabdomyolysis, disseminated intravascular coagulation and renal failure. Most cases will resolve within 24–48 hours once the precipitating agents are withdrawn. Even in severe cases the underlying biochemical abnormality rapidly improves. The morbidity and mortality in these cases is caused by the complications that develop while the syndrome is active.

Neuroleptic malignant syndrome

This syndrome manifests in patients who have recently been started on neuroleptic treatment, or in whom the dose of a neuroleptic agent has been increased. It has also been reported in patients in whom a dopaminergic agent has been rapidly withdrawn (e.g. in parkinsonism). There is a latent period of several days. Characteristically, there are four classic signs: fever, rigidity, altered mental state and autonomic instability. In practice, it may be very difficult to distinguish clinically from serotonin syndrome unless a good drug history is obtained. As in serotonin syndrome the spectrum of severity may be very broad, with only the more severe cases developing hyperthermia and its complications.[11]

Malignant hyperthermia

This occurs when a triggering agent is given to a susceptible individual, usually in the context of an anaesthetic. Triggering agents identified include inhalational anaesthetic agents such as halothane, isoflurane and enflurane, as well as succinylcholine and ketamine. The first signs are failure to achieve muscle relaxation following succinylcholine, tachypnoea and tachycardia. If not recognized and treated, acidosis, rhabdomyolysis and hyperthermia will ensue. In some cases signs and symptoms may be delayed, or even reappear after apparently successful treatment, so that malignant hyperthermia may even present as a postoperative fever. Untreated, the mortality is as high as 70%, but this can be reduced tenfold by appropriate management.

INVESTIGATION

Diagnosis of the hyperthermic disorders is based on the history, clinical picture and exclusion of alternative diagnoses. Investigations are, thus, directed towards excluding other possible causes of temperature elevation (e.g. infection, metabolic disorders) and evaluation of the specific complications of hyperthermia.

Patients with a presumed clinical diagnosis of heat exhaustion should still have serum electrolytes and creatinine kinase measured, together with a dipstick urinalysis. Measurement of serum electrolytes will detect dilutional hyponatraemia and other electrolyte disorders. In heat exhaustion there should be no myoglobin in the urine and, at most, only minor elevation of serum muscle enzymes.

All other heat disorders warrant a far more extensive laboratory and radiological work-up, as multiorgan system dysfunction is the rule.[12] Tests should include ECG, serum electrolytes, arterial blood gases, DIC screen, liver function tests, muscle enzyme assays, renal function and urinalysis, serum glucose and a chest X-ray.

MANAGEMENT

Heat exhaustion

Heat exhaustion and exercise associated collapse respond rapidly to rest and fluids. Oral fluids such as commercial glucose/electrolyte solutions are ideal if they can be tolerated. Intravenous normal saline will provide more rapid recovery in severe cases. Heat exhaustion is a diagnosis of exclusion: should any doubt exist the patient should be treated as for heatstroke.

Heatstroke

This is a true medical emergency. Early recognition and aggressive therapy in the field and in hospital can prevent substantial morbidity and mortality. The key management is aggressive cooling. Cooling rates of at least 0.1°C/min should be achievable. Several cooling methods have been proposed, including evaporative cooling, iced water immersion, ice slush, cool water immersion, iced peritoneal lavage and pharmacological methods.[5,13–16] A combination of a number of these methods seems the most practical and applicable. All of the patient's clothing should be removed and the patient sprayed with a fine mist of tepid water while gentle fanning is commenced (a ceiling fan is ideal). At the same time, vascular beds close to the surface (neck, axillae and groins) should be packed with ice bags. One advantage of this form of treatment is that the same technique can be applied in a field setting, such as a sporting event. This technique also allows more ready patient access and monitoring than methods such as ice-bath immersion.

In hospital, shivering, seizures and muscle activity may need to be controlled with pharmacologic agents such as chlorpromazine, benzodiazepines and paralyzing agents. Aspirin and paracetamol are ineffective and should be avoided. Intravenous fluids need to be used cautiously and may need titrating to CVP or PCWP measures. High-flow oxygen should be routine and ventilatory support may be required. Urine flow needs to be maintained with initial volume loading, and later with mannitol or furosemide, to prevent secondary renal injury, especially from rhabdomyolysis. Electrolyte, acid-base and clotting disturbances should be closely monitored and treated by standard measures.

Serotonin syndrome

Treatment of the drug-related hyperthermias involves both specific pharmacological therapy and full supportive and cooling measures, as described above. The objective is to recognize and treat before serious complications occur. In mild cases of the serotonin syndrome benzodiazepines may be all that is required while awaiting spontaneous resolution. In severe cases neuromuscular paralysis should be considered early, especially in cases of altered mental state. Specific antiserotoninergic drugs that have been used include chlorpromazine (12.5–50 mg IM/IV),[17,18] methysergide (2 mg bd orally), cyproheptadine (4 mg orally 4-hourly, max 20 mg in 24 hours),[7,8] and propranolol (1–3 mg IV as required, to a max of 0.1 mg/kg).[7] Nitroglycerin has been successfully used in some case reports.[19]

Neuroleptic malignant syndrome

Again early recognition and full supportive care, combined with specific therapy, is the mainstay of treatment. Dopamine agonists such as bromocriptine may reduce the duration of the syndrome which, in contrast to serotonin syndrome, takes several days to resolve spontaneously. It can be administered orally or by nasogastric tube at an initial dose of 2.5–10 mg tds.[9] Dantrolene has been used as a muscle relaxant, although it has no effect on the central aspects of the disorder.

Malignant hyperthermia

Dantrolene is the specific agent used in the treatment of malignant hyperthermia and should be given in addition to full supportive care and discontinuing the triggering agents. The dose is 1–2 mg/kg IV initially, repeated up to a maximum of 10 mg/kg/24 hours if needed. It acts by inhibiting release of Ca^{2+} from the sarcoplasmic reticulum.

PROGNOSIS AND DISPOSITION

In heatstroke both the maximum core temperature and the duration of temperature elevation are predictors of outcome.[15] Prolonged coma and oliguric renal failure are poor prognostic signs.[5] Mortality is still of the order of 10%, but most survivors will not suffer long-term sequelae.[5] Any patient with suspected heatstroke should routinely be referred to the intensive care unit for ongoing care. Most cases of heat exhaustion will be suitable for short-stay emergency department treatment.

Prevention of exertional heatstroke should focus on the education of at-risk groups. Dehydration limits the body's cooling ability, so the value of maintaining fluid intake during extreme exertion should be stressed. As high ambient temperatures and high humidity predispose to exertional heatstroke, exertion in these environments should be limited.

Prognosis in the drug-related group of hyperthermia is dependent largely on the degree to which the complications have progressed before definitive and aggressive treatment is begun. Again, early referral to intensive care is indicated. Even

CONTROVERSIES

❶ Although debate is likely to continue about the most effective cooling therapy in heatstroke, this is largely of academic interest as all methods seem to achieve the desired outcome of rapid temperature drop. Of more interest will be research that focuses on the cellular mechanisms of the damage seen with hyperthermia. Such research may lead to the development of pharmacologic agents that can prevent or treat heatstroke and other heat-related illnesses.

❷ There are as yet no trials comparing the various antiserotoninergic drugs available for the treatment of serotonin syndrome.

with appropriate treatment, mortality for malignant hyperthermia approaches 7%. After recovery the patient's medication regimen will need to be reassessed, though in the case of neuroleptic malignant syndrome it may be possible to slowly reintroduce a neuroleptic agent at a lower dose. With malignant hyperthermia future anaesthesia will need to be modified to avoid precipitating agents. In addition, family members should be tested for susceptibility.

REFERENCES

1. Tom PA 1994 Environment dependent sports emergencies. Medical Clinics of North America 78(2): 305–25

2. Hubbard RW 1990 Heat stroke pathophysiology: the energy depletion model. Medicine and Science in Sports and Exercise 22(1): 19–28
3. Francesconi RP, Willis JS, Gaffin SL, Hubbard RW 1997 On the trail of potassium in heat injury. Wilderness and Environmental Medicine 8: 105–10
4. Hubbard RW 1990 An introduction: the role of exercise in the aetiology of exertional heat stroke. Medicine and Science in Sports and Exercise 22(1): 2–5
5. Shapiro Y, Seidman DS 1990 Field and clinical observations of exertional heat stroke patients. Medical Science and Sports Exercise 22(1): 6–14
6. Sporer KA 1995 The serotonin syndrome. Drug Safety 13(2): 94–104
7. Brown T, Skop B, Mareth T 1996 Pathophysiology and management of the serotonin syndrome. Annals of Pharmacotherapy 30: 527–33
8. Bodner R, Lynch T, Lewis L, Katin D 1995 Serotonin syndrome. Neurology 45: 219–23
9. Heimann-Patterson TD 1993 Neuroleptic malignant syndrome and malignant hyperthermia. Medical Clinics of North America 77(2): 477–92
10. Sternbach H 1991 The serotonin syndrome. American Journal of Psychiatry 148: 705–13
11. Bristow MF, Kohen D 1993 How malignant is the neuroleptic malignant syndrome? British Medical Journal 307: 1223–4
12. Dematte JE, O'Mara K, Buescher J, et al 1998 Near fatal heat stroke during the 1995 heat wave in Chicago. Annals of Internal Medicine 130(7): 173–81
13. Costrini A 1990 Emergency treatment of exertional heat stroke and comparison of whole body cooling techniques. Medicine and Science in Sports and Exercise 22(1): 15–8
14. White JD, Kamath R, Nucci, R, Johnson C, Shepherd S 1993 Evaporation versus ice peritoneal lavage treatment of heat stroke: comparative efficacy in a canine model. American Journal of Emergency Medicine 11: 1–3
15. Tek D, Olshaker JS 1992 Heat illness. Emergency Medicine Clinics of North America 10(2): 299–310
16. Slovis CM 1999 Features and outcomes of classical heat stroke. Annals of Internal Medicine 130(7): 614
17. Gillman P 1996 Successful treatment of serotonin syndrome with chlorpromazine. Medical Journal of Australia 165: 345
18. Chan BSH, Graudins A, Whyte IM, et al 1998 Serotonin syndrome resulting from drug interactions. Medical Journal of Australia 169: 523–5
19. Brown T 1996 Nitroglycerin in the treatment of the serotonin syndrome. Annals of Pharmacotherapy 30: 191

27.2 HYPOTHERMIA

IAN ROGERS

ESSENTIALS

1 Hypothermia is categorized into mild (32–35°C), moderate (29–32°C) and severe (<29°C) on the basis of a rectal core temperature reading.

2 Moderate-to-severe hypothermia produces progressive delirium and coma, hypotension, bradycardia, and failure of thermogenesis.

3 The ECG will often show slow atrial fibrillation and an extra positive deflection in the QRS (the J or Osborn wave) in leads II and V_3–V_6 with worsening hypothermia.

4 Endotracheal intubation is safe in hypothermia. Ventilation and acid-base status should be manipulated to maintain uncorrected blood gases within the normal range.

5 Endogenous rewarming should form part of all rewarming protocols. In most cases of moderate-to-severe hypothermia rewarming can be achieved with forced-air blankets and warm, humidified inhalation.

6 In the arrested hypothermic patient rewarming should be with cardiopulmonary bypass or warm left pleural lavage.

INTRODUCTION

Hypothermia is defined as a core temperature of less than 35°C. This can be measured at a number of sites (including oesophageal, right heart, tympanic and bladder). Rectal remains the routine in most emergency departments, despite concerns at how rapidly it equilibrates to and reflects true core temperature. Conventionally, hypothermia is divided into three groups: mild (32–35°C), moderate (29–32°C) and severe (<29°C) on the basis of measured core tempe-

rature. In a field setting, where core temperature measurements may not be possible, moderate and severe are often grouped together as they typically share the clinical features of absence of shivering and altered mental state. These categorization systems can be used both out of and in hospital as a guide to selecting rewarming therapies and prognosis. Mild hypothermia is considered the stage where thermogenesis is still possible; moderate is characterized by a progressive failure of thermogenesis; and severe by adoption of the temperature of the surrounding environment (poikilothermia) and an increasing risk of malignant cardiac arrhythmias. Nevertheless, there are substantial differences between individuals in their response to hypothermia.

EPIDEMIOLOGY

Hypothermia may occur in any setting or season.[1] True environmental hypothermia occurring in a healthy patient in an adverse physical environment is less common in clinical practice than that

secondary to an underlying disorder. Common precipitants include injury, systemic illness, drug overdose and immersion, and are outlined in more detail in Table 27.2.1. The elderly are at greater risk of hypothermia because of reduced metabolic heat production and impaired responses to a cold environment.[2] Alcohol is a common aetiological factor[1,3] and probably acts by a number of mechanisms, including cutaneous vasodilatation, altered behavioural responses, impaired shivering and hypothalamic dysfunction. Hypothermia is more common in men than women.[1]

CLINICAL PRESENTATION

Despite substantial individual variations it is still possible to describe the typical patient in each category of hypothermia. The clinical manifestations of hypothermia also depend on the underlying aetiology and any associated features. To guide management in a field setting, where rectal temperature measurements are impractical or dangerous, moderate

Table 27.2.1 Hypothermia aetiologies	
Environmental	Cold, wet, windy ambient conditions Cold water immersion Exhaustion
Trauma	Multitrauma (entrapment, resuscitation, head injury) Minor trauma and immobility (e.g. #NOF, #NOH) Major burns
Drugs	Ethanol Sedatives (e.g. benzodiazepines) in overdose Phenothiazines (impaired shivering)
Neurological	CVA Paraplegia Parkinson's disease
Endocrine	Hypoglycaemia Hypothyroidism Hypoadrenalism
Systemic illness	Sepsis Malnutrition

and severe hypothermia are grouped together as 'profound'.[4]

Mild hypothermia manifests clinically as shivering, apathy, ataxia, dysarthria and tachycardia. Moderate hypothermia is typically marked by a loss of shivering, altered mental state, muscular rigidity, bradycardia and hypotension. In severe hypothermia signs of life may become almost undetectable, with coma, fixed and dilated pupils, areflexia and profound bradycardia and hypotension. The typical cardiac rhythm of severe hypothermia is slow atrial fibrillation. This may degenerate spontaneously, or with rough handling, into ventricular fibrillation and eventually asystole.

Many complications may also manifest as part of a hypothermia presentation, although at times it may be difficult to separate cause from effect. These include cardiac arrhythmias, thromboembolism, rhabdomyolysis, renal failure, disseminated intravascular coagulation and pancreatitis.

INVESTIGATION

Mild hypothermia with shivering and without underlying illness needs no investigation in the emergency department.

Moderate or severe hypothermia mandates a comprehensive work-up to seek common precipitants and complications that may not be clinically apparent.

Biochemical and haematological abnormalities are frequently associated with hypothermia,[1] although there is no consistent pattern. Blood tests that are indicated include sodium, potassium, glucose, renal function, calcium, phosphate, magnesium, amylase, creatine kinase, ethanol, full blood count, clotting profile and arterial blood gases. It is currently recommended to interpret blood gas results at face value, rather than adjusting for the patient's temperature.[5]

Impaired ciliary function, stasis of respiratory secretions or aspiration may be expected in moderate-to-severe hypothermia, so chest radiography should be routine. Other radiology may be indicated if a trauma-related aetiology is suspected.

A 12-lead ECG and continuous ECG monitoring should be routine in moderate-to-severe hypothermia. The typical appearance is slow atrial fibrillation, with J or Osborn waves most prominent in leads II and V_3–V_6 (Fig. 27.2.1). The J wave is the extra positive deflection after the normal S wave, and is more obvious and more commonly seen with increasing severity of hypothermia.

MANAGEMENT
General

The general and supportive management of hypothermia victims largely follows that of other critically ill patients. However, some syndrome-specific issues demand careful attention.

Muscle glycogen is the substrate preferentially used by the body to generate heat by shivering. All hypothermics, therefore, need glucose. In mild cases this can be given orally as sweetened drinks or easily palatable food. With more severe hypothermia gastric stasis and ileus are common, and glucose should be given intravenously: 5% dextrose can be infused at 200 mL/h. Additional volume resuscitation with normal saline or colloid should be gentle, bearing in mind the contracted intravascular space in severe hypothermia, and that hypotension that would be classified as severe at a core temperature of 37°C is a normal physiological state at 27°C. All intravenous fluids should be warmed to minimize ongoing cooling. Current opinion is that endotracheal intubation by a skilled operator is safe in severe hypothermia. Intubation is indicated as in any other clinical condition to provide airway protection or to assist in ventilation.

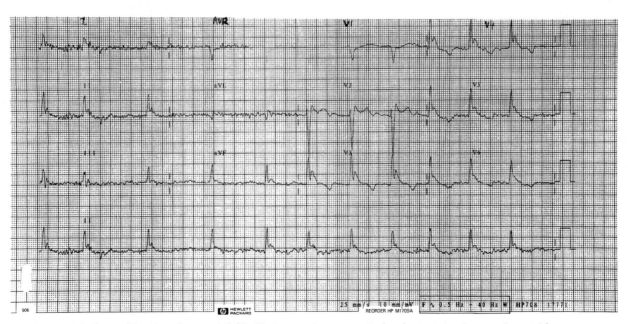

Fig. 27.2.1 ECG in hypothermia: slow atrial fibrillation and J waves in leads II, V_3–V_6 in a patient with a core temperature of 23.9°C.

Ventilatory support and, where necessary, manipulation of acid–base status, should be titrated to maintain uncorrected blood gas pH and P_{CO_2} within the normal range.

The slow atrial fibrillation so common in more severe hypothermia is a benign rhythm and requires no chemical or electrical correction. It will revert spontaneously with rewarming. Pulseless ventricular tachycardia and ventricular fibrillation should largely be managed along conventional lines. However, if the first 200J DC shock is unsuccessful, then others are unlikely to be so until the patient is warmer. Repeat countershocks are generally reapplied with every 1°C increase in core temperature.

Magnesium and, in particular, bretylium, have been suggested to possibly 'chemically cardiovert' VT and VF in hypothermia. However, bretylium production by the sole manufacturer in Australia ceased in May 1997, and at the time of writing no alternative source is available.

The pharmacokinetics and dynamics of most drugs are substantially altered at low body core temperatures. Indeed, for many of the common drugs used in an emergency department they are unknown. Insulin is known to be inactive at <30°C. Hyperglycaemia, due in part to loss of insulin activity, is common in hypothermia, but should probably be managed expectantly until sufficient rewarming has occurred to ensure full endogenous insulin activity.

Rewarming therapies

Rewarming therapies in hypothermia have generated substantial debate. Unfortunately, there are only limited clinical trials on which to base recommendations. Although more invasive and rapid techniques are advocated for more severe hypothermia, there is little evidence to support this advice. The traditional concern of afterdrop (a paradoxical initial drop in core temperature with rewarming) is probably of little or no relevance in a clinical setting.[6]

Rewarming therapies are broadly divided into three groups: endogenous rewarming, which allows the body to rewarm by its own endogenous heat production; external exogenous rewarming, which supplies heat to the outside of the body; and core exogenous rewarming, which applies the heat centrally. The classification of the common rewarming therapies is outlined in Table 27.2.2.

Endogenous rewarming is a mandatory component of any emergency department rewarming protocol. It consists of drying the patient, covering them with blankets, placing them in a warm and wind-free environment, and warming any intravenous or oral fluids that are administered. Endogenous rewarming alone can be expected to rewarm at a rate of about 0.75°C/h. For most patients above 32°C (the level at which shivering thermogenesis is typically preserved), endogenous rewarming is the only therapy required. The exception is the exhausted patient in whom shivering has ceased at a core temperature higher than expected. Although more sophisticated techniques, such as bath immersion, will more rapidly rewarm a mildly hypothermic patient, there is no evidence that an increased rewarming rate improves prognosis in this group.

In moderate hypothermia endogenous heat production is likely to progressively fail and more aggressive exogenous rewarming therapies are indicated. Hot-bath immersion has the theoretical disadvantage of causing peripheral vasodilatation, with shunting of cool blood to the core and convective heat loss. This might be expected to increase core afterdrop and produce circulatory collapse. In fact, rewarming rates of at least 2.5°C/h with minimal afterdrop have been achieved using baths at 43°C.[7] Nevertheless, substantial practical difficulties are obvious with monitoring a more seriously ill patient immersed in a bath. This method of rewarming can only be recommended for otherwise healthy patients who are expected to make a rapid recovery from accidental environmental hypothermia (e.g. immersion in very cold water).

The two therapies that have been best studied and are widely used in moderate hypothermia are forced-air rewarming and warm humidified inhalation.[8] Forced-air rewarming is achieved by covering the patient with a blanket filled with air at 43°C. These devices direct a continuous current of air over the patient's skin through a series of slits in the patient surface of the blanket. This method produces minimal if any afterdrop, is apparently without complication and, combined with warm humidified inhalation, should produce rewarming at about 2.5°C/h. Warm humidified inhalation has generated considerable debate in the literature.[9] Its value probably lies in preventing ongoing respiratory heat loss, and by heating both the mediastinum and the brain stem. Given its widespread availability and lack of complications, it seems reasonable to combine it with forced-air rewarming in moderate hypothermia. Body-to-body contact and chemical heat packs are often recommended as field treatments for all degrees of hypothermia. In mild hypothermia it seems that the benefit of any heat they deliver is negated by an inhibition of shivering thermogenesis. In more severe cases, where shivering is absent, it may be that even the small amount of exogenous heat they deliver is beneficial,

Table 27.2.2 Rewarming therapy classification	
Endogenous rewarming	Warm, dry, wind-free environment Warmed intravenous fluids
External exogenous rewarming	Hot bath immersion Forced-air blankets Heat packs Body-to-body contact

Core exogenous rewarming	Warmed, humidified inhalation
	Body cavity lavage
	    Peritoneal
	    Pleural
	Extracorporeal

but this remains unproven. Rapid rewarming rates have been reported with immersion of the limbs in warm water, potentially augmented by the use of negative pressure to distend the veins.[10] Although this method of rewarming has been used for many years by the Danish navy, its role both prehospital and in hospital requires further research.

In severe hypothermia more aggressive exogenous rewarming therapies may be indicated in order to rapidly achieve core temperature above 30°C, the threshold below which malignant cardiac arrhythmias may occur spontaneously. When available, full cardiopulmonary bypass achieves rewarming rates of about 7.5°C/h without core afterdrop. Pleural lavage using large volumes of fluid warmed to 40–45°C through an intercostal catheter may be nearly as effective. Both techniques are clearly invasive and carry associated risks. These risks are certainly acceptable in a hypothermic arrest, but in the non-arrested patient a slower rate of rewarming using forced-air and warm humidified inhalation may be more appropriate.

A suggested rewarming algorithm based on the evidence available to date is reproduced in Figure 27.2.2.

PROGNOSIS AND DISPOSITION

Attempts at developing a valid outcome prediction model for hypothermia are likely to be frustrated by its multifactorial aetiology.[11] Recovery with appropriate treatment is likely from accidental environmental hypothermia when there is no associated trauma. To date, the coldest patient to survive accidental hypothermia neurologically intact had an initial measured temperature of 13.7°C. Although increasing severity of hypothermia does worsen prognosis, the major determinant of outcome is the precipitating illness or injury. Reported mortality rates vary from 0 to 85%.

Mild hypothermics without associated illness or injury can be safely managed at home in the care of a responsible adult. Moderate hypothermia may be treatable in a short-stay observation ward, but often requires a longer inpatient stay to manage underlying illness or injury. Severe hypothermics are at risk of multiorgan system complications and should be considered for admission to an intensive care unit.

CONTROVERSIES

❶ Many questions remain unanswered in hypothermia, the major one being which rewarming therapy to use. This will only be answered when the focus moves to randomized clinical trials measuring clinically relevant outcomes, such as morbidity and mortality, rather than surrogate markers such as rewarming rate and core afterdrop.

❷ Should future research confirm the beneficial effects of mild therapeutic hypothermia post cardiac arrest shown in recent studies[12,13] then it is likely that hypothermia will come to be seen, not just as illness or syndrome, but as a therapy in its own right.

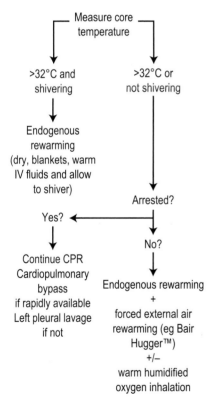

Fig. 27.2.2 A recommended rewarming algorithm in hypothermia.

REFERENCES

1. Danzl DF, Pozos RS, Auerbach PS, et al 1987 Multicentre hypothermia survey. Annals of Emergency Medicine 16: 1042–55

2. Weinberg AD 1993 Hypothermia. Annals of Emergency Medicine 22: 370–7
3. Jolly BT, Gherzzi KT 1992 Accidental hypothermia. Emergency Medicine Clinics of North America 10: 311–27
4. Forgey WM (ed.) 2001 Wilderness Medical Society Practice Guidelines for Wilderness Emergency Care. Globe Pequot, Guilford
5. Danzl DF 1998 Accidental hypothermia. In: Rosen P, Barkin R, et al (eds) Emergency Medicine: Concepts and Clinical Practice, 4th edn. Mosby, St Louis, pp 963–86
6. Rogers IR 1997 Which rewarming therapy in hypothermia? A review of the randomised trials. Emergency Medicine 9: 213–20
7. Hoskin RW, Melinshyn MG, Romet TT, Goode RC 1986 Bath rewarming from immersion hypothermia. Journal of Applied Physiology 61: 1518–22
8. Steele MT, Nelson MJ, Sessler DI, et al 1996 Forced air speeds rewarming in accidental hypothermia. Annals of Emergency Medicine 27: 479–84
9. Lloyd EL 1990 Airway rewarming in the treatment of accidental hypothermia: a review. Journal of Wilderness Medicine 1: 65–78
10. Giesbrecht GG 2001 Emergency treatment of hypothermia. Emergency Medicine 13: 9–16
11. Danzl DF, Hedges JR, Pozos RS 1989 Hypothermia outcome score: development and implications. Critical Care Medicine 17: 227–31
12. Bernard SA, Gray TW, Buist M, et al 2002 Treatment of comatose survivors of out-of-hospital cardiac arrest with induced hypothermia. New England Journal of Medicine 346: 557–63
13. The Hypothermia After Cardiac Arrest Study Group 2002 Mild therapeutic hypothermia to improve neurologic outcome after cardiac arrest. New England Journal of Medicine 346: 549–55

27.3 DYSBARISM

GREGORY M. EMERSON

ESSENTIALS

1 Dysbarism is the medical complications of exposure to gases at higher than normal atmospheric pressure. It includes barotrauma and decompression illness.

2 An understanding of the pathophysiology of dysbarism requires an understanding of the gas laws.

3 Barotrauma occurs as a consequence of excessive expansion or contraction of gas within enclosed body cavities. It principally affects the inner and middle ear, the sinuses and the lungs.

4 Decompression illness occurs when gas bubbles develop within the body. This may occur as a complication of pulmonary barotrauma, or when a diver whose tissues are supersaturated with nitrogen ascends too rapidly.

5 The clinical manifestations of decompression illness may affect many body systems, and are extremely variable in severity.

6 Once the clinical diagnosis of decompression illness is made, recompression in a hyperbaric chamber should be arranged as soon as possible.

INTRODUCTION

Scuba (self-contained underwater breathing apparatus) diving is becoming increasingly popular in Australasia. Emergency physicians will often be the first medical staff to assess the diver after a diving accident. It is therefore essential that they have an understanding of the potential risks and injuries of diving. This chapter focuses on diving problems secondary to breathing gases at higher than normal atmospheric pressure (dysbarism).

DIVING PHYSIOLOGY

Absolute pressure at sea level is 1 atmosphere (ATA). Pressure under water increases by 1 ATA for every 10 m of sea water. One ATA is equivalent to 760 mmHg. This pressure change alters gas within the body according to various laws. It does not affect the non-compressible fluid-filled compartments of the body. Knowledge of these gas laws is required in order to understand the pathophysiology of diving injuries.

Boyle's Law states that at a constant temperature the volume of a gas varies inversely to the pressure acting on it:

$$PV = k$$

where P = pressure, V = volume and k = constant.

Therefore, as a diver descends and pressure increases, gas-filled body cavities decrease in volume. The proportional change in volume is greatest near the surface (Table 27.3.1). As the diver ascends and pressure decreases, gas in the cavities increases in volume. If the body cavities such as the ears and lungs do not allow free movement of gas (for example, the eustachian tubes are

Table 27.3.1 Depth vs pressure and gas volume

Depth (m)	Absolute pressure (ATA)	Gas volume (%)
0	1	100
10	2	50
20	3	33
30	4	25

blocked or the diver holds their breath on ascent), then barotrauma will occur.

Dalton's Law states that the total pressure (P_t) exerted by a mixture of gases is equal to the sum of the pressures of the constituent gases (P_x, P_y, P_z):

$$P_t = P_x + P_y + P_z$$

Therefore, as divers breathe air at increasing atmospheric pressure, the partial pressures of nitrogen and oxygen increase:

surface = 1 ATA = 0.8 ATA N_2 + 0.2 ATA O_2
10 m = 2 ATA = 1.6 ATA N_2 + 0.4 ATA O_2
40 m = 5 ATA = 4.0 ATA N_2 + 1.0 ATA O_2

A diver breathing air at 40 m is inhaling a gas with a partial pressure of oxygen equivalent to breathing 100% oxygen at the surface.

Henry's Law states that at a constant temperature the amount of a gas that will dissolve in a liquid is proportional to the partial pressure of the gas in contact with the liquid.

$$Q = KP_{gas}$$

where Q = volume of gas dissolved in a liquid, K = constant and P_{gas} = partial pressure of the gas.

Therefore, as the partial pressures of inspired nitrogen and oxygen increase with increasing depth, so does the amount of nitrogen and oxygen dissolved in tissue fluid. This can lead to nitrogen narcosis and oxygen toxicity, respectively. When the diver ascends, the dissolved nitrogen comes out of solution as the ambient pressure decreases.

BAROTRAUMA

Barotrauma occurs when changes in ambient pressure lead to expansion or contraction of gas within enclosed body cavities.

Ear

Middle ear

Middle-ear barotrauma, the most common medical disorder of diving, almost always occurs on descent. Increased ambient pressure results in a reduction of middle-ear volume. If eustachian tube function is insufficient to allow compensation, a series of pathological changes results. The development of mucosal oedema is followed by vascular engorgement, haemorrhage and, finally, tympanic membrane (TM) rupture. Symptoms include pain, tinnitus and conductive hearing loss. Sensorineural hearing loss implies coexisting inner-ear barotrauma. Vertigo may occur if water enters the middle ear through a perforated TM. Severity is graded as shown in Table 27.3.2. An audiogram is useful to document any hearing loss. Treatment involves analgesia, decongestants, and ENT referral if there is TM perforation. Antibiotics are indicated for TM rupture because of potential contamination with water. The patient should not dive again until symptoms and signs have resolved, any TM perforation has healed, and the eustachian tube is patent.

Rarely, middle-ear barotrauma occurs on ascent. This occurs in divers using short-acting decongestants to clear their eustachian tubes that then wear off during the dive. Examination shows a bulging TM without haemorrhage.

Inner ear

Sudden pressure changes between the middle and inner ears can cause rupture of the round or oval windows. This usually occurs during rapid descent without equalizing or forceful Valsalva manoeuvres. Symptoms include sudden onset of tinnitus, vertigo, vestibular symptoms and hearing loss, which may not be apparent until the diver has left the water. Onset of symptoms after the dive while performing an activity that increases intracranial pressure suggests inner-ear barotrauma. There is usually coexistent middle-ear barotrauma.

The main differential diagnosis is decompression illness (DCI) involving the inner ear. Inner-ear DCI usually occurs on deep dives using helium and oxygen mixtures (heliox), and is typically accompanied by symptoms of cerebral DCI. Isolated inner-ear DCI has been reported in sports divers breathing air.[1]

Treatment of inner-ear barotrauma includes avoidance of activities which increase intracranial pressure, and urgent ENT referral for audiometry and surgical repair. If DCI cannot be excluded, the diver should have a trial of recompression.

It was thought that further diving was contraindicated after inner-ear barotrauma, but recent evidence suggests that diving can continue following surgical repair and appropriate counselling.[2]

External ear

Ear-canal barotrauma is very rare and only occurs if there is a complete obstruction of the canal (usually by wax, ear plugs or wetsuit hoods), creating a non-communicating gas cavity between the obstruction and the TM. Treatment is symptomatic.

Sinus

Mucosal swelling and haemorrhage occur if the communication of the sinuses with the nasopharynx is blocked. Symptoms, usually pain and epistaxis, most often occur on descent, but also can occur on ascent or at depth. The frontal sinuses are most commonly involved. Maxillary sinus involvement can refer pain to the upper teeth or cheek. Treatment includes analgesia, decongestants, antibiotics if secondary infection occurs, and recommendations to avoid diving until asymptomatic.

Pulmonary

In breath-hold diving lung volume decreases as the diver descends. It then returns to normal on ascent, in accordance with Boyle's Law. However, in scuba diving air is delivered at the pressure of the surrounding environment. This allows maintenance of normal lung volumes. At depth the lungs contain much more gas than they would on the surface. Divers are trained to breathe continuously on ascent or to exhale continuously if they have lost their air supply. If the breath is held, or they ascend faster than the lungs can empty, pulmonary barotrauma results and air can escape into the pulmonary circulation. This occurs most commonly when a diver runs out of air, panics and ascends too rapidly.[3] The change in pressure over 1 m near the surface is sufficient to cause barotrauma. It has been reported in student divers training in swimming pools[4] and in helicopter escape training.[5] It can also occur with a normal ascent if there is a localized area of lung that does not empty properly, as is possible in people with asthma, reduced pulmonary compliance or air trapping.[6]

Consequences depend on the sites at which the air escapes, and include pneumothorax, pneumomediastinum and arterial gas embolism (AGE). Each is managed differently. An isolated pneumothorax should be managed as for a non-diving-related pneumothorax, and recompression is not necessary. If recompression is required for coexisting DCI, a chest tube with a Heimlich valve should be placed before commencing recompression, because if more air escapes from the lung tear at depth, the size of the pneumothorax will increase markedly on ascent. Pneumomediastinum and surgical emphysema can be managed conservatively. If symptoms are severe, 100% oxygen can accelerate resolution of the trapped gas. Management of AGE is discussed later in this chapter. For unknown reasons the development of overt pulmonary barotrauma protects against AGE because few patients with

Table 27.3.2 Grading of severity of middle-ear barotrauma	
Grade 0	Symptoms without signs
Grade 1	Injection of TM along handle of malleus
Grade 2	Slight haemorrhage within the TM
Grade 3	Gross haemorrhage within the TM
Grade 4	Free blood in middle ear
Grade 5	Perforation of TM

pneumothorax or pneumomediastinum develop signs of AGE.[7]

Mask squeeze

If divers fail to exhale air into their masks on descent, the reduced volume inside the mask can cause pain, petechiae and conjunctival haemorrhage. Treatment is with analgesia alone.

Gastrointestinal

Expansion of gas within the gastrointestinal tract on ascent can occasionally cause colicky abdominal pain. Rupture of the stomach is rare but has occurred where panic or equipment failure has led to air swallowing and rapid ascent.[8] Presentation is with abdominal pain and distension. Shoulder pain may be due to diaphragmatic irritation or coexisting DCI.[9] Subdiaphragmatic free air may be visible on erect chest X-ray. The differential diagnosis includes pulmonary barotrauma, because air can enter the peritoneum via the mediastinum and oesophageal or aortic openings in the diaphragm.[10] The diagnosis is confirmed with endoscopy, and surgical repair is necessary.

Dental

Severe tooth pain may occur with descent or ascent if air is trapped under a decaying tooth or recent filling. Percussion of the involved tooth is painful. Treatment is with analgesia and dental repair.

DECOMPRESSION ILLNESS

Classification

Previously, diving accidents involving bubbles were divided into decompression sickness (due to nitrogen bubbles coming out of tissue) and AGE (due to pulmonary barotrauma releasing air into the circulation). Decompression sickness (DCS) was then classified as type I or II. Type I DCS involved the joints or skin only; type II involved all other pain, CNS, labyrinthine and pulmonary symptoms.

Recently, the term decompression illness (DCI) has been proposed to include both DCS and AGE, for the following reasons:

- It can be difficult to distinguish clinically between cerebral arterial gas embolism (CAGE) and severe DCS.
- AGE can be caused by arterialization of venous bubbles released from tissues.
- Pre-recompression management is identical.
- The division of DCS into type I and type II is felt to be inadequate for research purposes, and some divers classified as type I have been found to have subtle subclinical neurological manifestations.
- Symptomatic classification is adequate to guide management.

The new classification system has five components:

- Acute or chronic
- Evolution of symptoms (static/progressive/relapsing)
- Organ system involved
- DCI
- Presence/absence of barotrauma.

For example, a diver may be classified as having acute static musculoskeletal DCI with no evidence of barotrauma. The new classification has not been universally adopted. DCI is a satisfactory term from a management perspective, but from a scientific perspective it does not describe differing aetiologies and pathophysiologies. This text will use the term DCI but also describe the differing pathophysiology.

Pathophysiology

DCI is caused by intra- and extravascular bubbles of gas. These bubbles arise from inert gas diffusing out of tissues with a reduction in ambient pressure, or from pulmonary barotrauma.

As described by Henry's Law, body tissues absorb nitrogen while diving. Oxygen does not cause problems because it is rapidly metabolized by the tissues. The amount of nitrogen absorbed depends on both the depth (which determines the partial pressure of nitrogen) and the duration of the dive. Eventually, the tissues become saturated with nitrogen and no further absorption occurs. As the diver ascends and ambient pressure decreases, the partial pressure of nitrogen in some tissues will exceed ambient pressure, resulting in tissue supersaturation. If the diver ascends slowly enough, nitrogen diffuses out of the tissues and is transported, dissolved in the blood, to the lungs for elimination. This is known as 'off-gassing'.

DCI occurs if nitrogen comes out of solution as bubbles and gains access to the venous and lymphatic systems or if bubbles form within tissues themselves. The formation of bubbles requires both tissues to be supersaturated with nitrogen and ascent to be excessively rapid. Saturation divers can stay at great depths for days and decompress very slowly without precipitating DCI. A diver who ascends rapidly after a few minutes at 15 m will not have enough nitrogen dissolved in the tissues to result in DCI. A number of dive tables and computers have been developed in an attempt to avoid nitrogen supersaturation of tissues. However, one series has shown that 39% of DCI cases were within the limits of the table they were using, and 24% were within the limits of the conservative Canadian Defence and Civil Institute of Environmental Medicine (DCIEM) tables.[11] It is also frequently assumed that you cannot get DCI with dives under 10 m. Recent experience, however, has shown that it is possible, especially if there has been more than one dive per day, or multiple ascents.[12]

Bubbles entering the venous system via tissue capillaries are filtered out by the lung capillary system and do no harm. It is generally only when bubbles access the arterial system that they cause problems. This can occur under several circumstances. The bubbles may bypass the lungs via a right-to-left shunt. Up to one-third of the population may have a patent foramen ovale.[13] Under normal circumstances, the valve over the foramen is kept closed by the pressure difference between the left and right atria. However, during diving there are many instances where the pressure differential may be reversed, such as during a Valsalva manoeuvre.

Venous bubbles may also gain access to the arterial circulation if a massive shower of them overwhelms the pulmonary filter.

Bubbles can also occur if rupture of the alveolar-capillary wall allows air to escape into the pulmonary arterial or venous systems. If air enters the pulmonary arterial system it will be carried to the pulmonary capillaries, where it will be trapped and reabsorbed by the alveoli. Air tracking into the pulmonary venous system, however, will pass through the heart and result in arterial gas emboli.

Clinical presentation depends on the size and distribution of the bubbles. Gas bubbles entering the circulation (either from tissues or barotrauma) cause both mechanical and biochemical abnormalities. Trapping in the pulmonary circulation may result in elevation of right heart and pulmonary pressures, leading to increased venous pressures and impairment of tissue microcirculation. Arterial bubbles can cause end-organ ischaemia, although most pass through the capillaries and into the venous system. Most of the deleterious effects are a consequence of secondary inflammation of the vascular endothelium.

Bubble-endothelial interaction activates complement, kinin and coagulation systems, and precipitates leucocyte adherence. This results in increased vascular permeability, interstitial oedema and microvascular sludging.[14,15] The end result is ischaemia and haemoconcentration. Increased vascular permeability of the cerebral circulation will produce cerebral oedema. This explains the commonly observed clinical course of a diver with a CAGE having an initial deterioration (bubble emboli), followed by spontaneous improvement (bubbles pass through the cerebral capillaries) and then a subsequent deterioration (secondary inflammation).

Extravascular bubble formation causes pain by mechanical tissue distortion, and is probably responsible for most musculoskeletal symptoms.

Symptoms and signs

Any presentation within hours of a dive is assumed to be DCI until proved otherwise, often by an unsuccessful trial of recompression. Failure to recognize and treat doubtful cases can lead to permanent morbidity.

DCI caused by intravascular bubbles from barotrauma presents as a sudden onset of symptoms related to the organ with impaired blood supply. It can be rapidly fatal and has a mortality of 5% in sport divers who reach a recompression chamber alive.[3] In Australia it is the second most common cause of diving-related death, after drowning.[15] The brain is the organ most commonly affected, probably because of the vertical positioning of the diver on ascent. Cerebral gas emboli can cause sudden loss of consciousness, convulsions, visual disturbances, deafness, cranial nerve palsies, memory disturbance and asymmetric multiplegias. Hemiplegia is much less common than asymmetric multiplegias.[3] Symptoms almost always begin within 10 minutes of surfacing. Sudden loss of consciousness on surfacing should be assumed to be due to cerebral gas emboli. Spontaneous improvement may occur with first aid measures, but relapse is common.

Coronary arterial emboli may present as acute myocardial infarction or arrhythmia. Abdominal organs and skin may also be embolized. Elevation of serum creatine kinase (predominantly from skeletal muscle), serum transaminase and lactate dehydrogenase levels in divers with AGE suggests that emboli are distributed more extensively than previously recognized.[16,17] Peak CK may be a marker of the size and severity of AGE.[16,17]

DCI caused by bubbles released from tissues usually causes symptoms within 1 hour of completing a dive, and 90% of cases have symptoms within 6 hours.[15] In the absence of altitude exposure, onset of symptoms more than 24 hours post dive is unlikely to be due to DCI.[18] Onset within 10 minutes suggests the bubbles are due to barotrauma. In general, the earlier the onset of symptoms the more severe the injury. Common symptoms include profound fatigue, myalgia and periarticular pain. Shoulders and elbows are the joints most commonly involved. The pain is usually a dull ache, which may initially be intermittent and migrate from joint to joint, but later becomes constant. Movement aggravates the pain, but local pressure with an inflated sphygmomanometer cuff may improve it.

Spinal-cord involvement occurs in up to 60% of cases.[19] The exact cause of spinal DCI is still debated. It may be a result of venous infarction of the cord due to obstruction of the epidural vertebral venous plexus.[14] Other explanations include ischaemia and inflammation from bubble emboli or the formation of local bubbles within the spinal cord (autochthonous bubbles). Symptoms include back pain, paraesthesia and paraplegia, with bowel and bladder involvement. It is potentially disastrous to misdiagnose back pain coming on a few minutes after a dive as musculoskeletal pain and not spinal cord DCI.

Cerebral DCI may present as personality change, headache, memory loss, visual defects, convulsions, confusion and altered level of consciousness. A flat affect may be the only symptom. The vestibular system can also be involved, with vertigo, vomiting, nystagmus and tinnitus.

If the bubble load overwhelms the pulmonary filter a diver can present with dyspnoea, pleuritic substernal chest pain, cough, pulmonary oedema, cyanosis and haemoptysis (the 'chokes'). Salt water aspiration syndrome is the major differential diagnosis.

A variety of rashes can be caused by cutaneous bubbles. The most common presentations are pruritis with no rash, a scarlatiniform rash with pruritis, and cutis marmorata. Cutis marmorata begins as a spreading erythema but subsequently develops a marbled appearance of pale areas surrounded by cyanotic mottling.

Flying after diving can precipitate DCI. Even if there are no bubbles at the end of the dive, excess nitrogen will still be in the tissues and will be slowly off-gassed. A further reduction in ambient pressure with altitude can cause bubbles, or enlarge pre-existing asymptomatic ones. Current guidelines advise against flying for 12 hours after a single short no-decompression dive, and 24 hours for multiple dives and decompression dives.[20]

Assessment

The diagnosis of DCI is made on history and examination. A full dive history must be obtained, in addition to the medical history. Important details include the number of dives over recent days, depth, bottom time (the time from beginning descent to beginning direct ascent), performance of any decompression or safety stops, dive complications such as raid ascents, surface interval between dives, and the time interval between completing the dive and onset of symptoms. Previous dive experience, equipment used and gases breathed should also be recorded. Any exposure to altitude post dive should be inquired about. Cold water, hard exercise during the dive, increasing age, multiple ascents and repetitive dives are predisposing factors in the development of DCI.

A thorough examination, particularly of the neurological system, to detect subtle abnormalities is required. The sharpened Romberg's test is a valuable examination in patients with DCI.[21] It is performed by standing heel to toe with open palms on opposite shoulders. The eyes are closed once the patient is stable. They are then timed until they lose balance or achieve 60 seconds. The best score of four attempts is used. A best score of less than 60 seconds is suggestive of DCI in an injured diver. If symptoms are progressing rapidly, the examination should be brief so as to ensure rapid access to recompression. If the history suggests AGE, the patient should not be moved from the horizontal position to avoid reembolization.

INVESTIGATIONS

A full blood count is useful in that intravascular fluid depletion is common in severe DCI and the degree of haemoconcentration may correlate with eventual neurological outcome.[22] Electrolyte abnormalities are rare. The blood sugar should be checked in diabetic divers. A chest X-ray is indicated if pulmonary barotrauma is suspected, because a pneumothorax needs treatment before recompression. Although lung barotrauma is the cause of CAGE, only 5% of divers with CAGE have radiographic evidence of a pneumothorax.[23] However, subtle signs of extra-alveolar air suggesting pulmonary barotrauma are present in nearly half.[24]

CT and MRI are insensitive and have no role in the acute investigation of DCI. Recompression should only be delayed for investigations if they will directly alter management.

MANAGEMENT

First aid

Initial resuscitation is along standard basic and advanced life support protocols. If intubation is required, the endotracheal tube cuff should be filled with saline to avoid a change in volume on recompression.

One hundred per cent oxygen provides the maximum gradient for diffusion of nitrogen out of the bubbles. It should be administered immediately and continued during recompression. Failure to improve on oxygen does not rule out DCI. Conversely, complete improvement on oxygen does not obviate the need for recompression. The patient should be supine or in the left lateral position if unable to protect their airway. Traditionally, the Trendelenburg position has been advocated to reduce bubble embolization to the brain, but is now thought to increase the risk of cerebral oedema and should only be used if required to maintain blood pressure.[25] The diver should be prevented from sitting or standing up, to avoid bubbles redistributing from the left ventricle to the brain.

Intravenous isotonic crystalloids should be commenced and titrated to response. Glucose-containing fluids are to be avoided because they may exacerbate CNS injury. Divers who present after several days with mild symptoms may be adequately managed with oral fluids. A urinary catheter should be inserted for spinal cord DCI with bladder involvement. Hypothermia should be corrected.

Retrieval

Long-distance retrieval can either be by air transport pressurized to 1 ATA or by portable recompression chambers. There is little debate that the longer the delay in recompression of severe DCI, the worse the outcome. However, Australian experience suggests that the number of cases where a portable chamber would have made a difference is so small that their use is unwarranted.[26,27] Commercial aircraft are pressurized to 0.74 ATA (2440 m) and not appropriate to retrieve DCI patients. Road retrieval is not suitable over great distances, or where an altitude of 300 m will be exceeded. Consultation with a hyperbaric physician should occur if retrieval is difficult.

Recompression

Recompression in a hyperbaric chamber is indicated even if the diver becomes asymptomatic with first aid, because otherwise many will relapse. The relapse can be more severe than the original presentation, and waiting for this to occur will result in substantial delay to recompression. Response to recompression is determined mainly by initial severity, but also by time to recompression. Recompression should always be as soon as possible, but is particularly urgent for severe cases. Treatment commenced more than 12 hours after injury in this group is associated with a poor response. Mild cases often respond despite longer delays to recompression.[28]

In-water recompression is dangerous and difficult and should only be considered if retrieval is impossible. Supervision should be by a hyperbaric physician experienced in the technique.

Two types of hyperbaric chamber are available. Monoplace chambers accommodate the patient only and are compressed with 100% oxygen. Multiplace chambers can accommodate an attendant as well, and are compressed on air while the patient breathes 100% oxygen via a head hood, demand regulator or endotracheal tube. Air breaks to lessen the risks of oxygen toxicity are given by removing the head hood in a multiplace and by breathing air from a mask in a monoplace chamber. Full monitoring and mechanical ventilation are possible. All hyperbaric facilities in Australasia use multiplace chambers.

Hyperbaric oxygen has the following beneficial effects:

- Reduction in bubble size in accordance with Boyle's Law. Increased pressure also increases the partial pressure of nitrogen within the bubble. There is no nitrogen outside the bubble because of the 100% oxygen. This markedly increases the gradient for nitrogen to diffuse out. This relieves the obstruction caused by intravascular bubbles and the tissue distortion of extravascular bubbles.
- Reduction of endothelial inflammation caused by the bubbles.[29]
- Relief of ischaemia and hypoxia.

No published randomized trials compare recompression protocols, and therefore no international agreement on how to manage DCI exists. Even within Australasia practices differ markedly.[30] The general consensus is that initial treatments should begin with a standard 18 m (2.8 ATA) table breathing 100%

oxygen. Studies have shown no benefit in initially recompressing deeper.[31] This is likely to be because the greatest reduction in bubble volume occurs between 1 and 2 ATA (Table 27.3.1).

The identical Royal Navy 62 (RN62) and US Navy 6 are the most commonly used 18 m tables (see Fig. 27.3.1). Recompression is followed by gradual decompression. A response to treatment is usually evident by the second air break. If there is a partial response then the option of extending the table at 18 m does exist. If there is minimal or no response and there is no doubt about the diagnosis, then it is reasonable to proceed to a 30 m table (most units use the Comex 30 table). Because of the risks of oxygen toxicity at greater than 18 m, a combination of 50% helium and 50% oxygen (heliox) is used. Anecdotal evidence suggests that this technique is particularly effective for severe spinal cord DCI.[32,33]

Relapses can occur after initial recompression, and severe cases should be observed in hospital to allow immediate recompression if deterioration occurs. Otherwise, further daily recompression is carried out until the patient stops improving or becomes asymptomatic, and then one additional treatment is performed. Follow-up treatments are

usually at 18 m, using either the RN61 table (18 m for 45 minutes, ascent to 9 m over 30 minutes, 9 m for 30 minutes, then ascent over 30 minutes) or the 18:60:30 table (18 m for 60 minutes, then ascent over 30 minutes).

Residual symptoms occur in up to 30% of cases[11,34] and are more likely where recompression is delayed. This was not unusual with a mean time to recompression of 68 hours in one series.[11] It is not known whether there is a delay interval after which recompression is ineffective.

Lidocaine

Recent research in the use of lidocaine infusions in patients undergoing open heart surgery has demonstrated a significant benefit for the lidocaine group in terms of the incidence of postoperative neuropsychiatric abnormalities.[35] The mechanism of injury in open heart surgery is likely to be gas emboli and therefore provides a useful model for divers with AGE. There is now suffient evidence to recommend a 48 hour lidocaine infusion at standard anti-arrythmic doses to divers with unequivocal CAGE.

FURTHER DIVING

Recommendations for flying and diving after DCI vary greatly and are not evidence based. It is reasonable to permit resumption of diving after 4 weeks if there are no residual symptoms or signs. Flying should be avoided for at least 1 week after treatment to avoid relapse. Because of the risk of recurrence, further diving is contraindicated if the DCI is thought to be due to pulmonary barotrauma, or where there are residual neurological signs or symptoms.

ADVERSE EFFECTS OF HYPERBARIC OXYGEN

Middle-ear barotrauma is the most common adverse effect of hyperbaric therapy. Claustrophobia can occur.

The most serious adverse effect is oxygen toxicity, and the attendant must

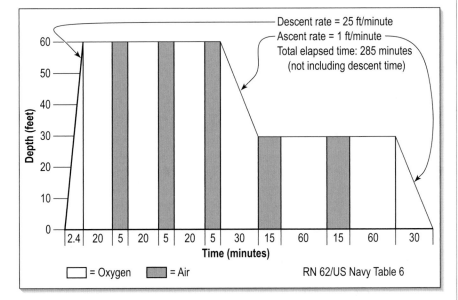

Fig. 27.3.1 US navy dive table.

Descent rate = 25 ft/minute
Ascent rate = 1 ft/minute
Total elapsed time: 285 minutes
(not including descent time)

☐ = Oxygen   ▨ = Air   RN 62/US Navy Table 6

continually watch for signs of its development. Toxicity is due to the formation of oxygen free radicals, which overwhelm the body's antioxidants. It can effect the brain and the lung.

Cerebral oxygen toxicity can occur with brief exposures to 2 ATA oxygen, and pulmonary toxicity may occur with prolonged exposure to 0.5 ATA or higher. The most common presentation of cerebral oxygen toxicity is muscle twitching, particularly of the lips and face. Other possible symptoms include apprehension, vertigo, visual disturbance, nausea, confusion and dizziness. If the oxygen is removed at this stage, progression to generalized convulsions may be avoided. Convulsions can, however, occur without premonitory symptoms. Treatment is as for any generalized convulsion, although removal of the oxygen will almost always stop it. Decompression should not be attempted during the convulsion as this may cause pulmonary barotrauma. Oxygen can be safely reinstituted 15 minutes after all symptoms have resolved. Predisposing factors to cerebral oxygen toxicity include fever, steroids, and a past history of epilepsy. Incidence is directly proportional to time of exposure and inspired oxygen partial pressure. The incidence of convulsions in divers treated at 2.8 ATA on the RN62 is approximately 1%.

Pulmonary oxygen toxicity manifests initially as an asymptomatic reduction in vital capacity, followed by cough and retrosternal pain. If the partial pressure of oxygen is not reduced at this stage, shortness of breath and eventual irreversible fibrotic changes will develop.

VERTIGO

There are several possible causes of vertigo in divers. Vertigo developing while the diver is underwater is extremely dangerous: it can induce panic and lead to a rapid ascent. It can disorientate the diver so that they do not know which way the surface is, and is often associated with vomiting.

The most common cause, alternobaric vertigo, begins just as divers commence their ascent, and is caused by a unilateral pressure difference between the middle and inner ears. It usually lasts only a few minutes. Other causes include inner-ear DCI, inner-ear barotrauma and TM rupture.

OXYGEN TOXICITY

Cerebral oxygen toxicity in the diver underwater causes the same problems as in the hyperbaric chamber. Divers are more likely to develop toxicity underwater than in the chamber because immersion, exercise and carbon-dioxide retention increase the risk. The use of oxygen-enriched gases such as nitrox increases the risk of cerebral oxygen toxicity. Enriched-air divers should ensure they stay below an oxygen partial pressure of 1.6 ATA.

NITROGEN NARCOSIS

Described by Jacques Cousteau as 'rapture of the deep', nitrogen narcosis is due to the anaesthetic effect of nitrogen dissolved in lipid membranes. Symptoms are similar to those of alcohol intoxication. Some divers experience it at 30 m and almost all by 50 m. Loss of consciousness occurs at 90 m. This condition will not present to the emergency department because it is immediately reversible on ascent. However, it may result in other diving accidents, such as rapid ascent or near-drowning. Those planning to dive deeper than 50 m should use an alternative to air, such as heliox.

GAS CONTAMINATION

Contaminants may be in the air before compression, added during compression, or already in the tanks. Common contaminants include carbon dioxide, carbon monoxide and oil. Increasing partial pressures of the contaminant gases at depth may result in toxicity. Contamination is rare but must always be included in the differential diagnosis of injured divers, particularly those presenting with headache, shortness of breath or loss of consciousness at depth.

PULMONARY OEDEMA

Pulmonary oedema in the diver may be caused by DCI, near-drowning or immersion itself. Preexisting cardiovascular disease and beta blockade appear to be risk factors for immersion-induced pulmonary oedema. Symptoms often begin while the diver is still at depth, distinguishing it from DCI. Treatment is supportive and recompression is not required as long as DCI has been excluded.

IMPORTANT PHONE NUMBERS

Twenty-four-hour services offering advice on management, retrieval and location of the nearest hyperbaric facility:

Divers Emergency Service (DES) Australia 1800 088200
+61 8 8373 5312 (outside Australia)
DES New Zealand (09) 4458454
Diving Accident Network (DAN) America (919) 6848111

UK numbers
Aberdeen Royal Infirmary
01224 681818
Diving Diseases Centre, Plymouth
01752 209999
Institute of Naval Medicine
02392 768026
Poole Hyperbaric Centre
01426 316636

REFERENCES

1. Shupak A, Doweck I, Greenberg E, et al 1991 Diving related inner ear injuries. Laryngoscope 101: 173–9
2. Roydhouse N 1997 Round window membrane rupture in scuba divers. SPUMS Journal 27(3): 148–51
3. Kizer KW 1987 Dysbaric cerebral air embolism in Hawaii. Annals of Emergency Medicine 16: 535–41
4. Weiss LD, Van Meter KW 1995 Cerebral air embolism in asthmatic scuba divers in a swimming pool. Chest 107: 1653–4
5. Benton PJ, Woodfine JD, Westwood PR 1996 Arterial gas embolism following a 1 metre ascent during helicopter escape training: a case report. Aviation Space and Environmental Medicine 67(1): 63–4
6. Williamson J 1988 Arterial gas embolism from pulmonary barotrauma: what happens in the lung? SPUMS Journal 18(3): 90–2
7. Gorman D 1984 Arterial gas embolism as a consequence of pulmonary barotrauma. SPUMS Journal 14(3): 8–16
8. Molenat FA, Boussuges AH 1995 Rupture of the stomach complicating diving accidents. Undersea and Hyperbaric Medicine 22(1): 87–94

9. Schriger DL, Rosenberg G, Wilder RJ 1987 Shoulder pain and pneumoperitoneum following a diving accident. Annals of Emergency Medicine 16: 1281–4

10. Rashleigh-Belcher HJ, Balham A 1984 Pneumoperitoneum in a sports diver. Injury 16: 47–8

11. Gardner M, Forbes C, Mitchell S 1996 One hundred divers with DCI treated in New Zealand during 1995. SPUMS Journal 26(4): 222–6

12. Goble SJ 1997 Is DCS possible if diving shallower than 10 metres? Presented at the 5th Annual Scientific Meeting on Diving and Hyperbaric Medicine, Sydney

13. Hagen PT, Scholz DG, Edwards WD 1984 Incidence and size of patent foramen ovale in the first ten decades of life: an autopsy study of 965 normal hearts. Mayo Clinic Proceedings 59: 17–20

14. Hallenbeck JM, Bove AA, Elliot DH 1975 Mechanisms underlying spinal cord damage in decompression sickness. Neurology 25: 308–16

15. Edmonds C, Lowry C, Pennefather J 1992 Diving and subaquatic medicine, 3rd edn. Butterworth Heinemann, Oxford

16. Smith RM, Neuman TS 1994 Elevation of serum creatine kinase in divers with arterial gas embolism. New England Journal of Medicine 330(1): 9–24

17. Smith RM, Neuman TS 1997 Abnormal serum biochemistries in association with arterial gas embolism. Journal of Emergency Medicine 15(3): 285–9

18. Divers Alert Network 1996 Report on diving accidents and facilities. Durham, NC

19. Divers Alert Network 1989 Report on 1988 diving accidents. Durham, NC

20. Sheffield PJ 1990 Flying after diving guidelines: a review. Aviation Space and Environmental Medicine 61: 1130–8

21. Fitzgerald B 1996 A review of the sharpened romberg test in diving medicine. SPUMS Journal 26(3): 142–6

22. Smith RM, Van Hosen KB, Neuman TS 1994 Arterial gas embolism and haemoconcentration. Journal of Emergency Medicine 12(2): 1147–53

23. Leitch D, Green R 1986 Pulmonary barotrauma in divers and the treatment of cerebral arterial gas embolism. Aviation Space and Environmental Medicine 57: 931–8

24. Harker CP, Neuman TS, Olson K, et al 1993 The roentographic findings associated with air embolism in sport scuba divers. Journal of Emergency Medicine 1(4): 443–9

25. Moon RE, Sheffield PJ 1997 Guidelines for treatment of decompression illness. Aviation Space and Environmental Medicine 68: 234–43

26. Butler C 1996 Hyperbaric retrievals in Townsville: is a portable chamber useful? SPUMS Journal 26(2): 66–70

27. Oxer HF 1987 Is transport of diving casualties under pressure worth it? Proceedings IX International Congress on Hyperbaric Medicine, Sydney, Australia, pp 137–8

28. Ball R 1993 Effect of severity, time to recompression with oxygen and retreatment on outcome in 49 cases of spinal cord decompression. Undersea and Hyperbaric Medicine 20(2): 133–45

29. Zamboni WA, Roth AC, Russell RC, Suchy H, Kucan J 1990 The effect of hyperbaric oxygen on the microcirculation of ischaemic skeletal muscle. Undersea Biomedical Research 17(Suppl): 26

30. Kluger M 1996 Initial treatment of decompression illness. A survey of Australian and New Zealand Hyperbaric Units. SPUMS Journal 26(1): 2–8

31. Bond JG, Moon RE, Morris DL 1990 Initial table treatment of decompression sickness and arterial gas embolism. Aviation Space and Environmental Medicine 611: 738–43

32. Kol S, Adir Y, Gordon CR, Melamed Y 1993 Oxy-helium treatment of severe spinal decompression sickness after air diving. Undersea and Hyperbaric Medicine 20(2): 147–54

33. Douglas JDM, Robinson C 1988 Heliox treatment for spinal decompression sickness following air dives. Undersea Biomedical Research 15(4): 315–9

34. Gorman DF, Pearce A, Webb RK 1988 Dysbaric illlness treated at the Royal Adelaide Hospital 1987: a factorial analysis. SPUMS Journal 18: 95–101

35. Mitchell SJ, Pellett O, Gorman DF 1999 Cerebral protection by lidocaine during cardiac operations. Annals of Thoracic Surgery 67: 1117–24

27.4 RADIATION ACCIDENTS

PAUL D. MARK

ESSENTIALS

1 Radiation accidents are very uncommon; however, the principles of management should be well understood by all emergency physicians.

2 The management of life-threatening illness or injury takes precedence over the radiation aspects of a patient's condition.

3 Contamination with radioactive material should be distinguished from exposure to ionizing radiation. It is very uncommon for both to occur in the same victim.

4 The management of contaminated patients follows the principles of barrier nursing, decontamination and contamination control used for pyogenic bacteria or toxic chemicals.

5 The presence of a qualified radiation physicist with appropriate radiation monitoring equipment is invaluable when dealing with (potentially) contaminated patients.

6 The principal risks of internal contamination arise from contamination of wounds and around body orifices.

7 Blocking and chelating agents can successfully reduce the incorporation of radioactive substances into body tissues.

8 Following whole-body irradiation, survival is likely only from the haemopoietic and milder gastrointestinal syndromes.

9 Effective triage can be based on early clinical symptoms and lymphocyte counts. Cytogenic analysis gives an accurate estimation of the dose received.

10 Authoritative and knowledgeable personnel and well considered hospital procedures, including media liaison, are essential to effectively manage these incidents.

INTRODUCTION

Until June 1990 there were 327 major radiation accidents worldwide, in which 91 individuals died.[1] Of these accidents, 18 were in nuclear installations, 84 involved unsealed radioactive sources (of which 38 involved medical applications), 147 involved sealed radioactive sources (mostly highly active industrial radiography sources), 62 were with X-ray devices, and 15 were with accelerators. These figures probably underestimate the true incidence by between 50 and 100%. Many accidents have occurred as a result of deliberate bypassing of safety procedures.[2]

In Australia, the Australian Radiation Incidence Registry records all accidents where exposures occur that are not 'within the limits known to be normal for the particular source of radiation and for the particular use being made of it'. Very few accidents are recorded in which individuals received exposure or contamination significant enough to cause health concerns.[3] Strict licensing and control systems, coupled with improving technology and training, have helped to minimize the number of Australian radiation incidents.

RADIATION SOURCES AND ACCIDENTS

Worldwide the most common radiation sources are:

- X-ray equipment: used for medical diagnosis and treatment, industrial and commercial inspections, quality control techniques, irradiations and research
- Accelerators: used for medical treatments, industrial irradiation, the production of radioisotopes and research
- Radioactive materials: used for medical diagnosis and treatment, industrial radiography, quality control and tracing techniques, soil density and moisture tests, and research. Radioactive material may be unsealed or contained within sealed containers.

- Nuclear processing and reactor plants: used for processing uranium and plutonium for fuel purposes and nuclear weapons, power production and research.

With X-ray equipment and accelerators the victim may be exposed to radiation but this does not make the tissues radioactive. These patients pose no threat to others, including medical attendants.

Unsealed radioactive material has the potential to cause radioactive contamination. This may be external on clothing or skin, or internal following ingestion, inhalation or absorption through body orifices, mucous membranes and wounds. Following internal contamination radioactive material may become incorporated into the patient's tissues.

Other than for accidents involving nuclear processing and reactor plants, accidents usually lead to either exposure or contamination. Contaminated patients rarely suffer significant radiation exposure, and exposed patients are seldom contaminated.[3]

EFFECTS OF RADIATION

The absorbed dose of radiation is the amount of ionization energy absorbed by exposed tissue. One gray (Gy) is equivalent to one joule per kilogram. The effect of a given dose of radiation depends on the rate of disintegration of the radionuclide, the type of radiation emitted, and the tissue type irradiated.

Rate of disintegration of the radionuclide

Radionuclide activity is the average number of nuclear disintegrations per second, and is a measure of the amount of radioactive material present. The becquerel (Bq) is the SI unit for one nuclear disintegration per second.

Type of radiation emitted

Different types of ionizing radiation transfer energy to tissue at different rates. The *equivalent dose* of radiation, measured by multiplying the absorbed radiation dose by a variable radiation weighting factor, is an indication of potential biological damage. α particles, consisting of two neutrons and two protons, rapidly lose energy to materials and only penetrate tissue to the thickness of the epidermis. β particles, with the mass and negative electric charge of an electron, penetrate tissue to only 1–2 mm. Photons, including γ-rays and X-rays, are the most common form of radiation. They lose energy as each successive layer of tissue is penetrated: the higher the initial energy, the greater the penetration.

Tissue type irradiated

Radiation damages tissue both directly and indirectly by the production of free radicals from water molecules. Direct damage to cell membranes may cause changes in permeability and the release of lysosomes. Germinal, haemopoietic and gastrointestinal epithelial cells are relatively radiosensitive. The cells of bone, liver, kidney, cartilage, muscle and nerve tissue are relatively radioresistant. The delayed effects of radiation depend on whether the dose is lethal or sublethal to the tissue involved.

Lethal (deterministic) injuries are threshold dependent. Cells are killed when they receive a radiation dose, which varies with different tissues. Clinical expression occurs when the amount of cell killing cannot be compensated for by proliferation of viable cells. The earliest delayed effect of radiation injury – cataract formation at about 10 months – is an example of this type of injury.

For sublethal (stochistic) injuries there is no threshold level of radiation. Sublethal injury to chromosomes is the most important effect of ionizing radiation. Double-strand breaks are not easily reparable, especially if the damage occurs simultaneously to both strands. This results in broken chromosomes with no template for repair. The exposed ends of chromosome fragments may join up at random, resulting in morphological chromosomal abnormalities. Clinical expression may occur not only in the affected individual, but also in future generations if gonadal cells have been involved. Although this occurs commonly

ENVIRONMENTAL

in laboratory animals, it is believed to be rare in humans.[4]

Sublethal damage to chromosomes is implicated in the development of tumours, including leukaemia, which may occur from 5 to 7 years after radiation exposure. Children are more prone to radiation-induced carcinogenesis. Although the incidence of malignancy is increased by radiation exposure, the age at which malignancies are clinically expressed does not change.

Radiation exposure to the gonads may produce temporary infertility in men, with preservation of secondary sexual characteristics. In the female, however, all ova are present at birth and larger radiation doses are required to produce sterility. Radiation-induced infertility in females is associated with premature menopause.

ACUTE RADIATION EXPOSURE

Radiation exposure accidents usually involve penetrating radiation such as high-energy X-rays or γ-rays. The effects are primarily due to the loss of cells in the body. Acute exposure is more dangerous than chronic, as it does not allow time for cell replacement or tissue recovery. Clinically, radiation exposure may produce a generalized acute radiation syndrome or a localized irradiation injury.

ACUTE RADIATION SYNDROME

Pathophysiology and clinical course

The term 'acute radiation syndrome' collectively refers to one or more of the haemopoietic syndrome, the gastrointestinal syndrome, the cardiovascular syndrome and the neurovascular syndrome. The symptoms arising depend on the part of the body irradiated, the dose, and the time over which it is delivered. Early symptoms are due to the effects of radiation on membranes and the release of vasoactive amines. The phase of manifest illness corresponds to loss of cells.[5]

The course of the illness can be divided into four phases. The higher the dose, the shorter the duration of each phase and the more severe the symptoms:

❶ The prodromal phase, which generally lasts up to 48 hours
❷ A latent period, lasting hours to weeks
❸ The manifest illness period, which may include bleeding and infection
❹ Death or recovery; the latter may take up to 10 weeks.

The prodromal period is non-specific, with anorexia, nausea, vomiting, weakness, fever, conjunctivitis, erythema and hyperaesthesia.

The haemopoietic syndrome occurs with whole-body radiation doses of between 1 and 10 Gy. The latent period lasts from 2 to 20 days and is followed by a rapid fall in the number of white blood cells and platelets. Recovery commences about 30 days after exposure, regardless of the dose.

The gastrointestinal syndrome predominates with radiation doses greater than 10 Gy. The prodromal symptoms are more severe. Bloody diarrhoea suggests death within 2 weeks. The prodromal symptoms recur during the manifest illness phase and can be very severe.

The cardiovascular syndrome occurs with doses of greater than 15 Gy and is characterized by leakage of fluid into tissues. Leakage into the brain causes neurological symptoms and consequent overlap with the neurovascular syndrome.

The neurovascular syndrome occurs with doses of greater than 50 Gy. There is incapacitation usually within the first few minutes and certainly within 40 minutes. The effects are largely due to disruption of cell membranes and electrochemical inactivation of neurons. Death can be anticipated within hours.

INVESTIGATION

Blood counts and chromosomal analyses may be used to estimate radiation dosage.[6] Lymphocyte counts made every 6–12 hours for the first 2 days after

exposure will give an indication of the radiation dose received and the prognosis. If the lymphocyte count does not fall below 1200/mm^3 within 24 hours the patient will probably not require clinical support. If it falls below 500/mm^3, a severe course can be anticipated. If lymphocytes disappear within 6 hours the dose is likely to be fatal.[7]

Cytogenetic studies examine the number and structure of chromosomes. Radiation dose is reflected in the number of excess acentric and dicentric forms.[8] This information is available after 48 hours, although a full analysis takes considerably longer. Importantly, T lymphocytes are relatively long-lived and reliable dose estimates can be made up to 5 weeks after collection of the sample.

A newer method involves electron spin resonance of tooth enamel, and can detect very low doses (0.1 Gy).[9]

TRIAGE

A patient presenting soon after an exposure or presumed exposure to ionizing radiation can be triaged on the basis of their symptoms and lymphocyte counts:[10]

- No symptoms and lymphocyte count above 1500/mm^3 at 48 hours: probably no life-threatening injury; observe periodically for any change in clinical status.
- Nausea, vomiting, possibly diarrhoea, conjunctival redness and erythema, lymphocyte count between 800 and 1500/mm^3 at 48 hours: probable serious injury; plan for therapy.
- Pronounced nausea and vomiting, diarrhoea, conjunctival redness and erythema, lymphocyte count between 100 and 800/mm^3 at 48 hours: probable life-threatening injury; plan for maximal therapy.
- Prompt severe vomiting and blood in diarrhoea, erythema and hypotension, lymphocyte count below 100/mm^3 at 48 hours: almost certainly lethal; give supportive therapy.

MANAGEMENT

Supportive treatment includes maintenance of fluid and electrolyte balance, nutritional supplementation and anti-emetics.

Control of infection commences in the prodromal phase, with identification and aggressive treatment of any potential infection, so that the patient is in optimal condition to survive a period of manifest haemopoietic depression. To reduce the infection risk patients may be kept home during the latent period and admitted to hospital when the haemopoietic syndrome develops. Hospital management involves strict isolation, lamina airflow units, and the administration of antibacterial, antiviral, antifungal and antihelminthic therapy as needed. Non-absorbable agents are commonly used to sterilize the gastrointestinal tract.

Management of the haemopoietic syndrome follows the principles established in the management of bone marrow suppression secondary to chemotherapeutic agents. If as many as 10% of the stem cells remain intact, the blood cells will repopulate. Therapeutic modalities include platelet transfusion, cytokines and colony-stimulating factor. The role of bone marrow transplantation is evolving.

PROGNOSIS

Survival from the cardiovascular and neurovascular syndromes does not occur. Survival is very unlikely from severe gastrointestinal syndrome.

Survival from the haemopoietic syndrome and the lower-dose gastrointestinal syndrome is much more likely, and appropriate supportive treatment should be provided.

COMBINED INJURIES

Combined injury occurs when there is additional trauma, either physical or thermal, in addition to the radiation injury. The effects of the radiation exposure may become apparent earlier and may be more severe when other injuries are present. Infection and haemorrhage remain the major problems, but may be multifactorial in nature. The lymphocyte count may drop as a result of physical trauma. All administered blood products should be irradiated to remove the T-cell population and minimize graft-versus-host reactions. Platelets should be transfused if the platelet count falls below $20 \times 10^9/L$ and, if surgery is anticipated, it should be maintained higher than $75 \times 10^9/L$. Major procedures should be carried out within 36–48 hours while some white blood cells remain. Elective surgery should be delayed as long as possible. For thermal burns, early excision of potentially septic tissue and skin grafting are indicated.

Early reintroduction of enteral nutrition is important to maintain gastric acidity and prevent infectious organisms spreading from the gut to the respiratory system. Antiulcer agents should be prescribed to reduce the risk of stress ulceration. Radiation pneumonitis may develop some time following the exposure and be confused with ARDS.

LOCAL IRRADIATION INJURIES

The majority of local irradiation injuries occur when operators of X-ray diffraction units inadvertently place their fingers or hands in the direct X-ray beam. Other accidents occur when radioactive sources, often from industrial radiography equipment, are detached and then picked up and placed in the pockets of workers. In addition, there have been misadministrations of doses to patients undergoing radiotherapy.

The higher the dose the greater the severity and the earlier the onset of the local injury. The smaller the area irradiated, the higher the dose required to produce a particular change.

Early skin effects include epilation, erythema, dry desquamation, wet desquamation, blisters and radionecrotic lesions. Symptoms may include tenderness, itching, tingling, and a changed sensitivity to heat and cold. If the area irradiated includes the epigastrium, nausea and vomiting may also occur.

The degree of radiosensitivity of the skin depends on the thickness of the epidermis. The most sensitive areas are those that are also moist and subject to friction, such as the axilla, groin and skin folds. The least sensitive areas are the nape of the neck, scalp, palms and soles.

Erythema may not appear for some days. If it occurs within 48 hours the lesion will probably progress to ulceration. If irradiated skin appears normal at 72 hours, the lesion is likely to be less severe but may still ulcerate in 1 or 2 weeks. Erythema may be delayed for up to 30 days. Pain is minimal unless ulceration occurs or the dose is extreme.

Late effects include progressive tissue atrophy, fibrosis and chronic radiodermatitis with tissue breakdown. There may be stiffness and tenderness and decreased sensitivity to temperature change.

Mild injuries may be simply observed. An effort should be made to protect the area from additional trauma. For more severe injuries, particularly with pain, local debridement and skin grafting may be necessary but should be delayed until the full extent of the lesion is known.[11] Methods of assessing the underlying circulation include arteriography, radionuclide perfusion studies and thermography. Amputation is reserved for gangrene. Skin grafts are indicated for areas of exposed cartilage or bone, or for severe scarring. Topical antibiotics are often prescribed in an attempt to reduce infection. Hyperbaric oxygen therapy may be useful.[12]

In the long term, an irradiated area must be watched for the possible development of neoplastic change.

CONTAMINATION WITH RADIOACTIVE MATERIAL

Prehospital phase

The care of individuals who are contaminated with radioactive material requires similar preparation and precautions as for those contaminated with hazardous chemicals. Radioactive contamination has the advantage that it can be readily detected by instruments when on the skin. With the exception of Chernobyl, survivors of radiation accidents have not been sufficiently contaminated so as to pose a threat to emergency or hospital personnel using appropriate precautions and procedures.[5]

Preparedness

Facilities using unshielded radioactive material must have procedures in place to deal with spillage and other accidents, and all workers must be adequately trained in those procedures. Emergency equipment must include adequate monitors for detecting ionizing radiation or contamination, facilities for decontaminating victims, and bags for containing biological and other samples. Appropriate blocking or chelating agents should be stocked at the facility.[13] Emergency planning must include early warning of the receiving hospital so that adequate preparations can be made prior to the arrival of patients.

Scene management

Serious illness or injury is not due to radiation per se, and should be treated on its own merits. Unless the patient's condition is serious, external decontamination begins at the scene so as to minimize internal contamination and incorporation of the radionuclide into the body tissues, and to reduce the risk of contaminating other persons and the hospital environment. As much as 80% of contaminating material may be on the clothing.[14] Accordingly, the victim's outer clothing should be removed at the earliest practicable stage. If monitoring is not available, it should be assumed that all outer clothing is contaminated. Clothing is cut from head to toe and down the sleeves, folded back over itself as it is cut, and then rolled up. The person removing the contaminated clothing must wear protective clothing and avoid contact with the outside of the victim's clothing. The victim is then wrapped in plain sheets and transferred to hospital.[15] If small contamination spots on the skin cannot be easily

removed at the scene, they should be dressed and the victim transported to hospital.

At large accidents, members of the rescue team should put on the protective clothing normally used by personnel working with radioactive material at that site. This includes gloves, facemask and cap. Gowns may be covered with large plastic aprons to make them waterproof. Additional measures, such as taping plastic bags over shoes, may be used if the normal protective clothing is judged inadequate. The implementation of life-saving procedures may make it necessary to forgo some of this protection. Contamination of the rescuer will be low and can be effectively removed later.

At larger accidents it is necessary to establish a controlled area, the periphery of which is located just beyond the region where contamination can be detected above background levels. Protective clothing worn by rescue teams should be removed at the perimeter of this area prior to both patient and rescuers leaving. Monitoring of all personnel leaving the area should be undertaken if facilities are available.[16]

Hospital phase

Preparedness

The elements of planning for the management of radiation accident patients are similar to those for other types of emergencies, namely prevention, preparedness, response and recovery.

Facilities using unsealed radioactive sources should be defined. These include nuclear medicine departments, scientific laboratories and nuclear facilities. An emergency response plan should be defined and emergency response team membership designated. Equipment for monitoring, decontamination and contamination control should be in place. Regular practice is essential.[17]

A decontamination area must be designated and be itself capable of adequate decontamination. Waste water may be legally discharged into normal draining systems if it does not exceed specified limits. In the clinical setting of a single patient this is unlikely.

Accidents involving contaminated or possibly contaminated patients rapidly deplete a receiving hospital's emergency response. If multiple patients with possible contamination are being managed, the hospital may need to be placed on temporary ambulance bypass.

Hospital protocols should include plans for dealing with relatives, the press and the public. The timely release of appropriate information is important. Persons issuing this information should be well versed in radiation medicine, as the avoidance of questions and confusion in answers may generate public uncertainty and panic. Security personnel will be required to restrict the entry of unauthorized persons to the treatment area.

Management

Life-saving procedures take priority over other actions related to the radiation aspects of the patient's condition, even if preparations to minimize the spread of contamination have not been completed. A radiation physicist with appropriate monitoring equipment should be present throughout the hospital management phase. However, if patients arrive before monitoring is available, treatment should proceed based on the patient's history, using the procedures for patients contaminated with pyogenic bacteria.

In the absence of significant injury patients from the incident should be monitored at triage and, if found to be contaminated, admitted to a controlled area for decontamination. The controlled area itself needs adequate preparation.[18] The entire floor should be covered with plastic and any non-essential items removed. Access to the controlled area must be strictly supervised, and there should preferably be a buffer zone. Staff should wear protective clothing of the type normally used in theatre. Gowns should be waterproof, but if not, large plastic aprons worn over them are satisfactory. Lead plastic aprons as used in X-ray departments are not satisfactory: these prevent exposure but not contamination. Plastic bags are taped over the shoes and the cuffs of trousers should be taped and secured to the outsides of overshoes. Facemasks are rarely required to protect against airborne contamination but they do protect the face from being touched by contaminated hands. Two pairs of gloves should be worn. The inner ones should be surgical gloves taped to the sleeves. The outer gloves are not taped down and should be changed whenever they become contaminated. Rubbish bins lined with garbage bags serve as waste receptacles.

Once the patient is in the controlled area, all clothing should be removed and other medical conditions assessed and treated. Blocking agents can be administered if they have not already been given. Excreta should be collected for later monitoring, and blood samples should be drawn for a baseline complete blood count, differential and absolute lymphocyte counts, and later cytogenic analysis.

External decontamination utilizes the principles of barrier nursing and contamination control. Staff should stand back from the patient except when actually examining them or performing procedures. Hospital personnel should be rotated during the decontamination procedure to minimize the perceived risk to any one individual. Pregnant staff should not be involved.

The priority areas for external decontamination are wounds and orifices, as it is through these that the risk of subsequent internal contamination is greatest. Other priority areas include the hands, face and head, as early contamination removal reduces spread. Decontamination of intact skin is the last priority.

If contamination is only discovered after patients are admitted to an emergency department, the entire area through which they have passed should be roped off, surveyed with the help of a radiation physicist and, if necessary, decontaminated. Staff should put on protective clothing and remove nearby patients so as to create a spacious treatment area.

External decontamination starts at the periphery of a contaminated area and works inwards. Wounds are decontaminated in the same manner as when removing dirt or bacteria. Deeper wounds should be opened up and thoroughly irrigated.

Deep debridement and excision of a wound may be necessary in extreme cases where highly toxic material is embedded in the tissues. The mouth is decontaminated by gentle irrigation and frequent rinsing with 30% hydrogen peroxide solution. Brushing of the teeth with toothpaste is helpful, as toothpaste contains chelating agents. External ear canals should be irrigated, and nasal douches can be effective. The eyes are rinsed by directing a stream of water or saline from the inner canthus to the outer canthus, so that material is not forced into the lacrimal duct. The skin is washed initially with warm water and mild soap. If this is ineffective, progressively stronger detergents can be used. If the skin becomes damaged or red and sore, cleansing should be discontinued. Hair should be shampooed several times with the head deflected backwards over a basin to keep water from the eyes and ears. A hair dryer is used to dry the hair. Clipping of hair may be necessary.

If whole-body contamination occurs, for example from a gaseous plume from a reactor accident, decontamination is best accomplished by showering.[3] Washing starts with the hair and works downwards. Wounds should be covered with a waterproof dressing.

Internal contamination causes no acute clinical effects and it is usually not feasible to confirm its presence before commencing treatment directed at the reduction of absorption, prevention of incorporation into tissues and promotion of elimination. Significant internal contamination usually occurs through wounds or body orifices, but can occur following inhalation or ingestion. Radionuclides, which have short effective half-lives, pose little danger unless the intake is large. Where internal contamination involves radionuclides with longer half-lives, there is a medical urgency to initiate treatment aimed at reducing uptake and enhancing elimination. Selection of the appropriate technique or drug depends on the radionuclide involved.[19] Uptake by the various organs can be reduced by the use of blocking agents, dilution techniques or chelating agents. Gastro-intestinal decontamination is accomplished by either gastric lavage or ipecac-induced emesis. In the absence of external contamination these are the only circumstances in which internal contamination poses any risk to hospital staff. Administration of stable iodine in the form of potassium iodate or potassium iodide tablets will reduce uptake by the thyroid gland by up to 90% if given less than 2 hours after intake, and by about 50% if in less than 3 hours. Chelating agents and mobilizing agents may be useful for up to 2 weeks. Mobilizing agents, such as antithyroid drugs, increase the natural rate of turnover of a biological molecule and thereby increase excretion.

CONCLUSION

Radiation-associated accidents are rare but require well planned protocols for successful management.[20] The main problems are with those patients who are potentially contaminated with radioactive particulate material. The principles of contamination control are little different from those already practised when dealing with patients contaminated with chemical or biological material.

The risks to hospital personnel are not great when dealing with contaminated patients. However, this is an emotive subject in the community and hospitals should be seen to be doing their utmost to protect all personnel and to limit the spread of any contamination.

The victims of radiation accidents may present with a variety of clinical syndromes, and their management requires a multidisciplinary approach and close liaison between clinical staff and health physicists.[21]

REFERENCES

1. Holmes JL, Mark PD 1991 Medical planning and emergency care in radiation accidents. Emergency Medicine 3(3) suppl: 136–48
2. Cardis E 1996 Epidemiology of accidental radiation exposures. Environmental Health Perspectives 104(3) suppl: 643–9
3. Swindon T 1991 Manual on the medical management of individuals involved in radiation accidents. Australian Radiation Laboratory

4. Rytoman T 1996 Ten years after Chernobyl. Annals of Medicine 28(2): 83–7
5. Mettler FD 1978 Emergency management of radiation accidents. JACEP 7: 302
6. Swindon T 1991 The management of individuals involved in radiation accidents. Emergency Medicine 3(3) suppl: 131–5
7. Goans RE, Holloway EC, Berger ME, Ricks RD 1997 Early dose assessment following severe radiation accidents. Health Physics 72(4): 513–8
8. Salassidis K, Schmid E, Peter RU, Braselmann H, Bauchinger M 1994 Dicentric and translocation analysis for retrospective dose estimation in humans exposed to ionising radiation during the Chernobyl nuclear power plant accident. Mutation Research 311(1): 39–48
9. Baranov AE, Guskova AK, Nadejini NM, Nugis Vyu 1995 Chernobyl experience: biological markers of exposure to ionising radiation. Stem Cells 13(1) suppl: 69–77
10. Anno GH, Baum SJ, Withers HR, et al 1989 Symptomatology of acute radiation effects in humans after exposure to doses of 0.5–30 Gray. Health Physics 56: 821–38
11. Oliveira AR, Brandao-Mello CE, Valverde NJ 1991 Localised lesions induced by 137 Cs during the Goiania accident. Health Physics 60: 25–9
12. Berger ME, Hurtado R, Dunlap J, et al 1997 Accidental radiation injury to the hand: anatomical and physiological considerations. Health Physics 72(3): 343–8
13. Lincoln TA 1976 Importance of initial management of persons internally contaminated with radionuclides. Journal of the American Industrial Hygiene Association 37: 16–21
14. Hugner KF, Fry SA (eds) 1980 The Medical Basis for Radiation Accident Preparedness. Elsevier, New York
15. Ricks RC 1983 Transport of irradiated or radioactively contaminated patients to the hospital. Bulletin of the New York Academy of Medicine 59: 1108–18
16. Hubner KF 1983 Symposium on the health aspects of nuclear power plant incidents. Decontamination procedures and risks to health care personnel. Bulletin of the New York Academy of Medicine 59: 1119–28
17. Fong F, Schrader DC 1996 Radiation disasters and emergency department preparedness. Emergency Medicine Clinics of North America 14(2): 349–70
18. Leonard RB, Ricks RD 1980 Emergency department radiation accident protocol. Annals of Emergency Medicine 9: 462–70
19. Zarzycki W, Zonenberg A, Telejko B, Kinalska I 1994 Iodide prophylaxis in the aftermath of the Chernobyl accident in the area of Senjy in north-eastern Poland. Hormone and Metabolic Research 26(6): 293–6
20. Swindon TN 2000 Medical Management of Individuals Involved in Radiation Accidents. Technical Report Series No. 131. Australian Radiation Protection and Nuclear Safety Agency,
21. Ricks RC 2002 Guidance for Radiation Accident Management. Radiation Emergency Assistance Centre/Training Site (REAC/TS) Oak Ridge Institute for Science and Education

27.5 NEAR-DROWNING

DAVID MOUNTAIN

ESSENTIALS

1 The incidence of near-drowning requiring medical assessment is estimated to be from two to 20 times greater than that of actual drowning.

2 The highest rates of near-drowning occur in children from 1 to 4 years of age and young adult males. Alcohol is associated with the majority of adult deaths.

3 From 10 to 20% of drownings are 'dry' with asphyxia, probably secondary to laryngospasm and mucus plug formation. Experimental differences between fresh and salt water drowning have been demonstrated but are unimportant in terms of management.

4 Hypothermia following warm-water (>10°C) near-drowning carries a poor prognosis. Hypothermia following cold-water (<10°C) near-drowning may be associated with improved outcome.

5 Initiation of good-quality CPR within 10 minutes of retrieval is associated with good outcome. Postural drainage procedures and the Heimlich manoeuvre are no longer recommended. PEEP/CPAP are useful therapies in hospital.

6 Newer therapies, such as artificial surfactant and inhaled nitric oxide, have so far shown equivocal results. Extracorporeal membrane oxygenation is used in some centres.

INTRODUCTION

Australia, the driest inhabited continent, has the highest reported incidence of drowning in the world. It is a major cause of death in those under 30 years of age.[1] This incidence probably reflects the proximity of major population centres to the coast and the popularity of aquatic activities in Australia. The increasing incidence of drowning in Australia over the past 30 years is likely to be related to increasing numbers of backyard pools and participation in aquatic activities.[2] Despite advances in the understanding of near-drowning, many questions remain unanswered, and mortality and morbidity from drowning continue to rise in most age groups.

EPIDEMIOLOGY

Overall, there is a marked preponderance of male over female deaths from drowning, and in adults the ratio is as great as 9:1.[3,4] Groups with high rates of drowning include young adult males (15–30 years), epileptics, overseas visitors and the mentally retarded. In young adult males, bravado, inexperience and alcohol lead to many deaths. Alcohol is found in up to 50% of all adult drownings and the majority of male adult drownings.[3,4,5] In the elderly, underlying medical illnesses and suicide attempts are common.

The ratio of near-drowning to drowning is not accurately known because of differences in nomenclature, definitions, and the inability to collect all attendances related to near-drowning, but is estimated at between 2 and 20:1.[5] In a well-conducted study from the Netherlands, the ratio of patients admitted to ICU following near-drowning compared to those who drowned was 2:1.[3]

DEFINITIONS AND TERMINOLOGY

Much confusion is caused by imprecise definitions of drowning, near-drowning, dry drowning, immersion, submersion, suffocation and asphyxia. Modell[6] gives succinct and precise definitions: drowning is defined as death due to suffocation (asphyxia) after submersion in a liquid medium. It is further divided into 'dry' or 'wet', depending on the presence or absence of aspirated fluid in the lungs. Near drowning is defined as survival, at least temporarily, after suffocation (asphyxia) due to submersion in a liquid medium. This includes those who later die from complications such as hypoxic encephalopathy and adult respiratory distress syndrome (ARDS). The term 'secondary' drowning is inaccurate and unnecessary, as it relates to a variety of late lung complications. The difference between submersion and immersion is only important in a small number of cases where the individual (normally elderly or with prolonged QT syndrome) suffers a cardiac event as a result of immersion in water, and does not suffocate.[7] This is known as the immersion syndrome.[6]

PATHOPHYSIOLOGY OF DROWNING/NEAR DROWNING

The sequential pathophysiology of drowning is well described:[8,5,9]

- Initial submersion leads to voluntary apnoea (except where drowning is due to initial loss of consciousness). Unless submersion is voluntary, most adult victims panic and struggle. This is associated with increases in blood pressure and pulse rate. Slowing of the pulse secondary to the primitive dive reflex or cold-induced reflex bradyarrhythmias, often accentuated by alcohol, may be observed.[9,10]

- After an interval that depends on presubmersion oxygenation, fitness levels and the degree of panic and struggle, the synergistic effects of hypercapnia and hypoxia lead to an involuntary breath. This is known as the 'breaking point'. If an individual hyperventilates before diving, plasma CO_2 concentrations may remain so low that unconsciousness from hypoxia occurs before the breaking point is reached.

- The initial inhalation of fluid leads to a sudden increase in airway pressure, bronchoconstriction and pulmonary hypertension. In 10–20% of cases laryngospasm prevents further aspiration, and a plug of mucus and foam forms ('dry-drowning').

- Secondary apnoea occurs and is closely followed by loss of consciousness. Vomiting of swallowed fluid is common and frequently results in pulmonary aspiration.

- Involuntary gasping respirations lead to flooding of the lungs and alveolar injury, surfactant loss and hypoxia.

- Hypoxia leads to marked bradycardia, hypotension and irreversible brain injury within 3–10 minutes, and culminates in cardiopulmonary arrest.

In patients who drown, the average amount of fluid retrieved from the lungs is from 3 to 4 mL/kg, or less than 10% of total lung volume. However, the effect on the lungs is dramatic. Experimentally, fresh water and sea water cause lung injury by different mechanisms. Fresh water denatures surfactant and damages the alveolar cells. Sea water tends to draw in fluid, wash out surfactant and lead to foam formation. The aspiration of vomitus and chemicals in the water further complicates the clinical picture. Soap and chlorine in water do not appear to affect outcome. Clinically, the type of fluid inhaled rarely makes a significant difference. Electrolyte disturbances are minimal and transient, owing to the small volumes aspirated (more than 20 mL/kg are required for major disturbances).[8,9]

ORGAN-SPECIFIC EFFECTS

Lungs

The major features are intense broncho-spasm and laryngospasm, pulmonary hypertension and marked V/Q mis-match with physiological shunt. Even in patients without respiratory embarrass-ment after near drowning, shunts of up to 70% may occur and take up to 1 week to resolve. In the alveoli there is surfactant loss, formation of protein-rich exudate and injury to alveolar cells, often exacerbated by pneumonitis from gastric aspiration and secondary infection.[9,11,12] These changes result in a marked reduction in pulmonary compliance and hypoxia.

Brain

The major effects on the brain are secondary to hypoxia. Cerebral oedema, convulsions and persistent vegetative states are all observed. The possibility of trauma or an underlying medical com-plaint should always be considered in the differential diagnosis of an altered mental state especially in unwitnessed events.

Cardiovascular

Most near-drowning patients are haemo-dynamically stable after resuscitation. Hypothermic patients may develop any arrhythmia and should be gently handled and aggressively rewarmed. In older patients underlying ischaemic heart disease should be considered. Congenital long QT syndrome is associated with arrythmia in some cold water immersions.[7,11,13]

Haematological

Haemolysis occurs occasionally in freshwater near-drownings.[5]

Renal

Acute tubular necrosis or tubular injury from hypoxia may occur. Electrolyte disturbances are rarely significant.[2,11]

Gastrointestinal

Vomiting is frequently observed. It is secondary to ingestion of large volumes of water and may be associated with aspiration. Diarrhoea is less frequent.

Orthopaedic

Cervical spine injury should always be considered and excluded in diving injuries. Coexistent trauma may complicate recreational drowning.[4,12]

MANAGEMENT

Prehospital

Rapid institution of effective prehospital care is the most important factor in determining good outcome following near-drowning.[13,14] All patients seen alive within 1 hour of removal from cold water should be transported for definitive care.[15] The level of prehospital care required varies with the clinical severity of the case, which may range from asymptomatic to cardiopulmonary arrest. Initial assessment of the airway, breathing and circulation should be followed by institution of cardiopulmonary resuscitation if respirations or pulse are absent. There is little role for in-water resuscitation except when performed by expert retrievers using snorkel equipment.[12] Drainage procedures and the Heimlich manoeuvre are dangerous because they increase the risk of aspiration. The Heimlich manoeuvre is only indicated for removal of a foreign body.[5,12] Victims often vomit upon resumption of spontaneous respiration, and obtunded, spontaneously breathing patients should be transported on their side to minimize the risk of aspiration.[2,11] Wet clothing should be removed and the patient wrapped to minimize further heat loss. If associated trauma is possible, the cervical spine should be immobilized.[12] All symptomatic patients should be given supplemental high-flow oxygen. Early access to emergency medical systems is essential to minimize time to definitive care.[16,17] A person with knowledge of the patient or witness to the drowning should be encouraged to go directly to the hospital or travel in the ambulance.[2,13]

Emergency department

History

Important factors in the history include duration of submersion (or time since last seen), time to institution of CPR, time to the first spontaneous breath, and time to return of spontaneous cardiac output. A collateral history regarding previous health problems, use of alcohol and drugs, occurrence of vomiting and likelihood of associated trauma is also useful.[2]

Initial resuscitation

Initial assessment and resuscitation, continuing the priorities established in the prehospital setting, is directed towards the assessment and maintenance of airway, breathing and circulation. Monitoring should include cardiac rhythm, blood pressure, pulse oximetry and core temperature.

Airway management may simply involve clearing and positioning the airway and the provision of supplemental oxygen via a non-rebreathing mask. Endotracheal intubation is indicated if respiration is ineffective or the patient is comatose. Patients who cannot maintain a P_aO_2 greater than 90 mmHg on a non-rebreathing mask should be considered for intubation, although continuous positive airway pressure (CPAP) ventilation is an alternative in the cooperative patient. In the unconscious patient a nasogastric tube should be placed early to minimize the risk of pulmonary aspiration.[2,13] All intubated patients require PEEP and end-tidal CO_2 monitoring. Patients with bronchospasm should be treated with nebulized β-agonists.

Cardiac complications should be managed according to standard treatment regimens except in patients with core temperatures less than 33°C. These hypothermic patients must be handled gently and administration of antiarrhythmic drugs avoided until rewarming has taken place. All rhythms without output require CPR.[13] In general, asystole following near-drowning has the same dire prognosis as from other causes. Hypotension is managed with inotropes and fluids, together with invasive monitoring if required.[2,11] This is particularly important in patients with pulmonary oedema.[2,16]

The management of hypothermia is described elsewhere in this book. Where cervical spine injury is a possibility (especially following diving and water sports accidents), cervical spine immobilization should be maintained until the injury can be excluded radiologically.

Investigations

Ordering of investigations in the emergency department is guided by the clinical status of the patient, in particular mental status. Using the Modell/Conn classification of mental status (Table 27.5.1),[18,19] patients in group A only require a chest X-ray and oximetry. Patients in group B also require a full blood count, electrolytes and creatinine, blood sugar, arterial blood gases and an ECG. If they do not improve rapidly

Table 27.5.1 Conn/Modell classification of mental status following near-drowning			
Grade	Description of mental status	Equivalent GCS	Expected likelihood of good outcome (neurologically intact) (%)
A	Awake/alert	14–15	100
B	Blunted	8–13	100
C	Comatose	6–7	>90
C1	Decerebrate	5	>90
C2	Decorticate	4	>90
C3/4	Flaccid coma or arrest	3	<20

after arrival and supplemental oxygen they should be investigated and managed like group C patients. Patients in group C should also have liver function tests, creatine kinase and troponin at 6 hours, coagulation profile, alcohol level, urine drug screen, urine dipstick and MSU, along with a CT scan of the head if coma persists. Cervical spine X-rays and other trauma films are indicated if trauma is suspected.

Ongoing management

Patients who require intubation for near-drowning, especially if pulmonary changes are present on chest X-ray, should be given positive end-expiratory pressure (PEEP). Commence with low pressures (5–7.5 cmH$_2$O) and then increase until adequate oxygenation is achieved or hypotension or high airway pressures prevent further increases. Pressure-controlled ventilation may be added. These modalities improve outcome for near-drowning patients with secondary lung injury. Ventilatory weaning should begin as soon as possible in order to minimize the risk of barotrauma.[2,11,13] Maintenance of normothermia, normo-glycaemia, normovolaemia, normocarbia, seizure control and avoidance of hypoxia and hypotension are important in optimizing cerebral outcome. Dehydration and prolonged hyperventilation are dangerous.

Experimental therapies

A number of other therapeutic modalities have been trialled in an effort to improve the outcome of lung and brain injuries caused by near-drowning. These include:

- Induced hypothermia. Popularized by Conn, this therapy offers the theoretical advantage of cerebral protection but is no longer recommended.[2,11]
- Pharmacological cerebral protection. Barbiturate infusions, steroids and chlorpromazine have all been trialled. None have been shown to be of benefit and all may have deleterious effects.[11,13]
- Intracranial pressure monitoring. Its use is controversial and lacking in

outcome data, and depends on which ICU cares for the patient.[2,11,13]
- Prophylactic antibiotics. These are of no value except following near drowning in polluted water. In such cases a second-generation cephalosporin is recommended. Near drownings in hot spas and tubs may require antipseudomonal cover.[5,11]
- Hyperbaric oxygen therapy and nitric oxide therapy.
- Exogenous surfactant therapy. No proven benefit and recent animal research has suggested that it may increase lung injury.
- Extracorporeal oxygenation. Has been used successfully in some centres for severe lung injury.[5,16]

PROGNOSIS

Potential prognostic features in near-drowning have been extensively evaluated in an effort to reduce the number of neurovegetative survivors, avoid prolonged CPR, and provide relatives and medical personnel with early accurate prognostic information.

The most useful predictors relate to the initial resuscitation (field predictors). Factors associated with good outcome include submersion time less than 5 minutes, good-quality CPR provided within 10 minutes, first spontaneous breath within 30 minutes of retrieval from the water, and return of spontaneous circulation before arrival at hospital.[13] The last two are associated with very good neurological outcome, provided secondary lung injury does not supervene. Prehospital factors associated with poor outcome include male sex, unwitnessed or prolonged submersion, asystole, fresh water submersion and prolonged resuscitation before arrival at hospital.[2,5,13] However, *absolute* field predictors of poor outcome have *not* been identified and all patients who arrive in the emergency department following near-drowning deserve full resuscitation efforts.

Emergency-department prognostic factors have also been identified, but again no combination of factors reliably

predicts all patients who will do badly. Emergency-department prognostic factors associated with good outcome are pupillary response on arrival, perfusing cardiac rhythm on arrival,[14] or any motor response to pain on arrival.[23] Asystole is predictive of very poor outcome and except in paediatric cold water drowning should lead to early cessation of CPR in the emergency department.[2,3,6] Hypothermia has been described as a favourable prognostic indicator. Although this may be true following near drowning of children in cold water, hypothermia is a marker of prolonged submersion and, as such, is associated with a poor prognosis in near drowning in warm water and in adults.[3,20]

In-hospital factors associated with poor outcome include GCS less than 5 on transfer to intensive care (less than 20% intact survival), fixed dilated pupils at 6 hours, and any abnormality on CT scan in the first 36 hours. However, a normal CT scan is of no prognostic value.

DISPOSITION

All near-drowning victims should be carefully observed for a minimum of 6 hours.[5,13] Monitoring during that time should include pulse oximetry. Any patient with an abnormal chest X-ray or respiratory examination or significant hypoxaemia after 6 hours should be admitted. Those requiring intubation, with a history of cardiorespiratory arrest, persistently altered mental status or significant hypoxaemia should be admitted to intensive care. Truly asymptomatic patients may be discharged home after 6 hours of observation, but should be instructed to return to hospital if they develop respiratory symptoms.[2,13]

PREVENTION

Prevention of drowning and near-drowning is a major area for ongoing research and it is important that emergency physicians act as advocates for preventative strategies of proven benefit.

Patrolled beaches and early CPR are associated with better outcome.[8,13] Important public educational initiatives include beach safety, CPR training, raising public awareness of the dangers of mixing alcohol and water activities,[4] and wearing of life vests. Enforcement of alcohol laws on the water and safety regulations pertaining to providers of water activities is also important.

CONCLUSION

Near-drowning is a major cause of mortality and morbidity, particularly in young adult males. Good outcome is mainly determined by prehospital factors, but an accurate history, a well-run resuscitation and informed judgement on prognosis will optimize outcome and aid management of the patient and their family. The most important strategies in reducing harm from near drowning will come from public health preventative strategies for which emergency physicians should be strong advocates.

CONTROVERSIES AND FUTURE DIRECTIONS

❶ The development of accurate prognostic indicators that decrease the burden of patients surviving in persistent vegetative states is very important. Currently, most authorities agree that all but the obviously dead should be aggressively resuscitated. However, of those patients admitted to ICU, up to 15% survive in a persistent vegetative state.[16]

❷ The role of new treatment modalities for secondary lung injury, including nitrous oxide, artificial surfactant and extracorporeal oxygenation, individually or sequentially, is yet to be delineated.

❸ Major reductions in the incidence of drowning and near-drowning are only likely to be achieved with new initiatives in the areas of public education and prehospital response.[2,5]

REFERENCES

1. Pearn J, Nixon J, Wilkey I 1976 Freshwater drowning and near-drowning accidents involving children: a five year total population study. Medical Journal of Australia 2: 942–6

2. Pearn J 1985 The management of near drowning. British Medical Journal 291: 1447–52
3. Bierens JJLM, van der Velde EA, van Berkel M, et al 1989 Submersion cases in the Netherlands. Annals of Emergency Medicine 18(4): 366–73
4. Plueckhahn VD 1984 Alcohol and accidental drowning. A 25 year study. Medical Journal of Australia 141: 22–5
5. Braun R 1997 Near Drowning. Emergency Medicine Clinics of North America 15(2): 461–4
6. Modell JH 1981 Drown versus near-drown: a discussion of definitions. Critical Care Medicine 9(4): 351–2
7. Ackerman MJ, Tester DJ, Porter CJ 1999 Swimming, a gene-specific arrhythmogenic trigger for inherited long QT syndrome. Mayo Clinical Proceedings 74(11): 1088–94
8. Martin TG 1984 Neardrowning and cold water immersion. Annals of Emergency Medicine 13: 263–73
9. Pearn J 1985 Pathophysiology of drowning. Medical Journal of Australia 142: 586–8
10. Gooden BA 1992 Why some people do not drown. Hypothermia versus the diving response. Medical Journal of Australia 157: 629–32
11. Oh TE 1997 Near-drowning. Intensive Care Manual, 4th edn. Butterworth-Heinemann, Oxford, pp 617–21
12. Ornato JP 1986 The resuscitation of near-drowning victims. Journal of the American Medical Association 256(1): 75–7
13. Olshaker JS 1992 Near drowning. Emergency Medicine Clinics of North America 10(2): 339–50
14. Quan L, Kinder D 1992 Paediatric submersions: Prehospital Predictors of Outcome. Pediatrics 90(6): 909–13
15. Wyatt JP, Tomlinson GS, Busuttil A 1999 Resuscitation of drowning victims in south-east Scotland. Resuscitation 41(2): 101–4
16. Maguire JE 1997 Advances in cardiac life support: sorting the science from the dogma. Emergency Medicine 9(Suppl): 1–21
17. Quan L 1993 Drowning issues in resuscitation. Annals of Emergency Medicine 22(2): 366–9
18. Conn AW, Montes JE, Barker GA, Edmonds JF 1980 Cerebral salvage in near-drowning following neurological classification by triage. Canadian Anaesthetic Society Journal 27(3): 211–5
19. Modell JH, Graves SA, Kuck EJ 1980 Near-drowning: correlation of level of consciousness and survival. Canadian Anaesthesia Society Journal 27(3): 211–5
20. Kemp AM 1991 Outcome in children who nearly drown : a British Isles study. British Medical Journal 302: 931–3

27.6 ELECTRIC SHOCK AND LIGHTNING INJURY

DANIEL M. FATOVICH

ESSENTIALS

1 Death from electric shock is due to ventricular fibrillation, the lethal arrhythmia occurring at the time of the exposure. Routine admission for ECG monitoring is unnecessary.

2 Most deaths are caused by low-voltage (<1000 V) exposures.

3 The amount of current passing through the body is determined mainly by tissue resistance, which is dramatically reduced by moisture.

4 Electrical injury resembles a crush injury more than a burn. The tissue damage below skin level is invariably more severe than the cutaneous wound would suggest.

5 There is a diversity of clinical manifestations seen with electrical injury.

6 Lightning injury is different from high-voltage electrical injury and has a unique range of clinical features. The management is predominantly expectant.

ELECTRIC SHOCK

INTRODUCTION AND EPIDEMIOLOGY

Electricity is an integral part of our everyday world and electric shock is common. Patients may present to the emergency department with resulting injuries that range from trivial to fatal (termed electrocution). Although permanent disability can occur, it is reassuring to note that if the initial exposure is survived, subsequent death is unlikely. For each death caused by electricity there

are two serious injuries and 36 reported electric shocks.[1]

There are approximately 80 electrical fatalities each year in Australia. Victims are predominantly male and relatively young. Death is just as likely to occur at home as in the workplace. Electricians and linesmen are most at risk. Almost three-quarters of deaths from electric shock occur in summer and spring, with the ratio of low-to-high-voltage deaths being 7:1. The presence of water is associated with fatality.[1]

Electrical burns represent 3–5% of admissions to burns units.[2]

PHYSICS OF ELECTRICITY AND PATHOPHYSIOLOGY OF ELECTRICAL INJURY

Electrical current passing through the body can cause damage in two ways:

❶ Thermal injury
❷ Physiological change.[3]

The threshold for perception of an electrical current is 1 mA, which results in a tingling sensation. Current greater than 10 mA can induce muscular tetany and prevent the patient letting go of the current source. Above about 50 mA extreme breathing difficulty and pain are experienced. The threshold for ventricular fibrillation is 100 mA.[4,5] (See Fig. 27.6.1) The maximum 'safe' current tolerable for 1 second is 50 mA.[4]

Ohm's Law is fundamental to the understanding of the physics of electricity. This states that:

$$\frac{\text{Resistance}}{\text{(Ohms)}} = \frac{\text{Voltage (Volts)}}{\text{Current (Amperes)}}$$

The amount of current passing through the body is directly proportional to voltage and inversely proportional to resistance. Factors that determine the

effects of an electrical current passing through the body are:

- Type of current
- Voltage
- Tissue resistance
- Current path
- Contact duration.

Type of current

The vast majority of serious electrical injuries result from alternating current, which is approximately three times as dangerous as direct current.[4] Alternating current can produce tetanic contraction of muscle such that the victim may not be able to let go of the current source. This is not a feature of direct current shock.[3]

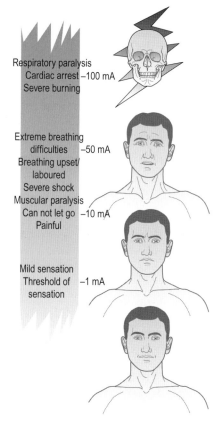

Respiratory paralysis
Cardiac arrest –100 mA
Severe burning

Extreme breathing
difficulties –50 mA
Breathing upset/laboured
Severe shock
Muscular paralysis
Can not let go –10 mA
Painful

Mild sensation
Threshold of –1 mA
sensation

Fig 27.6.1 The levels of electric shock and their effects.

Human muscular tissue is sensitive to frequencies between 40 and 150 Hz. As the frequency increases beyond 150 Hz, the response decreases and the current is less dangerous. In Australia, a frequency of 50 Hz is used for household current because this is optimal for the transmission and use of electricity, and also has advantages in terms of generation.[1] As such, household current lies directly within the dangerous frequency range. It also spans the vulnerable period of the cardiac electrical potential, and is thus capable of causing ventricular fibrillation.

Voltage

Voltage is the electromotive force in the system. In general terms, the greater the voltage the more extensive the injury, but it must be remembered that the amount of current passing through the body will also be determined by resistance (Ohm's Law). High voltage is defined as greater than 1000 V. Household voltage in Australia is 240 V. Voltages less than 50 V (50 Hz) have not been proved hazardous.[4] Survival has been reported following shocks of greater than 50 000 V.[3]

Resistance

Different tissues provide differing resistances to the passage of electrical current. Bone has the highest resistance, followed by, in decreasing order, fat, tendon, skin, muscle, blood vessels and nerves. Importantly, however, skin resistance varies greatly according to moisture, cleanliness, thickness and vascularity.[3] Moist skin may have a resistance of 1000 Ω and dry, thick, calloused skin a resistance of 100 000 Ω. By Ohm's Law, dry skin resistance to a contact with a 240 V potential results in a current of about 2.4 mA, which is just above the threshold for perception. However, the resistance of wet or sweat-soaked skin drops to 1000 Ω, increasing the current flow to 240 mA, which is easily enough to induce ventricular fibrillation. Not surprisingly, moisture has been identified as a key factor in over half of electrocutions.[1]

Current path

Prediction of injuries from a knowledge of the current path is unreliable.

Mortalities of 60% for hand-to-hand (transthoracic) and 20% for head-to-foot passage of current are quoted,[3] but have not been verified. When current passes hand-to-hand (or hand-to-foot), only about 5% of the total current passes through the heart. If current passes leg-to-leg, no current traverses the heart.[6]

Contact duration

The longer the duration of contact, the greater the potential for injury. Fortunately, most contacts are brief and frequently result in the victim being thrown back from the current source. This may result in a secondary injury, especially if the victim falls from a height.

Unfortunately, exposures to more than 10 mA of alternating current can induce sweating. Moisture decreases skin resistance and increases current flow, thereby reducing the ability to release the current source. This can progress to a fatal exposure.[4]

CLINICAL EFFECTS OF ELECTRICITY

Electrical injury resembles a crush injury more than a burn. Invariably the damage below skin level is more severe than the cutaneous wound suggests. The current passing through low-resistance structures produces massive necrosis of muscles, vessels, nerves and subcutaneous tissues.[3]

The clinical manifestations differ from thermal burns in the following ways:

- There are direct effects on the heart and nervous system.
- Electrical injury classically involves deep structures.
- The small entry and exit wounds do not accurately indicate the extent or depth of tissue damage.
- A diversity of clinical manifestations is seen with electrical injury.

Burns

As electricity traverses the skin, energy is converted to heat. The smaller the area of contact, the greater the current density, heat production, and the consequent skin and adjacent tissue destruction.

Electrothermal burns are best characterized by arc burns, which result from the external passage of current from the contact point to the ground. These may be associated with extensive damage to skin and underlying tissue. Secondary flame burns may occur when the current arc ignites clothing or nearby combustibles.[3]

Electrical burns may range from first degree to third degree. The typical appearance is of a central depressed charred black area surrounded by oedema and erythema. Single or multiple exit wounds may be present.

Cardiac

Ventricular fibrillation is the usual cause of immediate death from electric shock, and occurs at the time of the shock.[1] Delayed arrhythmia resulting in death is exceptionally rare. Sinus tachycardia is common, and non-specific ST- and T-wave changes may be observed. Atrial fibrillation occurs infrequently and usually resolves spontaneously. Acute myocardial infarction following electric shock has been reported.[7]

Nervous system

Both acute and delayed neurological sequelae have been described following electric shock. Acute complications include respiratory arrest, seizures, altered mental state, amnesia, coma, expressive dysphasia and motor deficits.[3] Reported delayed complications include spinal cord injury (myelopathy) with local amyotrophy and long tract signs, and reflex sympathetic dystrophy.[3]

Peripheral nerve injury is usually associated with significant soft-tissue injury. It has also been reported in the absence of soft-tissue injury, and such cases appear to have a good prognosis.[8]

Renal

Acute renal failure may occur secondary to myoglobinuria. Electric shock results in disruption of muscle cells with the release of myoglobin and creatine phosphokinase, similar to a crush injury. Transient oliguria, albuminuria, haemoglobinuria and renal casts are common, and there have been reports of high-output renal failure.[3,9]

Vascular

Large and small vessel arterial and venous thrombosis is responsible for the tissue damage in electrical injury. Vascular complications have included immediate and delayed major vessel haemorrhage, arterial thrombosis and deep vein thrombosis.[3,9]

Musculoskeletal

Tetanic muscle contractures can result in compression fractures of vertebral bodies, fractures of long bones, and dislocations of joints. Injuries may also result from a secondary fall, rather than from the electric shock.[3,9]

Other

Numerous complications involving other systems, including the eye (especially cataracts), have been reported following electric shock.[3,9]

ELECTRIC SHOCK IN PREGNANCY

Reports of electric shock in pregnancy are rare and the true incidence is unknown. A high mortality has been reported in the literature.[10] This may represent publication bias. It appears that the foetus is less resistant to electric shock than the mother. The hyperaemic pregnant uterus and amniotic fluid are excellent conductors of electricity. Foetal skin offers 200 times less resistance to the passage of current than does postnatal skin. Exposure of the foetus to 100–380 V, 25 mA for 0.3 s may be regarded as lethal.[11] This is much less than is required to produce significant injury to the mother.

The foetus exposed to an electric shock is at risk of immediate cardiac arrest. The mother may notice a sudden cessation of foetal movements. Other reported foetal complications of electric shock include intrauterine growth retardation, oligohydramnios and abortion.

Fortunately, therapeutic electric shocks such as DC cardioversion and electroconvulsive therapy are known to be safe in pregnancy. The critical factor is current path: accidental electric shocks include the uterus, whereas therapeutic shocks do not.[12–14]

MANAGEMENT

Prehospital

Everyone should be aware of the prehospital management of electric shock.[3] Most importantly, the rescuer should avoid becoming a further victim. The victim can be separated from the electrical source by using rubber, a wooden handle, a mat or any other non-conductive substance or, if possible, by turning off the electricity supply. Cardiopulmonary resuscitation should begin immediately, if indicated, and help summoned. Ventricular fibrillation is the most common lethal arrhythmia after electric shock, and early defibrillation provides the greatest chance for survival.[1]

Emergency department

The majority of patients who present to the emergency department after electric shock are relatively well. Following appropriate assessment to exclude primary or secondary injury, an ECG should be performed. Cardiac monitoring is not indicated if the patient is asymptomatic and has a normal ECG.[5] Most patients are able to be reassured and discharged directly from the emergency department. Measurement of creatine phosphokinase levels is not required. It should be remembered that exposure to an electric shock is a very unpleasant experience and this should be acknowledged. Tetanus status should be checked.

Some patients will have a degree of injury. This may be include a period of aphasia which requires simple observation. Many patients have a degree of muscle pain following electric shock owing to the tetanic nature of alternating current. Simple analgesia is appropriate. Any secondary injury, such as fractures or loss of consciousness, should be treated as dictated by the injury.

If an arrhythmia is present it will usually resolve spontaneously and not require specific treatment. Delayed lethal arrhythmias have not been reported in patients without initial arrhythmias.

Severe electrical injury with extensive soft-tissue damage should be managed as a crush injury. This is more likely following high-voltage exposure, which results in a large exudation and sequestration of fluids in the damaged area. Emergency management includes adequate volume replacement, and treatment of acidosis and myoglobinuria.[3,9]

Emergency physicians should be aware of the potential for fetal harm following electric shock in pregnancy. Apparently minor exposures can have profound effects. Urgent ultrasound and foetal monitoring with obstetric consultation is recommended.

PROGNOSIS

The prognosis for the majority of patients surviving the initial shock is excellent. Those with significant soft-tissue injury or secondary injury may be left with long-term deficits.

DISPOSITION

The majority of patients presenting to the emergency department following an electric shock will be suitable for discharge home following assessment and reassurance as detailed above. Those suffering muscle pain secondary to tetanic contractions should be given simple analgesia and instructed to follow-up with their general practitioner.

Patients with cardiac arrhythmias require admission for observation until the arrhythmia resolves. Those with evidence of neuropathy should be referred to a neurologist, as nerve conduction studies may be required.[8]

Severe electrical injuries with extensive soft-tissue damage require admission to hospital, and sometimes to an intensive care unit. All patients with electrical burns should be reviewed by a burns specialist, and referral to a specialist burns unit may be indicated. Minor burns may be suitable for elective review.

Secondary injuries such as loss of consciousness or fractures should be admitted or referred on their merits.

PREVENTION

All members of the community must be encouraged to treat electricity with respect and to practise electrical safety. Licensed electrical contractors should be used to carry out any electrical repairs or installations. Water and electricity should never be mixed.[15]

Residual current devices are useful in providing an additional level of personal protection from electric shock. These devices continuously compare current flow in both active and neutral conductors of an electrical circuit. If current flow becomes sufficiently unbalanced, then some of the current in the active conductor is not returned through the neutral conductor, and leaks to earth. These devices operate within 10–50 ms and disconnect the electricity supply when they sense harmful leakage, typically 30 mA.[4]

LIGHTNING INJURY

INTRODUCTION AND EPIDEMIOLOGY

There are two or three deaths each year in Australia from lightning. For each death there are five injuries. These events are always prominent and emergency physicians should be familiar with the pathophysiology. In addition, about 80 people each year report injuries caused by lightning surges while using the telephone during thunderstorms.

Many myths surround lightning injury; they include:

- Lightning strike is invariably fatal. In fact, the mortality is 30%. In addition, the probability of long-term impairment after recovery is low.
- A victim of lightning is charged and dangerous to touch. This false notion has led to the withholding of CPR, with fatal results.
- Lightning should be treated in the same way as high-voltage electrical injury. This is incorrect.[16]

PHYSICS OF LIGHTNING

Lightning occurs most commonly during thunderstorms. Particles moving up and down in a thunderstorm create static electricity, with a large negative charge building up at the bottom of clouds. Electrical discharge (lightning) occurs as a result of the great charge difference between the negatively charged thundercloud underside and the positively charged ground.[3] The duration of the lightning stroke is between 1 and 100 ms.

Lightning strike is very different from high-voltage electric shock (Table 27.6.1)[16] and produces different clinical effects, requiring a different management approach.

An interesting phenomenon called 'flashover' seems to save many victims from death by lightning. Current passes around and over, but not through the body. The victim's clothing and shoes may be blasted apart. Only cutaneous flame-type burns result.[3]

CLINICAL EFFECTS OF LIGHTNING INJURY

Immediate

- Cardiac arrest. This takes the form of asystole, as opposed to the ventricular fibrillation of high-voltage electrical injury.[16] The heart is thought to undergo massive depolarization. Although primary lightning-induced arrest may revert quickly, it can be followed by secondary hypoxic arrest.
- Chest pain and muscle aches.
- Neurological deficits. A person struck by lightning may be rendered unconscious. On first regaining consciousness they may be mute and unable to move. This is transient and usually resolves within minutes, but may take up to 24 hours.
- Contusions from shock waves.
- Tympanic membrane rupture.

Delayed

- Keraunoparalysis. Lightning-induced limb paralysis is extremely common. Flaccidity and complete loss of sensation of the affected limb are observed. Peripheral pulses are generally impalpable and the affected limb takes on a mottled, pale, blue appearance. The mechanism is unclear, but may be lightning-induced vasospasm. The condition is self-limiting and resolves within 1–6 hours.
- 'Feathery' cutaneous burns (Lichtenberg flowers). These burns, pathognomonic of lightning injury, may appear immediately but more often become visible a few hours after injury. Burns may be severe but heal remarkably easily.
- Cataracts. Occur more commonly than following electrical injuries.
- Myoglobinuria and haemoglobinuria are rare.

Other

- Sensorineural deafness
- Vestibular dysfunction

Table 27.6.1 Lightning versus high-voltage injury (*Adapted from:* Cooper MA 1983 Lightning injuries. In: Auerbach P, et al (eds) Management of wilderness and environmental emergencies. Macmillan, New York, pp 500–21)

Factor	Lightning	High voltage
Time of exposure	Brief instantaneous	Prolonged tetanic
Energy level	100 million V 200 000 Amp	Usually much lower
Type of current	Direct	Alternating
Shock wave	Yes	No
Flashover	Yes	No

- Retinal detachment
- Optic nerve damage.

Reports of lightning strike in pregnancy reveal a high rate of fetal death in utero, despite maternal survival.[10]

MANAGEMENT

Prehospital

The important principle is that those who appear dead should be resuscitated first. Immediate institution of basic cardiopulmonary resuscitation in the field for those in asystole prevents secondary hypoxic cardiac arrest during the interval until cardiac function resumes spontaneously. Fixed dilated pupils should not be taken as an indicator of death after lightning strike.

Emergency department

Most lightning strikes are unwitnessed, and diagnosis may be difficult in the unconscious or confused patient. The diagnosis should be considered where such patients were found outdoors in stormy weather. The presence of multiple victims, exploded clothing, linear or punctate burns, keraunic markings or tympanic membrane rupture all add weight to the diagnosis. The differential diagnosis includes cerebrovascular event, seizure disorder, spinal cord injury, closed-head injury, Stokes-Adams attack, myocardial infarction and toxin effects.[16]

Standard trauma resuscitation measures should be adopted. Examination of the ears for tympanic rupture and eyes for lens/corneal defects, retinal detachment and optic nerve injury is especially important. If the conscious state deteriorates after arrival, cranial CT scan is indicated. Examination of the cardiovascular system should include an ECG.

Burns are rarely more than superficial and are managed expectantly using standard treatments. Tetanus prophylaxis should be arranged.[16]

Treatment of lightning-induced limb paralysis is expectant. If it does not resolve within a few hours, other causes should be considered.[16] Fasciotomy is unnecessary.

Standard therapy for ocular complications such as retinal detachment or cataracts is indicated. Baseline visual acuity should be documented for future reference.

PROGNOSIS AND DISPOSITION

For survivors of the initial strike the prognosis is excellent, unless significant secondary trauma has occurred. Admission for observation is indicated for those with abnormal mental status or ECG, or with significant burns or traumatic complications. The burns usually heal well and grafting is rarely required.[16] For those with ocular complications, long-term ophthalmic follow-up is necessary.[16]

CONTROVERSIES

❶ Timing and extent of development of tissue necrosis associated with electrical injury.

REFERENCES

1. Fatovich DM 1992 Electrocution in Western Australia, 1976–1990. Medical Journal of Australia 157: 762–4
2. Walpole BG 1989 Electric shock. Australian Family Physician 18: 1252–6
3. Kobernick M 1982 Electrical injuries: pathophysiology and emergency management. Annals of Emergency Medicine 11: 633–8
4. Residual Current Devices. North Sydney, Standards Association of Australia 1991 (SEM 36–91)
5. Fatovich DM, Lee KY 1991 Household electric shocks: who should be monitored? Medical Journal of Australia 155: 301–3
6. Bruner JMR, Leonard PF 1989 Electricity, Safety and the Patient. Yearbook Medical Publishers, Chicago
7. Kinney TJ 1982 Myocardial infarction following electrical injury. Annals of Emergency Medicine 11: 622–5
8. Fatovich DM 1992 Neuropathy from household electric shock. Emergency Medicine 4: 63–5
9. Dixon GF 1983 The evaluation and management of electrical injuries. Critical Care Medicine 384–7
10. Fatovich DM 1993 Electric shock in pregnancy. Journal of Emergency Medicine 11: 175–7
11. Dordelmann P 1957 Intrauterin frucht tod. Zentralblatt für Gynaekologie 79: 1647
12. Abrams R 1988 Electroconvulsive Therapy. Oxford University Press, Oxford, pp 77–8
13. Schroeder JS, Harrison DC 1971 Repeated cardioversion during pregnancy. American Journal of Cardiology 27: 445–6
14. Finaly AY, Edmunds V 1979 DC cardioversion in pregnancy. British Journal of Clinical Practice 33: 88–94
15. Fatovich DM 1991 Household electric shocks (letter). Medical Journal of Australia 155: 852–3
16. Andrews CJ, Darveniza M, Mackerras D 1989 Lightning injury – a review of clinical aspects, pathophysiology, and treatment. Advances in Trauma 4: 241–88

27.7 ANAPHYLAXIS

ANTHONY F T BROWN

ESSENTIALS

1 The term anaphylaxis may be used to describe both IgE, immune-mediated reactions and non-immunologically triggered events, which present and are treated identically but have important aetiologic differences that will require elucidation in follow-up.

2 Parenteral penicillin, hymenopteran stings and food are the commonest causes of anaphylactic fatalities, with radiocontrast media, aspirin and other non-steroidal anti-inflammatory drugs most commonly responsible for anaphylactoid fatalities.

3 All patients with any features of acute anaphylaxis should initially be assessed in a monitored resuscitation area, as sudden deterioration may occur at any time. Never underestimate this potential for deterioration.

4 Oxygen, adrenaline (epinephrine) and fluids are the first-line treatment.

5 H$_1$ and H$_2$ antihistamines, steroids, glucagon and aminophylline are considered second-line therapies.

6 A careful discharge plan, including oral H$_1$ and H$_2$ antihistamines, oral steroids and a referral to an allergist for all significant or recurrent attacks, or when the stimulus is unknown or unavoidable, protects against further, often unheralded, attacks of anaphylaxis.

INTRODUCTION

Anaphylaxis is potentially the most severe of the immediate hypersensitivity reactions. It may be mild or severe, gradual in onset or fulminant, involve multiple organ systems, or cause isolated wheeze or shock. There is no immediate laboratory test to confirm the diagnosis, making the clinical recognition and prompt treatment a challenge.

DEFINITION

The term anaphylaxis was introduced by Richet and Portier in 1902, literally meaning 'against protection'. It is currently used to describe the rapid, generalized and often unheralded immunologically mediated events that follow exposure to certain foreign substances in previously sensitized persons. Anaphylactoid reactions are a clinically indistin-guishable syndrome involving similar mediators, but not triggered by IgE and thus not necessarily requiring previous exposure.[1] This chapter will use the clinical term 'anaphylaxis' to describe both of these syndromes, despite their important aetiological differences.

INCIDENCE AND EPIDEMIOLOGY

The true incidence of anaphylaxis is unknown. Figures vary internationally and are underestimated. Between 15 and 40 per 100 000 patients treated with penicillin will experience a significant reaction,[2] 0.3–0.5% of the population have allergic reactions to insect stings, and 1.5% of adults exhibit some form of food allergy.

Emergency department presentations with anaphylaxis range from 1 in 440 to 1 in 1500 attendances, that represents an incidence from 1 per 3400 to 1 per 10 000 catchment population per year.[3] Atopic patients are at increased risk from anaphylaxis due to ingested antigens, latex, radiocontrast media, exercise and idiopathic. Asthmatic patients are at overall greater risk of fatality, and patients taking β-blocker drugs develop generally more severe reactions that may prove resistant to treatment. Those taking angiotensin-converting enzyme inhibitor (ACEI) drugs are prone to potentially life-threatening angioedema, although the newer angiotensin-II receptor antagonists cause considerably fewer reactions.

Case fatality rates to anaphylactic reactions vary and may reach up to 3–9%, depending on the interval between exposures, route of administration and the amount of agent received. Parenteral penicillin, hymenopteran stings and food are the commonest causes of anaphylactic fatalities, whereas radiocontrast media and aspirin or other non-steroidal anti-inflammatory drugs are the most common causes of anaphylactoid fatalities.

PATHOPHYSIOLOGY

Triggering events

Most cases of anaphylaxis are IgE – or occasionally IgG$_4$ – mediated. Reaginic antibodies are released into the circulation by plasma cells derived from B lymphocytes, under the influence of helper T cells following previous exposure to an antigen. These antibodies bind to glycoprotein receptors on bloodborne basophils or tissue mast cells, sensitizing them. Re-exposure to the antigen cross-links the Fab portions of two surface-bound IgE molecules, activating the cell to release chemical mediators.

A huge variety of substances induce IgE antibody formation, ranging from drugs, including antibiotics and steroids, vaccines, foods such as peanuts, true nuts, shellfish and eggs, venoms from wasps, bees, fire ants and snakes, to chemicals, enzymes and latex (Table 27.7.1).

Anaphylactoid reactions are caused by mediator-release triggered independently of reaginic antibodies, leading to complement activation, the direct pharmacological release of mediators, or coagulation/fibrinolysis system activation (Table 27.7.2).

Cellular events

Irrespective of the triggering event, two main groups of mediators are released by mast cells and basophils. Preformed, granule-associated mediators include histamine, neutrophil and eosinophil chemotactic factors, enzymes such as tryptase and β-glucuronidase, and proteoglycans such as heparin and chondroitin sulphate.[4] Newly synthesized mediators include arachidonic acid metabolites of the cyclo-oxygenase pathway, such as prostaglandin D_2 and thromboxane A_2, or from the lipoxygenase pathway such as the leukotrienes LTB_4 (mast cells only) and LTC_4, LTD_4 and LTE_4, formerly called slow-reacting substance of anaphylaxis. In addition, platelet-activating factor (PAF) and cytokines such as the interleukins and TNF-α are also rapidly formed.

At the cellular level mediator release is modulated by the steady-state resting intracellular cyclic AMP (cAMP) levels. Substances that elevate cAMP, such as adrenaline (epinephrine), inhibit mediator release, partly explaining its essential role in treatment. Also, from knowledge of the complex array of mediators involved it is self-evident why antihistamines do not form the first line of therapy.

Mediator pharmacology

Primary mast cell and basophil mediators may be considered in three groups: those that induce vasodilatation and oedema, such as histamine, PAF, tryptase and bradykinin; those causing bronchoconstriction, mucosal oedema and mucus production, such as histamine, prostaglandin D_2, LTC_4 and LTD_4; and those that attract new cells to the area, such as neutrophil chemotactic factor, eosinophil chemotactic factor and LTB_4.

Neutrophils, eosinophils, lymphocytes, monocytes, platelets, mast cells and basophils are thus recruited to the area, releasing further mediators, leading to a vicious cycle of inflammation and increased vascular permeability.[4]

Table 27.7.1 Causes of IgE antibody formation

Drugs	Protein (hormones): insulin, ACTH, vasopressin Non-protein (haptens): penicillin, sulphonamides, muscle relaxants, thiamine, folic acid
Foods	Peanuts, true nuts, milk, eggs, chocolate, shellfish, fruits
Venoms	Wasp, bee, hornet, yellow jacket, fire ants, snakes, ticks
Vaccine and foreign protein agents	Influenza, yellow fever, tetanus toxoid, γ-globulin, protamine, venom antitoxin, semen
Enzymes and chemicals	Trypsin, chymopapain, streptokinase, penicillinase, formaldehyde, ethylene oxide gas
Allergen extracts and parasites	Pollen, mould, animal dander, hydatid cyst rupture
Latex	Surgical gloves, catheter tip

Note: Cross-reactivity may occur such as to egg protein in avian-based vaccines, or to certain foods with latex allergy.

Table 27.7.2 Causes of anaphylactoid reactions

Complement activation – classical pathway or alternate pathway	Blood transfusion including IgG anti-IgA immune complex formation, albumin, radiocontrast media, dialysis membranes, protamine, hereditary and acquired angioedema
Kinin production or potentiation; coagulation/fibrinolysis system activation	ACE inhibitors, radiocontrast media, plasma protein fraction
Direct pharmacological release of mediators	Histamine release: opiates, curare, radiocontrast media, Haemaccel®, N-acetylcysteine, muscle relaxants, fluorescein, mannitol, vancomycin, protamine Modulators of arachidonic acid metabolism: aspirin, NSAIDs
Sulphiting agents	Metabisulphite
Exercise induced ± foods or NSAIDs	
Idiopathic	

Note: More than one mechanism may exist
ACE, angiotensin-converting enzyme; NSAID, nonsteroidal anti-inflammatory drug

CLINICAL FEATURES

Anaphylaxis is characteristically a disease of fit patients, and is rarely seen or described in critically ill or shocked patients other than asthmatics.[2] The speed of onset of symptoms is related to the severity of the reaction. Parenteral antigen exposure may cause life-threatening anaphylaxis within minutes, although symptoms can be delayed for some hours, particularly with oral or topical exposure. However, most symptoms occur within 30 minutes.

Ninety five per cent of patients have cutaneous features that may assist the prompt, early diagnosis of anaphylaxis.[3] However, these alerting features can be absent due to prehospital treatment, their spontaneous resolution, or in cases presenting with the rapid onset of laryngeal oedema or circulatory shock alone.

Fatalities are principally caused by asphyxia from upper airway oedema and hypoxia from severe bronchospasm. One-quarter of deaths result from circulatory failure with shock related to hypovolaemia from plasma volume loss, arrhythmias, decreased myocardial contractility and pulmonary hypertension.[5]

Cutaneous reactions

A premonitory aura or a tingling and warmth sensation may precede generalized erythema, urticaria with pruritus, and angio-oedema. Erythematous wheals may spread rapidly, and rhinitis and conjunctivitis are also seen (Table 27.7.3).

Angioedema involves non-pruritic swelling of deeper tissues such as the face, neck and upper airway, leading to dyspnoea, odynophagia, and hoarseness or stridor if laryngeal oedema occurs.

Respiratory manifestations

Throat tightness and cough may precede mild-to-severe respiratory distress, due to oropharyngeal or laryngeal oedema and bronchospasm. Generalized wheeze may be the sole manifestation of anaphylaxis, or be accompanied by cardiovascular collapse and rash.

Cardiovascular reactions

Apprehension, light-headedness or syncope may precede or accompany cardiovascular collapse, with tachycardia, hypotension and cardiac arrhythmias, which can include apparently benign supraventricular rhythms but with an impalpable pulse. Transient or resistant hypotension exacerbated by hypoxia may cause myocardial infarction, cerebral ischaemia, incontinence, confusion and coma.

Gastrointestinal manifestations

Cramps, nausea, vomiting and diarrhoea are common, but usually overshadowed by the more immediately life-threatening manifestations.

Miscellaneous

Many other features have been described in anaphylaxis, including lacrimation, headache, generalized oedema, pulmonary odema, watery vaginal discharge and disseminated intravascular coagulation.[6]

DIFFERENTIAL DIAGNOSIS

Any of the preceding clinical features described may occur either in combination or alone. Thus the diagnosis may be obvious when generalized erythema, wheeze and hypotension follow parenteral drug exposure or a bee sting, or may be extremely difficult when isolated hypotension occurs.

Facial swelling or oedema may result from bacterial or viral infection, although fever and pain predominate, unlike in anaphylaxis.

Bronchial asthma, pulmonary oedema, chemical irritant exposure, foreign body airway obstruction and tension pneumothorax may all cause wheeze or difficulty in breathing.

Angioedema may be due to actual or functional C_1 esterase inhibitor deficiency, which can be hereditary with autosomal dominant characteristics or acquired associated with lymphoproliferative disorders, or be mimicked by venous or lymphatic obstruction.

Vasovagal reactions may be mistaken for anaphylaxis, but typically cause bradycardia, hyperventilation and a rapid response to a recumbent posture.

LABORATORY TESTING

There is no specific diagnostic or laboratory test immediately available for anaphylaxis. A blood glucose, full blood count, electrolyte and liver function test, arterial blood gas, chest X-ray and ECG may be indicated if there is a slow response to treatment or when there is doubt about the diagnosis.

A mast cell tryptase assay is available in specialized centres and is a highly sensitive indicator of anaphylaxis, becoming elevated from 1 to 6 hours following a reaction. It may be useful in complex presentations and has diagnosed anaphylaxis post mortem. If raised, it favours an IgE-mediated cause but does not distinguish between anaphylactic and anaphylactoid reactions.[7]

MANAGEMENT

A brief history of possible allergen exposure is obtained, causative drugs or fluids administered are ceased immediately, a rapid assessment of the extent and clinical severity is made and monitoring of vital signs and the ECG is commenced in a resuscitation area, even in apparently minor cases, as symptoms and signs may progress rapidly. A careful watch is kept for signs of laryngeal oedema, bronchospasm and circulatory collapse. Endotracheal intubation and mechanical ventilation may be needed, and rarely a surgical airway is necessary in the presence of severe upper airway swelling.

Shocked patients should be placed flat while rapid intravenous access is gained. Oxygen, adrenaline (epinephrine) and fluids are the mainstay of treatment,

Table 27.7.3	Clinical manifestations of anaphylaxis
Cutaneous	Erythema, urticaria, pruritus, angio-oedema, rhinitis, conjunctivitis
Respiratory	Tight throat, cough, hoarseness, stridor, wheeze
Cardiovascular	Dizziness, syncope, tachycardia, hypotension, arrhythymias, myocardial ischaemia, confusion, coma
Gastrointestinal	Cramps, nausea, vomiting, diarrhoea
Miscellaneous	Lacrimation, headache, generalized oedema, pulmonary oedema, vaginal discharge, DIC
DIC: disseminated intravascular coagulation	

whereas antihistamines, steroids, glucagon and aminophylline are second-line drugs.[8]

First-line treatment

Oxygen

Oxygen by face mask is given to all patients, aiming to keep the oxygen saturation above 92%. It may be discontinued if urticaria is the sole symptom.

Adrenaline (epinephrine)

Adrenaline (epinephrine) is the drug of choice and should be used in all but the most trivial cases, certainly in all patients with hypotension, airway swelling or bronchospasm.[9] It acts via α-adrenergic stimulation to increase peripheral vascular resistance, improving the blood pressure and coronary artery perfusion, reversing peripheral vasodilatation and decreasing angio-oedema and urticaria. β_1-adrenergic stimulation has positive inotropic and chronotropic effects, and β_2-adrenergic effects include bronchodilatation. In addition, β-adrenergic receptors cause a rise in intracellular cAMP, which inhibits further mast cell and basophil mediator release.

The dose, route and dilution of adrenaline (epinephrine) cause unnecessary confusion. When anaphylaxis is treated early, is mild or progressing slowly, if venous access is difficult or delayed, or if the patient is unmonitored, 0.3–0.5 mL of 1:1000 adrenaline (epinephrine) (0.3–0.5 mg) should be given intramuscular in adults (Table 27.7.4) and may be repeated every 5–10 minutes or longer, according to the response.[9]

However, in life-threatening or rapidly progressing cases, particularly in the presence of vascular collapse and shock, severe dyspnoea or airway compromise, intravenous adrenaline (epinephrine) is essential to achieve more rapid and reliable delivery. Adrenaline (epinephrine) 1:100 000 given at 1–2 mL (10–20 µg) per minute at an initial dose of 0.75–1.5 µg/kg combines immediate efficacy with a greater degree of safety,[8] but must only be given under ECG monitoring in a resuscitation area. Alternatively, an infusion may be prepared by putting 1 mg adrenaline (epinephrine) in 100 mL normal saline and running at 60–120 ml/h via an infusion device, again delivering 10–20 µg/min. The infusion rate may be altered or stopped according to the clinical response, although patients with persistent symptoms (protracted anaphylaxis) require a maintenance infusion of 1–5 µg/min and admission to a monitored intensive care area.

Whilst parenteral adrenaline (epinephrine) is being prepared, adenaline (epinephrine) may be given via an oxygen-driven nebulizer for acute upper airway oedema or bronchospasm at a dose of 1 to 4 mL (1 to 4 mg) of 1:1000 adrenaline (epinephrine).

Fluids

Crystalloid or colloid infusions are essential in anaphylactic shock to replace plasma losses of up to 50% of the circulatory volume. Gelatin preparations such as Haemaccel®, Gelofusine® or albumin given rapidly at 10–20 mL/kg are preferable to normal saline, although large quantities of fluid may be needed, guided by the packed cell volume and central venous pressure measurements.[8]

Second-line treatment

Once tissue oxygenation and the circulatory status have been restored with the use of oxygen, adrenaline (epinephrine) and fluids, other drugs, such as antihistamines, steroids, glucagon and aminophylline, play a supporting role (Table 27.7.5).

Antihistamines

Antihistamines are of greatest value when the allergic condition is not life-threatening and is progressing slowly, such as in angio-oedema and urticaria; to prevent the recrudescence of symptoms or signs; and as pretreatment for instance to prevent reactions to radiocontrast media.[10] New, second generation, non-sedating H_1 antihistamines such as loratadine and cetirizine are now available orally, but may still cause a degree of drowsiness.

H_2 antihistamines have been successful in protracted anaphylactic shock, and are now routinely used in combination with H_1 antihistamines. The H_1 and H_2 antihistamines given together improve outcome in both the prevention and the treatment of acute anaphylaxis, combined with steroids in certain circumstances.[11] Both may initially be given intravenously and changed to orally as soon as possible.

Steroids

Despite many theoretical beneficial effects, the role of steroids is limited to the prevention or shortening of protracted reactions, particularly bronchospasm. They are also used in discharge medication to reduce the likelihood of relapse of symptoms.

Hydrocortisone 5 mg/kg to a maximum of 200 mg, followed by 2.5 mg/kg 6-hourly intravenously is recommended

Table 27.7.4 First-line therapy for anaphylaxis	
Oxygen **Adrenaline** **(epinephrine)**	**Early, mild or progressing slowly, difficult venous access or unmonitored patient:** 0.3–0.5 mg (0.3–0.5 mL) 1:1000 adrenaline (epinephrine) IM repeated every 5–10 minutes according to response.
	Shock, severe dyspnoea, airway compromise or deteriorating patient. *Must* be monitored: 0.75–1.5 µg/kg 1:100 000 adrenaline (epinephrine) IV* at 10–20 µg/min (1–2 mL/min) initially, repeated as necessary.
	Stridor or severe wheeze, whilst preparing IV dose: 1–4 mg (1–4 mL) of 1:1000 adrenaline (epinephrine) nebulized with oxygen.
Colloid	10–20 mL/kg for shock

* Prepare 1:100 000 adrenaline (epinephrine) by drawing up 1 mg adrenaline (epinephrine) (1 mL of 1:1000) in a 20 mL syringe, plus 9 mL saline to give a total volume of 10 mL. Discard all but 2 mL (leaving 200 µg of adrenaline (epinephrine) in the syringe), and draw up saline again to a total volume of 20 mL, giving a final concentration of 10 µg/mL.

ENVIRONMENTAL

Table 27.7.5 Second-line therapy for anaphylaxis (after restoring cardiorespiratory stability first with oxygen, adrenaline (epinephrine) and fluids)	
Antihistamines	H_1 receptor blocker diphenhydramine 25–50 mg IV or promethazine 12.5–25 mg IV *plus* H_2 receptor blocker ranitidine 50 mg IV. Repeat 8-hourly. Change to orally when patient tolerates: diphenhydramine 25 mg orally 8-hourly or promethazine 10 mg orally 8-hourly, plus ranitidine 150 mg orally 12-hourly
Steroids (definitely for severe bronchospasm)	Hydrocortisone 5 mg/kg IV to maximum 200 mg, then 2.5 mg/kg IV 6-hourly or methylprednisolone 125 mg IV 6-hourly. Change to orally when patient tolerates: prednisone 40–50 mg orally per day
Glucagon (if patient on β-blockers)	1 mg IV every 5 minutes, then infusion at 5–15 µg/min
Aminophylline (refractory bronchospasm)	5 mg/kg IV over 30 minutes loading dose, then infusion at 0.5 mg/kg/h

Table 27.7.6 Discharge policy
Outpatient drug therapy for 3 days: Diphenhydramine 25 mg orally 8-hourly, or promethazine 10 mg orally 8-hourly *plus* ranitidine 150 mg orally 12-hourly. Prednisone 40–50 mg orally daily
Detailed discharge letter documenting reaction
Referral to allergist: All significant or recurrent attacks, or stimulus unavoidable or unknown

followed by oral prednisone as soon as the patient tolerates this. Side effects, including sodium and potassium ion flux changes and anaphylaxis itself, are more likely with intravenous steroid use.[8]

Glucagon

Glucagon has a particular role in patients taking β-blocking drugs, who appear to be at increased risk of anaphylaxis and have worse reactions that are then difficult to treat.[12] A dose of 1 mg IV repeated every 5 minutes, followed by an infusion at 5–15 µg/min, raises intracellular cAMP by a calcium-dependent non-adrenergic mechanism.

Aminophylline and other bronchodilators

Aminophylline may be used for severe bronchospasm resistant to adrenaline (epinephrine) and steroids, at a dose of 5 mg/kg IV over 30 minutes with ECG monitoring. It causes bronchodilatation, respiratory muscle stimulation, pulmonary vasodilatation and a rise in cAMP by inhibition of phosphodiesterase.

Nebulized salbutamol 5 mg (or nebulized 1:1000 adrenaline (epinephrine) 1–4 mg) may be used for predominant bronchospasm, particularly on arrival of a patient prior to venous access.

DISPOSITION

Patients with significant anaphylactic reactions, including all those who received adrenaline (epinephrine), should be admitted to a monitored observation area. If they remain unstable this should be to an intensive care area. All other patients who are stable and appear to have fully recovered must still be observed for a further 6–8 hours, as late deterioration may occur in around 1–5% (biphasic anaphylaxis).[13]

DISCHARGE POLICY

Drug treatment should be continued for 3 days after hospital discharge with combined oral H_1 and H_2 antihistamines and oral prednisone (Table 27.7.6). All patients are instructed to return immediately if symptoms recur. Patients on β-blockers and those on angiotensin-converting enzyme inhibitors (ACEI) or non-steroidal, anti-inflammatory drugs (NSAIDs) causally implicated in the anaphylactic reaction should have their medication urgently reassessed and changed by their regular physician.

Patients prescribed a self-treatment adrenaline regimen for home use, such as an EpiPen®, must be carefully instructed in its use, as must immediate family members.

Most patients should be referred for allergy testing, particularly if the attack of anaphylaxis was significant, recurrent, or the stimulus unavoidable or unknown.[8] Also refer any patients prescribed an EpiPen® and those who may be suitable

CONTROVERSIES

❶ Low-dose high-dilution 1:100 000 intravenous adrenaline (epinephrine) should be used in all moderate to severe cases, to avoid the inadvertently rapid or excessive delivery that has given IV adrenaline (epinephrine) its unwarranted bad reputation. Adrenaline (epinephrine) is safe and effective when used sensibly.

❷ All patients receiving adrenaline (epinephrine) need only be observed for 6–8 hours after an apparently full recovery, to avoid missing the late deterioration in 1–5% (biphasic anaphylaxis). Overnight admission is unnecessary.

❸ The mast cell tryptase assay available in specialized centres is the only useful laboratory marker, but will not distinguish between anaphylactic and anaphylactoid reactions. Anaphylaxis thus remains the quintessential medical emergency relying entirely on prompt clinical recognition and treatment.

for immunotheray following a wasp or bee sting. Expert knowledge is required to decide which cutaneous tests and radioimmunoassays for specific IgE are indicated. A detailed referral letter of the events leading up to the reaction is vital.[14]

CONCLUSION

Anaphylaxis is a common clinical and diagnostic challenge for emergency physicians. Prompt recognition and treatment with oxygen, adrenaline (epinephrine) and fluids to restore cardiorespiratory stability is followed by traditional second-line treatment, such as antihistamines and steroids. Proactive discharge planning, including allergy referral where appropriate, protects against further, often unheralded, attacks of anaphylaxis.

REFERENCES

1. Bochner BS, Lichtenstein LM 1991 Anaphylaxis. New England Journal of Medicine 324: 1785–90

2. Fisher MM 1987 Anaphylaxis. Disease a Month 33: 441–79
3. Brown AFT, McKinnon D, Chu K 2001 Emergency department anaphylaxis: A review of 142 patients in a single year. Journal of Allergy and Clinical Immunology 108: 861–6
4. Brown AFT 1995 Anaphylactic shock: mechanisms and treatment. Journal of Accident and Emergency Medicine 12: 89–100
5. Perkin RM, Anas NG 1985 Mechanisms and management of anaphylactic shock not responding to traditional therapy. Annals of Allergy 54: 202–8
6. Hollingsworth HM, Giansiracusa DF, Upchurch KS 1991 Anaphylaxis. Journal of Intensive Care Medicine 6: 55–70
7. Fisher MM, Baldo BA 1998 Mast cell tryptase in anaesthetic anaphylactoid reactions. British Journal of Anaesthesia 80: 26–9
8. Brown AFT 1998 Therapeutic controversies in the management of acute anaphylaxis. Journal of Accident and Emergency Medicine 15: 89–95

9. Fisher MM 1992 Treating anaphylaxis with sympathomimetic drugs. British Medical Journal 305: 1107–8
10. Lieberman PL 1998 Anaphylaxis and anaphylactoid reactions. In: Middleton E, Ellis EF, Yunginger J, et al (eds) Allergy: Principles and Practice, 5th edn. Mosby Year Book Inc, St Louis, pp 1079–92
11. Winbery SL, Lieberman PL 1996 Anaphylaxis and histamine antagonists. In: Estelle F, Simons R (eds) Histamine and H1 Receptor Antagonists in Allergic Disease. Clinical Allergy and Immunology, Marcel Decker Inc. Vol 7: 297–327
12. Toogood JH 1988 Risk of anaphylaxis in patients receiving beta blocker drugs. Journal of Allergy and Clinical Immunology 1: 1–5
13. Douglas DM, Sukenick E, Andrade P, Brown JS 1994 Biphasic systemic anaphylaxis: an inpatient and outpatient study. Journal of Allergy and Clinical Immunology 93: 977–85
14. Fisher M 1995 Treatment of acute anaphylaxis. British Medical Journal 311: 731–3

27.8 ALTITUDE ILLNESS

IAN ROGERS • DEBRA O'BRIEN

ESSENTIALS

1 The high-altitude syndromes – acute mountain sickness (AMS), high-altitude cerebral oedema (HACE) and high-altitude pulmonary oedema (HAPE) – are all clinical diagnoses, where management may need to be undertaken without access to diagnostic testing.

2 AMS and HACE represent stages along a continuum owing to cerebral vasodilatation and cerebral oedema.

3 Early recognition and descent are the keys to successful management.

4 Pharmacological agents are available to assist in the prevention and management of altitude syndromes, but are generally considered to be second line to physical therapy.

5 Prevention is best achieved by controlled ascent, with adequate time for acclimatization.

INTRODUCTION

Altitude illness comprises a number of syndromes that can occur on exposure to the hypobaric hypoxic environment of high altitude. At any altitude the partial pressure of inspired oxygen is equal to 0.21 times the barometric pressure minus water vapour pressure of 47 mmHg. At an altitude of 5500 m, barometric pressure is halved. On the summit of mount everest (8848 m), the P_iO_2 is only 43 mmHg, and a typical climber without oxygen can be expected to have a P_aO_2 of <30 mmHg and a P_aCO_2 of about 10 mmHg. In addition to the hypoxic stress of altitude, a subject may also be exposed to cold, low humidity, fatigue, poor diet and increased UV radiation. For the emergency physician the unique feature of altitude illness is that it requires recognition and treatment in the field, frequently without access to sophisticated diagnostic and imaging techniques, and often without access to rapid evacuation.

EPIDEMIOLOGY AND PATHOPHYSIOLOGY

The human body has the capacity to acclimatize to hypoxic environments. This is principally achieved by increasing ventilation (the hypoxic ventilatory response effected by the carotid body), increasing numbers of red blood cells (via stimulation of erythropoietin), increasing the diffusing capacity of the lungs (resulting from increased lung volume and pulmonary capillary blood volume), increasing vascularity of the tissues, and increasing the tissues' ability to use oxygen (possibly owing to increased numbers of mitochondria and oxidative enzyme systems).[1,2]

In some individuals exposure to low Po_2 initiates a sequence of pathophysiological changes, which result in oedema formation in the brain and lungs. The altitude illness syndromes, acute mountain sickness (AMS), high-altitude cerebral oedema (HACE) and high-altitude pulmonary oedema (HAPE), are the result of this oedema formation. The exact mechanism of these pathophysiologic changes is not known.

The traditional view is that arterial hypoxaemia initiates an increase in capillary permeability, and possibly also failure of the sodium-potassium pump.[2] More recent work has revealed that inappropriate ADH and aldosterone secretion may also have a role, and that eicosanoids, kinins and other inflammatory mediators contribute to increased vascular permeability.[3]

In the brain, the development of oedema causes intracranial pressure (ICP) to rise. Initially, this is partially compensated for by displacement of cerebrospinal fluid (CSF) into the spinal space, and adjustment of the balance between production and absorption of CSF. However, once these compensatory mechanisms are overwhelmed, ICP can rise beyond the cerebral perfusion pressure. Without intervention, cerebral blood flow ceases and the patient dies.

In the lung, non-cardiogenic pulmonary oedema develops. A significant rise in pulmonary artery pressure appears to be a crucial pathophysiologic factor.[4] Recent work suggests that impaired sodium driven clearance of alveolar fluid may contribute to HAPE.[5] Patients with a history of HAPE have an exaggerated pressor response to hypoxia, with increased secretion of noradrenaline (norepinephrine), adrenaline (epinephrine), renin, angiotensin, aldosterone and atrial natriuretic peptide.[2] It has been postulated that uneven pulmonary vasoconstriction increases the filtration pressure in non-vasoconstricted lung areas, worsening the interstitial and alveolar oedema.

The tendency to develop altitude illness is idiosyncratic. The major predisposing factors are the rate of ascent and the altitude reached. It is not related to physical fitness or gender. Individuals vary in their ability to compensate for changes in ICP, and in their pressor responses to hypoxia. This may explain the reproducibility of AMS, HACE and HAPE in susceptible individuals, and why some, and not others, develop symptoms at the same altitude. The risk is higher in those who have an impaired ventilatory response to hypoxia in normobaric conditions, and with dehydration, vigorous exercise and the use of depressant drugs.

CLINICAL SYNDROMES

AMS is common, occurring in about 30% of subjects exposed to moderate altitude (3500 m). HACE and HAPE are much less common, but a recent study in pilgrims at 4300 m reported AMS in 68%, HACE in 31% and HAPE in 5% of subjects.[6] The diagnosis is usually made on clinical assessment and setting.

Acute mountain sickness

AMS is primarily a neurological syndrome, associated with some degree of respiratory compromise. The onset is usually 6–24 hours after arrival at high altitude. The majority of patients present in the early stages when the symptoms are like those of a hangover, and include headache, nausea, anorexia, weakness and lassitude. At this stage there are no abnormalities on physical examination, and the oxygen saturation, if measured, should be no lower than that expected for a given altitude. Mild AMS is usually benign and self-limiting.

If the illness progresses, the more severe form of AMS is characterized by dyspnoea at rest, nausea and vomiting, altered mental state, headache and ataxia. Ataxia is the most useful sign of progression to serious illness. Retinal haemorrhages and venous dilatation may be seen on fundoscopy. Left untreated, severe AMS may progress to life-threatening HACE or HAPE.

High-altitude cerebral oedema

HACE is the progression of neurological signs and symptoms in the setting of AMS. There is a progressive decline in mental status and truncal ataxia is a prominent physical finding. Focal neurological signs, such as third and sixth cranial nerve palsies, may develop as a result of raised intracranial pressure. Unrecognized and untreated, there may be rapid progression to coma and death due to raised intracranial pressure.

High-altitude pulmonary oedema

HAPE occurs in susceptible individuals who may have no underlying pulmonary or cardiac disease. It most commonly manifests on the second night at high altitude. In the early stages the oedema is interstitial, and the patient may only have a dry cough and decreased exercise tolerance. Few abnormalities will be seen on examination at this stage. As more fluid accumulates the patient develops tachycardia, increasing dyspnoea, marked weakness, cough productive of frothy sputum, and cyanosis. Pulse oximetry, if available, confirms profound hypoxia. A chest X-ray will demonstrate widespread interstitial and alveolar infiltrates. It may occur in conjunction with AMS/HACE, or as an isolated clinical syndrome.

MANAGEMENT

Early recognition is an essential component of the management of all acute altitude syndromes. Developing symptoms in a party member may have substantial impact on route planning choices, particularly whether to halt ascent or descend. The goal is to stop the pathophysiological process (Table 27.8.1).

Table 27.8.1 Treatment of severe altitude syndromes	
HACE/Severe AMS	HAPE
Descent	Descent
Oxygen	Oxygen
Hyperbaric therapy (e.g. Gamow Bag)	Hyperbaric therapy (e.g. Gamow Bag)
Dexamethasone 4 mg qid	Nifedipine 10 mg 4-hourly

Acute mountain sickness and high-altitude cerebral oedema

A patient presenting with symptoms of mild AMS should be advised to halt ascent to allow time for acclimatization. They should rest, as physical exertion aggravates symptoms, and take simple analgesics and antiemetics if desired. It is important that the patient be closely observed for progression of symptoms.

With moderate symptoms the management is the same as for mild AMS, with the addition of oxygen 2–4 L/min and, possibly, pharmacologic agents. Acetazolamide, a carbonic anhydrase inhibitor, aids the normal process of ventilatory acclimatization by reducing the renal reabsorption of bicarbonate, resulting in metabolic acidosis and compensatory hyperventilation. It relieves symptoms, improves arterial oxygenation, and prevents further impairment of pulmonary gas exchange.[7] It also helps to maintain cerebral blood flow despite hypocapnia, and opposes the fluid retention of AMS. The recommended dose is 125–250 mg orally bd. Acetazolamide is a sulpha drug and contraindicated in those with allergy. Dexamethasone may also be used as it improves oxygen saturation and provides symptomatic relief.[8] This benefit may be derived from reduced capillary permeability and ICP. It does not aid in acclimatization. It may be given as an alternative, or in addition to acetazolamide. The dose recommended is 8 mg orally initially, followed by 4 mg every 6 hours.

If a patient shows signs of severe AMS progressing to HACE, then rapid and controlled descent is the highest priority. Oxygen 2–4 L/min should be administered. Additional therapy may be required if the illness is severe, the patient's condition must be improved to allow descent, or where immediate descent is not possible. Additional therapeutic options include dexamethasone 8 mg orally, IM or IV, and hyperbaric therapy using a portable fabric hyperbaric chamber (e.g. Gamow Bag). This device simulates descent and provides short-term relief for 1–3 hours. Long-term benefits have yet to be established.[9] The bags are expensive and need to be pumped continuously, but have the advantage of using air rather than oxygen. Acetazolamide does not have a role in the setting of severe AMS and HACE.

High-altitude pulmonary oedema

Rapid and controlled descent, with oxygen, is the mainstay of management in a patient suffering from HAPE. In a large proportion of cases this is sufficient. Oxygen flow should be titrated to maintain adequate oxygen saturation. Continuous positive airway pressure may be required. The patient should be rested and kept warm, as cold may further increase pulmonary hypertension through sympathetic stimulation.

Nifedipine should be considered as adjunctive therapy when oxygen is not available and descent is not possible. A calcium channel blocker, it lowers the raised pulmonary artery pressure that characterizes HAPE and results in clinical improvement, better oxygenation and progressive clearing of alveolar oedema on chest X-ray. The recommended dosage is 10 mg orally, followed by 20–30 mg slow-release every 8–12 hours. Other vasodilators, such as hydralazine and phentolamine, have been trialled and shown to be effective.[10] Furosemide 40 mg orally or IV can also be used as a single dose, if the patient is not dehydrated.

PREVENTION

The best form of prevention is gradual ascent to allow sufficient time for acclimatization. Although individuals vary in how quickly they acclimatize, a sensible recommendation is sleeping no more than 500 m higher than the previous day once above 2500 m. Keeping warm, avoiding alcohol, keeping well hydrated and eating a high-carbohydrate diet to improve the respiratory quotient, will all decrease the incidence of altitude illness. Modest exercise on acclimatization days should be encouraged.

Acclimatization is not always practical or possible, and so pharmacological agents may be required to enhance the physiological process. Acetazolamide reduces the incidence and severity of AMS/HACE when used prophylactically in subjects experiencing rapid ascent.[11] Chemoprophylaxis can be achieved with 125–250 mg bd, started 1 day before ascent and continued for 2 days after reaching high altitude. Dexamethasone 4 mg qid may be equally effective, and may be more so when a rapid onset is required, such as in unacclimatized personnel involved in high-altitude

CONTROVERSIES

❶ The effectiveness of acetazolamide and dexamethasone in AMS prophylaxis is now generally well accepted. Which agent is more effective, what doses should be used and which circumstances they should be used in, is less clear. Trial comparisons are difficult owing to a number of confounding factors. Methods of measuring the severity of AMS vary. The side effects of acetazolamide at recommended doses can mimic AMS and, conversely, the euphoriant effects of dexamethasone can interfere with a subject's ability to accurately report symptoms. Dexamethasone and acetazolamide appear to differ in their effectiveness when trialled in field conditions compared to simulated conditions in hypobaric chambers. The dose of each drug used is not the same across trials. The rate of ascent appears to influence the effectiveness of pharmacological prophylaxis. The current recommendation is that dexamethasone be used when individuals are required to ascend immediately and unexpectedly (e.g. for mountain rescues) and that acetazolamide be used when prophylaxis can be commenced greater than 24 hours prior to the ascent.[13] Further research is required to clarify these issues and the role of new preventive strategies such as ginkgo bilboa for AMS and salmeterol for HAPE.

rescue missions. Nifedipine 20 mg slow-release tds may provide protection against HAPE in susceptible individuals, but the wisdom of re-exposing patients to such an environment is questionable. Current research focuses on the value of ginkgo bilboa in prevention of AMS[12] and salmeterol in prevention of HAPE.[5]

REFERENCES

1. Guyton AC, Hall JE 1995 Aviation, high altitude and space physiology. In: Textbook of Medical Physiology, 9th edn. WB Saunders, Philadelphia
2. Hackett PH, Rabold M 1996 High altitude medical problems. In: Tintinalli J (ed) Emergency Medicine, 4th edn. McGraw-Hill, New York
3. Kleger GR, Bartsch P, Vock P, Heilig B, Roberts LJ II, Ballmer PE 1996 Evidence against an increase in capillary permeability in subjects exposed to high altitude. Journal of Applied Physiology 81(5): 1917–23
4. Bartsch P 1997 High altitude pulmonary oedema. Respiration 64(6): 435–43
5. Sartori C, Allemann Y, Duplain H, et al 2002 Salmeterol for the prevention of high altitude pulmonary edema. New England Journal of Medicine 346: 1631–6
6. Basnyat B, Subedi D, Sleggs J, et al 2000 Disorientated and ataxic pilgrims: an epidemiological study of acute mountain sickness and high altitude cerebral edema at a sacred lake at 4300 m in the Nepal Himalayas. Wilderness and Environmental Medicine 11: 89–93
7. Grissom CK, Roach RC, Sarnquist FH, Hackett PH 1992 Acetazolamide in the treatment of acute mountain sickness: clinical efficacy and effect on gas exchange. Annals of Internal Medicine 116(6): 461–5
8. Ferrazzini G, Maggiorini M, Kriemler S, Bartsch P, Oelz O 1987 Successful treatment of acute mountain sickness with dexamethasone. British Medical Journal (Clinical Research Edition) 294(6584): 1380–2
9. Bartsch P 1992 Treatment of high altitude diseases without drugs. International Journal of Sports Medicine 13(1): S71–S74
10. Hackett PH, Roach RC, Hartig GS, Greene ER, Levine BD 1992 The effect of vasodilators on pulmonary haemodynamics in high altitude pulmonary oedema: a comparison. International Journal of Sports Medicine 13(Suppl 1): S68–S71
11. Hackett PH, Rennie D 1976 The incidence, importance, and prophylaxis of acute mountain sickness. Lancet 2(7996): 1149–55
12. Maakestad K, Leadbetter G, Olson S, Hackett P 2001 Ginkgo bilboa reduces incidence and severity of acute mountain sickness. (abstract) Wilderness and Environmental Medicine 12: 51
13. Douglas Reid L, Carter KA, Ellsworth A 1994 Acetazolamide or dexamethasone for prevention of acute mountain sickness: a meta-analysis. Journal of Wilderness Medicine 5: 34–48

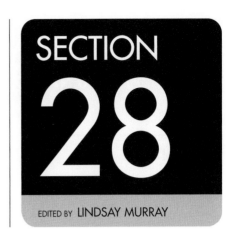

EDITED BY LINDSAY MURRAY

TOXICOLOGY

28.1 **General principles in the management of drug overdose** 790

28.2 **Antihistamine and anticholinergic poisoning** 797

28.3 **Cardiovascular drugs** 800

28.4 **Central nervous system drugs** 806

28.5 **Colchicine** 820

28.6 **Paracetamol** 823

28.7 **Salicylate** 827

28.8 **Theophylline** 830

28.9 **Carbon monoxide** 833

28.10 **Cyanide** 837

28.11 **Corrosive ingestion** 840

28.12 **Drugs of abuse** 844

28.13 **Methaemoglobinaemia** 854

28.14 **Pesticides** 857

28.15 **Hydrofluoric acid** 865

28.16 **Iron** 869

28.17 **Hypoglycaemic drugs** 872

28.18 **Lithium** 874

28.19 **Ethanol** 877

28.20 **Snakebite** 881

28.21 **Spider bite** 885

28.22 **Marine envenoming and poisoning** 890

28.1 GENERAL PRINCIPLES IN THE MANAGEMENT OF DRUG OVERDOSE

LINDSAY MURRAY

ESSENTIALS

1 Self-poisoning is symptomatic of an underlying psychiatric or social disorder.

2 A wide range of clinical manifestations of toxicity may be observed following drug overdose.

3 The mainstay of management is timely institution of an appropriate level of supportive care.

4 The role of gastrointestinal decontamination is controversial. Except in select cases it is unlikely that these procedures have a significant impact on clinical outcome when performed more than 1 hour following ingestion.

5 Specific antidotes and techniques of enhanced elimination are rarely indicated, but their timely use may be life-saving in specific instances.

INTRODUCTION

Drug overdose in adults usually occurs in the context of self-poisoning, which may be either recreational or an act of deliberate self-harm.

Deliberate self-poisoning is one of the commonest reasons for general hospital admission in the UK[1] and accounts for 1–5% of all public hospital admissions in Australia.[2,3] The bulk of the medical management of cases presenting to hospital is carried out in the emergency department, and the emergency physician is expected to be expert in the field. Although the management must vary considerably according to the nature and severity of the poisoning, some general principles apply.

Above all, it must be remembered that the acute overdose presentation is only a discrete time-limited event in the course of the underlying condition, which is usually psychiatric or social in origin.

PATHOPHYSIOLOGY AND CLINICAL PRESENTATION

The effects of ingestion of pharmaceuticals or illicit drugs range from the non-toxic to the life-threatening and may involve any system. Poisoning is a dynamic presentation and the patient may present at varying points in the time course of the poisoning. Consequently, rapid clinical deterioration or improvement may be observed after the initial presentation and assessment.

Acute morbidity and mortality from poisoning is usually a consequence of the cardiovascular, respiratory or CNS complications of the poisoning. Less commonly, hepatic, renal or metabolic effects are potentially life-threatening.

The most frequent life-threatening respiratory complication of poisoning is ventilatory failure, which is usually a consequence of CNS depression. Less commonly it is secondary to ventilatory muscle paralysis. The frequency and depth of respirations are reduced. Respiratory failure may also be caused by direct pulmonary toxicity, or complications such as pulmonary aspiration or non-cardiogenic pulmonary oedema (Table 28.1.1).

Cardiovascular manifestations of poisoning include tachycardia, bradycardia, hypertension, hypotension, conduction defects and arrhythmias (Table 28.1.2). Bradycardia is relatively rarely observed and is associated with a number of potentially life-threatening ingestions. Tachycardia is commonly observed and is usually benign. It may be due to intrinsic sympathomimetic or anticholinergic

Table 28.1.1 Toxic causes of respiratory failure

Central nervous system depression
Alcohols
Anticonvulsants
Antidepressants
Antihistamines
Barbiturates
Baclofen
Clonidine
Opioids
Phenothiazines
Sedative – hypnotics

Weakness of ventilatory muscles
Botulism
Carbamate pesticides
Muscle relaxants
Organophosphorus pesticides and warfare agents
Snakebite
Strychnine

Pulmonary
ARDS
Cardiogenic pulmonary oedema
Non-cardiogenic pulmonary oedema
Pulmonary aspiration and pneumonitis
    Activated charcoal
    Gastric contents
    Hydrocarbons
Paraquat

effects of a drug, or a reflex response to hypotension or hypoxia. Hypotension is also commonly observed and may be due to a number of different causes (Table 28.1.2). Hypertension is unusual. Severe hypertension is usually associated with illicit drug use and is important because it may produce complications such as intracerebral haemorrhage.

CNS manifestations of poisoning include decreased level of consciousness, agitation or delirium, seizures and disordered temperature regulation. A decreased level of consciousness is a common presentation of poisoning and is associated with many drugs, some of which are listed in Table 28.1.1. Although usually a direct drug effect, CNS depression is occasionally secondary to hypoglycaemia, hypoxia or hypotension.

Table 28.1.2 Cardiovascular effects of poisoning

Tachycardia
Anticholinergics
    Antihistamines
    Benztropine
    Phenothiazines
    Tricyclic antidepressants
Reflex response to hypotension
Sympathomimetics
    Amphetamines
    Caffeine
    Cocaine
    Theophylline

Bradycardia (includes AV block)
β-Blockers
Calcium channel blockers
Clonidine
Digoxin

Hypotension
Fluid loss/third spacing
Myocardial depressants
    β-Blockers
    Calcium channel blockers
Peripheral vasodilators

Hypertension
Anticholinergics
Sympathomimetics
    Amphetamines
    Cocaine
    MAO inhibitors

Rhythm/ECG abnormalities
QRS prolongation (fast sodium channel blockade)
    Class 1a and 1c antiarrhythmics
    Thioridazine
    Tricyclic antidepressants
    Propranolol
QT prolongation/torsades de pointes
    Chloroquine
    Citalopram
    Quinine
    Thioridazine
    Tricyclic antidepressants
Ventricular tachycardia/fibrillation
    Amphetamines
    Chloral hydrate
    Cocaine
    Digoxin
    Theophylline
    Tricyclic antidepressants

Ischaemia/infarction
Cocaine
Complication of hypoxia or hypotension

Table 28.1.3 Causes of drug-induced agitation or delirium

Amphetamines

Anticholinergics

Caffeine

Cocaine

Lithium

Theophylline

Table 28.1.4 Causes of drug-induced seizures

Amphetamines

Bupropion

Carbamazepine

Cocaine

Isoniazid

Mefenamic acid

Theophylline

Tricyclic antidepressants

Venlafaxine

Table 28.1.5 Toxic causes of hyperthermia

Amphetamines

Anticholinergics

Cocaine

MAO inhibitors

Salicylates

Serotonin syndrome

Common causes of agitation or delirium following overdose are listed in Table 28.1.3. Toxic seizures are potentially life threatening, and important causes are listed in Table 28.1.4.

Hypothermia is usually a complication of environmental exposure secondary to a decreased level of consciousness or altered behaviour. Hyperthermia is a direct toxic effect and causes are listed in Table 28.1.5. Severe hyperthermia is rapidly lethal if not corrected.

Metabolic and other manifestations of poisoning include hyper- and hypo-glycaemia, hyper- and hyponatraemia, acidosis and alkalosis, and hepatic failure.

Acute poisoning is distinguished from many other forms of acute illness in that, given appropriate supportive care over a relatively short period, a full recovery can usually be expected. A small number of potentially fatal poisonings may demonstrate progressive toxicity despite full supportive care. These are the so-called cellular toxins, and include colchicine, iron, salicylate, cyanide, paracetamol, theophylline and digoxin. In some of these cases timely administration of antidotes or the institution of techniques of enhanced elimination may be life saving.

Mortality or morbidity may also result from specific complications of a poisoning. These include trauma, pulmonary aspiration, adult respiratory distress syndrome, rhabdomyolysis, renal failure and hypoxic encephalopathy.

Pulmonary aspiration frequently complicates a period of decreased level of consciousness or a seizure. It is a leading cause of in-hospital morbidity and mortality following overdose. This complication is characterized by rapid onset of dyspnoea, cough, fever, wheeze and cyanosis.

Rhabdomyolysis occurs as a direct toxic effect (rare) or secondary to excessive muscular hyperactivity, seizures, hyperthermia, or prolonged coma with direct muscle compression. The urine is dark and acute renal failure can develop secondary to tubular deposition of myoglobin.

ASSESSMENT

Risk assessment

Assessment of the patient presenting after an overdose includes the need to make a risk assessment. This means the clinician makes an assessment of the likely time course, severity and nature of toxicity that will develop in that particular patient. Factors that need to be taken into account when formulating this risk assessment include: the substance(s) ingested, the dose ingested, the time since ingestion, the clinical features present, and the results of relevant investigations. Access to specialized poisons information in the form of a poisons information centre or in-house databases may be required to formulate an accurate risk assessment.

History

The history is invaluable in assisting the clinician to judge the likely clinical course and plan management of a case of poisoning. Every effort should be made to obtain information as to the type and dose of drug ingested, the time of ingestion, and the progression of symptoms since ingestion. History provided by the patient, if they are awake, is usually reliable and should not be dismissed.

Physical examination

The focused physical examination of the poisoned patient aims to:

- Identify any immediate threats to life and the need for intervention
- Establish a baseline clinical status
- Corroborate the history
- Identify intoxication syndromes
- Identify possible alternative diagnoses
- Identify any complications of the poisoning.

The initial physical examination of the overdose patient in many ways parallels the primary survey of the trauma patient. The airway, breathing and circulation are assessed and stabilized as necessary. The level of consciousness should be assessed, the presence of seizure activity noted, and the blood glucose and temperature measured.

A more complete examination is carried out when the patient is stable. This should include a full neurological examination, including assessment of the level of consciousness and mental status, pupil size, muscle tone and movements, and the presence or absence of focal neurological signs. Poisoning normally causes global CNS depression, and focal signs suggest an alternative diagnosis or a CNS complication such as cerebral haemorrhage.

Other features that should be specifically sought are any evidence of associated trauma, the state of hydration, the condition of the skin, in particular the presence of pressure areas, the presence or absence of bowel sounds and the condition of the urine.

Several toxic autonomic syndromes, or 'toxidromes', have been described in

Table 28.1.6 Toxic autonomic syndromes or 'toxidromes'

Toxidrome	Features	Common causes
Anticholinergic	Agitated delirium Tachycardia Hyperthermia Dilated pupils Dry flushed skin Urinary retention Ileus	Antihistamines Benztropine Carbamazepine Phenothiazines Plant poisonings Tricyclic antidepressants
Mixed cholinergic	Brady- or tachycardia Hypo- or hypertension Miosis or mydriasis Sweating Increased bronchial secretion Gastrointestinal hyperactivity Muscle weakness Fasciculations	Organophosphates Carbamates
Mixed α- and β-adrenergic	Hypertension Tachycardia Mydriasis Agitation	Amphetamines Cocaine
β-Adrenergic	Hypotension Tachycardia Hypokalaemia Hyperglycaemia	Caffeine Salbutamol Theophylline

Serotonin	Altered mental status
	Autonomic dysfunction
	  Fever
	  Hypertension
	  Sweating
	  Tachycardia
	Motor dysfunction
	  Hyperreflexia
	  Hypertonia (esp. lower limbs)
	  Myoclonus
		Amphetamines
		Antihistamines
		Monoamine oxidase inhibitors
		NSSRIs
		SSRIs
		Tricyclic antidepressants
		
		(Usually combined overdose)

relation to poisoning. The principal ones are listed in Table 28.1.6. Identification of these syndromes may narrow the differential diagnosis in cases of unknown poisoning.[4]

Poisons information

Information on the clinical course and toxic doses of specific pharmaceutical and non-pharmaceutical poisons is available on a 24-hour basis throughout Australia by telephoning 131126. The poison information centres are staffed by pharmacists and are also able to refer cases to clinical toxicologists for consultation.

INVESTIGATIONS

Investigations should only be performed if they are likely to affect the management of the patient. Investigations are useful to exclude important differential diagnoses, confirm a specific poisoning for which significant complications might be anticipated, assess the severity of intoxication, assess response to treatment, or assess the need for a specific antidote or enhanced elimination technique.

An ECG and serum paracetamol concentration measurement are indicated for virtually every patient who presents following acute overdose. The ECG is used to exclude conduction defects, which may predict potentially life-threatening cardiotoxicity. The serum paracetamol is useful to ensure that paracetamol poisoning is diagnosed within the time available for effective antidote treatment.

The patient with only minor manifestations of poisoning may require no other blood tests. More seriously ill patients may require electrolyte, renal and liver function tests and a full blood count, creatine kinase and arterial blood gases. Urinalysis reveals myoglobinuria in significant rhabdomyolysis. Pregnancy should be excluded in women of child-bearing age by serum or urine β-HCG if necessary.

Routine qualitative drug screening of urine or blood in the overdose patient is rarely useful in planning management.

Measurement of serum drug concentrations is only useful if this provides important diagnostic or prognostic information or assists in planning management. Some drug levels that may be useful are listed in Table 28.1.7. For most cases of drug overdose management is guided by clinical findings and not by drug levels. Some drugs commonly taken in overdose for which serum concentrations are of no value in planning management are listed in Table 28.1.8.

Radiology has a limited role in the management of overdose. A chest X-ray is indicated in any patient with a significantly decreased level of consciousness, seizures or hypoxia. It may show evidence of pulmonary aspiration. A CT scan of the head may be indicated to exclude other intracranial pathology in the patient with an altered mental status. The abdominal X-ray is useful in evaluating overdose of radioopaque metals

Table 28.1.7 Drug levels that may be helpful in the management of selected cases of overdose
Carbamazepine
Digoxin
Dilantin
Lithium
Iron
Paracetamol
Phenobarbitone
Salicylate
Theophylline
Valproate

Table 28.1.8 Drug levels that are not helpful in the management of overdose	
CNS drugs	Cardiovascular drugs
Antidepressants	ACE inhibitors
Benzodiazepines	Beta blockers
Benztropine	Calcium channel blockers
Cocaine	Clonidine
Newer antipsychotics	
Opiates	
Phenothiazines	

including iron, lithium, potassium, lead and arsenic.

DIFFERENTIAL DIAGNOSIS

It is essential to exclude important non-toxic diagnoses in the patient presenting with coma or altered mental status presumed to be due to drug overdose. These diagnoses include head injury, intracerebral haemorrhage or infarction, CNS infection, hyponatraemia, hypoglycaemia, hypo- or hyperthermia, post-ictal states and psychiatric disorders.

MANAGEMENT

Supportive care

Supportive care is the key element in the management of poisoning. The vast majority of poisonings result in temporary dysfunction of one or more of the body systems. If appropriate support of the system in question is instituted in a timely fashion and continued until the toxic substance is metabolized or excreted, a good outcome can be anticipated. In severe poisonings supportive care may be very aggressive, and possible interventions are listed in Table 28.1.9.

The specific supportive management of a number of manifestations or complications of poisoning warrants further mention insofar as it may differ from the

standard management of such conditions with other aetiologies.

Cardiopulmonary arrest from poisoning should be aggressively resuscitated. Direct current cardioversion is rarely successful in terminating toxic arrhythmias and should not take precedence over establishing adequate ventilation and oxygenation, cardiac compressions, correction of acidosis or hypovolaemia, and the administration of specific antidotes. Resuscitative efforts should be continued beyond the usual timeframe. In cardiac arrest due to drugs with direct cardiac toxicity, the use of cardiopulmonary bypass or extracorporeal membrane oxygenation (ECMO) until the drug is metabolized may be life saving.

In general, intravenous benzodiazepines are the drugs of choice for control of toxic seizures. Large doses may be required. Hypoxia and hypoglycaemia must be corrected if they are contributory factors. Patients with toxic seizures do not generally need long-term anticonvulsant therapy. Isoniazid-induced seizures are not controlled without administration of an adequate dose of the specific antidote, pyridoxine.

The management of pulmonary aspiration is essentially supportive, with supplemental oxygenation and intubation and mechanical ventilation if necessary. Neither prophylactic antibiotics nor corticosteroids have been shown to be helpful in the management of this condition, which is essentially a chemical pneumonitis.

Toxic hypertension rarely requires specific therapy. Most cases are mild and simple observation is sufficient. Agitation or delirium is a feature of many intoxications associated with hypertension, and adequate sedation with benzodiazepines usually lowers the blood pressure. Severe toxic hypertension is most likely in toxicity from cocaine or amphetamine-type drugs, and treatment may be indicated to avoid complications such as cardiac failure or intracerebral haemorrhage. The drug of choice in this situation is sodium nitroprusside by intravenous infusion. The extremely short duration of action of this vasodilator allows accurate control of hypertension during

Table 28.1.9 Supportive care measures for the poisoned patient

Airway	Endotracheal intubation
Breathing	Supplemental oxygen Ventilation
Circulation	Intravenous fluids Inotropes Antihypertensives Antiarrhythmics Defibrillation/cardioversion Cardiac pacing Cardiopulmonary bypass
Metabolic	Hypertonic dextrose Hypertonic saline Insulin/dextrose Calcium salts Sodium bicarbonate
Agitation/delirium	Benzodiazepines Butyrophenones
Seizures	Benzodiazepines Barbiturates
Body temperature	External rewarming External cooling
Impaired renal function	Rehydration Haemodialysis

Table 28.1.10 Materials that do not bind well to activated charcoal

Alcohols	Ethanol Ethylene glycol Isopropanol Methanol
Corrosives	Acids Alkalis
Hydrocarbons	
Metals and their salts	Iron Lead Lithium Potassium

the toxic phase, and avoids the development of hypotension once toxicity begins to wear off.

Management of rhabdomyolysis consists of treatment of the causative factors, fluid resuscitation and careful monitoring of fluids and electrolytes. The role of mannitol and urinary alkalinization in reducing the risk of renal failure is not clear. Established acute renal failure requires haemodialysis, often for up to 6 weeks.

Decontamination

The aim of decontamination of the gastrointestinal tract is to bind or remove ingested material before it is absorbed into the circulation and able to exert its toxic effects. This is a very attractive concept and has long been considered one of the fundamental interventions in management of the overdose patient.

However, gastrointestinal decontamination should not be regarded as a routine procedure in the management of the patient presenting to the emergency department following an overdose.

The decision to perform gastrointestinal decontamination and the choice of method should be based on an assessment of the likely benefit, the likely risk and the resources required. Performance of a gastric decontamination technique should never delay the institution of appropriate supportive care measures. Gastrointestinal decontamination should only be considered where there is likely to be a significant amount of a significantly toxic material remaining in the gut.

Three basic approaches to gastrointestinal decontamination are available: gastric emptying, administration of an adsorbent, and catharsis.

Gastric emptying can be attempted by the administration of an emetic, most commonly syrup of ipecac, or by gastric lavage. In volunteer studies both of these techniques removed highly variable amounts of marker substances from the stomach even if performed immediately after ingestion, and the effect diminished rapidly with time to the point of being negligible after one hour.[5,6] Clinical outcome trials have failed to demonstrate

improved outcome as a result of routine gastric emptying in addition to administration of activated charcoal, except, perhaps, in patients presenting unconscious within 1 hour of ingestion.[7–9]

The principal adsorbent available to clinicians is activated charcoal (AC), which effectively binds most pharmaceuticals and chemicals, and is currently the decontamination method of choice for most poisonings. Materials that do not bind well to charcoal are listed in Table 28.1.10.

Charcoal is 'activated' by treatment in acid and steam at high temperature. This process removes impurities and greatly increases the surface area available for binding. AC is packaged as a 50 g dose premixed with water or sorbitol, which is likely to be sufficient for the majority of ingestions. Adult patients are usually able to drink activated charcoal slurry from a cup. If the level of consciousness is too impaired to allow this, they should be intubated first. Administration of AC is absolutely contraindicated unless the patient has an intact or protected airway.

Volunteer studies demonstrate that the effect of AC diminishes rapidly with time and that the greatest benefit occurs if it is administered within one hour. There is as yet no evidence that AC improves clinical outcome.[10]

There is no evidence to suggest that the addition of a cathartic such as sorbitol to activated charcoal improves clinical outcome.[11,12]

Apart from rarely employed endoscopic and surgical techniques, whole-bowel irrigation (WBI) is the most aggressive form of gastrointestinal decontamination. Polyethylene glycol solution (Golytely™) is administered via a nasogastric tube at a rate of 2 L/h until a clear rectal effluent is produced. This usually takes about 6 hours and requires one-to-one nursing. In volunteer studies this technique reduced the absorption of slow-release pharmaceuticals and so may be of benefit in life threatening overdoses of these agents.[12,13] Again, clinical benefit has not yet been conclusively demonstrated.[14] The use of WBI has also been reported in the management of potentially toxic ingestions of iron, lead, and packets of illicit drugs. WBI is contraindicated if there is evidence of ileus or bowel obstruction, and in patients who have an unprotected airway or haemodynamic compromise.[14]

Enhanced elimination

A number of techniques are available to enhance the elimination of toxins from the body. Their use is rarely indicated as only a very few drugs, capable of causing severe poisoning, have pharmacokinetic parameters that render them amenable to these techniques (Table 28.1.11).

Repeat-dose activated charcoal (25–50 g every 3–4 hours) may enhance drug elimination by interrupting the enterohepatic circulation or by 'gastrointestinal dialysis'. Gastrointestinal dialysis is the movement of a toxin across the

gastrointestinal wall from the circulation into the gut down a concentration gradient that is maintained by charcoal binding. For this technique to be effective a drug must undergo considerable enterohepatic circulation or, in the case of 'gastrointestinal dialysis', have a small volume of distribution, small molecular weight, low protein binding, slow endogenous elimination, and bind to charcoal.[15,16] The advantages of this technique are that it is non-invasive and simple to carry out.

Alkalinization of the urine enhances urinary excretion of drugs that are filtered at the glomerulus and are unable to be reabsorbed across the tubular epithelium when in an ionized form at alkaline pH. For elimination to be effectively enhanced by this method, the drug must be predominantly eliminated by the kidneys in the unchanged form, have a low pKa, be distributed mainly to the extracellular fluid compartment, and be minimally protein bound.[17]

Haemodialysis (HD) and haemoperfusion (HP) are both very invasive techniques and for that reason are reserved for potentially life-threatening intoxications. Only a small number of drugs that have small volumes of distribution, slow endogenous clearance rates, small molecular weights (HD) and bind to charcoal (HP) will have their rates of elimination significantly enhanced by these procedures.

Use of antidotes

Very few drugs have effective antidotes. Occasionally, however, timely use of an antidote may be life saving or substantially reduce morbidity, time in hospital or resource requirements. Antidotes that may be indicated in the emergency department setting are listed in Table 28.1.12. However, it must be remembered that antidotes are also drugs, and are frequently associated with adverse effects of their own. An antidote should only be used where a specific indication exists, and then only at the correct dose, by the correct route, and with appropriate monitoring. Because many antidotes are so infrequently used, obtaining sufficient supplies when the need arises can be

difficult. Every emergency department must review its stocking of antidotes and have a plan for obtaining further supplies should the need arise.

DISPOSITION

Both the medical and the psychiatric disposition of the overdose patient must be considered. A good risk assessment is essential to determining timely and safe disposition.

The majority of overdose patients who remain stable at 4–6 hours after the ingestion do not need further close monitoring and may be admitted to a non-monitored bed until manifestations of toxicity completely resolve. An emergency observation ward is ideal for this purpose if one exists.

Any patient who develops clinical manifestations of intoxication severe enough to require the institution of specific supportive care measures requires admission to an intensive care environment. A few patients will require admission for prolonged monitoring based on the history of the ingestion. For example, anyone with a history of ingestion of colchicine, organophosphates, slow-release theophylline or slow-release calcium channel blockers requires admission because of the possibility of delayed onset of severe toxicity.

Psychiatric evaluation of deliberate self-poisoning cases is indicated as soon as the patient's medical condition permits. All such patients must be continuously supervised until the psychiatric evaluation has taken place.

CONCLUSION

Patients presenting to the emergency department following oral overdose may develop a wide range of clinical manifestations. The vast majority have a good clinical outcome with simple supportive care. Those who present within 1 hour of a potentially toxic ingestion should be decontaminated with oral activated charcoal. Some specific cases may benefit from delayed decontamination. Small numbers of

Table 28.1.11 Techniques of enhanced elimination	
Technique	*Suitable toxin*
Repeat-dose activated charcoal	Carbamazepine Dapsone Phenobarbitone Phenytoin Salicylate Theophylline
Urinary alkalinization	Phenobarbitone Salicylate
Haemodialysis	Ethylene glycol Lithium Methanol Salicylate Theophylline
Haemoperfusion	Theophylline

Table 28.1.12 Useful emergency antidotes

Poisoning	Antidote
Atropine	Physostigmine
Benzodiazepines	Flumazenil
β-Blockers	Glucagon
Chloroquine	Diazepam
Cyanide	Dicobalt edetate, hydroxocobalamin
Digoxin	Digoxin-specific *Fab* fragments
Insulin	Dextrose
Iron	Desferoxamine
Isoniazid	Pyridoxine
Methaemoglobinaemia	Methylene blue
Methanol and ethylene glycol	Ethanol, fomepizole
Organophosphates and carbamates	Atropine, oximes
Opioids	Naloxone
Paracetamol	N-acetyl cysteine
Sulphonylureas	Dextrose
Tricyclic antidepressants	Sodium bicarbonate
Warfarin, Brodifacoum	Vitamin K

CONTROVERSIES

❶ The role of, choice of method, and indications for gastric decontamination remain controversial. These procedures are no longer regarded as routine, but there are likely to be subgroups of overdose patients who may derive clinical benefit from gastrointestinal decontamination. These groups have not yet been precisely identified.

❷ Research is continuing into the development of new and safer antidotes for potentially life-threatening poisoning.

❸ The clinical and economic utility of establishing specialized toxicology treatment centres.[18,19]

patients may also benefit from the appropriate use of antidotes and methods of enhanced elimination.

Self-poisoning is merely a symptom of an underlying psychiatric or social disorder, and these must be carefully addressed in each case of overdose presenting to the emergency department.

REFERENCES

1. Hawton K, Fagg J 1992 Trends in deliberate self-poisoning and self-injury in Oxford. British Medical Journal 304: 1409–11
2. McGrath J 1989 A survey of deliberate self-poisoning. Medical Journal of Australia 150: 317–22
3. Pond SM 1995 Prescription for poisoning. Medical Journal of Australia 162: 174–5
4. Kulig K 1992 Initial management of ingestion of toxic substances. New England Journal of Medicine 326: 1677
5. Krenzelok EP, McGuigan M, Lheureux P 1997 Position statement: ipecac syrup. American Academy of Clinical Toxicology; European Association of Poisons Centres and Clinical Toxicologists. Journal of Toxicology – Clinical Toxicology 35(7): 699–709
6. Vale JA 1997 Position statement: gastric lavage. American Academy of Clinical Toxicology; European Association of Poisons Centres and Clinical Toxicologists. Journal of Toxicology – Clinical Toxicology 35(7): 711–9
7. Kulig K, Bar-Or D, Kantrill SV, et al 1990 Management of acutely poisoned patients without gastric emptying. Annals of Emergency Medicine 14: 562–7
8. Merigian KS, Woodard M, Hedges JR, et al 1990 Prospective evaluation of gastric emptying in the self-poisoned patient. American Journal of Emergency Medicine 8: 479–83
9. Pond SM, Lewis-Driver DJ, Williams G, et al 1995 Gastric emptying in acute overdose: a prospective randomised controlled trial. Medical Journal of Australia 163: 345–9
10. Chyka PA, Seger D 1997 Position statement: single-dose activated charcoal. American Academy of Clinical Toxicology; European Association of Poisons Centres and Clinical Toxicologists. Journal of Toxicology – Clinical Toxicology 35(7): 721–41
11. Barceloux D, McGuigan M, Hartigan-Go K 1997 Position statement: cathartics. American Academy of Clinical Toxicology; European Association of Poisons Centres and Clinical Toxicologists. Journal of Toxicology – Clinical Toxicology 35(7): 743–52
12. Kirshenbaum LA, Mathew SC, Sitar DS, Tenenbein M 1989 Whole-bowel irrigation versus activated charcoal in sorbitol for the ingestion of modified-release pharmaceuticals. Clinical Pharmacology Therapy 46: 264–71
13. Smith SW, Ling LJ, Halstenson CE 1991 Whole-bowel irrigation as a treatment for acute lithium overdose. Annals of Emergency Medicine 20: 536–9
14. Tenenbein M 1997 Position statement: whole bowel irrigation. American Academy of Clinical Toxicology; European Association of Poisons Centres and Clinical Toxicologists. Journal of Toxicology – Clinical Toxicology 35(7): 753–62
15. Pond SM 1986 Role of repeated oral doses of activated charcoal in clinical toxicology. Medical Toxicology 1: 3–11
16. Chyka PA 1995 Multiple-dose activated charcoal and enhancement of systemic drug clearance: summary of studies in animals and human volunteers. Clinical Toxicology 33: 399–405
17. Winchester JF 1998 Active methods for detoxification. In: Haddad LM, Shannon MW, Winchester JF (eds) Clinical Management of Poisoning and Drug Overdose, 3rd edn. WB Saunders, Philadelphia
18. Whyte IM, Dawson AH, Buckley NA et al 1997 A model for the management of self-poisoning. Medical Journal of Australia 167: 142–6
19. Lee V, Kerr JF, Braitberg G et al 2001 Impact of a toxicology service on a metropolitan teaching hospital. Emergency Medicine 13: 37–42

28.2 ANTIHISTAMINE AND ANTICHOLINERGIC POISONING

ANDIS GRAUDINS

ESSENTIALS

1 Anticholinergic toxicity is a relatively common and often unrecognized toxicologic problem in the emergency department.

2 H_1-receptor antagonists are readily accessible and a common cause of anticholinergic poisoning.

3 Significant CNS and CVS toxicity may infrequently complicate large ingestions of first-generation H_1-receptor antagonists.

4 H_2-receptor antagonist overdose produces insignificant clinical effects.

INTRODUCTION

Anticholinergic toxicity is a common side effect of many pharmaceutical agents, natural remedies, and plants both in therapeutic dosing and in overdose (see Table 28.2.1). Symptoms and signs may range from mild manifestations of the syndrome (e.g. dry mouth and blurred vision) to severe anticholinergic delirium with agitation, hallucinations and aggressive behaviour.

The antihistamine agents are a diverse group of drugs that can be broadly classified, based upon receptor specificity, into H_1- and H_2-receptor antagonists. The H_1-receptor antagonists are widely used in the treatment of allergic conditions and nasal congestion, as over-the-counter (OTC) sleep aids and as anti-emetics. This group can be further divided into the 'first-generation' agents, which tend to be more lipophilic and are more sedating, and the 'second-generation' or non-sedating agents. The H_2-receptor antagonists are primarily used in the treatment of peptic ulcer disease and gastroesophageal reflux, but are also used in conjunction with H_1 antagonists in the treatment of severe allergic reactions.

Antihistamine agents are relatively easy to obtain and frequently used in overdose for attempted suicide and abused recreationally for their sedating and anticholinergic effects. The incidence of antihistamine poisoning and abuse in Australia is not well characterized. Other prescription drugs may also result in anticholinergic toxicity both in therapeutic dosing and in overdose. These may also be intentionally abused for their anticholinergic effects.[1-4] Chinese and traditional herbal medicines may result in anticholinergic toxicity either directly from the herbal agent ingested or as a result of contamination with anticholinergic agents such as atropine or scopolamine.[5-7] The intentional abuse of botanicals (e.g. *Datura* spp.) may also present with anticholinergic toxicity.[8-10] In view of the easy availability of many of these pharmaceutical and herbal agents, the emergency physician should include a detailed drug history in the evaluation of any patient presenting with evidence of mental status change and anticholinergic symptoms and signs. In particular, polypharmacy and drug interactions between multiple agents with the potential for anticholinergic effects should be included in the differential diagnosis of elderly patients presenting with mental status changes.

PHARMACODYNAMICS AND PHARMACOKINETICS OF HISTAMINE RECEPTOR BLOCKING AGENTS

The H_1-antagonists are a diverse group of agents that reversibly block the action of histamine at H_1 receptors. High lipid solubility results in central nervous system (CNS) penetration and sedation. The first-generation agents also block muscarinic, α-adrenergic, and serotonergic receptors. Local anaesthetic effects due to sodium channel may mimic the antiarrhythmic properties of class 1A antiarrhythmic agents.[11] Diphenhydramine, dimenhydrinate and cyproheptadine, in particular, may prolong the cardiac muscle cell action potential duration by this mechanism.[12,13]

The second-generation H_1-antagonists (fexofenadine, loratadine) have much less CNS penetration and are more histamine receptor specific with little or no effect at

---

Table 28.2.1 Anticholinergic agents

Pharmaceuticals
Anticholinergic agents
    Atropine
    Benzhexol
    Benztropine
    Scopolamine
Cyclic antidepressants
    Amitriptyline
    Imipramine
    Dosulepin (dothiepin)
    Doxepin
Antipsychotics
    Phenothiazines
    Clozapine
    Risperidone
First-generation H_1-receptor blockers
    Cetirizine
    Cyproheptadine
    Dexchlorpheniramine
    Diphenhydramine
    Diphenylpyraline
    Hydroxyzine
    Methdilazine
    Pheniramine
    Promethazine
    Trimeprazine
Others
    Amantadine
    Carbamazepine

Botanicals
Datura spp.
Jimson weed or thorn apple
Angel's trumpet
Atropa belladona – deadly nightshade

---

other receptor subtypes.[11] Two agents in this group (astemizole and terfenadine) experimentally prolong cardiac muscle cell repolarization by blockade of inward potassium rectifier currents, L-type calcium channels, and voltage-dependent sodium channels.[14,15] In the presence of increased concentrations of the parent drug as occurs in overdose or where metabolism is impaired, this produces QT-interval prolongation and increased risk of polymorphic ventricular tachycardia.[15] These agents have been removed from the market because of this risk.

All the H$_1$-antagonists are well absorbed orally with peak serum concentrations occurring within 2 to 4 hours. Absorption may be delayed in overdose due to anticholinergic effects seen with the first-generation agents. Bioavailability is limited by significant first-pass metabolism. Some agents may be converted to active metabolites (e.g. terfenadine, hydroxyzine). Volume of distribution and protein binding are generally high. Elimination half-lives for the first generation agents are between 2 and 6 hours.[11] The second generation agents generally have longer half-lives (e.g. loratadine 8.3 hours).[11]

The H$_2$-antagonist agents are generally well tolerated with few side effects with therapeutic dosing. Cimetidine inhibits hepatic microsomal enzyme metabolism and reduces the metabolism of drugs eliminated by this pathway. This may result in increased serum concentrations and clinical effects of co-ingested medications.

All drugs with anticholinergic side effects have the potential to slow gastric emptying and produce gastrointestinal ileus when taken in overdose. As a result, absorption of these agents may be slowed and result in the potential for prolonged toxicity.

CLINICAL PRESENTATION

The anticholinergic syndrome is usually manifest by a combination of peripheral and central muscarinic, cholinergic receptor blockade. Peripheral effects may include sinus tachycardia, cutaneous vasodilatation and flushing, low-grade temperature, warm dry skin with an absence of axillary sweat, dry mucous membranes, gastrointestinal ileus, and urinary retention. Central nervous system effects include mydriasis with blurred vision due to the inhibition of visual accomodation, delirium, confusion, visual hallucinations, incoherent speech, agitation, combativeness, aggression, and coma.[16] Patients presenting with anticholinergic syndrome will often have an impaired perception of their environment. This may result in behaviour that could injure the patient. Anticholinergic symptoms and signs may be prominent with ingestion of first-generation antihistamines.[17–19] Even therapeutic doses of some of the H$_1$-antagonist agents may be sufficient to produce an anticholinergic delirium in susceptible individuals (especially the elderly and children). Topical use of these agents, particularly on broken skin surfaces, may also result in anticholinergic delirium.[20,21]

In patients who present to hospital several hours following poisoning with an anticholinergic agent, the peripheral features of the toxidrome may be absent.[22–24] This may also occur in elderly people with mild-to-moderate anticholinergic delirium resulting from the side effects of therapeutic drug administration.[24]

Other manifestations of H$_1$-antagonist toxicity may include CNS and cardiovascular effects, and rhabdomyolysis. Overdose of first-generation agents commonly produces drowsiness, sedation, confusion, agitation, and ataxia. Large ingestions may result in coma.[25, 26] Seizures may also occur. Pheniramine, a commonly abused antihistamine in Australia, appears to be more proconvulsant than other agents following overdose with a reported incidence of seizures of 30%.[19] Seizures have been reported with other first-generation H$_1$-antagonists, such as diphenhydramine, in doses as small as 150 mg in children.[25,27] Fatal doses of diphenhydramine in adults range from 20 to 40 mg/kg.[28] Doxylamine poisoning may result in non-traumatic rhabdomyolysis.[29,30] Hypotension, due to α-receptor blockade, can occur following large ingestions of first-generation agents. Conduction defects are infrequent following poisoning with first-generation H$_1$-antagonists. Diphenhydramine and dimenhydrinate poisoning can result in QRS-interval prolongation, broad-complex tachycardia, and ventricular arrhythmias similar to that seen in cyclic antidepressant poisoning.[12,13] This effect has not been reported with other first-generation H$_1$-antagonists.

Overdose with H$_2$-antagonists, such as cimetidine, usually results in little or no evidence of toxicity. Doses of up to 15 g have failed to produce clinical toxicity.[31]

INVESTIGATIONS

A 12-lead ECG should be performed to check for the presence of sinus tachycardia, QRS and QT-interval duration. A finger-stick blood glucose is necessary in all patients with changed mental state. Blood for serum electrolytes and paracetamol level should be collected. In patients with mental status changes that cannot be easily explained by drug intoxication, other organic causes for cognitive impairment should be ruled out. Serum antihistamine levels are not readily available and do not influence patient management. Standard 'drugs-of-abuse' urine screens do not detect antihistamines or most other agents with anticholinergic toxicity.

MANAGEMENT

The mainstay of therapy for poisoning with anticholinergic agents is supportive care in a safe environment. Comatose or hypoventilating patients should have appropriate airway intervention on arrival. Hypotension should be treated initially with intravenous colloid or crystalloid boluses. Hypotension refractory to fluids may necessitate the use of pressor agents such as noradrenaline (norepinephrine). Agitation and seizures can be controlled using parenteral benzodiazepines in the first instance.

Barbiturates (thiopental (thiopentone), phenobarbital (phenobarbitone)) may be considered in refractory cases.

Gastrointestinal decontamination should be performed with a single-dose of oral activated charcoal in most instances. The benefit of activated charcoal in patients presenting with minimal or no signs of toxicity more than 2 hours following ingestion is questionable. Methods of enhancing elimination of antihistamines are ineffective because of their large volumes of distribution and high protein binding.

The short-acting, reversible acetyl-cholinesterase inhibitors physostigmine and tacrine have been used in the management and diagnosis of anticholinergic agitation and delirium.[32-34] Both physostigmine and tacrine rapidly reverse the effects of anticholinergic delirium and may prevent the need for escalating doses of benzodiazepines to control agitation. Physostigmine may decrease the need for other interventions such as cerebral CT-scanning and lumbar puncture in patients with suspected anticholinergic delirium.[33]

When using physostigmine, an initial test dose 0.5 mg IV is followed by 1.0–2.0 mg over the following 3–5 minutes in an adult (0.02 mg/kg in a child to a maximum of 0.5 mg). A partial response may necessitate further 0.5–1.0 mg boluses. Clinical effects may last from 30 to 120 minutes. Tacrine has a significantly longer duration of action than physostigmine (4–6 hours vs 30–60 minutes). Consequently, physostigmine is a better agent to use initially when assessing the response of a patient to anticholinesterase therapy. Notably, these agents should *never* be used in patients with suspected acute cyclic antidepressant poisoning or ECG evidence of cardiac conduction delay because of the risk of precipitating cardiac asystole.[35]

Broad-complex tachycardia resulting from severe poisoning with diphenhydramine or dimenhydrinate should be treated with serum alkalinization with IV sodium bicarbonate boluses (0.5–1.0 mmol/kg) as for severe cyclic antidepressant poisoning.[12,13] Symptomatic bradycardia and high degree atrioventricular block should

be initially treated with atropine. Unresponsive cases may need cardiac pacing. Class-1a, -1c or -3 antiarrhythmic agents should be avoided in cases of antihistamine-induced arrhythmias.

DISPOSITION

Patients who present with minimal or no signs of toxicity require 4–6 hours of observation and monitoring. They may be medically cleared if, at the end of this period, they are alert and awake with a normal ECG. Patients with persistent mental status changes require further observation but, if the ECG is normal, do not require further cardiac monitoring. The duration of anticholinergic delirium may be from 12 hours to several days depending on the agent and dose ingested. Severe toxicity, if it is to develop, will be evident within 2–3 hours of ingestion. Those patients with poisoning complicated by coma, seizures, or CVS toxicity require admission and observation in an intensive-care or high-dependency setting.

All patients with intentional ingestions or suspicion of self-harm require psychiatric assessment prior to discharge.

CONCLUSIONS

Poisoning with a number of pharmaceutical agents, including the first-generation antihistamines may result in the development of anticholinergic symptoms and signs. Significant CNS and CVS toxicity may infrequently result following large ingestions of first-generation H_1-receptor blocking agents.

CONTROVERSIES

❶ The precise indications/contraindications for use of the anticholinesterase inhibitors, physostigmine and tacrine, are yet to be clearly delineated in the management of anticholinergic delirium.

H_2-receptor blocking drugs are intrinsically safe in overdose with few, if any, clinical effects even following large ingestions.

REFERENCES

1. Acri AA, Henretig FM 1998 Effects of risperidone in overdose. American Journal of Emergency Medicine 16: 498–501
2. Fisher RS, Cysyk B 1988 A fatal overdose of carbamazepine: case report and review of literature. Journal of Toxicology – Clinical Toxicology 26: 477–86
3. Graudins A, Peden G, Dowsett RP 2002 Massive overdose with controlled-release carbamazepine resulting in delayed peak serum concentrations and life-threatening toxicity. Emergency Medicine (Fremantle) 14: 89–94
4. Yang CC, Deng JF 1997 Anticholinergic syndrome with severe rhabdomyolysis—an unusual feature of amantadine toxicity. Intensive Care Medicine 23: 355–6
5. Chan TY 1995 Anticholinergic poisoning due to Chinese herbal medicines. Veterinary & Human Toxicology 37: 156–7
6. Chan JC, Chan TY, Chan KL, Leung NW, Tomlinson B, Critchley JA 1994 Anticholinergic poisoning from Chinese herbal medicines. Australian & New Zealand Journal of Medicine. 24: 317–8
7. Chan TY, Tang CH, Critchley JA 1995 Poisoning due to an over-the-counter hypnotic, Sleep-Qik (hyoscine, cyproheptadine, valerian). Postgraduate Medical Journal 71: 227–8
8. Finlay P 1998 Anticholinergic poisoning due to *Datura candida*. Tropical Doctor 28: 183–4
9. Hanna JP, Schmidley JW, Braselton WE, Jr 1992 Datura delirium. Clinical Neuropharmacology 15: 109–13
10. Mahler DA 1976 Anticholinergic poisoning from Jimson weed. Jacep 5: 440–2
11. Rimmer SJ, Church MK 1990 The pharmacology and mechanism of action of histamine H1 antagonists. Clinical and Experimental Allergy 20: 3
12. Clark RF, Vance MV 1992 Massive diphenhydramine poisoning resulting in a wide-complex tachycardia: successful treatment with sodium bicarbonate. Annals of Emergency Medicine 21: 318–21
13. Farrell M, Heinrichs M, Tilelli JA 1991 Response of life threatening dimenhydrinate intoxication to sodium bicarbonate administration. Journal of Toxicology – Clinical Toxicology 29: 527–35
14. Berul CI, Morad M 1995 Regulation of potassium channels by non-sedating antihistamines. Circulation 91: 2220–5
15. Woosley RL, Chen Y, Freiman JP, Gillis RA 1993 Mechanism of the cardiotoxic actions of terfenadine. Journal of the American Medical Association 269: 1532–6
16. Feldman MD 1986 The syndrome of anticholinergic intoxication. American Family Physician 34: 113–6
17. Jones IH, Stevenson J, Jordan A, Connell HM, Hetherington HD, Gibney GN 1973 Pheniramine as an hallucinogen. Medical Journal of Australia 1: 382–6
18. Jones J, Dougherty J, Cannon L 1986 Diphenhydramine-induced toxic psychosis. American Journal of Emergency Medicine 4: 369–71
19. Buckley NA, Whyte IM, Dawson AH, Cruickshank DA 1994 Pheniramine—a much abused drug. Medical Journal of Australia 160: 188–92
20. Schipior PG 1967 An unusual case of antihistamine intoxication. Journal of Pediatrics 71: 589–91
21. Reilly JF, Jr., Weisse ME 1990 Topically induced

diphenhydramine toxicity. Journal of Emergency Medicine 8: 59–61
22. Rupreht J, Dworacek B 1976 Central anticholinergic syndrome in anesthetic practice. Acta Anaesthesiologica Belgica 27: 45–60
23. Koppel C, Hopfe T, Menzel J 1990 Central anticholinergic syndrome after ofloxacin overdose and therapeutic doses of diphenhydramine and chlormezanone. Journal of Toxicology – Clinical Toxicology 28: 249–53
24. Feinberg M 1993 The problems of anticholinergic adverse effects in older patients. Drugs Aging 3: 335–48
25. Koppel C, Ibe K, Tenczer J 1987 Clinical symptomatology of diphenhydramine overdose: an evaluation of 136 cases in 1982 to 1985. Journal of Toxicology – Clinical Toxicology 25: 53–70
26. Koppel C, Tenczer J, Ibe K 1987 Poisoning with

over-the-counter doxylamine preparations: an evaluation of 109 cases. Human Toxicology 6: 355–9
27. Hestand HE, Teske DW 1977 Diphenhydramine hydrochloride intoxication. Journal of Paediatrics 90: 1017–8
28. Krenzelok EP, Anderson GM, Mirick M 1982 Massive diphenhydramine overdose resulting in death. Annals of Emergency Medicine 11: 212–3
29. Mendoza FS, Atiba JO, Krensky AM, Scannell LM 1987 Rhabdomyolysis complicating doxylamine overdose. Clinical Paediatrics 26: 595–7
30. Frankel D, Dolgin J, Murray BM 1990 Non-traumatic rhabdomyolysis complicating antihistamine overdosage. Clinical Toxicology 31: 493
31. Krenzelok EP, Litovitz T, Lippold KP, McNally CF 1987 Cimetidine toxicity: an assessment of 881

cases. Annals of Emergency Medicine 16: 1217–21
32. Beaver KM, Gavin TJ 1998 Treatment of acute anticholinergic poisoning with physostigmine. American Journal of Emergency Medicine 16: 505–7
33. Burns MJ, Linden CH, Graudins A, Brown RM, Fletcher KE 2000 A comparison of physostigmine and benzodiazepines for the treatment of anticholinergic poisoning. Annals of Emergency Medicine 35: 374–81
34. Mendelson G 1977 Pheniramine aminosalicylate overdosage. Reversal of delirium and choreiform movements with tacrine treatment. Archives of Neurology 34: 313
35. Pentel P, Peterson CD 1980 Asystole complicating physostigmine treatment of tricyclic antidepressant overdose. Annals of Emergency Medicine 9: 588–90

28.3 CARDIOVASCULAR DRUGS

BETTY CHAN • LINDSAY MURRAY

ESSENTIALS

1 Many cardiovascular medications, including the calcium channel blockers, the β-blockers and digoxin, are associated with potentially life-threatening toxicity.

2 The key to the management of calcium channel blocker and β-blocker toxicity rests with aggressive supportive care of the circulation.

3 The onset of toxicity following overdose with slow-release formulations of calcium channel blockers may be delayed.

4 Early aggressive decontamination with whole-bowel irrigation is important in the management of slow-release calcium channel blocker overdose.

5 Early identification of patients presenting with potentially severe digoxin toxicity and appropriate use of the specific Fab fragment antibody is life-saving.

CALCIUM CHANNEL BLOCKERS AND β-BLOCKERS

INTRODUCTION

The calcium channel blockers (CCBs) and β-blockers are widely prescribed in the community. In overdose, they present with similar clinical pictures of potentially life-threatening impairment of cardiac function. The management of both types of overdose is similar and they are discussed together.

PHARMACOKINETICS

Standard CCB preparations are rapidly absorbed from the gastrointestinal tract, with onset of action occurring within 30 minutes.[1] Pharmacokinetic parameters are shown in Table 28.3.1. Verapamil and diltiazem undergo significant first-pass hepatic clearance. Verapamil is metabolized to norverapamil, which possesses 15–20% of verapamil's pharmacological activity and is renally excreted. Diltiazem is metabolized to deacetyldiltiazem, which has half the potency of the parent compound and undergoes biliary

excretion. The elimination half-lives of all CCBs may be prolonged following massive overdose. Amlodipine has a longer plasma half-life (30–50 hours) than other CCBs.

Importantly, slow-release preparations of both verapamil and diltiazem are widely prescribed and are associated with much longer times to peak plasma concentration and clinical effect.

Absorption of β-blockers is rapid, with peak clinical effects occurring within 1–4 hours. Pharmacokinetic parameters of the principal β-blockers are detailed in Table 28.3.2. Agents with high lipid solubility, such as propranolol, penetrate the blood–brain barrier better than the water-soluble agents, and hence cause greater CNS toxicity.

PATHOPHYSIOLOGY

CCBs antagonize the entry of extracellular calcium into cardiac and smooth muscle, but not skeletal muscle. Upon entry into cells, calcium participates in mechanical, electrical and biochemical reactions. It is involved in excitation–contraction of cardiac and smooth muscles, as well as phase 0 depolarization in the sinus and atrioventricular (AV) nodes by calcium influx through channels.[2]

CCBs affect myocardial contractility and slow conduction through the sinus and AV nodes. Contraction of smooth muscle is mediated by calcium influx, which is inhibited by CCBs. This results in vasodilatation and secondary reflex tachycardia from an increase in sympathetic activity.

The different classes of CCB have somewhat different pharmacological and toxic effects, as a consequence of their different binding characteristics to the dihydropyridine (DHP) receptors. Verapamil, a phenylalkylamine, produces more profound cardiac conduction defects and equal reductions in systemic vascular resistance when compared with other CCBs on a mg/kg basis.[1] Verapamil is more likely to produce symptomatic decreases in blood pressure, heart rate and cardiac output than is diltiazem, a benzothiazepine. The dihydropyridines, which include nifedipine, felodipine, amlodipine and lercanidipine preferentially bind to vascular smooth muscle and predominantly decrease systemic and coronary vascular resistance. With the exception of felodipine, they also produce a reflex tachycardia by the unloading of baroreceptors.

β-blockers prevent the binding of catecholamines to β receptors (β_1, β_2). β_1 receptors are located in the myocardium, kidney and eye, and β_2 receptors in adipose tissue, pancreas, liver and both smooth and skeletal muscle. β_1 stimulation produces increased chronotropy and inotropy in the heart, increased renin secretion in the kidney and increased aqueous humor production. β_2 stimulation relaxes smooth muscle in the blood vessels, bronchial tree, intestinal tract and uterus.

Table 28.3.1 Pharmacological profiles of the calcium channel blockers (*Adapted from:* Kerns W II, Kline J, Ford MD 1994 β-blocker and calcium channel blocker toxicity. Emergency Medicine Clinics of North America 12: 365–389)

Class	Phenylalkylamines	Benzothiazepines	Dihydropyridines
Prototype	Verapamil	Diltiazem	Nifedipine
Hr to peak plasma concentration (NR/SR)	1.5/5–7	2.3/5–11	0.5/5
Half-life (h)	3–7/10–12	3–5/6–7	2–5/5–7
Half-life in massive overdose (h)	10–12	8–9	7–8
Absorption (%)	>90	>90	>90
Vd (L/kg)	4	5	1.2
Protein binding (%)	90	80–90	90
Predominant excretion route	(1) Hepatic (2) Renal	Hepatic	Renal
Active metabolite	Yes (20%)	Yes (25–50%)	No
Heart rate (%)	−10	−15	+10
Systemic vascular resistance (%)	−10	−10	−20
AV node conduction velocity (%)	−20	−25	+10

NR, normal release; SR, slow release

Table 28.3.2 Pharmacological profiles of the β-blockers (*Adapted from:* Kerns W II, Kline J, Ford MD 1994 β-blocker and calcium channel blocker toxicity. Emergency Medicine Clinics of North America 12: 365–389)

Agent	β_1 selective	Membrane stabilization	Absorption (%)	Protein binding (%)	Volume of distribution (L/kg)	Elimination/ half-life (h)	Lipophilic
Atenolol	Yes	No	50	<5	0.6–1.1	Renal/6–9	Weak
Carvedilol	No	Yes	25	98	2	Hepatic/6	Weak
Esmolol	Yes	No	NA	55	3.4	Blood esterase 9 min	Weak
Labetalol	No	No	90	50	5.1–9.4	Hepatic/3–4	Weak
Metoprolol	Yes	No	90	12	5.6	Hepatic/3–4	Moderate
Oxyprenolol	No	Yes	90	80	1.2	Hepatic/2–3	Moderate
Pindolol	No	Yes	90	57	1.2–2	Renal/3–4	Moderate
Propranolol	No	Yes	90	93	3.4–6	Hepatic/3–4	High
Sotalol	No	No	70	0	0.23–0.7	Renal/9–10	Weak
Timolol	No	No	90	10	1.3–3.6	Renal/4–5	Weak

Blockade of β-receptors results in increased intracellular cAMP concentrations, with a resultant blunting of the metabolic, chronotropic and inotropic effects of catecholamines. Some β-blockers, especially propranolol, may also impede sodium entry via myocardial fast inward sodium channels, thus slowing phase 0 of the action potential. This results in a prolonged QRS duration on the electrocardiogram and makes the drugs potentially more toxic in overdose.

The different β-blockers have slightly differing pharmacological properties, including selectivity for β-adrenoreceptors, intrinsic sympathomimetic activity, and membrane-stabilizing activity. The relative affinity for β-adrenoreceptors may influence expression of toxicity. Atenolol, esmolol and metoprolol are β_1-selective agents, and therapeutic use of these drugs is less likely to produce the peripheral vasoconstriction, bronchospasm and disturbances in glucose homoeostasis that result from β_2 inhibition. However, pharmacological specificity decreases with increasing dose.[3] Several β-blockers have partial agonist activity such that, although they block the β-receptor to catecholamines, they also weakly stimulate the receptor. This partial agonist activity may have a protective effect in overdose.

CLINICAL PRESENTATION

Calcium channel blockers

The severity of toxicity is determined by a number of factors, including the amount and characteristics of the drug ingested, the underlying health of the patient, coingestants, and delay until treatment. The majority of serious cases result from the ingestion of verapamil, the most toxic of the CCBs. Elderly patients and those with congestive cardiac failure are more prone to develop CCB poisoning. The principal clinical features are shown in Table 28.3.3. Ingestion of toxic amounts of standard preparations typically produces symptoms within 2 hours, although maximal toxicity may not occur for up to 6–8 hours. The slow-release preparations can produce significant toxicity, with onset of symptoms more than 6 hours post ingestion. The major threats to life are myocardial depression and hypotension. Nifedipine produces tachycardia with normal blood pressure during the first 30 minutes, followed later by hypotension and bradycardia in large ingestions (>10 mg/kg). With verapamil and diltiazem poisoning, nausea, vomiting, hyperglycaemia and metabolic acidosis can develop. All CCBs can cause symptoms of cerebral hypoperfusion, such as syncope, lethargy, lightheadedness, dizziness, altered mental status, seizures and coma.

β-blockers

In one large series of patients with β-blocker overdose, 30–40% of patients remained asymptomatic and only 20% developed severe toxicity.[4] Toxicity is more likely to develop after ingesiton of propranolol, in patients with pre-existing cardiac disease or where there is co-ingestion of other drugs with effects on the cardiovascular system, especially calcium channel blockers and cyclic antidepressants.[4,5] If β-blocker toxicity is to develop, it is usually observed within 6 hours of ingestion.[5,6]

Sinus node suppression and conduction abnormalities and decreased contractility are typical. First-degree AV block, AV dissociation, right bundle branch block and intraventricular conduction delay have been reported. Prolongation of the QRS interval may occur with those β-blocking drugs that have membrane-stabilizing effects, such as propranolol.

Sotalol has both β-blocker activity and class III antiarrhythmic properties. Class III drugs lengthen the duration of the QT interval owing to prolongation of the action potential in His-Purkinje tissue. Therefore, ventricular arrhythmias are more common with sotalol.

Hypotension occurs as a result of negative inotropic effect. In addition, CNS effects, such as depressed conscious level and seizures, can occur, especially with the more lipid-soluble and membrane-depressant agents such as propranolol. Hypoglycaemia is reported following atenolol overdose.

INVESTIGATIONS

The ECG is essential in evaluating and monitoring toxic conduction defects. Serum drug levels are unhelpful in management. Patients with severe toxicity require monitoring of serum electrolytes and glucose. Serum calcium must be closely monitored if calcium salts are administered therapeutically.

MANAGEMENT

The primary aim in both β-blocker and CCB toxicity is to restore perfusion to vital organs by increasing cardiac output, and the methods used are similar.

Supportive management may include airway and ventilatory support, intravenous fluid administration, transcutaneous or transvenous pacing, and administration of inotropes. Severe cases may require placement of a Swan-Ganz catheter and invasive blood pressure monitoring.

Oral activated charcoal should be administered as soon as practicable to all patients presenting within 2–4 hours of ingestion, and to all those presenting after ingestion of slow-release preparations. More aggressive decontamination, with whole-bowel irrigation, is indicated

---

Table 28.3.3 Clinical features of CCB overdose

Central nervous system
Lethargy, slurred speech, confusion, coma
Respiratory arrest
Coma

Gastrointestinal
Nausea, vomiting

Cardiovascular
Hypotension
Bradycardia and other arrhythmias
Sinus bradycardia
Accelerated AV nodal rhythm
2° AV block
3° AV block with AV nodal or ventricular escape rhythm
Sinus arrest with AV nodal escape rhythm
Asystole

Metabolic
Hyperglycaemia
Lactic acidosis

Table 28.3.4 Useful drugs in the management of CCB and β-blocker toxicity

	CCB	β-Blocker
Calcium	1–3 g CaCl$_2$ (10–30 mL 10%) followed by an infusion of 20–50 mg/kg/h of CaCl$_2$ in normal saline	
Catecholamines	Adrenaline (epinephrine) infusion started at 1 μg/kg/min and titrate to maintain organ perfusion	Isoprenaline or adrenaline (epinephrine) infusion titrated to maintain organ perfusion
Glucagon	A bolus dose of 5–10 mg followed by an infusion of 1–5 mg/h	A bolus dose of 5–10 mg followed by an infusion of 1–5 mg/h

following overdose with slow-release CCBs.[7]

A number of drugs play a role in the management of significant CCB or β-blocker poisoning, although none is a completely effective antidote. Suggested doses are shown in Table 28.3.4. Calcium, an inotropic agent, is the initial drug of choice for CCB toxicity. Administration must be closely monitored, with ionized calcium measured 30 minutes after commencing the infusion, and then second-hourly.[8] Catecholamines are useful in attempting to restore adequate tissue perfusion. Glucagon, a polypeptide hormone of pancreatic origin, enhances myocardial performance by increasing intracellular cAMP concentrations. This increase in cAMP triggers the release of cAMP-dependent protein kinase, which activates the calcium channels, causing an increase in heart rate and myocardial contractility. It works independently from that of the β-adrenoceptor stimulation of the heart.

There are no clinically effective methods of enhancing the elimination of CCBs or β-blockers.

DISPOSITION

Following overdose of β-blockers or standard CCBs, patients should be observed in a monitored environment for at least 6 hours. Overdoses of slow-release CCBs require monitoring for at least 16 hours from the time of ingestion. All symptomatic patients should be admitted to a monitored environment until toxicity resolves.

CONTROVERSIES

❶ Studies in canine models has suggested a role for high-dose insulin and dextrose therapy in both β-blocker and CCB toxicity.[9–11] Initial case reports of its use in human verapamil poisoning are encouraging.[12] The recommended initial dose of actrapid is 0.1–0.2 U/kg IV followed by an infusion of 0.2–1.0 U/kg/hour. This should be accompanied by an initial bolus dose of 25–50 mL 50% dextrose followed by an infusion to maintain euglycaemia.[12]

❷ There are reports of the successful use of cardiopulmonary bypass to maintain an adequate cardiac output until such time as hepatic metabolism of the drug occurs following severe β-blocker overdose.[13] Techniques such as this and extracorporeal membrane oxygenation (ECMO) may play a role in the management of otherwise fatal cases of cardiovascular collapse.

DIGOXIN

INTRODUCTION

Both chronic and acute digoxin toxicity are potentially life-threatening presentations to the emergency department. Early recognition and administration of the specific *Fab* fragment antidote, if indicated, usually results in a good outcome.

PHARMACOKINETICS

Digoxin is moderately well absorbed following oral administration, with a bio-availability in the range of 50–80%. The initial volume of distribution is relatively small, but it is then slowly redistributed, predominantly to skeletal muscle, to give a relatively large volume of distribution of approximately 8 L/kg. Digoxin is excreted predominantly unchanged by the kidney, with an elimination half-life of about 36 hours.

PATHOPHYSIOLOGY

At a subcellular level digoxin inhibits the function of Na-K ATPase, which leads to intracellular depletion of potassium and accumulation of sodium and calcium ions. Alteration of ionic fluxes affects cell membrane conduction. At toxic concentrations of digoxin the effects on the cardiac conducting system produce decreased conduction velocity throughout the system, increased refractoriness at the AV node, and enhanced automaticity of the Purkinje fibres. Vagal tone is also enhanced. In acute digoxin poisoning the sudden loss of Na-K ATPase function produces hyperkalaemia.

CLINICAL PRESENTATION

Two distinct clinical presentations of digoxin toxicity are observed: acute and chronic. Both are characterized by cardiac arrhythmias, and virtually all types of arrhythmia have been reported in the context of digoxin toxicity.[14]

Acute digoxin overdose in adults is usually intentional. The therapeutic margin for digoxin is relatively narrow, and any ingestion with suicidal intent is regarded as potentially life-threatening.

The non-cardiac manifestations of toxicity are nausea and vomiting and hypokalaemia. Nausea and vomiting occur early and may be the presenting complaint. The most common cardiac manifestations are sinus bradycardia, sinoatrial node arrest, and first-, second-, or third-degree heart block. Ventricular tachycardia and fibrillation may occur. In significant acute overdose progressive worsening of the conduction disturbance over a period of hours is usually observed.

Chronic digoxin toxicity may be precipitated by therapeutic errors, intercurrent illnesses that decrease renal elimination of digoxin, or by drug interactions. Common drug interactions include those with quinidine, calcium channel blockers, amiodarone and indometacin. The patient is commonly elderly. Reduced muscle mass and reduced renal function in the elderly mean that both the volume of distribution and rate of elimination of digoxin may be substantially reduced.

Nausea and vomiting are also common manifestations of chronic digoxin toxicity and are frequent presenting symptoms. Neurological manifestations are characteristic of chronic toxicity and include visual disturbances, weakness and fatigue. The most common cardiovascular manifestations of chronic digoxin toxicity are arrhythmias, and these may be sinus bradycardia, atrial fibrillation with slowed ventricular response or a junctional escape rhythm, atrial tachycardia with block, and ventricular tachycardia and fibrillation.

Death from digoxin toxicity results from pump failure, severe cardiac conduction impairment or ventricular arrhythmia.

INVESTIGATIONS

The most important investigations are the ECG, serum electrolytes and creatinine, and serum digoxin concentration.

The ECG is invaluable in documenting the type and severity of any cardiac conduction defect. Serial ECGs may demonstrate worsening of the cardiac conduction defects as toxicity progresses.

In acute poisoning the serum potassium rises as Na-K ATPase function is progressively impaired. Hyperkalaemia denotes significant acute digoxin toxicity. Prior to the availability of a specific antidote for digoxin poisoning, a serum

potassium concentration greater than 5.5 mEq/L was associated with a high probability of lethal outcome.[15] Hyperkalaemia is not usually observed in chronic digoxin toxicity. In fact, these patients are frequently hypokalaemic and hypomagnesaemic secondary to chronic diuretic use. Both these electrolyte disorders are important as they exacerbate digoxin toxicity.

Serum digoxin concentrations are extremely useful in assessing and confirming toxicity, but must be carefully interpreted in the context of the clinical presentation. They do not accurately correlate with clinical toxicity. Therapeutic concentrations are usually quoted as 0.6–2.3 nmol/L (0.5–1.8 µg/L). Significant chronic toxicity may be associated with relatively minor elevations of the serum digoxin concentration. This is particularly the case in the presence of pre-existing cardiac disease, hypokalaemia or hypomagnesaemia. Following acute overdose the serum digoxin concentration is relatively high compared to tissue concentrations, until distribution is completed by 6–12 hours post ingestion. However, early concentrations greater than 15 nmol/L indicate serious poisoning.

MANAGEMENT

The best outcome is associated with early recognition of digoxin toxicity.

For chronic non-life-threatening toxicity management may involve no more than observation, cessation of digoxin administration, correction of hypokalaemia and hypomagnesaemia, and appropriate management of any factors that contributed to the development of toxicity. However, presence of any haemodynamically significant cardiac arrhythmia is an indication for the administration of *Fab* fragments of digoxin-specific antibodies.

Following acute overdose the patient should be initially managed in a monitored area with full resuscitative equipment available. Immediate attention to the airway, breathing and circulation may be required. Intravenous access should be established and blood sent for

urgent electrolytes and serum digoxin concentration. Although digoxin is well bound by charcoal, administration is usually difficult because of repetitive vomiting, and attempts should not detract from other interventions.

The specific antidote to digoxin poisoning is *Fab* fragments of digoxin-specific antibodies, which should be administered as soon as possible in any potentially life-threatening digoxin intoxication. Commonly accepted indications for the administration of *Fab* fragments are listed in Table 28.3.5.

Fab fragments of digoxin-specific antibodies

These are derived from IgG antidigoxin antibodies produced in sheep. Removal of the *Fc* fragments of the antibodies greatly reduces the potential for hypersensitivity reactions and contributes to the remarkable safety profile of the product. Intravenously administered *Fab* fragments bind digoxin in the intravascular space on a mole-for-mole basis. As binding continues, digoxin moves down a concentration gradient from the tissue compartments to the intravascular compartment. Bound digoxin is inactive. A clinical response is usually observed within 20–30 minutes of administration. The *Fab*-digoxin complexes are excreted in the urine.

The extraordinary clinical efficacy of digoxin-specific fragments has been well documented in a multicentre study.[16] The same study also demonstrated the safety of the product, with the only adverse reactions reported being hypo-

Table 28.3.5 Indications for administration of *Fab* fragments of digoxin-specific antibodies
Hyperkalaemia (K >5.0 mmol/L) associated with digoxin toxicity
History of ingestion of more than 10 mg of digoxin
Haemodynamically unstable cardiac arrhythmia
Cardiac arrest from digoxin toxicity
Serum digoxin concentration greater than 15 mmol/L

kalaemia (4% incidence) and worsening of congestive cardiac failure (3%).

The correct dose of *Fab* fragments may be calculated on the basis that 40 mg (1 vial) will bind 0.6 mg of digoxin. If the dose ingested is unknown and/or a steady-state serum digoxin concentration is not available, dosing of *Fab* fragments must be empiric. Following acute overdose a reasonable approach to empiric dosing is to give 5 vials initially and then repeat until a clinical response is observed. Smaller doses (2–4 vials) are usually sufficient for chronic toxicity.

It is important that emergency department staff are aware of the amount and location of supplies of *Fab* fragments within their own institution, and know the most rapid way to acquire further stocks should the need arise.

Serum digoxin concentrations will be extremely high following the administration of *Fab* fragments because most assays measure both bound and unbound digoxin.

DISPOSITION

Patients with mild, chronic digoxin toxicity (gastrointestinal symptoms only) may be discharged after cessation of digoxin therapy provided there are no significant electrolyte disturbances, renal failure or other precipitating medical conditions. Following administration of *Fab* fragments, cases of chronic toxicity with conduction defects usually require medical admission for observation and treatment of intercurrent illness.

CONTROVERSIES AND FUTURE DIRECTIONS

❶ As experience with the use of digoxin-specific fragments increases, the threshold for administration has lowered. In the past, concerns about the safety and expense of treatment have limited their use. The cost of the fragments should be weighed against the costs of additional in-hospital care that may be incurred if they are withheld.

Acute overdoses require close observation for at least 12 hours. Those that develop toxicity require admission and an appropriate level of monitoring. Following successful administration of digoxin-specific *Fab* fragments, patients must be carefully monitored for hypokalaemia and worsening of any underlying medical conditions for which digoxin may have been prescribed therapeutically. All intentional ingestions require psychiatric evaluation prior to medical discharge.

REFERENCES

1. Robertson RM, Robertson D 1996 Drugs used for the treatment of myocardial ischaemia. In: Gilman AG, Hardman JG, Limbird LE, et al (eds) Goodman and Gilman's: The Pharmacological Basis of Therapeutics, 9th edn. Pergamon Press, New York, p. 770
2. Antman EM, Stone PH, Muller JE, Braunwald E 1980 Calcium channel blocking agents in the treatment of cardiovascular diseases: Part E Basic

and clinical electrophysiological effects. Annals of Internal Medicine 93: 875–85
3. Lewis RV, McDevitt DG 1986 Adverse reactions and interactions with beta-adrenoceptor blocking drugs. Medical Toxicology 1: 343–61
4. Taboulet P, Cariou A, Berdeaux A, Bismuth C 1993 Pathophysiology and management of self-poisoning with beta-blockers. Journal of Toxicology and Clinical Toxicology 31: 531–51
5. Reith DM, Dawson AH, Epid D, Whyte IM, Buckley NA, Sayer GP 1996 Relative toxicity of beta blockers in overdose. Journal of Toxicology and Clinical Toxicology 34: 273–8
6. Love J, Howell JM, Litovitz TL, Klein-Schwartz W 2000 Acute beta blocker overdose: Factors associated with the development of cardiovascular morbidity. Journal of Toxicology and Clinical Toxicology 38: 275–81
7. Buckley N, Dawson AH, Howarth D, Whyte IM 1993 Slow release verapamil poisoning. Use of polyethylene glycol whole bowel lavage and high dose calcium. Medical Journal of Australia 158: 202
8. Pertoldi F, D'Orlando L, Mercante WP 1998 Electromechanical dissociation 48 hours after atenolol overdose: usefulness of calcium chloride. Annuals of Emergency Medicine 31:777–81
9. Kerns W, Schroeder D, Williams C, Tomaszewski C, Raymond R 1997 Insulin improves survival in a canine model of acute beta-blocker toxicity. Annals of Emergency Medicine 29: 748–57
10. Kline JA, Tomaszewski CA, Schroeder JD, Raymond RM 1993 Insulin is a superior antidote for cardiovascualr toxicity induced by verapamil in the anesthetized canine. Journal of Pharmacology and Experimental Therapeutics 267: 744–50
11. Kline JA, Leonova E, Raymond RM 1995 Beneficial myocardial metabolic effects of insulin during verapamil toxicity in the anesthetized canine. Critical Care Medicine 23: 1251–63
12. Yuan I, Kerns WP, Tomaszewski CA, et al 1999 Insulin-glucose as adjunctive therapy for severe calcium channel antagonist poisoning. Journal of Toxicology and Clinical Toxicology 37: 463–74
13. McVey FK, Corke CF 1991 Extracorporeal circulation in the management of massive propranolol overdose. Anaesthesia 46: 744–6
14. Moorman JR, Pritchett ELC 1985 The arrhythmias of digitalis intoxication. Archives of Internal Medicine 145: 1289–92
15. Bismuth C, Gaultier M, Conso F, et al 1973 Hyperkalemia in acute digitalis poisoning: prognostic significance and therapeutic implications. Clinical Toxicology 6: 153–62
16. Antman EM, Wenger FL, Butler VP et al 1990 Treatment of 150 cases of life threatening digitalis intoxication with digoxin specific *Fab* antibody fragments: final report of multicenter study. Circulation 81: 1744–52

28.4 CENTRAL NERVOUS SYSTEM DRUGS

GEORGE BRAITBERG • FERGUS KERR

ESSENTIALS

1 Benzodiazepine overdose is associated with low lethality, with deaths limited to those cases involving coingestions.

2 The non-benzodiazepine sedatives and hypnotics exhibit a somewhat different toxicity profile.

3 The antipsychotics, at therapeutic doses, are associated with numerous adverse effects, including extrapyramidal movement, neuroleptic malignant syndrome, seizures, hypotension, agranulocytosis and priapism. They are generally associated with low lethality in overdose.

4 The newer atypical antipsychotics have an improved adverse effect profile and are relatively benign in overdose.

5 Tricyclic antidepressant (TCA) overdose remains a major cause of morbidity and death.

6 TCAs have multifactorial effects on the nervous and cardiovascular systems.

7 The specific treatment of TCA cardiotoxicity is sodium bicarbonate.

8 The selective serotonin reuptake inhibitors are associated with the serotonin syndrome, both following overdose and as an interaction with other serotonergic drugs.

9 The anticonvulsants, carbamazepine and sodium valproate, have specific toxicity and are potentially life-threatening in overdose.

INTRODUCTION

Pharmaceuticals used to treat CNS and psychiatric conditions are frequently taken in overdose. The manifestations of toxicity include systems other than the CNS. This chapter discusses those agents from this group most frequently taken in overdose including the sedative-hypnotics, antipsychotics, antidepressants and anticonvulsants.

BENZODIAZEPINES

PHARMACOLOGY

Benzodiazepines possess a shared structure comprising a benzene ring fused to a diazepine ring. The pharmacologically significant benzodiazepines also demonstrate a 5-aryl substituent.

Most benzodiazepines are highly lipid soluble and rapidly absorbed following oral administration. The more water-soluble agents, such as temazepam and oxazepam, are more slowly absorbed. Following ingestion, peak plasma concentrations are reached within 90 minutes for midazolam and diazepam, compared to 120–180 minutes for temazepam and oxazepam. Following intramuscular injection absorption of benzodiazepines is often erratic, except for lorazepam and midazolam.

Plasma protein binding is variable. Diazepam has the highest (99%) and alprazolam the lowest (70%) plasma protein binding. The unbound fraction is able to cross the blood–brain barrier and interact with specific receptors in the CNS. Benzodiazepines are widely distributed to the body tissues, with volumes of distribution ranging from 0.3 to 5.5 L/kg.

The duration of action for benzodiazepines depends on a number of factors, including the rate of redistribution from the CNS compartment to the body tissues, the metabolism and excretion of the drug, and the sensitivity of the benzodiazepine receptor to its agonist. Drugs that are lipophobic tend to have a shorter measured plasma half-life but a longer duration of action. This reflects slower redistribution from the CNS compartment. Lipophilic drugs rapidly redistribute, and, therefore, have a rapid onset of CNS effect, but of relatively short duration. Redistribution to body fat and muscle stores results in a relatively longer plasma half-life. Repeated dosing with lipophilic benzodiazepines eventually saturates peripheral body stores and this 'stored' drug may then leach out resulting in prolonged pharmacological activity.

The metabolism of most benzodiazepines includes both phase I oxidative and phase II conjugative processes, with phase I producing pharmacologically active metabolites. The major metabolite of diazepam is desmethyldiazepam, which is pharmacologically active and has a longer half-life than its parent compound. Lorazepam, temazepam and oxazepam only undergo phase II metabolism.

γ-Aminobutyric acid (GABA) is an inhibitory neurotransmitter found predominantly in the basal ganglia, the hippocampus, hypothalamus, cerebellum and the dorsal horn of the spinal cord.[1] GABA interacts with two receptors, GABA-A and GABA-B, resulting in the influx of chloride through a ligand-gated ion channel. The former receptor is the predominant site of benzodiazepine action. By binding to the GABA-A receptor complex at a specific site, benzodiazepines enhance the binding of GABA at GABA-A, which in turn opens more chloride channels, and hence produces their sedative, hypnotic, anxiolytic and anticonvulsant effects. GABA-B is mainly involved in feedback mechanisms and the control of muscle tone. GABA receptor subunits have been identified, and the sensitivity and specificity of individual benzodiazepines is determined by their interaction with these subunits. Tolerance develops to most of the effects of benzodiazepines, and may be associated with downregulation of GABA receptors.

CLINICAL PRESENTATION

Adverse effects

The various benzodiazepines share a common adverse effect profile. These effects vary in severity between individuals and tend to be more pronounced in the elderly. Common adverse effects include drowsiness, motor incoordination, amnesia, headache, nausea, vomiting and blurred vision. Long-acting agents such as diazepam may produce more residual lethargy and drowsiness. Conversely, rebound insomnia is associated with short-acting benzodiazepines such as temazepam. More unusual side effects include the unmasking of disinhibited and sometimes violent behaviour. Long-term use of benzodiazepines may also be associated with irreversible deficits in cognition. Parenteral admininstration of benzodiazepines has been associated with life-threatening reactions, including respiratory arrest, cardiac arrest and hypotension. This usually occurs following too-rapid parenteral administration of an excessive dose and may in part be related to the propylene glycol diluent.

Overdose

Death as a result of pure benzodiazepine overdose is very uncommon.[2] When death is reported, it is usually in the setting of a mixed overdose including other CNS depressants such as alcohol, antidepressants, phenothiazines and narcotics. The most common manifestation of overdose is drowsiness, which may progress to stupor depending on patient characteristics, coingestants and

dose. Coma is uncommon. Other features characteristic of benzodiazepine overdose are respiratory depression, hypothermia and hypotension, though these are not usually life threatening.[3] The duration of effect varies from 6 hours to 36 hours, depending on the drug.

Respiratory insufficiency in the setting of benzodiazepine overdose may be due to an increase in upper airway resistance and work of breathing rather than central apnoea.[4]

Acute alcohol ingestion tends to delay benzodiazepine metabolism whereas chronic alcohol ingestion induces metabolic pathways and may increase clearance rates of these drugs.[5]

MANAGEMENT

The management of benzodiazepine overdose is supportive, with careful attention to the patient's airway, ventilation and circulatory status. Consideration should be given to the administration of activated charcoal in those who present within 1 hour of ingestion. Patients should be assessed for the presence of coingestants, including paracetamol, alcohol and antidepressants. Those who are able to walk safely and who have normal vital signs can be medically cleared at 4–6 hours post ingestion, providing there are no complicating factors such as aspiration. Hypotension, if present, is usually mild and responds to intravenous fluid replacement.

Specific quantitative laboratory assays for individual benzodiazepines are available in some large centres, but they offer no clinical utility and should not be routinely performed. Clinical effects correlate very poorly with blood levels. Qualitative urine screens are readily available but are subject to a relatively high false-negative rate. They do offer some assistance in the setting of an unknown overdose or an unconscious patient.

Because of the high tissue-protein binding and high volume of distribution of most benzodiazepines, techniques of enhanced elimination such as haemodialysis and haemoperfusion are not

CONTROVERSIES

❶ The role of flumazenil, a specific benzodiazepine receptor antagonist, remains controversial. Flumazenil is reported to cause ventricular tachycardia, elevation of intracranial pressure in head-injured patients, precipitation of acute withdrawal in benzodiazepine-dependent patients, and seizures in those with coingestants that lower the seizure threshold.[6,7]

❷ Use of flumazenil is not associated with any reported change in the mortality or morbidity of benzodiazepine overdose.[8]

❸ Flumazenil may have a role as a diagnostic agent to confirm a benzodiazepine overdose, in the reversal of postoperative benzodiazepine-induced sedation, and in the management of patients with a pure benzodiazepine overdose who would otherwise require intubation.

effective. In any case, the relatively benign clinical course makes such aggressive intervention inappropriate.

CONCLUSION

Benzodiazepines have a wide safety margin, and death from isolated overdoses is very rare. The treatment is supportive.

NON-BENZODIAZEPINE SEDATIVE-HYPNOTICS

PHARMACOLOGY

Sedative and hypnotic effects are thought to be regulated through the GABA receptor complex, particularly GABA-A receptors. Agonist action at the GABA-A receptor results in longer and/or more frequent opening of the ligand-gated chloride ion channels. The subsequent influx of chloride hyperpolarises the neuron suppressing electrical excitability.

Barbiturates

Like benzodiazepines, barbiturates exert their action at the GABA-A receptor complex. However, barbiturates increase the length of time the chloride channel remains open, rather than increasing the frequency of opening. The CNS-depressant effect of barbiturates is stronger than that of the benzodiazepines. In combination these two types of drug have a synergistic effect.

Preparations of barbiturates are usually alkaline salts, which in turn dictates that the primary site of absorption is the small intestine. The more lipid-soluble barbiturates are taken up into the CNS more rapidly and produce a more rapid effect. Plasma protein binding varies from a high 80% for thiopental (thiopentone) to only 50% for phenobarbital (phenobarbitone). The volume of distribution ranges from 0.6 L/kg to 2.6 L/kg, depending on the agent. Elimination half-lives vary considerably, from only 6 hours for thiopental (thiopentone) to up to 100 hours for phenobarbital (phenobarbitone).

Clomethiazole (chlormethiazole)

Clomethiazole (chlormethiazole) also acts at the GABA-A receptor, but at a different site from that for barbiturates and benzodiazepines. It enhances the effects of glycine and GABA. The potentiation of the effect of glycine is thought to mediate its anticonvulsant properties. Clomethiazole (chlormethiazole) is rapidly absorbed, with peak plasma concentrations appearing within 1 hour of ingestion. There is, however, a large first-pass effect, with the oral bioavailability being as low as 10%. The volume of distribution is large, at between 4 and 12 L/kg. The plasma elimination half-life is approximately 6 hours, but in overdose may increase to as much as 17 hours.[9]

Chloral hydrate

The sedative effects of chloral hydrate are thought to be mediated through GABA-A receptors. Chloral hydrate is rapidly absorbed from the gastrointestinal tract and widely distributed throughout the body. A prodrug, it is metabolized almost entirely by alcohol dehydrogenase in the liver and red blood cells, with a half-life of only 4 minutes. Its active metabolite, trichloroethanol, begins to have a therapeutic effect within 30 minutes of dosing with the parent drug. Trichloroethanol is metabolized to an inactive compound via alcohol dehydrogenase and aldehyde dehydrogenase, with a half-life of approximately 8 hours.

Zopiclone

Zopiclone also acts on the GABA-A receptor complex, but at a separate site to that of the benzodiazepines and barbiturates. Furthermore, unlike the benzodiazepines where the binding to GABA-A receptors is modulated by the presence of GABA itself, the binding of zopiclone is not. It has also been suggested that zopiclone binds to the same receptor site as benzodiazepines, but the resulting conformational change is different.

Zopiclone is rapidly absorbed, with peak plasma concentrations occurring at about 1 hour postingestion. Its volume of distribution is approximately 1.5 L/kg, with a plasma protein binding of only 45%. Only 5% of an ingested dose is excreted unchanged by the kidneys, with most of the drug undergoing hepatic metabolism. The plasma elimination half-life varies between 4 and 7 hours.

Zolpidem

This drug is structurally unrelated to the other sedative-hyponotics, belonging to the imidazopyridine group. It selectively binds to the ω-1 receptor subtype of the GABA-A receptor complex in contrast to the benzodiazepines which bind all 3 ω subtypes. The modulation of the chloride anion channel at this receptor allows preservation of deep sleep. Zolpidem's effects are reversed by flumazenil. The elimination half-life of zolpidem is approximately 2.5 hours, with pharmacological effect lasting up to 6 hours. The volume of distribution in 0.5 L/kg, smaller in the elderly. The main cytochrome P450 enzyme involved in the hepatic biotransformation of zolpidem is CYP3A4. Its metabolites are pharmacologically inactive and are eliminated in the urine and faeces.

CLINICAL PRESENTATION

Barbiturates

Typical effects of barbiturate overdose include a depressed conscious state of varying degrees, including profound coma. Respiratory depression, hypotension, hypothermia and miosis are also observed. Cutaneous bullous lesions may be evident.

Clomethiazole (chlormethiazole)

As with barbiturates, the clinical effects following overdose with clomethiazole (chlormethiazole) include CNS depression including coma, respiratory depression, hypotension and, rarely, cutaneous bullous lesions. Other features more characteristic of clomethiazole (chlormethiazole) toxicity itself include increased salivation, sneezing and eye irritation.[9] Coingestion of ethanol potentiates the toxicity of clomethiazole (chlormethiazole).

Chloral hydrate

As well as CNS and respiratory depression, overdose with chloral hydrate may produce severe gastrointestinal irritation, with haematemesis, gastric ulceration and oesophageal stricture formation. More importantly, chloral hydrate overdose characteristically produces cardiac rhythm disturbances, including simple ventricular ectopics, ventricular tachycardia, torsades de pointes and ventricular fibrillation. Fatalities continue to be reported.[10]

Zopiclone

Overdose with zopiclone produces CNS depression and potentially respiratory depression. First-degree heart block[11] and fatalities are reported.[12,13]

Zolpidem

As with the other sedative-hyponotics, the primary clinical effects observed following zolpidem overdose are CNS and respiratory depression. Pure ingestions of less than 400 mg in adults tend to produce sedation and amnesia only.[14] Fatalities have been ascribed to zolpidem overdose on the basis of postmortem toxicological analyses.[15]

MANAGEMENT

As with the benzodiazepines, the most important aspect of management for patients presenting following an overdose of the other sedative-hypnotic drugs is good supportive care. Careful attention must be paid to maintaining an adequate airway, ventilation and blood pressure. Hypotension usually responds to intravenous fluid administration, but may require administration of inotropes. Activated charcoal should be considered if patients present within 1–2 hours of ingestion. Specific medications may be of use with certain types of overdose. Flumazenil has been shown to reverse the effect of zopiclone, and its use in pure zopiclone overdoses with respiratory depression that might otherwise require intubation should be considered.[16–18] In the setting of chloral hydrate overdose, ventricular arrhythmias may be resistant to usual therapies but will often respond to the use of β-blockers, such as intravenous propranolol.[19,20] Hypoxia and electrolyte disturbances should also be corrected.

Techniques to enhance elimination, such as haemodialysis and haemoperfusion, have been used in the past to manage barbiturate and chloral hydrate overdose. However, with more effective intensive care such techniques are rarely indicated. Alkalinization of the urine and repeat-dose activated charcoal enhance the elimination of phenobarbitone and may be useful in management of significant overdose of this drug.

ANTIPSYCHOTIC DRUGS

INTRODUCTION

The antipsychotics (neuroleptics, major tranquillisers) are a pharmacologically diverse group of drugs, used to treat a wide variety of disorders including psychoses, agitation, nausea, migraine, and extrapyramidal movement disorders.

Pharmacology

This large group of drugs can be classified as typical or atypical (Table 28.4.1), according to structure (Table 28.4.2) or according to neuroreceptor-binding affinity. The latter may offer the most reliable prediction of the risk of toxicity.[21]

Atypical drugs are defined as such on clinical and pharmacological grounds. Clinically, they produce fewer extrapyramidal side effects and tardive dyskinesias. For this reasons the newer atypical antipsychotic agents have largely replaced the traditional agents as first-line treatment of schizophrenia. Pharmacologically, they may be regarded as atypical for a variety of reasons including low D_2-dopamine receptor potency, low D_2-receptor occupancy in the mesolimbic and nigrostriatal areas, and high affinities for M_1-muscarinic, D_1- and D_4-dopamine and 5-HT1A- and 5-HT2A-serotonin receptors.[22] This produces three broad functional groups of atypical antipsychotics: the D_2-, D_3-receptor antagonists such as amisulpiride, the D_2, α_1, 5-HT2A-receptor antagonists such as risperidone, and the the broad spectrum multiple receptor antagonists such as clozapine, quetiapine and olanzapine.[22]

The therapeutic and predominant toxic effects of these drugs are related

Table 28.4.1 Typical and atypical antipsychotic drugs

Typical	Atypical
Chlorpromazine	Mesoridazine
Fluphenazine	Thioridazine
Perphenazine	Clozapine
Prochlorperazine	Olanzapine
Trifluoperazine	Risperidone
Haloperidol	Remoxipride
Thiothixene	Loxapine
Molindone	Quetiapine

Table 28.4.2 Structural classification of the antipsychotics

Structural class		Generic name
Phenothiazines		
	Aliphatic	Chlorpromazine Triflupromazine Promethazine
	Piperazine	Fluphenazine Perphenazine Prochlorperazine Trifluoperazine
	Piperidine	Mesoridazine Thioridazine
Butyrophenone		Haloperidol
Thioxanthene		Droperidol Chlorprothixene Thiothixene
Dihydroindolone		Molindone
Dibenzoxazepine		Loxapine Clozapine Olanzapine
Diphenylbutylpiperidine		Pimozide
Benzisoxazole		Risperidone
Benzamides		Sulpiride Remoxipride

to their blockade of the D_2-subtype dopamine receptors. These are located throughout the brain in the basal ganglia, hypothalamus, pituitary, medulla and the mesocortical and mesolimbic pathways. The antipsychotic effect of a drug is mediated by its blockade of D_2 receptors in the mesocortical and mesolimbic pathways. The development of extrapyramidal effects is closely related to a drug's affinity with D_2 receptors in the basal ganglia. D_2-receptor blockade in the pituitary can cause elevated prolactin levels, with resulting galactorrhoea and gynaecomastia. Blockade of D_2 receptors in the hypothalamus affects body temperature regulation: hypothermia or hyperthermia may result. The strong antiemetic effect of some antipsychotic agents is regulated through D_2-receptor blockade in the medulla.

The blockade of other neuroreceptors and the relative ratio to D_2-receptor blockade predicts the likelihood of adverse effects at therapeutic dosing and in overdose. Blockade of α_1-adrenergic receptors results in postural hypotension of varying degrees, depending on binding affinity. Significant α_2-receptor blockade occurs with clozapine but the clinical importance of this is not clear. H_1-histamine receptor blockade correlates with sedation and, to a lesser extent, hypotension. Sedation, along with delirium, hallucinations, mydriasis, flushing, dry skin, urinary retention and ileus, is seen with M_1-acetylcholine receptor blockade. Agents that possess a relatively higher anticholinergic activity compared to dopaminergic activity have a lower risk for inducing extrapyramidal side effects. Examples include chlorpromazine, thioridazine, clozapine and olanzapine. The reverse is also true: those drugs with a higher dopaminergic effect in relation to their anticholinergic activity have a higher risk of inducing extrapyramidal side effects, e.g. fluphenazine, prochlorperazine and haloperidol. Serotonin antagonism may be an important mechanism in the antipsychotic action and responsible for the low incidence of extrapyramidal side effects seen with the newer atypical antipsychotics such as clozapine and olanzapine. These drugs, which tend to

have a high 5-HT2A antagonism in relation to D_2 antagonism, can be given in smaller doses to produce the same therapeutic effect.

Phenothiazine antipsychotics also have a quinidine-like effect and can produce a variety of ECG changes, both at therapeutic doses and in overdose. Thioridazine and mesoridazine are considered to be the most cardioactive, and also possess calcium channel blocking ability, which may contribute to the cardiotoxicity observed in overdose of these agents.

Generally, the pharmacokinetics of this heterogeneous group of drugs are similar. They are rapidly and well absorbed after oral administration, with peak plasma concentrations occurring between 2 and 4 hours later. Greatly delayed absorption with levels peaking at greater than 100 hours is documented after overdose with thioridazine.[23] Most antipsychotics exhibit a relatively high plasma protein binding of between 75 and 99%, are widely distributed to the tissues, and have high volumes of distribution, ranging from 10 to 40 L/kg. Only about 1% of an ingested dose is excreted unchanged in the urine, with the majority of drug undergoing extensive hepatic metabolism, some with significant enterohepatic circulation.

CLINICAL PRESENTATION

Adverse effects

Adverse effects following therapeutic dosing may be both idiosyncratic or dose-related, and may occur after initiation of the medication in question or late into a course of treatment.

Extrapyramidal movement disorders

Up to 90% of patients receiving antipsychotic medication will experience some extrapyramidal side effects, and these often result in the cessation of treatment.[24] Of the four recognized extrapyramidal syndromes, acute dystonia, parkinsonism and akathisia are reversible and tend to occur early in a course of treatment. Tardive dyskinesia is irrevers-

ible but occurs after months to years of treatment. Clozapine, olanzapine and quetiapine are not associate with extrapyramidal syndromes.[22]

The pathophysiology of acute dystonic reactions is not fully understood, but involves disruption of the dopaminergic-cholinergic-GABA balance in the basal ganglia. Reactions are idiosyncratic and equally frequent following a single therapeutic ingestion or an overdose. Risk factors for developing an acute dystonic reaction following antipsychotic medication are the use of antipsychotic drugs with a high D_2-dopaminergic, low M_1-muscarinic and low 5-HT2A-serotonergic receptor binding affinity; young and male patients; the use of depot preparations; and the recent use of alcohol.[25,26] Reactions may present in varied forms and may be spasmodic or sustained, but are always involuntary. The muscles of the face, trunk and neck are commonly involved, but other sites may also be affected. About half of all cases occur within 48 hours of dosing.[24] The overall incidence of acute dystonic reactions varies considerably: rates of 3.5% have been reported for chlorpromazine, and 16% for haloperidol.[25]

Akathisia is dose-related, can occur at any age, and tends to appear some days after beginning treatment. It is thought to be due to D_2-dopaminergic blockade in the mesocortical pathways.[27] Drug-induced parkinsonism is more common in the elderly and tends to be seen with high-potency agents that block the postsynaptic D_2-dopaminergic receptors in the nigrostriatal area. Tardive dyskinesia appears after months or years of antipsychotic treatment. It is seen with all antipsychotics except clozapine, and has a prevalence of between 27 and 35 % in patients on long-term therapy.[28] It is thought to be the result of an increased number and sensitivity of dopaminergic receptors in the nigrostriatal area of the brain, a response to long-term blockade.

Seizures

Antipsychotic drugs lower the seizure threshold.[29] They also produce EEG changes that vary depending on the agent.[30] Organic brain disease, epilepsy, drug-associated seizures and polypharmacy are risk factors for the development of seizures. They are more likely with chlorpromazine, clozapine and loxapine.

Cardiovascular

Postural hypotension and ECG changes can occur with therapeutic dosing of antipsychotics. Postural hypotension is multifactorial, with α_1-adrenergic blockade, central vasomotor reflex depression and direct myocardial depression all playing a part. ECG changes can be diverse, with QRS and QT prolongation, a right axis shift, ST segment depression and T-wave inversion/flattening. QT prolongation is less evident with the newer atypical antipsychotics.[31] Torsades de pointes is reported following high therapeutic dosing with haloperidol, thioridazine and mesoridazine.

Neuroleptic malignant syndrome

This idiosyncratic adverse reaction to antipsychotic medication therapy is rare. It occurs early in the treatment course or after changes in dose. Neuroleptic malignant syndrome (NMS) has been reported with all typical antipsychotics but is particularly associated with higher potency drugs such as haloperidol and fluphenazine. In the atypical group, NMS has been reported with clozapine, olanzapine and risperidone.[32–34] Pooled data studies suggest the incidence is somewhere between 0.07% and 0.2%, although some have described incidences of up to 12.2%.

Typically, patients are male (male:female ratio 2:1), with symptoms developing over 1–3 days. Risk factors associated with the development of NMS include the use of high-potency agents and depot preparations, organic brain disease, past history of NMS, dehydration, and interactions with other drugs such as lithium and anticholinergics.[35] The characteristic clinical features are a temperature ≥38°C, muscle rigidity, altered consciousness and autonomic dysfunction. Other features that may be seen are an elevated creatine kinase, leucocytosis, elevated hepatic transaminases, renal failure and metabolic acidosis.

There is no specific test to confirm or exclude the diagnosis, which is reliant upon clinical and historical data. Alternative diagnoses must be excluded. The mortality rate has been reduced from ≤30% to 5–11% mainly as a result of improved intensive supportive care.[36] Death is usually secondary to respiratory or cardiovascular failure; however, renal failure secondary to myoglobinuria, arrhythmias, pulmonary embolism and disseminated intravascular coagulation are also reported.

Other

Clozapine is associated with idiosyncratic agranulocytosis. The incidence is between 0.6 and 2.0% and usually occurs within the first 18 weeks of therapy. The mortality rate of clozapine-induced agranulocytosis, once established, is up to 85%.[21] Other phenothiazines have also been associated with agranulocytosis, but with a much lower incidence.

Other unusual adverse effects seen with some phenothiazines include priapism, dermatitis, photosensitivity and cholestatic jaundice.

Overdose

Most patients with serious poisoning display manifestations of cardiovascular and/or CNS toxicity. Isolated antipsychotic overdose is rarely fatal. Peak toxicity is usually seen from 2 to 6 hours following ingestion but may be delayed especially after thioridazine overdose.[23,38] CNS effects vary greatly, depending on individual susceptibility, dose ingested and the presence of coingestants. Lethargy is common to most patients, with effects potentially progressing to confusion, ataxia, coma and seizures. Seizures are more often seen following overdose with loxapine or clozapine, and are usually generalized.[39] Paradoxically, agitation may also be observed, especially in the setting of mixed overdose, and following overdose with clozapine, olanzapine or thioridazine.

Life-threatening cardiotoxicity is unusual, except in the setting of piperidine phenothiazine overdoses, e.g. thioridazine, which is associated with QRS widening, QT prolongation, ventricular

tachycardia and torsade de pointes.[23,40,41] Common cardiovascular effects are hypotension (initially postural) and tachycardia. Uncommon effects are hypertension and bradycardia.

Temperature abnormalities may also occur, and commonly manifest as mild hypothermia. Hyperthermia may be seen in the setting of a high environmental temperature and seizures. Following ingestions of aliphatic and piperidine phenothiazines, clozapine and olanzapine, significant anticholinergic toxicity may occur.

The diagnosis of antipsychotic drug overdose is based on a history of ingestion and the presence of symptoms and signs in keeping with the expected findings, as outlined above. Qualitative serum and urine drug screening can be used to detect the presence of many of the antipsychotic drugs, but a high false-negative rate makes these screens notoriously unreliable. Quantitative levels may also be performed, but the results do not correlate with clinical findings and do affect management. The differential diagnosis of antipsychotic drug overdose includes meningitis and other CNS infections, stroke and head injury, as well as other drug toxicities, including tricyclic antidepressants, sedatives, alcohols, anticholinergic drugs and anticonvulsants. Many other agents have also been reported as causing acute dystonic reactions, including tricyclic antidepressants, antihistamines and anticonvulsants.

MANAGEMENT

The management of antipsychotic drug overdose is essentially supportive. Patients should undergo an initial resuscitation period with a careful airway assessment and, if necessary, endotracheal intubation. Ventilation should be supported with supplemental oxygen and mechanical ventilation if indicated. Hypotension should be treated with Trendelenburg positioning, intravenous fluids and, if resistant, inotropic agents, preferably with some α-agonist properties. All patients should be placed on a cardiac monitor, have a 12-lead ECG recorded and an intravenous cannula inserted, with blood being drawn for full blood examination, electrolytes, creatine kinase and renal function. If paracetamol overdose is suspected appropriate levels should be measured.

Activated charcoal should be administered to all patients unless there has been considerable delay in presentation. Multidose charcoal has not been shown to be of benefit in antipsychotic drug overdose. The use of extracorporeal blood purification techniques to enhance drug elimination are not effective, owing to the large volume of distribution and high tissue-protein binding of these drugs.

Seizures should be treated with benzodiazepines such as diazepam or clonazepam as the first-line agents. For resistant seizure activity phenobarbitone may be needed.

Cardiac arrhythmias should be treated according to advanced cardiac life support protocols. However, type IA antiarrhythmics should be avoided in the setting of QRS widening or conduction abnormalities, as they may exacerbate the toxicity. Serum alkalinization, to a pH of 7.45–7.55, should be performed in the presence of significant QRS widening or life-threatening arrhythmias. Intravenous magnesium and chemical or electrical overdrive pacing may be required to control torsade de pointes.

Acute dystonia

Acute dystonia is generally reversed by the use of an intravenous or intramuscular anticholinergic agent such as benztropine (1–2 mg IV or IM) or diphenhydramine (1 mg/kg IV or IM). Symptoms and signs usually resolve within 10–15 minutes. Repeated doses may be required for resistant cases. Following acute resolution of symptoms in the emergency department the patient should be discharged on oral medication for 2–3 days.

Neuroleptic malignant syndrome (NMS)

NMS is a diagnosis of exclusion, with a CT brain scan, lumbar puncture and routine blood analyses essential to exclude other pathology, especially CNS

CONTROVERSIES

❶ The use of specific agents in the treatment of neuroleptic malignant syndrome is controversial. Given the rarity of NMS, prospective controlled trials have not been, and are unlikely to be, conducted. Benzodiazepines, dantrolene, non-depolarizing muscle relaxants, nifedipine, amantadine and nitroprusside have all been tried, with anecdotal reports highlighting their efficacy. Dantrolene is used to treat NMS-related hyperthermia and rigidity, and is generally given intravenously in the emergency setting. Infusion rates are highly variable, and should be carefully titrated. Dopamine agonists such as bromocriptine and amantadine are often given in conjunction with dantrolene in an attempt to overcome the dopaminergic blockade. In the emergency department an intravenous benzodiazepine in association with cooling measures and rehydration is the most appropriate initial management.

infection. Empiric antibiotics are often necessary until a clearer picture can been gleaned and culture results have returned. Aggressive supportive care is life saving. Neuroleptic agents and other drugs, which may be contributing to the condition, should of course be ceased.

CONCLUSION

Generally, acute poisoning following antipsychotic drug overdose is not in itself life threatening. The management should focus on good supportive care and exclusion of non-toxicological causes of such presentations.

BUPROPION

INTRODUCTION

In Australia, bupropion is supplied in a slow-release preparation and is approved only for its use in smoking cessation. In other countries it has been marketed for many years as an atypical antidepressant with a relatively safe cardiovascular profile.

PHARMACOLOGY

Bupropion is a monocyclic antidepressant with structural similarities to amphetamine and diethylpropion. It is a selective inhibitor of the reuptake of catecholamines with minimal effect on the reuptake of serotonin. It also possesses mild anticholinergic activity.[42] Bupropion is metabolized to hydroxy-bupropion, with plasma protein binding of 84 and 77%, respectively. The elimination half-life of bupropion is between 13 and 20 hours, while that of hydroxy-bupropion is approximately 20 hours. Bupropion is widely distributed with an apparent volume of distribution of approximately 2000 L.[43]

The exact mechanism of action for its antidepressant effect and efficacy in aiding smoking cessation is unknown.

CLINICAL PRESENTATION

Adverse effects

The adverse effects of bupropion are relative mild compared to other antidepressants. Mild hypertension has been noted, but has usually occurred in that already hypertensive.[44] Postural hypotension was has also been observed in sporadic patients.[45] QRS or QT prolongation is not seen with bupropion at therapeutic doses.[46] Neurological side effects occur more commonly with headache, insomnia, agitation and seizures being reported.[46,48] Minor gastrointestinal irritation and priapism are also reported.

Overdose

In a series of 58 cases of bupropion overdose, lethargy, tremor, coma and seizures (21% of pure bupropion poisonings) were common findings.[49] In the same series, tachycardia was observed in 43% of patients but there were no

Table 28.4.3 Tricyclic antidepressants available in Australia
Amitriptyline
Clomipramine
Desipramine
Dothiepin
Doxepin
Imipramine
Nortriptyline
Trimipramine

ECG conduction abnormalities. A number of case reports describe conduction abnormalities, after bupropion overdose but none describe significant arrhythmias.[50–52] A wide complex tachycardia of 124 beats/minute, which resolved after administration of adenosine is described after ingestion of 13.5 g of bupropion.[53] Fatalities have been recorded following bupropion overdose. In one case a 26-year-old male who ingested 23 g of bupropion became hypoxic following recurrent seizure activity and died despite resuscitation after a cardiac arrest.[54] Other reported fatalities have involved co-ingestants including thioridazine, carbamazepine, diphenhydramine and benzodiazepines.[55]

MANAGEMENT

The management of bupropion overdose is essentially supportive, with attention to early gut decontamination with activated charcoal if appropriate. Patients should be monitored for a minimum of 6 hours after ingestion for evidence of QRS/QT prolongation. Seizures are treated along normal lines, with benzodiazepines being the drug of first choice.

CONCLUSION

Bupropion is generally a safe drug in moderate overdose amounts with the predominant complication being seizures. Treatment is supportive.

CONTROVERSIES

❶ The time of onset of first seizure after overdose of bupropion slow release preparations is not yet well established but is probably less than 12 hours. It is prudent to observe these patients in hospital for at least that period of time.

TRICYCLIC ANTIDEPRESSANTS

INTRODUCTION

Tricyclic antidepressants (TCAs) have long been the leading cause of death from prescription drug overdose. However, they are increasingly being replaced in clinical practice by newer agents, which appear to be significantly safer in overdose. The tricyclic antidepressant currently available in Australia are listed in Table 28.4.3. Reported mortality rates for intentional TCA overdose range from 2 to 5%.[56] The vast majority of successful TCA suicides do not reach hospital but die at home.[57] The ingestion of 15–20 mg/kg or more of a TCA is potentially fatal, though there are substantial differences in toxicity within the group. In Australia, doxepin is associated with the greatest lethality.[58]

PHARMACOLOGY

TCAs have a distinct chemical structure, comprised of three aromatic rings. TCAs are non-selective agents that exhibit a large number of pharmacological effects. The therapeutic effect is most likely due to the inhibition of amine reuptake in the CNS, particularly serotonin and dopamine.[59] This effect is not responsible for the toxicity of TCA overdose, but forms the basis of the role of TCAs in the development of serotonin syndrome.[60]

The major features of TCA overdose are related to the following pharmacological actions:

- Anticholinergic effects
- Antihistaminic effects
- Anti-α-adrenergic effects
- Anti-GABAminergic effects
- Sodium channel-blocking effects
- Potassium channel-blocking effects.

TCAs bind to inactivated sodium channels, producing a rate-dependent inhibition of fast sodium channel function. This is thought to be the principal mechanism of TCA-induced cardiotoxicity. Inhibition of sodium entry slows phase 0 depolarization in His-Purkinje and myocardial tissue, and this is reflected in widening of the QRS complex on the 12-lead ECG. This disturbed depolarization, if severe, can lead to cardiac rhythm disturbances and impaired myocardial contractility. TCAs also slow repolarization and phase 4 repolarization, and this is reflected in prolongation of the QT interval on the 12-lead ECG. Peripheral α-adrenergic blockade results in vasodilatation and contributes to the hypotension observed in TCA overdose.

CLINICAL PRESENTATION

The clinical features of TCA overdose include anticholinergic, cardiovascular and CNS effects. The onset of clinical manifestations is usually rapid and, following large ingestions, rapid deterioration in clinical status within 1–2 hours is characteristic.

The clinical features of central and peripheral anticholinergic toxicity are described elsewhere in this book. Anticholinergic delirium is most commonly observed following a modest TCA overdose or early in the course of more significant ingestions. Large overdoses usually lead to coma, which obscures any evidence of anticholinergic delirium. Seizures are characteristic of TCA overdose and usually occur early in the clinical course. Overall the rate is quoted to be 3–4%.[61] Myoclonic jerking is also associated with TCA overdose.

Sinus tachycardia is commonly observed following TCA overdose and is usually due to the anticholinergic effects of the TCA, rather than sodium channel blockade. More serious cardiac arrhythmias can develop as a consequence of the effects on the fast sodium channels and cardiac depolarization and conduction. These include supraventricular tachycardia (with or without aberrancy), ventricular tachycardia, torsades de pointes (augmented by potassium channel blocking effects) and ventricular fibrillation. Junctional or idioventricular rhythms, second- or third-degree heart block or asystole can also occur.[62] Hypotension is commonly observed and is due to both peripheral vasodilatation and impaired myocardial contractility.

INVESTIGATIONS

Serum TCA concentrations correlate poorly with the clinical severity of TCA intoxication. The single most important investigation in assessing the patient following a TCA overdose in the 12-lead ECG. The degree of prolongation of the QRS interval is predictive of the risk of both ventricular arrhythmias and seizures.[63] The positive and negative predictive value of ECG changes in TCA poisoning in one study were 66% and 100% respectively.[64] A QRS duration of greater than 120 ms in the setting of a TCA overdose indicates cardiotoxicity. A patient may exhibit significant CNS toxicity despite a normal ECG.

MANAGEMENT

The management of TCA poisoning is largely supportive. In particular, it involves maintenance of the airway, ventilation and blood pressure, and control of ventricular arrhythmias and seizures.

The potential for rapid deterioration in clinical status must be appreciated and patients with a history of recent TCA overdose should be managed in a closely monitored environment. Intravenous access should be established, supplemental oxygen administered, and cardiac monitoring commenced on arrival. There should be a relatively low threshold

for performing endotracheal intubation in the patient with deteriorating mental status, because hypoxia and acidosis exacerbate cardiotoxicity. Patients with a decreased level of consciousness or anticholinergic symptoms should undergo urinary catheterization.

Gastric emptying may be of value in patients with a significant or life-threatening ingestion and who present within 1 hour.[65,66] Oral activated charcoal should be administered to all patients with significant ingestions after the airway is secured (if necessary). All the TCAs have very large volumes of distribution, and so techniques of enhancing elimination are not helpful.

Hypotension should initially be managed with intravenous fluids. If blood pressure fails to respond to infusions of crystalloid or colloid, then sodium bicarbonate should be tried even in the presence of a normal QRS. If there is still no response inotropes should be started. The ideal inotrope is one that will overcome α-adrenergic blockade and have little stimulatory effect on β receptors. For these reasons, noradrenaline (norepinephrine) is usually regarded as the inotrope of choice. Dopamine is best avoided as it stimulates β receptors (and may lead to a paradoxical decrease in blood pressure) and, as an indirectly acting sympathomimetic, it will become ineffective when neuronal stores of noradrenaline (norepinephrine) are depleted in the presence of a potent reuptake pump inhibitor such as TCAs.[67]

Seizures, delirium and hyperthermia should be controlled using standard techniques.

Flumazenil should be avoided in the setting of a TCA overdose because its action may precipitate refractory seizures and increase morbidity and mortality.[68]

SODIUM BICARBONATE

Sodium bicarbonate is regarded as a specific antidote in the management of TCA poisoning. It offers a hypertonic source of sodium, which competitively overcomes sodium channel blockade. It

appears that the pH alteration also contributes to improved sodium channel function.[69,70] However, manipulation of pH by hyperventilation is not reliably effective in reducing QRS duration.

Sodium bicarbonate is absolutely indicated in the presence of cardiac arrhythmia and may be indicated as a prophylactic measure in the presence if significant widening of the QRS. A loading dose of 50–100 mmol should be given to achieve a pH of 7.50–7.55 (while maintaining PCO_2 below 40 mmHg with appropriate ventilation settings), followed by an infusion of 20–100 mmol/h.[56] Care must be taken to monitor sodium level and arterial blood gases. If arrhythmias persist despite adequate bicarbonate therapy, standard ACLS management should be instituted.

DISPOSITION

Patients with a history of TCA ingestion and who have received oral activated charcoal but show no signs of toxicity after 6 hours of observation are safe for medical discharge and ready for psychiatric evaluation.[71] Those with significant cardiovascular or CNS toxicity should be admitted to an intensive care environment. Those with mild CNS manifestations only should be observed in hospital until these resolve.

CONCLUSION

TCAs are still a major cause of morbidity and mortality. Management is largely supportive; however, specific management includes sodium bicarbonate for severe toxicity.

SELECTIVE SEROTONIN REUPTAKE INHIBITORS (AND ATYPICAL ANTIDEPRESSANTS)

INTRODUCTION

The selective serotonin reuptake inhibitors (SSRIs) have now replaced the

TCAs as the first-line drug therapy for depression bringing with them the advantages of fewer adverse effects and relative safety in overdose. These drugs are also used in the treatment of obsessive-compulsive disorder, panic disorders and bulimia nervosa. Currently available SSRIs together with the atypical antidepressants that modulate serotonin neurotransmission are listed in Table 28.4.4.

PHARMACOLOGY

SSRIs raise synaptic concentrations of serotonin by inhibiting serotonin uptake into presynaptic neurons. In addition, serotonin release from neurons, like other biogenic amines, is subject to autoregulation by presynaptic serotonin receptors that mediate negative feedback. SSRIs desensitize presynaptic serotonin autoreceptors, resulting in increased serotonin release. The rise in synaptic serotonin concentration and resultant stimulation of serotonin receptors (at least 14 different receptors discovered to date) is thought to explain SSRIs' antidepressant activity.[78]

The atypical antidepressants have other effects apart from those on serotonin neurotransmission and these are listed in Table 28.4.4.

The SSRIs and atypical antidepressants are generally rapidly and well absorbed after oral administration. Importantly, an extended release formulation of venlafaxine is widely prescribed. These drugs display diverse elimination patterns and have numerous active metabolites, which results in an extended therapeutic effect but also prolongs the time during which drug interactions and adverse effects can occur.

CLINICAL PRESENTATION

Adverse effects

The most common adverse effects attributed to the SSRIs are gastrointestinal symptoms, sexual dysfunction, headache, insomnia, jitteriness, dizziness and fatigue.[79] Inappropriate antidiuretic hormone secretion is also reported, particularly in the elderly.[80] The adverse effect most likely to result in presentation to the emergency department is the development of serotonin syndrome (see below) as a result of an interaction between two drugs that enhance serotonergic activity or where there has been an insufficient 'wash-out' period between ceasing one such drug and commencing another.

Overdose

Overdose of the SSRIs and atypical antidepressant generally follows a relatively benign course. These drugs have markedly less cardiovascular toxicity in overdose than the TCAs, with the exception of venlafaxine.[62] The major concerns with SSRIs are the adverse interactions and serotonin syndrome.

Serotonin syndrome

Previously known as serotonin behavioural syndrome, this was first described in the late 1960s and early 1970s when rats, after being given a combination of a non-selective monoamine oxidase inhibitor and L-tryptophan, developed resting tremor, rigidity, and abnormal limb, tail and head movements. Subsequent experiments showed that any drug capable of increasing synaptic levels of serotonin could induce a similar syndrome in larger animals. Human reports of recognized serotonin syndrome first appeared in the literature in the early 1980s.[82,83]

Clinically relevant drugs that can increase synaptic serotonin levels and have been implicated in the development of serotonin syndrome are listed in Table 28.4.5. The mechanisms by which these agents increase synaptic serotonin levels in the cortex, lower brain stem and spinal cord regions are variable and described elsewhere. The postsynaptic receptor subtype 5-HT$_{1A}$ appears to be mainly responsible.[78]

Symptoms usually begin shortly after the commencement of a serotoninergic drug, or the administration of two different classes of drugs that increase serotonin levels synergistically, for

Table 28.4.4 Seletive serotonin reuptake inhibitors and atypical antidepressants available in Australia

Selective serotonin reuptake inhibition
Citalopram
Fluoxetine
Fluvoxamine
Paroxetine
Sertraline

Serotonin, noradrenaline (norepinephrine) and dopamine reuptake inhibition
Venlafaxine

Serotonin reuptake inhibition with α-adrenergic antagonism
Nefazodone

Serotonin reuptake inhibition with α$_2$-adrenergic antagonism
Mirtazipine

Table 28.4.5 Serotonergically active drugs by mechanism

Increased serotonin production
Tryptophan

Increased release of stored serotonin
Amphetamines (including, 'ecstasy')
Bromocriptine
Cocaine
L-dopa

Impaired reuptake of serotonin into presynaptic nerve
Dextromethorphan
Mirtazipine
Nefazadone
Pethidine

Selective serotonin reuptake inhibition
Citalopram
Fluoxetine
Fluvoxamine
Paroxetine
Sertraline
Tricyclic antidepressants
Venlafaxine

Inhibition of serotonin metabolism
Monoamine oxidase (MAO) inhibitors
Moclobemide
Non-selective MAO inhibitors
  Phenelzine
  Tranylcypromine

Enhanced post-synaptic serotonin receptor stimulation
Lithium
Lysergic acid diethylamide (LSD)

example lithium and fluoxetine. In addition, potential drug interaction may arise when the appropriate 'change-over' period between drugs is not observed.[84] A severe form of the syndrome may develop some hours following overdose with an SSRI or, more commonly, following overdose with multiple serotonergically active drugs.[85–87]

The diagnosis of serotonin syndrome is clinical and based upon the presence of the triad of alteration in behaviour–cognitive ability, autonomic function and neuromuscular activity. In its most benign form the patient experiences anxiety and apprehension, but altered sensorium with confusion occurs in 50% of reported cases.[78] Seizures may occur.[86] Abnormal neuromuscular activity, caused by increased brain-stem and spinal-cord serotonin levels, manifests as increased rigidity (more in the lower than the upper limbs), hyperreflexia, involuntary jerks and resting extremity tremor. Hyperthermia secondary to increased muscle activity is a common feature and may lead to confusion with neuroleptic malignant syndrome (NMS). Diaphoresis, diarrhoea and rigors are common. Cardiovascular instability may occur. Although most patients recover, fatalities are reported.[86,87] There is no correlation with drug levels, and serotonin syndrome remains a clinical diagnosis.[78]

MANAGEMENT

Management is directed towards withdrawal of the causative agent and the administration of benzodiazepines to decrease muscular rigidity. Benzodiazepines have been reported to non-specifically inhibit serotonin neurotransmission. If hyperthermia is severe more aggressive treatment may be warranted, including neuromuscular paralysis. Seizures should be treated with benzodiazepines or barbiturates.

Non-specific $5\text{-}HT_1$ and $5\text{-}HT_2$ antagonists such as propranolol, cyproheptadine, chlorpromazine and methysergide have been tried.[88–90] There are no controlled trials using these agents, but anecdotally cyproheptadine appears to be effective without the adverse effects of the other drugs.[60] A dose of 4–8 mg 8-hourly is recommended.

Knowledge of this syndrome is important as an increasing number of selective serotonin reuptake inhibitors arrive on the market and the potential for drug interactions between serotoninergic drugs rises. It is important for the clinician to distinguish this syndrome from NMS, acute dystonia, hyperadrenergic states (e.g. cocaine toxicity), anticholinergic syndrome and malignant hyperthermia.

ANTICONVULSANTS

INTRODUCTION

Anticonvulsants are frequently taken in deliberate self-poisoning. Toxicity resulting in emergency department attendance also results as a consequence of therapeutic administration. The benzodiazepines and phenobarbitone are discussed earlier in this chapter. This section discusses the traditional anticonvulsants, carbamazepine, phenytoin and sodium valproate - all of which have important toxic syndromes, and the newer anticonvulsants.

CARBAMAZEPINE

Pharmacology

Carbamazepine is a carbamylated derivative of iminostilbene. It is structurally related to the tricyclic antidepressants but does not share the same cardiotoxicity profile. An extended-release preparation is widely prescribed.

Absorption from the gastrointestinal tract is slow and erractic because of the insoluble lipophillic nature of the drug. Peak concentrations usually occur at 4 to 8 hours but can be greatly delayed after overdose, particularly of the extended-release preparation. The volume of distribution is from 0.8 to 2.0 L/kg. Metabolism occurs in the liver with an active primary metabolite. The drug or metabolites may undergo entrohepatic circulation. Elimination half-life is normally 18–55 hours but may be longer following large overdoses.

Therapeutic carbamazepine concentrations are frequently quoted as 4–12 mcg/mL (17–51 mcmol/L) and are achieved after an oral loading dose of 18 mg/kg. Thus overdoses of greater than this amount may produce toxicity and ingestions of more than 100 mg/kg are likely to be associated with severe toxicity.

Clinical presentation

Onset of clinical features of carbamazepine toxicity may be delayed many hours following overdose due to delayed absorption.[91,92] The clinical features are predominantly neurological and include CNS depression with may progress to coma, drowsiness, ataxia, nystagmus and dystonia. Paradoxical seizures are also reported in severe poisoning.[93,94] Carbamezepine toxicity may also manifest as the anticholinergic syndrome, although the delirium may be masked by coma as the intoxication progresses.

Minor ECG changes may be observed in severe carbamazepine poisoning but significant cardiovascular effects are rare.[95]

Management

Management of carbamazepine toxicity is primarily supportive and in severe cases involving coma this will include intubation and ventilation. The potential for delayed absorption and deterioration must be considered when determining the period of observation and monitoring following carbamazepine overdose. Serial carbamazepine levels are very useful in determining that absorption is complete and that clinical deterioration will not take place. Carbamazepine levels are also useful in confirming the diagnosis of carbamazepine poisoning. Any elevation above the therapeutic range is significant and levels about 40 mg/L are usually associated with coma. Naturally, a low level early after presentation does not exclude carbamazepine overdose.

Administration of activated charcoal is indicated even after delayed presentation and repeat dose charcoal should be considered as it may enhance elimination of carbamazepine and shorten the duration of toxicity and medical care. Patients who present after carbamazepine overdose should be observed for at least 8 hours and have declining carbamazepine levels documented. They may then be medically cleared if asymptomatic. Patients with clinical evidence of poisoning require admission for further observation or supportive care as dictated by the clinical manifestations of poisoning.

PHENYTOIN

Pharmacology

Phenytoin, also known as diphenylhydantoin, is relatively slowly absorbed from the small intestine with peak levels occurring at about 8 hours after a single therapeutic dose but much later following overdose. The volume of distribution is from 0.4 to 0.6 L/kg and the drug is highly bound to plasma proteins. Metabolism occurs in the liver to form inactive metabolites and this metabolism is saturated at relatively low serum concentrations with the result that elimination half-lives are extremely variable.

Clinical presentation

Chronic toxicity

With a relatively low therapeutic index and multiple drug interactions phenytoin toxicity occurs relatively frequently with therapeutic dosing. This is most likely to occur after injudicious dose adjustment.[96,97] These patients usually present with neurological disturbance characterized by ataxia, dysarthria and nystagmus.

Overdose

Similar neurological disturbances are observed following acute overdose, although following large overdoses, a more severe neurological disturbance and even progressive CNS depression may develop. Paradoxical seizures may also occur.[98]

Oral phenytoin overdose is not associated with cardiovascular effects of clinical significance. Cardiotoxicity in the form of hypotension, dysrhythmias and death is only reported followed overrapid administration or excessive doses of intravenous phenytoin.[99] This cardiotoxicity is thought to be due to the propylene glycol diluent rather than the phenytoin *per se*.

Management

Management of chronic phenytoin toxicity consists of simply withdrawing the drug and maintaining the patient in a safe environment until toxicity resolves.

Table 28.4.6 Correlation between serum phenytoin concentration and clinical features	
Phenytoin concentration (mcmol/L)	Clinical features
80–120	Horizontal nystagmus
120–160	Vertical nystagmus, ataxia, dysathria
>160	CNS depression, coma, seizures

The management of phenytoin overdose is principally supportive. A single dose of activated charcoal should be administered in the patient who presents early. Cardiac monitoring is not required where phenytoin is the only agent ingested. Serial phenytoin levels may be useful to confirm the diagnosis and guide therapy. Therapeutic levels are 40–80 mcmol/L (10–20 mg/L). Progressive toxicity albeit with much individual variation is seen as levels extending above that range (Table 28.4.6).

VALPROIC ACID

Pharmacology

Valproic acid is a simple monocarboxylic acid, chemically unrelated to any other class of antiepileptic drug. Its mechanism of action is thought to involve but not be limited to a decrease in breakdown of $GABA_A$ and increased conversion of GABA from glutamate.[100]

Oral absorption of valproic acid is rapid with peak levels usually occurring within 4 hours but this may be delayed following overdose. The volume of distribution is very small at 0.13–0.23 L/kg and there is extensive plasma protein binding which may be saturated in overdose. The drug undergoes extensive hepatic metabolism and has active metabolites. The elimination half-life of 7–15 hours may be prolonged in overdose.

Clinical presentation

The clinical course following valproate overdose is dose-dependent. Ingestions of less than 200 mg/kg are usually asymptomatic or result in minor drowsiness only.[101] For ingestions greater than 200 mg/kg, coma may develop and, for ingestions greater than 400 mg/kg, there is a risk of prolonged profound coma and metabolic disorders including hyper-ammonaemia, hypernatraemia, hypocal-caemia, and bone-marrow depression.[102] Death from cerebral oedema is reported.

Management

Management is primarily supportive. Minor ingestions can usually be simply observed until drowsiness resolves. Ingestions of more than 200 mg/kg should be decontaminated with oral acti-vated charcoal if they present early and then observed closely for CNS depres-sion. This should occur within 4 hours. It is useful to monitor serum levels. Peak levels greater than 1000 mg/L are usually associated with coma. Patients who develop coma will require intuba-tion and intensive care management with careful attention to monitoring electro-lytes, renal function, blood counts and haemodynamics. The coma may persist days after valproate levels fall and in this instance, CT scanning of the head is indicated to look for cerebral oedema.

NEWER ANTIEPILEPTIC DRUGS

A number of new antiepileptic drugs with differing pharmacokinetic proper-ties and mechanisms of action have been introduced into clinical practice over the last decade. These include gabapentin, felbamate, vigabatrin, and topiramate and tiagabine. The toxicity profiles of these drugs in overdose is not yet well established. Gabapentin, felbamate and lamotrigine are reported to cause only minor CNS effects in overdose.[102–104] Vigabatrin overdose has resulted in severe agitation.[105]

REFERENCES

1. Goodchild CS 1993 GABA receptors and benzodiazepines. British Journal of Anaesthesia 71: 127–33
2. Greenblatt DJ, Allen MD, Noel BJ, et al 1977 Acute overdosage with benzodiazepine derivatives. Clinical Pharmacology and Therapy 21: 497–514
3. Busto U, Kaplan HL, Sellers EM 1980 Benzodiazepine-associated emergencies in Toronto. American Journal of Psychiatry 137: 224–7
4. Gueye PN, Lofaso F, Borron SW, et al 2002 Mechanism of respiratory insufficiency in pure or mixed drug-induced coma involving benzodiazepines. Clinical Toxicology 40: 35–47
5. Tanaka E 2002 Toxicological interactions between alcohol and benzodiazepines. Clinical Toxicology 40: 69–75
6. Sugarman JM, Paul RI 1994 Flumazenil: a review. Pediatric Emergency Care 10: 37-43
7. Haverkos GP, DiSalvo RP, Imhoff TE 1994 Fatal seizures after flumazenil administration in a patient with mixed overdose. Annals of Pharmacotherapy 28: 1347–9
8. Krenzelok EP 1993 Judicious use of flumazenil. Clinical Pharmacology 12: 691–2
9. Illingworth RN, Stewart MJ, Jarvie DR 1979 Severe poisoning with chlormethiazole. British Medical Journal 2: 902–3
10. Gaulier JM, Merle G, Lacassie E, et al 2001 Fatal intoxications with chloral hydrate. Journal of Forensic Sciences 46: 1507–9
11. Regouby Y, Delomez G, Tisserant A 1990 First-degree heart block caused by voluntary zopiclone poisoning. Therapie 45: 162
12. Bramness JG, Arnestad M, Karinen R, et al 2001 Fatal overdose of zopiclone in an elderly woman with bronchogenic coma. Journal of Forensic Sciences 46: 1247–9
13. Boniface PF, Russel SG 1996 Two cases of fatal zopiclone overdose. Journal of Analytical Toxicology 20: 131–3
14. Meram D, Descotes J 1989 Acute poisoning with zolpidem. Revue Medicine Interne 10: 466
15. Gock SB, Wong SHY, Nuwayhid N, et al 1999 Acute zolpidem overdose - report of two cases. Journal of Analytical Toxicology 23: 559–62
16. Ahmad Z, Herepath M Ebden P 1991 Diagnostic utility of flumazenil in coma with suspected poisoning. British Medical Journal 302: 292
17. Lheureux P, Debailleul G, De Witte O, et al 1990 Zolpidem intoxication mimicking narcotic overdoses: response to flumazenil. Human and Experimental Toxicology 9: 105–7
18. Lheureux P1998 Continuous flumazenil for zolpidem toxicity - commentary. Clinical Toxicology 36: 745–6
19. Graham SR, Day RO, Lee R, et al 1988 Overdose with chloral hydrate: a pharmacological and therapeutic review. Medical Journal of Australia 149: 686–8
20. Zahedi A, Grant MH, Wong DT Successful treatment of chloral hydrate cardiac toxicity with propranolol. American Journal of Emergency Medicine 17: 490–1
21. Black JL, Richelson E, Richardson JW 1985 Antipsychotic agents: a clinical update. Mayo Clinic Proceedings 60: 777
22. Burns MJ 2001 The pharmacology and toxicology of atypical antipsyhotic agents. Clinical Toxicology 39: 1–14
23. Murray LM Hackett LP, Illet KF 2001 Delayed absorption and peak cardiotoxicity following massive thioridazine overdose. Clinical Toxicology 39: 493
24. Casey DE, Keepers GA 1988 Neuroleptic side effects: acute extrapyramidal syndromes and tardive dyskinesia. In: Casey DE, Christensen AV (eds) Psychopharmacology: Current Trends. Springer-Verlag, New York, pp 74–83
25. Rupniak NJ, Jenner P, Marsden CD 1986 Acute dystonia induced by neuroleptic drugs. Psychopharmacology 88: 403
26. Swett C 1975 Drug induced dystonia. American Journal of Psychiatry 132: 532
27. Marsden CD, Jenner P 1980 The pathophysiology of extrapyramidal side effects of neuroleptic drugs. Psychological Medicine 10: 55
28. Yassa R, Ananth J, Cordozo S, et al 1983 Tardive dyskinesia in an outpatient population: prevalence and predisposing factors. Canadian Journal of Psychiatry 28: 391
29. Marks RC, Luchins DJ 1991 Antipsychotic medications and seizures. Psychiatric Medicine 9: 37
30. Logothetis J 1967 Spontaneous epileptic seizures and electroencephalographic changes in the course of phenothiazine therapy. Neurology 17: 869
31. Reilly JG, Ayis SA, Ferrier IN, et al 2000 QTc-interval abnormalities and psychotropic drug therapy in psychiatric patients. Lancet 355: 1048–52
32. Kariagianis JL, Phillips LC, Hogan KP, et al 1999 Clozapine-associated neuroleptic malignant syndrome: two new cases and a review of the literature. Annals of Pharmacotherapy 16: 192–3
33. Levin GM, Lazowick AL, Powell HS 1996 Neuroleptic malignant syndrome with risperidone. Journal of Clinical Psychopharmacology 16: 192–3
34. Burkhard PR, Vingerhoets FLG 1999 Olanzapine-induced neuroleptic malignant sydnorme (letter). Archives of General Psychiatry 56: 101–2
35. Nierenberg D, Disch M, Manheimer E, et al 1991 Facilitating prompt diagnosis and treatment of the neuroleptic malignant syndrome. Clinical Pharmacology and Therapy 50: 580
36. Shalev A, Hermesh H, Munitz H 1989 Mortality from neuroleptic malignant syndrome. Journal of Clinical Psychiatry 50: 18
37. Safferman A, Lieberman JA, Kane JM, et al 1991 Update on the clinical efficacy and side effects of clozapine. Schizophrenia Bulletin 17: 247
38. Blaye IL, Donatini B, Hall M, et al 1993 Acute overdosatge with thioridazine: a review of the available clinical exposure. Veterinary and Human Toxicology 35:147–50
39. Haag S, Spigset O, Edwardsson H, et al 1999 Prolonged sedation and slowly decreasing clozapine serum concentrations after an overdose. Journal of Clinical Psychopharmacology 19: 282–4
40. Buckley NA, Whyte IM, Dawson AH 1995 Cardiotoxicity is more common in thioridazine overdose than with other neuroleptics. Clinical Toxicology 33: 199–204

CONTROVERSIES AND FUTURE DIRECTIONS

❶ Haemodialysis and charcoal haemoperfusion enhance elimination of valproate but the the clinical value of these therapies has not been established.

❷ L-carnitine has been proposed as an antidote to valproate poisoning but again clinical value has not been established.

❸ Toxicity profiles for the newer anticonvulsants are yet to be established.

41. Schmidt W, Lang K 1997 Life-threatening dysrhythmias in severe thioridazine poisoning treated with physostigmine and transient atrial pacing. Critical Care Medicine 25: 1925–30

42. Bryant SG, Guernsey BG, Ingrim NB 1983 Review of bupropion. Clinical Pharmacology 2: 525–37

43. Lai AA, Schroeder DH 1983 Clinical pharmacokinetics of bupropion: a review. Journal of Clinical Psychiatry 44: 82–4

44. Roose SP, Dalack GW, Glassman AH, et al 1991 Cardiovascular effects of bupropion in depressed patients with heart disease. American Journal of Psychiatry 148: 512–6

45. Szuba MP, Leuchter AF 1992 Falling backward in two elderly patients taking bupropion. Journal of Clinical Psychiatry 53: 157–9

46. Wenger TL, Stern WC 1983 The cardiovascular profile of bupropion. Journal of Clinical Psychiatry 44:176–82

47. Settle EC, Stahl SM, Batey SR, et al 1999 Safety profile of sustained-release bupropion in depression: results of three clinical trials. Clinical Therapeutics 21: 454–63

48. Davidson J 1989 Seizures and bupropion: a review. Journal of Clinical Psychiatry 50: 256–61

49. Spiller HA, Ramoska EA, Krenzelok EP, et al 1994 Bupropion overdose: a 3-year multi-center retrospective analysis. American Journal of Emergency Medicine 12: 43–5

50. Paris PA, Saucier JR 1998 ECG conduction delays associated with massive bupropion overdose. Clinical Toxicology 36: 595–8

51. Shrier M, Diaz JE, Tsarouhas N 2000 Cardiotoxicity associated with bupropion overdose (letter). Annals of Emergerncy Medicine 35: 100

52. Fresh L, Donovan W, Burkhart K, et al 1999 Bupropion toxicity causes wide complex tachycardia (abstract). Clinical Toxicology 37: 635

53. Tracey JA, Ali I, Casey PB, et al 2002 Bupropion (Zyban) toxicity. Internet Medical Journal Toxicology 95: 23–4

54. Harris CR, Gualtieri J, Stark G 1997 Fatal bupropion overdose. Clinical Toxicology 35: 321–4

55. Friel PN, LoganBK, Fligner CL 1993 Three fatal drug overdoses involving bupropion. Journal of Analytical Toxicology 17: 436–8

56. Mills KC 1996 Tricyclic antidepressants. In: Tintinalli JE, Ruiz E, Krome RL (eds) Emergency Medicine: a Comprehensive Study Guide, 4th edn. pp 740

57. Buckley NA, Dawson AH, Whyte IM, McManus P, Ferguson N 1995 Six years of self-poisoning in Newcastle: 1987–1992. Medical Journal of Australia 162: 190–3

58. Buckley NA, Dawson AH, Whyte IM, Henry DA 1994 Greater toxicity of dothiepin in overdose than of other tricyclic antidepressants. Lancet 343: 159–62

59. Curry SC, et al 1994 Neurotransmitter principles. In: Goldfrank LR, Weissman RS, Flomenbaum NE, Howard MA, Lewin NA, Hoffman RS (eds) Goldfrank's Toxicologic Emergencies, 5th edn. Appleton and Lange, Norwalk, Connecticut, pp 231–57

60. Chan BC, Graudins A, Whyte IA, Dawson AH, Braitberg G, Duggan GG 1998 Serotonin syndrome resulting from drug interactions. Medical Journal of Australia 169: 523–5

61. Wedin GP, Odra GM, Klein-Schwartz W, et al 1986 Relative toxicity of cyclic antidepressants. Annals of Emergency Medicine 15: 797

62. Dzuikas LJ, Vohra J 1991 Tricyclic antidepressant poisoning. Medical Journal of Australia 154: 344–50

63. Boehnert MT, Lovejoy FH 1985 Value of the QRS duration versus the serum drug level in predicting seizures and ventricular arrhythmias after an acute overdose of tricyclic antidepresssant. New England Journal of Medicine 313: 474–9

64. Niemann JT et al 1986 Electrocardiographic criteria for tricyclic antidepressant cardiotoxicity. American Journal of Cardiology 57: 1154–9

65. Kulig KW, Bar-Or D et al 1985 Management of acutely poisoned patients without gastric emptying. Annals of Emergency Medicine 14: 562–7

66. Pond SM, Lewis-Driver DJ, Williams G, et al 1995 Gastric emptying in acute overdose: a prospective randomised controlled trial. Medical Journal of Australia 163(7): 345–9

67. Buchamn AL, Dauer J, Giederan J 1990 The use of vasoactive agents in the treatment of antidepressant overdose. Journal of Clinical Psychopharmacology 10: 409–13

68. Spivey WH 1992 Flumazenil and seizures. Analysis of 33 cases. Clinical Therapy 14: 292–305

69. Nattel S, Mittleman M 1984 Treatment of ventricular tachyarrhythmias from amitriptyline toxicity in dogs. Journal of Pharmacology and Experimental Therapy 1231: 430–5

70. Nattel S, Keable H, Sasyniuk BI 1984 Experimental amytriptyline intoxication: electrophysiologic manifestations and management. Journal of Cardiovascular Pharmacology 6: 83–9

71. Callaham M, Kassel D 1985 Epidemiology of fatal tricyclic antidepressant ingestion: implications for management. Annals of Emergency Medicine 14: 1–9

72. Blackman K, Brown SGA, Wilkes GJ 2001 Plasma alkalinisation for tricyclic antidepressant toxicity: a systematic review. Emergency Medicine 13: 204–10

73. Pentel P, Peterson CD 1980 Asystole complicating physostigmine treatment of tricyclic antidepressant overdose. Annals of Emergency Medicine 9: 588–90

74. Vance MA, Ross SM et al 1997 Potentiation of tricyclic antidepressant toxicity by physostigmine in rats. Clinical Toxicology 11: 413–21

75. Callaham M, Schumaker H, Pentel P 1988 Phenytoin prophylaxis of cardiotoxicity in experimental amitriptyline poisoning. Journal of Pharmacology and Experimental Therapy 245: 216–20

76. Pentel PR, Scarlett W, Ross CA, et al 1995 Reduction of desipramine cardiotoxicity and prolongation of survival in rats with the use of polyclonal drug-specific antibody fab fragments. Annals of Emergency Medicine 26: 334–41

77. Dart RC, Sidki A, Sullivan JD, et al 1996 Ovine desipramine antibody fragments reverse desipramine cardiovascular toxicity in the rat. Annals of Emergency Medicine 27: 309–15

78. Mills K. 1993 Serotonin toxicity: a comprehensive review for emergency medicine. Topics in Emergency Medicine 15(4): 54–73

79. Woodrum ST, Brown CS 1998 Management of SSRI-induced sexual dysfunction. Annals of Pharmacotherapy 32: 1209–15

80. Kirchner V, Silver LE, Kelly CA 1998 Selective serotonin reuptake inhiitors and hyponatremia: review and proposed mechanisms in the elderly. Journal of Psychopharmacology 12: 396–400

81. Fantaskey A, Burkhart KK 1995 A case report of venlafaxine toxicity. Clinical Toxicology 33: 359

82. Insel TR, Roy BF, Cohen RM, Murphy DL 1982 Possible development of the serotonin syndrome in man. American Journal of Psychiatry 139: 954–5

83. Sternbach H 1991 The serotonin syndrome. American Journal of Psychiatry 148: 705–14

84. DeVane DL 1992 Pharmacokinetics of the selective serotonin reuptake inhibitors. Journal of Clinical Psychiatry 53(Suppl): 13–19

85. Kaminski CA, Robbbins MS, et al 1994 Sertraline intoxication in a child. Annals of Emergency Medicine 23: 1371–4

86. Kline SS, Mauro LS, Scala-Barnett DM, Zuck D 1989 Serotonin syndrome versus neuroleptic malignant syndrome as a cause of death. Clinical Pharmacology 8: 510–4

87. Power BM, Pinder M, Hackett LP, Ilett KF1995 Fatal serotonin syndrome following a combined overdose of moclobemide, clomipramine and fluoxetine. Anaesthetics and Intensive Care 23: 499–502

88. Guze BH, Baxter LR Jr 1986 The serotonin syndrome: case responsive to propranolol (letter). Journal of Clinical Psychopharmacology 6: 119–20

89. Geer SC, Baldessarini RJ 1980 Motor effects of serotonin in the central nervous system. Life Sciences 27: 1435–51

90. Sandyk R 1980 L dopa induced 'serotonin syndrome' in a parkinsonian patient on bromocriptine (letter). Journal of Clinical Psychopharmacology 6: 194–5

91. Sullivan JB, Rumack BH, Peterson RG 1981 Acute carbamazepine toxicity resulting from overdose. Neurology 31: 621–4

92. Sethna M, Solomon G, Cedarbaum J, Kutt H 1989 Successful treatment of massive carbamazepine overdose. Epilepsia 30: 71–3

93. Hojer J, Malmlund HO, Berg A 1993 Clinical features in 28 consecutive cases of laboratory confirmed massive poisoning with carbamazepine alone. Clinical Toxicology 3: 449–58

94. Tibballs J 1992 Acute toxic reaction to carbamazepine: clinical effects and serum concentrations. Journal of Pediatrics 121: 295–9

95. Apfelbaum JD, Caravati EM, Kerns WP, et al 1995 Cardiovascular effects of carbamazepine toxicity. Annals of Emergency Medicine 25: 631–5

96. Morgan F 1999 Fortnightly review: drug treatment of epilepsy. British Medical Journal 318: 106–9

97. Maloteaux EG 1988 Pharmacological management of epilepsy. Mechanism of action, pharmacokinetic drug interactions, and new drug discovery possibilities. International Journal of Clinical Pharmacology and Therapeutics 36: 181–4

98. Peruca E, Gram L, Avanzi G, Dulac O 1998 Antiepileptic drugs as a cause of worsening seizures. Epilepsia 39: 5–17

99. Russell MA, Bousvaros G 1968 Fatal results from diphenylhydantoin administered intravenously. Journal of the American Medical Assoication 20: 2118–9

100. Curry SC, Mills KC, Graeme KA 1999 Neurotransmitters In: Goldfrank L, Flomenbaum N; Lewin, Howland M, Hoffman R, Nelson L (eds) Goldfranks Toxicologic Emergencies, 7th edn. pp 137–71

101. Garnier R, Boudignat O, Fournier PE 1982 Valproate poisoning. Lancet 2: 97

102. Anderson GO, Ritland S 1995 Lifethreatening intoxication with sodium valproate. Clinical Toxicology 33: 279–84

103. Fischer JH, Barr AN, Rogers SL, et al 1994 Lack of serious neurotoxicity following gabapentin overdose. Neurology 44: 982–3

104. Nagel TR, Schunk JE 1995 Felbamate overdose: a case report and discussion of a new antiepileptic drug. Pediatric Emergency Care 11: 369–71

105. O'Donnel J, Bateman ND 2000 Lamotrigine overdose in an adult. Clinical Toxicology 38: 659–60

28.5 COLCHICINE

LINDSAY MURRAY • ROGER HARRIS

ESSENTIALS

1 Even relatively small ingestions are potentially life-threatening.

2 Frequently presents during an initial asymptomatic phase.

3 Onset of gastrointestinal symptoms within 12–24 hours after acute overdose heralds significant toxicity.

4 Consider the diagnosis in patients presenting with gastrointestinal symptoms followed by development of multiorgan failure.

5 The key points in management of acute colchicine poisoning are early recognition of the potential severity of this intoxication, early gastrointestinal decontamination and aggressive supportive care.

INTRODUCTION

Colchicine is an alkaloid extracted from the plant *Colchicum autumnale*. It has traditionally been widely used in the treatment of acute gout but has also been prescribed for conditions including familial mediterranean fever, scleroderma, primary biliary cirrhosis and recurrent pericarditis.

Colchicine poisoning is relatively rare, most commonly occurring in the context of a suicide attempt or a therapeutic overdose. Severe toxicity from chronic administration of therapeutic doses of oral colchicine is also rare, but can occur in the elderly or patients with renal or hepatic disease. In this situation the appearance of gastrointestinal symptoms usually acts as a safety mechanism, and results in discontinuation of the drug before the appearance of more severe symptoms.

It is, however, important for the emergency physician to be familiar with the recognition and management of colchicine poisoning because it is associated with high mortality, and the potential seriousness of the intoxication is often underestimated at initial presentation.

PHARMACOKINETICS

Colchicine is rapidly absorbed following oral administration, with peak levels occurring from 0.5 to 2 hours post ingestion.[1] Absorption is not significantly delayed following overdose.[2] Bioavailability following oral administration ranges from 25 to 40% because of extensive first-pass hepatic metabolism.[3,4] Following absorption, colchicine rapidly distributes from plasma to tissues, where it binds with high affinity to intracellular binding sites. The distribution half-life is from 45 to 90 minutes and the apparent volume of distribution is 21 L/kg in patients with toxicity.[2] Terminal elimination half-lives in toxic patients range from 10.6 to 31.7 hours, elimination being primarily via hepatic metabolism.[2]

PATHOPHYSIOLOGY

Colchicine binds to tubulin and prevents its polymerization to form microtubules.[5] Microtubules are not only essential components of the cell cytoskeleton during mitosis, but are also integral to other cellular processes such as endocytosis, exocytosis, phagocytois, cell motility and protein assembly in the Golgi apparatus. This is the putative mechanism for colchicine's therapeutic action in acute gouty arthritis where disruption of microtubular-dependent neutrophil migration and phagocytosis results in a reduced inflammatory response. In toxic doses, colchicine causes mitosis to arrest in metaphase with serious consequences for the rapidly dividing cells of the gut mucosa and bone marrow. As colchicine-induced microtubular disruption continues it affects cell shape, intracellular transport and the secretion of hormones, enzymes and neurotransmitters resulting in toxicity to virtually every cell in the body.[6]

CLINICAL PRESENTATION (Table 28.5.1)

Severe colchicine poisoning presents as a relatively distinct clinical syndrome characterized by delayed onset of multiorgan toxicity and a high incidence of mortality.

In the largest reported series of colchicine poisoning (69 cases), ingestions estimated at less than 0.5 mg/kg were associated with gastrointestinal symptoms and coagulation disturbances only, and a mortality of 0%. Ingestions of 0.5–0.8 mg/kg were associated with bone-marrow aplasia and a mortality of 10%, and ingestions greater than 0.8 mg/kg with cardiovascular collapse and 100% mortality at 72 hours.[7] However, fatalities have been reported following ingestions of doses of colchicine as little as 7 mg and 12.5 mg respectively.[8,9] Therefore any overdose of colchicine should be regarded as potentially serious.

It is convenient to divide the clinical course of colchicine toxicity into three sequential (and usually overlapping) stages. Less severe cases may not progress beyond the first stage. The most severe cases die during the second stage.

Following a significant acute oral overdose the patient may remain asymptomatic for between 2 and 24 hours. The toxic patient then develops severe nausea, vomiting, diarrhoea and abdominal pain. This symptomatology corresponds to gastrointestinal mucosal damage and impairment of secretion of normal mucosal enzymes.[10] During this stage, fluid losses from vomiting and diarrhoea

Table 28.5.1 Clinical stages of significant colchicine toxicity

Stage 1: Gastrointestinal phase Time of onset: 2–24 hours post-ingestion	Nausea, vomiting, diarrhoea, abdominal pain Intravascular volume depletion Peripheral leucocytosis
Stage 2: Multiorgan failure phase Time of onset: 24–72 hours post-ingestion	Adult respiratory distress syndrome Bone marrow suppression Cardiac arrhythmias, failure, arrest Consumptive coagulopathy Fever Hypomagnesaemia Hyponatraemia Hypocalcaemia Hypophosphataemia Ileus Metabolic acidosis Mental status changes Neuromuscular abnormalities Oliguric renal failure Secondary sepsis Seizures
Stage 3: Recovery phase Time of onset: 6–8 days post-ingestion	Resolution of organ system derangements Rebound leucocytosis Alopecia

may be significant enough to result in hypovolaemic shock.

Multisystem organ failure is characteristic of the second stage, with onset from 24 to 72 hours following ingestion. Respiratory, neurologic, renal, haematologic and cardiovascular involvement is typical. Acute adult respiratory distress syndrome (ARDS) may be a consequence of hypovolaemic shock or sepsis, or occur as a result of direct damage to the pulmonary vasculature.[11] Bone marrow suppression is heralded by lymphopenia, followed by granulocytopenia, reticulocytopenia and thrombocytopenia, reaching a nadir at 4–8 days following ingestion.

Sepsis may complicate this stage of toxicity.[7] Disseminated intravascular coagulopathy was noted to be a frequent complication in one large series of patients with colchicine toxicity.[7] Fever occurs commonly, and may be a direct drug effect or a sign of complicating infection.[12] Shock, frequently observed during this phase, is cardiogenic and/or hypovolaemic in origin, and is strongly associated with death.[13] Cardiac rhythm disturbances, including sinus bradycardia and sinus arrest,[14] complete atrioventricular block,[10] and sudden cardiac arrest[6] have been reported. Renal failure in acute colchicine toxicity is multifactorial

and related to prolonged hypotension, hypoxia, sepsis and rhabdomyolysis.[6] Metabolic derangements described include metabolic acidosis, hyperglycaemia, hypokalaemia, hypocalcaemia, hypophosphataemia and hypomagnesaemia.[15] Neurological disturbances include delirium, coma, seizures, transverse myelitis and ascending paralysis.[6,16] Death is common during this period and usually occurs as a result of profound cardiogenic shock, sudden cardiac arrest or sepsis. Cardiac arrest has been observed as early as 36 hours following acute colchicine ingestion.[14]

In those who survive stage two, a rebound leucocytosis occurs at 7 or more days after initial symptoms and corresponds to the recovery of bone marrow function. Alopecia commonly occurs at about this time. Complete recovery is the rule in patients surviving stage two.

Myopathies and neuropathies have been observed as a reversible toxic reaction to long-term colchicine therapy.[17]

INVESTIGATIONS

Given the potential for severe multisystem organ failure as described above, extensive baseline laboratory studies should be performed upon presentation.

These include electrolytes, full blood count, coagulation profile, renal function tests, liver function tests, electrocardiography and chest radiography. These studies need to be repeated during a hospital admission at intervals dictated by the patient's clinical course. Although colchicine concentrations in biological fluids can be measured, they are not readily available and not useful in the management of colchicine poisoning.

MANAGEMENT

The key points in the management of acute colchicine toxicity are early recognition of the potential severity of this intoxication, early gastrointestinal decontamination and aggressive supportive care.

Decontamination of the gut by the administration of oral activated charcoal is the management priority for the patient presenting in the first (asymptomatic) stage of colchicine intoxication; prevention of absorption of even small amounts may favourably affect the severity of the intoxication and the ultimate outcome. In patients who present later (during the second stage) resuscitative efforts take precedence over gastrointestinal decontamination.

Careful monitoring of vital signs and cardiac rhythm should be instituted upon arrival. An IV cannula should be placed and IV fluid therapy commenced in any symptomatic patient. In those patients who present with substantial delay, immediate resuscitative measures may be required. Baseline laboratory studies as outlined above should be performed.

All patients with colchicine overdose require admission to hospital for a minimum of 24 hours' observation. Careful monitoring, not only of vital signs and cardiac rhythm but also of fluid and electrolyte status and blood cell counts, is mandatory. Further supportive therapy is dictated by clinical status, and may include intravenous crystalloid rehydration, plasma expansion, inotropes, artificial ventilation, correction of electrolyte and acid–base disturbances, correction of coagulation disorders, and antibiotic treatment of infectious complications.

Because of colchicine's large volume of distribution and high affinity to intracellular binding sites, attempts to enhance elimination by repeat-dose activated charcoal, haemodialysis or haemoperfusion are unlikely to be effective.

DISPOSITION

All patients in whom colchicine toxicity is diagnosed or even suspected require admission. The asymptomatic patient should be observed for a minimum of 24 hours. If no symptoms of intoxication (diarrhoea, vomiting or abdominal pain) are evident at the end of that period, colchicine toxicity may be confidently excluded and the patient discharged. The symptomatic patient should be admitted to an intensive care unit for careful monitoring and supportive care as outlined above.

PROGNOSIS

As noted above, a relatively high mortality is associated with colchicine overdose. However, in patients who survive stage two a complete recovery can be anticipated. The alopecia observed during the recovery phase is not permanent, with hair growth commencing after the first month.

REFERENCES

1. Wallace SL, Ertel NH 1973 Plasma levels of colchicine after administration of a single dose. Metabolism 22: 749–53

CONTROVERSIES/FUTURE DIRECTIONS

❶ The bone-marrow suppression associated with colchicine toxicity has been reported to respond to the administration of granulocyte colony-stimulating factor.[18–21] However, it is unclear whether these reports represent a true therapeutic response or the natural course of recovery.

❷ Colchicine-specific *Fab* fragments have been produced in goats immunized with a conjugate of colchicine and serum albumin, and effectively reverse colchicine toxicity in mice.[22] When administered to a patient with severe colchicine toxicity, rapid improvement in haemodynamic parameters and ultimate survival were observed.[23] Unfortunately, colchicine-specific *Fab* fragments are not yet commercially available.

2. Rochdi M, Sabouraud A, Baud FJ, et al 1992 Toxicokinetics of colchicine in humans: analysis of tissue, plasma and urine data in ten cases. Human Experimental Toxicology 11: 510–6
3. Hunter AL, Klaassen CD 1974 Biliary excretion of colchicine. Journal of Pharmacology and Experimental Therapy 192: 605–7
4. Thomas G, Girre C, Scherrmann JM, et al 1989 Zero-order absorption and linear disposition of oral colchicine in healthy volunteers. European Journal of Clinical Pharmacology 37: 79–84
5. Borizy GG, Taylor EW 1967 The mechanism of action of colchicine: binding of colchicine-H³ to cellular protein. Journal of Cell Biology 34: 525–33
6. Stapczynski JS, Rothstein RJ, Gaye WA, et al 1981 Colchicine overdose: report of two cases and a review of the literature. Annals of Emergency Medicine 10: 364–9

7. Bismuth C, Gautier M, Conso F 1977 Aplasie médullaire après intoxication aiguë á la colchicine. Nouvelle Presse Medicale 6: 1625–9
8. MacLeod JG, Phillips L 1947 Hypersensitivity to colchicine. Annals of Rheumatological Diseases 6: 224–9
9. Harris R, Gillet M 1998 Colchicine poisoning - overview and new directions. Emergency Medicine 10: 161–7
10. Stemmermann GN, Hayashi T 1971 Colchicine intoxication. A reappraisal of its pathology based on a study of three fatal cases. Human Pathology 2: 321–32
11. Heaney D, Derghazarian CB, Pineo GF, et al 1976 Massive colchicine overdose: report on the toxicity. American Journal of Medical Science 271: 233–8
12. Baldwin LR, Talber TL, Sampler R 1990 Accidental overdose of insufflated colchicine. Drug Safety 5: 305–12
13. Sauder P, Kopferschmitt J, Jaeger A, et al 1983 Haemodynamic studies in eight cases of acute colchicine poisoning. Human Toxicology 2: 169–79
14. Stahl N, Weinberger A, Benjamin D, et al 1976 Fatal colchicine poisoning in a boy with familial Mediterranean fever. American Journal of Medical Science 278: 77–81
15. Putterman C, Ben-Cherit E, Caraco Y, Levy M 1991 Colchicine intoxication: clinical pharmacology, risk factors, features and management. Seminars in Arthritis and Rheumatism 3: 143–55
16. Naidus R, Rodvien R, Nielke C 1977 Colchicine toxicity. A multisystem disease. Archives of Internal Medicine 137: 394–6
17. Kuncl RW, Duncan G, Watson D, et al 1987 Colchicine myopathy and neuropathy. New England Journal of Medicine 316: 1562–8
18. Katz R, Chuang LC, Sutton JD 1992 Use of granulocyte colony-stimulating factor in the treatment of pancytopenia secondary to colchicine overdose. Annals of Pharmacotherapy 26: 1087–8
19. Folpini A, Furfori P 1995 Colchicine toxicity - clinical features and treatment. Massive overdose case report. Clinical Toxicology 33: 71–7
20. Harris R, Marx G, Gillett M, Kark A 2000 Colchicine-induced bone marrow suppression: treatment with granulocyte colony-stimulating factor. Journal of Emrgency Medicine 18: 435–40
21. Yoon KH 2001 Colchicine induced toxicity and pancytopenia at usual doses and treatment with granulocyte colony-stimulating factor. Journal of Rheumatology 28: 1199–200
22. Sabouraud A, Urtizberea M, Grandgeorge M, et al 1991 Dose-dependent reversal of acute murine colchicine poisoning by goat colchicine-specific Fab fragments. Toxicology 68: 121–32
23. Baud FJ, Sabouraud A, Vicaut E, et al 1995 Brief report: treatment of severe colchicine overdose with colchicine-specific Fab fragments. New England Journal of Medicine 332: 642–5

28.6 PARACETAMOL

ANDIS GRAUDINS

ESSENTIALS

1 Paracetamol poisoning is a common toxicologic presentation to the emergency department.

2 The decision to treat patients with antidotal therapy following acute single ingestions should be made using the paracetamol treatment nomogram.

3 N-acetylcysteine, which acts a substrate for glutathione repletion, is an effective and safe antidote for paracetamol poisoning.

4 The threshold for antidotal therapy may need to be lowered in patients with hepatic impairment, malnourished states, or microsomal enzyme induction.

5 The efficacy of antidotal treatment decreases with time. Patients presenting more than 8 hours post-ingestion should have N-acetylcysteine commenced whilst waiting for the return of serum paracetamol concentrations.

6 The paracetamol treatment nomogram cannot be used to assess the risk of hepatotoxicity in staggered, sustained-release, or chronic ingestions.

7 Paracetamol overdose should be excluded in all patients with suicidal drug ingestion and anyone with evidence of unexplained hepatic impairment on liver function studies.

INTRODUCTION

Paracetamol is one of the most widely used over-the-counter analgesic and antipyretic medications in Australia, and a common cause of poisoning in Australia and other Western countries. Paracetamol exposure is the most common reason for calls to the New South Wales Poisons Information Centre.[1] In the USA, over a 100 000 potential paracetamol poisonings are reported annually to the American Association of Poison Control Centres.[2] In the UK, paracetamol poisoning accounts for up to 43% of poisonings presenting to emergency departments.[3]

PHARMACOKINETICS AND PATHOPHYSIOLOGY

Paracetamol (N-acetyl para-aminophenol, acetaminophen) is rapidly absorbed from the gastrointestinal tract following therapeutic doses with peak plasma concentrations occurring within 30–60 minutes with tablet formulations and less than 30 minutes with liquid preparations.[4] Oral bioavailability increases with size of the dose, ranging from 68% following 500 mg to 90% following 1 to 2 g.[5] Time to peak plasma concentration may be delayed in the presence of co-ingestants which delay gastric emptying such as dextropropoxyphene, antihistamines, and anticholinergic agents.[5–7] The volume of distribution for paracetamol is approximately 1 L/kg, with protein binding of less than 50%.

Metabolism occurs primarily in the liver with small amounts also metabolized in the kidneys. Metabolites are renally excreted with less than 4% excreted unchanged in the urine.[8] Elimination half-life is approximately 1.5 to 2.5 hours following therapeutic dosing.[8] Paracetamol is metabolized by three mechanisms. With therapeutic dosing approximately 60% is conjugated to glucuronide metabolites and 35% to sulphate metabolites.[5,8] Less than 5% is metabolized by microsomal enzymes, primarily CYP2E1, but also to a lesser degree CYP2A and CYP1A2. Microsomal metabolism produces a reactive intermediary metabolite N-acetyl para-benzoquinoneimine (NAPQI), which is rapidly conjugated with glutathione to produce non-toxic mercapturic acid and cysteine metabolites that are renally excreted.[8]

Recently, a sustained-release formulation of paracetamol (Panadol Extend™) was introduced in Australia for the management of arthritis pain. This formulation contains 665 mg of paracetamol in a bilayer tablet with one-third immediate-release and two-thirds sustained-release. It has been designed to release paracetamol slowly and maintain a therapeutic drug level for up to 8 hours.[9] Currently, there are no data on the toxicokinetics of this preparation in overdose.

In overdose, the glucuronidation and sulphation pathways of metabolism are rapidly saturated resulting in increased metabolism of paracetamol by the microsomal enzyme pathway. When glutathione stores are depleted by more than 70% of normal, NAPQI begins to accumulate within hepatocytes binding to intracellular proteins and producing cell death and a predominantly centrilobular hepatic necrosis.[10]

Microsomal metabolism of paracetamol may be enhanced by barbiturates, carbamazepine, oral contraceptives, chronic alcohol ingestion, or starvation.[11] Inhibition of microsomal metabolism may occur in the presence of acute alcohol ingestion and with 4-methylpyrazole treatment. Administration of large doses of cimetidine to rats has resulted in inhibition of CYP2E1 metabolism and reduction in subsequent paracetamol hepatotoxicity but therapeutic doses of cimetidine do not decrease excretion of mercapturate metabolites of paracetamol following therapeutic doses.[12] There are no human studies to support the use of cimetidine in prevention of hepatotoxicity following paracetamol poisoning.

An isolated small rise in INR has been observed in patients with paracetamol poisoning in the absence of hepatotoxicity. Mild elevations in INR and reduced levels of functional factor VII were found in 66% of patients with an extrapolated 4 hour paracetamol concentration greater or equal to 1000 μmol/L (150 mg/L).[13] This effect appears to be related to inhibition of vitamin-K-dependent activation of coagulation factors.[13]

CLINICAL PRESENTATION

The clinical features of early paracetamol poisoning are non-specific and do not permit diagnosis on clinical grounds. Classically, untreated poisoning progresses through four stages of toxicity.[10] Stage 1 (0–24 hours) is a subclinical period where the patient may exhibit only mild nausea, vomiting, and malaise. During this period paracetamol is being metabolized, glutathione stores are being depleted, and hepatotoxicity is in its early stages. In severe poisoning, mild elevations of hepatic aminotranferases may be apparent as early as 16 hours post-ingestion.[14] During stage 2 (24–48 hours post-ingestion) nausea and vomiting resolve and patients may develop right upper quadrant pain and hepatic tenderness. Liver function begins to deteriorate, with increasing serum aminotransferase and bilirubin concentrations, and prothrombin time. Stage 3 (48–96 hours post-ingestion) occurs in more severe cases only and is essentially a continuum of the above. Hepatic function deteriorates and chemical hepatitis, jaundice, and encephalopathy may develop. Peak aminotransferases are seen around 72–96 hours post ingestion.[14] Stage 4 is either the stage of resolution and fall in aminotransferase concentrations, or the development of fulminant hepatic failure. Patients with a prothrombin time greater than 180 seconds or with a rising prothrombin time on day 4 post-ingestion are at risk of developing fulminant liver failure with less than an 8% chance of survival.[15] Renal failure may also develop as a consequence of paracetamol toxicity. This may either be the result of direct hepatotoxicity due to renal microsomal enzymatic metabolism of paracetamol to NAPQI or as a consequence of liver-failure-induced hepatorenal syndrome.[16]

Other manifestations of paracetamol poisoning may include coma and myocardial damage. Coma may be observed following massive ingestions of paracetamol and is independent of any hepatic impairment. Serum paracetamol concentrations greater than 10 000 μmol/L (1000 mg/L) may present with coma.[17] Cardiac changes may include ST-T wave changes, bundle-branch block, and sinus bradycardia.[18]

In general, most patients recover fully from paracetamol toxicity. The overall untreated mortality is less than 1% and that of untreated patients with hepatotoxicity around 3.5%.[18]

There are currently a number of 'over-the-counter' cough and cold preparations that contain paracetamol in combination with other agents. These include sympathomimetics such as pseudoephedrine, antihistamines such as diphenhydramine, or cough suppressants such as dextromethorphan. Patients may present with symptoms and signs of an acute toxidrome from one or more of these agents. Compound analgesics may also be ingested. These may result in the development of salicylate and/or opioid toxicity. Ingestion of large amounts paracetamol/dextro-propoxyphene containing analgesics (e.g. Di-Gesic®, Capadex®, Paradex®) may also result in propoxyphene-induced cardiotoxicity. Dextro-propoxyphene is an opioid analgesic with cyclic antidepressant-like, type-1A anti-arrhythmic properties in overdose.[19]

ASSESSMENT OF RISK OF HEPATOTOXICITY

The risk of hepatotoxicity following acute ingestion of paracetamol is dose-dependent. In healthy adults, hepatotoxicity may result from ingestion of approximately 12 to 15 g or greater than 150 mg/kg.[20] The threshold for toxicity may be less in patients with underlying hepatic impairment (e.g. alcoholic liver disease, viral hepatitis), malnutrition, or in the presence of microsomal enzyme-inducing agents.[11, 21-23]

The Rumack-Matthews nomogram shows a clear relationship between the serum paracetamol concentration and the potential for subsequent hepatotoxicity.[10] The nomogram begins at 4 hours post-ingestion to allow for absorption and distribution of paracetamol. Serum concentrations taken less than 4 hours post-ingestion may be unreliable in predicting the potential for hepatotoxicity. The risk of hepatotoxicity from acute paracetamol ingestion can be estimated from this nomogram. Patients with a serum concentration falling above a line from 1300 μmol/L (200 mg/L) at 4 hours post ingestion to 170 μmol/L (25 mg/L) at 16 hours post ingestion (the 'probable toxicity' line) will have a 60% chance of developing hepatotoxicity if left untreated.[24] This risk increases to 87% in untreated patients with paracetamol concentrations above 2000 μmol/L (300 mg/L) 4 hours post ingestion.[24] Current recommendations in Australia, the UK and Europe are to treat any patient with a serum paracetamol concentration above the 'probable hepatotoxicity' line. In the USA a third 'possible hepatotoxicity' category was empirically added to the nomogram when antidotal treatment with N-acetylcysteine was being investigated during the 1980s. This line, 1000 μmol/L (150 mg/L) at 4 hours post-ingestion to 125 μmol/L (16 mg/L) at 16 hours post-ingestion, is still used as the treatment line in the USA.

It is widely recommended that the treatment line be dropped to 50% of the probable 'toxicity line' when treating certain 'at-risk' patients. This practice remains unvalidated. 'At-risk' groups include those with known chronic liver diseases, patients using drugs that enhance microsomal metabolism of paracetamol, and those at risk of glutathione depletion (malnutrition, acute illnesses with poor dietary intake).

Chronic over-medication or unintentional overdose with paracetamol may be associated with an increased risk of hepatotoxicity, particularly in those with the aforementioned risk factors. Liver failure has been reported in *retrospective* case series with chronic use of as little as 4 g a day in patients with underlying acute illnesses with associated decreased oral intake. Liver failure has been reported in alcoholic patients with chronic abdominal pain from gastritis or pancreatitis who chronically ingest supratherapeutic doses (up to 10 g daily) of paracetamol.[21,25] However, chronic alcoholics taking therapeutic doses of paracetamol have not been shown to be at increased risk of liver failure when studied *prospectively*.[26] In alcoholic patients, hepatic aminotransferases into the thousands suggest toxin-induced hepatitis as seen with paracetamol abuse. Neither alcoholic nor viral hepatitis commonly produce aminotransferase rises above 1000 IU/L.[21]

ANTIDOTAL THERAPY WITH N-ACETYLCYSTEINE

N-acetylcysteine (NAC) effectively prevents hepatotoxicity following paracetamol poisoning.[24,27-29] NAC is metabolized in the liver to cysteine a precursor to glutathione, necessary for the inactivation of the toxic metabolite NAPQI. Additionally, NAC may also act as a substrate for hepatic sulphation, thus reducing the amount of paracetamol being shunted to the microsomal metabolic pathway. NAC is usually administered according to the 24-hour IV protocol as described by Prescott (150 mg/kg over 15 minutes, 50 mg/kg over 4 hours, 100 mg/kg over 16 hours).[24] There is no need to empirically commence NAC therapy to patients presenting within 8 hours of ingestion. The incidence of hepatotoxicity following institution of therapy within 10 hours of ingestion is very small (1–6%) and independent of the route of dosing (IV versus oral) or length of NAC protocol.[24,27-29] The incidence of hepatotoxicity increases to 40% if NAC is commenced between 10 and 16 hours following ingestion and may be as high as 87% (same as no therapy at all) if commenced between 16 and 24 hours in patients.[24] A longer duration of intravenous NAC therapy may confer greater hepatoprotection following delayed presentation.[28,29]

Adverse reactions to intravenous NAC

are limited to allergic type phenomena such as urticaria, bronchospasm, and hypotension usually occurring during or soon after the administration of the IV loading dose.[29,30] These are not IgE mediated but anaphylactoid histamine release reactions, dose-dependent in nature, and usually respond to slowing or cessation of the infusion for a short period. Occasionally, antihistamine and adrenaline (epinephrine) therapy may be necessary to manage more severe reactions. The incidence of anaphylactoid reactions in retrospective observations may be as high as 14%.[29,31]

MANAGEMENT

Management of paracetamol poisoning varies according to the specific clinical scenario.

Acute poisoning presenting within 8 hours of ingestion

Gastrointestinal (GI) decontamination with activated charcoal should be performed if the patient presents within 1–2 hours of ingestion to limit any ongoing absorption. Early administration of charcoal may prevent the development of a toxic 4-hour paracetamol concentration and the need for subsequent antidotal therapy.[32] Administration of charcoal more than 2 hours post-ingestion is unlikely to affect serum paracetamol.[33] Patient history should be checked for the formulation of paracetamol ingested (immediate vs sustained-release) and the presence of risk factors for hepatic impairment. The threshold for antidotal therapy may be reduced by 50% in these patients. Blood for paracetamol concentration should be collected 4 hours post-ingestion. Antidotal therapy with N-acetylcysteine (NAC) should be commenced if the serum paracetamol concentration falls above the probable toxicity line.

Pregnant patients presenting with paracetamol poisoning should be treated in a similar fashion to other patients. Paracetamol crosses the placenta and in overdose may result in an increased risk of spontaneous abortion.[34] Cord blood

samples taken from newborns of mothers being treated with NAC for paracetamol poisoning have demonstrated therapeutic serum NAC concentrations in the fetal circulation.[35]

Acute poisoning presenting 8–24 hours post-ingestion

In view of the increased incidence of hepatotoxicity with delayed antidote administration, patients presenting greater than 8 hours post ingestion of more than 150 mg/kg of paracetamol should have NAC therapy commenced on presentation. Blood should be taken for serum paracetamol concentration and liver-function tests. Antidotal treatment may be ceased if the paracetamol level is non-toxic and liver function is normal. Otherwise, a full 20-hour course of NAC should be administered and LFTs and coagulation profile repeated at the completion of therapy.

Acute poisoning presenting more than 24 hours post-ingestion

Patients presenting more than 24 hours following paracetamol ingestion may still benefit from antidotal therapy with NAC. Therapy should be commenced whilst waiting for return of blood results. The nomogram cannot be used to assess potential toxicity. Therapy should be continued if there is clinical evidence of toxicity (right upper quadrant tenderness, nausea, vomiting), elevation of hepatic aminotranferases or a detectable serum paracetamol concentration indicating reduced hepatic clearance of paracetamol. These patients may benefit from prolonged duration of NAC therapy if serum aminotransferases and/or prothrombin time continue to rise after 20 hours of therapy.[28,29,36,37] NAC should be continued at a rate of 150 mg/kg/12 hours until prothrombin time and liver function begin to normalize or the patient requires liver transplantation.[37]

Patients with evidence of developing fulminant hepatic failure following paracetamol poisoning will exhibit clinical signs of liver failure associated with rising aminotransferases, bilirubin, and prothrombin time more than 72–96 hours post ingestion. NAC therapy may be of benefit in these patients along with supportive care in a dedicated tertiary hospital liver unit. A lower mortality may be seen in patients with hepatic failure treated with NAC. Early consultation with a liver transplantation unit should be sought in these patients.[36,37]

Acute poisoning with unknown time of ingestion

Where the time of ingestion of a single dose of paracetamol is unable to be determined as a result of altered mental status or any other reason, NAC should be commenced empirically in these patients to avoid delayed therapy. Serum paracetamol, liver-function tests, and prothrombin time should be collected. In view of the inherent safety of N-acetylcysteine, the most practical approach in this setting is empirical treatment with the standard 20 hour NAC protocol.

Chronic overdose

Patients presenting following supra-therapeutic doses of paracetamol over a 24-hour period or longer may be at risk of hepatotoxicity, particularly if they have underlying liver impairment, microsomal enzyme induction, or hepatic gluta-thione depletion. There is no consensus on an approach to treatment of these patients. A conservative approach should be adopted. NAC therapy should be commenced on presentation. Liver-function tests, prothrombin time, and serum paracetamol concentrations should be checked. Elevated aminotransferases and prothrombin time indicate hepato-toxicity and the need for continued NAC therapy. A detectable paracetamol concentration several hours following the last dose may indicate impaired parace-tamol elimination and the need to commence NAC. The nomogram is not helpful in this group of patients. If there is no history of hepatic impairment or enzyme-induction, a normal clinical examination, undetectable serum para-cetamol concentration and normal liver-function, NAC therapy may be stopped and the patient discharged.

Sustained-release paracetamol ingestion

No data exist for overdose with the Australian sustained-release formulation of paracetamol (Panadol Extend™). Although a similar preparation has been available in the USA for a number of years, the formulation of the two pro-ducts are not comparable and manage-ment recommendations for the US product are unlikely to be applicable.[38] The administration of activated charcoal more than 2 hours post ingestion may be of benefit in view of the sustained-release nature of this product. Additionally, the paracetamol treatment nomogram is also unlikely to be applicable to this prepara-tion in view of its delayed absorption profile. Recommendations for NAC therapy are currently empiric and should include the treatment of any patient with a history of ingestion of >150 mg/kg of paracetamol.

CONCLUSION

Paracetamol poisoning is a common toxicologic presentation to the emer-gency department with many possible variations. There is no need to empiri-cally treat patients with antidotal therapy if they present within 8 hours of an acute single ingestion. If patients present beyond this time frame or the return of paracetamol concentration results will be delayed beyond 8 hours NAC should be commenced empirically until results are available.

CONTROVERSIES AND FUTURE DIRECTIONS

❶ The value of NAC in patients who present late with clinical or biochemical evidence of hepatotoxicity.

❷ Predicting risk of hepatotoxicity and need for NAC following overdose with sustained-release paracetamol.

❸ Defining risk factors for paracetamol hepatotoxicity.

Patients with delayed presentations and staggered or multiple therapeutic ingestions are special groups which may benefit from early institution of antidotal therapy and consultation with a clinical toxicologist. Sustained-release parace-tamol provides a new conundrum in the management of poisoning with this analgesic.

REFERENCES

1. Kirby J 2001 Annual Report of the New South Wales Poison Information Centre. The New Children's Hospital, Sydney
2. Litovitz TL, Klein-Schwarz W, Dyer KS, Shannon M, Lee S, Powers M 1998 1997 Annual reports of the American Association of Poison Control Centers Toxic Exposure Surveillance System. American Journal of Emergency Medicine 16: 443–98
3. Thomas SH, Horner JE, Chew K, et al 1997 Paracetamol poisoning in the north east of England: presentation, early management and outcome. Human and Experimental Toxicology 16: 495–500
4. Rawlins MD, Henderson DB, Hijab AR 1977 Pharmacokinetics of paracetamol (acetaminophen) after intravenous and oral administration. European Journal of Clinical Pharmacology 11: 283–6
5. Forrest JA, Clements JA, Prescott LF 1982 Clinical pharmacokinetics of paracetamol. Clinical Pharmacokinetics 7: 93–107
6. Bizovi KE, Aks SE, Paloucek F, Gross R, Keys N, Rivas J 1996 Late increase in acetaminophen concentration after overdose of Tylenol Extended Relief. Annals of Emergency Medicine 28: 549–51
7. Tighe TV, Walter FG 1994 Delayed toxic acetaminophen level after initial four hour nontoxic level. Journal of Toxicology – Clinical Toxicology 32: 431–4
8. Prescott LF 1980 Kinetics and metabolism of paracetamol and phenacetin. British Journal of Clinical Pharmacology 10(Suppl 2): 291S–298S.
9. GlaxoSmithKline 2002 Panadol Extend Product Information
10. Rumack BH, Matthew H 1975 Acetaminophen poisoning and toxicity. Pediatrics 55: 871–6
11. Whitcomb DC, Block GD 1994 Association of acetaminophen hepatotoxicity with fasting and ethanol use. Journal of the American Medical Association 272: 1845–50
12. Burkhart KK, Janco N, Kulig KW, Rumack BH 1995 Cimetidine as adjunctive treatment for acetaminophen overdose. Human and Experimental Toxicology 14: 299–304
13. Whyte IM, Buckley NA, Reith DM, Goodhew I, Seldon M, Dawson AH 2000 Acetaminophen causes an increased International Normalized Ratio by reducing functional factor VII. Therapeutic Drug Monitoring 22: 742–8
14. Singer AJ, Carracio TR, Mofenson HC 1995 The temporal profile of increased transaminase levels in patients with acetaminophen-induced liver dysfunction. Annals of Emergency Medicine 26: 49–53
15. Harrison PM, O'Grady JG, Keays RT, Alexander GJ, Williams R 1990 Serial prothrombin time as prognostic indicator in paracetamol induced fulminant hepatic failure. British Medical Journal 301: 964–6
16. Eguia L, Materson BJ 1997 Acetaminophen-related acute renal failure without fulminant liver failure. Pharmacotherapy 17: 363–70
17. Flanagan RJ, Mant TG 1986 Coma and metabolic

acidosis early in severe acute paracetamol poisoning. Human Toxicology 5: 179–82

18. Hamlyn AN, Douglas AP, James O 1978 The spectrum of paracetamol (acetaminophen) overdose: clinical and epidemiological studies. Postgraduate Medicinne J 54: 400–4

19. Henry JA, Cassidy SL 1986 Membrane stabilising activity: a major cause of fatal poisoning. Lancet 1: 1414–7

20. Mitchell JR, Thorgeirsson SS, Potter WZ, Jollow DJ, Keiser H 1974 Acetaminophen-induced hepatic injury: protective role of glutathione in man and rationale for therapy. Clinical Pharmacology Ther 16: 676–84

21. Kumar S, Rex DK 1991 Failure of physicians to recognize acetaminophen hepatotoxicity in chronic alcoholics. Archives of Internal Medicine 151: 1189–91

22. Lauterburg BH, Velez ME 1988 Glutathione deficiency in alcoholics: risk factor for paracetamol hepatotoxicity. Gut 29: 1153–7

23. Bentur Y, Tannenbaum S, Yaffe Y, Halpert M 1993 The role of calcium gluconate in the treatment of hydrofluoric acid eye burn. Annals of Emergency Medicine 22: 1488–90

24. Prescott LF, Illingworth RN, Critchley JA, Stewart MJ, Adam RD, Proudfoot AT 1979 Intravenous N-acetylcystine: the treatment of choice for paracetamol poisoning. British Medical Journal 2: 1097–100

25. Benson GD 1983 Hepatotoxicity following the therapeutic use of antipyretic analgesics. American Journal of Medicine 75: 85–93

26. Palmer RB, Bogdan GM, Dart RC 2002 Alcohol-Acetaminophen syndrome: Maxin or myth? (abstract). Journal of Toxicology – Clinical Toxicology 40: 649–50

27. Rumack BH, Peterson RC, Koch GG, Amara IA 1981 Acetaminophen overdose. 662 cases with evaluation of oral acetylcysteine treatment. Archives of Internal Medicine 141: 380–5

28. Smilkstein MJ, Knapp GL, Kulig KW, Rumack BH 1988 Efficacy of oral N-acetylcysteine in the treatment of acetaminophen overdose. Analysis of the national multicenter study (1976 to 1985) [see comments]. New England Journal of Medicine 319: 1557–62

29. Smilkstein MJ, Bronstein AC, Linden C, Augenstein WL, Kulig KW, Rumack BH 1991 Acetaminophen overdose: a 48-hour intravenous N-acetylcysteine treatment protocol. Annals of Emergency Medicine 20: 1058–63

30. Prescott LF, Donovan JW, Jarvie DR, Proudfoot AT 1989 The disposition and kinetics of intravenous N-acetylcysteine in patients with paracetamol overdosage. European Journal of Clinical Pharmacology 37: 501–6

31. Brotodihardjo AE, Batey RG, Farrell GC, Byth K 1992 Hepatotoxicity from paracetamol self-poisoning in western Sydney: a continuing

challenge. Medical Journal of Australia 157: 382–5

32. Buckley NA, Whyte IM, O'Connell DL, Dawson AH 1999 Activated charcoal reduces the need for N-acetylcysteine treatment after acetaminophen (paracetamol) overdose. Journal of Toxicology – Clinical Toxicology 37: 753–7

33. Yeates PJ, Thomas SH 2000 Effectiveness of delayed activated charcoal administration in simulated paracetamol (acetaminophen) overdose. British Journal of Clinical Pharmacology 49: 11–4

34. Riggs BS, Bronstein AC, Kulig K, Archer PG, Rumack BH 1989 Acute acetaminophen overdose during pregnancy. Obstetrics and Gynecology 74: 247–53

35. Horowitz RS, Dart RC, Jarvie DR, Bearer CF, Gupta U 1997 Placental transfer of N-acetylcysteine following human maternal acetaminophen toxicity. Journal of Toxicology and Clinical Toxicology 35: 447–51

36. Harrison PM, Keays R, Bray GP, Alexander GJ, Williams R 1990 Improved outcome of paracetamol-induced fulminant hepatic failure by late administration of acetylcysteine. Lancet 335: 1572–3

37. Keays R, Harrison PM, Wendon JA, et al 1991 Intravenous acetylcysteine in paracetamol induced fulminant hepatic failure: a prospective controlled trial. British Medical Journal 303: 1026–9

38. Cetaruk EW, Dart RC, Hurlbut KM, Horowitz RS, Shih R 1997 Tylenol extended relief overdose. Annals of Emergency Medicine 30:104–8

28.7 SALICYLATE

ANDIS GRAUDINS

ESSENTIALS

1 Salicylate pharmacokinetics are complex and alter markedly following overdose.

2 Therapeutic serum salicylate concentrations range from 1.1 to 2.2 mmol/L (15 to 30 mg/dL).

3 Treatment and disposition decisions cannot be made on the basis of a single serum salicylate concentration.

4 The Done nomogram is unreliable and should not be used in the management of salicylate poisoning.

5 Urinary alkalinization is an effective method for enhancing elimination of salicylate. Haemodialysis in rarely indicated.

6 Chronic salicylate poisoning is an insidious condition, mostly seen in the elderly, with an unexplained metabolic acidosis that may be incorrectly attributed to another medical condition.

INTRODUCTION

Salicylate poisoning, once relatively common in Australia, is now rather infrequent. In 1996, only 332 (0.3%) calls to the New South Wales Poison Information Centre related to salicylate exposure.[1] This change largely reflects the change to paracetamol as the over-the-counter analgesic of choice. How-ever, salicylates remain widely available as pharmaceutical preparations and as over-the-counter herbal products, cough and cold remedies, ointments and topical rubefacients. The emergency physician must be able to recognize and manage significant salicylate poisoning, particularly in the very young or elderly patient, because of its significant morbidity and mortality.

PHARMACOLOGY AND PATHOPHYSIOLOGY

Aspirin (acetylsalicylic acid, ASA) is rapidly absorbed from the gastrointestinal tract, predominantly the upper small intestine,[2] and then undergoes rapid hydrolysis to form salicylic acid.[3] Peak serum salicylate levels usually occur within 2 hours of therapeutic dosing but may be delayed for up to 6 hours following administration of enteric-coated formulations.[2] Following overdose, absorption may be erratic and delayed.

This may be partly accounted for by pylorospasm and pharmacobezoar formation. Overdose with sustained-release or enteric-coated preparations may result in peak serum levels being delayed for up to 24 hours.[4]

Following therapeutic doses, salicylate is highly protein bound (85–90%) with a very small apparent volume of distribution (0.1–0.2 L/kg). Salicylic acid has a pKa of 3.0 and exists predominantly in the unionized form at a pH of 7.4. Following overdose, plasma protein binding is saturated and free salicylate concentrations rise. As pH falls, a greater proportion of salicylate exists in the unionized form, and movement into the extravascular compartments, including the CNS, is enhanced with resulting increases in the volume of distribution and tissue toxicity.[5]

Salicylic acid is metabolised in the liver and kidney to form salicyluric acid, glycine, glucuronic, acyl, and salicyl phenolic conjugates. These conjugates are excreted renally along with small amounts of free salicylate. The elimination half-life following therapeutic dosing is around 4 hours. Salicylate metabolism is saturated when plasma salicylate concentrations rise above therapeutic levels and the kinetics change from first-order to zero-order. As a consequence, elimination half-life increases dramatically.

Urinary excretion of unchanged salicylate in minimal when the urine pH is in the acidic range. As urine pH increases, a greater proportion of filtered salicylate is in an ionized state and is unavailable for reabsorption in the proximal convoluted tubule. An increase in urine pH from 5.0 to 8.0 results in an up to 1000-fold increase in ionized salicylate excretion.[2]

At therapeutic doses, salicylate acts as an analgesic, antipyretic, anti-platelet and anti-inflammatory agent primarily by way of its inhibitory effects on prostaglandin synthesis mediated by irreversible inhibition of cyclo-oxygenase enzymes one and two (COX-1 and COX-2). In overdose, the major toxic effects are on the CNS, acid–base balance, cellular metabolism, coagulation, lungs and the gastrointestinal tract.

CNS effects include an initial direct stimulation of the medullary respiratory centre producing an increase in rate and depth of respiration and a corresponding primary respiratory alkalosis, tinnitus, deafness, and confusion. In severe poisoning, where systemic acidaemia enhances cerebral penetration of unionized salicylate, coma, convulsions and cerebral oedema occur.[6]

Metabolic effects include direct uncoupling of oxidative phosphorylation and inhibition of Krebs cycle enzymes leading to systemic acidaemia, hyperglycaemia, hyperthermia, derangement of carbohydrate, amino acid, and lipid metabolism.[2,7] Increased oxygen consumption and carbon-dioxide production are also apparent. Dehydration results from increased insensible respiratory and cutaneous fluid losses, as well as from nausea and vomiting due to GI irritation. Inhibition of platelet aggregation as well as vitamin-K-sensitive clotting factor function may produce a mild coagulopathy. Haemorrhage rarely occurs in humans or animals following severe salicylate poisoning.[8] Salicylate-induced non-cardiogenic pulmonary oedema is also reported in association with severe poisoning.[9]

CLINICAL PRESENTATION

The degree of clinical toxicity following acute ingestion of salicylate is dose-related and may be predicted from the reported dose ingested. The most useful features in assessing the patient are the clinical signs and symptoms, the acid-base status and serum salicylate concentrations.

Acute ingestion of less than 150 mg/kg of salicylate is unlikely to produce significant toxicity. Ingestion of 150 to 300 mg/kg produces mild-to-moderate symptoms and signs including hyperpnoea, tinnitus, nausea, and vomiting. Ingestion of greater than 300 mg/kg is associated with severe toxicity including marked dehydration, hyperpyrexia, agitation, confusion, and mental status depression, which may progress to coma, seizures, and respiratory depression. Ingestion of greater than 500 mg/kg

may be fatal.[7] Cerebral and pulmonary oedema have been reported in association with severe acute poisoning but are more common with chronic salicylate intoxication.

The diagnosis of chronic salicylate poisoning, most common in the elderly, is frequently missed. Recurrent dosing with aspirin, usually in the context of a viral illness or chronic pain condition, results in accumulation of plasma salicylate and prolongation of the elimination half-life. Patients may present with non-specific symptoms or signs such as confusion, delirium, fever, dehydration, or hyperglycaemia. The history of excessive salicylate ingestion may not be elicited and the clinical findings erroneously attributed to other conditions such as septicaemia, cardiogenic pulmonary oedema, cerebrovascular accidents, or diabetic ketoacidosis. The presence of an unexplained metabolic acidosis may be the vital clue leading to the diagnosis.[10] Delay in the diagnosis of chronic salicylate poisoning is associated with an increased morbidity and mortality.[11,12]

INVESTIGATIONS AND ASSESSMENT OF SEVERITY

Salicylate intoxication should be suspected in any patient with clinical signs suggestive of poisoning, an unexplained respiratory alkalaemia or metabolic acidosis.[13] Patients in whom the diagnosis is suspected should have blood drawn for serum electrolytes, urea, creatinine, blood glucose, prothrombin time, paracetamol and salicylate concentration. An arterial blood gas is necessary to assess acid-base status and urine pH should be checked.

A qualitative screening test is available to assess the presence of salicylate in the urine. Addition of Trinder's reagent (ferric nitrate 0.1 molar, hydrochloric acid 0.1 molar, and mercuric chloride) in equal volumes with urine results in a deep purple discolouration of the urine in the presence of even trace quantities of salicylate. This test may be used to rapidly exclude the presence of salicylates in the urine in patients with unexplained metabolic acidosis thus obviating the need for a serum salicylate concentration.[14]

Patients with mild or early poisoning may present with a pure respiratory alkalosis due to respiratory centre stimulation and hypokalaemia. Urine pH may initially be alkaline as a response to hyperventilation. Adult patients with moderate-to-severe poisoning may present with a mixed acid–base disturbance of respiratory alkalosis and metabolic acidosis. Urine pH is commonly acidotic in this setting due to increased excretion of hydrogen ions. A pure metabolic acidosis signifies severe salicylate poisoning. Co-ingestion of sedatives may depress respiratory drive leading to loss of respiratory compensation for the metabolic acidosis and an earlier deterioration in acid–base status.

The Done nomogram was developed in 1960 in an attempt to relate peak serum salicylate concentration to clinical severity of salicylate poisoning.[15] It now appears that this nomogram is unreliable.[8] Combined use of clinical observation, acid-base status, and serial salicylate measurements to monitor ongoing absorption of aspirin appear to be a better approach.[15]

MANAGEMENT

Patients presenting following salicylate ingestion should have intravenous access established, blood drawn for serum salicylate levels, electrolytes, and blood sugar level. In moderate-to-severe poisoning these should be repeated every 2 to 3 hours in view of the potential for erratic salicylate absorption. Intravenous rehydration is often necessary in view of the increased insensible fluid losses due to hyperventilation and pyrexia, and vomiting from GI irritation. Strict attention to fluid balance should be observed particularly in the very young, elderly, or those with cardiac disease. Occasionally, central venous and arterial pressure monitoring may be necessary as well as urinary catherization and hourly urine measures.

Gastrointestinal decontamination with oral activated charcoal should be performed on presentation. It should *not* be withheld even when patients present several hours following ingestion in view of the potential for delayed aspirin absorption. Whole bowel irrigation with polyethylene glycol-electrolyte solution may be considered in patients with ingestion of sustained-release formulations of aspirin. Repeat-doses of activated charcoal may be of benefit where there is evidence of ongoing absorption of salicylate on serial serum levels. Multiple-dose activated charcoal does not enhance salicylate elimination but may inhibit ongoing GI absorption from pharmacobezoars or aspirin concretions.[16,17]

Pulmonary oedema should be treated with continuous positive pressure ventilation by mask or endotracheal intubation.[6,8,19] Ensure that of acidaemia is not exacerbated by institution of controlled ventilation. Seizures should be treated with parenteral benzodiazepines and/or barbiturates.

Urinary salicylate excretion can be enhanced by urinary alkalinization which may reduce salicylate elimination half-life from 20 hours to 5 hours. The aim of urinary alkalinization is to increase urine pH above 7.5 to enhance the trapping of ionized salicylate in the urine. Indications include the presence of symptoms, acid–base abnormalities, or serum salicylate levels greater than 2.2 mmol/L (30 mg/dL). In patients with clinical symptoms and signs of salicylate toxicity, urinary alkalinization can be commenced whilst awaiting the results of drug assays and electrolyte concentrations. Urinary alkalinization is accomplished by initially giving a bolus of intravenous sodium bicarbonate (0.5 to 1.0 mmol/kg) followed by an infusion of 100 to 150 mmol of sodium bicarbonate in 1 L of 5% dextrose solution at a rate of 100–250 mL/hour adjusted to urine pH. Urine output should be maintained between 1 and 2 mL/kg/hour. Serum potassium should be maintained within normal limits by the addition of supplemental potassium to the bicarbonate infusion (30 µmol per bag). In the presence of systemic hypokalaemia, the kidneys retain K^+ ions in preference to H^+ and it is extremely difficult to achieve urinary alkalinization.

Serial serum electrolytes, salicylate concentrations, and urinary pH should be measured every 2–4 hours. The end point for therapy is a serum salicylate concentration within the therapeutic range (1.1–2.2 µmol/L or 15–30 mg/dL), resolution of clinical signs of toxicity, and normalization of acid–base status.

Extracorporeal removal of salicylate is infrequently required. Intermittent high-flow haemodialysis (HD) is the preferred option as it can rapidly normalize acid–base, fluid balance, and electrolyte abnormalities as well as remove salicylate from the blood.[20] There is no case-controlled evidence to support the use of continuous artero-venous or veno-venous HD in severe salicylate poisoning.

Haemodialysis should be considered in those with evidence of altered mental status, persistent acidaemia, pulmonary oedema, or renal impairment. It should also be considered in those with persistently elevated serum levels despite adequate decontamination and urinary alkalinization.[8] Serum levels can be used as a guide for extracorporeal removal but these are not absolute. A salicylate concentration of 7.2 mmol/L (100 mg/dL) in acute poisoning has been suggested as an indication for HD.[21] In elderly patients, with chronic salicylate toxicity, the suggested serum threshold for HD is lower (2.2–4.4 mmol/L – 30–60 mg/dL).

DISPOSITION

In view of the potential for delayed and erratic salicylate absorption, patients require serial salicylate concentrations and observation for a minimum of 12 hours. Salicylate estimations earlier than 6 hours post-ingestion do not usually reflect peak serum concentrations.

Patients without clinical evidence of salicylate toxicity may be medically cleared in the presence of normal arterial blood gas and two falling serum salicylate levels in the therapeutic range (1.1–2.2 mmol/L; 15–30 mg/dL) 3–4 hours apart. Patients with evidence of acid–base abnormalities or end-organ dysfunction should be admitted to a high dependency or intensive care unit.

Transfer to a tertiary referral centre with facilities for haemodialysis should be considered if criteria for severe toxicity are present.

REFERENCES

1. Kirby J 2001 Annual Report of the New South Wales Poison Information Centre 2001. The New Children's Hospital, Sydney.
2. Notarianni L 1992 A reassessment of the treatment of salicylate poisoning. Drug Safety 7: 292–303
3. Kershaw RA, Mays DC, Bienchine JR 1987 Disposition of aspirin and its metabolites in the semen of man. Journal of Clinical Pharmacology 27: 304–9
4. Wortzman DJ, Grunfeld A 1987 Delayed absorption following enteric-coated aspirin overdose. Annals of Emergency Medicine 16: 434–6
5. Hill JB 1973 Salicylate intoxication. New England Journal of Medicine 288: 1110–3
6. Thisted B, Krantz T, Strom J, et al 1987 Acute salicylate self-poisoning in 177 consecutive patients treated in ICU. Acta Anaesthesiologica Scandinavica 31: 312–6
7. Temple AR 1981 Acute and chronic effects of aspirin toxicity and their treatment. Archives of Internal Medicine 141: 364–9
8. Yip L, Dart RC, Gabow PA 1994 Concepts and controversies in salicylate toxicity. Emergency Medicine Clinics of North America 12: 351–64
9. Heffner JE, Sahn SA 1981 Salicylate-induced pulmonary edema. Clinical features and prognosis. Annals of Internal Medicine 95: 405–9
10. Chalasani N, Roman J, Jurado RL 1996 Systemic inflammatory response syndrome caused by chronic salicylate intoxication. Southern Medical Journal 89: 479–82
11. Anderson RJ, Potts DE, Gabow PA, et al 1976 Unrecognized adult salicylate intoxication. Annals of Internal Medicine 85: 745–8
12. Gabow PA, Anderson RJ, Potts DE, et al 1978 Acid–base disturbances in the salicylate-intoxicated adult. Archives of Internal Medicine 138: 1481–4
13. Chan TYK, Chan AYW, Ho CS 1995 The clinical value of screening for salicylates in acute poisoning. Veterinary and Human Toxicology 37: 37–8
14. Asselin WM, Caughlin JD 1990 A rapid and simple color test for detection of salicylate in whole hemolyzed blood. Journal of Analytical Toxicology 14: 254–5
15. Dugandzic RM, Tierney MG, Dickinson GE, et al 1989 Evaluation of the validity of the Done nomogram in the management of acute salicylate intoxication. Annals of Emergency Medicine 18: 1186–90
16. Johnson D, Eppler J, Giesbrecht E, et al 1995 Effect of multiple-dose activated charcoal on the clearance of high-dose intravenous aspirin in a porcine model. Annals of Emergency Medicine 26: 569–74
17. Mayer AL, Sitar DS, Tenebein M 1992 Multiple-dose charcoal and whole-bowel irrigation do not increase clearance of absorbed salicylate. Archives of Internal Medicine 152: 393–6
18. Cohen DL, Post J, Ferroggiaro AA, et al 2000 Chronic salicylism resulting in noncardiogenic pulmonary edema requiring hemodialysis. American Journal of Kidney Diseases 36: E20
19. Woolley RJ 1993 Salicylate-induced pulmonary edema: a complication of chronic aspirin therapy. Journal of the American Board of Family Practice 6: 399–401
20. Jacobsen D, Wiik-Larsen E, Bredesen JE 1988 Haemodialysis or haemoperfusion in severe salicylate poisoning? Human Toxicology 7(2): 161–3
21. Flomenbaum NE 1998 Salicylates: In: Goldfrank LR, Flommenbaum NE, Lewin NA, et al (eds) Goldfranks toxicologic emergencies. Appleton and Lange, New York, pp 569–81

28.8 THEOPHYLLINE

LINDSAY MURRAY

ESSENTIALS

1 Theophylline toxicity is associated with life-threatening seizures and cardiac arrhythmias.

2 Serum theophylline levels are useful in assessing and managing acute theophylline toxicity.

3 Onset of maximal toxicity may be significantly delayed following overdose of sustained-release preparations.

4 Techniques of enhancing drug elimination play an important role in the management of severe theophylline toxicity.

5 Early identification of high-risk patients allows the institution of enhanced elimination techniques before life-threatening complications develop.

INTRODUCTION

Theophylline, a methylxanthine derivative related to caffeine, has long been used in the treatment of asthma and chronic airflow limitation. Although the use of the drug has declined in recent times, both acute and chronic theophylline toxicity continue to result in potentially life-threatening presentations to the emergency department.

Therapeutic blood concentrations of theophylline are generally regarded as being between 55 and 110 µmol/L (10 and 20 mg/L). A single ingestion of more than 10 mg/kg of theophylline by an adult is capable of producing a blood concentration above this range.

PHARMACOKINETICS

Theophylline is well absorbed orally, with a bioavailability of almost 100%. The rate of absorption depends on the pharmaceutical formulation. The most commonly prescribed preparations are sustained-release, and following overdose of these preparations peak absorption may be delayed up to 15 hours.

Once absorbed, theophylline is rapidly distributed with a relatively small volume of distribution (0.3–0.7 L/kg). Theophylline is metabolized via the cytochrome P450 system to produce active and inactive metabolites. Only about 10% of absorbed theophylline is excreted unchanged in the urine. The rate of metabolism is extremely variable and decreases with time. Theophylline metabolism exhibits saturable (Michaelis-Menten) kinetics. At higher doses of theophylline relatively small increments in dose are associated with disproportionate increases in serum concentration.[1] In cases of severe intoxication endogenous elimination of theophylline is very slow.

PATHOPHYSIOLOGY

The precise mechanism of toxicity of theophylline is unknown. Proposed mechanisms of action include inhibition of phosphodiesterase leading to elevated concentrations of intracellular cAMP, augmented plasma catecholamine activity, competitive antagonism of adenosine, and changes in intracellular calcium transport.[2]

CLINICAL PRESENTATION

Two different clinical syndromes of theophylline poisoning are recognized: acute and chronic. Both are potentially life-threatening, although the chronic form is associated with a greater incidence of morbidity and mortality.[3]

Chronic intoxication is the most common clinical presentation and occurs when excessive doses of theophylline are administered repeatedly, or where intercurrent illness or drug interaction interferes with hepatic metabolism. Theophylline has a notoriously narrow therapeutic index, and up to 15% of patients with a serum theophylline concentration in the therapeutic range have clinical manifestations of toxicity. Acute intoxication is usually the result of deliberate overdose with suicidal intent, but is occasionally observed following inadvertent iatrogenic overdose.

The clinical manifestations of theophylline intoxication are numerous and principally affect the gastrointestinal, cardiovascular, central nervous, musculoskeletal and metabolic systems.

The gastrointestinal tract is particularly sensitive to theophylline toxicity, the most prominent symptom being vomiting. This is usually severe and frequently refractory to treatment with antiemetics.

Sinus tachycardia is an almost universal manifestation of theophylline toxicity. However, severe intoxication is also associated with more unstable rhythms, including supraventricular tachycardia, atrial fibrillation, atrial flutter, multifocal atrial tachycardia and ventricular tachycardia.[4] Refractory hypotension may occur in severe toxicity as a result of β_2-mediated peripheral vasodilation.

CNS manifestations most commonly consist of anxiety and insomnia. With more severe intoxication, tachypnoea from respiratory centre stimulation and seizures occur. Seizures can develop suddenly, may be repetitive, are difficult to treat, and are associated with poor outcome.

Metabolic complications of theophylline poisoning include hypokalaemia, hypophosphataemia, hypomagnesaemia, hyperglycaemia and metabolic acidosis.[5] Hypokalaemia is frequent following acute overdose, occurs early and is a consequence of intracellular shift of potassium secondary to catecholamine excess.[6,7] Musculoskeletal manifestations include muscle aches, increased muscle tone and myoclonus.

Chronic intoxication usually occurs in elderly patients and is associated with vomiting and tachycardia. The metabolic abnormalities are less frequently observed. Seizures and cardiac arrhythmias occur more frequently and at much lower serum theophylline concentrations than in acute intoxication.[8,9]

Following acute overdose, especially where sustained-release preparations are involved, the clinical manifestations of severe toxicity may be delayed up to 12 hours. These patients usually present with severe vomiting before the onset of more severe toxicity, including seizures and arrhythmias.

INVESTIGATIONS

The diagnosis of theophylline toxicity is suspected on history and clinical presentation, and confirmed by documentation of a significant serum theophylline concentration. The serum theophylline concentration is also invaluable in the assessment of severity and ongoing management of theophylline poisoning. Although theophylline is readily measured, it is not detected on routine drug screens.

Patients with acute theophylline overdose generally exhibit signs of minor toxicity at serum concentrations from 110 to 220 μmol/L (20–40 mg/L), moderate toxicity with concentrations from 220 to 440 μmol/L (40–80 mg/L), and severe toxicity with concentrations >440 μmol/L (80 mg/L). Serum theophylline concentrations of >550 μmol/L (100 mg/L) are frequently fatal.[10] After an acute overdose serum theophylline should be measured every 3 hours or so until a plateau is documented, because of the risk of delayed absorption.

In chronic theophylline poisoning serious toxicity is observed at lower serum concentrations and the measured concentration is not predictive of the severity of poisoning.[11] Seizures, arrhythmias and fatalities can occur at concentrations as low as 220–330 μmol/L (20–30 mg/L).[12] In these patients the best predictor of poor outcome is age greater than 60 years.[13]

Other useful laboratory studies include electrolytes and creatinine, glucose, LFTs and ECG.

MANAGEMENT

The initial management of theophylline poisoning follows the principles of general supportive care. Specific attention may need to be directed towards control of the airway, hypotension, tachyarrhythmias and seizures.

Hypotension usually responds to intravenous fluid administration. A noradrenaline (norepinephrine) infusion may be necessary in resistant cases. Supraventricular arrhythmias can be treated with a β-blocker such as propranolol or esmolol intravenously,[14] but this may induce bronchospasm in susceptible individuals. Seizures must be treated aggressively with high-dose benzodiazepines. If this fails to control them, phenobarbitone and even general anaesthesia may be required. Phenytoin is ineffective and contraindicated. Metabolic disturbances do not generally require specific therapy. Severe hypokalaemia should be corrected with potassium supplementation.

Following acute overdose oral activated charcoal should be administered, even if presentation is delayed. Antiemetics are usually required for successful administration.

The pharmacokinetic properties of theophylline, especially the small volume of distribution, lend themselves to methods of enhanced elimination. Theophylline is relatively efficiently removed by haemodialysis, haemoperfusion and administration of repeat-dose activated charcoal.[15]

Theophylline clearance rates of 100 mL/min have been reported with multiple-dose activated charcoal.[15] Again, aggressive antiemetic therapy may be necessary if this non-invasive method of enhancing drug elimination is to be effective. Administration of a selective serotonin antagonist such as ondansetron has proved particularly effective in this setting.[16,17]

Both haemoperfusion and haemodialysis greatly increase the elimination of theophylline and highly effective in achieving a good clinical outcome. [3,18] Such invasive methods are only indicated in potentially life-threatening theophylline toxicity. Commonly accepted indications include acute intoxication, where the serum theophylline is greater than 550 µmol/L; chronic intoxication, where it is greater than 220–330 µmol/L; or in any patient with intractable hypotension, ventricular ectopy or resistant seizures.[8,10] Ideally, patients at greatest risk of developing arrhythmias or seizures should be identified early and haemodialysis or haemoperfusion instituted before these complications develop. Plasmapheresis has also been used to effectively enhance theophylline elimination.[3]

DISPOSITION

All patients with symptomatic theophylline toxicity require admission to

---

CONTROVERSIES AND FUTURE DIRECTIONS

❶ Although charcoal haemoperfusion has been recommended as the most effective way to enhance theophylline elimination, it has not yet been shown to be associated with any additional improvement in clinical outcome compared to haemodialysis.[19]

❷ Based on sound pharmacodynamic principles, adenosine infusion has been proposed as an antidote to theophylline toxicity. There are as yet no data to support the use of this therapy.[20]

---

hospital. Patients with acute overdose of sustained-release preparations should be admitted for monitoring and serial serum theophylline concentrations. Patients with moderate-to-severe theophylline toxicity require admission to a monitored bed.

REFERENCES

1. Weinberger M, Ginchansky E 1977 Dose-dependent kinetics of theophylline disposition in asthmatic children. Journal of Pediatrics 91: 820
2. Haddad L, Shannon MW, Winchester JF (eds) 1998 Clinical Management of Poisoning and Drug Overdose, 3rd edn. WB Saunders, Philadelphia
3. Shannon MW 1997 Comparative efficacy of hemodialysis and hemoperfusion in severe theophylline intoxication. Academic Emergency Medicine 4: 674–8
4. Bender PR, Brent J, Kulig K 1991 Cardiac arrhythmias during theophylline toxicity. Chest 100: 884–6
5. Hall KW, Dobson KE, Dalton JG, Chignone MC, Penner SB 1984 Metabolic abnormalities associated with intentional theophylline overdose. Annals of Internal Medicine 101: 457–62
6. Amitai Y, Lovejoy FH 1988 Hypokalaemia in acute theophylline poisoning. American Journal of Emergency Medicine 6: 214–8
7. Shannon M, Lovejoy FH 1989 Hypokalemia after theophylline intoxication. The effects of acute vs chronic poisoning. Archives of Internal Medicine 149: 2725–9
8. Olson KR, Benowitz NL, Woo OF, Pond SM 1984 Theophylline overdose: acute single ingestion versus chronic repeated overmedication. American Journal of Emergency Medicine 3: 386–94
9. Shannon M 1999 Life-threatening events after theophylline overdose: a 10-year prospective analysis. Archives of Internal Medicine 159: 989–4
10. Sessler C 1990 Theophylline toxicity: clinical features of 116 consecutive cases. American Journal of Medicine 88: 567–76
11. Shannon M, Lovejoy F 1992 Effect of acute versus chronic intoxication on clinical features of theophylline poisoning in children. Journal of Pediatrics 121: 125
12. Bahls F, Ma KK, Bird TD 1991 Theophylline-associated seizures with 'therapeutic' or low toxic serum concentrations: risk factors for serious outcome in adults. Neurology 41: 1309
13. Shannon M 1993 Predictors of major toxicity after theophylline overdose. Annals of Internal Medicine 119: 1161–7
14. Seneff M, Scott J, Friedman B, Smith M 1990 Acute theophylline toxicity and the use of esmolol to reverse cardiovascualr instability. Annals of Emergency Medicine 19: 671–3
15. Kulig KW, Bar-Or D, Rumack BH 1987 Intravenous theophylline poisoning and multiple-dose charcoal in an animal model. Annals of Emergency Medicine 16: 842
16. Brown S, Prentice D 1992 Ondansetron in the treatment of theophylline overdose. Medical Journal of Australia 156: 512
17. Sage TA, Jones WN, Clark RF 1993 Ondansetron in the treatment of intractable nausea associated with theophylline toxicity. Annals of Pharmacotherapy 27: 584–5
18. Heath A, Knudsen K 1987 Role of extracorporeal drug removal in acute theophylline poisoning - a review. Medical Toxicology 2: 294
19. Laussen P, Shann F, Butt W, Tibballs J 1991 Use of plasmapheresis in acute theophylline toxicity. Critical Care Medicine 12: 113–4
20. Blery JC, Kauflin MJ, Mauro VF 1995 Adenosine in acute theophylline intoxication. Annals of Pharmacotherapy 29: 1285–7

28.9 CARBON MONOXIDE

DAVID C. CRUSE

ESSENTIALS

1 Carbon monoxide is the commonest agent used in successful suicides in Australia and the UK.

2 Many cases of carbon monoxide poisoning remain undetected.

3 Carbon monoxide poisoning may result in significant long-term neuropsychological sequelae.

4 Oxygen is the single most effective treatment.

5 The optimal mode of oxygen delivery remains controversial.

INTRODUCTION

Carbon monoxide is the most common agent used for successful suicide in Australia,[1] the USA[2] and the UK.[3]

A colourless, odourless, tasteless and non-irritant gas, carbon monoxide is produced by the incomplete combustion of hydrocarbons. Small amounts are produced endogenously by normal metabolic processes. In our society the most common sources of significant exposure are car exhausts, fires, charcoal barbecues used in confined spaces, faulty home heaters and cigarette smoke. The introduction of catalytic converters has significantly reduced the production of carbon monoxide by recent-model cars. Consequently, attempted suicide using this method is often unsuccessful.

Carboxyhaemoglobin (COHb) concentrations in cigarette smokers range between 5 and 15%. Methylene chloride, the main ingredient in paint strippers, is readily absorbed through the skin and metabolized to produce carbon monoxide.

Because the gas is not detected by human senses and the initial symptoms of poisoning are non-specific, carbon monoxide poisoning frequently remains undiagnosed and, as a consequence, the incidence is underreported.[4]

The exact mechanism by which carbon monoxide exerts its toxic effects is still poorly understood, and the optimal treatment of poisoning is yet to be established.

PATHOPHYSIOLOGY

The principal toxic effects of carbon monoxide are thought to result from its ability to bind to haemoproteins.[5] Other important effects are the production of a relative hypoxia, a left shift of the oxygen-haemoglobin dissociation curve and direct cardiovascular depression.

The effects of carbon monoxide exposure are directly related to three important variables:[6]

- Length of exposure
- The partial pressure of carbon monoxide in the inspired air
- Alveolar ventilation.

Brief exposure to high concentrations of carbon monoxide produces minimal long-term effects, whereas a long exposure to low concentrations is associated with significant morbidity and mortality.

Effect on oxygen transport

Carbon monoxide rapidly crosses the alveolar capillary membrane and binds to haemoglobin 240 times more avidly than does oxygen. Once bound to carbon monoxide, haemoglobin is unavailable for oxygen transport.[7] In addition, binding shifts the oxygen-haemoglobin dissociation curve to the left. The decreased oxygen-carrying capacity of the blood produces a relative anaemia and hypoxaemic peripheral hypoxia. These effects are compounded if the patient has a pre-existing anaemia or associated cyanide exposure.

Carbon monoxide uptake is inversely related to the partial pressure of inspired oxygen. This fact contributes to the rapid demise of victims who suffer significant carbon monoxide exposure in confined spaces.

Effect on tissues

Carboxyhaemoglobin is not intrinsically toxic and COHb concentrations are a poor measure of both toxicity and patient outcome. This was demonstrated experimentally in dogs, where exposure to high concentrations of carbon monoxide resulted in death, whereas bleeding followed by transfusion with blood with a COHb concentration between 57% and 64% produced no deleterious effects.[8]

Extravascular uptake of carbon monoxide is estimated to be between 10 and 50% of the total body carbon monoxide.[9] It is thought that carbon monoxide reacts with a number of other haem compounds besides haemoglobin: myoglobin, hydroperoxidase, cytochrome A3 oxidase, and cytochrome P450.[10,11] As the blood oxygen level falls, a PO_2 is reached at which carbon monoxide avidly binds to these other haem proteins. Myoglobin is an oxygen carrier protein found in skeletal and cardiac muscle cells. The binding of carbon monoxide to myoglobin produces a nonfunctional form of myoglobin, which may explain the decrease in cardiac output observed even in mild carbon monoxide poisoning.

Cytochrome A3 is the terminal member of the mitochondrial electron transport chain and accounts for up to 90% of the total oxygen uptake of the body. As COHb concentrations rise and hypotension occurs, cytochrome A3 is inhibited.[12] Therefore, in addition to hypoxaemic hypoxia, carbon monoxide may also produce histotoxic hypoxia. Opponents of this theory contend that because oxygen has a nine-times higher affinity for cytochrome A3 than carbon monoxide, carbon monoxide binding to the cytochrome would be insufficient to inhibit cellular respiration.[13]

Consequences of reoxygenation

Dissociation of carbon monoxide from haemoproteins depends on the relative concentrations of oxygen, carbon monoxide and proteins, and their relative affinities. Dissociation of carbon monoxide from haemoglobin starts as soon as exposure ceases. The dissociation half-life depends upon inspired oxygen concentration being between 220 and 400 minutes in room air, approximately 90 minutes in 100% oxygen, and as little as 20 minutes in 100% oxygen at 3 ATA. As the major toxic effects of carbon monoxide are thought to occur at the cellular level, the effect of varying inspired oxygen concentrations to alter the dissociation rates of these proteins is not known.

Cytochrome A3 may remain inhibited as a patient is reoxygenated, and this could lead to free radical formation and reoxygenation injury. The cerebral pathology associated with carbon-monoxide poisoning is similar to that of postischaemic reperfusion injury. It has been postulated that the observed injury is caused by lipid peroxidation, and that hyperbaric oxygen at 3 ATA may antagonize this process by increasing the scavenging of oxygen free radicals by superoxide dismutase.[14]

Table 28.9.1 Signs and symptoms related to COHb level at time of exposure

COHb level (%)	Signs and symptoms
0	None
10	Frontal headache
20	Throbbing headache, shortness of breath on exertion
30	Impaired judgement, nausea, fatigue, visual disturbances, dizziness
40	Confusion, loss of consciousness
50	Seizures, coma
60	Hypotension, respiratory failure
70	Death

CLINICAL PRESENTATION

The signs and symptoms of acute carbon monoxide poisoning, as shown in Table 28.9.1, can be related to COHb concentration at the time of exposure. Acute exposure to carbon monoxide usually causes central nervous system and cardiovascular toxicity. These tissues have high blood flow and oxygen demand. Symptoms and signs reported after low-dose exposure reflect subtle central nervous system abnormalities, and may include fatigue, headache, dizziness, poor concentration, insomnia, language difficulties and psychomotor disturbances. Table 28.9.2 summarizes the clinical signs and symptoms, along with complications and useful investigations. The onset of some symptoms may be delayed from days to weeks, making detection difficult in the emergency setting. This in turn may result in potentially beneficial treatment being either delayed or withheld.

Central nervous system effects

The most commonly observed presenting signs and symptoms of carbon-monoxide poisoning relate to the central nervous system. There is a wide spectrum of effects. Headache is the most frequent symptom, and is usually accompanied by nausea and lightheadedness. Following low-level exposure the patient may experience difficulty in concentrating, appear vague, and have reproducible deficits on Mini Mental State Examination (MMSE), an example of which is provided in Table 28.9.3. A reproducible result of less than 27/30 indicates significant impairment. The MMSE is also

Table 28.9.2 Clinical features of carbon monoxide poisoning

System	Symptoms	Pathology	Diagnostic
CNS	Early: confusion, coma, seizures Late: psychoses, dementia, parkinsonism, ataxia, peripheral neuropathy, gait disturbance	Brain oedema, encephalopathy Cerebral atrophy, basal ganglia lesions	EEG CT scan
Cardiac	Arrhythmias, hypotension angina, tachycardia	Myocardial ischaemia	ECG, CK, CK-MB, Troponin
Pulmonary	Shortness of breath	Pulmonary oedema	CXR
Ophthalmological	Visual disturbances	Flame-shaped retinal haemorrhages, cerebral lesions, retrobulbar neuritis, papilloedema	Fundoscopy
Renal	Acute failure	Myoglobinuria	Renal function tests, serum myoglobin, urine myoglobin
Muscular	Ischaemia	Compartment syndrome, rhabdomyolysis	
Auditory and vestibular	Hearing loss, nystagmus, tinnitus		

Table 28.9.3 Mini Mental State Examination and Scoring

Orientation (time, day, date, month, year)	/5
Orientation (ward, hospital, state, country)	/5
Memorize three objects (dog, hat, book)	/3
Serial 7s (subtract 7 from 100, repeat five times)	/5
Recall the three memorized objects	/3
Visual recognition: name two objects	/2
Repeat sentence: NO IFS ANDS OR BUTS	/1
Perform a three-step command (show me your left index finger, then touch your chin and then touch your right ear)	/3
Read a sentence (CLOSE YOUR EYES)	/1
Write a sentence	/1
Draw a three-dimensional figure	/1
Total	/30
Mark on scale conscious state of patient: alert .... comatose	

useful to gauge treatment effect. Severe exposure produces gross neurological abnormalities, including lethargy, agitation and progressive depression of the conscious state. Regardless of the cause of exposure, these patients may be abusive, aggressive, or have psychotic features. Many of the symptoms due to lesions of the brain may be mistaken for psychiatric symptoms.

Delayed neuropsychiatric sequelae may manifest at a variable time interval following the acute exposure. These include minor manifestations such as headache, vertigo, motor impairment, sensory impairment and hypertonia, and major manifestations such as changes in behaviour, memory disturbance, motor paralysis and Parkinson's disease. The incidence of these sequelae has been estimated to be as great as 25–50% in patients with loss of consciousness or COHb levels greater than 25%.[15]

Cardiac effects

The heart is particularly vulnerable to carbon monoxide poisoning. Carbon monoxide binds to cardiac muscle myoglobin at a ratio of 3:1 compared to skeletal muscle myoglobin. S-T segment depression is the most commonly noted change. Myocardial depression can result in hypotension and further exacerbate cerebral ischaemia. Various arrhythmias and myocardial infarction may occur.

Pulmonary effects

Pulmonary oedema occurs in up to one-third of all severely poisoned patients and is due to hypoxia.

Vomiting in an unconscious patient may lead to aspiration pneumonia.

Other effects

Uncommonly reported sequelae of carbon monoxide poisoning include hepatitis, rhabdomyolysis, pancreatitis, thrombotic thrombocytopenic purpura and acute tubular necrosis.

Carbon monoxide exposure during pregnancy is reported to cause stillbirths, premature labour and severe fetal neurological impairment.

DIAGNOSIS

The most important factors in establishing the diagnosis are the history and a high index of clinical suspicion.

The differential diagnosis includes cerebrovascular disease, psychiatric illness, migraine and cardiovascular disease. These conditions may coexist with acute carbon monoxide poisoning. The diagnosis of carbon monoxide poisoning should be considered whenever multiple members of the same family or from the same workplace present with non-specific symptoms, especially headache, within 24 hours of each other.[16]

Measurement of an elevated COHb concentration confirms the diagnosis. However, a concentration within the normal range does not necessarily exclude carbon monoxide poisoning because of the effect of oxygen therapy and the time interval between exposure and sample collection. COHb concentration alone is a poor guide to the severity of toxicity.

Two methods of measuring the COHb concentration are in common use. The first involves spectrophotometric analysis of blood. The second analyses CO concentration in exhaled air and calculates a value for COHb.

Arterial blood gas analysis may demonstrate an acidosis, although alkalosis has also been reported.[17] Blood gas machines calculate the oxygen saturation from measured partial pressure and give a falsely elevated result in carbon monoxide poisoning. Similarly, pulse oximeters do not distinguish between oxy-Hb and COHb, and give falsely high readings.

MANAGEMENT

Initial management is directed towards securing the airway and stabilizing respiration and circulation. Hypotension, in the absence of an arrhythmia, usually responds to intravenous fluid administration. The patient should immediately be given oxygen therapy, ideally via a tight-fitting non-rebreathing face mask. In a comatose or agitated patient endotracheal intubation may be required to deliver 100% oxygen. If the only available oxygen delivery device is a Hudson mask, it should be remembered that at a flow rate of 15 L/min no more than 60% oxygen is delivered.

The patient should be placed on a cardiac monitor, a 12-lead ECG performed, an intravenous line inserted (if needed) and blood drawn for full blood count, electrolytes, urea and creatinine, COHb, blood sugar level and cardiac enzymes. Serum lactate is a better guide to tissue acidosis than arterial blood gases. A urinary catheter should be inserted in the unconscious patient to monitor urine output. Other investigations that may be clinically indicated include a chest X-ray and CT scan of the brain.

Oxygen therapy

Oxygen therapy has long been accepted as the treatment of choice in carbon-monoxide poisoning, the rationale for its use being that it decreases the effective elimination half-life of COHb.

Hyperbaric oxygen (HBO) has been purported to offer additional benefits over normobaric (NBO) therapy, in particular in reducing the risk of neuropsychological sequelae. HBO acts by increasing dissolved oxygen content in the blood, accelerating elimination of CO, and possibly by prevention of lipid peroxidation in the brain.

Randomized controlled studies comparing HBO with NBO in the treatment of CO poisoning report conflicting results in terms of outcome. Of the two most recent and rigorously conducted trials, one reported a deterioration in neuropsychological performance in the HBO group,[18] whereas the other reported improved neuropsychological performance in the HBO group.[19] However, it is difficult to draw firm conclusions from either study because of differences in patient population, treatment regimens, and neuropsychological evaluation. At this point it remains unclear whether HBO reduces the risk of neuropsychological sequelae in any subgroup of CO poisoned patients. The potential benefits of HBO for a particular patient must be weighed against the potential risks, which include those associated with transport to the HBO facility, barotrauma and hyperoxic seizures.

Indications for HBO commonly used by hyperbaric facilities include:

Table 28.9.4 Hyperbaric facilities in Australia and UK		
Australia		
Royal Adelaide Hospital	Phone	(08) 8222 4000
	Fax	(08) 8232 4207
The Alfred Hospital (Melbourne)	Phone	(03) 9276 2000
	Fax	(03) 9276 3052
Royal Darwin Hospital	Phone	(08) 8922 8888
	Fax	(08) 8922 8286
Fremantle Hospital	Phone	(08) 9431 3333
	Fax	(08) 9431 2819
Prince of Wales Hospital (Sydney)	Phone	(02) 9382 2222
	Fax	(02) 9382 3882
Royal Hobart Hospital	Phone	(03) 6238 8308
	Fax	(03) 6238 8322
Townsville General Hospital	Phone	(07) 4781 9211
	Fax	(07) 4781 9582
Broome District Hospital	Phone	(08) 9192 1401
	Fax	(08) 9192 2322
Christchurch Hyperbaric Medicine Unit	Phone	(03) 3640 045
	Fax	(03) 3640 187
Melanesian Hyperbaric Services (Boroko, Papua New Guinea)	Phone	(675) 321 7332
	Fax	(675) 321 7332
UK		
Aberdeen Royal Infirmary	Phone (+44)	02392 768026
Diving DiseasesCentre, Plymouth	Phone (+44)	01752 209999
Institute of Naval Medicine	Phone (+44)	02392 768026
Poole Hyperbaric Centre	Phone (+44)	01426 316636

- Coma
- Loss of consciousness during exposure
- Abnormal neuropsychiatric testing
- Pregnancy.

Completion of one of the batteries of neuropsychiatric tests that have been used to evaluate CO poisoning may be difficult in the emergency setting.

DISPOSITION

Remote areas

It is often impractical to transfer all but the most seriously ill to the nearest hyperbaric facility. Patients should be hospitalized and receive 100% normobaric oxygen for a minimum of 24 hours. If symptoms have not improved after this time, referral and transfer to the nearest hyperbaric facility should be considered. Table 28.9.4 lists hyperbaric facilities in Australasia and UK.

Follow-up

The hyperbaric medicine specialist will generally follow-up patients who receive hyperbaric oxygen therapy. Patients treated in the emergency setting should be reviewed at regular intervals to detect the development of delayed neuropsychiatric sequelae. A patient who suffers intentional carbon-monoxide poisoning should receive psychiatric review prior to discharge.

CONCLUSION

Carbon-monoxide poisoning is an important presentation to emergency departments in Australasia. An appreciation of the wide variation in symptomatology is required in the assessment of these patients. Early initiation of oxygen

CONTROVERSIES

❶ Controversy remains regarding the indications (if any) for HBO and the optimal duration of NBO. These are unlikely to be resolved anytime soon.

❷ Research continues into the mechanisms of CO poisoning and identification of accurate markers of poisoning severity.

therapy is essential. Consultation with the nearest hyperbaric medicine facility is often advisable.

REFERENCES

1. Australian Bureau of Statistics 1983 Suicides in Australia 1961–1981, Table 8. ABS, Canberra (Cat. no. 3309.0)
2. National Safety Council 1982 Accident Facts. National Safety Council, Chicago, pp 80–4
3. Office of Population Censuses and Surveys 1987 Mortality statistics 1985 – Cause, series DH2, Table 2, ICD code 986. HMSO, London
4. Meredith T, Vale A 1988 Carbon monoxide poisoning. British Medical Journal 296: 72–9
5. Walum E, Varnbo I, Peterson A 1985 Effects of dissolved carbon monoxide on the respiratory activity of perfused neuronal and muscle cell cultures. Clinical Toxicology 23(4–6): 299–308
6. Pace N, Consolazio W, White W 1946 Formulation of the principal factors affecting the rate of uptake of carbon monoxide by normal man. American Journal of Physiology 141: 17–31
7. Haldane J 1927 Carbon monoxide as a tissue poison. Biochemistry Journal 21: 1068–75
8. Goldbaum L, Orenallo T, Dergal E 1976 Mechanism of the toxic action of carbon monoxide. Annals of Clinical Laboratory Science 6: 372–6
9. Loumanmaki K, Coburn R 1969 Effects of metabolism and distribution of carbon monoxide on blood and body stores. American Journal of Physiology 217: 354–63
10. Coburn R, Mayers L 1971 Myoglobin oxygen tension determined from measurements of COHb in skeletal muscle. American Journal of Physiology 220: 66–74
11. Coburn R, Forman H Carbon monoxide toxicity. In: Fishman A (ed) Handbook of Physiology of the Respiratory System, vol 4. American Physiological Society, Bethesda, pp 439–56
12. Piantadosi C, Lee P, Sylvia A 1988 Direct effects of CO on cerebral energy metabolism in bloodless rats. Journal of Applied Physiology 65: 878–87
13. Ball EG, Strittmatter CF, Cooper O 1951 The reaction of cytochrome oxidase with carbon monoxide. Journal of Biology and Chemistry 193: 635–97
14. Thom S 1990 Carbon monoxide-mediated brain lipid peroxidation in the rat. Journal of Applied Physiology 68: 997–1003
15. Weaver LK 1999 Carbon monoxide poisoning. Critical Care Clinics 15: 297–317
16. Heckerling PS, Leikin JB, Maturen A 1988 Occult CO poisoning: validation of a prediction model. American Journal of Medicine 84: 251–6
17. Myers RAM, Britten JS 1987 Do arterial blood gases have value in prognosis and treatment decisions in carbon monoxide poisoning? Undersea Biomedical Research 14(2): Suppl 1
18. Scheinkestel, CD, Bailery M, Myles, et al 1999 Hyperbaric or normobaric oxygen for acute carbon monoxide poisoning: a randomised controlled clinical trial. Medical Journal of Australia 170: 203–10
19. Weaver LK, Hopkins RO, Chan KJ, et al 2002 Hyperbaric oxygen for acute carbon monoxide poisoning. New England Journal of Medicine 347: 1057–67

28.10 CYANIDE

GEORGE BRAITBERG

ESSENTIALS

1 Cyanide is a metabolic poison associated with a high mortality.

2 Cyanide exposure correlates well with serum lactate levels.

3 Cyanide treatment is controversial, with different treatment modalities being used in different parts of the world. The current recommended treatment in Australia is dicobalt edetate, Kelocyanor®. However, European data suggest that hydroxocobalamin is a far superior and safer antidote.

INTRODUCTION AND EPIDEMIOLOGY

Cyanide is used in a variety of commercial processes.[1] Exposure can be in the form of hydrogen cyanide (HCN) gas, produced when inorganic cyanide comes in contact with mineral acids as in electroplating, or accidentally when cyanide solutions are poured into acid waste containers. Cyanide is used in metal extraction and recovery, metal hardening, and in the production of agricultural and horticultural pest control compounds. Cyanide off-gassing in house fires is well documented, and in one study significant blood levels occurred in 59% of smoke inhalation patients.[2]

Death from cyanide poisoning is one of the most rapid and dramatic seen in medicine. A dose of 200 mg of ingested cyanide, or 3 minutes' exposure to HCN gas, is potentially lethal.[3]

Fortunately, serious acute cyanide poisoning is rare. Of 1 926 438 human poison exposures reported to the American Association of Poison Control Centers during 1994, only 360 involved cyanide poisoning. Of the 208 cases in which clinical outcome is known, only 13 were reported to develop major symptoms, and only nine patients died.[1] However, the incidence of cyanide poisoning may be significantly underestimated. Blood cyanide concentrations greater than 40 μmol/L were found in 74% of victims found dead at the scenes of fires.[2]

TOXICOKINETICS AND PATHOPHYSIOLOGY

The uptake of cyanide into cells is rapid and follows a first-order kinetic simple diffusion process. The half-life of cyanide is from 2 to 3 hours.

While the precise in vivo action of cyanide is yet to be determined, it is thought that its major effect is due to binding with the ferric ion (Fe^{3+}) of cytochrome oxidase, the last cytochrome in the respiratory chain. This results in inhibition of oxidative phosphorylation, leading to a net accumulation of hydrogen ions, a change in the NAD:NADH ratio, and greatly increased lactic acid production. Other enzymatic processes, involving antioxidant enzymes, catalase, superoxide dismutase and glutathione, may contribute to toxicity.[4] Cyanide is also a potent stimulator of neurotransmitter release, in both the central and the peripheral nervous systems.[5]

Humans detoxify cyanide by transferring sulphane sulphur, R-Sx-SH, to cyanide to form thiocyanate (SCN). The availability of R-Sx-SH is the rate-limiting step. This reaction is thought to be catalyzed by the liver enzyme rhodanese. However, other enzymes, such as β-mercaptopyruvate sulphur transferase, may be important. Other routes of biotransformation include oxidative detoxification.[4]

CLINICAL PRESENTATION

Cyanide toxicity is characterized by effects on the CNS, respiratory and cardiovascular systems, and by metabolic acidosis.[3]

CNS manifestations, in order of increasing severity of cyanide exposure, are headache, anxiety, disorientation, lethargy, seizures, respiratory depression, CNS depression and cerebral death. An initial tachypnoea gives way to respiratory depression as CNS depression develops.

Cardiovascular manifestations include hypertension followed by hypotension, tachycardia followed by bradycardia, arrhythmias, AV block and cardiovascular collapse. The classic finding of bright red skin and blood is not observed if significant myocardial, respiratory or CNS depression has already occurred: in these situations the patient may appear cyanotic. Other cardiovascular parameters of interest include decreased systemic vascular resistance, increased cardiac output, and decreased arterio-venous oxygen gradient.

INVESTIGATIONS

Arterial blood gas analysis and serum lactate measurements reveal metabolic acidosis with a raised lactate. Concentration decay curves suggest that serum lactate concentration is closely related to blood cyanide concentration. In smoke-inhalation victims without severe burns,

plasma lactate concentrations above 10 mmol/L correlate with blood cyanide concentrations above 40 μmol/L, with a sensitivity of 87%, a specificity of 94% and a positive predictive value of 95%.[6]

Cyanide is concentrated tenfold by erythrocytes and whole-blood cyanide concentrations are used as the benchmark when comparing levels. A level of 40 μmol/L is considered toxic, and a level of 100 μmol/L potentially lethal. Symptomatic intoxication starts at levels of about 20 μmol/L.[7]

MANAGEMENT

Attention to airway, breathing, circulation and other resuscitative measures must be instituted immediately.

In the case of cyanide poisoning from smoke inhalation or self-poisoning, with clinical signs and associated lactic acidosis, and where one is suspicious of cyanide poisoning as the cause of coma or cardiovascular instability, the following antidote regimen is recommended:

- 5–15 g of hydroxocobalamin IV over 30 minutes (but may be given as IV push if needed). Repeat if needed. PLUS
- Sodium thiosulphate 12.5 g IV (50 mL of a 25% solution at 2.5–5.0 mL/min).

Dicobalt edetate (Kelocyanor®)

Dicobalt edetate was introduced as a cyanide antidote in the late 1950s. It complexes with cyanide to form cobalt cyanide, thus removing cyanide from the circulation and reducing toxicity. However, unless cyanide is forced into the extracellular fluid, tissue levels are minimally affected.

Adverse effects are considerable and may be life-threatening.[7] Severe hypotension, cardiac arrhythmias, convulsions and gross oedema are reported.[8] These effects are exacerbated when individuals treated for suspected cyanide poisoning are, in fact, not cyanide poisoned. In life-threatening situations where cyanide poisoning is suspected the antidote must be given before confirmatory tests are

performed; the treating physician is, therefore, faced with a significant dilemma when the history of exposure is unclear. A semiquantitative bedside test for cyanide in blood is available and may be helpful in determining the need for antidotal therapy when time permits.[9] The recommended dose of dicobalt edetate is 300 mg intravenously.

Hydroxocobalamin

In Europe hydroxocobalamin is the antidote of choice in cyanide poisoning. Hydroxocobalamin (vitamin B_{12A}) complexes with cyanide, on a mole-for-mole ratio, to form cyanocobalamin. Antidotal doses of hydroxocobalamin are approximately 5000 times the physiological dose.

Hydroxocobalamin and cyanocobalamin are excreted by the kidney. The half-life of hydroxocobalamin in cyanide-exposed patients is 26.2 hours.[10] As the half-life of cyanide in smoke inhalation victims is calculated to be between 1.2 and 3.0 hours, it is suggested that hydroxocobalamin can be satisfactorily used as single-dose therapy. The amount of cyanocobalamin formed after a dose of 5 g hydroxocobalamin correlates linearly until a blood cyanide level of 40 μmol/L is reached. At higher blood cyanide concentrations there is little further rise in plasma cyanocobalamin, and it is suggested that the rate-limiting step in the formation of cyanocobalamin is the availability of antidote, not the absence of cyanide ions.[11]

Extensive research has demonstrated the safety of this drug.[12] In healthy adult smokers, 5 g of IV hydroxocobalamin is associated with a transient reddish discoloration of the skin, mucous membranes and urine, and a mean elevation in systolic blood pressure of 13.6%, with a concomitant 16.3% decrease in heart rate. No other clinical adverse effects are noted.[13] Allergic reactions are rare.[14] There is substantial experimental evidence to support the efficacy of hydroxocobalamin at lower levels of toxicity.[10,12] Hydroxocobalamin has been shown to be safe and efficacious in mild-to-moderate cyanide poisonings with levels up to 150 μmol/L and has been given successfully to patients with severe cyanide toxicity.[15] In cases of ingestion of cyanide with suicidal intent (where blood cyanide levels may be greater than 150 μmol/L or plasma lactate concentrations greater than 20 mmol/L), the usual dose of 5–10 g may be insufficient.

The paucity of scientific data comparing the efficacy of hydroxocobalamin with dicobalt edetate precludes any definitive conclusion about which antidote is best. However, in the emergency situation hydroxocobalamin appears to offer a greater margin of safety.

Limited volunteer studies suggest a synergistic effect of hydroxocobalamin and thiosulphate. Thiosulphate used on its own is limited by a slow onset of action and thus cannot be used as a first-line antidote. Case reports document successful outcomes in patients with extremely high levels of cyanide (494 μmol/L) with combination therapy.[15]

Hydroxocobalmin has recently been recommended as the treatment of choice for mass casualty chemical disasters where cyanide poisoning is suspected.[16]

Eli Lilly Cyanide kit

Administration of sodium nitrite followed by sodium thiosulphate is a long-accepted antidote for cyanide poisoning. The current Eli Lilly Cyanide kit was devised in 1970 and contains:

- Amyl nitrite perles
- Sodium nitrite 10 mL (30 mg/mL)
- Sodium thiosulphate 50 mL (250 mg/mL).

The kit is based upon the premise that humans can tolerate up to 30% methaemoglobinaemia.[17,18] Conversion of haemoglobin to methaemoglobin promotes the movement of cyanide out of the cytochrome system; 4 mg/kg of sodium nitrite takes 30 minutes to achieve 7–10.5% methaemoglobin.[15] The formation of sodium thiocyanate allows for the reformation of Hb^{2+}, restoring the oxygen-carrying capacity of haemoglobin. Cellular respiration can continue as normal with cyanide removed from the respiratory chain. The observation that dramatic improvements in symptoms have occurred well before methaemoglobin levels have peaked has led many authors to suggest different mechanisms of action, such as vasodilatation and extracellular redistribution of cyanide.[7,14] In smoke inhalation victims with suspected combined carbon monoxide and cyanide poisoning, the availability of an antidote that will not exacerbate any oxygen carriage or delivery problem, or cause toxicity by its own action, is highly desirable. The combination of 10% methaemoglobin with carboxyhaemoglobin has synergistic detrimental effects on the oxyhaemoglobin dissociation curve.

Hyperbaric oxygen

The role of hyperbaric medicine in the management of cyanide toxicity is controversial, with conflicting animal data. In most published human reports hyperbaric oxygen is offered after a combination of modalities, and it is not possible to determine the treatment effect specific to each.[19]

REFERENCES

1. Hall AH, Rumack BH 1998 Cyanide and related compounds. In: Haddad M, Shannon MW, Winchester JF (eds) Clinical Management Poisoning and Drug Overdose, 3rd edn. WB Saunders, pp 899–905
2. Baud FJ, Barriot P, Toffis V, et al 1991 Elevated blood cyanide levels in victims of smoke inhalation. New England Journal of Medicine 325: 1761–6
3. Gonzales J, Sabatini S 1989 Cyanide poisoning: pathophysiology and current approaches to therapy. International Journal of Artificial Organs 12(6): 347–55
4. Curry SC 1992 Hydrogen cyanide and inorganic salts. In: Sullivan JB, Krieger GR (eds) Hazardous Materials Toxicology. Clinical Principles of Environmental Health. Williams and Wilkins, pp 698–709
5. Isom GE, Borowitz JL 1995 Modification of cyanide toxicodynamics mechanistic based antidote development. Toxicology Letters 82/83: 795–9
6. Baud FJ, Borron SW, Bavoux E, et al 1996 Relationship between plasma lactate and blood cyanide concentrations in acute poisoning. British Medical Journal 312: 26–27
7. Marrs TC 1988 Anidotal treatment of acute cyanide poisoning. Advances in drug reaction. Acute Poisoning Review 4: 179–206
8. Dodds C, McKnight C 1985 Cyanide toxicity after immersion and the hazards of dicobalt edetate. British Medical Journal 291: 785–6
9. Fligner CL, Luthi R, Linkaityle-Weiss F, et al 1992 Paper strip screening method for detection of cyanide in blood using the CYANOTESTMO test paper. American Journal of Forensic Medical Pathology 13(1): 81–84
10. Houeto P, Borron SW, Sandauk P, et al 1996 Pharmacokinetics of hydroxocobalamin in smoke inhalation victims. Clinical Toxicology 34(4): 397–404
11. Houeto P, Hoffman JR, Imbert M, et al 1995 Relation of blood cyanide to plasma cyanocobalamin concentration after a fixed dose of hydroxocobalamin in cyanide poisoning. Lancet 346: 605–8
12. Riou B, Baud FJ, Borron SW, et al 1990 In vitro demonstration of the antidotal efficacy of hydroxocobalamin in cyanide poisoning. Journal of Neurosurgical Anaesthetics 2(4): 296–304
13. Forsyth JC, Mueller PD, et al 1993 Hydroxocobalamin as a cyanide antidote: safety, efficacy and pharamacokinetics in heavy smoking normal volunteers. Journal of Toxicology and Clinical Toxicology 31: 277–94
14. Borron SW, Baud FJ 1996 Acute cyanide poisoning: clinical spectrum, diagnosis and treatment. Arhiv za Higijenu Rada i Toksikologiju (Zagreb) 47: 307–22
15. Tassan H, Joyon D, Richard T, et al 1990 Potassium cyanide poisoning treated with hydroxocobalamin. Annales Françaises d'Anesthésie et réanimation 4: 383–5
16. Sauer SW, Keim ME 2001 Hydroxocobalamin: improved public health readiness fro cyanide disasters. Annals of Emergency Medicine 37: 635–41
17. Kirk MA, Gerace R, Kulig KW 1993 Cyanide and methaemoglobin kinetics in smoke inhalation victims treated with the cyanide antidote kit. Annals of Emergency Medicine 22: 1413–8
18. Kiese M, Weger N 1969 Formation of ferrihaemoglobin with aminophenols in the human for the treatment of cyanide poisoning. European Journal of Pharmacology 7: 97–105
19. Hart GB, Strauss MB, Lennon PA, et al 1985 Treatment of smoke inhalation by hyperbaric oxygen. Journal of Emergency Medicine 3: 111

28.11 CORROSIVE INGESTION

ROBERT DOWSETT

ESSENTIALS

1 Symptomatic patients may have burns to the airway or supraglottic tissues.

2 Decontamination has limited utility; care should be taken not to make patients vomit, and no attempt should be made to neutralize corrosives.

3 Serious injuries to the oesophagus or stomach may occur in the absence of visible burns to the lips, mouth or throat.

4 Admit all symptomatic patients.

5 Upper gastrointestinal endoscopy is the best guide to prognosis and management.

6 The major acute complications are perforation and necrosis, which may involve other intra-abdominal organs.

7 The major long-term complication is oesophageal stricture.

8 The value of corticosteroids for alkali ingestion is controversial.

INTRODUCTION

Corrosives are compounds capable of causing direct chemical injury to tissue. Most do so by acid–base reactions. Strong solutions, capable of causing significant injury, are those with a pH of less than 2 or greater than 12 (Table 28.11.1). The pH of a solution is dependant on the concentration and dissociation constant (pKa) of the chemical. Strong acids have a pKa =0 and strong alkalis have a pKa =14 (Table 28.11.2). The extent of injury also depends on the volume ingested, contact time and viscosity.

Domestic hypochlorite bleaches and ammonia products are the commonest substances ingested, but severe injury generally does not occur unless large amounts are swallowed.[1] Death results mainly from the ingestion of drain or toilet cleaners. Powdered automatic dishwasher detergents are also capable of causing severe injuries.[2,3]

PATHOPHYSIOLOGY

Acid–base reactions cause injury by disrupting organic macromolecules. Heat generation may cause thermal burns. Highly exothermic reactions occur between strong acids and bases, or between light metallic compounds and water. Chemical reactions may also result in the production of other compounds that can cause additional injury to the GI tract and lungs (Table 28.11.3).

Alkalis cause 'liquefactive' necrosis, a process that involves saponification of fats, dissolution of proteins and emulsification of lipid membranes. Disruption of cellular membranes enhances penetration of alkali through the tissues.

Acids cause 'coagulative' necrosis, a process that involves denaturation of protein. The denatured protein forms a

hard eschar that may limit further penetration of the acid.

In both settings, tissue injury progresses rapidly and can continue for several hours following ingestion. Granulation tissue develops after 3–4 days, but collagen deposition may not begin until the second week, making the healing tissue extremely fragile during this period. Complete repair of the epithelium may take weeks. From the third week, newly deposited collagen begins to contract and may produce strictures of the oesophagus, stomach and affected bowel.

Table 28.11.1 Approximate pH of some common solutions

Solution	pH
Battery acid (1% solution)	1.4
Domestic toilet cleaner (1%)	2.0
Bleach (1% solution)	9.5–10.2
Automatic dishwasher detergents	10.4–13
Laundry detergents	11.6–12.6
Domestic ammonium cleaners	11.9–12.4
Drain cleaner (containing NaOH, KOH)	13.3–14

Table 28.11.2 pKa of some common corrosives

Chemical	pKa	Highly corrosive?
Hydrochloric acid	−3	Yes
Bromic acid	<1	Yes
Nitric acid	<1	Yes
Sulphuric acid	1.9	
Arsenic acid	2.3	
Nitrous acid	3.3	
Hydrofluoric acid	3.4	
Ammonia	9.3	
Ammonium hydroxide	9.3	
Magnesium hydroxide	10	
Zinc hydroxide	11	
Calcium hydroxide	11.6	
Lithium hydroxide	>14	Yes
Potassium hydroxide	>14	Yes
Sodium hydroxide	>14	Yes
Calcium oxide	>14	Yes
Sodium carbonate	>14	Yes
Potassium carbonate	>14	Yes
Sodium hypochlorite	>14	Yes

Table 28.11.3 Chemical reactions resulting in the production of further toxic chemicals

Chemical	Plus	Produces
Chlorine	Water	Hydrochloric acid Hypochlorous acid Oxygen radicals Heat
Ammonia	Water	Ammonium hydroxide Heat
Nitrogen dioxide	Water	Nitric acid Nitrous acid
Ammonia	Hypochlorite	Chloramine gas (NH_2Cl and $NHCl_2$)
Hypochlorite	Acid	Chlorine gas Hydrogen sulphide
Sulphur compounds (e.g. plaster casts)	Acid	Sulphur oxide

Hydrocarbon compounds can produce injury by dissolving lipids and coagulating proteins. Other chemicals can injure tissues by redox reactions and alkylation.

Following corrosive ingestion tissue inflammation, necrosis and infection can result in hypovolaemia, acidosis and organ failure.

Sites that are most at risk from corrosive ingestion are the cricopharyngeal area, the diaphragmatic oesophagus, antrum and pylorus.[4] Up to 80% of patients have injuries at multiple sites.[5] Alkalis are more likely to produce oesophageal injury than are acids, which typically injure the stomach.[4,6–11] Solid corrosives are more likely to affect the mouth, pharynx and upper oesophagus, and to cause deeper burns.

The main acute complications of corrosive ingestion are haemorrhage, perforation and fistula formation. These result from severe burns causing full-thickness necrosis.

Full-thickness necrosis of the stomach may be associated with injury to the transverse colon, pancreas, spleen, small bowel, liver and kidneys. Perforation of the upper anterior oesophagus may lead to the formation of a tracheoesophageal fistula. Formation of an tracheoesophagoaortic-aortic fistula is a rapidly lethal complication.

CLINICAL PRESENTATION

Symptoms and signs associated with significant alkali ingestion include mouth and throat pain, drooling, pain on swallowing, vomiting, abdominal pain and haematemesis.[7] If the larynx is involved, local oedema may produce respiratory distress, stridor and a hoarse voice.[9,12,13]

Extensive tissue injury may be associated with fever, tachycardia, hypotension and tachypnoea.

Inspection of the oropharynx may reveal areas of mucosal burn. The absence of visible burns to the lips, mouth or throat does not imply an absence of significant burns to the oesophagus.[3,5,7,9–11,14–17]

Symptoms and signs associated with the life-threatening complications of oesophageal perforation and mediastinitis include chest pain, dyspnoea, fever, subcutaneous emphysema of the chest or neck, and a pleural rub. Perforation of the abdominal oesophagus or stomach is associated with the clinical features of chemical peritonitis, including abdominal pain, fever and ileus.[5,6,10,18] Septic shock, multi-organ failure and death may develop rapidly if perforation is not recognized.

The systemic effects of large acid ingestion include hypotension, metabolic acidosis, haemolysis, haemoglobinuria, nephrotoxicity, pulmonary oedema and hypotension. Features of systemic toxicity can result from the ingestion of arsenic, cyanide and other heavy metal salts, fluoride, ammonia, hydrazine, hydrochloric acid, nitrates, sulphuric acid and phosphoric acid. Ingestion of ammonia can cause coma, hypotension, acidosis, pulmonary oedema, liver dysfunction and coagulopathy.[19] Systemic effects of phenol and related compounds include haemolysis and renal failure.[20]

LONG-TERM COMPLICATIONS

The major late complication of corrosive ingestion is the development of an oesophageal stricture. All patients with full-thickness necrosis of the oesophageal wall develop strictures, as do 70% of those with deep ulceration.[5,10] Symptoms of oesophageal narrowing (principally dysphagia) may develop within 2 weeks; 80% occur within the first 2 months. Early onset of symptoms is associated with a more rapidly progressive and severe obstruction. Strictures do not develop in areas of superficial mucosal ulceration.[6,11,18,21–25] Strictures can also affect the mouth, pharynx and stomach. Only 40% of gastric outlet strictures become symptomatic.[5,10,11] A very late complication of alkali ingestion is the development of oesophageal carcinoma, reported to develop 22–81 years after exposure.[26]

INVESTIGATIONS

Initial investigations in symptomatic patients should include an ECG, arterial blood gas, blood count, type and crossmatch, coagulation profile, serum electrolytes, blood glucose, and liver and renal function.

A chest X-ray and upright abdominal film should be assessed for evidence of mediastinal widening, pleural effusions, pneumomediastinum, pneumothorax and subphrenic gas.

All patients who are symptomatic or have visible oropharyngeal burns should undergo upper gastrointestinal endoscopy within 24 hours.[5] Endoscopy should also be considered in any patient who has intentionally ingested a strong acid or alkali. Endoscopy is the only way to fully assess the extent of injury to the gastrointestinal tract, and the findings are the best guide to prognosis and subsequent management. The entire upper gastrointestinal tract may be safely examined with a small-diameter flexible endoscope, provided it is not retroflexed or forced through areas of narrowing.[4,5,27] It is not necessary to terminate the examination at the first circumferential or full-thickness lesion. The cricopharynx should be assessed initially to identify any laryngeal burns. If laryngeal oedema or ulceration is encountered, endotracheal intubation may be necessary before continuing with endoscopy.

Oesophageal burns can be graded according to the depth of ulceration and the presence of necrosis, as determined at endoscopy (Table 28.11.4). Some grading systems parallel those used for thermal skin burns whilst others differentiate several levels of ulceration and necrosis. Essentially, injuries can be divided into three main groups:

❶ Mucosal inflammation or superficial ulceration only. These injuries will heal completely and are not at risk of stricture formation.
❷ Areas of deep ulceration or discrete areas of necrosis or circumferential ulceration of any depth. Stricture formation may occur.
❸ Deep circumferential burns or extensive areas of necrosis. These patients are at high risk of perforation and stricture formation.

Contrast oesophagography with a water-soluble contrast agent is useful for the detection of perforation, but is less sensitive than endoscopy in evaluating ulceration.[28]

MANAGEMENT

Patients should initially be assessed for the presence of any symptomatic airway burns or respiratory distress. Urgent intubation is indicated in any patient with stridor or hypoxia.

Efforts at decontamination must not include induced vomiting, as this may exacerbate the oesophageal injury. The mouth should be rinsed thoroughly with water. Dilution of an ingested solid chemical by drinking 250 mL of water or milk is recommended. The value of administering oral fluids following ingestion of a liquid corrosive is controversial.[8,29] Patients should otherwise be given nothing by mouth. Neutralization, aspiration and administration of activated charcoal are all contraindicated.

Patients with persistent symptoms should be admitted for observation and undergo endoscopy within 24 hours. Further management is dictated by the findings at endoscopy.

Patients with endoscopic evidence of superficial injury only can be managed on a general medical ward with supportive care alone. Complete healing can be expected. Patients with deep discrete ulceration, circumferential ulceration or isolated areas of necrosis should be admitted to high-dependency or ICU and kept nil by mouth. IV fluid replacement, accurate fluid and electrolyte balance and symptom control are the mainstays of therapy. These patients may require prolonged IV access, and parenteral feeding and central venous access should be considered.

If perforation or penetration is suspected clinically or documented by endoscopy or contrast radiography, urgent laparotomy with or without thoracotomy must be considered. Early excision of areas with extensive full-thickness necrosis has been proposed, but this needs to be weighed against mortality rates of 40–50% for patients undergoing such emergency surgery.

Prophylactic broad-spectrum antibiotics are only indicated where there is evidence of gastrointestinal tract perforation.

Strictures are dilated by endoscopy 3–4 weeks after ingestion. Reconstructive surgery may be required if the oesophageal lumen becomes completely obstructed, or if perforation occurs.

DISPOSITION

Asymptomatic patients can be discharged after observation. They should be instructed to return if they develop pain, respiratory symptoms or difficulty swallowing. Symptomatic patients should be admitted for endoscopy with subsequent disposition dependent on the findings, as detailed above. Those patients that develop strictures will require long-term follow-up.

CONCLUSION

A wide variety of chemicals have the potential to cause corrosive injury to the gastrointestinal tract, and all symptomatic patients should be admitted for

Table 28.11.4 Classification of gastrointestinal corrosive burns	
Grade 1 Mucosal inflammation	**First-degree** Mucosal inflammation, oedema or superficial sloughing
Grade IIA Haemorrhages, erosions and superficial ulceration	**Second-degree** Damage extends to all layers of, but not through, the oesophagus
Grade IIB Isolated discrete or circumferential superficial ulceration	
Grade IIIA Small scattered areas of necrosis	**Third-degree** Ulceration through to perioesophageal tissues
Grade IIIB Extensive necrosis involving the whole oesophagus	

CONTROVERSIES AND FUTURE DIRECTIONS

❶ The use of corticosteroids to prevent oesophageal strictures following alkali ingestion is controversial. Clinical trials show contradictory results.[22,23,30,31] Steroids do not decrease stricture formation following extensive or deep ulceration or necrosis, and may increase the risk of perforation.

evaluation. Management is primarily supportive. Endoscopic evaluation is the best guide to prognosis and ongoing management.

REFERENCES

1. Litovitz TL, Klein-Schwartzt W, White S, et al 2001 2000 annual report of the American Association of Poison Control Centers Toxic Exposure Surveillance System. American Journal of Emergency Medicine 19: 337

2. Clausen JO, Nielsen TL, Fogh A 1994 Admission to Danish hospitals after suspected ingestion of corrosives. A nationwide survey (1984–1988) comprising children aged 0–14 years. Danish Medical Bulletin 41: 234

3. Kynaston JA, Patrick MK, Shepherd RW, et al 1989 The hazards of automatic-dishwasher detergent. Medical Journal of Australia 151: 5

4. Sugawa C, Lucas CE 1989 Caustic injury of the upper gastrointestinal tract in adults: a clinical and endoscopic study. Surgery 106: 802

5. Zargar SA, Kochhar R, Mehta S, et al 1991 The role of fiberoptic endoscopy in the management of corrosive ingestion and modified endoscopic classification of burns. Gastrointestinal Endoscopy 37: 165

6. Estrera A, Taylor W, Mills LJ 1986 Corrosive burns of the esophagus and stomach: a recommendation for an aggressive surgical approach. Annals of Thoracic Surgery 41: 276

7. Gorman RL, Khin-Maung-Gyi MT, Klein-Schwartz W, et al 1992 Initial symptoms as predictors of esophageal injury in alkaline corrosive ingestions. American Journal of Emergency Medicine 10: 189

8. Penner GE 1980 Acid ingestion: toxicology and treatment. Annals of Emergency Medicine 9: 374

9. Vergauwen P, Moulin D, Buts JP, et al 1991 Caustic burns of the upper digestive and respiratory tracts. European Journal of Pediatrics 150: 700

10. Zargar SA, Kochhar R, Nagi B, et al 1992 Ingestion of strong corrosive alkalis: spectrum of injury to upper gastrointestinal tract and natural history. American Journal of Gastroenterology 87: 337

11. Zargar SA, Kochhar R, Nagi B, et al 1989 Ingestion of corrosive acids: spectrum of injury to upper gastrointestinal tract and natural history. Gastroenterology 97: 702

12. Moulin D, Bertrand JM, Buts JP, et al 1985 Upper airway lesions in children after accidental ingestion of caustic substances. Journal of Pediatrics 106: 408

13. Scott JC, Jones B, Eisele DW, et al 1992 Caustic ingestion injuries of the upper aerodigestive tract. Laryngoscope 102: 1

14. Crain EF, Gershel JC, Mezey AP 1984 Caustic ingestions: symptoms as predictors of esophageal injury. American Journal of Diseases of Childhood 138: 863

15. Gaudreault P, Parent M, Mcguigan MA, et al 1983 Predictability of esophageal injury from symptoms and signs: a study of caustic ingestion in 378 children. Pediatrics 71: 767

16. Christesen-HB 1995 Prediction of complications following unintentional caustic ingestion in children. Is endoscopy always necessary? Acta Pediatrica 84(10): 1177–82

17. Muhlendahl KE, Oberdisse U, Krienke EG 1978 Local injuries by accidental ingestions of corrosive substances by children. Archives of Toxicology 39: 299

18. Ray JR, Meyers W, Lawton BR 1974 The natural history of liquid lye ingestion: rationale for aggressive surgical approach. Archives of Surgery 109: 436

19. Zitnik RS, Burchell HB, Shepherd JT 1969 Hemodynamic effects of inhalation of ammonia in man. American Journal of Cardiology 24: 187

20. Lin CH, Yang JY 1992 Chemical burn with cresol intoxication and multiple organ failure. Burns 18: 162

21. Middlekamp JN, Ferguson TB, Roper CL, et al 1969 The management and problems of caustic burns in children. Journal of Thoracic and Cardiovascular Surgery 57: 341

22. Hawkins DB, Demeter MJ, Barness TE 1980 Caustic ingestions: controversies in management - a review of 214 cases. Laryngoscope 90: 98

23. Anderson KD, Rouse TM, Randolph JG 1990 A controlled trial of corticosteroids in children with corrosive injury of the esophagus. New England Journal of Medicine 323: 637

24. Webb WR, Koutras P, Eckker RR, et al 1970 An evaluation of steroids and antibiotics in caustic burns of the esophagus. Annals of Thoracic Surgery 9: 95

25. Cannon S, Chandler JR 1963 Corrosive burns of the esophagus: analysis of 100 patients. Eye Ear Nose Throat Monthly 42: 35

26. Isolauri J, Markkula H 1989 Lye ingestion and carcinoma of the esophagus. Acta Chirurgica Scandinavica 155: 269

27. Chung RS, DenBestein L 1975 Fibreoptic endoscopy in the treatment of corrosive injury of the stomach. Archives of Surgery 110: 725

28. Mansson I 1978 Diagnosis of acute corrosive lesions of the esophagus. Journal of Laryngology and Otology 92: 499

29. Rumack BH, Burrington JD 1977 Caustic ingestions: a rational look at diluents. Clinical Toxicology 11: 27

30. Howell JM, Dalsey WC, Hartsell FW, et al 1992 Steroids for the treatment of corrosive esophageal injury: a statistical analysis of past studies. American Journal of Emergency Medicine 10: 421

31. Oakes DD, Sherck JP, Mark JB 1982 Lye ingestion: clinical patterns and therapeutic implications. Journal of Thoracic and Cardiovascular Surgery 83: 194

28.12 DRUGS OF ABUSE

FRANK DALY

ESSENTIALS

1 Heroin overdose is common in Australia.

2 Co-ingestion of other CNS depressant drugs, poor tolerance, high street purity and reluctance to seek medical care are associated with death from heroin overdose.

3 The diagnosis of the intoxication syndromes of the principal drugs of abuse is clinical, based on history and examination.

4 Good supportive care ensures optimal outcome for the majority of cases of overdose with drugs of abuse that present to the emergency department.

5 Naloxone, a short-acting opioid antagonist, is a useful adjunct in the management of opioid overdose.

6 Benzodiazepines are important in the management of CNS stimulation and seizures following intoxication with cocaine and amphetamines.

7 Gamma hydroxybutyrate (GHB) is an emerging drug of abuse. Central nervous system depression is the predominant effect and management is supportive.

8 Presentation to the emergency department following overdose with an illicit drug provides an important opportunity for intervention in terms of education to avoid future overdoses and referral to agencies specializing in drug detoxification and rehabilitation.

OPIOIDS

INTRODUCTION AND EPIDEMIOLOGY

Opioids are derivatives of the opium poppy, *Papaver somniferum*, which contains approximately 20 alkaloids, including morphine, codeine and thebaine.[1]

Between 1979 and 1995 the incidence of opioid-related deaths in Australia increased from 11 to 67 deaths per million population aged 15–44,[2] and in Western Australia the incidence of heroin-related death nearly doubled in 1995.[3] Forensic data indicate that 77% of opioid-related deaths in Western Australia are due to heroin (diacetylmorphine).[4]

Overseas longitudinal studies suggest that illicit drug abuse in teenagers is associated with mortality rates of 10–20 times that of their peers,[5] while heroin users have an annual mortality rate of between 1% and 3%, 6–20 times that of their peers.[6] The predominant cause of this excess mortality is overdose, rather than trauma, infectious disease or suicide.[5,6]

Factors that contribute to the clinical syndrome of non-fatal and fatal overdose include the coingestion of other CNS depressant drugs,[6,7,8] poor tolerance,[7] high street purity,[9] and reluctance to seek medical care.[6]

Heroin overdose is a common occurrence among Australian heroin users, with 68% experiencing overdose and 86% witnessing an overdose in one study.[7] It occurred in experienced addicts who used multiple drugs: the mean period of heroin use until a non-fatal overdose was 30 months, and overdose was related to an increased use and dependency on other drugs. Sixty per cent reported using alcohol or benzodiazepines at the time of their last overdose. Of all heroin-related deaths in New South Wales in 1992, two or more drug classes were detected in 71% of subjects.[8] Alcohol was detected in 45% and the mean blood alcohol concentration was 30 mmol/L (140 mg/dL).

PHARMACOLOGY AND PATHOPHYSIOLOGY

Most opioids are well absorbed across mucous membranes and from subcutaneous and intramuscular sites. Opioids absorbed from the gastrointestinal tract are subject to extensive first-pass metabolism. They are converted to polar metabolites for excretion in the urine. Tissue hydrolysis (diacetylmorphine/heroin to morphine) also occurs in addition to glucuronidation (morphine), demethylation (a minor pathway) and oxidative metabolism in the liver. Active metabolites (e.g. morphine-6-glucuronide) may accumulate in renal failure. The demethylated metabolite of pethidine may also accumulate and cause seizures.[1]

Opioids produce their effects by binding to specific receptors found in the brain and spinal cord, and are usually classified as agonists, partial agonists or antagonists. The receptors are classified as μ (mu), δ (delta) and κ (kappa). The principal effects of opioids on the CNS, such as analgesia, euphoria, sedation and respiratory depression, are due to their action on μ receptors. All opioids cause miosis, to which tolerance does not develop. Naloxone, an opioid antagonist, reverses the miosis of opioids. Other CNS effects include cough suppression, nausea and vomiting. In addition, opioids cause constipation, increased gastric tone, contraction of biliary smooth muscle and prolongation of labour.[1]

CLINICAL PRESENTATION

Patients may present to the emergency department following acute opioid intoxication, with symptoms of opioid withdrawal, or with complications of illicit opioid use. Illicit opioid use may be via the parenteral, inhalational, oral or rectal routes. Venepuncture (track) marks are not always evident.

The clinical signs of pure opioid intoxication are related to their well-known effects on the CNS. With increasing dose euphoria, miosis, sedation, coma, respiratory depression and apnoea may occur. Death is due to respiratory depression.

The signs of opioid intoxication may be altered by factors such as coingested drugs, trauma, or medical complications of illicit opioid use. Drugs such as alcohol, benzodiazepines, amphetamines and hallucinogenics may cloud the clinical picture. The purity of heroin purchased 'on the street' may vary from less than 20% to greater than 50%,[3] and the drug is 'cut' with a variety of adulterant agents,[6] which may have their own clinical effects. Hypoxia, hypercarbia and acidaemia may lead to tachycardia, hypertension and variable pupillary responses. Finally, bradycardia, hypotension and cardiac arrest occur as terminal events.

Differing opioid pharmacokinetics affect presentation and management. Morphine and heroin (diacetylmorphine) taken parenterally reach peak serum levels and have clinical effect within minutes, and have a relatively short half-life of 3 hours. In contrast, methadone and slow-release morphine preparations taken orally frequently have slow and erratic absorption, reach peak plasma concentrations after several hours, and have much longer durations of effect. The duration of clinical CNS depression also depends on any coingested drugs.

DIAGNOSIS

The diagnosis of opioid intoxication is clinical, based on history and examination. A Glasgow Coma Scale less than 12 associated with respirations of 12 breaths/min or less, miotic pupils, or circumstantial evidence of drug use had a sensitivity of 92% and specificity of 76% for diagnosing opiate overdose in one cohort of patients.[10] A thorough physical examination of all systems is usually adequate to exclude complications such as non-cardiogenic pulmonary oedema, aspiration and compartment syndrome. Investigations are directed at excluding alternative diagnoses and complications as clinically indicated. The differential diagnosis is that of any patient with an altered level of consciousness, and includes toxicological and metabolic causes, sepsis, neurotrauma, stroke and postictal state. The presence of fever without localizing symptoms and signs should direct the emergency physician to consider bacteraemia secondary to parenteral drug abuse.

COMPLICATIONS

The complications of opioid abuse may be classified into three main groups: those due to the opioid, those secondary to the intoxicated state, and those due to poor injection technique. The prevalence of complications in patients who present to emergency departments with non-fatal opioid intoxication is not known, but a recent Australian study suggests it is underestimated.[11] The emergency physician should always exercise a high degree of suspicion.

The complications of the opioid intoxicated state are myriad and depend on individual patient circumstances. Loss of airway protective reflexes may lead to aspiration pneumonitis or pneumonia. Respiratory depression may lead to hypoxic encephalopathy. Dependent areas may suffer peripheral neuropathy, compartment syndrome or rhabdomyolysis, which in turn may combine with hypovolaemia and hypoxia to produce renal failure and hyperkalaemia. Hypothermia or hyperthermia may occur depending on prevailing environmental conditions. Trauma must be considered in all intoxicated patients.

Heroin-induced non-cardiogenic pulmonary oedema is a rare complication of heroin abuse. The aetiology is poorly understood and its relevance to the disposition of patients from the emergency department is controversial.[12,13] It is usually recognized in the context of resuscitation from severe respiratory depression or apnoea, when hypoxia, high levels of catecholamines and other metabolic derangements are present.

Complications of poor injection technique include cellulitis, thrombophlebitis, inadvertent intra-arterial injection and possible embolization, mycotic aneurysm, staphylococcal pneumonia, endocarditis, anaerobic clostridial infection, and viral infections such as hepatitis B, C and HIV.

MANAGEMENT AND DISPOSITION

Initial care is directed at assessing and managing the immediate threats to airway, breathing and circulation in a conventional manner. All patients should receive oxygen and have a bed-side blood glucose estimation. Patients with an altered level of consciousness should be closely monitored in a resuscitation area, positioned to minimize the chances of aspiration, and moved frequently to prevent dependent injuries.

Physical examination and investigations are directed toward exclusion of complications and alternative diagnoses, as detailed above. Intravenous access plus laboratory and radiological investigation should be reserved for those in whom they are clinically indicated.

Naloxone is a short-acting opioid antagonist useful in the management of opioid intoxication. There are no data to suggest that naloxone alone decreases mortality or the duration of emergency department care, but it has a role as an important adjunct to the support of airway and ventilation. It may be given via the intravenous, intramuscular, subcutaneous or endotracheal routes. Naloxone is safe and rarely associated with serious complications. There are case reports of cardiac arrest following the administration of naloxone to deeply comatose patients.[14] However, such reports probably represent the complications of hypoxia rather than the naloxone itself. In general, naloxone should not be withheld for fear of complications, especially if the airway and breathing cannot be secured by other means.

Bolus therapy quickly reverses the respiratory depression of opioid intoxication, but may be complicated by rapid wakening, agitation and, rarely, an acute withdrawal state. This may lead to the patient's premature departure from the emergency department before appropriate assessment and management. A bolus dose of 0.4–2.0 mg intravenously or intramuscularly may be given in an adult. The dose for a neonate or child is 0.01 mg/kg.

An alternative approach to bolus therapy is the use of small intravenous doses (e.g. 0.1 mg) titrated to achieve airway control and adequate ventilation. The aim is to prevent abrupt emergence and behavioural difficulties. Intravenous doses of naloxone are usually effective within a few minutes. However, the serum half-life of naloxone (approximately 1 hour) is less than that of most opioids, therefore patients must be carefully monitored for resedation.[15]

Naloxone infusions may be useful in patients who are intoxicated by long-acting opioids. They may prevent airway compromise or intubation, but the rate of infusion must be carefully titrated to maintain a clinical effect. Naloxone infusions should not offer a false sense of security to those monitoring the patient: absorption and elimination of opioids may be unpredictable, and undulating levels of CNS depression may occur despite a continuous naloxone infusion. All patients, regardless of the use of opioid antagonists, must be closely observed.

The duration of observation in the emergency department and the need for admission depends on the opioid taken, the route of administration, the influence of coingested drugs and the presence of comorbidity or complications. Accidental or deliberate self-poisoning with long-acting opioids will generally require observation for a minimum of 6 hours. There is a paucity of data regarding the minimum period of observation required in the emergency department to exclude all complications of heroin overdose. Most patients may be safely discharged when they are ambulant and competent. Following naloxone, patients may be considered for discharge after 1 hour if they are ambulant, alert, have normal vital signs and normal oxygen saturation.[16]

Heroin overdose is a life-threatening event and represents a signifcant point for an illicit drug user. Australian data suggest that the 18-month mortality following presentation to an emergency department with non-fatal opioid overdose may be as high as 20% for recidivist patients.[17] Therefore, although patients may be medically fit for early discharge, presentation to an emergency department must also provide an opportunity for preventative intervention. Patients should be counselled regarding strategies to avoid future overdose. Such strategies include minimizing coingestion of other CNS depressants, not using heroin alone, awareness of tolerance levels, and early activation of emergency medical services. In addition, the patient may be referred to agencies specializing in drug detoxification and rehabilitation.

OPIOID WITHDRAWAL SYNDROME

The development of physiological dependence with repeated doses of opioid agonists leads to an abstinence or withdrawal syndrome when opioids are ceased. The symptoms represent the reverse of the central and peripheral effects of opioid administration, and may include anxiety, insomnia, apprehension, hyperventilation, mydriasis, nausea, vomiting, diarrhoea and abdominal pain. Opioid withdrawal is not associated with delirium, seizures or high fever unless there is concomitant pathology, such as alcohol/benzodiazepine withdrawal or sepsis. The onset of symptoms depends on the half-life of the opioid used. Symptoms usually occur 12 hours after the last dose of morphine or heroin, reach a peak at approximately 2 days, and abate after approximately 5 days.

Withdrawal from methadone may take several weeks. Psychological craving for opioids may persist for months.

Unlike the benzodiazepine and alcohol withdrawal syndromes, seizures do not occur and the prognosis is good, even without medical intervention. However, patients in opioid withdrawal may present to emergency departments seeking symptomatic relief. A multifaceted approach should include an attempt to exclude concomitant pathology, treatment of dehydration, palliation of symptoms, and referral to agencies specializing in withdrawal services.

The short-term use of small doses of benzodiazepine may alleviate anxiety and hyperventilation. Clonidine, an α_2-receptor adrenergic agonist, has been used to decrease symptoms of autonomic dysfunction.[18] An initial dose of 1–2 µg/kg, 2–3 times per day, can be increased depending on tolerance of side effects, such as dry mouth and orthostatic hypotension.

Methadone has an established role in the management of withdrawal and maintenance therapy, but non-compliance rates are high. Australian and international studies indicate that maintenance on a methadone program decreases the rate of mortality to approximately 25% that of opioid addicts not on a methadone programme.[19] Patients in such programmes are less likely to die of heroin overdose or suicide, but methadone maintenance does not seem to have a measurable effect on the risk of death from non-heroin overdose, violence, trauma or natural causes.

The efficacy and safety of rapid opioid detoxification under general anaesthetic and the use of the long-acting opioid antagonist naltrexone remain controversial and have yet to be established.

COCAINE

INTRODUCTION AND EPIDEMIOLOGY

Coca leaves have been chewed by the natives of the South American Andes for approximately 1200 years, and were exported to Europe in 1580. The local anaesthetic properties of cocaine were recognized in the second half of the 19th century. Cocaine has been used as a local anaesthetic with vasoconstrictive properties for over a century.

In Australia the prevalence of cocaine abuse is low in the general population (around 2% in NSW),[20] and few people present to Australian emergency departments with primary cocaine-related problems. However, the use of cocaine seems to have increased among inner Sydney intravenous drug users, and there have recently been large police seizures of the drug, possibly reflecting greater general availability.[21] In the USA the recreational use of cocaine has reached epidemic proportions.[22]

PHARMACOLOGY AND PATHOPHYSIOLOGY

Cocaine hydrochloride, or benzoyl-methylecgonine hydrochloride, is a fine white powder prepared from the leaves of the *Erythroxylon coca* plant. This form of cocaine is not heat stable and cannot be smoked. 'Freebase' cocaine is an alkaloid that melts at 98°C and may be smoked. It is prepared by mixing cocaine hydrochloride, water and baking soda. The precipitate is separated by a filter or by dissolution in ether or alcohol. If the solvent is allowed to evaporate pure cocaine crystals remain, known as 'rock' cocaine or 'crack' because of the sound they make when they are heated.[23]

Cocaine reaches the cerebral circulation 6–8 seconds after smoking, 16–20 seconds after intravenous injection, and 3–5 minutes after nasal insufflation.[23] Gastrointestinal peak absorption may be delayed for up to 90 minutes.[22]

Cocaine is an ester-type local anaesthetic and is hydrolyzed by plasma and liver cholinesterases to produce an active metabolite, ecgonine methyl ester.[22] From 5–10% of cocaine is excreted in the urine unchanged.[22] The half-life of cocaine in the blood is 60–90 minutes.[23] In animal models cocaine is metabolized in the presence of ethanol to ethylecgonine. This is a myocardial depressant more potent than the sum of the depressant effects of cocaine and ethanol alone.[24]

The pathophysiology of cocaine is complex and incompletely understood. It is a CNS stimulant acting via enhanced release of noradrenaline (norepinephrine), plus blockade of noradrenaline (norepinephrine), dopamine and serotonin reuptake. Cocaine is also a local anaesthetic that blocks fast sodium channels.

With increasing doses euphoria is followed by dysphoria, agitation, seizures and coma. Considerable tachyphylaxis may occur. Cocaine stimulates the medullary vasomotor centre resulting in hypertension and tachycardia. Small doses may produce transient bradycardia (rarely clinically significant) owing to a vagotonic effect on the cardiovascular system.[22] At high levels the medullary centres may be depressed, leading to respiratory depression. In severe toxicity hypotension may occur and is probably due to a direct toxic effect on the myocardium mediated by sodium channel blockade.

Peripherally, cocaine inhibits the reuptake of adrenaline (epinephrine) and noradrenaline (norepinephrine), while at the same time stimulating the presynaptic release of noradrenaline (norepinephrine). This leads to a sympathomimetic response mediated through both α- and β-adrenoreceptors, leading to tachycardia, diaphoresis, vasoconstriction and hypertension.

A model to explain the clinical effects of cocaine toxicity and provide a rationale for management has been proposed.[22] CNS stimulation leads to seizures, hyperthermia and increased sympathetic drive. This sympathetic drive is augmented by the peripheral synaptic effects of cocaine, and produces many of the cardiovascular manifestations of cocaine toxicity. The exaggerated peripheral sympathetic response in turn also has a positive feedback effect on the brain, increasing the likelihood of hyperthermia and seizures.

Increased psychomotor activity, vasoconstriction and direct hypothalamic toxicity, possibly mediated by dopamine receptors, contribute to hyperpyrexia.[25]

Cocaine-induced myocardial ischaemia and infarction may occur. The pathophysiology is complex, but it appears that cocaine increases myocardial oxygen demand while decreasing myocardial oxygen supply. Contributing factors include immediate or delayed coronary artery vasospasm, increased platelet aggregation, accelerated atherosclerosis and dilated cardiomyopathy.[22]

Wide complex tachyarrhythmias, including ventricular tachycardia and fibrillation, are observed with cocaine toxicity. There are reports of prolongation of QRS and QT intervals, plus terminal right axis deviation (large R wave in aVR), implicating sodium channel blockade in addition to the sympathomimetic, ischaemic and cardiomyopathic factors mentioned above.[22,26] Transient arrhythmias may account for the syncope noted by some patients not attributable to seizures.

CLINICAL PRESENTATION

The predominant symptoms are those of CNS excitation and peripheral sympathomimetic response. The wide variety of manifestations and complications may include palpitations, agitation, altered mental state, chest pain, syncope, seizures, dyspnoea, abdominal pain, transient focal neurological signs, urticaria, intracranial haemorrhage and cardiac arrest.[27]

The spectrum of neurological changes may include euphoria, apprehension, agitation, altered mental state, seizures and coma. Tachypnoea, mydriasis, tremor, diaphoresis and hyperpyrexia may also be seen. Cardiovascular manifestations may include tachycardia, hypertension, any supraventricular or ventricular tachydysrrhythmia, syncope and chest pain. Rhabdomyolysis has been reported in cocaine intoxication complicated by renal failure and hyperkalaemia.[22,28]

Chest pain may be due to musculoskeletal, pulmonary or cardiovascular causes. A retrospective study of patients intoxicated with cocaine presenting with chest pain consistent with ischaemia found that 6% suffered acute myocardial infarction.[29]

Aortic dissection associated with cocaine use has been reported.[30]

Smoking cocaine may lead to a number of respiratory complications, including thermal airway injury, pneumothorax and pneumomediastinum, non-cardiac pulmonary oedema, interstitial pneumonitis and bronchiolitis obliterans.[23]

Several CNS complications have been attributed to cocaine, in addition to the phenomena described above. Cerebral infarction, transient ischaemic attacks, subarachnoid haemorrhage, cerebral vasculitis and migraine-like headache have been described.[22] Contributing pathophysiological mechanisms include hypertension, vasoconstriction, vasculitis, increased coagulability, altered cerebrovascular autoregulation and embolization of particulate matter. Patients with headache or focal neurological signs should be referred urgently for CT scanning to exclude cerebral infarction, intracerebral haemorrhage or subarachnoid haemorrhage. Emergency physicians should have a high index of suspicion when assessing patients with abdominal pain, especially when it seems to be out of proportion to physical signs. Mesenteric vasoconstriction and vasculitis may lead to bowel ischaemia and infarction.[22]

DIAGNOSIS

The diagnosis of cocaine intoxication is usually clinical, based on history or clinical suspicion, the presence of sympathomimetic symptoms and signs, and the exclusion of other life-threatening conditions. The differential diagnosis includes other sympathomimetic agents such as amphetamines or hallucinogenic agents, anticholinergic delirium, serotonin syndrome, monoamine oxidase inhibitors, theophylline, alcohol and benzodiazepine withdrawal, sepsis, hypoglycaemia, thyrotoxicosis and phaeochromocytoma.

Rapid urine screening qualitative tests are commercially available to identify the presence of drugs of abuse. They should be interpreted with caution, as metabolites may be present for several days and not be relevant to the patient's presentation. Most commercially available urine qualitative tests detect metabolites of cocaine. The tests rarely alter management in emergencies, and may give false-negative results in cases where the cocaine was taken only a short time before the test is performed.

Physical examination and investigations should be directed at excluding complications and alternative diagnoses, as detailed above. Laboratory and radiological investigations should be reserved for those patients in whom they are clinically indicated. All patients with altered vital signs should have ECG monitoring in the emergency department, and all patients should have at least one 12-lead ECG.

MANAGEMENT AND DISPOSITION

Initial care is directed towards the assessment and management of immediate threats to airway, breathing and circulation, in a conventional manner. All patients should receive oxygen and have a bed-side blood glucose estimation. Patients with an altered level of consciousness should be closely monitored in a resuscitation area.

A direct relationship between the neuropsychiatric and cardiovascular complications of cocaine toxicity has been proposed.[22] Patients exhibiting CNS agitation or sympathomimetic cardiovascular effects should receive an intravenous benzodiazepine titrated to achieve sedation. In the majority of patients this will reduce most manifestations of cocaine toxicity. Seizures should be managed in the standard manner. Benzodiazepines are considered first-line therapy, followed by barbiturates, general anaesthesia and paralysis if required.

Atrial tachycardia and hypertension usually respond to sedation with benzodiazepines. Hypertension need not be treated specifically unless there is evidence of acute end-organ failure. If titrated benzodiazpine sedation fails to adequately control blood pressure vasodilators such as nitroprusside, intravenous nitrates or phentolamine have been recommended. Atrial tachyarrhythmias are usually benign and rarely require specific treatment other than benzodiazepine sedation. The use of β-adrenergic receptor blockers in cocaine intoxication is controversial and not recommended. There are no experimental data to show improved mortality in animal models with their use. In addition, there is the theoretical potential to produce 'unopposed' α-adrenergic receptor effects, leading to paradoxical hypertension.

Ventricular arrhythmias should be treated according to advanced cardiac life support guidelines. Those occurring within minutes of cocaine use are presumed to be secondary to excess catecholamines, myocardial ischaemia and a direct cocaine-mediated myocardial sodium channel blockade. The use of lidocaine in this setting is controversial. In addition to defibrillation or cardioversion, benzodiazepine sedation and intravenous bolus bicarbonate (1–2 mEq/kg) have been used in this setting. Ventricular arrhythmias occurring after the acute phase are presumed to be secondary to myocardial ischaemia and should, therefore, be treated in a standard manner.[22]

If myocardial ischaemia or infarction is suspected, management should be as for non-ischaemic chest pain of non-toxicological aetiology. Benzodiazepine sedation, nitrates and verapamil are recommended to decrease heart rate, reduce hypertension and reduce cocaine-induced coronary vasoconstriction,[31] but β-adrenergic blocking agents should be avoided as they increase coronary vasospasm.[32] Primary angioplasty is considered the treatment of choice for cocaine-induced acute myocardial infarction.[31] Thrombolytic therapy may be considered if angioplasty is not available, maximal medical management has failed and there is no evidence of intracranial haemorrhage.[31] In patients with non-diagnostic electrocardiograms short-term admission may be required to exclude myocardial infarction.

Hyperthermia is an important contributing factor to morbidity and mortality following cocaine intoxication.[25] A core temperature should be measured in all patients and core temperature monitoring is recommended if the temperature is elevated. Mild hyperthermia (<39°C) often responds to benzodiazepine sedation and aggressive fluid resuscitation. If this is unsuccessful, then cooling by convection, ice packs or intubation and paralysis may be required. Further study is required to delineate the role of dopamine receptor antagonists in the management of hyperthermia. There is no evidence that dantrolene has a role in the management of hyperthermia associated with psychostimulants.[25]

The duration of observation in the emergency department and the need for admission depends on the severity of toxicity, the influence of coingested drugs and the presence of comorbidity or complications. Patients with mild intoxication (without severe hyperthermia or ischaemic chest pain) may be observed in the emergency department and discharged when vital signs and mental status have returned to normal.

Presentation to an emergency department provides an opportunity for preventative intervention. Patients should be counselled and offered strategies to avoid future toxicity or overdose. Alternatively, the patient may be referred to agencies specializing in drug detoxification and rehabilitation.

AMPHETAMINE AND RELATED 'DESIGNER DRUGS'

INTRODUCTION AND EPIDEMIOLOGY

Amphetamine refers to β-phenylisopropylamine, but the term 'amphetamines' refers to a broad group of related derivatives characterized clinically by CNS stimulatory and peripheral sympathomimetic responses. Amphetamine was first synthesized in 1887, and marketed as a nasal decongestant in 1932.[33]

The potential for abuse was recognized as people became dependent on the euphoric and stimulant effects of these drugs.

The use of amphetamine as a drug of abuse has been prevalent since its introduction. Amphetamine, amphetamine derivatives and fentanyl derivatives (together often called the 'designer drugs'), plus the hallucinogenic drugs, have become increasingly popular in the recent past. In the Northern Territory, 7% of a survey of the general population over 14-years admitted using amphetamines in the 12-months prior to 1998.[20]

PHARMACOLOGY AND PATHOPHYSIOLOGY

Amphetamine is structurally related to ephedrine and resembles the catecholamines, but is effective when given orally.[34] The amphetamine group are characterized by substitutions on the basic structure of amphetamine, and include metamphetamine ('ice', 'speed'), 3,4-methylenedioxymethamphetamine (MDMA, 'Ecstasy', 'Adam' or 'E'), 3,4-methylenedioxyethamphetamine (MDEA, 'Eve'), and 3,4-methylenedioxyamphetamine (MDA, 'love drug').[33]

Amphetamines may be ingested, smoked, insufflated or injected parenterally.

All are absorbed from the gastrointestinal system, with peak serum levels within 3 hours. They are weak bases, 20% bound to plasma proteins and tend to have large volumes of distribution. Half-lives vary from 8 to 30 hours, with hepatic transformation being the major route of elimination. However, up to 30% of amphetamine and metamphetamine may be eliminated in the urine.[33]

Amphetamines enhance the release of catecholamines and block their subsequent reuptake. This causes increased stimulation of central and peripheral adrenergic receptors, leading to CNS excitation and a sympathomimetic syndrome. Higher doses also lead to central serotonin release. Increased dopaminergic action in the mesolimbic system leads to automatic behaviours, altered perception and psychosis. Different substitutions

on the basic amphetamine structure (the amphetamine derivatives) alter the relative hallucinogenic, behavioural and cardiovascular effects of the drugs at low doses. At high doses, the toxic effects of the group are more uniform and can be discussed as a single entity.

Considerable tolerance may develop, so that patients repeatedly take increasing doses to achieve euphoria and a stimulant effect. An acute organic psychosis, similar to paranoid schizophrenia, may develop during and after these binges.[34]

Severe hyponatraemia, associated with cerebral oedema is reported following MDMA use.[35,36] Mechanisms contributing to hyponatraemia may include psychogenic polydipsia[36] and inappropriate secretion of antidiuretic hormone.[36,37]

Animal models of MDMA abuse demonstrate destruction of serotonergic and dopaminergic neurons.[38] This has also been reported in humans and raises the concern of permanent neurological damage associated with chronic MDMA use, which in turn carries enormous public health implications.[39]

CLINICAL PRESENTATION

The clinical signs, symptoms and complications of amphetamine intoxication are similar to those of cocaine. However, amphetamine effects may last up to 24 hours. In addition, the spectrum of signs and symptoms is influenced by other drugs that may be coingested by the patient, such as opioids, alcohol, benzodiazepines or cannabis.

The predominant symptoms are those of CNS excitation and peripheral sympathomimetic response. Following euphoria, apprehension, agitation, altered mental state, seizures and coma may ensue. Tachypnoea, mydriasis, tremor, diaphoresis and hyperpyrexia may also be seen. After acute intoxication, with or without delirium, amphetamine-induced psychosis may occur[40] with frightening visual and tactile hallucinations, severe agitation and paranoia. MDMA-induced hyponatraemia may present with altered mental status and seizures.

Death is commonly secondary to hyperpyrexia, seizures, arrhythmia or intracerebral haemorrhage.[33] Myocardial infarction,[41] aortic dissection,[42] rhabdomyolysis, acidosis, shock, renal failure[25] and coagulopathy[33] are documented.

Parenteral amphetamine abuse may be complicated by cellulitis, thrombophlebitis, inadvertent intra-arterial injection and possible subsequent embolization, mycotic aneurysm, staphylococcal pneumonia, endocarditis, anaerobic clostridial infection, and viral infections such as hepatitis B, C and HIV. In addition, chronic abuse of amphetamines may be complicated by a necrotizing vasculitis that leads to a characteristic beading of small and medium arteries on angiography. The vasculitis may involve multiple organ systems and lead to renal failure, myocardial ischaemia and cerebrovascular disease.[33]

An amphetamine withdrawal state is recognized, during which the patient may sleep for long periods, feel depressed, and experience intense cravings for amphetamines.[34]

DIAGNOSIS

The diagnosis of amphetamine intoxication is clinical, based on history or clinical suspicion, the presence of sympathomimetic symptoms and signs, and the exclusion of other life-threatening conditions. In overdose it may be impossible to distinguish the exact amphetamine derivative involved, but this is unlikely to be clinically significant. Intoxication by an amphetamine derivative may not be discernible clinically from cocaine, except for the increased propensity for psychotic features and the longer duration of action. The differential diagnosis includes cocaine abuse, anticholinergic delirium, serotonin syndrome, monoamine oxidase inhibitors, theophylline, alcohol and benzodiazepine withdrawal, sepsis, hypoglycaemia, thyrotoxicosis and phaeochromocytoma.

Physical examination and investigations should be directed at excluding complications and alternative diagnoses, as detailed above. Laboratory and radiological investigations should be reserved for those in whom they are clinically indicated.

MANAGEMENT AND DISPOSITION

Initial attention must be directed at assessing and managing immediate threats to airway, breathing and circulation in a conventional manner. All patients should receive oxygen and have a bed-side blood glucose estimation. Close monitoring of the patient in a quiet area away from excessive stimulation may be advantageous.

Patients exhibiting psychomotor acceleration or psychosis should be managed with an intravenous benzodiazepine titrated to achieve adequate sedation. As with cocaine, hyperthermia, seizures and fluid resuscitation should be managed aggressively. The organ-specific effects of amphetamines are similar to those of cocaine, and management should follow that detailed above. Following resolution of the acute intoxication phase, patients with persistent psychotic features may respond to an antipsychotic agent such as olanzapine.[43]

The duration of observation in the emergency department and the need for admission will depend on the severity of intoxication, the influence of coingested drugs, and the presence of comorbidity or complications. Patients with mild intoxication (e.g. without severe hyperthermia or ischaemic chest pain) may be observed in the emergency department and discharged when vital signs and mental status have returned to normal. The longer half-lives of the amphetamines may dictate inpatient care if symptoms or abnormal vital signs do not resolve within a few hours.

Presentation to an emergency department provides an opportunity for preventative intervention. Patients should be counselled and offered strategies to avoid future toxicity or overdose. Alternatively, the patient may be referred to agencies specializing in drug detoxification and rehabilitation.

GAMMA-HYDROXYBUTYRATE

INTRODUCTION AND EPIDEMIOLOGY

Gamma-hydroxybutyrate (GHB) (4-hydroxybutanoate; sodium oxybate) is an emerging drug of abuse that acts as a central nervous system depressant. It has significant psychotropic effects and has the ability to lead to addiction. GHB was originally developed as short-acting anaesthetic agent in the 1960s, but lost favour due to poor analgesic properties and a propensity to cause seizure-like activity at the onset of coma.[44] GHB has also been used as a treatment for opioid withdrawal,[45] alcohol dependence and narcolepsy.[46,47]

In the last 15 years GHB (and its congeners gamma-butyrolactone-GBL and 1,4 butanediol) has become a popular recreational drug, being advocated as a bodybuilding agent, euphoric agent, sleep enhancer and sexual stimulant. Street names for GHB include 'grievous bodily harm', 'fantasy', 'scoop', 'liquid X', 'liquid E' and 'somatomax'.[48] Although forensic data are scarce, GHB has also been implicated as a 'date rape' agent.[49] Recreational use of GHB in Australia has not been assessed in large studies of illicit drug abuse, but small reports of epidemics of GHB use and anecdotal reports of emergency department presentations suggest that its use in Australia may be increasing.[50]

PHARMACOLOGY AND PATHOPHYSIOLOGY

GHB is a short-chain fatty acid that occurs naturally in the brain and possibly acts as a neurotransmitter. It is one of the breakdown products of gamma amino butyric acid (GABA), the primary inhibitory neurotransmitter in the CNS. The mechanisms by which GHB causes its effects are unclear, but it may be a combination of intrinsic effects via specific GHB receptors and effects mediated through $GABA_b$ receptors.[49] GHB also has dopaminergic activity, increases acetylcholine and serotonin levels, and may interact with endogenous opioids.[49]

GHB is usually ingested as a liquid and is rapidly absorbed by the gastrointestinal tract; peak plasma levels occur within 15–45 minutes.[49] It is rapidly metabolized to succinate, which then enters the Krebs cycle. The average half-life is usually 20–50 minutes.[49]

CLINICAL PRESENTATION

Most patients present to the emergency department following acute GHB intoxication. The major clinical signs of GHB intoxication are related to their effects on the CNS. With increasing dose there is euphoria followed rapidly by sedation and coma. Co-ingestion of ethanol or other illcit drugs is common.[44,49] Respiratory depression and apnoea may occur following GHB ingestion, but this is usually reported in the context of multiple co-ingestants. Profond coma may occur but the patient may resist instrumentation of the airway or rouse rapidly when stimulated, only to relapse again when the stimulus is removed. The duration of CNS depression is usually short. Most patients recover abruptly within 1–2 hours and persistent CNS depression beyond 6 hours should prompt the emergency physician to search for alternative causes.

Agitation, myoclonus and generalized seizures have also been reported. Generalized seizures have not been seen during EEG monitoring of human volunteers given sedative doses of GHB.[49] In animal studies, GHB causes an abnormal EEG pattern similar to that seen in absence seizures, and GHB has been used as a tool for the study of the neurophysiological mechanisms of this disorder.[51] It is possible that the seizures noted in some patients represent the clonic movements commonly seen with GHB intoxication, or they may be generalized seizures due to hypoxia or a co-ingested agent.[49,52]

Severe degrees of CNS depression may be associated with mild bradycardia and/or hypotension. There does not appear to be any consistent pattern of ECG changes seen with GHB intoxication.[49] GHB intoxication may be associated with vomiting in up to 40% of cases.[49]

DIAGNOSIS

The diagnosis of GHB intoxication is clinical. Abrupt resolution of coma within 1–2 hours of presentation is characteristic of GHB intoxication. However, other agents are frequently co-ingested (ethanol, amphetamines, cannabis, opiates) and may cloud the clinical picture. A thorough physical examination of all systems is usually adequate to exclude complications such as pulmonary aspiration. Investigations are directed at excluding alternative diagnoses and complications as clinically indicated. The differential diagnosis is that of any patient with an altered level of consciousness, and includes toxicological and metabolic causes, sepsis, neurotrauma, stroke and postictal state.

MANAGEMENT AND DISPOSITION

Initial care is directed at assessing and managing the immediate threats to airway, breathing and circulation in a conventional manner. All patients should receive oxygen and have a bed-side blood glucose estimation. Patients with an altered level of consciousness should be closely monitored in a resuscitation area, positioned to minimize the chances of aspiration, and moved frequently to prevent dependent injuries. Physical examination and investigations are directed toward exclusion of complications and alternative diagnoses, as detailed above. Intravenous access plus laboratory and radiological investigation should be reserved for those in whom they are clinically indicated. Persistent CNS depression beyond 6 hours should prompt the emergency physician to search for alternative causes.

As GHB is rapidly absorbed, may be associated with rapid onset of coma, has a short-clinical effect and has good prognosis with thorough supportive care, activated charcoal is not routinely indicated.

There is no specific antidote for GHB. Naloxone does not appear to reverse the CNS depression or respiratory depression associated with GHB intoxication.[49] The administration of physostigmine may attenuate the CNS depression of GHB intoxication.[53] However, as GHB intoxication is frequently associated with co-ingestants, has a short-clinical effect and has good prognosis with thorough supportive care, its routine use is not recommended.[49,54]

The duration of observation in the emergency department or the need for admission will depend on the need for intubation, co-ingested agents, or the presence of complications. Most patients recover within a few hours and may be safely discharged from the emergency department when they are ambulant and competent.[49]

Although patients may be medically fit for early discharge, presentation to an emergency department must also provide an opportunity for preventative intervention. Patients should be counselled regarding strategies to avoid future overdose. In addition, the patient may be referred to agencies specializing in drug detoxification and rehabilitation.

'BODY-PACKERS' AND 'BODY STUFFERS'

Body-packers and body-stuffers are people who conceal illicit drugs within body cavities. Their management can present a vexing problem for emergency physicians. Patients may ingest many times the lethal dose of an illicit drug, conceal the nature of their problem, and appear completely asymptomatic. In addition, there is a paucity of data regarding the efficacy of various imaging, decontamination and treatment modalities.

A body-packer attempts to conceal a large quantity of an illicit drug inside a body cavity, usually the gastrointestinal tract, in an attempt to smuggle it across an international border. The drugs are usually carefully packaged in plastic, latex, condoms or balloons, often layered with wax. By the time these patients reach the emergency department almost all of the packets will have entered the small or large intestine, making decontamination problematic. The vagina and rectum are less popular sites to conceal drugs as they are more likely to be discovered on physical examination.

A body-stuffer hurriedly ingests smaller quantities of illicit drugs just before they are apprehended by the authorities in order to avoid conviction. This haste means that the package is poorly constructed and may easily leak. Time from ingestion to hospital arrival is likely to be shorter and the drug may still be within the stomach at the time of presentation. The vagina and rectum are alternative sites for drug concealment in the body-stuffer.

In view of the potential sudden lethality of both these practices, regardless of presenting symptoms or signs, all patients should receive a high triage priority and be managed in a resuscitation setting. They should receive supplemental oxygen and intravenous access.

Police may bring the patient to the emergency department and request physical examination and/or investigation. When a history is taken in the presence of police many patients deny the practice and resist treatment. The emergency physician should remember the potential threat to the patient's life, and his or her primary duty of care to the patient.

Whenever possible a detailed history should be obtained, noting the exact type and amount of drug ingested, the method of packaging, symptoms of drug intoxication, and any factors that may increase the likelihood of bowel obstruction or ileus. A thorough physical examination should include speculum examination of the vagina, digital examination of the rectum, and a search for any signs of drug intoxication.

All cooperative patients should immediately receive activated charcoal to adsorb intraluminal drug.[55] In body-packers this should be followed by whole-bowel irrigation with polyethylene glycol solution.[56] Whole-bowel irrigation should be continued until all packages are retrieved.

Abdominal radiographs of body-stuffers are unlikely to show the packages clearly,[57] and a negative abdominal radiograph does not exclude the diagnosis. Fortunately, most patients remain asymptomatic or exhibit only mild symptoms, although deaths are reported.[58] Following a dose of activated charcoal, asymptomatic body-stuffers should be observed in the emergency department or emergency observation unit for a minimum of 8 hours. Those who remain asymptomatic at the end of the observation period may be discharged. If a patient becomes symptomatic they should be treated as outlined above for the individual substance.

Imaging of the potential body-packer is controversial. Abdominal radiographs are positive in a higher percentage of body-packers, where multiple package-air interfaces may be seen. In a prospective study of 75 suspected cocaine body-packers,[59] abdominal radiographs were positive in 35 of 48 patients (73%) subsequently known to have ingested packages. Radiographs were negative in two patients with rectal packages and negative in 12 who later passed between 15 and 135 packages. Again, a negative abdominal radiograph does not exclude the diagnosis. Plain abdominal films with oral contrast and abdominal CT scanning with oral contrast have been advocated as alternative diagnostic stategies,[33] however, no studies have been performed to compare imaging modalities and false-negative studies have been reported.[60] Given the need to confidently exclude the diagnosis of body-packing and the poor sensitivity of these modalities it has been suggested two imaging modalities (e.g. plain abdominal radiograph plus abdominal CT scanning) be used to exclude the diagnosis.[33]

All body-packer patients, even the asymptomatic, should remain monitored, either in the emergency department, observation unit , or intensive care unit, until there is satisfactory evidence that all packages have been retrieved. An individual risk assessment should dictate management in each case. Evidence of drug intoxication, either at presentation or during decontamination, is a medical emergency and should be treated aggressively. Initial care must be directed at assessing and managing immediate threats to airway, breathing, circulation, and the control of seizures in a standard manner. If a cocaine body-packer exhibits toxicity, immediate endoscopy or surgical exploration to remove all packages has been advocated.[56,61] Such interventions may also be indicated if there is evidence of bowel or gastric outflow obstruction, concretion formation, ileus or bowel perforation.[61] Such an aggressive approach is probably not necessary in the heroin body-packer where adequate resuscitation, supportive care and antidote therapy should ensure a favourable outcome.

If the exact number of packages is known, and all packages have been accounted for in the whole-bowel irrigation effluent, the effluent is clear and the patient exhibits no evidence of toxicity, decontamination efforts may cease. If there is any doubt about the total number of packages, barium swallow and small bowel follow-through examination after whole-bowel irrigation have been advocated to confirm that all packages have been removed.[56]

REFERENCES

1. Katzung BG 1998 Basic and Clinical Pharmacology, 7th edn. Prentice Hall, Australia
2. Hall W, Darke S 1998 Trends in opiate deaths in Australia 1979–1995. Drug and Alcohol Dependence 52(1): 71–77
3. Swensen G 1997 Opioid deaths in Western Australia, 1996. WA Drug Abuse Strategy Office, Statistical Bulletin No 4

CONTROVERSIES AND FUTURE DIRECTIONS

❶ The optimal decontamination methods and imaging modalites for management of the body packer remain controversial.

4. Swensen G 1996 Mortality caused by opioids Western Australia 1996. Task Force on Drug Abuse, Statistical Bulletin No 2

5. Oyefeso A, Ghodse H, Clancy C, Corkery J, Goldfinch R 1999 Drug abuse-related mortality: a study of teenage addicts over a 20-year period. Social Psychiatry and Psychiatric Epidemiology 34(8): 437–41

6. Darke S, Zador D 1996 Fatal heroin 'overdose': a review. Addiction 91(12): 1765–72

7. Darke S, Ross J, Hall W 1996 Overdose among heroin users in Sydney, Australia: I. Prevalence and correlates of non-fatal overdose. Addiction 91(3): 405–11

8. Zador D, Sunjic S, Darke S 1996 Heroin-related deaths in New South Wales, 1992: toxicological findings and circumstances. Medical Journal of Australia 164: 204–7

9. Darke S, Ross J, Hall W 1996 Overdose among heroin users in Sydney, Australia: II. Responses to overdose. Addiction 91(3): 413–7

10. Hoffman JR, Schriger DL, Luo JS 1991 The empiric use of naloxone in patients with altered mental status: a reappraisal. Annals of Emergency Medicine 20: 246–52

11. Warner-Smith M, Darke S, Day C 2002 Morbidity associated with non-fatal heroin overdose. Addiction 97(8): 927–8

12. Smith DA, Leake L, Loflin JR, Yealy DM 1992 Is admission after intravenous heroin overdose necessary? Annals of Emergency Medicine 21(11): 1326–30

13. Brzozowski M, Shih RD, Bania TC, Hoffman RS 1993 Discharging heroin overdose patients after observation (letter). Annals of Emergency Medicine 22(19): 1638

14. Osterwalder JJ 1996 Naloxone for intoxications with intravenous heroin and heroin mixtures - harmless or hazardous? A prospective clinical study. Clinical Toxicology 34(4): 409–16

15. Watson WA, Steele MT, Muelleman RL, Rush MD 1998 Opiod toxicity recurrence after an initial response to naloxone. Journal of Toxicology-Clinical Toxicology 36(1–2): 11–7

16. Christenson J, Etherington J, Grafstein E, et al 2000 Early discharge of patients with presumed opioid overdose: development of a clinical prediction rule. Academic Emergency Medicine 7(10): 1110–8

17. Morgan D, Daly FFS, Fatovich DM, Bartu A, Quigley A 2002 Eighteen-month mortality in a cohort of patients presenting to an emergency department with non-fatal opioid overdose (abstract). Emergency Medicine 14(1): A23

18. Braunwald E, Fauci A, Hauser S, Jameson J, Kasper D, Longo D 1991 Harrison's Principles of Internal Medicine, 12th edn. McGraw-Hill, New York, p 2153

19. Caplehorn JRM, Dalton MSYN, Haldar F, Petrenas AM, Nisbet JG 1996 Methadone maintenance and addicts risk of fatal heroin overdose. Substance Abuse and Misuse 31(2): 177–96

20. Miller M, Draper G. Statistics on drug use in Australia 2000. Australian Instititute of Health and Welfare Canberra, www.aihw.gov.au.

21. Hando J, Flaherty B, Rutter S 1997 An Australian profile on the use of cocaine. Addiction 92(2): 173–82

22. Goldfrank LR, Hoffman RS 1991 The cardiovascular effects of cocaine. Annals of Emergency Medicine 20(2): 165–75

23. Haim DY, Lippmann ML, Goldberg SK, Walkenstein MD 1995 The pulmonary complications of crack cocaine, a comprehensive review. Chest 107(1): 233–40

24. Henning RJ, Wilson LD, Glauser JM 1994 Cocaine plus ethanol is more cardiotoxic than cocaine or ethanol alone. Critical Care Medicine 2(12): 1896–906

25. Callaway CW, Clark RF 1994 Hyperthermia in psycho-stimulant overdose. Annals of Emergency Medicine 24(1): 68–76

26. Kerns W, Garvey L, Owens J 1997 Cocaine-induced wide complex dysrhythmia. Journal of Emergency Medicine 15(3): 321–9

27. Derlet RW, Albertson TE 1989 Emergency department presentation of cocaine intoxication. Annals of Emergency Medicine 18(2): 182–6

28. Skluth HA, Clark JE, Ehringer GL 1988 Rhabdomyolysis associated with cocaine intoxication. Drug Intelligence and Clinical Pharmacy 22: 778–80

29. Zimmerman JL, Dellinger RP, Majid PA 1991 Cocaine associated chest pain. Annals of Emergency Medicine 20(6): 611–5

30. Perron AD, Gibbs M 1997 Thoracic aortic dissection secondary to crack cocaine ingestion. American Journal of Emergency Medicine 15: 507–9

31. Lange RA, Hillis LD 2001 Medical progress: Cardiovascular complications of cocaine use. New England Journal of Medicine 345(5): 351–8

32. Lange RA, Cigarroa RG, Flores ED, et al 1990 Potentiation of cocaine-induced coronary vasoconstriction by beta-adrenergic blockade. Annals of Internal Medicine 112: 897–903

33. Goldfrank's Toxicologic Emergencies

34. Morgan JP 1992 Amphetamine and metamphetamine during the 1990s. Paediatric Review 13(9): 330–3

35. Maxwell DL, Polkey MI, Henry JA 1993 Hyponatraemia and catatonic stupor after taking "ecstacy." British Medical Journal 307(6916): 1399

36. Sue YM, Lee, YL, Huang, JJ 2002 Acute hyponatremia, seizure and rhabdomyolysis after ecstasy use. Journal of Toxicology – Clinical Toxicology 40(7): 931–2

37. Henry JA, Fallon JK, Kicman AT, Hutt AJ, Cowan DA, Forsling M 1998 Low-dose MDMA ("ecstasy") induces vasopressin secretion. Lancet 351(9118): 1784

38. Ricuarte G, Yuan J Hatzidimitriou G, Cord BJ, McCann UD 2002 Severe dopaminergic neurotoxicity in primates after a common recreational dose regimen of MDMA ("ecstacy"). Science 2260–3

39. McCann UD, Szabo Z, Scheffel U, Dannals RF, Ricaurte GA 1998 Positron emission tomographic evidence of toxic effect of MDMA ("Ecstasy") on brain serotonin neurons in human beings. Lancet 352(9138): 1433–7

40. Murray JB 1998 Psychophysiological aspects of amphetamine-methamphetamineabuse. Journal of Psychology 132(2): 227–37

41. Waksman J, Taylor RN Jnr, Bodor GS, Daly FFS, Jolliff HA, Dart RC 2001 Acute myocardial infarction associated with amphetamine use. Mayo Clinic Proceedings 76(3): 323–6

42. Dihmis WC. Ridley P. Dhasmana JP. Wisheart JD 1997 Acute dissection of the aorta with amphetamine misuse. British Medical Journal 314(7095): 1665

43. Landabaso MA, Iraurgi I, Jimenez-Lerma JM, Calle R, Sanz J, Gutierrez-Fraile M 2002 Ecstasy-induced psychotic disorder: six-month follow-up study. European Addiction Research 8(3): 133–40

44. Miró, Nogué S, Espinosa G, To-Figueras J, Sánchez M 2002 Trends in illicit drug emergencies: the emerging role of gamma-hydroxybutyrate. Journal of Toxicology – Clinical Toxicology 40(2): 129–35

45. Gallimberti L, Schifano F, Forza G, Miconi L, Ferrara SD 1994 Clinical efficacy of gamma-hydroxybutyric acid in treatment of opiate withdrawal. European Archives of Psychiatry and Clinical Neuroscience 244(3): 113–4

46. Li J, Stokes SA, Woeckener A 1998 A tale of novel intoxication: seven cases of g-hydroxybutyric acid overdose. Annals of Emergency Medicine 31(6): 723–8

47. Anonymous 2002 A randomized, double blind, placebo-controlled multicenter trial comparing the effects of three doses of orally administered sodium oxybate with placebo for the treatment of narcolepsy. Sleep 25(1): 42–9

48. Chin RL, Sporer KA, Cullison B, Dyer JE, Wu TD 1998 Clinical course of g-hydroxybutyrate overdose. Annals of Emergency Medicine 31(6): 716–22

49. Mason PE, Kerns WP 2002 Gamma-hydroxybutyrate (GHB) intoxication. Academic Emergency Medicine 9(7): 730–9

50. Harrayway T, Stephenson L 1999 Gamma hydroxybutyrate intoxication: The Gold Coast experience. Emergency Medicine 11: 45–8

51. Snead OC 1988 Gamma-Hydroxybutyrate model of generalized absence seizures: further characterization and comparison with other absence models. Epilepsia. 29(4): 361–8

52. Daly FFS 1999 Gamma hydroxybutyrate (letter). Emergency Medicine 11(4): 300

53. Caldicott DG, Kuhn M 2001 Gamma-hydroxybutyrate overdose and physostigmine: Teaching new tricks to an old drug? Annals of Emergency Medicine 37: 99–102

54. Traub SJ, Nelson LS, Hoffman RS 2002 Physostigmine as a treatment for gamma-hydroxybutyrate toxicity: a review. Journal of Toxicology – Clinical Toxicology 40(6): 781–7

55. Tomaszewski C, McKinney P, Phillips S, Brent J, Kulig K 1993 Prevention of toxicity from oral cocaine by activated charcoal in mice. Annals of Emergency Medicine 22(12): 1804–6

56. Hoffman RS, Smilkstein MJ, Goldfrank LR 1990 Whole bowel irrigation and the cocaine body-packer: a new approach to a common problem. American Journal of Emergency Medicine 8(6): 523–7

57. Hoffman RS, Chiang WK, Weisman RS, Goldfrank LR 1990 Prospective evaluation of 'crack-vial' ingestions. Veterinary and Human Toxicology 32(2): 164–7

58. June R, Aks SE, Keys N, Wahl M 2000 Medical outcome of cocaine bodystuffers. Journal of Emergency Medicine 18(2): 221–4

59. McCarron MM, Wood JD 1983 The cocaine 'body packer' syndrome. Diagnosis and treatment. Journal of the American Medical Association 250: 1417–20

60. Eng JG, Aks SE, Waldron R, Marcus C, Issleib S 1999 False-negative abdominal CT scan in a cocaine body stuffer. American Journal of Emergency Medicine 17(7): 702–4

61. Beck NE, Hale JE 1993 Cocaine 'body packers'. British Journal of Surgery 80: 1513–6

28.13 METHAEMOGLOBINAEMIA

ROBERT EDWARDS

ESSENTIALS

1 Consider the diagnosis of methaemoglobinaemia in patients with cyanosis unresponsive to oxygen therapy.

2 Pulse oximetry may be normal in methaemoglobinaemia and readings do not usually fall below 85% even in severe cases.

3 Administer methylene blue to symptomatic patients with elevated methaemoglobin levels and to unstable patients with a history of exposure to an agent known to cause methaemoglobinaemia.

4 Methylene blue can cause haemolysis and methaemoglobinaemia if given to patients who do not have methaemoglobinaemia or who are glucose-6-phosphate dehydrogenase deficient, or if more than 5 mg/kg is used.

5 Failure of response to methylene blue may result from too small or too large a dose, congenital enzyme or haemoglobin defects, or an incorrect diagnosis.

INTRODUCTION

Although it is an uncommon presentation, the emergency physician must be able to diagnose methaemoglobinaemia because it is potentially fatal and can be readily treated with the antidote, methylene blue.

AETIOLOGY AND PATHOPHYSIOLOGY

Under normal conditions, methaemoglobin is continuously produced from haemoglobin by the oxidation of the

iron molecule from the ferrous (Fe^{2+}) to the ferric (Fe^{3+}) state. In the normal physiological state, less than 1% of haemoglobin is methaemoglobin because it is continually being reduced, predominantly by the enzyme NADH methaemoglobin reductase (Fig. 28.13.1).

Excessive methaemoglobinaemia causes tissue hypoxia because methaemoglobin is incapable of carrying oxygen[1] and causes a shift of the oxygen–haemoglobin dissociation curve to the left.[2]

Methaemoglobinaemia may be acquired or congenital. Congenital methaemoglobinaemia is due either to a deficiency of the enzyme NADH methaemoglobin reductase (a rare autosomal recessive disorder) or the haemoglobinopathy, haemoglobin M. The latter is transmitted with an autosomal dominant pattern of inheritance. Homozygotes usually do not survive and heterozygotes live with a methemoglobin level of around 20–30%.[3]

Acquired methaemoglobinaemia in adults arises as a consequence of accidental or intentional exposure to a therapeutic drug or other oxidizing agent. Oxidants that commonly result in excessive methaemoglobin production are listed in Table 28.13.1. Nitrates and nitrites are well-known causes of methaemoglobinaemia. Nitrites are more powerful oxidants than nitrates. Recreational use of amyl, butyl or isobutyl nitrite can cause severe methaemoglobinaemia.[1,4] Transdermal absorption of industrial nitrate solutions, ingestion of food and water contaminated with nitrates, and intravenous use or inhalation of nitrates may all cause methaemoglobinaemia.[5] Therapeutic use of glyceryl trinitrate (GTN) has been reported to increase methaemoglobin levels up to 38% but is more likely to cause severe hypotension

Table 28.13.1 Agents causing acquired methaemoglobinaemia[1]

Nitrites
Amyl nitrite
Isobutyl (amyl) nitrite

Nitrates
Glyceryl trinitrate
Sodium nitrate
Nitrate food preservatives
Water contaminated with nitrates
Silver nitrate burns treatments

Local anaesthetics
Benzocaine
Prilocaine
Lidocaine

Aniline dyes and related compounds
Aniline
Toluidine
Nitroethane

Antimicrobial agents
Sulfonamides
Dapsone
Quinones (chloroquine, primaquine)

Others
Cetrimide
Chlorates
Copper sulphates
Methylene blue
Naphthalene
Combustion products

before methaemoglobinaemia develops. Prolonged use of high doses of GTN (>10 µg/kg/min) and the presence of renal or hepatic dysfunction make this complication more likely.[6]

Local anaesthetics, prilocaine and benzocaine in particular, can cause methaemoglobinaemia even when applied topically and administered in standard doses.[7,8]

Risk factors for the development of methaemoglobinaemia from topically applied local anaesthetics include excessive dosing, a break in the mucosal barrier

NADH + Methaemoglobin → NAD+ + Haemoglobin
NADH Methaemoglobin reductase

Fig. 28.13.1 Major pathway for the reduction of methaemoglobin under physiological conditions.

and a partial deficiency of the enzyme NADH methaemoglobin reductase.[8]

Aniline (aminobenzene), and its major metabolite, phenylhydroxylamine, are potent methaemoglobin-forming agents, even after transdermal exposure.[9] Aniline and related compounds such as nitrobenzene are widely used in industry, especially the chemical and rubber industries.

CLINICAL PRESENTATION

The symptoms and signs of methaemoglobinaemia are attributable to the effects of cellular hypoxia on the CNS and the heart. At levels between 20–45%, headache, weakness, anxiety, lethargy, syncope, tachycardia and dyspnoea are observed. Further elevations are associated with decreasing level of consciousness (45–55%) leading to coma, seizures, arrhythmias and cardiac conduction disturbances (55–70%). Levels above 70% are associated with mortality, but deaths can occur at lower levels.[10,11]

The hallmark of methaemoglobinaemia is a deep cyanosis that is unresponsive to oxygen therapy. The cyanosis may be so deep that it is more brown than blue and has been termed 'chocolate cyanosis'.[4] A useful diagnostic clue is the classic chocolate brown appearance of the patient's blood. This may be observed at methaemoglobin levels as low as 15–20% and is best appreciated by placing a drop of blood on filter paper and comparing it to a normal sample.

INVESTIGATIONS

The diagnosis of methaemoglobinaemia is confirmed by spectrophotometric measurement of methaemoglobin. The result is expressed as a percentage of the total haemoglobin level. Analysis of the blood sample should be performed as soon as possible because methaemoglobin levels decrease with time.[12] The indications for spectrophotometry are:

- Cyanosis unresponsive to O_2
- Tachypnoea or other features of hypoxia and history of exposure to methaemoglobin-inducing agents

- Normal or raised PaO_2 and low pulse oximetry
- Chocolate brown appearance of arterial blood.

Methaemoglobin interferes with the accuracy of pulse oximetry. With increasing levels of methaemoglobin, pulse oximetry readings approach 85% (at around 30% methaemoglobin) and remain in the mid eighties.[7,12] Methaemoglobin has a maximal light absorption at a wavelength similar to oxyhaemoglobin (660 nm) and it is, therefore, not differentiated from oxyhaemoglobin.[13]

Arterial blood gas analysis often demonstrates a metabolic acidosis with a normal oxygen tension. Other important investigations include a chest X-ray to exclude pulmonary pathology which might contribute to the hypoxia, and an ECG to assess cardiac rhythm and look for evidence of myocardial ischaemia or infarction. A FBC to check the haemoglobin level and electrolytes, urea, creatinine and liver function tests should also be performed.

MANAGEMENT

Initial management includes assessment of the airway, breathing and circulation and institution of appropriate measures of care. Administration of supplemental oxygen therapy is often not associated with any clinical benefit but the presence of cyanosis not responsive to oxygen is a diagnostic clue.

Decontamination of the gastro-intestinal tract or skin may be indicated.

Methylene blue (tetramethylthionine) is a specific antidote for methaemoglobinaemia. Whilst under normal conditions, 95% of methaemoglobin is reduced by the NADH methaemoglobin reductase system, a greater proportion is reduced by a second enzyme system, NADPH methaemoglobin reductase when methylene blue is present, acting as a cofactor to NADPH methaemoglobin reductase.

NADPH is produced by the Embden-Meyerhoff pathway and requires adequate G6PD activity. Thus, in states of G6PD deficiency, methylene blue may

not be as effective.

Methylene blue is indicated for symptomatic patients with an elevated methaemoglobin level. Patients who are blue but asymptomatic do not require methylene blue. Symptoms can normally be expected in patients with levels greater than 15%, less if the patient is anaemic.

The dose of methylene blue is 1–2 mg/kg intravenously over 5 minutes. Unstable patients with cyanosis unresponsive to high-flow oxygen and a history of oxidant exposure or 'chocolate brown' blood should be given methylene blue, even if the methaemoglobin level is not available. A reduction in the methaemoglobin level and accompanying clinical improvement usually occur over 30–60 minutes. A further dose of 1 mg/kg can be given after 1 hour if the methaemoglobin level remains elevated. Factors that may result in failure to respond to methylene blue are listed in Table 28.13.2.

The side effects of methylene blue include dyspnoea, a feeling of pressure on the chest, restlessness, apprehension, tremor, nausea and vomiting.[14] Paradoxically, methaemoglobin itself can oxidize haemoglobin to methaemoglobin if given in high doses (greater than 5–7 mg/kg).[15] Adverse effects are minimized if the correct dose is used.[16] Methylene blue

Table 28.13.2 Reasons for failure of methaemoglobinaemia to respond to methylene blue

Excessive oxidant
  Ongoing exposure
  Inadequate decontamination

Insufficient methylene blue
  Inadequate dose

Excessive methylene blue
  Excessive methylene blue acts as an oxidant in high doses (>7 mg/kg)

Methylene blue ineffective
  G-6-PD deficiency
  NADPH metHb reductase deficiency
  Hb M

Incorrect diagnosis
  Sulphaemoglobinaemia
  Carbon monoxide poisoning
  Cyanosis unresponsive to oxygen: cardiac shunt

occasionally causes persistent blue discolouration of the patient or haemolytic anaemia.[17] G6PD-deficient patients should not be given methylene blue as it may precipitate massive haemolysis.

Exchange transfusion is indicated for patients with G6-PD deficiency or where there is failure to respond to methylene blue.[5,9,12, 18, 19]

CONCLUSION

Methaemoglobinaemia is usually an acquired condition that develops following exposure to a wide range of chemicals that act as oxidants. Of particular concern are nitrites, nitrates used in industry, nitrates contaminating food and water, aniline derivatives, local anaesthetics and some antimicrobials. Pharmaceutical nitrates are an uncommon cause. The aim of management is to maintain adequate oxygenation. Symptomatic patients require intravenous administration of methylene blue, 1–2 mg/kg. In severe cases, treatment may need to begin without waiting for the methaemoglobin levels.

CONTROVERSIES AND FUTURE DIRECTIONS

❶ A methylene blue infusion has been used to treat recurrent methaemoglobinaemia due to dapsone ingestion.[18] A dose of 1 mg/hour was used and monitored with frequent methaemoglobin levels.

❷ Hyperbaric oxygen treatment has been recommended as an alternative to methylene blue. The partial pressure of oxygen in plasma can be increased to such a degree so as to ensure adequate oxygen transport in the absence of functioning haemoglobin.

❸ Ascorbic acid (vitamin C) reacts directly to reduce methaemoglobin. The dose is 0.5–1.0 g/6 hourly, either orally or intravenously, but the response is too slow to be used as a primary treatment for methaemoglobinaemia.[2]

REFERENCES

1. Edwards RJ, Ujma J 1995 Extreme methaemoglobinaemia secondary to recreational use of amyl nitrite. Journal of Accident and Emergency Medicine 12: 134–7

2. Curry S 1982 Methemoglobinemia. Annals of Emergency Medicine 11: 214–21
3. Babbit CJ, Garrett JS 2000 Diarrhea and methemoglobinemia in an infant. Paediatric Emergency Care 16: 416–7
4. Forsythe RJ, Moulden A 1991 Methaemoglobinaemia after ingestion of amyl nitrite. Archives of Diseases in Children 66: 152
5. Harris JC, Rumack BH, Peterson RG, McGuire BM 1979 Methemoglobinemia resulting from

absorption of nitrates. Journal of American Medical Association 242: 2869–70
6. Bojar RM, Rastegar H, Payne DP, et al 1987 Methemoglobinemia from intravenous nitroglycerin. A word of caution. Annals of Thoracic Surgery 43: 332–4
7. Anderson ST, Hadjucek J, Barker SJ 1988 Benzocaine induced methemoglobinemia. Anaesthesia and Analgesia 67: 1096–8
8. Dineen SF, Mohr DN, Fairbanks VF 1994 Methemoglobinemia from topically applied anaesthetic spray. Mayo Clinical Proceedings 69: 886–8
9. Mier RJ 1988 Treatment of aniline poisoning with exchange transfusion. Clinical Toxicology 26: 357–64
10. Gowans WJ 1990 Fatal methaemoglobinaemia in a dental nurse. A case of sodium nitrite poisoning. British Journal of General Practice 40: 470–1
11. Shesser R, Dixon D, Allen Y, et al 1980 Fatal methemoglobinemia from butyl nitrite ingestion. Annals of Internal Medicine 92: 131–2
12. Schimelman MA, Soler JM, Muller HA 1978 Methemoglobinemia: nitrobenzene. Journal of American College of Emergency Physicians 7: 406–8
13. Reider HU, Frei FJ, Zbinden AM, Thomson DA 1989 Pulse oximetry in methaemoglobinaemia. Failure to detect low oxygen saturation. Anaesthesia 44: 326–7
14. Rosen PL, Johnson C, McGehee WG 1971 Failure of methylene blue in toxic methaemoglobinaemia. Association with glucose-6-phosphate dehydrogenase deficiency. Annals of Internal Medicine 75: 83–6
15. Bodansky O 1951 Methaemoglobinaemia and methaemoglobin producing compounds. Pharmacological Review 3: 144–96
16. Harvey JW, Keith AS 1983 Studies of efficacy of methylene blue therapy in aniline induced methaemoglobinaemia. British Journal of Haematology 54: 29–41
17. Goluboff N, Wheaton R 1961 Methylene Blue induced cyanosis and acute haemolytic anaemia complicating treatment of methaemoglobinaemia. Journal of Paediatrics 58: 86–90
18. Berlin G, Brod AB, Hilden JO, et al 1984 Acute dapsone intoxication: a case treated with continuous infusion of methylene blue, forced diuresis and plasma exchange. Clinical Toxicology 22: 537–48
19. Kellet PB, Copeland CS 1983 Methemoglobinemia associated with benzocaine containing lubricant. Anesthesiology 59: 463–4

28.14 PESTICIDES

IAN WHYTE • ANDREW DAWSON

ESSENTIALS

1 The organophosphate pesticides are extremely toxic when ingested, producing muscarinic, nicotinic and CNS manifestations.

2 Management of organophosphate poisoning consists of general supportive care, together with administration of specific antidotes such as atropine and pralidoxime.

3 Carbamate poisoning is associated with a similar clinical presentation to organophosphate poisoning, but is generally more rapid in onset, less severe and of shorter duration.

4 Glyphosate toxicity is different from that of the organophosphates: gastrointestinal manifestations are common and large ingestions are associated with profound shock and death.

5 Paraquat is an extremely toxic herbicide and any ingestion should be regarded as potentially fatal. Toxicity is dose-related, with progressive pulmonary fibrosis occurring at smaller doses and rapid onset of multiorgan failure and death with larger doses.

ORGANOPHOSPHATES

INTRODUCTION

There are more than one hundred organophosphate compounds in regular use. Obtaining even clinically relevant data such as the lipid solubility, the half-life, the conversion to active metabolites, binding to antidotes and whether they are associated with delayed neuropathy or neuropsychiatric effects is difficult or impossible for many of these compounds.

Some of the organophosphate compounds commonly encountered in Australia include chlorpyrifos, coumaphos, diazinon, dichlorvos, dimethoate, famphur, fenthion, malathion, mevinphos and parathion.

The organophosphate insecticides are an extremely toxic group of compounds, which are rapidly absorbed via the dermal, oral and pulmonary routes. Ingestion of organophosphate concentrates may involve doses 100 to 1000 times greater than those following dermal or inhalational exposures, is much more likely to be associated with severe toxicity, and requires an entirely different approach to management.

MECHANISM OF TOXICITY

The organophosphate compounds phosphorylate and inactivate acetylcholinesterases. This causes an increase in acetylcholine concentration with stimulation of autonomic receptors and depolarizing block of neuromuscular junction receptors. This produces a large number of clinical effects in the CNS and autonomic nervous system and leads to paralysis.

After the initial formation of the organophosphate-acetylcholinesterase bond, a conformational change in the molecular structure of the organophosphate takes place and leads to irreversibility of the binding. This process is called 'ageing' and occurs within 12 to 36 hours of initial binding.

In addition to the inactivation of acetylcholinesterase and subsequent acetylcholine accumulation, there is also some inhibition of CNS GABA and dopaminergic neurons.

TOXICOKINETICS

All organophosphates are rapidly absorbed from the small intestine or through the skin (although less so than following oral exposure). Peak serum levels may occur within a few hours. There is a wide range of lipid/water solubility characteristics within this diverse group of compounds. As a consequence, volumes of distribution vary considerably but are usually large.

The major route of elimination is metabolism by paraoxonase, an enzyme found in serum bound to lipoproteins (HDL). Some organophosphates (-thions) are metabolized in the liver to much more active metabolites (-oxons). These agents (e.g. parathion, fenthion, chlorpyrifos) are also usually highly lipid soluble. The slow conversion of these substances, which are widely distributed into fat, may lead to delayed and/or prolonged cholinesterase inhibition and toxicity.

CLINICAL PRESENTATION

Four clinical syndromes have been described in relation to organophosphate exposure. These include an acute presentation, an intermediate syndrome and two later manifestations of toxicity.

Acute cholinergic symptoms and paralysis

This is the most commonly described clinical syndrome and is a result of the muscarinic, nicotinic and CNS effects of acetylcholine excess (Fig. 28.14.1).

Symptoms of toxicity generally occur within 4 hours ingestion. The exception to this is following exposure to extremely lipid soluble agents (e.g. fenthion and dichlofenthion), which are rapidly taken up into fat stores and subsequently slowly and intermittently released and

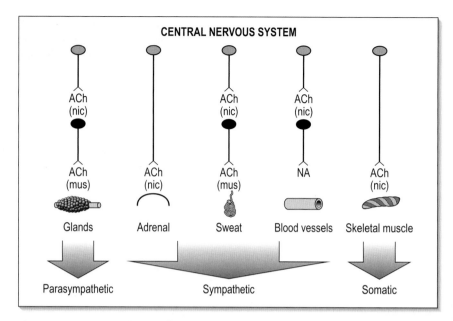

Fig. 28.14.1 Muscarinic and nicotinic effects of acetylcholine excess.

metabolized to more active compounds. With these agents, onset of toxic symptoms may be delayed up to 48 hours and symptoms may continue for weeks.

Muscarinic effects are those mediated by stimulation of the parasympathetic nervous system and include contraction of intestinal and bronchial smooth muscles, miosis, increased secretions from all secretory glands, decreased sinus node activity (bradycardia), AV conduction defects and occasionally ventricular arrhythmias. The most significant muscarinic features are described by the mnemonic DUMBELS: diarrhoea, urination, miosis, bronchospasm, emesis, lacrimation and salivation.

Nicotinic effects are due to the accumulation of acetylcholine both at the neuromuscular junction and at the preganglionic synapses of the autonomic nervous system. At the neuromuscular junction, this produces initial stimulation followed by depolarization and paralysis. Stimulation of the sympathetic nervous system may produce sweating, hypertension and tachycardia.

CNS effects include initial cerebral stimulation followed by increasing CNS depression progressing to coma and, occasionally, seizure activity.

Hypotension and tachycardia often complicate severe organophosphate poisoning. In addition, ischaemic sequelae may develop in patients with pre-existing vascular disease.

Symptomatology varies between individuals and within the same individual over time. This relates to a varying balance of muscarinic and nicotinic effects.

Subacute proximal weakness (intermediate syndrome)

A subacute syndrome is described in which patients develop proximal muscle weakness and cranial nerve lesions after recovery from the cholinergic effects. This may be caused by primary motor endplate degeneration due to prolonged inhibition of acetylcholinesterase. It has not been reported following high-dose pralidoxime therapy.

Late axonal degeneration: organophosphate-induced delayed neuropathy

Late neurological sequelae include a peripheral neuropathy caused by axonal degeneration. This may be due to the inhibition of the enzyme, neurotoxic target esterase (NTE). It is more common with (but not limited to) certain organophosphates that have a higher affinity for this enzyme.

Chronic organophosphate-induced neuropsychiatric disorder

Long-term neuropsychiatric sequelae have been described for all degrees of exposure. Formal neuropsychological testing and regular follow-up should be performed after all acute exposures. Use of benzodiazepines during the acute poisoning may reduce the severity of long-term neuropsychiatric sequelae.

INVESTIGATIONS

Plasma cholinesterase activity (PChE) is a sensitive marker of exposure but a poor indicator of severity. The normal range is from 3000 to 7000 U/L. This test has proved useful in documenting mild exposures, assessing adequacy of pralidoxime dose and determining the appropriate time to cease pralidoxime therapy.

The test can be done sequentially to confirm exposure in patients whose results fall within the low part of the normal range. Repeating the test a few weeks later will show whether the levels rebound.

In addition, some special tests involving assay of plasma cholinesterase activity are useful in guiding pralidoxime therapy.

Mixed cholinesterase test

This test is useful to determine whether sufficient pralidoxime is being given. PChE is measured in the patient's plasma, in a normal plasma sample, and in a 50/50 mixture of the two samples. If adequate doses of pralidoxime are being given, there will be no free organophosphate in the patient's plasma and the mixed sample will have a PChE value equal to the mean of the other two samples. A lower value indicates inadequate pralidoxime therapy.

Serial cholinesterase test

This test is useful to determine whether pralidoxime therapy can be ceased. If the patient appears clinically well on a pralidoxime infusion (after atropine has been ceased), it is difficult to judge when to cease the infusion. In this scenario,

PChE is measured in the patient's plasma, the pralidoxime is ceased and the PChE is measured 4 to 8 hours later. Pralidoxime may be recommended while awaiting results. If there is no residual organophosphate, the second measurement will be similar to the first. A lower second PChE value indicates continuing exposure to organophosphates, probably due to lipid soluble organophosphates stored in the patients fat.

Red blood cell cholinesterase activity correlates well with severity and prognosis but is not available at many centres. It is a better indicator of tissue acetylcholinesterase inhibition but is much less sensitive than plasma cholinesterase.

In moderate-to-severe poisonings, an ECG is useful to evaluate brady- and tachyarrhythmias. A chest X-ray and arterial blood gases are indicated in all severe poisonings, as aspiration pneumonia from the hydrocarbon solvents is not uncommon.

DIFFERENTIAL DIAGNOSIS

Difficulties in diagnosis usually arise when an unconscious or delirious patient is known to have ingested an unknown chemical from the garden shed. The absence of miosis does not exclude significant organophosphate poisoning. The presence of muscle fasciculations and associated weakness strongly supports the diagnosis. Organophosphates often have an odour similar to garlic, although this may be masked by hydrocarbon solvents. Significant poisoning is almost invariably associated with a low plasma cholinesterase. Similar, but usually milder, clinical features may occur with poisoning with carbamate insecticides.

DIFFERENCES IN TOXICITY

Organophosphates are often listed as being of low, moderate or high toxicity according to their lethal dose in animals. Such lists do not indicate the likelihood of developing clinical toxicity following human exposure because they are usually

prepared in concentrations that take into account their relative potencies. Following deliberate ingestion, organophosphate concentrates vary from being very poisonous to extremely poisonous. The major differences are that a number of these poisons require metabolic activation and thus may have a delayed or prolonged course.

DETERMINATION OF SEVERITY

Poisoning may be graded as mild, moderate or severe based on clinical findings and plasma cholinesterase activity (Table 28.14.1). However, in the presence of paralysis or any CNS signs or following ingestion of a concentrated preparation, poisoning is likely to be severe irrespective of the initial signs.

MANAGEMENT

The initial priority is the assessment and maintenance of airway, ventilation and circulation. Administration of supplemental oxygen, establishment of intravenous access and institution of appropriate monitoring should commence on arrival at hospital because patients may deteriorate rapidly. Mild acidosis is common in significant poisonings, the correction of the serum bicarbonate to normal concentrations with sodium bicarbonate has been suggested to be clinically useful.

Following dermal exposure, staff should wear gown and gloves, remove and destroy patient clothing and wash the patient a number of times (soap, alcohol and soap). While staff will often notice eye and upper respiratory symptoms while looking after these patients it has been shown that plasma cholinesterase concentrations in health-care workers do not change, indicating the symptoms are most likely from exposure to the irritant hydrocarbon solvent rather than to the organophosphate itself.

Oral activated charcoal should be given to all patients who have ingested organophosphates who present within 1–2 hours.

Complications of organophosphate poisoning that require specific therapy include seizures, hypotension, myocardial ischaemia, and ventricular tachycardia.

Seizures should initially be treated with diazepam 10–20 mg IV followed by phenobarbitone 15 mg/kg IV and elective intubation and ventilation (without paralysis).

Patients who become hypotensive often have an extremely low peripheral vascular resistance that will respond to very large doses of atropine. These patients should have a Swan-Ganz catheter inserted to monitor the effects of therapy. Such patients may appear adequately atropinized on standard clinical criteria. Paradoxical vasoconstriction can occur at atheromatous sites due to endothelial dysfunction at these sites and the unopposed action of acetyl-

Table 28.14.1 Severity grading of organophosphate poisoning		
Mild	Moderate	Severe
Walks & talks	Unable to walk	Unconscious
Headache & dizziness	Soft voice	No pupillary reflex
Nausea & vomiting	Muscle vesiculation	Muscle fasciculation
Abdominal pain	Small pupils	Flaccid paralysis
Sweating		Increased bronchial secretions
Salivation		Dyspnoea Crackles or wheeze Respiratory failure
Plasma cholinesterase 20%–50% of normal	Plasma cholinesterase 10%–20% of normal	Plasma cholinesterase <10% of normal

choline receptors on the arterial smooth muscle. In theory, this vasoconstriction should respond to atropine and be exacerbated by adrenaline (epinephrine) and dopamine. Also, most patients have high rather than low cardiac output. Thus atropine, rather than inotropic drugs, should be used for the treatment of hypotension.

Magnesium, isoprenaline or overdrive pacing (rate 120 to 140) are indicated for torsade de pointes and should be considered for all tachyarrhythmias. Magnesium is normally the drug of choice for treating torsade de pointes but its calcium channel blocking activity may aggravate the hypotension and heart block that can also complicate organophosphate poisoning.

Specific antidotes for organophosphate poisoning include atropine, pralidoxime and benzodiazepines.

Atropine is used to block muscarinic effects due to excessive acetylcholine. Initial treatment is to give a test dose of 1–2 mg of atropine over 10 minutes. If the patient exhibits signs of atropinization after this test dose, it is likely that they have mild poisoning. Otherwise, this dose should be repeated at 5–10 minute intervals until the patient is atropinized. Traditionally, the end point of atropinization is considered to be the absence of oropharyngeal secretions and this may require large doses. An atropine infusion of up to 10–20 mg/hour or even more may then be necessary to maintain atropinization in severe poisoning.

In severe poisoning, measurement of peripheral vascular resistance may be a better method of measuring adequate atropinization as, in some circumstances, cholinergic features may be surprisingly minimal (perhaps due to a depolarizing block of the muscarinic receptors), and hypotension and tachycardia due to circulating acetylcholine are the dominant clinical features.

Pralidoxime binds to organophosphates and removes them from acetylcholinesterase if ageing has not occurred. The pralidoxime-organophosphate complex is water-soluble and rapidly excreted by the kidneys. Patients with mild-to-moderate poisoning should receive pralidoxime with an initial dose of 2 g (30 mg/kg) intravenously over 15 minutes followed by 1 g every 8 hours for a minimum of 48 hours. Severe poisonings or oral exposures should have an infusion of 500 mg/hour (8 mg/kg/hour) after the initial dose. The adequacy of pralidoxime therapy may be determined by the mixed plasma cholinesterase test and the infusion adjusted accordingly. For the majority of organophosphate poisonings, this treatment is only of use in the first 36 hours but pralidoxime should be used in severe poisonings regardless of the time since exposure. For poisonings with highly lipid soluble organophosphates, pralidoxime may be commenced later and may need to be continued for up to 2–3 weeks. Pralidoxime undergoes renal excretion and in patients with renal failure, the dose may need to be reduced.

All patients with significant organophosphate poisoning should receive adjunctive treatment with benzodiazepines. There are no clinical trials to define the appropriate dose. In the absence of any other indications for benzodiazepines, the authors aim for a daily dose equivalent to 40 mg diazepam.

There are no effective methods of enhancing the elimination of organophosphates.

DISPOSITION

Patients with moderate or severe poisoning should be transferred to an intensive care facility. Asymptomatic patients who have ingested organophosphate concentrate should also be observed in an intensive care setting.

CARBAMATES

INTRODUCTION

Carbamates are found in numerous commercial products used as agricultural and household insect sprays. Carbamate insecticides available in Australia are listed in Table 28.14.2. Although less toxic than organophosphates, the carbamates result in poisoning with similar clinical features and deliberate ingestions have resulted in death. As with organophosphates, much written in textbooks relates to dermal or occupational exposure. Oral ingestion of carbamate concentrates may involve doses many times greater and requires a different approach to management.

MECHANISM OF TOXICITY

The carbamates, like organophosphates, inhibit acetylcholinesterase thus increasing acetylcholine concentration at autonomic receptors and neuromuscular junctions. However, unlike organophosphates, this inhibition is reversible and short-lived.

TOXICOKINETICS

The carbamate insecticides are rapidly absorbed by the oral and pulmonary

Table 28.14.2 Carbamates in use in Australia			
Extremely toxic (LD$_{50}$ <11 mg/kg)	*Highly toxic (LD$_{50}$ 11–50 mg/kg)*	*Moderately toxic (LD$_{50}$ 51–200 mg/kg)*	*Low toxicity (LD$_{50}$ >200 mg/kg)*
Aldicarb	Methiocarb	Thiodicarb	Carbaryl
Oxamyl	Aminocarb	Promecarb	
Carbofuran	Mecarban	Pirimicarb	
Methomyl	Bendiocarb		
Formetanate	Dimetilan		
	Propoxur		

routes, although most carbamates (the exception is Aldicarb) are relatively poorly absorbed through the skin compared with organophosphates. Following significant exposure, symptoms of toxicity generally occur early, within 30 minutes, but may be delayed for up to 1–2 hours. There is a wide range of lipid/water solubility characteristics resulting in variable, but usually large, volumes of distribution. Most of the carbamates are metabolized in the liver and then excreted in the urine within several days. Aldicarb undergoes extensive enterohepatic recirculation.

CLINICAL PRESENTATION

The clinical manifestations are similar to those seen with organophosphate poisoning, but are usually less severe, more rapid in onset and of shorter duration. Symptoms beyond 24 hours are unlikely to be due to carbamate intoxication. The most common clinical syndrome is acute cholinergic symptoms with or without paralysis. As with organophosphates, symptoms and signs vary between individuals and within the same individual at different points in time depending on the varying balance of muscarinic and nicotinic effects. Penetration of the blood–brain barrier by carbamates is very low and, for this reason, CNS symptoms are unusual. Case reports of late axonal degeneration exist. There does not appear to be an intermediate syndrome as is reported with organophosphates.

INVESTIGATIONS

Plasma cholinesterase and red cell cholinesterase activities are not reliable indicators of carbamate poisoning because the carbamate–cholinesterase complex spontaneously hydrolyses *in vivo* within minutes to hours. Thus, normal levels do not rule out intoxication. In a similar fashion to organophosphates, intoxication may be present despite normal cholinesterase activity because of the wide range of normal enzyme activity. However, a depression of 25% or more from an individual's baseline level of plasma cholinesterase activity is indicative of exposure. Samples need to be analysed immediately as *in vitro* hydrolysis of the carbamate-cholinesterase complex can occur.

As with organophosphate poisoning, an ECG, chest X-ray and arterial blood gas analysis may be useful in evaluating the patient.

DIFFERENTIAL DIAGNOSIS

The presence of CNS signs or muscle fasciculation and associated weakness suggests organophosphate rather than carbamate poisoning. The absence of significant reduction in plasma cholinesterase in the presence of a typical cholinergic syndrome suggests carbamate rather than organophosphate poisoning.

DIFFERENCES IN TOXICITY

Although carbamates may be classified according to their lethal dose in animals as in Table 28.14.2, these compounds are usually prepared in concentrations that take into account this relative potency. Deliberate ingestion of any carbamate concentrate produces significant poisoning and deaths have been recorded.

DETERMINATION OF SEVERITY

The same clinical features described for organophosphate poisoning in Table 28.14.1, may also be used to grade the severity of carbamate poisoning.

MANAGEMENT

The initial priority is the assessment and maintenance of airway, ventilation and circulation. Administration of supplemental oxygen, establishment of intravenous access and institution of appropriate monitoring should commence on arrival at hospital because patients may deteriorate rapidly.

Following dermal exposure, staff should wear gown and gloves, remove and destroy patient clothing and wash the patient a number of times (soap, alcohol and soap). Oral activated charcoal should be given to all patients who have ingested and who present within 1–2 hours.

Specific complications such as seizures, hypotension and myocardial ischaemia are less common with carbamate poisoning than with organophosphate poisoning but should be managed in the same manner if they occur.

Atropine should be administered to block muscarinic effects due to excess acetylcholine in the manner described for organophosphate poisoning. It is unlikely that an atropine infusion will be required to manage carbamate poisoning. Most patients with significant carbamate poisoning require approximately 6–12 hours of atropine treatment, but should be observed for a further 24 hours after the last atropine dose.

Pralidoxime binds to organophosphates, but does not bind particularly well to carbamates. In fact, animal work suggests that, with carbaryl poisoning, pralidoxime may actually increase acetyl-cholinesterase inactivation. However, if a combination of carbamate and organophosphate poisoning has occurred, pralidoxime should be given as described for organophosphate poisoning.

Some carbamates undergo enterohepatic circulation and repeated doses of activated charcoal may theoretically enhance their elimination. Invasive methods of enhanced elimination are not useful.

DISPOSITION

Patients with moderate or severe poisoning should be admitted to intensive care. Asymptomatic patients who have ingested carbamate concentrate should also be considered for observation in an intensive care setting.

GLYPHOSATE

INTRODUCTION

Glyphosate is a herbicide that is supplied as a concentrate with surfactant (Roundup®). The concentrate is 41% glyphosate, 10–20% polyoxyethylamine (surfactant) and water. The concentrate is diluted 40-fold before use. Glyphosate is also available as a 10% solution (Zero Weed Killer®).

It is unclear whether glyphosate itself is toxic but the surfactant certainly appears to be so. It is likely that both components contribute to the observed toxicity.

MECHANISM OF TOXICITY

Glyphosate is an organophosphate compound, however, it does not act as an acetylcholinesterase inhibitor in man. There is some evidence that glyphosate has a direct cardiotoxic effect and it is locally toxic to the gastrointestinal tract. The surfactant is approximately three times as toxic weight-for-weight as glyphosate and it may be responsible for the pulmonary complications.

TOXICOKINETICS

The extent of absorption following human ingestion is unknown, but only one-fifth to one-third of glyphosate appears to be absorbed in animals. The volume of distribution is low in dogs (0.28 L/kg). There is one major metabolite of unknown toxicity (aminomethyl phosphonic acid) and both glyphosate and its metabolite are excreted in the urine.

CLINICAL PRESENTATION

Glyphosate concentrate is locally irritating and the initial presentation is with gastrointestinal toxicity. In severe poisoning, hypotension, pulmonary dysfunction, renal failure, cardiac arrest, coma, repeated seizures or death may occur.

Manifestations of gastrointestinal toxicity include nausea, vomiting, epigastric and abdominal pain and diarrhoea. Corrosive injury to the pharynx, larynx, oesophagus and stomach may be evident clinically or on endoscopy.

Initial mild hypoxaemia may be followed by evidence of acute pulmonary oedema and respiratory failure requiring intubation and ventilation. Hypotension is frequently observed and, in severe cases, may be refractory to fluid and inotrope administration. This suggests a direct myocardial depressant effect. Evidence of renal dysfunction may include oliguria and elevated serum creatinine. Liver enzyme abnormalities may be observed but are rarely severe. Confusion, coma and seizures may occur. In seriously poisoned patients, a metabolic acidosis is frequent. Acute pancreatitis has been reported. Leucocytosis and hyperglycaemia are not infrequent.

DETERMINATION OF SEVERITY

The assessment of severity of toxicity is determined by dose ingested and clinical grading of toxicity (Table 28.14.3).

Ingestion of from 5 to 50 mL of concentrate usually results in either no symptoms or minor gastrointestinal symptoms only. Moderate symptoms occur with ingestions of from 50 to 100 mL and severe symptoms are likely when greater than 100 mL are ingested.

MANAGEMENT

Management of glyphosate poisoning is principally supportive. Corrosive injury to the upper airway may dictate a need for immediate airway control. Hypotension may develop within hours of ingestion and should be treated initially with intravenous fluids and, if unresponsive, inotropes. There is a risk of pulmonary oedema so over-aggressive fluid resuscitation should be avoided. Respiratory function should be monitored closely, oxygenation assured and intubation with assisted ventilation

Table 28.14.3 Clinical grading of glyphosate poisoning
Asymptomatic No abnormalities on physical or laboratory examination
Mild Predominantly gastrointestinal symptoms with stable vital signs and no other organ involvement
Moderate Gastrointestinal symptoms lasting longer than 24 hours Hypotension, responsive to intravenous fluids Pulmonary dysfunction not requiring intubation Acid–base disturbance Evidence of transient hepatic renal damage or temporary oliguria
Severe Pulmonary dysfunction requiring intubation Renal failure requiring dialysis Hypotension requiring inotropes Cardiac arrest Coma Repeated seizures Death

performed if necessary. If pulmonary oedema occurs, positive respiratory pressure may be of value. Urine output should be monitored and prevention of hypovolaemia and hypotension made a priority. Acidosis usually responds to bicarbonate therapy but may on occasions be resistant.

Gastrointestinal decontamination with oral activated charcoal is indicated in those patients who present within 1 hour of ingestion. There are no specific antidotes to glyphosate poisoning. Although the pharmacokinetic parameters of glyphosate suggest that haemodialysis may be useful to enhance elimination, there are no data to support its use. Haemodialysis may be of value for renal failure or acidosis unresponsive to bicarbonate administration.

PARAQUAT

INTRODUCTION

Paraquat is an extremely toxic herbicide capable of producing multisystem organ failure and pulmonary toxicity from as little as one mouthful of 20% concentrate. There is no specific treatment and any hope of survival rests on preventing absorption.

MECHANISM OF TOXICITY

Ingestion of paraquat leads to the generation of free oxygen radicals. These free oxygen radicals cause lipid peroxidation damaging cell membranes and leading to cell death. Free radical scavengers such as glutathione are rapidly overwhelmed due to the efficiency of paraquat in generating free radicals. Paraquat is actively taken up into type II pneumocytes and renal tubular cells. Thus in less severe poisonings, renal and pulmonary toxicity as well as direct gastrointestinal effects are the major clinical manifestations. In poisonings that are not fatal within days, the pulmonary fibrosis that develops is due to an acute pneumonitis that leads inevitably to generalized alveolar fibrosis. Increasing concentrations of inhaled oxygen increase pulmonary toxicity presumably by enhancing oxygen radical generation.

TOXICOKINETICS

Paraquat is poorly absorbed following oral administration. Despite this, peak plasma levels occur within 1 hour of ingestion. Absorption is decreased in the presence of food. There is little absorption through skin or via inhalation. The volume of distribution is large, as it is concentrated within cells, particularly pneumocytes. Distribution is rapid and substantially complete within the first few hours. Renal excretion is the major route of elimination and the development of renal toxicity reduces the rate of elimination. A substantial proportion of paraquat remains bound, especially within pneumocytes, even after serum levels are unmeasurable.

CLINICAL PRESENTATION

Systemic paraquat toxicity develops only after ingestion and not after inhalational or dermal exposure. Dermal or eye exposures can produce local corrosive effects.

The initial presentation of paraquat ingestion is with gastrointestinal toxicity. In severe poisoning, this is followed by multiorgan failure and, if patients survive this phase, by the slow development of pulmonary fibrosis leading to hypoxia and death.

Concentrated paraquat (20%) is corrosive and, when ingested, produces oesophageal and gastric erosions as well as burns in the mouth and throat. These corrosive effects are similar to those observed with alkali ingestion.

If more than 5–10 g of paraquat is ingested, multiorgan failure rapidly ensues. The major manifestations are acute renal failure, hepatic necrosis, myocardial necrosis, acute pneumonitis, internal haemorrhages, pulmonary fibrosis and death.

Ingestion of smaller quantities leads to gastrointestinal symptoms followed by progressive respiratory failure. The onset of pulmonary fibrosis may be delayed for days to weeks and death may occur up to 6 weeks later.

INVESTIGATIONS

Plasma levels of paraquat are important indicators of prognosis. A plasma level >5 mg/L at any time indicates an invariably fatal outcome. Nomograms have been developed which indicate the chance of survival (Fig. 28.14.2). Paraquat blood levels are performed by certain specialist laboratories.

A simple qualitative urine test for paraquat is available: 1 mL of a 1% sodium dithionate solution (found in haematology labs) is added to 10 mL of urine. A blue colour change indicates paraquat ingestion. If the test is negative on urine passed 2–6 hours after ingestion, a significant exposure is unlikely.

Numerous investigations including the full blood count, coagulation studies, electrolyte, LFTs, chest X-ray and ECG, are likely to be abnormal in paraquat poisoning. However, the inevitable failure of supportive care in the presence of multiorgan failure and the lack of

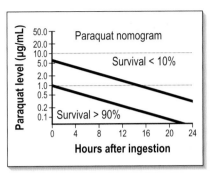

Fig. 28.14.2 Paraquat nomogram.

specific antidotes make the detection of these abnormalities largely unhelpful.

DETERMINATION OF SEVERITY

The following have been associated with fatal outcome:

- Oesophageal and gastric erosions
- Renal failure
- Ingestion of more than one mouthful of 20% concentrate
- Multi-organ failure
- Development of pulmonary opacities on chest X-ray
- Decreasing lung volumes on spirometry
- Paraquat level >3–5 mg/L.

The rate of increase in plasma creatinine over time (5 hours) is also correlated with outcome and can give prognostic information.

MANAGEMENT

The initial management priority is gastrointestinal decontamination. Activated charcoal or Fuller's earth (if available) should be given immediately. Emesis and lavage are contraindicated due to the corrosive nature of paraquat.

Patients with moderate poisoning may benefit from good supportive care. Oxygen should only be administered if the arterial oxygen saturation falls below 90%. In patients with high paraquat levels and/or multi-organ failure, it can be argued that palliative care is the only rational treatment due to the extremely poor prognosis.

LONG TERM SEQUELAE AND FOLLOW-UP

Patients who do not develop multi-organ failure and therefore do not die within the first week may still develop progressive pulmonary fibrosis. This may slowly develop up to 6 weeks later. Patients in this situation who have confirmed exposure to paraquat should have regular clinical follow-up and chest X-rays. Paraquat has only occasionally been reported to cause chronic non-fatal pulmonary fibrosis, i.e. the development of pulmonary fibrosis appears to lead almost inevitably to death.

ACKNOWLEDGEMENT

The material in this chapter has been adapted with permission from HyperTox 2002 (available from http://www.hypertox.com).

FURTHER READING

Adam A, Marzuki A, Rahman HA, Aziz MA 1997 The oral and intratracheal toxicities of Roundup and its components to rats. Veterinary and Human Toxicology 39(3): 147–51

Bolognesi C, Bonatti S, Degan P, et al 1997 Genotoxic activity of glyphosate and its technical formulation roundup. Journal of Agriculture and Food Chemistry 45(5): 1957–62

Bradberry SM, Vale JA 1999 How toxic are carbamate insecticides? EAPCCT XIX International Congress abstract. Journal of Toxicology – Clinical Toxicology 37(3): 372–3

Buckley NA 2001 Pulse corticosteroids and cyclophosphamide in paraquat poisoning. American Journal of Respiratory Critical Care Medicine 163(2): 585

CONTROVERSIES AND FUTURE DIRECTIONS

❶ Patients with borderline paraquat levels or ingestions around the potentially lethal dose (i.e. 5 g), may benefit from early charcoal haemoperfusion. This will only be useful if it can be given prior to the distribution of the majority of paraquat into pneumocytes (within 2–4 hours).

❷ Corticosteroids and cyclophosphamide has been suggested in the treatment of paraquat poisoning. There are two non-randomized trials with opposite results. Other theoretically appealing treatments include N-acetylcysteine, lung transplantation and superoxide dismutase, however, there is insufficient animal or human work to support their use.

Buckley NA, Dawson AH, Whyte IM 1994 Organophosphate poisoning: Peripheral vascular resistance – a measure of adequate atropinization. Journal of Toxicology – Clinical Toxicology 32(1): 61–8

Butera R, Locatelli C, Baretta S, Arrigoni S, Bernareggi G, Casorati P, Carli M, Manzo L 2002 Secondary exposure to malathion in emergency department healthcare workers. Journal of Toxicology – Clinical Toxicology 40(3) EAPCCT abstract 191

Casey PB 1999 Carbamate insecticides: are oximes harmful, beneficial or unnecessary? EAPCCT XIX International Congress abstract. Journal of Toxicology – Clinical Toxicology 37(3): 373–4

Chang C-Y, Peng Y-C, Hung D-Z, Hu W-H, Yang D-Y, Lin T-J 1999 Clinical impact of upper gastrointestinal tract injuries in glyphosate-surfactant oral intoxication. Human and Experimental Toxicology 18(8): 475–8

Dawson AH, Buckley NA, Whyte IM 1997 What target pralidoxime concentration? (letter). Journal of Toxicology – Clinical Toxicology 35(2): 227–8

Hart TB, Nevill A, Whitehead A 1984 A statistical approach to the prognostic significance of plasma paraquat concentrations. Lancet 2: 1222–3

Hung D-Z, Deng J-F, Wu T-C 1997 Laryngeal survey in glyphosate intoxication: a pathophysiological investigation. Human and Experimental Toxicology 16(10): 596–9

Jones AL, Elton R, Flanagan R 1999 Multiple logistic regression analysis of plasma paraquat concentrations as a predictor of outcome in 375 cases of paraquat poisoning. QJM 92: 573–8

Keifer MC, Mahurin RK 1997 Chronic neurologic effects of pesticide exposure. Occupational Medicine 12(2): 291–304

Kurtz PH 1990 Pralidoxime in the treatment of carbamate intoxication American Journal of Emergency Medicine 8(1): 68–70

Lee HL, Chen KW, Chi C-H 2000 Clinical presentations and prognostic factors of a glyphosate – surfactant herbicide intoxication: a review of 131 Cases. Academic Emergency Medicine 7: 906–10

Lin C-M, Lai C-P, Fang T-C, Lin C-L 1999 Cardiogenic shock in a patient with glyphosate-surfactant poisoning. Journal of the Formosan Medical Association 98(10): 698–700

Lin JL, Leu ML, Liu YC, Chen GH 1999 A prospective clinical trial of pulse therapy with glucocorticoid and cyclophosphamide in moderate to severe paraquat-poisoned patients. American Journal of Respiratory and Critical Care Medicine 159: 357–60

Lotti M 1991 Treatment of acute organophosphate poisoning. Medical Journal of Australia 154: 51–5

Pond SM 1990 Manifestations and management of paraquat poisoning. Medical Journal of Australia 152: 256–9

Pushnoy LA, Avnon LS, Carel RS 1998 Herbicide (Roundup) pneumonitis. Chest 114(6): 1769–71

Ragoucy-Sengler C, Pileire B 1996 A biological index to predict patient outcome in acute paraquat poisoning. Human Experimental Toxicology 15: 265–8

Thompson DF, Thompson GD, Greenwood RB, Trammel HL 1987 Therapeutic dosing of pralidoxime chloride. Drug Intelligence & Clinical Pharmacy 21(7–8): 590–3

Tominack R 1999 Glyphosate – contemporary clinical features. EAPCCT XIX International Congress abstract. Journal of Toxicology – Clinical Toxicology 37(3): 374–5

Wagner SL 1997 Diagnosis and treatment of organophosphate and carbamate intoxication. Occupational Medicine 12(2): 239–49

28.15 HYDROFLUORIC ACID

ANDIS GRAUDINS

ESSENTIALS

1 Patients and medical staff are often unaware of the presence of hydrofluoric acid (HF) in household cleaning products.

2 Topical HF exposures may result in the gradual onset of severe local pain out of proportion to any clinical signs evident on presentation.

3 Patients may not relate their dermal symptoms to HF exposure due to the delay in onset of pain.

4 Ingestion and inhalation of HF may result in gastrointestinal or respiratory burns, severe hypocalcaemia, hyperkalaemia and ventricular arrhythmias.

INTRODUCTION

The inorganic acid of fluoride, hydrofluoric acid (HF), is a moderately corrosive chemical widely used in industry for the etching of glass, metal and stone, and in the preparation of silicon computer chips. HF is also a common constituent of rust and scale removers, car wheel cleaners, brick cleaners and solder flux mixtures. These products may be for either commercial or home use and are often found in containers with inadequate labelling in regard to the potential toxicity. Concentrations of commercially available HF may vary from 50 to 100%. Products containing HF for domestic use generally have a concentration of less than 10% but higher concentration products may be obtained illicitly for home use.

The most common route of accidental exposure to HF is topical. This may occur when high-concentration HF leaks through damaged gloves in the industrial setting or when HF products are used in the home without gloves. Massive topical HF exposure and inhalational exposure to HF may also occur in the industrial setting.[1–3] Finally, ingestion of HF products may occur accidentally in the home in the paediatric age group or as a result of deliberate self-harm in adults.[4]

PATHOPHYSIOLOGY

HF is a relatively weak acid with less corrosive effects than other stronger acids such as hydrochloric or sulfuric. In particular, low concentrations of HF (<20%) may result in little or no perceptible corrosive injury to the skin immediately following exposure. This is due to the relatively small dissociation constant (pK_a = 3.8), which limits the concentration of free hydrogen ions on the skin surface.[4] As HF tends to remain in an undissociated, neutral state its ability to penetrate through the skin into deeper tissues is enhanced. Gradual dissociation of HF into free fluoride ions in the tissues leads to the characteristic local tissue injury. As the concentration of HF increases so does the potential for corrosive injury.[5] Nevertheless, chemical burns may result from exposures to dilute (<5%) solutions of HF, and fatal systemic poisoning has resulted from relatively small (<5% total body surface area) burns caused by more concentrated solutions.[3,6–9]

The primary mechanism of tissue damage resulting from exposure to HF is related to fluoride toxicity resulting from dissociation of the acid in exposed tissues. A number of pathologic mechanisms may be involved in both local and systemic fluoride poisoning. Fluoride binds divalent cations, especially calcium and magnesium, to form insoluble fluoride salts. The resulting hypocalcaemia and hypomagnesaemia may have profound local and systemic effects on cellular and organ functions. Fluoride is a cellular poison. It inhibits both aerobic and anaerobic metabolic enzyme systems and interferes with cellular respiration.[3] Fluoride also interferes with Na^+/K^+-ATPase activity and opens calcium-dependent potassium channels in cell membranes, resulting in the leak of potassium into the extracellular space with the potential for systemic hyperkalaemia.[10] Precipitation of calcium may also interfere with calcium-dependent clotting factors, resulting in coagulopathy. Finally, exposure to HF may produce direct corrosive injury.

Fatal systemic fluoride poisonings have also been reported following inhalational and gastrointestinal exposures.[2,3] Once absorbed, fluoride ions are distributed to virtually every tissue and organ resulting in widespread disruption of organ function. Fluoride is slowly eliminated in the urine and elevations of urinary fluoride excretion can be detected following exposure to HF although these do not correlate with clinical toxicity.[11]

CLINICAL PRESENTATION

Exposure to HF in the industrial setting is usually recognized as such and patients will often arrive with appropriate information in the form of material safety data sheets. Acute dermal exposures in the domestic setting may present a more difficult diagnostic dilemma. Domestic product labels may be incomplete and offer no advice regarding the use of protective apparel such as gloves.[12] Additionally, the onset of the signs and symptoms of HF injury may be delayed after exposure to low concentration domestic products and the patient may not recognize that the symptoms are related to chemical exposure.[12]

Highly concentrated (>70%) HF contains enough free hydrogen ions to produce a burning sensation on the skin providing some degree of warning of an acute exposure with symptom onset within 1–2 hours.[5] However, low concentrations of HF (<10%), found in products such as over-the-counter rust removers, often produce no symptoms at the time of contact and patients can present with gradually increasing pain from 6 to 12 hours following exposure.[13]

The primary presenting complaint of acute topical HF injury is pain out of all proportion to any physical signs. HF exposure should always be considered in this situation. The pain is usually described as a tingling sensation that progresses to a burning pain and, then to a typical deep, throbbing and severe pain.[5,13–15]

Visible evidence of HF burns also follows a fairly common pattern. Initially, the burn site is erythematous and may be oedematous. As tissue injury progresses, the site becomes pale and blanched.[16] Local vesiculation and frank tissue necrosis may ensue. This process can progress over several days in untreated patients, resulting in the development of deep ulceration and extensive tissue loss.

Dermal exposure to HF commonly occurs on the hands or feet with relatively small areas of the skin being exposed. Systemic fluoride poisoning is rarely a problem under these circumstances. The risk of systemic toxicity increases with the percentage of body surface area (BSA) exposed to HF and the concentration of HF. In general, if more than 3–5% BSA has been exposed to HF, there is a risk of hypocalcaemia.[17] Systemic fluoride toxicity is more likely following large dermal exposures, ingestion or inhalation of HF.[17,18]

Systemic fluoride toxicity is manifest by various effects, the most lethal of which are the severe electrolyte abnormalities produced by direct interaction with fluoride or effects on cell membranes.[3,10] Hypocalcaemia, is due to the complexing of calcium by fluoride ions. Hypomagnesaemia may also occur. However, the primary cause of the lethal arrhythmias (refractory ventricular tachycardia, ventricular fibrillation, and pulseless idioventricular rhythm) is the development of hyperkalaemia.[4,10] Patients with systemic fluoride poisoning

also develop a significant metabolic acidosis.[4] This is the result of fluoride interference with intracellular metabolism. The systemic manifestations of significant hypocalcaemia include carpopedal spasm, hyperreflexia, tetany, and coagulopathy. Headache, paraesthesiae, and visual complaints may be noted. In severe cases coma, seizures, shock, and dysrhythmias often precede death.

Fluoride inhalation is associated with pulmonary injury, including the development of non-cardiogenic pulmonary oedema, adult respiratory distress syndrome, and the potential for systemic fluoride toxicity.[19]

INVESTIGATIONS

No investigations are necessary following minor dermal exposures. Following significant dermal exposures to HF or any ingestion or inhalational exposure, serum electrolytes including magnesium and calcium, baseline coagulation studies and a 12-lead ECG (looking for evidence of hypocalcaemia or hyperkalaemia) are indicated. A chest radiograph should be performed in any patient with respiratory symptoms or severe systemic toxicity.

MANAGEMENT

All patients with significant dermal HF exposures (>5% body surface area) or any ingestion or inhalation exposures should have continuous cardiac monitoring and intravenous access established on arrival.

The initial management of an acute topical HF exposure is thorough skin decontamination with a water flush. This ideally should be performed as a first aid measure as soon as possible following the exposure as the delayed presentation of most patients makes it unlikely that significant amounts of HF still remain on the surface of the skin. Other first-aid measures in the work place, for known or suspected HF burns include topical treatments such as calcium gluconate gel (2.5–10%) or soaks with quaternary ammonium salts such as benzalkonium or benzethonium chloride. Topical

therapies are intended to form insoluble complexes with any surface fluoride ion thus preventing tissue penetration and minimizing deeper injury. Topical therapy is probably of little value once fluoride ions penetrate to deeper tissues but should be initiated on presentation to the emergency department. Calcium gluconate gel can be applied to the hand in a rubber glove. It may provide relief to some patients with low concentration HF exposures to the digits. In most cases topical therapy is a temporizing measure until more invasive methods of calcium administration can be employed. If calcium gluconate gel is not readily available, a 4.8% preparation can be rapidly prepared by mixing one ampoule of calcium gluconate injection BP in 10 g of KY jelly.

The definitive treatment of dermal HF burns involves the administration of calcium gluconate into the tissues affected by the exposure.[5,14,20–22] This may be achieved by a number of methods; direct tissue infiltration, regional intravenous infusion using a Bier's block technique, and intra-arterial infusion.[5,14,20–22] The choice of method depends upon the site and concentration of HF involved.

Direct injection of approximately 0.5 mL per square centimeter of 10% calcium gluconate solution at the burn site can be considered in areas with little skin tension such as the trunk, forearms, and legs. A small needle (25 gauge) should be used to minimize discomfort and care should be taken to infiltrate into, around, and beneath the burn area as completely as possible. Only calcium gluconate should be used for local infiltration as calcium chloride is more concentrated and produces direct injury when injected into tissues.[22]

HF burns to the hands are relatively common. In view of the lack of loose tissues to the digits, direct dermal injection may be extremely painful to perform and only small amounts of calcium gluconate may be injected. HF may also penetrate beneath the fingernails. In the past, removal of fingernails was advocated to allow for injection of calcium gluconate into the nail bed.[22,23] Fortunately, the advent of focused, parenteral calcium administration techniques to the affected limb have meant that nail removal is rarely, if ever indicated.

Two techniques are available as an alternative to direct injection of calcium gluconate into digital HF burns. The first is intra-arterial infusion of calcium gluconate to the involved digit(s). This technique involves inserting an arterial canula into the radial or brachial artery of the involved extremity and slowly infusing a dilute solution of calcium gluconate utilizing an infusion pump. This allows the calcium to be delivered to the affected tissues through the vascular supply and avoids the pain and tissue distention associated with direct injection.[14,23,24] A typical dose is 10–20 mL of 10% calcium gluconate in 50–100 mL of dextrose 5% in water infused over 4 hours and repeated as necessary. The end point for therapy should be the absence of pain. The number of intra-arterial infusions required for pain relief may vary from one to four or five, and depends on the concentration of HF to which exposure occurred.[13]

Regional intravenous calcium gluconate infusion using a Bier's block technique has also been employed in the treatment of HF burns to the limbs.[5,20,25] Success has been observed for digital, hand and forearm exposures as well as for exposures to the leg.[5,20,25] The technique is similar to that described by Bier for regional limb anesthesia and has the advantages of relative simplicity and of not requiring arterial canulation.[26] An intravenous canula is inserted in the dorsum of the hand of the affected limb and the arm is raised to exsanguinate the superficial venous system. A pneumatic tourniquet is applied to the upper arm and inflated to a pressure 100 mmHg above systolic blood pressure. Ten to 15 mL of 10% calcium gluconate is diluted to a total volume of 50 mL with normal saline and injected via the canula into the ischaemic arm. The tourniquet is sequentially released after 20 to 25 minutes.[5] Pain relief is usually apparent within 30 minutes of tourniquet release.

There have been no controlled studies comparing any of these techniques in the treatment of HF burns. However, intra-arterial calcium infusion appears to be a better technique for distal digital exposures, particularly in cases where exposure has been to high concentrations (>20%) or where multiple digits are involved.[5] Intra-arterial infusion of calcium has the advantages of more focal provision of calcium to the site of digital exposures and the potential for multiple infusions in patients with ongoing pain. If the intravenous route is selected as the primary therapy and is unsuccessful following one treatment, intra-arterial calcium infusion should then be used. The use of intra-arterial magnesium sulfate in place of calcium gluconate has resulted in tissue necrosis requiring surgical debridement in a small case series and cannot be recommended.[27]

It is sometimes difficult to determine whether ongoing pain at the exposure site is due to continued tissue destruction from fluoride still present in the tissues, or to established tissue damage. This is particularly the case with patients who have had digital exposures to high concentrations of HF and received multiple infusions of intraarterial calcium which do not seem to produce further pain relief. It also applies to patients who present more than 24 hours postexposure with ongoing pain despite calcium therapy. In both instances, failure to achieve pain relief with repeated infusions of calcium gluconate suggests that pain may be related to established tissue damage rather than ongoing tissue destruction.

Ocular HF exposures can result in serious consequences if left untreated. Patients should be treated as for other chemical exposures to the eye with copious saline irrigation, and local anesthetic drops for pain relief. Calcium gluconate (10–20 mL/L) may be added to saline irrigation fluid although animal studies suggest that calcium gluconate eye drops are no better than copious irrigation with normal saline and may, in fact, result in delayed corneal healing.[28] Clinical case reports of calcium gluconate eye drop use suggest that this treatment is not harmful but controlled studies are lacking.[29,30]

Systemic fluoride poisoning resulting from HF ingestion, inhalation, or large dermal exposures is potentially life threatening. Patients with HF ingestion should receive rapid GI decontamination. Aspiration of HF through a small bore nasogastric tube may limit absorption if the patient presents within 1 hour of ingestion. Calcium or magnesium containing antacids can complex intragastric HF and prevent some systemic absorption of fluoride ions. Nebulized calcium gluconate has been administered acutely to patients following HF inhalation.[31] Serum calcium, magnesium, and potassium levels should be closely monitored. Intravenous calcium and magnesium replacement should be commenced prior to any fall in serum Ca^{2+} or Mg^{2+} concentrations and replacement doses may be guided by the calculated dose of fluoride ingested. Large amounts of calcium (200–300 mmol) have been used in severe cases of systemic HF poisoning with hypocalcaemia.[4,8] Hyperkalaemia may be recognized on the 12-lead ECG, but close monitoring of serum potassium levels is warranted. Hyperkalaemia in systemic fluoride poisoning is resistant to standard measures of potassium reduction, such as insulin, glucose, and bicarbonate infusions. Ventricular arrhythmias associated with systemic fluoride poisoning are refractory to cardioversion and defibrillation.[10] Hemodialysis is indicated for severe or refractory hypocalcaemia, hyperkalaemia, or clinical toxicity (e.g. arrhythmias) and may be useful for the removal of fluoride ions. Calcium and magnesium monitoring and replacement should continue during this procedure. Endoscopy should be performed following HF ingestion as soon as the patient is clinically stable to assess the extent of any upper GI corrosive injury.

DISPOSITION

Patients with minor dermal exposures in whom emergency department treatment produces complete resolution of symptoms may be discharged home with follow-up arranged within 24 hours or should pain return. Those patients in whom tissue damage is evident, require referral to a plastic or hand surgeon.

Patients at risk of systemic fluoride poisoning require admission to an intensive care unit for ongoing monitoring and management of the electrolyte disturbances and other complications of systemic toxicity.

All patients with eye exposures require early ophthalmological referral.

CONCLUSION

HF exposures present a unique management challenge for the emergency physician. Early recognition of HF exposure and institution of appropriate therapy may result in the avoidance of significant morbidity from dermal exposures and potential mortality from more serious ingestions and inhalational toxicity.

CONTROVERSIES AND FUTURE DIRECTIONS

❶ Relative value of intra-arterial versus regional intravenous calcium gluconate administration.

REFERENCES

1. Blodgett DW, Suruda AJ, Crouch BI 2001 Fatal unintentional occupational poisonings by hydrofluoric acid in the U.S. American Journal of Industrial Medicine 40: 215–20

2. Kono K, Watanabe T, Dote T, et al 2000 Successful treatments of lung injury and skin burn due to hydrofluoric acid exposure. International Archives of Occupational and Environmental Health 73(Suppl): S93–S97

3. Caravati EM 1988 Acute hydrofluoric acid exposure. American Journal of Emergency Medicine 6: 143–50

4. Chan BS, Duggin GG 1997 Survival after a massive hydrofluoric acid ingestion. Journal of Toxicology – Clinical Toxicology 35: 307–9

5. Graudins A, Burns MJ, Aaron CK 1997 Regional intravenous infusion of calcium gluconate for hydrofluoric acid burns of the upper extremity. Annals of Emergency Medicine 30: 604–7

6. Chan KM, Svancarek WP, Creer M 1987 Fatality due to acute hydrofluoric acid exposure. Journal of Toxicology – Clinical Toxicology 25: 333–9

7. Manoguerra AS, Neuman TS 1988 Fatal poisoning from acute HF ingestion. American Journal of Emergency Medicine 4: 362

8. Mayer TG, Gross PL 1985 Fatal systemic fluorosis due to hydrofluoric acid burns. Annals of Emergency Medicine 14: 149–53

9. Bordelon BM, Saffle JR, Morris SE 1993 Systemic fluoride toxicity in a child with hydrofluoric acid burns: case report. Journal of Trauma 34: 437–9

10. Cummings CC, McIvor ME 1988 Fluoride-induced hyperkalemia: the role of Ca++-dependent K+ channels. American Journal of Emergency Medicine 6: 1

11. Saady JJ, Rose CS 1988 A case of non-fatal sodium fluoride ingestion. Journal of Analytical Toxicology 12: 270–1

12. Smith MA 1992 A hand burn from unmarked hydrofluoric acid [letter]. Medical Journal of Australia 157: 431

13. Siegel DC, Heard JM 1992 Intra-arterial calcium infusion for hydrofluoric acid burns. Aviation Space and Environmental Medicine 63: 206–11

14. Vance MV, Curry SC, Kunkel DB, Ryan PJ, Ruggeri SB 1986 Digital hydrofluoric acid burns: treatment with intraarterial calcium infusion. Annals of Emergency Medicine 15: 890–6

15. Wilkes GJ 1993 Intravenous regional calcium gluconate for hydrofluoric acid burns of the digits. Emergency Medicine 5: 149–244

16. Anderson WJ, Anderson JR 1988 Hydrofluoric acid burns of the hand: mechanism of injury and treatment. Journal of Hand Surgery [Am] 13: 52–7

17. Mullett T, Zoeller T, Bingham H, et al 1987 Fatal hydrofluoric acid cutaneous exposure with refractory ventricular fibrillation. Journal of Burn Care Rehabilitation 8: 216–9

18. Sadove R, Hainsworth D, Van Meter W 1990 Total body immersion in hydrofluoric acid. Southern Medical Journal 83: 698–700

19. Watson AA, Oliver JS, Thorpe JW 1973 Accidental death due to inhalation of hydrofluoric acid. Medicine Science and the Law 13: 277–9

20. Ryan JM, McCarthy GM, Plunkett PK 1997 Regional intravenous calcium—an effective method of treating hydrofluoric acid burns to limb peripheries. Journal of Accident and Emergency Medicine 14: 401–4

21. Murao M 1989 Studies on the treatment of hydrofluoric acid burn. Bulletin of the Osaka Medical College 35: 39–48

22. Bracken WM, Cuppage F, McLaury RL, Kirwin C, Klaassen CD 1985 Comparative effectiveness of topical treatments for hydrofluoric acid burns. Journal of Occupational Medicine 27: 733–9

23. Trevino MA, Herrmann GH, Sprout WL 1983 Treatment of severe hydrofluoric acid exposures. Journal of Occupational Medicine 25: 861–3

24. Kohnlein HE, Achinger R 1982 A new method of treatment of HF burns of the extremities. Chirurgie Plastica 6: 298

25. Henry JA, Hla KK 1992 Intravenous regional calcium gluconate perfusion for hydrofluoric acid burns. Journal of Toxicology – Clinical Toxicology 30: 203–7

26. Bier A 1908 Concerning a new method of local anaesthesia of the extremities. Arch Klin Chir 86: 123

27. Vance M, Curry S, Gerkin R, Kunkel D, Ryan P 1986 An update on the treatment of digital hydrofluoric acid burns with intra-arterial infusion techniques. Veterinary and Human Toxicology 28: 486

28. Beiran I, Miller B, Bentur Y 1997 The efficacy of calcium gluconate in ocular hydrofluoric acid burns. Human and Experimental Toxicology 16: 223–8

29. Bentur Y, Tannenbaum S, Yaffe Y, Halpert M 1993 The role of calcium gluconate in the treatment of hydrofluoric acid eye burn. Annals of Emergency Medicine 22: 1488–90

30. Rubinfeld RS, Silbert DI, Arentsen JJ, Laibson PR 1992 Ocular hydrofluoric acid burns. American Journal of Ophthalmology 114: 420–3

31. Lee DC, Wiley JFd, Synder JWd 1993 Treatment of inhalational exposure to hydrofluoric acid with nebulized calcium gluconate [letter]. Journal of Occupational Medicine 35: 470

28.16 IRON

ZEFF KOUTSOGIANNIS

ESSENTIALS

1 Acute iron poisoning is a potentially life-threatening condition.

2 The risk of severe toxicity is determined by the dose of elemental iron ingested.

3 Iron poisoning has both local (gastrointestinal) and systemic effects.

4 Early effective gastrointestinal decontamination, usually with whole bowel irrigation, is important in the management of high-risk cases.

5 Chelation therapy with IV desferrioxamine is the definitive treatment for severe poisoning.

6 Generally, most patients recover, although presence of shock or coma indicate a poor prognosis.

7 Long-term sequelae are gastrointestinal scarring and obstruction.

INTRODUCTION

Although the majority of exposures to iron occur in small children, significant iron ingestions also occur in adults as a result of deliberate self poisoning. It is one of the most commonly ingested agents in self-poisoning during pregnancy as a result of its ready availability to obstetric patients.[1]

PATHOPHYSIOLOGY

Iron is an essential element in red blood cell production, haemoglobin and myoglobin oxygenation, cytochrome function, and many enzyme cofactor catalytic activities.[2,3] Under normal circumstances, absorption of iron from the gastrointestinal (GI) tract is finely regulated according to the requirements of the body. After absorption across the GI mucosa in the ferrous form (Fe^{2+}), iron is oxidised to the ferric state (Fe^{3+}) and then stored bound to ferritin or transported across the cell membrane into the blood, where it binds to transferrin.[2] Iron is extracted from transferrin in the bone marrow and used for haemoglobin synthesis. It is also removed from transferrin by the reticuloendothelial system and hepatocytes and stored as haemosiderin and ferritin.[4] Total iron binding capacity (TIBC) is a measurement of the total amount of iron that transferrin can bind and normally exceeds serum iron by two- to threefold.[3] Ferritin is a large storage protein that reversibly binds to iron. When an iron deficit exists, iron is transported from ferritin and the GI tract to the liver, spleen and bone marrow where it is incorporated into appropriate molecules.[5] If the body's iron requirements have been met, iron remains stored in the intestinal cell rather than bind to transferrin. Eventually, the intestinal cell dies and sloughs off into the lumen for elimination.[3] This is the main mechanism limiting excessive iron absorption and the mechanism by which the body regulates iron balance.[5]

Iron rarely exists as an unbound or 'free' element.[9] It is free iron that is toxic to cellular processes. Iron toxicity manifests as both local (GI) and systemic effects.

Local effects

Iron preparations, like other metal salts, have a direct corrosive effect on the GI mucosa. In overdose this can lead to irritation, ulceration, bleeding, ischaemia, infarction, and perforation.[6] Associated profound fluid losses can result in hypotension, shock, and lactate formation leading to metabolic acidosis. The long-term sequelae of this corrosive action include GI scarring and obstruction.[6,7] As the mucosal surface is disrupted iron is absorbed passively down concentration gradients.[3,7] When the transferrin binding capacity is exhausted, free iron becomes available.

Systemic effects

Free iron is an intracellular toxin and localizes in the mitochondria, which in turn catalyses free radical formation, disrupts oxidative phosphorylation and lipid peroxidation.[8] The resultant mitochondrial dysfunction and destruction leads to cell death and can occur in any organ. Other systemic findings of iron poisoning include cardiovascular collapse, anion-gap metabolic acidosis, coagulopathy and encephalopathy.[3,8] The cardiovascular collapse has been attributed to decreased intravascular volume from GI haemorrhage, third space losses from increased capillary membrane permeability and iron-induced venodilation.[7] Metabolic acidosis persisting after hypovolaemia and hypoperfusion have been corrected probably results from the mitochondrial toxicity of iron.[8] Coagulopathy developing early in iron poisoning results from inhibition of serum proteases while in the later stages it is due to hepatic dysfunction.[9]

Toxic dose

In general, the risk of developing iron toxicity can be predicted from the dose of elemental iron ingested per kilogram body weight (Table 28.16.1).[8,10] It

Table 28.16.1 Risk assessment based on dose of elemental iron ingested

Risk assessment	Dose ingested (mg/kg)
Asymptomatic	<20
Local (GI) symptoms only	20–60
Risk of systemic iron poisoning	60–120
Potentially lethal	>120

essential to calculate the dose of *elemental* iron rather than dose of iron salt.

CLINICAL PRESENTATION

The clinical course of iron poisoning is traditionally described as comprising five stages.[7,11,12] Not all patients will experience all stages; they can die at any stage; can present at any stage and the time frames for each stage are imprecise and may overlap.

A more practical approach is to consider iron poisoning as comprising two clinical stages with a pathophysiological basis: GI toxicity and systemic toxicity.

Stage 1 (0–6 hours)

This stage is dominated by symptoms and signs of GI injury particularly vomiting, but also abdominal pain, diarrhoea and GI bleeding. In severe cases, hypovolaemic shock secondary to gastrointestinal losses can develop.[8] The failure to develop any GI symptoms within 6 hours of ingestion effectively excludes significant iron poisoning.[3,13,14]

Stage 2 (2–24 hours)

Also known as the 'latent' or 'quiescent' phase, this stage represents the period between resolution of GI symptoms and appearance of overt systemic toxicity. It is not always seen and, indeed, may represent a failure to recognize development of toxicity rather than a true quiescent phase. Most patients will recover and not progress to Stage 3. Those with significant poisoning remain clinically ill with subtle signs and progress to Stage 3.

Stage 3 (6–48 hours)

This is the stage of systemic toxicity characterized by shock and multiorgan system failure. By definition, it represents severe toxicity. The shock is multi-factorial arising from hypovolaemia, vasodilation and poor cardiac output. There is evidence of poor peripheral perfusion, worsening acidosis and acute renal failure. A coagulopathy may develop and lead to recurrent GI bleeding. CNS effects include lethargy, coma and convulsions.

Stage 4 (2–5 days)

This is the hepatic phase of iron toxicity and is relatively uncommon.[2] It is characterized by acute hepatic failure with jaundice, hepatic coma, hypoglycaemia, coagulopathy and elevated transaminase and ammonia levels. It has a high mortality.[15]

Stage 5 (2–6 weeks)

This stage is relatively rare and represents the delayed sequelae from the corrosive effects of iron resulting in GI scarring. This results in gastric outlet and small bowel obstructions.

INVESTIGATIONS

Acute iron poisoning is a clinical diagnosis and all symptomatic patients require treatment regardless of the iron level or results of other tests. However serum iron levels, abdominal X-rays and other tests do play a role in determing management.

Serum iron concentration

Normal serum iron concentrations are between 10 and 30 µmol/L. Peak iron levels usually occur between 2 and 6 hours after overdose, although they may sometimes be delayed.[3,16] Frequent levels may need to be taken to determine the true peak. Nevertheless, iron levels have been used to determine toxicity and direct management.[7] A serum iron concentration greater than 90 µmol/L at 4–6 hours after an overdose is associated with a greater risk of subsequently developing systemic iron toxicity. However, it is intracellular not serum iron that is responsible for systemic toxicity and thus during stages 2 or 3, the iron level may be decreasing or even normal while the patient deteriorates. In the presence of desferrioxamine, the serum iron level is artificially lowered.

The total iron binding capacity (TIBC) is falsely elevated in the presence of high iron concentrations or desferrioxamine and is no longer regarded as useful in the assessment of iron poisoning.[17]

Plain abdominal X-rays

Most iron preparations are radioopaque and an early abdominal X-ray is useful in confirming ingestion of iron, and in subsequently guiding gastric decontamination and the risk of continued iron absorption. A negative X-ray does not exclude iron ingestion as the tablets may have disintegrated or not be radiopaque.

Other laboratory tests

Although leucocytosis and hyperglycaemia are frequently observed in iron poisoning they are not useful in terms of diagnosis or management.[14] The presence of a anion gap metabolic acidosis is a useful marker of systemic iron poisoning. Other tests that are useful in managing patients with established iron poisoning include serum electrolytes, renal function, liver function, arterial blood gases, cross match and clotting profile.

MANAGEMENT

The approach to management of a patient presenting following an iron overdose is determined by the initial assessment of the risk of iron poisoning. This risk assessment is based on the dose ingested and the presence or absence of GI and/or systemic features of iron poisoning. For most patients, a period of observation and good supportive care, often including intravenous fluids will be sufficient. In those patients at risk of systemic poisoning or who present with established iron poisoning, aggressive decontamination measures and chelation therapy may be necessary to achieve a good outcome. The aim is to prevent the development of systemic toxicity in those patients at risk.

Observation and supportive care

All patients demonstrating signs and symptoms consistent with clinical toxicity of Stages 1, 2, or 3 warrant further treatment. Enthusiastic fluid replacement with isotonic fluid is essential. An initial bolus of 20 ml/kg should be given, followed by boluses as needed to replace fluid losses and maintain urine output. Patients with established iron poisoning may require more advanced supportive care including inotropic support, blood transfusions, correction of coagulopathy with fresh frozen plasma, and correction of acidosis.

Gastrointestinal decontamination

Iron is not well adsorbed to activated charcoal and so alternative methods of gastrointestinal decontamination must be considered in patients who present following ingestion of more than 60 mg/kg of elemental iron, especially where unabsorbed iron is evident on abdominal X-ray.

Inducing emesis with syrup of ipecac is not recommended because it may mask the symptoms produced by iron and can lead to an underestimation of the severity of the toxicity.[10] Gastric lavage may be a useful option if performed early but is often technically difficult in that the tablets tend to clump together, form pharmacobezoars and attach to the gastric mucosa.[2] Endoscopy has been used to remove large iron loads but this is also technically difficult.[8] Surgical removal is reported.[18,19]

Whole bowel irrigation (WBI) is widely advocated as the gastrointestinal decontamination method of choice in the setting of iron poisoning, although there are no controlled trials.[31] It should be initiated in any patient who has ingested more than 60 mg/kg of elemental iron and still has iron present in the GI tract on X-ray. The procedure should continue until there is a clear rectal effluent and no visible iron on X-ray.

Chelation therapy

Desferrioxamine is the parenteral chelating agent of choice for iron poisoning. It binds Fe^{3+} to form ferrioxamine which is water soluble, red-to-orange in colour and renally excreted.[3] Desferrioxamine binds free iron and iron in transit between transferrin and ferritin thus effecting a redistribution of iron from tissue sites back into plasma. It does not chelate iron bound to transferrin, haemoglobin, myoglobin, or cytochrome enzymes.[3]

Chelation therapy is indicated in any patient with established systemic iron toxicity or at risk of developing such toxicity. Clinical features and laboratory results may be useful in identifying these patients. The presence of gastrointestinal bleeding, coma, shock or metabolic acidosis are indications for immediate desferrioxamine therapy irrespective of iron levels. Serum iron levels greater than 90 μmol/L are generally regarded as being predictive of subsequent systemic toxicity and an indication to commence chelation therapy.

Ferrioxamine's red-to-orange colour is responsible for the classically described *vin rose* urine in patients given desferrioxamine but this colour change is an insensitive marker of the presence of free iron and the desferrioxamine IM challenge test is no longer used.[21]

Desferrioxamine is given as a continuous intravenous infusion starting slowly and aiming for a rate of 15 mg/kg/hour.[7,10] Administration rate may be limited by hypotension, the principal adverse effect. Intramuscular administration is not recommended as it is painful, requires multiple injections, has erratic absorption and higher side effect profile.[10] The precise endpoints for chelation therapy are unclear but therapy can be safely discontinued once the serum iron level is normal or low, the patient clinically well, the anion gap resolved and there is no further urine colour change.[3,22] Except under exceptional circumstances, desferrioxamine should not be continued greater than 24 hours because of the risk of pulmonary toxicity and ARDS.[23]

The approach to iron poisoning is not altered in the pregnant patient. Symptomatic iron overdose in pregnancy is associated with preterm labour, spontaneous abortion, and maternal death.[1] Desferrioxamine does not cause perinatal complications or foetal toxicity and is potentially life saving.[24]

CONTROVERSIES AND FUTURE DIRECTIONS

❶ An oral iron chelator, deferiprone, has been widely studied and shown to be effective in patients with chronic iron overload states such as thalassaemia. It has shown promise in acute iron poisoning in animal studies, but no human data are as yet available.[25,26]

DISPOSITION

Patients who have ingested less than 60 mg/kg of elemental iron and remain asymptomatic at 6 hours may be medically discharged. Those with gastrointestinal symptoms or requiring WBI because of large ingestion require admission for supportive care and ongoing observation and monitoring. Those with systemic toxicity and/or requiring chelation therapy require intensive care admission. All patients where deliberate self-poisoning is suspected require psychosocial assessment.

PROGNOSIS

Most patients with iron overdose remain asymptomatic or develop minor GI toxicity only and do well with supportive care. Those with large ingestions should have an excellent outcome if recognized early, and appropriate and timely decontamination and/or chelation therapy is instituted. Patients presenting late with established severe systemic toxicity have a poorer prognosis.[2] Gastrointestinal stricture formation is a potential long-term sequela.

REFERENCES

1. Tran T, Wax JR, Philput C, et al 2000 Intentional iron overdose in pregnancy-management and outcome. Journal of Emergency Medicine 18(2): 225–8
2. Gruber J 1998 Acute iron and lead poisoning. In: Rosen P, Barkin R (eds) Emergency medicine. St. Louis, Mosby, pp 1367–78
3. Mills KC, Curry SC 1994 Acute iron poisoning. Emergency Medical Clinics of North America 12(2): 397–413

4. Henretig FM, Temple AR 1984 Acute iron poisoning in children. Emergency Medical Clinics of North America 2(1): 121
5. Finch CA, Huebers H 1982 Perspectives in iron metabolism. New England Journal of Medicine 306: 1520
6. Tenenbein M, Littman C, Stimpson RE, et al 1990 Gastrointestinal pathology in adult iron overdose. Journal of Toxicology – Clinical Toxicology 28: 311–20
7. Banner W, Tong TG 1986 Iron poisoning. Pediatrics Clinics of North America 33: 393–409
8. Rella JG, Nelson LS 1997 Iron. In: Tintinalli, et al (eds) Emergency Medicine. New York, McGraw Hill, pp 1159–62
9. Tenenbein M, Israels SJ 1988 Early coagulopathy in severe iron poisoning. Journal of Pediatrics 113: 695
10. Curry SC 1993 Iron. In: Reisdorff EJ, et al (eds) Paediatric Emergency Medicine, Philadelphia, WB Saunders, pp 673–9
11. Jacobs J, Greene H 1965 Acute iron intoxication. New England Journal of Medicine 273: 1124–7
12. Schauben JL, Augenstein WL, Cox J, et al 1990 Iron poisoning: Report of 3 cases and review of therapeutic intervention. Journal of Emergency Medicine 8: 309–19
13. Chyka PA, Butler AY 1993 Assessment of acute iron poisoning by laboratory and clinical observations. American Journal of Emergency Medicine 11: 99
14. Palatnick W, Tenenbein M 1996 Leukocytosis, hyperglycaemia, vomiting, and positive X-rays are not indicators of severity of iron poisoning. American Journal of Emergency Medicine 14: 454–5
15. Tenenbein M 2001 Hepatotoxicity in acute iron poisoning. Journal of Toxicology – Clinical Toxicology 39(7): 721–6
16. Ling LJ, Hornfeldt CS 1991 Absorption of iron after experimental overdose of chewable vitamins. American Journal of Emergency Medicine 9: 24–6
17. Siff JE, Meldon SW 1999 Usefulness of the total iron binding capacity in the evaluation and treatment of acute iron overdose. Annals of Emergency Medicine 34(1): 567–8
18. Foxford R, Goldfrank L 1985 Gastrotomy: a surgical approach to iron overdose. Annals of Emergency Medicine 14: 1223–6
19. Peterson CD, Fifeld GS 1980 Emergency gastrotomy for acute iron poisoning. Annals of Emergency Medicine 9: 262–4
20. Tenenbein M 1993 Position statement: whole bowel irrigation. American Academy of Clinical Toxicology; European Association of Poisons Centres and Clinical Toxicologists. Journal of Toxology – Clinical Toxicology 35(7): 753–62
21. Yatscoff RW, Wayne EA, Tenenbein M, et al 1991 An objective criterion for the cessation of deferoxamine therapy in the acutely iron poisoned patient. Journal of Toxicology – Clinical Toxicology 29: 1–10
22. Howland MA 1996 Risks of parenteral deferoxamine for acute iron poisoning. Journal of Toxicology – Clinical Toxicology 35(5): 491–7
23. Tenenbein M, Kowalski S, Stenko A, et al 1992 Pulmonary toxic effects of continuous administration in acute iron poisoning. Lancet 34: 485–9
24. Tran T, Wax JR, Steinfeld, et al 1998 Acute intentional overdose in pregnancy. Obstetrics and Gynecology 92: 678–80
25. Diav-Citrin O, Koren G 1997 Oral iron chelation with deferiprone. Pediatric Clinics of North America 44(1): 236–47
26. Berkovitch M, Livne A, Lushkov G, et al 2000 The efficacy of oral deferiprone in acute iron poisoning. American Journal of Emergency Medicine 18(1): 36–40

28.17 HYPOGLYCAEMIC DRUGS

LINDSAY MURRAY • MARK LITTLE

ESSENTIALS

1 Both insulin and sulphonylurea overdose can result in profound prolonged hypoglycaemia.

2 The key to management of insulin and sulphonylurea overdoses lies in early recognition, correction of hypoglycaemia and maintenance of euglycaemia with dextrose supplementation.

3 Octreotide is useful adjunctive therapy in the management of sulphonylurea overdose.

4 Metformin overdose does not cause significant hypoglycaemia but may rarely result in life-threatening lactic acidosis.

INTRODUCTION

Diabetes is a common medical condition with the result that there is ready access to hypoglycaemic medications. The major groups of hypoglycaemic agents available are the insulins, the sulfonylureas and metformin (a biguanide). In overdose, with the exception of metformin, these agents cause profound prolonged hypoglycaemia that can provide a management challenge to the emergency physician.

INSULIN

Insulin is naturally secreted from the β cells as pro insulin which is then cleaved *in vivo* to produce insulin and C peptide. A number of preparations with variable durations of action are available for the management of diabetes but in overdose they are all capable of causing profound and prolonged hypoglycaemia. This is because the subcutaneous injection of a large mass of insulin acts as a 'depot' from which ongoing absorption occurs.[1]

The clinical features of insulin overdose are the neurological and autonomic manifestations of hypoglycaemia with which all emergency physicians are familiar. These are usually evident within hours of self-administration of an insulin overdose and the patient frequently presents in coma. The suspicion of deliberate overdose is aroused when recurrent profound hypoglycaemia occurs after initial response to dextrose administration. If the history of deliberate overdose is known at time of presentation, then profound prolonged hypoglycaemia should be anticipated. Insulin also effects the flow of electrolytes across cellular membranes and other electrolyte abnormalities, in particular hypokalaemia, may develop.

Management of insulin overdose is essentially supportive and involves administration of sufficient concentrated dextrose solution so as to maintain euglycaemia until all the insulin is absorbed from the depot site and its hypoglycaemic action terminated. After initial correction of hypoglycaemia with 50% dextrose, a 10% dextrose infusion should be commenced and blood sugar levels followed closely with appropriate further boluses of dextrose and titration of infusion rate. Very large doses of dextrose may be required sometimes for days. Frequently it will be necessary to administer a 50% dextrose infusion and this requires a central line because concentrated glucose solutions are irritating to the veins. Electrolyte abnormalities also need to be monitored and corrected. Admission to an intensive care or high-dependency unit is usually necessary to ensure adequate monitoring of blood glucose, serum potassium and adjustment of the dextrose infusion rate.

Exogenous insulin overdose may be distinguished from endogenous hyperinsulinaemia by measurement of the C peptide concentration. This will be low in the presence of exogenous insulin.

METFORMIN

Metformin is the only biguanide currently in use in Australasia. Phenformin was removed due to a high incidence of lactic acidosis: 66 cases per 100 000 patient years. Metformin has a rate of lactic acidosis of only three cases per 100 000 patient years.[2]

Metformin is rapidly and well absorbed from the GIT, undergoes little hepatic metabolism and is nearly completely excreted renally. It acts by increasing cellular insulin sensitivity, which results in increased uptake of glucose. It will not decrease the blood glucose level in a non-diabetic.

Lactic acidosis may develop with therapeutic dosing of metformin where deteriorating renal function leads to drug accumulation. This potentially lethal complication usually has an insidious and non-specific presentation including nausea, vomiting, diarrhoea, lethargy and tachypnoea.[3]

There is limited published experience of acute metformin overdose as most cases are uneventful. In particular, significant hypoglycaemia is not observed following metformin overdose. However, fatal lactic acidosis has been reported following metformin overdose.[4] Although this complication is unusual, any patient who becomes symptomatic following a metformin overdose should have their acid–base status and serum lactate concentration checked. Emergency haemodialysis is indicated for metformin-induced lactic acidosis.[5]

SULPHONYLUREAS

These are the most commonly prescribed oral hypoglycaemics in Australasia. Currently available agents include glibenclamide, glicizide, gliclazide, glimepiride and glipizide. Sulphonylurea drugs acts by increasing insulin secretion from the β cells of the pancreas, as well as decreasing hepatic clearance of insulin. This, in turn, increases serum insulin levels. Most sulphonylurea drugs have 12–24-hour duration of action but this is prolonged following overdose. All are metabolized in the liver.[2]

Sulphonylurea-induced hypoglycaemia may occur as a complication of therapy, inadvertent administration of a sulphonylurea to a non-diabetic patient, or as a consequence of deliberate self-poisoning. The hypoglycaemia observed after deliberate self-poisoning is likely to particularly profound and prolonged.

Hypoglycaemia should always be corrected immediately with a 50% dextrose bolus. All patients with sulphonylurea-induced hypoglycaemia should have the medication ceased and be admitted to hospital for monitoring of blood sugar levels and appropriate dextrose supplementation. Elderly patients with sulphonylurea-induced hypoglycaemia will often have intercurrent medical illnesses that need treatment.

Patients with an intentional sulphonylurea overdose will usually require large doses of dextrose, often receiving 50% dextrose via a central line, for a prolonged period of time. The hypoglycaemia may be particularly refractory to dextrose supplementation and early addition of octreotide to the therapeutic regimen may greatly reduce the dextrose requirement, obviate the need for central access and facilitate subsequent management and disposition. Gastric decontamination with activated charcoal should be undertaken in patients who present early following intentional ingestion of sulphonylureas but does not take precedence over supportive care and correction of hypoglycaemica. All intentional overdoses need psychiatric assessment once medically cleared.

CONTROVERSIES AND FUTURE DIRECTIONS

❶ Surgical excision of insulin overdose injection sites has been previously advocated but few would now recommend such aggressive management for a condition so amenable to medical management.

❷ The correct dose and route of administration of octreotide in the management of sulphonylurea overdose is undefined. Greater doses than quoted above may be necessary to effectively suppress insulin secretion following large sulphonylurea overdoses in non-diabetic patients.

Octreotide

Octreotide is a long-acting synthetic analogue of somatostatin and acts by blocking the release of insulin from the β cells in the pancreas. It effectively blocks the effect of sulphonylurea agents. Octreotide has minimal side effects, mainly gastrointestinal in nature. The currently recommended dose is recommended is 50 mcg 6 hourly sci.

In eight healthy volunteers with glipizide-induced hypoglycaemia, octreotide effectively suppressed serum insulin levels and reduced glucose requirement compared to diazoxide and dextrose infusions.[6] In a case series of nine sulphonylurea overdoses, the use of octreotide was associated with a significant reduction the number of hypoglycaemic episodes and amount of 50 % dextrose infused.[7]

REFERENCES

1. Arem R, Zoghbi W 1985 Insulin overdose in eight patients: insulin pharmcokinetics and review of the literature. Medicine (Baltimore) 64: 323–32
2. Harrigan RA, Nathan MS, Beattie P 2001 Oral agents for the treatment of type 2 diabetes: pharmacology, toxicity and treatment. Annals of Emergency Medicine 38: 68–78
3. Luft D, Schmulling RM, Eggstein M 1978 Lactic acidosis in biguanide-treated diabetics: a review of 330 case. Diabetologica 14: 75–87
4. Teale KFH, Devine A, Stewart H, Harper NJ 1998 The management of metformin overdose. Anaesthesia 53: 698–701
5. Lalau JD, Westeel PF, Debussche X, et al 1987 Bicarbonate haemodialysis: An adequate treatment for lactic acidosis in diabetics treated by metformin. Intensive Care Medicine 13: 383–7

6. Boyle PJ, Justice K, Krentz AJ, et al 1993 Octreotide reverses hyperinsulinemia and prevents hypoglycaemia induced by sulfonylurea overdoses. Journal of Clinical Endocrinology & Metabolism 76: 752–6

7. McLaughin SA, Crandall CS McKinney PE 2000 Octreotide: an antidote for sulphonylurea induced hypoglycaemia. Annals of Emergency Medicine 36: 133–8

28.18 LITHIUM

LINDSAY MURRAY

ESSENTIALS

1 Chronic lithium toxicity is associated with significant morbidity and mortality especially where diagnosis and treatment are delayed. Acute lithium overdose, unless massive, has a more benign course.

2 Chronic lithium poisoning presents with neurological dysfunction. Acute lithium overdose presents with gastrointestinal dysfunction.

3 Consider the diagnosis of lithium intoxication and check a serum lithium concentration in any patient on lithium therapy who presents unwell.

4 Chronic lithium intoxication usually develops because of impaired lithium excretion. The underlying factors must be identified and corrected.

5 Serum lithium levels correlate with clinical severity in chronic but not acute intoxication.

6 Haemodialysis effectively enhances lithium elimination. This intervention is more likely to be necessary in chronic intoxication than acute overdose.

INTRODUCTION

Lithium, the metal with the lowest molecular weight, is usually dispensed as the carbonate salt. It is widely used in the therapy of bipolar disorder and a number of other conditions. Both immediate-release and sustained-release preparations are available. This drug has a relatively narrow therapeutic index and chronic intoxication develops relatively frequently. Acute overdose is less common.

PHARMACOKINETICS

Standard lithium preparations are rapidly and completely absorbed after oral administration with peak serum levels occurring at 2–4 hours. Absorption and time to peak level is delayed after administration of sustained-release preparations and following overdose. Once absorbed, lithium is slowly re-distributed from the intravascular space to the total body water. Lithium is not metabolized and its elimination is almost exclusively renal. Lithium is freely filtered at the glomerulus but, under normal circumstances, approximately 80% of filtered ions are reabsorbed in the proximal tubule and only 20% are excreted in the urine. Under these circumstances, renal clearance of lithium is approximately 10–40 mL/min and its elimination half-life is 20–24 hours. The renal elimination of lithium is greatly affected by sodium and water balance and by the presence of drugs that affect renal tubular reabsorption of sodium. In the early stages following acute overdose, renal elimination is much greater because lithium is relatively concentrated in the intravascular compartment and available for filtration at the glomerulus.

CLINICAL PRESENTATION

Chronic lithium toxicity

Chronic lithium toxicity may develop in association with prolonged excessive dosing or, more commonly, as a result of impaired lithium excretion due to intercurrent illness or a drug interaction. Lithium excretion is impaired in renal failure and congestive cardiac failure because of reduced filtration at the glomerulus and also in water or sodium depletion states because of increased reabsorption of sodium (and lithium) in the proximal tubule. A number of drugs including NSAIDs, SSRIs, ACE inhibitors and diuretics may also impair lithium excretion.

The clinical features of chronic lithium toxicity are almost exclusively neurological and the following severity grading system is widely used:[1]

- Grade I (mild): nausea, vomiting, tremor, hyperreflexia, agitation, muscle weakness, ataxia
- Grade II (serious): stupor, rigidity, hypotonia, hypotension
- Grade III (life threatening): coma, seizures, myoclonia, cardiovascular collapse.

Lithium toxicity is not associated with significant cardiovascular effects. Minor benign ECG changes are sometimes observed.[2]

Chronic lithium therapy is also associated with nephrogenic diabetes insipidus and hypothyroidism, which may complicate the clinical presentation of toxicity.

Acute lithium overdose

Patients who take a significant overdose of lithium carbonate as with any other metal salt, develop rapid onset of gastro-intestinal toxicity characterized by nausea, vomiting, abdominal pain and diarrhoea. This gastrointestinal disturbance can be very severe and may result in significant fluid and electrolyte losses. It is usually observed where more than 25 g are ingested but can occur following smaller doses. Gastrointestinal upset is not a prominent feature of chronic lithium toxicity.

Acute lithium overdose is much less likely to result in significant neurotoxicity than is chronic lithium toxicity.[3] Neurotoxicity could theoretically slowly develop following acute overdose if renal clearance were sufficiently impaired so as to allow redistribution of sufficient lithium from the intravascular compartment to tissue compartments before it could be excreted. This situation may develop if there is pre-existing renal failure or if inadequate fluid resuscitation leads to dehydration, sodium depletion or renal impairment as a consequence of the fluid losses from gastrointestinal toxicity.

INVESTIGATIONS

Essential laboratory investigations in the assessment of lithium toxicity are serum electrolytes, renal function and serum lithium concentration. Serial serum lithium concentrations may be required. Other investigations are performed as indicated to evaluate and manage intercurrent disease processes and to exclude important differential diagnoses.

Therapeutic serum lithium concentrations are generally quoted as 0.6–1.2 mEq/L. although clinical evidence of lithium toxicity can be observed at concentrations within this range, particularly in the elderly.[4] More commonly in cases of chronic intoxication, mild toxicity is observed at lithium concentrations of 1.5–2.5 mEq/L, severe toxicity at concentrations of 2.5 to 3.5 mEq/L, and life-threatening toxicity at concentrations greater than 3.5 mEq/L. Following acute overdose, serum lithium concentrations do not correlate with clinical severity as they do not reflect CNS concentrations, however, when performed serially, they are useful in guiding management. Peak serum lithium concentrations greater than 4.0 mEq/L are frequently observed following acute overdose in patients who do not go on to develop neurotoxicity.

MANAGEMENT

Chronic lithium toxicity

The diagnosis of lithium toxicity should be considered in any individual on lithium therapy who presents to the emergency department unwell, in particular with evidence of neurological dysfunction. The diagnosis should be confirmed or excluded by ordering a serum lithium concentration as part of the initial work-up. A precipitating illness that has resulted in impaired lithium excretion will usually be present and require assessment and treatment on its own merits.

Appropriate supportive care measures should be instituted on arrival. Once the diagnosis of chronic lithium toxicity is confirmed, further care is oriented towards management of the precipitating medical condition and enhancing lithium excretion by optimizing renal function and correcting any water or sodium deficits with intravenous normal saline. Therapy with lithium carbonate and any drugs contributing to lithium toxicity should be immediately discontinued.

The definitive treatment of established chronic lithium neurotoxicity is haemodialysis. The aim of enhancing lithium elimination by this method is to minimize the duration of neurological dysfunction and avoid permanent neurological sequelae. Lithium has physicochemical and pharmacokinetic properties that render it very suitable for enhancing elimination by haemodialysis: low molecular weight, high water solubility, small volume of distribution, no plasma protein binding and an endogenous renal clearance rate much lower than that achieved by haemodialysis.[5] The indications for haemodialysis are difficult to define. It should be performed in any patient with an elevated serum lithium concentration and severe or life-threatening neurotoxicity. It should be considered in the patient with less severe toxicity in whom adequate renal function and a falling lithium concentration are unable to be established with initial fluid resuscitation. Once instituted haemodialysis should be continued until the serum lithium is <1 mEq/L. Some rebound in serum lithium may be noted after haemodialysis is discontinued. The decision to dialyse can usually be made some 8–12 hours after admission.[5]

Acute lithium overdose

Intravenous access should be established and infusion of normal saline commenced during the initial assessment. Administration should be sufficient to correct any sodium or water deficits arising as a result of the toxic gastroenteritis and to ensure a good urine output. Excessive administration of normal saline or attempts at forced diuresis do not further enhance lithium excretion.[6] A serum lithium concentration, renal function and electrolytes should be performed as part of the initial assessment and repeated as necessary to guide further management. In particular, the serum lithium should be followed until falling and less than 2 mEq/L.

Activated charcoal does not bind lithium well and need not be administered unless there has been a significant co-ingestion. Sodium polystyrene sulfonate has been proposed as an effective alternative absorbent but is not widely used and repeated administration can cause hypokalaemia.[7] On the basis of a single volunteer study, whole bowel irrigation has been recommended for overdose of extended-release preparations[8] but the gastrointestinal upset renders this intervention technically difficult in patients with large ingestions.

Haemodialysis is rarely indicated following acute overdose in the patient with normal renal function who receives good supportive care. It may be necessary in the presence of renal failure or in the patient who goes on to develop neurotoxicity in the presence of a slowly falling serum lithium concentration.

DISPOSITION AND PROGNOSIS

Patients with chronic lithium intoxication require admission for management

CONTROVERSIES AND FUTURE DIRECTIONS

❶ The indications for and preferred method of gastrointestinal decontamination following acute lithium overdose remain undefined.

❷ Precise criteria for haemodialysis in chronic lithium intoxication remain undefined.

❸ Continuous arterio- or venovenous haemofiltration have been proposed as alternatives to haemodialyis for enhancement of lithium elimination. Although lower clearances are achieved with these methods, they are often easier to institute and may minimize rapid transcellular fluid and electrolyte shifts.[11] At the moment they can only be recommended where haemodialysis is not available.

of their fluid and electrolyte status, monitoring of renal function and serum lithium concentration, and management of intercurrent illnesses. Ideally, admission should be to an institution with a capacity to perform haemodialysis where toxicity is moderate or severe. Following haemodialysis, neurological recovery may be delayed well beyond the removal of lithium and permanent neurological deficits are reported.[9,10]

Acute lithium overdose usually has an excellent outcome with good supportive care and may be admitted to a non-monitored setting for intravenous fluids and monitoring of fluid and electrolytes, and lithium concentrations. The asymptomatic patient with normal renal function and lithium level falling to below 2 mEq/L is fit for medical discharge. This usually occurs within 24 hours. Psychiatric evaluation is mandatory and may take place whilst waiting for lithium levels to fall.

REFERENCES

1. Hansen HE, Amdisen A 1978 Lithium intoxication. Quarterly Journal of Medicine (new series) 47: 123–44
2. Tilkian AG, Schroeder JS, Kao JJ 1976 Cardiovascular effects of lithium in man: a review of the literature. American Journal of Medicine 61: 665–70
3. Oakley PW, Whyte IM, Carter GL 2001 Lithium toxicity: an iatrogenic problem in susceptible individuals. Australian & New Zealand Journal of Psychiatry 35: 833–40
4. Strayhorn JM, Nash JL 1977 Severe neurotoxicity despite 'therapeutic' serum lithium levels. Diseases of the Nervous System 38: 107–11
5. Jaeger A, Saunder P, Koopferschmidt J, et al 1993 When should dialysis be performed in lithium poisoning? A kinetic study in 14 cases of lithium poisoning. Clinical Toxicology 31(3): 429–47
6. Amidsen A 1988 Clinical features and management of lithium poisoning. Medical and Toxicological Adverse Drug Experiences 3: 18–32
7. Roberge RJ, Martin TG, Schneider SM 1993 Use of sodium polystyrene sulfonate in a lithium overdose. Annals of Emergency Medicine 22: 1911–5
8. Smith S, Ling L, Halstenson C 1991 Whole-bowel irrigation as a treatment for acute lithium overdose. Annals of Emergency Medicine 20: 536–9
9. Shou M 1984 Long lasting neurological sequelae after lithium intoxication. Acta Psychiatrica Scandinavica 70: 594
10. Verdoux H, Bougeois ML 1990 A case of lithium neurotoxicity with irreversible cerebellar syndrome. Journal of Nervous and Mental Disorders 178: 761
11. LeBlanc M, Raymond M, Bonnardeau A, et al 1996 Lithium poisoning treated by high-performance continuous arteriovenous and venovenous hemodiafiltration. American Journal of Kidney Disease 27: 365–72

28.19 ETHANOL

MARK LITTLE • LINDSAY MURRAY

ESSENTIALS

1 Ethanol is a major cause of morbidity, mortality and emergency department presentation in all Western societies.

2 Presentations may be due to acute intoxication, withdrawal or medical complications of chronic ethanol ingestion.

3 Ethanol intoxication is frequently implicated in emergency department presentations related to trauma, drowning, fire, and acute behavioural disturbance.

4 Ethanol withdrawal has a mortality of 5% and may require inpatient management.

5 Wernicke's encephalopathy is a clinical diagnosis and requires prompt recognition and treatment with thiamine.

INTRODUCTION

Ethanol is the most commonly used drug in Australasia and elsewhere in the Western world. Ethanol misuse is a major cause of mortality and morbidity both directly and indirectly and emergency departments deal with the result of this misuse on a daily basis. It was estimated that in 1997, 3290 Australians died from injury due to high risk drinking and there were 72 302 hospitalizations.[1]

Chronic alcohol consumption contributes to the development of a number of medical and surgical conditions, all of which may result in emergency department presentation and are dealt with elsewhere in this text. This chapter confines its discussion to acute ethanol intoxication, ethanol withdrawal and two important emergency presentations that occur exclusively in alcoholics – Wernicke's encephalopathy and alcoholic ketoacidosis.

PHARMACOLOGY

Ethanol is a small molecule that is rapidly and almost completely absorbed from the stomach and small intestine. Ethanol is both water and lipid soluble and rapidly crosses lipid membranes to distribute uniformly throughout the total body water. Ethanol is principally eliminated by hepatic metabolism with smaller amounts (5–10%) excreted unchanged by the kidneys, lungs and in sweat.

The principal pathway for hepatic metabolism of ethanol is via the cytosolic enzyme, alcohol dehydrogenase (ADH). In this three-step oxidation process ethanol is initially metabolized to acetaldehyde by ADH. Acetaldehyde is in turn metabolized to acetate by aldehyde dehydrogenase. Acetate is converted to acetyl-CoA and enters the Krebs cycle to be finally metabolized to carbon dioxide and water. Entry of acetyl-CoA in the Krebs cycle is dependent on adequate thiamine stores.[2] Importantly, the ADH system is saturated at relatively low blood ethanol concentrations that results in blood ethanol elimination moving from first-order to zero-order kinetics. The rate of ethanol metabolism in non-tolerant adults is approximately 10 g/hour and blood ethanol level falls by about 0.02 g/dL/hour.[3]

An alternative pathway for ethanol metabolism is via the microsomal ethanol oxidizing system (MEOS), the activity of which increased in response to chronic alcohol exposure. Metabolism by this route is relatively important at very high blood ethanol concentrations and in chronic alcoholics.

The mechanism of action of ethanol is poorly understood. However, ethanol acts as a CNS depressant, at least partially by enhancing the effect of GABA at GABA$_A$ receptors. Tolerance to the CNS depressant effect develops with chronic exposure.

CLINICAL PRESENTATION

Acute ethanol intoxication

The clinical features associated with acute ethanol intoxication predominantly relate to the CNS and progress with increasing blood alcohol level, although there is remarkable inter-individual variation, most commonly as a function of tolerance. Initial features include a sense of well-being, increased self-confidence, and disinhibition. With increasing blood concentrations, impaired judgement, impaired coordination and emotional lability develop. At very high concentrations, ethanol is a non-specific CNS depressant and can cause coma, respiratory depression, loss of airway protective reflexes and death.

Presentation to the emergency department is usually as a result of the social and behavioural consequences of the alteration in higher CNS functions. Ethanol is frequently implicated in trauma, drowning, violence, self-harm, domestic and sexual abuse, and other acute social and psychiatric emergencies. Ethanol is a common co-ingestant in overdose. Less commonly the emergency presentation is a direct result of the CNS depressant effects of ethanol.

Many other important medical and surgical conditions that cause altered mental status may be incorrectly ascribed to ethanol intoxication or co-exist with ethanol intoxication. Table 28.19.1 lists an (incomplete) differential diagnosis.

In the absence of a clear history, the diagnosis of ethanol intoxication is only confirmed upon determination of a breath or blood ethanol concentration. Because ethanol consumption is so ubiquitous, a positive reading does not exclude co-existing pathology.

Table 28.19.1 Differential diagnosis of acute ethanol intoxication

Encephalopathy
Hepatic
Wernicke's

Head injury
Hypo-/hyperthermia
Intracranial infarction or haemorrhage
Metabolic
Hypoglycaemia
Hyponatraemia
Hypoxia
Hypocarbia

Overdose or other toxin
Post-ictal state
Psychosis
Sepsis

Ethanol withdrawal syndrome

Ethanol withdrawal can only occur in the ethanol-dependent individual. Although the pathophysiology is not well-understood, the syndrome presents as unopposed sympathetic and CNS stimulation. It is associated with a mortality of 5% and early clinical recognition of this syndrome is important.[4]

Classically symptoms occur within 8–24 hours of a reduction or cessation of ethanol consumption.[4] Symptoms can begin any time after the blood ethanol concentration begins to fall and blood ethanol is frequently still measurable in withdrawing patients. The duration of the syndrome may be from 2 to 7 days.

Patients may present to the emergency department already in withdrawal after deliberately abstaining from alcohol or after stopping drinking due to intercurrent illness or lack of funds to buy alcohol. Alternatively, ethanol-dependent patients may begin to withdraw whilst being treated in the emergency department, particularly where their stay is prolonged.

Clinical features of mild ethanol withdrawal are those of mild autonomic hyperactivity and include nausea, anorexia, coarse tremor, tachycardia, hypertension, hyperreflexia, insomnia and anxiety.[5] In more severe cases, the patient goes on to develop more pronounced anxiety, insomnia, irritability, tremor, tachycardia, hyperreflexia, hypertension, fever, visual hallucinations, decreased seizure threshold and finally delirium. Symptoms usually peak by 50 hours.[6] Delirium tremens represents the extreme end of the spectrum of ethanol withdrawal. It is an uncommon but frequently lethal complication.

Wernicke's encephalopathy

This condition develops in certain alcoholics as a complication of thiamine deficiency. The classical clinical presentation is a triad of:

❶ Oculomotor disturbance (usually nystagmus and ocular palsies)
❷ Abnormal mentation (usually confusion)
❸ Ataxia.[7]

It is a clinical diagnosis and constitutes a medical emergency with a mortality of 10–20 %. For this reason the emergency physician must maintain high index of suspicion in patients with long-term heavy ethanol intake.

Alcoholic ketoacidosis

Alcoholic ketoacidosis is a life-threatening medical condition that develops in the alcoholic patient in response to starvation and depletion of glycogen stores. The normal response to starvation is increased gluconeogenesis from pyruvate. In the alcoholic patient, pyruvate is preferentially converted to lactate. In response, fatty-acid metabolism is increased as an alternative source of energy resulting in the production of acetyl-CoA and acetoacetate, which in turn is reduced to β hydroxybutyrate producing the ketoacidotic state.

Alcoholic ketoacidosis usually develops within 24–72 hours of oral intake (including ethanol) being reduced as a result of gastritis, hepatitis, pancreatitis or other intercurrent acute medical illness such as meningitis, pyelonephritis or pneumonia.[8] The patient usually has a known history of heavy ethanol intake and presents very unwell with nausea, vomiting, and altered mental status. They are usually dehydrated, tachypnoeic, tachycardic and hypotensive. The clinical presentation may be complicated by the clinical features of the precipitating illness and of ethanol withdrawal.

The diagnosis is supported by the presence of the typical anion gap metabolic acidosis and urinary ketones. The blood glucose will be low or only mildly elevated and this helps distinguish the condition from diabetic ketoacidosis.

INVESTIGATIONS

The excretion of ethanol by the lungs, although relatively unimportant in terms of ethanol elimination, obeys Henry's law, i.e the ratio between the concentration of ethanol in the alveolar air and blood is constant. This allows breath sampling of ethanol to reliably estimate blood ethanol concentration.

For any individual, the clinical severity of intoxication progresses with increasing blood ethanol concentration, although, as consequence of tolerance, there is significant interindividual variation. Most non-tolerant adults would be expected to develop some impairment of higher functions at blood ethanol concentrations in the range of 0.025–0.05 mg/dL (5–11 mmol/L) and to develop significant CNS depression in the range of 0.25–0.4 mg/L (55–88 mmol/L).

In a patient presenting with acute intoxication no investigations may be necessary, however, blood or breath ethanol level (BAL) are frequently useful to confirm the diagnosis. A BAL of zero is highly significant in a patient with an altered level of consciousness, as ethanol intoxication is excluded, and other diagnoses need to be considered. A positive blood ethanol level does not exclude alternative diagnoses.

Other investigations should be performed as clinically indicated in an effort to exclude co-existing pathologies and alternative diagnoses as detailed above.

MANAGEMENT

Acute ethanol intoxication

Severe ethanol intoxication with CNS depression is life-threatening but a good outcome is assured by timely institution of supportive care. In particular, attention may need to be given to the airway and ventilation. Hypotension generally responds to intravenous crystalloid infusion. The blood sugar level must be checked and normoglycaemia maintained. Intravenous thiamine should be administered. There is no specific antidote to ethanol intoxication.

Less severe ethanol intoxication presents a management challenge to the emergency physician when it results in a combative or violent patient threatening harm to self or staff, or threatening to discharge against medical advice. Such patients frequently require chemical sedation with titrated doses of intravenous benzodiazepines or butyrophenones in order to facilitate assessment and observation, ensure safety for patient and staff and prevent unsafe discharge.

Ethanol withdrawal

The key to management of this condition is early recognition and institution of adequate dosing of benzodiazepines. Very large doses of benzodiazepines may be required to control symptoms. The risk and likely severity of ethanol withdrawal can usually be anticipated if an accurate history of alcohol intake and previous withdrawals is obtained. Co-existing conditions should be managed on their own merits. It is important to exclude hypoglycaemia and correct if present. Thiamine 100 mg p.o. or IV should be immediately given to any

chronic alcoholic patient who presents with or develops an altered mental status.

The management of ethanol withdrawal in the emergency department or observation ward is greatly facilitated by the use of ethanol withdrawal charts. These charts facilitate recognition of the first signs of ethanol withdrawal and timely administration of benzodiazepine in adequate doses. An example of such a chart is shown in Figure 28.22.1. Benzo-

diazepine, usually diazepam, administration is titrated to the clinical features of withdrawal. The total dose required to manage withdrawal is highly variable. Benzodiazepines are usually given orally but can be administered intravenously to the uncooperative or severely withdrawing patient. In cases of very severe agitation, carefully titrated intravenous doses of a butyrophenone may be used in addition to a benzodiazepine.

Table 28.19.2 Differential diagnosis of ethanol withdrawal
Anticholinergic syndrome
Acute schizophrenia
Benzodiazepine withdrawal
CNS infection
Hypoglycaemia
Neuroleptic malignant syndrome
Sepsis
Serotonin syndrome
Thyrotoxicosis

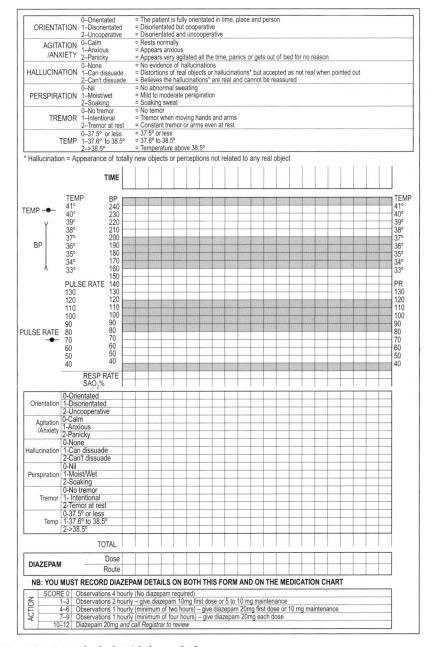

Fig. 28.19.1 Alcohol Withdrawal Chart.

Wernicke's encecephalopathy

As Wernicke's encephalopathy is a clinical diagnosis with high mortality if untreated, any known or suspected alcoholic patient who presents with altered mental status should receive thiamine 100 mg IV during the initial assessment. Giving dextrose to the thiamine-deficient patient may acutely worsen the neurological status of the patient. Magnesium is a cofactor for thiamine-dependent transketolase and so any magnesium deficiency should be corrected.[9]

Ethanol-induced ketoacidosis

Initial resuscitation should include administration of adequate crystalloid, dextrose and thiamine. Potassium and magnesium supplementation should be given according to serum electrolyte results. Administration of dextrose is essential as it stimulates insulin release, inhibits glucagon release and so inhibits fatty acid oxidation. Thiamine will facilitate entry of pyruvate into the Krebs cycle. Administration of insulin or bicarbonate is not necessary.[8]

Fluid, electrolyte and acid–base status should be closely monitored and further therapy tailored to the clinical response. Careful evaluation and treatment of the coexisting medical disorders is essential.

DISPOSITION

The disposition of many ethanol-intoxicated patients presenting to the emergency department is determined by the associated medical, surgical, psychiatric or social issues. Ethanol intoxicated patients should only be discharged from the emergency department where their subsequent safety can be ensured. Discharge into the care of a competent relative or friend is sometimes appropriate. Other patients, particularly if aggressive or neurologically impaired, require admission to a safe environment until such time as the intoxication resolves and they can be reassessed. An observation ward attached to the emergency department may be the most appropriate place if available. More severely intoxicated patients requiring airway control and support of ventilation should be admitted to the intensive care unit.

Patients in ethanol withdrawal may require admission for management of the precipitating medical or surgical illness. For those patients who wish to complete withdrawal with a view to abstinence, the remainder of the withdrawal may be managed in a general medical ward, specialized medical or non-medical detoxification centre, or at home. Medical detoxification is mandatory where a severe withdrawal syndrome is anticipated. In any case, ongoing psychosocial support will be required and it is important for emergency departments to have a good knowledge of the locally available drug and alcohol services to ensure appropriate referral.

Patients with Wernicke's encephalopathy should be admitted for ongoing care and thiamine and magnesium supplementation. The ophthalmoplegia and nystagmus usually have a good response to thiamine within hours to days. Ataxia and mental changes improve more slowly if at all and have a poorer prognosis. Up to 50% of cases will show no response despite thiamine therapy.[9]

Patients with ethanol-induced ketoacidosis also require admission for ongoing dextrose and thiamine, monitoring of fluids and electrolytes and management of the precipitating medical condition. Mortality from ethanol-induced ketoacidosis *per se* is rare with early recognition and treatment, but death may occur as a result of the underlying medical condition, particularly if unrecognized.

Ideally, any patient with an ethanol-related presentation should offered referral to drug and alcohol rehabilitation services for counselling.

CONTROVERSIES AND FUTURE DIRECTIONS

❶ It has been suggested that emergency departments could play a pivotal role in reducing ethanol-related morbidity by adopting procedures to detect and refer individuals who misuse ethanol. A number of centres have successfully trialled screening and brief intervention strategies for hazardous ethanol consumption.[11]

REFERENCES

1. Commonwealth of Australia 2001 Alcohol in Australia: Issues and Strategies 2001, A background paper to the National Alcohol Strategy: A plan for Action 2001 to 2004.
2. Abdulla A, Badawy B 1978 The metabolism of alcohol. Clinical and Endocrinological Metabolism 7: 247–52
3. Brennan DF, Bertzelos S, Reed R, Falk JL 1995 Ethanol elimination rates in an ED population. American Journal of Emergency Medicine 13: 276–80
4. Adinoff B, Bone GH, Linnoila M 1988 Acute ethanol poisoning and the ethanol withdrawal syndrome. Medical Toxicology 3: 172–96
5. Turner RC, Lichstein PR, Peden JG, Busher JT, Waivers LE 1989 Alcohol withdrawal syndromes: a review of pathophysiology, clinical presentation and treatment. Journal of General Internal Medicine 4: 432–44
6. Berk WA, Todd K 1993 Relationship of abstinence to the presentation and peak intensity of signs and alcohol withdrawal. Annals of Emergency Medicine 22: 339–45
7. Reuler JB, Girard DE, Cooney TG 1985 Current concepts. Wernicke's encephalopathy. New England Journal of Medicine. 312: 1035–9
8. Fulop M 1993 Alcoholic ketoacidosis. Endocrinological and Metabolic Clinics of North America 22: 209–19
9. Zuburan C, Fernandes JG, Rodnight R 1997 Wernicke-Korsakoff syndrome. Postgraduate Medical Journal 73: 27
10. Huntley JS, Blain C, Hood S, Touquet R 2001 Improving detection of alcohol misuse in patients presenting to an accident and emergency department. Emergency Medicine Journal 18: 99–104
11. Hungerford DW, Pollock DA, Todd KT 2000 Acceptability of emergency department-based screening and brief intervention for alcohol problems. Academic Emergency Medicine 7: 1383–92

28.20 SNAKEBITE

GEORGE JELINEK • PETER SPRIVULIS

ESSENTIALS

1 Australia has some of the most venomous snakes in the world. All are elapids (front-fanged). New Zealand has no snakes of medical importance.

2 Fatalities from snakebite are either immediate or delayed. Immediate deaths are usually a result of brown snake envenomation, presumably due to myocardial depression. Delayed deaths are mostly a consequence of the consumption coagulopathy caused by the procoagulant action of either brown or tiger snakes, or the taipan.

3 Pressure-immobilization first aid appears highly effective in retarding the spread of venom via the lymphatics. No fatality has been reported when first aid has been applied promptly and correctly.

4 All clinically important effects of snakebite can be treated by the prompt administration of appropriate antivenom. The indication for antivenom is clinical or laboratory evidence of envenomation.

5 Commonwealth Serum Laboratories make antivenoms to the five main genera of snakes in Australia: brown snake, black snake, tiger snake, taipan and death adder, as well as a polyvalent antivenom containing antivenoms to all five. The correct antivenom is polyvalent (except in certain geographical areas where there are only one or two genera of snakes) unless the snake is positively identified, usually by a venom detection kit test of a urine or bite-site swab or fang swab. Incorrect visual identification is a factor in a number of reported preventable deaths.

6 Antivenom is currently derived from horse serum, although in some parts of the world much less antigenic sheep serum antivenoms are available. It should be given intravenously. The correct dose is enough to neutralize the venom. Multiple doses may be needed, especially for bites by the brown and tiger snakes.

7 Concerns about an adverse reaction to antivenom should not delay administration in the clearly envenomed patient. Adrenaline (epinephrine) may be given subcutaneously as premedication. A short course of oral steroids may reduce the incidence of serum sickness, particularly for children and patients receiving polyvalent antivenom or multiple doses of monovalent antivenom.

8 Patients with a severe coagulopathy (fibrinogen <0.5 mg/L) following brown snake envenoming require large doses of antivenom (five times the manufacturer's recommended initial dose or more).

INTRODUCTION

Australia has the most venomous snakes in the world, in terms of the potency of their venoms.[1] All those that are dangerous to humans are elapids, which have permanently erect front fangs, one on each side at the front of fixed maxillary bones. The two fangs are typically 0.9–1.6 cm apart.[2] Non-venomous Australian snakes in contrast can leave a diagnostic semi-circular row of fang marks. Viperid snakes (vipers), such as the North American rattlesnake and the African puff adder, are also front fanged but the longer fangs can fold up against a relatively mobile maxilla. These snakes are not found in Australia, but are common in other parts of the world. Colubrid snakes, such as the African boomslang, have fangs at the back of the mouth. Some colubrids are found in Australia but none is harmful to humans.

Interestingly, all the dangerous Australian snakes can swim and climb trees. Contrary to popular mythology, snakes are relatively slow-moving and in most instances can be outrun by humans. New Zealand has no snakes of medical importance.[2]

Despite the potential lethality of Australian snakes, fatalities are uncommon. Prior to antivenom introduction in the 1930s, there were 11–12 deaths a year, falling to about half that after the introduction of antivenom. It has been estimated that around 3000 Australians are bitten by snakes every year, yet over the last 20 years or so there have been only two deaths per year,[3] the further fall probably a consequence of the introduction of effective pressure-immobilization first aid. Most of the deaths now occurring have in common inadequate first aid and delays in receiving the correct antivenom.[2,3] There has been a recent worrying increase in fatalities to about four per year,[4] although it remains to be seen whether this will be sustained.

TOXINOLOGY[5]

The top 10 venomous snakes in the world are all Australian; of the top 25, only four are not Australian. Venom is injected from venom glands, which are modified parotid glands. Less venom is injected in a quick strike than when the snake holds on and chews, or strikes many times. Australian snake venoms are almost completely absorbed from the site of injection, in contrast to North American viperids, where as much as 80% of the venom may remain in the affected limb.[2]

Their distribution and mode of excretion is as yet undetermined, however, Australian snake venoms are concentrated in urine.

Many Australian snake venoms (brown, tiger and taipan) possess potent prothrombin activators that catalyse the activation of prothrombin to thrombin, resulting in clot formation *in vitro* from the conversion of fibrinogen to fibrin. *In vivo* this manifests as a consumption coagulopathy, leading to afibrinogenaemia and secondary activation of the fibrinolytic system. Some venoms are weakly anticoagulant (black, death adder). Thrombocytopenia sometimes occurs, particulary after envenoming by brown snakes, and haemolysis has also been seen, usually associated with black snake envenoming.

Tiger and taipan venoms possess powerful presynaptic neurotoxins, which may result clinically in a descending paralysis with early involvement of the cranial nerves. Paralysis once established becomes difficult to reverse with antivenom. Death adder venom has principally postsynaptic neurotoxins and paralysis is readily reversible with antivenom.

Several Australian snakes (tiger, black, taipan) cause rhabdomyolysis, which can be profound, and lead to renal failure.

In addition, a syndrome of sudden collapse and death may occur, the aetiology of which is uncertain. This may be due to widespread intravascular clot formation following prothrombin activation, contributed to by myocardial depression, which has been demonstrated in dogs envenomed by brown snakes.[6] Renal failure may also occur, possibly due to the consumptive coagulopathy, a direct effect of venom (brown snake) or secondary to rhabdomyolysis (tiger snake and taipan). Australian snakes have few local bite site effects, although tiger snakes and sometimes black snakes may cause local pain and sometimes bruising. Surprisingly, elapids elsewhere in the world, such as the African cobras, cause significant local tissue necrosis. These effects are also important in viper envenomation. The clinical effects of Australian snake venoms are summarized in Table 28.20.1.

Table 28.20.1 Clinical toxicity of snake venoms, in typical order of appearance

Genus	Minutes	Hours	Days
Death adder	Paralysis		
Brown	Sudden collapse frequent Consumption coagulopathy	Paralysis unusual Mild anaemia	Renal failure Thrombocytopenia
Black	Mild anticoagulant	Bite site swelling	
Tiger	Consumption coagulopathy Sudden collapse possible	Bite site pain/bruising Paralysis	Rhabdomyolysis Renal failure
Taipan	Consumption coagulopathy	Paralysis	Rhabdomyolysis Renal failure

Most snakebite deaths now occur early as the result of sudden collapse and are caused by the brown snake. There are a few late deaths from intracerebral haemorrhage due to coagulopathy (brown, tiger and taipan), or multi-system failure following early cardiac arrest. Death has also been recorded due to respiratory failure as a result of neurotoxicity. Other possible causes include acute renal failure, hyperkalaemia due to rhabdomyolysis, and anaphylaxis due to venom or antivenom therapy, although this is extremely uncommon.

FIRST AID

Australian snake venoms are absorbed by the lymphatic system. The absorption is enhanced by exercise. The aim of first aid is to reduce lymphatic flow from the bitten part. A pressure bandage (crepe bandage, strips of clothing) is applied over the whole limb, with a similar pressure to that used for a sprain. If the bandage is applied too tightly, wiggling of fingers or toes can increase lymph flow and render the first aid ineffective. Bandaging begins distally on the limb and progresses proximally over the bite site until the whole limb is bandaged. This is a modification of Sutherland's original technique where the bite site was bandaged first, and is designed to make it more comfortable for the patient by emptying distal vessels first. There appears to be no disadvantage in practice related to this theoretical expulsion of some venom from the limb into the central circulation.[2] The part must be immobilized or the first aid is ineffective.[7] Immobilization consists of splinting and complete prevention of movement or exercise of the bitten part. It has been shown that movement of all limbs, not just the affected one, needs to be minimized for first aid to be optimally effective.[8] This means that transport should be brought to the patient rather than vice versa, and walking must be avoided. Prompt, properly applied first aid probably prevents significant absorption of venom for many hours. There appears to be some venom inactivation in the bandaged limb.[2] Occasionally bites are not to the extremities and pressure immobilization is impractical. Infiltration around the bite site with diluted adrenaline (epinephrine) may retard spread of the venom in these cases.

The bite site should not be washed, as it may prevent venom being identified from the wound swab. At this time there are no reports of the death of any patient who received prompt, effective first aid immediately after a snakebite.

The aim of antivenom treatment is to bring venom into contact with antivenom. First aid must, therefore, eventually be removed. This should take place only in a resuscitation area of a facility with the means to definitively treat envenoming. The first aid is removed when:

- No evidence of envenoming has been identified after thorough clinical and laboratory assessment. In these patients further clinical and laboratory evaluation for suspected envenoming is needed following removal of the bandage.

- There is definite clinical or laboratory evidence of envenoming. The bandage is removed after commencement of treatment with intravenous antivenom. There is some debate about the exact timing of first-aid removal in this situation, but no evidence of any difference in outcome related to timing. In massive life-threatening envenoming it may be prudent to leave the first aid in place until a reasonable proportion of the dose of antivenom has been administered.

INITIAL EMERGENCY DEPARTMENT MANAGEMENT

The patient is managed in an area with full resuscitation facilities. Assessment and management proceed simultaneously. The airway, breathing and circulation are assessed and stabilized. Signs of paralysis, such as ptosis, may be subtle and should be carefully sought. Oxygen may be commenced, the electrocardiogram and oxygen saturation monitored and intravenous access obtained. Investigations should be ordered as listed below:

- Urinalysis for myoglobin
- Full blood count
- Coagulation profile, including fibrinogen, fibrinogen degradation products, prothrombin time, activated partial thromboplastin times
- Urea, creatinine and electrolytes
- Creatine kinase
- Blood grouping and cross-matching.

CLINICAL EVALUATION

The important question is whether envenoming has occurred. Most patients (as many as 90% in some regions of Australia) bitten by snakes do not become systemically envenomed. The diagnosis of envenomation is made on history, examination and the investigations listed above. The features conventionally held to indicate definite envenoming are: a history of vomiting, abdominal pain or neurotoxic symptoms, including paralysis (difficulty swallowing, diplopia) and convulsions; on examination – neurotoxic effects, including paralysis (ptosis, drooling, weakness), or prolonged clotting time clinically as suggested by abnormal bleeding (ooze from venepuncture sites, gums); and, on investigation – the presence of coagulopathy (including raised FDPs), rhabdomyolysis (elevated CK, myoglobinuria), or acute renal failure. Nausea, giddiness, headache, sweating or regional lymphadenopathy without any of the above features are not generally taken as sufficient evidence of envenoming to warrant antivenom administration.

Examination of the bite site and the presence or absence of puncture marks does not add to the evaluation[9] except that a semi-circular array of fang marks indicates a non-venomous snake. Asymptomatic patients, particularly those seen early after a brown snake bite, may still be severely envenomed.

MANAGEMENT

The patient without evidence of envenoming

Following thorough clinical and laboratory evaluation, if no evidence of envenoming is detected the first-aid bandage is removed. The patient requires continued close monitoring for the development of envenoming including repeated investigation (listed above) within one hour of bandage removal, and at 6 and 12 hours later.

The envenomed patient

The definitive treatment of envenoming is antivenom. The aim of treatment is to bring antivenom in contact with circulating venom. In the absence of a definitely positive venom detection kit (VDK) result, except in certain geographical parts of Australia, the choice is polyvalent antivenom. In Victoria and metropolitan Perth[9], tiger and brown snake antivenom should be given, and in Tasmania tiger snake only.

The VDK allows identification of the genus of snake responsible for envenoming and testing should be reserved for the patient with a high likelihood or definite evidence of envenoming. The test is conducted on a urine specimen and a saline swab taken from the wound. VDK results on blood specimens are unreliable and should be avoided. The bandage should not be removed to swab the wound: a window should be cut to obtain access. If the snake responsible for the envenoming accompanies the patient, a swab of the fangs may also be tested. The venom sample may require considerable dilution or it may be so concentrated that it overwhelms the VDK and all wells change colour. Visual identification can only be accepted from qualified herpetologists. Many 'experts' are no such thing.

Commonwealth Serum Laboratories still recommend a prophylactic dose of adrenaline (epinephrine) subcutaneously, 0.25 mg for an adult, 0.1 mg for a child. There is now evidence that adrenaline (epinephrine) is effective in reducing the incidence of allergic reactions to antivenom,[10] but many emergency physicians do not premedicate as the risk of allergic reaction is so low without premedication. With monovalent antivenom the risk is around 1%, and 5% for polyvalent.[11] Antihistamines such as promethazine are ineffective[12] and should be avoided. They may also cloud neurological assessment. Children and patients who have received polyvalent or multiple doses of monovalent antivenom should receive a short course of oral steroids (prednisolone 50 mg/day for 5 days) to minimize the likelihood of serum sickness. Skin testing of antivenoms does not predict the occurrence of allergic reactions and should be avoided.

The dose of antivenom for children is the same as for adults. If the snake has been identified by VDK the appropriate monovalent antivenom is given, diluted tenfold in saline over 30 minutes, unless the patient is desperately ill and needs it faster. In an arrest situation it may need to be given as a bolus, undiluted. The correct dose of antivenom is enough to completely neutralize the venom. All antivenom ampoules carry information regarding the recommended inital dose. Further doses may be required, titrated against clinical effect. This may be difficult in patients who are asymptomatic. There is good evidence that the CSL-recommended starting dose of antivenom for tiger snake (1 ampoule) and brown snake (2 ampoules) envenomation is too low.[13] In cases of severe coagulopathy due to brown snake envenomation (fibrinogen <0.5 g/L) 5000 units (5 ampoules) is recommended as the minimum initial dose, and many emergency physicians are using 10 000 units as a starting dose. A further dose of 5000 units may be needed if coagulation studies do not show rapid improvement to normal.

GUIDELINES FOR TREATMENT

- Apply pressure immobilization if not already carried out
- Establish IV access
- Commence cardiac monitoring
- Consider adrenaline (epinephrine) 0.25 mg IM
- Give appropriate antivenom IV diluted 1:10 with saline over 30 minutes
- Administer tetanus prophylaxis as appropriate
- Treat children and patients receiving polyvalent or multiple doses of monovalent antivenom with prednisolone 50 mg daily for 5 days to prevent serum sickness.

ADDITIONAL TREATMENT

The use of fresh frozen plasma (FFP) is controversial, although it is widely used. There is no evidence to settle this issue, however, many emergency physicians believe that adequate antivenom is all that is required to treat a consumption coagulopathy. Logically FFP should only be given once venom has been adequately neutralized with antivenom, or the consumption coagulopathy may be worsened.

DISPOSITION

Patients with suspected snakebite but no evidence of envenoming 1 hour after the removal of first aid may be admitted to an observation area. Envenomed patients requiring ventilatory support should have continued management in ICU, but patients with coagulopathy only are commonly managed in emergency-department observation wards.

CONCLUSION

The risk of death, even after apparently trivial contact with Australian snakes, is significant and must be appreciated. The treatment of snake envenoming includes early pressure and immobilization of the entire length of the affected limb. Multiple doses of antivenom may be required, especially to treat coagulopathy, and should be given early, intravenously and repeatedly, until the venom effects are completely reversed. Australian antivenoms are safe and effective and there should be no hesitation in using them very promptly in envenomed patients. All patients giving a history of possible snakebite should be admitted to hospital.

REFERENCES

1. Broad AJ, Sutherland SK, Coulter AR 1979 The lethality in mice of dangerous Australian and other snake venoms. Toxicon 17: 661–4
2. Sutherland SK, Tibballs J 2001 Australian Animal Toxins. The Creatures, Their Toxins and Care of the Poisoned Patient. Oxford University Press, Oxford
3. Sutherland SK 1992 Deaths from snakebite in Australia, 1981–1991. Medical Journal of Australia 157: 740–64
4. Sutherland SK, Leonard RL 1995 Snakebite deaths in Australia 1992–1994 and a management update. Medical Journal of Australia 163: 616–8
5. White J 1987 Elapid envenomation. In: Covacevich J, Davie P, Pearn J (eds) Toxic Plants and Animals: a Guide for Australia. University of Queensland Press, Brisbane, pp 391–429

CONTROVERSIES

❶ Opinion is divided over whether fresh frozen plasma hastens or retards resolution of the consumption coagulopathy after elapid envenomation. It is still widely used.

❷ It is unclear why the fatality rate from snakebite in Australia is beginning to rise again. Some would argue that snakes are becoming 'urbanized' and are coming into contact with humans more frequently.

❸ The initial dose of brown snake antivenom is controversial. While CSL have gradually increased the recommended dose over recent years, many emergency physicians and toxicologists treating such envenomings are commencing with 10 ampoules of antivenom.

6. Tibballs J, Sutherland SK, Rivera RA, Masci PP 1992 The cardiovascular and haematological effects of purified prothrombin activator from the common brown snake (Pseudonaja textilis) and their antagonism with heparin. Anaesthesia and Intensive Care 20: 28–32
7. Sutherland SK, Coulter AR, Harris RD 1979 Rationalisation of first-aid measures for elapid snakebite. Lancet 1(8109): 183–5
8. Howarth DM, Southee AE, Whyte IM 1994 Lymphatic flow rates and first-aid in simulated peripheral snake or spider envenomation. Medical Journal of Australia 161: 695–700
9. Jelinek GA, Hamilton T, Hirsch RL 1991 Admissions for suspected snake-bite to the Perth adult teaching hospitals, 1979–1988. Medical Journal of Australia 155: 761–4
10. Premawardhena AP, de Silva CE, Fonseka MM, Gunatilake SB, de Silva HJ 1999 Low dose subcutaneous adrenaline to prevent acute adverse reactions to antivenom serum in people bitten by snakes: randomised, placebo controlled trial. British Medical Journal 318: 1041–3
11. Sutherland SK 1992 Antivenom use in Australia: premedication, adverse reactions and the use of venom detection kits. Medical Journal of Australia 157: 734–9
12. Fan HW, Marcopito LF, Cardoso JL, et al 1999 Sequential randomised and double blind trial of promethazine prophylaxis against early anaphylactic reactions to antivenom for bothrops snake bites. British Medical Journal 318: 1451–2
13. Sprivulis PC, Jelinek GA, Marshall LJ 1996 Efficacy and potency of antivenoms in neutralising the procoagulant effects of Australian snake venoms in dog and human plasma. Anaesthetics and Intensive Care 24: 379–81

ESSENTIALS

1 Bites by the majority of Australian spiders cause only minor problems. Redback (a widow spider) bite can cause severe and persistent pain, and less often systemic effects, while funnel web spider bite can cause life-threatening neurotoxic envenoming.

2 Fatalities have been recorded in Australia after bites by the redback and the funnel web spiders.

3 Australia appears to have the highest rate of widow spider envenoming (latrodectism) in the world.

4 Redback antivenom is a horse derived F(ab')₂ antivenom and causes relatively few allergic reactions (0.5–0.8%). The antivenom is usually given intramuscularly but may be given intravenously.

5 Antivenom has been at least partially effective months after a bite by the redback spider.

6 Antivenom to the funnel web spider is rabbit serum based and so less antigenic. No premedication is necessary and it is given intravenously.

28.21 SPIDER BITE

GEORGE JELINEK • GEOFFREY ISBISTER

INTRODUCTION

Australasia is home to a variety of spiders as well as some species that have been introduced, probably including the redback spider.[1] The majority of spiders have small jaws which are too small to penetrate human skin. Larger spiders with toxic venom, and habits and distribution that promote human encounters, can cause medically significant envenoming. Although there are over 2000 characterized species of spiders in Australia, a much smaller group is responsible for the majority of human bites with 6 families of spiders being responsible for over 80% of bites.[2] Spiders commonly responsible for human bites include huntsman spiders (*Sparassidae*), orb weaving spiders (*Araneidae*), white-tail spiders (*Lampona* spp.), redback spiders and the closely related *Steatoda* spp. (*Theridiidae*), wolf spiders (*Lycosidae*) and jumping spiders (*Salticidae*).[2] Fatalities have occurred in Australia after bites by the redback and the funnel web spider.[3]

REDBACK SPIDER (*LATRODECTUS HASSELTI*)

Distribution and taxonomy

The redback spider is a member of the widow group of spiders (*Latrodectus* spp.). The widow spider group is the single most medically important group of spiders worldwide and belongs to the family of comb-footed spiders (*Theridiidae*). Widow spiders are distributed throughout the world and thrive in urban environments, ensuring that they frequently come into contact with humans.[4] The taxonomy is not settled, and until recently only six species were recognized, but there are probably around 40 species,[5] including the North American black widow (*L. mactans*), the Australian redback (*L. hasselti*), the New Zealand katipo (*L. katipo*) and the brown widow (*L. geometricus*), which is found on most continents including Australia.[6] All species produce venom with similar properties and cause a similar clinical syndrome (latrodectism). Australia probably has the highest rate of latrodectism in the world, with at least 2000 definite bites per annum.[7] New Zealand reports few cases of envenoming by its widow spider, the katipo. The Australian redback spider is probably an introduced species, with the first reports of sightings from around the ports of Rockhampton and Bowen in 1870.[1] There is at least one other important genus of spiders in this family, *Steatoda* spp., that is responsible for human envenoming. There are both native and introduced *Steatoda* spp. in Australia. They are black spiders with the same body shape and size as widow spiders, but without the red markings.

Venom

The components toxic to humans in the venom of widow spiders are α-latrotoxins. These are closely related proteins of MW 130 000 daltons, toxic to vertebrates, which cause massive release of neurotransmitters and deplete synaptic vesicles at nerve endings. α-Latrotoxin was first isolated from the venom of *L. tredecimguttatus*, the European widow spider, but recent work suggests that all widow spiders have a similar toxin based on *in vitro* effects.[8] The massive release of neurotransmitters appears to cause autonomic effects with acetylcholine and catecholamine release from autonomic nerve terminals, and can also cause depletion of acetylcholine at the neuromuscular junction, resulting in patchy paralysis.

Epidemiology

In Australia more males than females are bitten (60:40), more patients are bitten in the warmer months of January, February and March (45–60%), and most are bitten on the extremities (74–85%).[7] Although early data showed a high proportion of bites to the genitalia (up to 80%),[9] recent series suggest this has all but disappeared (1%), along with outdoor lavatories.[7] Western

Australia reports the most cases annually (25%), followed by New South Wales and Queensland.[10] Most bites occur when the spider is disturbed in human-made objects, such as clothes, shoes, gloves, furniture, building materials and sheds.

There have been at least 14 deaths in Australia attributed to redback spider bite, 13 being before the introduction of antivenom in 1956[11] and one in 1999 due to gastric perforation after prolonged vomiting.[3] Reported mortality rates of more than 6% in the USA[12] and 5–10% in the Middle East[13] are likely to be over-estimates due to reporting bias. Prior to antivenom introduction in Australia the reported death rate was 6%,[9] but this too was almost certainly an overestimate.

Clinical syndrome

There are only reports of female redback spider envenomings, as the fangs of the much smaller male are far less able penetrate human skin.[3] Probably around one-third of patients bitten develop systemic features and two-thirds have significant pain lasting longer than 24 hours.[2] The initial bite may be painless, or may feel like a pinprick or a burning sensation. Usually within 1 hour the victim develops local pain which gradually worsens. There is often local sweating and less commonly piloerection. These signs are virtually pathognomonic of redback spider bite. They occur much less commonly with other species, especially *L. geometricus*.[6,14] There may be no signs at the bite site. The pain can then spread to regional lymph nodes and in a minority of cases may subsequently appear in remote sites, or become generalized. Sweating may follow a similar pattern, and lower limb sweating or sweating on one limb is characteristic. Muscle cramps, spasms and patchy paralysis have been noted in some series,[11] but not others,[7,15] so are likely to be rare.

General associated features include malaise, lethargy, nausea and vomiting, headache, fever, hypertension and tremor. A wide array of clinical manifestations have been reported. Although children are often said to be at risk of more severe morbidity from latrodectism, this is not substantiated in the literature

and indeed, in the one large study reported, children received less antivenom on average than adults.[15]

Untreated, patients may develop only minimal local signs and symptoms which resolve over hours to days. Most, however, experience pain persisting longer than 24 hours.[2] Some develop marked local features over a period of hours, but do not progress to generalized latrodectism. The severe local pain that occurs with the bite often necessitates the use of antivenom, although some settle with symptomatic treatment. About one in three patients progress to systemic envenoming.[7,15] This usually occurs within 12 hours or so, but can sometimes be delayed for days. Debilitating symptoms may continue for months if untreated,[16] although the vast majority of patients get better within a week.

Of the 14 deaths reported from Australia, details are available for only seven patients. Of the 13 deaths prior to antivenom introduction, the time to death was from 1 to 30 days, with a mean of 9 days, except for a 3-month-old infant who died within 6 hours.[9] The 1999 death occurred at 7 days.[3] It is difficult to be certain what the precise cause of death was in most of these reports: some died from complications of latrodectism such as hypertension, or from cardiac and renal effects. This information is from cases reported sometimes more than 50 years ago with very few details, and may not be particularly useful to emergency physicians. Death is not really an important consideration in redback bites. Of greater concern are systemic envenoming and severe and persistent pain.

Diagnosis

The diagnosis is clinical and based on history, typically one of persistent increasing pain that can radiate, and may be associated with local sweating. The findings of localized sweating and piloerection are almost pathognomonic. There are no tests to confirm latrodectism. As the bite may not be felt or may be painless, doctors should suspect the condition in circumstances where patients have been working in sheds,

potting plants, or where contact with widow spiders is possible. In these situations, if the clinical syndrome is suggestive, a trial of antivenom is commonly used to confirm the diagnosis.

Treatment

First aid

Ice has been recommended, although it remains unproven.[3] Pressure-immobilization bandaging is not appropriate.

Supportive treatment

The pain may be so intense that standard narcotic analgesics are often unhelpful and tend to produce more sedation that actual analgesia.[17] The most effective pain relief is a sufficient dose of redback spider antivenom.

Antivenom therapy

The definitive treatment of latrodectism is neutralization of venom with specific antivenom. Although the Commonwealth Serum Laboratory recommends that all patients except those with trivial symptoms receive the antivenom, most would suggest that only those with systemic envenoming or severe uncontrolled local symptoms be treated. However, this may represent more than two-thirds of all patients.[2]

Antivenom is conventionally given by the intramuscular (IM) route unless the patient is *in extremis*, when it is more quickly effective intravenously (IV). The IV route appears to carry a greater risk of precipitating allergic phenomena, but probably only if given undiluted as an intravenous bolus.[18] Anecdotal experience suggests that the IM route is not as effective as IV antivenom, and in one small series cases unresponsive to IM antivenom were subsequently treated rapidly and effectively with IV antivenom.[19] This is consistent with work on snake and scorpion antivenoms that demonstrate IM administration leads to delayed and only partial neutralization of venom.[20] A number of Australian multicentre studies are in progress to determine whether the most appropriate routine route is IM or IV. IM antivenom is said to be rapidly effective, usually within 1 hour, with a very low rate of allergic reactions, but this may be because IM antivenom gets into the intravascular space so slowly that it is unlikely to cause allergic reactions. Of the 0.5% of patients developing anaphylaxis in Sutherland's large series,[18] about half received the antivenom undiluted IV.

The use of premedication remains controversial. While adrenaline (epinephrine) has been shown to be effective in reducing the rate of allergic reactions to snake antivenom from 43% to 11% in Sri Lanka,[21] in latrodectism it probably should be reserved for those with allergic diatheses and who have previously received horse serum, given the very low rate of reactions.[18] Antihistamines have been shown to be ineffective in reducing the rate of allergic reactions from snake antivenom[22] and should be avoided.

Adequate antivenom should be given to neutralize the venom as judged by reversal of the clinical features of envenoming. If the patient is still significantly symptomatic 2 hours after antivenom, a further ampoule should be given. The use of multiple doses of antivenom is increasing in Australia.[10] However, this may be because latrodectism has been historically undertreated in Australia,[2] or that so little of an IM dose is absorbed.[20] In one series, 34% of patients received more than one ampoule.[7] As for all antivenoms, the dose for children is the same as for adults. Antivenom appears to be effective even when given up to months after the bite.[16]

STEATODA SPECIES (CUPBOARD OR BUTTON SPIDERS)

There have been a number of reports of bites by *Steatoda* spp., mainly in Australia over the last 20 years.[2,23] They appear to cause a similar syndrome to latrodectism with persistent local pain but fewer systemic features. *In vitro* studies of the venom of these spiders demonstrates they cause similar but far less potent effects compared to α-latrotoxin. These studies also demonstrate *in vitro* neutralization of *Steatoda* venom with redback antivenom.[23] The majority

of bites by this group of spiders cause only minor effects, although the patient may have annoying pain for a period of hours.[2] Uncommonly, they can cause more severe and persistent pain, similar to widow spiders. In the latter case it has been postulated that redback antivenom may be an appropriate treatment. This has been used in two cases by the IM route with equivocal results.[23]

FUNNEL WEB SPIDER (*ATRAX* AND *HADRONYCHE* SPECIES)

Distribution and taxonomy

At least 39 species of funnel web spiders occur on the east coast of Australia, including the Sydney funnel web (*Atrax robustus*), other *Atrax* species and numerous *Hadronyche* species. The Sydney funnel web has been responsible for most bites and fatalities, but bites by other species may cause significant illness and appear to be increasing.[24] This increase in bites by other species may be due to increasing population density in their area of distribution. Funnel web spiders are burrowing spiders and most encounters with humans occur when males are looking for mates. The male spiders can be aggressive if disturbed and probably cause 30–40 cases of envenoming annually in Australia.[25] Another group of spiders, the mouse spiders (*Missulena* spp.), has been reported to cause similar effects to funnel web spiders.[26] These spiders belong to the family *Actinopodidae*, and occur in most parts of Australia.

Venom

The males have a more potent venom than the females and only males have been reported to cause significant illness in humans.[3,25] In the case of the Sydney funnel web, the important toxin in human envenoming appears to be δ-atracotoxin-Ar1 (previously robustoxin), a low-molecular-weight neurotoxin that prevents inactivation of sodium channels. In other species the venoms appear to be similar in their *in-vitro* effects, and

reported bites by other species are consistent with this.[24,27] The main effect of the neurotoxin is an autonomic storm that can be predominantly sympathetic or parasympathetic, or mixed in effect, associated with initial excitation at neuromuscular junctions, followed by paralysis.[3,24,25]

Epidemiology

Most bites occur during summer to autumn. Although *Atrax robustus* is restricted to an area in a radius of around 160 km from the centre of Sydney, *Hadronyche* species can be found in Tasmania, South Australia, Victoria, New South Wales and Queensland.[3,24,25] However, significant envenoming from funnel web spiders has only been reported in NSW and southern Queensland.[24] Most bites, perhaps as many as 90%, do not cause severe systemic envenoming.[24,25]

Clinical syndrome

The bite is usually painful due to the size of the fangs and the acidity of the venom. Fang marks are usually present but other local signs are uncommon. Unlike with redback spiders, severe envenoming develops rapidly and usually occurs within 1 hour. Local fasciculations progress to generalized fasciculations. Fasciculation of the tongue is a classic finding. Perioral and distal paraesthesia may develop. Generalized autonomic features are typical of systemic envenoming with salivation, lacrimation and generalized sweating. This is often associated with nausea, vomiting and abdominal pain. Other autonomic features can include miosis, mydriasis, tachycardia or bradycardia and hypertension. Initially, the patient is usually agitated and anxious. Decreased level of consciousness and coma are late signs.[3,24,25]

Non-cardiogenic pulmonary oedema may develop and is thought to result from venom induced capillary leakage. Prior to antivenom treatment this occurred early, but is now more commonly reported as a delayed effect.

Diagnosis

As with redback spider bite the diagnosis is clinical.

Treatment

First aid

Pressure-immobilization first aid has been shown to be successful in retarding spread of the venom in an animal model.[3] If not applied at the scene, it should be applied in hospital on arrival.

Supportive treatment

With the introduction of antivenom therapy the requirement for intensive care therapy is far less than in the past. Attention to basic resuscitation is essential, but usually does not require more than IV fluid therapy after assessment and stabilization of the airway and ventilation. Atropine can be used to treat cholinergic features, but this is not a substitute for antivenom. The use of inotropes and other pharmacological agents is unnecessary except in the rare instance of delayed presentation with severe envenoming not responding to antivenom. If pulmonary oedema occurs this can be treated with diuretics and continuous positive airways pressure ventilation in association with antivenom therapy.[3,24,25]

Antivenom therapy

Definitive treatment is venom neutralization with specific funnel web spider antivenom. The antivenom is derived from rabbit serum and appears to be less antigenic to humans than horse serum antivenoms. Accordingly, premedication with adrenaline (epinephrine) is not recommended. Antivenom is indicated for systemic envenoming as defined above.[3,24,25] Initially, two ampoules should be given (four if severe), and repeated every 15 minutes if there is no improvement. Early immediate allergic reactions have not been reported. Delayed serum sickness reactions have been reported in at least one case.[28]

MOUSE SPIDERS (*MISSULENA SPP.*)

There are at least 11 species of mouse spiders that occur in various parts of Australia. Most bites are by wandering male spiders. The bite usually causes significant pain and fang marks, due to the size of the fangs.[6] There is one report of a bite by the eastern mouse spider (*Missulena bradleyi*) that caused a syndrome similar to funnel web envenoming in a 19-month-old child.[26] In this case the child was given both redback antivenom and funnel web spider antivenom and the symptoms resolved over a period of hours. Recent work on the venom of the eastern mouse spider has demonstrated that the venom causes similar effects *in vitro* to funnel web spider venom, and it is neutralized *in vitro* by funnel web antivenom.[29] However, the clinical significance of this remains unclear. There have only been between 10 and 20 reports of bites by mouse spiders,[6] and in none of these cases was there severe envenoming.

OTHER AUSTRALASIAN SPIDERS

There are a number of other Australian spiders that can and do cause human bites. In the majority of cases they cause only minor effects and symptomatic treatment is all that is required. In a large study of definite spider bites there were no cases of necrotic lesions or allergic reactions, suggesting these effects are either rare or do not occur.[2] The incidence of secondary infection is also low, and occurred in less than 1% of cases in the same study.[2]

NECROTIC ARACHNIDISM

Necrotic arachnidism is generally defined as necrotic lesions or ulcers that occur following a spider bite and are a result of venom effects. Significant skin necrosis following bites from recluse spiders (*Loxosceles* species) is well reported in many parts of the world. *Loxosceles rufescens* has been introduced to South Australia[30] and been responsible for a few bites, but there is no evidence that it has spread beyond this distribution.

The white-tailed spider (*Lampona cylindrata/murina* group) has been implicated in the development of necrotic arachnidism.[3] However, recent work suggests that this is not the case with over 120 definite bites by this spiders from this family causing no cases of necrotic lesions.[2] Other spiders have been implicated in this condition, including wolf spiders, sac spiders and the black house spiders. There is similarly little evidence to support this and prospective cases of definite bites by these groups of spiders have not demonstrated necrotic lesions.[2]

AN APPROACH TO THE PATIENT WITH SPIDER BITE

The first step is to take a careful history so as to determine whether the case is a definite spider bite or only a suspected spider bite. The diagnosis of definite spider bite requires sighting of the spider at the time of the bite and usually some initial symptoms such as local pain. If there is no history of bite or no spider was seen, then other diagnoses must be excluded. This is particularly important in persons presenting with ulcers or skin lesions with suspected spider bites. It is important in these cases that appropriate investigations are done and the case treated as a necrotic ulcer of unknown aetiology. In the majority of these cases an infective cause is found, although less commonly they are a result of pyoderma gangrenosum or a vasculitis.[31]

If the patient has a definite history of a spider bite and has either captured the spider or has a good description of the spider, a simple approach can be taken. Health professionals should not attempt to identify spiders beyond the following simple classification:

- Redback spider
- Moderate to large black spider that is potentially a funnel web spider in eastern Australia where funnel web spiders are known to occur
- All other spiders.

The majority of redback spiders are likely to be identified correctly and with supporting clinical features this diagnosis is usually fairly easy. The second group is only important in regions where funnel web spiders are known to occur and cause significant effects (east coast of Australia from southern Queensland to southern NSW). If the spider is large and black then the patient should be managed as a funnel web. Pressure-immobilization is the appropriate first aid measure. Once in the emergency department they should be observed for at least 2 hours, although 4 hours is recommended. If patients are asymptomatic at this time, they can be safely discharged. No attempt should be made to identify the spider because the distinction between some funnel web spiders and the less significant trapdoor spiders is impossible for non-experts.

The third group includes all other spiders. Despite previous concerns about particular spiders, such as the badged huntsman (*Neosparassus* spp.) and white-tail spiders,[3] all other spiders are very unlikely to cause more than minor effects.[2] Patients can be reassured, their tetanus status confirmed and updated, if required, and symptomatic treatment with ice and analgesia can be offered. These patients do not need to be observed in hospital.

CONCLUSION

Australasia has a number of venomous spiders. Redback spider bite is the most common and medically significant spider causing human envenoming in Australia. Funnel web spider bite can cause life-threatening neurotoxicity, but is restricted to eastern Australia and is uncommon. Antivenom is available for the redback and funnel web spiders, and emergency physicians can feel confident of the safety and efficacy of these products. All other spiders rarely cause more than minor effects and do not require medical treatment.

REFERENCES

1. Raven R 1987 The redback spider. In: Covacevich J, Davie P, Pearn J (eds) Toxic Plants and Animals. Queensland Museum Press, Queensland, pp 307–11

CONTROVERSIES AND FUTURE DIRECTIONS

❶ There is still some debate over whether adrenaline (epinephrine) premedication should be used before giving redback spider antivenom. With an incidence of allergic reactions of between 0.5 and 0.8%, there is probably no reason to give adrenaline (epinephrine) before intramuscular antivenom, except when there is a history of exposure to horse serum or marked atopy.

❷ The optimal route of administration of redback spider antivenom is being increasingly debated. Almost no other antivenom is given IM and there are theoretical reasons why this route should be relatively ineffective. Many emergency physicians are routinely giving the antivenom IV, although there is still no clinical study to support this practice. Trials underway in Australasia should answer this question. The IM route may explain the impression that insufficient doses of antivenom are currently being used.

❸ Enough antivenom should be given to eradicate all symptoms in patients with redback spider envenoming. Patients with residual symptoms are at risk of prolonged morbidity. Late antivenom has been used successfully in this situation.

2. Isbister G K, Gray MR 2002 A prospective study of 750 definite spider bites with expert spider identification. Quarterly Journal of Medicine 95: 723–31
3. Sutherland SK, Tibballs J 2001 Australian Animal Toxins. Oxford University Press, Melbourne
4. Jelinek GA 1997 Widow spider envenomation (latrodectism): a worldwide problem. Wilderness Environmental Medicine 8: 226–31
5. Platnick N 1990 Advances in Spider Taxonomy, 1981–1987. A Supplement to Brignoli's 'A Catalogue of the Araneae Described Between 1940–1981'. Manchester University Press, Manchester
6. Isbister GK, Churchill TB, Hirst DB, Gray MR, Currie BJ 2001 Clinical effects in bites from formally identified spiders in tropical. Northern Territory Medical Journal of Australia 174: 79–82
7. Jelinek GA, Banham NG, Dunjey SJ 1989 Red-back spider-bites at Fremantle Hospital, 1982–1987. Medical Journal of Australia 150: 693–5
8. Graudins A, Padula M, Broady K, Nicholson GM 2001 Red-back spider (*Latrodectus hasselti*) antivenom prevents the toxicity of widow spider venoms. Annals of Emergency Medicine 37: 154–60
9. Ingram WW, Musgrave A 1933 Spider bite (arachnidism): a survey of its occurrence in Australia, with case histories. Medical Journal of Australia 2: 10–5
10. Sutherland SK 1992 Antivenom use in Australia. Premedication, adverse reactions and the use of venom detection kits. Medical Journal of Australia 157: 734–9
11. Wiener S 1961 Redback spider bite in Australia: an analysis of 167 cases. Medical Journal of Australia II: 44–9
12. Bogen E 1932 Poisonous spider bites. Annals of International Medicine 6: 375–88
13. Press J, Gedalia A 1989 [Spider bite in a child]. Harefuah 116: 466–8
14. Muller GJ 1993 Black and brown widow spider bites in South Africa. A series of 45 cases. South African Medical Journal 83: 399–405
15. Mead HJ, Jelinek GA 1993 Red-back spider bites to Perth children, 1979–1988. Journal of Paediatrics & Child Health 29: 305–8
16. Banham ND, Jelinek GA, Finch PM 1994 Late treatment with antivenom in prolonged red-back spider envenomation. Medical Journal of Australia 161: 379–81
17. Clark RF, Wethern-Kestner S, Vance MV, Gerkin R 1992 Clinical presentation and treatment of black widow spider envenomation: a review of 163 cases. Annals of Emergency Medicine 21: 782–7
18. Sutherland SK, Trinca JC 1978 Survey of 2144 cases of red-back spider bites: Australia and New Zealand, 1963—1976. Medical Journal of Australia 2: 620–3
19. Isbister GK 2002 Failure of intramuscular antivenom in redback spider envenomation. Emergency Medicine 14(4): 436–9
20. Riviere G, Choumet V, Audebert F, et al 1997 Effect of antivenom on venom pharmacokinetics in experimentally envenomed rabbits: toward an optimization of antivenom therapy. Journal of Pharmacology and Experimental Therapeutics 281: 1–8
21. Premawardhena AP, de Silva CE, Fonseka MMD, Gunatilake SB, de Silva HJ 1999 Low dose subcutaneous adrenaline to prevent acute adverse reactions to antivenom serum in people bitten by snakes: randomised, placebo controlled trial. British Medical Journal 318: 1041–3
22. Fan HW, et al 1999 Sequential randomised and double blind trial of promethazine prophylaxis against early anaphylactic reactions to antivenom for bothrops snake bites. British Medical Journal 318: 1451–2
23. Graudins A, Gunja N, Broady KW, Nicholson GM 2002 Clinical and in vitro evidence for the efficacy of Australian red-back spider (*Latrodectus hasselti*) antivenom in the treatment of envenomation by a Cupboard spider (*Steatoda grossa*). Toxicon 40: 767–75
24. Miller MK, Whyte IM, White J, Keir PM 2000 Clinical features and management of Hadronyche envenomation in man. Toxicon 38: 409–27
25. White J, Cardoso JL, Hui WF 1995 Clinical toxicology of spider bites. In: Meier J, White J (eds.) Handbook of Clinical Toxicology of Animal Venoms and Poisons. CRC Press, Boca Raton, pp 259–330
26. Rendle Short H 1985 Mouse spider envenomation (Abstract). Proceedings of Australian and New Zealand Intensive Care Society Scientific Meeting, 25. Australian and New Zealand Intensive Care Society
27. Graudins A, Wilson D, Alewood P, Broady K, Nicholson G 2002 Cross-reactivity of Sydney funnel-web spider antivenom: neutralization of the in vitro toxicity of other Australian funnel-web (Atrax and Hadronyche) spider venoms. Toxicon 40: 259–66

28. Miller MK, Whyte IM, Dawson AH 1999 Serum sickness from funnelweb spider antivenom. Medical Journal of Australia 171: 54
29. Rash LD, Birinyi-Strachan LC, Nicholson GM, Hodgson WC 2000 Neurotoxic activity of venom from the Australian Eastern mouse spider (Missulena bradleyi) involves modulation of sodium channel gating. British Journal of Pharmacology 130: 1817–24
30. Southcott RV 1976 Spiders of the genus Loxosceles in Australia. Medical Journal of Australia 1: 406–8
31. Isbister GK 2001 Spider mythology across the world. Western Journal of Medicine 175: 86–87

28.22 MARINE ENVENOMING AND POISONING

NEIL BANHAM • MARK LITTLE

ESSENTIALS

1 The management of jellyfish stings includes the provision of basic life support, application of vinegar to the sting site, and transporting the patient to a hospital. Supportive and symptomatic care is adequate for most patients. Box jellyfish antivenom is available, but is rarely required.

2 The management of sea-snake envenoming is the same as for that by terrestrial snakes. If sea-snake antivenom is unavailable, then tiger-snake antivenom can be used.

3 Blue ringed octopus and cone-shell envenomation can present with a rapid onset of flaccid paralysis. Pressure-immobilization bandaging and supportive care are indicated.

4 The management of a fish spine injury includes immersion of the limb in hot water, regional analgesia and wound care. Antivenom is available for stonefish envenomation.

INTRODUCTION

Australia's coastline has numerous creatures with the potential to envenom those who venture into their habitat. Although many of these envenomations may cause only discomfort, some have the potential to cause death.

JELLYFISH ENVENOMING

Many jellyfish may cause painful stings, however, only the box jellyfish (*Chironex fleckeri*) and the species of jellyfish responsible for Irukandji syndrome have been documented to cause deaths. Approximately 70 deaths have been attributed to *Chironex* in Australian waters, and children are particularly prone to a fatal outcome.[1] The last ten *Chironex fleckeri* deaths in the Northern Territory have been children. *Chiropsalmus quadrigatus* is closely related to the box jellyfish, and although no deaths have been recorded, serious envenomation may occur and recommended management is as for *Chironex*.

In the summer of 2001/2002 two deaths were attributed to the Irukandji syndrome in north Queensland.

First aid for all Australian jellyfish stings consists of locally applied vinegar, as this will inactivate undischarged nematocysts; however, it will not inactivate venom from discharged nematocysts and hence will be ineffective in providing analgesia.[1–3] Vinegar should be applied liberally for at least 30 seconds. The role of pressure immobilization bandaging is controversial. There is no uniform recommendation and a recent review found no good scientific evidence to support the use of pressure immobilization bandaging in the management of jellyfish stings in Australia.[4] Animal work has demonstrated that naturally discharged *Chironex fleckeri* nematocysts treated with vinegar still have venom within them when pressure is applied to the nematocysts.

Box jellyfish envenomation

The box jellyfish, also known as the sea wasp (*Chironex fleckeri*), is found in the tropical, particularly shallow coastal and estuarine, waters of northern Australia, predominantly between November and April. In this environment the jellyfish may be extremely difficult to see and the sudden severe pain of a sting may be the first indication of its presence. Often tentacles will still be adherent to the victim's skin on removal from the water. These tentacles have a typical banded, ladder appearance and leave similar marks on the skin. Shock and loss of consciousness from cardiorespiratory depression may occur and victims, especially children, have died within minutes of being stung. However, in a prospective study of jellyfish stings presentating to the Royal Darwin Hospital over a 12-month period, of 23 patients with nematocyst proven *Chironex fleckeri* sting, only one required parenteral analgesia and none received antivenom.[5]

The injected venom has numerous effects, including, cardiotoxicity and dermatonecrosis. *Chironex* stings can be prevented by avoiding swimming in their known habitat during the dangerous months of the year, usually November to April but varying depending on the region, swimming within netted areas on beaches (mainly in Queensland), the wearing of lycra protective suits or pantyhose when swimming, and entering the water slowly as the jellyfish may take evasive action to avoid a swimmer.

Management of box jellyfish envenoming

- Remove the victim from the water
- Commence CPR if indicated and continue until adequate antivenom administered
- Apply vinegar to the affected areas for at least 30 seconds
- Scrape off adherent tentacles
- Box jellyfish antivenom if indicated by:
  - severe pain not relieved by parenteral opiates
  - any cardiorespiratory compromise, including arrythmias.
  Premedication is not recommended because allergic reactions are uncommon. It is preferably given diluted 1 in 10 in normal saline by slow intravenous injection, but may also be given by paramedics or surf lifesavers by intramuscular injection (3 ampoules). **In cardiac arrest the use of up to 6 ampoules given consecutively undiluted has been advocated.**[2]
- General and supportive management, usually in intensive care
- Treat sting as a burn. Watch for and treat any secondary infection
- A delayed hypersensitivity rash may develop 1–2 weeks after the sting and responds to corticosteroid cream.

Irukandji syndrome

The Irukandji jellyfish(*Carukia barnesi*) consists of a bell measuring only 2 cm across, but with tentacles up to 75 cm long. It is found in waters north of Geraldton, Western Australia, and Mackay, Queensland. This jellyfish is almost invisible in the water. It was first captured in 1961 in Cairns by Dr Jack Barnes, who proved this jellyfish was responsible for the Irukandji syndrome by reproducing the symptoms by stinging himself, his 9-year-old son and the local lifeguard.[6] All three were taken to hospital for treatment! Evidence is emerging that more than one jellyfish species may be responsible for this syndrome.

Patients with Irukandji syndrome often have minimal symptoms at the time of the sting. After a latent period of approximately half an hour the 'Irukandji syndrome' may develop, with clinical features that include vomiting, abdominal, chest and back pain, sweats, blood pressure lability, and tachycardia.[7] Occasionally these cases go on to develop pulmonary oedema. Pulmonary oedema usually occurs within 10 hours of a sting but can occur within 3 hours. All patients developing cardiac dysfunction have ongoing pain. There have now been two deaths from Irukandji syndrome, although these were as a result of cerebral haemorrhage rather than pulmonary oedema.[8] There is no antivenom.

Vinegar has been recommended as first aid, and again pressure immobilization bandaging is unproven. These patients are in pain and may require large doses of opioids to relieve their symptoms. In a review of 62 cases of Irukandji syndrome presenting to Cairns hospitals in one year, 38 required parenteral analgesia.[9] Fentanyl has been recommended. Patients should be observed in hospital for 6 hours after their last dose of opioid and, if asymptomatic, may then be discharged. Those patients who go on to develop pulmonary oedema usually require intensive care admission for supportive care of ventilation and blood pressure. Global cardiac hypokinesis has been documented in this situation and inotropes may be necessary.

SEA SNAKE ENVENOMING

Sea snakes are readily distinguished from terrestrial snakes by their flat oarlike tail. It is important to remember that terrestrial snakes may also take to the water, but swim on the surface. Sea snakes, like terrestrial snakes, are air-breathing reptiles and in Australia are found in tropical or temperate waters. They do not survive long out of water but bites have been recorded from handling animals that have been washed ashore.

The bite of a sea snake typically causes minimal pain,[3] in contrast to fish stings which tend to cause intense pain. Symptoms include progressive muscle pain and tenderness, with pain and stiffness on passive movement. Neuromuscular paralysis of the affected limb and rhabdomyolysis are common, but coagulopathy is rare.[3] Fortunately, as for terrestrial snakes, not all bitten victims are envenomed.

Management

- Apply pressure-immobilization bandaging
- Antivenom and resuscitative facilities should be available before pressure-immobilization bandaging is removed
- Give antivenom if there is clinical or biochemical evidence of envenomation. Specific sea snake antivenom is preferred but, if unavailable, tiger snake antivenom is an alternative.[2]
- One ampoule of sea snake antivenom (1000 units), or alternatively, 3 ampoules of tiger snake antivenom, is diluted 1 in 10 with crystalloid and infused over 30 minutes. Further doses may be required and, as with any antivenom, the dose is titrated to effect.
- Supportive care including airway management, ventilatory assistance and treatment of rhabdomyolysis may be required.
- If the patient is asymptomatic after 4 hours without first-aid measures being instituted, envenomation is unlikely. As with terrestrial snakebite, it is recommended that patients with confirmed or suspected sea snake bite be observed for a minimum of 12 hours prior to discharge.

BLUE-RINGED OCTOPUS ENVENOMING

This small octopus, which may weigh only 10–100 g and measure 12–20 cm across the tentacles, is common along the Australian coastline. It is normally brown in colour, but the characteristic bright blue rings become apparent when the animal is agitated. Humans are at risk of envenomation when they disturb the animal. There have been two deaths documented from the blue-ringed octopus (*Hapalochlaena maculosa*) in Australia,[1] and several other cases of potentially fatal envenomings that were successfully managed. The active component of the venom, maculotoxin, is similar or identical to tetrodotoxin (Sutherland). It acts as a paralyzing agent by preventing conduction in motor nerves via sodium channel blockade.[3] Death occurs from respiratory failure due to paralysis. The bite is typically painless, but a small lesion with bleeding may occasionally be visible. There is a spectrum of envenomation, from no symptoms to rapid onset of paralysis, during which time the patient remains conscious until succumbing to the effects of hypoxia.

Management

- Apply pressure-immobilization bandaging after washing the bite site
- Supportive management as required, which may include artificial ventilation with sedation and inotropes for up to 12 hours
- No antivenom is available.

CONE SHELL ENVENOMATION

Of the many species of cone shell, about 18 have been implicated in human envenomation. The sole Australian fatality reported was caused by *Conus geographus* in 1936.[11] The cone shell animal injects venom from a radular tooth harpoon carried on a proboscis that protrudes from the narrow end of the shell. The venom consists of peptitoxins called conotoxins. Pain is usually felt at the site of the bite and, in serious envenomation, evidence of muscular weakness may rapidly develop and occasionally progress to respiratory paralysis.

Management

- Apply pressure-immobilization bandaging
- Be prepared to commence expired air resuscitation
- Supportive ventilation and sedation may be required

- Antivenom is not available
- Clinical recovery has been documented after 4 hours of assisted ventilation.

STONEFISH ENVENOMING

Although the stonefish (*Synanceia* species) has caused deaths elsewhere, there are no confirmed Australian fatalities,[1] although Sutherland reports the death of an Army doctor on Thursday Island in 1915.[10] The stonefish possesses 13 dorsal fin spines, each with paired venom glands. These spines become erect when the fish is trodden on and venom is discharged deep into the wound. The venom has neurotoxic, myotoxic, vascular and myocardial effects. Because of their excellent camouflage stonefish are not often seen, and the first indication of their presence may be the excruciating pain of a sting.

Management

- Immerse the limb in hot water (approximately 40–45°C)[1,2]
- Pressure-immobilization bandaging is not indicated as it is likely to exacerbate the intense pain
- Opioid analgesics are often ineffective. Regional anaesthesia with bupivacaine may be required
- Stonefish antivenom, 1 ampoule (2000 units) per two puncture wounds via intramuscular injection should be given if there is significant envenomation. Intravenous use is not recommended
- Debride the wound. Consider radiography to exclude retained foreign body
- Tetanus prophylaxis should be given as needed
- Contaminated wounds may require appropriate antibiotic treatment.

MANAGEMENT OF VENOMOUS FISH STINGS

The following generalizations may apply to the management of any fish spine wound:

- The appropriate first aid is immersion of the affected limb in hot water (40–45°C). Scalding may be prevented by placing the unaffected limb in the water as well
- Pressure-immobilization bandaging is not indicated
- Regional nerve blockade is preferable to local infiltration
- Radiography should be considered to exclude retained foreign body. This is much less common with fish spine injuries than with sea urchin spines
- Wound debridement may be necessary
- Consider appropriate antibiotics for contaminated wounds
- Tetanus prophylaxis as needed
- If the wound fails to heal or becomes infected then a retained foreign body is likely.

STINGRAY INJURY

Stingrays possess a barbed spine with an enveloping integumentary sheath and associated venom glands on the tail. Human injury usually occurs when the animal is trodden on and a wound occurs from slashing of the tail. Two deaths have been documented in Australia as a result of stingray injury, both from penetrating cardiac wounds.[1,12] In one of these cases, cardiac tamponade occurred 5 days post injury, secondary to myonecrosis of myocardium at the site of the wound. Part of the spine is not infrequently left in the wound. Injury occurs from both direct trauma and envenomation. Treatment is symptomatic, as for any fish spine injury. No antivenom is available.

CIGUATERA POISONING

Ciguatera is a disease caused by eating tropical fish contaminated with ciguatoxin, a lipid-soluble toxin that accumulates up the food chain. The toxin originates in dynoflagellate algae. Humans are exposed to the toxin when they eat contaminated fish. The toxin is heat stable and, therefore, not inactivated by cooking. There is no test that will readily detect it in fish. In Australia, ciguatoxic fish are particularly found between Mackay and Cairns, but also occur around Fraser Island, Rockhampton, Groote Eylandt and Gove.

Poisoning is characterized by an acute gastrointestinal illness and a subsequent neurological illness classically involving reversal of heat and cold sensation.[3] Gastrointestinal and neurological symptoms usually begin within 1 and 24 hours of eating contaminated fish. Gastrointestinal symptoms include nausea, vomiting, abdominal pain and diarrhoea, and neurological symptoms include myalgia, paraesthesiae, a burning sensation on contact with cold, mood disorders and disturbance of balance. Alcohol classically exacerbates symptoms, which may recur on eating contaminated fish. Treatment until recently was supportive, but there are now several reports of the effectiveness of mannitol given at a dose of 1 g/kg IV over 20–30 minutes, following adequate hydration of the patient.[1,3,13] The usual osmotic diuresis expected following an infusion of mannitol is said not to occur when mannitol is used to treat ciguatera poisoning.

SCOMBROID POISONING

Scombroid is an allergic-type reaction to a toxin that develops in the flesh of fish after they have been landed. It typically occurs from eating the flesh of mackerel, bonito and tuna. If the fish is not immediately refrigerated upon being caught, microorganisms may break down histidine in the flesh to form histamine-like substances. Following the ingestion of fish affected by this toxin, the features of histamine ingestion appear, including an urticarial rash with associated weakness and lethargy. Associated features may include bronchospasm, diarrhoea and vomiting. Less severe reactions may be treated with antihistamines but more severe reactions should be treated as for anaphylaxis.[14]

PARALYTIC SHELLFISH POISONING

Paralytic shellfish poisoning is similar to ciguatera in that it occurs as a result of the concentration of a toxin produced by a dynoflagellate microorganism. The toxin, known as saxitoxin, becomes concentrated in the flesh of bivalve molluscs and has similar effects to tetrodotoxin. Treatment is supportive. Death may result from respiratory failure in untreated cases.

TETRODOTOXIN POISONING

Tetrodotoxin (TTX) is a paralytic toxin that occurs in the flesh, skin and viscera of puffer fish. TTX acts by selectively blocking voltage-sensitive sodium channels and thus preventing conduction in motor and sensory nerves. In Australia TTX poisoning is rare and usually occurs in those who do not know the puffer fish to be poisonous. In Japan, where such fish are a delicacy called 'fugu', numerous cases and deaths occur every year. Toxicity usually manifests soon after eating the fish with typical features including perioral paraesthesiae followed by numbness of the mouth, tongue and face, and then widespread paralysis. Severe cases can progress to death from respiratory failure. Management is supportive as there is no antidote.[1,3] All cases should be admitted for observation until peak clinical effects have passed. It is extremely unlikely that life-threatening effects will occur after 24 hours in patients who have not already developed severe effects.[15]

REFERENCES

1. Williamson JA, Fenner PJ, Burnett JW, Rifkin JF (eds) 1996 Venomous and Poisonous Marine Animals – a Medical and Biological Handbook.

CONTROVERSIES AND FUTURE DIRECTIONS

❶ The biology and venoms of potentially lethal Australian jellyfish remain poorly understood. Further basic research in this area is needed to help prevent and treat envenomations more effectively.

❷ The most effective first aid for jellyfish stings, particularly in tropical Australia, remains controversial. A recent laboratory study demonstrated that heat inactivates box jellyfish venom and the role of hot showers in first aid merits further investigation.[16]

University of New South Wales Press, Sydney
2. White J 1995 CSL Antivenom Handbook. CSL Ltd.
3. Edmonds C 1989 Dangerous Marine Creatures. Reed Books
4. Little M 2002 Is there a role for the use of immobilisation bandages in the treatment of jellyfish envenomation in Australia? Emergency Medicine 14: 171–4
5. O'Rielly G, Isbister GK, Lawrie PM, et al 2001 Prospective study of jellyfish stings from tropical Australia, including the major box jellyfish Chironex fleckeri. Medical Journal of Australia 175: 652–5
6. Barnes J 1964 Cause and effect in Irukandji stingings. Medical Journal of Australia 177: 654–5
7. Hawdon GM 1997 Venomous marine creatures. Australian Family Physician 26(12): 1369–74
8. Fenner PJ, Hadok JC 2002 Fatal envenomation by jellyfish causing Irukandji syndrome. Medical Journal of Australia 177: 362–3
9. Little M, Mulcahy R 1998 A years experience of Irukandji envenomation in far north Queensland. Medical Journal of Australia;169: 638–41
10. Sutherland SK, Tibballs J (eds) 2001 Australian Animal Toxins, 2nd edn. Oxford University Press, Melbourne, Victoria
11. Flecker H 1936 Cone shell mollusc poisoning with report of a fatal case. Medical Journal of Australia 1: 464–6
12. Fenner PJ, Williamson JA, Skinner RA 1989 Fatal and non-fatal stingray envenomation. Medical Journal of Australia 151: 621–5
13. Palafox NA, Jain LG, Pinano AZ, et al 1988 Successful treatment of ciguatera fish poisoning with intravenous mannitol. Journal of the American Medical Association 259: 2740–2
14. Smart DR 1992 Scombroid poisoning: a report of seven cases involving the Western Australian salmon Arripis truttaceus. Medical Journal of Australia 157: 748–51
15. Isbister GK, Son J, Wang F, et al 2002 Puffer fish poisoning: a potentially life-threatening condition. Medical Journal of Australia 177: 650–3
16. Carrette TJ, Cullen P, Little M, Peiera PL, Seymour JE 2002 Temperature effects on box jellyfish venom: a possible treatment for envenomed patients? Medical Journal of Australia 177: 654–5

Note: Page numbers in *italics* refer to either tables or figures.

A

Abacavir, HIV/AIDS 422
Abbreviated Injury Scale 45–46
Abdomen
  distension 307
  examination, pelvic pain 573
  pain *see* Abdominal pain
  trauma *see* Abdominal trauma
Abdominal aortic aneurysm(s) 248–251
  differential diagnosis 641
  ultrasound 636, 641, *641*
Abdominal migraine 350
Abdominal pain
  acute appendicitis 332
  adrenocortical insufficiency 470
  barotrauma 756
  bowel obstruction 307
  HIV/AIDS 420, 421
  inflammatory bowel disease 336
  pelvic inflammatory disease 570
  right upper quadrant 326
Abdominal trauma 71–75
  blunt *72*
  diagnostic peritoneal lavage 72, 73, 96
  elderly patients 107
  examination 71–72
  history 71
  initial management 72–73, *74*
  investigations 72–73
    comparisons *73*
  laparoscopy 73
  laparotomy 72
    indications *72*
  penetrating *72*, *72*, 73–74
  radiology 96–99
  risk factors *71*
Abdominal X-ray(s) 96–99
  bowel obstruction 307
  drug 'body-packers'/'body-stuffers' 852
  inflammatory bowel disease 336
  iron overdose 870
  nephrolithiasis 458
  trauma 96–99
ABO blood group system *494*
Abscess(es)
  anal canal 345
  anorectal 344–345
  cerebral 383, 551
  cutaneous 406
    bacterial pathogens 405
    investigations 403
    management 406
  epidural 523
  febrile patients 383
  retropharyngeal 269, 408, 554
  submandibular 408
  supralevator 345
  ultrasound 644
Absence seizure(s) 371, 374, 375
Acarbose 464

ACE inhibitors *see* Angiotensin-converting
  enzyme (ACE) inhibitors
Acetabulum, fractures 151
Acetaminophen *see* Paracetamol
  (acetaminophen)
Acetazolamide
  altitude illness 785, 786
  central retinal artery occlusion 541
N-Acetylcysteine *see* N-acetylcysteine (NAC)
Achilles tendon rupture 170–171
Achronobacter 29
Aciclovir 432
Acid-base disturbance(s) 476–480
  arterial blood gases 479
  crush syndrome 85
  drug overdose 791
  management 450
  renal failure 450
Acid-base values 476
Acid corrosives injury 840, 841
Acidosis 477–479
  definition 477
  management 478
  metabolic *see* Lactic acidosis; Metabolic
    acidosis
  renal tubular acidosis 478
  respiratory 478–479
Acinetobacter 29
Acquired immunodeficiency syndrome
  (AIDS) *see* Human immunodeficiency
  virus (HIV)/AIDS
Acromioclavicular joint injuries 130
Actinomyces israeli, penicillin 427
Activated charcoal, in drug overdose *794*,
  794–795, 825
  antihistamines 799
  antipsychotic drugs 812
  beta-blockers 802–803
  bupropion 813
  calcium channel blocker drugs 802–803
  carbamazepine 817
  colchicine 821
  drugs of abuse 852
  glyphosate 862
  paraquat 863
  pesticides 859
  phenytoin 817
  salicylate 829
  sodium valproate 817
  sulphonylurea 873
  tricyclic antidepressant drugs 814
Acute acalculous cholecystitis 328
Acute angle-closure glaucoma 538–539
Acute generalized exanthematous pustulosis
  (AGEP) 533
Acute interstitial nephritis (ATIN) 445
Acute management area 717
Acute pelvic pain *see* Pelvis, pain
Acute-phase reactants 333
Acute pulmonary oedema *see* Pulmonary
  oedema, acute
Acute tubular necrosis (ATN) 442–443
Acute uraemic syndrome 450
Acyclovir 180
  herpes simples keratitis 540
  meningitis *389*

viral rashes 531
Addisonian crisis, conscious state 368
Addison's disease 470
Adenomyosis
  chronic pelvic pain 576
  uterine pain 573
Adenosine 206–207
Adenosine diphosphate inhibitor(s)
  188–189
  see also individual drugs
Adenovirus
  arthritis 523
  gastroenteritis 312, *313*
Adhesions, chronic pelvic pain 573, 576
Administration, complaints 735–736
Adnexae, torsion of 575
Adolescents, consent
  Australia 674–676
  UK 678
Adrenal emergencies 470–471
Adrenaline 201, 213
  advanced life support 11, 13
  anaphylaxis 782, *782*
  cardiogenic shock 28
  redback spider (*Latrodectus hasseltii*) bite
    886
  self-management for home use 783
  severe asthma 273
  snakebite envenoming 883
Adrenocortical insufficiency 470–471
Adrenocorticotrophic hormone analogues
  51
Adult respiratory distress syndrome (ARDS)
  femoral shaft fracture 157
  hydrofluoric acid burns 866
  iron overdose 871
Advance directive(s) 35–36
  UK 678
Advanced life support 6–14, 203, 208
  airway management 10, 15–20
    oxygenation/ventilation 10–11
  algorithm *7*
  cardiac arrhythmias *205*, 205–207
  defibrillation 6, 7–10, *205*
  discontinuation 13
  drug therapy 11–12
  guidelines 6–7
  haemodynamic monitoring 13
  prehospital emergency services 683
Adverse incident(s) 739–740, *741*, *742*
  complaints 737–738
Adverse outcome(s) *742*
Aerial transport *688*, *689*
  after diving 760
  airway management 692
  contraindications *689*, *693*
  decompression illness 760, 761
  defibrillation 689
  equipment 690
  helicopter *688*, *689*
Aeromonas 29
Aeromonas hydrophila 408
Affect assessment 581
Affective disorders, suicide/deliberate
  self-harm 598
Age-related macular degeneration 542–543

Aggression control team(s) 590, 592
Agitation
    drug overdose 791
    gamma-hydroxybutyrate abuse 851
    sedation 43
    trauma patients 43
AIDS *see* Human immunodeficiency virus
    (HIV)/AIDS
Airbag(s) 104
Aircraft *see* Aerial transport
Air viva® 259, *259*
Airway management
    advanced life support 10, 15–20
    aircraft 692
    basic life support 3–4
    facial trauma 67, 69
    head injury 49, 50–51
    massive haemoptysis 301
    near-drowning 771
    prehospital emergency services 683–684
    retrieval 691–692
    shock 25
    spinal cord injury 55, 57, 63
    trauma 41, 42
    see also Ventilation; *individual methods*
Alarms, retrieval 690
Alcohol abuse 516, 877
    avascular necrosis 152
    domestic violence 620, 622
    fever 382, 384
    hepatitis 410, 415
    hypomagnesaemia 490
    meningitis 387, 388
    observation wards 711
    suicide/deliberate self-harm 598
    upper gastrointestinal haemorrhage 317
    see also Alcohol intake
Alcohol dehydrogenase (ADH) 877
Alcoholic ketoacidosis 471–473, 878
    differential diagnosis 473
    investigations 472
    management 473, 880
    presentation 472
Alcohol intake 190, 322, 877–880
    acute intoxication 877
        differential diagnosis *878*
        management/disposition 880
    alcoholic ketoacidosis *see* Alcoholic
        ketoacidosis
    clinical toxicity 877–878
    conscious state alteration 367
    consent issues (Australia) 675
    consent issues (UK) 678
    hypothermia 752
    management 878–880
    mental health legislation (Australia) 663
    toxicity-related seizures 375
    withdrawal syndrome 878
        management 878
    see also Alcohol abuse
Aldosterone 442
Alkali corrosives injury 840
Alkalosis 479
Allen's test 476–477, *477*
Allergic reaction(s)
    antihistamines 797
    thrombolytic therapy 186–187
    see also Anaphylaxis
Allis manoeuvre, hip dislocation 155
Allopurinol
    acute interstitial nephritis 445
    gout 517
Alpha 1-antitrypsin deficiency 286

Alpha-glucosidase inhibitor(s) 464
Alphavirus arthritis 522–523
Alprazolam, pharmacology 806
Altitude illness 784–787
    cerebral oedema 784–785, *785*
        management 785–786
    clinical syndromes 785
    epidemiology 784–785
    management *785*, 785–786
    pathophysiology 784–785
    predictors 785
    prevention 786–787
    pulmonary oedema 784, 785
        management 786
Alvardo score, acute appendicitis 333
Alveolar gas equation 479–480
Alveolar gases 476
Alveolar hypoventilation, respiratory acidosis
    478–479
Alveolar osteitis 546
Alveolar process injury 67–68
Amanita phalloides poisoning 339
    hepatitis 411
Ambulance service 698–699
Amenorrhoea 567
Aminoglycoside(s) 425, 430
    adverse reactions 430
    bacterial resistance 430
    cellulitis 405–406
    gangrene 406–407
    necrotizing fasciitis 406
    nosocomial pneumonia 284
    septic shock 30
    see also individual drugs
Aminopenicillin(s) 427
    see also individual drugs
Aminophylline
    anaphylaxis 782, 783, *783*
    severe asthma 273
Aminosalicylate(s)
    inflammatory bowel disease 337
    see also individual drugs
Amiodarone 12, 204, 208
    antiretroviral drug interactions 423
    epididymo-orchitis 455
    hepatitis *412*
Amisulpride, pharmacology 809
Amlodipine, pharmacology 801
Ammonia products ingestion 840
Amoebiasis *see Entamoeba histolytica*
Amoebic hepatitis 410
Amoxicillin
    acute pyelonephritis 400
    HIV/AIDS 422
    otitis media 551
    in pregnancy 401
    sexually-transmitted diseases 614
    sinusitis 552
    streptococcal pneumonia 280
Amoxicillin-clavulanate 428
    endometritis 566
    epididymo-orchitis 456
    facial cellulitis 405–406
    HIV/AIDS 422
    pelvic inflammatory disease 571
    urinary tract infection 399, 400–401
AMPA receptors 21
Amphetamines
    abuse 849–850
    acute intoxication 376, 850
    pharmacology 849
    withdrawal state 850
    see also individual drugs

Amphotericin
    HIV/AIDS 422
    meningitis *389*
    neutropenia 500
Ampicillin 428
    acute cholecystitis 327
    bacterial resistance 428
    biliary tract disease 327
    bowel obstruction 308
    cholangitis 328
    chronic obstructive airway disease 290
    induced fever 381
    inflammatory bowel disease 337
    meningitis *389*
    peptic ulcer disease 324
    septic shock 31
Amprenavir, HIV/AIDS 422
Amylase 257
    acute pancreatitis 329, *330*
Amyloid angiopathy 353, 357
Anaemia 503–510
    aplastic 506
    causes *504*
    of chronic disorders 506
    haemolytic *see* Haemolytic anaemia
    haemorrhage-associated 503–505
    iron-deficiency 505–506
    megaloblastic *505*, 505–506
    pernicious 505–506
    red cell production deficit 505–507
    renal failure
        acute 448
        chronic 506–507
    sickle cell *see* Sickle cell anaemia
Anaesthesia, sensory function documentation
    60, *60*, 61
Anaesthetic, local *see* Local anaesthesia
Anaesthetic deaths 668
Anal canal, abscesses/fistula 345
Analgesia 626–633
    acute pancreatitis 331
    acute pulmonary oedema 195
    ankle injury 168
    aortic dissection 247
    burns 126
        hydrofluoric acid 128
    children 630
    disasters management 700
    dislocation
        patella 162
        proximal tibiofibular joint 162
        shoulder 131
    fractures
        Colles' fracture 140
        femur 153, 157, 160
        humerus 134
        radius 138
        tibia 167
    general principles 627
    hydrofluoric acid burns 867
    labour 558
    limb trauma 82
    local anaesthesia 630
    non-pharmacologic therapies 629–630
    in pregnancy 629
    prehospital emergency services 684
    renal colic 458
    sickle cell crisis 508
    spinal cord injury 63
    trauma patients 43
Anaphylactic shock 43, 780–781, 782
Anaphylaxis 779–784
    biphasic 783

Anaphylaxis (*cont.*)
    causes 779–780, *780*
    cellular events 780
    clinical features 780–781
    definition 779
    differential diagnosis 781
    epidemiology 779
    follow-up 783
    hospital admission/discharge 783, *783*
    laboratory tests 781
    management 781–783
        first-line 782, *782*
        second-line 782–783, *783*
    mediator pharmacology 780
    monitoring 783
    prehospital emergency services 685
    second-line 782–783
    triggering events 186–187, 779–780
Ancillary staff 715
Aneurysm(s) 248–251
    abdominal aorta *see* Abdominal aortic
        aneurysm(s)
    carotid artery 251
    cerebral *see* Cerebral aneurysm(s)
    peripheral arteries 251
    ruptures 357
    subclavian artery 234, 251
    thoracic aorta 305
    visceral 251
Angina 183–184
    cardiogenic shock 27
    clinical features 183
    management 183–184
    severity classification 178
    therapeutic challenge response 178–179
    unstable *see* Unstable angina
    variant (Prinzmetal) 183
Angiodysplasia 342, 343
Angioedema 533
    anaphylaxis 781
    upper airway obstruction 266
Angiography
    acute arterial limb ischaemia 232
    aortic dissection 246
    cerebral 88
    facial penetrating trauma 69
    haemoptysis 301
    limb trauma 81, 99
        arterial injury 83
    pelvic trauma 98
    pulmonary embolism 212
    rectal bleeding 343
    stroke 357
    thoracic aortic transection 78
    transient ischaemic attack 356–357
Angiotensin-converting enzyme (ACE)
        inhibitors
    acute renal failure 445
    acute tubular necrosis 443
    anaphylactic reaction 779
    diabetes mellitus 464
    hypertension in stroke 240
    ischaemic heart disease 188
    lithium excretion 874
    post-myocardial infarction cardiac failure
        189
    see also individual drugs
Aniline, methaemoglobinaemia 855
Anistreplase 186
Ankle, anatomy 168
Ankle injury 168–171
    Achilles tendon rupture 170–171
    dislocations 170

examination 168
    fractures 169–170
        pillion 170
    radiography 168–169
    soft tissue 170–171
    sprained 170
Anorectal disorder(s) 342
    abscesses 344–345
Anserine bursitis 525
Antacids, peptic ulcer disease 324
Antepartum haemorrhage(s) 564–565
Anterior cervical cord syndrome, acute *53,
    54*
Anterior chamber paracentesis 541
Anterior cruciate ligament injury 163–164
Anterior dislocation
    hip 156
    shoulder 131
Anterior drawer test, anterior cruciate
        ligaments 163
Anterior inferior iliac spine fracture(s) 150
Anterior ischaemic optic neuropathy
        541–542
Anterior superior iliac spine fracture(s) 150
Antibiotic prophylaxis 425, 427
    AIDS opportunistic infection 423
    infective endocarditis 226
    near-drowning 772
    sickle cell crisis 508
    wound management 114, 403
        facial penetrating trauma 69–70
        hand injuries 145
        skull fracture 51
        tibial shaft fracture 167
Antibiotic resistance 425
    community-acquired pneumonia 282
Antibiotic therapy 424–434
    acute liver failure 340
    acute renal failure 450
    administration routes 425
    AIDS opportunistic infections 422
    bacterial keratitis 539–540
    biliary tract disease 327
        cholangitis 328
    bowel obstruction 308
    cellulitis 405–406
    chronic obstructive airway disease 290
    community-acquired pneumonia 279–281
    conscious state alteration 370
    cutaneous abscess 406
    diabetic foot infections 408–409
    epiglottitis 270
    fever 384
    gastroenteritis 314, 315, *315*
    host factors 425
    infective endocarditis 226
    inflammatory bowel disease 337
    limb trauma 82
    Ludwig's angina 269
    mastitis 408
    meningitis 390, *390*
    micro-organism susceptibility 424–425,
        426
    necrotizing fasciitis 406
    neutropenia 500
    osteomyelitis 394–395
    otitis externa 551
    otitis media 551
    outpatient parenteral 433–434
    pelvic inflammatory disease 571
    peptic ulcer perforation 324
    pharyngitis/tonsillitis 268–269
    principles 424

quinsy (peritonsillar abscess) 269
    rape 614
    septic arthritis 393
    septic shock 31
    sinusitis 552
    skin/soft tissue infection 404
    unnecessary, airway infections 268
    urinary tract infection 399
    see also individual drugs
Anticholinergic drug, toxicity
    antihistamines *see* Antihistamines
    antipsychotic drug overdose 811
    carbamates poisoning 860–861
    organophosphates toxicity 857–858
    tricyclic antidepressant overdose 814
Anticholinergic drugs 306
    see also individual drugs
Anticholinergic syndrome 797–800
Anticoagulation therapy
    atrial fibrillation 353
    axillary vein thrombosis 237
    deep vein thrombosis 235–236
    haemorrhagic stroke 352
    mitral incompetence 229
    myocardial infarction 189–190
    prevention 213
    pulmonary embolism 210, 213
    stroke 357
    subarachnoid haemorrhage 364
    transient ischaemic attacks 358
    see also individual drugs
Anticonvulsant drugs 816–818
    analgesia 630
    conscious state alteration 370
    head injury 51
    in pregnancy 376
    status epilepticus 374
    see also individual drugs
Antidepressant drugs
    analgesia 630
    deliberate self-harm/suicide 601
    see also individual drugs
Antidiuretic hormone (ADH) 484–485
    ischaemic acute tubular necrosis 442
    syndrome of inappropriate ADH secretion
        482–483
Antidotes, drug overdose 795, *796*
Antiemetic drugs
    acute pancreatitis 331
    gastroenteritis 314–315
    ocular trauma 538
    see also individual drugs
Antiendotoxin antibodies, septic shock 31
Antiglobulin (Coombs') test 507
Antiglomerular basement membrane
        antibodies *444*
Antihistamines
    allergic reactions 797
    anaphylaxis 782, *782*
    antiretroviral drug interactions 423
    clinical features 376, 670
    overdose/poisoning 669–671, *670*,
        797–800
        management 798–799
    pharmacodynamics 669, 797–798
    redback spider (*Latrodectus hasseltii*) bite
        886
    sinusitis 552
    urticaria 533
    see also H$_1$-antagonists; H$_2$-antagonists;
        individual drugs
Antihypertensive drugs
    aortic dissection 247

Antihypertensive drugs (cont.)
  cerebrovascular disease prevention 353–354
  hypertensive emergencies 239–241
  stroke 358
  see also individual drugs
Antimalarial drugs
  rheumatoid arthritis 520
  systemic lupus erythematosus 521
  see also individual drugs
Antimotility agents 314–315
Anti-neutrophil cytoplasmic antibody
    (ANCA), acute renal failure 447
Antiphospholipid antibody syndrome 356,
    357
Antiplatelet agents
  ischaemic heart disease 189
  stroke 359
  transient ischaemic attacks 358
  see also individual drugs
Antipsychotic drugs 809
  adverse effects 810–812
  chemical restraint 592, 592–593, 593
  classification 809
  overdose 810–812
  pharmacology 809–810
  see also individual drugs
Antiretroviral drugs 422–423, 432–433
  acute liver failure 339
  adverse reactions 432–433
  interactions 433
  side effects 423
  see also individual drugs
Antithrombin III, stroke 357
Antithrombotic therapy, complications 230
Antivenom therapy
  funnel web spider (Atrax/Hadronyche)
      bite 887
  redback spider (Latrodectus hasseltii)
      bite 886
  snakebite 882–883, 883
Antiviral drugs 432
  adverse reactions 432
  analgesia 630
  conscious state alteration 370
  see also individual drugs
Anxiolytic drugs
  analgesia 630
  see also individual drugs
AO classification, ankle fractures 169
Aorta
  acute incompetence 226–227, 243
  blood flow monitoring 44
  chronic incompetence 226–227
  coarctation 29
  thoracic see Thoracic aorta
  trauma 78–79, 94–96
Aortic aneurysm(s)
  abdominal see Abdominal aortic
      aneurysm(s)
  infrarenal 248–251
  thoracic 305
Aortic dissection 29, 242–248
  classification 243
    anatomical 243
    pathophysiology 244
  clinical features 243–244
  differential diagnosis 246, 246
  epidemiology 242
  examination 244
  hypertension 239
  imaging 245–246
    sensitivity/specificity 245
  management 246–247

  mortality 242, 247–248
  pathophysiology 242–243
  predisposing factors 29, 242, 242
  prognosis 247–248
Aortic stenosis 229
Aortoenteric fistula 317, 342
Aortography 93, 95–96
APACHE, septic shock 31
Apathetic hyperthyroidism 469
Aplastic anaemia 506
Apley's test, knee injury 160
Apologies, complaints procedure 736, 738
Appearance assessment 582, 582
Appendicectomy 334
Appendicitis
  acute 332–334
    differential diagnosis 333
  Mantrel's criteria 644
  pelvic pain 572
  ultrasound 644
Arrhythmias 183, 197–209
  anaphylaxis 781
  carbon monoxide poisoning 835
  cardiogenic shock 27, 28
  drug overdose 790, 791
    amphetamines 849–850
    antihistamines 670
    antipsychotic drugs 811
    beta-blockers 802
    cocaine 848
    theophylline 831
    tricyclic antidepressants 814
  electric shock injury 774, 775, 776
  hydrofluoric acid burns 866
  hypocalcaemia 488
  hypokalaemia 486
  hypothermia 754
  management 199–209
    prehospital emergency services 685
  near-drowning 770, 771
  organophosphates poisoning 859–860
  pathogenesis 198
  preterminal 208–209
  sternal fracture 93
  thyroid storm 468–469
  thyrotoxicosis 467
  see also Bradyarrhythmia(s);
      Tachyarrhythmia(s)
Arterial blood gases 476–477
  acid-base disorders 479
  alveolar gas equation 479–480
  asthma 272
  chronic obstructive airway disease 287
  community-acquired pneumonia 279
  hypothermia 753
  interpretation 479–480
  pulmonary embolism 210–211
  specimen collection 476–477
  trauma management 42
Arterial catheter insertion 477
Arterial gas embolism 758, 759
  oxygen therapy 261
Arterial limb ischaemia
  acute (limb-threatening) 232–233
  chronic 232
  upper limb 233
Arterial puncture 476–477
Arteriography, femoral shaft fracture 157
Arteriovenous malformation 88
  haemorrhagic stroke 353
  lobar haemorrhage 357
  rectal bleeding 341
  subarachnoid haemorrhage 364

Arthritis
  degenerative, Lisfranc fractures 174
  gonococcal 519, 521
  post-traumatic
    ankle fractures 170
    femoral head fracture 152
    hip dislocation 156
  rheumatoid see Rheumatoid arthritis
Arthroscopy, meniscal injury 165
Artefacts, ultrasound 637
Ascending cholangitis 326, 328
  gallstones 327
Aseptic meningitis 389
Aspergillus, cutaneous infection 405
Asphyxia 3–4
Aspiration of gastric contents
  drug overdose 791, 793
  spinal cord injury 55, 57
Aspiration pneumonia 276
  opioid abuse 845
Aspirin 49–50, 181, 184, 250
  as analgesic 628
    arthritis 522
      rheumatoid arthritis 520
      tension headache 349
  anaphylactic reaction 779
  ischaemic heart disease 187, 190
  overdose see Salicylates, poisoning
  peptic ulcer disease 322
  pharmacokinetics 827–828
  prosthetic valves 230
  stroke 359
  transient ischaemic attacks 358
Astemizole
  overdose 670
  pharmacodynamics 798
Asthma 271–274
  clinical features 271–272
  disposition 274
  epidemiology 271
  Hudson face masks 262
  mild 272, 272
  moderate 272, 272
  observation wards 710
  oxygen therapy 262
  severe 272, 272–273
  severity categories 272
Asymptomatic bacteriuria 396
Asystole 8, 10, 208–209
  lightning injury 777
Ataxia, phenytoin overdose 817
Atenolol
  aortic dissection 247
  pharmacology 801, 802
Atheroembolic disease, acute renal failure
    444–445
Atherosclerosis
  aneurysms 249
  cerebrovascular disease 352–353, 353–354
  chronic limb ischaemia 232
  ischaemic heart disease 182–183
ATLANTIS trials, ischaemic stroke therapy
    359
Atlanto-axial bony injury 91–92
Atlanto-occipital bony injury 91–92
Atlas (C1) fracture 56
Atopic eczema 529
Atrax (funnel web spider) 887–888
Atrial ectopic beat(s) 208
Atrial fibrillation 198, 207–208, 228, 229
  causes 207
  clinical features 207–208
  electrocardiogram 208

Atrial fibrillation (*cont.*)
  mitral incompetence 228, 229
  stroke risk/anticoagulation 353
Atrial flutter 198, 206, 208, 228, 229
  electrocardiogram *208*
Atrial natriuretic peptide 442
Atrial tachycardia 206–207
Atrioventricular (first degree) heart block 199–200
Atrioventricular node 197–198
Atrioventricular re-entry tachycardia 206
Atropine 200, 201
  advanced life support 12, 13
  carbamates poisoning 861
  funnel web spider (*Atrax/Hadronyche*) bite 887
  neurogenic shock 32
  pesticides poisoning 860
Attitude assessment 582
Audit(s)
  clinical risk management 743, 744–745, 745, *746*
  observation wards 712
  trauma management 45–46
Australasian College for Emergency Medicine (ACEM) 727–728
  ultrasound training 644–645
Australian Council on Healthcare Standards (ACHS) 721, 725
Australian Radiation Incidents Registry 764
Australian Triage Scale 703, 721, 724
Autoimmune blistering disorder(s) 530–534, 532
Autoimmune chronic active hepatitis 411, 416
Autoimmune haemolytic anaemias 508–509
Autoimmune (Hashimoto's) thyroiditis 469
Automated external defibrillator(s) (AEDs) 9
Autonomic nervous system
  spinal cord damage 54–55
  toxic syndromes ('toxidromes') 792, *792*
Autonomy of patient 33, 35–36, 36, 676
  mandated choice 37
Autopsy/postmortem(s)
  Australia 668–669
  UK 672–673
Avascular necrosis (AVN)
  chronic pancreatitis 152
  haemarthrosis 152
  hip disorders 152, 156
  navicular fractures 174
  sickle cell anaemia 152
  vasculitis 152
Axial ultrasound 637
Axillary artery aneurysm 234, 251
Axillary nerve injury 84
  proximal humerus fracture 133
Axillary vein thrombosis 236
Axis (C2) fracture 56
Axonotmesis 83
Azathioprine
  inflammatory bowel disease 337
  psoriasis 530
  rheumatoid arthritis 520
Azithromycin 429
  otitis media 551

B

Babinski response 367
Bacillus anthracis, penicillin susceptibility 427

Bacillus cereus, gastroenteritis 312, *313*
Bacillus subtilis, macrolide resistance 429
Back pain 523–524
  clinical features 523
  decompression illness 758
  management 524
  pathology 523
Bacteraemia 29
  febrile patient 381–382, 383
  infective endocarditis 224, 225
Bacterial keratitis 539–540
Bacterial meningitis *see* Meningitis
Bacteriuria
  asymptomatic 396
  significant 396
  urinary tract infection 398
Bacteroides
  antibiotic susceptibility 427, 431, 432
  cholangitis 328
  Ludwig's angina 269
Bacteroides fragilis
  cephalosporin susceptibility 349
  cutaneous infection 405
Bad news, breaking 609–610
Bag/mask ventilation 18, 42
Baker's cyst 525
Barbiturates 51
  antihistamine overdose 798–799
  near-drowning 772
  overdose 808
  pharmacology 808
  status epilepticus 374
  see also individual drugs
Barium studies
  oesophageal/diaphragmatic injury 96
  rectal bleeding 343
Barotrauma 756–758
  dental pain 758
  ear 757
  gastrointestinal 758
  mask squeeze 758
  pulmonary 757–758
  sinus 757
Bartholin's abscess 406
Barton's fracture 141
Bartter's syndrome 479
Base deficit 25
Base excess 476
Basic life support 2–5, 7, 8
  algorithm 3
  call for help 4
  defibrillation 4–5
  defibrillation relationship 8, 10
  initial evaluation 2–4
  near-drowning 771
  prehospital emergency services 683
  see also First aid
Behaviour assessment 582, *582*
Below elbow plaster (BEPOP) 139
Benchmarking 721
Beneficence principle 33, 676
Benign early depolarization 216
Bennett's fracture 146
Benzocaine, methaemoglobinaemia 854
Benzodiazepines 51, 106
  adverse effects 807
  alcohol abuse 879
  amphetamine abuse 850
  antihistamine overdose 798
  antipsychotic drug overdose 812
  back pain 524
  chemical restraint *592*, 592–593, *593*
  cocaine abuse 848, 849

conscious sedation 629
heatstroke 750
labyrinthitis 551
non-convulsive seizures 375
opioid withdrawal syndrome 846
overdose *793*, 807
pesticides poisoning 860
pharmacology 806–807
in pregnancy 376
prehospital emergency services 685
status epilepticus 374
see also individual drugs
Benzylpenicillin, community-acquired pneumonia 280
Bereavement 611
Beta-adrenergic agonists
  asthma 273
  chronic obstructive airway disease 289
  hyperkalaemia 487
Beta-blockers
  analgesia 630
  anaphylactic reaction 779
  angina 183–184
  aortic dissection 247
  atrial fibrillation 207
  ischaemic heart disease 187–188, 191
  overdose 800–803
    clinical features 802
    management 802–803, *803*
    pathophysiology 800–802
  pharmacokinetics 800
  pharmacology *801*
  post-myocardial infarction cardiac failure 189
  thyroid storm 468–469
  see also individual drugs
Beverage-making facilities 719
Bicarbonate values 476
Bicipital tendinitis/rupture 524
Bicuspid aortic valve 29
Bier's block (intravenous regional anaesthesia) 632–633
  hydrofluoric acid burns 867
Bifascicular block 202–203
Biguanides 464
  see also individual drugs
Bi-level positive airway pressure (Bi-PAP)
  acute pulmonary oedema 195
  chronic obstructive airway disease 288–289
  complications 195
Biliary tract disease 178, 323, 326–328
  calculus 330
  complications 326–327
  disposition 327
  management 327
  ultrasound 642
  see also Gallbladder disease; *individual diseases/disorders*
Bimalleolar fractures 169
Biological agents
  decontamination 699
  disasters 698
Bisphosphonates
  hypercalcaemia 489
  see also individual drugs
Bites 145, 530
Bladder injuries 149
Bladder instrumentation 397
Bleach ingestion 840
Blinding, clinical trials 650–651
Blind nasotracheal intubation 18
Blisters *528*

Blood culture
  community-acquired pneumonia 278
  febrile patient 384
Blood ethanol level (BAL) 878
Blood gas analysis, conscious state alteration 368
Blood group antigen secretor status 397
Blood tests
  acute pulmonary oedema 194
  gallbladder disease 326
  inflammatory bowel disease 336
  pelvic pain 574
  primary HIV infection 421
Blood transfusion(s) 494–498
  adverse reactions 496–497
  anaemia 506, 507
  consent 495
  cross-matching precautions 495–496
  femoral shaft fracture 157
  gastrointestinal bleeding 319
  granulocytes 497
  guidelines *495*
  haemorrhage 505
  indications 44, *494*
  massive 497
    thrombocytopenia 513
  micropore blood filters 44
  packed red blood cells 494–495, *495*, 509
  platelets *495*, 497, 509
  risks *497*
  transmissible pathogens *496*, 496–497
  unstable pelvic fracture 149
Blood urea nitrogen (BUN), acute renal failure 440
Blue bloaters 287
Blue-ringed octopus (*Hapalochlaena maculosa*) envenomation 891–892
Blunt trauma
  abdomen, ultrasound 639–640
  ear 550–551
  eyes 537–538
  testicles 456
  upper airway 267, *268*
B-mode (brightness modulation) ultrasound 636, 637
'Body-packer(s)' 851–852
'Body-stuffer(s)' 851–852
Bone marrow failure, anaemia 506
Bone scans, foot injury 172
Bordetella pertussis, antibiotic susceptibility 429
Bornholm disease (epidemic myalgia) 180
Borrelia, antibiotic susceptibility 429
Botulism 407
Bowel neoplasia 342
Bowel obstruction 306–309
  causes *306*, 306–307
  clinical features 307
  management 308–309
  strangulation 307, 308, 310
Bowel pseudo-obstruction 306
Box jellyfish (*Chironex fleckeri*) envenomation 890–891
Brachial artery
  aneurysm 251
  embolization 232
  injury 83
  puncture 477
Brachial plexus injuries 560
Bradyarrhythmia(s) 198
  gamma-hydroxybutyrate abuse 851
  management principles 199

opioid abuse 845
paracetamol poisoning 824
vaginal bleeding 561
see also Arrhythmias
Bradycardia-tachycardia (sick sinus) syndrome 199
Brain death 608
Branch retinal vein occlusion 543
Breaking bad news 609–610
Breast(s)
  abscesses 180, 408
  disorders 180
  tumours 180
Breath ethanol level (BAL) 878
Breech delivery 559–560
Bretylium
  advanced life support 13
  hypothermia 754
Broad complex tachycardia 203
Bronchial artery embolization 302
Bronchitis 268, 286–287
  continuous positive airway pressure 264
  see also Chronic obstructive airway disease (COAD)
Bronchodilators
  anaphylaxis 783
  asthma 273
  chronic obstructive airway disease 289
Bronchoscopy
  cavitating lesions 283
  haemoptysis 300–301
  upper airway penetrating trauma 267–268
Bronchospasm
  anaphylaxis 781, 782
  near-drowning 770
Brown–Sequard syndrome *53*, 54
Brucella, antibiotic therapy *426*, 429, 432
Brucella abortus, antibiotic susceptibility 431
Brudzinski's sign 388
Bruising, proximal humerus fracture 133
Buck splints, femoral shaft fracture 157
Budd–Chiari syndrome 339
'Buddy strapping', phalangeal fracture/dislocation 175
Bullae *528*
Bullous pemphigoid 530
Bundle branch block
  paracetamol poisoning 824
  see also Left bundle branch block; Right bundle branch block
Bupivacaine, radial head/neck fractures 138
Bupropion 812–813
Burn(s) 123–128
  area evaluation 124, *125*
  chemical *see* Chemical burn(s)
  classification 124
  compartment syndrome 84
  corrosives ingestion 840, 842
  elderly patients 106, 107
  electric shock injury 775
  examination 124
  eye 538
  facial trauma 67
  history taking 124
  hypernatraemia 485
  infection 126–127
  investigations 124
  lightning injury 777, 778
  management 126–127
    analgesia 126
    emergency department care *125*, 126–127

escharotomy 126
fluid resuscitation 126
prehospital care 124–125
special burns unit transfer 126, 127
respiratory tract 264
  inhalation injury 127
shock 127
skin injury zones 123–124
stress ulcers 317
Business planning 723–726
  activity data 724
  equipment 725
  facility maintenance 725
  financial aspects 723, 724
  implementation 726
  monitoring 726
  plan content 724
  process 723–725
  projections 725
  projects 725
  quality indicators 724–725
  timing 723–724
Button spider (*Steatoda*) 885
Butyrophenones, alcohol intoxication 879

C

Caesarean section(s) 104
Calcaneus, fractures 99, 173, *173*
Calcitriol 488
Calcium 487
  advanced life support 12
  hyperkalaemia 487
  imbalance *see* Hypercalcaemia; Hypocalcaemia
Calcium channel blockers (CCBs)
  antiretroviral drug interactions 423
  atrial fibrillation 207
  cerebral protection 51
  ischaemic heart disease 183–184, 188
  migraine 350
  overdose 800–803
    clinical features 802
    management 802–803, *803*
    pathophysiology 800–802
  pharmacokinetics 800
  pharmacology *801*
  renal insufficiency 240
  see also individual drugs
Calcium chloride
  hyperkalaemia 487
  hypocalcaemia 488
Calcium gluconate
  analgesia 630
  hydrofluoric acid burns 866–867
  hyperkalaemia 487
  hypocalcaemia 488
Calcium pyrophosphate dihydrate deposition disease 517–518
Calcivirus gastroenteritis 312, *313*
Campylobacter
  arthritis 522
  erythromycin resistance 430
  gastroenteritis 312, 314, 315, *313*
  traveller's diarrhoea 313
Campylobacter jejuni
  antibiotic therapy *426*
    susceptibility 429
  gastroenteritis 312
Canadian Emergency Department Triage and Acuity Scale (CTAS) 704

Candida
  HIV/AIDS 418–419, 420, 422
  paronychia 406
  pustular lesions 532
Carbamates *860*
  poisoning 860–861
    management 861
  see also individual drugs
Carbamazepine 816–817
  acute interstitial nephritis 445
  therapeutic concentrations 817
Carbenicillin, cellulitis 406
Carbimazole 468
Carbon dioxide narcosis 263
Carbon monoxide poisoning 124, 833–837
  alkalosis 479
  clinical features *834*, 834–835
  with cyanide poisoning 839
  investigations 124, 836
  management 835–836
  pathophysiology 833–834
    carboxyhaemoglobin levels 833, *834*
  reoxygenation response 834, 836
  smoke inhalation 268
Carbon tetrachloride, hepatitis 410
Carbuncle(s) 405
Cardiac arrest
  aetiology 6
  diagnosis of rhythm 8
  discontinuation 13
  drug overdose 793
  endotracheal intubation 10
  immersion syndrome 769
  incidence 6
  lightning injury 777
  management
    basic life support 4–5
    bicarbonate therapy 478
    defibrillation 6, 7, 8–10
    drug therapy 11–12, 12–13
    prehospital emergency services 684–685
    ventilation 10–11
  neurological injury 21
  post-arrest hyperglycaemia 13
  prognosis 13–14
    determinants 6
  research reporting 14
  systems management approach 6–7
  vascular access 12–13
Cardiac arrhythmias *see* Arrhythmias
Cardiac tamponade 78, 79, 217–219
  causes *218*
  differential diagnosis 218–219
  echocardiography 643
  management 219
  post-myocardial infarction 189
  shock 27, 28
Cardiogenic pulmonary oedema 193, *193*
Cardiogenic shock 24–25, 27–29, 43, 189,
    229–230
  definition 27
  management 28–29
  myocarditis 219, 220
  trauma 43
Cardiotocography 104
  antepartum haemorrhage 565
Cardiovascular changes of pregnancy 102
Cardiovascular disease, risk factors 183
Cardiovascular drug(s), toxicity 800–805
Cardiovascular response
  spinal autonomic nervous system damage
    55, 57–58
  trauma 43

Carotid artery, aneurysms 251
Carotid artery disease 354
  haemorrhagic stroke 353
Carotid artery dissection 88
Carotid stenosis surgery, transient ischaemic
    attacks 358
Carpal bone fracture(s) 99
Carpal tunnel syndrome 525
Carukia barnesi (irukandji) envenomation
  891
Carvedilol, pharmacology *801*
Case-control studies 650
Case report studies 650
Casting 119
  hand injuries 146
  patellar fractures 162
  tibial plateau fractures 161
  tibial shaft fracture 167
  tibia tubercle fracture 167
  see also Immobilization
Cataract(s)
  electric shock injury 776
  lightning injury 778
Catheter aspiration
  pleural effusion 299
  pneumothorax 293–294
Catheter placement, ultrasound 644
Catheters, urinary *see* Urinary catheterization
Cation exchange resins, hyperkalaemia 487
Cauliflower ear (ot haematoma) 550, 551
Caval interruption techniques 214
Cavitating lesion(s) 283, *283*
Cefaclor 428
Cefepime 429
  septic shock 31
Cefotaxime 428
  acute cholecystitis 327–328
  facial cellulitis 405
  meningitis 389
  pelvic inflammatory disease 571
  septic arthritis 393
  septic shock 31
  systemic lupus erythematosus 521
Cefotetan 428
Cefoxitin 428
Cefpirome 428
  septic shock 31
Ceftazidime 428
  HIV/AIDS 422
  septic shock 31
  urinary tract infection 400, 401
Ceftriaxone 428
  acute cholecystitis 327–328
  cellulitis 405–406
  chronic obstructive airway disease 290
  epididymo-orchitis 456
  gonococcal arthritis 521
  HIV/AIDS 422
  meningitis 389, *389*
  septic arthritis 393
  septic shock 31
  sexually-transmitted diseases 614
Cefuroxime 428
Cellulitis 405–406
Centor's criteria 269
Central cervical cord syndrome, acute 54
Central nervous system drug toxicity
    806–819
Central pontine myelinosis 483, 484
Central retinal artery occlusion 541
Central retinal vein occlusion 542–543
Central venous pressure monitoring 12, 13
  crush syndrome 85

gastrointestinal bleeding 318–319
  shock 24, 30
  trauma 44
  ultrasound placement 642–643
Cephalexin 428
  mastitis 408
  tibial shaft fracture 167
  urinary tract infection 399, 400, 401
Cephalosporin(s) 425, 428–429
  adverse reactions 429
  bacterial keratitis 540
  bacterial resistance 429
  cellulitis 405–406
  chronic obstructive airway disease 290
  classification 428–429
  Haemophilus influenzae pneumonia 280
  mastitis 408
  meningitis 390, *390*
  near-drowning 772
  necrotizing fasciitis 406
  otitis media 551
  septic shock 31
  submandibular abscess 408
  toxic shock syndrome 407
  urinary tract infection 399–401
  wound infection prophylaxis 403
  see also individual drugs
Cephalothin 51, 82, 428
  cellulitis 405–406
  septic shock 31
Cephamandole 428
Cephamycin(s) 428
Cephazolin 428
  cellulitis 405–406
  septic shock 31
Cerebral abscess(es) 383, 551
Cerebral aneurysm(s) 87–88
  haemorrhagic stroke 353
Cerebral angiography 88
  subarachnoid haemorrhage 362–363
Cerebral artery
  dissection 356
  gas embolism 758, 759
  thromboembolism 352
Cerebral contusions 48
Cerebral ischaemia 21
  anaphylaxis 781
  head injury 48–49
  neuroprotective drugs 21
  neurotrauma 48–49
  pathophysiology 20, 21
  reperfusion injury 20–21
Cerebral monitoring 22
Cerebral oedema
  alkalosis 479
  Ecstasy (MDMA) abuse 849
  high altitude 784–785, 785–786
  near-drowning 770
  stroke 356
Cerebral perfusion pressure
  head injury 49–50, 51
  monitoring 22
Cerebral resuscitation 20–23
  drug therapy 21
  hypothermia 21–22
  ischaemic stroke 359
  near-drowning 772
  neurotrauma 50–51
Cerebral thromboembolism 20
  ischaemic stroke 352
Cerebral vasospasm, subarachnoid
    haemorrhage 363
Cerebrospinal fluid (CSF), meningitis *389*

Cerebrospinal fluid (CSF) otorrhoea 66
Cerebrospinal fluid (CSF) rhinorrhoea 66, 69, 552
Cerebrovascular disease 352–360
  acidosis 478
Cervical cord syndrome 53
  acute anterior 53, 54
  acute central 54, 61
Cervical spine
  fracture 55–57, 89–90
    atlas (C1) 56
    axis (C2) 56
    C3–C7 56
    distraction 56
    flexion-rotation 56
    hyperextension 56
    hyperflexion 55–56
    lateral flexion 56
    vertical compression 56
  immobilization 54
    trauma management 41, 42
  injury
    elderly patients 107
    fracture see also Fractures
    near-drowning 771
    radiology 86–91
    tracheal intubation 16
    without radiological abnormality (SCIWORA) 89–90
  rheumatoid arthritis 519
  X-ray 50, 86–91, 87, 92
Chain of evidence in rape 615–616
Chain of survival concept 6–7
Chance fracture(s) 57, 72, 92–93
  lumbar vertebrae 93
  radiology 93
Charcoal, activated see Activated charcoal
Charcot's triad 326
  cholangitis 328
Chauffeur's fracture 141, 141
Chelation therapy, iron overdose 870, 871
Chemical agent(s)
  decontamination 699
  disasters 698
Chemical burn(s) 127–128
  corrosives ingestion 840, 841
  eye 538
    caustic injury 538
  management principles 128
Chemical hepatitis 410
Chemical restraint 591, 592–593
  administration route 593
  agents 592, 592–593, 593
  alcohol intoxication 878–880
  deliberate self-harm 600
  see also Sedation
Chest pain 178–182
  aortic dissection 242, 243–244, 245
  decompression illness 759
  differential diagnosis 180, 183
  disposition 181, 190
  examination 178
  history taking 178
  investigations 179
  management 180–181
  pneumothorax 292
  therapeutic challenge response 178–179
Chest trauma 76–80, 227
  elderly patients 107
  emergency thoracotomy 79
  lung injury 78
  mediastinal injury 78–79
  penetrating injury 94

pleural injury 77–78
  radiology 93–95
  resuscitative thoracotomy 79
  spinal injury 79
  subcutaneous emphysema 94
  tracheobronchial injury 78
  wall injury 76–77
Chest wall disorders
  acidosis 478–479
  trauma 76–77
Chest X-ray 93–95
  acute pulmonary oedema 194
  aortic dissection 245, 245
  aortic incompetence 226–227
  asthma 272
  cardiac tamponade 217–219
  chest pain differential diagnosis 179
  chronic obstructive airway disease 288
  community-acquired pneumonia 277
  conscious state alteration 369
  corrosives ingestion 841
  drug overdose 793
  febrile patient 384
  gastrointestinal bleeding 318, 323
  haemoptysis 300
  hydrofluoric acid burns 866
  hypertension 239
  hypothermia 753
  mitral stenosis 230
  mitral valve incompetence 227, 229
  myocardial infarction 185
  myocarditis 220
  oesophageal obstruction 302–305
  pericarditis 215
  pleural effusion 298
  pneumothorax 292
  pulmonary embolism 210
  thoracic aortic injury 94–95, 95, 95
  tracheal laceration 94
  trauma 87, 93–95
Childbirth see Delivery
Children
  abuse 619
  consent (Australia) 674–676
  consent (UK) 678
  oxygen therapy 260–261
  oxygen toxicity 261
Chinese medicine, anticholinergic effects 797
Chin lift 2, 3, 42
Chironex fleckeri (box jellyfish) envenomation 890–891
Chlamydia
  acute epididymo-orchitis 455, 456
  antibiotic therapy 426
    susceptibility 429, 432
  Bartholin's abscess 406
  pelvic inflammatory disease 570, 571
  pelvic pain 574
  post-partum haemorrhage 566
  Reiter's syndrome 522
  urinary tract infection 401
Chloral hydrate 808
Chloramphenicol 425
  anterior chamber paracentesis 541
  meningitis 389
Chloride shift 476
Chlormethiazole
  overdose 808
  pharmacology 808
  status epilepticus 374
Chlorpromazine
  chemical restraint 593
  heatstroke 750

hepatitis 410
  meningitis 390
  migraine 351
  near-drowning 772
  pharmacology 809
  serotonin syndrome 750
Cholangitis 328, 383
Cholecystectomy 327, 328
Cholecystitis 327–328
  acute 327–328
  acute acalculous 328
  ultrasound 642, 642
Choledocholithiasis 328
Cholelithiasis 327
Cholestyramine 338
Cholinesterase test 858–859
Christmas disease see Haemophilia B (Christmas disease)
Chronic obstructive airway disease (COAD) 286–291
  acute respiratory failure 287
  clinical features 287
  definitions 286
  management 288–289
  oxygen therapy 257, 262–263
Chronic pelvic pain see Pelvis, pain
Chvostek's sign
  hypocalcaemia 488
  hypomagnesaemia 490
Cicatricial pemphigoid 530
Ciclosporin 516
  autoimmune blistering disease 530
Ciguatera poisoning 892–893
Cimetidine
  anaphylaxis 783
  overdose 670, 798
  peptic ulcer disease 324
  pharmacodynamics 798
Ciprofloxacin 431–432
  HIV/AIDS 422
  inflammatory bowel disease 337
  meningitis 389
  neutropenia 500
  otitis externa 551
  sexually-transmitted diseases 614
Cirrhosis, liver 411
  alkalosis 479
  hypervolaemic hyponatraemia 481
  meningitis 387, 388
Cisapride, HIV/AIDS 422
Citrobacter 29
  antibiotic susceptibility 432
Civamide 350
Civilian triage 702
Clarithromycin 428, 429
  HIV/AIDS 422
  otitis media 551
Claudication 232, 233
Clavicle fracture 93, 130
Clavulanate 428
  with amoxicillin see Amoxicillin-clavulanate
  chronic obstructive airway disease 290
  epididymo-orchitis 456
  HIV/AIDS 422
  septic shock 31
  urinary tract infection 399, 400–401
Clay shoveler's fracture 55, 56
Clerical office 719
Clerical staff 715
Clindamycin
  community-acquired pneumonia 280
  quinsy 408
  septic shock 31

Clinical care problems, complaints 734–735
Clinical guidelines, clinical risk management 742
Clinical indicator(s) 721
Clinical performance measure(s) 721
Clinical research 648–657
  benefits forgone 656
  concepts 651
  confounding 649, 653–654
  data collection 649, 652–653, 655
    proformas 653
  data management 649, 655
  endpoints 649, 651
  ethics 649, 655–656
  external validity 651
  informed consent 656
  initiation 648
  internal validity 651
  repeatability 651
  response rate 651
  sampling 651–652
    size 654
  statistics 649, 654–655
  study design 649–651
    case-control studies 650
    case report studies 650
    cohort studies 649–650
    cross-sectional studies 649
    ecological studies 649
    experimental (clinical trials) 650–651
    observational 649–650
  study protocol 649
  systematic errors (bias) 649, 653
  validity 651
  variables 651
Clinical risk management 739–746
  audit 744–745
  cause and effect 740–741, *742*
  definitions 739–740, *741, 742*
  indicators 743–744, *744, 745*
  phase of care strategies *744*
  practical applications 741–743
    audit 743, 745, *746*
    clinical guidelines 742
    facilities 743
    major incidents/disasters 742, *744*
    quality assurance 743
    reference databases 742
    reverse triage 742, *744*
    reviews 743
  process strategies *743*
  system strategies *743*
Clonazepam 374
Clonidine 846
Clopidogrel
  ischaemic heart disease 188
  transient ischaemic attacks 358
Closed-circuits, pure oxygen therapy 260
Closed dislocations, ankle 170
Closed (simple) fracture(s) 81
Closed reduction
  hip dislocation 155
  Lisfranc fractures 174
  talar fractures 172
  tibial plateau fractures 161
Clostridium
  antibiotic susceptibility 427, 428, 431
  cholangitis 328
Clostridium botulinum 407
Clostridium difficile
  antibiotic therapy *426*
  HIV/AIDS 420, *420*
  hospital-acquired infections 313

Clostridium novyi, gangrene 406–407
Clostridium perfringens
  antibiotic susceptibility 429
  antibiotic therapy *426*
  erythromycin resistance 430
  gangrene 406–407
  gastroenteritis 312, *313*
Clostridium septicum, gangrene 406–407
Clostridium tetani, antibiotic therapy *426*
'Clothesline injuries', upper airway trauma 267
Cloxacillin 427
Clozapine
  agranulocytosis 811
  overdose 811–812
  pharmacology 809
COAD *see* Chronic obstructive airway disease (COAD)
Coagulation cascade 502
Coagulopathy
  gastrointestinal bleeding 317, 319
  hepatic failure 338, 339
  trauma 44
Coarctation of aorta 29
Cocaine 28, 180
  abuse 846–849
    'body-packers'/'body-stuffers' 852
    clinical features 847–848
    clinical presentation 847–848
    diagnosis 848
    epidemiology 846–847
    management 848–849
    overdose 847–848
    pathophysiology 847
  clinical features 376
  haemorrhagic stroke 353
  pharmacology 847
Coccidioides, cutaneous infection 405
Coccyx fracture(s) 93, 151
Codeine 844
  analgesia 628
  renal colic 458
Cognitive function assessment(s) 583, 587
  carbon monoxide poisoning 834–835
Cohort studies 649–650
Colchicine
  gout 517
  pharmacokinetics 820
  poisoning 791, 800, 820–822
    clinical stages 820–821, *821*
    management 821–822
    pathophysiology 820
Cold autoimmune haemolytic anaemia 508–509
Coliform bacteria 276
Colitis 342
Collateral ligament injury 163
Colles' fracture 106, *140*, 140–141
Colloidal bismuth subcitrate 324
Colloid volume replacement
  acute liver failure 339
  anaphylaxis 782, *782*
  burns patients 126
  gastrointestinal bleeding 318
  hypovolaemic shock 26–27
  trauma 44
Colonoscopy 343
Colour Doppler imaging 454
Coma
  anaphylaxis 781
  electric shock injury 775
  gamma-hydroxybutyrate abuse 851
  neurological assessment 48–49

paracetamol poisoning 824
position 3
prognosis 51
spinal cord injury 61–64
see also Conscious state alteration
Comminuted fractures
  femoral shaft 157
  radial head/neck 138
Communication
  complaints 735, 738
  retrieval 691
Community-acquired pneumonia 275–285
  classification 279–280
  clinical features 276–277
    cavitating lesions 283, *283*
    empyema 284–285
  concomitant disease/infections 276, 277
  differential diagnosis 282
  disposition 282
  infection routes 275–276
  investigations 277–279
    sputum analysis 277–278, *279*
  management 279–282, *280*
    antibiotics 279–281
    response 281–282
  pathogens *276, 280, 281*
    see also individual organisms
  pathophysiology 275–276
  prognosis 282
    mortality *278, 281*
    severity markings *278*
  zoonoses 276
  see also individual infections
Compartment syndrome 84–85
  haemophilia 501
  knee dislocation 162
  opioid abuse 845
  retrieval 692
  tibial plateau fractures 161
Compensation, complaints 735, 736
Competence
  Australia 675
  UK 677
    guidelines *677*
    lack of 679–680
    questions *677*
Complaint(s) 733–738
  documentation 735, 738
  incidence 734
  investigations 737
  litigation/compensation 735, 736
  misdiagnosis 737
  prevention 737–738
  procedures 736–737
    apologies 736, 738
  reasons *734*, 734–736
    administration 735–736
    clinical care problems 734–735
    communication problems 735, 738
    delays 735
    resolution 737
    verbal 736
    written 736
Complement, acute renal failure 447
Complete heart block 201
Compound fracture(s) 81
Computed tomography (CT)
  abdomen
    acute appendicitis 333
    bowel obstruction 308
    inflammatory bowel disease 336
    pelvic inflammatory disease 571
    pelvic pain 574

Computed tomography (CT) (cont.)
  pelvic trauma 98
  peptic ulcer disease 323
  trauma see below
  trauma in pregnancy 104
 abdominal trauma 72, 73, 96–97, 107
  advantages/disadvantages 73
  focused assessment by sonography for
   trauma (FAST) vs. 639–640
 brain
  cavitating lesions 283
  conscious state alteration 369
  dysphagia 305
  head injury 49, 87, 87, 89, 89
  meningitis 389
  seizures 373
  spinal cord injury 62
  stroke 357
  subarachnoid haemorrhage 362
  thoracolumbar spine injury 93
  transient ischaemic attack (TIA) 357
 chest
  aortic dissection 245
  cardiac tamponade 219
  chronic obstructive airway disease 288
  community-acquired pneumonia 277
  haemoptysis 300
  pneumothorax 77, 292
  pulmonary embolism 212
  thoracic aortic injury 78, 79, 95
  trauma 93
 facial trauma 66, 69, 88
 limbs
  ankle injury 169
  calcaneal fractures 173
  distal humerus fracture 135
  foot injury 172
  hip dislocation 156
  knee injury 160
  navicular fractures 174
  odontoid fracture 91–92
  radial head/neck fractures 138
  scapula fracture 131
  talar fractures 172
  tibial plateau fractures 161
  trauma 81–82, 99
 lumbar spinal fractures 57
 upper airway
  obstruction 266
  trauma 268
Computed tomography (CT) angiography
  300
Concussion 47
 spinal cord 54
Cone shell envenomation 892
Confounding, clinical research 649,
  653–654
Confusion Assessment Method (CAM)
  587–588
Congestive heart failure 27
Connective tissue disease 387
 meningitis 388
Conn/Modell classification of mental status
  771, 771
Conscious sedation 629
Conscious state alteration 365–370
 causes 366, 366, 368–370
  drug overdose 790
  electric shock injury 775
  febrile patients 383
  HIV/AIDS 419–420, 421, 422
  lightning injury 777
  meningitis 387–388

 near-drowning (Conn/Modell
  classification) 771, 771–772
 clinical assessment 366–368
 differential diagnosis 366
 disposition 370
 examination 367–368
 history taking 367
 investigations 368–369
 management 369, 369–370
 pathophysiology 365
 primary survey 366–367
 prognosis 370
 secondary survey 367–368
Consent 674–676
 blood transfusion 495
 children/adolescents 675
 clinical research 656
 construed 36
 documentation 674–675
 drug/alcohol intoxication 675
 emergency patient 676
 failure, complaints 735
 forensic examination in rape cases 615
 Guardianship Boards 676
 implied 674
 intellectually disabled patients 675
 medical substituted judgment 36, 675
 mentally ill patients 675
 parental refusal of management 675
 post mortems 673
 presumed/implied 35, 36, 37
 proxy 35–36, 37, 675
 resuscitation 34, 35–36
  practising procedures on newly dead
   36–37, 37
 United Kingdom 676–680
  advance directives/statements 678
  children/adolescents 678, 678
  competence 677
  documentation 679
  drug/alcohol intoxication 678
  emergency management 679–680, 680
  incompetency 679
  information needed 678–679, 679
  intellectual impairment 678
  Mental Health Act detainees 678
  parental responsibility 678
  proxy 678
  temporary impairment 678
  verbal 679
  voluntariness 679
  written 679
 verbal 674
 written 675
Constipation 307
Consultant staff 714, 715
Consultation area(s) 718
Contact allergic dermatitis 531
Continuous arteriovenous haemodiafiltration
  (CAVHDF) 451
Continuous arteriovenous haemofiltration
  (CAVH) 451
Continuous positive airway pressure (CPAP)
  264
 acute pulmonary oedema 195
 acute renal failure 450
 acute respiratory failure 264
 bronchitis 264
 chronic obstructive airway disease 288–289
 near-drowning 771
 pneumonia 264
 pulmonary oedema 263, 264
  high altitude 786

 respiratory tract burns 264
 severe asthma 273
Continuous quality improvement (CQI)
  720–721, 721
Continuous venovenous haemodiafiltration
  (CVVHDF) 451
Continuous venovenous haemodialysis
  (CVVHD) 451
Continuous venovenous haemofiltration
  (CVVH) 451
Contraception
 diaphragm/spermicide 397
 emergency 615
 oral see Oral contraception
Convulsion(s) 371
 HIV/AIDS 419–420, 421, 422
 see also Seizures
Coombs' (antiglobulin) test 507
Co-ordination
 refugee health 707–708
 retrieval 691
Copper toxicosis 339
Core exogenous rewarming 754
Cornea 537
Coronary arterial gas emboli 758
Coronary artery bypass grafting (CABG)
 cardiogenic shock 27, 29
 ischaemic heart disease 187
Coronaviruses, chronic obstructive airway
  disease 288
Coroner (Australia) 667–670
 inquests 669–670
 investigations 668–669
 legislation 667–668
 reportable deaths 668
  reporting process 669
 use of expert opinion 669
Coroner (UK) 670–673
 bodies, handling of 672
 documentation 672
 family information 672
 history 671
 inquests 673–674
 post mortems 673
 preparing statements 669
 reportable deaths 672
 Scotland 672
 structure 671
Coroners' Acts (Australia) 668
Corrosives ingestion 840–843
 burns classification 842, 842
 clinical features 841
 common corrosives 840, 841
 complications, long-term 841
 investigations 841–842
 management 842
 oesophageal trauma see Oesophagus
 paraquat 862–864
 pathophysiology 840–841
Corticosteroid therapy
 Achilles tendon rupture 170
 adrenocortical insufficiency 471
 anaphylaxis 782–783, 783
 asthma 272–273
 autoimmune blistering disease 530
 avascular necrosis 152
 cerebral ischaemia 21
 chronic obstructive airway disease
  289–290
 conscious state alteration 370
 epiglottitis 270
 femoral neck fracture 153
 giant cell (temporal) arteritis 542

Corticosteroid therapy (*cont.*)
  gout 517
  head injury 51
  high altitude cerebral oedema 786
  hypercalcaemia 489–490
  inflammatory bowel disease 337
  meningitis 390, *390*
  myxoedema coma 470
  near-drowning 772
  psoriatic arthritis 522
  rheumatoid arthritis 520
  septic shock 30
  snakebite envenoming 883
  spinal cord injury 63
  subarachnoid haemorrhage 363
  systemic lupus erythematosus 521
  thyroid storm 469
Corynebacterium diphtheriae 407
  antibiotic susceptibility 427, 429, 431
  antibiotic therapy *426*
Costochondritis 180
Co-trimoxazole 431
  adverse reactions 431
  bacterial resistance 431
  HIV/AIDS 422
  induced fever 381
Counseling services
  domestic violence 622
  observation wards 711
Coxiella burnetii
  antibiotic susceptibility 430
  pneumonia 276
Coxsackie virus 180, 339
  arthritis 523
C-reactive protein
  conscious state alteration 368
  pelvic pain 574
Creatine kinase 185
  acute renal failure 447
Creatinine
  acute renal failure 447
  conscious state alteration 368
Crepitus, proximal humerus fracture 132
Creutzfeldt–Jakob disease *see* Variant Creutzfeldt–Jakob disease (vCJD)
Cricoid pressure 15, 16
Cricothyroidectomy
  epiglottitis 408
  prehospital emergency services 683
Cricothyroidotomy 19, 42, 67, 69
Cricothyrostomy 268
Crisis intervention 604–607
  assessment 605
  family/friends support 606
  follow-up 606
  goals 605
  implementation 606
  planning 605–606
  staff support 590, 606–607
Crisis process 604–605
Critical Incident Monitoring Study (CIMS) 739
Cross-infection control 312
  universal precautions 110, 593–594
Cross-sectional studies 649
Cruciate ligament injury 163–164
Crush syndrome 85
Cryoglobulin 447
Cryoprecipitate *495*, 499, 509
Cryptococcus neoformans
  cutaneous infection 405
  epididymo-orchitis 455

  meningitis 386, 387, 389, 419, 420, *420*, 422
Cryptosporidium
  gastroenteritis *313*
  immunocompromised patients 313
Cryptosporidium parvum
  gastroenteritis 312
  HIV/AIDS *420*
Crystalloid volume replacement
  alcoholic ketoacidosis 880
  anaphylaxis 782
  antihistamine overdose 798
  bowel obstruction 308
  burns patients 126
  gastrointestinal bleeding 318
  hypovolaemia 26–27, 449
  trauma 44
CSF otorrhoea 66
CSF rhinorrhoea 66, 69, 552
Cuboid fracture(s) 174
Cuneiform fracture(s) 174
Cupboard spider (*Steatoda*) 885
Curved-array transducer(s) 639
Cushing's syndrome 485
Cutaneous abscess(es) *see* Abscess(es)
Cyanide poisoning 791, 837–839
  clinical features 838
  conscious state alteration 367
  epidemiology 837
  management 838–839
  pathophysiology 837–838
  toxicokinetics 837–838
Cyclo-oxygenase inhibitor(s)
  COX-2 specific, acute liver failure 339
  dysfunctional uterine bleeding 568
  selective *vs.* non-selective 628
  see also individual drugs
Cyclophosphamide
  autoimmune blistering disease 530
  rheumatoid arthritis 520
Cyproheptadine 670, 797
  serotonin syndrome 750
Cystitis 396–397
  antibiotic management *400*
Cystography 98
Cytokine inhibitor(s)
  septic shock 31
  see also individual drugs
Cytomegalovirus
  acute interstitial nephritis 445
  arthritis 523
  granulocyte transfusions 497
  hepatitis 410
  HIV/AIDS 420, *420*, 422
  immunocompromised patients 313
  needlestick injuries 434–435
Cytoprotective agent(s), peptic ulcer disease 324

D

Danazol 569
Danis–Weber classification 169
Dantrolene
  malignant hyperthermia 750–751
  neuroleptic malignant syndrome 750
Dapsone 532
'Dashboard injuries', upper airway trauma 267
Data collection, clinical research 649, 652–653, 655
  proformas 653

Data management
  clinical research 649, 655
  clinical risk management 742
D-dimer 211
  acute renal failure 447
  deep vein thrombosis 234
Death 608
  aftercare 611
  breaking news 609–610
  definition 608
  documentation 669
  family/friends' support 609
  involuntary mental patients 666
  legal aspects 610–611
  organ donation 610–611
  process 608–609
  reactions to news 610
  reportable to coroner 668
  staff support 611
  viewing body 610
Death certificate 610, 668, 669
De Bakey classification 243
Decompression illness 758–761
  aerial transport
    following 761
    precipitating 759–760
  assessment 760
  avascular necrosis 152
  classification 758
  clinical features 759–760
  first aid 760
  further diving 761
  lidocaine 761
  oxygen therapy 261
  pathophysiology 758–759
  recompression 760–761
    portable recompression chambers 760
  retrieval 760
Decongestant(s), sinusitis 552
Decontamination rooms 718
Decubitus ulcer(s) 408–409
Deep vein thrombosis 178, 234–236
  clinical assessment 234–235
  differential diagnosis 235
  electric shock injury 776
  investigations 235
  management 213, 235–236
    thrombolytic therapy 236
  risk factors 234
  ultrasound 643
Defibrillation 8–10
  advanced life support 6, 7–10
  aircraft 689
  automated equipment 9
  basic life support 4–5, 8, 10
  biphasic waveform 10
  complications 9
  current-based 9–10
  electric shock injury 775
  failure 10
  retrieval 689
  technical problems 9
  technique 8–9
    paddle placement 8–9
    timing/energy of shocks 9
  torsades de pointes 205
  transthoracic impedance reduction 8
Delavirdine *see* Nevirapine (delavirdine)
Delayed transfusion reaction(s) 496–497
Deliberate self-harm 597–602
  aetiology 597–598
    alcohol intoxication 877
    drug overdose 795–796

Deliberate self-harm (*cont.*)
  assessment 599
  definition 597
  examination 599
  management/disposition 599–601
  patient characteristics 598–599
  repeated episodes 601
  risk assessment 601
  see also Suicide
Delirium 586, 587
  drug overdose 791, *791*
Delirium tremens 878
Delivery (childbirth)
  complications 559–560
    breech 559–560
    post-partum haemorrhage 560
    shoulder dyscrasia 560
  emergency 556–560
  equipment/drugs *558*
  examination 557
  history taking 556–557
  labour 557–559
    first stage 558
    second stage 558–559
    third stage 559
  post-delivery disposition 559
  post-delivery procedures 559
  preparations 557, *558*
  transfer to delivery suite 556, 557
  see also Labour
Delivery pack 557, 558, *558*
Delusion(s) 581–582
Dengue fever, thrombocytopenia 513
Dental caries 546
Dental trauma *see* Teeth, trauma
Depression
  domestic violence 620
  suicide/deliberate self-harm 598
De Quervain's tenosynovitis 524–525
Dermatitis, exfoliative 532, 533
Dermatology 528–534
  lesion definitions *528*
  skin disorder patterns *528*
  see also individual diseases/disorders
Dermatomyositis 519
Desferrioxamine 871
Dextromoramide 844
Dextrose
  alcoholic ketoacidosis 880
  hypoglycaemia 872–873
  sulphonylurea overdose 873
Diabetes insipidus
  central 485
  lithium toxicity 874
  nephrogenic 485
    of hypokalaemia *486*
Diabetes mellitus 462–466
  complications
    cellulitis 405–406
    foot infections 409
    ischaemic heart disease 183
    prevention 464
    stroke risk 353
    urinary tract infection 397
    Vibrio soft tissue infection 409
  differential diagnosis 464
  fever 382, 384
  gestational, shoulder dyscrasia 560
  management 464–465
    insulin therapy 464–465
    pancreatic transplantation 465
  open wound injury 109
  presentation 463

see also Hyperglycaemia; Hypoglycaemia
Diabetic hypoglycaemia 463
  management 465
  presentation 463
Diabetic ketoacidosis 462–463, 478
  differential diagnosis *463*, 464
  hypomagnesaemia 490
  investigations 463–464
  management 465
  presentation 463
  prognosis 466
Diacetylmorphine *see* Heroin
    (diacetylmorphine)
Diagnosis-related groups 724
Diagnostic peritoneal lavage
  abdominal trauma 72, 73, 96
    advantages/disadvantages *73*
  trauma in pregnancy 104
Dialysis *see* Haemodialysis
Diaphragm
  rupture 77
  trauma 94, *95*
Diarrhoea
  anaphylaxis 781
  differential diagnosis 314
  febrile patient 381
  gastroenteritis 312
  HIV/AIDS 418, 420, 421, 422
  hypernatraemia 485
  hypomagnesaemia 490
  inflammatory bowel disease 336
Diazepam
  alcohol withdrawal 879, *879*
  antipsychotic drug overdose 812
  antiretroviral drug interactions 423
  chemical restraint 593
  meningitis 390
  pharmacology 806
  status epilepticus 374
Diclofenac 322
Dicloxacillin 427
  cellulitis 405–406
  mastitis 408
  osteomyelitis 395
  septic arthritis 393
Dicobalt edetate (Kelocyanor) 838
Didanosine 432
  HIV/AIDS 422
Difficult intubation 16–18
  failed intubation drill *17*
Diffuse axonal injury 48, 51
Digital nerve block 631
Digital subtraction angiography (DSA) 96
Digoxin 208
  overdose 791, 803–805
    Fab fragment management *804*,
      804–805
    management 804–805
  pharmacokinetics 803
  serum level measurement 804
  thyroid storm 469
Dilated cardiomyopathy (DCM) 221
Diltiazem
  overdose 802
  pharmacokinetics 800
  pharmacology 801
Dimenhydrinate 670, 797
  overdose 670, 798
Diphenhydramine 670, 797
  overdose 670, 798
Diphenoxalate 315
Diphtheria *see Corynebacterium diphtheriae*
Dipyridamole 358

Disabilities, retrieval 692
Disasters 694–701
  all agencies (integrated) management
    approach 697
  all hazards management approach 697
  classification 694, *695*, *695*
  clinical risk management 742, *744*
  comprehensive management approach 697
  contamination with radioactive materials
    766–768
  definitions 695, *695*
  epidemiology 695–696
    incidence *696*
  exercises 697
  hazard-specific issues 698
    decontamination 699
  hospital care 700
  incident management 694, 697–698
    communications 698
    scene assessment 697
    site arrangements 698
  mass gatherings 700
  medical management 699
    casualty flow plan 699
    personnel 698–699
    stabilization 699
    trapped patients 699
    triage 699
  mental health issues 590
  planning 591, 697–698
  prepared community approach 697
  public health issues 591
  socioeconomic impact 696–697
  transportation of patients 699–700
  triage 704–705
  Urban Search and Rescue 700
Discitis, back pain 523
Discogenic sciatica, back pain 523
Disease-modifying antirheumatic drugs
    (DMARDs) 520
Dislocation(s) *see individual joints*
Disodium pamidronate, hypercalcaemia 489
Disseminated intravascular coagulation
    (DIC) 509, 512–513
  acute renal failure 448
Dissociation, domestic violence 620
Distal humerus fracture(s) 134–135
Distressed relatives' room 718–719
Diuretic drugs
  acute interstitial nephritis 445
  acute renal failure 445–446, 449
  funnel web spider *(Atrax/Hadronyche)*
    bite 887
  hypernatraemia 485
  hypokalaemia *484*
  hypomagnesaemia 490
  hypovolaemia 449
  lithium excretion 874
  renal insufficiency 240
  see also individual drugs
Dive reflex 770
Diverticulosis
  colonoscopic management 343
  rectal bleeding 341–342
Diving 756–625
  after decompression illness 761
  barotrauma *see* Barotrauma
  decompression illness *see* Decompression
    illness
  emergency phone numbers 762
  gas contamination 762
  mask squeeze 758
  nitrogen narcosis 762

Diving (*cont.*)
oxygen toxicity 762
physiology 756–758
pulmonary oedema 762
vertigo 762
DNA testing in rape 616
Dobutamine 28
septic shock 30
Documentation
complaints 735, 738
consent (UK) 679
domestic violence 622
retrieval 692
Domestic violence 619–623
alcohol intoxication 877
definition 619
detection, barriers to 621
incidence 619
management 622
physical injury/illness 620
predictors of 619–620
psychological effects 620–621
screening 621
social effects 621
Do not resuscitate (DNR) order(s) 34
Donway splint(s)
femoral shaft fracture 157
subtrochanteric femur fracture 155
Dopamine 28
crush syndrome 85
septic shock 30
Doppler ultrasound 637
arterial limb ischaemia 232
cerebral vascular injury 88
femoral shaft fracture 157
foot injury 172
Doxycycline
community-acquired pneumonia 280
pelvic inflammatory disease 571
sexually-transmitted diseases 614
Doxylamine poisoning 670, 798
Dressings 119
Droperidol
chemical restraint 593
migraine 350
Drowning 769
alcohol intoxication 877
pathophysiology 770
reportable deaths 668
wet/dry 770
see also Near-drowning
Drug abuse 844–853
'body-packers' 851–852
'body-stuffers' 852
conscious state alteration 367–368
consent while intoxicated (Australia) 675
consent while intoxicated (UK) 678
domestic violence 620, 622
intravenous *see* Intravenous drug abusers
mental health legislation (Australia) 663
overdose 790–796
agitation/delirium 791, *791*
antidotes 795, *796*
cardiovascular effects *791*
cellular toxins 791
disposition 795
drug level measurements 792–793,
793, 793
enhanced elimination 795, *795*
examination 792
gastrointestinal decontamination
794–795
history taking 792

investigations 792–793
pathophysiology 790–791
poisons information 792
prehospital emergency services 685
respiratory failure 790, *790*
seizures 376
subarachnoid haemorrhage 364
supportive care 793–794
toxic autonomic syndromes
('toxidromes') 792, *792*
suicide/deliberate self-harm 598
see also individual drugs
Drug-induced fever 381
Drug-induced haemolysis 510, *510*
Drug-induced hepatitis 410, *412*
Drug-induced rash 381
Drug-induced serotonin syndrome
748–749, *749*
Dry drowning 770
Duke criteria 225
Duverney fracture(s) 151
Dying patient(s) 608–612
Dysarthria, phenytoin overdose 817
Dysbarism *see* Barotrauma; Decompression
illness; Diving
Dysfunctional uterine bleeding (DUB) 567
management 568–569
Dysmenorrhoea
adenomyosis 576
chronic pelvic pain 576
Dyspareunia 567
Dysphagia 302–305
anaphylaxis 781
causes *302*
disposition 305
febrile patients 383
HIV/AIDS 420, 421, 422
management 305

E

Ear 550–551
barotrauma 757
hyperbaric oxygen 761
middle ear *see* Middle-ear barotrauma
foreign body removal 550
infection 551
otitis externa 551
otitis media 551
otitis media with effusion (glue ear) 551
trauma 550–551
lightning injury 777
wound repair 117
Ebstein's anomaly 29
ECASS 2 study 359
Echocardiography
aortic dissection 245–246
aortic incompetence 226–227
cardiac tamponade 217–219, 643
chest pain differential diagnosis 179
chronic aortic incompetence 226–227
mitral incompetence 227, 229
myocardial contusion 78
myocardial laceration 78
myocarditis 220
pericardial effusions 643
pericarditis 216
pulmonary embolism 643
stroke 357
subarachnoid haemorrhage 363
transient ischaemic attacks 357

transoesophageal *see* Transoesophageal
echocardiography (TOE)
transthoracic *see* Transthoracic
echocardiography (TTE)
ultrasound 643
Echo virus 180
Eclampsia 376
management 240
Ecological studies 649
Economics
domestic violence 621
suicide/deliberate self-harm 598
Ecstasy (MDMA) 180, 849
acute hyponatraemia 482
acute liver failure 339
Ectopic pregnancy 561–563
diagnosis 561
ultrasound 640
management 562–563
ultrasound 640
Ectopic tachyarrhythmias 198
Edinburgh face masks 257
Efavirenz 422
Effusions, knee injury 159
Ehlers–Danlos syndrome 29
Elbow disorders 524
dislocations 136–137
fractures 99
Elderly patients
acute appendicitis 332, 333, *333*
bed rest complications 106, 108
burns 107
cerebrovascular disease 353–354
classification 105
co-morbidity 105–106, 108
disposition 107
fever 382
fractures 106–107
Colles' fracture 140
gastrointestinal bleeding 317–318, 319
haemorrhage management 505
meningitis 387
observation wards 711
osteoporosis 106, 107, 108
outcomes 108
trauma 105–108
abdominal injuries 107
causes 106
fractures *see also Fractures*
head injury 106–107, 108
pathophysiology 106
pelvic injury 107
penetrating injuries 107
prevention 108
resuscitation management 106, 107
spinal injuries 107
thoracic injuries 107
urinary tract infection 396
management 401
Electricity 774
retrieval 690
Electric shock injury 774–777
clinical effects 84, 775–776
emergency department management 776
physical determinants 774–775
physiological changes 774
in pregnancy 776
prehospital management 776
prevention 777
prognosis 776
thermal injury 774
ventricular fibrillation 774, 776
see also Lightning injury

Electrocardiography (ECG)
  acute pulmonary oedema 194
  antihistamine overdose 798
  aortic dissection 242–245
  atrial fibrillation *207*
  atrial flutter *208*
  beta-blocker overdose 802
  bradycardia-tachycardia (sick sinus)
      syndrome 199
  cardiac tamponade 219
  chest pain differential diagnosis 179,
      180
  chronic obstructive airway disease 287
  conscious state alteration 369
  drug overdose 792
  electric shock injury 776
  gastrointestinal bleeding 318–319
  heart block
    first degree atrioventricular *199,*
        199–200
    left anterior fascicular 202, *203*
    left bundle branch *see* Left bundle
        branch block
    left posterior fascicular 202
    right bundle branch *202, 203*
    second degree Mobitz I (Wenkebach)
        200, *200*
    second degree Mobitz II 200, *200*
    third degree (complete) 201, *201*
  hydrofluoric acid burns 866
  hyperkalaemia 487
  hypertension 239
  hypocalcaemia 488
  hypokalaemia 486
  hypomagnesaemia 490
  hypothermia 753, *753*
  myocardial infarction 185–186
  myocarditis 220
  paroxysmal supraventricular tachycardia
      206
  pericarditis 215–216
  pulmonary embolism 210
  rapid sequence intubation 15
  sinus bradycardia 199
  torsades de pointes 205, *206*
  ventricular tachycardia 203–205, *204*
  Wolff-Parkinson-White syndrome *206*
Electroencephalography (EEG)
  pseudoseizures 375
  seizures 373
Electrolyte balance
  acute renal failure 447
  conscious state alteration 368
  disturbances 481–491
    crush syndrome 85
    hypertension 239
  imbalance correction 449–450
  see also individual diseases/disorders
Electromechanical dissociation 8, 10, 208
  causes 208
Eli Lilly Cyanide kit 839
ELISA (enzyme-linked immunoabsorbent
    assays) 235
Ellis classification 547, *547*
Embolization
  gastro-oesophageal varices 320
  peptic ulcer bleeding 318
  unstable pelvic fracture 149
Emergency contraception, rape 615
Emesis, iron overdose 871
Emphysema 286–287
Employment, suicide/deliberate self-harm
    598

Empyema, community-acquired pneumonia
    284–285
Encephalopathy, opioid abuse 845
Endocarditis, infectious *see* Infective
    endocarditis
Endogenous rewarming 754
Endometriosis, pelvic pain 573
  acute 574
  chronic 575, 576
Endometritis, post-partum haemorrhage *vs.*
    566
Endomyocardial biopsy 220–221
Endoscopic retrograde
    cholangiopancreatography (ERCP),
    choledocholithiasis 328
Endoscopy
  bowel obstruction 308
  corrosives ingestion 842
  dysphagia 302
  gastrointestinal bleeding 318, *318*
  gastro-oesophageal varices
    ligation 320
    sclerotherapy 319, 320
  inflammatory bowel disease 336
  iron overdose 871
  peptic ulcer disease 323
    haemorrhage management 319
  upper airway obstruction 266
  upper airway trauma 268
Endothelin antagonists 196
Endotracheal intubation *see* Tracheal
    intubation
Endpoints, clinical research 649, 651
End-tidal CO_2
  advanced life support 13
  rapid sequence intubation 15
  shock 25
Enflurane 43
  malignant hyperthermia 751
Enhanced elimination procedure, drug
    overdose 795
Enhancement, ultrasound 637
Enkephalins 626
Entamoeba histolytica
  antibiotic susceptibility 431
  gastroenteritis 312, *313*
  HIV/AIDS 420, *420*
  traveller's diarrhoea 313
Enteral decontamination 340
Enterobacter 29
  antibiotic resistance 351, 428
  antibiotic therapy *426*
  cholangitis 328
Enterococcus
  antibiotic therapy *426*
  infective endocarditis *224*
Enterococcus faecalis
  ampicillin susceptibility 428
  antibiotic susceptibility 431
Enteroinvasive *Escherichia coli* (EIEC) *313*
Enteropathogenic *Escherichia coli* (EPEC)
    313
Enterotoxigenic *Escherichia coli* (ETEC)
    313, *313*
Enzyme-linked immunoabsorbent assays
    (ELISAs) 235
Ephedrine, neurogenic shock 32
Epicondylitis 524
Epidemic myalgia (Bornholm disease) 180
Epidermolysis bullosa acquisita 530, 532,
    534
Epididymo-orchitis 455–456
  ultrasound 643

Epidural abscess(es), back pain 523
Epigastric hernia 310
Epiglottitis 269–270, 408
  adult 383
  antibiotic therapy 270
  corticosteroid therapy 270
  radiology 266
  Vallecula sign *266*
Epilepsy 373
  management strategy 371–372
  post-traumatic 376
  in pregnancy 376
  seizure types 371
Epinephrine *see* Adrenaline
Epistaxis 552–553
Epsilon-aminocaproic acid 363
  haemophilia 502
Epstein–Barr virus (EBV)
  acute interstitial nephritis 445
  arthritis 523
  hepatitis 410
  thrombocytopenia 513
EquIP (Evaluation and Quality Improvement
    Program) 721
Equipment
  business planning 725
  emergency delivery *558*
Erbs palsy, shoulder dyscrasia 560
Ergotamine, analgesia 630
Erysipelas 405
Erysipelothrix, antibiotic susceptibility 428
Erythema multiforme 531, *532*, 533
Erythema nodosum 531
Erythrocyte sedimentation rate (ESR)
  conscious state alteration 368
  pelvic pain 574
  subarachnoid haemorrhage 363
Erythroderma 529, 532
  management 534
Erythromycin 178, 429
  bacterial resistance 429–430
  community-acquired pneumonia 280
  drug interactions 429
  endometritis 566
  gonococcal arthritis 521
  infective arthritis 522
  mastitis 408
  sexually-transmitted diseases 614
Erythropoiesis, anaemia 506–507
Escharotomy 126
Escherichia coli 29, 126
  acute epididymo-orchitis 455
  antibiotic resistance 428, 430
    aminoglycosides 430
    co-trimoxazole 432
    erythromycin 429–430
  antibiotic susceptibility 431–432
    ampicillin 428
    cephalosporin 349
  antibiotic therapy *426*
  cholangitis 328
  cutaneous infection 405
  enteroinvasive (EIEC) *313*
  enteropathogenic (EPEC) *313*
  enterotoxigenic (ETEC) 313, *313*
  gangrene 406–407
  gastroenteritis 312, 315, *313*
  meningitis 389
  pneumonia, mortality 282
  thrombotic thrombocytopenic purpura
      512
  urinary tract infection 396, 397, *400*
ESI Triage Algorithm 704

Esmolol 468
  aortic dissection 247
  pharmacology *801*, 802
Essex–Lopressti fracture-dislocation 138
Ethambutol 516
  HIV/AIDS 422
Ethanol, pharmacology 877
Ethanol toxicity *see* Alcohol abuse; Alcohol
    intake
Ethics 33–37
  clinical research 649, 655–656
  mandated choice 37
  medical decision-making principles 34
  resuscitation 34–37
    benefits 34
    consent 34, 35–36
    futility 35
    harms 34–35
    practising procedures on newly dead 36–37
    withdrawing 36–37
    withholding 37
  violent patient 594–595
Ethylene glycol toxicity
  acidosis 478
  hepatitis 410
Etidronate, hypercalcaemia 489
Etomidate 43
Euvolaemic hypernatraemia 485
Euvolaemic hyponatraemia 482, *482*
Exchange transfusion(s), sickle cell anaemia
    508, *508*
Exercise testing 179
Exfoliative dermatitis 532, 533
Expert opinion 669
Expired air resuscitation (EAR) 4
Exposure, retrieval 692
External cardiac massage (ECM) 4
External ear barotrauma 757
External exogenous rewarming 754
External fixation, unstable pelvic fracture 149
External validity, clinical research 651
Extracapsular hip fracture(s) 153–154, *154*
Extracorporeal oxygenation
  near-drowning 772
  retrieval 687
Extracorporeal shockwave lithotripsy 458
Extradural intracranial haematoma 48
Eye
  emergencies 536–543
  inflammatory conditions 538–540
  movements, conscious state alteration
      367, *368*
  trauma 536–538
    blunt 537–538
    chemical burns 538
    facial trauma 66, 69
    history taking 536
    investigations 537
    management 537–538
    penetrating 537, *537*
    prevention 538
    superficial 537
    visual acuity assessment 536–537
Eyelid injury 67
  wound repair 117

F

FABER test 150
Fab fragments of digoxin-specific antibodies
    804, 804–805

Face mask oxygenation 18, 42, 257, *257*
Facial cellulitis 405
Facial nerve injury 67
Facial trauma 65–70
  central facial smash 89
  dental trauma 546, 547
  examination 66
  fractures 68–69
  history 66
  management
    haemorrhage control 67
    immediate 66–67
    wound repair 116–117, *120*
  medicolegal aspects 67
  penetrating injuries 69
  radiology 66, 88–89
  soft tissue injuries 67–68, 403
  temporomandibular joint dislocation 69
Factor VIII replacement therapy 502
Factor IX replacement therapy 502
Faecal occult blood testing 317
Faeces culture 314
Falls (in elderly) 106
Famciclovir 432
  hepatitis B 414
Family/friends
  bereavement aftercare 611
  breaking news of death 609–610
  crisis intervention 606
  emergency department facilities 718–719
  grief management 608, 610
  information concerning death 669
  reactions to news of death 610
  viewing body 610
Famotidine, peptic ulcer disease 319, 324
Fasciotomy 84
Fat embolism 84
  femoral shaft fracture 157
Fatty liver of pregnancy, acute 340
Federal Privacy Act (1988) 735–736
Feedback, observation wards 712
Feet
  anatomy 171
  fractures
    calcaneus 173, *173*
    cuboid 174
    cuneiform 174
    forefoot 174–175
    Lisfranc 174
    metatarsus 174–175
    midfoot 173–174
    navicular 173–174
    phalanges 175
    subtalar dislocations 172–173
    talar fractures 172
  injury 171–175
    examination 171–172
    fractures *see also* Fractures
    history 171
    radiography 172
  nerve blocks at ankle 632
Felbamate 818
Felodipine 801
Femoral artery
  aneurysms 251
  injury 83
    femoral shaft fracture 157
Femoral hernia 310
Femoral nerve block 82, 632
  femoral neck fracture 153
Femoral vein cannulation 643
Femur fracture 82
  distal 160

  head 152–153
  intertrochanteric 153–154, *154*
  neck fracture in elderly 106, 153
  shaft 157–158, *158*
  subtrochanteric 155
  see also Hip, fractures
Fenoldapam
  hypertension in stroke 240
  renal insufficiency 240
Fentanyl 43
  analgesia 628
  dosage *628*
Fetal heart rate monitoring 557
Fetomaternal haemorrhage 103
Fetor hepaticus 367
Fever 380–309, 380–385
  'at-risk' patient groups 382
    alcoholic patients 382, 384
    elderly people 382
    HIV/AIDS 418, 420, 421, 422
    immunocompromised patients
        382–383, 384
    intravenous drug users 382, 384
    splenectomized patients 382
  diabetes mellitus 382, 384
  disposition 384–385
  evolution of illness 383
  examination 381–382
  follow-up 384–385
  history taking 380–381
  investigations 381–382
  localized infections 381–382
  management 381–384
  meningococcal meningitis 383–384, 387
  neutropenia 382, 499, 500
  non-specific clinical features 383
  thyroid storm 468, 469
  travellers' 383, 384
  urgent intervention *380*, 380–381, *384*
  zoonoses 383
  see also Hyperthermia
Fexofenadine 797–798
Fibreoptic bronchoscope-assisted intubation
    18–19
Fibroids *see* Leiomyoma (fibroids)
Fibula
  anatomy 165–166
  fractures 167
Filarial epididymo-orchitis *455*
Finger injuries, occupational 146
Finkelstein's test 524–525
First aid
  box jellyfish *(Chironex fleckeri)*
      envenomation 890–891
  electric shock injury 776
  funnel web spider *(Atrax/Hadronyche)*
      bite 887
  irukandji *(Carukia barnesi)* envenomation
      891
  lightning injury 778
  near-drowning 771
  radioactive materials contamination
      766–768
  redback spider *(Latrodectus hasseltii)* bite
      886
  snakebite 882–883
    sea snake 891
  see also Basic life support; Prehospital
      emergency services
First medical responders 698–699
Fish fancier's finger 407
Fish spine wounds 892
Fissure in ano 346

Fit(s) 371
  see also Seizures
Fitz–Hugh–Curtis syndrome 570
Fixation
  external, unstable pelvic fracture 149
  internal *see* Internal fixation
Fixed drug eruption(s) 531
Flail chest 77
Flecainide 207, 208
Fleck sign, Lisfranc fractures 174
Flucloxacillin 51, 82, 427
  facial cellulitis 405
  infective endocarditis 226
  osteomyelitis 395
  otitis externa 551
  septic arthritis 393
  septic shock 31
  Staphylococcus aureus pneumonia 280
Fluconazole, HIV/AIDS 422
Flucytosine, meningitis *389*
Fluid attenuated inversion recover (FLAIR) 362
Fluid balance *see* Volume replacement
Fluoride toxicity *see* Hydrofluoric acid burns
5-Fluorocytosine 34
Fluoroquinolones 431–432
  urinary tract infection 399, 400–401
  see also individual drugs
Fluphenazine, overdose 810
Focused trauma ultrasound 73
Focussed assessment by sonography for
  trauma (FAST) 97, *97, 639*, 639–640
Folate deficiency 505–506
Folliculitis 405
Food allergy 779
Forced-air rewarming 754–755
Forearm fracture(s) 138–141
  Colles' fracture 106, *140*, 140–141
  distal radius/ulna 140–141
  Galeazzi fracture-dislocation 139–140, *140*
  Monteggia fracture-dislocation 139
  radial head 138
  radial neck 138
  radial shaft 139
  radius/ulna shaft 138–139
  ulna shaft 139
Foreign bodies
  cornea 537
  cutaneous abscess 403
  dysphagia 302–305
  ear 550
  hand injuries 146
  nose 551–552
  ocular trauma 537
  throat 302–305, 553
  ultrasound 644
  upper airway obstruction 266, 267,
    302–305
  wound contamination 110
Forensic examination
  consent 615
  sexual assault 615–616
Formality, lack of, complaints 735–736
Foscarnet, HIV/AIDS 422
'F pieces' 257
Fracture(s)
  closed reduction *see* Closed reduction
  comminuted *see* Comminuted fractures
  compartment syndrome 84
  compound 81
  elderly patients 106–107
  electric shock injury 776
  limb trauma 81, 82

open reduction *see* Open reduction with
  internal fixation (ORIF)
  reduction 82
  simple (closed) 81
  see also individual bones
Free-flowing circuits, pure oxygen therapy
  258, *258*
Free radical-mediated damage
  cerebral reperfusion injury 20–21
  paraquat poisoning 863
Freidrich–Waterhouse syndrome 470
Frequency dysuria syndrome 399
Fresh frozen plasma *495*, 498–499
Frontal sinus fracture 88–89
Furosemide
  acute pulmonary oedema 194–195
  hypercalcaemia 489
  hyperkalaemia 487
  hypernatraemia 485
Full blood count (FBC) *503*
  hypertension 239
  thrombocytopenia 513
  vaginal bleeding 568
Fuller's Earth, paraquat poisoning 863
Funding, retrieval 690
Fungal meningitis 386, 388
Funnel web spider (*Atrax/Hadronyche*)
  887–888
Furuncle 405, 551
Fusobacterium, antibiotic susceptibility 428,
  431
Futility concept 35

G

Gabapentin 818
Galeazzi fracture-dislocation 139–140, *140*
Gallbladder disease 326–328
  ultrasound 642
  see also Biliary tract disease
Gallstones 327
  ultrasound 642
Gamekeeper's thumb (ulnar collateral
  ligament rupture) 99, 145
Gamma-hydroxybutyrate abuse 850–851
  management 851
Ganciclovir, HIV/AIDS 422
Gangrene 406–407
Garden classification, femoral neck fracture
  153
Gas embolism 356
Gas expansion, diving physiology 756
Gas gangrene 406–407
Gas supplies 716
Gastric outlet obstruction 841
  peptic ulcer disease 325, 326
  perforation 325
Gastritis 322–325
Gastroenteritis 311–316
  clinical examination 313–314
  clinical features 312, 314
  differential diagnosis 314
  hospital acquired 313
  immunocompromised patients 313
  investigations 314
  management 314–315
    antibiotic regimen *315*
    cross-infection control 312
  microbiology 312, *313*
  observation wards 710
  traveller's diarrhoea 313

Gastrograffin
  dysphagia 305
  oesophagus/diaphragm injury 79, 96
Gastrointestinal system
  barotrauma 758
  bleeding 316–322
    acuity of blood loss 317
    co-morbidities 317–318
    determining site 316
    inflammatory bowel disease 336
    initial management 318–319
    investigations 318
    nasogastric aspiration 316–317, *317*
    outpatient management criteria 321,
      321
    peptic ulcer disease 323–324
    rectal bleeding 341–344
    upper gastrointestinal tract 317, *317*
  changes in pregnancy 102
  decontamination 825
    antihistamine overdose 799
    glyphosphate poisoning 862
    iron overdose 871
    paraquat poisoning 863
    salicylate overdose 829
  dialysis, drug overdose 794
  see also Stomach
Gastro-oesophageal varices 317, 319–320
  endoscopic therapy 318, *318*
Gender, suicide/deliberate self-harm 598
Genitourinary injuries, pelvic fracture
  149–150
Gentamicin 82, 429, 430
  acute cholecystitis 327
  adverse reactions 430
  biliary tract disease 327
  bowel obstruction 308
  cholangitis 328
  infective endocarditis 226
  peptic ulcer disease 324
  septic shock 31
Gestational age estimation 556
Gestational diabetes, shoulder dyscrasia 560
Giant cell (temporal) arteritis 541–542
  headache *349*
Giardia lamblia 312, 314
  antibiotic susceptibility 431
  gastroenteritis 312, 315, *313*
  traveller's diarrhoea 313
Gitelman's syndrome, alkalosis 479
Glasgow Coma Scale 49, *49*, 51, 365, *365*
  elderly head injured patients 107
  prehospital emergency services 683
Glasgow Outcome Scale 45
Glaucoma
  acute angle-closure 538–539
  headache *349*
Glenohumeral dislocations, with proximal
  humerus fracture 134
Glibenclamide, overdose 873
Gliclazide, overdose 873
Glimepriride, overdose 873
Glipizide, overdose 873
Globus 302
Glomerular filtration rate (GFR), acute renal
  failure 440
Glomerulonephritis 443–444, 445
  proteinuria 443
  signs/symptoms 446
  urinary tests 448
Gloves, protective 110
Glucagon 465
  anaphylaxis 782, 783, *783*

Glucose-6-phosphate dehydrogenase
    deficiency 507
    methaemoglobinaemia 855, 855–856
Glue ear (otitis media with effusion) 551
Glyceryl trinitrate (GTN)
    analgesia 630
    aortic dissection 247
    hypertensive encephalopathy 240
Glycoprotein IIb/IIIa receptor inhibitors
    188
Glyphosphate poisoning 862
    clinical grading 862
Gold salts, rheumatoid arthritis 520
Gonorrhoea see Neisseria gonorrhoeae
Gout 516–517
    Achilles tendon rupture 170
    clinical features 517
    investigations 517
        synovial fluid findings 517, 518
    management 517
Gram-negative organisms
    nosocomial pneumonia 284
    sepsis 29–30
Granulocytes transfusion 497
    neutropenia 500
Graves' disease (toxic diffuse goitre) 467
    idiopathic thrombocytopenic purpura 512
Gravitational traction, shoulder dislocation
    131
Greater trochanteric fracture(s) 154
Great vessel injury 96
Grief 608, 610
    reactions to situational loss 604, 605
    resolution 611
Guardianship Boards (Australia) 675
Guedel airway 19
Guidelines 720–721
    advanced life support 6–7
    antibiotic therapy, gastroenteritis 315
    antihypertensives in stroke 358
    myocardial infarction early management
        186
    resuscitation 2, 3
    snakebite management 883–884
Guillain–Barré syndrome, acidosis 478
Gunshot wounds, subtrochanteric femur
    fracture 155

H

H₁-antagonists 669
    anaphylaxis 782
    applications 797
    overdose 670, 798
    pharmacodynamics 669, 797–798
    see also Antihistamines
H₂-antagonists 669
    applications 797
        acute liver failure 340
        anaphylaxis 782
        NSAID-induced ulcer management 325
        peptic ulcer disease 324
    haemorrhage 319
    overdose 670, 798
    pharmacodynamics 669, 798
    see also Antihistamines
Hadronyche (funnel web spider) 887–888
Haemarthrosis 518–519
    avascular necrosis 152
    haemophilia 501
    knee injury 159, 160

tibial plateau fractures 160–161
tibia tubercule fracture 167
Haematemesis 316, 342
Haematocrit see Full blood count (FBC)
Haematology
    changes in pregnancy 102
    conscious state alteration 368
    early pregnancy 562
Haematoma
    ear 550, 551
    extradural intracranial 48
    femoral shaft fracture 157
    intertrochanteric femur fracture 153
    mediastinal 79, 95
    radial head/neck fractures 138
    subdural intracranial 48, 51
    upper airway obstruction 266
Haematuria 457
    glomerulonephritis 443
    pelvic fractures 149
    urinary tract infection 398
Haemodiafiltration, acute renal failure 451
Haemodialysis
    acute renal failure 451
    crush syndrome 85
    drug overdose 795, 795
        salicylates 829
    hydrofluoric acid burns 867
    hyperkalaemia 487
    lithium toxicity 875
    metformin overdose 873
Haemodynamic monitoring
    advanced life support 13
    asthma 272
    cardiac tamponade 219
    shock 25
    trauma 44
        elderly patients 107
Haemoglobin C disease 508
Haemoglobin H disease 508
Haemoglobin–oxygen dissociation curves
    255, 255
Haemoglobin sickle cell disease 508
    see also Sickle cell anaemia
Haemoglobinuria, acute tubular necrosis
    443
Haemolysis 516
    associated infections 510, 510
    drug/toxins-induced 510, 510
    mechanical trauma 509–510
    near-drowning 770
    transfusion reactions 496
Haemolytic anaemia 506–510
    acquired 508–509
    aplastic crisis 507
    cold autoimmune 508–509
Haemolytic uremic syndrome (HUS) 445,
    509
Haemoperfusion, drug overdose 795, 795
Haemophilia 501–503
    clinical presentation 501–502
    inhibitors 502–503
    management 502–503
Haemophilia A 501
    management 502–503
Haemophilia B (Christmas disease) 501
    management 503
Haemophilus, antibiotic
    resistance/susceptibility 425, 430,
    432
Haemophilus influenzae
    antibiotic resistance 428
    antibiotic susceptibility 429, 430, 431

ampicillin 428
cephalosporin 349
antibiotic therapy 426
cellulitis 405–406
chronic obstructive airway disease 288,
    290
epiglottitis 270, 383
erysipelas 405
facial cellulitis 405
infection routes 276
meningitis 383, 387, 389, 390, 390, 389
otitis media 551
pelvic inflammatory disease 570
pneumonia 276
    cavitating lesions 283
    management 280
    sputum analysis 277–278
quinsy (peritonsillar abscess) 269
sinusitis 552
vaccination 389
Haemophilus parainfluenzae
    chronic obstructive airway disease 288
    epiglottitis 270
Haemoptysis 300–302
    aetiology 300, 300
    clinical assessment 300
    massive 301–302
Haemorrhage(s)
    anaemia 503–505
        clinical features 504
        investigations 504–505
    causes 503, 504
        electric shock injury 776
        thrombocytopenia 513
    chronic 505
    fetomaternal 103
    intra-abdominal 71–72, 73
    management 505
        coagulation factors replacement 44
        hypovolaemic shock 25, 26
        surgical ligation of source 45
    trauma 43
        facial 67
        femoral shaft fracture 157
        limb 81
        pelvic fracture 149
        uterine in pregnancy 103
    see also individual haemorrhages
Haemorrhagic shock 24
    elderly fracture patients 107
    femoral shaft fracture 157
Haemorrhoid(s) 342, 345–346
Haemothorax 77–78, 79, 93
Hairline radial head/neck fractures 138
Hallucination(s) 581–582, 583, 586, 587,
    591
Haloperidol
    chemical restraint 593
    meningitis 390
    overdose 810
Halothane 43
    acute liver failure 339
    hepatitis 410, 412
    malignant hyperthermia 751
Hamman's crunch 292
Hand injuries
    antibiotic prophylaxis 145
    disposition 146
    dorsum/dorsal tendon repair 146
    foreign bodies 146
    hydrofluoric acid burns 128
    metacarpal 145–146
    metacarpophalangeal joints 145

Hand injuries (*cont.*)
  occupational 146
  palmar wounds 146
  penetrating wounds 146
  prevention 146
  prognosis 146
  radiography 146
Handling of patient 54
Handover, retrieval 691
Hangman's fracture 55, 56
Hantavirus, acute interstitial nephritis 445
Hapalochlaena maculosa (blue-ringed
    octopus) envenomation 891–892
Hare splints, femoral shaft fracture 157
Hashimoto's (autoimmune) thyroiditis 469
Hawkin's classification, talar fractures 172
Hb-Barts hydrops syndrome 508
HCO_3-values 476
Headache 348–351
  analgesia 630
  assessment 349
  bacterial meningitis 387
  carbon monoxide poisoning 834
  classic clinical complexes *349*
  febrile patients 383
  HIV/AIDS 420, 422
  investigations 349
  pathophysiological causes 348, *348*
  subarachnoid haemorrhage 361, 363
  see also Migraine
Head injury
  airway management 16, 49
  cerebral hypoxia 20, 48
  elderly patients 106–107, *107*
  haemophilia 501
  investigations 49–50
  management 50–51
  mild 49–50
    patient advice 49, *50*
  moderate to severe 50–51
  post-traumatic epilepsy 376
  radiology 87
  stress ulcers 317
  volume replacement 49
Head and neck
  secondary survey 58, 59
  wound repair outcome 119, 121
Heart
  conducting system 197–198
    accessory tracts 198
  enzymes 179, 185
  failure 183
    hypervolaemic hyponatraemia 482
    Killip classification 189
    post-myocardial infarction 189
    see also Left ventricular failure
  pacing 200, 203
    organophosphates poisoning 859–860
  pain 178
  rehabilitation 190
  rupture 189
  troponin 185
  valve emergencies 223–231
    infective endocarditis 223–226
  see also under Cardiac
Heart block 199–200
  combination blocks 203
  electrocardiography *see*
    Electrocardiography (ECG)
  first degree atrioventricular 199–200
  left anterior fascicular 202
  left bundle branch *see* Left bundle branch
    block

left posterior fascicular 202
right bundle branch 201
second degree
  Mobitz I (Wenkebach) 200, *200*
  Mobitz II 200
third degree (complete) 200–201
Heat exhaustion 748, 749
  management 750
Heat-related illness 748–751
  diagnosis 750
  hyperthermia *see* Hyperthermia
  hypothermia *see* Hypothermia
  management 750–751
Heatstroke 748, 749
  classic 748
  exertional 748
  management 750
  prognosis 751
  risk factors *748*
Heimlich manoeuvre 3, 267, 771
Helicobacter pylori
  antibiotic susceptibility 431
  diagnostic tests 323
  eradication therapy 324
  peptic ulcer disease 322
Helicopter services
  disasters management 698–699, 699–700
  retrieval *688*, 689
Heliox, asthma 273
HELLP syndrome 239, 509
  acute renal failure 445
  thrombocytopenia 512
Henderson classification 169
Heparin
  deep vein thrombosis 235
  ischaemic heart disease 189
  ischaemic stroke 359
  prosthetic valves 230
  pulmonary embolism 213
  thrombocytopenia 512
  transient ischaemic attacks 358
Hepatic artery aneurysm 250
Hepatic encephalopathy 338, 339
  conscious state alteration 367
  grading 338
  management 340
  thiamine 367
Hepatitis 410–416
  alcoholic 415–416
  chronic 411
    autoimmune 416
  drug-induced 410, *412*
  viral 339, 381, 411–415
    acute liver failure 339, 411–412
    characteristics 411–412
    fever 381
    needlestick injury transmission 435,
      435
    see also individual types below
Hepatitis A 339, *411*, 412–413
  acute interstitial nephritis 445
  acute liver failure 410
  immunization 413
  management 413
Hepatitis B 410, *411*, 413–414
  acute liver failure 339, 340, 410
  arthritis 522
  chronic hepatitis 410, 414
  clinical course 413–414
  epidemiology 413
  immunization 414, 435, 614
  laboratory tests 413
  management 414

needlestick injuries 434, 435
  postexposure management *435*
serology 413–414
Hepatitis B immune globulin (HBIG) 435,
    435
Hepatitis C 410, *411*, 414–415
  acute liver failure 339
  chronic hepatitis 410, 414
  management 415
  needlestick injuries 434, 435
Hepatitis D 410, *411*, 415
  acute liver failure 339
Hepatitis E 339, 410, *411*, 415
Hepatitis F 410
Hepatitis G 410, *411*, 415
Hepatitis GB 410, *411*, 415
Hepatorenal syndrome 447
Herbal medicine, anticholinergic effects 797
Hereditary haemorrhagic telangiectasia
    (Osler-Rendu-Weber syndrome) 342
Hereditary spherocytosis 507
Hernia 309–311
  bowel obstruction 306, 307, 308
  complications 310
  epigastric 310
  femoral 310
  management 310–311
  Richter's 310
  sportsman's 310
Heroin (diacetylmorphine) 844
  abuse 598
  'body-packers'/'body-stuffers' 852
  complications 845
Herpes simplex virus (HSV)
  acute liver failure 339
  arthritis 523
  HIV/AIDS 419, 420
  keratitis 540
  vesicles 531
Herpes zoster 180
  analgesia 630
  antiviral agents 432
  rashes 531
Heterotopic pregnancy 562
Hidroadenitis suppurativa 406
High altitude *see* Altitude illness
Highly-active antiretroviral therapy
    (HAART) 432
Hip
  anatomy 152
  dislocation 155–156
    anterior 156
    knee injuries 156
  disorders 525
    avascular necrosis 152
    posterior dislocation 99
  fractures 152–155
    extracapsular 153–154, *154*
    greater trochanter 154
    intracapsular 152–153
    lesser trochanter 154–155
    see also Femur fracture
Hirudin 189
Histoplasma capsulatum, HIV/AIDS 420
HIV antibody tests *see under* Human
    immunodeficiency virus
    (HIV)/AIDS
Homan's sign, deep vein thrombosis 234
Homatropine, acute iritis 539
Homelessness, domestic violence 621
Homicide 586, 610
  with rape 614, 616
Homocystine 354

Horizontal fissure fracture of vertebral body 57
Horizontal mattress suture *119*
Hormone replacement therapy (HRT) 190–191
Horner's syndrome 58
Hospital acquired infections *see* Nosocomial infections
Hospital disaster plans 700
Hudson face masks 257
  asthma 262
Human chorionic gonadotrophin (hCG) 562
Human immunodeficiency virus (HIV)/AIDS 417–424
  abdominal pain 420, 421, 422
  acute interstitial nephritis 445
  acute renal failure 446–447
  antibody tests
    postexposure 435
    primary HIV infection 421
  arthritis 523
  clinical presentation 417–420
  diarrhoea 418, 420, 421, 422
  disposition 423
  epidemiology 417
  fever 420, 421, 422
  hyponatraemia 482
  investigations 420–421
  management 421–423
    antiretroviral drugs 422–423
    postexposure 435–436
  natural history 418, *418*
  neurological features 419–420, 421, 422
    behavioural disturbances 586
    meningitis 386, 387, 388, 420, 421, 422
    neuropsychiatric disorders 420
  opportunistic infections 419, 420
    prophylaxis 423
  pathogenesis 417–418
  prevention 423
    prophylactic retrovirals 614–615
  previously undiagnosed infection 418
  primary infection 418, *419*
  prognosis 423
  rape victims 614–615
  rectal bleeding 342
  respiratory complications 418, 419, *419*, 421
  skin/soft tissue infections 409
  swallowing difficulty 420, 421, 422
  transmission 415
    needlestick injuries 435–436
  visual complaints 420
Humerus fracture(s) 132–136
  distal 134–135
  neck/articular surface 106, 133–134
  proximal 132–134
    classification/management *133*, 133–134, *134*
    dislocations 134
  shaft 134
Humidification, oxygen therapy 263–264
Hutchison fracture 141, *141*
Hydralazine
  altitude illness 786
  chronic aortic incompetence 226–227
  hypertension in stroke 240
  preeclampsia 240
  renal insufficiency 240
Hydrocarbon compounds ingestion 840
Hydrocephalus, subarachnoid haemorrhage 363

Hydrocoele, ultrasound 643
Hydrofluoric acid burns 128, 865–868
  clinical presentation 865–866
  disposition 867–868
  investigations 866
  management 866–867
  pathophysiology 865
Hydronephrosis, ultrasound 642
Hydroxycobalamin 838–839
Hydroxyzine 670
Hymenopteran stings 779
Hyperactivity 590
Hyperaesthesia 61
Hyperaldosteronism
  alkalosis 479
  hypernatraemia 485
Hyperalgesia 61
Hyperbaric oxygen therapy 264
  adverse effects 761–762
  altitude illness 786
  carbon monoxide poisoning 836, *836*
  cyanide poisoning 839
  decompression illness 761–762
  facilities in Australia 708
  gangrene 406–407
  indications *264*
  local irradiation injuries 766
  near-drowning 772
  necrotizing fasciitis 406
  spinal cord injury 64–65
Hyperbilirubinaemia, *Streptococcus pneumoniae* pneumonia 283
Hypercalcaemia 488–490
  causes 489, *489*
  malignant 488–489, 490
  management 489–490
    bone resorption inhibition 489–490
Hypercholesterolaemia
  ischaemic heart disease 182–183, 183, 190, 191
  stroke risk 353–354
Hypercoagulable states 356
  stroke 357
Hyperglycaemia 482
  cerebral ischaemia 21, 22
  drug overdose 791
  hypothermia 754
  post-cardiac arrest 13
  stroke 357, 358
  see also Diabetes mellitus
Hyperglycaemic, hyperosmotic non-ketotic syndrome (HHNS) 463
  differential diagnosis *463*, 464
  investigations 463–464
  management 465
  presentation 463
  prognosis 466
Hyperkalaemia 485–486
  acute renal failure 448
  bicarbonate therapy 478
  causes *486*
  clinical features 486
  crush syndrome 85
  definition 486
  denervation injury 63
  hydrofluoric acid burns 865, 867
  management 487
  metabolic acidosis 486
  transfusion reactions 496, 497
Hypermagnesaemia 491
  acute renal failure 450
  management 450
Hypernatraemia 484–485

causes *484*
  definition 484
  drug overdose 791
  euvolaemic 485
  hypervolaemic 484–485, *485*
  hypovolaemic 484–485, *485*
  management 485
  pathophysiology 484
  at risk groups 484–485, *485*
Hyperparathyroidism, Achilles tendon rupture 170
Hyperphosphataemia 450
Hypersplenism, thrombocytopenia 513
Hypertension 237–241, 516
  acute aortic dissection 238
  acute pulmonary oedema 193, 194–196, 238
  aortic dissection 242
  cardiovascular complications 238–239
  cerebrovascular disease 352–353, 353–354
  clinical assessment 238–239
  drug overdose 790, *791*, 793–794
  encephalopathy 238
    management 239–240
  epistaxis 552
  induction in cerebral resuscitation 21
  investigations 239
  ischaemic heart disease 182–183, 183, 190
  management 239–240
  microangiopathic haemolytic anaemia 239
  myocardial ischaemia 238–239
  neurological complications 238
  pathophysiology 237–238
  preeclampsia 239
    management 240
  renal failure 238
    management 240
  stroke 358
  subarachnoid haemorrhage 363
  unstable angina 238
Hypertensive crisis 237–238
Hyperthermia
  cocaine abuse 848–849
  drug overdose *791*, 849–850
  hepatitis 410
  malignant 750–751
  opioid abuse 845
  pathophysiology 748
  see also Fever
Hyperthyroidism 467–469
  apathetic 469
Hypertonic hyponatraemia 481
Hypertonic volume replacement 26–27
  burns patients 126
  head injury 49
  hypernatraemia 485
  hyponatraemia management 483, 484
Hypertrophic scarring 121
Hyperuricaemia 516
  acute renal failure 450
  management 450
Hyperventilation
  alkalosis 479
  head injury 49, 50–51
  meningitis 390
Hypervolaemia
  acute renal failure 450
  management 450
Hypervolaemic hypernatraemia 485
Hypervolaemic hyponatraemia 482, *482*
Hyphema, ocular trauma 537–538

Hypnotics overdose 808–809
Hypoaesthesia 61
Hypoalgesia 61
Hypocalcaemia 487–488
  acute renal failure 450
  causes 488
  hydrofluoric acid burns 866, 867
  hypomagnesaemia 490
  management 450, 488
Hypochlorite, decontamination 699
Hypoglycaemia
  community-acquired pneumonia 279
  conscious state alteration 366, 368
  diabetes mellitus 463
  drug overdose 791, 793, 872–873
  insulin overdose 872
  prehospital emergency services 685
  see also Diabetes mellitus; Diabetic
    hypoglycaemia
Hypokalaemia
  acute renal failure 449
  alkalosis 479
  causes 486
  hypomagnesaemia 490
  management 449, 486
Hypomagnesaemia 490, 491
  causes 490
  clinical effects 491
  hydrofluoric acid burns 866
  management 491
Hyponatraemia 481–484
  assessment 483, 483
  clinical features 482, 482
    acute renal failure 447–448, 450
  definition 481
  drug overdose 791
    Ecstasy (MDMA) abuse 849
  encephalopathy 482
    management 483, 484
    at risk groups 482, 482
  euvolaemic 482, 482
  hypertonic 481
  hypervolaemic 482, 482
  hypovolaemic 481–482, 482
  lithium toxicity 875
  management 450, 483–484
    acute symptomatic hyponatraemia 483
    central pontine myelinosis 483, 484
    chronic asymptomatic hyponatraemia
      484
    chronic symptomatic hyponatraemia
      483–484
  normotonic 481
  normotonic (pseudohyponatraemia) 481
  pathophysiology 481
  at risk groups 482, 482
Hypoperfusion (prerenal), acute renal failure
    440–441, 441, 442
Hypopharyngeal puncture 180
Hypotension
  acute renal failure 440–441, 449
  alcohol intoxication 879
  antihistamine overdose 798
  drug overdose 790, 791
  gamma-hydroxybutyrate abuse 851
  glyphosphate poisoning 862
  H_1-antagonist overdose 798
  management 449
  opioid abuse 845
  organophosphates poisoning 859
  postural, bupropion 813
  secondary spinal cord damage 55
  vaginal bleeding 561

Hypotensive resuscitation 44–45
  limb trauma 82
Hypothermia 752–755
  aetiology 752
    drug overdose 791
    major trauma 44
    near-drowning 770, 771, 772
    opioid abuse 845
  clinical presentation 752–753
  complications 753
  epidemiology 752
  induced 21–22, 772
  investigations 753
  management 753–754
    rewarming therapies 754, 754–755, 755
  mild 753
  moderate 753
  prognosis 755
  severe 753
Hypothyroidism 469–470
  lithium toxicity 874
Hypotonia, conscious state alteration 367
Hypovolaemia
  acute renal failure 446, 449
  diuretics 449
  management 449
  signs/symptoms 446
Hypovolaemic hypernatraemia 484–485
Hypovolaemic hyponatraemia 481–482, 482
Hypovolaemic shock 24, 24, 25–27, 81
  clinical features 26
  investigations 26
  iron overdose 870
  limb trauma 81
  management 26–27
  subtrochanteric femur fracture 155
  volume losses 26
Hypoxia 254
  secondary spinal cord damage 55
  tissue 255–256
Hysterectomy, post-partum haemorrhage
    560

I

Ibuprofen 628
  dysfunctional uterine bleeding 568
  peptic ulcer disease 322
  rheumatoid arthritis 520
  septic shock 31
  tension headache 349
Idiopathic thrombocytopenic purpura (ITP)
    512
  Graves' disease 512
Iliac spine fracture(s) 150
Iliac wing fracture(s) 151
Iliopsoas bursitis 525
Imipenem/cilastatin
  acute pancreatitis 331
  urinary tract infection 400–401
Immersion syndrome 770
Immobilization
  ankle injury 170
  complications in elderly patients 106, 108
  decubitus ulcer 408–409
  distal femoral fractures 160
  femoral shaft fracture 157
  hand injuries 146
  intertrochanteric femur fracture 153
  limb trauma 82–83
  snakebite first aid 882

tibial shaft fracture 167
tibia tubercule fracture 167
unstable pelvic fracture 149
wound management 119
  see also Casting; Splinting
Immune complexes, glomerular deposition
    443
Immune-related thrombocytopenia 512
Immunocompromised patients
  community-acquired pneumonia 276
  fever 382–383, 384
  gastroenteritis 313
  meningitis 389
    fungal 386
  septic arthritis 392
  Vibrio soft tissue infections 407
Immunoglobulin A, community-acquired
    pneumonia 275
Immunosuppressive therapy
  autoimmune blistering disease 530
  inflammatory bowel disease 337
  rheumatoid arthritis 520
  systemic lupus erythematosus 521
Impairment, intellectual, consent (UK) 678
Impairment, temporary, consent (UK) 678
Impetigo 532
Impulse control 582
Incisional hernia 310
Incompetence, complaints 734–735
Indicators, clinical risk management
    743–744, 744, 745
Indinavir 432
  HIV/AIDS 422
  postexposure prophylaxis 436, 436
Indomethacin
  renal colic 458
  rheumatoid arthritis 520
Induced hypothermia, near-drowning 772
Infection, barriers to 275–276
Infective endocarditis 223–226
  clinical features 224–225
  diagnosis 225
  febrile patient 382, 383
  intravenous drug users 409
  investigations 225–226
  management 226
    antibiotic therapy 226
  mortality/prognosis 226
  pathogenesis 224
  pathogens 223–224, 224
  pathology 223–224
  prophylaxis 226
  stroke risk 354
  surgery 226
Inferior alveolar nerve injury 66
Inferior dislocation, shoulder 132
Inflammatory bowel disease 335–338
  clinical features 336, 342
  course 335–336
  epidemiology/pathogenesis 335
  extraintestinal manifestations 335–336
  management 336–337
Inflammatory breast disease 180
Infliximab, inflammatory bowel disease 337
Influenza 288
Information for patients
  mild head injury 49
  plaster splints 83
Infusion pumps, retrieval 690
Infusions, retrieval 692
Inguinal hernia 310
Inhibitors, haemophilia 502–503
Injury Severity Score 45–46

Inner-ear barotrauma 757
Inotropic support
   cardiac tamponade 219
   cardiogenic shock 28
   near-drowning 771
   pulmonary embolism 213
   right ventricular myocardial infarction 184
   septic shock 30
   spinal cord injury 64
Inquests (UK) 673–674
Insect(s)
   removal from ear 550
   stings 779
Insight assessment 582
Insulin therapy 464–465
   diabetic ketoacidosis 465
   hyperglycaemic, hyperosmotic non-ketotic
      syndrome 465
   hyperkalaemia 487
   overdose 872–873
   pharmacokinetics 464
Intellectual impairment, consent (UK) 678
Intensive care unit, acute renal failure
      450–451
Intercondylar humerus fracture(s) 135, 160
Interferon
   hepatitis B 414
   hepatitis C 435
Interhospital neurotrauma patient transfer 51
Interleukin-1 receptor antagonists, septic
      shock 31
Intermittent haemodialysis (IHD) 451
Internal fixation
   navicular fractures 174
   radius/ulnar shaft fractures 139
Internal validity, clinical research 651
International Liaison Committee on
      Resuscitation (ILCOR) 3
Interpretation bias 653
Intertrochanteric femoral fracture 153–154,
      154
Interviewer bias 653
Interview room 718
Intracapsular hip fracture(s) 152–153
Intracerebral haemorrhage(s) 355
   location 357
   management 359
Intracerebral intracranial haematoma 48
Intracranial haematoma 48
Intracranial pressure elevation
   high altitude illness 785
   hyponatraemic encephalopathy 482
   meningitis 390
   neurotrauma 49
   stroke 356
Intraocular pressure reduction, central retinal
      artery occlusion 541
Intraovarian haemorrhage, acute pelvic pain
      575
Intrauterine contraceptive device
   pelvic inflammatory disease 570
   rape 615
Intravenous drug abusers
   fever 382, 384
   infective endocarditis 223, 409
   injection complications 845, 850
Intravenous pyelogram
   nephrolithiasis 458
   urinary tract infection 398
Intravenous regional anaesthesia
      (Bier's block) see Bier's block
      (intravenous regional anaesthesia)
Intraventricular haemorrhage 48

Intubation see Tracheal intubation
Ipratropium bromide
   asthma 273
   chronic obstructive airway disease 289
Iritis, acute 539
Iron-deficiency anaemia 505–506
Iron overdose 791, 793–794, 869–871
   clinical presentation 870
   investigations 870
   local effects 869
   management 870–871
   systemic effects 869
   toxic dose 869–870
Iron supplements 506
Irukandji (Carukia barnesi) envenomation
      891
Ischaemic acute tubular necrosis 442–443
Ischaemic heart disease 182–196
   cardiac rehabilitation 190
   clinical manifestations 183
   complications 189–190
   definition 182
   disposition 190
   epidemiology 182
   medical therapy 187–189
   pathogenesis 182–183
   prevention
      primary 190–191
      secondary 191
   prognosis 190
   revascularization 187
      angioplasty 187
      cardiac bypass surgery 187
   risk factors 183
   silent ischaemia 183
   see also Myocardial ischaemia
Ischaemic spinal cord damage 55
Ischaemic stroke see Stroke
Ischial bursitis 525
Ischial tuberosity fracture(s) 150
Ischiorectal abscess 345
Isolated avulsion fracture(s), pelvis 150
Isolated pubic ramus fracture(s) 150
Isolation areas 717
Isoniazid
   hepatitis 410, 412
   HIV/AIDS 422
   poisoning 376, 793
Isopora, immunocompromised patients 313
Isoprenaline 201, 206, 213
   pesticides poisoning 860

J

Jackson–Rees systems, paediatric oxygenation
      261
Jaundice
   febrile patients 383
   Streptococcus pneumoniae pneumonia 283
   viral hepatitis 411
Jaw thrust 2, 3, 42
JC virus, HIV/AIDS 420
Jefferson fracture 56
Jellyfish stings 890–891
Joint dislocation 99
Jones fracture 175
Judgment assessment 582
Jugular venous oxygen saturation 22
Jugular venous pressure 28
Junior medical staff 715
Justice principle 34, 676

K

Kaposi's sarcoma 419
Kelocyanor (dicobalt edetate) 838
Keloid scarring 121
Keratitis, acute infectious 539–540
Keraunoparalysis 777
Kernig's sign, meningitis 387
Kessler tendon repair technique 146
Ketamine 43
   analgesia 629
   conscious sedation 629
   malignant hyperthermia 750
   severe asthma 272–273, 273
Ketoacidosis, alcoholic see Alcoholic
      ketoacidosis
Ketoconazole, HIV/AIDS 422
Ketoprofen, tension headache 349
Ketorolac 628–629
   migraine 350
Ketosis, conscious state alteration 367
Kidneys
   replacement therapy 451
   transplant patients, acute renal failure 445
   ultrasound 642
   see also under Renal
Klebsiella 29, 126
   antibiotic susceptibility 432
      cephalosporin 349
   cholangitis 328
   cutaneous infection 405
   epididymo-orchitis 455
   pneumonia 277
      mortality 282
   renal colic 458
Klebsiella pneumoniae
   antibiotic therapy 426
      susceptibility 430
   meningitis 387
Kleihauer-Betke test 103
Knee, anatomy 159
Knee disorders 159–165, 525
   clinical assessment 159–160
   dislocation 162–163
      posterior 99
      proximal tibiofibular joint 162
   examination 159–160
   fractures 160–162
      supracondylar humerus 160
      tibia plateau 160–161, 161
   hip dislocation 156
   ligament injury 163–164
   menisci injury 164–165
   quadriceps tendinitis 164
   quadriceps tendon injury 164
   radiography 160
   soft tissue 163–165
Kocher's manoeuvre, shoulder dislocation 131
Kub film 458
Kussmaul respiration, diabetic ketoacidosis
      463
Kussmaul's sign 29

L

Labetalol
   hypertensive encephalopathy 240
   pharmacology 801, 802
   preeclampsia 240
   stroke 240, 358

Labour 556, 557–559
  first stage 558
  second stage 558–559
  third stage 559
  see also Delivery
Labyrinthitis 551
Lachman's test
  anterior cruciate ligaments 163
  knee injury 159
Lactic acidosis 478
  metformin overdose 873
Lactulose, acute liver failure 340
Laerdal® system 259, 259
  paediatric use 261
Lamivudine 432
  HIV/AIDS 422
    postexposure prophylaxis 436, 436
Lampona cylindrata (white-tailed spider) 888
Laparoscopy
  abdominal trauma 73
  pelvic inflammatory disease 571
  pelvic pain 573
Laparotomy
  abdominal trauma 72
  indications 72
Large bowel obstruction 306, 306
Laryngeal mask airway (LMA) 18, 42
  tracheal intubation 18
Laryngeal oedema
  anaphylaxis 781, 782
  burns 124, 126
Laryngeal tube airway 18
Laryngospasm, near-drowning 770
Lasegue's sign, back pain 523
Lateral collateral ligament injury 163
Lateral resolution, ultrasound 637
Latrodectus hasseltii spider see Redback spider (Latrodectus hasseltii)
Lauge–Hansen classification 169
Layout of emergency department 716–720
  acute management area 717
  clinical areas 717–718
  clinical support areas 718
  configurations 716
  consultation areas 718
  decontamination rooms 718
  design 716–717
  isolation areas 717
  management rooms 717
  non-clinical areas 718–719
  plaster room 718
  procedure room 718
  resuscitation area 717
  seclusion rooms 717–718
  size considerations 717
  staff station 718
  utility areas 718
Lead poisoning 516
Left anterior fascicular block 202–203
Left bundle branch block 201, 201, 202, 202–203
  myocardial infarction 185
Left posterior fascicular block 202
Left ventricular aneurysm 354
Left ventricular failure 189
  aortic incompetence 226–227
  mitral incompetence 227
  transfusion reactions 496
  wall motion defects 189
Legal aspects
  coroners' functions 667–668
  death 610–611

definition 608
erythromycin resistance 429–430
facial trauma 67
mental health legislation see Mental Health Acts (Australia); Mental Health Acts (UK)
violent patient 594–595
Legal services, domestic violence 622
Legionella pneumophila 276, 283
  antibiotic therapy 426
    resistance/susceptibility 430, 432
  pneumonia, management 280, 281
Leiomyoma (fibroids)
  chronic pelvic pain 576
  uterine pain 573
Leishmaniasis 531
Leprosy 522
Leptospirosis
  acute interstitial nephritis 445
  hepatitis 411
Lercanidipine 801
Lesion(s), cavitating 283, 283
Lesser trochanteric fracture(s) 154–155
Leucocyte esterase strip screening test 399
Leucopenia, community-acquired pneumonia 278
Leucotriene inhibitors, asthma 274
Lichtenberg flowers 777
Lighting
  emergency department 716
  retrieval 690
Lightning injury 777–778
  management 778
  physical aspects 777
  in pregnancy 777
  see also Electric shock injury
Lidocaine 11–12, 13, 205
  decompression illness 761
  migraine 350
  status epilepticus 374
Limb, lower see Lower limb
Limb trauma 83–85
  analgesia 82
  antibiotic therapy 82
  complications 83–84
  crush syndrome 85
  examination 81
  fractures see Fracture(s); individual bones
  history taking 81
  immobilization 82–83
  lightning-induced paralysis 777
  management 82–83
  radiology 81, 99
  rehabilitation 83
  wound decontamination 82
Linear IgA bullous disease 530, 532, 533
Lipase 330
Lipid-lowering drugs 191
Lisfranc fractures 174
Listeria monocytogenes
  antibiotic susceptibility 429
    ampicillin 428
  antibiotic therapy 426
  erythromycin resistance 429
  fever 381
  meningitis 387
Lithium
  pharmacokinetics 874
  thyroid storm 469
Lithium overdose 874–876
  clinical presentation 874–875
  disposition/prognosis 875–876
  management 875

Litigation, complaints 735, 736
Liver
  cirrhosis see Cirrhosis
  failure 338–340
    acute, iron overdose 870
    aetiology 338–339
    disposition 340
    drug overdose 791
    investigations 339
    management 339–340
    prevention 340
    prognosis 340
    viral hepatitis 411
  hepatitis see Hepatitis
  injury 71–72
  transplantation 338, 340
    paracetamol poisoning 825
  see also under Hepatic
Liver function tests
  community-acquired pneumonia 279
  conscious state alteration 368
Lobar pneumonia 277
  Streptococcus pneumoniae 276
Local anaesthesia 630
  adverse reactions 630–631, 631
  dosage 631
  duration of action 630
  limb trauma 82
  methaemoglobinaemia 854–855
  pharmacology 630
  specific nerve blocks 631–633
  systemic toxicity 630–631
  wound cleansing 110
'Locked-in syndrome' 365
'Locked knee' 165
Loop sutures 119
Loperamide
  gastroenteritis 315
  HIV/AIDS 422
  inflammatory bowel disease 337
Lopinavir, HIV/AIDS 422
Loratadine, pharmacodynamics 797–798
Lorraine–Smith effect 263
Loss to follow-up, clinical research 651–652
Lovastatin, acute liver failure 339
Lower limb
  anatomy 165–166
  compartments 166, 166
  rheumatoid arthritis 519
  see also individual components
Low-molecular weight heparins (LMWHs) 184, 213
  deep vein thrombosis 236
  ischaemic heart disease 189
Loxapine, overdose 810, 811–812
Loxosceles (recluse spider) 888
Ludloff's sign, lesser trochanteric fracture 154
Ludwig's angina 269, 408
  antibiotic therapy 269
  upper airway obstruction 266
Lumbar puncture
  meningitis 388–389, 389
  subarachnoid haemorrhage 362
Lumbar spine injury
  fracture 57
  radiology 93
Lunate/perilunate dislocation 99
Lund and Browder chart 124, 125
Lung function tests 272
Lungs
  angiography
    haemoptysis 300
    pulmonary embolism 212

Lungs (*cont.*)
 barotrauma 180, 757
 embolectomy 213–214
 gas exchange 254–255
 injury 78
  contusion 78, 94
 see also under Pulmonary
Lyme disease 519
Lymphocytosis, community-acquired
   pneumonia 278
Lymphoma 531
 acute liver failure 339
 HIV/AIDS 419, 420
 hypercalcaemia 490
Lymphoproliferative disorders 516

M

Macrolides 428–429
 adverse reactions 429
 bacterial resistance 429–430
 community-acquired pneumonia 280
 Legionella pneumophilia pneumonia 283
 see also individual drugs
Mafenide 127
Magnesium 12, 189, 205, 754
 asthma 273–274
 imbalance *see* Hypermagnesaemia;
   Hypomagnesaemia
 pesticides poisoning 860
 preeclampsia 240
Magnesium sulphate, migraine 350
Magnetic resonance angiography (MRA)
   357
 subarachnoid haemorrhage 362–363
 transient ischaemic attacks 356–357
Magnetic resonance imaging (MRI)
 aortic dissection 246
 cardiac tamponade 219
 contraindications *94*
 head trauma 88
  conscious state alteration 369
 knee injury 160
  anterior cruciate ligaments 163
  posterior cruciate ligaments 164
  tibial plateau fractures 161
 limb trauma 82
  distal humerus fracture 135
  elbow dislocations 136
  femoral neck fracture 153
  quadriceps tendon injury 164
 pelvic inflammatory disease 571
 pelvic pain 574
 pulmonary embolism 212
 spinal trauma
  cervical spine injury 92
  SCIWORA 93
  spinal cord injury 62–63, *63*
  thoracolumbar spine injury 93
 stroke 357
 transient ischaemic attacks 356
Maintenance expenditure 725
Maisonneuve fractures 167
Major incidents, clinical risk management
   742, *744*
Malaria 383
Male rape 617
Malgaigne fracture(s) 149
Malignant hypercalcaemia 488–489, 490
Malignant hyperthermia 750–751
Malignant pleural effusion 297

Mallory-Weiss tears 317
Malnutrition, refugees 707, 708
Malpractice *742*
Malunion
 ankle fractures 170
 Colles' fracture 141
Management rooms 717
Manchester Triage Scale 704
Mandible fracture 66, 67, 68
 radiology 88–89
Mania 590, 591
Mannitol 49, 50
 conscious state alteration 369–370
 crush syndrome 85
 drug overdose 794
 hypervolaemia 450
 meningitis 390
Mannose, hypervolaemia 450
MANTRELS criteria 333, 644
Mapleson circuits *258, 259–260*
 paediatric use 261
March haemoglobinuria 509–510
Marfan's syndrome 29
 aortic dissection surgery 247
Marginal radial head/neck fractures 138
Marine envenomation 890–893
Marital status, suicide/deliberate self-harm
   598
Mason–Hotchkiss classification *139*
Massive blood transfusion 497
Massive haemoptysis 301–302
Mastalgia 180
Mastitis 180, 408
Mastoiditis 551
Mast suits 26, 44
Matching, as confounder 654
Maxillary fracture 66, 67, 69
 Le Fort classification 69, 88–89, 89, *90*
 radiology 88–89, 89
McMurray's test
 knee injury 159–160
 meniscal injury 165
MCPJ injuries *see* Metacarpophalangeal joint
   injuries
McRoberts manoeuvre, shoulder dyscrasia
   560
MDA 849
MDEA 849
MDMA *see* Ecstasy (MDMA)
Mean cell volume (MCV) elevation 506
Measles
 fever 381
 immunization, refugees 707
Measurement bias 653
Medial collateral ligament injury 163
Median nerve
 injury 84
  Colles' fracture 141
  elbow dislocations 136
  wrist block 631–632
Mediastinal emphysema 180
Mediastinal haematoma 79, 95
Mediastinal injury 78–79
Medical errors 739–740, *742*
Medical ethics *see* Ethics
Medical staff *see* Staffing
Medical substituted judgment 36
Medishield mask 257
Medroxyprogesterone acetate 568
Mefenamic acid 568
Megaloblastic anaemia *505*, 505–506
Melaena 316–322
Meningism 387

Meningitis 386–392
 aseptic 386, 389
 bacterial 386, 387
  clinical features 387–388
  fever 381, 383, 387
  mortality 389
  Neisseria meningitidis see Neisseria
    meningitidis
 causes *386*, 386–387
 classification 386
 differential diagnosis 389–390
 disposition 390–389
 epidemiology 387
 examination 388
 febrile patient 381, 382
 fungal 386, 388
 headache 348, *349*
 history taking 387–388
 immunocompromised host 389
  HIV/AIDS 420, 421, 422
 investigations 388–389
  microbiological diagnosis 389
 management 390–389
  antibiotic therapy 390, *390, 389*
  corticosteroid therapy 390
 meningism 387
 pathogenesis 387
 prevention 389
 prognosis 389
 risk factors 388
 spinal 387
 tuberculous 386–387, 387, 388, 420,
   422
 viral 386, 387, 388, 389
Menorrhagia 567, 570
 adenomyosis 576
Mental disorders
 classification *584*
 community-acquired pneumonia 279
 consent to management (Australia) 675
 diagnosis 584–589
  examination 586–588
  general approach 584–585
  history taking 586
  investigations 588
  mental state examination 587
 disasters impact 590
 DSM-IV terminology 584, *584*
 HIV/AIDS 420
 interview environment 581, 586
 legislation *see* Mental Health Acts
   (Australia); Mental Health Acts (UK)
 medical illness differentiation 588–589,
   589, 660
 triage *585*, 585–586, 586, *586*
 violent patients 590
Mental Health Acts (Australia) 662
 alcohol/drug-related behaviours 663
 emergency medical/surgical management
   665
 involuntary admissions 663–664
  absconding patients 665–666
  admission criteria 663
  amendment of documents 666
  certification offenses 666
  deliberate self-harm 601
  patient deaths 666
  status of recommending doctor
    664–665
 mental illness definitions 662
 physical restraint 665
 police powers 665–666
 prejudice safeguards 662–663

Mental Health Acts (Australia) (cont.)
  protection from suit/liability 666
  removal to a place of safety 665–666
  sedation 665
Mental Health Acts (UK) 660–661
  involuntary admissions 660–662
    consent issues 678
    deliberate self-harm 601
    for emergency assessment 661
  physical restraint 661
  police powers 661–662
  removal to a place of safety 661–662
  sedation 661
Mental state assessment/examination
    580–583, 585, 586–588
  physical examination 583
  problems in emergency department 585
  psychiatric interview 581–583
    concomitant observations 582–583
  security/safety 581
  seizures 372–373
Meralgia paraesthetica 525
  6-mercaptopurine 337
Mesalamine, inflammatory bowel disease
    337
Mesoridazine, overdose 810
Metabolic acidosis 477–478
  anion gap 477–478
  hyperkalaemia 486
  non-anion gap 478
  renal failure 450
  see also Lactic acidosis
Metabolic alkalosis 479
Metacarpal injuries 145–146
  fractures/dislocation 99
Metacarpophalangeal joint injuries 145
Metal burns 128
Metatarsus, fractures 174–175
Metformin
  diabetes mellitus 464
  overdose 873
Methadone 846
Methaemoglobinaemia 854–856
  aetiology 854, 854–855
  clinical syndrome 855
  investigations 855
  methylene blue management 855–856
  pathophysiology 854–855
Methamphetamine 849
Methicillin 427
Methicillin-resistant Staphylococcus aureus
    (MRSA) 425
  cephalosporin susceptibility 349
  pneumonia 280
  septic shock 31
Methotrexate
  hepatitis 410
  psoriatic arthritis 522
  rheumatoid arthritis 520
Methylene blue, methaemoglobinaemia
    855–856
Methylprednisolone, spinal cord injury 63
Methylsergine, serotonin syndrome 750
Metoclopramide 50
  gastroenteritis 315
  migraine 350
Metoprolol 208
  aortic dissection 247
  pharmacology 801, 802
Metromenorrhagia 568
Metronidazole 82, 430–431
  acute liver failure 340
  adverse reactions 431

bacterial resistance 431
bowel obstruction 308
cellulitis 405–406
cholangitis 328
community-acquired pneumonia 280
inflammatory bowel disease 337
pelvic inflammatory disease 571
peptic ulcer disease 324
septic shock 31
submandibular abscess 408
Microangiopathic haemolytic anaemia 509,
    509
  hypertension 239
Microbiology
  conscious state alteration 368–369
  gastroenteritis 312, 313
  inflammatory bowel disease 336
  meningitis 389
  osteomyelitis 394
Micropore blood filters 44
Microsomal ethanol oxidizing system
    (MEOS) 877
Microsporidium, immunocompromised
    patients 313
Midazolam 43
  analgesia 629, 630
  antiretroviral drug interactions 423
  chemical restraint 593
  meningitis 390
  pharmacology 806
  status epilepticus 374, 374
Middle-ear barotrauma 757
  hyperbaric oxygen 761–762
Middle-grade staff 714, 715
Mifepristone, rape 615
Migraine 348, 349, 349–351
  ischaemic stroke 352
  management 350–351, 630
  observation wards 710
  pathophysiology 350
Military triage 704–705
Milker's nodules 531
Mini-mental state examination 587–588,
    587–588, 835
Minocycline 532
Misconduct, complaints 735
Misdiagnosis, complaints 734, 737
Misoprostol, peptic ulcer disease 325
Missulena occatoria (mouse spider) 888
Mitral stenosis 229–230
Mitral valve
  disorders 223, 227–229
    acute 227
    chronic 227–229
    post-myocardial infarction 189
    stroke risk 354
  prolapse 227
  replacement 229
Mittelschmerz 567, 575–576
M-mode ultrasound 637
Mobitz I (Wenkebach) second degree heart
    block 200, 200
Mobitz II second degree heart block 200
Molluscum contagiosum 531
Monitors, retrieval 689
Monoamine oxidase inhibitors
  hepatitis 410
  serotonin syndrome 749
Monoarticular arthritis, acute 516
Monteggia fracture-dislocation
  elbow dislocations 136
  forearm 139
  management 136

Montelukast, asthma 274
Mood assessment 581
Moraxella catarrhalis
  antibiotic therapy 426
    susceptibility 429, 431–432
  chronic obstructive airway disease 288,
    289
  otitis media 551
Morganella, antibiotic susceptibility 432
Morphine 126, 844, 845
  acute pulmonary oedema 195
  dosage 628
  prehospital emergency services 684
  renal colic 458
  sickle cell anaemia 508
Motor function assessment, spinal cord
    injury 59, 61
  documentation conventions 61, 61
Motor vehicle accidents
  basic life support 2–3
  in elderly 106
  pelvic fractures 148
  tibial shaft fracture 166
Mountain sickness 784, 785
  management 785–786
Mouse spider (Missulena occatoria) 888
Mouth-to-mask ventilation 3–4
Mouth-to-mouth ventilation 3–4
Multifocal atrial tachycardia 198, 209
Multiple myeloma
  back pain 523
  hypercalcaemia 490
Multiple organ dysfunction syndrome
    (MODS) 29
Multiple Trauma Outcome Scale (MTOS) 45
Mumps
  arthritis 523
  epididymo-orchitis 455
Munchausen's syndrome 375
  renal colic 458
Murphy's sign, acute cholecystitis 327
Muscle trauma 85
Muscular dystrophy, respiratory acidosis
    478–479
Musculoskeletal chest pain 180
Mushroom poisoning 339
  hepatitis 411
Myasthenia gravis, respiratory acidosis
    478–479
Mycobacterium, antibiotic susceptibility 429,
    430, 432
Mycobacterium avium complex (MAC) 422
  HIV/AIDS 420
Mycobacterium catarrhalis, cephalosporin
    susceptibility 349
Mycobacterium chelonei 407
Mycobacterium fortuitum 407
Mycobacterium gordanae 407
Mycobacterium kansasii, cutaneous infection
    405
Mycobacterium marinum 531
Mycobacterium tuberculosis
  antibiotic resistance 425
  cutaneous infection 405
  epididymo-orchitis 455
  meningitis 387
  pneumonia 277
  see also Tuberculosis
Mycoplasma, antibiotic susceptibility
    431–432
Mycoplasma pneumoniae
  antibiotic therapy 426
    susceptibility 429, 430

Mycoplasma pneumoniae (*cont.*)
arthritis 522
pneumonia 276–277
cavitating lesions 283
management 280, *280*
mortality 282
response to management 281
Myelodysplastic syndromes 506
classification *506*
Myeloma, multiple *see* Multiple myeloma
Myeloproliferative disorders 516
Myocardial contusion 78
hypovolaemic shock 26
Myocardial infarction 183, 184–186
aetiology
anaphylaxis 781
carbon monoxide poisoning 835
cardiogenic shock 27, 28–29, 189
cocaine overdose 847, 848
mechanical defects 189
anterior 184
clinical features 185
chest pain 178, 179, 181, 185
complete heart block 203
disposition 190
emergency department assessment 185–186
inferior 184
investigations 179, 185–186
cardiac enzymes 185
chest X-ray 185
electrocardiogram 185–186
left bundle branch block 185
left ventricular failure 189
Killip classification 189
management 189
management 180–181, 186
analgesia 630
guidelines 186
oxygen therapy 263
thrombolytic therapy 181, 186–187
myocarditis differentiation *vs.* 221
pathophysiology 184–185
pericarditis *vs.* 190, 216
posterior 184
prognosis 190
morbidity 183
right ventricular 184
stroke risk 354
thromboembolism 189–190
Myocardial ischaemia
chest pain 178, 180–181
hypertension 238
management 240
investigations 179
physiological changes 182–183
silent ischaemia 183
see also Ischaemic heart disease
Myocardial laceration 78
Myocarditis 220–221
causes 220
diagnosis 221
management 221
natural history 221, *221*
pathophysiology 220
Myoclonus, gamma-hydroxybutyrate abuse 851
Myoglobin 185
Myoglobinuria
acute tubular necrosis 443
conscious state alteration 368
Myositis 383
Myositis ossificans, femoral head fracture 152
Myxoedema coma 470

N

N-acetylcysteine (NAC)
acute liver failure 339
paracetamol poisoning 825–826
Naloxone 65
gamma-hydroxybutyrate abuse 851
opioid overdose management 844, 845–846
prehospital emergency services 685
Naproxen 517
rheumatoid arthritis 520
Nasal cannulae, oxygen therapy 256–257, *257*
Nasogastric intubation
abdominal trauma 72
bowel obstruction 308
burns patients 126
gastrointestinal bleeding 316–317
spinal cord injury 57
Nasolacrimal apparatus injury 68
Nasopharyngeal airway 42
National Emergency X-Radiography Utilization Study (NEXUS) 58, *59*, 90
National Service Framework for Mental Health (UK) 661
Navicular bone, fractures 173–174
Near-drowning 3, 769–773
Conn/Modell classification of mental status *771*, 771–772
definitions 770
emergency department management 771–772
epidemiology 769–770
hypothermia 770, 771, 772
investigations 771
organ-specific effects 770–771
pathophysiology 770
pre-hospital management 771
field predictors of outcome 772
prevention 772–773
prognosis 772
Neck X-ray
dysphagia 302
epiglottitis *266*
oesophageal foreign body 553
upper airway obstruction 266, *266*
Necrotic arachnidism 888
Necrotizing fasciitis 383, 406
Needle holders 113–114
Needle pericardiocentesis 219
Needles, surgical 113–114, 115, *115*
Needlestick injuries 114, 434–437
hepatitis B 413–414
hepatitis transmission 435, *435*
HIV transmission 435–436
Neer classification 133, *133, 134*
Negligence *742*
Neisseria
antibiotic susceptibility 428, 429, 430, 431
cephalosporin 349
co-trimoxazole resistance 431
Neisseria gonorrhoeae
acute epididymo-orchitis 455, 456
antibiotic therapy *426*
resistance 425, 428
susceptibility 427, 429, 430
arthritis 519, 521
Bartholin's abscess 406
pelvic inflammatory disease 570, 571

pelvic pain 574
rape 614
Neisseria meningitidis 429
antibiotic therapy *426*
penicillin susceptibility 427
susceptibility 429, 430, 431
bacteraemia 383–384
adrenocortical insufficiency 470
rate of progression 383
clinical presentation *384*
febrile patient 381, 383
meningitis 386, 387, 389
antigenic studies 389
course 388
prophylaxis 389
rash 383, 384, 387, 531, 533
Nelfinavir, HIV/AIDS 422
Neomycin, acute liver failure 340
Nephrolithiasis 457–459
hyperuricaemia 516
Nephrotic syndrome, hypervolaemic hyponatraemia 482
Nerve blocks 631–633
see also individual types
Nerve injury 83–84
see also individual nerves
Nesiritide, acute pulmonary oedema 195–196
Neuralgia, headache *349*
Neurogenic shock (spinal sympathetic interruption) 31–32, 43, 55
Neuroleptic malignant syndrome 748, 749–750
antipsychotic drugs 811
management 750
risk factors *749*
Neurological assessment
initial trauma management 41
primary survey 48–49
secondary survey 49
seizures 372–373
specific examination 49
spinal injury *see* Spinal cord injury
stroke 355
subarachnoid haemorrhage 361
trauma 49
Neuropathy, peripheral, opioid abuse 845
Neuropraxia 83
Neuroprotective drugs 21
Neuroses, suicide/deliberate self-harm 598–599
Neurotmesis 83
Neurotrauma 47–52
cerebral protection 51
clinical presentation 48–49
interhospital transfer 51
pathogenesis 48
primary injury classification 47–48
primary spinal cord damage 53–54
prognosis 51
resuscitation 49
severity *47*
see also Head injury
Neutropenia 499–500
causes *499*
drugs *500*
fever 382
infection risk 499
management 500
Nevirapine (delavirdine) 432
HIV/AIDS 422
Nicardipine, hypertension in stroke 240

Nifedipine
  altitude illness 786
  chronic aortic incompetence 226–227
  hypertension in stroke 240
  overdose 802
  pharmacology 801
  stroke 358
'Nightstick' fractures 139
Nimodipine
  ischaemic stroke 359
  subarachnoid haemorrhage 363
Nitrates 183–184
  acute pulmonary oedema 194
  cocaine abuse 848
  ischaemic heart disease 188
  methaemoglobinaemia 854
  myocardial ischaemia 240
  pulmonary oedema 240
  stroke 358
Nitrazine paper 103
Nitric oxide
  hypertension 238
  septic shock 30
Nitrofurantoin 432
  adverse reactions 432
  recurrent urinary tract infection 399
  urinary tract infection 400–401
Nitrogen narcosis 756, 762
Nitroprusside
  aortic dissection 247
  cocaine abuse 848
  drug overdose 793
  hypertension in stroke 240
  hypertensive encephalopathy 240
  renal insufficiency 240
  stroke 358
Nitroprusside test, diabetic ketoacidosis
    463–464
Nitrous oxide
  analgesia 629
  conscious sedation 629
  prehospital emergency services 684
Nizatidine, peptic ulcer disease 324
NMDA receptors 21, 350
N-methyl-D-aspartate (NMDA) receptors
    21, 350
Nociceptors 626
Nodules 528, 531
'No intensive care' directive 35–36
Non-bacterial thrombotic endocarditis 224
Non-cardiogenic pulmonary oedema see
    Pulmonary oedema
Non-invasive ventilation (NIV), severe
    asthma 273
Non-maleficence principle 34, 676
Non-nucleoside reverse transcriptase
    inhibitors 432–433
  HIV/AIDS 422–423
  side effects 423
  see also individual drugs
Non-pharmacologic analgesia 629–630
Non-probability sampling, clinical research
    652
Non-response bias 653
Non-steroidal anti-inflammatory drugs
    (NSAIDs) 628–629
  acute interstitial nephritis 445
  acute renal failure 445
  acute tubular necrosis 443
  anaphylactic reaction 779
  back pain 524
  cyclo-oxygenase selectivity 628
  dysfunctional uterine bleeding 568

dysmenorrhoea 576
gout 517
lithium excretion 874
Mittelschmerz 576
peptic ulcer disease 317, 322
  prevention of 324–325
pseudogout 518
psoriatic arthritis 522
rectal bleeding 342
Reiter's syndrome 522
renal colic 458
rheumatic fever 522
rheumatoid arthritis 520
sprained ankle 170
systemic lupus erythematosus 521
tension headache 349
see also individual drugs
Noradrenaline (norepinephrine) 28
  antihistamine overdose 798
  neurogenic shock 32
  septic shock 30
Normaesthesia 61
Normalgesia 61
Normotonic hyponatraemia
    (pseudohyponatraemia) 481
Norwalk virus gastroenteritis 312
Nose 551–553
  foreign body 551–552
  fracture 68, 69, 552
  packing 553
  septal abscess 552
  septum blood supply 553
  trauma 552
Nosocomial infections
  gastroenteritis 314
  pneumonia 284, 284
Nucleoside reverse transcriptase inhibitors
    432–433
  HIV/AIDS 422–423
  side effects 423
  see also individual drugs
Nutritional support
  inflammatory bowel disease 336–337
  refugees 707, 708
Nystagmus, phenytoin overdose 817

O

Obesity 190
Observational studies 649–650
Observation wards 710–712
  admission
    criteria 710–711
    process 710
  audit/feedback 712
  exclusion criteria 711
  patient care 711
  roles 710
  short-stay medicine 712
  staffing 711–712
Obstetric examination 103
Obstructive airway disease, chronic see
    Chronic obstructive airway disease
    (COAD)
Obturator dislocations 156
Obturator hernia 310
Occupational hand injuries 146
Occupational therapy 715
Octreotide
  gastro-oesophageal varices 319
  overdose 873

Odontoid fracture 91–92
Odynophagia 302, 305, 553
  anaphylaxis 781
Oesophageal tracheal combitube
    (Combitube™) 18
Oesophagitis, HIV/AIDS 420
Oesophagus
  carcinoma 841
  corrosives burns 840, 841–842
    grading 842, 842
    management 842
  foreign body 553
  obstructive lesions 305
  perforation 79, 842
    corrosives ingestion 842
    radiology 95
  reflux 180
  spasm 180
  strictures 842
    corrosives ingestion 842
Oestrogens, dysfunctional uterine bleeding
    568
Office facilities 719
Olanzapine
  amphetamine abuse 850
  overdose 810, 811
  pharmacology 809
Olecranon bursitis 524
Oligomenorrhoea 567
Omeprazole, peptic ulcer disease 324
Open dislocations, ankle 170
Open reduction, radius/ulnar shaft fractures
    139
Open reduction with internal fixation
    (ORIF)
  intertrochanteric femur fracture 153
  patellar fractures 162
Ophthalmoplegic migraine 350
Opioid antagonists
  septic shock 30
  spinal cord injury 65
Opioid drug(s) 627–628, 629
  abuse see below
  acute pancreatitis 331
  administration route 628
  conscious sedation 629
  doses 628
  duration of effects 628
  leiomyoma (fibroids) 576
  limb trauma 82
  meningitis 390
  ocular trauma 537, 538
  paralytic ileus 306
  pharmacology 844
  renal colic 458
  side effects 628
  tibial shaft fracture 167
  see also individual drugs
Opioid drug abuse 844–846
  clinical presentation 845
  complications 845
  conscious state alteration 366–367
  overdose 845
    epidemiology 844
    management 845–846
  withdrawal syndrome 846
Optic neuritis 543
Oral contraception
  dysfunctional uterine bleeding 568
  dysmenorrhoea 576
  emergency post-rape 615
Oral hypoglycaemic agents 464
  see also individual drugs

Oral rehydration solution 314, 750
Orbital blowout fracture 68–69
  radiology 88
Orbital cellulitis 405
Organ donation 610–611
Organic mental disorders 584
Organophosphates, toxicity 478, 668,
    857–860
  clinical presentation 857–858
  differential diagnosis 859
  investigations 858–859
  long-term neuropsychiatric sequelae 858,
    860
  management 859–860
  mechanism 857
  severity determination 859, *859*
  toxicokinetics 857
Orientation assessment 583
Oropharyngeal airway 42
Osgood–Schlatter disease 167
Osler-Rendu-Weber syndrome (hereditary
    haemorrhagic telangiectasia) 342
Osmotic diuresis, hypernatraemia 485
Osteoarthritis, tibial plateau fractures 161
Osteomyelitis 394–395
  ankle fractures 170
  antibiotic therapy 395
  back pain 523
  microbiology 395
Osteoporosis
  back pain 523
  Colles' fracture 140
Ot haematoma (cauliflower ear) 550, 551
Otitis externa 551
Otitis media 551
Otitis media with effusion (glue ear) 551
Ottowa Ankle Rules (OAR) 168–169
Outcome measures 722
  trauma 45–46
Outpatient parenteral antibiotic therapy
    (OPAT) *433,* 433–434
Ovaries, acute pelvic pain
  cysts 574
  infection 575
Oxacillin 427
Oxazepam, pharmacology 806
Oxprenolol, pharmacology *801, 802*
Oxycodone 844
Oxygen, retrieval 689, 692
Oxygen blenders, oxygen therapy 258
Oxygen physiology 254–256
  blood transport 255
  pulmonary gas exchange 254–255
  tissue perfusion/diffusion 255–256
  tissue utilization 256
  ventilation 254
Oxygen-powered resuscitators *258,* 259
Oxygen therapy 254–264
  acute pulmonary oedema 195
  advanced life support 10–11
  altitude illness 786
  analgesia 630
  anaphylaxis 782, *782*
  arterial gas embolism 261
  asthma 262, 272–273
  carbon monoxide poisoning 836
  childbirth 557
  chronic obstructive airway disease 257,
    262–263, 288–289
  complications 263
  decompression illness 261, 760
  failed intubation 18–19
  fixed performance systems 256, 257–258

oxygen blenders 258
  Venturi mask 257–258
gamma-hydroxybutyrate abuse 851
gastrointestinal bleeding 318
humidification 263–264
hyperbaric *see* Hyperbaric oxygen therapy
myocardial infarction 263
near-drowning 771
oxygenation measurement 260
paediatric considerations 260–261
pneumothorax 292
pulmonary oedema 263
pure oxygen 256, *258,* 258–260
  closed-circuits 260
  free-flowing circuits 258, *258*
  Mapleson circuits *258,* 259–260
  oxygen-powered resuscitators *258,* 259
  self-refilling, non-rebreathing 259, *259*
  soft reservoirs *258,* 259
sepsis 263
shock 263
system definitions 256, *256*
transfers 261
trauma management 42
variable performance systems 256–257,
    257
  face masks 257, *257*
  nasal cannulae 256–257, *257*
Oxygen toxicity 263
  children 261
  divers 756, 762
  hyperbaric oxygen 761–762
Oxytocin
  emergency delivery 559
  post-partum haemorrhage 560
OxyViva® system 259

P

P24 antigen tests, primary HIV infection
    421
Paget's disease, back pain 523
Pain
  assessment 627
  definition 626
  perception documentation conventions 61
  physiology 626–627
  relief *see* Analgesia
Pain scales 627
Palmar wounds 146
Pancreatic injury 71–72
Pancreatic transplantation 465
Pancreatitis 323
  acute 329–331
    causes *329*
    complications 330
    management 331
    necrotizing 331
    severity markers 330, *330*
  chest pain 178
  chronic 331
    avascular necrosis 152
  hypomagnesaemia 490
Papillary muscle rupture 189
Papule *528,* 530–531
Paracetamol (acetaminophen) 50
  analgesia 628, 630
  ocular trauma 538
  pharmacokinetics 823–824
  poisoning 791, 792, 823–827
    acute liver failure 338–339, 339, 340

clinical features 824
  hepatitis 410, *412*
  hepatotoxicity risk assessment 824–825,
    825
  management 339–340, 825–826
  N-acetylcysteine therapy 339,
    825–826
  pathophysiology 823–824
  pregnancy 825
  prevention 340
  renal colic 458
  tension headache 349
Paradoxical breathing 57, 58, 62
Paraldehyde, status epilepticus *374*
Parallel group clinical trials 650
Paralysing agents 43
Paralytic ileus 306
  spinal cord damage 55
Paramedical staff 715
Para-ovarian cysts, acute pelvic pain 574
Paraquat poisoning 862–864
  long-term sequelae 864
  management 863
Parathyroid crisis, hypercalcaemia 489
Parathyroid hormone (PTH), hypercalcaemia
    489
Paratubal cysts, acute pelvic pain 574
Paronychia 406
Parotid injury 67
Paroxysmal nocturnal haemoglobinuria 509
Paroxysmal supraventricular tachycardia,
    electrocardiogram 198, 206–207,
    207
Parvovirus
  arthritis 522
  gastroenteritis 312
Pasteurella haemolytica, antibiotic
    susceptibility 431
Pasteurella multocida
  antibiotic susceptibility 429
  antibiotic therapy *426*
  penicillin susceptibility 427
Patella
  fracture 161–162
  tendinitis 164
  tendon rupture 164, 525
PATHOS 599
PCO$_2$ values 476
Pelvic inflammatory disease 570–572
  acute pelvic pain 574
  bacterial pathogens 570
  differential diagnosis 571
  epidemiology 570
  management 571
Pelvis
  anatomy 148
  congestion syndrome 577
  pain *see below*
  trauma 97–99
    fracture *see below*
    X-ray 87, 97–98
Pelvis, fracture 148–151
  clinical assessment 149
  complications 149–150
  elderly patients 107
  management 150–151
  MAST suits 44
  open 150
  in pregnancy 103
  radiological classification 98
  urethral rupture 98
  Young and Ressnick classification
    148–149

Pelvis, pain 572–577
  acute 574–575
    causes *573*
  chronic 575–577
    acyclic 576–577
    causes *575*
    cyclic 575–576
    psychosocial factors 573
  differential diagnosis 574–577
  examination 573
  history 572–573
  imaging 574
  laboratory investigations 573–574
Pemphigoid *530,* 532, 533
Pemphigus 530, 532, 533
Penetrating trauma
  abdomen 72, *72,* 73–74
  chest trauma 94
  elderly patients 107
  eye 537, *537*
  facial injuries 69
  femoral shaft fracture 157
  hand 146
  upper airway 267–268
Penicillin(s) 424, 425, 427–428
  acute liver failure 339
  adverse reactions 428
    anaphylactic reaction 779
  arthritis 522
  bacterial resistance 425
  cellulitis 405–406
  cutaneous infection 403
  erysipelas 405
  fever 384
  Haemophilus influenzae pneumonia 280
  HIV/AIDS 422
  necrotizing fasciitis 406
  penicillinase-resistant 427
  quinsy 408, 553–554
  resistance to, community-acquired
    pneumonia 282
  tonsillitis 553
  toxic shock syndrome 407
Penicillin G (benzylpenicillin) 82, 427
  gangrene 406–407
  infective endocarditis 226
  meningitis 390, *389*
  necrotizing fasciitis 406
Penicillin V (phenoxymethyl penicillin) 427
Pentobarbitone, status epilepticus *374*
Peptic ulcer disease 322–325
  clinical features 323
  chest pain 178
  complications 325
  gastrointestinal bleeding 317, 318,
    318–319, 323–324
  investigations 323
  management 324–325
    antihistamines 797
  pathophysiology 322
  risk factors 322–323
Peptococcus, antibiotic susceptibility 431
Peptostreptococcus, antibiotic susceptibility
    428, 431
Percutaneous inferior vena cava umbrellas 214
Percutaneous nephrolithotomy 458
Percutaneous transcoronary angioplasty
    (PTCA)
  cardiogenic shock 27, 29
  ischaemic heart disease 187
Perforation
  gastric outlet obstruction 325
  oesophagus *see* Oesophagus

Performance indicators 744, *744*
Perhexaline, hepatitis *412*
Perianal abscess 345, 403, 405, 406
Perianal disorders 344–346
Perianal haematoma 345–346
Perianal injuries 346
Pericardial effusions, echocardiography 643
Pericarditis 215–216
  clinical features 178, 215
    management 216
  post-myocardial infarction 190
Periorbital cellulitis 405
Peripheral artery aneurysm 251
Peripheral neuropathy, opioid abuse 845
Peripheral vascular disease 231–237
    arterial 232–233
    venous 234
Peripheral venous cannulae 13
Peritoneal dialysis (PD) 451
Peritonitis, uterine pain 573
Peritonsillar abscess (quinsy) *see* Quinsy
Pernicious anaemia 505–506
Peroneal nerve injury 84
    knee dislocation 162
    tibial plateau fractures 161
Personality disorder(s) 590
    suicide/deliberate self-harm 598–599
Pesticide poisoning 857–864
    see also individual pesticides
Pethidine 558
    analgesia 628, 629
    antiretroviral drug interactions 423
    dosage *628*
    migraine 350
    renal colic 458
    serotonin syndrome *749*
Phalanges, fractures/dislocations 99, 175
Phalen's sign 524
Pharmacy room 718
Pharyngeal foreign bodies 305
Pharyngitis 268–269, 383
Phased-array transducers, ultrasound 639
Phase of care strategies, clinical risk
    management *744*
Pheniramine, overdose 798
Phenobarbitone
    antihistamine overdose 798–799
    meningitis 390
    pesticides poisoning 859
Phenothiazines 106
    overdose 810–812
    paralytic ileus 306
    pharmacology 809
    see also individual drugs
Phenoxybarbitone, status epilepticus *374*
Phentolamine
    altitude illness 786
    cocaine abuse 848
Phenylephrine, neurogenic shock 32
Phenylhydroxylamine, methaemoglobinaemia
    855
Phenytoin 51, 817
    acute interstitial nephritis 445
    hepatitis *412*
    meningitis 390
    status epilepticus 374, *374*
    therapeutic levels 817
Phosphate imbalance 450
PH range 476
    common corrosive solutions 840, *840*
Physical restraint 591, 592
    deliberate self-harm 600
    mental health legislation 665

Physiotherapy 715
Physostigmine
    antihistamine overdose 799
    gamma-hydroxybutyrate abuse 851
    tricyclic antidepressant overdose 814
Pillion fractures 170
Pilonidal abscess 344, 406
Pilonidal sinus 344
Pindolol, pharmacology *801,* 802
Pink puffers 287
Piperacillin
    septic shock 31
    urinary tract infection 400–401
Piperidine, antipsychotic drug overdose
    811–812
Pituitary apoplexy, subarachnoid
    haemorrhage 364
Pityriasis rubra pilaris 532
PKa range, common corrosive solutions *840*
Placental abruption 103
Placenta praevia, antepartum haemorrhage
    564
Plaque *528*
Plasmodium, antibiotic susceptibility 430
Plaster room 718
Platelets
    thrombocytopenia 513
    transfusion *495,* 497, 507
Pleura
    biopsy 298
    effusions *see* Pleural effusion
    injury 77–78
    pain 178
    respiratory acidosis 478–479
Pleural effusion 296–299
    aetiology 296, *297*
      community-acquired pneumonia 278
    classification 296
    clinical features 296–297
    complications 299
    examination 297
    exudates 298, *298*
    history 296–297
    investigations 298
    malignant 297
    management 299
    pathophysiology 296
    transudates *297*
Pleurisy 180
    differential diagnosis *181*
Pneumatic anti-shock garments (PASG)
    149
Pneumocephalus 51
Pneumococcus
    antibiotic susceptibility 428
    pneumonia 277
Pneumocystis carinii 419
    antibiotic susceptibility 431
    antibiotic therapy *426*
    HIV/AIDS 420, 421, 422
Pneumomediastinum 94–95, 180
    pulmonary barotrauma 757–758
Pneumonia
    community-acquired *see*
      Community-acquired pneumonia
    continuous positive airway pressure 264
    HIV/AIDS 419
    lobar 277
    *Mycoplasma pneumoniae see Mycoplasma
      pneumoniae*
    nosocomial 284, *284*
    opioid abuse 845
    pneumococcal 277

Pneumonia (*cont.*)
  *Pseudomonas aeruginosa see Pseudomonas
    aeruginosa*
  *Streptococcus pneumoniae see Streptococcus
    pneumoniae*
Pneumothorax 77, 180, 291–295
  clinical features 292
  differential diagnosis 292
  disposition 295
  grading 292
  iatrogenic 291
  immediate decompression 292
  investigations
    chest X-ray 93, 94
    size determination 292, 293, *293*
  management 292–293, 294
    simple aspiration 293
  observation 293
  open 77
  prognosis 295
  pulmonary barotrauma 757–758
  small-lumen catheters 294
  spontaneous 291
  tension *see* Tension pneumothorax
  thoracocentesis 299
Poisoning
  observation wards 710–711
  pesticides 857–864
  see also Drug abuse, overdose
Poisons information 792
Polyarthritis, acute 519
Polydipsia 463
  hypercalcaemia 489
  hypernatraemia 486
Polyethylene glycol 852
  drug overdose 795
  salicylate overdose 829
Polymenorrhoea 567
Polymerase chain reaction (PCR), meningitis
    389
Polyuria 463
  hypercalcaemia 489
  hypernatraemia 486
Popliteal artery
  aneurysm 251
  injury 83, 98
    knee dislocation 162
Position of patient
  decompression illness 760
  head injury 49–50, 50–51
  hypovolaemic shock 26
  massive haemoptysis 301
Positive end expiratory pressure (PEEP)
  chronic obstructive airway disease
    288–289
  near-drowning 772
Posterior cord syndrome 54
Posterior cruciate ligament injury 164
Posterior dislocation, shoulder 132
Posterior vitreous detachment 542
Posthypercapneoic alkalosis 479
Postmortem procedures
  caesarian section 104
  resuscitation practice 36–37
Post-partum haemorrhage 559, 565–566
Post-transfusion purpura 512
Post-traumatic epilepsy 376
Post-traumatic seizures 376
Post-traumatic stress disorder 611
  deliberate self-harm/suicide 601
  disasters 590
  domestic violence 622
  rape 616

Postural hypotension, bupropion 813
Potassium imbalance *see* Hyperkalaemia;
    Hypokalaemia
Poverty
  domestic violence 621
  suicide/deliberate self-harm 598
Povidone-iodine 82
Power Doppler transvaginal ultrasound,
    pelvic inflammatory disease 571
Power supplies 716
Pralidoxime
  carbamates poisoning 861
  pesticides poisoning 860
Precipitous birth ('born before arrival') 556
Prednisolone
  acute iritis 539
  chronic obstructive airway disease
    289–290
Preeclampsia 238–239
  antepartum haemorrhage 565
  management 240
  stroke 353
Pregnancy
  analgesia 628, 629
  anatomical/physiological changes 102
  concealed 556
  delivery *see* Delivery
  diseases/disorders
    acute appendicitis 334
    acute pelvic pain 574
    aortic dissection 29
    epilepsy 376
    folate deficiency 506
    hepatitis 411
    hypertensive emergencies 238–239, 241
    paracetamol poisoning 825
    seizures 376
    thrombocytopenia 512
  ectopic *see* Ectopic pregnancy
  following rape 615, 616
  heterotopic 562
  labour *see* Labour
  Rhesus (Rh) factor 562–563
  trauma 102–105
    domestic violence 619, 620
    electric shock injury 776
    fetal death 103
    lightning injury 777
    management 104
    primary/secondary survey 103
  ultrasound 562, 640–641
    interstitial diagnosis 641
    timings *640*
  unrecognized 556
  urinary tract infection 396, 397
    antibiotic management *400*
    management 400–401
  vaginal bleeding *see* Vaginal bleeding
Pregnancy test 793
  pelvic inflammatory disease 571
  pelvic pain 574
  vaginal bleeding 568
Prehospital emergency services 682–686
  acute coronary syndromes 685
  anaphylaxis 685
  arrhythmias 685
  cardiac arrest 684–685
  clinical skills 682
  disasters management 698–699
  dispatch 682
  drug overdose 685
  hypoglycaemia 685
  pulmonary oedema 685

seizures 685
spinal immobilization 683
trauma care 682–684
  advanced life support 683
  airway management 683–684
  analgesia 684
  basic life support 683
  fluid resuscitation 684
triage 704
see also First aid
Premature labour 104
Prepatellar bursitis 525
Prerenal azotemia 441, *442*
Prevarication bias 653
Priapism 58, 62
Prilocaine, methaemoglobinaemia 854
Prinzmetal's (variant) angina 183
Prions, blood transfusions 496–497
Private emergency departments 725
Probability sampling, clinical research 652
Probenecid, sexually-transmitted diseases
    614
Procainamide 203
Procedure room 718
Process indicators 745, *745*
Process strategies, clinical risk management
    743
Prochlorperazine 50
  analgesia 630
  gastroenteritis 315
  overdose 810
Proctalgia fugax 346
Proctoscopy 342–343
Progesterone agents, dysfunctional uterine
    bleeding 568
Progressive multifocal leucoencephalopathy,
    HIV/AIDS 420
Project plans 723
Propanolol
  pharmacology *801*
  serotonin syndrome 750
Propofol, status epilepticus *374*
Propoxyphene 844
Propranolol 208
  aortic dissection 247
  overdose 802
  pharmacokinetics 800
  pharmacology 802
  thyrotoxicosis 468
Propylthiouracil
  thyroid storm 469
  thyrotoxicosis 468
Prostacyclin, hypertension 238
Prostaglandin F2a, post-partum haemorrhage
    560
Prostaglandins 457
Prosthetic valve complications 230
  stroke risk 354
Prosthetic valve endocarditis 224, *224*
PROTACT 2 study, ischaemic stroke therapy
    359
Protease inhibitors 432–433
  HIV/AIDS 422–423
  side effects *423*
Protective clothing 110
  radiation contamination 767
Protein C
  septic shock 31
  stroke 357
Protein S, stroke 357
Proteinuria
  glomerulonephritis 443
  urinary tract infection 398

Proteus 29, 126
  antibiotic susceptibility 431, 432
    cephalosporin 349
  antibiotic therapy *426*
  cutaneous infection 405
  hidradenitis suppurativa 406
  otitis externa 551
  renal colic 458
Proteus mirabilis
  ampicillin susceptibility 428
  antibiotic therapy *426*
Prothrombinex HT 499
Proton pump inhibitors (PPIs)
  NSAID-induced ulcer management 325
  peptic ulcer disease 324
  see also individual drugs
Providencia, antibiotic susceptibility 432
Proximal humerus fracture(s) *see* Humerus
  fracture(s)
Proximal tibiofibular joint dislocation 162
Pruritus ani 346
Pseudogout, acute 517–518
Pseudohyponatraemia (normotonic
  hyponatraemia) 481
Pseudomonas
  antibiotic susceptibility 432
  co-trimoxazole resistance 431
  erythromycin resistance 429
Pseudomonas aeruginosa 29, 126
  antibiotic resistance 431
    aminoglycosides 430
  antibiotic susceptibility 431
    cephalosporin 349
  antibiotic therapy *426*
  cellulitis 405–406
  epididymo-orchitis *455*
  folliculitis 405
  otitis externa 551
  pneumonia
    management *280*
    mortality 282
Pseudoseizures (psychogenic seizures) 375
Psoriasis 516, 529, *529*, 532
  arthritis 519, 521–522
  HIV/AIDS 419
  management 529
Psychiatric factors, suicide/deliberate self-
  harm 598
Psychiatric interview *see* Mental state
  assessment/examination
Psychogenic polydipsia 482
Psychogenic seizures (pseudoseizures) 375
Pubic ramus fracture(s), isolated 150
Public health surveillance, refugees 707, 708
Pulmonary embolism 43, 179, 210–214
  cardiogenic 193, *193*
  clinical features 210
    Wells criteria *211*
  echocardiography 643
  investigations 179, 210–213
    algorithm *211, 213*
  management 213–214
  mortality 210, 214
  prognosis 214
  risk factors 210
Pulmonary oedema 229
  acute *see* Pulmonary oedema, acute
  carbon monoxide poisoning 835
  continuous positive airway pressure 263,
    264
  divers 762
  funnel web spider (*Atrax/Hadronyche*)
    bite 887

glyphosphate poisoning 862
high altitude 784, 785, 786
hypertension 238–239
  management 240
near-drowning 771
non-cardiogenic 193, *194*
  hydrofluoric acid burns 866
oxygen therapy 263
prehospital emergency services 685
respiratory acidosis 478–479
salicylates poisoning 828, 829
Pulmonary oedema, acute 193–196
  cardiogenic 193, *193*
  examination 193–194
  history 193
  investigation 194
  management 194–196
    hypotensive patients 193, 196
    normotensive/hypertensive patients
      193, 194–196
  non-cardiogenic 193, *194*
  pathophysiology 193
Pulse oximetry
  acute pulmonary oedema 194
  asthma 272
  chronic obstructive airway disease 287
  community-acquired pneumonia 278–279
  gastrointestinal bleeding 318–319
  interference 260, *260*
  rapid sequence intubation 15
Pulsus paradoxus 218
Pupillary responses, neurological assessment
  49
Pure red cell aplasia 507
Purkinje cells 198
Purpuric papular lesions *528*, 530–531
Pustular lesions *528*, 531–532
Pustular psoriasis 529
Pyelonephritis
  acute 397, 399–400, 401, 458
    antibiotic management *400*
  chronic 397
  febrile patients 383
  investigations 398–399
Pyoderma gangrenosum 531–532
Pyogenic liver abscess 383
Pyrazinamide 516
  HIV/AIDS 422
Pyridoxine, drug overdose 793
Pyuria 399
  urinary tract infection 398

Q

Q fever 276
Quadriceps tendon 164
  rupture 525
  tendinitis 164
Quality 720–722, 723
Quality assurance 720–722
  clinical performance measures 722
  clinical risk management 743
  definition 720–721
  historical aspects 720
  national bodies 721
Quality improvement 720
Quality in Australian Health Care Study
  (QAHS) 739
Quality indicators (QIs) 724–725, 743–744,
  744, *744,* 745
  categories 745

Quality of life 34
Quetiapine, pharmacology 809
Quinidine, HIV/AIDS 422
Quinolones 431–432
  see also individual drugs
Quinsy (peritonsillar abscess) 268, 269,
  408, 553–554
  antibiotic therapy 269

R

Racemic salbutamol 274
Radial artery
  embolization 233
  puncture 476–477
Radial nerve
  injury 84
    elbow dislocations 136
    humerus shaft fracture 134
  wrist block 632
Radial styloid fracture 141, *141*
Radiation 763–769
  acute exposure 765
  acute radiation syndrome 765
  biological effects 764–765
  colitis 342
  contamination 764, 766–768
    hospital management 767–768
    hospital preparations 767
    prehospital care 766–767
  decontamination 699
  disasters 698
  equivalent dose 764
  hazards 86
  induced infertility 765
  local irradiation injuries 766
  pneumonitis 766
  sources 764
  whole-body effective radiation doses 86,
    86
Radiation syndrome 764–765
  combined injuries 766
  investigations 765
  management 766
  prognosis 766
  triage 765
Radiocontrast agents
  acute tubular necrosis 443
  anaphylactic reaction 779
Radiography
  abdominal *see* Abdominal X-ray
  acromioclavicular joint injuries 130
  acute renal failure 448
  ankle/foot injury 168–169, 172
    calcaneal fractures 173
    navicular fractures 174
    subtalar dislocations 173
    talar fractures 172
  chest *see* Chest X-ray
  femoral fractures
    distal 160
    head 152
    neck 153
    shaft 157
  Galeazzi fracture 140, *140*
  head injuries 87–88
    facial trauma 66, 88–89
  hip injury
    acetabular fractures 151
    dislocation 155
    intertrochanteric femur fracture 153

Radiography (*cont.*)
  lesser trochanteric fracture 154
  pelvic fractures 149
  knee injury 160
    anterior cruciate ligaments 163
    collateral ligament injury 163
    dislocation 162
    meniscal injury 165
    patellar dislocation 162
    posterior cruciate ligaments 164
    quadriceps tendon injury 164
    tibial plateau fractures 161
  limb trauma 99
    see also individual limbs
  Lisfranc fractures 174
  major trauma 86–101
  multi-trauma patient *90*
  neck *see* Neck X-ray
  open wound injury 110
  osteomyelitis 395
  pelvic trauma 97–99
  radiation hazards 86
  septic arthritis 392–393
  spinal trauma 89–93, *90, 91*
    spinal cord injury 62
  tibial shaft fracture 166
  trauma in pregnancy 103
  trauma series 45, 87
    elderly patients 106
  upper airway trauma 268
  upper limb injury
    Colles' fracture 140
    distal humerus fracture 135
    elbow dislocations 136
    hand injuries 146
    humerus shaft fracture 134
    Monteggia fracture-dislocation 139
    proximal humerus fracture 133
    radius/ulnar shaft fractures 139
    scapula fracture 131
    shoulder dislocation 131
    Smith fracture 141
    sternoclavicular injury 130
Radiolabelled antimyosin 220
Radiolabelled leucocyte scans, pelvic
    inflammatory disease 571
Radius fracture(s)
  distal 140–141
  head 138
  neck 138
  shaft 139
Randomization
  clinical trials 650
  as confounder 654
Randomness, clinical research sampling 651
Ranitidine, peptic ulcer disease 324
Ranson criteria, pancreatitis 330, *330*
Rape 612–618
  barriers to care 613
  definition 612–613
  epidemiology 613
  forensic examination 615–616
  incidence 613
  male 617
  management
    medical care 613–615
    options 615
  physical injury 613–614, 616
  postmenopausal women 617
  in pregnancy 616–617
  pregnancy risk 615
  psychological impact 616
  reporting incidence 613

sexually transmitted disease risk 613–615
  victim-blaming myths 613
Rape trauma syndrome 616
Rapidly progressing glomerulonephritis
    (RPG) 443–444, *444*
Rapid sequence intubation 15–16
  drugs *16*
Rash
  acute on chronic 528
  anaphylaxis 781
  decompression illness 759
  drug-induced 381
  febrile patient 381, 383, 384–385
  localized 531
  meningococcal bacteraemia 383,
    384–385, 387, 531, 533
  new generalized 532–534
Reactive oxygen species, acute tubular
    necrosis 443
Recall bias 653
Reception area 719
Recluse spider (*Loxosceles*) 888
Rectal bleeding 341–344, 345–346
  aetiology 341–342
  clinical features 342
  investigations 342–343
  management 343
Rectal examination
  abdominal trauma 71
  acute appendicitis 332
  pelvic fractures 149
  rectal bleeding 342–343
  trauma in pregnancy 103
  upper gastrointestinal haemorrhage 317
Rectal ulcers 342
Rectal varices 342
Rectovaginal examination, pelvic pain 573
Redback spider (*Latrodectus hasseltii*)
    885–887
  antivenom therapy 886
  characteristics 885
  clinical features 885–886
  diagnosis 886
  epidemiology 885
  first aid 886
  venom 885
Red cell count, subarachnoid haemorrhage
    362
Reduction
  closed *see* Closed reduction
  Colles' fracture 140
  femoral shaft fracture 157
  hernia 310–311
  open
    with internal fixation *see* Open reduction
      with internal fixation (ORIF)
    radius/ulnar shaft fractures 139
Re-entry tachyarrhythmias *see*
    Tachyarrhythmia(s)
Reflexes assessment, spinal cord injury 59
  documentation 61, *61*
Reflex sympathetic dystrophy, ankle fractures
    170
Refraction, ultrasound 637
Refugee health 706–709
  at-risk groups *708*
  camps 706–707
  emergency phase 707–708
  innovations 708–709
  permanent solutions 708
  post-emergency phase 708
  responsibility 706
  staff attributes 709

Registrars 715
Regurgitation
  dysphagia 302
  spinal cord injury 55, 57
Reiter's syndrome 519, 522
Renal artery aneurysm 251
Renal colic 457–459
  analgesia 458
  management 458
  observation wards 710
  pain pathophysiology 457
  presentation 457–458
  radiology 458
Renal failure
  acid-base disturbance(s) 450
  anaemia 506–507
  chronic, Achilles tendon rupture 170
  drug overdose 793
  electric shock injury 775
  hepatic failure 340
  hypertension 230
    management 239–240
  hypervolaemic hyponatraemia 482
  meningitis 387, 388
  paraquat poisoning 863
  upper gastrointestinal haemorrhage 317
Renal failure, acute 440–452
  causes 440–445
    acute tubular necrosis 442–443
    glomerular disease 443–444
    hypoperfusion (prerenal) 440–441,
      441, 442
    interstitial disease 445
    postrenal 440–441
    renal causes 442, *443*
    vascular disease 444–445
  clinical features 447
  clinical presentation 445
  examination 446–447
  history 445–446
  hypervolaemia 450
  hypovolaemia 446
  incidence 440
  investigations 447–448
  liver damage 446
  management 448–451
    emergency department 449–450
    intensive care unit 450–451
  prevention 448–449
  prognosis 451
  risk factors *441*, 445, *446*
  in transplant patients 445
  urinary tract obstruction 441–442, 446
Renal function tests, conscious state
    alteration 368
Renal replacement therapy 451
  see also individual techniques
Renal tubular acidosis 478
Renin, ischaemic acute tubular necrosis 442
Renin–angiotensin–aldosterone (RAS) system
    238
Repatriation 708
Repeatability, clinical research 651
Reperfusion injury 20–21
Reporting, domestic violence 622
Representation, clinical research sampling
    651
Resettlement 708
Resolution, ultrasound 637
Resonium, hyperkalaemia 487
Respiratory acidosis 478–479
Respiratory alkalosis 479
Respiratory changes in pregnancy 102

Respiratory failure
acute, continuous positive airway pressure
264
basic life support 3–4
drug overdose 790, *790*
Response checks, basic life support 3
Response rate, clinical research 651
Restraint 591, 592–593
physical *see* Physical restraint
sedation *see* Chemical restraint
Restriction, as confounder 654
Resuscitation
advanced life support 6–14, 209
anaphylaxis 782–783
basic life support *see* Basic life support
bowel obstruction 308
cardiac arrhythmias 198–199
cardiac tamponade 218
cerebral *see* Cerebral resuscitation
consent 34, 35–36
decompression illness 760
discontinuation 36–37
drug overdose 793–794
elderly patients 106
emergency department layout 717
ethical aspects 33–37
gastrointestinal bleeding 318–319
guidelines development 2
near-drowning 771
practising procedures on newly dead
36–37
shock 23–32
snakebite 883
status epilepticus 373–374
trauma
burns patients *125*, 126–127
disasters management 699
electric shock injury 776
hypotensive 44–45
initial management 41–42
lightning injury 778
neurotrauma 49
in pregnancy 104
resuscitation bay layout *41*
team member roles *42*
Resuscitation area 717
Resuscitators, oxygen-powered *258*, *259*
Retinal detachment 542
Retinal migraine 350
Retrieval 686–693
aircraft *see* Aerial transport
airway management 691–692
ambulance service 698–699
assessment/stabilization 691–692
circulatory management 692
communication 691
co-ordination 691
decompression illness 760
definition 686–687
disabilities 692
disasters management 698–699, 699–700
triage 699–700
documentation 692
equipment 689–690
exposure 692
extremities 692
funding 690
handover 691
indications for 687
infusions 692
level of care 687–688
limitations 692
organization 690

patient preparation 691
risks, associated 692–693
road *688*, 688–689
spinal cord injury 64
staffing 690
team composition 687–688
training 690–691
types *688*, 688–689
Retrograde intubation 18
Retrograde urethrogram, pelvic fractures
149
Retroperitoneal bleeding 501
Retropharyngeal abscess(es) 269, 408, 554
Reverse triage, clinical risk management
742, *744*
Revised Trauma Score 45–46, 49
Rewarming therapies 754–755
near-drowning 771
Rhabdomyolysis
acute renal failure 448
acute tubular necrosis 443
crush syndrome 85
drug overdose 791, 792, 794
H$_1$-antagonist overdose 798
opioid abuse 845
Streptococcus pneumoniae pneumonia 283
Rhesus (Rh) factor 103, 562–563
Rheumatic fever 519, 522
management 522
Rheumatic heart disease 223–224, 226–229
Rheumatoid arthritis 519–520
Achilles tendon rupture 170
acute complications 521
extrarticular manifestations 520
femoral neck fracture 153
management 520
Rheumatoid emergencies 516–525
Rhinoviruses, chronic obstructive airway
disease 288
Ribavirin 435
Rib fracture(s) 76, 93, 94, 180
elderly patients 107
Richards' splint 163
Richter's hernia 310
Rickettsia
antibiotic susceptibility 430
antibiotic therapy *426*
Rifabutin
antiretroviral drug interactions 423
HIV/AIDS 422
Rifampicin 421
antiretroviral drug interactions 423
hepatitis 410
HIV/AIDS 422
meningitis 389
Right bundle branch block 201, 202–203
Rigors 383
Risperidone, pharmacology 809
Ritonavir 422, 423
Road transport retrieval systems *688*,
688–689
decompression illness 760
Rocuronium 43
Romberg's test, decompression illness 760
Ross River virus, arthritis 523
Rotator cuff tear 131, 524
with proximal humerus fracture 134
Rotator cuff tendinitis 524
Rotavirus gastroenteritis 312, 314, *313*
Rovsing's sign 332–333
Roxithromycin 429
community-acquired pneumonia 280
pelvic inflammatory disease 571

Rubella
arthritis 523
thrombocytopenia 513
Rule of nines 124, *125*

S

Sad Person's Scale 599, *600*
Safety, domestic violence 622
Salbutamol 104, 346
asthma 272
chronic obstructive airway disease 289
hyperkalaemia 487
racemic 274
severe asthma 274
Salicylates 516
mode of action 828
pharmacokinetics 827–828
poisoning 478, 479, 791, 827–830
assessment 828–829
clinical presentation 828
management 829
see also individual drugs
Salmonella 29
antibiotic resistance 428
co-trimoxazole 431
antibiotic susceptibility 431, 432
ampicillin 428
antibiotic therapy *426*
arthritis 522
gastroenteritis 312, 314, 315, *313*
traveller's diarrhoea 313
Salmonella enteritidis, gastroenteritis 312
Salmonella typhi, ampicillin susceptibility
428
Sampling, clinical research *see* Clinical
research
Sanitation, refugees 707
Saquinavir, HIV/AIDS 422, 423
Sarcoidosis, hypercalcaemia 490
Scabies 532
Scapula fracture 93, 130–131
Scapular rotation, shoulder dislocation
131–132
Schilling's test 506
Schizophrenia 590, 591
suicide/deliberate self-harm 598
Sciatic nerve injury 84, 98
Scintigraphic testicular scanning 454
SCIWORA 89–90, 93
Scleroderma 519, 522
Scromboid poisoning 893
Scrotum, acute 453–456
Sea snake envenomation 891
Seatbelts in pregnancy 104
Seating, retrieval 690
Sebaceous cyst infection 406
Seborrhoeic dermatitis, HIV/AIDS 419
Seclusion rooms 717–718
Sedation
alcohol intoxication 879
conscious 629
meningitis 390
mental health legislation 665
overdose 808–809
reportable deaths 668
trauma patients 43
see also Chemical restraint
Segmental radial head/neck fractures 138
Seizures 371–377
aetiology *372*

Seizures (*cont.*)
alcohol-related 375
convulsive 371
drug overdose 376, 790, *791, 793*
amphetamines 849
antipsychotic drugs 810–811, 811
cocaine 848
gamma-hydroxybutyrate abuse 851
H₁-antagonist overdose 798
isoniazid 376, 793
electric shock injury 775
examination 372–373
generalized 371, 372
history taking 371–372
hypocalcaemia 488
investigations 373
management 371–372
follow-up 373
prehospital emergency services 685
meningitis 387–388, 390
non-convulsive 371, 374–375
organophosphates poisoning 859
partial 371, 372
post-traumatic 376
in pregnancy 376
subarachnoid haemorrhage 361, 363
types 371–372
see also Convulsion(s)
Selection bias 653
Selective serotonin reuptake inhibitors
(SSRIs) *813,* 814–817
adverse effects 815
deliberate self-harm/suicide 601
lithium excretion 874
overdose 815
management 816
pharmacology 815
serotonin syndrome *749*
Semi-automatic external defibrillation
(SAED) 4–5
Senior house officers (SHOs) 714
Sensory function assessment
burns 124
definition 29
spinal cord injury 59–60
documentation conventions *60*
stress ulcers 317
Sepsis
acute renal failure 446
adrenocortical insufficiency 470
conscious state alteration 368–369
febrile patient 381–382, 383, 384
hepatic failure 339–340
oxygen therapy 263
peptic ulcer perforation 324
respiratory alkalosis 479
Septic arthritis 392–393, 521
Septic shock 29–31, 43, 390, 407
APACHE 31
clinical features 30
high-risk groups 30
management 30–31
meningitis 390
methicillin-resistant *Staphylococcus aureus*
(MRSA) 31
Serotonin, migraine 350
Serotonin syndrome 748–749, 815–816
drugs causing *749*
features *749*
management 750
Serratia 29
aminoglycoside resistance 431
antibiotic susceptibility 431, 432

cephalosporin susceptibility 349
Severe sepsis 29
Sexual abuse 612–613, 617
alcohol intoxication 877
definition 619
Sexual assault 612–618
definition 612–613
epidemiology 613
management options 615
medical care 613–615
physical injury 616
psychological impact 616
reporting incidence 613
see also Rape
Sexual intercourse, pain 572
Sexually-transmitted diseases (STDs)
pelvic pain 573
see also individual diseases/disorders
Sexual misconduct, complaints 735
Sezary's syndrome 534
Sf36 (Short Form-36 Questions) 45
Shadowing, ultrasound 637
Shaving 82
Shellfish poisoning, paralytic 893
Shelters, refugees 707
Shigella 29
antibiotic resistance 428
co-trimoxazole 431
antibiotic susceptibility 430, 431, 432
antibiotic therapy *426*
arthritis 522
gastroenteritis 312, 315, *313*
traveller's diarrhoea 313
Shigella dysenteriae
gastroenteritis 312
thrombotic thrombocytopenic purpura
512
Shingles *see* Herpes zoster
Shock 23–32
anaphylactic 43, 781, 782
bowel obstruction 307
burns 127
cardiac tamponade 218, 219
cardiogenic *see* Cardiogenic shock
classification *24,* 25
clinical signs 24–25
definition 23
elderly fracture patients 106
emergency department monitoring 25
gastrointestinal bleeding 318
haemorrhagic *see* Haemorrhagic shock
hepatic failure 339
hypovolaemic *see* Hypovolaemic shock
management 25
oxygen therapy 263
neurogenic (spinal sympathetic
interruption) 31–32, 43, 55
pathophysiology 24
peptic ulcer perforation 324
septic *see* Septic shock
spinal (acute cord confusion) 55
trauma 43
Short-stay medicine, observation wards 712
Shoulder
dislocation 99, 131–132
recurrence 132
injuries 130–132
pain 524
Shoulder dyscrasia, delivery complications
560
Sickle cell anaemia 507–508
avascular necrosis 152
subarachnoid haemorrhage 364

Sick sinus (bradycardia-tachycardia)
syndrome 199
Sigmoidoscopy 343
Significant bacteriuria 396
Silibinin, acute liver failure 339
Silver nitrate 127
Silver sulphadiazine 126–127
Simmonds' test 171
Simple (closed) fracture(s) 81
Simple random sampling, clinical research
652
Simvastatin, diabetes mellitus 464
Sinoatrial node 197
Sinus barotrauma 757
Sinus bradycardia 199
Sinusitis 552
headache 348, *349*
Sinus tachycardia 205
Skier's thumb 99
Skin
anatomy *124*
examination, conscious state alteration
367
infection 403–409
antibiotic therapy 404
superficial 405–406
water-related 407–408
lesions, meningitis 389
protection of 64
Skull fracture
neurotrauma 47
radiology 87–88
Skull X-ray 50, 87–88
Towne view *88*
Waters view *88*
Small bowel
injury 71–72
obstruction 306, *306*
Smith fracture 57, 141
Smoke inhalation 127, 268
carbon monoxide poisoning 268
cyanide poisoning 837, 838, 839
Smoking 232, 361
chronic obstructive airway disease 286
ischaemic heart disease 182, 183, 190
peptic ulcer disease 322
stroke risk 353
Snakebite 881–884
compartment syndrome 84
emergency department management 883
first aid 882–883
management guidelines 883–884
sea snakes 891
systemic envenomation
detection 882–883
management 883
toxicology 881–882
venom detection kit 369, 883
Social factors, suicide/deliberate self-harm
598
Sodium bicarbonate
acidosis 478
advanced life support 12
crush syndrome 85
hyperkalaemia 487
hypernatraemia 485
tricyclic antidepressants overdose 814
Sodium clodronate, hypercalcaemia 489
Sodium imbalance *see* Hypernatraemia;
Hyponatraemia
Sodium polystyrene sulphonate
lithium toxicity 875
tricyclic antidepressant overdose 814

Sodium valproate 818
  migraine 350
  overdose 818
  pharmacology 818
Soft tissue(s)
  infection 403–409
    antibiotic therapy 404
    deep 406–407
  injuries
    electric shock injury 775
    facial trauma 67–68
  rheumatic conditions 524–525
Somatostatin, gastro-oesophageal varices 319
Sore throats 268–269, *269*
Sotalol 208
  overdose 802
  pharmacology *801*
Spaso technique 131
Spermatic cord (testicular) torsion 453–455
  differential diagnosis 453–454
  intermittent 453
  investigations 454
  management 454–455
  ultrasound 643
Spider bites 885–889
  cupboard/button spider (*Steatoda*) 887
  funnel web spider (*Atrax/Hadronyche*)
      887–888
  mouse spider (*Missulena occatoria*) 888
  necrotic arachnidism 888
  recluse spider (*Loxosceles*) 888
  redback spider (*Latrodectus hasseltii*) *see*
      Redback spider (*Latrodectus hasseltii*)
  white-tailed spider (*Lampona cylindrata*)
      888
Spigelian hernia 310
Spinal cord injury 53–55
  autonomic nervous system effects 54–55
  concussion 54
  documentation conventions 61–62
  electric shock injury 775
  hyperbaric oxygen 64–65
  incomplete spinal cord syndromes 54
  investigations 62–63
    imaging consideration algorithm *62*
    magnetic resonance imaging 62–63, *63*
  ischaemic 55
  management 57–60, 63–64
    primary survey 57–58
    secondary survey 58–60
  neurological assessment 58–59
    motor function 59
    reflexes 59, 61, *61*
    sensory function 59–60
  primary 53–54
  referral 64
  secondary 54
  skin protection 64
  thoracic 79
  transverse spinal cord syndrome 53–54
  unconscious patients 60–64
Spinal meningitis 387
Spinal stenosis, back pain 523
Spine
  cervical *see* Cervical spine
  immobilization
    in pregnancy 103
    prehospital emergency services 683
    spinal cord injury 63
  lumbar *see* Lumbar spine injury
  shock 55
  thoracolumbar *see* Thoracolumbar spine
      injury

trauma 52–65
  associated injuries 52–53
  elderly patients 107
  radiology 89–93
  vertebral injury 55–57
  vertebral level 52
  see also Spinal cord injury
tumours, back pain 523
Spirometry, chronic obstructive airway
    disease 287
Splenectomized patients 382
Splenic artery aneurysm 250
Splenic injury 71–72
Splinting 119
  collateral ligament injury 163
  Colles' fracture 140
  femoral shaft fracture 157
  hand injuries 146
  limb immobilization 82–83
  subtrochanteric femur fracture 155
  see also Immobilization
Spondylosis, back pain 523
Sportsman's hernia 310
Sprained ankle 170
Sputum analysis
  chronic obstructive airway disease 288
  community-acquired pneumonia
      277–278, *279*
  Haemophilus influenzae pneumonia
      277–278
  haemoptysis 301
  Streptococcus pneumoniae pneumonia 277
Stabilization, retrieval 691–692
Stable pelvic fracture, management 150–151
Staff facilities 719
Staffing 714–715, *715*
  ancillary 715
  clerical 715
  costs 724
  medical 714–715
  observation wards 711–712
  retrieval 690
  workload calculation 714
  work practices optimization 715
Staff station 718
Stanford classification 243
Staphylococcus 383
  co-trimoxazole resistance 431
  cutaneous abscess 404–405
  decubitus/varicose ulcer 408–409
  diabetic foot infections 409
  furuncle 405
  gangrene 406–407
  toxic shock syndrome 381, 407
Staphylococcus aureus 126
  antibiotic resistance/susceptibility 431,
      432
    aminoglycosides 431
    erythromycin 429–430
    methicillin *see* Methicillin-resistant
        Staphylococcus aureus (MRSA)
  antibiotic therapy *426*
  cellulitis 405
  cutaneous abscess/infections 404–405
  diabetic foot infections 409
  endocarditis 224, 225, 226
  erysipelas 405
  facial cellulitis 405
  folliculitis 405
  gastroenteritis 312, *313*
  hidradenitis suppurativa 406
  infection routes 276
  infective endocarditis *224*

Ludwig's angina 269
  meningitis 387
  necrotizing fasciitis 406
  otitis externa 551
  paronychia 406
  pneumonia 276
    cavitating lesions 283
    management *280*
  pustules 532
  quinsy (peritonsillar abscess) 269
  toxic shock syndrome 407
Staphylococcus epidermidis
  antibiotic susceptibility 431
  cutaneous infection 404–405
  Ludwig's angina 269
Staphylococcus hominis, cutaneous infection
    405
Staphylococcus saprophyticus
  antibiotic susceptibility 432
  urinary tract infection 396
Staples 112
Statins
  acute liver failure 339
  see also individual drugs
Statistics, clinical research 649, 654–655
Status epilepticus 373–374
  non-convulsive 374–375
Stavudine 422
Steatoda (cupboard/button spiders) 887
Stenting, aortic dissection 247
Steristrips 113, *113*
Sternoclavicular injury 130
Sternum fracture 76–77, 93
Stingray injury 892
Stomach
  corrosives burns 840–841, 842
  decompression 72
  erosions 317
  lavage
    drug overdose 794–795
    iron overdose 871
    sulphonylurea overdose 873
  *see also under Gastric; Gastrointestinal
      system*
Stonefish (*Synanceia*) envenomation 892
Storage space 718
Strategic plans 723
Stratification, as confounder 654
Stratified sampling, clinical research 652
Streptococcus 126, 224, 383
  antibiotic therapy *426*
  cellulitis 405
  co-trimoxazole resistance 431
  decubitus/varicose ulcer 408–409
  diabetic foot infections 409
  gangrene 406–407
  infective endocarditis *224*
  necrotizing fasciitis 406
  pelvic inflammatory disease 570
  pharyngitis/tonsilitis 268–269
  toxic shock syndrome 381, 407
Streptococcus agalactiae, meningitis 389
Streptococcus influenzae, epiglottitis 270
Streptococcus pneumoniae 224
  antibiotic resistance/susceptibility 429,
      430, 431, 432
    erythromycin 429–430
    penicillin 390, 425, 427
  antibiotic therapy *426*
  cellulitis 405
  chronic obstructive airway disease 288,
      290
  erysipelas 405

Streptococcus pneumoniae (*cont.*)
  infection routes 276
  meningitis 386, 387, 388, 389, 390, 389
  otitis media 551
  pneumonia 282–283
    cavitating lesions 283
    clinical features 276
    lobar 276
    management 280, *280*
    mortality 282
    response to management 281
    sputum analysis 277
  sinusitis 552
Streptococcus pyogenes 407
  antibiotic resistance/susceptibility 429, 431, 432
    erythromycin 429–430
    penicillin 427
  erysipelas 405
  pharyngitis 268
  pustules 532
Streptococcus viridans 224
  antibiotic susceptibility 431
  antibiotic therapy *426*
  cutaneous abscess 405
  cutaneous infection 405
  hidradenitis suppurativa 406
Streptokinase 186–187
  allergic reactions 186–187
  hypotensive response 186
  pulmonary embolism 213
Stress
  emotional fatigue 611
  occupational 590, 606–607
  staff support 611
  structural collapses 590
Stress ulcers 317
Stroke 352–360
  cardiovascular examination 355–356
  causes 352–353, *353*
    amphetamines intoxication 849–850
    cocaine overdose 848
  central nervous system examination 355
  complications 356
  definition 352
  differential diagnosis 356, *356*
  haemorrhagic 353, 355
  history taking 355
  hypertension induction 21
  imaging 357
  ischaemic 352–353
    anterior circulation 354–355
    anticoagulation 359
    antiplatelet therapy 359
    hypertension management 240
    lacunar infarction 355
    posterior circulation 355
    surgical procedures 359
    thrombolytic therapy 359
  management 358–359
    neuroprotective drugs 21, 359
  risk factors 353–354
Structural collapses 700
Subacute combined degeneration of spinal cord 505–506
Subarachnoid haemorrhage 48, 361–364
  aneurysmal surgery 363–364
  causes 364
  cerebral hypoxia 21, 48–49
  clinical grading scheme 361, *362*
  complications 363
  examination 361
  haemorrhagic stroke 353

headache 348, *349*
  history taking 361
  imaging 357
  investigations 361–393
  management 359, 363–364
  prognosis 364
  risk factors 361
Subclavian artery aneurysm(s) 234, 250
Subcutaneous emphysema 94
Subdural intracranial haematoma 48, 51
Submandibular abscess(es) 408
Substance P 626
  migraine 350
Subtalar dislocation(s) 172–173
Subtrochanteric femoral fracture(s) 155
Subxiphoid pericardiotomy 219
Sucralfate, peptic ulcer disease 324
Suction drains 118–119, *122*
  retrieval 119
Suicidal Intent Scale 599
Suicide 597–602, 610
  aetiology 597–598
  common methods 597
  definition 597
  incidence 597
  patient characteristics 598–599, *600*
  prevention 601–602
  risk assessment 599, 601, *601*
  risk factors 586
  see also Deliberate self-harm
Sulbactam 428
Sulphadiazine, HIV/AIDS 422
Sulphasalazine
  inflammatory bowel disease 337
  psoriatic arthritis 522
  rheumatoid arthritis 520
Sulphonylureas
  diabetes mellitus 464
  overdose 873
  see also individual drugs
Sumatriptan
  analgesia 629, 630
  migraine 351
Superficial venous thrombosis 234
Superior mesenteric artery aneurysm 250
Superoxide dismutase 51
Supracondylar humerus fracture(s) 135, 160
Supralevator abscess(es) 345
Suprapubic bladder aspiration, ultrasound 644
Suprasternal ultrasound 44
Supraventricular tachycardia 203
Surfactant therapy 772
Sustained low-efficiency dialysis (SLED) 451
Suture(s)
  absorbable 113
  continuous 115
  dead space obliteration 115–116, 119, *120*
  interrupted 115
  intradermal 115
  removal 119, *120*, 121
  technique 114–116, 118, *118*
    'dog ear' avoidance/removal 117, *122*
    horizontal mattress sutures 117, *119*
    loop sutures *119*
    special 117
  types 112–113, 114, *114*
Suxamethonium 43
  malignant hyperthermia 750
  prehospital emergency services 683
  tracheal intubation 63

Swan-Ganz catheterization
  acute liver failure 339
  pesticides poisoning 859–860
Sweet syndrome 531, 532, 533, *533*
Swelling, knee injury 159
Sympathomimetic toxicity, haemorrhagic stroke 353
Synanceia (stonefish) envenomation 892
Syndrome of inappropriate ADH secretion (SIADH) 482–483
Synovial fluid analysis
  gout 517, *518*
  septic arthritis 392
Syphilis see *Treponema pallidum*
Syrup of ipecac, drug overdose 794–795
Systematic errors (bias), clinical research 649, 653
Systematic sampling, clinical research 652
Systemic inflammatory response syndrome (SIRS) 29
Systemic lupus erythematosus (SLE) 519, 521
  Achilles tendon rupture 170
  clinical features 521
  idiopathic thrombocytopenic purpura 512
  management 521
System indicators 745, *745*
System strategies, clinical risk management *743*

T

Tachyarrhythmia(s) 198, 203–209
  antihistamine overdose 798
  broad complex 203
  bupropion 813
  narrow complex 205
  opioid abuse 845
  re-entry 198
    supraventricular tachycardias 206–207
  ventricular see Ventricular tachycardia
  see also Arrhythmias
Tacrine, antihistamine overdose 799
Talar, fractures 172
Tape
  wound closure 112, 113, *113*
  wound support 121
Technetium-99m scan
  acute appendicitis 333
  chest pain differential diagnosis 179
  rectal bleeding 343
Teeth
  anatomy 546, *546*
  avulsion 546–547
  emergencies 546–548
  fractures 547, *547*
  pain in barotrauma 758
  reimplantation 547
  trauma 68, 546–547
    Ellis classification 547, *547*
Teicoplanin, neutropenia 500
Telemedicine area 719
Temazepam, pharmacology 806
Temporal arteritis, headache *349*
Temporary impairment, consent (UK) 678
Temporomandibular joint dislocation 69, 547–548
Tendon injury 110
Tension headache 348, *348*, 349
Tension pneumopericardium 78

Tension pneumothorax 43, 77, 292
  neurogenic shock 31–32
  shock 27, 28
Terfenadine 670
  pharmacodynamics 798
Testicles
  appendage torsion 455
  blunt trauma 456
  pain
    acute epididymo-orchitis 455–456
    differential diagnosis 454
    spermatic cord torsion see Spermatic
      cord (testicular) torsion
  ultrasound 643
Tetanic muscle contraction
  electric shock injury 776
  hypocalcaemia 488
Tetanus 407
Tetanus prophylaxis 51, 68, 69–70, 404, 776
  burns patients 126
  immunization schedule 112
  limb trauma 81, 82
  open wound management 111, 112
    at risk wounds 112
  snakebite 883
  tibial shaft fracture 167
Tetracycline 429
  adverse reactions 429
  bacterial resistance 429
  epididymo-orchitis 456
Tetrodotoxin poisoning 893
Thalassaemias 508
Thallium scan 179
Theophylline
  chronic obstructive airway disease 288, 289
  pharmacokinetics 830
  poisoning 479, 668, 830–832
    clinical features 376, 830–831
    management 831–832
Thermal trauma, upper airway 268
Thermoregulation with spinal cord damage 55, 63
Thiamine
  alcoholic ketoacidosis 473, 880
  alcohol intoxication 879
  hepatic encephalopathy 367
Thiazolidinediones 464
  see also individual drugs
Thiopentone 43
  antihistamine overdose 798–799
  status epilepticus 374
Thioridazine
  antipsychotic drug overdose 811
  overdose 810
  pharmacology 809
Thirst 484
  hypernatraemia 484
Thomas splints
  femoral shaft fracture 157
  subtrochanteric femur fracture 155
Thoracic aorta
  aneurysm 305
  injury 94–96
  transection 78–79
Thoracic outlet decompression 236
Thoracic outlet syndrome 233
Thoracic spinal fracture 56–57, 79
Thoracocentesis, pleural effusion 298
Thoracolumbar spine injury
  classification 92
  fractures 56
  radiology 92–93

Thoracoscopy 294
  pleural effusion 298
Thoracostomy 294
  pleural effusion 299
Thoracotomy 79, 213–214, 219, 294
  resuscitative 79
Thought content 583
Thought disorder 582–583, 583
Throat 553–554
  foreign body 553
  infection 383, 553–554
Thrombocytopenia 511–514
  acute renal failure 448
  aetiology 511, 511
    artifactual 511–512
    hypersplenism 513
    immune-related 512
    impaired platelet production 513
    massive blood transfusion 513
    non-immune 512–513
    in pregnancy 512
  clinical presentation 513
  disposition 514
  investigations 513
  management 513–514
  see also individual types
Thromboembolism, cerebral see Cerebral
    thromboembolism
Thrombolectomy, deep vein thrombosis 235–236
Thrombolysis
  acute arterial limb ischaemia 232–233
  allergic reactions 186–187
  axillary vein thrombosis 237
  bleeding complications 186
  cardiogenic shock 27, 28
  deep vein thrombosis 213, 235–236
  hypotension complications 187
  ischaemic stroke 359
  myocardial infarction 181, 186–187
    indications/contraindications 186
    reperfusion arrhythmias 187
  pulmonary embolism 213
Thrombotic thrombocytopenic purpura
    (TTP) 445, 509, 512
  Escherichia coli 512
'Thumb sign', epiglottitis 266
Thyroid-blocking drugs
  thyroid storm 468–469
  thyrotoxicosis 468
  see also individual drugs
Thyroid function tests, conscious state
    alteration 368
Thyroid gland
  autoantibodies 469
  disorders 467–471
    conscious state alteration 368
Thyroid hormone replacement 469, 470
Thyroiditis 467
Thyroid stimulating hormone (TSH) assay
    467, 469
Thyroid storm 468–469
Thyrotoxicosis 467–469
  clinical features 467, 468
  thyroid-blocking drugs 468
Thyroxine (free T4) assay 467, 469
Tibia, anatomy 165–166
Tibia, fracture 99
  plateau 160–161, 161
  shaft 166, 166–167
    fibula fractures 167
  spine/intercondylar eminence 161
  tubercule 167

Tibial artery injury 83
Ticarcillin 428
  septic shock 31
  urinary tract infection 400–401
Ticlopidine
  ischaemic heart disease 188
  ischaemic stroke 359
Tietze's syndrome 180
Tigabine 818
Timolol, pharmacology 801
Tinel's sign 524
Tissue adhesive 112, 113
Tissue hypoxia 255–256
Tissue plasminogen activator (tPA) 186
  ischaemic stroke 359
  pulmonary embolism 213
Tocolytics 104
Tonsillitis 268–269, 553
Topiramate 818
Torsades de pointes
  antihistamine poisoning 670
  electrocardiogram 198, 205–206, 206
    causes 205
  organophosphates poisoning 860
Total quality management (TQM) 721
Towne view, skull X-ray 88
Toxic acute tubular necrosis 443
Toxic autonomic syndromes ('toxidromes')
    792, 792
Toxic diffuse goitre (Graves' disease) 467
Toxic epidermolysis necrolysis 532, 532,
    533, 534
Toxic erythema 532
Toxic megacolon 335, 336
Toxic multinodular goitre 467
Toxicology, observation wards 710–711
Toxic shock syndrome 381, 407
Toxic thyroid adenoma 467
Toxin-induced haemolysis 509–510
Toxin-related hepatitis 411
Toxoplasmosis, cerebral 420, 422
'T pieces' 257
Trachea, laceration 94
Tracheal intubation 15–16
  advanced life support 10
    drug delivery 13
  asthma 272
  blind nasotracheal 18
  cardiogenic shock 28
  conscious state alteration 366
  difficult 16–18, 42, 67
    failed intubation drill 17
  facial trauma 67, 69
  fibreoptic bronchoscope-assisted 18–19
  hypotension 16
  laryngeal mask airway 18
  laryngeal oedema 124, 126
  massive haemoptysis 301
  near-drowning 771
  neurotrauma 49
  practising procedures on newly dead 37
  prehospital emergency services 683
  rapid sequence 15–16
  retrieval 691–692
  retrograde 18
  shock 25
  spinal cord injury 63
  tracheal placement confirmation 16
  trauma management 42
    emergency procedure 42
    paralysing agents 43
  upper airway obstruction 267
Tracheobronchial injury 78

Tracheomalacia, upper airway obstruction 266
Tracheostomy 19, 67
  epiglottitis 408
  upper airway penetrating trauma 268
Traction splints 82–83
Training (emergency medicine) 726–730
  overseas 728–730
  refugee health 707
  retrieval 690–691
Tramadol, analgesia 628
Tranexamic acid
  dysfunctional uterine bleeding 568–569
  haemophilia 502
Transabdominal ultrasound 640
Transducers, ultrasound 638–639
Transient ischaemic attacks (TIAs) 352–360
  cocaine overdose 848
  definition 352
  imaging 356–357
  locations 354
  management 358
  risk factors 353–354
Transjugular intrahepatic portosystemic
    stent-shunt (TIPS) 320
Transoesophageal echocardiography (TOE)
    93
  aortic blood flow monitoring 44
  aortic dissection 246
  chest pain differential diagnosis 179
  infective endocarditis 225–226
  pulmonary embolism 212–213
  thoracic aortic injury 96
    transection 79
  transient ischaemic attacks 357
Transthoracic echocardiography (TTE)
  aortic dissection 245–246
  infective endocarditis 225
  transient ischaemic attacks 357
Transvaginal ultrasound 640
Transverse spinal cord syndrome 53–54, 61
  sacral sparing 53–54
Trapped patients 699
  structural collapses 590
Trauma 40–46
  abdominal see Abdominal trauma
  alcohol abuse 877
  audit 45–46
  care systems 40–41, 41
  chest see Chest trauma
  clinical presentation 43–44
  coagulation factors 44
  conscious state alteration 367, 369
  dental see Teeth, trauma
  ear see Ear, trauma
  elderly patients 105–108
  eye see Eye, trauma
  facial see Facial trauma
  fluid replacement 44–45
  hypotensive resuscitation 44–45
  hypothermia 44
  initial management 41–42
    resuscitation bay layout 41
    team member roles 42
  injury patterns, domestic violence 620
  life-threatening features 41
  limb see Limb trauma
  MAST suits 26, 44
  monitoring 44
  mortality/morbidity 40
  neurotrauma see Neurotrauma
  nose 552
  paralysing agents 43

perianal 346
pregnant patients 102–105
radiology 45, 86–101, 103, 106
  trauma series X-rays 87
sedation 43
shock 43
specialist management needs 45
spinal see Spine, trauma
spinal immobilization 41, 42, 54, 58
staff debriefing 611
stress ulcers 317
surgery 44
testicular 456
tracheal intubation 42
trapped patients 699
triage 40–41
venous access 44
ventilation 42–43
Trauma Score 49
Trauma series X-rays 87
Traveller's diarrhoea, gastroenteritis 314
Traveller's fever 382–383, 384
Trendelenburg position 26, 301
  decompression illness 760
Treponema pallidum
  antibiotic therapy 426
  arthritis 522
  meningitis 387, 420
  mental disorders 588
  penicillin susceptibility 427
  rape 614
Triage 40–41, 702–705
  Australian National Triage Scale 721,
    724
  business planning 724, 725
  civilian development 702
  delays, complaints 735
  deliberate self-harm 599
  disasters management 699
  drug 'body-packers'/'body-stuffers' 852
  hospital emergency department 718
  military/disaster 704–705
  origins 702
  pre-hospital 704
  process 702–703
  psychiatric disorders 585, 585–586, 586,
    586
  radiation accidents
    acute exposure 765
    contamination with radioactive materials
      767
  reverse 742, 744
  scale categories 714, 714
  structure/function 704
  upper airway 265–266
  waiting time 704, 715
  waiting times 744, 745
Triazolam, HIV/AIDS 422
Trichomonas vaginalis, antibiotic
    susceptibility 430–431
Tricyclic antidepressants (TCAs) 812
  overdose 478, 813–815
    management 814
  paralytic ileus 306
  pharmacology 813
  seizures 376
  serotonin syndrome 749
  see also individual drugs
Tri-iodothyronine (free T3) assay 467
Trimalleolar fractures 169
Trimethoprim
  epididymo-orchitis 456
  otitis media 551

recurrent urinary tract infection 399
urinary tract infection 399
TRISS 45–46, 49
Trochanteric bursitis 525
Troglitazone, diabetes mellitus 464
Trousseau's sign
  hypocalcaemia 488
  hypomagnesaemia 490
Trusses 310
Tuberculosis 305
  adrenocortical insufficiency 470
  arthritis 522
  HIV/AIDS 419, 420, 422
  meningitis 386–387, 387, 388, 420, 422
  see also Mycobacterium tuberculosis
Tubular necrosis, near-drowning 770
Tubulo-interstitial nephritis, acute (ATIN)
    445
Tumour markers, pelvic pain 574
Tutorial room 719
Two-period crossover clinical trials 650
Typhoid fever 383

U

Ulna fracture(s)
  distal 140–141
  shaft 139
Ulnar artery embolization 232
Ulnar collateral ligament rupture
    (gamekeeper's thumb) 99, 145
Ulnar nerve
  injury 84, 136
  wrist block 631
Ultrasound 636–646
  abdominal aortic aneurysms 636, 641,
    641
  abdominal trauma 72–73, 73
    advantages/disadvantages 73
    FAST examination 97, 97, 639,
      639–640
  abscesses 644
  acute renal failure 448
  antepartum haemorrhage 565
  appendicitis 333, 644
  artifacts 637
  axial 637
  B-mode (brightness modulation) 636, 637
  bowel obstruction 307–308
  catheter placement 644
  central line placement 642–643
  cholecystitis 327, 642, 642
  cholelithiasis 327
  deep vein thrombosis 235, 643
  distal humerus fracture 135
  Doppler see Doppler ultrasound
  early pregnancy 562
  echocardiography 643
  ectopic pregnancy 640
  epididymo-orchitis 643
  femoral vein cannulation 643
  fetal heart assessment 103
  foreign bodies 644
  gallbladder 326, 642
  gallstones 642
  hydrocoele 643
  hydronephrosis 642
  indications for 637
  interstitial pregnancy 641
  intravascular, aortic dissection 245–246
  kidneys 642

Ultrasound (*cont.*)
  limb trauma 82
  M-mode 637
  nephrolithiasis 458
  open wound injury 110
  pelvic pain 573, 574
  physics 636–637
  post-partum haemorrhage 566
  pregnancy 640–641
    gestational age estimation 556
    timings *640*
    trauma 103, 104
  septic arthritis 392
  spermatic cord (testicular) torsion 643
  suprapubic bladder aspiration 644
  terminology 637
  testicles 643
  training/credentialing 644–645
  transabdominal 640
  transducers 638–639
  transient ischaemic attacks 356
  transvaginal 640
  urinary tract infection 399
  vaginal bleeding 568
Umbilical hernia 310
Unimalleolar fractures 169
Universal precautions 110, 593–594
Unstable angina 179, 181, 183, 470
  disposition 190
  hypertension 238–239
  management 183
  thallium scan 179
Unstable pelvic fracture, management 150
Upper airway 265–270
  infections 268–270
    non-specific 268
    see also individual infections
  management *see* Airway management
  obstruction 266–267
    causes *265*
    respiratory acidosis 478–479
  trauma
    blunt trauma 267, *268*
    investigations 268
    penetrating trauma 267–268
    thermal trauma 268
  triage 265–266
Upper gastrointestinal tract *see*
    Gastrointestinal system
Upper limb, rheumatoid arthritis 519
Uraemic syndrome, acute 450
Urban Search and Rescue (USAR) 700
Urea, plasma levels
  acute renal failure 447
  pelvic pain 574
Urease breath test 323
Ureteroscopic stone removal 458
Urethra
  epididymo-orchitis 455
  injury 72
    pelvic fracture 149–150
  rupture 98
Urethral syndrome 397, 398
Urethritis 397, 398
Urethrography 98
Urinalysis
  acute epididymo-orchitis 455
  acute renal failure 448, *448*
  bowel obstruction 307
  drug overdose 792–793
  febrile patient 381, 384
  glomerulonephritis 448
  hypertension 239

infective endocarditis 225
  pelvic pain 574
  renal colic 458
  trauma in pregnancy 103
  urinary tract infection 398–399
Urinary catheterization
  abdominal trauma 72
  acute liver failure 339
  burns patients 126
  spinal cord damage 55, 57–58
  urinary tract infection 397
    management *400*, 401
Urinary tract infections (UTIs) 396–402,
    458
  aetiology 396–397
    catheter-associated 397, 401
  bladder defence mechanisms 397
  definitions 396
  disposition 401–402
  epidemiology 396
  examination 398
  frequency dysuria syndrome 399
  history taking 398
  imaging 399
  investigations 398–399
  management 399–401
    antibiotic therapy 399
  pathogenesis 397
    bacterial factors 397
    host factors 397
  in pregnancy 396, 397, 400–401
  prognosis 402
  recurrent 399
  urinary tract instrumentation 397
  urinary tract obstruction 397
Urinary tract obstruction
  acute renal failure 441–442, 446
  urinary tract infection 397
Urine
  alkalinization
    drug overdose 795, *795*
    renal failure 449
    salicylate poisoning 829
  nitrites 398
  retention 55
Urokinase
  ischaemic stroke 359
  pulmonary embolism 213
Urticaria 532, *532*
  anaphylaxis 781
  management 533
Urticarial vasculitis 533
Uterine changes in pregnancy 102
Uterine rupture, traumatic 103
Utility areas 718

V

Vaginal bleeding 567–569
  antepartum haemorrhage 564–565
  causes 567, *567*
  definitions 567
  early pregnancy 561–563
    examination 561–562
    history 561
    investigations 562
    management 562–563, *563*
    prognosis 563
  examination 568
  history 567–568
  hypotension 561

investigations 568
  late pregnancy 564–566
    antepartum haemorrhage 564–565
    see also Post-partum haemorrhage
  management 568–569
  pregnancy test 568
  structural lesions 569
Vaginal examination
  abdominal trauma 71
  childbirth 557
Valaciclovir 432
Validity, clinical research 651
Vallecula sign, epiglottitis *266*
Valsalva manoeuvre 758
Vancomycin
  infective endocarditis 226
  meningitis 390, *389*
  neutropenia 500
  osteomyelitis 395
  septic arthritis 393
  septic shock 31
  Staphylococcus aureus pneumonia 280
Vanilloid receptor agonists, migraine 350
Variant (Prinzmetal's) angina 183
Variant Creutzfeldt–Jakob disease (vCJD)
  496–497
  haemophilia, blood products 501–502
  needlestick injuries 435
Varicella zoster *see* Herpes zoster
Varicose ulcer 408–409
Varicose veins 234
Vasa praevia, antepartum haemorrhage 564
Vascular access
  burns patients 126
  cardiac arrest 12–13
  trauma 44
Vascular disease, acute renal failure 444–445
Vasculitis *443*, 445, *530*, 530–531, 532, 533
  avascular necrosis 152
  signs/symptoms 446
  stroke 356, 357
Vasoactive hormone, ischaemic acute tubular
  necrosis 442
Vasodilator drugs
  aortic dissection 247
  chronic aortic incompetence 226–227
  mitral incompetence 229
  myocardial ischaemia 240
  pulmonary oedema 240
  see also individual drugs
Vasopressin
  advanced life support 11
  gastro-oesophageal varices 320
  rectal bleeding 343
Vasospasm, cerebral, subarachnoid
  haemorrhage 363
Vecuronium 43
Venography 235–236
  deep vein thrombosis 235
Venom detection kits (VDKs) 883
  conscious state alteration 369
Venous blood gas values 476
Venous disease
  lower limb 233–236
  upper limb 235–236
Ventilation 254
  acute pulmonary oedema 195
  advanced life support 10–11
  asthma 272–273
  basic life support 3–4
  chronic obstructive airway disease 288–289
  failure, respiratory acidosis 478–479
  hypothermia 753–754

Ventilation (*cont.*)
near-drowning 771, 772
neurotrauma 49
prehospital emergency services 683
pulmonary embolism 213
respiratory acidosis 479
retrieval 689
spinal cord injury 57, 63
trauma 42–43
see also Airway management; *individual*
techniques
Ventilation/perfusion (V/Q) scan
chest pain differential diagnosis 179
haemoptysis 300
pulmonary embolism 211–212
Ventricular fibrillation 198
advanced life support protocol 205–206
cardiac arrest 7–8
defibrillation failure 10
electric shock injury 774, 776
torsades de pointes 205
Ventricular septal defect 190
Ventricular tachycardia 203–205
advanced life support 203–205
protocol 205–207
cardiac arrest 7–8
Venturi mask 257–258
Verapamil 205, 206, 207, 208
overdose 802
pharmacokinetics 800
pharmacology 801
Verbal abuse 590
Verbal complaints 736
Vertebral artery dissection 88
Vertebral injury 52–53, 55–57
cervical fractures 55–57
lumbar spine 57
thoracic spinal fractures 56–57
thoracolumbar spine 56
Vertical mattress suture 118, *118*
Vertigo in divers 762
Vesicles *528*, 530–531
Vesicoureteric reflux 397
Vibrio, soft tissue infections 407
Vibrio cholerae
antibiotic susceptibility 429, 430
antibiotic therapy *426*
gastroenteritis 312, *313*
Vibrio parahaemolyticus, gastroenteritis *313*
Vigabatrin 818
Violent crime 106
Violent patient 590–596
assessment 591
common errors *595*
diagnosis 590–591
disposition 594
impact on staff 595
legal aspects 594–595
management 591–593
chemical restraint 591, 592–593
physical restraint 591, 592
post-incident 594
organic disease diagnosis 590
prediction of violence 590
preventive approach 595
psychiatric disorders 590
staff training/preparation 592, 593–594
verbal intervention 591–592
weapons 593
Viral arthritis 519, 522–523
Viral epididymo-orchitis *455*
Viral gastroenteritis 312, *313*
Viral haemorrhagic fever 383

Viral hepatitis *see* Hepatitis, viral
Viral meningitis 386, 387, 388, 389
Viral rhinosinusitis 552
Visceral aneurysms 250–251
Visual failure
acute 540–543
therapeutic options *540*
age-related macular degeneration 542–543
AIDS patients 420
anterior ischaemic optic neuropathy
541–542
central retinal artery occlusion 541
central retinal vein occlusion 543
clinical assessment *540*, 540–541
examination 541
history taking 540
optic neuritis 543
posterior vitreous detachment 542
retinal detachment 542
vitreous haemorrhage 542
Vitamin B$_{12}$ deficiency 505–506
Vitamin D toxicity, hypercalcaemia 489
Vitreous haemorrhage 542
Volume replacement
acute liver failure 339
adrenocortical insufficiency 471
anaphylaxis 782
bowel obstruction 308
burns 123, 126
cardiac tamponade 219
cardiogenic shock 28
colloids *see* Colloid volume replacement
crush syndrome 85
crystalloids *see* Crystalloid volume
replacement
decompression illness 760
gastroenteritis 314
gastrointestinal bleeding 318
hypercalcaemia 489
hypothermia 44, 753
hypovolaemic hypernatraemia 485
hypovolaemic shock 26–27
lithium toxicity 875
prehospital emergency services 684
receptors 58
rectal bleeding 343
renal colic 458
septic shock 30
trauma 44
head injury 49
hypotensive resuscitation 44–45
spinal cord injury 63–64
unstable pelvic fracture 149
Voluntariness, consent (UK) 679
Volvulus 306, 307, 308
Vomiting
acute appendicitis 332
alkalosis 479
anaphylaxis 781
bowel obstruction 307
differential diagnosis 314
febrile patients 383
gastroenteritis 312
near-drowning 771
Von Willebrand disease 502
V-Y flap advancement *121*

Warfarin 213
prosthetic valves 230
stroke 353
transient ischaemic attacks 358
Warm autoimmune haemolytic anaemia
508–509
Warm humidified inhalation 754–755
Water-related skin infections 407–408
Water supplies, refugees 707, 708
Waters view, skull X-ray *88*
Wells criteria, pulmonary embolism *211*
Wenkebach (Mobitz I) second degree heart
block 200
electrocardiogram *200*
Wernicke's encephalopathy
clinical presentation 877–878
disposition 880
management 878–880
Wet drowning 770
White cell count (WCC), community-
acquired pneumonia 278
White phosphorus burns 128
White-tailed spider (*Lampona cylindrata*)
888
Whole-body effective radiation doses 86, *86*
Whole bowel irrigation
drug overdose 795, 852
iron overdose 871
lithium toxicity 875
salicylates poisoning 829
Withdrawing management 36
Withholding management 36
Wolff-Parkinson-White syndrome 206
electrocardiogram *206*
Woods corkscrew manoeuvre, shoulder
dyscrasia 560
Workload calculation 714
Work practices optimization 715
Wound(s)
clinical presentation 109–110
epidemiology 109
healing 111–112
infection 403–404
Wound management 109–122, 403
antibiotic prophylaxis 403
cleansing 110–111, 403
facial wounds 116
irrigation 110, 111, *111*
limb trauma 82
solutions *110*
closure/repair
delayed 111, *112*
facial wounds 116–117, *120*
needles 113–114
surgical instruments *115*
sutures *see* Suture(s)
V-Y flap advancement *121*
debridement 110–111, 403
dehiscence 121
drainage 118–119
suction drains 119, *122*
dressings 119
immobilization 119
tetanus prophylaxis 111, *112*
Wrist disorders 524–525
Written complaints 736

W

Waiting areas 718–719
Waiting times, triage 704, 744, *745*

X

Xanthomonas 29
X-rays *see* Radiography

Y

Yellow fever, hepatitis 410
Yersinia
    antibiotic susceptibility 431
    arthritis 522
    gastroenteritis 312, 315, *313*
Yersinia enterocolitica
    cutaneous infection 404–405
    gastroenteritis 312
Young and Ressnick classification *see* Pelvis,
    fracture

Z

Zalcitabine, HIV/AIDS 422, 423
Zavanelli's procedure, shoulder dyscrasia
    560
Zidovudine 432
    HIV/AIDS 422, 423
        postexposure prophylaxis 435–436,
            436, *436*
    rape 615
Zollinger-Ellison syndrome 323
Zolpidem 808

Zoonoses
    community-acquired pneumonia 276
    fever 383
    skin/soft tissue infection 408–409
Zopiclone 808
Zygomatic arch fracture 67, 68, 88, 89
Zygomaticomaxillary complex fracture 68,
    88